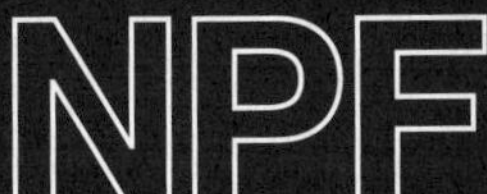

NURSE PRESCRIBERS' FORMULARY

FOR COMMUNITY PRACTITIONERS

2005-2007

Incorporating

BNF 50

SEPTEMBER 2005

and including

Nurse Prescribers' Extended Formulary List

•

British Medical Association

Royal Pharmaceutical Society of Great Britain

In association with

Community Practitioners' and Health Visitors' Association

Royal College of Nursing

Published by the BMJ Publishing Group Ltd

Tavistock Square, London WC1H 9JP, UK

and the **Royal Pharmaceutical Society of Great Britain**

1 Lambeth High Street, London, SE1 7JN, UK

ISBN: 0 85369 651 9

ISSN: 1468-4853

Printed in Germany by Clausen & Bosse, CPI Books, Leck

A catalogue record for this book is available from the British Library.

Copies may be obtained through any bookseller or direct from the publishers:

Pharmaceutical Press
c/o Turpin Distribution
Stratton Business Park
Pegasus Drive
Biggleswade
Bedfordshire
SG18 8TQ
UK
Tel: +44 (0) 1767 604 971
Fax:+44 (0) 1767 601 604
E-mail: custserv@turpin-distribution.com
www.pharmpress.com

For detailed advice on medicines used for children consult *BNF for Children*

Contents

Preface

The Nurse Prescribers' Formulary for Community Practitioners (formerly the Nurse Prescribers' Formulary for District Nurses and Health Visitors) is for use by District Nurses and Specialist Community Public Health Nurses (Health Visitors) who have received nurse prescriber training. It provides details of preparations that can be prescribed for patients receiving NHS treatment on form FP10P (form HS21(N) in Northern Ireland, form FP10(N) in Scotland, form WP10(PN) in Wales or, when available, WP10CN and WP10PN in Wales). This current edition incorporates BNF No. 50.

Nurses who have received specific preparation and training (distinct from that provided to Community Practitioner nurse prescribers) are able to prescribe from the *Nurse Prescribers' Extended Formulary*, which includes certain prescription-only medicines. The current edition of the NPF includes a list of the prescription-only medicines and of the conditions that are covered by the Nurse Prescribers' Extended Formulary. Further details may be found on the Department of Health website www.dh.gov.uk

Community Practitioner nurse prescribers should prescribe only from the list of preparations in the Nurse Prescribers' Formulary for Community Practitioners (for conditions specified in the NPF); extended formulary nurse prescribers can additionally prescribe for conditions specified in the Nurse Prescribers' Extended Formulary. Nurses must not prescribe independently for conditions other than those in the nurse formularies.

The Nurse Prescribers' Formulary Subcommittee (p. v) oversees the preparation of the NPF for Community Practitioners and advises the UK health ministers on the list of preparations that may be prescribed by Community Practitioner nurse prescribers. The Subcommittee is responsible for the interpretation of the recommendations made by the Advisory Group on Nurse Prescribing (as outlined in the Group's report published in 1989).

The list of preparations from which Community Practitioner nurse prescribers may prescribe is reviewed constantly in the light of comments from nurse prescribers and applications from manufacturers. The Department of Health and MHRA have made separate arrangements for the Nurse Prescribers' Extended Formulary.

The NPF forms an appendix to the BNF and as such is termed the Nurse Prescribers' Formulary Appendix (Appendix NPF).

The Subcommittee records its thanks to C. Dalton, R. Blessing, M. Hamilton, M.G.V. Jenkins, K. Mann, and P. Robinson, for their help with the preparation of this edition. The Subcommittee is grateful to those who have commented on previous editions of the NPF. In order that future editions of the NPF for Community Practitioners are able to reflect the requirements of nurse prescribers, users are urged to send comments and constructive criticism to:

Executive Editor, NPF/BNF,
Royal Pharmaceutical Society of Great Britain
1 Lambeth High Street, London SE1 7JN
Email: editor@bnf.org

Acknowledgements

The Joint Formulary Committee and the Nurse Prescribers' Formulary Subcommittee are grateful to individuals and organisations that have provided advice and information to the NPF/BNF.

The principal contributors for this edition were:

I.H. Ahmed-Jushuf, K.W. Ah-See, S.P. Allison, M.N. Badminton, T.P. Baglin, P.R.J. Barnes, D.N. Bateman, D. Bowsher, R.J. Buckley, I.F. Burgess, D.J. Burn, A.J. Camm, D. Chamberlain, G. Clayden, G.M.Cooper, R. Dinwiddie, P.N. Durrington, T.S.J. Elliott, B.G. Gazzard, A.M. Geretti, A.H. Ghodse, N.J.L. Gittoes, P.J. Goadsby, E.C. Gordon-Smith, I.A. Greer, J. Guillebaud, C.H. Hawkes, C.J. Hawkey, S.H.D. Jackson, A. Jones, J.R. Kirwan, P.G. Kopelman, L. Lane, M.J.S. Langman, T.H. Lee, P.Mason, K.E.L. McColl, G.M. Mead, E. Miller, N.S. Morton, J.M. Neuberger, C.G. Newstead, D.J. Nutt, D.J. Oliver, L.P. Ormerod, P.A. Poole-Wilson, D.J. Rowbotham, P.C. Rubin, P.G. Ryan, R.S. Sawers, P. Simmonds, C.H. Smith, A.E. Tattersfield, S. Thomas, D.G. Waller, L.D. Watkins, A. Wilcock.

Expert advice on the management of oral and dental conditions was kindly provided by M. Addy, M.A.O. Lewis, J.G. Meechan, N.D. Robb, C. Scully, R.A. Seymour, and R. Welbury.

Members of the British Association of Dermatologists Therapy Guidelines and Audit Subcommittee, A.V. Anstey, D.J. Eedy, F. Humphreys, K.J. Jackson, S.K. Jones, D. Mitchell, A.D.Ormerod, and M. Donoghue (Secretariat) have provided valuable advice.

Members of the Advisory Committee on Malaria Prevention, B.A. Bannister, R.H. Behrens, P.L. Chiodini, A.D.Green, D.Hill, G. Kassianos, D.G. Lalloo, G. Lea, J. Leese, G. Pasvol, M. Powell, E. Stewart, E. Walker, D.A. Warrell, C.J.M. Whitty, P.A. Winstanley, and C. Swales (Secretariat) have provided valuable advice.

The Joint British Societies' Coronary Risk Prediction Charts have been reproduced with the kind permission of P.N. Durrington who has also provided the BNF with access to the computer program for assessing coronary and stroke risk.

Correspondents in the pharmaceutical industry have provided information on new products and commented on products in the BNF. The Prescription Pricing Authority has supplied the prices of products in the BNF.

Numerous doctors, pharmacists, nurses and others have sent comments and suggestions.

The BNF has valuable access to the *Martindale* data banks by courtesy of S. Sweetman and staff.

A. Breewood, E. Carranza-Pitcher, M. Davis, C.L. Iskander, and J. Mehta provided considerable assistance during the production of this edition of the NPF/BNF.

Xpage and CSW Informatics Ltd have provided technical assistance with the editorial database and typesetting software.

Joint Formulary Committee 2004–2005

Chairman
Martin J. Kendall
MB, ChB, MD, FRCP

Deputy Chairman
Nicholas L. Wood
BPharm, FRPharmS

Committee Members
Nigel S. Baber
BSc, MB, FRCP, FRCP(Ed), FFPM, DipClinPharmacol

Alison Blenkinsopp
PhD, BPharm, FRPharmS

Michael J. Goodman
MA, BM, BCh, DPhil, FRCP

W. Moira Kinnear
BSc, MSc, MRPharmS

Frank P. Marsh
MA, MB, BChir, FRCP

Roopendra K. Prasad
MB BS, MS, FRCS, FRCGP

Ewen Sim
BSc, MB, ChB, DipHlthMgmt

James Smith
BPharm, PhD, FRPharmS, MCPP, MIInfSc

Executive Secretary
Tracy L. South
BTEC

Editorial Staff

Executive Editor
Dinesh K. Mehta, *BPharm, MSc, FRPharmS*

Senior Assistant Editor
John Martin, *BPharm, PhD, MRPharmS*

Assistant Editors
Ian Costello, *BPharm, MSc, MRPharmS*
Bryony Jordan, *BSc, DipPharmPract, MRPharmS*
Colin R. Macfarlane, *BPharm, MSc, MRPharmS*
Rachel S. M. Ryan, *BPharm, MRPharmS*
Shama M. S. Wagle, *BPharm, DipPharmPract, MRPharmS*

Staff Editors
Leigh Anne Claase, *BSc, PhD, MRPharmS*
Allison F. Corbett, *BPharm, MRPharmS*
Laura K. Glancy, *MPharm, MRPharmS*
Trinh Huynh, *BPharm, MRPharmS*
Sangeeta Kakar, *BSc, MRPharmS*
Maria Kouimtzi, *BPharm, PhD, MRPharmS*
Sukeshi A. Makhecha, *BSc, DipPharmPract, MRPharmS*
Helen M. N. Neill, *MPharm, MRPharmS*
Elizabeth Nix, *DipPharm(NZ), MRPharmS*
Shaistah J. Qureshi, *MPharm, MRPharmS*
Benjamin Rehman, *BPharm, MRPharmS*
Vinaya K. Sharma, *BPharm, MSc, PGDipPIM, MRPharmS*

Editorial Assistant
Gerard P. Gallagher, *MSc, MRSH, MRIPH*

Nurse Prescribers' Formulary Subcommittee 2004–2005

Chairman
Nicky Cullum
PhD, RGN

Committee Members
Paul B. Anderson
MA, BM, BCh, FRCP

David J.D. Sleator
MB, BCh, BAO, BA, MSc

Maureen P. Morgan
RN, RHV, MBA

Peter J. Curphey
BPharm, FRPharmS

Susan Dewar
MA, BSc, RGN, DN Cert, RNT

Judith Moreton
RGN, RHV, MSc

George Rae
MB, ChB, BSc

Nicholas L. Wood
BPharm, FRPharmS

Joint Secretaries

Molly Courtenay
BSc, MSc, PhD, CertEd, RGN

Philip E. Green
BSc, MSc, LLM, MRPharmS

Matthew T. Griffiths
RGN, A&E Cert, FAETC

Mark Jones
BSc, RGN, RHV, MSc

Vivienne H. Nathanson
MB, BS

Head of Publishing Services
John Wilson

Director of Publications
Charles Fry

Knowledge Systems
Eric I. Connor
BSc(Econ), *MSc, DIC, MBCS*
Knowledge Systems Manager
Simon N. Dunton
BA, PhDr
Editorial Production Assistant
Philip D. Lee
BSc, PhD
Digital Development Assistant
Karl A. Parsons
BSc
Knowledge Systems Administrator
Candace C. Partridge
BA
Digital Quality Specialist

How to use the NPF/BNF

Nurse Prescribers' Formulary

The NPF part provides information of special relevance to the nurse prescriber. This section includes notes on preparations on the Nurse Prescribers' Formulary for Community Practitioners (formerly the Nurse Prescribers' Formulary for District Nurses and Health Visitors), followed by details of the preparations.

Guidance on prescribing

This part includes information on prescription writing, controlled drugs and dependence, prescribing for children and the elderly, prescribing in palliative care, and prescribing in dental practice. Advice is given on the reporting of adverse reactions (see also p. N2).

Emergency treatment of poisoning

This chapter provides information on the management of acute poisoning when first seen in the home, although aspects of hospital-based treatment are mentioned.

Notes on conditions, drugs and preparations

The main text consists of classified notes on clinical conditions, drugs and preparations. These notes are divided into 15 chapters, each of which is related to a particular system of the body or to an aspect of medical care. Each chapter is then divided into sections which begin with appropriate *notes for prescribers*. These notes are intended to provide information to doctors, dental surgeons, pharmacists, nurses, and other healthcare professionals to facilitate the selection of suitable treatment. The notes are followed by details of relevant drugs and preparations.

DRUG NAME [▬]

Indications: details of uses and indications

Cautions: details of precautions required (with cross-references to appropriate Appendixes) and also any monitoring required

COUNSELLING. Verbal explanation to the patient of specific details of the drug treatment (e.g. posture when taking a medicine)

Contra-indications: details of any contra-indications to use of drug

Side-effects: details of common and more serious side-effects

Dose: dose and frequency of administration (max. dose); CHILD and ELDERLY details of dose for specific age group

By alternative route, dose and frequency

* **Approved Name** (Non-proprietary) [PoM]
Pharmaceutical form, colour, coating, active ingredient and amount in dosage form, net price, pack size = basic NHS price. Label: (as in Appendix 9)

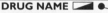

Proprietary Name® (Manufacturer) [PoM] [NHS]
Pharmaceutical form, sugar-free, active ingredient mg/mL, net price, pack size = basic NHS price. Label: (as in Appendix 9)
Excipients: include clinically important excipients or electrolytes

* exceptions to the prescribing status indicated by a footnote.

Note. Specific notes about the product e.g. handling

Preparations

Preparations usually follow immediately after the drug which is their main ingredient.

Preparations are included under a non-proprietary title, if they are marketed under such a title, if they are not otherwise prescribable under the NHS, or if they may be prepared extemporaneously.

If proprietary preparations are of a distinctive colour this is stated.

In the case of compound preparations the indications, cautions, contra-indications, side-effects, and interactions of all constituents should be taken into account for prescribing.

Note. The presentation of preparations in the NPF is slightly different because of the requirements of nurse prescribing.

Drugs

Drugs appear under pharmacopoeial or other non-proprietary titles. When there is an *appropriate current monograph* (Medicines Act 1968, Section 65) preference is given to a name at the head of that monograph; otherwise a British Approved Name (BAN), if available, is used see also p. viii

The symbol [▬] is used to denote those preparations that are considered by the Joint Formulary Committee to be less suitable for prescribing. Although such preparations may not be considered as drugs of first choice, their use may be justifiable in certain circumstances

Prescription-only medicines [PoM]

This symbol has been placed against those preparations that are available only on prescription issued by an appropriate practitioner. For more detailed information see *Medicines, Ethics and Practice*, No. 29, London, Pharmaceutical Press, 2005 (and subsequent editions as available).

The symbol [CD] indicates that the preparation is subject to the prescription requirements of the Misuse of Drugs Act. For regulations governing prescriptions for such preparations see pages 7–9.

Preparations not available for NHS prescription [NHS]

This symbol has been placed against those preparations included in the BNF that are not prescribable under the NHS. Those prescribable only for specific disorders have a footnote specifying the condition(s) for which the preparation remains available. Some preparations which are not *prescribable* by brand name under the NHS may nevertheless be *dispensed* using the brand name providing that the prescription shows an appropriate non-proprietary name.

Prices

Prices have been calculated from the basic cost used in pricing NHS prescriptions dispensed in May 2005 or later, see p. vii for further details.

Appendixes and indexes

The appendixes include information on interactions, liver disease, renal impairment, pregnancy, breast-feeding, intravenous additives, borderline substances, wound management products, and cautionary and advisory labels for dispensed medicines. They are designed for use in association with the main body of the text.

The Dental Practitioners' List and the Nurse Prescribers' List are also included in this section. The indexes consist of the Index of Manufacturers and the Main Index.

Prices in the NPF/BNF

Basic **net prices** are given in the NPF/BNF to provide an indication of relative cost. Where there is a choice of suitable preparations for a particular disease or condition the relative cost may be used in making a selection. Cost-effective prescribing must, however, take into account other factors (such as dose frequency and duration of treatment) that affect the total cost. The use of more expensive drugs is justified if it will result in better treatment of the patient or a reduction of the length of an illness or the time spent in hospital.

Prices have generally been calculated from the net cost used in pricing NHS prescriptions dispensed in May 2005. Unless an original pack is available these prices are based on the largest pack size of the preparation in use in community pharmacies. The price for an extemporaneously prepared preparation has been omitted where the net cost of the ingredients used to make it would give a misleadingly low impression of the final price. In Appendix 8 prices stated are for for a single dressing or bandage.

The unit of 20 is still sometimes used as a basis for comparison, but where suitable original packs or patient packs are available these are priced instead.

Gross prices vary as follows:

1. Costs to the NHS are greater than the net prices quoted and include professional fees and overhead allowances;
2. Private prescription charges are calculated on a separate basis;
3. Over-the-counter sales are at retail price, as opposed to basic net price, and include VAT.

NPF/BNF prices are **not**, therefore, suitable for quoting to patients seeking private prescriptions or contemplating over-the-counter purchases.

A fuller explanation of costs to the NHS may be obtained from the Drug Tariff.

It should be noted that separate Drug Tariffs are applicable in England and Wales, Scotland, and Northern Ireland. Prices in the different tariffs may vary.

Patient Packs

On January 1 1994, EC Directive 92/27/EEC came into force, outlining requirements for the labelling of medicines and for the format and content of patient information leaflets to be supplied with each medicine. The directive also requires the use of Recommended International Nonproprietary Names for drugs (see p. viii)

All medicines now have approved labelling and patient information leaflets; anyone who supplies a medicine is responsible for providing the relevant information to the patient (see also Appendix 9).

Many medicines are available in manufacturers' original packs complete with patient information leaflets. Where patient packs are available, the NPF/BNF shows the number of dose units in the packs. In particular clinical circumstances, where patient packs need to be split or medicines are provided in bulk dispensing packs, manufacturers will provide additional supplies of patient information leaflets on request.

During the revision of each edition of the NPF/BNF careful note is taken of the information that appears on the patient information leaflets. Where it is considered appropriate to alert a prescriber to some specific limitation appearing on the patient information leaflet (for example, in relation to pregnancy) this advice now appears in the NPF/BNF.

The patient information leaflet also includes details of all inactive ingredients in the medicine. A list of common E numbers and the inactive ingredients to which they correspond is now therefore included in the NPF/BNF (see inside back cover).

Name changes

European Law requires use of the Recommended International Nonproprietary Name (rINN) for medicinal substances. In most cases the British Approved Name (BAN) and rINN were identical. Where the two differed, the BAN has been modified to accord with the rINN.

The following list shows those substances for which the former BAN has been modified to accord with the rINN. Former BANs have been retained as synonyms in the NPF/BNF.

ADRENALINE AND NORADRENALINE. Adrenaline and noradrenaline are the terms used in the titles of monographs in the European Pharmacopoeia and are thus the official names in the member states. For these substances, BP 2004 shows the European Pharmacopoeia names and the rINNs at the head of the monographs; the NPF/BNF has adopted a similar style.

Former BAN	New BAN
adrenaline	*see above*
amethocaine	tetracaine
aminacrine	aminoacridine
amoxycillin	amoxicillin
amphetamine	amfetamine
amylobarbitone	amobarbital
amylobarbitone sodium	amobarbital sodium
beclomethasone	beclometasone
bendrofluazide	bendroflumethiazide
benzhexol	trihexyphenidyl
benzphetamine	benzfetamine
benztropine	benzatropine
busulphan	busulfan
butobarbitone	butobarbital
carticaine	articaine
cephalexin	cefalexin
cephradine	cefradine
chloral betaine	cloral betaine
chlorbutol	chlorobutanol
chlormethiazole	clomethiazole
chlorpheniramine	chlorphenamine
chlorthalidone	chlortalidone
cholecalciferol	colecalciferol
cholestyramine	colestyramine
clomiphene	clomifene
colistin sulphomethate sodium	colistimethate sodium
corticotrophin	corticotropin
cyclosporin	ciclosporin
cysteamine	mercaptamine
danthron	dantron
dexamphetamine	dexamfetamine
dibromopropamidine	dibrompropamidine
dicyclomine	dicycloverine
dienoestrol	dienestrol
dimethicone(s)	dimeticone
dimethyl sulphoxide	dimethyl sulfoxide
dothiepin	dosulepin
doxycycline hydrochloride (hemihydrate hemiethanolate)	doxycycline hyclate

Former BAN	New BAN
eformoterol	formoterol
ethamsylate	etamsylate
ethinyloestradiol	ethinylestradiol
ethynodiol	etynodiol
flumethasone	flumetasone
flupenthixol	flupentixol
flurandrenolone	fludroxycortide
frusemide	furosemide
guaiphenesin	guaifenesin
hexachlorophane	hexachlorophene
hexamine hippurate	methenamine hippurate
hydroxyurea	hydroxycarbamide
indomethacin	indometacin
lignocaine	lidocaine
lysuride	lisuride
methicillin	meticillin
methotrimeprazine	levomepromazine
methyl cysteine	mecysteine
methylene blue	methylthioninium chloride
mitozantrone	mitoxantrone
nicoumalone	acenocoumarol
noradrenaline	*see above*
oestradiol	estradiol
oestriol	estriol
oestrone	estrone
oxpentifylline	pentoxifylline
phenobarbitone	phenobarbital
pipothiazine	pipotiazine
polyhexanide	polihexanide
potassium clorazepate	dipotassium clorazepate
pramoxine	pramocaine
procaine penicillin	procaine benzylpenicillin
prothionamide	protionamide
quinalbarbitone	secobarbital
riboflavine	riboflavin
salcatonin	calcitonin (salmon)
sodium calciumedetate	sodium calcium edetate
sodium cromoglycate	sodium cromoglicate
sodium ironedetate	sodium feredetate
sodium picosulphate	sodium picosulfate
sorbitan monostearate	sorbitan stearate
stibocaptate	sodium stibocaptate
stilboestrol	diethylstilbestrol
sulphacetamide	sulfacetamide
sulphadiazine	sulfadiazine
sulphamethoxazole	sulfamethoxazole
sulphapyridine	sulfapyridine
sulphasalazine	sulfasalazine
sulphathiazole	sulfathiazole
sulphinpyrazone	sulfinpyrazone
tetracosactrin	tetracosactide
thiabendazole	tiabendazole
thioguanine	tioguanine
thiopentone	thiopental
thymoxamine	moxisylyte
thyroxine sodium	levothyroxine sodium
tribavirin	ribavirin
trimeprazine	alimemazine
urofollitrophin	urofollitropin

Nurse Prescribers' Formulary

for Community Practitioners

This edition of the NPF/BNF is intended as a pocket book for rapid reference and so cannot contain all the information necessary for patient management. For additional information the nurse prescriber should refer to the doctor who will have access to further information including manufacturers' product literature. Supplementary information is also available from pharmacists. Information can also be found in authoritative websites (follow links from http://bnf.org).

Prescription Writing

Further information may be found in BNF pp. 1–5

Prescriptions written by nurse prescribers should:

- be written legibly in ink;
- be dated;
- state patient's full name and address;
- be signed in ink by the prescriber;
- include age and date of birth of patient.

Also recommended:

- Dose and the dose frequency should be stated. For preparations to be taken 'as required' *a minimum dose interval* should be specified, e.g. 'every 4 hours'.
- The unnecessary use of decimal points should be avoided, e.g. 3 mg, not 3.0 mg.
- Strength of the preparation should be stated, e.g. Paracetamol Tablets 500 mg.
- Quantities of 1 gram or more should be written as 1 g etc.
- Quantities of less than 1 gram should be written in milligrams, e.g. 500 mg, not 0.5 g (see inside back cover for conversion guide). It is, however, acceptable to express a range in the decimal form, e.g. 0.5 to 1 g.
- Quantity prescribed should generally be the pack size specified in the NPF under each preparation.
- Names of medicines should be written clearly using approved (generic) titles or proprietary names as specified throughout the NPF and should **not** be abbreviated.
- Directions should be in *English* and should **not** be abbreviated.

Security and validity of prescriptions

In order to ensure the security and validity of prescriptions nurse prescribers should:

- not leave them unattended;
- not leave them in a car where they may be visible;
- keep them locked up when not in use.

When there is any doubt about the authenticity of a prescription, the pharmacist will contact the nurse prescriber; see also Incomplete Prescriptions, below.

Children

Prescriptions should be written according to the guidelines above, stating the child's age.

Children's doses are stated in the NPF where appropriate but nurse prescribers should exercise **special caution** when contemplating prescribing for children and, for laxatives in particular, should consider discussing with the child's medical practitioner before initiating a prescription.

Where a single dose is stated for a given age range, it applies to the middle of the age range and may need to be adjusted to obtain doses for ages at the lower and upper limits of the stated range. Nurse prescribers are advised to err on the side of caution.

The pharmacist will supply an **oral syringe** with oral liquid preparations if the dose prescribed is less than 5 mL. The oral syringe is marked in 0.5-mL divisions from 1 to 5 mL to measure doses of less than 5 mL. It is provided with an adaptor and an instruction leaflet. A 5-mL spoon will be given for doses of 5 or 10 mL.

Excipients

Where an oral liquid medicine in the NPF is available in a form free of *fructose, glucose,* or *sucrose* a note has been added to say that a sugar-free version may be requested by adding 'sugar free' to the prescription. Preparations containing hydrogenated glucose syrup, mannitol, maltitol, sorbitol, or xylitol are also marked 'sugar-free' because there is evidence that they do not cause dental caries. Whenever possible sugar-free preparations should be requested for children to reduce the risk of dental decay.

Where information on the presence of *aspartame, gluten, tartrazine, arachis (peanut) oil* or *sesame oil* is available, this is indicated against the relevant product entry; if it is essential to check details and the information is not available in the NPF or in the product literature, then the manufacturer should be contacted.

Information is provided on *selected excipients* in skin preparations (see BNF section 13.1.3).

Prevention of adverse reactions

Adverse reactions may be prevented as follows:

- Never prescribe any medicine unless there is a good indication.
- A Community Practitioner nurse prescriber should **not** prescribe medicines for pregnant women (except folic acid and, in some circumstances, nicotine replacement therapy); the patient should be referred to her doctor.
- It is very important to recognise allergy as a cause of adverse drug reactions. Ask if the patient has had any previous reactions, particularly when prescribing aspirin or dressings impregnated with iodine.
- Ask if the patient is taking any other medicines **including self medication**; remember that aspirin interacts with warfarin.
- Check whether there are any special instructions in relation to hepatic or renal disease.
- Prescribe as few medicines as possible and give very clear instructions to the elderly or any patient likely to misunderstand complicated instructions. Elderly patients cannot normally cope with more than three different medicines (and ideally they should not need to be taken more than twice daily).

Reporting of adverse reactions. If a patient has an adverse reaction to a medicine or dressing, the nurse prescriber should consider reporting it to the Committee on Safety of Medicines using the 'yellow card' scheme for reporting adverse reactions (see BNF p. 10).

Incomplete prescriptions

A pharmacist may need to contact the nurse prescriber if the *quantity, strength* or *dose* are missing from the prescription. The pharmacist will then arrange for the missing details to be added. Under some circumstances the pharmacist will use professional judgement as to what to give and will endorse the prescription.

Labelling of dispensed medicine

The following will appear on the label of a dispensed medicine:

- name of product
- name of patient
- date of dispensing
- name and address of pharmacy
- directions for use
- total quantity of product dispensed
- advice to keep out of reach of children.

Other information (e.g. 'flammable') will be added by the pharmacist as appropriate. Preparation entries in the NPF provide details of any additional cautionary advice that the pharmacist will add.

The *name of the product* will be that which is written on the prescription.

Safety in the home

Patients must be warned to keep all medicines out of the reach of children. Medicines will be dispensed in reclosable *child-resistant containers* unless:

- they are in manufacturers' original packs designed for supplying to the patient
- the patient would have difficulty in opening a child-resistant container.

In the latter case the pharmacist will make a particular point of advising that the medicines be kept out of reach of children. The nurse prescriber could usefully *reinforce this advice*.

Patients should be advised to dispose of *unwanted medicines* by returning them to a pharmacist for destruction.

Duplicate medicines

Nurses are well placed to check on whether patients are at risk of taking two medicines with the same action (or which contain the same ingredient) at the same time. This is of special concern in the case of medicines that can also be bought over the counter (e.g. aspirin and paracetamol). Pharmacists reduce this risk to some extent by making sure that the words 'aspirin' *or* 'aspirin and paracetamol' appear on relevant preparations. A check on the patient's medicines (including cough and cold cures) might prevent the patient inadvertently taking duplicate doses of aspirin or paracetamol. A list of preparations on sale to the public that contain aspirin or paracetamol alone or with other ingredients can be found in the BNF (section 4.7.1).

Prices

Net prices have been included in the NPF to provide an indication of relative cost. These prices are **not** suitable for quoting to patients since they do not include the pharmacist's professional fee and other allowances, nor do they include VAT.

PACT and SPA

PACT (Prescribing Analyses and Cost) and SPA (Scottish Prescribing Analysis) provide prescribers with information about their prescribing in comparison with the prescribing figures for the local Primary Care Trust equivalent practice and with a national equivalent.

Changes to the Nurse Prescribers' List for Community Practitioners

Additions

***Medicinal preparations, appliances, and reagents added to Nurse Prescribers' List since 2003*[1]**

Chemical Reagents as listed below:
- Detection Strips for Blood Ketones
- Detection Strips for Determination of International Normalised Ratio (INR)

Dry Mouth Products

Emollients as listed below:
- Zerobase® Cream

Emollient Bath Additives as listed below:
- Cetraben® Emollient Bath Additive

Emollients (as listed in the Drug Tariff)

Macrogol Oral Powder, Compound, Half-strength

Oral Film Forming Agents

Phosphate Suppositories

Spermicidal Contraceptives as listed below:
- Gynol II® Jelly
- Ortho-Creme® Cream
- Orthoforms® Pessaries

Vaginal Moisturisers

Wound Management and Related Products as listed below:
- Gauze Dressings (Impregnated)
- Venous Ulcer Compression System
- Wound Management Dressings (including collagen dressings)

Zinc Cream, BP

Zinc Ointment, BP

Zinc Paste Bandage, BP 1993

Zinc Paste and Calamine Bandage

Zinc Paste, Calamine and Clioquinol Bandage, BP 1993

Zinc Paste and Ichthammol Bandage, BP 1993

Deletions

Preparations deleted from the Nurse Prescribers' List since 2003

Catheter Maintenance Solution, Mandelic Acid, NPF

Detection Tablets for Glycosuria

Detection Strips for Ketonuria

Dextranomer Beads, NPF

Dextranomer Paste, NPF

Elastic Diachylon Bandage, Ventilated, BPC

Eurax® Dermatological Bath Oil

Permethrin Cream Rinse, NPF

Phenothrin Foam Application, NPF

Reagent Solutions

Saliva Stimulating Tablets (now included under Dry Mouth Products)

Urine Sugar Analysis Equipment

Nurse Prescribers' Extended Formulary

Nurses who have received specific training (distinct from that provided to Community Practitioner Nurse Prescribers) may prescribe from the Nurse Prescribers' Extended Formulary, see p. N8

1. Some appliances and reagents are not prescribable by nurses in Northern Ireland and Scotland—see full amended list

Nurse Prescribers' Formulary

for Community Practitioners

List of preparations approved by the Secretary of State which may be prescribed on form FP10P (form HS21(N) in Northern Ireland, form GP10(N) in Scotland, forms FP10(CN) and FP10(PN) in Wales or, when available, WP10CN and WP10PN in Wales) by Nurses for National Health Service patients.

Community Practitioners who have completed the necessary training may only prescribe items appearing in the nurse prescribers' list set out below.

Medicinal Preparations

Almond Oil Ear Drops, BP
Arachis Oil Enema, NPF
[1]Aspirin Tablets, Dispersible, 300 mg, BP
Bisacodyl Suppositories, BP (includes 5-mg and 10-mg strengths)
Bisacodyl Tablets, BP
Cadexomer-Iodine Ointment, NPF
Cadexomer-Iodine Paste, NPF
Cadexomer-Iodine Powder, NPF
Catheter Maintenance Solution, Chlorhexidine, NPF
Catheter Maintenance Solution, Sodium Chloride, NPF
Catheter Maintenance Solution, 'Solution G', NPF
Catheter Maintenance Solution, 'Solution R', NPF
Choline Salicylate Dental Gel, BP
Clotrimazole Cream 1%, BP
Co-danthramer Capsules, NPF
Co-danthramer Capsules, Strong, NPF
Co-danthramer Oral Suspension, NPF
Co-danthramer Oral Suspension, Strong, NPF
Co-danthrusate Capsules, BP
Co-danthrusate Oral Suspension, NPF
Crotamiton Cream, BP
Crotamiton Lotion, BP
Dimeticone barrier creams containing at least 10%
Docusate Capsules, BP
Docusate Enema, NPF
Docusate Enema, Compound, BP
Docusate Oral Solution, BP
Docusate Oral Solution, Paediatric, BP
Econazole Cream 1%, BP
Emollients as listed below:
- Aqueous Cream, BP
- Arachis Oil, BP
- Cetraben® Emollient Cream
- Decubal® Clinic
- Dermamist®
- Diprobase® Cream
- Diprobase® Ointment
- Doublebase®
- E45® Cream
- Emulsifying Ointment, BP
- [2]Epaderm®
- Gammaderm® Cream
- Hydromol® Cream
- Hydromol® Ointment
- Hydrous Ointment, BP
- Keri® Therapeutic Lotion
- LactiCare® Lotion
- Lipobase®
- Liquid and White Soft Paraffin Ointment, NPF
- Neutrogena1 Dermatological Cream
- Oilatum® Cream
- Paraffin, White Soft, BP
- Paraffin, Yellow Soft, BP
- Ultrabase®
- Unguentum M®
- Zerobase® Cream

Emollient Bath Additives as listed below:
- Alpha Keri® Bath Oil
- Ashbourne Emollient Medicinal Bath Oil
- [3]Balneum®
- Cetraben® Emollient Bath Additive
- Dermalo® Bath Emollient
- Diprobath®
- Hydromol® Emollient
- Imuderm® Bath Oil
- Oilatum® Emollient
- Oilatum® Fragrance Free Junior
- Oilatum® Gel

Folic Acid 400 micrograms/5mL Oral Solution, NPF
Folic Acid Tablets 400 micrograms, BP
Glycerol Suppositories, BP
[4]Ibuprofen Oral Suspension, BP
[4]Ibuprofen Tablets, BP
Ispaghula Husk Granules, BP
Ispaghula Husk Granules, Effervescent, BP
Ispaghula Husk Oral Powder, BP
Lactulose Solution, BP
Lidocaine Gel, BP
Lidocaine Ointment, BP
Lidocaine and Chlorhexidine Gel, BP
Macrogol Oral Powder, NPF
Macrogol Oral Powder, Compound, NPF
Macrogol Oral Powder, Compound, Half-strength, NPF
Magnesium Hydroxide Mixture, BP
Magnesium Sulphate Paste, BP
Malathion alcoholic lotions containing at least 0.5%
Malathion aqueous lotions containing at least 0.5%
Mebendazole Oral Suspension, NPF
Mebendazole Tablets, NPF
Methylcellulose Tablets, BP
Miconazole Cream 2%, BP
Miconazole Oromucosal Gel, BP
Mouthwash Solution-tablets, NPF
Nicotine Inhalation Cartridge for Oromucosal Use, NPF
Nicotine Lozenge, NPF
Nicotine Medicated Chewing Gum, NPF
Nicotine Nasal Spray, NPF
Nicotine Sublingual Tablets, NPF
Nicotine Transdermal Patches, NPF
Nystatin Oral Suspension, BP
Nystatin Pastilles, BP
Olive Oil Ear Drops, BP
Paracetamol Oral Suspension, BP (includes 120 mg/5 mL and 250 mg/5 mL strengths—both of which are available as sugar-free formulations)
[1]Paracetamol Tablets, BP
[1]Paracetamol Tablets, Soluble, BP (includes 120-mg and 500-mg tablets)
Permethrin Cream, NPF
Phenothrin Alcoholic Lotion, NPF
Phenothrin Aqueous Lotion, NPF
Phosphate Suppositories, NPF
Phosphates Enema, BP
Piperazine and Senna Powder, NPF
Povidone–Iodine Solution, BP
Senna Granules, Standardised, BP
Senna Oral Solution, NPF
Senna Tablets, BP
Senna and Ispaghula Granules, NPF
Sodium Chloride Solution, Sterile, BP
Sodium Citrate Compound Enema, NPF
Sodium Picosulfate Capsules, NPF
Sodium Picosulfate Elixir, NPF

---

1. Max. 96 tablets; max. pack size 32 tablets
2. Included in the Drug Tariff, Scottish Drug Tariff, and Northern Ireland Drug Tariff
3. Except pack sizes that are not to be prescribed under the NHS (see Part XVIIIA of the Drug Tariff, Part XI of the Northern Ireland Drug Tariff)
4. Except for indications and doses that are PoM

Spermicidal Contraceptives as listed below:
- Gynol II® Jelly
- Ortho-Creme® Cream
- Orthoforms® Pessaries

Sterculia Granules, NPF
Sterculia and Frangula Granules, NPF
Streptokinase and Streptodornase Topical Powder, NPF
Thymol Glycerin, Compound, BP 1988
Titanium Ointment, BP
Water for Injections, BP
Zinc and Castor Oil Ointment, BP
Zinc Cream, BP
Zinc Ointment, BP
Zinc Oxide and Dimeticone Spray, NPF
Zinc Oxide Impregnated Medicated Stocking, NPF
Zinc Paste Bandage, BP 1993
Zinc Paste and Calamine Bandage
Zinc Paste, Calamine and Clioquinol Bandage BP 1993
Zinc Paste and Ichthammol Bandage, BP 1993

Appliances and Reagents (including Wound Management Products)

In the Drug Tariff Appliances and Reagents which may not be prescribed by Nurses are annotated ⊗ (**Nx** in the Scottish Drug Tariff and N̸ in the Northern Ireland Drug Tariff)

Applicators, Vaginal as listed in Part IXA of the Drug Tariff (Part 3 of the Scottish Drug Tariff, not prescribable by nurses in Northern Ireland)

Atomizers, Hand Operated as listed in Part IXA of the Drug Tariff (Part 3 of the Scottish Drug Tariff, not prescribable by nurses in Northern Ireland)

Auto Inflation Device (for treatment of glue ear) as listed in Part IXA of the Drug Tariff (Part 3 of the Scottish Drug Tariff, Part III of the Northern Ireland Drug Tariff)

Breast Reliever as listed in Part IXA of the Drug Tariff (Part 3 of the Scottish Drug Tariff, not prescribable by nurses in Northern Ireland)

Breast Shields as listed in Part IXA of the Drug Tariff (not prescribable by nurses in Scotland or Northern Ireland)

Chemical Reagents

The following as listed in Part IXR of the Drug Tariff (Part 9 of the Scottish Drug Tariff, Part II of the Northern Ireland Drug Tariff):
- Detection Strips for Glycosuria
- Detection Strips for Ketonuria
- Detection Strips for Proteinuria
- Detection Strips for Blood Glucose
- Detection Strips for Blood Ketones (not prescribable by nurses in Northern Ireland)
- Detection Strips for Determination of International Normalised Ratio (INR) (not prescribable by nurses in Northern Ireland)

Also in BNF section 6.1.6. Items not in the Drug Tariff (and thus not prescribable) are described as NHS *in the BNF. Although glucose for glucose tolerance test is in section 6.1.6 it is not on the Nurse Prescribers' List*

Catheter Accessories as listed in Part IXA of the Drug Tariff (Part 3 of the Scottish Drug Tariff, Part III of the Northern Ireland Drug Tariff)

Catheter Maintenance Solutions as listed in Part IXA of the Drug Tariff (Part 3 of the Scottish Drug Tariff, Part III of the Northern Ireland Drug Tariff)

Note. See also under Medicinal Preparations

Catheters, Urethral Sterile as listed under Catheters in Part IXA of the Drug Tariff (Part 3 of the Scottish Drug Tariff, Part III of the Northern Ireland Drug Tariff)

Cervical Collar, Soft Foam as listed in Part IXA of the Drug Tariff (Part 3 of the Scottish Drug Tariff, not prescribable by nurses in Northern Ireland)

Chiropody Appliances as listed in Part IXA of the Drug Tariff (Part 2 of the Scottish Drug Tariff (except for Corn Plasters), not prescribable by nurses in Northern Ireland)

Contraceptive Devices as listed in Part IXA of the Drug Tariff (Part 3 of the Scottish Drug Tariff, Part III of the Northern Ireland Drug Tariff (fertility (ovulation) thermometers only))

Also in BNF section 7.3.4

Douches (with vaginal and rectal fittings) as listed in Part IXA of the Drug Tariff (Part 3 of the Scottish Drug Tariff, not prescribable by nurses in Northern Ireland)

Droppers as listed in Part IXA of the Drug Tariff (Part 3 of the Scottish Drug Tariff, not prescribable by nurses in Northern Ireland)

Dry Mouth Products as listed in Part IXA of the Drug Tariff (Part 3 of the Scottish Drug Tariff, not prescribable by nurses in Northern Ireland)

Ear Wax Softening Medical Devices as listed in Part IXA of the Drug Tariff

Elastic Hosiery including accessories as listed in Part IXA of the Drug Tariff (Part 4 of the Scottish Drug Tariff, Part III of the Northern Ireland Drug Tariff)

Also in BNF Appendix 8 (section A8.3)

Emollients as listed in Part IXA of the Drug Tariff (Part 3 of the Scottish Drug Tariff, Part III of the Northern Ireland Drug Tariff)

Note. See also under Medicinal Preparations

Eye Baths as listed in Part IXA of the Drug Tariff (Part 3 of the Scottish Drug Tariff, not prescribable by nurses in Northern Ireland)

Eye-drop Dispensers as listed in Part IXA of the Drug Tariff (Part 3 of the Scottish Drug Tariff, Part III of the Northern Ireland Drug Tariff)

Eye Shades as listed in Part IXA of the Drug Tariff (Part 3 of the Scottish Drug Tariff, not prescribable by nurses in Northern Ireland)

Finger Cots as listed in Part IXA of the Drug Tariff (Part 3 of the Scottish Drug Tariff, not prescribable by nurses in Northern Ireland)

Finger Stalls as listed in Part IXA of the Drug Tariff (Part 3 of the Scottish Drug Tariff, not prescribable by nurses in Northern Ireland)

Head Lice Device as listed in Part IXA of the Drug Tariff (Part 3 of the Scottish Drug Tariff, Part III of the Northern Ireland Drug Tariff)

Hypodermic Equipment as listed in Part IXA of the Drug Tariff (Part 3 of the Scottish Drug Tariff, Part III of the Northern Ireland Drug Tariff (with some exceptions))

Also in BNF section 6.1.1.3. Items not in the Drug Tariff (and thus not prescribable) are described as NHS *in the BNF*

Incontinence Appliances as listed in Part IXB of the Drug Tariff (Part 5 of the Scottish Drug Tariff, Part III of the Northern Ireland Drug Tariff)

Inhaler, Spare Tops as listed in Part IXA of the Drug Tariff (Part 3 of the Scottish Drug Tariff, not prescribable by nurses in Northern Ireland)

Insufflators as listed in Part IXA of the Drug Tariff (Part 3 of the Scottish Drug Tariff, not prescribable by nurses in Northern Ireland)

Irrigation Fluids as listed in Part IXA of the Drug Tariff (Part 2 of the Scottish Drug Tariff, Part III of the Northern Ireland Drug Tariff)

Note. See also under Medicinal Preparations (Sodium Chloride Solution, Sterile)

Latex Foam, Adhesive as listed in Part IXA of the Drug Tariff (not prescribable by nurses in Scotland or Northern Ireland)

Lubricating Jelly as listed in Part IXA of the Drug Tariff (Part 2 of the Scottish Drug Tariff, not prescribable by nurses in Northern Ireland)

Nasal Device (nasal dilator) as listed in Part IXA of the Druf Tariff (Part 3 of the Scottish Drug Tariff, Part III of the Northern Ireland Drug Tariff)

Nipple Shields, Plastic as listed in Part IXA of the Drug Tariff (Part 3 of the Scottish Drug Tariff, not prescribable by nurses in Northern Ireland)

Oral Film Forming Agents as listed in Part IXA of the Drug Tariff (Part 3 of the Scottish Drug Tariff, not prescribable by nurses in Northern Ireland)

Peak Flow Meters as listed in Part IXA of the Drug Tariff (Part 3 of the Scottish Drug Tariff, not prescribable by nurses in Northern Ireland)

Also in BNF section 3.1.5

Pessaries as listed in Part IXA of the Drug Tariff (Part 3 of the Scottish Drug Tariff, Part III of the Northern Ireland Drug Tariff (with some exceptions))

Protectives as listed in Part IXA of the Drug Tariff (Part 2 of the Scottish Drug Tariff, Part III of the Northern Ireland Drug Tariff (EMA Disposable Film Gloves only))

Stoma Appliances and Associated Products as listed in Part IXC of the Drug Tariff (Part 6 of the Scottish Drug Tariff, Part III of the Northern Ireland Drug Tariff)

Suprapubic Belts (replacements only) as listed in Part IXA of the Drug Tariff (Part 3 of the Scottish Drug Tariff, not prescribable by nurses in Northern Ireland)

Suprapubic Catheters as listed in Part IXA of the Drug Tariff (Part 3 of the Scottish Drug Tariff, not prescribable by nurses in Northern Ireland)

Synovial Fluid as listed in Part IXA of the Drug Tariff (Part 3 of the Scottish Drug Tariff, not prescribable by nurses in Northern Ireland)

Note. Mentioned in text of BNF section 10.1

Syringes (Bladder/Irrigating, Ear, Enema, Spare Vaginal Pipes) as listed in Part IXA of the Drug Tariff (Part 3 of the Scottish Drug Tariff, not prescribable by nurses in Northern Ireland)

Test Tubes as listed in Part IXA of the Drug Tariff (Part 3 of the Scottish Drug Tariff, not prescribable by nurses in Northern Ireland)

Tracheostomy and Laryngectomy Appliances as listed in Part IXA of the Drug Tariff (Part 2 of the Scottish Drug Tariff, not prescribable by nurses in Northern Ireland)

Trusses as listed in Part IXA of the Drug Tariff (Part 3 of the Scottish Drug Tariff, not prescribable by nurses in Northern Ireland)

Vacuum Pumps and Constrictor Rings for Erectile Dysfunction as listed in Part IXA of the Drug Tariff (Parts 3 of the Scottish Drug Tariff, Part III of the Northern Ireland Drug Tariff)—prescribing restrictions may apply (see Drug Tariff)

Vaginal Moisturisers as listed in Part IXA of the Drug Tariff (Part 3 of the Scottish Drug Tariff)

Wound Management and Related Products (including bandages, dressings, gauzes, lint, stockinette, etc)

The following as listed in Part IXA of the Drug Tariff (Part 2 of the Scottish Drug Tariff, Part III of the Northern Ireland Drug Tariff):

- Absorbent Cellulose Dressing with Fluid Repellent Backing
- Absorbent Cottons
- Absorbent Cotton Gauzes
- Absorbent Cotton and Viscose Ribbon Gauze, BP 1988
- Absorbent Dressing Pads, Sterile
- Absorbent Lint, BPC
- Absorbent Perforated Dressing with Adhesive Border
- Absorbent Perforated Plastic Film Faced Dressing
- Arm Slings
- Belladonna Adhesive Plaster, BP 1980
- Boil Dressing Pack
- Cellulose Wadding, BP 1988
- Chlorhexidine Gauze Dressing, BP
- Conforming Bandage (Synthetic)
- Cotton Conforming Bandage, BP 1988
- Cotton Crêpe Bandage, BP 1988
- Cotton Crêpe Bandage, Hospicrepe 239
- Cotton, Polyamide and Elastane Bandage
- Cotton Stretch Bandage, BP 1988
- Crêpe Bandage, BP 1988
- Elastic Adhesive Bandage, BP
- Elastic Web Bandages
- Elastomer and Viscose Bandage, Knitted
- Gauze and Cotton Tissues
- Gauze Dressings (Impregnated)
- Heavy Cotton and Rubber Elastic Bandage, BP
- High Compression Bandages (Extensible)
- Knitted Polyamide and Cellulose Contour Bandage, BP 1988
- Knitted Viscose Primary Dressing, BP, Type 1
- Multi-layer Compression Bandaging
- Multiple Pack Dressing No. 1
- Open-wove Bandage, BP 1988, Type 1
- Paraffin Gauze Dressing, BP
- Plaster of Paris Bandage, BP 1988
- Polyamide and Cellulose Contour Bandage, BP 1988
- Polyester Primary Dressing with Neutral Triglycerides, Knitted
- Povidone–Iodine Fabric Dressing, Sterile
- Short Stretch Compression Bandage
- Skin Adhesive, Sterile
- Skin Closure Strips, Sterile
- Standard Dressings
- Sterile Dressing Packs
- Stockinettes
- Sub-compression Wadding Bandage
- Surgical Adhesive Tapes
- Surgical Sutures (absorbable and non-absorbable)
- Suspensory Bandages, Cotton
- Swabs
- Triangular Calico Bandage, BP 1980
- Vapour-permeable Adhesive Film Dressing, BP (including with absorbent pad)
- Vapour-permeable Waterproof Plastic Wound Dressing, BP, Sterile

Venous Ulcer Compression System
Wound Drainage Pouch
Wound Management Dressings (including activated charcoal, alginate, capillary-action, cavity, collagen, hydrocolloid, hydrogel, foam, polyurethane matrix, protease modulating matrix, silicone, silver-coated and silver-impregnated, and soft polymer dressings)
Zinc Paste Bandages (including both plain and with additional ingredients)—see also under Medicinal Preparations

Also in BNF Appendix 8. Items not in the Drug Tariff (and thus not prescribable) are described as NHS *in the BNF.*

In the Drug Tariff Appliances and Reagents which may **not** be prescribed by Nurses are annotated Ⓝ

(**Nx** in the Scottish Drug Tariff and N in the Northern Ireland Drug Tariff)

Nurse Prescribers' Extended Formulary

List of preparations which may be prescribed by Extended Formulary Nurse Prescribers on Form FP10P, for NHS patients in England (Form HS21(N) in Northern Ireland, Form GP10(N2) in Scotland)

Independent nurse prescribers who have completed the necessary training and are authorised to prescribe from the Nurse Prescribers' Extended Formulary list may prescribe all General Sales List and Pharmacy medicines currently prescribable by GPs, together with specified Prescription Only Medicines. In addition they may prescribe all items in the nurse prescribing list for Community Practitioners on pp. N4–7.

The Committee on Safety of Medicines advises that Extended Formulary Nurse Prescribers should prescribe medicines (including pharmacy-only and General Sales List medicines) **only** for the medical conditions specified below. This advice is reinforced in Extending Independent Nurse Prescribing within the NHS in England: a guide for implementation (available on the Department of Health website, www.dh.gov.uk). Nurses should **not** prescribe independently for conditions other than those on the list.

Medical Conditions

	BNF section[1]
Central Nervous System	
Acute dystonias	4.9.2
Acute severe pain after trauma	4.7.2
Changing painful dressings	15.2
Nausea and vomiting	4.6
Prophylaxis and treatment of nausea and vomiting in the postoperative period	4.6
Recurrent generalised tonic-clonic seizures	4.8.2
Circulatory	
Acute myocardial infarction	2.10
Acute pulmonary oedema associated with cardiac failure	2.2.2
Angina pectoris	2.6
Fluid replacement and potassium replacement (hypovolaemia and dehydration)	9.2.2.1
Haemorrhoids	1.7.1, 1.7.2
Phlebitis, superficial	–
Plasma substitutes for patients with a low blood volume	9.2.2.2
Thromboprophylaxis—defined as prophylaxis against venous thrombosis (including congestive heart failure, in bed-bound patients, and perioperatively) and for acute coronary syndrome	2.8.1
Ventricular fibrillation or pulseless ventricular tachycardia	2.7.3
Ear	
Furuncle	–
Otitis externa	12.1.1
Otitis media	12.1.2
Wax in ear	12.1.3
Endocrine	
Hyperglycaemia	6.1.1
Hypoglycaemia	6.1.4
Eye	
Blepharitis	11.3.1
Conjunctivitis, allergic	11.4.2
Conjunctivitis, infective	11.3.1
Corneal trauma	11.7
Diagnostic use in ophthalmology	11.5
Local anaesthetic for ophthalmic conditions	11.7
Tear deficiency	11.8.1
Gastro-intestinal conditions	
Constipation	1.6
Gastro-enteritis	1.4
Heartburn	1.1
Infantile colic	1.1.1
Pre-surgery prophylaxis against acid aspiration	1.3.1, 1.3.5
Worms, threadworms	5.5.1
Immunisations	
Routine childhood and specific vaccinations	14.1, 14.4
Infections	
Emergency treatment of suspected meningococcal septicaemia or meningococcal meningitis	5.1 (table 1)
Spreading cellulitis usually of a limb with a risk of, or an established lymphangitis	5.1 (table 1)
Tetanus prophylaxis and treatment	14.4, 14.5
Musculoskeletal	
Back pain, acute uncomplicated	4.7.1, 10.1.1
Neck pain, acute uncomplicated	4.7.1, 10.1.1
Pain and inflammation	10.1.1
Soft tissue injuries	4.7.1, 10.1.1, 10.3.2
Sprains	4.7.1, 10.1.1, 10.3.2
Oral conditions	
Aphthous ulcer	12.3.1
Candidiasis, oral	12.3.2
Dental abscess	4.7.1, 10.1.1
Dental infections	5.1 (table 1)
Gingivitis	12.3.4
Stomatitis	–
Poisoning	
Poisoning	Emergency treatment of poisoning
Respiratory	
Acute attacks of asthma	3.1
Acute exacerbation of chronic bronchitis	5.1 (table 1)
Acute nasopharyngitis (coryza)	12.2.2
Acute reversible airways obstruction (acute severe asthma or acute exacerbation of chronic obstructive pulmonary disease)	3.1
Anaphylaxis	3.4.3
Conditions requiring oxygen supplementation (e.g. hypoxaemia)	3.6
Croup	3.1
Laryngitis	12.3.1
Pharyngitis	12.3.1
Rhinitis, allergic	3.4.1, 12.2.1, 12.2.2
Sinusitis, acute	12.2.2
Tonsillitis	12.3.1

1. BNF sections appropriate to the listed conditions are shown. However, not all drugs in these sections are prescribable by nurses. Also, in some cases preparations (including General Sales List and Pharmacy medicines) in other BNF sections may be suitable. Before choosing a Prescription Only Medicine, nurses need to check the Nurse Prescribers' Extended Formulary list and to satisfy themselves that the product is licensed for the condition they wish to prescribe for and that the condition falls within the remit of the Nurse Prescribers' Extended Formulary.

Medical Conditions (*—continued*)	BNF section[1]
Skin	
Abrasions	13.10.5
Acne	13.6
Animal and human bites	5.1 (table 1)
Boil/carbuncle	13.10.5
Burn/scald	13.11, App. 8
Candidiasis, skin	13.10.2
Chronic skin ulcer	13.11.7, 13.10.1
Dermatitis, atopic	13.5.1
Dermatitis, contact	13.5.1
Dermatitis, seborrhoeic	13.5.1
Dermatophytosis of the skin (ringworm)	13.10.2
Herpes labialis	13.10.3
Impetigo	5.1 (table 1), 13.10.1
Insect bite/sting	13.3
Lacerations	13.11, App. 8
Local anaesthetic for occasions when procedure requires it	15.2
Local anaesthetic for suturing of lacerations	15.2
Molluscum contagiosum	–
Nappy rash	13.2.2
Pediculosis (head lice)	13.10.4
Pruritus in chickenpox	13.3
Psoriasis	13.5.2
Scabies	13.10.4
Urticaria	3.4.1
Warts (including verrucas)	13.7
Substance dependance	
Acute alcohol withdrawal	4.10
Smoking cessation	4.10
Urinary system	
Urinary tract infection (women) —lower, uncomplicated	5.1 (table 1), 7.4.3
Female genital system	
Bacterial vaginosis	5.1.11, 7.2.2
Candidiasis, vulvovaginal	7.2.2
Contraception	7.3
Dysmenorrhoea	4.7.1, 10.1.1
Emergency contraception	7.3
Laboratory-confirmed uncomplicated genital chlamydia infection (and the sexual partners of these patients)	5.1 (table 1)
Menopausal vaginal atrophy	7.2.1
Preconceptual counselling	9.1.2
Trichomonas vaginalis infection (and the sexual partners of these patients)	5.4.3
Male genital system	
Balanitis	13.10.2

Palliative Care of patients with advanced progressive illness

Anxiety	4.1.2
Bowel colic	Prescribing in palliative care
Candidiasis, oral	12.3.2
Confusion	Prescribing in palliative care
Constipation	Prescribing in palliative care
Convulsions and restlessness	Prescribing in palliative care
Cough	Prescribing in palliative care
Dry mouth	Prescribing in palliative care
Excessive respiratory secretions	Prescribing in palliative care
Fungating malodorous tumours	13.10.1.2
Muscle spasm	Prescribing in palliative care
Nausea and vomiting	Prescribing in palliative care
Neuropathic pain in palliative care	Prescribing in palliative care
Pain control	Prescribing in palliative care

1. BNF sections appropriate to the listed conditions are shown. However, not all drugs in these sections are prescribable by nurses. Also, in some cases preparations (including General Sales List and Pharmacy medicines) in other BNF sections may be suitable. Before choosing a Prescription Only Medicine, nurses need to check the Nurse Prescribers' Extended Formulary list and to satisfy themselves that the product is licensed for the condition they wish to prescribe for and that the condition falls within the remit of the Nurse Prescribers' Extended Formulary.

Nurse Prescribers' Extended Formulary

- All licensed P and GSL Medicines prescribable on the NHS for the specified list of medical conditions
- Prescription Only Medicines from the list below by the route or form specified
- See above for the list of those medical conditions for which nurses may prescribe independently

List of prescription only medicines for prescribing by extended formulary nurse prescribers

Oral antibacterials marked * —see separate list below for indications

Drug	Route of administration, use or pharmaceutical form
Acetylcysteine	Parenteral
Aciclovir	External
Acrivastine	Oral
Adapalene	External
Adrenaline	Parenteral
Alclometasone dipropionate	External
Alimemazine tartrate (trimeprazine tartrate)	Oral
Alteplase	Parenteral
Amiodarone	Parenteral
Amitriptyline hydrochloride	Palliative care—oral
Amorolfine hydrochloride	External
Amoxicillin trihydrate*	Oral
Aspirin	Oral
Azelaic acid	External
Azelastine hydrochloride	Ophthalmic, nasal
Azithromycin dihydrate*	Oral
Baclofen	Palliative care—oral
Beclometasone dipropionate	External, inhalation, nasal
Bemiparin sodium	Parenteral
Benzatropine mesilate	Parenteral
Benzylpenicillin sodium	Parenteral
Betamethasone sodium phosphate	Aural, nasal
Betamethasone valerate	External, rectal
Budesonide	Inhalation, nasal
Calcipotriol	External
Calcitriol	External
Carbamazepine	Palliative care—oral, rectal
Carbaryl	External
Carbenoxolone sodium	Mouthwash
Cefotaxime sodium	Parenteral
Ceftriaxone sodium	Parenteral
Certoparin sodium	Parenteral
Cetirizine hydrochloride	Oral
Chloramphenicol	Ophthalmic
Chlorphenamine maleate	Parenteral
Cimetidine	Oral, parenteral
Cinchocaine hydrochloride	Rectal
[1]Clavulanic acid	Oral
Clindamycin phosphate	External, vaginal
Clobetasone butyrate	External
Clotrimazole	External
Codeine phosphate	Oral
Conjugated oestrogens (equine)	External
Co-phenotrope	Oral
Cyclizine hydrochloride	Oral
Cyclizine lactate	Parenteral
Dalteparin sodium	Parenteral
Dantrolene sodium	Palliative care—oral
Dantron	Oral
[2]Desogestrel	Oral
Desoximetasone	External
Dexamethasone	Aural
Dexamethasone isonicotinate	Nasal
Dexamethasone sodium phosphate	Oral
Dextran 70	Parenteral
Diazepam	Oral, parenteral and rectal
Diclofenac diethylammonium	External
Diclofenac potassium	Oral
Diclofenac sodium	Oral, rectal, ophthalmic
Dihydrocodeine tartrate	Oral
Dolasetron mesilate	Oral and parenteral
Domperidone	Oral and rectal
Domperidone maleate	Oral
Doxycycline*	Oral
Doxycycline hyclate*	Oral
Econazole nitrate	External, vaginal
Emedastine	Ophthalmic
Enoxaparin	Parenteral
Erythromycin*	External, oral
Erythromycin ethyl succinate*	Oral
Erythromycin stearate*	Oral
Estradiol	External
Estriol	External
[2]Ethinylestradiol	Oral
Etonogestrel	Implant
[2]Etynodiol diacetate	Oral
Famotidine	Oral
Felbinac	External
Fenticonazole nitrate	Vaginal
Fexofenadine hydrochloride	Oral
Flucloxacillin magnesium*	Oral
Flucloxacillin sodium*	Oral, parenteral
Fluconazole	Oral
Fludroxycortide (flurandrenolone)	External
Flumazenil	Parenteral
Flumetasone pivalate	Aural
Flunisolide	Nasal
Fluocinolone acetonide	External
Fluocinonide	External
Fluocortolone hexanoate	External, rectal
Fluocortolone pivalate	External, rectal
Flurbiprofen	Lozenges
Fluticasone propionate	External, nasal
Furosemide	Oral, parenteral
Fusidic acid	External
Gabapentin	Palliative care—oral
Gelatin 3.5–4%	Parenteral
Gentamicin sulphate	Aural
[2]Gestodene	Oral
Glucagon hydrochloride	Parenteral
Glucose intravenous infusion	Parenteral
Glucose 5% intravenous infusion	Parenteral
Granisetron hydrochloride	Parenteral
Heparin	Parenteral
Heparin sodium	Parenteral for the purpose of cannulae flushing
Hexastarch	Parenteral
Human soluble insulin	Parenteral
Hydrocortisone	External including rectal
Hydrocortisone acetate	Aural, external
Hydrocortisone butyrate	External

Footnotes—see page N12

Drug	Route of administration, use or pharmaceutical form
Hydrocortisone sodium succinate	Lozenges, parenteral
Hydroxyethyl starch	Parenteral
Hyoscine	Palliative care—transdermal
Hyoscine butylbromide	Palliative care—parenteral
Hyoscine hydrobromide	Palliative care—oral, parenteral
Ibuprofen	External, oral
Ibuprofen lysine	Oral
Imipramine hydrochloride	Palliative care—oral
Ipratropium bromide	Inhalation, nasal
Isotretinoin	External
Ketoconazole	External
Ketoprofen	External
Levocabastine hydrochloride	Nasal and ophthalmic
Levomepromazine (including levomepromazine (methotrimeprazine) maleate and levomepromazine (methotrimeprazine) hydrochloride)	Oral, parenteral
[2]Levonorgestrel	Oral
Lidocaine hydrochloride	External, parenteral
Lithium succinate	External
Lodoxamide trometamol	Ophthalmic
Loperamide hydrochloride	Oral
Loratadine	Oral
Lorazepam	Oral, parenteral
Lymecycline*	Oral
Mebendazole	Oral
[2]Medroxyprogesterone acetate	Injection
[2]Mestranol	Oral
Metoclopramide hydrochloride	Oral, parenteral
Metronidazole*	Oral, external, rectal, vaginal
Metronidazole benzoate*	Oral
Miconazole	Dental lacquer
Miconazole nitrate	External, vaginal
Midazolam	Parenteral
Minocycline hydrochloride*	Oral
Mizolastine	Oral
Mometasone furoate	External, nasal
Naloxone	Parenteral
Nedocromil sodium	Ophthalmic
Nefopam hydrochloride	Oral
Neomycin sulphate	Aural
Neomycin undecanoate	Aural
Nitrofuratoin*	Oral
Nizatidine	Oral
[2]Norethisterone	Oral
[2]Norethisterone acetate	Oral
[2]Norethisterone enanthate	Parenteral
[2]Norgestimate	Oral
[2]Norgestrel	Oral
Nortriptyline hydrochloride	Palliative care—oral
Nystatin	External, local mouth treatment, vaginal
Omeprazole	Oral
Omeprazole sodium	Parenteral
Ondansetron hydrochloride	Oral, parenteral
Oxybuprocaine hydrochloride	Ophthalmic
Oxytetracycline dihydrate*	Oral
Paracetamol	Oral
Penciclovir	External
Pentastarch	Parenteral
Piroxicam	External
Potassium chloride 0.3% and glucose 5% intravenous infusion (K^+ 40 mmol/litre)	Parenteral
Potassium chloride 0.3% and sodium chloride 0.9% intravenous infusion	Parenteral
Potassium chloride 0.3%, sodium chloride 0.45% and glucose 5% intravenous infusion (K+ 40 mmol/litre	Parenteral
Prednisolone	Oral
Prednisolone hexanoate	Rectal
Prednisolone sodium phosphate	Aural, oral
Prilocaine	External, parenteral
Prochlorperazine mesilate	Oral, rectal
Prochlorperazine maleate	Oral, rectal, buccal
Proxymetacaine hydrochloride	Ophthalmic
Ranitidine hydrochloride	Oral, parenteral
Reteplase	Parenteral
Salbutamol sulphate	Inhalation
Silver sulfadiazine	External
Sodium chloride 0.45% and glucose 5% intravenous infusion	Parenteral
Sodium chloride 0.9% and glucose 5% intravenous infusion	Parenteral
Sodium chloride 0.9% intravenous infusion	Parenteral
Sodium cromoglicate	Ophthalmic
Sodium fusidate	External
Streptodornase	External
Streptokinase	External, parenteral
Sulconazole nitrate	External
Tacalcitol	External
Tenecteplase	Parenteral
Terbinafine hydrochloride	External
Terbutaline sulphate	Inhalation
Tetanus immunoglobulin	Parenteral
Tetracaine	External
Tetracycline hydrochloride*	External, oral
Tinzaparin sodium	Parenteral
Tretinoin	External
Triamcinolone acetonide	Aural, external, nasal, oral paste
Trimethoprim*	Oral
Tropicamide	Ophthalmic
Tropisetron hydrochloride	Parenteral
[3]Tuberculin PPD	Injection
[3]Vaccine, Adsorbed Diphtheria	Injection
[3]Vaccine, Adsorbed Diphtheria and Tetanus	Injection
[3]Vaccine, Adsorbed Diphtheria and Tetanus for Adults and Adolescents	Injection
[3]Vaccine, Adsorbed Diphtheria for Adults and Adolescents	Injection
[3]Vaccine, Adsorbed Diphtheria, Tetanus and Pertussis	Injection
[3]Vaccine, Adsorbed Diphtheria, Tetanus Toxoid and Pertussis (Acellular Component)	Injection
[3]Vaccine, BCG	Injection
Vaccine, BCG Percutaneous	Injection
Vaccine, Combined Tetanus, Diphtheria, Acellular Pertussis, Inactivated Poliomyelitis and Haemophilus Influenza Type B	Parenteral

Footnotes—see next page

Drug	Route of administration, use or pharmaceutical form
[3]Vaccine, Haemophilus Influenzae Type B (Hib)	Injection
[3]Vaccine, Haemophilus Influenzae Type B (Hib) with Diphtheria, Tetanus and Pertussis	Injection
[3]Vaccine, Haemophilus Influenzae Type B, (Hib) with Diphtheria, Tetanus and Acellular Pertussis	Injection
[4]Vaccine, Hepatitis A	Injection
[4]Vaccine, Hepatitis A with Typhoid	Injection
[4]Vaccine, Hepatitis A, Inactivated, with recombinant (DNA) Hepatitis B	Injection
[4]Vaccine, Hepatitis B	Injection
Vaccine, Inactivated Poliomyelitis	Parenteral
[4]Vaccine, Influenza	Injection
[3]Vaccine, Live Measles, Mumps and Rubella (MMR)	Injection
[3]Vaccine, Meningococcal Group C Conjugate	Injection
[3 or 4]Vaccine, Meningococcal Polysaccharide A and C	Injection
Vaccine, Meningococcal Polysaccharide A, C, W135 and Y	Injection
[4]Vaccine, Pneumococcal	Injection
[3]Vaccine, Poliomyelitis, Live (Oral)	Oral
[3]Vaccine, Rubella, Live	Injection
[4]Vaccine, Tetanus, Adsorbed	Injection
Vaccine, Typhoid, Live Attenuated (Oral)	Oral
[4]Vaccine, Typhoid, Polysaccharide	Injection
Water for injections	Parenteral

* Oral antibacterials and indications considered suitable for nurse prescribing

Drug	Indication
[5]Amoxicillin trihydrate	Lower urinary-tract infection (women), animal and human, bites, acute exacerbation of chronic bronchitis, dental infections
Azithromycin dihydrate	Laboratory-confirmed uncomplicated genital chlamydial infection, plus sexual partners of these patients
Doxycycline hyclate	Acne, animal and human bites, laboratory-confirmed uncomplicated genital chlamydial infection, plus sexual partners of these patients
Doxycycline monohydrate	Acne, animal and human bites, laboratory-confirmed uncomplicated genital chlamydial infection, plus sexual partners of these patients
Erythromycin	Impetigo, animal and human bites, laboratory-confirmed uncomplicated genital chlamydial infection, plus sexual partners of these patients, spreading cellulitis usually of a limb with a risk of, or an established lymphangitis, dental infections
Erythromycin ethyl succinate	Impetigo, animal and human bites, laboratory-confirmed uncomplicated genital chlamydial infection, plus sexual partners of these patients, spreading cellulitis usually of a limb with a risk of, or an established lymphangitis, dental infections
Erythromycin stearate	Impetigo, animal and human bites, laboratory-confirmed uncomplicated genital chlamydial infection, plus sexual partners of these patients, spreading cellulitis usually of a limb with a risk of, or an established lymphangitis, dental infections
Flucloxacillin magnesium	Impetigo, spreading cellulitis usually of a limb with a risk of, or an established lymphangitis
Flucloxacillin sodium	Impetigo, spreading cellulitis usually of a limb with a risk of, or an established lymphangitis
Lymecycline	Acne
Metronidazole	Animal and human bites; fungating malodorous tumours; bacterial vaginosis; *trichomonas vaginalis* infection plus sexual partners of these patients, dental infections
Metronidazole benzoate	Animal and human bites, dental infections
Minocycline hydrochloride	Acne
Nitrofurantoin	Lower urinary-tract infection (women)
Oxytetracycline dihydrate	Acne, animal and human bites, acute exacerbation of chronic bronchitis
Tetracycline hydrochloride	Acne
Trimethoprim	Lower urinary-tract infection (women)

1. Present as potassium clavulanate in co-amoxiclav
2. Nurse Prescribers in Family Planning Clinics—where it is not appropriate for nurse prescribers in family planning clinics to prescribe contraceptive drugs using form FP10(P) (forms FP10(CN) and FP10(PN), or when available WP10CN and WP10PN, in Wales), they may prescribe using the same system as doctors in the clinic.
3. Centrally supplied vaccine excluded from reimbursement via prescription route
4. High Volume Personally Administered Vaccine. Claims for these vaccines should be ordered on form FP34D
5. With Clavulanic acid (as co-amoxiclav) for animal and human bites

Laxatives

Corresponds to BNF section 1.6.

Before prescribing laxatives it is important to be sure that the patient *is* constipated and that the constipation is *not* secondary to an underlying undiagnosed complaint.

It is also important for those who complain of constipation to understand that bowel habit can vary considerably in frequency without doing harm. Some people may consider themselves constipated if they do not have a bowel movement each day. A useful definition of constipation is the passage of hard stools less frequently than the patient's own normal pattern and this can be explained to the patient.

Misconceptions about bowel habits have led to excessive laxative use. Abuse may lead to hypokalaemia and an atonic non-functioning colon. *Simple constipation* is usually relieved by increasing the intake of dietary fibre.

Laxatives should generally be **avoided** except where straining will exacerbate a condition (such as angina) or increase the risk of rectal bleeding as in haemorrhoids. Laxatives are also of value in *drug-induced constipation*, for the *expulsion of parasites* after anthelmintic treatment, and to clear the alimentary tract *before surgery and radiological procedures*. Prolonged treatment of constipation is seldom necessary except occasionally in the elderly.

CHILDREN. The use of laxatives in children should be discouraged unless prescribed by a doctor. Infrequent defaecation may be normal in breast-fed babies or in response to poor intake of fluid or fibre. Delays of greater than 3 days between stools may increase the likelihood of pain on passing hard stools leading to anal fissure, anal spasm and eventually to a learned response to avoid defaecation. Increased fluid and fibre intake may be sufficient to regulate bowel action.

Nurse prescribers should discuss with the doctor before prescribing a laxative for a child

Laxatives can be divided into four main groups: *bulk-forming laxatives*, *stimulant laxatives*, *faecal softeners*, and *osmotic laxatives*. This simple classification, however, disguises the fact that some laxatives have complex actions.

Bulk-forming laxatives

Bulk-forming laxatives relieve constipation by increasing faecal mass which stimulates peristalsis. Patients should be told that the full effect may take some days to develop. In nursing practice they are particularly useful in the management of patients with *colostomy, ileostomy, haemorrhoids,* and *anal fissure.* Methylcellulose tablets are licensed for other indications including diarrhoea and obesity but nurse prescribers should prescribe them **only** for constipation.

BULK-FORMING LAXATIVES

Indications: constipation, see also notes above

Cautions: adequate fluid intake should be maintained to avoid intestinal obstruction—it may be necessary to supervise elderly or debilitated patients or those with intestinal narrowing or decreased motility

Contra-indications: difficulty in swallowing, intestinal obstruction, colonic atony, faecal impaction; avoid methylcellulose in infective bowel disease

Side-effects: flatulence, abdominal distension; gastro-intestinal obstruction or impaction; hypersensitivity reported

Dose: see preparations, below

COUNSELLING. Preparations that swell in contact with liquid should always be carefully swallowed with water and should not be taken immediately before going to bed

Prescribe as:

Ispaghula Husk Granules

Granules, brown, sugar- and gluten-free, ispaghula husk 90%, net price 200 g = £2.67. *Proprietary product: Isogel*

Dose: 2 teaspoonfuls in water once or twice daily, preferably at mealtimes; CHILD (but see notes above) 1 teaspoonful

Ispaghula Husk Oral Powder (*Ispagel*)

Powder, beige, effervescent, sugar- and gluten-free, ispaghula husk 3.5 g/sachet (orange flavour), net price 30 sachets = £2.10.

Excipients: include aspartame (see BNF section 9.4.1)

Dose: 1 sachet in water 1–3 times daily; CHILD (but see notes above) 6–12 years ½ adult dose

Ispaghula Husk Oral Powder (*Regulan*)

Powder, beige, sugar- and gluten-free, ispaghula husk 3.4 g/5.85-g sachet (orange or lemon/lime flavour), net price 30 sachets = £2.12.

Excipients: include aspartame (see BNF section 9.4.1)

Dose: 1 sachet in 150 mL water 1–3 times daily; CHILD (but see notes above) 6–12 years 2.5–5 mL

Effervescent Ispaghula Husk Granules

Granules, buff, effervescent, sugar- and gluten-free, ispaghula husk 3.5 g/sachet, net price 30 sachets (lemon or orange flavour or plain) = £2.12, 150 g (orange flavour) = £3.44. *Proprietary product: Fybogel*

Excipients: include aspartame 16 mg/sachet (see BNF section 9.4.1)

Dose: 1 sachet or 2 level 5-mL spoonfuls in water twice daily, preferably after meals; CHILD (but see notes above) 6–12 years ½–1 level 5 mL spoonful

Methylcellulose Tablets

Tablets, pink, scored, methylcellulose '450' 500 mg, net price 112-tab pack = £2.69. *Proprietary products*: *Celevac* tablets

Dose: 3–6 tablets twice daily with at least 300 mL of liquid

Sterculia Granules

Granules, coated, gluten-free, sterculia 62%, net price 500 g = £6.18; 60 × 7-g sachets = £5.19. *Proprietary product: Normacol*

Dose: 1–2 heaped 5-mL spoonfuls or contents of 1–2 sachets, washed down without chewing with plenty of liquid once or twice daily after meals; CHILD (but see notes above) 6–12 years half adult dose

Sterculia and Frangula Granules
Granules, brown, coated, gluten-free, sterculia 62%, frangula (standardised) 8%, net price 500 g = £6.60; 60 × 7-g sachets = £5.56. *Proprietary product: Normacol Plus*
Dose: 1–2 heaped 5-mL spoonfuls or contents of 1–2 sachets, washed down without chewing with plenty of liquid once or twice daily after meals

Stimulant laxatives

Stimulant laxatives increase intestinal motility and are used in functional constipation that has not responded to dietary measures.

Stimulant laxatives often cause abdominal cramp. They should be avoided in intestinal obstruction, and prolonged use can cause diarrhoea and related effects such as hypokalaemia. They should preferably be avoided in children.

BISACODYL

Indications: constipation; tablets act in 10–12 hours; suppositories act in 20–60 minutes
Cautions: see notes on stimulant laxatives
Contra-indications: see notes on stimulant laxatives; acute surgical abdominal conditions, acute inflammatory bowel disease, severe dehydration
Side-effects: see notes on stimulant laxatives; tablets, griping; suppositories, local irritation
Dose: see under preparations, below

Prescribe as:

Bisacodyl Tablets 5 mg
Tablets, enteric coated, bisacodyl 5 mg. Net price 20 = 45p
Dose: 1–2 tablets at night; CHILD (but see notes above) 4–10 years (on doctor's advice only) 1 tablet at night, over 10 years 1–2 tablets at night

Bisacodyl Suppositories 10 mg
Suppositories, bisacodyl 10 mg. Net price 12 = 77p
Dose: 1 suppository rectally in the morning; CHILD over 10 years (but see notes above) 1 suppository rectally in the morning

Bisacodyl Paediatric Suppositories 5 mg
Paediatric suppositories, bisacodyl 5 mg. Net price 5 = 94p
Dose: CHILD (but see notes above) under 10 years 1 suppository rectally in the morning (on doctor's advice only)

> Nurse prescribers should discuss with the doctor before prescribing a laxative for a child

DANTRON

(Danthron)

Indications: in consultation with doctor, only for: constipation in terminally ill patients of all ages; acts within 6–12 hours
Cautions: see notes on stimulant laxatives; avoid prolonged contact with skin (as in incontinent patients)—risk of irritation and excoriation; *rodent* studies indicate potential carcinogenic risk
Contra-indications: see notes on stimulant laxatives; pregnancy (BNF Appendix 4); breast-feeding (BNF Appendix 5)
Side-effects: see notes on stimulant laxatives; urine may be coloured red
Dose: see under preparations

Prescribe as:

Co-danthramer Capsules PoM
Capsules, co-danthramer 25/200 (dantron 25 mg, poloxamer '188' 200 mg). Net price 60-cap pack = £12.86
Dose: (restricted indications, see above) 1–2 capsules at bedtime; CHILD 1 capsule at bedtime

Strong Co-danthramer Capsules PoM
Capsules, co-danthramer 37.5/500 (dantron 37.5 mg, poloxamer '188' 500 mg). Net price 60-cap pack = £15.55
Dose: (restricted indications, see above) 1–2 capsules at bedtime; CHILD under 12 years not recommended

Co-danthramer Oral Suspension PoM
Oral suspension, co-danthramer 25/200 in 5 mL (dantron 25 mg, poloxamer '188' 200 mg/5 mL). Net price 300 mL = £11.27, 1 litre = £37.57
Dose: (restricted indications, see above) 5–10 mL at night; CHILD 2.5–5 mL

Strong Co-danthramer Oral Suspension PoM
Strong oral suspension, co-danthramer 75/1000 in 5 mL (dantron 75 mg, poloxamer '188' 1 g/5 mL). Net price 300 mL = £30.13
Dose: (restricted indications, see above) 5 mL at night; CHILD under 12 years not recommended

Co-danthrusate Capsules PoM
Capsules, co-danthrusate 50/60 (dantron 50 mg, docusate sodium 60 mg). Net price 63-cap pack = £13.45
Dose: (restricted indications, see above) 1–3 capsules, usually at night; CHILD 6–12 years 1 capsule at night

Co-danthrusate Oral Suspension PoM
Oral suspension, yellow, co-danthrusate 50/60 in 5 mL (dantron 50 mg, docusate sodium 60 mg/5 mL). Net price 200 mL = £8.75. *Proprietary product: Normax*
Dose: (restricted indications, see above) 5–15 mL at night; CHILD 6–12 years 5 mL at night

> Cross-references to the BNF are provided but nurse prescribers may only prescribe those items that are listed on the Nurse Prescribers' List.

DOCUSATE SODIUM

(Dioctyl Sodium Sulphosuccinate)

Indications: constipation (oral preparations act within 1–2 days)
Cautions: see notes on stimulant laxatives; do not give with liquid paraffin; rectal preparations not indicated if haemorrhoids or anal fissure; pregnancy (BNF Appendix 4); breast-feeding (BNF Appendix 5)

Contra-indications: see notes on stimulant laxatives
Side-effects: see notes on stimulant laxatives
Dose: see under preparations
Note. Docusate preparations probably also have faecal softening effect.

Prescribe as:

Docusate Capsules 100 mg
Capsules, yellow/white, docusate sodium 100 mg, net price 30-cap pack = £2.40, 100-cap pack = £8.00. *Proprietary product: Dioctyl Capsules*
Dose: (acts within 1–2 days) up to 5 capsules daily in divided doses

Docusate Oral Solution 50 mg/5 mL
Oral solution, sugar-free, docusate sodium 50 mg/5 mL. Net price 300-mL = £2.48. *Proprietary product: Docusol Adult Solution*
Dose: (acts within 1–2 days) up to 50 mL daily in divided doses

Paediatric Docusate Oral Solution 12.5 mg/5 mL
Paediatric oral solution, sugar-free, docusate sodium 12.5 mg/5 mL. Net price 300 mL = £1.63. *Proprietary product: Docusol Paediatric Solution*
Dose: (acts within 1–2 days) CHILD (but see notes above) over 6 months 5 mL 3 times daily, 2–12 years 5–10 mL 3 times daily

Docusate Enema
Enema, docusate sodium 120 mg in 10-g single-dose disposable packs. Net price 10-g unit = 60p. *Proprietary product: Norgalax Micro-enema*
Dose: ADULT and CHILD (but see notes above) over 12 years, 10-g unit

GLYCEROL

(Glycerin)
Indications: constipation
Dose: see under preparations

Prescribe as:

Glycerol Suppositories
(Synonym: Glycerin Suppositories)
Suppositories, gelatin 140 mg, glycerol (glycerin) 700 mg/g. Net price 12 × 1-g size (for infants) = 81p; 12 × 2-g size (for children) = 82p; 12 × 4-g size (for adults) = £1.83
Dose: 1 suppository moistened with water before use
The usual sizes are for INFANT under 1 year, small (1-g mould), 1–2 years medium (2-g mould), CHILD medium (2-g mould), ADULT large (4-g mould)

SENNA

Indications: constipation (acts within 8–12 hours)
Cautions: see notes on stimulant laxatives
Contra-indications: see notes on stimulant laxatives; breast-feeding (BNF Appendix 5)
Side-effects: see notes on stimulant laxatives
Dose: see under preparations

Prescribe as:

Senna Tablets
Tablets, total sennosides (calculated as sennoside B) 7.5 mg. Net price 20 = 30p
Dose: (acts in 8–12 hours) 2–4 tablets, usually at bedtime; initial dose should be low and then gradually increased; CHILD (but see notes above) over 6 years, half adult dose in the morning (on doctor's advice only)
Note. For senna tablets on general sale to the public lower dose recommended

Senna Granules
Granules, brown, total sennosides (calculated as sennoside B) 15 mg/5 mL or 5.5 mg/g (one 5-mL spoonful = 2.7 g). Net price 100 g = £3.10. *Proprietary product: Senokot Granules*
Dose: (acts in 8–12 hours) 5–10 mL, usually at bedtime; CHILD (but see notes above) over 6 years 2.5–5 mL in the morning
Note. For senna granules on general sale to the public lower dose recommended

Senna Oral Solution
Syrup, brown, total sennosides (calculated as sennoside B) 7.5 mg/5 mL. Net price 100 mL = £2.37. *Proprietary product: Senokot Syrup*
Dose: (acts in 8–12 hours) 10–20 mL, usually at bedtime; CHILD (but see notes above) 2–6 years 2.5–5 mL in the morning (on doctor's advice only), over 6 years, 5–10 mL in the morning
Note. For senna oral solution on general sale to the public lower dose recommended

Senna and Ispaghula Granules
Granules, coated, senna fruit 12.4%, ispaghula 54.2%. Contain ispaghula as a bulk laxative. Net price 400 g = £7.45. *Proprietary product: Manevac Granules*
Dose: (acts in 8–12 hours) 1–2 level 5-mL spoonfuls with water or warm drink after supper and, if necessary, before breakfast *or* every 6 hours in resistant cases for 1–3 days; CHILD (but see notes above) 5–12 years 1 level 5-mL spoonful daily
COUNSELLING. Preparations that swell in contact with liquid should always be carefully swallowed with water and should not be taken immediately before going to bed

SODIUM PICOSULFATE

(Sodium Picosulphate)
Indications: constipation (acts within 6–12 hours)
Cautions: see notes on stimulant laxatives; active inflammatory bowel disease (avoid if fulminant); breast-feeding (see BNF Appendix 5)
Contra-indications: see notes on stimulant laxatives; severe dehydration
Side-effects: see notes on stimulant laxatives
Dose: see under preparations

Prescribe as:

Sodium Picosulfate Capsules
Capsules, sodium picosulfate 2.5 mg, net price 20-cap pack = £1.93, 50-cap pack = £2.73. *Proprietary product*: [1]*Dulco–lax Perles*
Dose: 2–4 capsules at night; CHILD (but see notes above) 4–10 years 1–2 capsules at night, over 10 years 2–4 capsules at night

1. The brand name *Dulco-lax*® is also used for bisacodyl tablets and suppositories

Sodium Picosulfate Elixir

Elixir, sodium picosulfate 5 mg/5 mL. Net price 100 mL = £1.85. *Proprietary products:* [2]*Dulco-lax Liquid, Laxoberal* NHS

Dose: 5–10 mL at night; CHILD (but see notes above), under 4 years 250 micrograms/kg, 4–10 years 2.5–5 mL at night, over 10 years 5–10 mL at night

2. The brand name *Dulco-lax*® is also used for bisacodyl tablets and suppositories

Nurse prescribers should discuss with the doctor before prescribing a laxative for a child

Faecal softeners

Faecal softeners, such as enemas containing arachis oil (ground-nut oil, peanut oil), lubricate and soften impacted faeces and promote a bowel movement.

ARACHIS OIL

Indications: constipation, see also notes above

Dose: see under preparation

Prescribe as:

Arachis Oil Enema

Enema, arachis (peanut) oil in 130-mL single-dose disposable packs. Net price 130 mL = 96p. *Proprietary product: Fletchers' Arachis Oil Retention Enema*

Dose: to soften impacted faeces, 130 mL; the enema should be warmed before use; CHILD on doctor's advice only

Osmotic laxatives

Osmotic laxatives increase the amount of water in the large bowel, either by drawing fluid from the body into the bowel or by retaining the fluid they were administered with.

Lactulose is a semi-synthetic disaccharide which is not absorbed from the gastro-intestinal tract. It is contra-indicated in galactosaemia and in intestinal obstruction; side-effects include flatulence, abdominal cramps and discomfort.

Macrogol (polyethylene glycol) may be used by mouth for constipation and the short-term treatment of faecal impaction. It is important that the initial assessment of faecal impaction is undertaken by a doctor. Macrogols sequester fluid in the bowel; giving fluid with macrogols may reduce the dehydrating effect sometimes seen with osmotic laxatives.

Magnesium hydroxide mixture is suitable for occasional use provided an adequate fluid intake is maintained after it has been given. It may be used when a rapid action is required but should be prescribed with caution because it is often abused.

Phosphate enemas are useful in bowel clearance before radiology, endoscopy, and surgery.

LACTULOSE

Indications: constipation (may take up to 48 hours to act)

Cautions: lactose intolerance

Contra-indications: galactosaemia, intestinal obstruction

Side-effects: flatulence, cramps, and abdominal discomfort

Dose: see under preparation

Prescribe as:

Lactulose Solution

Solution, lactulose 3.1–3.7 g/5 mL with other ketoses. Net price 500-mL pack = £2.85

Dose: initially 15 mL twice daily, adjusted according to patient's needs; CHILD (but see notes above) under 1 year 2.5 mL twice daily, 1–5 years 5 mL twice daily, 5–10 years 10 mL twice daily

MACROGOLS

(Polyethylene glycols)

Indications: constipation; faecal impaction (**only after** initial assessment by medical practitioner)

Cautions: pregnancy and breast-feeding (see BNF Appendix 5); discontinue if symptoms of fluid and electrolyte disturbance

Contra-indications: intestinal perforation or obstruction, paralytic ileus, severe inflammatory conditions of the intestinal tract (such as Crohn's disease, ulcerative colitis, and toxic megacolon)

Side-effects: abdominal distension and pain, nausea

Dose: see under preparation below

Prescribe as:

Macrogol Oral Powder

Oral powder, macrogol '4000' (polyethylene glycol '4000') 10 g/sachet, net price 20-sachet pack (orange-grapefruit flavour) = £4.84. *Proprietary product: Idrolax*

Dose: constipation, 1–2 sachets as a single dose in the morning; content of each sachet dissolved in a glass of water; CHILD over 8 years, as adult dose for max. 3 months

Compound Macrogol Oral Powder

Oral powder, macrogol '3350' (polyethylene glycol '3350') 13.125 g, sodium bicarbonate 178.5 mg, sodium chloride 350.7 mg, potassium chloride 46.6 mg/sachet. Net price 20-sachet pack (lime and lemon flavour) = £4.63, 30-sachet pack = £6.95. *Proprietary product: Movicol*

Note. Not to be confused with a preparation also containing sodium sulphate which is used for bowel cleansing before surgery and bowel procedures

Dose: chronic constipation, 1–3 sachets daily in divided doses usually for up to 2 weeks; content of each sachet dissolved in half a glass (approx. 125 mL) water; maintenance, 1–2 sachets daily; CHILD not recommended

Faecal impaction (**important**: initial assessment by doctor), 8 sachets daily dissolved in 1 litre of water; the solution should be drunk within 6 hours, usually for max. 3 days; CHILD not recommended.

After reconstitution the solution should be kept in a refrigerator and discarded if unused after 6 hours

Caution: patients with cardiovascular impairment should not take more than 2 sachets in any 1 hour

Compound Macrogol Oral Powder. Half-Strength

Oral powder, macrogol '3350' (polyethylene glycol '3350') 6.563 g, sodium bicarbonate 89.3 mg, sodium chloride 175.4 mg, potassium chloride 23.3 mg/sachet, net price 20-sachet pack (lime and lemon flavour) = £2.78, 30-sachet pack = £4.17.

Dose: chronic constipation, 2–6 sachets daily in divided doses usually for up to 2 weeks; content of each sachet dissolved in quarter of a glass (approx. 60–65 mL) water; maintenance, 2–4 sachets daily; CHILD not recommended

Faecal impaction (**important**: initial assessment by doctor), 16 sachets daily dissolved in 1 litre of water and drunk within 6 hours, usually for max. 3 days; CHILD not recommended.

After reconstitution the solution should be kept in a refrigerator and discarded if unused after 6 hours

Caution: patients with cardiovascular impairment should not take more than 4 sachets in any 1 hour

MAGNESIUM HYDROXIDE

Indications: constipation

Cautions: renal impairment (see BNF Appendix 3; risk of magnesium accumulation); hepatic impairment (see BNF Appendix 2); elderly and debilitated; see also notes above; **interactions:** see BNF Appendix 1 (antacids)

Contra-indications: acute gastro-intestinal conditions

Side-effects: colic

Dose: see under preparation

Prescribe as:

Magnesium Hydroxide Mixture

(Synonym: Cream of Magnesia)

Mixture, aqueous suspension containing about 8% of hydrated magnesium oxide. Do not store in a cold place

Dose: constipation, 25–50 mL when required

PHOSPHATES (RECTAL)

Indications: rectal use in constipation, see also notes above

Cautions: elderly and debilitated; see also notes above

Contra-indications: acute gastro-intestinal conditions

Side-effects: local irritation

Dose: see under preparations

Prescribe as:

Phosphate Suppositories

Suppositories, sodium acid phosphate (anhydrous) 1.3 g, sodium bicarbonate 1.08 g, net price 12 = £2.01. *Proprietary product: Carbalax*

Dose: constipation, 1 suppository, inserted 30 minutes before evacuation required; moisten with water before use; CHILD under 12 years not recommended

Phosphates Enema (Formula B)

Enema, sodium acid phosphate 12.8 g, sodium phosphate 10.24 g/128 mL. Net price 128 mL with standard tube = 44p, with long rectal tube = 61p.

Dose: 128 mL; CHILD (but see notes above) over 3 years, reduced according to body weight (under 3 years not recommended)

Phosphates Enema (*Fleet*)

Enema, sodium acid phosphate 21.4 g, sodium phosphate 9.4 g/118 mL. Net price single-dose pack (standard tube) = 46p

Dose: ADULT and CHILD over 12 years, 118 mL; CHILD (but see notes above) 3–12 years, on doctor's advice only (under 3 years not recommended)

Nurse prescribers should discuss with the doctor before prescribing a laxative for a child

SODIUM CITRATE (RECTAL)

Indications: rectal use in constipation

Cautions: elderly and debilitated; see also notes above

Contra-indications: acute gastro-intestinal conditions

Dose: see under preparations

Prescribe as:

Sodium Citrate Compound Enema

Enema, sodium citrate 450 mg with other ingredients including glycerol, sorbitol and an anionic surfactant in a 5-mL single-dose disposable pack. *Proprietary products: Micolette Micro-enema* (net price 5-mL pack = 31p), *Micralax Micro-enema* (5-mL pack = 41p), *Relaxit Micro-enema* (5-mL pack = 32p)

Dose: ADULT and CHILD (but see notes above) over 3 years, 5 mL (under 3 years not recommended)

Gloves

GLOVES

EMA Film Gloves, Disposable

Gloves, small, medium, or large. Net price pack of 30 = £2.26. *Proprietary product: Dispos-A-Gloves*

For use as a barrier during manual evacuation of the bowel

Polythene Gloves

Gloves, net price pack of 25 = 52p.

For use as occlusives with medicated creams

Analgesics

Corresponds to BNF section 4.7.1 (non-opioid analgesics) and 10.1.1 (non-steroidal anti-inflammatory drugs)

The **non-opioid** analgesics **aspirin, ibuprofen** and **paracetamol** are particularly suitable for pain in musculoskeletal conditions, whereas the opioid analgesics are more suitable for severe visceral pain. Aspirin, ibuprofen, and paracetamol are effective analgesics for the relief of *mild to moderate pain*. Their familiar role as household remedies should not detract from their considerable value as analgesics; they are also of value in some forms of *severe chronic pain*.

Combinations of aspirin or paracetamol with an opioid analgesic (such as codeine) are commonly used but their advantages have not been substantiated (and they are not on the Nurse Prescribers' List). Any additional pain relief that they might provide can be at the cost of *increased side-effects caused by the opioid component* (constipation, in particular).

> When prescribing aspirin or paracetamol it is important to make sure that the patient is not already taking an aspirin- or a paracetamol-containing preparation (possibly bought over-the-counter). The BNF (section 4.7.1) includes a list of preparations on sale to the public that contain aspirin or paracetamol alone or with other ingredients.

Aspirin

Aspirin is indicated for mild to moderate pain including headache, transient musculoskeletal pain, and dysmenorrhoea; it has anti-inflammatory properties which may be useful, and is an antipyretic. The main side-effect is gastric irritation; rarely, gastric bleeding can be a serious complication. Aspirin increases bleeding time and must **not** be prescribed as an analgesic to patients receiving anticoagulants such as warfarin. Aspirin is also associated with bronchospasm and allergic reactions, particularly in patients with asthma. It should **not** be prescribed for patients with a history of hypersensitivity to aspirin or any other non-steroidal anti-inflammatory drug (NSAID)—which includes those in whom asthma, angioedema, urticaria or rhinitis have been precipitated by aspirin or another NSAID. Aspirin should **not** be prescribed for children and adolescents **under the age of 16 years** owing to its association with Reye's syndrome.

> OTHER USES. Since aspirin decreases platelet aggregation, it is prescribed *by doctors* in low doses (e.g. 75–150 mg daily) to prevent cerebrovascular or cardiovascular disease. Aspirin is also occasionally prescribed *by doctors* for rheumatic conditions. Nurse prescribers should **not** prescribe aspirin for these conditions.

ASPIRIN

Indications: mild to moderate pain, pyrexia

Cautions: asthma, allergic disease, impaired hepatic or renal function (avoid if severe; see BNF appendixes 2 and 3), dehydration; preferably avoid during fever or viral infection in adolescents (risk of Reye's syndrome, see below); pregnancy (BNF Appendix 4); elderly; G6PD-deficiency (acceptable in a dose of 1 g daily in most G6PD-deficient individuals); **interactions:** see BNF Appendix 1 (aspirin)

Contra-indications: children and adolescents under 16 years and in breast-feeding (Reye's syndrome—see below and BNF Appendix 5); previous or active peptic ulceration, haemophilia; not for treatment of gout

HYPERSENSITIVITY. Aspirin and other NSAIDs are **contra-indicated** in patients with a history of hypersensitivity to aspirin or any other NSAID—*which includes those* in whom attacks of *asthma, angioedema, urticaria or rhinitis* have been precipitated by aspirin or any other NSAID

REYE'S SYNDROME. Owing to an association with Reye's syndrome, the CSM has advised that aspirin-containing preparations should not be given to children and adolescents under 16 years, unless specifically indicated, e.g. for Kawasaki syndrome.

Side-effects: generally mild and infrequent but high incidence of gastro-intestinal irritation with slight asymptomatic blood loss, increased bleeding time, bronchospasm and skin reactions in hypersensitive patients

Dose: usual, 300–600 mg every 4–6 hours when necessary, not more than 2.4 g daily without doctor's advice; CHILD and ADOLESCENT not recommended (see Reye's syndrome above)

Prescribe as:

[1]**Dispersible Aspirin Tablets 300 mg** PoM

Dispersible tablets, aspirin 300 mg. Net price 20 = 22p

Cautionary label added by pharmacist: dissolve or mix with water before taking and take with or after food

1. Nurse prescribers should prescribe packs containing no more than **32 tablets**, a max. of **3** packs of 32 tablets may be prescribed on each occasion; PoM but may be sold to the public under certain circumstances—for details see *Medicines, Ethics and Practice*, No. 29, London, Pharmaceutical Press, 2005 (and subsequent editions as available)

Ibuprofen

In single doses **ibuprofen** has analgesic activity comparable to that of paracetamol, but paracetamol is preferred for the management of pain, particularly in the elderly. Ibuprofen also has antipyretic properties. In regular dosage ibuprofen has a lasting analgesic and anti-inflammatory effect which makes it particularly useful for the treatment of pain associated with inflammation.

Like aspirin, ibuprofen has been associated with bronchospasm and allergic disorders; it is contra-indicated in patients with a history of hypersensitivity to aspirin or any other NSAID—which includes those in whom attacks of asthma, angioedema, urticaria or rhinitis have been precipitated by aspirin or any other NSAID.

The side-effects of ibuprofen include gastro-intestinal discomfort, nausea, diarrhoea, and occasionally bleeding and ulceration occur.

OTHER USES. Ibuprofen is prescribed by doctors for chronic inflammatory diseases. However, nurse prescribers should not prescribe ibuprofen for indications or at doses other than those listed below.

IBUPROFEN

Indications: rheumatic and muscular pain, headache, dental pain, feverishness, symptoms of colds and influenza; in adults also backache, neuralgia, migraine, dysmenorrhoea

Cautions: pregnancy and breast-feeding (see BNF Appendixes 4 and 5); coagulation defects; renal, cardiac or hepatic impairment (risk of deterioration of renal function—see also BNF Appendixes 2 and 3), elderly (risk of serious side-effects); **interactions**: see BNF Appendix 1 (NSAIDS)

Contra-indications: previous or active peptic ulceration

HYPERSENSITIVITY. **Contra-indicated** in patients with a history of hypersensitivity to aspirin or any other NSAID—which includes those in whom attacks of *asthma, angioedema, urticaria, or rhinitis* have been precipitated by aspirin or any other NSAID

Side-effects: gastro-intestinal discomfort including pain, indigestion and nausea; gastro-intestinal bleeding, bruising, bronchospasm, rashes, oedema, raised blood pressure, renal impairment; blood disorders reported; see BNF section 10.1.1 for other side-effects

Dose: initially 400 mg, then 200–400 mg every 4 hours, max. 1.2 g daily; if symptoms persist for more than 3 days refer to doctor

Fever and pain in children, CHILD over 6 months and over 7 kg body-weight, 20 mg/kg daily in divided doses (max. 800 mg daily) *or* 1–2 years 50 mg 3–4 times daily; 3–7 years 100 mg 3–4 times daily, 8–12 years 200 mg 3–4 times daily; if symptoms persist for more than 3 days refer to doctor

Post-immunisation pyrexia, CHILD over 6 months 50 mg followed if necessary by second dose after 6 hours; if pyrexia persists refer to doctor

Prescribe as:

[1]Ibuprofen PoM

Tablets, coated, ibuprofen 200 mg, net price 16 = 32p

Oral suspension, ibuprofen 100 mg/5 mL, net price 100 mL = £2.65

Note. Sugar-free versions are available and can be ordered by specifying 'sugar-free' on the prescription

1. May be sold to the public under certain circumstances—for details see *Medicines, Ethics and Practice*, No. 29, London, Pharmaceutical Press, 2005 (and subsequent editions as available)

Community Practitioner nurse prescribers should not prescribe outside the indications and doses above, other indications and doses are PoM

Paracetamol

Paracetamol is similar in efficacy to aspirin, but has no demonstrable anti-inflammatory activity. It is less irritant to the stomach and for that reason paracetamol is now generally preferred to aspirin, particularly in the elderly. It must be remembered, however, that overdosage with paracetamol (alone or as an ingredient of a combination product) is particularly dangerous.

PARACETAMOL

Indications: mild to moderate pain, pyrexia

Cautions: hepatic impairment (see BNF Appendix 2), alcohol dependence; **interactions**: see BNF Appendix 1 (paracetamol)

Side-effects: side-effects rare, but rashes and blood disorders (including thrombocytopenia, leucopenia, neutropenia) reported; **important:** liver damage (and less frequently renal damage) following **overdosage**, immediate transfer to hospital essential

Dose: 0.5–1 g every 4–6 hours; max. 4 g daily

CHILD under 3 months on doctor's advice only, 10 mg/kg (5 mg/kg if jaundiced)—post-immunisation pyrexia, see below; 3 months–1 year 60–120 mg; 1–5 years 120–250 mg; 6–12 years 250–500 mg; these doses may be repeated every 4–6 hours when necessary; max. 4 doses in 24 hours

Post-immunisation pyrexia, INFANT 2–3 months, 60 mg followed, if necessary, by second dose after 6 hours; if pyrexia persists refer to doctor

Prescribe as:

[2]Paracetamol Tablets 500 mg PoM

Tablets, paracetamol 500 mg. Net price 20 = 21p

Cautionary label added by pharmacist: Do not take more than 2 tablets at any one time. Do not take more than 8 in 24 hours. Do not take with any other paracetamol products

2. Nurse prescribers should prescribe packs containing no more than **32 tablets**, a max. of **3** packs of 32 tablets may be prescribed on each occasion; PoM but may be sold to the public under certain circumstances—for details see *Medicines, Ethics and Practice*, No. 29, London, Pharmaceutical Press, 2005 (and subsequent editions as available)

[3]Soluble Paracetamol Tablets 500 mg PoM

Soluble tablets, paracetamol 500 mg. Net price 20 = 77p

Cautionary label added by pharmacist: Do not take more than 2 tablets at any one time, do not take more than 8 in 24 hours, dissolve in water. Do not take with any other paracetamol products

3. Nurse prescribers should prescribe packs containing no more than **32 tablets**, a max. of **3** packs of 32 tablets may be prescribed on each occasion; PoM but may be sold to the public under certain circumstances—for details see *Medicines, Ethics and Practice*, No. 29, London, Pharmaceutical Press, 2005 (and subsequent editions as available)

Soluble Paracetamol Tablets 120 mg

Tablets (= paediatric dispersible tablets), paracetamol 120 mg. Net price 16-tab pack = 91p

Cautionary label added by pharmacist: Dissolve or mix with water before taking. Do not take with any other paracetamol products

Paracetamol Oral Suspension 120 mg/5 mL

Oral suspension (= paediatric mixture), paracetamol 120 mg/5 mL. Net price 100 mL = 42p

Note. Sugar-free version can be ordered by specifying 'sugar-free' on the prescription

Cautionary label added by pharmacist: Do not take with any other paracetamol products. If a 60-mg dose is required the pharmacist will supply an oral syringe and advise on how to give a 2.5-mL dose

Paracetamol Oral Suspension 250 mg/5 mL

Oral suspension (= mixture), paracetamol 250 mg/5 mL. Net price 100 mL = 73p

Note. Sugar-free version can be ordered by specifying 'sugar-free' on the prescription

Cautionary label added by pharmacist: Do not take with any other paracetamol products.

Lidocaine and Chlorhexidine Gel

Gel, anhydrous lidocaine hydrochloride 1% or 2%, chlorhexidine gluconate solution 0.25% in a sterile lubricant basis. Net price 15 g = 70p.

Administration: into urethra at least 5 minutes before catheter insertion, men 10 mL followed by 3–5 mL; women 3–5 mL; CHILD 1–5 mL

Gel in disposable syringe, lidocaine hydrochloride 2%, chlorhexidine gluconate solution 0.25%, in a sterile lubricant basis in disposable syringe. Net price 6-mL syringe = £1.41, 11-mL syringe = £1.58. *Proprietary product: Instillagel* (6 mL, 11 mL)

Administration: into urethra, 6–11 mL

Local anaesthetics

Corresponds to BNF section 15.2.

Lidocaine

Lidocaine (lignocaine) is effectively absorbed from mucous membranes and is a useful surface anaesthetic in concentrations of 2 to 4%. Except for surface anaesthesia, solutions should not usually exceed 1% in strength.

LIDOCAINE HYDROCHLORIDE

(Lignocaine Hydrochloride)

Indications: surface anaesthesia (**important:** consult with doctor), see notes above

Cautions: absorbed through mucosa therefore special care if history of epilepsy, cardiac disease, respiratory disease, hepatic or renal impairment, myasthenia gravis, or porphyria (BNF section 9.8.2) and in pregnancy; do **not** use in mouth (risk of choking); also **special care** in infants or young children

Side-effects: include confusion, convulsions, respiratory depression, and cardiac depressant effects; allergic reactions (rarely anaphylaxis)

Administration: see under preparations

Prescribe as:

Lidocaine Gel

Gel, anhydrous lidocaine hydrochloride in a sterile water-miscible lubricant basis. Net price 1%, 15 mL = £1.30; 2%,15 mL = £1.30

Administration: into urethra at least 5 minutes before catheter insertion, men 10 mL followed by further 3–5 mL; women 3–5 mL; CHILD 1–5 mL

Lidocaine Ointment

Ointment, lidocaine hydrochloride 5% in a water-miscible basis. Net price 15 g = 88p.

Administration: sore nipples from breast-feeding, apply using gauze and wash off immediately before feed

Prevention of neural tube defects

Corresponds to BNF section 9.1.2.

PREVENTION OF NEURAL TUBE DEFECTS. Recommendations of an expert advisory group of the Department of Health include the advice that:

> To prevent *first occurrence of neural tube defect* women who are planning a pregnancy should be advised to take folic acid as a medicinal or food supplement at a dose of 400 micrograms daily before conception and during the first 12 weeks of pregnancy. Women who have not been taking supplements and who suspect they are pregnant should start at once and continue until week 12 of pregnancy.

Women at risk of a recurrence of neural tube defect (in a child of a man or woman with spina bifida or if there is a history of neural tube defect in a previous child) should be referred to a doctor because a higher dose of folic acid is appropriate. Women receiving antiepileptic therapy need individual counselling by their doctor before starting folic acid.

FOLIC ACID

Indications: prevention of neural tube defects, see notes above

Dose: see notes above

Prescribe as:

[1] **Folic Acid Tablets, 400 micrograms**

Tablets, folic acid 400 micrograms, net price 90-tab pack = £2.24. *Proprietary product: Preconceive and possibly others*

[1] **Folic Acid Oral Solution 400 micrograms/5 mL**

Oral solution, folic acid 400 micrograms/5 mL, net price 150 mL = £1.40. *Proprietary product: Folicare*

1. Can be sold to the public provided daily doses do not exceed 500 micrograms

Nicotine replacement therapy

Corresponds to BNF section 4.10

Smoking cessation interventions are a cost-effective way of reducing ill health and prolonging life. Smokers should be advised to stop and offered help if interested in doing so, with follow-up where appropriate.

Where possible, smokers should have access to a smoking cessation clinic for behavioural support. **Nicotine replacement therapy** is an effective aid to smoking cessation for those smoking more than 10 cigarettes a day. The form of nicotine replacement therapy chosen should take into account individual preference and tolerance of side-effects. Smokers who are pregnant or breast-feeding should discuss the use of nicotine replacement therapy with a healthcare professional trained in smoking cessation; nicotine replacement therapy should be used only if other measures have failed.

Nicotine replacement therapy should be prescribed for short durations at a time and the prescriptions repeated only if the attempt at stopping smoking is continuing (see also NICE guidance, BNF section 4.10).

NICOTINE PRODUCTS

Indications: adjunct to smoking cessation

Cautions: cardiovascular disease (avoid if severe); peripheral vascular disease; hyperthyroidism; diabetes mellitus; phaeochromocytoma, renal impairment (see BNF Appendix 3); hepatic impairment; history of gastritis and peptic ulcers; should not smoke or use nicotine replacement products in combination; pregnancy and breast-feeding (see BNF Appendixes 4 and 5); *patches*, exercise may increase absorption and side-effects, skin disorders (patches should not be placed on broken skin)

Contra-indications: severe cardiovascular disease (including severe arrhythmias or immediate post-myocardial infarction period); recent cerebrovascular accident (including transient ischaemic attacks)

Side-effects: nausea, dizziness, headache and cold and influenza-like symptoms, palpitations, dyspepsia and other gastro-intestinal disturbances, hiccups, insomnia, vivid dreams, myalgia; other side-effects reported include chest pain, blood pressure changes, anxiety and irritability, somnolence and impaired concentration, abnormal hunger, dysmenorrhoea, rash; *with patches*, skin reactions (discontinue if severe)—vasculitis also reported; *with spray*, nasal irritation, nose bleeds, watering eyes, ear sensations; *with gum, sublingual tablets* or *inhalator*, aphthous ulceration (sometimes with swelling of tongue); *with spray, inhalator, lozenges, sublingual tablets* or *gum*, throat irritation; *with inhalator*, cough, rhinitis, pharyngitis, stomatitis, sinusitis, dry mouth; *with lozenges* or *sublingual tablets*, unpleasant taste

Dose: see under preparations, below

Prescribe as:

[1]Nicotine Inhalation Cartridge for Oromucosal Use

Cartridge (for oromucosal use), nicotine 10 mg, net price 6-cartridge (starter) pack = £3.39, 42-cartridge (refill) pack = £11.37. *Proprietary products*: *Nicorette Inhalator, Boots Nicotine Inhalator*

1. For use with inhalation mouthpiece; starter pack contains 6 cartridges with inhalator device and holder, refill pack contains 42 cartridges with inhalator device

ADMINISTRATION: Inhale when urge to smoke occurs; initially use 6–12 cartridges daily for up to 8 weeks, then reduce number of cartridges used by half over next 2 weeks and then stop altogether after further 2 weeks; review treatment if abstinence not achieved in 3 months

Nicotine Lozenge

Lozenge, nicotine (as bitartrate) 1 mg, net price pack of 12 = £1.71, pack of 36 = £4.27, pack of 96 = £9.12, 2 mg pack of 12 = £1.99, pack of 36 = £4.95, pack of 96 = £10.60 (*proprietary product*: *Nicotinell Mint Lozenge*) *or* nicotine (as polacrilex) 2 mg, net price pack of 36 = £5.12, pack of 72 = £9.97, 4 mg pack of 36 = £5.12, pack of 72 = £9.97 (*proprietary product*: *NiQuitin CQ Lozenge*)

Excipients: include aspartame (BNF section 9.4.1)

Dose: initially suck 1 lozenge every 1–2 hours, when urge to smoke occurs; max. 30 mg daily for lozenges of 1 mg or 2 mg, or 60 mg daily for lozenges of 4 mg; withdraw gradually after 3 months; usual max. period of treatment 6 months

Nicotine Sublingual Tablets

Sublingual tablet, nicotine (as a cyclodextrin complex) 2 mg, net price starter pack of 2 × 15-tablet discs with dispenser = £3.57, refill pack of 7 × 15-tablet discs = £9.84. *Proprietary product*: *Nicorette Microtab*

Dose: individuals smoking 20 cigarettes or fewer daily, *sublingually*, 2 mg each hour; patients who fail to stop smoking or have significant withdrawal symptoms, consider increasing to 4 mg each hour

Individuals smoking more than 20 cigarettes daily, 4 mg each hour

Max. 80 mg daily; treatment should be continued for at least 3 months followed by a gradual reduction in dosage; max. period of treatment 6 months

Nicotine Medicated Chewing Gum

Chewing gum, nicotine 2 mg, net price pack of 12 = £1.59, pack of 15 = £1.71, pack of 24 = £2.85, pack of 96 = £8.55, pack of 105 = £8.89; 4 mg, net price pack of 12 = £1.70, pack of 15 = £2.11, pack of 24 = £2.85, pack of 96 = £8.55, pack of 105 = £10.83. *Proprietary products*: *Nicorette Gum, Nicorette Plus Gum, Nicotinell Gum, Nicotinell Plus Gum, NiQuitin CQ Gum, Boots Nicotine Gum*

Note. Available in various flavours

Dose: individuals smoking 20 cigarettes or fewer daily, initially one 2-mg piece chewed slowly for approx. 30 minutes, when urge to smoke occurs; individuals smoking more than 20 cigarettes daily or needing more than 15 pieces of 2-mg gum daily may need 4-mg strength; max. 15 pieces of 4-mg strength daily; withdraw gradually after 3 months

Nicotine Nasal Spray

Nasal spray, nicotine 500 micrograms/metered spray, net price 200-spray unit = £10.99. *Proprietary product*: *Nicorette Nasal Spray*

ADMINISTRATION: Apply 1 spray into each nostril as required to max. twice an hour for 16 hours daily (max. 64 sprays daily) for 8 weeks, then reduce gradually over next 4 weeks (reduce by half at end of first 2 weeks, stop altogether after further 2 weeks); max. treatment period of 3 months

[1]Nicotine Transdermal Patches

Patches, self-adhesive, releasing in each 16 hours, nicotine approx. 5 mg, 10 mg, or 15 mg (*proprietary product*: *Nicorette Patch*) *or* releasing in each 24 hours nicotine approx. 7 mg, 14 mg, or 21 mg (*proprietary products*: *Nicotinell TTS, NiQuitin CQ, Boots NRT Patch*)

Note. for pack sizes and prices, see individual products in BNF section 4.10

1. Prescriber should specify the brand to be dispensed

ADMINISTRATION: see individual products in BNF section 4.10

> Cross-references to the BNF are provided but nurse prescribers may only prescribe those items that are listed on the Nurse Prescribers' List.

Drugs for the mouth

Corresponds to BNF sections 12.3.2, 12.3.1, 12.3.4 and 12.3.5

Candida albicans may cause thrush and other forms of stomatitis which sometimes follow the use of broad-spectrum antibacterials or cytotoxics; withdrawal of the causative drug may lead to rapid resolution; alternatively antifungal treatment may be required. Infants may develop thrush which responds to use of an antifungal mouth preparation.

Patients with denture stomatitis may also respond to the use of an antifungal mouth preparation. They should be instructed to cleanse their dentures thoroughly to prevent reinfection; ideally they should leave their dentures out as often as possible during the treatment period. Proper dental appraisal may be necessary.

> Patients with an unexplained mouth ulcer of more than 3 weeks' duration require urgent referral to exclude oral cancer.

Oral antifungal drugs

Miconazole and **nystatin** are suitable for the treatment of oral thrush.

MICONAZOLE

Indications: prevention and treatment of oral fungal infections

Cautions: pregnancy (see BNF Appendix 4) and breast-feeding; avoid in porphyria (BNF section 9.8.2); **interactions:** see BNF Appendix 1 (antifungals, imidazole); oral gel may be absorbed enough for interactions to occur after application to the oral mucosa

Contra-indications: hepatic impairment

Side-effects: nausea and vomiting, diarrhoea (with long-term treatment); rarely allergic reactions; isolated reports of hepatitis

Dose: see under preparation

Prescribe as:

[2]Miconazole Oromucosal Gel PoM

Oral gel, sugar-free, orange-flavoured, miconazole 24 mg/mL (20 mg/g). Net price 15-g tube = £2.45, 80-g tube = £4.75. *Proprietary product: Daktarin Oral Gel*

Dose: place 5–10 mL in the mouth after food and retain near lesions, 4 times daily; CHILD under 2 years 2.5 mL twice daily, 2–6 years 5 mL twice daily, over 6 years 5 mL 4 times daily; treatment continued for 48 hours after lesions have resolved

Localised lesions, smear small amount of gel on affected area with clean finger 4 times daily (dentures should be removed at night and brushed with gel) (prescribe 15-g tube)

Note. Not licensed for use in NEONATES

2. The 15-g tube can be sold to the public

NYSTATIN

Indications: oral and perioral fungal infections

Side-effects: oral irritation and sensitisation, nausea reported; see also BNF section 5.2

Dose: see under preparations, below

Prescribe as:

Nystatin Oral Suspension PoM

Oral suspension, nystatin 100 000 units/mL. Net price 30 mL (with pipette) = £1.95

Note. A sugar-free formulation can be requested

Dose: ADULT and CHILD over 1 month, place 1 mL in the mouth after food and retain near the lesions 4 times daily, usually for 7 days (continued for 48 hours after lesions have resolved); prophylaxis in newborn 1 mL once daily

Note. Not licensed for treating candidiasis in NEONATE under 1 month. Only medical practitioners should prescribe for immunosuppressed patients

Nystatin Pastilles PoM
Pastilles, nystatin 100 000 units. Net price 28-pastille pack = £3.24. *Proprietary product: Nystan Pastilles*
Dose: suck 1 pastille slowly 4 times daily after food usually for 7 days (continued for 48 hours after lesions have resolved)
Note. Only medical practitioners should prescribe for immunosuppressed patients

Thymol

Compound thymol glycerin is a refreshing mouthwash which has a mechanical cleansing action, and helps to alleviate the pain of oral ulceration.

Mouthwash solution-tablets may contain thymol as well as an antimicrobial; they are used to remove unpleasant tastes.

THYMOL

Indications: oral hygiene, see notes above

Dose: see under preparation, below

Prescribe as:

Compound Thymol Glycerin
Mouthwash, glycerol 10%, thymol 0.05% with colouring and flavouring. Net price 100 mL = 24p
Dose: to be used up to 3–4 times daily when necessary; may be used undiluted or diluted with 3 volumes of warm water

Mouthwash Solution-tablets, consist of tablets which may contain antimicrobial, colouring, and flavouring agents in a suitable soluble effervescent basis to make a mouthwash. Net price, 100 = £3.79
Dissolve 1 tablet in a glass of warm water

Drugs for oral ulceration and inflammation

Choline salicylate dental gel has some analgesic action and may provide relief for recurrent mouth ulcers, but excessive application or confinement under a denture irritates the mucosa and can itself cause ulceration. Benefit in teething may merely be due to pressure of application (comparable with biting a teething ring); excessive use can lead to salicylate poisoning.

> Patients with an unexplained mouth ulcer of more than 3 weeks' duration require urgent referral to exclude oral cancer.

SALICYLATES

Indications: mild oral and perioral lesions
Cautions: not to be applied to dentures–leave at least 30 minutes before re-insertion of dentures; frequent application, especially in children, may give rise to salicylate poisoning
Note. CSM warning on aspirin and Reye's syndrome does not apply to non-aspirin salicylates or to topical preparations such as teething gels
Dose: Apply ½-inch of gel with gentle massage not more often than every 3 hours; CHILD over 4 months ¼-inch of gel not more often than every 3 hours; max. 6 applications daily

Prescribe as:

Choline Salicylate Dental Gel
Oral gel, choline salicylate 8.7% in a flavoured gel basis, net price 15 g = £1.79. *Proprietary products*: *Bonjela* (sugar-free)

Treatment of dry mouth

Dry mouth may be relieved in many patients by simple measures such as frequent sips of cool drinks or sucking pieces of ice or sugar-free fruit pastilles. Sugar-free chewing gum stimulates salivation in patients with residual salivary function.

Saliva stimulating tablets may be prescribed for dry mouth in patients with salivary gland impairment (and patent salivary ducts).

Prescribe as:

Saliva Stimulating Tablets
Tablets, sugar-free, citric acid, malic acid and other ingredients in a sorbitol base, net price 100-tab pack = £4.86. *Proprietary product*: *SST tablets*
Dose: allow 1 tablet to dissolve slowly in the mouth when required

> Cross-references to the BNF are provided but nurse prescribers may only prescribe those items that are listed on the Nurse Prescribers' List.

Removal of earwax

Corresponds to BNF section 12.1.3

Wax is a normal bodily secretion which provides a protective film on the meatal skin and need only be removed if it causes deafness or interferes with a proper view of the ear drum. Syringing is generally best avoided in young children and in patients with a history of recurring otitis externa, a history of ear drum perforation, or previous ear surgery. A person who has hearing only in one ear should not have that ear syringed because even a very slight risk of damage is unacceptable in this situation.

Wax may be removed by syringing with water (warmed to body temperature). If necessary, wax can be softened before syringing with simple remedies such as **sodium bicarbonate** ear drops, **olive oil** ear drops or **almond oil** ear drops, which are safe, effective and inexpensive. If the wax is hard and impacted the drops may be used twice daily for a few days before syringing; otherwise the wax may be softened on the day of syringing. The patient should lie with the affected ear uppermost for 5 to 10 minutes after a generous amount of the softening remedy has been introduced into the ear.

Prescribe as:

Almond Oil Ear Drops

Ear drops, almond oil in a suitable container. Net price 10 mL = 50p

Application: allow to warm to room temperature and use as indicated above

Note. Do not heat

Olive Oil Ear Drops

Ear drops, olive oil in a suitable container. Net price 10 mL = 50p

Application: allow to warm to room temperature and use as indicated above

Note. Do not heat

Sodium Bicarbonate Ear Drops

Ear drops, sodium bicarbonate 5%. Net price 10 mL = £1.25

Application: allow to warm to room temperature and use as indicated above

Drugs for threadworms

Corresponds to BNF section 5.5.1.

Anthelmintics are effective for threadworm infections (enterobiasis) but their use needs to be combined with hygiene measures to break the cycle of auto-infection. Threadworms are highly infectious therefore all members of the family need to be treated at the same time.

Adult threadworms do not live for longer than 6 weeks; eggs need to be swallowed and subjected to the action of digestive juices for the development of the worms. Adult females lay eggs on the perianal skin, which causes pruritus. Scratching the area leads to eggs being transferred to the fingers and thence to the mouth, starting the cycle afresh. It is therefore important to advise patients to wash their hands and scrub their nails before each meal and after each visit to the toilet. A bath taken immediately after rising will remove eggs laid during the night. Advice for patients is included in the packaging of most preparations, but it is useful to reinforce this advice verbally.

Mebendazole

Mebendazole is the drug of choice for patients over 2 years of age. It is given as a single dose but as reinfection is very common a second dose may be given after 2 weeks.

MEBENDAZOLE

Indications: threadworm infection; other infections, on doctor's prescription only

Cautions: pregnancy (toxicity found in *rats*), see package insert information below; breast-feeding (see BNF Appendix 5); **interactions:** BNF Appendix 1 (mebendazole)

Side-effects: rarely abdominal pain, diarrhoea; allergic reactions including rash and angioedema reported

Dose: threadworms, ADULT and CHILD over 2 years, 100 mg as a single dose; if reinfection occurs second dose may be needed after 2 weeks; CHILD under 2 years not recommended

Prescribe as:

[1] **Mebendazole Tablets 100 mg** PoM

Tablets, flavoured, chewable, mebendazole 100 mg. Net price 6-tab pack = £1.45.

Note. The package insert includes the information that the tablets are not suitable for women known to be pregnant or for children under 2 years

1. Packs containing no more than 800 mg and labelled to show a max. single dose of 100 mg are on sale to the public for the treatment of threadworm infection

[1] **Mebendazole Oral Suspension 100 mg/5 mL** PoM

Oral Suspension, mebendazole 100 mg/5 mL. Net price 30 mL = £1.68. *Proprietary product: Vermox*

Note. The package insert includes the information that the suspension is not suitable for women known to be pregnant or for children under 2 years

1. Packs containing no more than 800 mg and labelled to show a max. single dose of 100 mg are on sale to the public for the treatment of threadworm infection

Piperazine

Piperazine is available in combination with sennosides; 2 doses are given for threadworm infection with an interval of 2 weeks between them.

> Mebendazole and piperazine are also prescribed by doctors for other infections (e.g. roundworms). Nurse prescribers should, however, prescribe them for threadworm infection **only**.

PIPERAZINE

Indications: threadworm infection; other infections, on doctor's prescription only

Cautions: renal impairment (avoid if severe), liver impairment (BNF Appendix 2); epilepsy, pregnancy (see below for warnings in packs and BNF Appendix 4)

Side-effects: nausea, vomiting, colic, diarrhoea; allergic reactions including urticaria, bronchospasm, and rare reports of arthralgia, fever, Stevens-Johnson syndrome and angioedema; rarely dizziness, muscular incoordination ('worm wobble'); drowsiness, nystagmus, vertigo, blurred vision, confusion and clonic contractions in patients with neurological or renal abnormalities

Dose: threadworms, see under preparation, below

Prescribe as:

Piperazine and Senna Powder

Oral powder, piperazine phosphate 4 g sennosides (calculated as sennoside B) 15.3 mg/sachet. Net price two-dose sachet pack = £1.36. *Proprietary product: Pripsen*

Dose: stirred into a small glass of milk or water and drunk immediately, ADULT and CHILD over 6 years, content of 1 sachet as a single dose (bedtime in adults or morning in children), repeated after 14 days; INFANT 3 months–1 year 1 level 2.5-mL spoonful in the morning, repeated after 14 days; CHILD 1–6 years, 1 level 5-mL spoonful in

the morning, repeated after 14 days
Cautionary label added by pharmacist: dissolve or mix with water before taking
Note. For children under 10 years, only one dual-dose treatment should be given in any 28-day period without medical advice. Packs on sale to the public carry a warning to avoid in epilepsy and in pregnancy

Drugs for scabies and head lice

Corresponds to BNF section 13.10.4

Scabies

Malathion, and **permethrin** are used for *scabies* (*Sarcoptes scabiei*).

The following should be noted:

- *alcoholic lotions* are not recommended (owing to irritation of excoriated skin and genitalia);
- it is not necessary to apply preparations *after a hot bath* (a hot bath may even increase absorption into the blood, removing the drug from its site of action on the skin).

All members of the affected household should be treated simultaneously. Treatment should be applied to the whole body including the scalp, neck, face, and ears. Particular attention should be paid to the webs of the fingers and toes, and lotion brushed under the ends of the nails. It is now recommended that malathion and permethrin should be applied twice, one week apart. Patients with hyperkeratotic (crusted or 'Norwegian') scabies may require 2 or 3 applications on consecutive days to ensure that enough penetrates the skin crusts to kill all the mites.

It is important to warn users **not** to wash their hands since this would require re-application.

The itch of scabies persists for some weeks after the infestation has been eliminated and antipruritic treatment may be required. Application of **crotamiton** can be used to control itching after treatment with more effective acaricides, but caution is necessary if the skin is excoriated.

Head lice

Malathion, and the **pyrethroids** (permethrin and phenothrin) are effective against *head lice* (*Pediculus humanus capitis*) but lice in some districts have developed resistance; resistance to two or more parasiticidal preparations has also been reported. Lotion or liquid formulations should be used. Shampoos are diluted too much in use to be effective. Aqueous formulations are preferred in severe eczema and for asthmatic patients and small children, to avoid alcoholic fumes. A contact time of 12 hours or overnight treatment is recommended for lotions and liquids. A 2-hour treatment is not sufficient to kill eggs.

In general, a course of treatment for head lice should be 2 applications of product 7 days apart to prevent lice emerging from any eggs that survive the first application.

The policy of rotating insecticides on a district-wide basis is now considered outmoded. To overcome the development of resistance, a mosaic strategy is required whereby, if a course of treatment fails to cure, a different insecticide is used for the next course. If a course of treatment with either permethrin or phenothrin fails, then a non-pyrethroid parasiticidal product should be used for the next course.

Carbaryl is also effective against head lice but in the light of data from animal studies, it would be prudent to consider carbaryl as a human carcinogen. Carbaryl preparations are now restricted to **prescription-only** use although the Department of Health has emphasised that the risk is theoretical (and for intermittent use in head lice, it is likely to be exceedingly small).

WET COMBING METHODS. Several products are available which require the use of a plastic detection comb and hair conditioner; some head lice devices are prescribable on the NHS (consult Drug Tariff). The methods typically involve meticulous combing with the detection comb (probably for at least 30 minutes each time) over the whole scalp at 4-day intervals for a minimum of 2 weeks.

Not all preparations included here are licensed for *crab lice* therefore advice on crab lice has not been included

Individuals can rarely react to certain ingredients in preparations applied to the skin. Special care is required when prescribing skin and scalp products for these individuals—see BNF section 13.1.3. Excipients associated with sensitisation are shown under individual product entries

Malathion

Malathion is recommended for *scabies* and *head lice* (for details see notes above).

The risk of systemic effects associated with 1–2 applications of malathion is considered to be very low; however applications of lotions repeated at intervals of less than 1 week *or* application for more than 3 consecutive weeks should be **avoided** since the likelihood of eradication of lice is not increased.

MALATHION

Indications: scabies, head lice

Cautions: avoid contact with eyes; do not use on broken or infected skin; do not use lotion more than once a week for 3 consecutive weeks; use in children under 6 months on doctor's advice only; alcoholic lotions **not** recommended for head lice in severe eczema, asthma or in small children, or for scabies or crab lice (see notes above)

Side-effects: skin irritation

Administration:

Head lice, rub into dry hair and scalp, allow to dry naturally, remove by washing 12 hours later (see also notes above); repeat application after 7 days [unlicensed use]

Scabies, apply over whole body, wash off after 24 hours; if hands are washed with soap within 24 hours, they should be retreated; see also notes above; repeat application after 7 days [unlicensed use]

Note. For scabies, manufacturer recommends application to the body but not necessarily to the head and neck. However, application should be extended to the scalp, neck, face, and ears.

Prescribe as:

Malathion Alcoholic Lotion 0.5%

Alcoholic lotion, malathion 0.5% in an alcoholic basis. Flammable. *Proprietary products: Prioderm Lotion* (net price 50 mL = £2.22, 200 mL = £5.70), *Suleo-M Lotion* (50 mL = £2.22, 200 mL = £5.70)

Alcohol: alcoholic lotion not recommended for head lice in those with severe eczema, or asthmatics or in young children, or for scabies (for details see notes above)

Excipients: include fragrance

Malathion Aqueous Lotion 0.5%

Aqueous lotion, malathion 0.5% in an aqueous basis. *Proprietary products: Derbac-M Liquid* (net price 50 mL = £2.22, 200 mL = £5.70), *Quellada M* (50 mL = £1.85, 200 mL = £4.62)

Excipients: include cetostearyl alcohol, fragrance, hydroxybenzoates (parabens)

Permethrin

Permethrin is effective for *scabies* (for details see notes above). Permethrin is active against *head lice* but the formulation and licensed methods of application of the current products make them unsuitable for the treatment of head lice.

PERMETHRIN

Indications: scabies

Cautions: avoid contact with eyes; do not use on broken or infected skin; use for scabies in children under 2 years on doctor's advice only

Side-effects: pruritus, erythema, and stinging; rarely rashes and oedema

Administration: scabies, apply over whole body and wash off after 8–12 hours; CHILD (see also Cautions above) apply over whole body including face, neck, scalp, and ears; cream should be reapplied to hands if they are washed with soap and water within 8 hours of application (see notes above); repeat application after 7 days

Note. Manufacturer recommends application to the body but to exclude the head and neck. However, application should be extended to the scalp, neck, face, and ears.

Larger patients may require up to two 30-g packs for adequate treatment

Prescribe as:

Permethrin Cream 5%

Cream, permethrin 5%. Net price 30 g = £5.52. *Proprietary product: Lyclear Dermal Cream*

Excipients: may *include* butylated hydroxytoluene, wool fat derivative

Cross-references to the BNF are provided but nurse prescribers may only prescribe those items that are listed on the Nurse Prescribers' List.

Phenothrin

Phenothrin is recommended for *head lice* (for details see notes above).

PHENOTHRIN

Indications: head lice

Cautions: avoid contact with eyes; do not use on broken or infected skin; do not use more than once a week for 3 weeks at a time; use for children under 6 months on doctor's advice only; alcoholic preparations **not** recommended for head lice in severe eczema, or in small children

Side-effects: skin irritation

Administration: see under preparations

Prescribe as:

Phenothrin Alcoholic Lotion 0.2%

Lotion, phenothrin 0.2% in basis containing isopropyl alcohol 69.3%. Net price 50 mL = £2.22, 200 mL = £5.70. Flammable. *Proprietary product: Full Marks Lotion*

Excipients: include fragrance

Administration: head lice, apply to dry hair and allow to dry naturally; shampoo after 12 hours [unlicensed contact duration]; comb hair while still wet; repeat application after 7 days [unlicensed use]

Alcohol: alcoholic lotion not recommended for head lice in severe eczema, asthmatics or small children

Phenothrin Aqueous Lotion

Liquid, phenothrin 0.5% in an aqueous basis. Net price 50 mL = £2.22; 200 mL = £5.70. *Proprietary product: Full Marks Liquid*

Excipients: include cetostearyl alcohol, fragrance, hydroxybenzoates (parabens)

Administration: head lice, apply to dry hair, allow to dry naturally; shampoo after 12 hours or next day, comb hair while still wet; repeat application after 7 days [unlicensed use]

Skin preparations

Emollients

Corresponds to BNF section 13.2.1 and 13.2.1.1.

Emollients soothe, smooth and hydrate the skin and are indicated for all dry or scaling disorders. Their effects are short-lived and they should be applied frequently even after improvement occurs. They are useful in dry and eczematous disorders, and to a lesser extent in psoriasis. Light emollients such as **aqueous cream** are suitable for many patients with dry skin but a wide range of more greasy preparations including **white soft paraffin**, **emulsifying ointment**, and **liquid and white soft paraffin ointment** are available; the severity of the condition, patient preference and site of application will often guide the choice of emollient; emollients should be applied in the direction of hair growth. Some ingredients may occasionally cause sensitisation (BNF section 13.1.3) and this should be suspected if an eczematous reaction occurs.

Preparations such as **aqueous cream** and **emulsifying ointment** can be used as soap substitutes for hand washing and in the bath; the preparation is rubbed on the skin before rinsing off completely. The addition of a bath oil may also be helpful; several proprietary emollient bath additives are available (see below).

Arachis oil (peanut oil) is used for cleansing in dry skin conditions (see also BNF section 13.9).

> Individuals can rarely react to certain ingredients in preparations applied to the skin. Special care is required when prescribing skin and scalp products for these individuals—see BNF section 13.1.3. Excipients associated with sensitisation are shown under individual product entries

EMOLLIENTS

Prescribe as:

Aqueous Cream
Cream, emulsifying ointment 30%, [1]phenoxyethanol 1%, in freshly boiled and cooled purified water. Net price 100 g = 50p

1. The BP permits use of alternative antimicrobials provided their identity and concentration are stated on the label

Excipients: include cetostearyl alcohol

Emulsifying Ointment
Ointment, emulsifying wax 30%, white soft paraffin 50%, liquid paraffin 20%. Net price 100 g = 65p

Excipients: include cetostearyl alcohol

Hydrous Ointment
(Also known as Oily Cream)
Ointment, dried magnesium sulphate 0.5%, phenoxyethanol 1%, wool alcohols ointment 50% in freshly boiled and cooled purified water. Net price 100 g = 40p

Liquid and White Soft Paraffin Ointment
Ointment, liquid paraffin 50%, white soft paraffin 50%. Net price 250 g = £3.24

Paraffin, White Soft (white petroleum jelly). Net price 100 g = 52p

Paraffin, Yellow Soft (yellow petroleum jelly). Net price 100 g = 33p

Proprietary emollients, prescribe as:

Cetraben® Emollient Cream (Sankyo)
Cream, white soft paraffin 13.2 %, light liquid paraffin 10.5 %. Net price 50 g = £1.17, 125 g = £2.38, 500-g pump pack = £5.61

For inflamed, damaged, dry or chapped skin including eczema

Excipients: include cetostearyl alcohol, hydroxybenzoates (parabens)

Decubal® Clinic (Alpharma)
Cream, isopropyl myristate 17%, glycerol 8.5%, wool fat 6 %, dimeticone 5%, net price 50 g = £1.02, 100 g = £1.98

Excipients: include cetyl alcohol, polysorbates, sorbic acid, wool fat

For dry skin conditions including ichthyosis, psoriasis, dermatitis and hyperkeratosis

Dermamist® (Yamanouchi)
Spray application, white soft paraffin 10% in a basis containing liquid paraffin, fractionated coconut oil. Net price 250-mL pressurised aerosol unit = £9.22

For dry skin conditions including eczema, ichthyosis, pruritus of the elderly

Caution: flammable

Diprobase® Cream (Schering-Plough)
Cream, cetomacrogol 2.25%, cetostearyl alcohol 7.2%, liquid paraffin 6%, white soft paraffin 15%, water-miscible basis used for *Diprosone®* cream. Net price 50 g = £1.43; 500-g dispenser = £6.15

For dry skin conditions

Excipients: include cetostearyl alcohol, chlorocresol

Diprobase® Ointment (Schering-Plough)
Ointment, liquid paraffin 5%, white soft paraffin 95%, basis used for *Diprosone®* ointment. Net price 50 g = £1.54

For dry skin conditions

Doublebase® (Dermal)
Gel, isopropyl myristate 15 %, liquid paraffin 15%, net price 100 g = £2.77; 500 g = £6.09

For dry chapped or itchy skin conditions

E45® Cream (Crookes)
Cream, light liquid paraffin 12.6%, white soft paraffin 14.5%, hypoallergenic hydrous wool fat (hypoallergenic lanolin) 1% in self-emulsifying monostearin. Net price 50 g = £1.18, 125 g = £2.39, 350 g = £4.14, 500-g pump pack = £6.20

For dry skin conditions

Excipients: include cetyl alcohol, cetostearyl alcohol, hydroxybenzoates (parabens)

Epaderm® (Medlock)
Ointment, emulsifying wax 30%, yellow soft paraffin 30%, liquid paraffin 40%, net price 125 g = £3.67; 500 g = £6.21

For use as an emollient or soap substitute

Excipients: include cetostearyl alcohol

Gammaderm® Cream (Linderma)

Cream, evening primrose oil 20%, net price 50 g = £2.83, 250 g = £8.20

Excipients: include beeswax, hydroxybenzoates (parabens), propylene glycol

Cautions: epilepsy (but hazard unlikely with topical preparations)

For dry skin conditions

Hydromol® Cream (Ferndale)

Cream, sodium pidolate 2.5%, net price 50 g = £2.04, 100 g = £3.80, 500 g = £12.60

For dry skin conditions

Excipients: include cetostearyl alcohol, hydroxybenzoates (parabens)

Hydromol® Ointment (Ferndale)

Ointment, yellow soft paraffin 30%, emulsifying wax 30%, net price 125 g = £2.79, 500 g = £4.74

For use as an emollient or as a bath additive

Excipients: include cetostearyl alcohol

Keri® Therapeutic Lotion (Bristol-Myers Squibb)

Lotion, mineral oil 16%, with lanolin oil. Net price 190-mL pump pack = £3.56; 380-mL pump pack = £5.81

For dry skin conditions and nappy rash

Excipients: include fragrance, hydroxybenzoates (parabens), *N*-(3-chloroallyl) hexaminium chloride (quaternium 15), propylene glycol

LactiCare® Lotion (Stiefel)

Lotion, lactic acid 5%, sodium pidolate 2.5%. Net price 150 mL = £3.19

For dry skin conditions

Excipients: include cetostearyl alcohol, imidurea, isopropyl palmitate, fragrance

Lipobase® (Yamanouchi)

Cream, fatty cream basis used for *Locoid Lipocream®*. Net price 50 g = £2.08

For dry skin conditions

Excipients: include cetostearyl alcohol, hydroxybenzoates (parabens)

Neutrogena® Dermatological Cream (J&J)

Cream, glycerol 40% in an emollient basis. Net price 100 g = £3.77

For dry skin conditions

Excipients: include cetostearyl alcohol, hydroxybenzoates (parabens)

Oilatum® Cream (Stiefel)

Cream, light liquid paraffin 6%, white soft paraffin 15%. Net price 40 g = £1.79, 150 g = £3.38

For dry skin conditions

Excipients: include benzyl alcohol, cetostearyl alcohol

Ultrabase® (Schering Health)

Cream, water-miscible, containing liquid paraffin and white soft paraffin. Net price 50 g = 89p; 500-g dispenser = £6.44

For dry skin conditions

Excipients: include fragrance, hydroxybenzoates (parabens), disodium edetate, stearyl alcohol

Unguentum M® (Crookes)

Cream, saturated neutral oil, liquid paraffin, white soft paraffin. Net price 50 g = £1.59, 100 g = £3.13, 200-mL dispenser = £6.19, 500 g = £9.55

For dry skin conditions and nappy rash

Excipients: include cetostearyl alcohol, polysorbate 40, propylene glycol, sorbic acid

Zerobase® Cream (Zeroderma)

Cream, liquid paraffin 11%, net price 500 g = £5.99

For dry skin conditions

Excipients: include cetostearyl alcohol, chlorocresol

Proprietary emollient bath additives, prescribe as:

Alpha Keri Bath® Oil (Bristol-Myers Squibb)

Bath oil, liquid paraffin 91.7%, oil-soluble fraction of wool fat 3%. Net price 240 mL = £3.45; 480 mL = £6.43

For dry skin conditions including ichthyosis and pruritus of the elderly, add 10–20 mL /bath (INFANT 5 mL)

Excipients: include fragrance

Ashbourne Emollient Medicinal Bath Oil (Ashbourne)

Emollient bath oil, liquid paraffin 65%, acetylated wool alcohols 5%, net price 250 mL = £2.75; 500 mL = £5.46

For dry skin conditions including dermatitis, pruritus of the elderly, and ichthyosis, add 15–20 mL /bath (INFANT and CHILD 5–10 mL added to a small bath or washbasin)

[1]Balneum® (Crookes)

Balneum® bath oil, soya oil 84.75%. Net price 200 mL = £2.79, 500 mL = £6.06, 1 litre = £11.70

For dry skin conditions including those associated with dermatitis and eczema; add 20 mL/bath (INFANT 5 mL)

Excipients: include butylated hydroxytoluene, propylene glycol, fragrance

Cetraben® Emollient Bath Additive (Sankyo)

Emollient bath additive, light liquid paraffin 82.8%, net price 500 mL = £5.25

For dry skin conditions, including eczema, add 1–2 capfuls/bath (CHILD ½ –1 capful)

Dermalo® (Dermal)

Bath emollient, acetylated wool alcohols 5%, liquid paraffin 65%. Net price 500 mL = £3.60

For dermatitis, dry skin conditions including ichthyosis and pruritus of the elderly; add 15–20 mL/bath (INFANT and CHILD 5–10 mL)

Diprobath® (Schering-Plough)

Bath additive, isopropyl myristate 39%, light liquid paraffin 46%. Net price 500 mL = £6.97

For dry skin conditions including dermatitis and eczema; add 25 mL/bath (INFANT 10 mL)

Hydromol Emollient® (Ferndale)

Bath additive, isopropyl myristate 13%, light liquid paraffin 37.8%. Net price 150 mL = £1.87; 350 mL = £3.80; 1 litre = £9.00

For dry skin conditions including eczema, ichthyosis and pruritus of the elderly; add 1–3 capfuls/bath (INFANT 0.5–2 capfuls)

Imuderm® Bath Oil (Goldshield)

Bath oil, almond oil 30%, light liquid paraffin 69.6%, net price 250 mL = £3.75

Excipients: include butylated hydroxyanisole

For dry skin conditions including dermatitis, eczema, pruritus of the elderly, and ichthyosis, add 15–30 mL/bath (INFANT and CHILD 7.5–15 mL)

---

1. Some pack sizes may not be prescribed on the NHS and are not listed here

Oilatum® Emollient (Stiefel)

Bath additive (emulsion), acetylated wool alcohols 5%, liquid paraffin 63.4%. Net price 250 mL = £2.75; 500 mL = £4.57

For dry skin conditions including dermatitis, pruritus of the elderly and ichthyosis; add 1–3 capfuls/bath (INFANT 0.5–2 capfuls)

Excipients: include isopropyl palmitate, fragrance

Oilatum® Fragrance Free Junior (Stiefel)

Bath additive, light liquid paraffin 63.4%, net price 250 mL = £3.25, 500 mL = £5.75, 1 litre = £11.50

For dry skin conditions including dermatitis, pruritus of the elderly and ichthyosis; add 1–3 capfuls/bath (INFANT 0.5–2 capfuls)

Excipients: include wool fat, isopropyl palmitate

Oilatum® Gel (Stiefel)

Shower emollient (gel), light liquid paraffin 70%. Net price 150 g = £5.15

For dry skin conditions including dermatitis

Excipients: include fragrance

Barrier preparations

Corresponds to BNF section 13.2.2.

Barrier preparations often contain water-repellent substances such as **dimeticone** (dimethicone) or other silicones. They are used on the skin around stomas, bedsores, and pressure areas in the elderly where the skin is intact. Where the skin has broken down, barrier preparations have a limited role in protecting adjacent skin. They are no substitute for adequate nursing care and it is doubtful if they are any more effective than the traditional compound **zinc ointments**. A spray preparation, **zinc oxide and dimeticone spray**, is also available.

NAPPY RASH. Barrier creams and ointments are used for protection against nappy rash which is usually a local dermatitis. The first line of treatment is to ensure that nappies are changed frequently and that tightly fitting water-proof pants are avoided. The rash may clear when left exposed to the air, and a barrier preparation may be helpful. If the rash is associated with a fungal infection, an antifungal cream such as clotrimazole cream is useful.

DIMETICONE (SILICONE)

Dimeticone barrier creams containing at least 10%

Prescribe as:

Dimeticone Cream (*Conotrane*)

Cream, benzalkonium chloride 0.1%, dimeticone '350' 22%. Net price 100 g = 74p; 500 g = £3.51.

For nappy and urinary rash and pressure sores

Excipients: include cetostearyl alcohol, fragrance

Dimeticone Cream (*Siopel*)

Barrier cream, dimeticone '1000' 10%, cetrimide 0.3%, arachis (peanut) oil. Net price 50 g = £1.66.

For protection against water-soluble irritants

Excipients: include butylated hydroxytoluene, cetostearyl alcohol, hydroxybenzoates (parabens)

Dimeticone Cream (*Vasogen*)

Barrier cream, dimeticone 20%, calamine 1.5%, zinc oxide 7.5%. Net price 50 g = 80p; 100 g = £1.36.

For nappy rash, pressure sores, ileostomy and colostomy care

Excipients: include hydroxybenzoates (parabens), wool fat

TITANIUM or ZINC

Prescribe as:

Titanium Ointment

Ointment, titanium dioxide 20%, titanium peroxide 5%, titanium salicylate 3% in a basis containing dimeticone, light liquid paraffin, white soft paraffin, and benzoin tincture. Net price 30 g = £2.01.

For nappy rash and related disorders.

Proprietary product: Metanium Ointment

Zinc Cream

Cream, zinc oxide 32%, arachis (peanut) oil 32%, calcium hydroxide 0.045%, oleic acid 0.5%, wool fat 8%, in freshly boiled and cooled purified water, net price 50 g = 50p.

For nappy and urinary rash and eczematous conditions

Zinc Ointment

Cream, zinc oxide 15%, in Simple Ointment BP 1988 (which contains wool fat 5%, hard paraffin 5%, cetostearyl alcohol 5%, white soft paraffin 85%), net price 25 g = 16p.

For nappy and urinary rash and eczematous conditions

Zinc and Castor Oil Ointment

Ointment, zinc oxide 7.5%, castor oil 50%, arachis (peanut) oil 30.5%, white beeswax 10%, cetostearyl alcohol 2%. Net price 25 g = 14p.

For nappy and urinary rash

Zinc Oxide and Dimeticone Spray

Spray application, dimeticone 1.04%, zinc oxide 12.5%, in a basis containing wool alcohols, cetostearyl alcohol, dextran, white soft paraffin, liquid paraffin, propellants. Net price 115-g pressurised aerosol unit = £3.54.

For urinary rash, pressure sores, leg ulcers, moist eczema, fissures, fistulae and ileostomy care

Caution: flammable

Excipients: include cetostearyl alcohol, hydroxybenzoates (parabens), wool fat

Proprietary product: Sprilon

Pruritus

Corresponds to BNF section 13.3.

Pruritus may be caused by systemic disease (such as drug hypersensitivity, obstructive jaundice, endocrine disease, and certain malignant diseases) as well as by skin disease (e.g. psoriasis, eczema, urticaria, and scabies). Where possible the underlying causes should be treated. An **emollient** may be of value where the pruritus is associated with dry skin (which is common in otherwise healthy elderly people).

Preparations containing **crotamiton** are sometimes used in pruritus but are of uncertain value.

Crotamiton can be used to control itching after treatment with a parasiticidal preparation for scabies (NPF p. N25).

Preparations containing calamine are often ineffective and therefore these preparations are no longer included in the NPF.

CROTAMITON

Indications: pruritus (including pruritus after scabies); see notes above
Cautions: avoid use near eyes and broken skin; use on doctor's advice for children under 3 years
Contra-indications: acute exudative dermatoses
Administration: pruritus, apply 2–3 times daily; CHILD below 3 years, apply once daily

Precribe as:

Crotamiton Cream 10%
Cream, crotamiton 10%. Net price 30 g = £2.27; 100 g = £3.95
Excipients: include beeswax, fragrance, hydroxybenzoates (parabens), stearyl alcohol

Crotamiton Lotion10%
Lotion, crotamiton 10%. Net price 100 mL = £2.99
Excipients: include cetyl alcohol, fragrance, propylene glycol, sorbic acid, stearyl alcohol

Fungal infections

Corresponds to BNF section 13.10.2.

Fungal skin infections can be prevented by keeping the susceptible area as clean and dry as possible. Established fungal infections such as ringworm infection and candidal skin infection may be treated with **clotrimazole cream, econazole cream** or **miconazole cream.**

CLOTRIMAZOLE

Indications: fungal skin infections
Cautions: avoid contact with eyes and mucous membranes
Side-effects: occasional skin irritation or sensitivity including mild burning sensation, erythema, and itching (discontinue if severe)
Administration: apply 2–3 times daily

Prescribe as:

Clotrimazole Cream 1%
Cream, clotrimazole 1%. Net price 20 g = £2.12.
Excipients: not shown because preparation available from several sources; for sensitised individuals, check that version dispensed is free from the sensitising ingredient

ECONAZOLE NITRATE

Indications; Cautions; Side-effects: see under Clotrimazole
Administration: apply twice daily

Prescribe as:

Econazole Cream 1%
Cream, econazole nitrate 1%. *Proprietary products: Ecostatin Cream* (net price 15 g = £1.49, 30 g = £2.75), *Pevaryl Cream* (net price 30 g = £2.65)
Excipients: include butylated hydroxyanisole, fragrance

MICONAZOLE NITRATE

Indications; Cautions; Side-effects: see under Clotrimazole
Administration: apply twice daily continuing for 10 days after lesions have healed

Prescribe as:

Miconazole Cream 2%
Cream, miconazole nitrate 2%. Net price 20 g = £2.05, 45 g = £1.97
Excipients: not shown because preparation available from several sources; for sensitised individuals, check that version dispensed is free from the sensitising ingredient

Boils

Boils are generally treated with an antibacterial, but **magnesium sulphate paste** is a traditional adjunct.

MAGNESIUM SULPHATE

Indications: paste used as an adjunct in the management of boils
Administration: apply under dressing

Prescribe as:

Magnesium Sulphate Paste
Paste, dried magnesium sulphate 45 g, glycerol 55 g, phenol 500 mg. Net price 25 g = 59p, 50 g = 72p
Note. Stir before use

Disinfection and cleansing

Corresponds to BNF section 13.11.

Physiological saline

Sterile **sodium chloride solution 0.9%** is suitable for general cleansing of skin and wounds but tap water is often appropriate.

SODIUM CHLORIDE

Indications: skin cleansing

Prescribe as:

Sterile Sodium Chloride Solution 0.9%
Sterile solution, sodium chloride 0.9%. To be used undiluted for topical irrigation of wounds. Net price 10 × 10-mL unit = £3.60; 10 × 20-mL unit = £10.36; 10 × 30-mL unit = £3.00; 25 × 20-mL unit = £5.50 (*Proprietary brands: Irripod, Steripod and possibly others); 25 ×* 25-mL sachets = £5.95, 10 × 100-mL sachets = £7.28 (*Proprietary brands: Normasol and possibly others*); 30 × 45-mL bottles = £15.00, 30 × 100-mL bottles = £21.30 (*Proprietary brand: Miniversol*); 1 × 240-

mL aerosol can = £3.00 (*Proprietary brand: Irriclens*); 1 × 200-mL can = £2.65 (*Proprietary brand: Nine Lives*); 1 × 120-mL bellows pack = £1.50 (*Proprietary brand: Flowfusor*); 1 × 500-mL bottle = 90p, 1 × 1-litre bottle = 95p (*Proprietary brand: Versol*); other sizes also prescribable if available

Povidone–iodine

Povidone–iodine aqueous solution 10% is useful where skin disinfection is required.

POVIDONE–IODINE

Indications: skin disinfection

Cautions: pregnancy (BNF Appendix 4), breast-feeding (BNF Appendix 5), broken skin (see below), renal impairment (avoid regular application to inflamed or broken skin or mucosa)

LARGE OPEN WOUNDS. The application of povidone–iodine to large wounds or severe burns may produce systemic adverse effects such as metabolic acidosis, hypernatraemia and impairment of renal function

Contra-indications: avoid regular use in patients with thyroid disorders or those receiving lithium therapy

Side-effects: rarely sensitivity; may interfere with thyroid function tests

Prescribe as:

Povidone–Iodine Solution 10%

Solution, povidone–iodine 10% in aqueous solution. Net price 500 mL = £1.75. *Proprietary preparation: Betadine Antiseptic Solution.*

Administration: apply undiluted in pre- and post-operative skin disinfection; NEONATE not recommended for regular use (and contra-indicated if birth-weight below 1.5 kg)

Note. Not for body cavity irrigation

Wound management products

See BNF Appendix 8

The following items in BNF Appendix 8 are not on the Nurse Prescribers' List:

- Items not in the Drug Tariff (described as NHS in the BNF)

Desloughing agents

Corresponds to BNF section 13.11.7 and Appendix 8.

Preparations have been included here because they are licensed as medicinal products. Details of all other wound management products are in BNF Appendix 8.

CADEXOMER–IODINE

Indications; Administration: see under preparations below

Cautions: patients with severe renal impairment or history of thyroid disorders; iodine may be absorbed particularly if large wounds treated

Contra-indications: avoid in thyroid disorders, in those receiving lithium, in pregnancy and breast-feeding and in children

Prescribe as:

Cadexomer–Iodine Ointment

Ointment, iodine 0.9% as cadexomer–iodine in an ointment basis. Net price 4 × 10-g tubes = £17.24, 2 × 20-g tubes = £17.24. *Proprietary product: Iodosorb Ointment*

Administration: for treatment of chronic exuding wounds, such as leg ulcers, apply to wound surface to depth of approx. 3 mm and cover; renew when saturated (usually 2–3 times weekly, daily for heavily exuding wounds); max. single application 50 g, max. weekly application 150 g; max. duration up to 3 months in any single course of treatment

Cadexomer–Iodine Paste

Paste, iodine 0.9% as cadexomer–iodine in a paste basis with gauze backing. Net price 5 × 5-g units = £19.48, 3 × 10-g units = £23.40, 2 × 17-g units = £24.68. *Proprietary product: Iodoflex*

Administration: for treatment of chronic exuding wounds, such as leg ulcers, apply to wound surface, remove gauze backing and cover; renew when saturated (usually 2–3 times weekly, daily for heavily exuding wounds); max. single application 50 g, max. weekly application 150 g; max. duration up to 3 months in any single course of treatment

Cadexomer–Iodine Powder

Powder, iodine 0.9% as cadexomer–iodine microbeads. Net price 7 x 3-g sachets = £12.89. *Proprietary product: Iodosorb Powder*

Administration: for treatment of chronic exuding wounds, such as leg ulcers, apply to wound surface to depth of approx. 3 mm and cover; renew when saturated (usually 2–3 times weekly, daily for heavily exuding wounds); max. single application 50 g, max. weekly application 150 g; max. duration up to 3 months in any single course of treatment

STREPTOKINASE WITH STREPTODORNASE

Indications: removal of clotted blood, fibrinous or purulent accumulation from suppurative surface lesions such as ulcers, pressure ulcers, amputation sites, diabetic gangrene, radiation necrosis, infected wounds, and surgical incisions

Contra-indications: active haemorrhage, severe hypertension

Side-effects: infrequent allergic reactions (reduced by careful and frequent removal of exudate and thorough irrigation with physiological saline); fever, transient burning, haemorrhage, and hypersensitivity reactions including shock reported

Administration: reconstitute with 20 mL sterile physiological saline (or water for injections) and apply as wet dressing 1–2 times daily; cover with semi-occlusive dressing; irrigate lesion thoroughly with physiological saline and remove loosened material before next application

Prescribe as:

Streptokinase and Streptodornase Topical Powder PoM

Powder, streptokinase 100 000 units, streptodornase 25 000 units. For preparing solutions for topical use. Net price with sterile physiological saline 20 mL (combi-pack) = £10.06. *Proprietary product: Varidase Topical*

Medicated stocking

Corresponds to BNF Appendix 8.

Zinc Paste Bandage remains one of the standard treatments for leg ulcers and can be left on undisturbed for up to a week; it is often used in association with compression for treatment of venous ulcers.

Zinc paste bandages are also used with **coal tar** or **ichthammol** in chronic lichenified skin conditions such as chronic eczema (ichthammol often being preferred since its action is considered to be milder). They are also used with calamine in milder eczematous skin conditions (but the inclusion of **clioquinol** may lead to irritation in susceptible subjects).

ZINC OXIDE

Indications; Administration: see notes above and under preparations below

Prescribe as:

Zinc Paste Bandage, BP 1993

Cotton fabric, plain weave, impregnated with suitable paste containing zinc oxide; requires additional bandaging. Net price 6 m × 7.5 cm = £3.28 (*proprietary product: Steripaste* (15%), excipients: include polysorbate 80); £3.23 (*proprietary product: Zincaband* (15%), *excipients: include* hydroxybenzoates); £3.37 (*proprietary product: Viscopaste PB7* (10%), *excipients: include* hydroxybenzoates)

Zinc Paste and Calamine Bandage

(Drug Tariff specification 5). Cotton fabric, plain weave, impregnated with suitable paste containing calamine and zinc oxide; requires additional bandaging. Net price 6 m × 7.5 cm = £3.33 (*proprietary product: Calaband*)

Zinc Paste, Calamine, and Clioquinol Bandage, BP 1993

Cotton fabric, plain weave, impregnated with suitable paste containing calamine, clioquinol, and zinc oxide; requires additional bandaging. Net price 6 m × 7.5 cm = £3.33 (*proprietary product: Quinaband, excipients: include* hydroxybenzoates)

Zinc Paste and Ichthammol Bandage, BP 1993

Cotton fabric, plain weave, impregnated with suitable paste containing zinc oxide and ichthammol; requires additional bandaging. Net price 6 m × 7.5 cm = £3.24 (*proprietary product: Icthaband* (15/2%), *excipients: include* hydroxybenzoates; *proprietary product: Ichthopaste* (6/2%)
Uses: see BNF section 13.5

Zinc Oxide Impregnated Medicated Stocking

Stocking, sterile rayon, impregnated with ointment containing zinc oxide 20%. Net price 4-pouch carton = £12.50; 10-pouch carton = £31.26. *Proprietary product: Zipzoc*
Administration: chronic leg ulcers; can be used under appropriate compression bandages or hosiery in chronic venous insufficiency

Cross-references to the BNF are provided but nurse prescribers may only prescribe those items that are listed on the Nurse Prescribers' List.

Elastic hosiery

Corresponds to BNF Appendix 8.

Before elastic hosiery can be dispensed, the quantity (single or pair), article (including accessories), and compression class (I, II, or III) must be specified by the prescriber; for further details see Drug Tariff.

Note. Graduated compression tights are not prescribable on the NHS

Peak flow meters

Corresponds to BNF section 3.1.5

Measurement of peak flow is particularly helpful for patients who are 'poor perceivers' and hence slow to detect deterioration in their asthma, and for those with moderate or severe asthma. Standard-range peak flow meters are suitable for both adults and children; low-range peak flow meters are appropriate for severely restricted airflow in adults and children. Patients must be given clear guidance on the action they should take if the peak flow falls below a specified level.

Prescribe as:

Standard-range peak flow meter

Conforms to standard EN 13826

Peak flow meter, range 60–800 litres/minute, net price = £6.50 (*proprietary product*: *Micropeak*), 60–800 litres/minute = £6.86 (*proprietary product*: *Mini-Wright*), 60–800 litres/minute = £6.53 (*proprietary product*: *Ferraris Pocketpeak*); 50–800 litres/minute = £5.95 (*proprietary product*: *Vitalograph*); replacement mouthpieces available (not interchangeable between brands)

Note. Readings from new peak flow meters are often lower than those obtained from old Wright-scale peak flow meters and the correct chart should be used

Low-range peak flow meter

Conforms to standard EN 13826 except for reduced measurement range

Peak flow meter, range 30–400 litres/minute, net price = £6.90 (*proprietary product*: *Mini-Wright*), 50–400 litres/minute = £6.53 (*proprietary product*: *Ferraris Pocketpeak*) 50–400 litres/minute = £5.95 (*proprietary product*: *Vitalograph*); replacement mouthpieces available (not interchangeable between brands)

Note. Readings from new peak flow meters are often lower than those obtained from old Wright-scale peak flow meters and the correct chart should be used

Urinary catheters and appliances

Urinary appliances

These are listed in Part IXB of the Drug Tariff (Part 5 of the Scottish Drug Tariff, Part III of the Northern Ireland Drug Tariff).

Urethral catheters

These are listed in Part IXA of the Drug Tariff (Part 3 of the Scottish Drug Tariff, Part III of the Northern Ireland Drug Tariff).

Catheter patency

Corresponds to BNF section 7.4.4.

The deposition which occurs on catheters is usually chiefly composed of phosphate and to minimise this the catheter (if latex) should be changed at least as often as every 6 weeks. If the catheter is to be left for longer periods a silicone catheter should be used together with the appropriate use of catheter maintenance solutions. Repeated blockage usually indicates that the catheter needs to be changed.

CATHETER PATENCY SOLUTIONS

Indications: catheter care; see also under preparations, below

Administration: to be warmed to body temperature and instilled as required, see also under preparations, below

Prescribe as:

Chlorhexidine 0.02% Catheter Maintenance Solution

Sterile solution, chlorhexidine 0.02%. *Proprietary products: Uro-Tainer Chlorhexidine* (net price 100-mL sachet = £2.60), *Uriflex C* (100-mL sachet = £2.40)

For mechanical cleansing and prevention of bacterial contamination (but not effective against *Pseudomonas* species); discontinue if burning or haematuria occur

Sodium Chloride 0.9% Catheter Maintenance Solution

Sterile solution, sodium chloride 0.9%. *Proprietary products: OptiFlo S* (Net price 50- and 100-mL sachets = £3.15), *Uro-Tainer Sodium Chloride* (50- and 100-mL sachets = £3.05), *Uriflex S* (100-mL sachet = £3.23)

For removal of clots and other debris, to be instilled as required

'Solution G' Catheter Maintenance Solution

Sterile solution, citric acid 3.23%, magnesium oxide 0.38%, sodium bicarbonate 0.7%, disodium edetate 0.01%. *Proprietary products: OptiFlo G* (Net price 50- and 100-mL sachets = £3.34), *Uriflex G* (100-mL sachet = £3.23); *Uro-Tainer Twin Suby G* (2 × 30mL = £4.17)

For prevention of catheter encrustation and crystallisation, to be instilled once daily to once weekly according to severity; in very severe cases use 'Solution R'

'Solution R' Catheter Maintenance Solution

Sterile solution, citric acid 6%, gluconolactone 0.6%, magnesium carbonate 2.8%, disodium edetate 0.01%. *Proprietary products: OptiFlo R* (Net price 50- and 100-mL sachets = £3.23), *Uriflex R* (100-mL sachet = £3.23), *Uro-Tainer Twin Solutio R* (2 × 30mL = £4.17),

For prevention of catheter encrustation and dissolution of crystallisation if 'Solution G' unsuccessful, to be instilled once weekly or more frequently up to once daily according to severity

Water

Corresponds to BNF section 9.2.2.1
Prescribe as:

Water for Injections. PoM Net price 1-mL amp = 18p; 2-mL amp = 17p; 5-mL amp = 28p; 10-mL amp = 31p; 20-mL amp = 55p; 50-mL amp = £1.91; 100-mL vial = 23p

Stoma care products

Corresponds to BNF section 1.8.

The 3 major types of abdominal stoma are:
- colostomy
- ileostomy
- urostomy

Each requires the collection of body waste into an artificial appliance (the 'bag') attached to the body. The bags and accessories are tailored for the different types of stoma.

COLOSTOMY. In a colostomy, a stoma is formed from a cut end of colon. The output depends on the position along the colon from which the stoma is created; the further down the colon's length from which the colostomy is formed, the greater the volume of fluid that can be reabsorbed. The discharge changes from a liquid or paste-like consistency to a nearly fully formed stool mass. The nature of the discharge determines whether the bag can be drainable or non-drainable.

A *permanent colostomy* is formed by surgical removal of the diseased part of the colon. A *temporary colostomy* may be created to allow a distal part of the colon to recover from trauma (e.g. a gunshot wound, stabbing, or road traffic accident). On healing, the colon is surgically rejoined to permit normal faecal output.

ILEOSTOMY. In an ileostomy, a piece of ileum is brought to the abdominal surface following removal of varying lengths of the colon:
- pan-procto colectomy—removal of all parts of the colon
- total colectomy—removal of all of the colon apart from the rectal stump. Later, it may be possible to create an artificial pouch in the abdominal cavity which rejoins the ileum to the rectal stump, permitting normal discharge of faeces.

UROSTOMY. A urostomy (ileal conduit) is created by the diversion of the two ureters into a piece of colon or, more commonly, ileum. The piece of intestine is brought to the abdominal surface to form a stoma. Normal gastro-intestinal function is resumed after removal of the piece to form the stoma.

Stoma appliances

The only essential prerequisites for stoma management are the collection receptacle (the 'bag') and a means of attaching it to the abdominal wall. However, practical and successful management demands, and the *Drug Tariff* permits, the supply of a range of other components.

STOMA BAGS AND FLANGES. Modern stoma bags are oblong or tapered, rectangular, plastic receptacles. A circular opening is placed over the stoma. Around the opening is a flange that is used to attach the bag to the abdominal wall. A bag may be non-drainable, for use with a descending colostomy with a solid and predictable action; or it may be drainable, having a wide-necked opening with a **bag closure**, for all other types of colostomy and for an ileostomy. A bag for a urostomy has a tap for regular drainage of urine.

A bag may be one- or two-piece, depending on whether the flange is integral with the bag, or separate.

The **flange** may be attached to the abdominal wall by double-sided adhesive rings, or by the separate use of plasters or other adhesives. Skin care is important in stoma management, and a varied range of karaya-based flanges is also available. Non-adhesive flanges are available for stomas that have a solid output only.

As a colostomy stoma is much larger than that formed from ileum, a range of flange sizes is available. However, most flanges have to be cut to size by the patient, for which measuring cards are commonly provided.

A **two-piece bag** is one in which the flange is separate from the bag, and from which the bag can be detached without removing the flange from the skin. The bag is clipped to the flange, and a waist belt can be clipped to the bag. The two-piece bag permits rapid changing should the bag develop a leak.

ACCESSORIES. **Adhesive removers** are available to assist in cleaning the skin after the flange has been removed. Care must be taken to ensure that their use does not cause or aggravate skin soreness.

Bag covers of a wide range of designs and colours are available. They are particularly useful for bags that are made of transparent or semi-transparent material.

Belts are available for use with one- or two-piece bags. Their use may aid the confidence of wearers in the ability of the adhesive to keep the bag attached to the abdomen, and be necessary in wearers with irregularly shaped or distended abdomens.

Deodorants can be placed in the bag to minimise the odour from the discharge.

Filters are integral to many colostomy and ileostomy bags, and are useful for the removal of flatus from the bag. Replacement filters can be incorporated into some designs.

Irrigation/wash-out appliances are available for colostomy patients who evacuate the bowel once every 24 to 48 hours as an alternative to uncontrolled, irregular evacuation through the stoma. A cone-shaped irrigation system is inserted into the stoma, and the distal colon filled with 1–1.5 litres of warm water. Only replacement parts can be prescribed on the NHS; complete systems have to be supplied by a hospital.

Skin fillers and protectives comprise a range of aerosols, barrier creams, gels, lotions, pastes, and wipes. Fillers are used if the abdominal wall is distorted and needs levelling to allow successful attachment of the flange. Protectives are used in cases of skin soreness, but care must be taken to ensure that their use does not compromise the adhesiveness of the flange.

Stoma caps can be clipped to the flange of a two-piece bag for short periods (e.g. during swimming or sports). Their use is practicable only with colostomies that have regular faecal movements.

Tubing that may be prescribed consists of drainage tubing for urostomy bags, for use by immobile patients, or for overnight attachment to night drainage bags.

PRESCRIBING MEDICINES. Prescribing for patients with stoma calls for special care. The following is a brief account of some of the main points to be borne in mind.

Enemas and washouts should **not** be prescribed for patients with ileostomies as they may cause rapid and severe dehydration.

Colostomy patients may suffer from constipation and whenever possible should be treated by increasing fluid intake or dietary fibre. **Bulk-forming drugs** (see p. N13) should be tried. If they are insufficient, as small a dose as possible of senna (see under Stimulant Laxatives, p. N14) should be used.

The doctor's advice should be obtained for other complications such as diarrhoea.

New patients should be given advice about the use of *cleansing agents, protective creams, lotions, deodorants,* or *sealants.*

Stoma appliances and associated products

These are listed in Part IXC of the Drug Tariff (Part 6 of the Scottish Drug Tariff, Part III of the Northern Ireland Drug Tariff).

Urostomy pouches

These are listed in Part IXC of the Drug Tariff (Part 6 of the Scottish Drug Tariff, Part III of the Northern Ireland Drug Tariff).

Appliances and reagents for diabetes

Hypodermic equipment

Corresponds to BNF section 6.1.1.3.

Patients should be advised on the safe disposal of lancets, single-use syringes, and needles. Suitable arrangements for the safe disposal of contaminated waste must be made before these products are prescribed for patients who are carriers of infectious diseases.

Lancets may be used on their own or in an automatic 'finger pricking' device such as *Autolet* [NHS] or *Glucolet* [NHS]. Various devices take different lancets; see BNF section 6.1.1.3 for further details

HYPODERMIC EQUIPMENT

See BNF section 6.1.1.3
The following items in BNF section 6.1.1.3 are not on the Nurse Prescribers' List:

- Items not in the Drug Tariff (described as [NHS] in the BNF)

Monitoring agents

Corresponds to BNF section 6.1.6.

Glucose (for glucose tolerance test) is **not** on the Nurse Prescribers' List.

URINALYSIS

Urine testing for glucose is useful in patients who find blood glucose monitoring difficult. Tests for glucose employ reagent strips specific to glucose; *Clinistix* is suitable for screening purposes only.

Reagents are also available to test for ketones and protein in urine but these are usually used in clinics; patients are rarely required to do these tests for themselves unless they become unwell.

■ Reagents
See BNF section 6.1.6
The following items in BNF section 6.1.6 are not on the Nurse Prescribers' List:

- Items not in the Drug Tariff (described as [NHS] in the BNF)

BLOOD GLUCOSE MONITORING

Blood glucose monitoring gives a direct measure of the glucose concentration at the time of the test and can detect hypoglycaemia as well as hyperglycaemia. Patients should be properly trained in the use of blood glucose monitoring systems and to take appropriate action on the results obtained. Inadequate understanding of the normal fluctuations in blood glucose may lead to confusion and inappropriate action.

Blood glucose monitoring is best carried out by means of a meter. Visual colour comparison is sometimes used but is much less satisfactory. Meters give a more precise reading and are useful for patients with poor eyesight or who are colour blind

Note. In the UK blood glucose concentration is expressed in mmol/litre and Diabetes UK advises that these units should be used for self-monitoring of blood glucose. In other European countries units of mg/100 mL (or mg/dL) are commonly used.
It is advisable to check that the meter is pre-set in the correct units.

■ Reagents

See BNF section 6.1.6

The following items in BNF section 6.1.6 are not on the Nurse Prescribers' List:

- Items not in the Drug Tariff (described as NHS in the BNF)

Eye-drop dispensers

Eye-drop dispensers are available to aid the instillation of eye drops especially amongst the elderly, visually impaired, arthritic, or otherwise physically limited patients. Eye-drop dispensers are for use with plastic eye drop bottles, for repeat use by individual patients. Details of products available may be found in the Drug Tariff section IXA (Part 3 of the Scottish Drug Tariff, Part III of the Northern Ireland Drug Tariff).

Fertility and gynaecological products

Fertility (Ovulation) Thermometer
Mercury in glass thermometer, range 35 to 39°C (graduated in 0.1°C). Net price = £1.83
For monitoring ovulation for the fertility awareness method of contraception

Hodges Pessaries
Pessaries, perspex, 8 mm thick, net price 1 pessary, 60 mm = £4.08, 65 mm = £4.18, 68 mm = £4.27, 73 mm = £4.39, 78 mm = £4.49, 80 mm = £4.60, 82 mm = £4.69, 85 mm = £4.80, 88 mm = £4.91, 90 mm = £5.01, 95 mm = £5.10, 100 mm = £5.23
Antiseptics: phenols or cresols should be avoided because absorption may cause severe irritation; pessaries may be washed in soapy water or boiled

Polythene Ring Pessaries
Pessaries, 7.5 mm thick, 50–80 mm (rising in 3 mm), 85–100 mm (rising in 5 mm), and 110 mm. Net price 1 pessary = £1.78
Antiseptics: phenols or cresols should be avoided because absorption may cause severe irritation; pessaries may be washed in soapy water or boiled

PVC Ring Pessaries
Pessaries, 1.25 cm thick, 50–80 mm (rising in 3 mm), 85–100 mm (rising in 5 mm), and 110 mm. Net price 1 pessary = £1.93
Antiseptics: phenols or cresols should be avoided as these may be absorbed causing irritation in use

Contraceptive devices

Corresponds to BNF section 7.3.4

Intra-uterine devices

The intra-uterine device (IUD) is suitable for older parous women and as a second-line contraceptive in young nulliparous women who should be carefully screened because they have an increased background risk of pelvic inflammatory disease.

The healthcare professional inserting (or removing) the device should be fully trained in the technique and should provide full counselling backed by the manufacturer's approved leaflet.

INTRA-UTERINE CONTRACEPTIVE DEVICES

Indications: contraception, see BNF section 7.3.4
Cautions: anaemia, heavy menses (progestogen intra-uterine system might be preferable, BNF section 7.3.2.3), endometriosis, severe primary dysmenorrhoea, history of pelvic inflammatory disease, history of ectopic pregnancy or tubal surgery, diabetes, fertility problems, nulliparity and young age, severely scarred uterus (including after endometrial resection) or severe cervical stenosis, valvular heart disease (antibacterial cover

needed—BNF section 5.1 table 2); drug- or disease-induced immunosuppression (risk of infection—avoid if marked immunosuppression); epilepsy; increased risk of expulsion if inserted before uterine involution; gynaecological examination before insertion, 6–8 weeks after then annually but counsel women to see doctor promptly in case of significant symptoms, especially pain; anticoagulant therapy (avoid if possible); remove if pregnancy occurs; if pregnancy occurs, increased likelihood that it may be ectopic

Contra-indications: pregnancy, severe anaemia, recent sexually transmitted infection (if not fully investigated and treated), unexplained uterine bleeding, distorted or small uterine cavity, genital malignancy, active trophoblastic disease, pelvic inflammatory disease, established or marked immunosuppression; *copper devices:* copper allergy, Wilson's disease, medical diathermy

Side-effects: uterine or cervical perforation, displacement, expulsion; pelvic infection may be exacerbated, menorrhagia, dysmenorrhoea, allergy; *on insertion*: pain (alleviated by NSAID such as ibuprofen 30 minutes before insertion) and bleeding, occasionally epileptic seizure and vasovagal attack

Prescribe as:

Flexi-T® 300
Intra-uterine device, copper wire, surface area approx. 300 mm² wound on vertical stem of T-shaped plastic carrier, impregnated with barium sulphate for radio-opacity, monofilament thread attached to base of vertical stem; preloaded in inserter, net price = £8.95
For uterine length over 5 cm; replacement every 5 years (see also notes in BNF section 7.3.4)

GyneFix®
Intra-uterine device, 6 copper sleeves with surface area of 330 mm² on polypropylene thread, net price = £25.19
Suitable for all uterine sizes; replacement every 5 years; fitting technique requires additional training

Multiload® Cu375
Intra-uterine device, copper wire, surface area approx. 375 mm² vertical stem length 3.5 cm, net price = £9.24
For uterine length 6–9 cm; replacement every 5 years (see also notes in BNF section 7.3.4)

Nova-T® 380
Intra-uterine device, copper wire with silver core, surface area approx. 380 mm² wound on vertical stem of T-shaped plastic carrier, impregnated with barium sulphate for radio-opacity, threads attached to base of vertical stem, net price = £13.50
For uterine length 6.5–9 cm; replacement every 5 years (see also notes in BNF section 7.3.4)

T-Safe® CU 380 A
Intra-uterine device, copper wire, wound on vertical stem of T-shaped plastic carrier with copper collar on the distal portion of each arm, total surface area approx. 380 mm², impregnated with barium sulphate for radio-opacity, threads attached to base of vertical stem, net price = £9.73
For uterine length 6.5–9 cm; replacement every 8 years (see also notes in BNF section 7.3.4)

Other contraceptive devices

■ Contraceptive caps

Prescribe as:

Soft Silicone cap
Silicone, sizes 22 mm, 26 mm, and 30 mm, net price = £14.75. *Proprietary product*: *FemCap*

Type A contraceptive cap (pessary)
Opaque rubber, sizes 1 to 5 (55–75 mm rising in steps of 5 mm), net price = £6.61. *Proprietary product*: *Dumas Vault Cap*

Type B contraceptive cap (pessary)
Opaque rubber, sizes 22 to 31 mm (rising in steps of 3 mm), net price = £7.81. *Proprietary product*: *Prentif Cavity Rim Cervical Cap*

Type C contraceptive cap (pessary)
Opaque rubber, sizes 1 to 3 (42, 48 and 54 mm), net price = £6.61. *Proprietary product*: *Vimule Cap*

■ Contraceptive diaphragms

Prescribe as:

Reflexions Flat Spring Diaphragm
Transparent rubber with flat metal spring, sizes 55–95 mm (rising in steps of 5 mm), net price = £5.78. *Proprietary product*: *Reflexions*

Type B Diaphragm with coiled metal rim
Opaque rubber with coiled metal rim, sizes 60–100 mm (rising in steps of 5 mm), net price = £6.35. *Proprietary product*: *Ortho*

Type C Arcing Spring Diaphragm
Opaque rubber with arcing spring, sizes 60–95 mm (rising in steps of 5 mm), net price = £7.23. *Proprietary product*: *All-Flex*

Spermicidal contraceptives

Corresponds to BNF section 7.3.3

Spermicidal contraceptives are useful additional safeguards but do **not** give adequate protection if used alone except where fertility is already significantly diminished; they are suitable for use with barrier methods. They have two components: a spermicide and a vehicle which itself may have some inhibiting effect on sperm activity.

CSM advice. Products such as petroleum jelly (*Vaseline®*), baby oil and oil-based vaginal and rectal preparations are likely to damage condoms and contraceptive diaphragms made from latex rubber, and may render them less effective as a barrier method of contraception and as a protection from sexually transmitted diseases (including HIV).

Condoms: no evidence of harm to latex condoms and diaphragms with the products listed below:

Gynol II® (Janssen-Cilag)
Jelly, nonoxinol '9' 2% in a water-soluble basis. Net price 81 g = £2.61; applicator = 75p
Excipients: include hydroxybenzoates (parabens), propylene glycol, ascorbic acid

Ortho-Creme® (Janssen-Cilag)
Cream, nonoxinol '9' 2% in a water-miscible basis. Net price 70 g = £2.44; applicator = 75p
Excipients: include cetyl alcohol, hydroxybenzoates (parabens), propylene glycol, sorbic acid, fragrance

Orthoforms® (Janssen-Cilag)
Pessaries, nonoxinol '9' 5% in a water-soluble basis. Net price 15 pessaries = £2.40

NPF Index

Guidance on prescribing

General guidance

Medicines should be prescribed only when they are necessary, and in all cases the benefit of administering the medicine should be considered in relation to the risk involved. This is particularly important during pregnancy where the risk to both mother and fetus must be considered (for further details see Prescribing in Pregnancy, Appendix 4).

It is important to discuss treatment options carefully with the patient to ensure that the patient is content to take the medicine as prescribed (see also Taking Medicines to Best Effect, below). In particular, the patient should be helped to distinguish the side-effects of prescribed drugs from the effects of the medical disorder. Where the beneficial effects of the medicine are likely to be delayed, the patient should be advised of this.

TAKING MEDICINES TO BEST EFFECT. Difficulties in compliance with drug treatment occur regardless of age. Factors contributing to poor compliance with prescribed medicines include:

- Prescription not collected or not dispensed
- Purpose of medicine not clear
- Perceived lack of efficacy
- Real or perceived side-effects
- Patients' perception of the risk and severity of side-effects may differ from that of the prescriber
- Instructions for administration not clear
- Physical difficulty in taking medicines (e.g. with swallowing the medicine, with handling small tablets, or with opening medicine containers)
- Unattractive formulation (e.g. unpleasant taste)
- Complicated regimen

The prescriber and the patient should agree on the health outcomes that the patient desires and on the strategy for achieving them ('concordance'). The prescriber should be sensitive to religious, cultural, and personal beliefs that can affect patients' acceptance of medicines. Further information on concordance is available on the Internet (www.medicines-partnership.org).

Taking the time to explain to the patient (and relatives) the rationale and the potential adverse effects of treatment may improve compliance. Reinforcement and elaboration of the physician's instructions by the pharmacist also helps. Advising the patient of the possibility of alternative treatments may encourage the patient to seek advice rather than merely abandon unacceptable treatment.

Simplifying the drug regimen may help; the need for frequent administration may reduce compliance although there appears to be little difference in compliance between once-daily and twice-daily administration. Combination products reduce the number of drugs taken but this may be at the expense of the ability to titrate individual doses.

COMPLEMENTARY MEDICINE. An increasing amount of information on complementary ('alternative') medicine is becoming available. However, the BNF's scope is restricted to the discussion of conventional medicines but reference is made to complementary treatments if they affect conventional therapy (e.g. interactions with St John's wort—see Appendix 1). Further information on herbal medicines is available at www.mhra.gov.uk

ABBREVIATION OF TITLES. In general, titles of drugs and preparations should be written *in full*. Unofficial abbreviations should not be used as they may be misinterpreted; obsolete titles, such as Mist. Expect. should not be used.

NON-PROPRIETARY TITLES. Where non-proprietary ('generic') titles are given, they should be used in prescribing. This will enable any suitable product to be dispensed, thereby saving delay to the patient and sometimes expense to the health service. The only exception is where bioavailability problems are so important that the patient should always receive the same brand; in such cases, the brand name or the manufacturer should be stated. Non-proprietary titles should **not** be invented for the purposes of prescribing generically since this can lead to confusion, particularly in the case of compound and modified-release preparations.

Titles used as headings for monographs may be used freely in the United Kingdom but in other countries may be subject to restriction.

Many of the non-proprietary titles used in this book are titles of monographs in the European Pharmacopoeia, British Pharmacopoeia or British Pharmaceutical Codex 1973. In such cases the preparations must comply with the standard (if any) in the appropriate publication, as required by the Medicines Act (Section 65).

PROPRIETARY TITLES. Names followed by the symbol® are or have been used as proprietary names in the United Kingdom. These names may in general be applied only to products supplied by the owners of the trade marks.

MARKETING AUTHORISATION AND BNF ADVICE. In general the *doses, indications, cautions, contra-indications and side-effects* in the BNF reflect those in the manufacturers' data sheets or Summaries of Product Characteristics (SPCs) which, in turn, reflect those in the corresponding Marketing Authorisations (formerly known as Product Licences). Where an unlicensed drug is included in the BNF, this is indicated in brackets after the entry. Where the BNF suggests a use (or route) that is outside the licensed indication of a product ('off-label' use), this too is indicated. Unlicensed use of medicines becomes necessary if the clinical need cannot be met by licensed medicines; such use should be supported by appropriate evidence and experience. When a preparation is available from more than one manufacturer, the BNF reflects advice that is the most clinically relevant regardless of any variation in the marketing authorisations.

The doses stated in the BNF are intended for general guidance and represent, unless otherwise stated, the usual range of doses that are generally regarded as being suitable for adults.

Prescribing medicines outside the recommendations of their Marketing Authorisation alters (and probably increases) the doctor's professional responsibility.

ORAL SYRINGES. An **oral syringe** is supplied when oral liquid medicines are prescribed in doses other than multiples of 5 mL. The oral syringe is marked in 0.5-mL divisions from 1 to 5 mL to measure doses of less than 5 mL. It is provided with an adaptor and an instruction leaflet. The *5-mL spoon* is used for doses of 5 mL (or multiples thereof).

STRENGTHS AND QUANTITIES. The strength or quantity to be contained in capsules, lozenges, tablets, etc. should be stated by the prescriber.

If a pharmacist receives an incomplete prescription for a systemically administered preparation[1] and considers it would not be appropriate for the patient to return to the doctor, the following procedures will apply:

(a) an attempt must always be made to contact the prescriber to ascertain the intention;
(b) if the attempt is successful the pharmacist must, where practicable, subsequently arrange for details of quantity, strength where applicable, and dosage to be inserted by the prescriber on the incomplete form;
(c) where, although the prescriber has been contacted, it has not proved possible to obtain the written intention regarding an incomplete prescription, the pharmacist may endorse the form 'p.c.' (prescriber contacted) and add details of the quantity and strength where applicable of the preparation supplied, and of the dose indicated. The endorsement should be initialled and dated by the pharmacist;
(d) where the prescriber cannot be contacted and the pharmacist has sufficient information to make a professional judgment the preparation may be dispensed. If the quantity is missing the pharmacist may supply sufficient to complete up to 5 days' treatment; except that where a combination pack (i.e. a proprietary pack containing more than one medicinal product) or oral contraceptive is prescribed by name only, the smallest pack shall be dispensed. In all cases the prescription must be endorsed 'p.n.c.' (prescriber not contacted), the quantity, the dose, and the strength (where applicable) of the preparation supplied must be indicated, and the endorsement must be initialled and dated;
(e) if the pharmacist has any doubt about exercising discretion, an incomplete prescription must be referred back to the prescriber.

EXCIPIENTS. Oral liquid preparations that do not contain *fructose, glucose* or *sucrose* are described as 'sugar-free' in the BNF. Preparations containing hydrogenated glucose syrup, mannitol, maltitol, sorbitol or xylitol are also marked 'sugar-free' since there is evidence that they do not cause dental caries. Patients receiving medicines containing cariogenic sugars should be advised of appropriate dental hygiene measures to prevent caries. Sugar-free preparations should be used whenever possible.

Where information on the presence of *aspartame, gluten, tartrazine, arachis (peanut) oil* or *sesame oil* is available, this is indicated in the BNF against the relevant preparation.

Information is provided on *selected excipients* in skin preparations (see section 13.1.3), vaccines (see section 14.1), and on *selected preservatives* and *excipients* in eye drops and injections. Pressurised metered aerosols containing *chlorofluorocarbons* (CFCs) have also been identified throughout the BNF (see section 3.1.1.1).

The presence of *benzyl alcohol* and *polyoxyl castor oil* (polyethoxylated castor oil) in injections is indicated in the BNF. Benzyl alcohol has been associated with a fatal toxic syndrome in preterm neonates, and therefore, parenteral preparations containing the preservative should not be used in neonates. Polyoxyl castor oils, used as vehicles in intravenous injections, have been associated with severe anaphylactoid reactions.

The presence of *propylene glycol* in oral or parenteral medicines is indicated in the BNF; it can cause adverse effects if its elimination is impaired, e.g. in renal failure, in neonates and young children, and in slow metabolisers of the substance. It may interact with disulfiram and metronidazole.

In the absence of information on excipients in the BNF and in the product literature, contact the manufacturer (see Index of Manufacturers) if it is essential to check details.

EXTEMPORANEOUS PREPARATION. A product should be dispensed extemporaneously only when no product with a marketing authorisation is available.

The BP direction that a preparation must be *freshly prepared* indicates that it must be made not more than 24 hours before it is issued for use. The direction that a preparation should be *recently prepared* indicates that deterioration is likely if the preparation is stored for longer than about 4 weeks at 15–25° C.

The term **water** used without qualification means either potable water freshly drawn direct from the public supply and suitable for drinking or freshly boiled and cooled purified water. The latter should be used if the public supply is from a local storage tank or if the potable water is unsuitable for a particular preparation (Water for injections, section 9.2.2).

DRUGS AND DRIVING. Prescribers should advise patients if treatment is likely to affect their ability to drive motor vehicles. This applies especially to drugs with sedative effects; patients should be warned that these effects are increased by alcohol. General information about a patient's fitness to drive is available from the Driver and Vehicle Licensing Agency at www.dvla.gov.uk (see also Appendix 9).

PATENTS. In the BNF, certain drugs have been included notwithstanding the existence of actual or potential patent rights. In so far as such substances are protected by Letters Patent, their inclusion in this

1. With the exception of temazepam, an incomplete prescription is **not** acceptable for controlled drugs in schedules 2 and 3 of the Misuse of Drugs Regulations 2001

Formulary neither conveys, nor implies, licence to manufacture.

HEALTH AND SAFETY. When handling chemical or biological materials particular attention should be given to the possibility of allergy, fire, explosion, radiation, or poisoning. Substances, including corticosteroids, some antimicrobials, phenothiazines, and many cytotoxics, are irritant or very potent and should be handled with caution. Contact with the skin and inhalation of dust should be avoided.

SAFETY IN THE HOME. Patients must be warned to keep all medicines out of the reach of children. All solid dose and all oral and external liquid preparations must be dispensed in a reclosable *child-resistant container* unless:

- the medicine is in an original pack or patient pack such as to make this inadvisable;
- the patient will have difficulty in opening a child-resistant container;
- a specific request is made that the product shall not be dispensed in a child-resistant container;
- no suitable child-resistant container exists for a particular liquid preparation.

All patients should be advised to dispose of *unwanted medicines* by returning them to a supplier for destruction.

NAME OF MEDICINE. The name of the medicine should appear on the label unless the prescriber indicates otherwise.

(a) The strength is also stated on the label in the case of tablets, capsules, and similar preparations that are available in different strengths.
(b) If it is the wish of the prescriber that a description such as 'The Sedative Tablets' should appear on the label, the prescriber should write the desired description on the prescription form.
(c) The arrangement will extend to approved names, proprietary names or titles given in the BP, BPC, BNF, DPF, or NPF. The arrangement does not apply when a prescription is written so that several ingredients are given.
(d) The name written on the label is that used by the prescriber on the prescription.
(e) When a prescription is written other than on an NHS prescription form the name of the prescribed preparation will be stated on the label of the dispensed medicine unless the prescriber indicates otherwise.
(f) The Council of the Royal Pharmaceutical Society advises that the labels of dispensed medicines should indicate the total quantity of the product dispensed in the container to which the label refers. This requirement applies equally to solid, liquid, internal, and external preparations. If a product is dispensed in more than one container, the reference should be to the amount in each container.

> Non-proprietary names of **compound preparations** which appear in the BNF are those that have been compiled by the British Pharmacopoeia Commission or another recognised body; whenever possible they reflect the names of the active ingredients.
> Prescribers should avoid creating their own compound names for the purposes of generic prescribing; such names do not have an approved definition and can be misinterpreted.
> Special care should be taken to avoid errors when prescribing compound preparations; in particular the hyphen in the prefix 'co-' should be retained.
> Special care should also be taken to avoid creating generic names for **modified-release** preparations where the use of these names could lead to confusion between formulations with different lengths of action.

SECURITY AND VALIDITY OF PRESCRIPTIONS. The Councils of the British Medical Association and the Royal Pharmaceutical Society have issued a joint statement on the security and validity of prescriptions.

In particular, prescription forms should:

- not be left unattended at reception desks;
- not be left in a car where they may be visible; and
- when not in use, be kept in a locked drawer within the surgery and at home.

Where there is any doubt about the authenticity of a prescription, the pharmacist should contact the prescriber. If this is done by telephone, the number should be obtained from the directory rather than relying on the information on the prescription form, which may be false.

PATIENT GROUP DIRECTION (PGD). In most cases, the most appropriate clinical care will be provided on an individual basis by a prescriber to a specific individual patient. However, a Patient Group Direction for supply and administration of medicines by other healthcare professionals can be used where it would benefit patient care without compromising safety.

A Patient Group Direction is a written direction relating to supply and administration (or administration only) of a prescription-only medicine by certain classes of healthcare professionals; the Direction is signed by a doctor (or dentist), and by a pharmacist. Further information on Patient Group Directions is available in Health Service Circular HSC 2000/026 (England), HDL (2001) 7 (Scotland), and WHC (2000) 116 (Wales).

Prescription writing

Shared care. In its guidelines on responsibility for prescribing (circular EL (91) 127) between hospitals and general practitioners, the Department of Health has advised that legal responsibility for prescribing lies with the doctor who signs the prescription.

Prescriptions[1] should be written legibly in ink or otherwise so as to be indelible[2], should be dated, should state the full name and address of the patient, and should be signed in ink by the prescriber[3]. The age and the date of birth of the patient should preferably be stated, and it is a legal requirement in the case of prescription-only medicines to state the age for children under 12 years.

The following should be noted:

(a) The unnecessary use of decimal points should be avoided, e.g. 3 mg, not 3.0 mg.
Quantities of 1 gram or more should be written as 1 g etc.
Quantities less than 1 gram should be written in milligrams, e.g. 500 mg, not 0.5 g.
Quantities less than 1 mg should be written in micrograms, e.g. 100 micrograms, not 0.1 mg.
When decimals are unavoidable a zero should be written in front of the decimal point where there is no other figure, e.g. 0.5 mL, not .5 mL.
Use of the decimal point is acceptable to express a range, e.g. 0.5 to 1 g.

(b) 'Micrograms' and 'nanograms' should **not** be abbreviated. Similarly 'units' should **not** be abbreviated.

(c) The term 'millilitre' (ml or mL)[4] is used in medicine and pharmacy, and cubic centimetre, c.c., or cm^3 should not be used.

Pharmacy Stamp | Age: 1yr 3mths | Title, Forename, Surname & Address: Master Peter Patient
D.o.B 2/4/2004 | Flat 1, 50 Stanhope Street, Newtown TE22 1ST
Please don't stamp over age box
Number of days' treatment N.B. Ensure dose is stated: 5
Endorsements
Amoxicillin oral suspension
125mg/5ml sugar-free
125mg three times daily
Supply 100ml
[No more items on this prescription]

SAMPLE

Signature of Prescriber | Date 02/07/05

For dispenser No. of Prescns. on form
Anyborough Health Authority
Dr D O Good 345543
7 High Street
Anytown KB1 CD2
Tel: 0111 222 333

NHS FP10NC0105

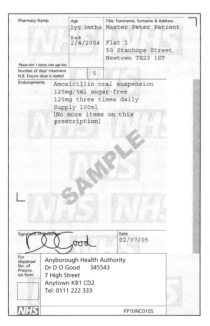

(d) Dose and dose frequency should be stated; in the case of preparations to be taken 'as required' a **minimum dose interval** should be specified.
When doses other than multiples of 5 mL are prescribed for *oral liquid preparations* the dose-volume will be provided by means of an **oral syringe**, see p. 2 (except for preparations intended to be measured with a pipette).
Suitable quantities:
Elixirs, Linctuses, and Paediatric Mixtures (5-mL dose), 50, 100, or 150 mL
Adult Mixtures (10-mL dose), 200 or 300 mL
Ear Drops, Eye drops, and Nasal Drops, 10 mL (or the manufacturer's pack)
Eye Lotions, Gargles, and Mouthwashes, 200 mL

(e) For suitable quantities of dermatological preparations, see section 13.1.2.

(f) The names of drugs and preparations should be written clearly and **not** abbreviated, using approved titles **only** (see also advice in box on p. 3 to **avoid** creating generic titles for modified-release preparations).

(g) The quantity to be supplied may be stated by indicating the number of days of treatment required in the box provided on NHS forms. In most cases the exact amount will be supplied. This does not apply to items directed to be used as required—if the dose and frequency are not given the quantity to be supplied needs to be stated.
When several items are ordered on one form the box can be marked with the number of days of treatment provided the quantity is added for any item for which the amount cannot be calculated.

(h) Although directions should preferably be in **English without abbreviation**, it is recognised that some Latin abbreviations are used (for details see Inside Back Cover).

(i) Medical and dental practitioners may prescribe unlicensed medicines (i.e. those without marketing authorisation) or withdrawn medicines. The prescriber should inform the patient or the patient's carer that the product does not have a marketing authorisation.

PRESCRIBING BY DENTAL SURGEONS. Until new prescribing arrangements are in place for NHS prescriptions dental surgeons should use form FP10D (GP14 in Scotland, WP10D in Wales) to prescribe only those items listed in the Dental Practitioners' Formulary. The Act and Regulations do not set any limitations upon the number and variety of substances which the dental surgeon may administer to patients in the surgery or may order by

1. The above recommendations are acceptable for **prescription-only medicines** (PoM). For items marked CD see also Controlled Drugs and Drug Dependence p. 7.

2. It is permissible to issue carbon copies of NHS prescriptions as long as they are signed in ink.

3. Computer-generated facsimile signatures do not meet the legal requirement.

4. The use of capital 'L' in mL is a printing convention throughout the BNF; both 'mL' and 'ml' are recognised SI abbreviations.

private prescription—provided the relevant legal requirements are observed the dental surgeon may use or order whatever is required for the clinical situation. There is no statutory requirement for the dental surgeon to communicate with a patient's medical practitioner when prescribing for dental use. There are, however, occasions when this would be in the patient's interest and such communication is to be encouraged.

Computer-issued prescriptions

For computer-issued prescriptions the following recommendations of the Joint GP Information Technology Committee should also be noted:

1. The computer must print out the date,[1] the patient's surname, one forename, other initials, and address, and may also print out the patient's title and date of birth. The age of children under 12 years and of adults over 60 years must be printed in the box available; the age of children under 5 years should be printed in years and months. A facility may also exist to print out the age of patients between 12 and 60 years.
2. The doctor's name must be printed at the bottom of the prescription form; this will be the name of the doctor responsible for the prescription (who will normally sign it). The doctor's surgery address, reference number, and Primary Care Trust (PCT[2]) are also necessary. In addition, the surgery telephone number should be printed.
3. When prescriptions are to be signed by general practitioner registrars, assistants, locums, or deputising doctors, the name of the doctor printed at the bottom of the form must still be that of the responsible principal.
4. Names of medicines must come from a dictionary held in the computer memory, to provide a check on the spelling and to ensure that the name is written in full. The computer can be programmed to recognise both the non-proprietary and the proprietary name of a particular drug and to print out the preferred choice, but must not print out both names. For medicines not in the dictionary, separate checks are required—the user must be warned that no check was possible and the entire prescription must be entered in the lexicon.
5. The dictionary may contain information on the usual doses, formulations, and pack sizes to produce standard predetermined prescriptions for common preparations, and to provide a check on the validity of an individual prescription on entry.
6. The prescription must be printed in English without abbreviation; information may be entered or stored in abbreviated form. The dose must be in numbers, the frequency in words, and the quantity in numbers in brackets, thus: 40 mg four times daily (112). It must also be possible to prescribe by indicating the length of treatment required, see (h) above.
7. The BNF recommendations should be followed as in (a), (b), (c), (d), and (e) above.
8. Checks may be incorporated to ensure that all the information required for dispensing a particular drug has been filled in. For instructions such as 'as directed' and 'when required', the maximum daily dose should normally be specified.
9. Numbers and codes used in the system for organising and retrieving data must never appear on the form.
10. Supplementary warnings or advice should be written in full, should not interfere with the clarity of the prescription itself, and should be in line with any warnings or advice in the BNF; numerical codes should not be used.
11. A mechanism (such as printing a series of non-specific characters) should be incorporated to cancel out unused space, or wording such as 'no more items on this prescription' may be added after the last item. Otherwise the doctor should delete the space manually.
12. To avoid forgery the computer may print on the form the number of items to be dispensed (somewhere separate from the box for the pharmacist). The number of items per form need be limited only by the ability of the printer to produce clear and well-demarcated instructions with sufficient space for each item and a spacer line before each fresh item.
13. Handwritten alterations should only be made in exceptional circumstances—it is preferable to print out a new prescription. Any alterations must be made in the doctor's own handwriting and countersigned; computer records should be updated to fully reflect any alteration. Prescriptions for drugs used for contraceptive purposes (but which are not promoted as contraceptives) may need to be marked in handwriting with the symbol ♀ (or endorsed in another way to indicate that the item is prescribed for contraceptive purposes).
14. Prescriptions for controlled drugs must not be printed from the computer. Blank forms may be computer-printed with the doctor's name, surgery address and telephone number, reference number and Primary Care Trust (PCT[2]); the remaining details must be handwritten.[3]
15. The strip of paper on the side of the FP10SS[4] may be used for various purposes but care should be taken to avoid including confidential information. It may be advisable for the patient's name to appear at the top, but this should be preceded by 'confidential'.
16. In rural dispensing practices prescription requests (or details of medicines dispensed) will normally be entered in one surgery. The prescriptions (or dispensed medicines) may then need to be delivered to another surgery or location; if possible the computer should hold up to 10 alternatives.
17. Prescription forms that are reprinted or issued as a duplicate should be labelled clearly as such.

1. The exemption for own handwriting regulations for phenobarbital does not apply to the date; a computer-generated date need not be deleted but the date must also be added by the prescriber.

2. Health Board in Scotland, Local Health Board in Wales.

3. Except in the case of phenobarbital (but see also footnote 1) or where the prescriber has been exempted from handwriting requirements, for details see Controlled Drugs and Drug Dependence p. 7

4. GP10(COMP) and GP10SS in Scotland, WP10SS in Wales

Emergency supply of medicines

For details of emergency supply at the request of a doctor, see *Medicines, Ethics and Practice*, No. 29, London, Pharmaceutical Press, 2005 (and subsequent editions).

Pharmacists are sometimes called upon by members of the public to make an emergency supply of medicines. The Medicines (Products Other Than Veterinary Drugs) (Prescription Only) Order 1983, as amended, allows exemptions from the Prescription Only requirements for emergency supply to be made by a person lawfully conducting a retail pharmacy business provided:

(a) that the pharmacist has interviewed the person requesting the prescription-only medicine and is satisfied:
  (i) that there is immediate need for the prescription-only medicine and that it is impracticable in the circumstances to obtain a prescription without undue delay;
  (ii) that treatment with the prescription-only medicine has on a previous occasion been prescribed by a doctor,[1] a supplementary prescriber, a district nurse or health visitor prescriber or an extended formulary nurse prescriber for the person requesting it;
  (iii) as to the dose which it would be appropriate for the person to take;
(b) that no greater quantity shall be supplied than will provide 5 days' treatment except when the prescription-only medicine is:
  (i) insulin, an ointment or cream, or a preparation for the relief of asthma in an aerosol dispenser when the smallest pack can be supplied;
  (ii) an oral contraceptive when a full cycle may be supplied;
  (iii) an antibiotic in liquid form for oral administration when the smallest quantity that will provide a full course of treatment can be supplied;
(c) that an entry shall be made in the prescription book stating:
  (i) the date of supply;
  (ii) the name, quantity and, where appropriate, the pharmaceutical form and strength;
  (iii) the name and address of the patient;
  (iv) the nature of the emergency;
(d) that the container or package must be labelled to show:
  (i) the date of supply;
  (ii) the name, quantity and, where appropriate, the pharmaceutical form and strength;
  (iii) the name of the patient;
  (iv) the name and address of the pharmacy;
  (v) the words 'Emergency supply';
  (vi) the words 'Keep out of the reach of children' (or similar warning).
(e) that the prescription-only medicine is not a substance specifically excluded from the emergency supply provision, and does not contain a Controlled Drug specified in schedules 1, 2, or 3 to the Misuse of Drugs Regulations 2001 except for phenobarbital or phenobarbital sodium for the treatment of epilepsy: for details see *Medicines, Ethics and Practice*, No. 29, London, Pharmaceutical Press, 2005 (and subsequent editions as available).

Royal Pharmaceutical Society's Guidelines

1. The pharmacist should consider the medical consequences of *not* supplying a medicine in an emergency.
2. If the pharmacist is unable to make an emergency supply of a medicine the pharmacist should advise the patient how to obtain essential medical care.

For conditions that apply to supplies made at the request of a patient see *Medicines, Ethics and Practice*, No. 29, London Pharmaceutical Press, 2005 (and subsequent editions).

1. The doctor must be a UK-registered doctor.

Controlled drugs and drug dependence

PRESCRIPTIONS. Preparations which are subject to the prescription requirements of the Misuse of Drugs Regulations 2001, i.e. preparations specified in schedules 2 and 3, are distinguished throughout the BNF by the symbol CD (Controlled Drugs). The principal legal requirements relating to medical prescriptions are listed below.

Prescriptions for Controlled Drugs, which are subject to prescription requirements, must be in ink or otherwise indelible and must be *signed* and *dated*[1] by the prescriber and specify the prescriber's *address*. The prescription must always state *in the prescriber's own handwriting*:[2]

- The name and address of the patient;
- In the case of a preparation, the form[3] and where appropriate the strength[4] of the preparation;
- The total quantity of the preparation, or the number of dose units, *in both words and figures;*[5]
- The dose;[6]
- The words 'for dental treatment only' if issued by a dentist.

A prescription may order a Controlled Drug to be dispensed by instalments; the amount of the instalments and the intervals to be observed must be specified.[7] Prescriptions ordering 'repeats' on the same form are **not** permitted. A prescription is valid for 13 weeks from the date stated thereon.

It is an offence for a prescriber to issue an incomplete prescription and a pharmacist is **not** allowed to dispense a Controlled Drug unless all the information required by law is given on the prescription. Failure to comply with the regulations concerning the writing of prescriptions will result in inconvenience to patients and delay in supplying the necessary medicine.

DEPENDENCE AND MISUSE. The most serious drugs of addiction are **cocaine**, **diamorphine** (heroin), **morphine**, and the **synthetic opioids**. For arrangements for prescribing of diamorphine, dipipanone or cocaine for addicts, see p. 9.

Despite marked reduction in the prescribing of **amphetamines** there is concern that abuse of illicit amfetamine and related compounds is widespread.

Temazepam is subject to the requirement for safe custody of controlled drugs because of problems with abuse, but it is exempt from the prescription and handwriting requirements for controlled drugs. A prescription for temazepam is valid for 13 weeks from the date stated thereon.

The principal **barbiturates** are now Controlled Drugs, but phenobarbital (phenobarbitone) and phenobarbital sodium (phenobarbitone sodium) or a preparation containing either of these are exempt from the handwriting requirement but must fulfil all other controlled drug prescription requirements (**important:** the own handwriting exemption does **not** apply to the date; a computer-generated date need not be deleted but the date must also be added by the prescriber). Moreover, for the treatment of epilepsy phenobarbital and phenobarbital sodium are available under the emergency supply regulations (p. 6).

Cannabis (Indian hemp) has no approved medicinal use and cannot be prescribed by doctors. Its use is illegal but has become widespread. Cannabis is a mild hallucinogen seldom accompanied by a desire to increase the dose; withdrawal symptoms are unusual. **Lysergide** (lysergic acid diethylamide, LSD) is a much more potent hallucinogen; its use

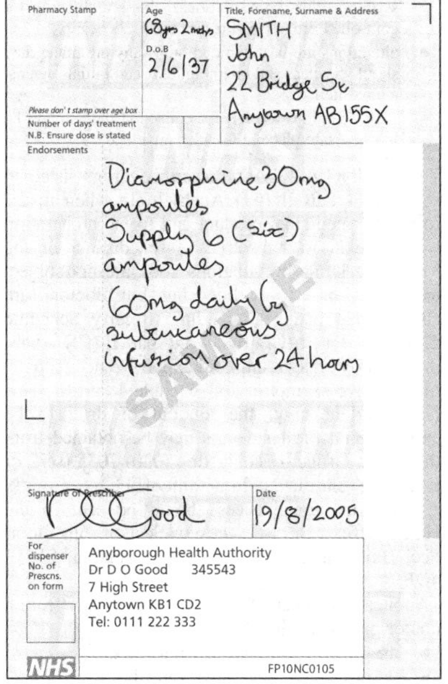

Pharmacy Stamp | Age: 68yrs 2mths | D.O.B: 2/6/37 | Title, Forename, Surname & Address: SMITH John 22 Bridge St Anytown AB155X

Please don't stamp over age box

Number of days' treatment
N.B. Ensure dose is stated

Endorsements

Diamorphine 30mg ampoules
Supply 6 (six) ampoules
60mg daily by subcutaneous infusion over 24 hours

SAMPLE

Signature of Prescriber: D O Good | Date: 19/8/2005

For dispenser
No. of Prescns. on form

Anyborough Health Authority
Dr D O Good 345543
7 High Street
Anytown KB1 CD2
Tel: 0111 222 333

NHS FP10NC0105

1. A computer-generated date is **not** acceptable; however, the prescriber may use a date stamp.

2. Does not apply to prescriptions for temazepam. Otherwise applies unless the prescriber has been specifically exempted from this requirement or unless the prescription contains no controlled drug other than phenobarbital or phenobarbital sodium or a preparation containing either of these; the exemption does **not** apply to the date—a computer-generated date need not be deleted but the date must also be added by the prescriber.

3. The dosage form (e.g. tablets) must be included on a Controlled Drugs prescription irrespective of whether it is implicit in the proprietary name (e.g. *MST Continus*) or of whether only one form is available.

4. When more than one strength of a preparation exists the strength required must be specified.

5. Does not apply to prescriptions for temazepam.

6. The instruction 'one as directed' constitutes a dose but 'as directed' does not.

7. A total of 14 days' treatment by instalment of any drug listed in Schedule 2 of the Misuse of Drugs Regulations and buprenorphine may be prescribed in England. In *England*, form FP10MDA-SS (blue) or occasionally form FP10MDA (blue) should be used; in hospital, form FP10HP(AD) is being replaced by form FP10MDA-SS. In *Scotland* forms HBP(A) (hospital-based prescribers) or GP10 (general practitioners) should be used. In *Wales* a total of 14 days treatment by instalment of any drug listed in Schedules 2–5 of the Misuse of Drugs Regulations may be prescribed. In Wales form WP10(MDA) or form WP10HP(AD) for hospital prescribers should be used when available; in the meantime existing stocks of FP10(MDA) for general practice prescribers, or FP10HP(AD) for hospital prescribers should continue to be used.

can lead to severe psychotic states in which life may be at risk.

PRESCRIBING DRUGS LIKELY TO CAUSE DEPENDENCE OR MISUSE. The prescriber has three main responsibilities:

- To avoid creating dependence by introducing drugs to patients without sufficient reason. In this context, the proper use of the morphine-like drugs is well understood. The dangers of other controlled drugs are less clear because recognition of dependence is not easy and its effects, and those of withdrawal, are less obvious.
- To see that the patient does not gradually increase the dose of a drug, given for good medical reasons, to the point where dependence becomes more likely. This tendency is seen especially with hypnotics and anxiolytics (for CSM advice see section 4.1). The prescriber should keep a close eye on the amount prescribed to prevent patients from accumulating stocks. A minimal amount should be prescribed in the first instance, or when seeing a new patient for the first time.
- To avoid being used as an unwitting source of supply for addicts. Methods include visiting more than one doctor, fabricating stories, and forging prescriptions.

Patients under temporary care should be given only small supplies of drugs unless they present an unequivocal letter from their own doctors. Doctors should also remember that their own patients may be doing a collecting round with other doctors, especially in hospitals. It is sensible to decrease dosages steadily or to issue weekly or even daily prescriptions for small amounts if it is apparent that dependence is occurring.

The stealing and misuse of prescription forms could be minimised by the following precautions:

- do not leave unattended if called away from the consulting room or at reception desks; do not leave in a car where they may be visible; when not in use, keep in a locked drawer within the surgery and at home;
- draw a diagonal line across the blank part of the form under the prescription;
- write the quantity in words and figures when prescribing drugs prone to abuse; this is obligatory for controlled drugs (see Prescriptions, above);
- alterations are best avoided but if any are made they should be clear and unambiguous; add initials against altered items;
- if prescriptions are left for collection they should be left in a safe place in a sealed envelope.

TRAVELLING ABROAD. Prescribed drugs listed in schedule 4 Part II (CD Anab) [only when in the form of a medicinal product and for administration by a person to himself] and schedule 5 of the Misuse of Drugs Regulations 2001 are not subject to import or export licensing but doctors are advised that patients intending to carry Schedule 2, 3 and 4 Part I (CD Benz) and part II (CD Anab) drugs abroad may require an export licence (subject to the above exemption for schedule 4 Part II). This is dependent upon the amount of drug to be exported and further details may be obtained from the Home Office by contacting (020) 7035 0472 or licensing_enquiry.aadu@homeoffice.gsi.gov.uk. Applications for licences should be sent to the Home Office, Drugs Licensing Section, 6th Floor, Peel Building, 2 Marsham Street, London, SW1P 4DF.

Applications must be supported by a letter from a doctor giving details of:

- the patient's name and current address;
- the quantities of drugs to be carried;
- the strength and form in which the drugs will be dispensed;
- the dates of travel to and from the United Kingdom.

Ten days should be allowed for processing the application.

Individual doctors who wish to take Controlled Drugs abroad while accompanying patients may similarly be issued with licences. Licences are not normally issued to doctors who wish to take Controlled Drugs abroad solely in case a family emergency should arise.

These import/export licences for named individuals do not have any legal status outside the UK and are only issued to comply with the Misuse of Drugs Act and facilitate passage through UK Customs and Excise control. For clearance in the country to be visited it would be necessary to approach that country's consulate in the UK.

Misuse of Drugs Act

The Misuse of Drugs Act, 1971 prohibits certain activities in relation to 'Controlled Drugs', in particular their manufacture, supply, and possession. The penalties applicable to offences involving the different drugs are graded broadly according to the *harmfulness attributable to a drug when it is misused* and for this purpose the drugs are defined in the following three classes:

Class A includes: alfentanil, cocaine, diamorphine (heroin), dipipanone, lysergide (LSD), methadone, methylenedioxymethamfetamine (MDMA, 'ecstasy'), morphine, opium, pethidine, phencyclidine, remifentanil, and class B substances when prepared for injection

Class B includes: oral amphetamines, barbiturates, codeine, ethylmorphine, glutethimide, pentazocine, phenmetrazine, and pholcodine

Class C includes: certain drugs related to the amphetamines such as benzfetamine and chlorphentermine, buprenorphine, cannabis, cannabis resin, diethylpropion, mazindol, meprobamate, pemoline, pipradrol, most benzodiazepines, zolpidem, androgenic and anabolic steroids, clenbuterol, chorionic gonadotrophin (HCG), non-human chorionic gonadotrophin, somatotropin, somatrem, and somatropin

The Misuse of Drugs Regulations 2001 define the classes of person who are authorised to supply and possess controlled drugs while acting in their professional capacities and lay down the conditions under which these activities may be carried out. In the regulations drugs are divided into five schedules each specifying the requirements governing such activities as import, export, production, supply, possession, prescribing, and record keeping which apply to them.

Schedule 1 includes drugs such as cannabis and lysergide which are not used medicinally. Possession and supply are prohibited except in accordance with Home Office authority.

Schedule 2 includes drugs such as diamorphine (heroin), morphine, remifentanil, pethidine, secobarbital, glutethimide, amfetamine, and cocaine and are subject to the full controlled drug requirements relating to prescriptions, safe custody (except for secobarbital), the need to keep registers, etc. (unless exempted in schedule 5).

Schedule 3 includes the barbiturates (except secobarbital, now schedule 2), buprenorphine, diethylpropion, mazindol, meprobamate, pentazocine, phentermine, and temazepam. They are subject to the special prescription requirements (except for phenobarbital and temazepam, see p. 7) but not to the safe custody requirements (except for buprenorphine, diethylpropion, and temazepam) nor to the need to keep registers (although there are requirements for the retention of invoices for 2 years).

Schedule 4 includes in Part I benzodiazepines (except temazepam which is in schedule 3) and zolpidem, which are subject to minimal control. Part II includes androgenic and anabolic steroids, clenbuterol, chorionic gonadotrophin (HCG), non-human chorionic gonadotrophin, somatotropin, somatrem, and somatropin. Controlled drug prescription requirements do not apply and Schedule 4 Controlled Drugs are not subject to safe custody requirements.

Schedule 5 includes those preparations which, because of their strength, are exempt from virtually all Controlled Drug requirements other than retention of invoices for two years.

Notification of drug misusers

Doctors are expected to report cases of drug misuse to their regional or national drug misuse database or centre—see below for contact telephone numbers. The National Drugs Treatment Monitoring System (NDTMS) was introduced in England in April 2001; regional (NDTMS) centres replace the Regional Drug Misuse Databases. A similar system has been introduced in Wales.

Notification to regional (NDTMS) or national centre should be made when a patient starts treatment for drug misuse. All types of problem drug misuse should be reported including opioid, benzodiazepine, and CNS stimulant.

The regional (NDTMS) or national centres are now the only national and local source of epidemiological data on people presenting with problem drug misuse; they provide valuable information to those working with drug misusers and those planning services for them. The databases cannot, however be used as a check on multiple prescribing for drug addicts because the data are anonymised.

Enquiries about the regional (NDTMS) or national centres (including information on how to submit data) can be made to one of the centres listed below:

ENGLAND

Eastern
Tel: (01223) 597 598
Fax: (01223) 597 601

South East
Tel: (01865) 334 734
Fax: (01865) 334 733

London
Tel: (020) 7261 8801
Fax: (020) 7261 8883

North West
Tel: (0151) 231 4533
Fax: (0151) 231 4515

North East
Tel: (0191) 334 0372
Fax: (0191) 334 0391

Yorkshire and the Humber
Tel: (0113) 295 3714
Fax: (0113) 295 3720

South Western
Tel: (0117) 970 6474 ext 311
Fax: (0117) 970 7021

East Midlands
Tel: (0115) 971 2738
Fax: (0115) 971 2740

West Midlands
Tel: (0121) 415 8556
Fax: (0121) 414 8197

SCOTLAND
Tel: (0131) 275 6193
Fax: (0131) 275 7511

WALES
Tel: (029) 2050 3343
Fax: (029) 2050 2330

In **Northern Ireland**, the Misuse of Drugs (Notification of and Supply to Addicts) (Northern Ireland) Regulations 1973 require doctors to send particulars of persons whom they consider to be addicted to certain controlled drugs to the Chief Medical Officer of the Department of Health and Social Services. The Northern Ireland contacts are:

Medical contact:

Dr Ian McMaster
C3 Castle Buildings
Belfast BT4 3FQ
Tel: (028) 9052 2421
Fax: (028) 9052 0718

Administrative contact:

Drug & Alcohol Information & Research Unit
Annex 2
Castle Building
Belfast BT4 3SQ
Tel: (028) 9052 2520

The Drug & Alcohol Information & Research Unit also maintains the Northern Ireland Drug Misuse Database (NIDMD) which collects detailed information on those presenting for treatment, on drugs misused and injecting behaviour; participation is not a statutory requirement.

Prescribing of diamorphine (heroin), dipipanone, and cocaine for addicts

The Misuse of Drugs (Supply to Addicts) Regulations 1997 require that only medical practitioners who hold a special licence issued by the Home Secretary may prescribe, administer or supply diamorphine, dipipanone[1] (*Diconal*®) or cocaine in the treatment of drug addiction; other practitioners must refer any addict who requires these drugs to a treatment centre. Whenever possible the addict will be introduced by a member of staff from the treatment centre to a pharmacist whose agreement has been obtained and whose pharmacy is conveniently sited for the patient. Prescriptions for weekly supplies will be sent to the pharmacy by post and will be dispensed on a daily basis as indicated by the doctor. If any alterations of the arrangements are requested by the addict, the portion of the prescription affected must be represcribed and not merely altered.

General practitioners and other doctors do not require a special licence for prescribing diamorphine, dipipanone, and cocaine for patients (including addicts) for *relieving pain* from organic disease or injury.

For guidance on prescription writing, see p. 7.

---

1. Dipipanone in *Diconal*® tablets has been much misused by opioid addicts in recent years. Doctors and others should be suspicious of people who ask for the tablets, especially if temporary residents.

Adverse reactions to drugs

Any drug may produce unwanted or unexpected adverse reactions. Detection and recording of these is of vital importance. Doctors, dentists, coroners, pharmacists and nurses are urged to help by reporting suspected adverse reactions on yellow cards to:

Medicines and Healthcare products Regulatory Agency
CSM
Freepost
London SW8 5BR
Tel: (0800 731 6789)

Suspected adverse reactions to *any* therapeutic agent should be reported, including drugs *(self-medication* as well as those *prescribed)*, blood products, vaccines, radiographic contrast media and herbal products. Prepaid Yellow Cards for reporting are available from the above address and are also bound in this book (inside back cover). Adverse reactions can also be reported at: www.yellowcard.gov.uk.

A 24-hour Freefone service is available to all parts of the UK for advice and information on suspected adverse drug reactions; contact the National Yellow Card Information Service at the MHRA (formerly MCA) on 0800 731 6789. Outside office hours a telephone-answering machine will take messages.

The following regional centres also collect data:

CSM Mersey
Freepost
Liverpool L3 3AB
Tel: (0151) 794 8206

CSM Wales
Freepost
Cardiff CF4 1ZZ
Tel: (029) 2074 4181 (direct line)

CSM Northern & Yorkshire
Freepost 1085
Newcastle upon Tyne
NE1 1BR
Tel: (0191) 232 1525 (direct line)

CSM West Midlands
Freepost SW2991
Birmingham B18 7BR
Tel: (0121) 507 5672

CSM Scotland
CARDS
Freepost NAT3271
Edinburgh EH16 4BR
Tel: (0131) 242 2919

The MHRA's Adverse Drug Reactions On-line Information Tracking (ADROIT) facilitates the monitoring of adverse drug reactions.

More detailed information on reporting and a list of products currently under intensive monitoring can be found on the CSM homepage: medicines.mhra.gov.uk.

PRESCRIPTION-EVENT MONITORING. In addition to the CSM's Yellow Card scheme, an independent scheme monitors the safety of new medicines using a different approach. The Drug Safety Research Unit identifies patients who have been prescribed selected new medicines and collects data on clinical events in these patients. The data are submitted on a voluntary basis by general practitioners on green forms. More information about the scheme and the Unit's educational material is available from www.dsru.org.

NEWER DRUGS AND VACCINES. Only limited information is available from clinical trials on the safety of new medicines. Further understanding about the safety of medicines depends on the availability of information from routine clinical practice.

The black triangle symbol (▼) identifies newly licensed medicines that are monitored intensively by the MHRA/CSM. Such medicines include those that have been licensed for administration by a new route or drug delivery system, or for significant new indications which may alter the established risks and benefits of that drug. There is no standard time for which products retain a black triangle; safety data are usually reviewed after 2 years.

Spontaneous reporting is particularly valuable for recognising possible new hazards rapidly. For medicines showing the black triangle symbol, the MHRA/CSM asks that **all** suspected reactions (including those considered not to be serious) are reported through the Yellow Card scheme. An adverse reaction should be reported even if it is not certain that the drug has caused it, or if the reaction is well recognised, or if other drugs have been given at the same time.

ESTABLISHED DRUGS AND VACCINES. Doctors, dentists, coroners, pharmacists and nurses are asked to report *all* serious suspected reactions, including those that are fatal, life-threatening, disabling, incapacitating, or which result in or prolong hospitalisation; they should be reported even if the effect is well recognised. Examples include anaphylaxis, blood disorders, endocrine disturbances, effects on fertility, haemorrhage from any site, renal impairment, jaundice, ophthalmic disorders, severe CNS effects, severe skin reactions, reactions in pregnant women, and any drug interactions. Reports of serious adverse reactions are required to enable comparison with other drugs of a similar class. Reports of overdoses (deliberate or accidental) can complicate the assessment of adverse drug reactions, but provides important information on the potential toxicity of drugs.

For established drugs there is no need to report well-known, relatively minor side-effects, such as dry mouth with tricyclic antidepressants or constipation with opioids.

ADVERSE REACTIONS TO MEDICAL DEVICES. Suspected adverse reactions to medical devices including dental or surgical materials, intra-uterine devices and contact lens fluids should be reported. Information on reporting these can be found at: devices.mhra.gov.uk

SIDE-EFFECTS IN THE BNF. The BNF includes clinically relevant side-effects for most drugs; an exhaustive list is not included for drugs that are used by specialists (e.g. cytotoxics and drugs used in anaesthesia). Side-effects in the manufacturers' literature whose causality has not been established may be omitted from the BNF.

Side-effects are generally listed in order of frequency and arranged broadly by body systems. Occasionally a rare side-effect might be listed first if it is considered to be particularly important because of its seriousness.

In the product literature the frequency of side-effects is generally described as follows:

Very common	greater than 1 in 10
Common	1 in 100 to 1 in 10
Uncommon	1 in 1000 to 1 in 100
Rare	1 in 10 000 to 1 in 1000
Very rare	less than 1 in 10 000

Special problems

Delayed drug effects. Some reactions (e.g. cancers, chloroquine retinopathy, and retroperitoneal fibrosis) may become manifest months or years after exposure. Any suspicion of such an association should be reported.

The elderly. Particular vigilance is required to identify adverse reactions in the elderly.

Congenital abnormalities. When an infant is born with a congenital abnormality or there is a malformed aborted fetus doctors are asked to consider whether this might be an adverse reaction to a drug and to report all drugs (including self-medication) taken during pregnancy.

Children. Particular vigilance is required to identify and report adverse reactions in children, including those resulting from the unlicensed use of medicines; **all** suspected reactions should be reported (see p. 12).

Prevention of adverse reactions

Adverse reactions may be prevented as follows:

- Never use any drug unless there is a good indication. If the patient is pregnant do not use a drug unless the need for it is imperative.
- Allergy and idiosyncrasy are important causes of adverse drug reactions. Ask if the patient had previous reactions.
- Ask if the patient is already taking other drugs *including self-medication drugs, health supplements, herbal and complementary therapies*; interactions may occur.
- Age and hepatic or renal disease may alter the metabolism or excretion of drugs, so that much smaller doses may be needed. Genetic factors may also be responsible for variations in metabolism, notably of isoniazid and the tricyclic antidepressants.
- Prescribe as few drugs as possible and give very clear instructions to the elderly or any patient likely to misunderstand complicated instructions.
- When possible use a familiar drug. With a new drug be particularly alert for adverse reactions or unexpected events.
- If serious adverse reactions are liable to occur warn the patient.

Oral side-effects of drugs

Drug-induced disorders of the mouth may be due to a local action on the mouth or to a systemic effect manifested by oral changes. In the latter case urgent referral to the patient's medical practitioner may be necessary.

Oral mucosa

Medicaments left in contact with or applied directly to the oral mucosa can lead to inflammation or ulceration; the possibility of allergy should also be borne in mind.

Aspirin tablets allowed to dissolve in the sulcus for the treatment of toothache can lead to a white patch followed by ulceration.

Flavouring agents, particularly **essential oils**, may sensitise the skin, but mucosal swelling is not usually prominent.

The oral mucosa is particularly vulnerable to ulceration in patients treated with cytotoxic drugs, e.g. **methotrexate**. Other drugs capable of causing oral ulceration include **gold**, **nicorandil**, **NSAIDs**, **pancreatin**, **penicillamine**, and **proguanil**. **Captopril** (and other ACE inhibitors) can cause *stomatitis*.

Erythema multiforme (including Stevens-Johnson syndrome) may follow the use of a wide range of drugs including **antibacterials**, **sulphonamide derivatives**, and **anticonvulsants**; the oral mucosa may be extensively ulcerated, with characteristic target lesions on the skin. Oral lesions of *toxic epidermal necrolysis* (Lyell's syndrome) have been reported with a similar range of drugs.

Lichenoid eruptions are associated with **NSAIDs**, **methyldopa**, **chloroquine**, **oral antidiabetics**, **thiazide diuretics**, and **gold**.

Candidiasis can complicate treatment with **antibacterials** and **immunosuppressants** and is an occasional side-effect of **corticosteroid inhalers**, see also p. 154.

Teeth

Brown staining of the teeth frequently follows the use of **chlorhexidine** mouthwash, spray or gel, but can readily be removed by polishing. **Iron** salts in liquid form can stain the enamel black. Superficial staining has been reported rarely with **co-amoxiclav** suspension.

Intrinsic staining of the teeth is most commonly caused by **tetracyclines**. They will affect the teeth if given at any time from about the fourth month *in utero* until the age of twelve years; they are contra-indicated in pregnancy, breast-feeding women, and in children under 12 years. All tetracyclines can cause permanent, unsightly staining in children, the colour varying from yellow to grey.

Excessive ingestion of **fluoride** leads to *dental fluorosis* with mottling of the enamel and areas of hypoplasia or pitting; fluoride supplements may occasionally cause mild mottling (white patches) if the dose is too large for the child's age, taking into account the fluoride content of the local drinking water.

Periodontium

Gingival overgrowth (gingival hyperplasia) is a side-effect of **phenytoin** and sometimes of **ciclosporin** or of **nifedipine** (and some other calcium-channel blockers).

Thrombocytopenia may be drug related and may cause bleeding at the gingival margins, which may be spontaneous or may follow mild trauma (such as toothbrushing).

Salivary glands

The most common effect that drugs have on the salivary glands is to *reduce flow* (xerostomia). Patients with a persistently dry mouth may have poor oral hygiene; they may develop increased dental caries, and oral infections (particularly candidiasis). Many drugs have been implicated in xerostomia, particularly **antimuscarinics** (anticholinergics), **antidepressants** (including tricyclic antidepressants, and selective serotonin re-uptake inhibitors), **baclofen**, **clonidine**, and **tizanidine**. Excessive use of **diuretics** can also result in xerostomia.

Some drugs (e.g. clozapine, neostigmine) can *increase saliva production* but this is rarely a problem unless the patient has associated difficulty in swallowing.

Pain in the salivary glands has been reported with some **antihypertensives** (e.g. clonidine, methyldopa) and with **vinca alkaloids**.

Swelling of the salivary glands can occur with **iodides**, **antithyroid drugs**, **phenothiazines**, **ritodrine**, and **sulphonamides**.

Taste

There can be *decreased* taste acuity or *alteration* in taste sensation. Drugs implicated include **amiodarone**, **captopril** (and other ACE inhibitors), **carbimazole**, **gold**, **griseofulvin**, **lithium salts**, **metronidazole**, **penicillamine**, **phenindione**, **propafenone**, **terbinafine**, and **zopiclone**.

Defective medicines

During the manufacture or distribution of a medicine an error or accident may occur whereby the finished product does not conform to its specification. While such a defect may impair the therapeutic effect of the product and could adversely affect the health of a patient, it should **not** be confused with an Adverse Drug Reaction where the product conforms to its specification.

The Defective Medicines Report Centre assists with the investigation of problems arising from licensed medicinal products thought to be defective and co-ordinates any necessary protective action. Reports on suspect defective medicinal products should include the brand or the non-proprietary name, the name of the manufacturer or supplier, the strength and dosage form of the product, the product licence number, the batch number or numbers of the product, the nature of the defect, and an account of any action already taken in consequence. The Centre can be contacted at:

The Defective Medicines Report Centre
Medicines and Healthcare products Regulatory Agency
Room 18–159
1 Nine Elms Lane
London SW8 5NQ
(020) 7084 2574 (weekdays 9.00 am–5.00 pm)
or (020) 7210 3000 (outside office hours)

Prescribing for children

For further information on the use of drugs in children, see *BNF for Children*.

Children, and particularly neonates, differ from adults in their response to drugs. Special care is needed in the neonatal period (first 30 days of life) and doses should always be calculated with care. At this age, the risk of toxicity is increased by inefficient renal filtration, relative enzyme deficiencies, differing target organ sensitivity, and inadequate detoxifying systems causing delayed excretion.

Whenever possible, painful intramuscular injections should be **avoided** in children.

Where possible, medicines for children should be prescribed within the terms of the marketing authorisation (product licence) However, many children may require medicines not specifically licensed for paediatric use.

Although medicines cannot be promoted outside the limits of the licence, the Medicines Act does not prohibit the use of unlicensed medicines. It is recognised that the informed use of unlicensed medicines or of licensed medicines for unlicensed applications ('off-label' use) is often necessary in paediatric practice.

ADVERSE DRUG REACTIONS IN CHILDREN. The reporting of all suspected adverse drug reactions in children is **strongly encouraged** through the Yellow Card scheme (see p. 10) even if the intensive monitoring symbol (▼) has been removed, because experience in children may still be limited.

The identification and reporting of adverse reactions to drugs in children is particularly important because:

- the action of the drug and its pharmacokinetics in children (especially in the very young) may be different from that in adults
- drugs are not extensively tested in children
- many drugs are not specifically licensed for use in children and are used 'off-label'
- suitable formulations may not be available to allow precise dosing in children
- the nature and course of illnesses and adverse drug reactions may differ between adults and children.

PRESCRIPTION WRITING. Prescriptions should be written according to the guidelines in Prescription Writing (p. 4) Inclusion of age is a legal requirement in the case of prescription-only medicines for children under 12 years of age, but it is preferable to state the age for **all** prescriptions for children.

It is particularly important to state the strengths of capsules or tablets. Although liquid preparations are particularly suitable for children, they may contain sugar which encourages dental decay. Sugar-free medicines are preferred for long-term treatment.

Many children are able to swallow tablets or capsules and may prefer a solid dose form; involving the child and parents in choosing the formulation is helpful.

When a prescription for a liquid oral preparation is written and the dose ordered is smaller than 5 mL an **oral syringe** will be supplied (for details, see p. 2). Parents should be advised not to add any medicines to the infant's feed, since the drug may interact with the milk or other liquid in it; moreover the ingested dosage may be reduced if the child does not drink all the contents.

Parents must be warned to keep **all** medicines out of reach of children, see Safety in the Home, p. 3

Rare paediatric conditions

Information on substances such as *biotin* and *sodium benzoate* used in rare metabolic conditions is included in *BNF for Children*; further information can be obtained from:

Alder Hey Children's Hospital
Drug Information Centre
Liverpool L12 2AP
Tel: (0151) 252 5381

Great Ormond Street Hospital for Children
Pharmacy
Great Ormond St
London WC1N 3JH
Tel: (020) 7405 9200

Dosage in Children

Children's doses in the BNF are stated in the individual drug entries as far as possible, except where paediatric use is not recommended, information is not available, or there are special hazards.

Doses are generally based on body-weight (in kilograms) or the following age ranges:

first month (neonate)
up to 1 year (infant)
1–5 years
6–12 years

Unless the age is specified, the term 'child' in the BNF includes persons aged 12 years and younger.

DOSE CALCULATION. Children's doses may be calculated from adult doses by using age, body-weight, or body-surface area, or by a combination of these factors. The most reliable methods are those based on body-surface area.

Body-weight may be used to calculate doses expressed in mg/kg. Young children may require a higher dose per kilogram than adults because of their higher metabolic rates. Other problems need to be considered. For example, calculation by body-weight in the overweight child may result in much higher doses being administered than necessary; in such cases, dose should be calculated from an ideal weight, related to height and age (see inside back cover).

Body-surface area (BSA) estimates are more accurate for calculation of paediatric doses than body-weight since many physiological phenomena correlate better to body-surface area. Body-surface area may be calculated from height and weight by means of a nomogram. For more information, refer to *BNF for Children*.

Where the dose for children is not stated, prescribers should consult *BNF for Children* or seek advice from a medicines information centre.

DOSE FREQUENCY. Antibacterials are generally given at regular intervals throughout the day. Some flexibility should be allowed in children to avoid waking them during the night. For example, the night-time dose may be given at the parent's bed-time.

Where new or potentially toxic drugs are used, the manufacturers' recommended doses should be carefully followed.

Prescribing in palliative care

Palliative care is the active total care of patients whose disease is not responsive to curative treatment. Control of pain, of other symptoms, and of psychological, social and spiritual problems, is paramount to provide the best quality of life for patients and their families. Careful assessment of symptoms and needs of the patient should be undertaken by a multidisciplinary team.

Specialist palliative care is available in most areas as day hospice care, home care teams (often known as Macmillan teams), in-patient hospice care, and hospital teams. Many acute hospitals and teaching centres now have consultative, hospital-based teams.

Hospice care of terminally ill patients has shown the importance of symptom control and psychosocial support of the patient and family. Families should be included in the care of the patient if they wish.

Many patients wish to remain at home with their families. Although some families may at first be afraid of caring for the patient at home, support can be provided by community nursing services, social services, voluntary agencies and hospices together with the general practitioner. The family may be reassured by the knowledge that the patient will be admitted to a hospital or hospice if the family cannot cope.

DRUG TREATMENT. The number of drugs should be as few as possible, for even the taking of medicine may be an effort. Oral medication is usually satisfactory unless there is severe nausea and vomiting, dysphagia, weakness, or coma, in which case parenteral medication may be necessary.

Pain

Analgesics are more effective in preventing pain than in the relief of established pain; it is important that they are given regularly.

The non-opioid analgesics **paracetamol** or an **NSAID** (section 10.1.1) given regularly will often make the use of opioids unnecessary. The NSAID may also control the pain of *bone secondaries*; if necessary, flurbiprofen or indometacin can be given rectally. Radiotherapy, bisphosphonates (section 6.6.2) and radioactive isotopes of **strontium** (*Metastron*® available from GE Healthcare) may also be useful for pain due to bone metastases.

An opioid such as **codeine**, alone or in combination with a non-opioid analgesic at adequate dosage, may be helpful in the control of moderate pain if non-opioids alone are not sufficient. Alternatively, **tramadol** can be considered for moderate pain. If these preparations are not controlling the pain, **morphine** is the most useful opioid analgesic. Alternatives to morphine include **hydromorphone**, **methadone**, **oxycodone** (section 4.7.2) and transdermal **fentanyl** (see below and section 4.7.2); these drugs are best initiated by those with experience in palliative care. Initiation of an opioid analgesic should not be delayed by concern over a theoretical likelihood of psychological dependence (addiction).

Equivalent single doses of strong analgesics

These equivalences are intended **only** as an approximate guide; patients should be carefully monitored after **any** change in medication and dose titration may be required

Analgesic	Dose
Morphine salts (oral)	10 mg
Diamorphine hydrochloride (intramuscular)	3 mg
Hydromorphone hydrochloride	1.3 mg
Oxycodone (oral)	5 mg

ORAL ROUTE. Morphine is given *by mouth* as an oral solution or as standard ('immediate release') tablets regularly every 4 hours, the initial dose depending largely on the patient's previous treatment. A dose of 5–10 mg is enough to replace a weaker analgesic (such as paracetamol or co-proxamol), but 10–20 mg or more is required to replace a strong one (comparable to morphine itself). If the first dose of morphine is no more effective than the previous analgesic, the next dose should be increased by 50%, the aim being to choose the lowest dose which prevents pain. The dose should be adjusted with careful assessment of the pain and the use of adjuvant analgesics (such as NSAIDs) should also be considered. Although morphine in a dose of 5–20 mg is usually adequate there should be no hesitation in increasing it stepwise according to response to 100 mg or occasionally up to 500 mg or higher if necessary. It may be possible to omit the overnight dose if double the usual dose is given at bedtime.

If pain occurs between regular doses of morphine ('breakthrough pain'), an additional dose ('rescue dose') should be given. An additional dose should also be given 30 minutes before an activity that causes pain (e.g. wound dressing). Fentanyl lozenges are also licensed for breakthrough pain.

When the pain is controlled and the patient's 24-hour morphine requirement is established, the daily dose can be given as a single dose or in 2 divided doses as a *modified-release preparation*.

Preparations suitable for twice daily administration include *MST Continus*® tablets or suspension, and *Zomorph*® capsules. Preparations that allow administration of the total daily morphine requirement as a single dose include *MXL*® capsules. *Morcap SR*® capsules may be given either twice daily or as a single daily dose.

The starting dose of modified-release preparations designed for twice daily administration is usually 10–20 mg every 12 hours if no other analgesic (or only paracetamol) has been taken previously, but to replace a weaker opioid analgesic (such as co-proxamol) the starting dose is usually 20–30 mg every 12 hours. Increments should be made to the dose, not to the frequency of administration, which should remain at every 12 hours.

The effective dose of modified-release preparations can alternatively be determined by giving the oral solution of morphine every 4 hours in increasing doses until the pain has been controlled, and then transferring the patient to the same total 24-hour dose of morphine given as the modified-release preparation (divided into two portions for 12-hourly administration). The first dose of the modified-release preparation is given 4 hours after the last dose of the oral solution.[1]

Morphine, as oral solution or standard formulation tablets, should be prescribed for breakthrough pain; the dose should be about one-sixth of the total daily dose of oral morphine repeated every 4 hours if necessary (review pain management if analgesic required more frequently).

PARENTERAL ROUTE. If the patient becomes unable to swallow, the equivalent intramuscular dose of morphine is half the oral solution dose; in the case of the modified-release tablets it is half the total 24-hour dose (which is then divided into 6 portions to be given every 4 hours). **Diamorphine** is preferred for injection because, being more soluble, it can be given in a smaller volume. The equivalent intramuscular (or subcutaneous) is approximately a third of the oral dose of morphine. *Subcutaneous infusion* of diamorphine via syringe driver can be useful (for details, see p. 16).

If the patient can resume taking medicines by mouth, then oral morphine may be substituted for subcutaneous infusion of diamorphine; see table of equivalent doses of morphine (p. 18) for equivalences between the two opioids.

RECTAL ROUTE. Morphine is also available for *rectal administration* as suppositories; alternatively **oxycodone** suppositories can be obtained on special order.

TRANSDERMAL ROUTE. Transdermal preparations of fentanyl are available (section 4.7.2). Careful conversion from oral morphine to transdermal fentanyl is necessary. The following 24-hour doses of morphine are considered to be equivalent to the fentanyl patches shown:

Morphine salt 90 mg daily ≡ fentanyl '25' patch
Morphine salt 180 mg daily ≡ fentanyl '50' patch
Morphine salt 270 mg daily ≡ fentanyl '75' patch
Morphine salt 360 mg daily ≡ fentanyl '100' patch

Morphine (as oral solution or standard formulation tablets) is given for breakthrough pain.

GASTRO-INTESTINAL PAIN. The pain of *bowel colic* may be reduced by loperamide 2–4 mg 4 times daily. Hyoscine hydrobromide may also be helpful, given sublingually at a dose of 300 micrograms 3 times daily as *Kwells*® (Roche Consumer Health) tablets. For the dose by subcutaneous infusion using a syringe driver, see p. 17).

Gastric distension pain due to pressure on the stomach may be helped by a preparation incorporating an antacid with an antiflatulent (section 1.1.1) and by domperidone 10 mg 3 times daily before meals.

MUSCLE SPASM. The pain of muscle spasm can be helped by a muscle relaxant such as diazepam 5–10 mg daily or baclofen 5–10 mg 3 times daily.

NEUROPATHIC PAIN. Patients with neuropathic pain (section 4.7.3) may benefit from a trial of a tricyclic antidepressant for several weeks. An anticonvulsant may be added or substituted if pain persists; gabapentin and pregabalin (both section 4.8.1) are licensed for neuropathic pain.

Pain due to nerve compression may be reduced by a corticosteroid such as dexamethasone 8 mg daily, which reduces oedema around the tumour, thus reducing compression.

Nerve blocks may be considered when pain is localised to a specific area. **Transcutaneous electrical nerve stimulation** (TENS) may also help.

Miscellaneous conditions

Non-licensed indications or routes. Several recommendations in this section involve non-licensed indications or routes.

RAISED INTRACRANIAL PRESSURE. Headache due to raised intracranial pressure often responds to a high dose of a corticosteroid, such as dexamethasone 16 mg daily for 4 to 5 days, subsequently reduced to 4–6 mg daily if possible; dexamethasone should be given before 6 p.m. to reduce the risk of insomnia.

INTRACTABLE COUGH. Intractable cough may be relieved by moist inhalations or by regular administration of oral morphine in an initial dose of 5 mg every 4 hours. Methadone linctus should be avoided because it has a long duration of action and tends to accumulate.

DYSPNOEA. Breathlessness at rest may be relieved by regular oral morphine in carefully titrated doses, starting at 5 mg every 4 hours. Diazepam 5–10 mg daily may be helpful for dyspnoea associated with anxiety. A corticosteroid, such as dexamethasone 4–8 mg daily, may also be helpful if there is bronchospasm or partial obstruction.

EXCESSIVE RESPIRATORY SECRETION. Excessive respiratory secretion (death rattle) may be reduced by subcutaneous injection of hyoscine hydrobromide 400–600 micrograms every 4 to 8 hours; care must however be taken to avoid the discomfort of dry mouth. Alternatively glycopyrronium may be given by subcutaneous or intramuscular injection in a dose of 200 micrograms every 4 hours. For the dose by subcutaneous infusion using a syringe driver, see p. 17.

RESTLESSNESS AND CONFUSION. Restlessness and confusion may require treatment with haloperidol 1–3 mg by mouth every 8 hours. Chlorpromazine 25–50 mg by mouth every 8 hours is an alternative, but causes more sedation. Levomepromazine (methotrimeprazine) is also used occasionally for restlessness. For the dose by subcutaneous infusion using a syringe driver, see p. 17.

HICCUP. Hiccup due to gastric distension may be helped by a preparation incorporating an antacid with an antiflatulent (section 1.1). If this fails, metoclopramide 10 mg every 6 to 8 hours by mouth or by subcutaneous or intramuscular injection can be added; if this also fails baclofen 5 mg twice daily, or nifedipine 10 mg three times daily, or chlorpromazine 10–25 mg every 6 to 8 hours can be tried.

ANOREXIA. Anorexia may be helped by prednisolone 15–30 mg daily or dexamethasone 2–4 mg daily.

1. Studies have indicated that administration of the last dose of the *oral solution* with the first dose of the *modified-release tablets* is not necessary.

CONSTIPATION. Constipation is a very common cause of distress and is almost invariable after administration of an opioid. It should be prevented if possible by the regular administration of laxatives; a faecal softener with a peristaltic stimulant (e.g. co-danthramer), or lactulose solution with a senna preparation should be used (section 1.6.2 and section 1.6.3).

FUNGATING GROWTH. Fungating growth may be treated by regular dressing and oral administration of metronidazole; topical application of metronidazole is also used.

CAPILLARY BLEEDING. Capillary bleeding may be reduced by applying gauze soaked in adrenaline (epinephrine) solution 1 mg/mL (1 in 1000).

DRY MOUTH. Dry mouth may be relieved by good mouth care and measures such as the sucking of ice or pineapple chunks or the use of artificial saliva (section 12.3.5); dry mouth associated with candidiasis can be treated by oral preparations of nystatin or miconazole (section 12.3.2); alternatively, fluconazole can be given by mouth (section 5.2). Dry mouth may be caused by certain medication including opioids, antimuscarinic drugs (e.g. hyoscine), antidepressants and some anti-emetics; if possible, an alternative preparation should be considered.

PRURITUS. Pruritus, even when associated with obstructive jaundice, often responds to simple measures such as application of emollients (section 13.2.1). In the case of obstructive jaundice, further measures include administration of colestyramine (section 1.9.2).

CONVULSIONS. Patients with cerebral tumours or uraemia may be susceptible to convulsions. Prophylactic treatment with phenytoin or carbamazepine (section 4.8.1) should be considered. When oral medication is no longer possible, diazepam as suppositories 10–20 mg every 4 to 8 hours, or phenobarbital by injection 50–200 mg twice daily is continued as prophylaxis. For the use of midazolam by subcutaneous infusion using a syringe driver, see below.

DYSPHAGIA. A corticosteroid such as dexamethasone 8 mg daily may help, temporarily, if there is an obstruction due to tumour. See also under Dry Mouth.

NAUSEA AND VOMITING. Nausea and vomiting are common in patients with advanced cancer. Ideally, the cause should be determined before treatment with an anti-emetic (section 4.6) is started.

Nausea and vomiting may occur with opioid therapy particularly in the initial stages but can be prevented by giving an anti-emetic such as haloperidol or metoclopramide. An anti-emetic is usually necessary only for the first 4 or 5 days and therefore combined preparations containing an opioid with an anti-emetic are not recommended because they lead to unnecessary anti-emetic therapy (and associated side-effects when used long-term).

Metoclopramide has a prokinetic action and is used in a dose of 10 mg 3 times daily by mouth for nausea and vomiting associated with gastritis, gastric stasis, and functional bowel obstruction. Drugs with antimuscarinic effects antagonise prokinetic drugs and, where possible, should not therefore be used concurrently.

Haloperidol is used in a dose of 1.5 mg daily (or twice daily if nausea continues) by mouth for most chemical causes of vomiting (e.g. hypercalcaemia, renal failure).

Cyclizine is given in a dose of 50 mg up to 3 times daily by mouth. It is used for nausea and vomiting due to mechanical bowel obstruction, raised intracranial pressure, and motion sickness.

Anti-emetic therapy should be reviewed every 24 hours; it may be necessary to substitute the anti-emetic or to add another one.

Levomepromazine (methotrimeprazine) may be used if first-line anti-emetics are inadequate; it is given by mouth in a dose of 6–25 mg daily [6-mg tablets available on named-patient basis]. Dexamethasone 8–16 mg daily by mouth may be used as an adjunct.

For the administration of anti-emetics by subcutaneous infusion using a syringe driver, see below.

For the treatment of nausea and vomiting associated with cancer chemotherapy, see section 8.1.

INSOMNIA. Patients with advanced cancer may not sleep because of discomfort, cramps, night sweats, joint stiffness, or fear. There should be appropriate treatment of these problems before hypnotics are used. Benzodiazepines, such as temazepam, may be useful (section 4.1.1).

HYPERCALCAEMIA. See section 9.5.1.2.

Syringe drivers

Although drugs can usually be administered *by mouth* to control the symptoms of advanced cancer, the parenteral route may sometimes be necessary. If the parenteral route is necessary, repeated administration of *intramuscular injections* can be difficult in a cachectic patient. This has led to the use of a portable syringe driver to give a *continuous subcutaneous infusion*, which can provide good control of symptoms with little discomfort or inconvenience to the patient.

> **Syringe driver rate settings.** Staff using syringe drivers should be **adequately trained** and different rate settings should be **clearly identified** and **differentiated**; incorrect use of syringe drivers is a common cause of drug errors.

Indications for the **parenteral route** are:

- the patient is unable to take medicines by mouth owing to *nausea and vomiting, dysphagia, severe weakness,* or *coma;*
- there is *malignant bowel obstruction* in patients for whom further surgery is inappropriate (avoiding the need for an intravenous infusion or for insertion of a nasogastric tube);
- occasionally when the patient *does not wish* to take regular medication by mouth.

NAUSEA AND VOMITING. Haloperidol is given in a *subcutaneous infusion dose* of 2.5–10 mg/24 hours.

Levomepromazine (methotrimeprazine) causes sedation in about 50% of patients; it is given in a *subcutaneous infusion dose* of 25–200 mg/24 hours, although lower doses of 5–25 mg/24 hours may be effective with less sedation.

Cyclizine is particularly liable to precipitate if mixed with diamorphine or other drugs (see under Mixing and Compatibility, below); it is given in a *subcutaneous infusion dose* of 150 mg/24 hours.

Metoclopramide may cause skin reactions; it is given in a *subcutaneous infusion dose* of 30–100 mg/24 hours.

Octreotide (section 8.3.4.3), which stimulates water and electrolyte absorption and inhibits water secretion in the small bowel, can be used by subcutaneous infusion, in a dose of 300–600 micrograms/24 hours to reduce intestinal secretions and vomiting.

BOWEL COLIC AND EXCESSIVE RESPIRATORY SECRETIONS. Hyoscine hydrobromide effectively reduces respiratory secretions and is sedative (but occasionally causes paradoxical agitation); it is given in a *subcutaneous infusion dose* of 0.6–2.4 mg/24 hours.

Hyoscine butylbromide is effective in bowel colic, is less sedative than hyoscine hydrobromide, but is not always adequate for the control of respiratory secretions; it is given in a *subcutaneous infusion dose* of 20–60 mg/24 hours (**important:** this dose of *hyoscine butylbromide* must not be confused with the much lower dose of *hyoscine hydrobromide*, above).

Glycopyrronium 0.6–1.2 mg/24 hours may also be used.

RESTLESSNESS AND CONFUSION. Haloperidol has little sedative effect; it is given in a *subcutaneous infusion dose* of 5–15 mg/24 hours.

Levomepromazine (methotrimeprazine) has a sedative effect; it is given in a *subcutaneous infusion dose* of 50–200 mg/24 hours.

Midazolam is a sedative and an antiepileptic which may be suitable for a very restless patient; it is given in a *subcutaneous infusion dose* of 20–100 mg/24 hours.

CONVULSIONS. If a patient has previously been receiving an antiepileptic *or* has a primary or secondary cerebral tumour *or* is at risk of convulsion (e.g. owing to uraemia) antiepileptic medication should not be stopped. Midazolam is the benzodiazepine antiepileptic of choice for *continuous subcutaneous infusion*, and it is given intially in a dose of 20–40 mg/24 hours.

PAIN CONTROL. Diamorphine is the preferred opioid since its high solubility permits a large dose to be given in a small volume (see under Mixing and Compatibility, below). The table below gives the approximate doses of *morphine by mouth* (as oral solution or standard formulation tablets or as modified-release tablets) equivalent to *diamorphine by injection* (intramuscularly or by subcutaneous infusion).

MIXING AND COMPATIBILITY. The general principle that injections should be given into separate sites (and should not be mixed) does not apply to the use of syringe drivers in palliative care. Provided that there is evidence of compatibility, selected injections can be mixed in syringe drivers. Not all types of medication can be used in a subcutaneous infusion. In particular, chlorpromazine, prochlorperazine and diazepam are **contra-indicated** as they cause skin reactions at the injection site; to a lesser extent cyclizine and levomepromazine (methotrimeprazine) may also sometimes cause local irritation.

In theory injections dissolved in water for injections are more likely to be associated with pain (possibly owing to their hypotonicity). The use of physiological saline (sodium chloride 0.9%) however increases the likelihood of precipitation when more than one drug is used; moreover subcutaneous infusion rates are so slow (0.1–0.3 mL/hour) that pain is not usually a problem when water is used as a diluent.

Diamorphine can be given by subcutaneous infusion in a strength of up to 250 mg/mL; up to a strength of 40 mg/mL either *water for injections* or *physiological saline* (sodium chloride 0.9%) is a suitable diluent—above that strength only *water for injections* is used (to avoid precipitation).

The following can be mixed with *diamorphine*:

Cyclizine[1]	Hyoscine hydrobromide
Dexamethasone[2]	Levomepromazine
Haloperidol[3]	Metoclopramide[4]
Hyoscine butylbromide	Midazolam

Subcutaneous infusion solution should be monitored regularly both to check for precipitation (and discoloration) and to ensure that the infusion is running at the correct rate

PROBLEMS ENCOUNTERED WITH SYRINGE DRIVERS. The following are problems that may be encountered with syringe drivers and the action that should be taken:

- if the subcutaneous infusion runs *too quickly* check the rate setting and the calculation;
- if the subcutaneous infusion runs *too slowly* check the start button, the battery, the syringe driver, the cannula, and make sure that the injection site is not inflamed;
- if there is an *injection site reaction* make sure that the site does not need to be changed—firmness or swelling at the site of injection is not in itself an indication for change, but pain or obvious inflammation is.

1. Cyclizine may precipitate at concentrations above 10 mg/mL *or* in the presence of sodium chloride 0.9% *or* as the concentration of diamorphine relative to cyclizine increases; mixtures of diamorphine and cyclizine are also liable to precipitate after 24 hours.

2. Special care is needed to avoid precipitation of dexamethasone when preparing.

3. Mixtures of haloperidol and diamorphine are liable to precipitate after 24 hours if haloperidol concentration is above 2 mg/mL.

4. Under some conditions metoclopramide may become discoloured; such solutions should be discarded.

Equivalent doses of morphine sulphate by mouth (as oral solution or standard tablets or as modified-release tablets) or of diamorphine hydrochloride by intramuscular injection or by subcutaneous infusion

These equivalences are approximate only and may need to be adjusted according to response

ORAL MORPHINE		PARENTERAL DIAMORPHINE	
Morphine sulphate oral solution or standard tablets	Morphine sulphate modified-release tablets	Diamorphine hydrochloride by intramuscular injection	Diamorphine hydrochloride by subcutaneous infusion
every 4 hours	every 12 hours	every 4 hours	every 24 hours
5 mg	20 mg	2.5 mg	15 mg
10 mg	30 mg	5 mg	20 mg
15 mg	50 mg	5 mg	30 mg
20 mg	60 mg	7.5 mg	45 mg
30 mg	90 mg	10 mg	60 mg
40 mg	120 mg	15 mg	90 mg
60 mg	180 mg	20 mg	120 mg
80 mg	240 mg	30 mg	180 mg
100 mg	300 mg	40 mg	240 mg
130 mg	400 mg	50 mg	300 mg
160 mg	500 mg	60 mg	360 mg
200 mg	600 mg	70 mg	400 mg

If breakthrough pain occurs give a subcutaneous (preferable) or intramuscular injection of diamorphine equivalent to one-sixth of the total 24-hour subcutaneous infusion dose. It is kinder to give an intermittent bolus injection *subcutaneously*—absorption is smoother so that the risk of adverse effects at peak absorption is avoided (an even better method is to use a subcutaneous butterfly needle).

To minimise the risk of infection no individual subcutaneous infusion solution should be used for longer than 24 hours.

Prescribing for the elderly

Old people, especially the very old, require special care and consideration from prescribers. *Medicines for Older People*, a component document of the National Service Framework for Older People,[1] describes how to maximise the benefits of medicines and how to avoid excessive, inappropriate, or inadequate consumption of medicines by older people.

APPROPRIATE PRESCRIBING. Elderly patients often receive multiple drugs for their multiple diseases. This greatly increases the risk of drug interactions as well as adverse reactions, and may affect compliance (see Taking medicines to best effect under General guidance). The balance of benefit and harm of some medicines may be altered in the elderly. Therefore, elderly patients' medicines should be reviewed regularly and medicines which are not of benefit should be stopped.

Non-pharmacological measures may be more appropriate for symptoms such as headache, sleeplessness and lightheadedness when associated with social stress as in widowhood, loneliness, and family dispersal.

In some cases prophylactic drugs may be inappropriate if they are likely to complicate existing treatment or introduce unnecessary side-effects, especially in elderly patients with poor prognosis or with poor overall health. However, elderly patients should not be denied medicines which may help them, such as anticoagulants or antiplatelet drugs for atrial fibrillation, antihypertensives, statins, and drugs for osteoporosis.

FORM OF MEDICINE. Frail elderly patients may have difficulty swallowing tablets; if left in the mouth, ulceration may develop. They should always be encouraged to take their tablets or capsules with enough fluid, and whilst in an upright position to avoid the possibility of oesophageal ulceration. It may be helpful to discuss with the patient the possibility of taking the drug as a liquid if available.

MANIFESTATIONS OF AGEING. In the very old, manifestations of normal ageing may be mistaken for disease and lead to inappropriate prescribing. In addition, age-related muscle weakness and difficulty in maintaining balance should not be confused with neurological disease. Disorders such as lightheadedness not associated with postural or postprandial hypotension are unlikely to be helped by drugs.

SELF-MEDICATION. Just as in a younger patient self-medication with over-the-counter products or with drugs prescribed for a previous illness (or even for another person) may be an added complication. Discussion with both the patient and relatives as well as a home visit may be needed to establish exactly what is being taken.

SENSITIVITY. The ageing nervous system shows increased *susceptibility* to many commonly used drugs, such as opioid analgesics, benzodiazepines, antipsychotics, and antiparkinsonian drugs, all of which must be used with caution. Similarly, other organs may also be more susceptible to the effects of drugs such as antihypertensives and NSAIDs.

1. Department of Health. National Service Framework for Older People. London: Department of Health, March 2001

Pharmacokinetics

The most important effect of age is reduction in renal clearance. Many aged patients thus *excrete drugs slowly*, and are *highly susceptible to nephrotoxic drugs*. Acute illness may lead to rapid reduction in renal clearance, especially if accompanied by dehydration. Hence, a patient stabilised on a drug with a narrow margin between the therapeutic and the toxic dose (e.g. digoxin) may rapidly develop adverse effects in the aftermath of a myocardial infarction or a respiratory-tract infection. The metabolism of some drugs may be reduced in the elderly.

Pharmacokinetic changes may markedly increase the tissue concentration of a drug in the elderly, especially in debilitated patients.

Adverse reactions

Adverse reactions often present in the elderly in a vague and non-specific fashion. *Confusion* is often the presenting symptom (caused by almost any of the commonly used drugs). Other common manifestations are *constipation* (with antimuscarinics and many tranquillisers) and postural *hypotension* and *falls* (with diuretics and many psychotropics).

HYPNOTICS. Many hypnotics with long half-lives have serious hangover effects of drowsiness, unsteady gait, and even slurred speech and confusion. Those with short half-lives should be used but they too can present problems (section 4.1.1). Short courses of hypnotics are occasionally useful for helping a patient through an acute illness or some other crisis but every effort must be made to avoid dependence. Benzodiazepines impair balance, which may result in falls.

DIURETICS. Diuretics are overprescribed in old age and should **not** be used on a long-term basis to treat simple gravitational oedema which will usually respond to increased movement, raising the legs, and support stockings. A few days of diuretic treatment may speed the clearing of the oedema but it should rarely need continued drug therapy.

NSAIDs. Bleeding associated with *aspirin* and *other NSAIDs* is more common in the elderly who are more likely to have a fatal or serious outcome. NSAIDs are also a special hazard in patients with cardiac disease or renal impairment which may again place older patients at particular risk.

Owing to the *increased susceptibilty of the elderly* to the *side-effects of NSAIDs* the following recommendations are made:

- for *osteoarthritis, soft-tissue lesions* and *back pain* first try measures such as weight reduction (if obese), warmth, exercise and use of a walking stick;
- for *osteoarthritis, soft-tissue lesions, back pain* and *pain in rheumatoid arthritis*, paracetamol should be used first and can often provide adequate pain relief;
- alternatively, a low-dose NSAID (e.g. ibuprofen up to 1.2 g daily may be given;
- for pain relief when either drug is inadequate, paracetamol in a full dose plus a low-dose NSAID may be given;
- if necessary, the NSAID dose can be increased or an opioid analgesic given with paracetamol;
- do not give two NSAIDs at the same time.

For advice on prophylaxis of NSAID-induced peptic ulcers if continued NSAID treatment is necessary, see section 1.3.

OTHER DRUGS. Other drugs which commonly cause adverse reactions are *antiparkinsonian drugs, antihypertensives, psychotropics*, and *digoxin*. The usual maintenance dose of digoxin in very old patients is 125 micrograms daily (62.5 micrograms in those with renal disease); lower doses are often inadequate but toxicity is common in those given 250 micrograms daily.

Drug-induced blood disorders are much more common in the elderly. Therefore drugs with a tendency to cause bone marrow depression (e.g. *co-trimoxazole, mianserin*) should be avoided unless there is no acceptable alternative.

The elderly generally require a lower maintenance dose of *warfarin* than younger adults; once again, the outcome of bleeding tends to be more serious.

Guidelines

Always consider whether a drug is indicated at all.

LIMIT RANGE. It is a sensible policy to prescribe from a limited range of drugs and to be thoroughly familiar with their effects in the elderly.

REDUCE DOSE. Dosage should generally be substantially lower than for younger patients and it is common to start with about 50% of the adult dose. Some drugs (e.g. long-acting antidiabetic drugs such as glibenclamide and chlorpropamide) should be avoided altogether.

REVIEW REGULARLY. Review repeat prescriptions regularly. In many patients it may be possible to stop some drugs, provided that clinical progress is monitored. It may be necessary to reduce the dose of some drugs as renal function declines.

SIMPLIFY REGIMENS. Elderly patients benefit from simple treatment regimens. Only drugs with a clear indication should be prescribed and whenever possible given once or twice daily. In particular, regimens which call for a confusing array of dosage intervals should be avoided.

EXPLAIN CLEARLY. Write full instructions on every prescription (*including* repeat prescriptions) so that containers can be properly labelled with full directions. Avoid imprecisions like 'as directed'. Child-resistant containers may be unsuitable.

REPEATS AND DISPOSAL. Instruct patients what to do when drugs run out, and also how to dispose of any that are no longer necessary. Try to prescribe matching quantities.

If these guidelines are followed most elderly people will cope adequately with their own medicines. If not then it is essential to enrol the help of a third party, usually a relative or a friend.

Prescribing in dental practice

The following is a list of topics of particular relevance to dental surgeons.

> Advice on the drug management of dental and oral conditions has been integrated into the BNF. For ease of access, guidance on such conditions is usually identified by means of a relevant heading (e.g. Dental and Orofacial Pain) in the appropriate sections of the BNF.

Medical emergencies in dental practice

This section provides guidelines on the management of the more common medical emergencies which may arise in dental practice. Dental surgeons and their staff should be familiar with standard resuscitation procedures, but in all circumstances it is advisable to summon medical assistance as soon as possible. For an **algorithm** of the procedure for **cardiopulmonary resuscitation**, see inside back cover.

> **The drugs referred to in this section include:**
> Adrenaline Injection (Epinephrine Injection), adrenaline 1 in 1000, (adrenaline 1 mg/mL as acid tartrate), 1-mL amps
> Aspirin Dispersible Tablets 300 mg
> Chlorphenamine Injection (Chlorpheniramine Injection), chlorphenamine maleate 10 mg/mL, 1-mL amps
> Diazepam Injection, diazepam 5 mg/mL, 2-mL amps
> Glucagon Injection, glucagon (as hydrochloride), 1-unit vial (with solvent)
> Glucose Powder
> Glucose Intravenous Infusion, glucose 20% (200 mg/mL), 500-mL pack or glucose 50% (500 mg/mL), 50-mL prefilled syringe
> Glyceryl Trinitrate Tablets and Sprays
> Hydrocortisone Injection, hydrocortisone 100 mg (preferably as sodium succinate vials with 2-mL solvent)
> Oxygen
> Salbutamol Aerosol Inhalation, salbutamol 100 micrograms/metered inhalation
> Salbutamol Injection, salbutamol (as sulphate) 500 micrograms/mL, 1-mL amps

Adrenal insufficiency

Adrenal insufficiency may be caused by administration of corticosteroids and can persist for years after stopping long-term therapy. A patient with adrenal insufficiency may become hypotensive under the stress of a dental visit (important: see also p. 361 for details of cover for anaesthesia or surgery).

Management

- Lay the patient flat
- Give hydrocortisone (as sodium succinate) 100 mg intravenously
- Give oxygen
- Call for medical assistance

Anaphylaxis

A severe allergic reaction may follow oral or parenteral administration of a drug. Anaphylactic reactions in dentistry may follow the administration of a drug or contact with substances such as latex in surgical gloves. In general, the more rapid the onset of the reaction the more profound it tends to be. Symptoms may develop within minutes and rapid treatment is essential.

Anaphylactic reactions may also be associated with *additives* and *excipients* in foods and medicines (see Excipients, p. 2). Refined arachis (peanut) oil, which may be present in some medicinal products, is

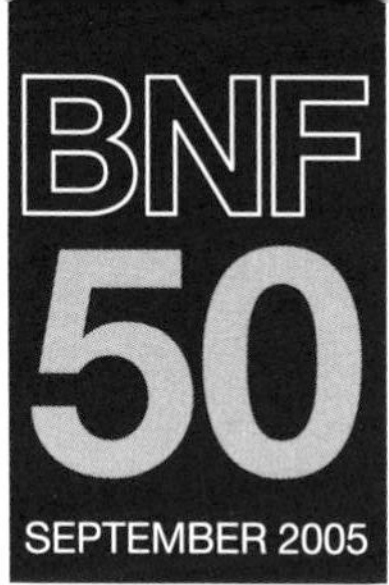

Publication of this the 50th edition seems an opportune moment to reflect on how the BNF has evolved.

Some readers may still remember the hard-backed BNF that *did* fit easily into the white coat pocket, but because it appeared not to have kept up with medicinal advances, it fell out of use. The BNF was therefore completely redesigned – from the composition of its committee to the scope and format of its content. The new-style, more comprehensive BNF, which was much more in touch with professional needs, was born in 1981. It included details on virtually all prescribed medicines. Information on individual drugs was preceded by a commentary on the drug therapy of a particular condition and a summary of the principal clinical properties of the drugs used for treating the condition.

Features such as the table of suggested therapy for bacterial infections made the new-style BNF particularly popular. The first edition also took the bold step of identifying products that were less suitable for prescribing; the BNF was distinctly cool about preparations such as reserpine tablets and combinations of barbiturates with bronchodilators and of tetracyclines with ephedrine and ipecacuanha extracts. Over the years these preparations have been withdrawn from the UK market.

The BNF is used by busy practitioners, often at the point of care. Careful organisation of the text allows rapid retrieval of the information (including warnings) relevant to any medicine-related decision. Comments from numerous users have helped to shape the BNF into its current form. For example, in response to readers' requests, BNF No. 14 introduced actual net prices (in place of price bands); BNF No. 18 saw a complete revision of the presentation of interactions; and, from BNF No. 22, changes to interactions entries were identified.

A great deal of new information continues to be added, especially about practical advice on the drug management of specific conditions, and to make way for it, the BNF has jettisoned less useful information. Like its antecedents, early editions of the new-style BNF included a section on formulations, but with a shift from the use of compounded medicines to commercially manufactured products, this section was removed from BNF No. 20. For the editors, the greatest challenge is to maintain the compactness of the BNF whilst providing the user with all the information necessary to make effective use of medicines.

The layout of the BNF underwent an extensive makeover in 1998 (BNF No. 36). The more contemporary design also allowed the BNF to squeeze in a few extra words on each page, while the second print colour has improved navigation and eased information retrieval.

Licensed translations of the BNF have been undertaken in a number of countries including Spain, Turkey and Italy. A number of independent national formularies are modelled on the BNF and derive a great deal of their core information from the BNF.

The first digital version of the BNF was launched 10 years ago and numerous improvements have been made since. The digital medium improves information retrieval, removes the constraints of space, and allows the BNF to interact with other digital systems. The BNF has recently embarked on an intense programme to develop a new generation of digital services.

Perhaps one of the most important developments of recent months is the launch of *BNF for Children*. The publication has applied well-established BNF processes to construct information on the use of medicines for childhood disorders. The result is an up-to-date and authoritative resource that helps overcome the handicap of scarce and variable paediatric drug information.

New in this edition

For a list of significant changes for this edition, turn to page xii.

Malaria prophylaxis for southern Africa

In line with the Health Protection Agency's advice, the BNF no longer recommends prophylaxis with chloroquine plus proguanil for parts of Botswana, Namibia and Zimbabwe (BNF section 5.4.1). Travellers are now advised to use the same regimen as that for the rest of sub-Saharan Africa where the risk of malaria transmission is intense and high-level chloroquine resistance very prevalent. Appropriate prophylactic antimalarials for these areas are mefloquine, or doxycycline, or the combination of atovaquone with proguanil.

The BNF works closely with the Health Protection Agency's Advisory Committee on Malaria Prevention to provide up-to-date advice. Expert members of the Committee also advise the BNF on the treatment of malaria in returning travellers.

Tricyclic antidepressants

Following reports of fatalities from overdose of certain tricyclic antidepressants, the BNF has further emphasised the dangers of using particular antidepressants for the management of depression (BNF section 4.3.1). Readers are advised that limited quantities of tricyclic antidepressants should be prescribed at any one time because their cardiovascular effects are dangerous in overdosage. An overview of the management of antidepressant poisoning is presented in the BNF section on emergency treatment of poisoning (pp. 31–2).

Advice on vaccination

Changes to the BCG vaccination programme announced by the Chief Medical Officer (PL/CMO/2005/3) are reflected in BNF 50 (pp. 606–7). The new programme is better targeted and no longer requires routine vaccination of all children; vaccination is required only for individuals at highest risk (because of local prevalence or prevalence in the region of their origin). The Heaf test for determining tuberculin reactivity is being phased out and is being replaced by the Mantoux test.

The advice on rabies vaccination has been completely revised. More detail is now provided on post-exposure prophylaxis of rabies (BNF 50 p. 617)

Feedback

We welcome constructive comments from readers. If you have suggestions on how the content of the BNF might be improved, please write to:

The Executive Editor
BNF
Royal Pharmaceutical Society of Great Britain
1 Lambeth High Street
LONDON SE1 7JN
Email: editor@bnf.org

To report a fault with your printed copy of the BNF please contact John Wilson on 020 7572 2354 or email john.wilson@rpsgb.org

Distribution of BNFs

The UK health departments distribute BNFs to NHS hospitals, doctors, dental surgeons, and community pharmacies. In England, BNFs are mailed individually to NHS general practitioners and community pharmacies; contact the NHS Responseline on 08701 555 455 for extra copies or changes relating to mailed BNFs.

Pharmaid

BNFs—even those that are 6–12 months old—are much in demand in many developing countries. The Pharmaid scheme of the Commonwealth Pharmaceutical Association dispatches old BNFs to Commonwealth countries. BNFs are collected from certain community pharmacies each year in November. For further details check the health press or contact:

Betty Falconbridge
Tel: 020 7572 2364
Email: admin@commonwealthpharmacy.org

unlikely to cause an allergic reaction—nevertheless it is wise to check the full formula of preparations which may contain allergenic fats or oils (including those for topical application, particularly if they are intended for use in the mouth or for application to the nasal mucosa).

Symptoms and signs

- Paraesthesia, flushing, and swelling of face
- Generalised itching, especially of hands and feet
- Bronchospasm and laryngospasm (with wheezing and difficulty in breathing)
- Rapid weak pulse together with fall in blood pressure and pallor; finally cardiac arrest

Management
First-line treatment includes securing the airway, restoration of blood pressure (laying the patient flat, raising the feet), and administration of **adrenaline** (epinephrine) injection. This is given **intramuscularly** in a dose of 500 micrograms (0.5 mL adrenaline injection 1 in 1000); a preparation delivering a dose of 300 micrograms (0.3 mL adrenaline injection 1 in 1000) is available for immediate *self-administration*. The dose is repeated if necessary at 5-minute intervals according to blood pressure, pulse and respiratory function. **Oxygen** administration is also of primary importance. An antihistamine (e.g. **chlorphenamine** (chlorpheniramine), given by slow intravenous injection in a dose of 10–20 mg, see p. 162) is a useful adjunctive treatment, given after adrenaline injection and continued for 24 to 48 hours to prevent relapse; chlorphenamine can alternatively be given by intramuscular injection. In patients receiving non-cardioselective beta-blockers severe anaphylaxis may not respond to adrenaline injection, calling for administration of **salbutamol** by intravenous injection (alternatively it can be given by intramuscular or subcutaneous injection); adrenaline may also cause severe hypertension in those receiving beta-blockers. Patients on tricyclic antidepressants are considerably more susceptible to cardiac arrhythmias calling for a much reduced dose of adrenaline (for other interactions, see Appendix 1 (sympathomimetics)).

An intravenous corticosteroid e.g. **hydrocortisone** (as sodium succinate) (section 6.3.2) in a dose of 100–300 mg is of secondary value in the initial management of anaphylactic shock because the onset of action is delayed for several hours, but it should be given to prevent further deterioration in severely affected patients.

> For further details on the management of anaphylaxis including details of paediatric doses of adrenaline, see p. 164

Asthma

Patients with asthma may have an attack while at the dental surgery. Most attacks will respond to 2 puffs of the patient's short-acting beta$_2$-adrenoceptor stimulant inhaler such as **salbutamol** 100 micrograms/puff (or **terbutaline** 250 micrograms/puff); further puffs are required if the patient does not respond rapidly. If the patient is unable to use the inhaler effectively further puffs should be given through a large-volume spacer device (or, if not available, through a plastic or paper cup with a hole in the bottom for the inhaler mouthpiece). If the response remains unsatisfactory, or if the patient develops tachycardia, then arrangements should be made to transfer the patient urgently to hospital. Whilst awaiting transfer, **oxygen** should be given with salbutamol 2.5–5 mg by nebuliser. If a nebuliser is unavailable, then 4–6 puffs of salbutamol inhaler or terbutaline inhaler should be given (preferably by a large-volume spacer device), and repeated every 10 minutes if necessary. Hydrocortisone (preferably as sodium succinate) 200 mg may be given by intravenous injection. If asthma is part of a more generalised anaphylactic reaction, an intramuscular injection of **adrenaline** (as detailed under Anaphylaxis above) should be given.

For a table describing the management of Acute Severe Asthma, see p. 141

Patients with severe chronic asthma or whose asthma has deteriorated previously during a dental procedure may require an increase in their prophylactic medication before a dental procedure. This should be discussed with the patient's medical practitioner and may include increasing the dose of inhaled or oral corticosteroid.

Cardiac emergencies

If there is a history of *angina* the patient will probably carry **glyceryl trinitrate** spray or tablets (or isosorbide dinitrate tablets) and should be allowed to use them. See also Coronary Artery Disease on p. 23.

Arrhythmias may lead to a sudden reduction in cardiac output with loss of consciousness. Medical assistance should be summoned. For advice on pacemaker interference, see also Pacemakers, p. 24.

The pain of *myocardial infarction* is similar to that of angina but generally more severe and more prolonged. For general advice see also Coronary Artery Disease on p. 23

Symptoms and signs of myocardial infarction

- Progressive onset of severe, crushing pain across front of chest; pain may radiate towards the shoulder and down arm, or into neck and jaw
- Skin becomes pale and clammy
- Nausea and vomiting are common
- Pulse may be weak and blood pressure may fall

Initial management of myocardial infarction
Call immediately for medical assistance and an ambulance, as appropriate.

Allow the patient to rest in the position that feels most comfortable; in the presence of breathlessness this is likely to be sitting position, whereas the syncopal patient should be laid flat; often an intermediate position (dictated by the patient) will be most appropriate.

Intramuscular injection of drugs does not provide useful relief of pain because absorption is too slow (particularly when cardiac output is reduced) but a mixture of **nitrous oxide** 50% and **oxygen** 50% can be effective if given continuously; it is safe in this situation.

Reassure the patient as much as possible to relieve

further anxiety. If available, aspirin in a single dose of 150–300 mg should be given. A note (to say that aspirin has been given) should be sent with the patient to the hospital. For further details on the initial management of myocardial infarction, see p. 127.

If the patient collapses and loses consciousness attempt standard resuscitation measures. For an **algorithm** of the procedure for **cardiopulmonary resuscitation**, see inside back cover.

Epileptic seizures

Patients with epilepsy must continue with their normal dosage of anticonvulsant drugs when attending for dental treatment. It is not uncommon for epileptic patients not to volunteer the information that they are epileptic but there should be little difficulty in recognising a tonic-clonic (grand mal) seizure.

Symptoms and signs

- There may be a brief warning (but variable)
- Sudden loss of consciousness, the patient becomes rigid, falls, may give a cry, and becomes cyanotic (tonic phase)
- After 30 seconds, there are jerking movements of the limbs; the tongue may be bitten (clonic phase)
- There may be frothing from mouth and urinary incontinence
- The seizure typically lasts a few minutes; the patient may then become flaccid but remain unconscious. After a variable time the patient regains consciousness but may remain confused for a while

Management

During a convulsion try to ensure that the patient is not at risk from injury but make no attempt to put anything in the mouth or between the teeth (in mistaken belief that this will protect the tongue).

Do not attempt to restrain convulsive movements.

After convulsive movements have subsided place the patient in the coma (recovery) position and check the airway.

After the convulsion the patient may be confused ('post-ictal confusion') and may need reassurance and sympathy. The patient should not be sent home until fully recovered but it is not necessary to seek medical attention or transfer to hospital unless the convulsion was atypical, prolonged (or repeated), or if injury occurred.

Medication should only be given if convulsive seizures are prolonged (convulsive movements lasting 5 minutes or longer) or repeated rapidly.

Intravenous administration of **diazepam** 10 mg is often effective but should be used with caution because of the risk of respiratory depression (for further details see p. 248). Alternatively, in prolonged or recurrent seizures, **midazolam** (section 15.1.4.1) can be given intranasally [unlicensed use] in a single dose of 200 micrograms/kg.

Partial seizures similarly need very little active management (in an automatism only a minimum amount of restraint should be applied to prevent injury). Again, the patient should be observed until post-ictal confusion has completely resolved.

Hypoglycaemia

Insulin-treated diabetic patients attending for dental treatment under general anaesthesia normally require admission to hospital; those only needing local anaesthesia should inject insulin and eat meals as normal. If food is omitted the blood glucose will fall to an abnormally low level (hypoglycaemia). Patients can often recognise the symptoms themselves and this state responds to sugar in water or a few lumps of sugar. Children may not have such prominent changes but may appear unduly lethargic.

Symptoms and signs

- Shaking and trembling
- Sweating
- 'Pins and needles' in lips and tongue
- Hunger
- Palpitation
- Headache (occasionally)
- Double vision
- Difficulty in concentration
- Slurring of speech
- Confusion
- Change of behaviour; truculence
- Unconsciousness

Management

Initially glucose 10–20 g is given by mouth either in liquid form or as granulated sugar or sugar lumps. Glucose 10 g is available from 2 teaspoons sugar, 3 sugar lumps, *GlucoGel*® (formerly known as *Hypostop*® *Gel*; glucose 9.2 g/23-g oral ampoule, available from British BioCell International), milk 200 mL, and non-diet versions of *Lucozade*® *Sparkling Glucose Drink* 50–55 mL, *Coca-Cola*® 90 mL, *Ribena*® *Original* 15 mL (to be diluted). If necessary this may be repeated in 10–15 minutes.

If hypoglycaemia causes unconsciousness, **glucagon** 1 mg (1 unit) should be given by intramuscular (or subcutaneous) injection; a child under 8 years or of body-weight under 25 kg should be given 500 micrograms. If glucagon is ineffective or contra-indicated, 50 mL of **glucose intravenous infusion 20%** can be given (for further details see p. 355). Alternatively, 25 mL of glucose intravenous infusion 50% may be given, but this higher concentration is viscous, making administration difficult; it is also more irritant. Once the patient regains consciousness oral glucose should be administered as above. The patient must be admitted to hospital if hypoglycaemia is caused by an oral antidiabetic drug.

Syncope

Insufficient blood supply to the brain results in loss of consciousness. The commonest cause is a vasovagal attack or simple faint (syncope) due to emotional stress.

Symptoms and signs

- Patient feels faint
- Pallor and sweating
- Yawning and slow pulse
- Nausea and vomiting
- Dilated pupils
- Muscular twitching

Management

- Lay the patient as flat as is reasonably comfortable and, in the absence of associated breathlessness, raise the legs to improve cerebral circulation
- Loosen any tight clothing around the neck
- Once consciousness is regained, give sugar in water or a cup of sweet tea

Other possible causes

Postural hypotension can be a consequence of rising abruptly or of standing upright for too long; antihypertensive drugs predispose to this. When rising, susceptible patients should take their time. Management is as for a vasovagal attack.

Under stressful circumstances, some patients hyperventilate. This gives rise to feelings of faintness but does not usually result in syncope. In most cases reassurance is all that is necessary; rebreathing from cupped hands or a bag may be helpful but calls for careful supervision.

Adrenal insufficiency or Arrhythmias are other possible causes, see p. 20 and below.

Medical problems in dental practice

Individuals presenting at the dental surgery may also suffer from an unrelated medical condition; this may require modification to the management of their dental condition. If the patient has systemic disease or is taking other medication, the matter may need to be discussed with the patient's general practitioner or hospital consultant.

For advice on adrenal insufficiency, anaphylaxis, asthma, cardiac emergencies, epileptic seizures, hypoglycaemia and syncope see under Medical Emergencies in Dental Practice.

Allergy

Patients should be asked about any history of allergy; those with a history of atopic allergy (asthma, eczema, hay fever, etc.) are at special risk. Those with a history of a severe allergy or of anaphylactic reactions are at high risk—it is essential to confirm that they are not allergic to any medication, or to any dental materials or equipment (including latex gloves). See also Anaphylaxis on p. 20.

Arrhythmias

Patients, especially those who suffer from heart failure or who have sustained a myocardial infarction, may have irregular cardiac rhythm. Atrial fibrillation is a common arrhythmia even in patients with normal hearts and is of little concern except that dental surgeons should be aware that such patients may be receiving anticoagulant therapy. The patient's medical practitioner should be asked whether any special precautions are necessary. Premedication (e.g. with temazepam) may be useful in some instances for very anxious patients.

See also Cardiac emergencies, p. 21 and Local Anaesthetics with Vasoconstrictors for Dental Anaesthesia, p. 640).

Breast-feeding

Evidence on the use of medicines during breast-feeding is often inadequate and care is required in choosing appropriate treatment. Appendix 5 includes information on drug treatment and breast-feeding.

Cardiac prostheses

For an account of the risk of infective endocarditis in patients with prosthetic heart valves and the recommendations of a Working Party of the British Society for Antimicrobial Chemotherapy, see Infective endocarditis, below. For advice on patients receiving anticoagulants, see Thromboembolic disease, below.

Coronary artery disease

Patients are vulnerable for at least 4 weeks following a myocardial infarction or following any sudden increase in the symptoms of angina. It would be advisable to check with the patient's medical practitioner before commencing treatment. See also Cardiac Emergencies on p. 21.

Treatment with low-dose aspirin (75–300 mg daily), clopidogrel, or dipyridamole should not be stopped routinely nor should the dose be altered before dental procedures.

A Working Party of the British Society for Antimicrobial Chemotherapy has not recommended antibiotic prophylaxis for patients following coronary artery bypass surgery.

Cyanotic heart disease

Patients with cyanotic heart disease are at risk in the dental chair, particularly if they have pulmonary hypertension. In such patients a syncopal reaction increases the shunt away from the lungs, causing more hypoxia which worsens the syncopal reaction—a vicious circle that may prove fatal. The advice of the cardiologist should be sought on any patient with congenital cyanotic heart disease. Treatment in hospital is more appropriate for some patients with this condition.

Hypertension

Patients with hypertension are likely to be receiving antihypertensive drugs such as those described in section 2.5. Their blood pressure may fall dangerously low under general anaesthesia, which should only be administered in hospital where appropriate precautions can be taken. See also under Local Anaesthetics with Vasoconstrictors for Dental Anaesthesia on p. 640.

Immunosuppression and indwelling intraperitoneal catheters

See Table 2, section 5.1

Infective endocarditis

Although almost any dental procedure is capable of causing bacteraemia, infective endocarditis is a rare complication even in susceptible patients. It is virtually impossible, therefore, to assess the relative effectiveness of different prophylactic regimens; nevertheless, there is now some consensus among cardiologists and microbiologists. The recommendations of a Working Party of the British Society for Antimicrobial Chemotherapy are reflected in Table

2, section 5.1. Alternative guidelines have been produced and may be in use in some settings.

PATIENTS AT RISK. Patients with *cardiac defects* (congenital, rheumatic, etc.) are at risk from infective endocarditis following dental procedures. Those who have a *history of infective endocarditis* in the past are particularly at risk. There is no evidence that patients with *prosthetic heart valves* are any more susceptible to infective endocarditis after dental operations than those with damaged natural valves, but if it develops treatment may be more difficult.

All patients must be questioned about any history of heart defects or rheumatic fever and especially whether they have previously had infective endocarditis. Turbulence around the valves has been identified as a risk factor. Heart murmurs in children are often of no significance but whenever there is any doubt a cardiologist should be consulted. The peak incidence of infective endocarditis is after the sixth decade.

The following patients, who are considered to be at *special risk* should be referred to hospital for endocarditis prophylaxis:

- patients with prosthetic valves who are to have a general anaesthetic;
- patients who are allergic to penicillin who are to have a general anaesthetic;
- patients who have had more than a single dose of a penicillin in the previous month who are to have a general anaesthetic;
- all patients who have had a previous episode of endocarditis.

PROCEDURES THAT NEED COVER. Dental procedures that require antibacterial prophylaxis include:

- extractions
- scaling[1]
- surgery involving gingival tissues

REDUCTION OF ORAL SEPSIS. The frequency and severity of bacteraemia is related to the severity of the gingival inflammation. The highest possible standards of oral hygiene in patients at risk reduces:

- need for dental extractions or other surgery;
- chances of severe bacteraemia if dental surgery is needed;
- possibility of 'spontaneous' bacteraemia.

Application of an antiseptic such as chlorhexidine gluconate gel 1% to the dry gingival margin or the use of a chlorhexidine gluconate mouthwash (0.2%) 5 minutes before the dental procedure may reduce the possibility of bacteraemia and may be used to supplement antibiotic prophylaxis in those at risk.

Intraligamentary (periodontal) injection of local anaesthetic solutions may carry a risk of severe bacteraemia and is best avoided in patients susceptible to endocarditis.

POSTOPERATIVE CARE. Patients at risk of endocarditis should be warned to report to the doctor or dental surgeon any minor illness that develops after dental treatment, whether or not antibacterials have been given, because infective endocarditis has an insidious onset and treatment may fail if diagnosis is delayed. If endocarditis develops it is likely to be within a month of dental treatment.

PATIENTS ON ANTICOAGULANT THERAPY. The prophylactic doses of the antibacterials (see Table 2, section 5.1) are unlikely to alter the International Normalised Ratio (INR) in patients receiving oral anticoagulants. Nevertheless, it is prudent to measure the INR again a few days after the procedure especially if a general anaesthetic was used.

For general advice on dental surgery in patients receiving oral anticoagulant therapy see Thromboembolic Disease, below.

Joint prostheses

See Table 2, section 5.1

Liver disease

Liver disease may alter the response to drugs and drug prescribing should be kept to a minimum in patients with severe liver disease. Problems are likely mainly in patients with *jaundice*, *ascites*, or evidence of *encephalopathy*.

For a table of drugs to be avoided or used with caution in liver disease see Appendix 2.

Pacemakers

Pacemakers prevent asystole or severe bradycardia. Some ultrasonic scalers, electronic apex locators, electro-analgesic devices, and electrocautery devices interfere with the normal function of pacemakers (including shielded pacemakers) and should not be used. The manufacturer's literature should be consulted whenever possible. If severe bradycardia occurs in a patient fitted with a pacemaker, electrical equipment should be switched off and the patient placed supine with the legs elevated. If the patient loses consciousness and the pulse remains slow or is absent, cardiopulmonary resuscitation (see inside back cover) may be needed. Call immediately for medical assistance and an ambulance, as appropriate.

A Working Party of the British Society for Antimicrobial Chemotherapy does not recommend antibacterial prophylaxis for patients with pacemakers.

Pregnancy

Drugs taken during pregnancy can be harmful to the fetus and should be prescribed only if the expected benefit to the mother is thought to be greater than the risk to the fetus; all drugs should be avoided if possible during the first trimester.

Appendix 4 includes information on drug treatment during pregnancy

Renal impairment

The use of drugs in patients with reduced renal function can give rise to many problems. Many of these problems can be avoided by reducing the dose or by using alternative drugs.

Special care is required in renal transplantation and immunosuppressed patients; if necessary such patients should be referred to specialists.

For a table of drugs to be avoided or used with caution in renal impairment see Appendix 3.

1. Prophylaxis is considered appropriate for all scaling and other procedures involving the periodontium

Thromboembolic disease

Patients receiving **heparin** or oral anticoagulants such as **warfarin**, **acenocoumarol** (nicoumalone), or **phenindione** may be liable to excessive bleeding after extraction of teeth or other dental surgery. Often dental surgery can be delayed until the anticoagulant therapy has been completed.

For a patient requiring long-term oral anticoagulant therapy, the patient's medical practitioner should be consulted and the International Normalised Ratio (INR) should be assessed preferably no more than 24 hours before the dental procedure (no more than 72 hours beforehand if INR stable). Patients requiring minor dental procedures *without extractions* who have an INR below 4.0 may continue warfarin without dose adjustment. Patients requiring *extractions* and who have an INR below 3.0 may continue warfarin without dose adjustment. If possible, a single extraction should be done first; if this goes well further teeth may be extracted at subsequent visits (two or three at a time). Measures should be taken to minimise bleeding during and after the procedure. Scaling and root planing should initially be restricted to a limited area to assess the potential for bleeding. Some dental surgeons suture the gum over the socket to hold in place a haemostatic such as oxidised cellulose, collagen sponge or resorbable gelatin sponge. For a patient on long-term anticoagulation treatment, the advice of the clinician responsible for the patients's anticoagulation should be sought if:

- the INR is unstable, or if the INR is greater than 4.0, or for minor dental procedures with extractions if the INR is greater than 3.0;
- the patient has thrombocytopenia, haemophilia, or other disorders of haemostasis, or suffers from liver impairment, alcoholism, or renal failure;
- the patient is receiving cytotoxic drugs or radiotherapy.

Intramuscular injections are *contra-indicated* in patients on anticoagulant therapy, and in those with any disorder of haemostasis.

A local anaesthetic containing a vasoconstrictor should be given by infiltration or by intraligamentary injection if possible. If regional nerve blocks cannot be avoided the local anaesthetic should be given cautiously using an aspirating syringe.

Drugs which have potentially serious interactions with anticoagulants include aspirin and other NSAIDs, carbamazepine, imidazole and triazole antifungals (including miconazole), erythromycin, clarithromycin, and metronidazole; for details of these and other interactions with anticoagulants, see Appendix 1 (heparin, phenindione, warfarin and other coumarins). Although studies have failed to demonstrate an interaction, common experience in anticoagulant clinics is that the INR can be altered following a course of an oral broad-spectrum antibiotic, such as ampicillin or amoxicillin.

Drugs and sport

UK Sport advises that athletes are personally responsible should a prohibited substance be detected in their body. Information and advice, including the status of specific drugs in sport, can be obtained at www.uksport.gov.uk An advice card listing examples of permitted and prohibited substances is available from:

Drug-Free Sport
UK Sport
40 Bernard Street
London WC1N 1ST
drug-free@uksport.gov.uk

A similar card detailing classes of drugs and doping methods prohibited in football is available from the Football Association.

General Medical Council's advice. Doctors who prescribe or collude in the provision of drugs or treatment with the intention of improperly enhancing an individual's performance in sport would be contravening the GMC's guidance, and such actions would usually raise a question of a doctor's continued registration. This does not preclude the provision of any care or treatment where the doctor's intention is to protect or improve the patient's health.

Emergency treatment of poisoning

These notes provide only an overview of the treatment of poisoning and it is strongly recommended that either a **poisons information centre** or **TOXBASE** (see below) be consulted where there is doubt about the degree of risk or about management.

HOSPITAL ADMISSION. All patients who show features of poisoning should generally be admitted to hospital. Patients who have taken poisons with delayed action should also be admitted, even if they appear well. Delayed-action poisons include aspirin, iron, paracetamol, tricyclic antidepressants, co-phenotrope (diphenoxylate with atropine, *Lomotil*®), and paraquat; the effects of modified-release preparations are also delayed. A note of all relevant information including what treatment has been given should accompany the patient to hospital.

Further information and advice

TOXBASE, the primary clinical toxicology database of the National Poisons Information Service, is available on the Internet to registered users at www.spib.axl.co.uk. It provides information about routine diagnosis, treatment and management of patients exposed to drugs, household products, and industrial and agricultural chemicals.

Specialist information and advice on the treatment of poisoning is available from the **UK National Poisons Information Service** through the local poisons information centre on the following number:
Tel: 0870 600 6266

Advice on laboratory analytical services can be obtained from TOXBASE or from a poisons information centre.

Help on identifying capsules or tablets may be available from a regional medicines information centre (see inside front cover).

> The **poisons information centres** (Tel: 0870 600 6266) will provide specialist advice on all aspects of poisoning day and night

General care

It is often impossible to establish with certainty the identity of the poison and the size of the dose. Fortunately this is not usually important because only a few poisons (such as opioids, paracetamol, and iron) have specific antidotes; few patients require active removal of the poison. In most patients, treatment is directed at managing symptoms as they arise. Nevertheless, knowledge of the type and timing of poisoning can help in anticipating the course of events. All relevant information should be sought from the poisoned individual and from carers or parents. However, such information should be interpreted with care because it may not be complete or entirely reliable. Sometimes symptoms arise from other illnesses and patients should be assessed carefully. Accidents may involve a number of domestic and industrial products (the contents of which are not generally known). A **poisons information centre** should be consulted where there is doubt about any aspect of suspected poisoning.

Respiration

Respiration is often impaired in unconscious patients. An obstructed airway requires immediate attention. In the absence of trauma, the airway should be opened with simple measures such as chin lift or jaw thrust. An oropharyngeal or nasopharyngeal airway may be useful in patients with reduced consciousness to prevent obstruction, provided ventilation is adequate. Intubation and ventilation should be considered in patients whose airway cannot be protected or who have inadequate ventilation because of respiratory acidosis; such patients should be monitored in a critical care area.

Most poisons that impair consciousness also depress respiration. Assisted ventilation by mouth-to-mouth or *Ambu-bag* inflation may be needed. Oxygen is not a substitute for adequate ventilation, though it should be given in the highest concentration possible in poisoning with carbon monoxide and irritant gases.

Respiratory stimulants do not help and should be **avoided**.

Blood pressure

Hypotension is common in severe poisoning with central nervous system depressants. A systolic blood pressure of less than 70 mmHg may lead to irreversible brain damage or renal tubular necrosis. Hypotension should be corrected initially by tilting down the head of the bed and administration of either sodium chloride intravenous infusion or a colloidal infusion. Vasoconstrictor sympathomimetics (section 2.7.2) are rarely required and their use may be discussed with a poisons information centre.

Fluid depletion without hypotension is common after prolonged coma and after aspirin poisoning due to vomiting, sweating, and hyperpnoea.

Hypertension, often transient, occurs less frequently than hypotension in poisoning; it may be associated with sympathomimetic drugs such as amphetamines, phencyclidine, and cocaine.

Heart

Cardiac conduction defects and arrhythmias may occur in acute poisoning, notably with tricyclic antidepressants, some antipsychotics, some antihistamines, and co-proxamol. Arrhythmias often respond to correction of underlying hypoxia, acidosis, or other biochemical abnormalities. Ventricular arrhythmias that have been confirmed by ECG and which are causing serious hypotension require treatment. If the QT interval is prolonged, specialist advice should be sought because the use of some anti-arrhythmic drugs may be inappropriate. Supraventricular arrhythmias are seldom life-threatening and drug treatment is best withheld until the patient reaches hospital.

Body temperature

Hypothermia may develop in patients of any age who have been deeply unconscious for some hours particularly following overdose with barbiturates or phenothiazines. It may be missed unless core temperature is measured using a low-reading rectal thermometer or by some other means. Hypothermia is best treated by wrapping the patient (e.g. in a 'space blanket') to conserve body heat.

Hyperthermia can develop in patients taking CNS stimulants; children and the elderly are also at risk when taking therapeutic doses of drugs with antimuscarinic properties. Hyperthermia is initially managed by removing all unnecessary clothing and using a fan. Sponging with tepid water will promote evaporation; iced water should **not** be used. Advice should be sought from a poisons information centre on the management of severe hyperthermia resulting from conditions such as the serotonin syndrome.

Both hypothermia and hyperthermia require **urgent** hospitalisation for assessment and supportive treatment.

Convulsions

Single short-lived convulsions do not require treatment. If convulsions are protracted or recur frequently, lorazepam 4 mg or diazepam (preferably as emulsion) up to 10 mg should be given by slow intravenous injection into a large vein; the benzodiazepines should not be given intramuscularly.

Removal and elimination

Removal from the gastro-intestinal tract

Gastric lavage is rarely required and for substances that cannot be removed effectively by other means (e.g. iron), it should be considered only if a life-threatening amount has been ingested within the previous hour. It should be carried out only if the airway can be protected adequately. Gastric lavage is contra-indicated if a corrosive substance or a petroleum distillate has been ingested but it may occasionally be considered in patients who have ingested drugs that are not absorbed by charcoal, such as iron or lithium. Induction of *emesis* (e.g. with ipecacuanha) is **not** recommended because there is no evidence that it affects absorption and it may increase the risk of aspiration.

Whole bowel irrigation (by means of a bowel cleansing solution) has been used in poisoning with certain modified-release or enteric-coated formulations, in severe poisoning with iron and lithium salts, and if illicit drugs are carried in the gastro-intestinal tract ('body-packing'). However, it is not clear that the procedure improves outcome and advice should be sought from a poisons information centre.

Prevention of absorption

Given by mouth, **activated charcoal** can bind many poisons in the gastro-intestinal system, thereby *reducing their absorption*. The **sooner** it is given the **more effective** it is, but it may still be effective up to 1 hour after ingestion of the poison—longer in the case of modified-release preparations or of drugs with antimuscarinic (anticholinergic) properties. It is relatively safe and is particularly useful for the prevention of absorption of poisons which are toxic in small amounts, e.g. antidepressants.

For the use of charcoal in active elimination techniques, see below.

CHARCOAL, ACTIVATED

Indications: adsorption of poisons in the gastro-intestinal system; see also active elimination techniques, below

Cautions: drowsy or comatose patient (risk of aspiration); reduced gastro-intestinal motility (risk of obstruction); not for poisoning with petroleum distillates, corrosive substances, alcohols, clofenotane (dicophane, DDT), malathion, and metal salts including iron and lithium salts

Side-effects: black stools

Dose: see under preparations below

Actidose-Aqua® Advance (Cambridge)
Oral suspension, activated charcoal, net price 50-g pack (240 mL) = £11.63
NOTE. The brand name *Actidose-Aqua®* was formerly used
Dose: reduction of absorption, 50–100 g; INFANT under 1 year 1 g/kg (approx. 5 mL/kg), CHILD 1–12 years 25–50 g
Active elimination (see below for ADULT dose); INFANT under 1 year, 1 g/kg (approx. 5 mL/kg) every 4–6 hours; CHILD 1–12 years, 25–50 g every 4–6 hours

Carbomix® (Meadow)
Powder, activated charcoal, net price 25-g pack = £8.50, 50-g pack = £11.90
Dose: reduction of absorption, 50 g, repeated if necessary; CHILD under 12 years 25 g (50 g in severe poisoning)
Active elimination, see below

Charcodote® (PLIVA)
Oral suspension, activated charcoal, net price 50-g pack = £11.88
Dose: reduction of absorption, 50 g; CHILD under 12 years 25 g (50 g in severe poisoning)
Active elimination, see below

Active elimination techniques

Repeated doses of **activated charcoal** by mouth *enhance the elimination* of some drugs after they have been absorbed; repeated doses are given after overdosage with:

Carbamazepine
Dapsone
Phenobarbital
Quinine
Theophylline

The usual adult dose of activated charcoal is 50 g initially then 50 g every 4 hours. Vomiting should be treated (e.g. with an anti-emetic drug) since it may reduce the efficacy of charcoal treatment. In cases of intolerance, the dose may be reduced and the frequency increased (e.g. 25 g every 2 hours *or*

12.5 g every hour) but this may compromise efficacy.

Other techniques intended to enhance the elimination of poisons after absorption are only practicable in hospital and are only suitable for a small number of severely poisoned patients. Moreover, they only apply to a limited number of poisons. Examples include:

- haemodialysis for salicylates, phenobarbital, methyl alcohol (methanol), ethylene glycol, and lithium;
- alkanisation of the urine for salicylates and phenoxyacetate herbicides (e.g. 2,4-dichlorophenoxyacetic acid).

Forced alkaline diuresis is no longer recommended.

Specific drugs

Alcohol

Acute intoxication with alcohol (ethanol) is common in adults but also occurs in children. The features include ataxia, dysarthria, nystagmus, and drowsiness, which may progress to coma, with hypotension and acidosis. Aspiration of vomit is a special hazard and hypoglycaemia may occur in children and some adults. Patients are managed supportively with particular attention to maintaining a clear airway and measures to reduce the risk of aspiration of gastric contents. The blood glucose is measured and glucose given if indicated.

> The **poisons information centres** (Tel: 0870 600 6266) will provide specialist advice on all aspects of poisoning day and night

Analgesics (non-opioid)

ASPIRIN. The chief features of salicylate poisoning are hyperventilation, tinnitus, deafness, vasodilatation, and sweating. Coma is uncommon but indicates very severe poisoning. The associated acid-base disturbances are complex.

Treatment must be in hospital where plasma salicylate, pH, and electrolytes can be measured; absorption of aspirin may be slow and the plasma-salicylate concentration may continue to rise for several hours, requiring repeated measurement of plasma-salicylate concentration. Fluid losses are replaced and sodium bicarbonate (1.26%) given to enhance urinary salicylate excretion when the plasma-salicylate concentration is greater than:

500 mg/litre (3.6 mmol/litre) in adults *or*
350 mg/litre (2.5 mmol/litre) in children.

Haemodialysis is the treatment of choice for severe salicylate poisoning and should be considered when the plasma-salicylate concentration exceeds 700 mg/litre (5.1 mmol/litre) or in the presence of severe metabolic acidosis.

NSAIDS. Mefenamic acid has important consequences in overdosage because it can cause convulsions, which if prolonged or recurrent, require treatment with intravenous lorazepam or diazepam.

Ibuprofen may cause nausea, vomiting, and tinnitus, but more serious toxicity is very uncommon. Activated charcoal followed by symptomatic measures are indicated if more than 400 mg/kg has been ingested within the preceding hour, followed by symptomatic measures.

PARACETAMOL. As little as 10–15 g (20–30 tablets) or 150 mg/kg of paracetamol taken within 24 hours may cause severe hepatocellular necrosis and, much less frequently, renal tubular necrosis. Nausea and vomiting, the only early features of poisoning, usually settle within 24 hours. Persistence beyond this time, often associated with the onset of right subcostal pain and tenderness, usually indicates development of hepatic necrosis. Liver damage is maximal 3–4 days after ingestion and may lead to encephalopathy, haemorrhage, hypoglycaemia, cerebral oedema, and death.

Therefore, despite a lack of significant early symptoms, patients who have taken an overdose of paracetamol should be transferred to hospital urgently.

Administration of activated charcoal should be considered if paracetamol in excess of 150 mg/kg or 12 g **whichever is the smaller**, is thought to have been ingested within the previous hour.

Acetylcysteine protects the liver if infused within 24 hours of ingesting paracetamol. It is most effective if given within 8 hours of ingestion after which effectiveness declines sharply and if more than 24 hours have elapsed advice should be sought from a poisons information centre or from a liver unit on the management of serious liver damage. In remote areas **methionine** (2.5 g) by mouth is an alternative if acetylcysteine cannot be given promptly. Once the patient reaches hospital the need to continue treatment with the antidote will be assessed from the plasma-paracetamol concentration (related to the time from ingestion).

Patients at risk of liver damage and therefore requiring treatment can be identified from a single measurement of the plasma-paracetamol concentration, related to the time from ingestion, provided this time interval is not less than 4 hours; earlier samples may be misleading. The concentration is plotted on a paracetamol treatment graph of a reference line ('normal treatment line') joining plots of 200 mg/litre (1.32 mmol/litre) at 4 hours and 6.25 mg/litre (0.04 mmol/litre) at 24 hours (see p. 30). Those whose plasma-paracetamol concentration is above the *normal treatment line* are treated with acetylcysteine by intravenous infusion (or, if acetylcysteine is not available, with methionine by mouth, provided the overdose has been taken **within 10–12 hours** *and* the patient is not vomiting).

Patients on enzyme-inducing drugs (e.g. carbamazepine, phenobarbital, phenytoin, primidone, rifampicin, alcohol, and St John's wort) or who are malnourished (e.g. in anorexia, in alcoholism, or those who are HIV-positive) may develop toxicity at **lower** plasma-paracetamol concentration and should be treated if the concentration is above the *high-risk treatment line* (which joins plots that are at 50% of the plasma-paracetamol concentrations of the normal treatment line).

The prognostic accuracy of plasma-paracetamol concentration taken after 15 hours is uncertain but a concentration above the relevant treatment line should be regarded as carrying a serious risk of liver damage.

Plasma-paracetamol concentration may be difficult to interpret when paracetamol has been ingested over

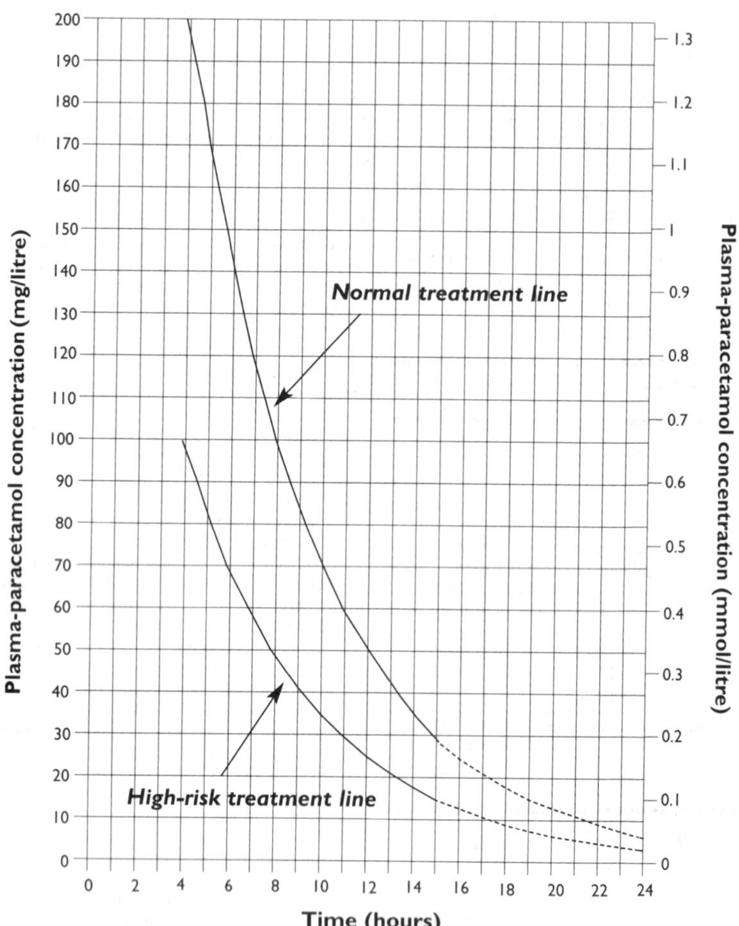

Patients whose plasma-paracetamol concentrations are above the **normal treatment line** should be treated with acetylcysteine by intravenous infusion (or, if acetylcysteine cannot be used, with methionine by mouth, provided the overdose has been taken **within 10–12 hours** and the patient is not vomiting).

Patients on enzyme-inducing drugs (e.g. carbamazepine, phenobarbital, phenytoin, primidone, rifampicin, alcohol, and St John's wort) or who are malnourished (e.g. in anorexia, in alcoholism, or those who are HIV-positive) should be treated if their plasma-paracetamol concentration is above the **high-risk treatment line**.

The prognostic accuracy after 15 hours is uncertain but a plasma-paracetamol concentration above the relevant treatment line should be regarded as carrying a serious risk of liver damage.

Graph reproduced courtesy of University of Wales College of Medicine Therapeutics and Toxicology Centre

several hours. If there is doubt about timing or the need for treatment then the patient should be treated with an antidote.

See also Co-proxamol, under Analgesics (opioid).

ACETYLCYSTEINE

Indications: paracetamol overdosage, see notes above

Cautions: asthma (see side-effects below but do not delay treatment)

Side-effects: hypersensitivity-like reactions managed by reducing infusion rate or suspending until reaction settled—contact poisons information centre (rash also managed by giving antihistamine and acute asthma by giving a short-acting $beta_2$ agonist)

Dose: *by intravenous infusion*, ADULT and CHILD, initially 150 mg/kg over 15 minutes, then 50 mg/kg over 4 hours then 100 mg/kg over 16 hours

ADMINISTRATION. Dilute requisite dose in glucose intravenous infusion 5% as follows: ADULT and CHILD over 12 years, initially 200 mL given over 15 minutes, then 500 mL over 4 hours, then 1 litre over 16 hours; CHILD under 12 years body-weight over 20 kg, initially 100 mL given over 15 minutes, then 250 mL over 4 hours, then 500 mL over 16 hours; CHILD body-weight under 20 kg, initially 3 mL/kg given over 15 minutes, then 7 mL/kg over 4 hours, then 14 mL/kg over 16 hours

NOTE. Manufacturer also recommends other infusion fluids, but glucose 5% is preferable

Acetylcysteine (Non-proprietary) PoM
Injection, acetylcysteine 200 mg/mL, net price 10-mL amp = £2.50

Parvolex® (Celltech) PoM
Injection, acetylcysteine 200 mg/mL, net price 10-mL amp = £2.50

METHIONINE

Indications: paracetamol overdosage, see notes above
Cautions: hepatic impairment (Appendix 2)
Side-effects: nausea, vomiting, drowsiness, irritability
Dose: ADULT and CHILD over 6 years initially 2.5 g, followed by 3 further doses of 2.5 g every 4 hours, CHILD under 6 years initially 1 g, followed by 3 further doses of 1 g every 4 hours

Methionine (Celltech)
Tablets, DL-methionine 250 mg, net price 200-tab pack = £66.05

Analgesics (opioid)

Opioids (narcotic analgesics) cause coma, respiratory depression, and pinpoint pupils. The specific antidote **naloxone** is indicated if there is coma or bradypnoea. Since naloxone has a shorter duration of action than many opioids, close monitoring and repeated injections are necessary according to the respiratory rate and depth of coma. Where repeated administration of naloxone is required, it may be given by continuous intravenous infusion instead and the rate of infusion adjusted according to vital signs. The effects of some opioids, such as buprenorphine, are only partially reversed by naloxone. Dextropropoxyphene and methadone have very long durations of action; patients may need to be monitored for long periods following large overdoses.

CO-PROXAMOL. A combination of dextropropoxyphene and paracetamol (co-proxamol) is frequently taken in overdosage and is the most frequent prescription product to cause death. The initial features are those of acute opioid overdosage with coma, respiratory depression, and pinpoint pupils. Patients may die of acute cardiovascular collapse before reaching hospital (particularly if alcohol has also been consumed) unless adequately resuscitated.

Naloxone reverses the opioid effects of dextropropoxyphene; the long duration of action of dextropropoxyphene calls for prolonged monitoring and further doses of naloxone may be required . Norpropoxyphene, a metabolite of dextropropoxyphene, also has cardiotoxic effects which may require treatment with **sodium bicarbonate**, or **magnesium sulphate**, or both; arrhythmias may occur for up to 12 hours. Paracetamol hepatotoxicity may develop later and should be anticipated and treated as indicated above.

NALOXONE HYDROCHLORIDE

Indications: overdosage with opioids; postoperative respiratory depression (section 15.1.7)
Cautions: physical dependence on opioids; cardiac irritability; naloxone is short-acting, see notes above
Dose: *by intravenous injection*, 0.4–2 mg repeated at intervals of 2–3 minutes to a max. of 10 mg if respiratory function does not improve (then question diagnosis); CHILD 10 micrograms/kg; subsequent dose of 100 micrograms/kg if no response

By subcutaneous or intramuscular injection, ADULT and CHILD dose as for intravenous injection but use only if intravenous route not feasible (onset of action slower)

By continuous intravenous infusion using an infusion pump, 10 mg diluted in 50 mL intravenous infusion solution [unlicensed concentration] at a rate adjusted according to response (initial rate may be set at 60% of initial intravenous injection dose (see above) and infused over 1 hour)

IMPORTANT. Doses used in acute opioid overdosage may not be appropriate for the management of opioid-induced respiratory depression and sedation in those receiving palliative care and in chronic opioid use, see also section 15.1.7 for management of postoperative respiratory depression

Naloxone (Non-proprietary) PoM
Injection, naloxone hydrochloride 400 micrograms/mL, net price 1-mL amp = £4.10; 1 mg/mL, 2-mL prefilled syringe = £6.61

Minijet® **Naloxone** (Celltech) PoM
Injection, naloxone hydrochloride 400 micrograms/mL, net price 1-mL disposable syringe = £5.57; 2-mL disposable syringe = £10.71

Narcan® (Bristol-Myers Squibb) PoM
Injection, naloxone hydrochloride 400 micrograms/mL, net price 1-mL amp = £5.12

■ Neonatal preparations
Section 15.1.7

The **poisons information centres** (Tel: 0870 600 6266) will provide specialist advice on all aspects of poisoning day and night

Antidepressants

Tricyclic and related antidepressants cause dry mouth, coma of varying degree, hypotension, hypothermia, hyperreflexia, extensor plantar responses, convulsions, respiratory failure, cardiac conduction defects, and arrhythmias. Dilated pupils and urinary retention also occur. Metabolic acidosis may complicate severe poisoning; delirium with confusion, agitation, and visual and auditory hallucinations, are common during recovery.

Transfer to hospital is strongly advised in case of poisoning by *tricyclic and related antidepressants* but symptomatic treatment and activated charcoal may be given before transfer. Supportive measures to ensure a clear airway and adequate ventilation during transfer are mandatory. Intravenous diazepam (preferably in emulsion form) may be required for control of convulsions. Although arrhythmias are worrying, some will respond to correction of hypoxia and acidosis. The use of anti-arrhythmic drugs is best avoided but intravenous infusion of sodium bicarbonate can arrest arrythmias or prevent them in those with an extended QRS duration. Diazepam given by mouth is usually adequate to sedate delirious patients but large doses may be required.

Antimalarials

Overdosage with chloroquine and hydroxychloroquine is extremely hazardous and difficult to treat. Urgent advice from a poisons information centre is essential. Life-threatening features include arrhythmias (which can have a very rapid onset) and convulsions (which can be intractable). Quinine overdosage is also a severe hazard and calls for urgent advice from a poisons information centre.

Beta-blockers

Therapeutic overdosages with beta-blockers may cause lightheadedness, dizziness, and possibly syncope as a result of bradycardia and hypotension; heart failure may be precipitated or exacerbated. These complications are most likely in patients with conduction system disorders or impaired myocardial function. Bradycardia is the most common arrhythmia caused by beta-blockers, but sotalol may induce ventricular tachyarrhythmias (sometimes of the torsades de pointes type). The effects of massive overdosage may vary from one beta-blocker to another; propranolol overdosage in particular may cause coma and convulsions.

Acute massive overdosage must be managed in hospital and expert advice should be obtained. Maintenance of a clear airway and adequate ventilation is mandatory. An intravenous injection of atropine is required to treat bradycardia and hypotension (3 mg for an adult, 40 micrograms/kg for a child). Cardiogenic shock unresponsive to atropine is probably best treated with an intravenous injection of glucagon 2–10 mg (CHILD 50–150 micrograms/kg) [unlicensed indication and dose] in glucose 5% (with precautions to protect the airway in case of vomiting) followed by an intravenous infusion of 50 micrograms/kg/hour. If glucagon is not available, intravenous isoprenaline [special order only] is an alternative. A cardiac pacemaker may be used to increase the heart rate.

Calcium-channel blockers

Features of calcium-channel blocker poisoning include nausea, vomiting, dizziness, agitation, confusion, and coma in severe poisoning. Metabolic acidosis and hyperglycaemia may occur. Verapamil and diltiazem have a profound cardiac depressant effect causing hypotension and arrhythmias including complete heart block and asystole. The dihydropyridine calcium-channel blockers cause severe hypotension secondary to profound peripheral vasodilatation.

Activated charcoal is given if the patient presents within 1 hour of overdosage with a calcium-channel blocker; repeated doses of activated charcoal are considered if a modified-release preparation is involved. In patients with significant features of poisoning, calcium chloride or calcium gluconate (section 9.5.1.1) is given by injection; atropine is given to correct symptomatic bradycardia. For the management of hypotension, the choice of inotropic sympathomimetic depends on whether hypotension is secondary to vasodilation or to myocardial depression and advice should be sought from a poisons information centre.

Hypnotics and anxiolytics

BENZODIAZEPINES. Benzodiazepines taken alone cause drowsiness, ataxia, dysarthria, and occasionally minor and short-lived depression of consciousness. They potentiate the effects of other central nervous system depressants taken concomitantly. Use of the benzodiazepine antagonist flumazenil can be hazardous, particularly in mixed overdoses involving tricyclic antidepressants or in benzodiazepine-dependent patients. Flumazenil should be used on **expert advice** only.

Iron salts

Iron poisoning is commonest in childhood and is usually accidental. The symptoms are nausea, vomiting, abdominal pain, diarrhoea, haematemesis, and rectal bleeding. Hypotension, coma, and hepatocellular necrosis occur later. Mortality is reduced with intensive and specific therapy with **desferrioxamine**, which chelates iron. The stomach should be emptied by gastric lavage (with a wide-bore tube) within 1 hour of ingesting a significant quantity of iron or if radiography reveals tablets in the stomach; whole bowel irrigation may be considered in severe poisoning but advice should be sought from a poisons information centre. The serum-iron concentration is measured as an emergency and intravenous desferrioxamine given to chelate absorbed iron in excess of the expected iron binding capacity. In **severe toxicity** intravenous desferrioxamine should be given *immediately* without waiting for the result of the serum-iron measurement (contact a poisons information centre for advice).

DESFERRIOXAMINE MESILATE

(Deferoxamine Mesilate)

Indications: iron poisoning; chronic iron overload (section 9.1.3)

Cautions: section 9.1.3

Side-effects: section 9.1.3

Dose: *by continuous intravenous infusion*, ADULT and CHILD up to 15 mg/kg/hour; max. 80 mg/kg in 24 hours (in severe cases, higher doses on advice from a poisons information centre)

■ Preparations

Section 9.1.3

Lithium

Most cases of lithium intoxication occur as a complication of long-term therapy and are caused by reduced excretion of the drug due to a variety of factors including dehydration, deterioration of renal function, infections, and co-administration of diuretics or NSAIDs (or other drugs that interact). Acute deliberate overdoses may also occur with delayed onset of symptoms (12 hours or more) due to slow entry of lithium into the tissues and continuing absorption from modified-release formulations.

The early clinical features are non-specific and may include apathy and restlessness which could be confused with mental changes due to the patient's depressive illness. Vomiting, diarrhoea, ataxia, weakness, dysarthria, muscle twitching, and tremor may follow. Severe poisoning is associated with convulsions, coma, renal failure, electrolyte imbalance, dehydration, and hypotension.

Therapeutic lithium concentrations are within the range of 0.4–1.0 mmol/litre; concentrations in excess of 2.0 mmol/litre are usually associated with serious toxicity and such cases may need treatment with haemodialysis (if there is renal failure). In acute overdosage much higher serum concentrations may be present without features of toxicity and all that is usually necessary is to take measures to increase urine production (e.g. by ensuring adequate fluid intake; but avoid diuretics). Otherwise treatment is supportive with special regard to electrolyte balance, renal function, and control of convulsions. Whole bowel irrigation should be considered for significant ingestion, but advice should be sought from a poisons information centre.

Phenothiazines and related drugs

Phenothiazines cause less depression of consciousness and respiration than other sedatives. Hypotension, hypothermia, sinus tachycardia, and arrhythmias (particularly with thioridazine) may complicate poisoning. Dystonic reactions can occur with therapeutic doses, (particularly with prochlorperazine and trifluoperazine) and convulsions may occur in severe cases. Arrhythmias may respond to correction of hypoxia, acidosis and other biochemical abnormalities but specialist advice should be sought if arrhythmias result from a prolonged QT interval; the use of some anti-arrhythmic drugs may worsen such arrhythmias. Dystonic reactions are rapidly abolished by injection of drugs such as benzatropine or diazepam (section 4.8.2, emulsion preferred).

Stimulants

AMPHETAMINES. These cause wakefulness, excessive activity, paranoia, hallucinations, and hypertension followed by exhaustion, convulsions, hyperthermia, and coma. The early stages can be controlled by diazepam or lorazepam; advice should be sought from a poisons information centre on the management of hypertension. Later, tepid sponging, anticonvulsants, and artificial respiration may be needed.

COCAINE. Cocaine stimulates the central nervous system, causing agitation, dilated pupils, tachycardia, hypertension, hallucinations, hyperthermia, hypertonia, and hyperreflexia; cardiac effects include chest pain, myocardial infarction, and arrhythmias.

Initial treatment of cocaine poisoning involves intravenous administration of diazepam to control agitation and cooling measures for hyperthermia (see Body temperature, p. 28); hypertension and cardiac effects require specific treatment and expert advice should be sought.

ECSTASY. Ecstasy (methylenedioxymethamfetamine, MDMA) may cause severe reactions, even at doses that were previously tolerated. The most serious effects are delirium, coma, convulsions, ventricular arrhythmias, hyperpyrexia, rhabdomyolysis, acute renal failure, acute hepatitis, disseminated intravascular coagulation, adult respiratory distress syndrome, hyperreflexia, hypotension and intracerebral haemorrhage; hyponatraemia has also been associated with ecstasy use.

Treatment is supportive, with diazepam to control severe agitation or persistent convulsions and close monitoring including ECG. Self-induced water intoxication should be considered in patients with ecstasy poisoning.

Theophylline

Theophylline and related drugs are often prescribed as modified-release formulations and toxicity may therefore be delayed. They cause vomiting (which may be severe and intractable), agitation, restlessness, dilated pupils, sinus tachycardia, and hyperglycaemia. More serious effects are haematemesis, convulsions, and supraventricular and ventricular arrhythmias. Profound **hypokalaemia** may develop rapidly.

The stomach should be emptied if the patient presents within 2 hours. Elimination of theophylline is enhanced by repeated doses of activated charcoal by mouth (see also under Active Elimination Techniques). Hypokalaemia is corrected by intravenous infusion of potassium chloride and may be so severe as to require 60 mmol/hour (high doses under ECG monitoring). Convulsions should be controlled by intravenous administration of diazepam (emulsion preferred). Sedation with diazepam may be necessary in agitated patients.

Provided the patient does **not** suffer from asthma, **propranolol** (section 2.4) may be administered intravenously to reverse extreme tachycardia, hypokalaemia, and hyperglycaemia.

Other poisons

Consult either a poisons information centre day and night or TOXBASE, see p. 27.

> The **poisons information centres** (Tel: 0870 600 6266) will provide specialist advice on all aspects of poisoning day and night

Cyanides

Cyanide antidotes include dicobalt edetate, given alone, and sodium nitrite followed by sodium thiosulphate. These antidotes are held for emergency use in hospitals as well as in centres where cyanide poisoning is a risk such as factories and laboratories. Hydroxocobalamin is an alternative antidote but its use should ideally be discussed with a poisons information centre; the usual dose is hydroxocobalamin 70 mg/kg by intravenous infusion (repeated once or twice according to severity). *Cyanokit*®, which provides hydroxocobalamin 2.5 g/bottle, is available but it is not licensed for use in the UK.

DICOBALT EDETATE

Indications: acute poisoning with cyanides

Cautions: owing to toxicity to be used only when patient tending to lose, or has lost, consciousness; not to be used as a precautionary measure

Side-effects: hypotension, tachycardia, and vomiting

Dose: *by intravenous injection*, ADULT 300 mg over 1 minute (5 minutes if condition less serious) followed immediately by 50 mL of glucose intravenous infusion 50%; if response inadequate a second dose of both may be given; if no response after further 5 minutes a third dose of both may be given; CHILD consult a poisons information centre

[1]**Dicobalt Edetate** (Cambridge) PoM
Injection, dicobalt edetate 15 mg/mL, net price 20-mL (300-mg) amp = £10.58

1. PoM restriction does not apply where administration is for saving life in emergency

SODIUM NITRITE

Indications: poisoning with cyanides (used in conjunction with sodium thiosulphate)

Side-effects: flushing and headache due to vasodilatation

Dose: *by intravenous injection* over 5–20 minutes (as sodium nitrite injection 30 mg/mL), 300 mg (CHILD 4–10 mg/kg) followed by sodium thiosulphate (as sodium thiosulphate injection 500 mg/mL) *by intravenous injection* over 10 minutes 12.5 g (CHILD 400 mg/kg)

[1]**Sodium Nitrite** PoM
Injection, sodium nitrite 3% (30 mg/mL) in water for injections
'Special-order' [unlicensed] product: contact Martindale, or regional hospital manufacturing unit

1. PoM restriction does not apply where administration is for saving life in emergency

SODIUM THIOSULPHATE

Indications: poisoning with cyanides (used in conjunction with sodium nitrite)

Dose: see above under Sodium Nitrite

[1]**Sodium Thiosulphate** PoM
Injection, sodium thiosulphate 50% (500 mg/mL) in water for injections
'Special-order' [unlicensed] product: contact Martindale, or regional hospital manufacturing unit

1. PoM restriction does not apply where administration is for saving life in emergency

Ethylene glycol and methanol

Ethanol (by mouth or by intravenous infusion) is used for the treatment of ethylene glycol or methanol (methyl alcohol) poisoning. Fomepizole (*Antizol*®, available on named-patient basis from IDIS) has also been used for the treatment of ethylene glycol or methanol poisoning. Advice on the treatment of ethylene glycol or methanol poisoning should be obtained from a poisons information centre.

Heavy metals

Heavy metal antidotes include dimercaprol, penicillamine, and sodium calcium edetate. Other antidotes for heavy metal poisoning include succimer (DMSA) and unithiol (DMPS) [both unlicensed]; their use may be valuable in certain cases and the advice of a poisons information centre should be sought.

DIMERCAPROL

(BAL)

Indications: poisoning by antimony, arsenic, bismuth, gold, mercury, possibly thallium; adjunct (with sodium calcium edetate) in lead poisoning

Cautions: hypertension, renal impairment (discontinue or use with extreme caution if impairment develops during treatment), elderly, pregnancy and breast-feeding; **interactions:** Appendix 1 (dimercaprol)

Contra-indications: not indicated for iron, cadmium, or selenium poisoning; severe hepatic impairment (unless due to arsenic poisoning)

Side-effects: hypertension, tachycardia, malaise, nausea, vomiting, salivation, lacrimation, sweating, burning sensation (mouth, throat, and eyes), feeling of constriction of throat and chest, headache, muscle spasm, abdominal pain, tingling of extremities; pyrexia in children; local pain and abscess at injection site

Dose: *by intramuscular injection*, ADULT and CHILD 2.5–3 mg/kg every 4 hours for 2 days, 2–4 times on the third day, then 1–2 times daily for 10 days or until recovery

Dimercaprol (Sovereign) PoM
Injection, dimercaprol 50 mg/mL. Net price 2-mL amp = £42.73
NOTE. Contains arachis (peanut) oil as solvent

PENICILLAMINE

Indications: lead poisoning

Cautions: see section 10.1.3

Contra-indications: see section 10.1.3

Side-effects: see section 10.1.3

Dose: 1–2 g daily in divided doses before food until urinary lead is stabilised at less than 500 micrograms/day; CHILD 20 mg/kg daily

- Preparations

Section 10.1.3

SODIUM CALCIUM EDETATE

(Sodium Calciumedetate)

Indications: poisoning by heavy metals, especially lead

Cautions: renal impairment

Side-effects: nausea, diarrhoea, abdominal pain, pain at site of injection, thrombophlebitis if given too rapidly, renal damage particularly in overdosage; hypotension, lacrimation, myalgia, nasal congestion, sneezing, malaise, thirst, fever, chills, headache also reported

Dose: *by intravenous infusion*, ADULT and CHILD up to 40 mg/kg twice daily for up to 5 days, repeated if necessary after 48 hours

Ledclair® (Durbin) PoM
Injection, sodium calcium edetate 200 mg/mL, net price 5-mL amp = £7.29

Noxious gases

CARBON MONOXIDE. Carbon monoxide poisoning is usually due to inhalation of smoke, car exhaust, or fumes caused by blocked flues or incomplete combustion of fuel gases in confined spaces. Its toxic effects are entirely due to hypoxia.

Immediate treatment of carbon monoxide poisoning is essential. The person should be moved to fresh air, the airway cleared, and **oxygen** 100% administered through a tight-fitting mask with an inflated face seal. Artificial respiration should be given as necessary and continued until adequate spontaneous breathing starts, or stopped only after persistent and efficient treatment of cardiac arrest has failed. The patient should be admitted to hospital because complications may arise after a delay of hours or days. Cerebral oedema should be anticipated in severe poisoning and is treated with an intravenous infusion of mannitol (section 2.2.5). Referral for hyperbaric oxygen treatment should be discussed with the poisons information services if the victim is or has been unconscious, or has psychiatric or neurological features other than a headache, or has myocardial ischaemia or an arrhythmia, or has a blood carboxyhaemoglobin concentration of more than 20%, or is pregnant.

SULPHUR DIOXIDE, CHLORINE, PHOSGENE, AMMONIA. All of these gases can cause upper respiratory tract and conjunctival irritation. Pulmonary oedema, with severe breathlessness and cyanosis may develop suddenly up to 36 hours after exposure. Death may occur. Patients are kept under observation and those who develop pulmonary oedema are given oxygen. Assisted ventilation may be necessary in the most serious cases.

CS Spray

CS spray, which is used for riot control, irritates the eyes (hence 'tear gas') and the respiratory tract; symptoms normally settle spontaneously within 15 minutes. If symptoms persist, the patient should be removed to a well-ventilated area, and the exposed skin washed with soap and water after removal of contaminated clothing. Contact lenses should be removed and hard ones washed (soft ones should be discarded). Eye symptoms should be treated by irrigating the eyes with physiological saline (or water if saline not available) and advice sought from an ophthalmologist. Patients with features of severe poisoning, particularly respiratory complications, should be admitted to hospital for symptomatic treatment.

Nerve agents

Treatment of nerve agent poisoning is similar to organophosphorus insecticide poisoning (see below), but advice must be sought from a poisons information centre. The risk of cross-contamination is significant; adequate decontamination and protective clothing for healthcare personnel are essential. In emergencies involving the release of nerve agents, kits ('NAAS pods') which contain **pralidoxime** may be obtained through the Ambulance Service from the National Blood Service (or the Welsh Blood Service in South Wales or designated hospital pharmacies in Northern Ireland and Scotland—see TOXBASE for list of designated centres). In the very rare circumstances where the nerve agent is tabun (GA), **obidoxime** will also be supplied as part of the pod.

> The **poisons information centres** (Tel: 0870 600 6266) will provide specialist advice on all aspects of poisoning day and night

Pesticides

PARAQUAT. Concentrated liquid paraquat preparations (e.g. *Gramoxone*®), available to farmers and horticulturists, contain 10–20% paraquat and are extremely toxic. Granular preparations, for garden use, contain only 2.5% paraquat and have caused few deaths.

Paraquat has local and systemic effects. Splashes in the eyes irritate and ulcerate the cornea and conjunctiva. Copious washing of the eye should aid healing but it may be a long process. Skin irritation, blistering, and ulceration can occur from prolonged contact both with the concentrated and dilute forms. Inhalation of spray, mist, or dust containing paraquat may cause nose bleeding and sore throat but not systemic toxicity.

Ingestion of concentrated paraquat solutions is followed by nausea, vomiting, and diarrhoea. Painful ulceration of the tongue, lips, and fauces may appear after 36 to 48 hours together with renal failure. Some days later there may be dyspnoea with pulmonary fibrosis due to proliferative alveolitis and bronchiolitis.

Treatment should be started immediately. The single most useful measure is oral administration of **activated charcoal**. Vomiting may preclude the use of activated charcoal and an anti-emetic may be required. Gastric lavage is of doubtful value. Intravenous fluids and analgesics are given as necessary. Oxygen therapy should be avoided in the early stages of management since this may exacerbate damage to the lungs, but oxygen may be required in the late stages to palliate symptoms. Measures to enhance elimination of absorbed paraquat are probably valueless but should be discussed with the poisons information centres who will also give guidance on predicting the likely outcome from plasma concentrations. Paraquat absorption can be confirmed by a simple qualitative urine test.

ORGANOPHOSPHORUS INSECTICIDES. Organophosphorus insecticides are usually supplied as powders or dissolved in organic solvents. All are absorbed through the bronchi and intact skin as well as through the gut and inhibit cholinesterase activity thereby prolonging and intensifying the effects of acetylcholine. Toxicity between different compounds varies considerably, and onset may be delayed after skin exposure.

Anxiety, restlessness, dizziness, headache, miosis, nausea, hypersalivation, vomiting, abdominal colic, diarrhoea, bradycardia, and sweating are common features of organophosphorus poisoning. Muscle weakness and fasciculation may develop and progress to generalised flaccid paralysis including the ocular and respiratory muscles. Convulsions, coma, pulmonary oedema with copious bronchial secretions, hypoxia, and arrhythmias occur in severe cases. Hyperglycaemia and glycosuria without ketonuria may also be present.

Further absorption of the organophosphorus insecticide should be prevented by moving the patient to fresh air, removing soiled clothing, and washing contaminated skin. In severe poisoning it is vital to ensure a clear airway, frequent removal of bronchial secretions, and adequate ventilation and oxygenation; gastric lavage may be considered provided that the airway is protected. **Atropine** will reverse the muscarinic effects of acetylcholine and is given in a dose of 2 mg (20 micrograms/kg in a child) as atropine sulphate (intramuscularly or intravenously according to the severity of poisoning) every 5 to 10 minutes until the skin becomes flushed and dry, the pupils dilate, and tachycardia develops.

Pralidoxime mesilate (P2S), a cholinesterase reactivator, is used as an adjunct to atropine in moderate or severe poisoning. It improves muscle tone within 30 minutes of administration. Repeated doses are required; an intravenous infusion is required in severe cases. Pralidoxime mesilate may be obtained from designated centres, the names of which are held by the poisons information centres (see p. 27).

PRALIDOXIME MESILATE

(P2S)

Indications: adjunct to atropine in the treatment of poisoning by organophosphorus insecticide or nerve agent

Cautions: renal impairment, myasthenia gravis

Contra-indications: poisoning due to carbamates and to organophosphorus compounds without anticholinesterase activity

Side-effects: drowsiness, dizziness, disturbances of vision, nausea, tachycardia, headache, hyperventilation, and muscular weakness

Dose: *by slow intravenous injection* (diluted to 10–15 mL with water for injections) over 5–10 minutes, initially 30 mg/kg repeated every 4–6 hours *or by intravenous infusion*, 8 mg/kg/hour; usual max. 12 g in 24 hours

NOTE. Pralidoxime mesilate doses in BNF may differ from those in product literature

[1]**Pralidoxime Mesilate** PoM

Injection, pralidoxime mesilate 200 mg/mL

Available as 5-mL amps (from designated centres for organophosphorus insecticide poisoning or from the National Blood Service and the Welsh Blood Service for nerve agent poisoning—see TOXBASE for list of designated centres)

1. PoM restriction does not apply where administration is for saving life in emergency

Snake bites and animal stings

SNAKE BITES. Envenoming from snake bite is uncommon in the UK. Many exotic snakes are kept, some illegally, but the only indigenous venomous snake is the adder (*Vipera berus*). The bite may cause local and systemic effects. Local effects include pain, swelling, bruising, and tender enlargement of regional lymph nodes. Systemic effects include early anaphylactoid symptoms (transient hypotension with syncope, angioedema, urticaria, abdominal colic, diarrhoea, and vomiting), with later persistent or recurrent hypotension, ECG abnormalities, spontaneous systemic bleeding, coagulopathy, adult respiratory distress syndrome, and acute renal failure. Fatal envenoming is rare but the potential for severe envenoming must not be underestimated.

Early anaphylactoid symptoms should be treated with **adrenaline (epinephrine)** (section 3.4.3). Indications for antivenom treatment include systemic envenoming, especially hypotension (see above), ECG abnormalities, vomiting, haemostatic abnormalities, and marked local envenoming such that after bites on the hand or foot, swelling extends beyond the wrist or ankle within 4 hours of the bite. For both **adults** and **children**, the contents of one vial (10 mL) of **European viper venom antiserum** (available from Farillon) is given *by intravenous injection* over 10–15 minutes or *by intravenous infusion* over 30 minutes after diluting in sodium chloride intravenous infusion 0.9% (use 5 mL diluent/kg body-weight). The **same dose** should be used for **adults** and **children**. The dose can be repeated in 1–2 hours if symptoms of **systemic envenoming** persist. Adrenaline (epinephrine) injection must be immediately to hand for treatment of anaphylactic reactions to the antivenom (for the management of anaphylaxis see section 3.4.3).

Antivenom is available for certain foreign snakes, spiders and scorpions. For information on identification, management, and supply, telephone:

Oxford	(01865) 220 968
	or (01865) 221 332
	or (01865) 741 166
Liverpool	(0151) 708 9393
Liverpool (Royal Liverpool University Hospital) (emergency supply only)	(0151) 706 2000
London (emergency supply only)	(020) 7771 5394

INSECT STINGS. Stings from ants, wasps, hornets, and bees cause local pain and swelling but seldom cause severe direct toxicity unless many stings are inflicted at the same time. If the sting is in the mouth or on the tongue local swelling may threaten the upper airway. The stings from these insects are usually treated by cleaning the area. Bee stings should be removed as quickly as possible. Anaphylactic reactions require immediate treatment with intramuscular **adrenaline (epinephrine)**; self-administered intramuscular adrenaline (e.g. *EpiPen*®) is the best first-aid treatment for patients with severe hypersensitivity. An inhaled bronchodilator should be used for asthmatic reactions. For the management of anaphylaxis, see section 3.4.3. A short course of an **oral antihistamine** or a **topical corticosteroid** may help to reduce inflammation and relieve itching.

MARINE STINGS. The severe pain of weeverfish (*Trachinus vipera*) stings can be relieved by immersing the stung area in uncomfortably hot, but not scalding, water (not more than 45° C). People stung by jellyfish and Portuguese man-o'-war around the UK coast should be removed from the sea as soon as possible. Adherent tentacles should be lifted off carefully (wearing gloves or using tweezers) or washed off with seawater. Alcoholic solutions including suntan lotions should **not** be applied because they may cause further discharge of stinging hairs. Ice packs will reduce pain and a slurry of baking soda (sodium bicarbonate), but not vinegar, may be useful for treating stings from UK species.

1: Gastro-intestinal system

1.1 Dyspepsia and gastro-oesophageal reflux disease

1.1.1 Antacids and simeticone
1.1.2 Compound alginates and proprietary indigestion preparations

Dyspepsia

Dyspepsia covers pain, fullness, early satiety, bloating, and nausea. It can occur with gastric and duodenal ulceration (section 1.3) and gastric cancer but most commonly it is of uncertain origin.

Helicobacter pylori may be present in patients with dyspepsia. *H. pylori* eradication therapy (section 1.3) should be considered for dyspepsia if it is ulcer-like. However, most individuals with functional (investigated, non-ulcer) dyspepsia do not benefit symptomatically from *H. pylori* eradication. Urgent investigation is required if the dyspepsia is accompanied by 'alarm features' (e.g. bleeding, dysphagia, recurrent vomiting, and weight loss).

Gastro-oesophageal reflux disease

Gastro-oesophageal reflux disease (including non-erosive gastro-oesophageal reflux and erosive oesophagitis) is associated with heartburn, acid regurgitation, and sometimes, difficulty in swallowing (dysphagia); oesophageal inflammation (oesophagitis), ulceration, and stricture formation may occur and there is an association with asthma.

The management of gastro-oesophageal reflux disease includes drug treatment, lifestyle changes and, in some cases, surgery. Initial treatment is guided by the severity of symptoms and treatment is then adjusted according to response. The extent of healing depends on the severity of the disease, the treatment chosen, and the duration of therapy.

For *mild symptoms* of gastro-oesophageal reflux disease, initial management may include the use of **antacids** and **alginates**. Alginate-containing antacids form a 'raft' that floats on the surface of the stomach contents to reduce reflux and protect the oesophageal mucosa. **Histamine H_2-receptor antagonists** (section 1.3.1) suppress acid secretion. They may relieve symptoms and permit reduction in antacid consumption. For refractory cases, a course of a **proton pump inhibitor** (section 1.3.5) may be considered (as described for severe symptoms, below).

For *severe symptoms* of gastro-oesophageal reflux disease or for patients with a proven or severe pathology (e.g. *oesophagitis, oesophageal ulceration, oesophagopharyngeal reflux, Barrett's oesophagus*), initial management involves the use of a **proton pump inhibitor** (section 1.3.5); patients need to be reassessed if symptoms persist despite treatment for 4–6 weeks with a proton pump inhibitor. When symptoms abate, treatment is titrated down to a level which maintains remission (e.g. by reducing the dose of the proton pump inhibitor or by giving it intermittently, or by substituting treatment with a histamine H_2-receptor antagonist). However, for endoscopically confirmed *erosive, ulcerative*, or *stricturing* disease, treatment with a proton pump inhibitor usually needs to be maintained at the minimum effective dose.

A prokinetic drug such as **metoclopramide** (section 4.6) may improve gastro-oesophageal sphincter function and accelerate gastric emptying.

Patients with gastro-oesophageal reflux disease need to be advised about lifestyle changes (avoidance of excess alcohol and of aggravating foods such as fats); other measures include weight reduction, smoking cessation, and raising the head of the bed.

CHILDREN. Gastro-oesophageal reflux disease is common in infancy but most symptoms resolve between 12 and 18 months of age. Mild or moderate reflux without complications can be managed initially by changes in posture and thickening of liquid feeds (see Appendix 7 for suitable products) followed if necessary by treatment with an alginate-containing product (low sodium and low aluminium content for infants). For older children, life-style changes similar to those for adults (see above) may be helpful followed if necessary by treatment with an alginate-containing product.

Children who do not respond to these measures or who have problems such as respiratory disorders or suspected oesophagitis need to be referred to hospital; an H_2-receptor antagonist (section 1.3.1) may be needed to reduce acid secretion. If the oesophagitis is resistant to H_2-receptor blockade, the proton pump inhibitor omeprazole (section 1.3.5) can be tried.

1.1.1 Antacids and simeticone

Antacids (usually containing aluminium or magnesium compounds) can often relieve symptoms in *ulcer dyspepsia* and in *non-erosive gastro-oesophageal reflux* (see also section 1.1); they are also sometimes used in functional (non-ulcer) dyspepsia but the evidence of benefit is uncertain. Antacids are best given when symptoms occur or are expected, usually between meals and at bedtime, 4 or more times daily; additional doses may be required up to once an hour. Conventional doses e.g. 10 mL 3 or 4 times daily of liquid magnesium–aluminium antacids promote ulcer healing, but less well than antisecretory drugs (section 1.3); proof of a relationship between healing and neutralising capacity is lacking. Liquid preparations are more effective than solids.

Aluminium- and **magnesium-containing** antacids (e.g. aluminium hydroxide, and magnesium carbonate, hydroxide and trisilicate), being relatively insoluble in water, are long-acting if retained in the stomach. They are suitable for most antacid purposes. Magnesium-containing antacids tend to be laxative whereas aluminium-containing antacids may be constipating; antacids containing both magnesium and aluminium may reduce these colonic side-effects. Aluminium accumulation does not appear to be a risk if renal function is normal (see also Appendix 3).

The acid-neutralising capacity of preparations that contain more than one antacid may be the same as simpler preparations. Complexes such as **hydrotalcite** confer no special advantage.

Sodium bicarbonate should no longer be prescribed alone for the relief of dyspepsia but it is present as an ingredient in many indigestion remedies. However, it retains a place in the management of urinary-tract disorders (section 7.4.3) and acidosis (section 9.2.1.3 and section 9.2.2). Sodium bicarbonate should be avoided in patients on salt-restricted diets.

Bismuth-containing antacids (unless chelates) are not recommended because absorbed bismuth can be neurotoxic, causing encephalopathy; they tend to be constipating. **Calcium-containing** antacids (section 1.1.2) can induce rebound acid secretion: with modest doses the clinical significance is doubtful, but prolonged high doses also cause hypercalcaemia and alkalosis, and can precipitate the milk-alkali syndrome.

Simeticone (activated dimeticone) is added to an antacid as an antifoaming agent to relieve flatulence. These preparations may be useful for the relief of hiccup in palliative care. **Alginates**, added as protectants, may be useful in gastro-oesophageal reflux disease (section 1.1). The amount of additional ingredient or antacid in individual preparations varies widely, as does their sodium content, so that preparations may not be freely interchangeable.

For **preparations** on sale to the public (not prescribable on the NHS), see p. 40.

See also section 1.3 for drugs used in the treatment of peptic ulceration.

INTERACTIONS. Antacids should preferably not be taken at the same time as other drugs since they may impair absorption. Antacids may also damage enteric coatings designed to prevent dissolution in the stomach. See also **Appendix 1** (antacids, calcium salts).

Low Na^+. The words low Na^+ added after some preparations indicate a sodium content of less than 1 mmol per tablet or 10-mL dose.

Aluminium- and magnesium-containing antacids

ALUMINIUM HYDROXIDE

Indications: dyspepsia; hyperphosphataemia (section 9.5.2.2)

Cautions: see notes above; renal impairment (Appendix 3); **interactions:** Appendix 1 (antacids)

Contra-indications: hypophosphataemia; porphyria (section 9.8.2)

Side-effects: see notes above

■ Aluminium-only preparations

Aluminium Hydroxide (Non-proprietary)
Tablets, dried aluminium hydroxide 500 mg. Net price 20 = 28p
Dose: 1–2 tablets chewed 4 times daily and at bedtime or as required

Oral suspension, about 4% w/w Al_2O_3 in water, with a peppermint flavour. Net price 200 mL = 41p
Dose: antacid, 5–10 mL 4 times daily between meals and at bedtime or as required; CHILD 6–12 years, up to 5 mL 3 times daily
NOTE. The brand name *Aludrox*® NHS (Pfizer Consumer) is used for aluminium hydroxide mixture; net price 200 mL = £1.42. *Aludrox*® NHS tablets also contain magnesium.

Alu-Cap® (3M)
Capsules, green/red, dried aluminium hydroxide 475 mg (low Na^+). Net price 120-cap pack = £3.75
Dose: antacid, 1 capsule 4 times daily and at bedtime; CHILD not recommended for antacid therapy

■ Co-magaldrox

Co-magaldrox is a mixture of aluminium hydroxide and magnesium hydroxide; the proportions are expressed in the form *x*/*y* where *x* and *y* are the strengths in milligrams per unit dose of magnesium hydroxide and aluminium hydroxide respectively

Maalox® (Rhône-Poulenc Rorer)
Suspension, sugar-free, co-magaldrox 195/220 (magnesium hydroxide 195 mg, dried aluminium hydroxide 220 mg/5 mL (low Na^+)). Net price 500 mL = £2.59
Dose: 10–20 mL 20–60 minutes after meals and at bedtime or when required; CHILD under 14 years not recommended

Mucogel® (Forest)
Suspension, sugar-free, co-magaldrox 195/220 (magnesium hydroxide 195 mg, dried aluminium hydroxide 220 mg/5 mL (low Na^+)). Net price 500 mL = £1.71
Dose: 10–20 mL 3 times daily, 20–60 minutes after meals, and at bedtime or when required; CHILD under 12 years not recommended

MAGNESIUM CARBONATE

Indications: dyspepsia
Cautions: renal impairment (Appendix 3); see also notes above; **interactions:** Appendix 1 (antacids)
Contra-indications: hypophosphataemia
Side-effects: diarrhoea; belching due to liberated carbon dioxide

Aromatic Magnesium Carbonate Mixture, BP
(Aromatic Magnesium Carbonate Oral Suspension)
Oral suspension, light magnesium carbonate 3%, sodium bicarbonate 5%, in a suitable vehicle containing aromatic cardamom tincture. Contains about 6 mmol Na^+/10 mL. Net price 200 mL = 64p
Dose: 10 mL 3 times daily in water

For **preparations** also containing aluminium, see above and section 1.1.2.

MAGNESIUM TRISILICATE

Indications: dyspepsia
Cautions: see under Magnesium Carbonate
Contra-indications: see under Magnesium Carbonate
Side-effects: diarrhoea, belching due to liberated carbon dioxide; silica-based renal stones reported on long-term treatment

Magnesium Trisilicate Tablets, Compound, BP
Tablets, magnesium trisilicate 250 mg, dried aluminium hydroxide 120 mg
Dose: 1–2 tablets chewed when required

Magnesium Trisilicate Mixture, BP
(Magnesium Trisilicate Oral Suspension)
Oral suspension, 5% each of magnesium trisilicate, light magnesium carbonate, and sodium bicarbonate in a suitable vehicle with a peppermint flavour. Contains about 6 mmol Na^+/10 mL
Dose: 10 mL 3 times daily in water

For **preparations** also containing aluminium, see above and section 1.1.2.

Aluminium-magnesium complexes

HYDROTALCITE

Aluminium magnesium carbonate hydroxide hydrate
Indications: dyspepsia
Cautions: see notes above; **interactions:** Appendix 1 (antacids)
Side-effects: see notes above

Hydrotalcite (Peckforton)
Suspension, hydrotalcite 500 mg/5 mL (low Na^+). Net price 500-mL pack = £1.96
Dose: 10 mL between meals and at bedtime; CHILD under 6 years not recommended, 6–12 years 5 mL
NOTE. The brand name *Altacite*® NHS is used for hydrotalcite suspension; for *Altacite Plus*® suspension, see below

Antacid preparations containing simeticone

Altacite Plus® (Peckforton)
Suspension, sugar-free, co-simalcite 125/500 (simeticone 125 mg, hydrotalcite 500 mg)/5 mL (low Na^+). Net price 500 mL = £1.96
Dose: 10 mL between meals and at bedtime when required; CHILD 8–12 years 5 mL
Tablets NHS, see p. 40

Asilone® (Thornton & Ross)
Suspension, sugar-free, dried aluminium hydroxide 420 mg, simeticone 135 mg, light magnesium oxide 70 mg/5 mL (low Na^+). Net price 500 mL = £1.95
Dose: 5–10 mL after meals and at bedtime or when required up to 4 times daily; CHILD under 12 years not recommended
Tablets NHS, see p. 40
Liquid NHS, see p. 40

Maalox Plus® (Rhône-Poulenc Rorer)
Suspension, sugar-free, dried aluminium hydroxide 220 mg, simeticone 25 mg, magnesium hydroxide 195 mg/5 mL (low Na^+). Net price 500 mL = £2.59
Dose: 5–10 mL 4 times daily (after meals and at bedtime or when required); CHILD under 5 years 5 mL 3 times daily, over 5 years appropriate proportion of adult dose
Tablets NHS, see p. 41

Simeticone alone

Simeticone (activated dimeticone) is an antifoaming agent. It is licensed for infantile colic but evidence of benefit is uncertain.

Dentinox® (DDD)
Colic drops (= emulsion), simeticone 21 mg/2.5-mL dose. Net price 100 mL = £1.73
Dose: gripes, colic or wind pains, INFANT 2.5 mL with or after each feed (max. 6 doses in 24 hours); may be added to bottle feed
NOTE. The brand name *Dentinox*® is also used for other preparations including teething gel

Infacol® (Forest)
Liquid, sugar-free, simeticone 40 mg/mL (low Na^+). Net price 50 mL = £2.03 Counselling, use of dropper
Dose: gripes, colic or wind pains, INFANT 0.5–1 mL before feeds

1.1.2 Compound alginates and proprietary indigestion preparations

Alginate-containing antacids form a 'raft' that floats on the surface of the stomach contents to reduce reflux and protect the oesophageal mucosa; they are used in the management of mild symptoms of gastro-oesophageal reflux disease.

Indigestion preparations on sale to the public include antacids with other ingredients such as alginates, calcium salts, simeticone, and peppermint oil.

Compound alginate preparations

Algicon® (Rhône-Poulenc Rorer)
Suspension, yellow, aluminium hydroxide-magnesium carbonate co-gel 140 mg, magnesium alginate 250 mg, magnesium carbonate 175 mg, potassium bicarbonate 50 mg/5 mL (low Na^+). Net price 500 mL (lemon- or mint-flavoured) = £3.07
Dose: 10–20 mL 4 times daily (after meals and at bedtime); CHILD under 12 years not recommended

Gastrocote® (Thornton & Ross)
Tablets, alginic acid 200 mg, dried aluminium hydroxide 80 mg, magnesium trisilicate 40 mg, sodium bicarbonate 70 mg. Contains about 1 mmol Na^+/tablet. Net price 100-tab pack = £3.51
Cautions: diabetes mellitus (high sugar content)
Dose: 1–2 tablets chewed 4 times daily (after meals and at bedtime); CHILD under 6 years not recommended
Liquid, sugar-free, peach-coloured, dried aluminium hydroxide 80 mg, magnesium trisilicate 40 mg, sodium alginate 220 mg, sodium bicarbonate 70 mg/5 mL. Contains 1.8 mmol Na^+/5 mL. Net price 500 mL = £2.67
Dose: 5–15 mL 4 times daily (after meals and at bedtime)

Gaviscon® (R&C)
Tablets, sugar-free, alginic acid 500 mg, dried aluminium hydroxide 100 mg, magnesium trisilicate 25 mg, sodium bicarbonate 170 mg. Contains 2 mmol Na^+/tablet. Net price 60-tab pack (peppermint- or lemon-flavoured) = £2.25
Dose: 1–2 tablets chewed after meals and at bedtime, followed by water; CHILD 2–6 years 1 tablet (on doctor's advice only) and 6–12 years 1 tablet
Liquid, sugar-free, sodium alginate 250 mg, sodium bicarbonate 133.5 mg, calcium carbonate 80 mg/5 mL. Contains about 3 mmol Na^+/5 mL. Net price 500 mL (aniseed- or peppermint-flavour) = £2.70
Dose: 10–20 mL after meals and at bedtime; CHILD 2–6 years (on doctor's advice only) and 6–12 years 5–10 mL
Gaviscon 250® NHS and *Gaviscon 500*® *Tablets*, see p. 41

Gaviscon® **Advance** (R&C)
Suspension, sugar-free, sodium alginate 500 mg, potassium bicarbonate 100 mg/5 mL. Contains 2.3 mmol Na^+, 1 mmol K^+/5 mL. Net price 500 mL (aniseed- or peppermint-flavour) = £5.40
Dose: ADULT and CHILD over 12 years, 5–10 mL after meals and at bedtime

Gaviscon® **Infant** (R&C)
Oral powder, sugar-free, sodium alginate 225 mg, magnesium alginate 87.5 mg, with colloidal silica and mannitol/dose (half dual-sachet). Contains 0.92 mmol Na^+/dose. Net price 15 dual-sachets (30 doses) = £2.46
Dose: INFANT under 4.5 kg 1 dose (half dual-sachet) mixed with feeds (or water in breast-fed infants) when required; over 4.5 kg 2 doses (1 dual-sachet); CHILD 2 doses (1 dual-sachet) in water after each meal
NOTE. Not to be used in preterm neonates, or where excessive water loss likely (e.g. fever, diarrhoea, vomiting, high room temperature), or if intestinal obstruction. Not to be used with other preparations containing thickening agents
IMPORTANT. Each half of the dual-sachet is identified as 'one dose'. To avoid errors prescribe as 'dual-sachet' with directions in terms of 'dose'

Peptac® (IVAX)
Suspension, sugar-free, sodium bicarbonate 133.5 mg, sodium alginate 250 mg, calcium carbonate 80 mg/5 mL. Contains 3.1 mmol Na^+/5mL. Net price 500 mL (aniseed-flavoured) = £2.16
Dose: 10–20 mL after meals and at bedtime; CHILD 6–12 years 5–10 mL

Rennie® **Duo** (Roche Consumer Health)
Suspension, sugar-free, calcium carbonate 600 mg, magnesium carbonate 70 mg, sodium alginate 150 mg/5 mL. Contains 2.6 mmol Na^+/5 mL. Net price 500 mL (mint flavour) = £2.67
Dose: ADULT and CHILD over 12 years, 10 mL after meals and at bedtime; an additional 10 mL may be taken between doses for heartburn if necessary, max. 80 mL daily
Excipients: include propylene glycol
Rennie® NHS and *Rennie Deflatine*®, see p. 41

Topal® (Ceuta)
Tablets, alginic acid 200 mg, dried aluminium hydroxide 30 mg, light magnesium carbonate 40 mg with lactose 220 mg, sucrose 880 mg, sodium bicarbonate 40 mg (low Na^+). Net price 42-tab pack = £1.67
Cautions: diabetes mellitus (high sugar content)
Dose: 1–3 tablets chewed 4 times daily (after meals and at bedtime); CHILD half adult dose

Indigestion preparations

Indigestion **preparations** on sale to the public (may not be prescribable on the NHS) include:
Actal® (alexitol sodium), **Actonorm Gel**® (aluminium hydroxide, magnesium hydroxide, peppermint oil, simeticone), **Actonorm Powder**® (section 1.2), **Altacite Plus**® (hydrotalcite), **Andrews Antacid**® (calcium carbonate, magnesium carbonate), **Asilone Antacid Liquid**® (aluminium hydroxide, magnesium oxide, simeticone), **Asilone Antacid Tablets**® (aluminium hydroxide, simeticone), **Asilone Heartburn Liquid**® (aluminium hydroxide, magnesium trisilicate, sodium alginate, sodium bicarbonate), **Asilone Heartburn Tablets**® (alginic acid, aluminium hydroxide, magnesium trisilicate, sodium bicarbonate), **Asilone Windcheaters**® **Capsules** (simeticone)
Bisodol Heartburn Relief Tablets® (alginic acid, magaldrate, sodium bicarbonate), **Bisodol Indigestion Relief Powder**® (magnesium carbonate, sodium bicarbonate), **Bisodol Indigestion Relief Tablets**® and **Bisodol Extra Strong Mint Tablets**® (calcium carbonate,

magnesium carbonate, sodium bicarbonate), **Bisodol Wind Relief Tablets**® (calcium carbonate, magnesium carbonate, simeticone, sodium bicarbonate), **Boots Heartburn Relief**® (calcium carbonate sodium alginate, sodium bicarbonate), **Boots Indigestion Relief Tablets Original**® (calcium carbonate, ginger, magnesium carbonate, magnesium trisilicate, sodium bicarbonate), **Boots Gripe Mixture I Month Plus**® (sodium bicarbonate)
Carbellon® (charcoal, magnesium hydroxide, peppermint oil)
Eno® (citric acid, sodium bicarbonate, sodium carbonate)
Gaviscon 250® **Tablets** (alginic acid, aluminium hydroxide, magnesium trisilicate, sodium bicarbonate; (**Gaviscon**® and **Gaviscon 500**® **Tablets** are prescribable)
Maalox Plus Tablets® (aluminium hydroxide, magnesium hydroxide, simeticone), **Moorland**® (aluminium hydroxide, bismuth aluminate, calcium carbonate, magnesium carbonate, light kaolin)
Original Andrews Salts® (citric acid, magnesium sulphate, sodium bicarbonate)
Pepto-Bismol® (bismuth), **Phillips' Milk of Magnesia**® (magnesium hydroxide)
Rap-eze® (calcium carbonate), **Remegel**® (calcium carbonate), **Remegel Wind Relief**® (calcium carbonate, simeticone), **Rennie**® (calcium carbonate, magnesium carbonate), **Rennie Deflatine**® (calcium carbonate, magnesium carbonate, simeticone)
Setlers Antacid® (calcium carbonate)
Tums® (calcium carbonate)
Wind-eze® (simeticone)

1.2 Antispasmodics and other drugs altering gut motility

Drugs in this section include antimuscarinic compounds and drugs believed to be direct relaxants of intestinal smooth muscle. The smooth muscle relaxant properties of antimuscarinic and other antispasmodic drugs may be useful in *irritable bowel syndrome* and in *diverticular disease*.

The dopamine-receptor antagonists metoclopramide and domperidone (section 4.6) stimulate transit in the gut.

Antimuscarinics

Antimuscarinics (formerly termed 'anticholinergics') reduce intestinal motility. They are used for the management of *irritable bowel syndrome* and *diverticular disease*. However, their value has not been established and response varies. Other indications for antimuscarinic drugs include arrhythmias (section 2.3.1), asthma and airways disease (section 3.1.2), motion sickness (section 4.6), parkinsonism (section 4.9.2), urinary incontinence (section 7.4.2), mydriasis and cycloplegia (section 11.5), premedication (section 15.1.3) and as an antidote to organophosphorus poisoning (p. 36).

Antimuscarinics that are used for gastro-intestinal smooth muscle spasm include the tertiary amines **atropine sulphate** and **dicycloverine hydrochloride** (dicyclomine hydrochloride) and the quaternary ammonium compounds **propantheline bromide** and **hyoscine butylbromide**. The quaternary ammonium compounds are less lipid soluble than atropine and are less likely to cross the blood–brain barrier; they are also less well absorbed.

Dicycloverine hydrochloride has a much less marked antimuscarinic action than atropine and may also have some direct action on smooth muscle. Hyoscine butylbromide is advocated as a gastro-intestinal antispasmodic, but it is poorly absorbed; the injection is useful in endoscopy and radiology. Atropine and the belladonna alkaloids are outmoded treatments, any clinical virtues being outweighed by atropinic side-effects.

CAUTIONS. Antimuscarinics should be used with caution in Down's syndrome, in children and in the elderly; they should also be used with caution in gastro-oesophageal reflux disease, diarrhoea, ulcerative colitis, acute myocardial infarction, hypertension, conditions characterised by tachycardia (including hyperthyroidism, cardiac insufficiency, cardiac surgery), pyrexia, pregnancy and breast-feeding. **Interactions:** Appendix 1 (antimuscarinics).

CONTRA-INDICATIONS. Antimuscarinics are contra-indicated in angle-closure glaucoma, myasthenia gravis (but may be used to decrease muscarinic side-effects of anticholinesterases—section 10.2.1), paralytic ileus, pyloric stenosis and prostatic enlargement.

SIDE-EFFECTS. Side-effects of antimuscarinics include constipation, transient bradycardia (followed by tachycardia, palpitations and arrhythmias), reduced bronchial secretions, urinary urgency and retention, dilatation of the pupils with loss of accommodation, photophobia, dry mouth, flushing and dryness of the skin. Side-effects that occur occasionally include confusion (particularly in the elderly), nausea, vomiting, and giddiness.

ATROPINE SULPHATE

Indications: symptomatic relief of gastro-intestinal disorders characterised by smooth muscle spasm; mydriasis and cycloplegia (section 11.5); premedication (section 15.1.3); see also notes above
Cautions: see notes above
Contra-indications: see notes above
Side-effects: see notes above

Atropine (Non-proprietary) PoM
Tablets, atropine sulphate 600 micrograms. Net price 28-tab pack = £6.60
Available from CP
Dose: 0.6–1.2 mg at night

■ Preparations on sale to the public
Preparations on sale to the public (not prescribable on the NHS) containing atropine or related compounds include **Actonorm Powder**® (atropine, aluminium, calcium carbonate, magnesium, sodium bicarbonate, peppermint oil)

DICYCLOVERINE HYDROCHLORIDE

(Dicyclomine hydrochloride)
Indications: symptomatic relief of gastro-intestinal disorders characterised by smooth muscle spasm
Cautions: see notes above
Contra-indications: see notes above; infants under 6 months
Side-effects: see notes above
Dose: 10–20 mg 3 times daily; INFANT 6–24 months 5–10 mg up to 3–4 times daily, 15 minutes before feeds; CHILD 2–12 years 10 mg 3 times daily

[1]**Merbentyl**® (Florizel) PoM
Tablets, dicycloverine hydrochloride 10 mg, net price 20 = £1.01; 20 mg (*Merbentyl 20*®), 84-tab pack = £8.47
Syrup, dicycloverine hydrochloride 10 mg/5 mL, net price 120 mL = £1.84

1. Dicycloverine hydrochloride can be sold to the public provided that max. single dose is 10 mg and max. daily dose is 60 mg

■ Compound preparations

Kolanticon® (Peckforton)
Gel, sugar-free, dicycloverine hydrochloride 2.5 mg, dried aluminium hydroxide 200 mg, light magnesium oxide 100 mg, simeticone 20 mg/5 mL, net price 200 mL = £1.69, 500 mL = £1.85
Dose: 10–20 mL every 4 hours when required

HYOSCINE BUTYLBROMIDE

Indications: symptomatic relief of gastro-intestinal or genito-urinary disorders characterised by smooth muscle spasm
Cautions: see notes above
Contra-indications: see notes above; avoid in porphyria (section 9.8.2)
Side-effects: see notes above
Dose: *by mouth* (but poorly absorbed, see notes above), 20 mg 4 times daily; CHILD 6–12 years, 10 mg 3 times daily
Irritable bowel syndrome, 10 mg 3 times daily, increased if required up to 20 mg 4 times daily
By intramuscular or slow intravenous injection, acute spasm and spasm in diagnostic procedures, 20 mg repeated after 30 minutes if necessary (may be repeated more frequently in endoscopy), max. 100 mg daily; CHILD not recommended

Buscopan® (Boehringer Ingelheim) PoM
[1]*Tablets,* coated, hyoscine butylbromide 10 mg. Net price 56-tab pack = £2.59
Injection, hyoscine butylbromide 20 mg/mL. Net price 1-mL amp = 20p

1. Hyoscine butylbromide can be sold to the public provided single dose does not exceed 20 mg, daily dose does not exceed 80 mg, and pack does not contain a total of more than 240 mg; brands include *Buscopan*® *IBS Relief*

PROPANTHELINE BROMIDE

Indications: symptomatic relief of gastro-intestinal disorders characterised by smooth muscle spasm; urinary frequency (section 7.4.2); gustatory sweating (section 6.1.5)
Cautions: see notes above
Contra-indications: see notes above
Side-effects: see notes above
Dose: 15 mg 3 times daily at least 1 hour before meals and 30 mg at night, max. 120 mg daily; CHILD not recommended

Pro-Banthine® (Concord) PoM
Tablets, pink, s/c, propantheline bromide 15 mg, net price 112-tab pack = £15.32. Label: 23

Other antispasmodics

Alverine, **mebeverine**, and **peppermint oil** are believed to be direct relaxants of intestinal smooth muscle and may relieve pain in *irritable bowel syndrome* and *diverticular disease*. They have no serious adverse effects but, like all antispasmodics, should be avoided in paralytic ileus. Peppermint oil occasionally causes heartburn.

ALVERINE CITRATE

Indications: adjunct in gastro-intestinal disorders characterised by smooth muscle spasm; dysmenorrhoea
Cautions: pregnancy; breast-feeding (Appendix 5)
Contra-indications: paralytic ileus; when combined with sterculia, intestinal obstruction, faecal impaction, colonic atony
Side-effects: nausea, headache, pruritus, rash and dizziness reported
Dose: 60–120 mg 1–3 times daily; CHILD under 12 years not recommended

Spasmonal® (Norgine)
Capsules, alverine citrate 60 mg (blue/grey), net price 100-cap pack = £11.95; 120 mg (*Spasmonal*® *Forte*, blue/grey), 60-cap pack = £13.80

MEBEVERINE HYDROCHLORIDE

Indications: adjunct in gastro-intestinal disorders characterised by smooth muscle spasm
Cautions: pregnancy (Appendix 4); avoid in porphyria (section 9.8.2.)
Contra-indications: paralytic ileus
Side-effects: rarely allergic reactions (including rash, urticaria, angioedema)
Dose: ADULT and CHILD over 10 years 135–150 mg 3 times daily preferably 20 minutes before meals

[1]**Mebeverine Hydrochloride** (Non-proprietary) PoM
Tablets, mebeverine hydrochloride 135 mg, net price 20 = £1.58

1. Mebeverine hydrochloride can be sold to the public for symptomatic relief of irritable bowel syndrome provided that max. single dose is 135 mg and max. daily dose is 405 mg; for uses other than symptomatic relief of irritable bowel syndrome provided that max. single dose is 100 mg and max. daily dose is 300 mg; proprietary brands on sale to the public include *Colofac IBS*® (135 mg), *Equilon*® (135 mg), *IBS Relief*®

Colofac® (Solvay) PoM
Tablets, s/c, mebeverine hydrochloride 135 mg. Net price 20 = £1.50

■ Modified release

Colofac® **MR** (Solvay) PoM
Capsules, m/r, mebeverine hydrochloride 200 mg, net price 60-cap pack = £6.67. Label: 25
Dose: irritable bowel syndrome, 1 capsule twice daily preferably 20 minutes before meals; CHILD not recommended

■ Compound preparations

[1]**Fybogel**® **Mebeverine** (R&C) PoM
Granules, buff, effervescent, ispaghula husk 3.5 g, mebeverine hydrochloride 135 mg/sachet. Contains 7 mmol K^+/sachet (caution in renal impairment). Net price 60 sachets = £15.00. Label: 13, 22, counselling, see below
Dose: irritable bowel syndrome, ADULT, 1 sachet in water, morning and evening 30 minutes before food; an

additional sachet may also be taken before the midday meal if necessary; CHILD not recommended

COUNSELLING. Preparations that swell in contact with liquid should always be carefully swallowed with water and should not be taken immediately before going to bed

1. 10-sachet pack can be sold to the public

PEPPERMINT OIL

Indications: relief of abdominal colic and distension, particularly in irritable bowel syndrome

Cautions: rarely sensitivity to menthol

Side-effects: heartburn, perianal irritation; rarely, allergic reactions (including rash, headache, bradycardia, muscle tremor, ataxia)

LOCAL IRRITATION. Capsules should not be broken or chewed because peppermint oil may irritate mouth or oesophagus

Colpermin® (Pharmacia)

Capsules, m/r, e/c, light blue/dark blue, blue band, peppermint oil 0.2 mL. Net price 100-cap pack = £12.05. Label: 5, 25

Excipients: include arachis (peanut) oil

Dose: 1–2 capsules, swallowed whole with water, 3 times daily for up to 2–3 months if necessary; CHILD under 15 years not recommended

Mintec® (Shire)

Capsules, e/c, green/ivory, peppermint oil 0.2 mL. Net price 84-cap pack = £7.04. Label: 5, 22, 25

Dose: 1–2 capsules swallowed whole with water, 3 times daily before meals for up to 2–3 months if necessary; CHILD not recommended

Motility stimulants

Metoclopramide and **domperidone** (section 4.6) are dopamine antagonists which stimulate gastric emptying and small intestinal transit, and enhance the strength of oesophageal sphincter contraction. They are used in some patients with *non-ulcer dyspepsia*. Metoclopramide is also used to speed the transit of barium during intestinal follow-through examination, and as accessory treatment for *gastro-oesophageal reflux disease*. Metoclopramide and domperidone are useful in non-specific and in cytotoxic-induced nausea and vomiting. Metoclopramide and occasionally domperidone may induce an acute dystonic reaction, particularly in young women and children—for further details of this and other side-effects, see section 4.6.

1.3 Ulcer-healing drugs

Peptic ulceration commonly involves the stomach, duodenum, and lower oesophagus; after gastric surgery it involves the gastro-enterostomy stoma.

Healing can be promoted by general measures, stopping smoking and taking antacids and by antisecretory drug treatment, but relapse is common when treatment ceases. Nearly all duodenal ulcers and most gastric ulcers not associated with NSAIDs are caused by *Helicobacter pylori*.

The management of *H. pylori* infection and of NSAID-associated ulcers is discussed below.

Helicobacter pylori infection

Long-term healing of gastric and duodenal ulcers can be achieved rapidly by eradicating *Helicobacter pylori*; it is recommended that the presence of *H. pylori* is confirmed before starting eradication treatment. Acid inhibition combined with antibacterial treatment is highly effective in the eradication of *H. pylori*; reinfection is rare. Antibiotic-induced colitis is an uncommon risk.

One-week triple-therapy regimens that comprise a proton pump inhibitor, amoxicillin, and either clarithromycin or metronidazole, eradicate *H. pylori* in over 90% of cases. There is normally no need to continue antisecretory treatment (with a proton pump inhibitor or H_2-receptor antagonist) unless the ulcer is complicated by haemorrhage or perforation. Resistance to clarithromycin or to metronidazole is much more common than to amoxicillin and can develop during treatment. A regimen containing amoxicillin and clarithromycin is therefore recommended for initial therapy and one containing amoxicillin and metronidazole for eradication failure. Ranitidine bismuth citrate may be substituted for a proton pump inhibitor. Other regimens, including those combining clarithromycin and metronidazole are best used in specialist settings. Treatment failure usually indicates antibacterial resistance or poor compliance.

Two-week triple-therapy regimens offer the possibility of higher eradication rates compared to one-week regimens, but adverse effects are common and poor compliance is likely to offset any possible gain.

Two-week dual-therapy regimens using a proton pump inhibitor and a single antibacterial are licensed, but produce low rates of *H. pylori* eradication and are **not** recommended.

A two-week regimen using tripotassium dicitratobismuthate *plus* a proton pump inhibitor *plus* two antibacterials may have a role in the treatment of resistant cases after confirmation of the presence of *H. pylori*.

Tinidazole or tetracycline are also used occasionally for *H. pylori* eradication; they should be used in combination with antisecretory drugs and other antibacterials.

There is insufficient evidence to support eradication therapy in patients infected with *H. pylori* who continue to take NSAIDs.

Test for *Helicobacter pylori*

^{13}C-Urea breath test kits are available for the diagnosis of gastro-duodenal infection with *Helicobacter pylori*. The test involves collection of breath samples before and after ingestion of an oral solution of ^{13}C-urea; the samples are sent for analysis by an appropriate laboratory. The test should not be performed within 4 weeks of treatment with an antibacterial or within 2 weeks of treatment with an antisecretory drug. A specific ^{13}C-urea breath test kit for children is available (*Helicobacter Test INFAI for children of the age 3–11®*). However, the appropriateness of testing for *H.pylori* infection in children has not been established.

diabact UBT® (MDE) PoM
Tablets, ^{13}C-urea 50 mg, net price 1 kit (including 1 tablet, 4 breath-sample containers, straws) = £15.25 (analysis included), 10-kit pack (hosp. only) = £68.50 (analysis not included)

Helicobacter Test Hp-Plus® (Espire) PoM
Soluble tablets, ^{13}C-urea 100 mg, net price 1 kit (including 4 breath-sample containers, straws, citric acid test meal) = £19.75 (analysis included)

Helicobacter Test INFAI® (Infai) PoM
Oral powder, ^{13}C-urea 75 mg, net price 1 kit (including 4 breath-sample containers, straws) = £19.20 (spectrometric analysis included), 1 kit (including 2 breath bags) = £14.20 (spectroscopic analysis not included), 50-test set = £855.00 (spectrometric analysis included); 45 mg (*Helicobacter Test INFAI for children of the age 3–11*®), 1 kit (including 4 breath-sample containers, straws) = £19.20 (spectrometric analysis included)

Pylobactell® (Torbet) PoM
Soluble tablets, ^{13}C-urea 100 mg, net price 1 kit (including 6 breath-sample containers, 30-mL mixing and administration vial, straws) = £20.75 (analysis included)

NSAID-associated ulcers

Gastro-intestinal bleeding and ulceration can occur with NSAID use (section 10.1.1). Wherever possible, NSAIDs should be **withdrawn** if an ulcer occurs.

In those at risk of ulceration a proton pump inhibitor, an H_2-receptor antagonist such as ranitidine given at twice the usual dose, or misoprostol may be considered for protection against NSAID-associated gastric and duodenal ulcers; colic and diarrhoea may limit the dose of misoprostol.

NSAID use and *H. pylori* infection are independent risk factors for gastro-intestinal bleeding and ulceration. In patients already on a NSAID, eradication of *H. pylori* is not recommended because it is unlikely to reduce the risk of NSAID-induced bleeding or ulceration. However, in patients about to start long-term NSAID treatment who are *H. pylori* positive and have dyspepsia or a history of gastric or duodenal ulcer, eradication of *H. pylori* may reduce the overall risk of ulceration.

If the *NSAID can be discontinued* in a patient who has developed an ulcer, a proton pump inhibitor usually produces the most rapid healing, but the ulcer can be treated with an H_2-receptor antagonist or misoprostol.

If *NSAID treatment needs to continue*, the following options are suitable (see also NICE guidance, section 1.3.5):

- Treat ulcer with a proton pump inhibitor and on healing continue the proton pump inhibitor (dose not normally reduced because asymptomatic ulcer deterioration may occur);
- Treat ulcer with a proton pump inhibitor and on healing switch to misoprostol for maintenance therapy (colic and diarrhoea may limit the dose of misoprostol);
- Treat ulcer with a proton pump inhibitor and switch NSAID to a cyclo-oxygenase-2 selective inhibitor.

1.3.1 H_2-receptor antagonists

All H_2-receptor antagonists heal *gastric and duodenal ulcers* by reducing gastric acid output as a result of histamine H_2-receptor blockade; they can also be expected to relieve *gastro-oesophageal reflux disease* (section 1.1). High doses of

Recommended regimens for *Helicobacter pylori* eradication

Acid suppressant	Antibacterial			Price for 7–day course
	Amoxicillin	Clarithromycin	Metronidazole	
Esomeprazole	1 g twice daily	500 mg twice daily	—	£32.59
20 mg twice daily	—	500 mg twice daily	400 mg twice daily	£31.73
Lansoprazole	1 g twice daily	500 mg twice daily	—	£35.15
30 mg twice daily	1 g twice daily	—	400 mg twice daily	£13.83
	—	500 mg twice daily	400 mg twice daily	£34.29
Omeprazole	1 g twice daily	500 mg twice daily	—	£29.71
20 mg twice daily	500 mg 3 times daily	—	400 mg 3 times daily	£8.03
	—	500 mg twice daily	400 mg twice daily	£28.85
Pantoprazole	1 g twice daily	500 mg twice daily	—	£34.18
40 mg twice daily	—	500 mg twice daily	400 mg twice daily	£33.32
Rabeprazole	1 g twice daily	500 mg twice daily	—	£33.92
20 mg twice daily	—	500 mg twice daily	400 mg twice daily	£33.06
Ranitidine bismuth	1 g twice daily	500 mg twice daily	—	£35.43
citrate	1 g twice daily	—	400 mg twice daily	£14.11
400 mg twice daily	—	500 mg twice daily	400 mg twice daily	£34.57

Regimens that include amoxicillin with either clarithromycin or metronidazole are suitable for use in the community. Regimens that combine clarithromycin with metronidazole are best used in specialist settings (see also notes above)

H_2-receptor antagonists have been used in *Zollinger–Ellison syndrome*, but a proton pump inhibitor is preferred.

Maintenance treatment with low doses has largely been replaced in *Helicobacter pylori* positive patients by eradication regimens (section 1.3). Maintenance treatment may occasionally be used for those with frequent severe recurrences and for the elderly who suffer ulcer complications.

Treatment of *undiagnosed dyspepsia* with H_2-receptor antagonists may be acceptable in younger patients but care is required in older people because of the possibility of gastric cancer in these patients.

H_2-receptor antagonist therapy can promote healing of *NSAID-associated ulcers* (particularly duodenal) (section 1.3).

Treatment has not been shown to be beneficial in haematemesis and melaena, but prophylactic use reduces the frequency of bleeding from *gastroduodenal erosions in hepatic coma*, and possibly in other conditions requiring intensive care. Treatment also reduces the risk of *acid aspiration* in obstetric patients at delivery (Mendelson's syndrome).

CAUTIONS. H_2-receptor antagonists should be used with caution in renal impairment (Appendix 3), pregnancy (Appendix 4), and in breast-feeding (Appendix 5). H_2-receptor antagonists might mask symptoms of gastric cancer; particular care is required in those whose symptoms change and in those who are middle-aged or older.

SIDE-EFFECTS. Side-effects of the H_2-receptor antagonists include diarrhoea and other gastro-intestinal disturbances, altered liver function tests (rarely liver damage), headache, dizziness, rash, and tiredness. Rare side-effects include acute pancreatitis, bradycardia, AV block, confusion, depression, and hallucinations particularly in the elderly or the very ill, hypersensitivity reactions (including fever, arthralgia, myalgia, anaphylaxis), blood disorders (including agranulocytosis, leucopenia, pancytopenia, thrombocytopenia), and skin reactions (including erythema multiforme and toxic epidermal necrolysis). There have been occasional reports of gynaecomastia and impotence.

INTERACTIONS. Cimetidine retards oxidative hepatic drug metabolism by binding to microsomal cytochrome P450. It should be avoided in patients stabilised on warfarin, phenytoin, and theophylline (or aminophylline), but other interactions (see **Appendix 1**) may be of less clinical relevance. Famotidine, nizatidine, and ranitidine do not share the drug metabolism inhibitory properties of cimetidine.

CIMETIDINE

Indications: benign gastric and duodenal ulceration, stomal ulcer, reflux oesophagitis, Zollinger–Ellison syndrome, other conditions where gastric acid reduction is beneficial (see notes above and section 1.9.4)

Cautions: see notes above; also preferably avoid intravenous injection (use intravenous infusion) particularly in high dosage and in cardiovascular impairment (risk of arrhythmias); hepatic impairment (Appendix 2); **interactions:** Appendix 1 (histamine H_2-antagonists) and notes above

Side-effects: see notes above; also alopecia; very rarely tachycardia, interstitial nephritis

Dose: *by mouth*, 400 mg twice daily (with breakfast and at night) *or* 800 mg at night (benign gastric and duodenal ulceration) for at least 4 weeks (6 weeks in gastric ulceration, 8 weeks in NSAID-associated ulceration); when necessary the dose may be increased to 400 mg 4 times daily; INFANT under 1 year 20 mg/kg daily in divided doses has been used; CHILD over 1 year 25–30 mg/kg daily in divided doses

Maintenance, 400 mg at night *or* 400 mg morning and night

Reflux oesophagitis, 400 mg 4 times daily for 4–8 weeks

Zollinger–Ellison syndrome (but see notes above), 400 mg 4 times daily or occasionally more (max. 2.4 g daily)

Prophylaxis of stress ulceration, 200–400 mg every 4–6 hours

Gastric acid reduction (prophylaxis of acid aspiration; do not use syrup), obstetrics 400 mg at start of labour, then up to 400 mg every 4 hours if required (max. 2.4 g daily); surgical procedures 400 mg 90–120 minutes before induction of general anaesthesia

Short-bowel syndrome, 400 mg twice daily (with breakfast and at bedtime) adjusted according to response

To reduce degradation of pancreatic enzyme supplements, 0.8–1.6 g daily in 4 divided doses 1–1½ hours before meals

By intramuscular injection, 200 mg every 4–6 hours

By slow intravenous injection (but see Cautions above) over at least 5 minutes, 200 mg; may be repeated every 4–6 hours; if larger dose needed or if cardiovascular impairment, dilute and give injection over at least 10 minutes (infusion preferable); max. 2.4 g daily

By intravenous infusion, 200–400 mg (may be repeated every 4–6 hours) *or by continuous intravenous infusion* usually at a rate of 50–100 mg/hour over 24 hours, max. 2.4 g daily; INFANT under 1 year, *by slow intravenous injection or by intravenous infusion*, 20 mg/kg daily in divided doses has been used; CHILD over 1 year, 25–30 mg/kg daily in divided doses

[1]**Cimetidine** (Non-proprietary) PoM

Tablets, cimetidine 200 mg, net price 60-tab pack = £2.35; 400 mg, 60-tab pack = £2.98; 800 mg, 30-tab pack = £2.98

Brands include *Peptimax*®

Oral solution, cimetidine 200 mg/5 mL, net price 300 mL = £14.25

1. Cimetidine can be sold to the public for adults and children over 16 years (provided packs do not contain more than 2 weeks' supply) for the short-term symptomatic relief of heartburn, dyspepsia, and hyperacidity (max. single dose 200 mg, max. daily dose 800 mg), and for the prophylactic management of nocturnal heartburn (single night-time dose 100 mg); a proprietary brand (*Tagamet 100*® containing cimetidine 100 mg) is on sale to the public

Dyspamet® (Goldshield) PoM

Suspension, sugar-free, cimetidine 200 mg/5 mL. Contains sorbitol 2.79 g/5 mL. Net price 600 mL = £24.08

Tagamet® (Chemidex) PoM
Tablets, all green, f/c, cimetidine 200 mg, net price 120-tab pack = £19.58; 400 mg, 60-tab pack = £22.62; 800 mg, 30-tab pack = £22.62
Syrup, orange, cimetidine 200 mg/5 mL. Net price 600 mL = £28.49

Tagamet® (GSK) PoM
Injection, cimetidine 100 mg/mL. Net price 2-mL amp = 33p

FAMOTIDINE

Indications: see under Dose
Cautions: see notes above; **interactions:** Appendix 1 (histamine H_2-antagonists) and notes above
Side-effects: see notes above; also very rarely anxiety, anorexia, dry mouth, cholestatic jaundice
Dose: benign gastric and duodenal ulceration, treatment, 40 mg at night for 4–8 weeks; maintenance (duodenal ulceration), 20 mg at night; CHILD not recommended
Reflux oesophagitis, 20–40 mg twice daily for 6–12 weeks; maintenance, 20 mg twice daily
Zollinger–Ellison syndrome (but see notes above), 20 mg every 6 hours (higher dose in those who have previously been receiving another H_2-receptor antagonist); up to 800 mg daily in divided doses has been used

[1]**Famotidine** (Non-proprietary) PoM
Tablets, famotidine 20 mg, net price 28-tab pack = £5.97; 40 mg, 28-tab pack = £9.90

1. Famotidine can be sold to the public for adults and children over 16 years (provided packs do not contain more than 2 weeks' supply) for the short-term symptomatic relief of heartburn, dyspepsia, and hyperacidity, and for the prevention of these symptoms when associated with consumption of food or drink including when they cause sleep disturbance (max. single dose 10 mg, max. daily dose 20 mg); proprietary brands (*Boots Excess Acid Control®*, *Pepcid® AC*, *Pepcid®AC Chewable* all containing famotidine 10 mg) are on sale to the public; a combination of famotidine and antacids (*Pepcidtwo®*) is also available for sale to the public

Pepcid® (MSD) PoM
Tablets, f/c, famotidine 20 mg (beige), net price 28-tab pack = £13.37; 40 mg (brown), 28-tab pack = £25.40

NIZATIDINE

Indications: see under Dose
Cautions: see notes above; also avoid rapid intravenous injection (risk of arrhythmias and postural hypotension); hepatic impairment (Appendix 2); **interactions:** Appendix 1 (histamine H_2-antagonists) and notes above
Side-effects: see notes above; also sweating; rarely hyperuricaemia
Dose: *by mouth*, benign gastric, duodenal or NSAID-associated ulceration, treatment, 300 mg in the evening *or* 150 mg twice daily for 4–8 weeks; maintenance, 150 mg at night; CHILD not recommended
Gastro-oesophageal reflux disease, 150–300 mg twice daily for up to 12 weeks; CHILD not recommended
By intravenous infusion, for short-term use in peptic ulcer as alternative to oral route (for hospital inpatients), *by intermittent intravenous infusion* over 15 minutes, 100 mg 3 times daily, *or by continuous intravenous infusion*, 10 mg/hour; max. 480 mg daily; CHILD not recommended

[1]**Nizatidine** (Non-proprietary) PoM
Capsules, nizatidine 150 mg, net price 30-cap pack = £4.86; 300 mg, 30-cap pack = £7.77

1. Nizatidine can be sold to the public for the prevention and treatment of symptoms of food-related heartburn and meal-induced indigestion in adults and children over 16 years; max. single dose 75 mg, max. daily dose 150 mg for max. 14 days

Axid® (Flynn) PoM
Capsules, nizatidine 150 mg (pale yellow/dark yellow), net price 28-cap pack (hosp. only) = £6.87, 30-cap pack = £7.97; 300 mg (pale yellow/brown), 30-cap pack = £15.80
Injection, nizatidine 25 mg/mL. For dilution and use as an intravenous infusion. Net price 4-mL amp = £1.14

RANITIDINE

Indications: see under Dose, other conditions where reduction of gastric acidity is beneficial (see notes above and section 1.9.4)
Cautions: see notes above; also avoid in porphyria (section 9.8.2); **interactions:** Appendix 1 (histamine H_2-antagonists) and notes above
Side-effects: see notes above; also rarely tachycardia, agitation, visual disturbances, alopecia; very rarely interstitial nephritis
Dose: *by mouth*, 150 mg twice daily *or* 300 mg at night for 4 to 8 weeks in benign gastric and duodenal ulceration, up to 6 weeks in chronic episodic dyspepsia, and up to 8 weeks in NSAID-associated ulceration (in duodenal ulcer 300 mg can be given twice daily for 4 weeks to achieve a higher healing rate); CHILD (peptic ulcer) 2–4 mg/kg twice daily, max. 300 mg daily
Duodenal ulceration associated with *H. pylori*, see eradication regimens on p. 44
Prophylaxis of NSAID-associated gastric or duodenal ulcer [unlicensed dose], 300 mg twice daily
Gastro-oesophageal reflux disease, 150 mg twice daily *or* 300 mg at night for up to 8 weeks or if necessary 12 weeks (moderate to severe, 600 mg daily in 2–4 divided doses for up to 12 weeks); long-term treatment of healed gastro-oesophageal reflux disease, 150 mg twice daily
Zollinger–Ellison syndrome (but see notes above), 150 mg 3 times daily; doses up to 6 g daily in divided doses have been used
Gastric acid reduction (prophylaxis of acid aspiration) in obstetrics, *by mouth*, 150 mg at onset of labour, then every 6 hours; surgical procedures, *by intramuscular or slow intravenous injection*, 50 mg 45–60 minutes before induction of anaesthesia (intravenous injection diluted to 20 mL and given over at least 2 minutes), or *by mouth*, 150 mg 2 hours before induction of anaesthesia and also when possible on the preceding evening
By intramuscular injection, 50 mg every 6–8 hours
By slow intravenous injection, 50 mg diluted to 20 mL and given over at least 2 minutes; may be repeated every 6–8 hours
By intravenous infusion, 25 mg/hour for 2 hours; may be repeated every 6–8 hours
Prophylaxis of stress ulceration, initial *slow intra-*

venous injection of 50 mg (as above) then *continuous infusion*, 125–250 micrograms/kg per hour (may be followed by 150 mg twice daily *by mouth* when oral feeding commences)

[1]**Ranitidine** (Non-proprietary) PoM
Tablets, ranitidine (as hydrochloride) 150 mg, net price 60-tab pack = £7.19; 300 mg, 30-tab pack = £7.19
Brands include *Ranitic*®, *Rantec*®,
Effervescent tablets, ranitidine (as hydrochloride) 150 mg, net price 60-tab pack = £24.93; 300 mg, 30-tab pack = £24.04. Label: 13
Excipients: may include sodium (check with supplier)
Oral solution, ranitidine (as hydrochloride) 75 mg/5 mL, net price 300 mL = £22.32

1. Ranitidine can be sold to the public for adults and children over 16 years (provided packs do not contain more than 2 weeks' supply) for the short-term symptomatic relief of heartburn, dyspepsia, and hyperacidity, and for the prevention of these symptoms when associated with consumption of food or drink (max. single dose 75 mg, max. daily dose 300 mg); proprietary brands (*Gavilast-P*®, *Zantac*® *75*, *Ranzac*® containing ranitidine (as hydrochloride) 75 mg) are on sale to the public

Zantac® (GSK) PoM
Tablets, f/c, ranitidine (as hydrochloride) 150 mg, net price 60-tab pack = £1.30; 300 mg, 30-tab pack = £1.30
Effervescent tablets, pale yellow, ranitidine (as hydrochloride) 150 mg (contains 14.3 mmol Na^+/tablet), net price 60-tab pack = £25.94; 300 mg (contains 20.8 mmol Na^+/tablet), 30-tab pack = £25.51. Label: 13
Excipients: include aspartame (section 9.4.1)
Syrup, sugar-free, ranitidine (as hydrochloride) 75 mg/5 mL. Net price 300 mL = £20.76
Excipients: include alcohol 8%
Injection, ranitidine (as hydrochloride) 25 mg/mL. Net price 2-mL amp = 60p

RANITIDINE BISMUTH CITRATE

(Ranitidine bismutrex)

Indications: see under Dose

Cautions: see notes above; see also under Tripotassium Dicitratobismuthate; renal impairment (Appendix 3); **interactions:** Appendix 1 (histamine H_2-antagonists) and notes above

Contra-indications: pregnancy (Appendix 4); breast-feeding (Appendix 5); porphyria (section 9.8.2)

Side-effects: see notes above; may darken tongue or blacken faeces; rarely tachycardia, agitation, visual disturbances, erythema multiforme, alopecia

Dose: 400 mg twice daily, preferably with food, for 8 weeks in benign gastric ulceration or 4–8 weeks in duodenal ulceration; CHILD not recommended
Eradication of *Helicobacter pylori*, see eradication regimens on p. 44; ranitidine bismuth citrate treatment may be continued for a total of 4 weeks; long-term (maintenance) treatment not recommended (max. total of 16 weeks treatment in any 1 year); CHILD not recommended
COUNSELLING. May darken tongue and blacken faeces

Pylorid® (GSK) PoM
Tablets, blue, f/c, ranitidine bismuth citrate 400 mg. Net price 14-tab pack = £12.09; Counselling (discoloration of tongue and faeces)

1.3.2 Selective antimuscarinics

Pirenzepine is a selective antimuscarinic drug which was used for the treatment of gastric and duodenal ulcers. It has been discontinued.

1.3.3 Chelates and complexes

Tripotassium dicitratobismuthate is a bismuth chelate effective in healing gastric and duodenal ulcers. For the role of tripotassium dicitratobismuthate in a *Helicobacter pylori* eradication regimen for those who have not responded to first-line regimens, see section 1.3.

The bismuth content of tripotassium dicitratobismuthate is low but absorption has been reported; encephalopathy (described with older high-dose bismuth preparations) has not been reported.

Ranitidine bismuth citrate (section 1.3.1) is used in the management of gastric and duodenal ulcers, and in combination with two antibacterials for the eradication of *H. pylori* (section 1.3).

Sucralfate may act by protecting the mucosa from acid-pepsin attack in gastric and duodenal ulcers. It is a complex of aluminium hydroxide and sulphated sucrose but has minimal antacid properties. It should be used with caution in patients under intensive care (**important:** reports of bezoar formation, see CSM advice below)

TRIPOTASSIUM DICITRATOBISMUTHATE

Indications: benign gastric and duodenal ulceration; see also *Helicobacter pylori* infection, section 1.3

Cautions: see notes above; **interactions:** Appendix 1 (tripotassium dicitratobismuthate)

Contra-indications: severe renal impairment; pregnancy (Appendix 4)

Side-effects: may darken tongue and blacken faeces; nausea and vomiting reported

De-Noltab® (Yamanouchi)
Tablets, f/c, tripotassium dicitratobismuthate 120 mg. Net price 112-tab pack = £7.27. Counselling, see below
Dose: 2 tablets twice daily *or* 1 tablet 4 times daily; taken for 28 days followed by further 28 days if necessary; maintenance not indicated but course may be repeated after interval of 1 month; CHILD not recommended
COUNSELLING. To be swallowed with half a glass of water; twice-daily dosage to be taken 30 minutes before breakfast and main evening meal; four-times-daily dosage to be taken as follows: one dose 30 minutes before breakfast, midday meal and main evening meal, and one dose 2 hours after main evening meal; milk should not be drunk by itself during treatment but small quantities may be taken in tea or coffee or on cereal; antacids should not be taken half an hour before or after a dose; may darken tongue and blacken faeces

SUCRALFATE

Indications: see under Dose

Cautions: renal impairment (avoid if severe, see Appendix 3); pregnancy and breast-feeding; administration of sucralfate and enteral feeds should be separated by 1 hour; **interactions:** Appendix 1 (sucralfate)

BEZOAR FORMATION. Following reports of bezoar formation associated with sucralfate, the **CSM** has advised caution in seriously ill patients, especially those receiving concomitant enteral feeds or those with predisposing conditions such as delayed gastric emptying

Side-effects: constipation, diarrhoea, nausea, indigestion, gastric discomfort, dry mouth, rash, hypersensitivity reactions, back pain, dizziness, headache, vertigo and drowsiness, bezoar formation (see above)

Dose: benign gastric and duodenal ulceration and chronic gastritis, 2 g twice daily (on rising and at bedtime) *or* 1 g 4 times daily 1 hour before meals and at bedtime, taken for 4–6 weeks or in resistant cases up to 12 weeks; max. 8 g daily

Prophylaxis of stress ulceration, 1 g 6 times daily (max. 8 g daily)

CHILD not recommended

Antepsin® (Chugai) PoM

Tablets, scored, sucralfate 1 g, net price 50-tab pack = £4.37. Label: 5

COUNSELLING. Tablets may be dispersed in water

Suspension, sucralfate, 1 g/5 mL, net price 250 mL (aniseed- and caramel-flavoured) = £4.37. Label: 5

1.3.4 Prostaglandin analogues

Misoprostol, a synthetic prostaglandin analogue has antisecretory and protective properties, promoting healing of *gastric and duodenal ulcers*. It can prevent NSAID-associated ulcers, its use being most appropriate for the frail or very elderly from whom NSAIDs cannot be withdrawn.

For comment on the use of misoprostol to induce abortion or labour [unlicensed indications], see section 7.1.1.

MISOPROSTOL

Indications: see notes above and under Dose

Cautions: conditions where hypotension might precipitate severe complications (e.g. cerebrovascular disease, cardiovascular disease)

Contra-indications: pregnancy or planning pregnancy (Appendix 4), (increases uterine tone)—**important:** women of childbearing age, see also below, and breast-feeding (Appendix 5)

WOMEN OF CHILDBEARING AGE. Manufacturer advises that misoprostol should not be used in women of childbearing age unless the patient requires non-steroidal anti-inflammatory (NSAID) therapy and is at high risk of complications from NSAID-induced ulceration. In such patients it is advised that misoprostol should only be used if the patient takes *effective contraceptive measures* and has been advised of the *risks of taking misoprostol if pregnant*.

Side-effects: diarrhoea (may occasionally be severe and require withdrawal, reduced by giving single doses not exceeding 200 micrograms and by avoiding magnesium-containing antacids); also reported: abdominal pain, dyspepsia, flatulence, nausea and vomiting, abnormal vaginal bleeding (including intermenstrual bleeding, menorrhagia, and postmenopausal bleeding), rashes, dizziness

Dose: benign gastric and duodenal ulceration and NSAID-associated ulceration, 800 micrograms daily (in 2–4 divided doses) with breakfast (or main meals) and at bedtime; treatment should be continued for at least 4 weeks and may be continued for up to 8 weeks if required

Prophylaxis of NSAID-induced gastric and duodenal ulcer, 200 micrograms 2–4 times daily taken with the NSAID

CHILD not recommended

Cytotec® (Pharmacia) PoM

Tablets, scored, misoprostol 200 micrograms, net price 60-tab pack = £10.03, 140-tab pack = £23.40. Label: 21

■ With diclofenac or naproxen

Section 10.1.1

1.3.5 Proton pump inhibitors

The proton pump inhibitors **omeprazole**, **esomeprazole**, **lansoprazole**, **pantoprazole** and **rabeprazole** inhibit gastric acid by blocking the hydrogen-potassium adenosine triphosphatase enzyme system (the 'proton pump') of the gastric parietal cell. Proton pump inhibitors are effective short-term treatments for *gastric and duodenal ulcers*; they are also used in combination with antibacterials for the eradication of *Helicobacter pylori* (see p. 44 for specific regimens). An initial short course of a proton pump inhibitor is the treatment of choice in *gastro-oesophageal reflux disease* with severe symptoms; patients with endoscopically confirmed *erosive*, *ulcerative*, or *stricturing oesophagitis* usually need to be maintained on a proton pump inhibitor (section 1.1).

Proton pump inhibitors are also used in the prevention and treatment of NSAID-associated ulcers (see p. 44 and guidance issued by NICE, below). In patients who need to continue NSAID treatment after an ulcer has healed, the dose of proton pump inhibitor should normally not be reduced because asymptomatic ulcer deterioration may occur.

Omeprazole is effective in the treatment of *Zollinger-Ellison syndrome* (including cases resistant to other treatment); lansoprazole is also indicated for this condition.

CAUTIONS. Proton pump inhibitors should be used with caution in patients with liver disease (Appendix 2), in pregnancy (Appendix 4) and in breast-feeding (Appendix 5). Proton pump inhibitors may mask the symptoms of gastric cancer; particular care is required in those presenting with 'alarm features' (see p. 37), in such cases gastric malignancy should be ruled out before treatment.

SIDE-EFFECTS. Side-effects of the proton pump inhibitors include gastro-intestinal disturbances (including nausea, vomiting, abdominal pain, flatulence, diarrhoea, constipation), headache, and dizziness. Less frequent side-effects include dry mouth, insomnia, drowsiness, malaise, blurred vision, rash, and pruritus. Other side-effects reported rarely or very rarely include taste disturbance, liver dysfunction, peripheral oedema, hypersensitivity reactions (including urticaria, angioedema, bronchospasm, anaphylaxis), photosensitivity, fever, sweating, depression, interstitial nephritis, blood disorders (including leucopenia, leucocytosis, pancytopenia, thrombocytopenia), arthralgia, myalgia and skin reactions (including Stevens-Johnson syndrome, toxic epidermal necrolysis, bullous eruption). Proton pump inhibitors, by decreasing gastric acidity, may increase the risk of gastro-intestinal infections.

NICE advice (proton pump inhibitors). NICE has provided guidance (July 2000) on the use of proton pump inhibitors for the following indications:

- Gastro-oesophageal reflux disease—use only for severe symptoms (reduce dose when symptoms abate) and in disease complicated by stricture, ulceration, or haemorrhage (full dose should be maintained);
- NSAID-associated ulceration in patients who need to continue NSAID treatment—on healing of the ulcer a lower dose of proton pump inhibitor may be used [but see notes above].

ESOMEPRAZOLE

Indications: see under Dose

Cautions: see notes above; renal impairment (Appendix 3); **interactions:** Appendix 1 (proton pump inhibitors)

Side-effects: see notes above; also reported, dermatitis

Dose: *by mouth* duodenal ulcer associated with *Helicobacter pylori*, see eradication regimens on p. 44

NSAID-associated gastric ulcer, 20 mg once daily for 4–8 weeks; prophylaxis in patients with an increased risk of gastroduodenal complications who require continued NSAID treatment, 20 mg daily

Gastro-oesophageal reflux disease, 40 mg once daily for 4 weeks, continued for further 4 weeks if not fully healed or symptoms persist; maintenance 20 mg daily; symptomatic treatment in the absence of oesophagitis, 20 mg daily for up to 4 weeks, then 20 mg daily when required

CHILD not recommended

COUNSELLING. Swallow whole *or* disperse in water

By intravenous injection over at least 3 minutes or *by intravenous infusion*, gastro-oesophageal reflux disease, 40 mg once daily; symptomatic reflux disease without oesophagitis, 20 mg daily; continue until oral administration possible

CHILD not recommended

Nexium® (AstraZeneca) PoM

Tablets, f/c, esomeprazole (as magnesium trihydrate) 20 mg (light pink), net price 28-tab pack = £18.50 (also 7-tab pack, hosp. only); 40 mg (pink), 28-tab pack = £25.19 (also 7-tab pack, hosp. only). Counselling, administration

Injection▼, powder for reconstitution, esomeprazole (as sodium salt), net price 40-mg vial = £5.21

LANSOPRAZOLE

Indications: see under Dose

Cautions: see notes above; **interactions:** Appendix 1 (proton pump inhibitors)

Side-effects: see notes above; also reported, alopecia, paraesthesia, bruising, purpura, petechiae, fatigue, vertigo, hallucinations, confusion; rarely gynaecomastia, impotence

Dose: benign gastric ulcer, 30 mg daily in the morning for 8 weeks

Duodenal ulcer, 30 mg daily in the morning for 4 weeks; maintenance 15 mg daily

NSAID-associated duodenal or gastric ulcer, 15–30 mg once daily for 4 weeks, continued for further 4 weeks if not fully healed; prophylaxis, 15–30 mg once daily

Duodenal ulcer associated with *Helicobacter pylori*, see eradication regimens on p. 44

Zollinger-Ellison syndrome (and other hypersecretory conditions), initially 60 mg once daily adjusted according to response; daily doses of 120 mg or more given in two divided doses

Gastro-oesophageal reflux disease, 30 mg daily in the morning for 4 weeks, continued for further 4 weeks if not fully healed; maintenance 15–30 mg daily

Acid-related dyspepsia, 15–30 mg daily in the morning for 2–4 weeks

CHILD not recommended

Zoton® (Wyeth) PoM

Capsules, enclosing e/c granules, lansoprazole 15 mg (yellow), net price 28-cap pack = £12.92; 30 mg (lilac/purple), 28-cap pack = £23.63. Label: 5, 25

FasTab® (= orodispersible tablet), lansoprazole 15 mg, net price 28-tab pack = £10.86; 30 mg, 7-tab pack = £4.98, 14-tab pack = £9.94, 28-tab pack = £19.88. Label: 5, counselling, administration

Excipients: include aspartame (section 9.4.1)

COUNSELLING. Tablets should be placed on the tongue, allowed to disperse and swallowed, or may be swallowed whole with a glass of water; tablets should not be crushed or chewed.

Suspension, pink, powder for reconstitution, lansoprazole 30 mg/sachet (strawberry flavour), net price 28-sachet pack = £33.97. Label: 5, 13

■ With antibacterials

For additional cautions, contra-indications and side-effects see Amoxicillin (section 5.1.1), and Clarithromycin (section 5.1.5)

HeliClear® (Wyeth) PoM

Triple pack, lansoprazole capsules 30 mg (*Zoton*®), amoxicillin (as trihydrate) capsules 500 mg, clarithromycin tablets 500 mg (*Klaricid*®). Net price 7-day pack (14 × lansoprazole caps, 28 × amoxicillin caps, 14 × clarithromycin tabs) = £35.01. Label: 5, 9, 25

Dose: eradication of *Helicobacter pylori* in patients with duodenal ulcer, lansoprazole 30 mg twice daily, clarithromycin 500 mg twice daily, and amoxicillin 1 g twice daily for 7–14 days; CHILD not recommended

OMEPRAZOLE

Indications: see under Dose

Cautions: see notes above; **interactions:** Appendix 1 (proton pump inhibitors)

Side-effects: see notes above; also reported, paraesthesia, vertigo, alopecia, gynaecomastia, impotence, stomatitis, encephalopathy in severe liver disease; hyponatraemia; reversible confusion, agitation, and hallucinations in the severely ill; visual impairment reported with high-dose injection

Dose: *by mouth*, benign gastric and duodenal ulcers, 20 mg once daily for 4 weeks in duodenal ulceration or 8 weeks in gastric ulceration; in severe or recurrent cases increase to 40 mg daily; maintenance for recurrent duodenal ulcer, 20 mg once daily; prevention of relapse in duodenal ulcer, 10 mg daily increasing to 20 mg once daily if symptoms return

NSAID-associated duodenal or gastric ulcer and gastroduodenal erosions, 20 mg once daily for 4 weeks, continued for further 4 weeks if not fully healed; prophylaxis in patients with a history of NSAID-associated duodenal or gastric ulcers, gastroduodenal lesions, or dyspeptic symptoms who require continued NSAID treatment, 20 mg once daily

Duodenal or benign gastric ulcer associated with *Helicobacter pylori*, see eradication regimens on p. 44

Zollinger–Ellison syndrome, initially 60 mg once daily; usual range 20–120 mg daily (above 80 mg in 2 divided doses)

Gastric acid reduction during general anaesthesia (prophylaxis of acid aspiration), 40 mg on the preceding evening then 40 mg 2–6 hours before surgery

Gastro-oesophageal reflux disease, 20 mg once daily for 4 weeks, continued for further 4–8 weeks if not fully healed; 40 mg once daily has been given for 8 weeks in gastro-oesophageal reflux disease refractory to other treatment; maintenance 20 mg once daily

Acid reflux disease (long-term management), 10 mg daily increasing to 20 mg once daily if symptoms return

Acid-related dyspepsia, 10–20 mg once daily for 2–4 weeks according to response

Severe ulcerating reflux oesophagitis (treat for 4–12 weeks), CHILD over 1 year, body-weight 10–20 kg, 10 mg once daily increased if necessary to 20 mg once daily; body-weight over 20 kg, 20 mg once daily increased if necessary to 40 mg once daily; to be initiated by hospital paediatrician

By intravenous injection over 5 minutes *or by intravenous infusion*, prophylaxis of acid aspiration, 40 mg completed 1 hour before surgery

Benign gastric ulcer, duodenal ulcer and gastro-oesophageal reflux, 40 mg once daily until oral administration possible

CHILD not recommended

COUNSELLING. Swallow whole, *or* disperse *MUPS*® tablets in water, *or* mix capsule contents or *MUPS*® tablets with fruit juice or yoghurt

Omeprazole (Non-proprietary) PoM

Capsules, enclosing e/c granules, omeprazole 10 mg, net price 28-cap pack = £7.72; 20 mg, 28-cap pack = £12.75; 40 mg, 7-cap pack = £10.05. Label: 5, counselling, administration

[1]*Tablets*, e/c, omeprazole 10 mg, net price 28-tab pack = £11.40; 20 mg, 28-tab pack = £12.75; 40 mg, 7-tab pack = £10.05. Label: 25

1. Omeprazole 10 mg tablets can be sold to the public for the short-term relief of reflux-like symptoms (e.g. heartburn) in adults over 18 years, max. daily dose 20 mg for max. 4 weeks, and a pack size of 28 tablets; proprietary brands on sale to the public include *Zanprol*®

Losec® (AstraZeneca) PoM

MUPS® (multiple-unit pellet system = dispersible tablets), f/c, omeprazole 10 mg (light pink), net price 28-tab pack = £19.34; 20 mg (pink), 28-tab pack = £29.22; 40 mg (red-brown), 7-tab pack = £14.61. Counselling, administration

Capsules, enclosing e/c granules, omeprazole 10 mg (pink), net price 28-cap pack = £19.34; 20 mg (pink/brown), 28-cap pack = £29.22; 40 mg (brown), 7-cap pack = £14.61. Counselling, administration

Intravenous infusion, powder for reconstitution, omeprazole (as sodium salt), net price 40-mg vial = £5.21

Injection, powder for reconstitution, omeprazole (as sodium salt), net price 40-mg vial (with solvent) = £5.21

PANTOPRAZOLE

Indications: see under Dose

Cautions: see notes above; also renal impairment (Appendix 3); **interactions:** Appendix 1 (proton pump inhibitors)

Side-effects: see notes above; also reported, raised triglycerides

Dose: *by mouth*, benign gastric ulcer, 40 mg daily in the morning for 4 weeks, continued for further 4 weeks if not fully healed

Gastro-oesophageal reflux disease, 20–40 mg daily in the morning for 4 weeks, continued for further 4 weeks if not fully healed; maintenance 20 mg daily, increased to 40 mg daily if symptoms return

Duodenal ulcer, 40 mg daily in the morning for 2 weeks, continued for further 2 weeks if not fully healed

Duodenal ulcer associated with *Helicobacter pylori*, see eradication regimens on p. 44

Prophylaxis of NSAID-associated gastric or duodenal ulcer in patients with an increased risk of gastroduodenal complications who require continued NSAID treatment, 20 mg daily

Zollinger–Ellison syndrome (and other hypersecretory conditions), initially 80 mg once daily adjusted according to response (ELDERLY max. 40 mg daily); daily doses above 80 mg given in 2 divided doses

CHILD not recommended

By intravenous injection over at least 2 minutes *or by intravenous infusion*, duodenal ulcer, gastric ulcer, and gastro-oesophageal reflux, 40 mg daily until oral administration can be resumed

Zollinger–Ellison syndrome (and other hypersecretory conditions), initially 80 mg (160 mg if rapid acid control required) then 80 mg once daily adjusted according to response; daily doses above 80 mg given in 2 divided doses

CHILD not recommended

Protium® (Altana) PoM

Tablets, yellow, e/c, pantoprazole (as sodium sesquihydrate) 20 mg, net price 28-tab pack = £12.31; 40 mg, 28-tab pack = £21.69. Label: 25

Injection, powder for reconstitution, pantoprazole (as sodium sesquihydrate), net price 40-mg vial = £5.71

RABEPRAZOLE SODIUM

Indications: see under Dose

Cautions: see notes above; **interactions:** Appendix 1 (proton pump inhibitors)

Side-effects: see notes above; also reported, cough, pharyngitis, rhinitis, asthenia, influenza-like syndrome; less commonly chest pain, sinusitis, nervousness, urinary tract infection; rarely stomatitis, encephalopathy in severe liver disease, anorexia, weight gain

Dose: benign gastric ulcer, 20 mg daily in the morning for 6 weeks, continued for further 6 weeks if not fully healed
Duodenal ulcer, 20 mg daily in the morning for 4 weeks, continued for further 4 weeks if not fully healed
Gastro-oesophageal reflux disease, 20 mg once daily for 4–8 weeks; maintenance 10–20 mg daily; symptomatic treatment in the absence of oesophagitis, 10 mg daily for up to 4 weeks, then 10 mg daily when required
Duodenal and benign gastric ulcer associated with *Helicobacter pylori*, see eradication regimens on p. 44
Zollinger–Ellison syndrome, initially 60 mg once daily adjusted according to response (max. 120 mg daily); doses above 100 mg daily given in 2 divided doses
CHILD not recommended

Pariet® (Janssen-Cilag, Eisai) PoM
Tablets, e/c, rabeprazole sodium 10 mg (pink), net price 28-tab pack = £11.56; 20 mg (yellow), 28-tab pack = £21.16. Label: 25

1.3.6 Other ulcer-healing drugs

Carbenoxolone is a synthetic derivative of glycyrrhizinic acid (a constituent of liquorice) which was used for the treatment of oesophageal ulceration and inflammation. It has been discontinued.

1.4 Acute diarrhoea

The priority in acute diarrhoea, as in gastro-enteritis, is the prevention or reversal of fluid and electrolyte depletion. This is particularly important in infants and in frail and elderly patients. For details of **oral rehydration preparations**, see section 9.2.1.2. Severe depletion of fluid and electrolytes requires immediate admission to hospital and urgent replacement.

Antimotility drugs (section 1.4.2) relieve symptoms of acute diarrhoea. They are used in the management of uncomplicated acute diarrhoea in adults; fluid and electrolyte replacement may be necessary in case of dehydration. However, antimotility drugs are **not** recommended for acute diarrhoea in young children.

Antispasmodics (section 1.2) are occasionally of value in treating abdominal cramp associated with diarrhoea but they should **not** be used for primary treatment. Antispasmodics and antiemetics should be **avoided** in young children with gastro-enteritis because they are rarely effective and have troublesome side-effects.

Antibacterial drugs are generally unnecessary in simple gastro-enteritis because the complaint usually resolves quickly without them, and infective diarrhoeas in the UK often have a viral cause. Systemic bacterial infection does, however, need appropriate systemic treatment; for drugs used in campylobacter enteritis, shigellosis, and salmonellosis, see section 5.1, table 1. **Ciprofloxacin** is occasionally used for prophylaxis against travellers' diarrhoea, but routine use is **not** recommended. Lactobacillus preparations have not been shown to be effective.

Colestyramine (cholestyramine, section 1.9.2) and **aluminium hydroxide mixture** (section 1.1.1), bind unabsorbed bile salts and provide symptomatic relief of diarrhoea following ileal disease or resection.

1.4.1 Adsorbents and bulk-forming drugs

Adsorbents such as kaolin are **not** recommended for *acute diarrhoeas*. Bulk-forming drugs, such as ispaghula, methylcellulose, and sterculia (section 1.6.1) are useful in controlling faecal consistency in ileostomy and colostomy, and in controlling diarrhoea associated with diverticular disease.

KAOLIN, LIGHT

Indications: diarrhoea but see notes above
Cautions: interactions: Appendix 1 (kaolin)

Kaolin Mixture, BP
(Kaolin Oral Suspension)
Oral suspension, light kaolin or light kaolin (natural) 20%, light magnesium carbonate 5%, sodium bicarbonate 5% in a suitable vehicle with a peppermint flavour.
Dose: 10–20 mL every 4 hours
NOTE. Kaolin-containing preparations on sale to the public include *KLN*®

1.4.2 Antimotility drugs

Antimotility drugs have a role in the management of uncomplicated *acute diarrhoea* in adults but not in young children; see also section 1.4. However, in severe cases, fluid and electrolyte replacement (section 9.2.1.2) are of primary importance.

For comments on the role of antimotility drugs in *chronic diarrhoea* see section 1.5. For their role in *stoma care* see section 1.8.

CODEINE PHOSPHATE

Indications: see notes above; cough suppression (section 3.9.1); pain (section 4.7.2)
Cautions: see section 4.7.2; also not recommended for children; tolerance and dependence may occur with prolonged use; **interactions:** Appendix 1 (opioid analgesics)
Contra-indications: see section 4.7.2; also conditions where inhibition of peristalsis should be avoided, where abdominal distension develops, or in acute diarrhoeal conditions such as acute ulcerative colitis or antibiotic-associated colitis
Side-effects: see section 4.7.2
Dose: see preparations

Codeine Phosphate (Non-proprietary) PoM
Tablets, codeine phosphate 15 mg, net price 28 = £1.66; 30 mg, 28 = £2.29; 60 mg, 28 = £3.46. Label: 2
Dose: acute diarrhoea, 30 mg 3–4 times daily (range 15–60 mg); CHILD not recommended
NOTE. Travellers needing to take codeine phosphate tablets abroad may require a doctor's letter explaining why they are necessary.

Kaodene® (Sovereign) NHS
Suspension, codeine phosphate 5 mg, light kaolin 1.5 g/5 mL. Net price 250 mL = £2.06
Dose: 20 mL 3–4 times daily; CHILD under 5 years not recommended, over 5 years 10 mL but see cautions and notes above

CO-PHENOTROPE

A mixture of diphenoxylate hydrochloride and atropine sulphate in the mass proportions 100 parts to 1 part respectively

Indications: adjunct to rehydration in acute diarrhoea (but see notes above); chronic mild ulcerative colitis; control of faecal consistency after colostomy or ileostomy (section 1.8)

Cautions: see under Codeine Phosphate; also young children are particularly susceptible to **overdosage** and symptoms may be delayed and observation is needed for at least 48 hours after ingestion; presence of subclinical doses of atropine may give rise to atropine side-effects in susceptible individuals or in overdosage; **interactions:** Appendix 1 (opioid analgesics)

Contra-indications: see under Codeine Phosphate; jaundice

Side-effects: see under Codeine Phosphate, section 4.7.2

Dose: see preparation

[1]**Lomotil**® (Goldshield) PoM
Tablets, co-phenotrope 2.5/0.025 (diphenoxylate hydrochloride 2.5 mg, atropine sulphate 25 micrograms), net price 20 = £1.63
Dose: initially 4 tablets, followed by 2 tablets every 6 hours until diarrhoea controlled; CHILD under 4 years not recommended, 4–8 years 1 tablet 3 times daily, 9–12 years 1 tablet 4 times daily, 13–16 years 2 tablets 3 times daily, but see also notes above

1. Co-phenotrope 2.5/0.025 can be sold to the public for adults and adolescents over 16 years (provided packs do not contain more than 20 tablets) as an adjunct to rehydration in acute diarrhoea (max. daily dose 10 tablets); proprietary brands on sale to public include *Dymotil*®

LOPERAMIDE HYDROCHLORIDE

Indications: symptomatic treatment of acute diarrhoea; adjunct to rehydration in acute diarrhoea in adults and children over 4 years (but see notes above); chronic diarrhoea in adults only

Cautions: see notes above; also liver disease; pregnancy (Appendix 4); **interactions:** Appendix 1 (loperamide)

Contra-indications: conditions where inhibition of peristalsis should be avoided, where abdominal distension develops, or in conditions such as active ulcerative colitis or antibiotic-associated colitis

Side-effects: abdominal cramps, dizziness, drowsiness, and skin reactions including urticaria; paralytic ileus and abdominal bloating also reported

Dose: acute diarrhoea, 4 mg initially followed by 2 mg after each loose stool for up to 5 days; usual dose 6–8 mg daily; max. 16 mg daily; CHILD under 4 years not recommended, 4–8 years 1 mg 3–4 times daily for up to *3 days only*, 9–12 years 2 mg 4 times daily for up to 5 days
Chronic diarrhoea in adults, initially, 4–8 mg daily in divided doses, subsequently adjusted according to response and given in 2 divided doses for maintenance; max. 16 mg daily

[1]**Loperamide** (Non-proprietary) PoM
Capsules, loperamide hydrochloride 2 mg. Net price 30-cap pack = £1.59
Brands include *Norimode*®

[1]**Imodium**® (Janssen-Cilag) PoM
Capsules, green/grey, loperamide hydrochloride 2 mg. Net price 30-cap pack = £1.16
Syrup, red, sugar-free, loperamide hydrochloride 1 mg/5 mL. Net price 100 mL = £1.00

■ Compound preparations

Imodium® **Plus** (J&J MSD)
Tablets (chewable), scored, loperamide hydrochloride 2 mg, simeticone 125 mg, net price 6-tab pack = £1.97, 12-tab pack = £3.40, 18-tab pack = £4.54. Label: 24
Caplets (= tablets), loperamide hydrochloride 2 mg, simeticone 125 mg, net price 6-tab pack = £2.14, 12-tab pack = £3.40
Dose: acute diarrhoea with abdominal colic, initially 2 tablets or caplets (ADOLESCENT 12–18 years 1 tablet or caplet) then 1 tablet or caplet after each loose stool; max. 4 tablets or caplets daily for up to 2 days; CHILD not recommended

MORPHINE

Indications: see notes above

Cautions: see notes above and under Codeine Phosphate (section 4.7.2)

Contra-indications: see notes above and under Codeine Phosphate

Side-effects: see notes above and under Codeine Phosphate (section 4.7.2); sedation and the risk of dependence are greater

Dose: see preparation

Kaolin and Morphine Mixture, BP
(Kaolin and Morphine Oral Suspension)
Oral suspension, light kaolin or light kaolin (natural) 20%, sodium bicarbonate 5%, and chloroform and morphine tincture 4% in a suitable vehicle. Contains anhydrous morphine 550–800 micrograms/10 mL.
Dose: 10 mL every 4 hours in water

■ Preparations on sale to the public

Preparations on sale to the public containing morphine include:
Diocalm® (attapulgite, morphine)
Opazimes® (belladonna, morphine, aluminium, kaolin)

1.5 Chronic bowel disorders

Once tumours are ruled out individual symptoms of chronic bowel disorders need specific treatment including dietary manipulation as well as drug treatment and the maintenance of a liberal fluid intake.

1. Loperamide can be sold to the public, for adults and children over 12 years, provided it is licensed and labelled for the treatment of acute diarrhoea; proprietary brands including *Arret*® capsules NHS, *Boots Diareze Diarrhoea Relief*® capsules, *Diasorb*® capsules, *Diocalm Ultra*® capsules NHS and *Imodium*® NHS (8- and 12-cap packs), *Imodium*® liquid and *Normaloe*® tablets are on sale to the public

Irritable bowel syndrome

Irritable bowel syndrome can present with pain, constipation, or diarrhoea. In some patients there may be important psychological aggravating factors which respond to reassurance and possibly specific treatment e.g. with an antidepressant. A laxative (section 1.6) may be needed to relieve constipation. Antimotility drugs such as loperamide (section 1.4.2) may relieve diarrhoea and antispasmodic drugs (section 1.2) may relieve pain. Opioids with a central action such as codeine are better avoided because of the risk of dependence.

Malabsorption syndromes

Individual conditions need specific management and also general nutritional consideration. Thus coeliac disease (gluten enteropathy) usually needs a gluten-free diet (Appendix 7) and pancreatic insufficiency needs pancreatin supplements (section 1.9.4).

Inflammatory bowel disease

Chronic inflammatory bowel diseases include *ulcerative colitis* and *Crohn's disease*. Effective management requires drug therapy, attention to nutrition, and in severe or chronic active disease, surgery.

Aminosalicylates (balsalazide, mesalazine, olsalazine, and sulfasalazine), and **corticosteroids** (hydrocortisone, budesonide, and prednisolone) form the basis of drug treatment.

TREATMENT OF ACUTE ULCERATIVE COLITIS AND CROHN'S DISEASE. Acute mild to moderate disease affecting the rectum (proctitis) or the recto-sigmoid (distal colitis) is treated initially with local application of a corticosteroid or an aminosalicylate; foam preparations and suppositories are especially useful where patients have difficulty retaining liquid enemas.

Diffuse inflammatory bowel disease or disease that does not respond to local therapy requires oral treatment; mild disease affecting the colon may be treated with an aminosalicylate alone but refractory or moderate disease usually requires adjunctive use of an oral corticosteroid such as **prednisolone** for 4–8 weeks. Modified-release **budesonide** is licensed for Crohn's disease affecting the ileum and the ascending colon; it causes fewer systemic side-effects than oral prednisolone but may be less effective.

Severe inflammatory bowel disease calls for hospital admission and treatment with intravenous corticosteroid; other therapy may include intravenous fluid and electrolyte replacement, blood transfusion, and possibly parenteral nutrition and antibiotics. Specialist supervision is required for patients who fail to respond adequately to these measures. Patients with ulcerative colitis may benefit from a short course of ciclosporin (section 8.2.2) [unlicensed indication]. Patients with unresponsive or chronically active Crohn's disease may benefit from azathioprine (section 8.2.1), mercaptopurine (see below), or once-weekly methotrexate (section 10.1.3) [all unlicensed indications].

Infliximab is licensed for the management of severe active Crohn's disease in patients whose condition has not responded adequately to treatment with a corticosteroid and a conventional immunosuppressant or who are intolerant of them. Infliximab is also licensed for the management of refractory fistulating Crohn's disease. Maintenance therapy with infliximab should be considered for patients who respond to the initial induction course; fixed-interval dosing may be superior to intermittent dosing.

> **NICE guidance (infliximab for Crohn's disease).** NICE has recommended (April 2002) that infliximab is used only for the treatment of severe active Crohn's disease (with or without fistulae) when treatment with immunomodulating drugs and corticosteroids has failed or is not tolerated and when surgery is inappropriate. Treatment may be repeated if the condition responded to the initial course but relapsed subsequently. Infliximab should be prescribed only by a gastroenterologist.

Metronidazole (section 5.1.11) may be beneficial for the treatment of active Crohn's disease with perianal involvement, possibly through its antibacterial activity. Metronidazole in doses of 0.6–1.5 g daily in divided doses has been used; it is usually given for a month but no longer than 3 months because of concerns about developing peripheral neuropathy. Other antibacterials should be given if specifically indicated (e.g. sepsis associated with fistulas and perianal disease) and for managing bacterial overgrowth in the small bowel.

MAINTENANCE OF REMISSION OF ACUTE ULCERATIVE COLITIS AND CROHN'S DISEASE. **Aminosalicylates** are of great value in the maintenance of remission of ulcerative colitis. They are of less value in the maintenance of remission of Crohn's disease; an oral formulation of mesalazine is licensed for the long-term management of ileal disease. Corticosteroids are **not** suitable for maintenance treatment because of side-effects. In resistant or frequently relapsing cases either **azathioprine** (section 8.2.1) 2–2.5 mg/kg daily [unlicensed indication] or **mercaptopurine** (section 8.1.3) 1–1.5 mg/kg daily [unlicensed indication], given under close supervision may be helpful; some patients may respond to lower doses of these drugs. Methotrexate (section 10.1.3) is tried in Crohn's disease if azathioprine or mercaptopurine cannot be used [unlicensed indication]; a dose of methotrexate 15 mg *weekly* is used. **Infliximab** is licensed for maintenance therapy in Crohn's disease (but see notes above).

ADJUNCTIVE TREATMENT OF INFLAMMATORY BOWEL DISEASE. Due attention should be paid to diet; high-fibre or low-residue diets should be used as appropriate. Irritable bowel syndrome during remission of ulcerative colitis calls for avoidance of a high-fibre diet and possible treatment with an antispasmodic (section 1.2).

Antimotility drugs such as codeine and loperamide, and antispasmodic drugs may precipitate paralytic ileus and megacolon in active ulcerative colitis; treatment of the inflammation is more logical. Laxatives may be required in proctitis. Diarrhoea resulting from the loss of bile-salt absorption (e.g. in terminal ileal disease or bowel resection) may improve with **colestyramine** (section 1.9.2), which binds bile salts.

Antibiotic-associated colitis

Antibiotic-associated colitis (pseudomembranous colitis) is caused by colonisation of the colon with *Clostridium difficile* which may follow antibiotic therapy. It is usually of acute onset, but may run a chronic course; it is a particular hazard of clindamycin but few antibiotics are free of this side-effect. Oral **vancomycin** (see section 5.1.7) or **metronidazole** (see section 5.1.11) are used as specific treatment; vancomycin may be preferred for very sick patients.

Diverticular disease

Diverticular disease is treated with a high-fibre diet, **bran supplements**, and **bulk-forming drugs**. **Antispasmodics** may provide symptomatic relief when colic is a problem (section 1.2). **Antibacterials** are used only when the diverticula in the intestinal wall become infected (specialist referral). **Antimotility** drugs which slow intestinal motility, e.g. codeine, diphenoxylate, and loperamide could possibly exacerbate the symptoms of diverticular disease and are **contra-indicated**.

Aminosalicylates

Sulfasalazine is a combination of 5-aminosalicylic acid ('5-ASA') and sulfapyridine; sulfapyridine acts only as a carrier to the colonic site of action but still causes side-effects. In the newer aminosalicylates, **mesalazine** (5-aminosalicylic acid), **balsalazide** (a prodrug of 5-aminosalicylic acid) and **olsalazine** (a dimer of 5-aminosalicylic acid which cleaves in the lower bowel), the sulphonamide-related side-effects of sulfasalazine are avoided, but 5-aminosalicylic acid alone can still cause side-effects including blood disorders (see recommendation below) and lupoid phenomenon also seen with sulfasalazine.

CAUTIONS. Aminosalicylates should be used with caution in renal impairment (Appendix 3), during pregnancy (Appendix 4) and breast-feeding (Appendix 5); blood disorders can occur (see recommendation below).

Blood disorders
Patients receiving aminosalicylates should be advised to report any unexplained bleeding, bruising, purpura, sore throat, fever or malaise that occurs during treatment. A blood count should be performed and the drug stopped immediately if there is suspicion of a blood dyscrasia.

CONTRA-INDICATIONS. Aminosalicylates should be avoided in salicylate hypersensitivity.

SIDE-EFFECTS. Side-effects of the aminosalicylates include diarrhoea, nausea, vomiting, abdominal pain, exacerbation of symptoms of colitis, headache, hypersensitivity reactions (including rash and urticaria); side-effects that occur rarely include acute pancreatitis, hepatitis, myocarditis, pericarditis, lung disorders (including eosinophilia and fibrosing alveolitis), peripheral neuropathy, blood disorders (including agranulocytosis, aplastic anaemia, leucopenia, methaemoglobinaemia, neutropenia, and thrombocytopenia—see also recommendation above), renal dysfunction (interstitial nephritis, nephrotic syndrome), myalgia, arthralgia, skin reactions (including lupus erythematosus-like syndrome, Stevens-Johnson syndrome), alopecia.

BALSALAZIDE SODIUM

Indications: treatment of mild to moderate ulcerative colitis and maintenance of remission
Cautions: see notes above; also history of asthma; **interactions:** Appendix 1 (aminosalicylates)
BLOOD DISORDERS. See recommendation above
Contra-indications: see notes above; also severe hepatic impairment
Side-effects: see notes above; also cholelithiasis
Dose: acute attack, 2.25 g 3 times daily until remission occurs or for up to max. 12 weeks
Maintenance, 1.5 g twice daily, adjusted according to response (max. 6 g daily)
CHILD not recommended

Colazide® (Shire) PoM
Capsules, beige, balsalazide sodium 750 mg. Net price 130-cap pack = £39.00. Label: 21, 25, counselling, blood disorder symptoms (see recommendation above)

MESALAZINE

Indications: treatment of mild to moderate ulcerative colitis and maintenance of remission; see also under preparations
Cautions: see notes above; elderly; with oral preparations, test renal function initially and every 3 months for first year then every 6 months for next 4 years and annually thereafter (risk of serious renal toxicity); **interactions:** Appendix 1 (aminosalicylates)
BLOOD DISORDERS. See recommendation above
Contra-indications: see notes above; also severe hepatic impairment
Side-effects: see notes above
Dose: see under preparations, below
NOTE. The delivery characteristics of enteric-coated mesalazine preparations may vary; these preparations should not be considered interchangeable

Asacol® (Procter & Gamble Pharm.) PoM
Foam enema, mesalazine 1 g/metered application, net price 14-application cannister with disposable applicators and plastic bags = £35.17. Counselling, blood disorder symptoms (see recommendation above)
Dose: acute attack affecting the rectosigmoid region, 1 metered application (mesalazine 1 g) into the rectum daily for 4–6 weeks; acute attack affecting the descending colon, 2 metered applications (mesalazine 2 g) once daily for 4–6 weeks; CHILD not recommended
Suppositories, mesalazine 250 mg, net price 20-suppos pack = £6.35; 500 mg, 10 suppos pack = £6.35. Counselling, blood disorder symptoms (see recommendation above)
Dose: 0.75–1.5 g daily in divided doses, with last dose at bedtime; CHILD not recommended

Asacol® **MR** (Procter & Gamble Pharm.) PoM
Tablets, red, e/c, mesalazine 400 mg, net price 90-tab pack = £29.03, 120-tab pack = £38.71. Label: 5, 25, counselling, blood disorder symptoms (see recommendation above)
Dose: ulcerative colitis, acute attack, 6 tablets daily in divided doses; maintenance of remission of ulcerative

colitis and Crohn's ileo-colitis, 3–6 tablets daily in divided doses; CHILD not recommended
NOTE. Preparations that lower stool pH (e.g. lactulose) may prevent release of mesalazine

Ipocol® (Sandoz) PoM
Tablets, e/c, mesalazine 400 mg, net price 120-tab pack = £35.20. Label: 5, 25, counselling, blood disorder symptoms (see recommendation above)
Dose: acute attack, 6 tablets daily in divided doses; maintenance of remission, 3–6 tablets daily in divided doses; CHILD not recommended
NOTE. Preparations that lower stool pH (e.g. lactulose) may prevent release of mesalazine

Mesren MR® (IVAX) PoM
Tablets, red-brown, e/c, mesalazine 400 mg, net price 90-tab pack = £20.29, 120-tab pack = £27.05. Label: 5, 25, counselling, blood disorder symptoms (see recommendation above)
Dose: acute attack, 6 tablets daily in divided doses; maintenance of remission, 3–6 tablets daily in divided doses; CHILD not recommended
NOTE. Preparations that lower stool pH (e.g. lactulose) may prevent release of mesalazine

Pentasa® (Ferring) PoM
Slow release tablets, m/r, scored, mesalazine 500 mg (grey), net price 100-tab pack = £25.48. Counselling, administration, see dose, blood disorder symptoms (see recommendation above)
Dose: acute attack, up to 4 g daily in 2–3 divided doses; maintenance, 1.5 g daily in 2–3 divided doses; tablets may be dispersed in water, but should not be chewed; CHILD under 15 years not recommended
Prolonged release granules, m/r, pale brown, mesalazine 1 g/sachet, net price 50-sachet pack = £30.02. Counselling, administration, see dose, blood disorder symptoms (see recommendation above)
Dose: acute attack, up to 4 g daily in 2–4 divided doses; maintenance, 2 g daily in 2 divided doses; granules should be placed on tongue and washed down with water or orange juice without chewing; CHILD under 12 years not recommended
Retention enema, mesalazine 1 g in 100-mL pack. Net price 7 enemas = £18.09. Counselling, blood disorder symptoms (see recommendation above)
Dose: 1 enema at bedtime; CHILD not recommended
Suppositories, mesalazine 1 g. Net price 28-suppos pack = £41.55. Counselling, blood disorder symptoms (see recommendation above)
Dose: ulcerative proctitis, acute attack, 1 suppository daily for 2–4 weeks; maintenance, 1 suppository daily; CHILD under 15 years not recommended

Salofalk® (Dr Falk) PoM
Tablets, e/c, yellow, mesalazine 250 mg. Net price 100-tab pack = £17.40. Label: 5, 25, counselling, blood disorder symptoms (see recommendation above)
Dose: acute attack, 6 tablets daily in 3 divided doses; maintenance 3–6 tablets daily in divided doses; CHILD not recommended
Granules, m/r, grey, mesalazine 500 mg/sachet, net price 100-sachet pack = £29.30; 1 g/sachet, 50-sachet pack = £29.30. Counselling, administration, see dose, blood disorder symptoms (see recommendation above)
Excipients: include aspartame (section 9.4.1)
Dose: acute attack, 0.5–1 g 3 times daily; maintenance, 500 mg 3 times daily; CHILD over 6 years, body-weight under 40 kg half adult dose, body-weight over 40 kg, adult dose; granules should be placed on tongue and washed down with water without chewing
NOTE. Preparations that lower stool pH (e.g. lactulose) may prevent release of mesalazine
Suppositories, mesalazine 500 mg. Net price 30-suppos pack = £15.90. Counselling, blood disorder symptoms (see recommendation above)
Dose: acute attack, 1–2 suppositories 2–3 times daily adjusted according to response; CHILD not recommended
Enema, mesalazine 2 g in 59-mL pack. Net price 7 enemas = £31.20. Counselling, blood disorder symptoms (see recommendation above)
Dose: acute attack *or* maintenance, 1 enema daily at bedtime; CHILD not recommended
Rectal foam, mesalazine 1 g/metered application, net price 14-application cannister with disposable applicators and plastic bags = £31.10. Counselling, blood disorder symptoms (see recommendation above)
Dose: mild ulcerative colitis affecting sigmoid colon and rectum, 2 metered applications (mesalazine 2 g) into the rectum at bedtime increased if necessary to 2 metered applications (mesalazine 2 g) twice daily; CHILD not recommended

OLSALAZINE SODIUM

Indications: treatment of mild ulcerative colitis and maintenance of remission
Cautions: see notes above; **interactions:** Appendix 1 (aminosalicylates)
BLOOD DISORDERS. See recommendation above
Contra-indications: see notes above
Side-effects: see notes above; also watery diarrhoea
Dose: acute attack, 1 g daily in divided doses after meals increased if necessary over 1 week to max. 3 g daily (max. single dose 1 g)
Maintenance, 500 mg twice daily after meals; CHILD not recommended

Dipentum® (Celltech) PoM
Capsules, brown, olsalazine sodium 250 mg. Net price 112-cap pack = £20.57. Label: 21, counselling, blood disorder symptoms (see recommendation above)
Tablets, yellow, scored, olsalazine sodium 500 mg. Net price 60-tab pack = £22.04. Label: 21, counselling, blood disorder symptoms (see recommendation above)

SULFASALAZINE

(Sulphasalazine)

Indications: treatment of mild to moderate and severe ulcerative colitis and maintenance of remission; active Crohn's disease; rheumatoid arthritis (section 10.1.3)
Cautions: see notes above; also history of allergy; hepatic impairment; G6PD deficiency (section 9.1.5); slow acetylator status; risk of haematological and hepatic toxicity (differential white cell, red cell and platelet counts initially and at monthly intervals for first 3 months, liver function tests at monthly intervals for first 3 months); kidney function tests at regular intervals; upper gastro-intestinal side-effects common over 4 g daily; porphyria (section 9.8.2); **interactions:** Appendix 1 (aminosalicylates)
BLOOD DISORDERS. See recommendation above
Contra-indications: see notes above; also sulphonamide hypersensitivity; CHILD under 2 years of age

Side-effects: see notes above; also loss of appetite; fever; blood disorders (including Heinz body anaemia, megaloblastic anaemia); hypersensitivity reactions (including exfoliative dermatitis, epidermal necrolysis, pruritus, photosensitisation, anaphylaxis, serum sickness); ocular complications (including periorbital oedema); stomatitis, parotitis; ataxia, aseptic meningitis, vertigo, tinnitus, insomnia, depression, hallucinations; kidney reactions (including proteinuria, crystalluria, haematuria); oligospermia; urine may be coloured orange; some soft contact lenses may be stained

Dose: *by mouth*, acute attack 1–2 g 4 times daily (but see **cautions**) until remission occurs (if necessary corticosteroids may also be given), reducing to a maintenance dose of 500 mg 4 times daily; CHILD over 2 years, acute attack 40–60 mg/kg daily, maintenance dose 20–30 mg/kg daily

By rectum, in suppositories, alone or in conjunction with oral treatment 0.5–1 g morning and night after a bowel movement. As an enema, 3 g at night, retained for at least 1 hour

Sulfasalazine (Non-proprietary) PoM

Tablets, sulfasalazine 500 mg. Net price 112 = £10.51. Label: 14, counselling, blood disorder symptoms (see recommendation above), contact lenses may be stained

Available from Generics, Hillcross

Tablets, e/c, sulfasalazine 500 mg. Net price 112-tab pack = £8.43. Label: 5, 14, 25, counselling, blood disorder symptoms (see recommendation above), contact lenses may be stained

Available from Alpharma (*Sulazine EC*®)

Salazopyrin® (Pharmacia) PoM

Tablets, yellow, scored, sulfasalazine 500 mg. Net price 112-tab pack = £6.97. Label: 14, counselling, blood disorder symptoms (see recommendation above), contact lenses may be stained

EN-Tabs® (= tablets e/c), yellow, f/c, sulfasalazine 500 mg. Net price 112-tab pack = £8.43. Label: 5, 14, 25, counselling, blood disorder symptoms (see recommendation above), contact lenses may be stained

Suspension, yellow, sulfasalazine 250 mg/5 mL. Net price 500 mL = £18.84. Label: 14, counselling, blood disorder symptoms (see recommendation above), contact lenses may be stained

Suppositories, yellow, sulfasalazine 500 mg. Net price 10 = £3.30. Label: 14, counselling, blood disorder symptoms (see recommendation above), contact lenses may be stained

Retention enema, sulfasalazine 3 g in 100-mL single-dose disposable packs fitted with a nozzle. Net price 7× 100 mL = £11.87. Label: 14, counselling, blood disorder symptoms (see recommendation above), contact lenses may be stained

Corticosteroids

BUDESONIDE

Indications: see preparations
Cautions: see section 6.3.2
Contra-indications: see section 6.3.2
Side-effects: see section 6.3.2
Dose: see preparations

Budenofalk® (Dr Falk) PoM

Capsules, pink, enclosing e/c pellets, budesonide 3 mg, net price 100-cap pack = £76.70. Label: 5, 10, steroid card, 22, 25

Dose: mild to moderate Crohn's disease affecting the ileum or ascending colon, collagenous colitis, ADULT over 18 years, 3 mg 3 times daily for up to 8 weeks; reduce dose for the last 2 weeks of treatment. See also section 6.3.2

Entocort® (AstraZeneca) PoM

CR Capsules, grey/pink, enclosing e/c, m/r granules, budesonide 3 mg, net price 100-cap pack = £99.00. Label: 5, 10, steroid card, 22, 25

NOTE. Dispense in original container (contains dessicant)

Dose: mild to moderate Crohn's disease affecting the ileum or ascending colon, 9 mg once daily in the morning before breakfast for up to 8 weeks; reduce dose for the last 2–4 weeks of treatment. See also section 6.3.2

CHILD not recommended

Enema, budesonide 2 mg/100 mL when dispersible tablet reconstituted in isotonic saline vehicle, net price pack of 7 dispersible tablets and bottles of vehicle = £33.00

Dose: ulcerative colitis involving rectal and recto-sigmoid disease, 1 enema at bedtime for 4 weeks; CHILD not recommended

HYDROCORTISONE

Indications: ulcerative colitis, proctitis, proctosigmoiditis
Cautions: see section 6.3.2; systemic absorption may occur; prolonged use should be avoided
Contra-indications: use of enemas and rectal foams in obstruction, bowel perforation, and extensive fistulas; untreated infection
Side-effects: see section 6.3.2; local irritation
Dose: rectal, see preparations

Colifoam® (Meda) PoM

Foam in aerosol pack, hydrocortisone acetate 10%, net price 14-application cannister with applicator = £8.21

Dose: initially 1 metered application (125 mg hydrocortisone acetate) inserted into the rectum once or twice daily for 2–3 weeks, then once on alternate days

PREDNISOLONE

Indications: ulcerative colitis, and Crohn's disease; other indications, see section 6.3.2, see also preparations
Cautions: see under Hydrocortisone and section 6.3.2
Contra-indications: see under Hydrocortisone and section 6.3.2
Side-effects: see under Hydrocortisone and section 6.3.2
Dose: *by mouth*, initially 20–40 mg daily in single or divided doses, until remission occurs, followed by reducing doses

By rectum, see under preparations

■ Oral preparations

Section 6.3.2

■ Rectal preparations

Predenema® (Forest) PoM

Retention enema, prednisolone 20 mg (as sodium metasulphobenzoate) in 100-mL single-dose disposable pack. Net price 1 (standard tube) = 71p, 1 (long tube) = £1.21

Dose: ulcerative colitis, initially 1 enema at bedtime for 2–4 weeks, continued if good response; CHILD not recommended

Predfoam® (Forest) PoM

Foam in aerosol pack, prednisolone 20 mg (as metasulphobenzoate sodium)/metered application, net price 14-application cannister with disposable applicators = £6.32

Dose: proctitis and distal ulcerative colitis, 1 metered application (20 mg prednisolone) inserted into the rectum once or twice daily for 2 weeks, continued for further 2 weeks if good response; CHILD not recommended

Predsol® (Celltech) PoM

Retention enema, prednisolone 20 mg (as sodium phosphate) in 100-mL single-dose disposable packs fitted with a nozzle. Net price 7 = £7.50

Dose: rectal and rectosigmoidal ulcerative colitis and Crohn's disease, initially 1 enema at bedtime for 2–4 weeks, continued if good response; CHILD not recommended

Suppositories, prednisolone 5 mg (as sodium phosphate). Net price 10 = £1.40

Dose: ADULT and CHILD proctitis and rectal complications of Crohn's disease, 1 suppository inserted night and morning after a bowel movement

Cytokine inhibitors

Infliximab is a monoclonal antibody which inhibits the pro-inflammatory cytokine, tumour necrosis factor α. It should be used by specialists where adequate resuscitation facilities are available.

INFLIXIMAB

Indications: see under Inflammatory Bowel Disease above; ankylosing spondylitis, rhematoid arthritis (section 10.1.3)

Cautions: see section 10.1.3

HYPERSENSITIVITY REACTIONS. Risk of delayed hypersensitivity if drug-free interval exceeds 16 weeks

Contra-indications: see section 10.1.3

Side-effects: see section 10.1.3

Dose: *by intravenous infusion*, severe active Crohn's disease, ADULT and ADOLESCENT over 17 years, initially 5 mg/kg, then if the condition responds within 2 weeks of initial dose, either 5 mg/kg 2 weeks and 6 weeks after initial dose, then 5 mg/kg every 8 weeks *or* after initial dose, further dose of 5 mg/kg if signs and symptoms recur

Fistulating Crohn's disease, ADULT and ADOLESCENT over 17 years, initially 5 mg/kg, then 5 mg/kg 2 weeks and 6 weeks after initial dose, then if condition has responded, consult literature for guidance on further doses

■ Preparations

Section 10.1.3

Food allergy

Allergy with classical symptoms of vomiting, colic and diarrhoea caused by specific foods such as shellfish should be managed by strict avoidance. The condition should be distinguished from symptoms of occasional food intolerance in those with irritable bowel syndrome. **Sodium cromoglicate** (sodium cromoglycate) may be helpful as an adjunct to dietary avoidance.

SODIUM CROMOGLICATE

(Sodium cromoglycate)

Indications: food allergy (in conjunction with dietary restriction); asthma (section 3.3); allergic conjunctivitis (section 11.4.2); allergic rhinitis (section 12.2.1)

Side-effects: occasional nausea, rashes, and joint pain

Dose: 200 mg 4 times daily before meals; CHILD 2–14 years 100 mg; capsules may be swallowed whole or the contents dissolved in hot water and diluted with cold water before taking. May be increased if necessary after 2–3 weeks to a max. of 40 mg/kg daily and then reduced according to the response

Nalcrom® (Sanofi-Aventis) PoM

Capsules, sodium cromoglicate 100 mg. Net price 100-cap pack = £62.17. Label: 22, counselling, see dose above

1.6 Laxatives

Before prescribing laxatives it is important to be sure that the patient *is* constipated and that the constipation is *not* secondary to an underlying undiagnosed complaint.

It is also important for those who complain of constipation to understand that bowel habit can vary considerably in frequency without doing harm. Some people tend to consider themselves constipated if they do not have a bowel movement each day. A useful definition of constipation is the passage of hard stools less frequently than the patient's own normal pattern and this can be explained to the patient.

Misconceptions about bowel habits have led to excessive laxative use. Abuse may lead to hypokalaemia.

Thus, laxatives should generally be **avoided** except where straining will exacerbate a condition (such as angina) or increase the risk of rectal bleeding as in haemorrhoids. Laxatives are also of value in *drug-induced constipation*, for the expulsion of *parasites* after anthelmintic treatment, and to clear the alimentary tract before *surgery and radiological procedures*. Prolonged treatment of constipation is sometimes necessary.

CHILDREN. The use of laxatives in children should be discouraged unless prescribed by a doctor. Infrequent defaecation may be normal in breast-fed babies or in response to poor intake of fluid or fibre. Delays of greater than 3 days between stools may increase the likelihood of pain on passing hard stools leading to anal fissure, anal spasm and eventually to a learned response to avoid defaecation.

If increased fluid and fibre intake is insufficient, an osmotic laxative such as lactulose or a bulk-forming laxative such as methylcellulose may be effective; methylcellulose is given in a dose of 0.5–1 g twice daily for a child over 7 years [unlicensed use]—an appropriate formulation for a younger child is not readily available. If there is evidence of minor faecal retention, the addition of a stimulant laxative such as senna may overcome withholding but may lead to colic or, in the presence of faecal impaction in the rectum, an increase of faecal overflow. Referral to hospital may be needed unless the child evacuates the impacted mass spontaneously. In hospital, use of a macrogol preparation by mouth or the use of enemas or suppositories may clear the mass but the use of rectal preparations is frequently distressing for the child and may lead to a persistence of withholding. Enemas may be administered under heavy sedation in hospital or alternatively, a bowel cleansing solution (section 1.6.5) may be tried. In severe cases or where the child is afraid, a manual evacuation under anaesthetic may be appropriate.

Long-term use of stimulant laxatives such as senna or sodium picosulfate (sodium picosulphate, section 1.6.2) is essential to prevent recurrence of the faecal impaction. Parents should be encouraged to use them regularly for many months; intermittent use may provoke a series of relapses.

PREGNANCY. If dietary and lifestyle changes fail to control constipation in pregnancy, moderate doses of poorly absorbed laxatives may be used. A bulk-forming laxative should be tried first. An osmotic laxative, such as lactulose, can also be used. Bisacodyl or senna may be suitable, if a stimulant effect is necessary.

> The laxatives that follow have been divided into 5 main groups (sections 1.6.1–1.6.5). This simple classification disguises the fact that some laxatives have a complex action.

1.6.1 Bulk-forming laxatives

Bulk-forming laxatives relieve constipation by increasing faecal mass which stimulates peristalsis; patients should be advised that the full effect may take some days to develop.

Bulk-forming laxatives are of particular value in those with small hard stools, but should not be required unless fibre cannot be increased in the diet. A balanced diet, including adequate fluid intake and fibre is of value in preventing constipation.

Bulk-forming laxatives are useful in the management of patients with *colostomy*, *ileostomy*, *haemorrhoids*, *anal fissure*, *chronic diarrhoea associated with diverticular disease*, *irritable bowel syndrome*, and as adjuncts in *ulcerative colitis* (section 1.5). Adequate fluid intake must be maintained to avoid intestinal obstruction. Unprocessed wheat **bran**, taken with food or fruit juice, is a most effective bulk-forming preparation. Finely ground bran, though more palatable, has poorer water-retaining properties, but can be taken as bran bread or biscuits in appropriately increased quantities. Oat bran is also used.

Methylcellulose, **ispaghula**, and **sterculia** are useful in patients who cannot tolerate bran. Methylcellulose also acts as a faecal softener.

ISPAGHULA HUSK

Indications: see notes above; hypercholesterolaemia (section 2.12)

Cautions: adequate fluid intake should be maintained to avoid intestinal obstruction—it may be necessary to supervise elderly or debilitated patients or those with intestinal narrowing or decreased motility

Contra-indications: difficulty in swallowing, intestinal obstruction, colonic atony, faecal impaction

Side-effects: flatulence, abdominal distension, gastro-intestinal obstruction or impaction; hypersensitivity reported

Dose: see preparations below

COUNSELLING. Preparations that swell in contact with liquid should always be carefully swallowed with water and should not be taken immediately before going to bed

Fibrelief® (Manx)

Granules, sugar- and gluten-free, ispaghula husk 3.5 g/sachet (natural or orange flavour), net price 10 sachets = £1.23, 30 sachets = £2.07. Label: 13, counselling, see above

Excipients: include aspartame (section 9.4.1)

Dose: 1–6 sachets daily in water in 1–3 divided doses

Fybogel® (R&C)

Granules, buff, effervescent, sugar- and gluten-free, ispaghula husk 3.5 g/sachet (low Na^+), net price 30 sachets (plain, lemon, or orange flavour) = £2.12, 150 g (orange flavour) = £3.44. Label: 13, counselling, see above

Excipients: include aspartame 16 mg/sachet (see section 9.4.1)

Dose: 1 sachet or 2 level 5-mL spoonfuls in water twice daily preferably after meals; CHILD (but see section 1.6) 6–12 years ½–1 level 5-mL spoonful (children under 6 years on doctor's advice only)

Isogel® (Pfizer Consumer)

Granules, brown, sugar- and gluten-free, ispaghula husk 90%. Net price 200 g = £2.67. Label: 13, counselling, see above

Dose: constipation, 2 teaspoonfuls in water once or twice daily, preferably at mealtimes; CHILD (but see section 1.6) 1 teaspoonful

Diarrhoea (section 1.4.1), 1 teaspoonful 3 times daily

Ispagel Orange® (LPC)

Granules, beige, effervescent, sugar- and gluten-free, ispaghula husk 3.5 g/sachet, net price 30 sachets = £2.10. Label: 13, counselling, see above

Excipients: include aspartame (section 9.4.1)

Dose: 1 sachet in water 1–3 times daily; CHILD (but see section 1.6) 6–12 years ½ adult dose (children under 6 years on doctor's advice only)

Regulan® (Procter & Gamble)

Powder, beige, sugar- and gluten-free, ispaghula husk 3.4 g/5.85-g sachet (orange or lemon/lime flavour). Net price 30 sachets = £2.12. Label: 13, counselling, see above

Excipients: include aspartame (section 9.4.1)

Dose: 1 sachet in 150 mL water 1–3 times daily; CHILD (but see section 1.6) 6–12 years 2.5–5 mL

METHYLCELLULOSE

Indications: see notes above and section 1.6 [unlicensed dose in children]; adjunct in obesity (but see section 4.5.1)

Cautions: see under Ispaghula Husk

Contra-indications: see under Ispaghula Husk; also infective bowel disease

Side-effects: see under Ispaghula Husk

Dose: see preparations below

COUNSELLING. Preparations that swell in contact with liquid should always be carefully swallowed with water and should not be taken immediately before going to bed

Celevac® (Shire)

Tablets, pink, scored, methylcellulose '450' 500 mg. Net price 112-tab pack = £2.69. Counselling, see above and dose

Dose: constipation and diarrhoea, 3–6 tablets twice daily. In constipation the dose should be taken with at least 300 mL liquid. In diarrhoea, ileostomy, and colostomy control, minimise liquid intake for 30 minutes before and after dose

Adjunct in obesity (but see section 4.5.1), 3 tablets with at least 300 mL warm liquid 30 minutes before food or when hungry

STERCULIA

Indications: see notes above
Cautions: see under Ispaghula Husk
Contra-indications: see under Ispaghula Husk
Side-effects: see under Ispaghula Husk
Dose: see under preparations below

COUNSELLING. Preparations that swell in contact with liquid should always be carefully swallowed with water and should not be taken immediately before going to bed

Normacol® (Norgine)

Granules, coated, gluten-free, sterculia 62%. Net price 500 g = £6.18; 60 × 7-g sachets = £5.19. Label: 25, 27, counselling, see above

Dose: 1–2 heaped 5-mL spoonfuls, or the contents of 1–2 sachets, washed down without chewing with plenty of liquid once or twice daily after meals; CHILD (but see section 1.6) 6–12 years half adult dose

Normacol Plus® (Norgine)

Granules, brown, coated, gluten-free, sterculia 62%, frangula (standardised) 8%. Net price 500 g = £6.60; 60 × 7 g sachets = £5.56. Label: 25, 27, counselling, see above

Dose: constipation and after haemorrhoidectomy, 1–2 heaped 5-mL spoonfuls or the contents of 1–2 sachets washed down without chewing with plenty of liquid once or twice daily after meals

1.6.2 Stimulant laxatives

Stimulant laxatives include **bisacodyl** and members of the **anthraquinone** group, **senna** and **dantron** (danthron). The indications for dantron are limited (see below) by its potential carcinogenicity (based on *rodent* carcinogenicity studies) and evidence of genotoxicity. Powerful stimulants such as **cascara** (an anthraquinone) and **castor oil** are obsolete. **Docusate** sodium probably acts both as a stimulant and as a softening agent.

Stimulant laxatives increase intestinal motility and often cause abdominal cramp; they should be avoided in intestinal obstruction. Prolonged use of stimulant laxatives can cause diarrhoea and related effects such as hypokalaemia; however, prolonged use may be justifiable in some circumstances (see section 1.6 for the use of stimulant laxatives in children).

Glycerol suppositories act as a rectal stimulant by virtue of the mildly irritant action of glycerol.

The **parasympathomimetics** bethanechol, distigmine, neostigmine, and pyridostigmine (see section 7.4.1 and section 10.2.1) enhance parasympathetic activity in the gut and increase intestinal motility. They are rarely used for their gastro-intestinal effects. Organic obstruction of the gut must first be excluded and they should not be used shortly after bowel anastomosis.

BISACODYL

Indications: see under Dose; tablets act in 10–12 hours; suppositories act in 20–60 minutes
Cautions: see notes above
Contra-indications: see notes above, acute surgical abdominal conditions, acute inflammatory bowel disease, severe dehydration
Side-effects: see notes above; tablets, griping; suppositories, local irritation
Dose: constipation, *by mouth*, 5–10 mg at night; CHILD (but see section 1.6) 4–10 years (on medical advice only) 5 mg at night, over 10 years, adult dose

By rectum in suppositories, 10 mg in the morning; CHILD (but see section 1.6) under 10 years (on medical advice only) 5 mg, over 10 years, adult dose

Before radiological procedures and surgery, *by mouth*, 10–20 mg the night before procedure and *by rectum* in suppositories, 10 mg the following morning; CHILD 4–10 years *by mouth*, 5 mg the night before procedure and *by rectum* in suppositories, 5 mg the following morning; over 10 years, adult dose

Bisacodyl (Non-proprietary)

Tablets, e/c, bisacodyl 5 mg. Net price 20 = 45p. Label: 5, 25

Suppositories, bisacodyl 10 mg. Net price 12 = 77p

Paediatric suppositories, bisacodyl 5 mg. Net price 5 = 94p

NOTE. The brand name *Dulco-lax*® NHS (Boehringer Ingelheim) is used for bisacodyl tablets, net price 10-tab pack = 74p; suppositories (10 mg), 10 = £1.57; paediatric suppositories (5 mg), 5 = 94p

The brand names *Dulco-lax*® *Liquid* and *Dulco-lax Perles*® are used for sodium picosulfate preparations

DANTRON

(Danthron)

Indications: only for constipation in terminally ill patients of all ages
Cautions: see notes above; avoid prolonged contact with skin (as in incontinent patients)—risk of irritation and excoriation; avoid in pregnancy (Appendix 4) and breast-feeding (Appendix 5); *rodent* studies indicate potential carcinogenic risk
Contra-indications: see notes above
Side-effects: see notes above; urine may be coloured red
Dose: see under preparations

■ With poloxamer '188' (as co-danthramer)

NOTE. Co-danthramer suspension 5 mL = one co-danthramer capsule, **but** strong co-danthramer suspension 5 mL = two strong co-danthramer capsules

Co-danthramer (Non-proprietary) PoM

Capsules, co-danthramer 25/200 (dantron 25 mg, poloxamer '188' 200 mg). Net price 60-cap pack = £12.86. Label: 14, (urine red)

Dose: 1–2 capsules at bedtime; CHILD 1 capsule at bedtime (restricted indications, see notes above)

Strong capsules, co-danthramer 37.5/500 (dantron 37.5 mg, poloxamer '188' 500 mg). Net price 60-cap pack = £15.55. Label: 14, (urine red)
Dose: 1–2 capsules at bedtime (restricted indications, see notes above); CHILD under 12 years not recommended

Suspension, co-danthramer 25/200 in 5 mL (dantron 25 mg, poloxamer '188' 200 mg/5 mL). Net price 300 mL = £11.27, 1 litre = £37.57. Label: 14, (urine red)
Dose: 5–10 mL at night; CHILD 2.5–5 mL (restricted indications, see notes above)
Brands include *Codalax*® NHS, *Danlax*®

Strong suspension, co-danthramer 75/1000 in 5 mL (dantron 75 mg, poloxamer '188' 1 g/5 mL). Net price 300 mL = £30.13. Label: 14, (urine red)
Dose: 5 mL at night (restricted indications, see notes above); CHILD under 12 years not recommended
Brands include *Codalax Forte*® NHS

■ With docusate sodium (as co-danthrusate)

Co-danthrusate (Non-proprietary) PoM
Capsules, co-danthrusate 50/60 (dantron 50 mg, docusate sodium 60 mg). Net price 63-cap pack = £13.46. Label: 14, (urine red)
Dose: 1–3 capsules, usually at night; CHILD 6–12 years 1 capsule at night (restricted indications, see notes above)
Brands include *Capsuvac*®, *Normax*® NHS

Suspension, yellow, co-danthrusate 50/60 (dantron 50 mg, docusate sodium 60 mg/5 mL). Net price 200 mL = £8.75. Label: 14, (urine red)
Dose: 5–15 mL at night; CHILD 6–12 years 5 mL at night (restricted indications, see notes above)
Brands include *Normax*®

DOCUSATE SODIUM

(Dioctyl sodium sulphosuccinate)

Indications: constipation (oral preparations act within 1–2 days); adjunct in abdominal radiological procedures
Cautions: see notes above; do not give with liquid paraffin; rectal preparations not indicated if haemorrhoids or anal fissure; pregnancy (Appendix 4); breast-feeding (Appendix 5)
Contra-indications: see notes above
Side-effects: see notes above
Dose: *by mouth*, chronic constipation, up to 500 mg daily in divided doses; CHILD (but see section 1.6) over 6 months 12.5 mg 3 times daily, 2–12 years 12.5–25 mg 3 times daily (use paediatric oral solution only)
With barium meal, 400 mg

Dioctyl® (Schwarz)
Capsules, yellow/white, docusate sodium 100 mg, net price 30-cap pack = £2.40, 100-cap pack = £8.00

Docusol® (Typharm)
Adult oral solution, sugar-free, docusate sodium 50 mg/5 mL, net price 300 mL = £2.48
Paediatric oral solution, sugar-free, docusate sodium 12.5 mg/5 mL, net price 300 mL = £1.63

■ Rectal preparations

Norgalax Micro-enema® (Norgine)
Enema, docusate sodium 120 mg in 10-g single-dose disposable packs. Net price 10-g unit = 60p
Dose: ADULT and CHILD (but see section 1.6) over 12 years, 10-g unit

GLYCEROL

(Glycerin)

Indications: constipation
Dose: see below

Glycerol Suppositories, BP
(Glycerin Suppositories)
Suppositories, gelatin 140 mg, glycerol 700 mg, purified water to 1 g. Net price 12 = 81p (infant), 82p (child), £1.83 (adult)
Dose: 1 suppository moistened with water before use. The usual sizes are for INFANT under 1 year, small (1-g mould) 1–2 years medium (2-g mould), CHILD medium (2-g mould), ADULT large (4-g mould)

SENNA

Indications: constipation; acts in 8–12 hours
Cautions: see notes above
Contra-indications: see notes above; breast-feeding (Appendix 5)
Side-effects: see notes above
Dose: see under preparations

Senna (Non-proprietary)
Tablets, total sennosides (calculated as sennoside B) 7.5 mg. Net price 20 = 30p
Dose: 2–4 tablets, usually at night; initial dose should be low then gradually increased; CHILD (but see section 1.6) over 6 years, half adult dose in the morning (on doctor's advice only)
NOTE. Lower dose on packs on sale to the public
Brands include *Senokot*® NHS

Manevac® (Galen)
Granules, coated, senna fruit 12.4%, ispaghula 54.2%, net price 400 g = £7.45. Label: 25, 27, counselling, see Ispaghula Husk
Dose: 1–2 level 5-mL spoonfuls with water or warm drink after supper and, if necessary, before breakfast *or* every 6 hours in resistant cases for 1–3 days; CHILD (but see section 1.6) 5–12 years 1 level 5-mL spoonful daily
COUNSELLING. Preparations that swell in contact with liquid should always be carefully swallowed with water and should not be taken immediately before going to bed

Senokot® (R&C)
Tablets NHS, see above
Granules, brown, total sennosides (calculated as sennoside B) 15 mg/5 mL or 5.5 mg/g (one 5-mL spoonful = 2.7 g). Net price 100 g = £3.10
Dose: 5–10 mL, usually at bedtime; CHILD (but see section 1.6) over 6 years 2.5–5 mL in the morning
NOTE. Lower dose on packs on sale to the public
Syrup, brown, total sennosides (calculated as sennoside B) 7.5 mg/5 mL. Net price 100 mL = £2.37
Dose: 10–20 mL, usually at bedtime; CHILD (but see section 1.6) 2–6 years 2.5–5 mL in the morning (doctor's advice only), over 6 years 5–10 mL
NOTE. Lower dose on packs on sale to the public; the brand name *Senokot*® is also used for glycerol suppositories

SODIUM PICOSULFATE

(Sodium picosulphate)

Indications: constipation; bowel evacuation before abdominal radiological and endoscopic procedures on the colon, and surgery (section 1.6.5); acts within 6–12 hours
Cautions: see notes above; active inflammatory bowel disease (avoid if fulminant); breast-feeding (Appendix 5)

Contra-indications: see notes above; severe dehydration
Side-effects: see notes above
Dose: 5–10 mg at night; CHILD (but see section 1.6) under 4 years 250 micrograms/kg, 4–10 years 2.5–5 mg at night, over 10 years, adult dose

Sodium Picosulfate (Non-proprietary)
Elixir, sodium picosulfate 5 mg/5 mL, net price 100 mL = £1.85
NOTE. The brand names *Laxoberal*® NHS and *Dulco-lax*® *Liquid* (both Boehringer Ingelheim) are used for sodium picosulfate elixir 5 mg/5 mL

Dulco-lax® (Boehringer Ingelheim)
Perles® (= capsules), sodium picosulfate 2.5 mg, net price 20-cap pack = £1.93, 50-cap pack = £2.73
NOTE. The brand name *Dulco-lax*® is also used for bisacodyl tablets and suppositories

■ Bowel cleansing solutions
Section 1.6.5

Other stimulant laxatives

Unstandardised preparations of cascara, frangula, rhubarb, and senna should be **avoided** as their laxative action is unpredictable. Aloes, colocynth, and jalap should be **avoided** as they have a drastic purgative action.

■ Preparations on sale to the public
Stimulant laxative preparations on sale to the public (not prescribable on the NHS) together with their significant ingredients:
Boots Syrup of Figs® (fig, senna), **Boots Natural Senna Laxative Tablets**® (senna)
Califig® (fig, senna), **Calsalettes**® (aloin)
Ex-lax Senna® (senna)
Fam-Lax Senna® (Irish moss, rhubarb, senna)
Jackson's Herbal Laxative® (cascara, rhubarb, senna)
Juno Junipah Salts® (juniper berry oil, sodium bicarbonate, sodium phosphate, sodium sulphate)
Nylax with Senna® (senna)
Potter's Cleansing Herb® (aloes, cascara, senna)

1.6.3 Faecal softeners

Liquid paraffin, the traditional lubricant, has disadvantages (see below). Bulk laxatives (section 1.6.1) and non-ionic surfactant 'wetting' agents e.g. docusate sodium (section 1.6.2) also have softening properties. Such drugs are useful for oral administration in the management of haemorrhoids and anal fissure; glycerol (section 1.6.2) is useful for rectal use.

Enemas containing **arachis oil** (ground-nut oil, peanut oil) lubricate and soften impacted faeces and promote a bowel movement.

ARACHIS OIL

Indications: see notes above
Dose: see below

Fletchers' Arachis Oil Retention Enema® (Forest)
Enema, arachis (peanut) oil in 130-mL single-dose disposable packs. Net price 130 mL = 96p
Dose: to soften impacted faeces, 130 mL; the enema should be warmed before use; CHILD (but see section 1.6) under 3 years not recommended; over 3 years reduce adult dose in proportion to body-weight (medical supervision only)

LIQUID PARAFFIN

Indications: constipation
Cautions: Avoid prolonged use; contra-indicated in children under 3 years
Side-effects: anal seepage of paraffin and consequent anal irritation after prolonged use, granulomatous reactions caused by absorption of small quantities of liquid paraffin (especially from the emulsion), lipoid pneumonia, and interference with the absorption of fat-soluble vitamins
Dose: see under preparation

Liquid Paraffin Oral Emulsion, BP
Oral emulsion, liquid paraffin 5 mL, vanillin 5 mg, chloroform 0.025 mL, benzoic acid solution 0.2 mL, methylcellulose-20 200 mg, saccharin sodium 500 micrograms, water to 10 mL
Dose: 10–30 mL at night when required
COUNSELLING. Should not be taken immediately before going to bed

1.6.4 Osmotic laxatives

Osmotic laxatives increase the amount of water in the large bowel, either by drawing fluid from the body into the bowel or by retaining the fluid they were administered with.

Lactulose is a semi-synthetic disaccharide which is not absorbed from the gastro-intestinal tract. It produces an osmotic diarrhoea of low faecal pH, and discourages the proliferation of ammonia-producing organisms. It is therefore useful in the treatment of *hepatic encephalopathy*.

Macrogols are inert polymers of ethylene glycol which sequester fluid in the bowel; giving fluid with macrogols may reduce the dehydrating effect sometimes seen with osmotic laxatives.

Saline purgatives such as **magnesium hydroxide** are commonly abused but are satisfactory for occasional use; adequate fluid intake should be maintained. **Magnesium salts** are useful where rapid bowel evacuation is required. **Sodium salts** should be avoided as they may give rise to sodium and water retention in susceptible individuals. **Phosphate enemas** are useful in bowel clearance before radiology, endoscopy, and surgery.

LACTULOSE

Indications: constipation (may take up to 48 hours to act), hepatic encephalopathy (portal systemic encephalopathy)
Cautions: lactose intolerance
Contra-indications: galactosaemia, intestinal obstruction
Side-effects: flatulence, cramps, and abdominal discomfort
Dose: see under preparations below

Lactulose (Non-proprietary)
Solution, lactulose 3.1–3.7 g/5 mL with other ketoses. Net price 500-mL pack = £2.85
Dose: constipation, initially 15 mL twice daily, adjusted according to patient's needs; CHILD (but see section 1.6) under 1 year 2.5 mL twice daily, 1–5 years 5 mL twice daily, 5–10 years 10 mL twice daily
Hepatic encephalopathy, 30–50 mL 3 times daily, subsequently adjusted to produce 2–3 soft stools daily

Brands include *Duphalac*® [NHS], *Lactugal*®, *Regulose*®
NOTE. A proprietary brand of lactulose 3.3 g/5 mL (*Regulose*®) is on sale to the public

MACROGOLS

(Polyethylene glycols)

Indications: see preparations below

Cautions: pregnancy and breast-feeding (Appendix 5); discontinue if symptoms of fluid and electrolyte disturbance

Contra-indications: intestinal perforation or obstruction, paralytic ileus, severe inflammatory conditions of the intestinal tract (such as Crohn's disease, ulcerative colitis, and toxic megacolon)

Side-effects: abdominal distension and pain, nausea

Dose: see preparations below

Idrolax® (Schwarz)
Oral powder, macrogol '4000' (polyethylene glycol '4000') 10 g/sachet, net price 20-sachet pack (orange-grapefruit flavour) = £4.84. Label: 13
Dose: constipation, 1–2 sachets preferably as a single dose in the morning; content of each sachet dissolved in a glass of water; CHILD over 8 years, as adult dose for max. 3 months

Movicol® (Norgine)
Oral powder, macrogol '3350' (polyethylene glycol '3350') 13.125 g, sodium bicarbonate 178.5 mg, sodium chloride 350.7 mg, potassium chloride 46.6 mg/sachet, net price 20-sachet pack (lime and lemon flavour) = £4.63, 30-sachet pack = £6.95. Label: 13
Cautions: patients with cardiovascular impairment should not take more than 2 sachets in any 1 hour
Dose: chronic constipation, 1–3 sachets daily in divided doses usually for up to 2 weeks; content of each sachet dissolved in half a glass (approx. 125 mL) of water; maintenance, 1–2 sachets daily; CHILD not recommended
Faecal impaction, 8 sachets daily dissolved in 1 litre water and drunk within 6 hours, usually for max. 3 days; CHILD not recommended.
After reconstitution the solution should be kept in a refrigerator and discarded if unused after 6 hours

Movicol®-Half (Norgine)
Oral powder, macrogol '3350' (polyethylene glycol '3350') 6.563 g, sodium bicarbonate 89.3 mg, sodium chloride 175.4 mg, potassium chloride 23.3 mg/sachet, net price 20-sachet pack (lime and lemon flavour) = £2.78, 30-sachet pack = £4.17. Label: 13
Cautions: patients with cardiovascular impairment should not take more than 4 sachets in any 1 hour
Dose: chronic constipation, 2–6 sachets daily in divided doses usually for up to 2 weeks; content of each sachet dissolved in quarter of a glass (approx. 60–65 mL) of water; maintenance, 2–4 sachets daily; CHILD not recommended
Faecal impaction, 16 sachets daily dissolved in 1 litre of water and drunk within 6 hours, usually for max. 3 days; CHILD not recommended
After reconstitution the solution should be kept in a refrigerator and discarded if unused after 6 hours

Movicol® Paediatric Plain (Norgine) [PoM]
Oral powder, macrogol '3350' (polyethylene glycol '3350') 6.563 g, sodium bicarbonate 89.3 mg, sodium chloride 175.4 mg, potassium chloride 25.1 mg/sachet, net price 30-sachet pack = £4.63. Label: 13
Contra-indications: cardiovascular impairment; renal impairment
Dose: chronic constipation, CHILD 2–6 years 1 sachet daily; 7–11 years 2 sachets daily; adjust according to response, max. 4 sachets daily
Faecal impaction, CHILD (taken in divided doses over 12 hours each day until impaction resolves or for max. 7 days) 2–4 years 2 sachets on first day, then 4 sachets daily for 2 days, then 6 sachets daily for 2 days, then 8 sachets daily for 2 days; 5–11 years 4 sachets on first day then increased in steps of 2 sachets daily to 12 sachets daily; content of each sachet dissolved in quarter of a glass (approx. 60–65 mL) of water
After reconstitution the solution should be kept in a refrigerator and discarded if unused after 24 hours

MAGNESIUM SALTS

Indications: see under preparations below

Cautions: renal impairment (Appendix 3; risk of magnesium accumulation); hepatic impairment (see Appendix 2); elderly and debilitated; see also notes above; **interactions:** Appendix 1 (antacids)

Contra-indications: acute gastro-intestinal conditions

Side-effects: colic

Dose: see under preparations below

■ Magnesium hydroxide

Magnesium Hydroxide Mixture, BP
Aqueous suspension containing about 8% hydrated magnesium oxide. Do not store in cold place
Dose: constipation, 25–50 mL when required

■ Magnesium hydroxide with liquid paraffin

Liquid Paraffin and Magnesium Hydroxide Oral Emulsion, BP
Oral emulsion, 25% liquid paraffin in aqueous suspension containing 6% hydrated magnesium oxide
Dose: constipation, 5–20 mL when required
NOTE. Liquid paraffin and magnesium hydroxide preparations on sale to the public include: *Milpar*® [NHS]

■ Magnesium sulphate

Magnesium Sulphate
Label: 13, 23
Dose: rapid bowel evacuation (acts in 2–4 hours) 5–10 g in a glass of water preferably before breakfast
NOTE. Magnesium sulphate is on sale to the public as Epsom Salts

■ Bowel cleansing solutions

Section 1.6.5

PHOSPHATES (RECTAL)

Indications: rectal use in constipation; bowel evacuation before abdominal radiological procedures, endoscopy, and surgery

Cautions: elderly and debilitated; see also notes above

Contra-indications: acute gastro-intestinal conditions

Side-effects: local irritation

Dose: see under preparations

Carbalax® (Forest)
Suppositories, sodium acid phosphate (anhydrous) 1.3 g, sodium bicarbonate 1.08 g, net price 12 = £2.01
Dose: constipation, 1 suppository, inserted 30 minutes before evacuation required; moisten with water before use; CHILD under 12 years not recommended

Fleet® Ready-to-use Enema (De Witt)
Enema, sodium acid phosphate 21.4 g, sodium phosphate 9.4 g/118 mL. Net price single-dose pack (standard tube) = 46p
Dose: ADULT and CHILD (but see section 1.6) over 12 years, 118 mL; CHILD 3–12 years, on doctor's advice only (under 3 years not recommended)

Fletchers' Phosphate Enema® (Forest)
Enema, sodium acid phosphate 12.8 g, sodium phosphate 10.24 g, purified water, freshly boiled and cooled, to 128 mL (corresponds to Phosphates Enema Formula B). Net price 128 mL with standard tube = 41p, with long rectal tube = 57p
Dose: 128 mL; CHILD (but see section 1.6) over 3 years, reduced according to body weight (under 3 years not recommended)

SODIUM CITRATE (RECTAL)

Indications: rectal use in constipation
Cautions: elderly and debilitated; see also notes above
Contra-indications: acute gastro-intestinal conditions
Dose: see under preparations

Micolette Micro-enema® (Pinewood)
Enema, sodium citrate 450 mg, sodium lauryl sulphoacetate 45 mg, glycerol 625 mg, together with citric acid, potassium sorbate, and sorbitol in a viscous solution, in 5-mL single-dose disposable packs with nozzle. Net price 5 mL = 31p
Dose: ADULT and CHILD over 3 years, 5–10 mL (but see section 1.6)

Micralax Micro-enema® (Celltech)
Enema, sodium citrate 450 mg, sodium alkylsulphoacetate 45 mg, sorbic acid 5 mg, together with glycerol and sorbitol in a viscous solution in 5-mL single-dose disposable packs with nozzle. Net price 5 mL = 41p
Dose: ADULT and CHILD over 3 years, 5 mL (but see section 1.6)

Relaxit Micro-enema® (Crawford)
Enema, sodium citrate 450 mg, sodium lauryl sulphate 75 mg, sorbic acid 5 mg, together with glycerol and sorbitol in a viscous solution in 5-mL single-dose disposable packs with nozzle. Net price 5 mL = 32p
Dose: ADULT and CHILD (but see section 1.6) 5 mL (insert only half nozzle length in child under 3 years)

1.6.5 Bowel cleansing solutions

Bowel cleansing solutions are used before colonic surgery, colonoscopy, or radiological examination to ensure the bowel is free of solid contents. They are **not** treatments for constipation.

BOWEL CLEANSING SOLUTIONS

Indications: see above
Cautions: pregnancy; renal impairment(avoid if severe—Appendix 3); heart disease; ulcerative colitis; diabetes mellitus; reflux oesophagitis; impaired gag reflex; unconscious or semiconscious or possibility of regurgitation or aspiration
Contra-indications: gastro-intestinal obstruction, gastric retention, gastro-intestinal ulceration, perforated bowel, congestive cardiac failure; toxic colitis, toxic megacolon or ileus
Side-effects: nausea and bloating; less frequently abdominal cramps (usually transient—reduced by taking more slowly); vomiting
Dose: see under preparations

Citramag® (Sanochemia)
Powder, effervescent, magnesium carbonate 11.57 g, anhydrous citric acid 17.79 g/sachet, net price 10-sachet pack (lemon and lime flavour) = £14.90. Label: 10, patient information leaflet, 13, counselling, see below
Dose: bowel evacuation for surgery, colonoscopy or radiological examination, on day before procedure, 1 sachet at 8 a.m. and 1 sachet between 2 and 4 p.m.; CHILD 5–9 years one-third adult dose; over 10 years and frail ELDERLY one-half adult dose
COUNSELLING. The patient information leaflet advises that hot water (200 mL) is needed to make the solution and provides guidance on the timing and procedure for reconstitution; it also mentions need for high fluid, low residue diet beforehand (according to hospital advice), and explains that only clear fluids can be taken after *Citramag®* until procedure completed

Fleet Phospho-soda® (De Witt)
Oral solution, sugar-free, sodium dihydrogen phosphate dihydrate 24.4 g, disodium phosphate dodecahydrate 10.8 g/45 mL. Net price 2 × 45-mL bottles = £4.79. Label: 10, patient information leaflet, counselling
Dose: 45 mL diluted with half a glass (120 mL) of cold water, followed by one full glass (240 mL) of cold water
Timing of doses is dependent on the time of the procedure
For morning procedure, first dose should be taken at 7 a.m. and second at 7 p.m. on day before the procedure
For afternoon procedure, first dose should be taken at 7 p.m. on day before and second dose at 7 a.m. on day of the procedure
Solid food must not be taken during dosing period; clear liquids or water should be substituted for meals
CHILD and ADOLESCENT under 15 years not recommended

Klean-Prep® (Norgine)
Oral powder, macrogol '3350' (polyethylene glycol '3350') 59 g, anhydrous sodium sulphate 5.685 g, sodium bicarbonate 1.685 g, sodium chloride 1.465 g, potassium chloride 743 mg/sachet, net price 4 sachets = £8.56. Label: 10, patient information leaflet, counselling
Excipients: include aspartame (section 9.4.1)
Four sachets when reconstituted with water to 4 litres provides an iso-osmotic solution for bowel cleansing before surgery, colonoscopy or radiological procedures
Dose: a glass (approx. 250 mL) of reconstituted solution every 10–15 minutes, or by nasogastric tube 20–30 mL/minute, until 4 litres have been consumed or watery stools are free of solid matter; CHILD not recommended
The solution from all 4 sachets should be drunk within 4–6 hours (250 mL drunk rapidly every 10–15 minutes); flavouring such as clear fruit cordials may be added if required; to facilitate gastric emptying domperidone or metoclopramide may be given 30 minutes before starting. Alternatively the administration may be divided into two, e.g. taking the solutions from 2 sachets on the evening before examination and the remaining 2 on the morning of the examination
After reconstitution the solution should be kept in a refrigerator and discarded if unused after 24 hours
NOTE. Allergic reactions reported

Picolax® (Ferring)
Oral powder, sugar-free, sodium picosulfate 10 mg/sachet, with magnesium citrate (for bowel eva-

cuation before radiological procedure, endoscopy, and surgery), net price 2-sachet pack = £3.53. Label: 10, patient information leaflet, 13, counselling, see below

Dose: ADULT and CHILD over 9 years, 1 sachet in water in morning (before 8 a.m.) and a second in afternoon (between 2 and 4 p.m.) of day preceding procedure; CHILD 1–2 years quarter sachet morning and afternoon, 2–4 years half sachet morning and afternoon, 4–9 years 1 sachet morning and half sachet afternoon

Acts within 3 hours of first dose

NOTE. Low residue diet recommended for 2 days before procedure and copious intake of water or other clear fluids recommended during treatment

COUNSELLING. Patients should be warned that heat is generated on addition to water; for this reason the powder should be added initially to 30 mL (2 tablespoonfuls) of water; after 5 minutes (when reaction complete) the solution should be further diluted to 150 mL (approx. half a glass)

1.7 Local preparations for anal and rectal disorders

Anal and perianal pruritus, soreness, and excoriation are best treated by application of bland ointments and suppositories (section 1.7.1). These conditions occur commonly in patients suffering from haemorrhoids, fistulas, and proctitis. Cleansing with attention to any minor faecal soiling, adjustment of the diet to avoid hard stools, the use of bulk-forming materials such as bran (section 1.6.1) and a high residue diet are helpful. In proctitis these measures may supplement treatment with corticosteroids or sulfasalazine (see section 1.5).

When necessary topical preparations containing **local anaesthetics** (section 1.7.1) or **corticosteroids** (section 1.7.2) are used provided perianal thrush has been excluded. Perianal thrush is best treated with **nystatin** by mouth and by local application (see section 5.2, section 7.2.2, and section 13.10.2).

For the management of *anal fissures*, see section 1.7.4.

1.7.1 Soothing haemorrhoidal preparations

Soothing preparations containing mild astringents such as bismuth subgallate, zinc oxide, and hamamelis may give symptomatic relief in haemorrhoids. Many proprietary preparations also contain lubricants, vasoconstrictors, or mild antiseptics.

Local anaesthetics are used to relieve pain associated with *haemorrhoids* and *pruritus ani* but good evidence is lacking. Lidocaine (lignocaine) ointment (section 15.2) is used before emptying the bowel to relieve pain associated with *anal fissure*. Alternative local anaesthetics include tetracaine (amethocaine), cinchocaine, and pramocaine (pramoxine), but they are more irritant. Local anaesthetic ointments can be absorbed through the rectal mucosa therefore excessive application should be **avoided**, particularly in infants and children. They should be used for short periods only (no longer than a few days) since they may cause sensitisation of the anal skin.

■ Preparations on sale to the public

Soothing haemorrhoidal preparations on sale to the public together with their significant ingredients include:

Anacal® (heparinoid, lauromacrogol '400'), **Anodesyn**® (allantoin, lidocaine), **Anusol**® **cream** (bismuth oxide, Peru balsam, zinc oxide), **Anusol**® **ointment** and **suppositories** (bismuth oxide, bismuth subgallate, Peru balsam, zinc oxide)

Boots Haemorrhoid Relief Ointment® (lidocaine, zinc oxide), **Boots Haemorrhoid Relief Suppositories**® (benzyl alcohol, glycol monosalicylate, methyl salicylate, zinc oxide)

Germoloids® (lidocaine, zinc oxide)

Hemocane® (benzoic acid, bismuth oxide, cinnamic acid, lidocaine, zinc oxide)

Lanacane® **cream** (benzocaine, chlorothymol)

Nupercainal® (cinchocaine)

Preparation H® **gel** (hamamelis water), **Preparation H**® **ointment and suppositories** (shark liver oil, yeast cell extract)

1.7.2 Compound haemorrhoidal preparations with corticosteroids

Corticosteroids are often combined with local anaesthetics and soothing agents in preparations for haemorrhoids. They are suitable for occasional short-term use after exclusion of infections, such as herpes simplex; prolonged use can cause atrophy of the anal skin. See section 13.4 for general comments on topical corticosteroids and section 1.7.1 for comment on local anaesthetics.

CHILDREN. Haemorrhoids in children are rare. Treatment is usually symptomatic and the use of a locally applied cream is appropriate for short periods; however, local anaesthetics can cause stinging initially and this may aggravate the child's fear of defaecation.

Anugesic-HC® (Pfizer) PoM

Cream, benzyl benzoate 1.2%, bismuth oxide 0.875%, hydrocortisone acetate 0.5%, Peru balsam 1.85%, pramocaine hydrochloride 1%, zinc oxide 12.35%. Net price 30 g (with rectal nozzle) = £3.71

Dose: apply night and morning and after a bowel movement; do not use for longer than 7 days; CHILD not recommended

Suppositories, buff, benzyl benzoate 33 mg, bismuth oxide 24 mg, bismuth subgallate 59 mg, hydrocortisone acetate 5 mg, Peru balsam 49 mg, pramocaine hydrochloride 27 mg, zinc oxide 296 mg, net price 12 = £2.69

Dose: insert 1 suppository night and morning and after a bowel movement; do not use for longer than 7 days; CHILD not recommended

Anusol-HC® (Pfizer Consumer) PoM

Ointment, benzyl benzoate 1.25%, bismuth oxide 0.875%, bismuth subgallate 2.25%, hydrocortisone acetate 0.25%, Peru balsam 1.875%, zinc oxide 10.75%. Net price 30 g (with rectal nozzle) = £3.50

Dose: apply night and morning and after a bowel movement; do not use for longer than 7 days; CHILD not recommended

NOTE. A proprietary brand (*Anusol Plus HC®* ointment) is on sale to the public

Suppositories, benzyl benzoate 33 mg, bismuth oxide 24 mg, bismuth subgallate 59 mg, hydrocortisone acetate 10 mg, Peru balsam 49 mg, zinc oxide 296 mg. Net price 12 = £2.46

Dose: insert 1 suppository night and morning and after a bowel movement; do not use for longer than 7 days; CHILD not recommended

NOTE. A proprietary brand (*Anusol Plus HC®* suppositories) is on sale to the public

Perinal® (Dermal)

Spray application, hydrocortisone 0.2%, lidocaine hydrochloride 1%. Net price 30-mL pack = £6.39

Dose: spray twice over the affected area up to 3 times daily; do not use for longer than 1–2 weeks; CHILD under 14 years not recommended

NOTE. Also available as *Germoloids® HC* (Bayer Consumer Care)

Proctofoam HC® (Meda) PoM

Foam in aerosol pack, hydrocortisone acetate 1%, pramocaine hydrochloride 1%. Net price 21.2-g pack (approx. 40 applications) with applicator = £5.06

Dose: haemorrhoids and proctitis, 1 applicatorful (4–6 mg hydrocortisone acetate, 4–6 mg pramocaine hydrochloride) by rectum 2–3 times daily and after a bowel movement (max. 4 times daily); do not use for longer than 7 days; CHILD not recommended

Proctosedyl® (Aventis Pharma) PoM

Ointment, cinchocaine (dibucaine) hydrochloride 0.5%, hydrocortisone 0.5%. Net price 30 g = £7.83 (with cannula)

Dose: apply morning and night and after a bowel movement, externally or by rectum; do not use for longer than 7 days

Suppositories, cinchocaine (dibucaine) hydrochloride 5 mg, hydrocortisone 5 mg. Net price 12 = £3.53

Dose: insert 1 suppository night and morning and after a bowel movement; do not use for longer than 7 days

Scheriproct® (Schering Health) PoM

Ointment, cinchocaine (dibucaine) hydrochloride 0.5%, prednisolone hexanoate 0.19%. Net price 30 g = £3.00

Dose: apply twice daily for 5–7 days (3–4 times daily on 1st day if necessary), then once daily for a few days after symptoms have cleared

Suppositories, cinchocaine (dibucaine) hydrochloride 1 mg, prednisolone hexanoate 1.3 mg. Net price 12 = £1.41

Dose: insert 1 suppository daily after a bowel movement, for 5–7 days (in severe cases initially 2–3 times daily)

Ultraproct® (Meadow) PoM

Ointment, cinchocaine (dibucaine) hydrochloride 0.5%, fluocortolone caproate 0.095%, fluocortolone pivalate 0.092%, net price 30 g (with rectal nozzle) = £4.57

Dose: apply twice daily for 5–7 days (3–4 times daily on 1st day if necessary), then once daily for a few days after symptoms have cleared

Suppositories, cinchocaine (dibucaine) hydrochloride 1 mg, fluocortolone caproate 630 micrograms, fluocortolone pivalate 610 micrograms, net price 12 = £2.15

Dose: insert 1 suppository daily after a bowel movement, for 5–7 days (in severe cases initially 2–3 times daily) then 1 suppository every other day for 1 week

Uniroid-HC® (Chemidex) PoM

Ointment, cinchocaine (dibucaine) hydrochloride 0.5%, hydrocortisone 0.5%. Net price 30 g (with applicator) = £4.23

Dose: apply twice daily and after a bowel movement, externally or by rectum; do not use for longer than 7 days; CHILD under 12 years not recommended

Suppositories, cinchocaine (dibucaine) hydrochloride 5 mg, hydrocortisone 5 mg. Net price 12 = £1.91

Dose: insert 1 suppository twice daily and after a bowel movement; do not use for longer than 7 days; CHILD under 12 years not recommended

Xyloproct® (AstraZeneca) PoM

Ointment (water-miscible), aluminium acetate 3.5%, hydrocortisone acetate 0.275%, lidocaine 5%, zinc oxide 18%, net price 20 g (with applicator) = £2.26

Dose: apply several times daily; short-term use only

1.7.3 Rectal sclerosants

Oily phenol injection is used to inject haemorrhoids particularly when unprolapsed.

PHENOL

Indications: see notes above

Side-effects: irritation, tissue necrosis

Oily Phenol Injection, BP PoM

phenol 5% in a suitable fixed oil. Net price 5-mL amp = £5.00

Dose: 2–3 mL into the submucosal layer at the base of the pile; several injections may be given at different sites, max. total injected 10 mL at any one time

Available from Celltech

1.7.4 Management of anal fissures

The management of *anal fissures* requires stool softening by increasing dietary fibre in the form of bran or by using a bulk-forming laxative. Short-term use of local anaesthetic preparations may help (section 1.7.1). If these measures are inadequate, the patient should be referred for specialist treatment in hospital; surgery or the use of a topical nitrate (e.g. glyceryl trinitrate 0.4% ointment) may be considered.

GLYCERYL TRINITRATE

Indications: anal fissure; angina, left ventricular failure (section 2.6.1)

Cautions: section 2.6.1

Contra-indications: section 2.6.1

Side-effects: section 2.6.1; also *less commonly* nausea, vomiting, burning and itching and rectal bleeding

Dose: see preparations

Rectogesic® (Strakan) PoM
Rectal ointment, glyceryl trinitrate 0.4%, net price 30 g = £32.80
Excipients: include lanolin, propylene glycol
Dose: apply 2.5 cm of ointment to anal canal every 12 hours until pain stops; max. duration of use 8 weeks
NOTE. 2.5 cm of ointment contains glyceryl trinitrate 1.5 mg

1.8 Stoma care

Prescribing for patients with stoma calls for special care. The following is a brief account of some of the main points to be borne in mind.

Enteric-coated and *modified-release* preparations are **unsuitable**, particularly in patients with ileostomies, as there may not be sufficient release of the active ingredient.

Laxatives. Enemas and washouts should **not** be prescribed for patients with ileostomies as they may cause rapid and severe loss of water and electrolytes.

Colostomy patients may suffer from constipation and whenever possible should be treated by increasing fluid intake or dietary fibre. **Bulk-forming drugs** (section 1.6.1) should be tried. If they are insufficient, as small a dose as possible of senna (section 1.6.2) should be used.

Antidiarrhoeals. Drugs such as **loperamide**, **codeine phosphate**, or **co-phenotrope** (diphenoxylate with atropine) are effective. Bulk-forming drugs (section 1.6.1) may be tried but it is often difficult to adjust the dose appropriately.

Antibacterials should **not** be given for an episode of acute diarrhoea.

Antacids. The tendency to diarrhoea from magnesium salts or constipation from aluminium salts may be increased in these patients.

Diuretics should be used with caution in patients with ileostomies as they may become excessively dehydrated and potassium depletion may easily occur. It is usually advisable to use a **potassium-sparing** diuretic (see section 2.2.3).

Digoxin. Patients with a stoma are particularly susceptible to hypokalaemia if on digoxin therapy and potassium supplements or a potassium-sparing diuretic may be advisable (for comment see section 9.2.1.1).

Potassium supplements. Liquid formulations are preferred to modified-release formulations (see above).

Analgesics. Opioid analgesics (see section 4.7.2) may cause troublesome constipation in colostomy patients. When a non-opioid analgesic is required **paracetamol** is usually suitable but anti-inflammatory analgesics may cause gastric irritation and bleeding.

Iron preparations may cause loose stools and sore skin in these patients. If this is troublesome and if iron is definitely indicated an intramuscular iron preparation (see section 9.1.1.2) should be used. Modified-release preparations should be **avoided** for the reasons given above.

Patients are usually given advice about the use of *cleansing agents*, *protective creams*, *lotions*, *deodorants*, or *sealants* whilst in hospital, either by the surgeon or by the health authority stoma care nurses. Voluntary organisations offer help and support to patients with stoma.

1.9 Drugs affecting intestinal secretions

1.9.1 Drugs affecting biliary composition and flow

The use of laparoscopic cholecystectomy and of endoscopic biliary techniques has limited the place of the bile acid **ursodeoxycholic acid** in gallstone disease. Ursodeoxycholic acid is suitable for patients with unimpaired gall bladder function, small or medium-sized radiolucent stones, and whose mild symptoms are not amenable to other treatment; it should be used cautiously in those with liver disease (but see below). Patients should be given dietary advice (including avoidance of excessive cholesterol and calories) and they require radiological monitoring. Long-term prophylaxis may be needed after complete dissolution of the gallstones has been confirmed because they may recur in up to 25% of patients within one year of stopping treatment.

Ursodeoxycholic acid is also used in primary biliary cirrhosis; liver tests improve in most patients but the effect on overall survival is uncertain. Ursodeoxycholic acid has also been tried in primary sclerosing cholangitis [unlicensed indication].

URSODEOXYCHOLIC ACID

Indications: see under Dose and under preparations
Cautions: see notes above; **interactions:** Appendix 1 (ursodeoxycholic acid)
Contra-indications: radio-opaque stones, pregnancy (Appendix 4), non-functioning gall bladder, inflammatory diseases and other conditions of the small intestine, colon and liver which interfere with entero-hepatic circulation of bile salts
Side-effects: nausea, vomiting, diarrhoea; gallstone calcification; pruritus
Dose: dissolution of gallstones, 8–12 mg/kg daily as a single dose at bedtime *or* in two divided doses, for up to 2 years; treatment is continued for 3–4 months after stones dissolve
Primary biliary cirrhosis, see under *Ursofalk*®

Ursodeoxycholic Acid (Non-proprietary) PoM
Tablets, ursodeoxycholic acid 150 mg, net price 60-tab pack = £18.51. Label: 21
Capsules, ursodeoxycholic acid 250 mg, net price 60-cap pack = £35.11. Label: 21

Destolit® (Norgine) PoM
Tablets, scored, ursodeoxycholic acid 150 mg, net price 60-tab pack = £18.39. Label: 21

Urdox® (CP) PoM
Tablets, f/c, ursodeoxycholic acid 300 mg, net price 60-tab pack = £30.24. Label: 21

Ursofalk® (Dr Falk) PoM
Capsules, ursodeoxycholic acid 250 mg, net price 60-cap pack = £31.10, 100-cap pack = £32.85. Label: 21
Suspension, sugar-free, ursodeoxycholic acid 250 mg/5 mL, net price 250 mL = £28.50. Label: 21
Dose: primary biliary cirrhosis, 10–15 mg/kg daily in 2–4 divided doses
Dissolution of gallstones, see Dose, above

Ursogal® (Galen) PoM
Tablets, scored, ursodeoxycholic acid 150 mg, net price 60-tab pack = £17.05. Label: 21
Capsules, ursodeoxycholic acid 250 mg, net price 60-cap pack = £30.50. Label: 21

Other preparations for biliary disorders

A **terpene** mixture (*Rowachol*®) raises biliary cholesterol solubility. It is not considered to be a useful adjunct.

Rowachol® (Rowa) PoM
Capsules, green, e/c, borneol 5 mg, camphene 5 mg, cineole 2 mg, menthol 32 mg, menthone 6 mg, pinene 17 mg in olive oil. Net price 50-cap pack = £7.35. Label: 22
Dose: 1–2 capsules 3 times daily before food (but see notes above)
Interactions: Appendix 1 (*Rowachol*®)

1.9.2 Bile acid sequestrants

Colestyramine (cholestyramine) is an anion-exchange resin that is not absorbed from the gastro-intestinal tract. It relieves diarrhoea and pruritus by forming an insoluble complex with bile acids in the intestine. Colestyramine can interfere with the absorption of a number of drugs. Colestyramine is also used in hypercholesterolaemia (section 2.12).

COLESTYRAMINE

(Cholestyramine)
Indications: pruritus associated with partial biliary obstruction and primary biliary cirrhosis; diarrhoea associated with Crohn's disease, ileal resection, vagotomy, diabetic vagal neuropathy, and radiation; hypercholesterolaemia (section 2.12)
Cautions: see section 2.12
Contra-indications: see section 2.12
Side-effects: see section 2.12
Dose: pruritus, 4–8 g daily in water (or other suitable liquid)
Diarrhoea, after initial introduction over 3–4 week period, 12–24 g daily mixed with water (or other suitable liquid) in 1–4 divided doses, then adjusted as required; max. 36 g daily
CHILD 6–12 years, consult product literature
COUNSELLING. Other drugs should be taken at least 1 hour before or 4–6 hours after colestyramine to reduce possible interference with absorption

■ Preparations
Section 2.12

1.9.3 Aprotinin

Section 2.11.

1.9.4 Pancreatin

Supplements of pancreatin are given by mouth to compensate for reduced or absent exocrine secretion in cystic fibrosis, and following pancreatectomy, gastrectomy, or chronic pancreatitis. They assist the digestion of starch, fat, and protein. Pancreatin may also be necessary if a tumour (e.g. pancreatic cancer) obstructs outflow from the pancreas.

Pancreatin is inactivated by gastric acid therefore pancreatin preparations are best taken with food (or immediately before or after food). Gastric acid secretion may be reduced by giving cimetidine or ranitidine an hour beforehand (section 1.3). Concurrent use of antacids also reduces gastric acidity. Enteric-coated preparations deliver a higher enzyme concentration in the duodenum (provided the capsule contents are swallowed whole without chewing). Higher-strength versions are also available (**important:** see CSM advice below).

Since pancreatin is also inactivated by heat, excessive heat should be avoided if preparations are mixed with liquids or food; the resulting mixtures should not be kept for more than one hour.

Dosage is adjusted according to size, number, and consistency of stools, so that the patient thrives; extra allowance may be needed if snacks are taken between meals.

Pancreatin can irritate the perioral skin and buccal mucosa if retained in the mouth, and excessive doses can cause perianal irritation. The most frequent side-effects are gastro-intestinal, including nausea, vomiting, and abdominal discomfort; hyperuricaemia and hyperuricosuria have been associated with very high doses. Hypersensitivity reactions occur occasionally and may affect those handling the powder.

PANCREATIN

NOTE. The pancreatin preparations which follow are all of porcine origin
Indications: see also above
Cautions: see also above and (for higher-strength preparations) see below
Side-effects: see also above and (for higher-strength preparations) see below
Dose: see preparations

Creon® **10 000** (Solvay)
Capsules, brown/clear, enclosing buff-coloured e/c granules of pancreatin, providing: protease 600 units, lipase 10 000 units, amylase 8000 units. Net price 100-cap pack = £16.66. Counselling, see dose
Dose: ADULT and CHILD initially 1–2 capsules with meals either taken whole or contents mixed with fluid or soft food (then swallowed immediately without chewing)

Creon® **Micro** (Solvay)
Gastro-resistant granules, brown, pancreatin, providing: protease 2000 units, lipase 50 000 units, amylase 36 000 units/g, net price 20 g = £31.50
Counselling, see dose
Dose: ADULT and CHILD initially 100 mg with meals either taken whole or mixed with acidic fluid or soft food (then swallowed immediately without chewing)

Nutrizym 10® (Merck)
Capsules, red/yellow, enclosing e/c minitablets of pancreatin providing minimum of: protease

500 units, lipase 10 000 units, amylase 9000 units. Net price 100 = £14.47. Counselling, see dose

Dose: ADULT and CHILD 1–2 capsules with meals and 1 capsule with snacks, swallowed whole or contents taken with water or sprinkled on soft food (then swallowed immediately without chewing); higher doses may be required according to response

Pancrease® (Janssen-Cilag)

Capsules, enclosing e/c beads of pancrelipase USP, providing minimum of: protease 330 units, lipase 5000 units, amylase 2900 units. Net price 100 = £16.22. Counselling, see dose

Dose: ADULT and CHILD 1–2 (occasionally 3) capsules during each meal and 1 capsule with snacks swallowed whole or contents sprinkled on liquid or soft food (then swallowed immediately without chewing); higher doses may be required according to response

Pancrex® (Paines & Byrne)

Granules, pancreatin, providing minimum of: protease 300 units, lipase 5000 units, amylase 4000 units/g. Net price 300 g = £20.39. Label: 25, counselling, see dose

Dose: ADULT and CHILD 5–10 g just before meals washed down or mixed with liquid

Pancrex V® (Paines & Byrne)

Capsules, pancreatin, providing minimum of: protease 430 units, lipase 8000 units, amylase 9000 units. Net price 300-cap pack = £15.80. Counselling, see dose

Dose: ADULT and CHILD over 1 year 2–6 capsules with meals, swallowed whole or sprinkled on food; INFANT up to 1 year 1–2 capsules mixed with feeds

Capsules '125', pancreatin, providing minimum of: protease 160 units, lipase 2950 units, amylase 3300 units. Net price 300-cap pack = £9.72. Counselling, see dose

Dose: NEONATE 1–2 capsules with feeds

Tablets, e/c, pancreatin, providing minimum of: protease 110 units, lipase 1900 units, amylase 1700 units. Net price 300-tab pack = £4.51. Label: 5, 25, counselling, see dose

Dose: ADULT and CHILD 5–15 tablets before meals

Tablets forte, e/c, pancreatin, providing minimum of: protease 330 units, lipase 5600 units, amylase 5000 units. Net price 300-tab pack = £13.74. Label: 5, 25, counselling, see dose

Dose: ADULT and CHILD 6–10 tablets before meals

Powder, pancreatin, providing minimum of: protease 1400 units, lipase 25 000 units, amylase 30 000 units/g. Net price 300 g = £24.28. Counselling, see dose

Dose: ADULT and CHILD 0.5–2 g with meals washed down or mixed with liquid; NEONATE 250–500 mg with each feed

■ Higher-strength preparations

The **CSM** has advised of data associating the high-strength pancreatin preparations *Nutrizym 22®* and *Pancreatin HL®* with the development of large bowel strictures (fibrosing colonopathy) in children with cystic fibrosis aged between 2 and 13 years. No association was found with *Creon® 25 000*. The following was recommended:

- *Pancrease HL®*, *Nutrizym 22®*, *Panzytrat® 25 000* [now discontinued] should not be used in children aged 15 years or less with cystic fibrosis;
- the total dose of pancreatic enzyme supplements used in patients with cystic fibrosis should not usually exceed 10 000 units of lipase per kg body-weight daily;
- if a patient on any pancreatin preparation develops new abdominal symptoms (or any change in existing abdominal symptoms) the patient should be reviewed to exclude the possibility of colonic damage.

Possible risk factors are gender (boys at greater risk than girls), more severe cystic fibrosis, and concomitant use of laxatives. The peak age for developing fibrosing colonopathy is between 2 and 8 years.

COUNSELLING. It is important to ensure adequate hydration at all times in patients receiving higher-strength pancreatin preparations.

Creon® 25 000 (Solvay) PoM

Capsules, orange/clear, enclosing brown-coloured e/c pellets of pancreatin, providing: protease (total) 1000 units, lipase 25 000 units, amylase 18 000 units, net price 100-cap pack = £30.03. Counselling, see above and under dose

Dose: ADULT and CHILD initially 1 capsule with meals either taken whole or contents mixed with fluid or soft food (then swallowed immediately without chewing)

Creon® 40 000 (Solvay) ▼ PoM

Capsules, brown/clear, enclosing brown-coloured e/c granules of pancreatin, providing: protease (total) 1600 units, lipase 40 000 units, amylase 25 000 units, net price 100-cap pack = £60.00. Counselling, see above and under dose

Dose: ADULT and CHILD initially 1–2 capsules with meals either taken whole or contents mixed with fluid or soft food (then swallowed immediately without chewing)

Nutrizym 22® (Merck) PoM

Capsules, red/yellow, enclosing e/c minitablets of pancreatin, providing minimum of: protease 1100 units, lipase 22 000 units, amylase 19 800 units. Net price 100-cap pack = £33.33. Counselling, see above and under dose

Dose: 1–2 capsules with meals and 1 capsule with snacks, swallowed whole or contents taken with water or sprinkled on soft food (then swallowed immediately without chewing)

CHILD under 15 years not recommended

Pancrease HL® (Janssen-Cilag) PoM

Capsules, enclosing light brown e/c minitablets of pancreatin, providing minimum of: protease 1250 units, lipase 25 000 units, amylase 22 500 units. Net price 100 = £34.37. Counselling, see above and under dose

Dose: 1–2 capsules during each meal and 1 capsule with snacks swallowed whole or contents sprinkled on liquid or soft food (then swallowed immediately without chewing)

CHILD under 15 years not recommended

2: Cardiovascular system

2.1 Positive inotropic drugs

Positive inotropic drugs increase the force of contraction of the myocardium; for sympathomimetics with inotropic activity see section 2.7.1.

2.1.1 Cardiac glycosides

Cardiac glycosides increase the force of myocardial contraction and reduce conductivity within the atrioventricular (AV) node. Digoxin is the most commonly used cardiac glycoside.

Cardiac glycosides are most useful in the treatment of supraventricular tachycardias, especially for controlling ventricular response in persistent atrial fibrillation (section 2.3.1). For reference to the role of digoxin in heart failure, see section 2.5.5.

For management of atrial fibrillation the maintenance dose of the cardiac glycoside can usually be determined by the ventricular rate at rest which should not be allowed to fall below 60 beats per minute except in special circumstances, e.g. with the concomitant administration of a beta-blocker.

Digoxin is now rarely used for rapid control of heart rate (see section 2.3 for the management of supraventricular arrhythmias). Even with intravenous administration, response may take many hours; persistence of tachycardia is therefore not an indication for exceeding the recommended dose. The intramuscular route is **not** recommended.

In patients with mild heart failure a loading dose is not required, and a satisfactory plasma-digoxin concentration can be achieved over a period of about a week, using a dose of digoxin 125 to 250 micrograms twice a day which is then reduced.

Digoxin has a long half-life and maintenance doses need to be given only once daily (although higher doses may be divided to avoid nausea). **Digitoxin** also has a long half-life and maintenance doses need to be given only once daily or on alternate days. Renal function is the most important determinant of digoxin dosage, whereas elimination of digitoxin depends on metabolism by the liver.

Unwanted effects depend both on the concentration of the cardiac glycoside in the plasma and on the sensitivity of the conducting system or of the myocardium, which is often increased in heart disease. It may sometimes be difficult to distinguish between toxic effects and clinical deterioration because symptoms of both are similar. Also, the plasma concentration alone cannot indicate toxicity reliably but the likelihood of toxicity increases progressively through the range 1.5 to 3 micrograms/litre for digoxin. Cardiac glycosides should be used with special care in the elderly who may be particularly susceptible to digitalis toxicity.

Regular monitoring of plasma-digoxin concentration during maintenance treatment is not necessary unless problems are suspected. Care should be taken to avoid hypokalaemia if a diuretic is used with a cardiac glycoside because hypokalaemia predisposes the patient to digitalis toxicity. Hypokalaemia is managed by giving a potassium-sparing diuretic or, if necessary, potassium supplements (or foods rich in potassium).

Toxicity can often be managed by discontinuing digoxin and correcting hypokalaemia if appropriate; serious manifestations require urgent specialist management. **Digoxin-specific antibody fragments** are available for reversal of life-threatening overdosage (see below).

CHILDREN. The dose is based on body-weight; children require a relatively larger dose of digoxin than adults.

DIGOXIN

Indications: heart failure (see also section 2.5.5), supraventricular arrhythmias (particularly atrial fibrillation; see also section 2.3.2)

Cautions: recent infarction; sick sinus syndrome; thyroid disease; reduce dose in the elderly; avoid hypokalaemia; avoid rapid intravenous administration (nausea and risk of arrhythmias); renal impairment (Appendix 3); pregnancy (Appendix 4); **interactions:** Appendix 1 (cardiac glycosides)

Contra-indications: intermittent complete heart block, second degree AV block; supraventricular arrhythmias caused by Wolff-Parkinson-White syndrome; ventricular tachycardia or fibrillation; hypertrophic obstructive cardiomyopathy (unless concomitant atrial fibrillation and heart failure — but with caution)

Side-effects: usually associated with excessive dosage, include: anorexia, nausea, vomiting, diarrhoea, abdominal pain; visual disturbances, headache, fatigue, drowsiness, confusion, dizziness, delirium, hallucinations, depression; arrhythmias, heart block; rarely rash, intestinal ischaemia; gynaecomastia on long-term use; thrombocytopenia reported; see also notes above

Dose: *by mouth*, rapid digitalisation, 1–1.5 mg in divided doses over 24 hours; less urgent digitalisation, 250–500 micrograms daily (higher dose may be divided)

Maintenance, 62.5–500 micrograms daily (higher dose may be divided) according to renal function and, in atrial fibrillation, on heart-rate response; usual range, 125–250 micrograms daily (lower dose may be appropriate in elderly)

Emergency loading dose *by intravenous infusion*, 0.75–1 mg over at least 2 hours (see also Cautions) then maintenance dose *by mouth* on the following day

NOTE. The above doses may need to be reduced if digoxin (or another cardiac glycoside) has been given in the preceding 2 weeks. Digoxin doses in the BNF may differ from those in product literature. For plasma concentration monitoring, blood should ideally be taken at least 6 hours after a dose

Digoxin (Non-proprietary) PoM

Tablets, digoxin 62.5 micrograms, net price 20 = £1.09; 125 micrograms, 20 = £1.04; 250 micrograms, 20 = £1.27

Injection, digoxin 250 micrograms/mL, net price 2-mL amp = 70p

Available from Antigen

Paediatric injection, digoxin 100 micrograms/mL

'Special order' [unlicensed] product

Lanoxin® (GSK) PoM

Tablets, digoxin 125 micrograms, net price 20 = 32p; 250 micrograms (scored), 20 = 32p

Injection, digoxin 250 micrograms/mL. Net price 2-mL amp = 66p

Lanoxin-PG® (GSK) PoM

Tablets, blue, digoxin 62.5 micrograms. Net price 20 = 32p

Elixir, yellow, digoxin 50 micrograms/mL. Do not dilute, measure with pipette. Net price 60 mL = £5.35. Counselling, use of pipette

DIGITOXIN

Indications: heart failure, supraventricular arrhythmias (particularly atrial fibrillation)

Cautions: see under Digoxin; renal impairment (Appendix 3)

Contra-indications: see under Digoxin

Side-effects: see under Digoxin

Dose: maintenance, 100 micrograms daily *or* on alternate days; may be increased to 200 micrograms daily if necessary

Digitoxin (Non-proprietary) PoM

Tablets, digitoxin 100 micrograms, net price 20 = £2.66

Digoxin-specific antibody

Digoxin-specific antibody fragments are indicated for the treatment of known or strongly suspected digoxin or digitoxin overdosage, where measures beyond the withdrawal of the cardiac glycoside and correction of any electrolyte abnormality are felt to be necessary (see also notes above).

Digibind® (GSK) PoM

Injection, powder for preparation of infusion, digoxin-specific antibody fragments (F(ab)) 38 mg. Net price per vial = £93.97 (hosp. and poisons centres only)

Dose: consult product literature

2.1.2 Phosphodiesterase inhibitors

Enoximone and **milrinone** are selective phosphodiesterase inhibitors which exert most of their effect on the myocardium. Sustained haemodynamic benefit has been observed after administration, but there is no evidence of any beneficial effect on survival.

ENOXIMONE

Indications: congestive heart failure where cardiac output reduced and filling pressures increased

Cautions: heart failure associated with hypertrophic cardiomyopathy, stenotic or obstructive valvular disease or other outlet obstruction; monitor blood pressure, heart rate, ECG, central venous pressure, fluid and electrolyte status, renal function, platelet count, hepatic enzymes; avoid extravasation; renal impairment (Appendix 3); pregnancy (Appendix 4); breast-feeding (Appendix 5)

Side-effects: ectopic beats; less frequently ventricular tachycardia or supraventricular arrhythmias (more likely in patients with pre-existing arrhythmias); hypotension; also headache, insomnia, nausea and vomiting, diarrhoea; occasionally, chills, oliguria, fever, urinary retention; upper and lower limb pain

Dose: *by slow intravenous injection* (rate not exceeding 12.5 mg/minute), diluted before use, initially 0.5–1 mg/kg, then 500 micrograms/kg every 30 minutes until satisfactory response or total of 3 mg/kg given; maintenance, initial dose of up to 3 mg/kg may be repeated every 3–6 hours as required

By intravenous infusion, initially 90 micrograms/kg/minute over 10–30 minutes, followed by continuous or intermittent infusion of 5–20 micrograms/kg/minute

Total dose over 24 hours should not usually exceed 24 mg/kg

Perfan® (Myogen) PoM
Injection, enoximone 5 mg/mL. For dilution before use. Net price 20-mL amp = £15.02
Excipients: include alcohol, propylene glycol
NOTE. Plastic apparatus should be used; crystal formation if glass used

MILRINONE

Indications: short-term treatment of severe congestive heart failure unresponsive to conventional maintenance therapy (not immediately after myocardial infarction); acute heart failure, including low output states, following heart surgery

Cautions: see under Enoximone; also correct hypokalaemia, monitor renal function; renal impairment (Appendix 3); pregnancy (Appendix 4); breast-feeding (Appendix 5)

Side-effects: see under Enoximone; also chest pain, tremor, bronchospasm, anaphylaxis and rash reported

Dose: *by intravenous injection* over 10 minutes, diluted before use, 50 micrograms/kg followed by *intravenous infusion* at a rate of 375–750 nanograms/kg/minute, usually for up to 12 hours following surgery or for 48–72 hours in congestive heart failure; max. daily dose 1.13 mg/kg

Primacor® (Sanofi-Synthelabo) PoM
Injection, milrinone (as lactate) 1 mg/mL. For dilution before use. Net price 10-mL amp = £16.61

2.2 Diuretics

Thiazides (section 2.2.1) are used to relieve oedema due to chronic heart failure (section 2.5.5) and, in lower doses, to reduce blood pressure.

Loop diuretics (section 2.2.2) are used in pulmonary oedema due to left ventricular failure and in patients with chronic heart failure (section 2.5.5).

Combination diuretic therapy may be effective in patients with oedema resistant to treatment with one diuretic. Vigorous diuresis, particularly with loop diuretics, may induce acute hypotension; rapid reduction of plasma volume should be avoided.

ELDERLY. Lower initial doses of diuretics should be used in the elderly because they are particularly susceptible to the side-effects. The dose should then be adjusted according to renal function. Diuretics should not be used continuously on a long-term basis to treat simple gravitational oedema (which will usually respond to increased movement, raising the legs, and support stockings).

POTASSIUM LOSS. Hypokalaemia may occur with both thiazide and loop diuretics. The risk of hypokalaemia depends on the duration of action as well as the potency and is thus greater with thiazides than with an equipotent dose of a loop diuretic.

Hypokalaemia is dangerous in severe coronary artery disease and in patients also being treated with cardiac glycosides. Often the use of potassium-sparing diuretics (section 2.2.3) avoids the need to take potassium supplements.

In hepatic failure hypokalaemia caused by diuretics can precipitate encephalopathy, particularly in alcoholic cirrhosis; diuretics may also increase the risk of hypomagnesaemia in alcoholic cirrhosis, leading to arrhythmias. Spironolactone, a potassium-sparing diuretic (section 2.2.3), is chosen for oedema arising from cirrhosis of the liver.

Potassium supplements or potassium-sparing diuretics are seldom necessary when thiazides are used in the routine treatment of hypertension (see also section 9.2.1.1).

2.2.1 Thiazides and related diuretics

Thiazides and related compounds are moderately potent diuretics; they inhibit sodium reabsorption at the beginning of the distal convoluted tubule. They act within 1 to 2 hours of oral administration and most have a duration of action of 12 to 24 hours; they are usually administered early in the day so that the diuresis does not interfere with sleep.

In the management of *hypertension* a low dose of a thiazide, e.g. bendroflumethiazide (bendrofluazide) 2.5 mg daily, produces a maximal or near-maximal blood pressure lowering effect, with very little biochemical disturbance. Higher doses cause more marked changes in plasma potassium, sodium, uric acid, glucose, and lipids, with little advantage in blood pressure control. For reference to the use of thiazides in chronic heart failure see section 2.5.5.

Bendroflumethiazide (bendrofluazide) is widely used for mild or moderate heart failure and for hypertension—alone in the treatment of mild hypertension or with other drugs in more severe hypertension.

Chlortalidone (chlorthalidone), a thiazide-related compound, has a longer duration of action than the thiazides and may be given on alternate days to control oedema. It is also useful if acute retention is liable to be precipitated by a more rapid diuresis or if patients dislike the altered pattern of micturition promoted by other diuretics.

Other thiazide diuretics (including benzthiazide, clopamide, cyclopenthiazide, hydrochlorothiazide and hydroflumethiazide) do not offer any significant advantage over bendroflumethiazide and chlortalidone.

Metolazone is particularly effective when combined with a loop diuretic (even in renal failure); profound diuresis may occur and the patient should therefore be monitored carefully.

Xipamide and **indapamide** are chemically related to chlortalidone. Indapamide is claimed to lower blood pressure with less metabolic disturbance, particularly less aggravation of diabetes mellitus.

BENDROFLUMETHIAZIDE

(Bendrofluazide)

Indications: oedema, hypertension (see also notes above)

Cautions: electrolytes may need to be monitored with high doses or in renal impairment, aggravates diabetes and gout; may exacerbate systemic lupus erythematosus; elderly; see also notes above; hepatic impairment (Appendix 2); renal impairment (Appendix 3); pregnancy (Appendix 4); breast-feeding (Appendix 5); **interactions:** Appendix 1 (diuretics)

Contra-indications: refractory hypokalaemia, hyponatraemia, hypercalcaemia; severe renal and hepatic impairment; symptomatic hyperuricaemia; Addison's disease

Side-effects: postural hypotension and mild gastro-intestinal effects; impotence (reversible on withdrawal of treatment); hypokalaemia (see also notes above), hypomagnesaemia, hyponatraemia, hypercalcaemia, hypochloraemic alkalosis, hyperuricaemia, gout, hyperglycaemia, and altered plasma lipid concentration; less commonly rashes, photosensitivity; blood disorders (including neutropenia and thrombocytopenia—when given in late pregnancy neonatal thrombocytopenia has been reported); pancreatitis, intrahepatic cholestasis, and hypersensitivity reactions (including pneumonitis, pulmonary oedema, severe skin reactions) also reported

Dose: oedema, initially 5–10 mg in the morning, daily *or* on alternate days; maintenance 5–10 mg 1–3 times weekly

Hypertension, 2.5 mg in the morning; higher doses rarely necessary (see notes above)

Bendroflumethiazide (Non-proprietary) [PoM]
Tablets, bendroflumethiazide 2.5 mg, net price 20 = 74p; 5 mg, 20 = 81p
Brands include *Aprinox*®, *Neo-NaClex*®

CHLORTALIDONE

(Chlorthalidone)

Indications: ascites due to cirrhosis in stable patients (under close supervision), oedema due to nephrotic syndrome, hypertension (see also notes above), mild to moderate chronic heart failure; diabetes insipidus (see section 6.5.2)

Cautions: see under Bendroflumethiazide

Contra-indications: see under Bendroflumethiazide

Side-effects: see under Bendroflumethiazide

Dose: oedema, up to 50 mg daily for limited period

Hypertension, 25 mg in the morning, increased to 50 mg if necessary (but see notes above)

Heart failure, 25–50 mg in the morning, increased if necessary to 100–200 mg daily

Hygroton® (Alliance) [PoM]
Tablets, yellow, scored, chlortalidone 50 mg, net price 28-tab pack = £1.64

CYCLOPENTHIAZIDE

Indications: oedema, hypertension (see also notes above)

Cautions: see under Bendroflumethiazide

Contra-indications: see under Bendroflumethiazide

Side-effects: see under Bendroflumethiazide

Dose: heart failure, 250–500 micrograms daily in the morning increased if necessary to 1 mg daily (reduce to lowest effective dose for maintenance)

Hypertension, initially 250 micrograms daily in the morning, increased if necessary to 500 micrograms daily (but see notes above)

Oedema, up to 500 micrograms daily for a short period

Navidrex® (Goldshield) [PoM]
Tablets, scored, cyclopenthiazide 500 micrograms. Net price 28-tab pack = £1.27
Excipients: include gluten

INDAPAMIDE

Indications: essential hypertension

Cautions: monitor plasma potassium and urate concentrations in elderly, hyperaldosteronism, gout, or with concomitant cardiac glycosides; hyperparathyroidism (discontinue if hypercalcaemia); porphyria (section 9.8.2); hepatic impairment (Appendix 2); renal impairment (Appendix 3—stop if deterioration); pregnancy (Appendix 4); breast-feeding (Appendix 5); **interactions:** Appendix 1 (diuretics)

Contra-indications: severe hepatic impairment

Side-effects: hypokalaemia, headache, dizziness, fatigue, muscular cramps, nausea, anorexia, diarrhoea, constipation, dyspepsia, rashes (erythema multiforme, epidermal necrolysis reported); rarely postural hypotension, palpitation, increase in liver enzymes, blood disorders (including thrombocytopenia), hyponatraemia, metabolic alkalosis, hyperglycaemia, increased plasma urate concentrations, paraesthesia, photosensitivity, impotence, renal impairment, reversible acute myopia; diuresis with doses above 2.5 mg daily

Dose: 2.5 mg in the morning

Indapamide (Non-proprietary) PoM
Tablets, s/c, indapamide 2.5 mg, net price 30-tab pack = £2.86, 56-tab pack = £6.65
Brands include *Nindaxa 2.5*®

Natrilix® (Servier) PoM
Tablets, f/c, indapamide 2.5 mg. Net price 30-tab pack = £4.50, 60-tab pack = £9.00

■ Modified release

Natrilix SR® (Servier) PoM
Tablets, m/r, indapamide 1.5 mg. Net price 30-tab pack = £4.50. Label: 25
Dose: hypertension, 1 tablet daily, preferably in the morning

METOLAZONE

Indications: oedema, hypertension (see also notes above)

Cautions: see under Bendroflumethiazide; also profound diuresis on concomitant administration with furosemide (monitor patient carefully); porphyria (section 9.8.2)

Contra-indications: see under Bendroflumethiazide

Side-effects: see under Bendroflumethiazide

Dose: oedema, 5–10 mg in the morning, increased if necessary to 20 mg daily in resistant oedema, max. 80 mg daily
Hypertension, initially 5 mg in the morning; maintenance 5 mg on alternate days

Metenix 5® (Borg) PoM
Tablets, blue, metolazone 5 mg. Net price 100-tab pack = £18.94

XIPAMIDE

Indications: oedema, hypertension (see also notes above)

Cautions: see under Bendroflumethiazide; also porphyria (section 9.8.2)

Contra-indications: see under Bendroflumethiazide

Side-effects: gastro-intestinal disturbances; mild dizziness; hypokalaemia, more rarely other electrolyte disturbances such as hyponatraemia

Dose: oedema, initially 40 mg in the morning, increased to 80 mg in resistant cases; maintenance 20 mg in the morning
Hypertension, 20 mg in the morning

Diurexan® (Viatris) PoM
Tablets, scored, xipamide 20 mg. Net price 140-tab pack = £19.46

2.2.2 Loop diuretics

Loop diuretics are used in pulmonary oedema due to left ventricular failure; intravenous administration produces relief of breathlessness and reduces preload sooner than would be expected from the time of onset of diuresis. Loop diuretics are also used in patients with chronic heart failure. Diuretic-resistant oedema (except lymphoedema and oedema due to peripheral venous stasis or calcium-channel blockers) can be treated with a loop diuretic combined with a thiazide or related diuretic (e.g. bendroflumethiazide 5–10 mg daily or metolazone 5–20 mg daily).

A loop diuretic is sometimes used to lower blood pressure especially in hypertension resistant to thiazide therapy.

Loop diuretics inhibit reabsorption from the ascending limb of the loop of Henlé in the renal tubule and are powerful diuretics. Hypokalaemia may develop, and care is needed to avoid hypotension. If there is an enlarged prostate, urinary retention may occur; this is less likely if small doses and less potent diuretics are used initially.

Furosemide (frusemide) and **bumetanide** are similar in activity; both act within 1 hour of oral administration and diuresis is complete within 6 hours so that, if necessary, they can be given twice in one day without interfering with sleep. Following intravenous administration they have a peak effect within 30 minutes. The diuresis associated with these drugs is dose related. In patients with impaired renal function very large doses may occasionally be needed; in such doses both drugs can cause deafness and bumetanide can cause myalgia.

Torasemide has properties similar to those of furosemide and bumetanide, and is indicated for oedema and for hypertension.

FUROSEMIDE

(Frusemide)

Indications: oedema (see notes above), oliguria due to renal failure

Cautions: hypotension; correct hypovolaemia before using in oliguria; prostatic enlargement; although manufacturer advises that rate of intravenous administration should not exceed 4 mg/minute, single doses of up to 80 mg may be administered more rapidly; hepatic impairment (Appendix 2); renal impairment (Appendix 3); pregnancy (Appendix 4); **interactions:** Appendix 1 (diuretics)

Contra-indications: precomatose states associated with liver cirrhosis; renal failure with anuria

Side-effects: hyponatraemia, hypokalaemia, and hypomagnesaemia (see also section 2.2), hypochloraemic alkalosis, increased calcium excretion, hypotension; less commonly nausea, gastro-intestinal disturbances, hyperuricaemia and gout; hyperglycaemia (less common than with thiazides); temporary increase in plasma cholesterol and triglyceride concentrations; rarely rashes, photosensitivity and bone marrow depression (withdraw treatment), pancreatitis (with large parenteral doses), tinnitus and deafness (usually with large parenteral doses and rapid administration and in renal impairment)

Dose: *by mouth*, oedema, initially 40 mg in the morning; maintenance 20–40 mg daily, increased in resistant oedema to 80 mg daily or more; CHILD 1–3 mg/kg daily, max. 40 mg daily
Oliguria, initially 250 mg daily; if necessary larger doses, increasing in steps of 250 mg, may be given every 4–6 hours to a max. of a single dose of 2 g (rarely used)
By intramuscular injection or slow intravenous injection (see Cautions, above), initially 20–50 mg; CHILD 0.5–1.5 mg/kg to a max. daily dose of 20 mg

By intravenous infusion (by syringe pump if necessary), in oliguria, initially 250 mg over 1 hour (rate not exceeding 4 mg/minute), if satisfactory urine output not obtained in the subsequent hour further 500 mg over 2 hours, then if no satisfactory response within subsequent hour, further 1 g over 4 hours, if no response obtained dialysis probably required; effective dose (up to 1 g) can be repeated every 24 hours

Furosemide (Non-proprietary) PoM
Tablets, furosemide 20 mg, net price 28 = 62p; 40 mg, 28-tab pack = £1.00; 500 mg, 28 = £9.22
Brands include *Froop*®, *Rusyde*®
Oral solution, sugar-free, furosemide, net price 20 mg/5 mL, 150 mL = £12.07; 40 mg/5 mL, 150 mL = £15.58; 50 mg/5 mL, 150 mL = £16.84
Brands include *Frusol*® (contains alcohol 10%)
Injection, furosemide 10 mg/mL, net price 2-mL amp = 55p; 5-mL amp = 66p

Lasix® (Sanofi-Aventis) PoM
Tablets, both scored, furosemide 40 mg, 28-tab pack = £2.11; 500 mg (yellow), 20 = £20.22
Injection, furosemide 10 mg/mL, net price 2-mL amp = 78p
NOTE. Large volume furosemide injections also available; brands include *Minijet*®

BUMETANIDE

Indications: oedema (see notes above), oliguria due to renal failure
Cautions: see under Furosemide; hepatic impairment (Appendix 2); renal impairment (Appendix 3); pregnancy (Appendix 4); breast-feeding (Appendix 5)
Contra-indications: see under Furosemide
Side-effects: see under Furosemide; also myalgia
Dose: *by mouth*, 1 mg in the morning, repeated after 6–8 hours if necessary; severe cases, increased up to 5 mg or more daily
ELDERLY, 500 micrograms daily may be sufficient
By intravenous injection, 1–2 mg, repeated after 20 minutes; when *intramuscular injection* considered necessary, 1 mg initially then adjusted according to response
By intravenous infusion, 2–5 mg over 30–60 minutes

Bumetanide (Non-proprietary) PoM
Tablets, bumetanide 1 mg, net price 28-tab pack = £1.10; 5 mg, 28-tab pack = £3.28
Liquid, bumetanide 1 mg/5 mL, net price 150 mL = £15.22
Injection, bumetanide 500 micrograms/mL, net price 4-mL amp = £1.79

Burinex® (Leo) PoM
Tablets, both scored, bumetanide 1 mg, net price 28-tab pack = £1.52; 5 mg, 28 = £9.67

TORASEMIDE

Indications: oedema (see notes above), hypertension
Cautions: see under Furosemide; hepatic impairment (Appendix 2); renal impairment (Appendix 3); pregnancy (Appendix 4)
Contra-indications: see under Furosemide
Side-effects: see under Furosemide; also dry mouth; rarely limb paraesthesia
Dose: oedema, 5 mg once daily, preferably in the morning, increased if required to 20 mg once daily; usual max. 40 mg daily
Hypertension, 2.5 mg daily, increased if necessary to 5 mg once daily

Torasemide (Non-proprietary) PoM
Tablets, torasemide 5 mg, net price 28-tab pack = £5.95; 10 mg, 28-tab pack = £8.14

Torem® (Roche) PoM
Tablets, torasemide 2.5 mg, net price 28-tab pack = £3.78; 5 mg (scored), 28-tab pack = £5.53; 10 mg (scored), 28-tab pack = £8.14

2.2.3 Potassium-sparing diuretics and aldosterone antagonists

Amiloride and **triamterene** on their own are weak diuretics. They cause retention of potassium and are therefore used as a more effective alternative to giving potassium supplements with thiazide or loop diuretics. (See section 2.2.4 for compound preparations with thiazides or loop diuretics.)

Potassium supplements must **not** be given with potassium-sparing diuretics. It is also important to bear in mind that administration of a potassium-sparing diuretic to a patient receiving an ACE inhibitor or an angiotensin-II receptor antagonist can cause severe hyperkalaemia.

AMILORIDE HYDROCHLORIDE

Indications: oedema, potassium conservation with thiazide and loop diuretics
Cautions: diabetes mellitus; elderly; renal impairment (Appendix 3); pregnancy (Appendix 4); breast-feeding (Appendix 5); **interactions:** Appendix 1 (diuretics)
Contra-indications: hyperkalaemia, renal failure
Side-effects: include gastro-intestinal disturbances, dry mouth, rashes, confusion, postural hypotension, hyperkalaemia, hyponatraemia
Dose: used alone, initially 10 mg daily *or* 5 mg twice daily, adjusted according to response; max. 20 mg daily
With other diuretics, congestive heart failure and hypertension, initially 5–10 mg daily; cirrhosis with ascites, initially 5 mg daily

Amiloride (Non-proprietary) PoM
Tablets, amiloride hydrochloride 5 mg, net price 28 = £1.18
Oral solution, sugar-free, amiloride hydrochloride 5 mg/5 mL, net price 150 mL = £37.35
Brands include *Amilamont*®

■ Compound preparations with thiazide or loop diuretics
See section 2.2.4

TRIAMTERENE

Indications: oedema, potassium conservation with thiazide and loop diuretics
Cautions: see under Amiloride Hydrochloride; may cause blue fluorescence of urine
Contra-indications: see under Amiloride Hydrochloride
Side-effects: include gastro-intestinal disturbances, dry mouth, rashes; slight decrease in blood pressure, hyperkalaemia, hyponatraemia; photosensit-

ivity and blood disorders also reported; triamterene found in kidney stones

Dose: initially 150–250 mg daily, reducing to alternate days after 1 week; taken in divided doses after breakfast and lunch; lower initial dose when given with other diuretics

COUNSELLING. Urine may look slightly blue in some lights

Dytac® (Goldshield) PoM

Capsules, maroon, triamterene 50 mg. Net price 30-cap pack = £17.35 Label: 14, (see above), 21

■ Compound preparations with thiazides or loop diuretics

See section 2.2.4

Aldosterone antagonists

Spironolactone potentiates thiazide or loop diuretics by antagonising aldosterone; it is a potassium-sparing diuretic. It is of value in the treatment of the oedema of cirrhosis of the liver. Low doses of spironolactone are beneficial in severe heart failure, see section 2.5.5.

Spironolactone is also used in primary hyperaldosteronism (Conn's syndrome). It is given before surgery or if surgery is not appropriate, in the lowest effective dose for maintenance.

Eplerenone is licensed for use as an adjunct in left ventricular dysfunction and heart failure after a myocardial infarction (see also section 2.5.5 and section 2.10.1). The *Scottish Medicines Consortium* has advised (December 2004) that the use of eplerenone should be restricted to patients who cannot tolerate the hormonal side-effects of spironolactone.

As with potassium-sparing diuretics, potassium supplements must **not** be given with aldosterone antagonists.

EPLERENONE

Indications: adjunct in stable patients with left ventricular dysfunction with evidence of heart failure, following myocardial infarction (start therapy within 3–14 days of event)

Cautions: measure plasma-potassium concentration before treatment, during initiation, and when dose changed; elderly; hepatic impairment (Appendix 2); renal impairment (Appendix 3); pregnancy; breast-feeding (Appendix 5); **interactions:** Appendix 1 (diuretics)

Contra-indications: hyperkalaemia; concomitant use of potassium-sparing diuretics or potassium supplements

Side-effects: diarrhoea, nausea; hypotension; dizziness; hyperkalaemia; *less commonly* flatulence, vomiting, atrial fibrillation, postural hypotension, arterial thrombosis, dyslipidaemia, pharyngitis, headache, insomnia, pyelonephritis, hyponatraemia, dehydration, eosinophilia, asthenia, malaise, back pain, leg cramps, impaired renal function, azotaemia, sweating and pruritus

Dose: initially 25 mg once daily, increased within 4 weeks to 50 mg once daily; CHILD not recommended

Inspra® (Pfizer) ▼ PoM

Tablets, yellow, f/c, eplerenone 25 mg, net price 28-tab pack = £42.72; 50 mg, 28-tab pack = £42.72

SPIRONOLACTONE

Indications: oedema and ascites in cirrhosis of the liver, malignant ascites, nephrotic syndrome, congestive heart failure (section 2.5.5); primary hyperaldosteronism

Cautions: potential metabolic products carcinogenic in *rodents*; elderly; monitor electrolytes (discontinue if hyperkalaemia); porphyria (section 9.8.2); hepatic impairment; renal impairment (Appendix 3); pregnancy (Appendix 4); breast-feeding (Appendix 5); **interactions:** Appendix 1 (diuretics)

Contra-indications: hyperkalaemia, hyponatraemia; Addison's disease

Side-effects: gastro-intestinal disturbances; impotence, gynaecomastia; menstrual irregularities; lethargy, headache, confusion; rashes; hyperkalaemia (discontinue); hyponatraemia; hepatotoxicity, osteomalacia, and blood disorders reported

Dose: 100–200 mg daily, increased to 400 mg if required; CHILD initially 3 mg/kg daily in divided doses

Heart failure, see section 2.5.5

Spironolactone (Non-proprietary) PoM

Tablets, spironolactone 25 mg, net price 28 = £3.00; 50 mg, 28 = £4.99; 100 mg, 28 = £5.02

Brands include *Spirospare*®

Oral suspensions, sugar-free, spironolactone 5 mg/5 mL, 10 mg/5 mL, 25 mg/5 mL, 50 mg/5 mL and 100 mg/5 mL available from Rosemont (special order)

Aldactone® (Searle) PoM

Tablets, all f/c, spironolactone 25 mg (buff), net price 100-tab pack = £8.89; 50 mg (off-white), 100-tab pack = £17.78; 100 mg (buff), 28-tab pack = £9.96

■ With thiazides or loop diuretics

See section 2.2.4

2.2.4 Potassium-sparing diuretics with other diuretics

Although it is preferable to prescribe thiazides (section 2.2.1) and potassium-sparing diuretics (section 2.2.3) separately, the use of fixed combinations may be justified if compliance is a problem. Potassium-sparing diuretics are not usually necessary in the routine treatment of hypertension, unless hypokalaemia develops. For **interactions**, see Appendix 1 (diuretics).

■ Amiloride with thiazides

Co-amilozide (Non-proprietary) PoM

Tablets, co-amilozide 2.5/25 (amiloride hydrochloride 2.5 mg, hydrochlorothiazide 25 mg), net price 28-tab pack = £1.85

Brands include *Moduret 25*®

Dose: hypertension, initially 1 tablet daily, increased if necessary to max. 2 tablets daily

Congestive heart failure, initially 1 tablet daily, increased if necessary to max. 4 tablets daily

Oedema and ascites in cirrhosis of the liver, initially 2 tablets daily, increased if necessary to max. 4 tablets daily; reduce for maintenance if possible

Tablets, co-amilozide 5/50 (amiloride hydrochloride 5 mg, hydrochlorothiazide 50 mg), net price 28 = £1.86
Brands include *Amil-Co*®, *Moduretic*®
Dose: hypertension, initially ½ tablet daily, increased if necessary to max. 1 tablet daily
Congestive heart failure, initially ½ tablet daily, increased if necessary to max. 2 tablets daily
Oedema and ascites in cirrhosis of the liver, initially 1 tablet daily, increased if necessary to max. 2 tablets daily; reduce for maintenance if possible

Navispare® (Novartis) PoM
Tablets, f/c, orange, amiloride hydrochloride 2.5 mg, cyclopenthiazide 250 micrograms. Net price 28-tab pack = £2.25
Excipients: include gluten
Dose: hypertension, 1–2 tablets in the morning

■ Amiloride with loop diuretics

Co-amilofruse (Non-proprietary) PoM
Tablets, co-amilofruse 2.5/20 (amiloride hydrochloride 2.5 mg, furosemide 20 mg). Net price 28-tab pack = £2.00, 56-tab pack = £2.97
Brands include *Frumil LS*®
Dose: oedema, 1 tablet in the morning
Tablets, co-amilofruse 5/40 (amiloride hydrochloride 5 mg, furosemide 40 mg). Net price 28-tab pack = £2.05
Brands include *Froop-Co*®, *Fru-Co*®, *Frumil*®, *Lasoride*®
Dose: oedema, 1–2 tablets in the morning
Tablets, co-amilofruse 10/80 (amiloride hydrochloride 10 mg, furosemide 80 mg). Net price 28-tab pack = £7.43, 56-tab pack = £14.86
Brands include *Aridil*®, *Frumil Forte*®
Dose: oedema, 1 tablet in the morning

Burinex A® (Leo) PoM
Tablets, ivory, scored, amiloride hydrochloride 5 mg, bumetanide 1 mg. Net price 28-tab pack = £2.63
Dose: oedema, 1–2 tablets daily

■ Triamterene with thiazides

COUNSELLING. Urine may look slightly blue in some lights

Co-triamterzide (Non-proprietary) PoM
Tablets, co-triamterzide 50/25 (triamterene 50 mg, hydrochlorothiazide 25 mg), net price 30-tab pack = 95p. Label: 14, (see above), 21
Dose: hypertension, 1 tablet daily after breakfast, increased if necessary, max. 4 daily
Oedema, 2 tablets daily (1 after breakfast and 1 after midday meal) increased to 3 daily if necessary (2 after breakfast and 1 after midday meal); usual maintenance in oedema, 1 daily or 2 on alternate days; max. 4 daily
Brands include *Triam-Co*®

Dyazide® (Goldshield) PoM
Tablets, peach, scored, co-triamterzide 50/25 (triamterene 50 mg, hydrochlorothiazide 25 mg). Net price 30-tab pack = 95p. Label: 14, (see above), 21
Dose: hypertension, 1 tablet daily after breakfast, increased if necessary, max. 4 daily
Oedema, 2 tablets daily (1 after breakfast and 1 after midday meal) increased to 3 daily if necessary (2 after breakfast and 1 after midday meal); usual maintenance in oedema, 1 daily or 2 on alternate days; max. 4 daily

Dytide® (Goldshield) PoM
Capsules, clear/maroon, triamterene 50 mg, benzthiazide 25 mg. Net price 30-cap pack = £17.35. Label: 14, (see above), 21
Dose: oedema, initially 3 capsules daily (2 after breakfast and 1 after midday meal) for 1 week then 1 or 2 on alternate days

Kalspare® (PLIVA) PoM
Tablets, orange, f/c, scored, triamterene 50 mg, chlortalidone 50 mg. Net price 28-tab pack = £3.05. Label: 14, (see above), 21
Dose: hypertension, oedema, 1–2 tablets in the morning

■ Triamterene with loop diuretics

COUNSELLING. Urine may look slightly blue in some lights

Frusene® (Orion) PoM
Tablets, yellow, scored, triamterene 50 mg, furosemide 40 mg. Net price 56-tab pack = £4.54. Label: 14, (see above), 21
Dose: oedema, ½–2 tablets daily in the morning

■ Spironolactone with thiazides

Co-flumactone (Non-proprietary) PoM
Tablets, co-flumactone 25/25 (hydroflumethiazide 25 mg, spironolactone 25 mg). Net price 100-tab pack = £20.23
Brands include *Aldactide 25*®
Dose: congestive heart failure, initially 4 tablets daily; range 1–8 daily (but not recommended because spironolactone generally given in lower dose)
Tablets, co-flumactone 50/50 (hydroflumethiazide 50 mg, spironolactone 50 mg). Net price 28-tab pack = £10.70
Brands include *Aldactide 50*®
Dose: congestive heart failure, initially 2 tablets daily; range 1–4 daily (but not recommended because spironolactone generally given in lower dose)

■ Spironolactone with loop diuretics

Lasilactone® (Borg) PoM
Capsules, blue/white, spironolactone 50 mg, furosemide 20 mg. Net price 28-cap pack = £8.29
Dose: resistant oedema, 1–4 capsules daily

2.2.5 Osmotic diuretics

Osmotic diuretics are rarely used in heart failure as they may acutely expand the blood volume. **Mannitol** is used in cerebral oedema—a typical dose is 1 g/kg as a 20% solution given by rapid intravenous infusion.

MANNITOL

Indications: see notes above; glaucoma (section 11.6)
Cautions: extravasation causes inflammation and thrombophlebitis
Contra-indications: congestive cardiac failure, pulmonary oedema
Side-effects: chills, fever
Dose: *by intravenous infusion*, diuresis, 50–200 g over 24 hours, preceded by a test dose of 200 mg/kg by slow intravenous injection
Cerebral oedema, see notes above

Mannitol (Baxter) PoM
Intravenous infusion, mannitol 10% and 20%

2.2.6 Mercurial diuretics

Mercurial diuretics are effective but are now almost never used because of their nephrotoxicity.

2.2.7 Carbonic anhydrase inhibitors

The carbonic anhydrase inhibitor **acetazolamide** is a weak diuretic and is little used for its diuretic effect. It is used for prophylaxis against mountain sickness [unlicensed indication] but is not a substitute for acclimatisation.

Acetazolamide and eye drops of dorzolamide and brinzolamide inhibit the formation of aqueous humour and are used in glaucoma (section 11.6).

2.2.8 Diuretics with potassium

Many patients on diuretics do not need potassium supplements (section 9.2.1.1). For many of those who do, the amount of potassium in combined preparations may not be enough, and for this reason their use is to be discouraged.

Diuretics with potassium and potassium-sparing diuretics should **not** usually be given together.

COUNSELLING. Modified-release potassium tablets should be swallowed whole with plenty of fluid during meals while sitting or standing

Burinex K® (Leo) PoM
Tablets, bumetanide 500 micrograms, potassium 7.7 mmol for modified release. Net price 20 = 80p. Label: 25, 27, counselling, see above

Centyl K® (Leo) PoM
Tablets, green, s/c, bendroflumethiazide 2.5 mg, potassium 7.7 mmol for modified release, net price 56-tab pack = £7.50. Label: 25, 27, counselling, see above

Lasikal® (Borg) PoM
Tablets, white/yellow, f/c, furosemide 20 mg, potassium 10 mmol for modified release. Net price 100-tab pack = £15.21. Label: 25, 27, counselling, see above

Neo-NaClex-K® (Goldshield) PoM
Tablets, pink/white, f/c, bendroflumethiazide 2.5 mg, potassium 8.4 mmol for modified release. Net price 20 = £1.59. Label: 25, 27, counselling, see above

2.3 Anti-arrhythmic drugs

2.3.1 Management of arrhythmias

Management of an arrhythmia requires precise diagnosis of the type of arrhythmia, and electrocardiography is essential; underlying causes such as heart failure require appropriate treatment.

ECTOPIC BEATS. If spontaneous with a normal heart, ectopic beats rarely require treatment beyond reassurance. If they are particularly troublesome, beta-blockers are sometimes effective and may be safer than other suppressant drugs.

ATRIAL FIBRILLATION. The ventricular rate in atrial fibrillation can be controlled with a beta-blocker, or diltiazem [unlicensed indication], or verapamil. Digoxin is usually effective for controlling the rate at rest; it is also appropriate if atrial fibrillation is accompanied by congestive heart failure. If the rate at rest or during exercise cannot be controlled, diltiazem or verapamil may be combined with digoxin, but care is required if the ventricular function is diminished. In some cases, e.g. acute atrial fibrillation or paroxysmal atrial fibrillation, diltiazem or verapamil or a beta-blocker may be more appropriate than digoxin (see also Paroxysmal Supraventricular Tachycardia and Supraventricular Arrhythmias below). Anticoagulants are indicated especially in valvular or myocardial disease, and in the elderly; in the very elderly the overall benefit and risk needs careful assessment. Younger patients with lone atrial fibrillation in the absence of heart disease probably do not need anticoagulation. Aspirin is less effective than warfarin at preventing emboli but may be appropriate if there are no other risk factors for stroke; aspirin 75 mg may be used.

ATRIAL FLUTTER. The ventricular rate at rest can sometimes be controlled with digoxin. Reversion to sinus rhythm (if indicated) may be achieved by appropriately synchronised d.c. shock. Alternatively, amiodarone may be used to restore sinus rhythm, and amiodarone or sotalol to maintain it. If the arrhythmia is long-standing a period of treatment with anticoagulants should be considered before cardioversion to avoid the complication of emboli.

PAROXYSMAL SUPRAVENTRICULAR TACHYCARDIA. In most patients this remits spontaneously or can be returned to sinus rhythm by reflex vagal stimulation with respiratory manoeuvres, prompt squatting, or pressure over one carotid sinus (**important:** pressure over carotid sinus should be restricted to monitored patients—it can be dangerous in recent ischaemia, digitalis toxicity, or the elderly).

If vagal stimulation fails, intravenous administration of adenosine is usually the treatment of choice. Intravenous administration of verapamil is useful for patients without myocardial or valvular disease (**important:** never in patients recently treated with beta-blockers, see p. 113). For arrhythmias that are poorly tolerated, synchronised d.c. shock usually provides rapid relief.

In cases of paroxysmal supraventricular tachycardia with block, digitalis toxicity should be suspected. In addition to stopping administration of the cardiac glycoside and giving potassium supplements, intravenous administration of a beta-blocker may be useful. Specific digoxin antibody is available if the toxicity is considered life-threatening (section 2.1.1).

ARRHYTHMIAS AFTER MYOCARDIAL INFARCTION. In patients with a paroxysmal tachycardia or rapid irregularity of the pulse it is best not to administer an antiarrhythmic until an ECG record has been obtained. Bradycardia, particularly if complicated by hypotension, should be treated with atropine sulphate, given intravenously in a dose of 0.3–1 mg. If the initial dose is effective it may be repeated if necessary.

VENTRICULAR TACHYCARDIA. Drug treatment is used both for the treatment of ventricular tachycardia and for prophylaxis of recurrent attacks that merit suppression. Ventricular tachycardia requires treatment most commonly in the acute stage of myocardial infarction, but the likelihood of this and other life-threatening arrhythmias diminishes sharply over the first 24 hours after the attack, especially in patients without heart failure or shock. Lidocaine (lignocaine) is the preferred drug for emergency use. Other drugs are best administered under specialist supervision. Very rapid ventricular tachycardia causes profound circulatory collapse and should be treated urgently with d.c. shock.

Torsades de pointes is a special form of ventricular tachycardia which tends to occur in the presence of a long QT interval (usually drug induced, but other factors including hypokalaemia, severe bradycardia, and genetic predisposition may also be implicated). The episodes are usually self-limiting, but are frequently recurrent and may cause impairment (or loss) of consciousness. If not controlled, the arrhythmia may progress to ventricular fibrillation. Intravenous infusion of magnesium sulphate (section 9.5.1.3) is usually effective. A beta-blocker (but not sotalol) and atrial (or ventricular) pacing may be considered. Anti-arrhythmics (including lidocaine) may further prolong the QT interval, thus worsening the condition.

2.3.2 Drugs for arrhythmias

Anti-arrhythmic drugs can be classified clinically into those that act on supraventricular arrhythmias (e.g. verapamil), those that act on both supraventricular and ventricular arrhythmias (e.g. disopyramide), and those that act on ventricular arrhythmias (e.g. lidocaine (lignocaine)).

They can also be classified according to their effects on the electrical behaviour of myocardial cells during activity:

Class Ia, b, c: membrane stabilising drugs (e.g. quinidine, lidocaine, flecainide respectively)
Class II: beta-blockers
Class III: amiodarone and sotalol (also Class II)
Class IV: calcium-channel blockers (includes verapamil but not dihydropyridines)

This latter classification (the Vaughan Williams classification) is of less clinical significance.

CAUTIONS. The negative inotropic effects of anti-arrhythmic drugs tend to be additive. Therefore special care should be taken if two or more are used, especially if myocardial function is impaired. Most or all drugs that are effective in countering arrhythmias can also provoke them in some circumstances; moreover, hypokalaemia enhances the arrhythmogenic (pro-arrhythmic) effect of many drugs.

Supraventricular arrhythmias

Adenosine is usually the treatment of choice for terminating paroxysmal supraventricular tachycardia. As it has a very short duration of action (half-life only about 8 to 10 seconds, but prolonged in those taking dipyridamole), most side-effects are short lived. Unlike verapamil, adenosine may be used after a beta-blocker. Verapamil may be preferable to adenosine in asthma.

Oral administration of a **cardiac glycoside** (such as digoxin, section 2.1.1) slows the ventricular response in cases of atrial fibrillation and atrial flutter. However, intravenous infusion of digoxin is rarely effective for rapid control of ventricular rate. Cardiac glycosides are contra-indicated in supraventricular arrhythmias associated with Wolff-Parkinson-White syndrome.

Verapamil (section 2.6.2) is usually effective for supraventricular tachycardias. An initial intravenous dose (**important**: serious beta-blocker interaction hazard, see p. 113) may be followed by oral treatment; hypotension may occur with larger doses. It should not be used for tachyarrhythmias where the QRS complex is wide (i.e. broad complex) unless a supraventricular origin has been established beyond reasonable doubt. It is also contra-indicated in atrial fibrillation with pre-excitation (e.g. Wolff-Parkinson-White syndrome). It should not be used in children with arrhythmias without specialist advice; some supraventricular arrhythmias in childhood can be accelerated by verapamil with dangerous consequences.

Intravenous administration of a **beta-blocker** (section 2.4) such as esmolol or propranolol, can achieve rapid control of the ventricular rate.

Drugs for both supraventricular and ventricular arrhythmias include **amiodarone**, **beta-blockers**, **disopyramide**, **flecainide**, **procainamide**, **propafenone** and **quinidine**, see below under Supraventricular and Ventricular Arrhythmias.

ADENOSINE

Indications: rapid reversion to sinus rhythm of paroxysmal supraventricular tachycardias, including those associated with accessory pathways (e.g. Wolff-Parkinson-White syndrome); aid to diagnosis of broad or narrow complex supraventricular tachycardias

Cautions: atrial fibrillation or flutter with accessory pathway (conduction down anomalous pathway may increase); heart transplant (see below); **interactions:** Appendix 1 (adenosine)

Contra-indications: second- or third-degree AV block and sick sinus syndrome (unless pacemaker fitted); asthma

Side-effects: include transient facial flush, chest pain, dyspnoea, bronchospasm, choking sensation, nausea, light-headedness; severe bradycardia reported (requiring temporary pacing); ECG may show transient rhythm disturbances

Dose: *by rapid intravenous injection* into central or large peripheral vein, 3 mg over 2 seconds with cardiac monitoring; if necessary followed by 6 mg after 1–2 minutes, and then by 12 mg after a further 1–2 minutes; increments should not be given if high level AV block develops at any particular dose

NOTE. 3-mg dose ineffective in a number of patients, therefore higher initial dose sometimes used but patients with *heart transplant* are **very sensitive** to effects of adenosine, and should **not** receive higher initial dose. Also if essential to give with dipyridamole reduce initial dose to 0.5–1 mg

Adenocor® (Sanofi-Synthelabo) PoM
Injection, adenosine 3 mg/mL in physiological saline. Net price 2-mL vial = £4.45 (hosp. only)
NOTE. Intravenous infusion of adenosine (*Adenoscan*®, Sanofi Winthrop) may be used in conjunction with

radionuclide myocardial perfusion imaging in patients who cannot exercise adequately or for whom exercise is inappropriate—consult product literature

Supraventricular and ventricular arrhythmias

Amiodarone is used in the treatment of arrhythmias particularly when other drugs are ineffective or contra-indicated. It may be used for paroxysmal supraventricular, nodal and ventricular tachycardias, atrial fibrillation and flutter, and ventricular fibrillation. It may also be used for tachyarrythmias associated with Wolff-Parkinson-White syndrome. It should be initiated only under hospital or specialist supervision. Amiodarone may be given by intravenous infusion as well as by mouth, and has the advantage of causing little or no myocardial depression. Unlike oral amiodarone, intravenous amiodarone may act relatively rapidly.

Intravenous injection of amiodarone may be used in cardiopulmonary resuscitation for ventricular fibrillation or pulseless tachycardia unresponsive to other interventions (section 2.7.3).

Amiodarone has a very long half-life (extending to several weeks) and only needs to be given once daily (but high doses may cause nausea unless divided). Many weeks or months may be required to achieve steady-state plasma-amiodarone concentration; this is particularly important when drug interactions are likely (see also Appendix 1).

Most patients taking amiodarone develop corneal microdeposits (reversible on withdrawal of treatment); these rarely interfere with vision, but drivers may be dazzled by headlights at night. Because of the possibility of phototoxic reactions, patients should be advised to shield the skin from light during treatment and for several months after discontinuing amiodarone; patients should use a wide-spectrum sunscreen (section 13.8.1) to protect against both long ultraviolet and visible light.

Amiodarone contains iodine and can cause disorders of thyroid function; both hypothyroidism and hyperthyroidism may occur. Clinical assessment alone is unreliable, and laboratory tests should be performed before treatment and every 6 months. Thyroxine (T4) may be raised in the absence of hyperthyroidism; therefore tri-iodothyronine (T3), T4, and thyroid-stimulating hormone (thyrotrophin, TSH) should all be measured. A raised T3 and T4 with a very low or undetectable TSH concentration suggests the development of thyrotoxicosis. The thyrotoxicosis may be very refractory, and amiodarone should usually be withdrawn at least temporarily to help achieve control; treatment with carbimazole may be required. Hypothyroidism can be treated with replacement therapy without withdrawing amiodarone if it is essential; careful supervision is required.

Pneumonitis should always be suspected if new or progressive shortness of breath or cough develops in a patient taking amiodarone. Fresh neurological symptoms should raise the possibility of peripheral neuropathy.

Amiodarone is also associated with hepatotoxicity and treatment should be discontinued if severe liver function abnormalities or clinical signs of liver disease develop.

Beta-blockers act as anti-arrhythmic drugs principally by attenuating the effects of the sympathetic system on automaticity and conductivity within the heart, for details see section 2.4. For special reference to the role of **sotalol** in ventricular arrhythmias, see also p. 84.

Disopyramide may be given by intravenous injection to control arrhythmias after myocardial infarction (including those not responding to lidocaine (lignocaine)), but it impairs cardiac contractility. Oral administration of disopyramide is useful but it has an antimuscarinic effect which limits its use in patients with glaucoma or prostatic hypertrophy.

Flecainide belongs to the same general class as lidocaine. It may be of value in serious symptomatic ventricular arrhythmias. It may also be indicated for junctional re-entry tachycardias and for paroxysmal atrial fibrillation. As with quinidine it may precipitate serious arrhythmias in a small minority of patients (including those with otherwise normal hearts).

Procainamide is given by intravenous injection to control ventricular arrhythmias.

Propafenone is used for the prophylaxis and treatment of ventricular arrhythmias and also for some supraventricular arrhythmias. It has complex mechanisms of action, including weak beta-blocking activity (therefore caution is needed in obstructive airways disease—contra-indicated if severe).

Quinidine can suppress supraventricular and ventricular arrhythmias but it may itself precipitate rhythm disorders and is best used on specialist advice; it is rarely used nowadays.

Drugs for supraventricular arrhythmias include **adenosine**, **cardiac glycosides** and **verapamil**, see above under Supraventricular Arrhythmias. Drugs for ventricular arrhythmias include **lidocaine**, **mexiletine**, and **phenytoin**, see below under Ventricular Arrhythmias.

AMIODARONE HYDROCHLORIDE

Indications: see notes above (should be initiated in hospital or under specialist supervision)

Cautions: liver-function and thyroid-function tests required before treatment and then every 6 months (see notes above for tests of thyroid function); serum potassium concentration and chest x-ray required before treatment; heart failure; elderly; severe bradycardia and conduction disturbances in excessive dosage; intravenous use may cause moderate and transient fall in blood pressure (circulatory collapse precipitated by rapid administration or overdosage) or severe hepatocellular toxicity (monitor transaminases closely); porphyria (section 9.8.2); **interactions:** Appendix 1 (amiodarone)

Contra-indications: sinus bradycardia, sino-atrial heart block; unless pacemaker fitted avoid in severe conduction disturbances or sinus node disease; thyroid dysfunction; iodine sensitivity; avoid *intravenous use* in severe respiratory failure, circulatory collapse (except in cardiac arrest, see section 2.7.3), severe arterial hypotension; avoid bolus injection in congestive heart failure or cardiomyopathy; pregnancy (Appendix 4); breast-feeding (Appendix 5)

Side-effects: nausea, vomiting, taste disturbances, raised serum transaminases (may require dose reduction or withdrawal if accompanied by acute liver disorders), jaundice; bradycardia (see Cautions); pulmonary toxicity (including pneumonitis and fibrosis); tremor, sleep disorders; hypothyroidism, hyperthyroidism; reversible corneal microdeposits (sometimes with night glare); phototoxicity, persistent slate-grey skin discoloration (see also notes above); *less commonly* onset or worsening of arrhythmia, conduction disturbances (see Cautions), peripheral neuropathy and myopathy (usually reversible on withdrawal); *very rarely* chronic liver disease including cirrhosis, sinus arrest, bronchospasm (in patients with severe respiratory failure), ataxia, benign intracranial hypertension, headache, vertigo, epididymo-orchitis, impotence, haemolytic or aplastic anaemia, thrombocytopenia, rash (including exfoliative dermatitis), hypersensitivity including vasculitis, alopecia, impaired vision due to optic neuritis, anaphylaxis on rapid injection, also hypotension, respiratory distress syndrome, sweating, and hot flushes

Dose: *by mouth*, 200 mg 3 times daily for 1 week reduced to 200 mg twice daily for a further week; maintenance, usually 200 mg daily or the minimum required to control the arrhythmia

By intravenous infusion via central venous catheter, initially 5 mg/kg over 20–120 minutes with ECG monitoring; subsequent infusion given if necessary according to response up to max. 1.2 g in 24 hours

Ventricular fibrillation or pulseless ventricular tachycardia, *by intravenous injection* over at least 3 minutes, 300 mg (section 2.7.3)

Amiodarone (Non-proprietary) PoM

Tablets, amiodarone hydrochloride 100 mg, net price 28-tab pack = £2.43; 200 mg, 28-tab pack = £2.67. Label: 11

Brands include *Amyben*®

Injection, amiodarone hydrochloride 30 mg/mL, net price 10-mL prefilled syringe = £10.25

Excipients: may include benzyl alcohol (avoid in neonates, see Excipients, p. 2)

Sterile concentrate, amiodarone hydrochloride 50 mg/mL, net price 3-mL amp = £1.33, 6-mL amp = £2.86. For dilution and use as an infusion

Excipients: may include benzyl alcohol (avoid in neonates, see Excipients, p. 2

Cordarone X® (Sanofi-Synthelabo) PoM

Tablets, both scored, amiodarone hydrochloride 100 mg, net price 28-tab pack = £4.45; 200 mg, 28-tab pack = £7.27. Label: 11

Sterile concentrate, amiodarone hydrochloride 50 mg/mL. Net price 3-mL amp = £1.33. For dilution and use as an infusion

Excipients: include benzyl alcohol (avoid in neonates, see Excipients, p. 2)

DISOPYRAMIDE

Indications: ventricular arrhythmias, especially after myocardial infarction; supraventricular arrhythmias

Cautions: discontinue if hypotension, hypoglycaemia, ventricular tachycardia, ventricular fibrillation or torsades de pointes develop; atrial flutter or tachycardia with partial block, bundle branch block, heart failure (avoid if severe); prostatic enlargement; glaucoma; hepatic impairment (Appendix 2); renal impairment (Appendix 3); pregnancy (Appendix 4); breast-feeding (Appendix 5); **interactions:** Appendix 1 (disopyramide)

Contra-indications: second-and third-degree heart block and sinus node dysfunction (unless pacemaker fitted); cardiogenic shock; severe uncompensated heart failure

Side-effects: ventricular tachycardia, ventricular fibrillation or torsades de pointes (usually associated with prolongation of QRS complex or QT interval—see Cautions above), myocardial depression, hypotension, AV block; antimuscarinic effects include dry mouth, blurred vision, urinary retention; gastro-intestinal irritation; psychosis, cholestatic jaundice, hypoglycaemia also reported (see Cautions above)

Dose: *by mouth*, 300–800 mg daily in divided doses

By slow intravenous injection, 2 mg/kg over at least 5 minutes to a max. of 150 mg, with ECG monitoring, followed immediately *either* by 200 mg *by mouth*, then 200 mg every 8 hours for 24 hours *or* 400 micrograms/kg/hour *by intravenous infusion*; max. 300 mg in first hour and 800 mg daily

Disopyramide (Non-proprietary) PoM

Capsules, disopyramide (as phosphate) 100 mg, net price 20 = £5.51; 150 mg, 20 = £7.83

Rythmodan® (Borg) PoM

Capsules, disopyramide 100 mg (green/beige), net price 84-cap pack = £14.71; 150 mg, 84-cap pack = £19.52

Injection, disopyramide (as phosphate) 10 mg/mL, net price 5-mL amp = £2.72

■ Modified release

Rythmodan Retard® (Borg) PoM

Tablets, m/r, scored, f/c, disopyramide (as phosphate) 250 mg. Net price 56-tab pack = £28.85. Label: 25

Dose: 250–375 mg every 12 hours

FLECAINIDE ACETATE

Indications: *Tablets and injection:* AV nodal reciprocating tachycardia, arrhythmias associated with Wolff-Parkinson-White syndrome and similar conditions with accessory pathways, disabling symptoms of paroxysmal atrial fibrillation in patients without left ventricular dysfunction (arrhythmias of recent onset will respond more readily)

Tablets only: symptomatic sustained ventricular tachycardia, disabling symptoms of premature ventricular contractions or non-sustained ventricular tachycardia in patients resistant to or intolerant of other therapy

Injection only: ventricular tachyarrhythmias resistant to other treatment

Cautions: patients with pacemakers (especially those who may be pacemaker dependent because stimulation threshold may rise appreciably); avoid in sinus node dysfunction, atrial conduction defects, second-degree or greater AV block, bundle branch block or distal block unless pacing rescue available; atrial fibrillation following heart surgery; elderly (accumulation may occur); hepatic impairment (Appendix 2); renal impairment (monitor plasma-flecainide concentration, see also Appendix 3); pregnancy (Appendix 4); breast-feeding (Appendix 5); **interactions:** Appendix 1 (flecainide)

Contra-indications: heart failure; history of myocardial infarction and either asymptomatic ventricular ectopics or asymptomatic non-sustained ventricular tachycardia; long-standing atrial fibrillation where conversion to sinus rhythm not attempted; haemodynamically significant valvular heart disease

Side-effects: nausea, vomiting; pro-arrhythmic effects; dyspnoea; visual disturbances; less commonly gastro-intestinal disturbances, jaundice, hepatic dysfunction, AV block, heart failure, myocardial infarction, hypotension, pneumonitis, hallucinations, depression, convulsions, peripheral neuropathy, paraesthesia, ataxia, dyskinesia, hypoaesthesia, tinnitus, vertigo, reduction in red blood cells, in white blood cells and in platelets, corneal deposits, rashes, alopecia, sweating, urticaria, photosensitivity, increased antinuclear antibodies

Dose: *by mouth* (initiated under direction of hospital consultant), ventricular arrhythmias, initially 100 mg twice daily (max. 400 mg daily usually reserved for rapid control or in heavily built patients), reduced after 3–5 days if possible

Supraventricular arrhythmias, 50 mg twice daily, increased if required to max. 300 mg daily

By slow intravenous injection (in hospital), 2 mg/kg over 10–30 minutes, max. 150 mg, with ECG monitoring; followed if required by *infusion* at a rate of 1.5 mg/kg/hour for 1 hour, subsequently reduced to 100–250 micrograms/kg/hour for up to 24 hours; max. cumulative dose in first 24 hours, 600 mg; transfer to *oral* treatment, as above

NOTE. Plasma-flecainide concentration for optimum response 0.2–1 mg/litre

Flecainide (Non-proprietary) PoM

Tablets, flecainide acetate 50 mg, net price 60-tab pack = £14.04; 100 mg, 60-tab pack = £18.09

Tambocor® (3M) PoM

Tablets, flecainide acetate 50 mg, net price 60-tab pack = £14.46; 100 mg (scored), 60-tab pack = £20.66

Injection, flecainide acetate 10 mg/mL. Net price 15-mL amp = £4.40

PROCAINAMIDE HYDROCHLORIDE

Indications: ventricular arrhythmias, especially after myocardial infarction; atrial tachycardia

Cautions: elderly; asthma, myasthenia gravis; hepatic impairment (Appendix 2); renal impairment (Appendix 3); pregnancy (Appendix 4); **interactions:** Appendix 1 (procainamide)

Contra-indications: heart block, heart failure, hypotension; systemic lupus erythematosus; not indicated for torsades de pointes (can exacerbate); breast-feeding (Appendix 5)

Side-effects: nausea, diarrhoea, rashes, fever, myocardial depression, heart failure, lupus erythematosus-like syndrome, agranulocytosis after prolonged treatment; psychosis and angioedema also reported

Dose: *by slow intravenous injection*, rate not exceeding 50 mg/minute, 100 mg with ECG monitoring, repeated at 5-minute intervals until arrhythmia controlled; max. 1 g

By intravenous infusion, 500–600 mg over 25–30 minutes with ECG monitoring, followed by maintenance at rate of 2–6 mg/minute, then if necessary oral anti-arrhythmic treatment starting 3–4 hours after infusion

NOTE. Serum procainamide concentration for optimum response 3–10 mg/litre

Pronestyl® (Squibb) PoM

Injection, procainamide hydrochloride 100 mg/mL. Net price 10-mL vial = £1.90

PROPAFENONE HYDROCHLORIDE

Indications: ventricular arrhythmias; paroxysmal supraventricular tachyarrhythmias which include paroxysmal atrial flutter or fibrillation and paroxysmal re-entrant tachycardias involving the AV node or accessory pathway, where standard therapy ineffective or contra-indicated

Cautions: heart failure; elderly; pacemaker patients; great caution in obstructive airways disease owing to beta-blocking activity (contra-indicated if severe); hepatic impairment (Appendix 2); renal impairment; pregnancy (Appendix 4); breast-feeding (Appendix 5); **interactions:** Appendix 1 (propafenone)

Contra-indications: uncontrolled congestive heart failure, cardiogenic shock (except arrhythmia induced), severe bradycardia, electrolyte disturbances, severe obstructive pulmonary disease, marked hypotension; myasthenia gravis; unless adequately paced avoid in sinus node dysfunction, atrial conduction defects, second degree or greater AV block, bundle branch block or distal block

Side-effects: antimuscarinic effects including constipation, blurred vision, and dry mouth; dizziness, nausea and vomiting, fatigue, bitter taste, diarrhoea, headache, and allergic skin reactions reported; postural hypotension, particularly in elderly; bradycardia, sino-atrial, atrioventricular, or intraventricular blocks; arrhythmogenic (pro-arrhythmic) effect; rarely hypersensitivity reactions (cholestasis, blood disorders, lupus syndrome), seizures; myoclonus also reported

Dose: 70 kg and over, initially 150 mg 3 times daily after food under direct hospital supervision with ECG monitoring and blood pressure control (if QRS interval prolonged by more than 20%, reduce dose or discontinue until ECG returns to normal limits); may be increased at intervals of at least 3 days to 300 mg twice daily and, if necessary, to max. 300 mg 3 times daily; under 70 kg, reduce dose

ELDERLY may respond to lower doses

Arythmol® (Abbott) PoM

Tablets, both f/c, propafenone hydrochloride 150 mg, net price 90-tab pack = £8.57; 300 mg (scored), 60-tab pack = £10.86. Label: 21, 25

QUINIDINE

Indications: suppression of supraventricular tachycardias and ventricular arrhythmias (see notes above)

Cautions: 200-mg test dose to detect hypersensitivity reactions; extreme care in uncompensated heart failure, first- or second-degree heart block, myocarditis, severe myocardial damage and in myasthenia gravis; pregnancy (Appendix 4); **interactions:** Appendix 1 (quinidine)

Contra-indications: heart block; pregnancy

Side-effects: see under Procainamide Hydrochloride; also ventricular arrhythmias, thrombocytopenia, haemolytic anaemia; rarely granulomatous hepatitis; also cinchonism (see Quinine, section 5.4.1)

Dose: quinidine sulphate 200–400 mg 3–4 times daily

NOTE. Quinidine sulphate 200 mg = quinidine bisulphate 250 mg

Quinidine Sulphate (Non-proprietary) PoM
Tablets, quinidine sulphate 200 mg, net price 100-tab pack = £32.95

■ Modified release

Kinidin Durules® (AstraZeneca) PoM
Tablets, m/r, f/c, quinidine bisulphate 250 mg. Net price 100-tab pack = £11.05. Label: 25
Dose: 500 mg every 12 hours, adjusted as required

Ventricular arrhythmias

Lidocaine (lignocaine) is relatively safe when used by slow intravenous injection and should be considered first for emergency use. Though effective in suppressing ventricular tachycardia and reducing the risk of ventricular fibrillation following myocardial infarction, it has not been shown to reduce mortality when used prophylactically in this condition. In patients with cardiac or hepatic failure doses may need to be reduced to avoid convulsions, depression of the central nervous system, or depression of the cardiovascular system.

Mexiletine may be given as a slow intravenous injection if lidocaine is ineffective; it has a similar action. Adverse cardiovascular and central nervous system effects may limit the dose tolerated; nausea and vomiting may prevent an effective dose being given by mouth.

Moracizine (*Ethmozine*®, Shire) is available on a named-patient basis for the prophylaxis and treatment of serious and life-threatening ventricular arrhythmias for patients already stabilised on moracizine.

Phenytoin (section 4.8.2) by slow intravenous injection was formerly used in ventricular arrhythmias particularly those caused by cardiac glycosides, but this use is now obsolete.

Drugs for both supraventricular and ventricular arrhythmias include **amiodarone**, **beta-blockers**, **disopyramide**, **flecainide**, **procainamide**, **propafenone** and **quinidine**, see above under Supraventricular and Ventricular Arrhythmias.

LIDOCAINE HYDROCHLORIDE

(Lignocaine hydrochloride)

Indications: ventricular arrhythmias, especially after myocardial infarction

Cautions: lower doses in congestive cardiac failure, and following cardiac surgery; elderly; hepatic impairment (Appendix 2); renal impairment (Appendix 3); pregnancy (Appendix 4); **interactions:** Appendix 1 (lidocaine)

Contra-indications: sino-atrial disorders, all grades of atrioventricular block, severe myocardial depression; porphyria (see section 9.8.2)

Side-effects: dizziness, paraesthesia, or drowsiness (particularly if injection too rapid); other CNS effects include confusion, respiratory depression and convulsions; hypotension and bradycardia (may lead to cardiac arrest); hypersensitivity reported

Dose: *by intravenous injection*, in patients without gross circulatory impairment, 100 mg as a bolus over a few minutes (50 mg in lighter patients or those whose circulation is severely impaired), followed immediately by *infusion* of 4 mg/minute for 30 minutes, 2 mg/minute for 2 hours, then 1 mg/minute; reduce concentration further if infusion continued beyond 24 hours (ECG monitoring and specialist advice for infusion)

IMPORTANT. Following intravenous injection lidocaine has a short duration of action (lasting for 15–20 minutes). If an *intravenous infusion* is not immediately available the initial *intravenous injection* of 50–100 mg can be repeated if necessary once or twice at intervals of not less than 10 minutes

Lidocaine (Non-proprietary) PoM
Injection 2%, lidocaine hydrochloride 20 mg/mL, net price 2-mL amp = 28p; 5-mL amp = 25p; 10-mL amp = 60p; 20-mL amp = 63p
Available from Braun
Infusion, lidocaine hydrochloride 0.1% (1 mg/mL) and 0.2% (2 mg/mL) in glucose intravenous infusion 5%. 500-mL containers
Available from Baxter

Minijet® **Lignocaine** (Celltech) PoM
Injection, lidocaine hydrochloride 1% (10 mg/mL), net price 10-mL disposable syringe = £4.40; 2% (20 mg/mL), 5-mL disposable syringe = £4.30

MEXILETINE HYDROCHLORIDE

Indications: ventricular arrhythmias, especially after myocardial infarction

Cautions: close monitoring on initiation of therapy (including ECG, blood pressure, etc.); hepatic impairment (Appendix 2); pregnancy (Appendix 4); **interactions:** Appendix 1 (mexiletine)

Contra-indications: bradycardia, cardiogenic shock; high degree AV block (unless pacemaker fitted)

Side-effects: nausea, vomiting, constipation; bradycardia, hypotension, atrial fibrillation, palpitation, conduction defects, exacerbation of arrhythmias, torsades de pointes; drowsiness, confusion, convulsions, psychiatric disorders, dysarthria, ataxia, paraesthesia, nystagmus, tremor; jaundice, hepatitis, and blood disorders reported; see also notes above

Dose: *by mouth*, initial dose 400 mg (may be increased to 600 mg if opioid analgesics also given), followed after 2 hours by 200–250 mg 3–4 times daily

By intravenous injection, 100–250 mg at a rate of 25 mg/minute with ECG monitoring followed by *infusion* of 250 mg as a 0.1% solution over 1 hour, 125 mg/hour for 2 hours, then 500 micrograms/minute

Mexitil® (Boehringer Ingelheim) PoM
Capsules, mexiletine hydrochloride 50 mg (purple/red), net price 100-cap pack = £4.95; 200 mg (red), 100-cap pack = £11.87
Injection, mexiletine hydrochloride 25 mg/mL. Net price 10-mL amp = £1.49

2.4 Beta-adrenoceptor blocking drugs

Beta-adrenoceptor blocking drugs (beta-blockers) block the beta-adrenoreceptors in the heart, peripheral vasculature, bronchi, pancreas, and liver.

Many beta-blockers are now available and in general they are all equally effective. There are, however, differences between them which may affect choice in treating particular diseases or individual patients.

Intrinsic sympathomimetic activity (ISA, partial agonist activity) represents the capacity of beta-blockers to stimulate as well as to block adrenergic receptors. **Oxprenolol**, **pindolol**, **acebutolol** and **celiprolol** have intrinsic sympathomimetic activity; they tend to cause less bradycardia than the other beta-blockers and may also cause less coldness of the extremities.

Some beta-blockers are lipid soluble and some are water soluble. **Atenolol**, **celiprolol**, **nadolol**, and **sotalol** are the most water-soluble; they are less likely to enter the brain, and may therefore cause less sleep disturbance and nightmares. Water-soluble beta-blockers are excreted by the kidneys; they accumulate in renal impairment and dosage reduction is therefore often necessary.

Beta-blockers with a relatively short duration of action have to be given two or three times daily. Many of these are, however, available in modified-release formulations so that administration once daily is adequate for hypertension. For angina twice-daily treatment may sometimes be needed even with a modified-release formulation. Some beta-blockers such as atenolol, bisoprolol, carvedilol, celiprolol, and nadolol have an intrinsically longer duration of action and need to be given only once daily.

Beta-blockers slow the heart and can depress the myocardium; they are contra-indicated in patients with second- or third-degree heart block. Beta-blockers should also be avoided in patients with worsening unstable heart failure; care is required when initiating a beta-blocker in those with stable heart failure (see also section 2.5.5). **Sotalol** may prolong the QT interval, and it occasionally causes life-threatening ventricular arrhythmias (**important:** particular care is required to avoid hypokalaemia in patients taking sotalol).

Labetalol, **celiprolol**, **carvedilol** and **nebivolol** are beta-blockers which have, in addition, an arteriolar vasodilating action, by diverse mechanisms, and thus lower peripheral resistance. There is no evidence that these drugs have important advantages over other beta-blockers in the treatment of hypertension.

Beta-blockers may precipitate asthma and this effect can be dangerous. Beta-blockers should be **avoided** in patients with a history of asthma or bronchospasm; if there is no alternative, a cardioselective beta-blocker may be used with extreme caution under specialist supervision. **Atenolol**, **bisoprolol**, **metoprolol**, **nebivolol** and (to a lesser extent) **acebutolol**, have less effect on the $beta_2$ (bronchial) receptors and are, therefore, relatively *cardioselective*, but they are **not** *cardiospecific*. They have a lesser effect on airways resistance but are **not** free of this side-effect.

Beta-blockers are also associated with fatigue, coldness of the extremities (may be less common with those with ISA, see above), and sleep disturbances with nightmares (may be less common with the water-soluble beta-blockers, see above).

Beta-blockers are not contra-indicated in diabetes; however, they can lead to a small deterioration of glucose tolerance and interfere with metabolic and autonomic responses to hypoglycaemia. Cardioselective beta-blockers (see above) may be preferable and beta-blockers should be avoided altogether in those with frequent episodes of hypoglycaemia.

HYPERTENSION. Beta-blockers are effective for reducing blood pressure (section 2.5), but their mode of action is not understood; they reduce cardiac output, alter baroceptor reflex sensitivity, and block peripheral adrenoceptors. Some beta-blockers depress plasma renin secretion. It is possible that a central effect may also explain their mode of action. Blood pressure can usually be controlled with relatively few side-effects. In general the dose of beta-blocker does not have to be high; for example, **atenolol** is given in a dose of 50 mg daily and it is usually not necessary to increase the dose to 100 mg.

Combined thiazide and beta-blocker preparations may help compliance but combined preparations should only be used when blood pressure is not adequately controlled by a thiazide or a beta-blocker alone. Beta-blockers reduce, but do not abolish, the tendency for diuretics to cause hypokalaemia.

Beta-blockers can be used to control the pulse rate in patients with *phaeochromocytoma* (section 2.5.4). However, they should never be used alone as beta-blockade without concurrent alpha-blockade may lead to a hypertensive crisis. For this reason phenoxybenzamine should always be used together with the beta-blocker.

ANGINA. By reducing cardiac work beta-blockers improve exercise tolerance and relieve symptoms in patients with *angina* (for further details on the management of stable and unstable angina see section 2.6). As with hypertension there is no good evidence of the superiority of any one drug, although occasionally a patient will respond better to one beta-blocker than to another. There is some evidence that sudden withdrawal may cause an exacerbation of angina and therefore gradual reduction of dose is preferable when beta-blockers are to be stopped. There is a risk of precipitating heart failure when beta-blockers and verapamil are used together in established ischaemic heart disease (**important**: see p. 113).

MYOCARDIAL INFARCTION. For advice on the management of myocardial infarction see section 2.10.1.

Several studies have shown that some beta-blockers can reduce the recurrence rate of *myocardial infarction*. However, uncontrolled heart failure, hypotension, bradyarrhythmias, and obstructive airways disease render beta-blockers unsuitable in some patients following a myocardial infarction. **Atenolol** and **metoprolol** may reduce early mortality after intravenous and subsequent oral administration in the acute phase, while **acebutolol**, **metoprolol**, **propranolol**, and **timolol** have protective value when started in the early convalescent phase. The evidence relating to other beta-blockers is less convincing; some have not been tested in trials of secondary protection. It is also not known whether the protective effect of beta-blockers continues after 2–3 years; it is possible that sudden cessation may cause a rebound worsening of myocardial ischaemia.

ARRHYTHMIAS. Beta-blockers act as *anti-arrhythmic drugs* principally by attenuating the effects of the sympathetic system on automaticity and conductivity within the heart. They may be used in conjunction with digoxin to control the ventricular response in atrial fibrillation, especially in patients with thyrotoxicosis. Beta-blockers are also useful in the management of supraventricular tachycardias, and are used to control those following myocardial infarction, see above.

Esmolol is a relatively cardioselective beta-blocker with a very short duration of action, used intravenously for the short-term treatment of supraventricular arrhythmias, sinus tachycardia, or hypertension, particularly in the peri-operative period. It may also be used in other situations, such as acute myocardial infarction, where sustained beta blockade might be hazardous.

Sotalol, a non-cardioselective beta-blocker with additional class III anti-arrhythmic activity, is used for prophylaxis in paroxysmal supraventricular arrhythmias. It also suppresses ventricular ectopic beats and non-sustained ventricular tachycardia. It has been shown to be more effective than lidocaine (lignocaine) in the termination of spontaneous sustained ventricular tachycardia due to coronary disease or cardiomyopathy. However, it may induce torsades de pointes in susceptible patients.

HEART FAILURE. Beta-blockers may produce benefit in heart failure by blocking sympathetic activity. **Bisoprolol** and **carvedilol** reduce mortality in any grade of stable heart failure. Treatment should be initiated by those experienced in the management of heart failure (see section 2.5.5 for details on heart failure).

THYROTOXICOSIS. Beta-blockers are used in pre-operative preparation for thyroidectomy. Administration of propranolol can reverse clinical symptoms of *thyrotoxicosis* within 4 days. Routine tests of increased thyroid function remain unaltered. The thyroid gland is rendered less vascular thus making surgery easier (section 6.2.2).

OTHER USES. Beta-blockers have been used to alleviate some symptoms of *anxiety*; probably patients with palpitation, tremor, and tachycardia respond best (see also section 4.1.2 and section 4.9.3). Beta-blockers are also used in the *prophylaxis of migraine* (section 4.7.4.2). Betaxolol, carteolol, levobunolol, metipranolol and timolol are used topically in *glaucoma* (section 11.6).

PROPRANOLOL HYDROCHLORIDE

Indications: see under Dose

Cautions: avoid abrupt withdrawal especially in ischaemic heart disease; first-degree AV block; portal hypertension (risk of deterioration in liver function); diabetes; history of obstructive airways disease (introduce cautiously and monitor lung function—see also Bronchospasm below); myasthenia gravis; history of hypersensitivity—may increase sensitivity to allergens and result in more serious hypersensitivity response, also may reduce response to adrenaline (epinephrine) (see also section 3.4.3); see also notes above; reduce dose of oral propranolol in hepatic impairment; renal impairment (Appendix 3); pregnancy (Appendix 4); breast-feeding (Appendix 5); **interactions:** Appendix 1 (beta-blockers), **important:** verapamil interaction, see also p. 113

Contra-indications: asthma (**important:** see Bronchospasm below), uncontrolled heart failure, Prinzmetal's angina, marked bradycardia, hypotension, sick sinus syndrome, second- or third-degree AV block, cardiogenic shock, metabolic acidosis, severe peripheral arterial disease; phaeochromocytoma (apart from specific use with alpha-blockers, see also notes above)

BRONCHOSPASM. The CSM has advised that beta-blockers, including those considered to be cardioselective, should not be given to patients with a history of asthma or bronchospasm. However, in rare situations where there is no alternative a cardioselective beta-blocker is given to these patients with extreme caution and under specialist supervision

Side-effects: bradycardia, heart failure, hypotension, conduction disorders, bronchospasm, peripheral vasoconstriction (including exacerbation of intermittent claudication and Raynaud's phenomenon), gastro-intestinal disturbances, fatigue, sleep disturbances; rare reports of rashes and dry eyes (reversible on withdrawal), sexual dysfunction, and exacerbation of psoriasis; see also notes above; **overdosage:** see Emergency Treatment of Poisoning, p. 32

Dose: *by mouth*, hypertension, initially 80 mg twice daily, increased at weekly intervals as required; maintenance 160–320 mg daily

Portal hypertension, initially 40 mg twice daily, increased to 80 mg twice daily according to heart-rate; max. 160 mg twice daily

Phaeochromocytoma (only with an alpha-blocker), 60 mg daily for 3 days before surgery *or* 30 mg daily in patients unsuitable for surgery

Angina, initially 40 mg 2–3 times daily; maintenance 120–240 mg daily

Arrhythmias, hypertrophic obstructive cardiomyopathy, anxiety tachycardia, and thyrotoxicosis (adjunct), 10–40 mg 3–4 times daily

Anxiety with symptoms such as palpitation, sweating, tremor, 40 mg once daily, increased to 40 mg 3 times daily if necessary

Prophylaxis after myocardial infarction, 40 mg 4 times daily for 2–3 days, then 80 mg twice daily, beginning 5 to 21 days after infarction

Migraine prophylaxis and essential tremor, initially 40 mg 2–3 times daily; maintenance 80–160 mg daily

By intravenous injection, arrhythmias and thyrotoxic crisis, 1 mg over 1 minute; if necessary repeat at 2-minute intervals; max. 10 mg (5 mg in anaesthesia)

NOTE. Excessive bradycardia can be countered with intravenous injection of atropine sulphate 0.6–2.4 mg in divided doses of 600 micrograms; for **overdosage** see Emergency Treatment of Poisoning, p. 32

Propranolol (Non-proprietary) PoM

Tablets, propranolol hydrochloride 10 mg, net price 28 = £1.46; 40 mg, 28 = £1.25; 80 mg, 56 = £1.45; 160 mg, 56 = £3.88. Label: 8

Brands include *Angilol*®

Oral solution, propranolol hydrochloride 5 mg/5 mL, net price 150 mL = £12.50; 10 mg/5 mL, 150 mL = £16.45; 50 mg/5 mL, 150 mL = £19.98
Brands include *Syprol*®

Inderal® (AstraZeneca) PoM
Injection, propranolol hydrochloride 1 mg/mL, net price 1-mL amp = 21p

■ Modified release

Half-Inderal LA® (AstraZeneca) PoM
Capsules, m/r, lavender/pink, propranolol hydrochloride 80 mg. Net price 28-cap pack = £5.40. Label: 8, 25
NOTE. Modified-release capsules containing propranolol hydrochloride 80 mg also available; brands include *Bedranol SR*®, *Half Beta Prograne*®

Inderal-LA® (AstraZeneca) PoM
Capsules, m/r, lavender/pink, propranolol hydrochloride 160 mg. Net price 28-cap pack = £6.67. Label: 8, 25
NOTE. Modified-release capsules containing propranolol hydrochloride 160 mg also available; brands include *Bedranol SR*®, *Beta Prograne*®, *Lopranol LA*®, *Slo-Pro*®

ACEBUTOLOL

Indications: see under Dose
Cautions: see under Propranolol Hydrochloride
Contra-indications: see under Propranolol Hydrochloride
Side-effects: see under Propranolol Hydrochloride
Dose: hypertension, initially 400 mg once daily *or* 200 mg twice daily, increased after 2 weeks to 400 mg twice daily if necessary
Angina, initially 400 mg once daily *or* 200 mg twice daily; 300 mg 3 times daily in severe angina; up to 1.2 g daily has been used
Arrhythmias, 0.4–1.2 g daily in 2–3 divided doses

Sectral® (Aventis Pharma) PoM
Capsules, acebutolol (as hydrochloride) 100 mg (buff/white), net price 84-cap pack = £14.97; 200 mg (buff/pink), 56-cap pack = £19.18. Label: 8
Tablets, f/c, acebutolol 400 mg (as hydrochloride). Net price 28-tab pack = £18.62. Label: 8

■ With diuretic

Secadrex® (Aventis Pharma) PoM
Tablets, f/c, acebutolol 200 mg (as hydrochloride), hydrochlorothiazide 12.5 mg. Net price 28-tab pack = £17.59. Label: 8
Dose: hypertension, 1 tablet daily, increased to 2 daily as a single dose if necessary

ATENOLOL

Indications: see under Dose
Cautions: see under Propranolol Hydrochloride
Contra-indications: see under Propranolol Hydrochloride
Side-effects: see under Propranolol Hydrochloride
Dose: *by mouth*,
Hypertension, 50 mg daily (higher doses rarely necessary)
Angina, 100 mg daily in 1 or 2 doses
Arrhythmias, 50–100 mg daily

By intravenous injection, arrhythmias, 2.5 mg at a rate of 1 mg/minute, repeated at 5-minute intervals to a max. of 10 mg
NOTE. Excessive bradycardia can be countered with intravenous injection of atropine sulphate 0.6–2.4 mg in divided doses of 600 micrograms; for **overdosage** see Emergency Treatment of Poisoning, p. 32

By intravenous infusion, arrhythmias, 150 micrograms/kg over 20 minutes, repeated every 12 hours if required
Early intervention within 12 hours of myocardial infarction (section 2.10.1), *by intravenous injection* over 5 minutes, 5 mg, then *by mouth*, 50 mg after 15 minutes, 50 mg after 12 hours, then 100 mg daily

Atenolol (Non-proprietary) PoM
Tablets, atenolol 25 mg, net price 28-tab pack = 73p; 50 mg, 28-tab pack = £1.02; 100 mg, 28-tab pack = 67p. Label: 8
Brands include *Atenix*®

Tenormin® (AstraZeneca) PoM
'25' tablets, f/c, atenolol 25 mg. Net price 28-tab pack = £4.41. Label: 8
LS tablets, orange, f/c, scored, atenolol 50 mg. Net price 28-tab pack = £5.11. Label: 8
Tablets, orange, f/c, scored, atenolol 100 mg. Net price 28-tab pack = £6.50. Label: 8
Syrup, sugar-free, atenolol 25 mg/5mL. Net price 300 mL = £8.55. Label: 8
Injection, atenolol 500 micrograms/mL. Net price 10-mL amp = 96p (hosp. only)

■ With diuretic

Co-tenidone (Non-proprietary) PoM
Tablets, co-tenidone 50/12.5 (atenolol 50 mg, chlortalidone 12.5 mg), net price 28-tab pack = £2.72; co-tenidone 100/25 (atenolol 100 mg, chlortalidone 25 mg), 28-tab pack = £2.51. Label: 8
Brands include *AtenixCo*®, *Totaretic*®
Dose: hypertension, 1 tablet daily (but see also under Dose above)

Kalten® (BPC 100) PoM
Capsules, red/ivory, atenolol 50 mg, co-amilozide 2.5/25 (anhydrous amiloride hydrochloride 2.5 mg, hydrochlorothiazide 25 mg). Net price 28-cap pack = £8.39. Label: 8
Dose: hypertension, 1 capsule daily

Tenoret 50® (AstraZeneca) PoM
Tablets, brown, f/c, co-tenidone 50/12.5 (atenolol 50 mg, chlortalidone 12.5 mg). Net price 28-tab pack = £5.70. Label: 8
Dose: hypertension, 1 tablet daily

Tenoretic® (AstraZeneca) PoM
Tablets, brown, f/c, co-tenidone 100/25 (atenolol 100 mg, chlortalidone 25 mg). Net price 28-tab pack = £8.12. Label: 8
Dose: hypertension, 1 tablet daily (but see also under Dose above)

■ With calcium-channel blocker

NOTE. Only indicated when calcium-channel blocker or beta-blocker alone proves inadequate

Beta-Adalat® (Bayer) PoM
Capsules, reddish-brown, atenolol 50 mg, nifedipine 20 mg (m/r). Net price 28-cap pack = £10.41. Label: 8, 25
Dose: hypertension, 1 capsule daily, increased if necessary to twice daily; elderly, 1 daily
Angina, 1 capsule twice daily

Tenif® (AstraZeneca) PoM
Capsules, reddish-brown, atenolol 50 mg, nifedipine 20 mg (m/r). Net price 28-cap pack = £10.63. Label: 8, 25
Dose: hypertension, 1 capsule daily, increased if necessary to twice daily; elderly, 1 daily
Angina, 1 capsule twice daily

BISOPROLOL FUMARATE

Indications: see under Dose
Cautions: see under Propranolol Hydrochloride; in heart failure monitor clinical status for 4 hours after initiation (with low dose) and ensure heart failure not worsening before increasing each dose; psoriasis; hepatic impairment (Appendix 2)
Contra-indications: see under Propranolol Hydrochloride; also acute or decompensated heart failure requiring intravenous inotropes; sino-atrial block
Side-effects: see under Propranolol Hydrochloride
Dose: hypertension and angina, usually 10 mg once daily (5 mg may be adequate in some patients); max. 20 mg daily
Adjunct in stable moderate to severe heart failure (section 2.5.5), initially 1.25 mg once daily (in the morning) for 1 week then, if well tolerated, increased to 2.5 mg once daily for 1 week, then 3.75 mg once daily for 1 week, then 5 mg once daily for 4 weeks, then 7.5 mg once daily for 4 weeks, then 10 mg once daily; max. 10 mg daily

Bisoprolol Fumarate (Non-proprietary) PoM
Tablets, bisoprolol fumarate 5 mg, net price 28-tab pack = £1.68; 10 mg, 28-tab pack = £2.69. Label: 8
Brands include *Bipranix*®, *Soloc*®, *Vivacor*®

Cardicor® (Merck) ▼ PoM
Tablets, f/c, bisoprolol fumarate 1.25 mg, net price 28-tab pack = £8.56; 2.5 mg (scored), 28-tab pack = £5.90; 3.75 mg (scored, white-yellow), 28-tab pack = £5.90; 5 mg (scored, light yellow), 28-tab pack = £5.90; 7.5 mg (scored, yellow), 28-tab pack = £5.90; 10 mg (scored, orange), 28-tab pack = £5.90. Label: 8

Emcor® (Merck) PoM
LS Tablets, yellow, f/c, scored, bisoprolol fumarate 5 mg. Net price 28-tab pack = £9.42. Label: 8
Tablets, orange, f/c, scored, bisoprolol fumarate 10 mg. Net price 28-tab pack = £10.57. Label: 8

Monocor® (Lederle) PoM
Tablets, both f/c, bisoprolol fumarate 5 mg (pink), net price 28-tab pack = £7.96; 10 mg, 28-tab pack £8.94. Label: 8

CARVEDILOL

Indications: hypertension; angina; adjunct to diuretics, digoxin, or ACE inhibitors in symptomatic chronic heart failure
Cautions: see under Propranolol Hydrochloride; before increasing dose ensure renal function and heart failure not deteriorating; severe heart failure, avoid in acute or decompensated heart failure requiring intravenous inotropes
Contra-indications: see under Propranolol Hydrochloride; severe chronic heart failure; hepatic impairment
Side-effects: postural hypotension, dizziness, headache, fatigue, gastro-intestinal disturbances, bradycardia; occasionally diminished peripheral circulation, peripheral oedema and painful extremities, dry mouth, dry eyes, eye irritation or disturbed vision, impotence, disturbances of micturition, influenza-like symptoms; rarely angina, AV block, exacerbation of intermittent claudication or Raynaud's phenomenon; allergic skin reactions, exacerbation of psoriasis, nasal stuffiness, wheezing, depressed mood, sleep disturbances, paraesthesia, heart failure, changes in liver enzymes, thrombocytopenia, leucopenia also reported
Dose: hypertension, initially 12.5 mg once daily, increased after 2 days to usual dose of 25 mg once daily; if necessary may be further increased at intervals of at least 2 weeks to max. 50 mg daily in single or divided doses; ELDERLY initial dose of 12.5 mg daily may provide satisfactory control
Angina, initially 12.5 mg twice daily, increased after 2 days to 25 mg twice daily
Adjunct in heart failure (section 2.5.5) initially 3.125 mg twice daily (with food), dose increased at intervals of at least 2 weeks to 6.25 mg twice daily, then to 12.5 mg twice daily, then to 25 mg twice daily; increase to highest dose tolerated, max. 25 mg twice daily in patients with severe heart failure or body-weight less than 85 kg and 50 mg twice daily in patients over 85 kg

Carvedilol (Non-proprietary) PoM
Tablets, carvedilol 3.125 mg, net price 28-tab pack = £6.85; 6.25 mg, 28-tab pack = £7.89; 12.5 mg, 28-tab pack = £8.89; 25 mg, 28-tab pack = £10.84. Label: 8

Eucardic® (Roche) ▼ PoM
Tablets, all scored, carvedilol 3.125 mg (pink), net price 28-tab pack = £7.57; 6.25 mg (yellow), 28-tab pack = £8.41; 12.5 mg (peach), 28-tab pack = £9.35; 25 mg, 28-tab pack = £11.68. Label: 8

CELIPROLOL HYDROCHLORIDE

Indications: mild to moderate hypertension
Cautions: see under Propranolol Hydrochloride
Contra-indications: see under Propranolol Hydrochloride
Side-effects: headache, dizziness, fatigue, nausea and somnolence; also bradycardia, bronchospasm; depression and pneumonitis reported rarely
Dose: 200 mg once daily in the morning, increased to 400 mg once daily if necessary

Celiprolol (Non-proprietary) PoM
Tablets, celiprolol hydrochloride 200 mg, net price 28-tab pack = £8.11; 400 mg, 28-tab pack = £19.21. Label: 8, 22

Celectol® (Sanofi-Aventis) PoM
Tablets, both f/c, scored, celiprolol hydrochloride 200 mg (yellow), net price 28-tab pack = £15.99; 400 mg, 28-tab pack = £31.97. Label: 8, 22

ESMOLOL HYDROCHLORIDE

Indications: short-term treatment of supraventricular arrhythmias (including atrial fibrillation, atrial flutter, sinus tachycardia); tachycardia and hypertension in peri-operative period
Cautions: see under Propranolol Hydrochloride; renal impairment
Contra-indications: see under Propranolol Hydrochloride
Side-effects: see under Propranolol Hydrochloride; also on infusion venous irritation and thrombophlebitis

Dose: *by intravenous infusion*, usually within range 50–200 micrograms/kg/minute (consult product literature for details of dose titration and doses during peri-operative period)

Brevibloc® (Baxter) PoM
Injection, esmolol hydrochloride 10 mg/mL, net price 10-mL vial = £7.79, 250-mL infusion bag = £81.54
Injection concentrate, esmolol hydrochloride 250 mg/mL (for dilution before infusion), 10-mL amp = £79.08

LABETALOL HYDROCHLORIDE

Indications: hypertension (including hypertension in pregnancy, hypertension with angina, and hypertension following acute myocardial infarction); hypertensive crisis (but see section 2.5); controlled hypotension in anaesthesia

Cautions: see under Propranolol Hydrochloride; interferes with laboratory tests for catecholamines; liver damage (see below)

LIVER DAMAGE. Severe hepatocellular damage reported after both short-term and long-term treatment. Appropriate laboratory testing needed at first symptom of liver dysfunction and if laboratory evidence of damage (or if jaundice) labetalol should be stopped and not restarted

Contra-indications: see under Propranolol Hydrochloride

Side-effects: postural hypotension (avoid upright position during and for 3 hours after intravenous administration), tiredness, weakness, headache, rashes, scalp tingling, difficulty in micturition, epigastric pain, nausea, vomiting; liver damage (see above); rarely lichenoid rash

Dose: *by mouth*, initially 100 mg (50 mg in elderly) twice daily with food, increased at intervals of 14 days to usual dose of 200 mg twice daily; up to 800 mg daily in 2 divided doses (3–4 divided doses if higher); max. 2.4 g daily

By intravenous injection, 50 mg over at least 1 minute, repeated after 5 minutes if necessary; max. total dose 200 mg

NOTE. Excessive bradycardia can be countered with intravenous injection of atropine sulphate 0.6–2.4 mg in divided doses of 600 micrograms; for **overdosage** see Emergency Treatment of Poisoning, p. 32

By intravenous infusion, 2 mg/minute until satisfactory response then discontinue; usual total dose 50–200 mg, (**not** recommended for phaeochromocytoma, see under Phaeochromocytoma, section 2.5.4)

Hypertension of pregnancy, 20 mg/hour, doubled every 30 minutes; usual max. 160 mg/hour

Hypertension following myocardial infarction, 15 mg/hour, gradually increased to max. 120 mg/hour

Labetalol Hydrochloride (Non-proprietary) PoM
Tablets, all f/c, labetalol hydrochloride 100 mg, net price 20 = £3.01; 200 mg, 20 = £4.13; 400 mg, 20 = £6.82. Label: 8, 21

Trandate® (Celltech) PoM
Tablets, all orange, f/c, labetalol hydrochloride 50 mg, net price 56-tab pack = £3.79; 100 mg, 56-tab pack = £4.17; 200 mg, 56-tab pack = £6.77; 400 mg, 56-tab pack = £9.42. Label: 8, 21
Injection, labetalol hydrochloride 5 mg/mL. Net price 20-mL amp = £2.12

METOPROLOL TARTRATE

Indications: see under Dose

Cautions: see under Propranolol Hydrochloride; reduce dose in hepatic impairment

Contra-indications: see under Propranolol Hydrochloride

Side-effects: see under Propranolol Hydrochloride

Dose: *by mouth*, hypertension, initially 100 mg daily, increased if necessary to 200 mg daily in 1–2 divided doses; max. 400 mg daily (but high doses rarely necessary)

Angina, 50–100 mg 2–3 times daily

Arrhythmias, usually 50 mg 2–3 times daily; up to 300 mg daily in divided doses if necessary

Migraine prophylaxis, 100–200 mg daily in divided doses

Hyperthyroidism (adjunct), 50 mg 4 times daily

By intravenous injection, arrhythmias, up to 5 mg at rate 1–2 mg/minute, repeated after 5 minutes if necessary, total dose 10–15 mg

NOTE. Excessive bradycardia can be countered with intravenous injection of atropine sulphate 0.6–2.4 mg in divided doses of 600 micrograms; for **overdosage** see Emergency Treatment of Poisoning, p. 32

In surgery, 2–4 mg *by slow intravenous injection* at induction or to control arrhythmias developing during anaesthesia; 2-mg doses may be repeated to a max. of 10 mg

Early intervention within 12 hours of infarction, 5 mg *by intravenous injection* every 2 minutes to a max. of 15 mg, followed after 15 minutes by 50 mg *by mouth* every 6 hours for 48 hours; maintenance 200 mg daily in divided doses

Metoprolol Tartrate (Non-proprietary) PoM
Tablets, metoprolol tartrate 50 mg, net price 28 = £1.07; 100 mg, 28 = £2.62. Label: 8

Betaloc® (AstraZeneca) PoM
Tablets, both scored, metoprolol tartrate 50 mg, net price 100-tab pack = £3.30; 100 mg, 100-tab pack = £6.13. Label: 8
Injection, metoprolol tartrate 1 mg/mL. Net price 5-mL amp = 42p

Lopresor® (Novartis) PoM
Tablets, both f/c, scored, metoprolol tartrate 50 mg (pink), net price 56-tab pack = £2.57; 100 mg (blue), 56-tab pack = £6.68. Label: 8

■ Modified release

Betaloc-SA® (AstraZeneca) PoM
Durules® (= tablets, m/r), metoprolol tartrate 200 mg, net price 28-tab pack = £4.56. Label: 8, 25
Dose: hypertension, angina, 200 mg daily in the morning, increased to 400 mg daily if necessary; migraine prophylaxis, 200 mg daily

Lopresor SR® (Novartis) PoM
Tablets, m/r, yellow, f/c, metoprolol tartrate 200 mg, net price 28-tab pack = £9.80. Label: 8, 25
Dose: hypertension, 200 mg daily; angina, 200-400 mg daily; migraine prophylaxis, 200 mg daily

■ With diuretic

Co-Betaloc® (Searle) PoM
Tablets, scored, metoprolol tartrate 100 mg, hydrochlorothiazide 12.5 mg, net price 28-tab pack = £5.59. Label: 8
Dose: hypertension, 1–3 tablets daily in single or divided doses

NADOLOL

Indications: see under Dose

Cautions: see under Propranolol Hydrochloride

Contra-indications: see under Propranolol Hydrochloride

Side-effects: see under Propranolol Hydrochloride

Dose: hypertension, 80 mg daily, increased at weekly intervals if required; max. 240 mg daily

Angina, 40 mg daily, increased at weekly intervals if required; usual max. 160 mg daily

Arrhythmias, initially 40 mg daily, increased to 160 mg if required; reduce to 40 mg if bradycardia occurs

Migraine prophylaxis, initially 40 mg daily, increased by 40 mg at weekly intervals; usual maintenance dose 80–160 mg daily

Thyrotoxicosis (adjunct), 80–160 mg daily

Corgard® (Sanofi-Synthelabo) PoM

Tablets, blue, scored, nadolol 80 mg, net price 28-tab pack = £5.20. Label: 8

NEBIVOLOL

Indications: essential hypertension

Cautions: see under Propranolol Hydrochloride; reduce dose in renal impairment (Appendix 3); elderly

Contra-indications: see under Propranolol Hydrochloride; hepatic impairment (Appendix 2)

Side-effects: see under Propranolol Hydrochloride; oedema, headache, depression, visual disturbances, paraesthesia, impotence

Dose: 5 mg daily; ELDERLY initially 2.5 mg daily, increased if necessary to 5 mg daily

Nebilet® (Menarini) PoM

Tablets, scored, nebivolol (as hydrochloride) 5 mg, net price 28-tab pack = £9.23. Label: 8

OXPRENOLOL HYDROCHLORIDE

Indications: see under Dose

Cautions: see under Propranolol Hydrochloride; reduce dose in hepatic impairment

Contra-indications: see under Propranolol Hydrochloride

Side-effects: see under Propranolol Hydrochloride

Dose: hypertension, 80–160 mg daily in 2–3 divided doses, increased as required; max. 320 mg daily

Angina, 80–160 mg daily in 2–3 divided doses; max. 320 mg daily

Arrhythmias, 40–240 mg daily in 2–3 divided doses; max. 240 mg daily

Anxiety symptoms (short-term use), 40–80 mg daily in 1–2 divided doses

Oxprenolol (Non-proprietary) PoM

Tablets, all coated, oxprenolol hydrochloride 20 mg, net price 56 = £1.55; 40 mg, 56 = £3.11; 80 mg, 56 = £6.20; 160 mg, 20 = £2.36. Label: 8

Trasicor® (Amdipharm) PoM

Tablets, all f/c, oxprenolol hydrochloride 20 mg (contain gluten), net price 56-tab pack = £1.55; 40 mg (contain gluten), 56-tab pack = £3.11; 80 mg (yellow), 56-tab pack = £6.20. Label: 8

■ Modified release

Slow-Trasicor® (Amdipharm) PoM

Tablets, m/r, f/c, oxprenolol hydrochloride 160 mg. Net price 28-tab pack = £6.63. Label: 8, 25

Dose: hypertension, angina, initially 160 mg once daily; if necessary may be increased to max. 320 mg daily

■ With diuretic

Trasidrex® (Novartis) PoM

Tablets, red, s/c, co-prenozide 160/0.25 (oxprenolol hydrochloride 160 mg (m/r), cyclopenthiazide 250 micrograms). Net price 28-tab pack = £8.88. Label: 8, 25

Dose: hypertension, 1 tablet daily, increased if necessary to 2 daily as a single dose

PINDOLOL

Indications: see under Dose

Cautions: see under Propranolol Hydrochloride

Contra-indications: see under Propranolol Hydrochloride

Side-effects: see under Propranolol Hydrochloride

Dose: hypertension, initially 5 mg 2–3 times daily *or* 15 mg once daily, increased as required at weekly intervals; usual maintenance 15–30 mg daily; max. 45 mg daily

Angina, 2.5–5 mg up to 3 times daily

Pindolol (Non-proprietary) PoM

Tablets, pindolol 5 mg, net price 100-tab pack = £7.10. Label: 8

Visken® (Amdipharm) PoM

Tablets, both scored, pindolol 5 mg, net price 56-tab pack = £4.88; 15 mg, 28-tab pack = £7.33. Label: 8

■ With diuretic

Viskaldix® (Amdipharm) PoM

Tablets, scored, pindolol 10 mg, clopamide 5 mg. Net price 28-tab pack = £6.70. Label: 8

Dose: hypertension, 1 tablet daily in the morning, increased if necessary to 2 daily; max. 3 daily

SOTALOL HYDROCHLORIDE

Indications: *Tablets and injection:* life-threatening arrhythmias including ventricular tachyarrhythmias, symptomatic non-sustained ventricular tachyarrhythmias

Tablets only: prophylaxis of paroxysmal atrial tachycardia or fibrillation, paroxysmal AV re-entrant tachycardias (both nodal and involving accessory pathways), paroxysmal supraventricular tachycardia after cardiac surgery, maintenance of sinus rhythm following cardioversion of atrial fibrillation or flutter

Injection only: electrophysiological study of inducible ventricular and supraventricular arrhythmias; temporary substitution for tablets

CSM advice. The use of sotalol should be limited to the treatment of ventricular arrhythmias or prophylaxis of supraventricular arrhythmias (see above). It should no longer be used for angina, hypertension, thyrotoxicosis or for secondary prevention after myocardial infarction; when stopping sotalol for these indications, the dose should be reduced gradually

Cautions: see under Propranolol Hydrochloride; reduce dose in renal impairment (avoid if severe); correct hypokalaemia, hypomagnesaemia, or other electrolyte disturbances; severe or prolonged diarrhoea; **interactions:** Appendix 1 (beta-blockers), **important:** verapamil interaction see also p. 113

Contra-indications: see under Propranolol Hydrochloride; congenital or acquired long QT syndrome; torsades de pointes; renal failure
Side-effects: see under Propranolol Hydrochloride; arrhythmogenic (pro-arrhythmic) effect (torsades de pointes—increased risk in women)
Dose: *by mouth* with ECG monitoring and measurement of corrected QT interval, arrhythmias, initially 80 mg daily in 1–2 divided doses increased gradually at intervals of 2–3 days to usual dose of 160–320 mg daily in 2 divided doses; higher doses of 480–640 mg daily for life-threatening ventricular arrhythmias under specialist supervision
By intravenous injection over 10 minutes, acute arrhythmias, 20–120 mg with ECG monitoring, repeated if necessary with 6-hour intervals between injections
Diagnostic use, see product literature
NOTE. Excessive bradycardia can be countered with intravenous injection of atropine sulphate 0.6–2.4 mg in divided doses of 600 micrograms; for **overdosage** see Emergency Treatment of Poisoning, p. 32

Sotalol (Non-proprietary) PoM
Tablets, sotalol hydrochloride 40 mg, net price 56 = £1.34; 80 mg, 56-tab pack = £1.99; 160 mg, 28-tab pack = £5.27. Label: 8

Beta-Cardone® (Celltech) PoM
Tablets, all scored, sotalol hydrochloride 40 mg (green), net price 56-tab pack = £1.34; 80 mg (pink), 56-tab pack = £1.99; 200 mg, 28-tab pack = £2.50. Label: 8

Sotacor® (Bristol-Myers Squibb) PoM
Tablets, both scored, sotalol hydrochloride 80 mg, net price 28-tab pack = £3.25; 160 mg, 28-tab pack = £6.41. Label: 8
Injection, sotalol hydrochloride 10 mg/mL. Net price 4-mL amp = £1.76

TIMOLOL MALEATE

Indications: see under Dose; glaucoma (section 11.6)
Cautions: see under Propranolol Hydrochloride; hepatic impairment (Appendix 2)
Contra-indications: see under Propranolol Hydrochloride
Side-effects: see under Propranolol Hydrochloride
Dose: hypertension, initially 5 mg twice daily *or* 10 mg once daily; gradually increased if necessary to max. 60 mg daily (given in divided doses above 20 mg daily)
Angina, initially 5 mg 2–3 times daily, usual maintenance 35–45 mg daily (range 15–45 mg daily)
Prophylaxis after myocardial infarction, initially 5 mg twice daily, increased after 2 days to 10 mg twice daily, starting 7 to 28 days after infarction
Migraine prophylaxis, 10–20 mg once daily

Betim® (Valeant) PoM
Tablets, scored, timolol maleate 10 mg. Net price 30-tab pack = £2.08. Label: 8

■ With diuretic

Moducren® (MSD) PoM
Tablets, blue, scored, timolol maleate 10 mg, co-amilozide 2.5/25 (amiloride hydrochloride 2.5 mg, hydrochlorothiazide 25 mg). Net price 28-tab pack = £8.00. Label: 8
Dose: hypertension, 1–2 tablets daily as a single dose

Prestim® (Valeant) PoM
Tablets, scored, timolol maleate 10 mg, bendroflumethiazide 2.5 mg. Net price 30-tab pack = £3.49. Label: 8
Dose: hypertension, 1–2 tablets daily; max. 4 daily

2.5 Drugs affecting the renin-angiotensin system and some other antihypertensive drugs

Lowering raised blood pressure decreases the frequency of stroke, coronary events, heart failure, and renal failure. Advice on antihypertensive therapy in this section takes into account the recommendations of the British Hypertension Society (Guidelines for management of hypertension: report of the fourth working party of the British Hypertension Society 2004—BHS IV. *J Hum Hypertens* 2004; **18:** 139–85).

Possible causes of hypertension (e.g. renal disease, endocrine causes), contributory factors, risk factors, and the presence of any complications of hypertension, such as left ventricular hypertrophy, should be established. Patients should be given advice on lifestyle changes to reduce blood pressure or cardiovascular risk; these include smoking cessation, weight reduction, reduction of excessive intake of alcohol, reduction of dietary salt, reduction of total and saturated fat, increasing exercise, and increasing fruit and vegetable intake.

THRESHOLDS AND TARGETS FOR TREATMENT. The following thresholds for treatment are recommended:

- Accelerated (malignant) hypertension (with papilloedema or fundal haemorrhages and exudates) *or* acute cardiovascular complications, admit for **immediate treatment**;
- Where the initial blood pressure is systolic ≥ 220 mmHg *or* diastolic ≥ 120 mmHg, **treat immediately**;
- Where the initial blood pressure is systolic 180–219 mmHg *or* diastolic 110–119 mmHg, confirm over 1–2 weeks then **treat** if these values are sustained;
- Where the initial blood pressure is systolic 160–179 mmHg *or* diastolic 100–109 mmHg, *and* the patient has cardiovascular complications, target-organ damage (e.g. left ventricular hypertrophy, renal impairment) or diabetes mellitus (type 1 or 2), confirm over 3–4 weeks then **treat** if these values are sustained;
- Where the initial blood pressure is systolic 160–179 mmHg *or* diastolic 100–109 mmHg, but the

patient has *no* cardiovascular complications, no target-organ damage, or no diabetes, advise lifestyle changes, reassess weekly initially and **treat** if these values are sustained on repeat measurements over 4–12 weeks;

- Where the initial blood pressure is systolic 140–159 mmHg *or* diastolic 90–99 mmHg *and* the patient has cardiovascular complications, target-organ damage or diabetes, confirm within 12 weeks and **treat** if these values are sustained;
- Where the initial blood pressure is systolic 140–159 mmHg *or* diastolic 90–99 mmHg and *no* cardiovascular complications, no target-organ damage, or no diabetes, advise lifestyle changes and **reassess** monthly; **treat** persistent mild hypertension if the 10-year cardiovascular disease risk is ≥ 20%[1].

An optimal target systolic blood pressure < 140 mmHg *and* diastolic blood pressure < 85 mmHg is suggested.[2] In some individuals it may not be possible to reduce blood pressure below the suggested targets despite the use of appropriate therapy.

DRUG TREATMENT OF HYPERTENSION. No consistent or important differences have been found between the major classes of antihypertensive drugs in terms of antihypertensive efficacy, side-effects or changes to quality of life (but there are differences in response related to age and ethnic group). The choice of antihypertensive drug will depend on the relevant indications or contra-indications for the individual patient; *some* indications and contra-indications for various antihypertensive drugs are shown below (see also under individual drug entries for details):

- **Thiazides** (section 2.2.1)—particularly indicated for hypertension in the elderly (see below); a contra-indication is gout;
- **Beta-blockers** (section 2.4)—indications include myocardial infarction, angina; compelling contra-indications include asthma, heart block;
- **ACE inhibitors** (section 2.5.5.1)—indications include heart failure, left ventricular dysfunction and diabetic nephropathy; contra-indications include renovascular disease (but see section 2.5.5.1) and pregnancy;
- **Angiotensin-II receptor antagonists** (section 2.5.5.2) are alternatives for those who cannot tolerate ACE inhibitors because of persistent dry cough, but they have the same contra-indications as ACE inhibitors;
- **Calcium-channel blockers**. There are important differences between calcium-channel blockers (section 2.6.2). **Dihydropyridine calcium-channel blockers** are valuable in isolated systolic hypertension in the elderly when a low-dose thiazide is contra-indicated or not tolerated (see below). **'Rate-limiting' calcium-channel blockers** (e.g. diltiazem, verapamil) may be valuable in angina; contra-indications include heart failure and heart block;
- **Alpha-blockers** (section 2.5.4)—a possible indication is prostatism; a contra-indication is urinary incontinence.

A single antihypertensive drug is often not adequate and other antihypertensive drugs are usually added in a step-wise manner until control is achieved. Unless it is necessary to lower the blood pressure urgently, an interval of at least 4 weeks should be allowed to determine response.

Where two antihypertensive drugs are needed, an ACE inhibitor *or* an angiotensin-II receptor antagonist *or* a beta-blocker may be combined with *either* a thiazide *or* a calcium-channel blocker.

If control is inadequate with 2 drugs, a thiazide *and* a calcium-channel blocker may be added. In patients at high risk of diabetes it is best to avoid a combination of a beta-blocker and a thiazide. In patients with *primary hyperaldosteronism*, spironolactone (section 2.2.3) is effective.

Response to drug treatment for hypertension may be affected by the patient's age and ethnic background. A beta-blocker or an ACE inhibitor may be the most appropriate initial drug in younger Caucasians; Afro-Caribbean patients respond less well to these drugs and a thiazide or a calcium-channel blocker may be chosen for initial treatment.

OTHER MEASURES TO REDUCE CARDIOVASCULAR RISK. **Aspirin** (section 2.9) in a dose of 75 mg daily reduces the risk of cardiovascular events and myocardial infarction; however, concerns about an increased risk of bleeding need to be considered. Unless it is contra-indicated, aspirin is recommended for *secondary prevention* in patients with cardiovascular complications (myocardial infarction, angina, non-haemorrhagic cerebrovascular disease, peripheral vascular disease, or atherosclerotic renovascular disease), and for *primary prevention* in patients aged over 50 years with controlled blood pressure (systolic pressure < 150 mmHg and diastolic pressure < 90 mmHg) who have end-organ damage, type 2 diabetes, or a cardiovascular disease risk ≥ 20% over 10 years[1].

A **statin** can be of benefit in those at high risk of cardiovascular disease and in those with hypercholesterolaemia (see section 2.12 for details).

HYPERTENSION IN THE ELDERLY. Benefit from antihypertensive therapy is evident up to at least 80 years of age, but it is probably inappropriate to apply a strict age limit when deciding on drug therapy. Elderly individuals who have a good outlook for longevity should have their blood pressure lowered if they are hypertensive. The thresholds for treatment are diastolic pressure averaging ≥ 90 mmHg *or* systolic pressure averaging ≥ 160 mmHg over 3 to 6 months' observation (despite appropriate non-drug treatment). A low dose of a thiazide is the clear drug of first choice, with addition of another antihypertensive drug when necessary.

ISOLATED SYSTOLIC HYPERTENSION. Isolated systolic hypertension (systolic pressure ≥ 160 mmHg, diastolic pressure < 90 mmHg) is associated with an increased cardiovascular disease risk, particularly in those aged over 60 years. Systolic blood

1. Cardiovascular disease risk may be determined from the chart issued by the British Hypertension Society (*J Hum Hypertens* 2004; **18**: 139–85)—see inside back cover. The Joint British Societies' 'Cardiac Risk Assessor' computer programme may also be used to determine cardiovascular disease risk by adding together the coronary heart disease risk and stroke risk.

2. A lower target for blood pressure should be considered for the secondary prevention of stroke, and for patients with diabetes and renal disease

pressure averaging 160 mmHg or higher over 3 to 6 months (despite appropriate non-drug treatment) should be lowered in those over 60 years, even if diastolic hypertension is absent. Treatment with a low dose of a thiazide, with addition of a beta-blocker when necessary is effective; a long-acting dihydropyridine calcium-channel blocker is recommended when a thiazide is contra-indicated or not tolerated. Patients with severe postural hypotension should not receive blood pressure lowering drugs.

Isolated systolic hypertension in younger patients is uncommon but treatment may be indicated in those with a threshold systolic pressure of 160 mmHg (or less if at increased risk of cardiovascular disease, see above).

HYPERTENSION IN DIABETES. For patients with diabetes, the aim should be to maintain systolic pressure < 130 mmHg and diastolic pressure < 80 mmHg. However, in some individuals, it may not be possible to achieve this level of control despite appropriate therapy. Low-dose thiazides, beta-blockers, ACE inhibitors (or angiotensin-II receptor antagonists) and long-acting dihydropyridine calcium-channel blockers are all beneficial. Most patients require a combination of antihypertensive drugs.

Hypertension is common in type 2 (non-insulin-dependent) diabetes and antihypertensive treatment prevents macrovascular and microvascular complications. In type 1 (insulin-dependent) diabetes, hypertension usually indicates the presence of diabetic nephropathy. An ACE inhibitor (or an angiotensin-II receptor antagonist) may have a specific role in the management of diabetic nephropathy (section 6.1.5); in patients with type 2 diabetes, an ACE inhibitor (or an angiotensin-II receptor antagonist) can delay progression of microalbuminuria to nephropathy.

HYPERTENSION IN RENAL DISEASE. The threshold for antihypertensive treatment in patients with renal impairment or persistent proteinuria is a systolic blood pressure ≥ 140 mmHg *or* a diastolic blood pressure ≥ 90 mmHg. Optimal blood pressure is a systolic blood pressure < 130 mmHg and a diastolic pressure < 80 mmHg, or lower if proteinuria exceeds 1 g in 24 hours. Thiazides may be ineffective and high doses of loop diuretics may be required. Specific cautions apply to the use of ACE inhibitors in renal impairment, see section 2.5.5.1, but ACE inhibitors may be effective. Dihydropyridine calcium-channel blockers may be added.

HYPERTENSION IN PREGNANCY. High blood pressure in pregnancy may usually be due to pre-existing essential hypertension or to pre-eclampsia. Methyldopa (section 2.5.2) is safe in pregnancy. Beta-blockers are effective and safe in the third trimester. Modified-release preparations of nifedipine [unlicensed] are also used for hypertension in pregnancy. Intravenous administration of labetalol (section 2.4) can be used to control hypertensive crises; alternatively, hydralazine (section 2.5.1) may be used by the intravenous route. For use of magnesium sulphate in pre-eclampsia and eclampsia, see section 9.5.1.3.

ACCELERATED OR VERY SEVERE HYPERTENSION. Accelerated (or malignant) hypertension or very severe hypertension (e.g. diastolic blood pressure > 140 mmHg) requires urgent treatment in hospital, but it is not an indication for parenteral antihypertensive therapy. Normally treatment should be by mouth with a beta-blocker (atenolol or labetalol) or a long-acting calcium-channel blocker (e.g. amlodipine or modified-release nifedipine). Within the first 24 hours the diastolic blood pressure should be reduced to 100–110 mmHg. Over the next 2 or 3 days blood pressure should be normalised by using beta-blockers, calcium-channel blockers, diuretics, vasodilators, or ACE inhibitors. Very rapid reduction in blood pressure can reduce organ perfusion leading to cerebral infarction and blindness, deterioration in renal function, and myocardial ischaemia. Parenteral antihypertensive drugs are rarely necessary; sodium nitroprusside by infusion is the drug of choice on the rare occasions when parenteral treatment is necessary.

For advice on short-term management of hypertensive episodes in phaeochromocytoma, see under Phaeochromocytoma, section 2.5.4.

2.5.1 Vasodilator antihypertensive drugs

These are potent drugs, especially when used in combination with a beta-blocker and a thiazide.

Important: for a warning on the hazards of a very rapid fall in blood pressure, see section 2.5.

Diazoxide has been used by intravenous injection in hypertensive emergencies.

Hydralazine given by mouth is a useful adjunct to other treatment, but when used alone causes tachycardia and fluid retention. Side-effects can be few if the dose is kept below 100 mg daily, but systemic lupus erythematosus should be suspected if there is unexplained weight loss, arthritis, or any other unexplained ill health.

Sodium nitroprusside is given by intravenous infusion to control severe hypertensive crises on the rare occasions when parenteral treatment is necessary.

Minoxidil should be reserved for the treatment of severe hypertension resistant to other drugs. Vasodilatation is accompanied by increased cardiac output and tachycardia and the patients develop fluid retention. For this reason the addition of a beta-blocker and a diuretic (usually furosemide, in high dosage) are mandatory. Hypertrichosis is troublesome and renders this drug unsuitable for women.

Prazosin, doxazosin, and terazosin (section 2.5.4) have alpha-blocking and vasodilator properties.

Bosentan and **iloprost** are licensed for the treatment of some types of pulmonary hypertension. **Epoprostenol** (section 2.8.1) is also used for the treatment of pulmonary hypertension.

BOSENTAN

Indications: pulmonary arterial hypertension

Cautions: not to be initiated if systemic systolic blood pressure is below 85 mmHg; monitor liver function before and during treatment (reduce dose or suspend treatment if liver enzymes raised significantly)—discontinue if symptoms of liver impairment; monitor haemoglobin; **interactions:** Appendix 1 (bosentan)

Contra-indications: hepatic impairment (Appendix 2); **avoid** pregnancy **during** and for **3 months after** treatment (Appendix 4); breast-feeding (Appendix 5)

Side-effects: dyspepsia, flushing, hypotension, palpitation, fatigue, oedema, anaemia, pruritus, nasopharyngitis, hepatic impairment (see Cautions above)

Dose: initially 62.5 mg twice daily increased after 4 weeks to 125 mg twice daily; max. 250 mg twice daily

Tracleer® (Actelion) ▼ PoM

Tablets, f/c, orange, bosentan (as monohydrate) 62.5 mg, net price 56-tab pack = £1541.00; 125 mg, 56-tab pack = £1541.00

DIAZOXIDE

Indications: hypertensive emergency including severe hypertension associated with renal disease (but see section 2.5); hypoglycaemia (section 6.1.4)

Cautions: ischaemic heart disease; renal impairment (Appendix 3); pregnancy and labour (Appendix 4); **interactions:** Appendix 1 (diazoxide)

Side-effects: tachycardia, hypotension, hyperglycaemia, sodium and water retention; *rarely* cardiomegaly, hyperosmolar non-ketotic coma, leucopenia, thrombocytopenia, and hirsuitism

Dose: *by rapid intravenous injection* (less than 30 seconds), 1–3 mg/kg to max. single dose of 150 mg (see below); may be repeated after 5–15 minutes if required

NOTE. Single doses of 300 mg have been associated with angina and with myocardial and cerebral infarction

Eudemine® (Goldshield) PoM

Injection, diazoxide 15 mg/mL. Net price 20-mL amp = £30.00

HYDRALAZINE HYDROCHLORIDE

Indications: moderate to severe hypertension (adjunct); heart failure (with long-acting nitrate, but see section 2.5.5); hypertensive crisis (including during pregnancy) (but see section 2.5)

Cautions: hepatic impairment (Appendix 2); renal impairment (Appendix 3); coronary artery disease (may provoke angina, avoid after myocardial infarction until stabilised), cerebrovascular disease; occasionally blood pressure reduction too rapid even with low parenteral doses; pregnancy (Appendix 4); breast-feeding (Appendix 5); manufacturer advises test for antinuclear factor and for proteinuria every 6 months and check acetylator status before increasing dose above 100 mg daily, but evidence of clinical value unsatisfactory; **interactions:** Appendix 1 (hydralazine)

Contra-indications: idiopathic systemic lupus erythematosus, severe tachycardia, high output heart failure, myocardial insufficiency due to mechanical obstruction, cor pulmonale, dissecting aortic aneurysm; porphyria (section 9.8.2)

Side-effects: tachycardia, palpitation, flushing, hypotension, fluid retention, gastro-intestinal disturbances; headache, dizziness; systemic lupus erythematosus-like syndrome after long-term therapy with over 100 mg daily (or less in women and in slow acetylator individuals) (see also notes above); rarely rashes, fever, peripheral neuritis, polyneuritis, paraesthesia, arthralgia, myalgia, increased lacrimation, nasal congestion, dyspnoea, agitation, anxiety, anorexia; blood disorders (including leucopenia, thrombocytopenia, haemolytic anaemia), abnormal liver function, jaundice, raised plasma creatinine, proteinuria and haematuria reported

Dose: *by mouth*, hypertension, 25 mg twice daily, increased to usual max. 50 mg twice daily (see notes above)

Heart failure (initiated in hospital) 25 mg 3–4 times daily, increased every 2 days if necessary; usual maintenance dose 50–75 mg 4 times daily

By slow intravenous injection, hypertension with renal complications and hypertensive crisis, 5–10 mg diluted with 10 mL sodium chloride 0.9%; may be repeated after 20–30 minutes (see Cautions)

By intravenous infusion, hypertension with renal complications and hypertensive crisis, initially 200–300 micrograms/minute; maintenance usually 50–150 micrograms/minute

Hydralazine (Non-proprietary) PoM

Tablets, hydralazine hydrochloride 25 mg, net price 20 = £1.18; 50 mg, 20 = £1.47

Apresoline® (Sovereign) PoM

Tablets, yellow, s/c, hydralazine hydrochloride 25 mg, net price 84-tab pack = £2.50

Excipients: include gluten

Injection, powder for reconstitution, hydralazine hydrochloride. Net price 20-mg amp = £1.64

ILOPROST

Indications: primary pulmonary hypertension

Cautions: unstable pulmonary hypertension with advanced right heart failure; hypotension (do not initiate if systolic blood pressure below 85 mmHg); hepatic impairment (Appendix 2); **interactions:** Appendix 1 (iloprost)

Contra-indications: unstable angina; within 6 months of myocardial infarction; decompensated cardiac failure (unless under close medical supervision); severe arrhythmias; congenital or acquired heart-valve defects; within 3 months of cerebrovascular events; pulmonary veno-occlusive disease; conditions which increase risk of bleeding; pregnancy (Appendix 4); breast-feeding (Appendix 5)

Side-effects: vasodilatation, hypotension, syncope, cough, headache, trismus

Dose: *by inhalation of nebulised solution*, 2.5–5 micrograms 6–9 times daily, adjusted according to response

Ventavis (Schering Health) ▼ PoM

Nebuliser solution, iloprost (as trometamol) 10 micrograms/mL, net price 30 x 2 mL (20 microgram) unit-dose vials = £425.00; 100 x 2-mL = £1415.08; 300 x 2-mL = £4243.88. For use with *Prodose*® NHS nebuliser

MINOXIDIL

Indications: severe hypertension, in addition to a diuretic and a beta-blocker

Cautions: see notes above; angina; after myocardial infarction (until stabilised); lower doses in dialysis patients; porphyria (section 9.8.2); pregnancy (Appendix 4); **interactions:** Appendix 1 (minoxidil)

Contra-indications: phaeochromocytoma
Side-effects: sodium and water retention; weight gain, peripheral oedema, tachycardia, hypertrichosis; reversible rise in creatinine and blood urea nitrogen; occasionally, gastro-intestinal disturbances, breast tenderness, rashes
Dose: initially 5 mg (elderly, 2.5 mg) daily, in 1–2 doses, increased by 5–10 mg every 3 or more days; max. usually 50 mg daily

Loniten® (Pharmacia) PoM
Tablets, all scored, minoxidil 2.5 mg, net price 60-tab pack = £8.88; 5 mg, 60-tab pack = £15.83; 10 mg, 60-tab pack = £30.68

SODIUM NITROPRUSSIDE

Indications: hypertensive crisis (but see section 2.5); controlled hypotension in anaesthesia; acute or chronic heart failure
Cautions: hypothyroidism, hyponatraemia, ischaemic heart disease, impaired cerebral circulation, elderly; hypothermia; monitor blood pressure and blood-cyanide concentration and if treatment exceeds 3 days, also blood-thiocyanate concentration; avoid sudden withdrawal—terminate infusion over 15–30 minutes; hepatic impairment (Appendix 2); renal impairment (Appendix 3); pregnancy (Appendix 4); breast-feeding; **interactions:** Appendix 1 (nitroprusside)
Contra-indications: severe vitamin B_{12} deficiency; Leber's optic atrophy; compensatory hypertension
Side-effects: associated with over rapid reduction in blood pressure (reduce infusion rate): headache, dizziness, nausea, retching, abdominal pain, perspiration, palpitation, apprehension, retrosternal discomfort; occasionally reduced platelet count, acute transient phlebitis
CYANIDE. Side-effects caused by excessive plasma concentration of the cyanide metabolite include tachycardia, sweating, hyperventilation, arrhythmias, marked metabolic acidosis (discontinue and give antidote, see p. 33)
Dose: hypertensive crisis, *by intravenous infusion*, initially 0.5–1.5 micrograms/kg/minute, then increased in steps of 500 nanograms/kg/minute every 5 minutes within range 0.5–8 micrograms/kg/minute (lower doses in patients already receiving other antihypertensives); stop if response unsatisfactory with max. dose in 10 minutes
NOTE. Lower initial dose of 300 nanograms/kg/minute has been used
Maintenance of blood pressure at 30–40% lower than pretreatment diastolic blood pressure, 20–400 micrograms/minute (lower doses for patients being treated with other antihypertensives)
Controlled hypotension in surgery, *by intravenous infusion*, max. 1.5 micrograms/kg/minute
Heart failure, *by intravenous infusion*, initially 10–15 micrograms/minute, increased every 5–10 minutes as necessary; usual range 10–200 micrograms/minute normally for max. 3 days

Sodium Nitroprusside (Mayne) PoM
Intravenous infusion, powder for reconstitution, sodium nitroprusside 10 mg/mL. For dilution and use as an infusion, net price 5-mL vial = £6.64

2.5.2 Centrally acting antihypertensive drugs

Methyldopa is a centrally acting antihypertensive; it may be used for the management of hypertension in pregnancy. Side-effects are minimised if the daily dose is kept below 1 g.

Clonidine has the disadvantage that sudden withdrawal may cause a hypertensive crisis.

Moxonidine, a centrally acting drug, is licensed for mild to moderate essential hypertension. It may have a role when thiazides, beta-blockers, ACE inhibitors and calcium-channel blockers are not appropriate or have failed to control blood pressure.

CLONIDINE HYDROCHLORIDE

Indications: hypertension; migraine (section 4.7.4.2); menopausal flushing (section 6.4.1.1)
Cautions: must be withdrawn gradually to avoid hypertensive crisis; Raynaud's syndrome or other occlusive peripheral vascular disease; history of depression; avoid in porphyria (section 9.8.2); pregnancy (Appendix 4); breast-feeding (Appendix 5); **interactions:** Appendix 1 (clonidine)
DRIVING. Drowsiness may affect performance of skilled tasks (e.g. driving); effects of alcohol may be enhanced
Side-effects: dry mouth, sedation, depression, fluid retention, bradycardia, Raynaud's phenomenon, headache, dizziness, euphoria, nocturnal unrest, rash, nausea, constipation, rarely impotence
Dose: *by mouth*, 50–100 micrograms 3 times daily, increased every second or third day; usual max. dose 1.2 mg daily
By slow intravenous injection, 150–300 micrograms; max. 750 micrograms in 24 hours

Catapres® (Boehringer Ingelheim) PoM
Tablets, both scored, clonidine hydrochloride 100 micrograms, net price 100-tab pack = £5.60; 300 micrograms, 100-tab pack = £13.04. Label: 3, 8
Injection, clonidine hydrochloride 150 micrograms/mL. Net price 1-mL amp = 29p

Dixarit® PoM
(migraine), section 4.7.4.2

METHYLDOPA

Indications: hypertension
Cautions: history of liver impairment (Appendix 2); renal impairment (Appendix 3); blood counts and liver-function tests advised; history of depression; positive direct Coombs' test in up to 20% of patients (may affect blood cross-matching); interference with laboratory tests; **interactions:** Appendix 1 (methyldopa)
DRIVING. Drowsiness may affect performance of skilled tasks (e.g. driving); effects of alcohol may be enhanced
Contra-indications: depression, active liver disease, phaeochromocytoma; porphyria (section 9.8.2)
Side-effects: gastro-intestinal disturbances, dry mouth, stomatitis, sialadenitis; bradycardia, exacerbation of angina, postural hypotension, oedema; sedation, headache, dizziness, asthenia, myalgia, arthralgia, paraesthesia, nightmares, mild psychosis, depression, impaired mental acuity, parkinsonism, Bell's palsy; abnormal liver

function tests, hepatitis, jaundice; pancreatitis; haemolytic anaemia; bone-marrow depression, leucopenia, thrombocytopenia, eosinophilia; hypersensitivity reactions including lupus erythematosus-like syndrome, drug fever, myocarditis, pericarditis; rashes (including toxic epidermal necrolysis); nasal congestion, failure of ejaculation, impotence, decreased libido, gynaecomastia, hyperprolactinaemia, amenorrhoea

Dose: initially 250 mg 2–3 times daily, increased gradually at intervals of 2 or more days, max. 3 g daily; ELDERLY initially 125 mg twice daily, increased gradually, max. 2 g daily

Methyldopa (Non-proprietary) PoM
Tablets, coated, methyldopa (anhydrous) 125 mg, net price 20 = 94p; 250 mg, 20 = £1.08; 500 mg, 20 = £1.67. Label: 3, 8

Aldomet® (MSD) PoM
Tablets, all yellow, f/c, methyldopa (anhydrous) 250 mg, net price 60 = £1.88; 500 mg, 30 = £1.90. Label: 3, 8

MOXONIDINE

Indications: mild to moderate essential hypertension

Cautions: renal impairment (Appendix 3); avoid abrupt withdrawal (if concomitant treatment with beta-blocker has to be stopped, discontinue beta-blocker first, then moxonidine after few days); **interactions:** see Appendix 1 (moxonidine)

Contra-indications: history of angioedema; conduction disorders (sick sinus syndrome, sino-atrial block, second- or third-degree AV block); bradycardia; life-threatening arrhythmia; severe heart failure; severe coronary artery disease, unstable angina; severe liver disease or severe renal impairment; also on theoretical grounds: Raynaud's syndrome, intermittent claudication, epilepsy, depression, Parkinson's disease, glaucoma; pregnancy (Appendix 4); breast-feeding (Appendix 5)

Side-effects: dry mouth; headache, fatigue, dizziness, nausea, sleep disturbance (rarely sedation), asthenia, vasodilatation; rarely skin reactions

Dose: 200 micrograms once daily in the morning, increased if necessary after 3 weeks to 400 micrograms daily in 1–2 divided doses; max. 600 micrograms daily in 2 divided doses (max. single dose 400 micrograms)

Moxonidine (Non-proprietary) PoM
Tablets, all f/c, moxonidine 200 micrograms, net price 28-tab pack = £9.86; 300 micrograms, net price 28-tab pack = £11.17; 400 micrograms, net price 28-tab pack = £13.44. Label: 3

Physiotens® (Solvay) PoM
Tablets, f/c, moxonidine 200 micrograms (pink), net price 28-tab pack = £9.72; 300 micrograms (red), 28-tab pack = £11.49; 400 micrograms (red), 28-tab pack = £13.26. Label: 3

2.5.3 Adrenergic neurone blocking drugs

Adrenergic neurone blocking drugs prevent the release of noradrenaline from postganglionic adrenergic neurones. These drugs do not control supine blood pressure and may cause postural hypotension. For this reason they have largely fallen from use, but may be necessary with other therapy in resistant hypertension.

Guanethidine, which also depletes the nerve endings of noradrenaline, is licensed for the rapid control of blood pressure.

GUANETHIDINE MONOSULPHATE

Indications: hypertensive crisis (but see section 2.5)

Cautions: renal impairment (avoid if creatinine clearance < 40 mL/minute; Appendix 3); coronary or cerebral arteriosclerosis, asthma, history of peptic ulceration; pregnancy (Appendix 4); **interactions:** Appendix 1 (adrenergic neurone blockers)

Contra-indications: phaeochromocytoma, heart failure

Side-effects: postural hypotension, failure of ejaculation, fluid retention, nasal congestion, headache, diarrhoea, drowsiness

Dose: *by intramuscular injection*, 10–20 mg, repeated after 3 hours if required

Ismelin® (Sovereign) PoM
Injection, guanethidine monosulphate 10 mg/mL. Net price 1-mL amp = £1.56

2.5.4 Alpha-adrenoceptor blocking drugs

Prazosin has post-synaptic alpha-blocking and vasodilator properties and rarely causes tachycardia. It may, however, cause a rapid reduction in blood pressure after the first dose and should be introduced with caution. **Doxazosin**, **indoramin**, and **terazosin** have properties similar to those of prazosin.

Alpha-blockers may be used with other antihypertensive drugs in the treatment of hypertension.

PROSTATIC HYPERPLASIA. Alfuzosin, doxazosin, indoramin, prazosin, tamsulosin and terazosin are indicated for benign prostatic hyperplasia (section 7.4.1).

DOXAZOSIN

Indications: hypertension; benign prostatic hyperplasia (section 7.4.1)

Cautions: care with initial dose (postural hypotension); hepatic impairment (Appendix 2); susceptibility to heart failure; pregnancy (Appendix 4); breast-feeding (Appendix 5); **interactions:** Appendix 1 (alpha-blockers)

Side-effects: postural hypotension; dizziness, vertigo, headache, fatigue, asthenia, oedema, sleep disturbance, nausea, rhinitis; less frequently abdominal discomfort, diarrhoea, vomiting, agitation, tremor, rash, pruritus; rarely blurred vision, epistaxis, haematuria, thrombocytopenia, purpura, leucopenia, hepatitis, jaundice, cholestasis, and urinary incontinence; isolated cases of priapism and impotence reported

Dose: hypertension, 1 mg daily, increased after 1–2 weeks to 2 mg once daily, and thereafter to 4 mg once daily, if necessary; max. 16 mg daily

Doxazosin (Non-proprietary) PoM
Tablets, doxazosin (as mesilate) 1 mg, net price 28-tab pack = £1.81; 2 mg, 28-tab pack = £2.61; 4 mg, 28-tab pack = £4.58
Brands include *Doxadura*®

Cardura® (Pfizer) PoM
Tablets, doxazosin (as mesilate) 1 mg, net price 28-tab pack = £10.56; 2 mg, 28-tab pack = £14.08

■ Modified-release

Cardura® **XL** (Pfizer) PoM
Tablets, m/r, doxazosin (as mesilate) 4 mg, net price 28-tab pack = £6.33; 8 mg, 28-tab pack = £12.67. Label: 25
Dose: 4 mg once daily, increased to 8 mg once daily after 4 weeks if necessary

INDORAMIN

Indications: hypertension; benign prostatic hyperplasia (section 7.4.1)
Cautions: avoid alcohol (enhances rate and extent of absorption); control incipient heart failure with diuretics and digoxin; hepatic or renal impairment; elderly patients; Parkinson's disease; epilepsy (convulsions in *animal* studies); history of depression; **interactions:** Appendix 1 (alpha-blockers)
DRIVING. Drowsiness may affect performance of skilled tasks (e.g. driving); effects of alcohol may be enhanced
Contra-indications: established heart failure; patients receiving MAOIs
Side-effects: sedation; also dizziness, depression, failure of ejaculation, dry mouth, nasal congestion, weight gain; rarely exacerbation of Parkinson's disease
Dose: hypertension, initially 25 mg twice daily, increased by 25–50 mg daily at intervals of 2 weeks; max. daily dose 200 mg in 2–3 divided doses

Baratol® (Shire) PoM
Tablets, blue, f/c, indoramin (as hydrochloride) 25 mg, net price 84-tab pack = £9.00. Label: 2

■ Prostatic hyperplasia

Doralese® PoM
See section 7.4.1

PRAZOSIN

Indications: see under Dose
Cautions: first dose may cause collapse due to hypotension (therefore should be taken on retiring to bed); elderly; hepatic impairment (Appendix 2); renal impairment (Appendix 3); pregnancy (Appendix 4); breast-feeding (Appendix 5); **interactions:** Appendix 1 (alpha-blockers)
Contra-indications: not recommended for congestive heart failure due to mechanical obstruction (e.g. aortic stenosis)
Side-effects: postural hypotension, drowsiness, weakness, dizziness, headache, lack of energy, nausea, palpitation; urinary frequency, incontinence and priapism reported
Dose: hypertension, 500 micrograms 2–3 times daily for 3–7 days, the initial dose on retiring to bed at night (to avoid collapse, see Cautions); increased to 1 mg 2–3 times daily for a further 3–7 days; further increased if necessary to max. 20 mg daily in divided doses
Congestive heart failure (but see section 2.5.5), 500 micrograms 2–4 times daily (initial dose at bedtime, see above), increasing to 4 mg daily in divided doses; maintenance 4–20 mg daily in divided doses (but rarely used)
Raynaud's syndrome (but efficacy not established, see section 2.6.4.1), initially 500 micrograms twice daily (initial dose at bedtime, see above) increased, if necessary, after 3–7 days to usual maintenance 1–2 mg twice daily
Benign prostatic hyperplasia, section 7.4.1

Prazosin (Non-proprietary) PoM
Tablets, prazosin (as hydrochloride) 500 micrograms, net price 56-tab pack = £2.51; 1 mg, 56-tab pack = £3.23; 2 mg, 56-tab pack = £4.39; 5 mg, 56-tab pack = £8.75. Label: 3, counselling, initial dose
Brands include *Kentovase*®

Hypovase® (Pfizer) PoM
Tablets, prazosin (as hydrochloride) 500 micrograms, net price 56-tab pack = £2.51; 1 mg (orange, scored), 56-tab pack = £3.23; 2 mg (scored), 56-tab pack = £4.39. Label: 3, counselling, initial dose

TERAZOSIN

Indications: mild to moderate hypertension; benign prostatic hyperplasia (section 7.4.1)
Cautions: first dose may cause collapse due to hypotension (within 30–90 minutes, therefore should be taken on retiring to bed) (may also occur with rapid dose increase); pregnancy (Appendix 4); **interactions:** Appendix 1 (alpha-blockers)
Side-effects: drowsiness, dizziness, lack of energy, peripheral oedema; urinary frequency and priapism reported; see also section 7.4.1
Dose: hypertension, 1 mg at bedtime (compliance with bedtime dose important, see Cautions); dose doubled after 7 days if necessary; usual maintenance dose 2–10 mg once daily; more than 20 mg daily rarely improves efficacy

Terazosin (Non-proprietary) PoM
Tablets, terazosin (as hydrochloride) 2 mg, net price 28-tab pack = £7.06; 5 mg, 28-tab pack = £12.72; 10 mg, 28-tab pack = £25.97. Label: 3, counselling, see dose above

Hytrin® (Abbott) PoM
Tablets, terazosin (as hydrochloride) 2 mg (yellow), net price 28-tab pack = £4.57; 5 mg (tan), 28-tab pack = £8.57; 10 mg (blue), 28-tab pack = £17.14; starter pack (for hypertension) of 7 × 1-mg tabs with 21 × 2-mg tabs = £13.00. Label: 3, counselling, see dose above

Phaeochromocytoma

Long-term management of phaeochromocytoma involves surgery. Alpha-blockers are used in the short-term management of hypertensive episodes in phaeochromocytoma. Once alpha blockade is established, tachycardia can be controlled by the cautious addition of a beta-blocker (section 2.4); a cardioselective beta-blocker is preferred.

Phenoxybenzamine, a powerful alpha-blocker, is effective in the management of phaeochromocytoma but it has many side-effects. **Phentolamine** is a short-acting alpha-blocker used mainly during surgery of phaeochromocytoma; its use for the diagnosis of phaeochromocytoma has been superseded by measurement of catecholamines in blood and urine.

PHENOXYBENZAMINE HYDROCHLORIDE

Indications: hypertensive episodes in phaeochromocytoma

Cautions: elderly; congestive heart failure; severe heart disease (see also Contra-indications); cerebrovascular disease (avoid if history of cerebrovascular accident); renal impairment; carcinogenic in *animals*; avoid in porphyria (section 9.8.2); avoid infusion in hypovolaemia; avoid extravasation (irritant to tissues); pregnancy (Appendix 4); breast-feeding (Appendix 5)

Contra-indications: history of cerebrovascular accident; during recovery period after myocardial infarction (usually 3–4 weeks)

Side-effects: postural hypotension with dizziness and marked compensatory tachycardia, lassitude, nasal congestion, miosis, inhibition of ejaculation; rarely gastro-intestinal disturbances; decreased sweating and dry mouth after intravenous infusion; idiosyncratic profound hypotension within few minutes of starting infusion

Dose: see under preparations

Phenoxybenzamine (Goldshield) PoM
Injection concentrate, phenoxybenzamine hydrochloride 50 mg/mL. To be diluted before use. Net price 3 × 2-mL amp = £94.88 (hosp. only)
Dose: by *intravenous infusion* (preferably through large vein), adjunct in severe shock (but rarely used) and phaeochromocytoma, 1 mg/kg daily over at least 2 hours; do not repeat within 24 hours (intensive care facilities needed)
CAUTION. Owing to risk of contact sensitisation healthcare professionals should avoid contamination of hands

Dibenyline® (Goldshield) PoM
Capsules, red/white, phenoxybenzamine hydrochloride 10 mg. Net price 30-cap pack = £10.84
Dose: phaeochromocytoma, 10 mg daily, increased by 10 mg daily; usual dose 1–2 mg/kg daily in 2 divided doses

PHENTOLAMINE MESILATE

Indications: hypertensive episodes due to phaeochromocytoma e.g. during surgery; diagnosis of phaeochromocytoma

Cautions: monitor blood pressure (avoid in hypotension), heart rate; renal impairment; gastritis, peptic ulcer; elderly; pregnancy (Appendix 4) and breast-feeding (Appendix 5); **interactions:** Appendix 1 (alpha-blockers)
ASTHMA. Presence of sulphites in ampoules may (especially in patients with asthma) lead to hypersensitivity (with bronchospasm and shock)

Contra-indications: hypotension; history of myocardial infarction; coronary insufficiency, angina, or other evidence of coronary artery disease

Side-effects: postural hypotension, tachycardia, dizziness, flushing; nausea and vomiting, diarrhoea, nasal congestion; also acute or prolonged hypotension, angina, chest pain, arrhythmias

Dose: hypertensive episodes, *by intravenous injection*, 2–5 mg repeated if necessary
Diagnosis of phaeochromocytoma, consult product literature

Rogitine® (Alliance) PoM
Injection, phentolamine mesilate 10 mg/mL. Net price 1-mL amp = £1.66

2.5.5 Drugs affecting the renin-angiotensin system

Heart failure

The treatment of chronic heart failure aims to relieve symptoms, improve exercise tolerance, reduce the incidence of acute exacerbations and reduce mortality. An **ACE inhibitor** given at an adequate dose[1] generally achieves these aims; a diuretic is also necessary in most patients to reduce symptoms of fluid overload. Digoxin improves symptoms and exercise tolerance and reduces hospitalisation due to acute exacerbations but it does not reduce mortality. Drug treatment of chronic systolic heart failure is covered below; optimal management of diastolic heart failure is less certain but digoxin should probably be avoided.

An ACE inhibitor (section 2.5.5.1) is generally advised for patients with asymptomatic left ventricular dysfunction or symptomatic heart failure.

Patients with fluid overload should also receive either a loop or a thiazide diuretic (with salt or fluid restriction where appropriate). A **thiazide diuretic** (section 2.2.1) may be of benefit in patients with mild heart failure and good renal function; however, thiazide diuretics are ineffective in patients with poor renal function (estimated creatinine clearance less than 30 mL/minute, see Appendix 3) and a **loop diuretic** (section 2.2.2) is preferred. If diuresis with a single diuretic is insufficient, a combination of a loop diuretic and a thiazide diuretic may be tried; addition of metolazone (section 2.2.1) may also be considered but the resulting diuresis may be profound and care is needed to avoid potentially dangerous electrolyte disturbances.

The aldosterone antagonist **spironolactone** (section 2.2.3) may be considered for patients with severe heart failure who are already receiving an ACE inhibitor and a diuretic; low doses of spironolactone (usually 25 mg daily) reduce symptoms and mortality in these patients. If spironolactone cannot be used, eplerenone (section 2.2.3) may be considered for the management of heart failure after an acute myocardial infarction with evidence of left ventricular dysfunction. Close monitoring of serum creatinine and potassium is necessary with any change in treatment or in the patient's condition.

1. For heart failure the dose of the ACE inhibitor is titrated to a 'target' dose (or to the maximum tolerated dose if lower). Target doses for some ACE inhibitors may exceed licensed ones, e.g. captopril (target dose 50 mg three times daily), enalapril (10–20 mg twice daily), lisinopril (30–35 mg daily), ramipril (5 mg twice daily), trandolapril (4 mg daily [unlicensed indication])

The **beta-blockers** bisoprolol and carvedilol (section 2.4) are of value in any grade of stable heart failure and left-ventricular systolic dysfunction. Beta-blocker treatment should be started by those experienced in the management of heart failure, at a very low dose and titrated very slowly over a period of weeks or months. Symptoms may deteriorate initially, calling for adjustment of concomitant therapy.

Digoxin (section 2.1) is given to patients with atrial fibrillation and also to selected patients in sinus rhythm who remain symptomatic despite treatment with an ACE inhibitor, a diuretic, and a beta-blocker.

Patients who cannot tolerate ACE inhibitors or in whom they are contra-indicated may be given **isosorbide dinitrate** (section 2.6.1) with **hydralazine** (section 2.5.1), but this combination may be poorly tolerated. **Angiotensin-II receptor antagonists** (section 2.5.5.2) may be useful alternatives for patients who, because of symptoms such as cough, cannot tolerate ACE inhibitors.

2.5.5.1 Angiotensin-converting enzyme inhibitors

Angiotensin-converting enzyme inhibitors (ACE inhibitors) inhibit the conversion of angiotensin I to angiotensin II. They are effective antihypertensives and generally well tolerated. The main indications of ACE inhibitors are shown below.

HEART FAILURE. ACE inhibitors are used in all grades of heart failure, usually combined with a diuretic (section 2.5.5). Potassium supplements and potassium-sparing diuretics should be discontinued before introducing an ACE inhibitor because of the risk of hyperkalaemia. However, a low dose of spironolactone may be beneficial in severe heart failure (section 2.5.5) and can be used with an ACE inhibitor provided serum potassium is monitored carefully. Profound first-dose hypotension may occur when ACE inhibitors are introduced to patients with heart failure who are already taking a high dose of a loop diuretic (e.g. furosemide 80 mg daily or more). Temporary withdrawal of the loop diuretic reduces the risk, but may cause severe rebound pulmonary oedema. Therefore, for patients on high doses of loop diuretics, the ACE inhibitor may need to be initiated under specialist supervision, see below. An ACE inhibitor can be initiated in the community in patients who are receiving a low dose of a diuretic or who are not otherwise at risk of serious hypotension; nevertheless, care is required and a very low dose of the ACE inhibitor is given initially.

HYPERTENSION. ACE inhibitors should be considered for hypertension when thiazides and beta-blockers are contra-indicated, not tolerated, or fail to control blood pressure; they are particularly indicated for hypertension in insulin-dependent diabetics with nephropathy (see also section 6.1.5). ACE inhibitors may cause very rapid falls of blood pressure in some patients particularly in those receiving diuretic therapy (see Cautions, below); the first dose should preferably be given at bedtime.

DIABETIC NEPHROPATHY. For comment on the role of ACE inhibitors in the management of diabetic nephropathy, see section 6.1.5.

PROPHYLAXIS OF CARDIOVASCULAR EVENTS. ACE inhibitors are used in the early and long-term management of patients who have had a myocardial infarction, see section 2.10.1. An ACE inhibitor may also have a role in preventing cardiovascular events and stroke in those at risk because of stable coronary heart disease.

INITIATION UNDER SPECIALIST SUPERVISION. ACE inhibitors should be initiated under specialist supervision and with careful clinical monitoring in those with severe heart failure or in those:

- receiving multiple or high-dose diuretic therapy (e.g. more than 80 mg of furosemide daily or its equivalent);
- with hypovolaemia;
- with hyponatraemia (plasma-sodium concentration below 130 mmol/litre);
- with pre-existing hypotension (systolic blood pressure below 90 mmHg);
- with unstable heart failure;
- with renal impairment (plasma-creatinine concentration above 150 micromol/litre);
- receiving high-dose vasodilator therapy;
- aged 70 years or more.

RENAL EFFECTS. In patients with severe bilateral renal artery stenosis (or severe stenosis of the artery supplying a single functioning kidney), ACE inhibitors reduce or abolish glomerular filtration and are likely to cause severe and progressive renal failure. They are thus contra-indicated in patients known to have these forms of critical renovascular disease.

ACE inhibitor treatment is unlikely to have an adverse effect on overall renal function in patients with severe unilateral renal artery stenosis and a normal contralateral kidney, but glomerular filtration is likely to be reduced (or even abolished) in the affected kidney and the long-term consequences are unknown.

In general, ACE inhibitors are therefore best avoided in patients with known or suspected renovascular disease, unless the blood pressure cannot be controlled by other drugs. If they are used in these circumstances renal function needs to be monitored.

ACE inhibitors should also be used with particular caution in patients who may have undiagnosed and clinically silent renovascular disease. This includes patients with peripheral vascular disease or those with severe generalised atherosclerosis.

Renal function and electrolytes should be checked before starting ACE inhibitors and monitored during treatment (more frequently if features mentioned above present). Although ACE inhibitors now have a specialised role in some forms of renal disease they also occasionally cause impairment of renal function which may progress and become severe in other circumstances (at particular risk are the elderly).

Concomitant treatment with NSAIDs increases the risk of renal damage, and potassium-sparing diuretics (or potassium-containing salt substitutes) increase the risk of hyperkalaemia.

CAUTIONS. ACE inhibitors need to be initiated with care in patients receiving diuretics (**important:** see Concomitant diuretics, below); first doses may cause hypotension especially in patients taking high doses of diuretics, on a low-sodium diet, on dialysis, dehydrated or with heart failure (see above). They should also be used with caution in peripheral vascular disease or generalised atherosclerosis owing to risk of clinically silent renovascular disease (see also above). Renal function should be monitored before and during treatment, and the dose reduced in renal impairment (see also above and Appendix 3). The risk of agranulocytosis is possibly increased in collagen vascular disease (blood counts recommended). ACE inhibitors should be used with care in patients with severe or symptomatic aortic stenosis (risk of hypotension). They should also be used with care (or avoided) in those with a history of idiopathic or hereditary angioedema. Use ACE inhibitors with caution in breast-feeding (see Appendix 5). **Interactions:** Appendix 1 (ACE inhibitors)

ANAPHYLACTOID REACTIONS. To prevent anaphylactoid reactions, ACE inhibitors should be avoided during dialysis with high-flux polyacrylonitrile membranes and during low-density lipoprotein apheresis with dextran sulphate; they should also be withheld before desensitisation with wasp or bee venom

Concomitant diuretics. ACE inhibitors can cause a very rapid fall in blood pressure in volume-depleted patients; treatment should therefore be initiated with very low doses. If the dose of diuretic is greater than 80 mg furosemide or equivalent, the ACE inhibitor should be initiated under close supervision and in some patients the diuretic dose may need to be reduced or the diuretic discontinued at least 24 hours beforehand. If high-dose diuretic therapy cannot be stopped, close observation is recommended after administration of the first dose of ACE inhibitor, for at least 2 hours or until the blood pressure has stabilised.

CONTRA-INDICATIONS. ACE inhibitors are contra-indicated in patients with hypersensitivity to ACE inhibitors (including angioedema) and in known or suspected renovascular disease (see also above). ACE inhibitors should not be used in pregnancy (Appendix 4).

SIDE-EFFECTS. ACE inhibitors can cause profound hypotension (see Cautions) and renal impairment (see Renal effects above), and a persistent dry cough. They may also cause angioedema (onset may be delayed), rash (which may be associated with pruritus and urticaria), pancreatitis and upper respiratory-tract symptoms such as sinusitis, rhinitis and sore throat. Gastro-intestinal effects reported with ACE inhibitors include nausea, vomiting, dyspepsia, diarrhoea and constipation. Altered liver function tests, cholestatic jaundice and hepatitis have been reported. Blood disorders including thrombocytopenia, leucopenia, neutropenia and haemolytic anaemia have also been reported. Other reported side-effects include headache, dizziness, fatigue, malaise, taste disturbance, paraesthesia, bronchospasm, fever, serositis, vasculitis, myalgia, arthralgia, positive antinuclear antibody, raised erythrocyte sedimentation rate, eosinophilia, leucocytosis and photosensitivity.

COMBINATION PRODUCTS. Products incorporating an ACE inhibitor with a thiazide diuretic are available for the treatment of hypertension. Use of these combination products should be reserved for patients whose blood pressure has not responded to a thiazide diuretic or an ACE inhibitor alone.

Products combining an ACE inhibitor with a calcium-channel blocker are also available for the management of hypertension. Such a combination product should be considered only for those patients who have been stabilised on the individual components in the same proportions.

CAPTOPRIL

Indications: mild to moderate essential hypertension alone or with thiazide therapy and severe hypertension resistant to other treatment; congestive heart failure (adjunct—see section 2.5.5); following myocardial infarction, see dose; diabetic nephropathy (microalbuminuria greater than 30 mg/day) in insulin-dependent diabetes

Cautions: see notes above

Contra-indications: see notes above

Side-effects: see notes above; tachycardia, serum sickness, weight loss, stomatitis, maculopapular rash, photosensitivity, flushing and acidosis

Dose: hypertension, used alone, initially 12.5 mg twice daily; if used in addition to diuretic (see notes above), or in elderly, initially 6.25 mg twice daily (first dose at bedtime); usual maintenance dose 25 mg twice daily; max. 50 mg twice daily (rarely 3 times daily in severe hypertension)

Heart failure (adjunct), initially 6.25–12.5 mg under close medical supervision (see notes above); usual maintenance dose 25 mg 2–3 times daily (but see section 2.5.5); usual max. 150 mg daily

Prophylaxis after infarction in clinically stable patients with asymptomatic or symptomatic left ventricular dysfunction (radionuclide ventriculography or echocardiography undertaken before initiation), initially 6.25 mg, starting as early as 3 days after infarction, then increased over several weeks to 150 mg daily (if tolerated) in divided doses

Diabetic nephropathy, 75–100 mg daily in divided doses; if further blood pressure reduction required, other antihypertensives may be used in conjunction with captopril; in severe renal impairment, initially 12.5 mg twice daily (if concomitant diuretic therapy required, loop diuretic rather than thiazide should be chosen)

Captopril (Non-proprietary) PoM
Tablets, captopril 12.5 mg, net price 56-tab pack = 85p; 25 mg, 56-tab pack = £1.83; 50 mg, 56-tab pack = £1.78
Brands include *Ecopace*®, *Kaplon*®, *Tensopril*®

Capoten® (Squibb) PoM
Tablets, captopril 12.5 mg (scored), net price 56-tab pack = £9.82; 25 mg, 56-tab pack = £11.19, 84-tab pack = £16.79; 50 mg (scored), 56-tab pack = £19.07, 84-tab pack = £28.60 (also available as *Acepril*®)

■ With diuretic

NOTE. For mild to moderate hypertension in patients stabilised on the individual components in the same proportions

Co-zidocapt (Non-proprietary) PoM
Tablets, co-zidocapt 12.5/25 (hydrochlorothiazide 12.5 mg, captopril 25 mg), net price 28-tab pack = £11.00
Brands include *Capto-co*®

Tablets, co-zidocapt 25/50 (hydrochlorothiazide 25 mg, captopril 50 mg), net price 28-tab pack = £14.00
Brands include *Capto-co*®

Capozide® (Squibb) PoM
LS tablets, scored, co-zidocapt 12.5/25 (hydrochlorothiazide 12.5 mg, captopril 25 mg). Net price 28-tab pack = £10.46
Tablets, scored, co-zidocapt 25/50 (hydrochlorothiazide 25 mg, captopril 50 mg). Net price 28-tab pack = £13.15 (also available as *Acezide*®)

CILAZAPRIL

Indications: essential hypertension; congestive heart failure (adjunct—see section 2.5.5)
Cautions: see notes above; severe hepatic impairment (Appendix 2)
Contra-indications: see notes above; ascites
Side-effects: see notes above; dyspnoea and bronchitis
Dose: hypertension, initially 1 mg once daily (reduced to 500 micrograms daily in those receiving a diuretic (see notes above), in the elderly, and in renal impairment), then adjusted according to response; usual maintenance dose 2.5–5 mg once daily; max. 5 mg daily
Heart failure (adjunct), initially 500 micrograms once daily under close medical supervision (see notes above), increased to 1 mg once daily; usual maintenance dose 1–2.5 mg daily; max. 5 mg daily

Vascace® (Roche) PoM
Tablets, f/c, cilazapril 500 micrograms (white), net price 28-tab pack = £3.65; 1 mg (yellow), 28-tab pack = £6.01; 2.5 mg (pink), 28-tab pack = £7.64; 5 mg (brown), 28-tab pack = £13.28

ENALAPRIL MALEATE

Indications: hypertension; symptomatic heart failure (adjunct—see section 2.5.5); prevention of symptomatic heart failure in patients with left ventricular dysfunction
Cautions: see notes above; hepatic impairment (Appendix 2)
Contra-indications: see notes above
Side-effects: see notes above; also palpitation, arrhythmias, angina, chest pain, Raynaud's syndrome, syncope, cerebrovascular accident, myocardial infarction; abdominal pain, dry mouth, peptic ulcer, anorexia, ileus, stomatitis, glossitis, hepatic failure; dermatological side-effects including Stevens-Johnson syndrome, toxic epidermal necrolysis, exfoliative dermatitis and pemphigus; gastro-intestinal angioedema, confusion, depression, nervousness, asthenia, drowsiness, insomnia, dream abnormalities, vertigo, blurred vision, tinnitus, flushing, impotence, gynaecomastia, alopecia, dyspnoea, asthma, pulmonary infiltrates, muscle cramps, and hyponatraemia
Dose: hypertension, used alone, initially 5 mg once daily; if used in addition to diuretic (see notes above), or in renal impairment, lower initial doses may be required; usual maintenance dose 20 mg once daily; max. 40 mg once daily
Heart failure (adjunct), asymptomatic left ventricular dysfunction, initially 2.5 mg daily under close medical supervision (see notes above); increased over 2–4 weeks to usual maintenance dose 20 mg daily in 1–2 divided doses (but see section 2.5.5); max. 40 mg daily

Enalapril Maleate (Non-proprietary) PoM
Tablets, enalapril maleate 2.5 mg, net price 28-tab pack = £1.00; 5 mg, 28-tab pack = £1.51; 10 mg, 28-tab pack = £1.46; 20 mg, 28-tab pack = £1.60
Brands include *Ednyt*®

Innovace® (MSD) PoM
Tablets, enalapril maleate 2.5 mg, net price 28-tab pack = £5.35; 5 mg (scored), 28-tab pack = £7.51; 10 mg (red), 28-tab pack = £10.53; 20 mg (peach), 28-tab pack = £12.51

■ With diuretic
NOTE. For mild to moderate hypertension in patients stabilised on the individual components in the same proportions

Innozide® (MSD) PoM
Tablets, yellow, scored, enalapril maleate 20 mg, hydrochlorothiazide 12.5 mg. Net price 28-tab pack = £13.90
NOTE. Non-proprietary tablets containing enalapril maleate (20 mg) and hydrochlorothiazide (12.5 mg) are available

FOSINOPRIL SODIUM

Indications: hypertension; congestive heart failure (adjunct—see section 2.5.5)
Cautions: see notes above; hepatic impairment (Appendix 2)
Contra-indications: see notes above
Side-effects: see notes above; abdominal pain; chest pain; musculoskeletal pain
Dose: hypertension, initially 10 mg daily, increased if necessary after 4 weeks; usual dose range 10–40 mg (doses over 40 mg not shown to increase efficacy); if used in addition to diuretic see notes above
Heart failure (adjunct), initially 10 mg daily under close medical supervision (see notes above); if initial dose well tolerated, may be increased to up to 40 mg once daily

Fosinopril sodium (Non-proprietary) PoM
Tablets, fosinopril sodium 10 mg, net price 28-tab pack = £8.45; 20 mg, 28-tab pack = £10.13

Staril® (Squibb) PoM
Tablets, fosinopril sodium 10 mg, net price 28-tab pack = £11.20; 20 mg, 28-tab pack = £12.09

IMIDAPRIL HYDROCHLORIDE

Indications: essential hypertension
Cautions: see notes above; hepatic impairment (Appendix 2)
Contra-indications: see notes above
Side-effects: see notes above; dry mouth, glossitis, abdominal pain, ileus; bronchitis, dyspnoea; sleep disturbances, depression, confusion, blurred vision, tinnitus, impotence
Dose: initially 5 mg daily before food; if used in addition to diuretic (see notes above), in elderly, in patients with heart failure, angina or cerebrovascular disease, or in renal or hepatic impairment, initially 2.5 mg daily; if necessary increase dose at intervals of at least 3 weeks; usual maintenance dose 10 mg once daily; max. 20 mg daily (elderly, 10 mg daily)

Tanatril (Trinity) PoM
Tablets, scored, imidapril hydrochloride 5 mg, net price 28-tab pack = £5.65; 10 mg, 28-tab pack = £6.39; 20 mg, 28-tab pack = £7.67

LISINOPRIL

Indications: essential and renovascular hypertension (but see notes above); congestive heart failure (adjunct—see section 2.5.5); following myocardial infarction in haemodynamically stable patients; diabetic nephropathy in normotensive insulin-dependent and hypertensive non-insulin-dependent diabetes mellitus

Cautions: see notes above

Contra-indications: see notes above

Side-effects: see notes above; tachycardia, cerebrovascular accident, myocardial infarction; dry mouth, blurred vision, confusion, mood changes, asthenia, sweating, impotence and alopecia

Dose: hypertension, initially 10 mg daily; if used in addition to diuretic (see notes above) or in renal impairment, initially 2.5–5 mg daily; usual maintenance dose 20 mg once daily; max. 80 mg daily

Heart failure (adjunct), initially 2.5 mg daily under close medical supervision (see notes above); usual maintenance dose 5–20 mg daily (but see section 2.5.5)

Prophylaxis after myocardial infarction, systolic blood pressure over 120 mmHg, 5 mg within 24 hours, followed by further 5 mg 24 hours later, then 10 mg after a further 24 hours, and continuing with 10 mg once daily for 6 weeks (or continued if heart failure); systolic blood pressure 100–120 mmHg, initially 2.5 mg, increasing to maintenance dose of 5 mg once daily

NOTE. Should not be started after myocardial infarction if systolic blood pressure less than 100 mmHg; temporarily reduce maintenance dose to 5 mg and if necessary 2.5 mg daily if systolic blood pressure 100 mmHg or less during treatment; withdraw if prolonged hypotension occurs (systolic blood pressure less than 90 mmHg for more than 1 hour)

Diabetic nephropathy, initially 2.5 mg daily adjusted to achieve a sitting diastolic blood pressure below 75 mmHg in normotensive insulin-dependent diabetes and below 90 mmHg in hypertensive non-insulin dependent diabetes; usual dose range 10–20 mg daily

Lisinopril (Non-proprietary) PoM
Tablets, lisinopril (as dihydrate) 2.5 mg, net price 28-tab pack = £1.76; 5 mg, 28-tab pack = £1.98; 10 mg, 28-tab pack = £1.78; 20 mg, 28-tab pack = £2.43

Carace® (Bristol-Myers Squibb) PoM
Tablets, lisinopril 2.5 mg (blue), net price 28-tab pack = £6.79; 5 mg (scored), 28-tab pack = £8.51; 10 mg (yellow, scored), 28-tab pack = £10.51; 20 mg (orange, scored), 28-tab pack = £11.89

Zestril® (AstraZeneca) PoM
Tablets, lisinopril (as dihydrate) 2.5 mg, net price 28-tab pack = £6.26; 5 mg (pink, scored), 28-tab pack = £7.86; 10 mg (pink), 28-tab pack = £9.70; 20 mg (pink), 28-tab pack = £10.97

■ With diuretic

NOTE. For mild to moderate hypertension in patients stabilised on the individual components in the same proportions

Carace Plus® (Bristol-Myers Squibb) PoM
Carace 10 Plus tablets, blue, lisinopril 10 mg, hydrochlorothiazide 12.5 mg. Net price 28-tab pack = £10.51
Carace 20 Plus tablets, yellow, scored, lisinopril 20 mg, hydrochlorothiazide 12.5 mg. Net price 28-tab pack = £11.89

Caralpha® (Alpharma) PoM
Caralpha 10/12.5 mg tablets, peach, lisinopril (as dihydrate) 10 mg, hydrochlorothiazide 12.5 mg, net price 28-tab pack = £10.51
Caralpha 20/12.5 mg tablets, scored, lisinopril (as dihydrate) 20 mg, hydrochlorothiazide 12.5 mg, net price 28-tab pack = £11.89

Lisicostad® (Genus) PoM
Lisicostad 10/12.5 mg tablets, scored, lisinopril (as dihydrate) 10 mg, hydrochlorothiazide 12.5 mg, net price 28-tab pack = £10.99
Lisicostad 20/12.5 mg tablets, scored, lisinopril (as dihydrate) 20 mg, hydrochlorothiazide 12.5 mg, net price 28-tab pack = £11.99

Zestoretic® (AstraZeneca) PoM
Zestoretic 10 tablets, peach, lisinopril (as dihydrate) 10 mg, hydrochlorothiazide 12.5 mg. Net price 28-tab pack = £13.01
Zestoretic 20 tablets, lisinopril (as dihydrate) 20 mg, hydrochlorothiazide 12.5 mg. Net price 28-tab pack = £14.72

MOEXIPRIL HYDROCHLORIDE

Indications: essential hypertension

Cautions: see notes above; hepatic impairment (Appendix 2)

Contra-indications: see notes above

Side-effects: see notes above; arrhythmias, angina, chest pain, syncope, cerebrovascular accident, myocardial infarction; appetite and weight changes; dry mouth, photosensitivity, flushing, nervousness, mood changes, anxiety, drowsiness, sleep disturbance, tinnitus, influenza-like syndrome, sweating and dyspnoea

Dose: used alone, initially 7.5 mg once daily; if used in addition to diuretic (see notes above), with nifedipine, in elderly, in renal or hepatic impairment, initially 3.75 mg once daily; usual range 15–30 mg once daily; doses above 30 mg daily not shown to increase efficacy

Perdix® (Schwarz) PoM
Tablets, f/c, both pink, scored, moexipril hydrochloride 7.5 mg, net price 28-tab pack = £7.55; 15 mg, 28-tab pack = £8.70

PERINDOPRIL ERBUMINE

Indications: hypertension (but see notes above); symptomatic heart failure (adjunct—see section 2.5.5)

Cautions: see notes above; hepatic impairment (Appendix 2)

Contra-indications: see notes above

Side-effects: see notes above; asthenia, mood and sleep disturbances

Dose: hypertension, initially 4 mg daily (before food); if used in addition to diuretic (see notes above), in elderly or in renal impairment, initially

2 mg daily; usual maintenance dose 4 mg once daily; max. 8 mg daily

Heart failure (adjunct), initial dose 2 mg in the morning under close medical supervision (see notes above); usual maintenance 4 mg once daily (before food)

Coversyl® (Servier) PoM

Tablets, perindopril erbumine (= *tert*-butylamine) 2 mg (white), net price 30-tab pack = £10.95; 4 mg (light green, scored), 30-tab pack = £10.95; 8 mg (green), 30-tab pack = £10.95

■ With diuretic

NOTE. For hypertension not adequately controlled by perindopril alone

Coversyl® Plus (Servier) PoM

Tablets, perindopril erbumine (= *tert*-butylamine) 4 mg, indapamide 1.25 mg, net price 30-tab pack = £13.96

QUINAPRIL

Indications: essential hypertension; congestive heart failure (adjunct—see section 2.5.5)

Cautions: see notes above; hepatic impairment (Appendix 2)

Contra-indications: see notes above

Side-effects: see notes above; asthenia, chest pain, oedema, flatulence, nervousness, depression, insomnia, blurred vision, impotence, back pain and myalgia

Dose: hypertension, initially 10 mg once daily; with a diuretic (see notes above), in elderly, or in renal impairment initially 2.5 mg daily; usual maintenance dose 20–40 mg daily in single or 2 divided doses; up to 80 mg daily has been given

Heart failure (adjunct), initial dose 2.5 mg under close medical supervision (see notes above); usual maintenance 10–20 mg daily in single or 2 divided doses; up to 40 mg daily has been given

Quinapril (Non-proprietary) PoM

Tablets, quinapril (as hydrochloride) 5 mg, net price 28-tab pack = £8.16; 10 mg, 28-tab pack = £5.32; 20 mg, 28-tab pack = £5.92; 40 mg, 28-tab pack = £6.15

Brands include *Quinil*®

Accupro® (Pfizer) PoM

Tablets, all brown, f/c, quinapril (as hydrochloride) 5 mg, net price 28-tab pack = £8.60; 10 mg, 28-tab pack = £8.60; 20 mg, 28-tab pack = £10.79; 40 mg, 28-tab pack = £9.75

■ With diuretic

NOTE. For hypertension in patients stabilised on the individual components in the same proportions

Accuretic® (Pfizer) PoM

Tablets, pink, f/c, scored, quinapril (as hydrochloride) 10 mg, hydrochlorothiazide 12.5 mg. Net price 28-tab pack = £11.75

RAMIPRIL

Indications: mild to moderate hypertension; congestive heart failure (adjunct—see section 2.5.5); following myocardial infarction in patients with clinical evidence of heart failure; susceptible patients over 55 years, prevention of myocardial infarction, stroke, cardiovascular death or need of revascularisation procedures (consult product literature)

Cautions: see notes above; hepatic impairment (Appendix 2)

Contra-indications: see notes above

Side-effects: see notes above; arrhythmias, angina, chest pain, syncope, cerebrovascular accident, myocardial infarction, loss of appetite, stomatitis, dry mouth, skin reactions including erythema multiforme and pemphigoid exanthema; precipitation or exacerbation of Raynaud's syndrome; conjunctivitis, onycholysis, confusion, nervousness, depression, anxiety, impotence, decreased libido, alopecia, bronchitis and muscle cramps

Dose: hypertension, initially 1.25 mg once daily, increased at intervals of 1–2 weeks; usual range 2.5–5 mg once daily; max. 10 mg once daily; if used in addition to diuretic see notes above

Heart failure (adjunct), initially 1.25 mg once daily under close medical supervision (see notes above), increased if necessary at intervals of 1–2 weeks; max. 10 mg daily (daily doses of 2.5 mg or more may be taken in 1–2 divided doses) (see also section 2.5.5)

Prophylaxis after myocardial infarction (started in hospital 3 to 10 days after infarction), initially 2.5 mg twice daily, increased after 2 days to 5 mg twice daily; maintenance 2.5–5 mg twice daily

NOTE. If initial 2.5-mg dose not tolerated, give 1.25 mg twice daily for 2 days before increasing to 2.5 mg twice daily, then 5 mg twice daily; withdraw if 2.5 mg twice daily not tolerated

Prophylaxis of cardiovascular events or stroke, initially 2.5 mg once daily, increased after 1 week to 5 mg once daily, then increased after a further 3 weeks to 10 mg once daily

Ramipril (Non-proprietary) PoM

Capsules, ramipril 2.5 mg, net price 28-cap pack = £3.74; 5 mg, 28-cap pack = £4.76; 10 mg, 28-cap pack = £6.42

Brands include *Lopace*®

Tritace® (Aventis Pharma) PoM

Tablets, all scored, ramipril 1.25 mg (white), net price 28-tab pack = £5.30; 2.5 mg (yellow), 28-tab pack = £7.51; 5 mg (red), 28-tab pack = £10.46; 10 mg (white), 28-tab pack = £14.24

Titration pack, capsules, 35-day starter pack of ramipril 7 × 2.5 mg with 21 × 5 mg and 7 × 10 mg, net price = £13.00

■ With calcium-channel blocker

NOTE. For hypertension in patients stabilised on the individual components in the same proportions. For cautions, contra-indications and side-effects of felodipine, see section 2.6.2

Triapin® (Aventis Pharma) ▼ PoM

Triapin® tablets, f/c, brown, ramipril 5 mg, felodipine 5 mg (m/r), net price 28-tab pack = £24.46. Label: 25

Triapin mite® tablets, f/c, orange, ramipril 2.5 mg, felodipine 2.5 mg (m/r), net price 28-tab pack = £19.37. Label: 25

TRANDOLAPRIL

Indications: mild to moderate hypertension; following myocardial infarction in patients with left ventricular dysfunction; heart failure [unlicensed] see section 2.5.5

Cautions: see notes above; hepatic impairment (Appendix 2)

Contra-indications: see notes above

Side-effects: see notes above; tachycardia, arrhythmias, angina, transient ischaemic attacks, cerebral haemorrhage, myocardial infarction; ileus, dry mouth; skin reactions including Stevens-Johnson syndrome, toxic epidermal necrolysis, psoriasis-like efflorescence; asthenia, alopecia, dyspnoea and bronchitis

Dose: hypertension, initially 500 micrograms once daily, increased at intervals of 2–4 weeks; usual range 1–2 mg once daily; max. 4 mg daily; if used in addition to diuretic see notes above

Prophylaxis after myocardial infarction (starting as early as 3 days after infarction), initially 500 micrograms daily, gradually increased to max. 4 mg once daily

NOTE. If symptomatic hypotension develops during titration, do not increase dose further; if possible, reduce dose of any adjunctive treatment and if this is not effective or feasible, reduce dose of trandolapril

Gopten® (Abbott) PoM

Capsules, trandolapril 500 micrograms (red/yellow), net price 14-cap pack = £1.71; 1 mg (red/orange), 28-cap pack = £12.28; 2 mg (red/red), 28-cap pack = £8.39; 4 mg (red/maroon), 28-cap pack = £14.24

Odrik® (Aventis Pharma) PoM

Capsules, trandolapril 500 micrograms (red/yellow), net price 28-cap pack = £7.62; 1 mg (red/orange), 28-cap pack = £9.62; 2 mg (red/red), 28-cap pack = £11.43

■ With calcium-channel blocker

NOTE. For hypertension in patients stabilised on the individual components in the same proportions. For cautions, contra-indications and side-effects of verapamil, see section 2.6.2

Tarka® (Abbott) ▼ PoM

Capsules, pink, trandolapril 2 mg, verapamil hydrochloride 180 mg (m/r). Net price 28 cap-pack = £17.85. Label: 25

2.5.5.2 Angiotensin-II receptor antagonists

Candesartan, **irbesartan**, **losartan**, and **valsartan** are specific angiotensin-II receptor antagonists with many properties similar to those of the ACE inhibitors; **eprosartan**, **olmesartan**, and **telmisartan** have been introduced more recently. However, unlike ACE inhibitors, they do not inhibit the breakdown of bradykinin and other kinins, and thus do not appear to cause the persistent dry cough which commonly complicates ACE inhibitor therapy. They are therefore a useful alternative for patients who have to discontinue an ACE inhibitor because of persistent cough.

An angiotensin-II receptor antagonist may be used as an alternative to an ACE inhibitor in the management of heart failure (section 2.5.5) or diabetic nephropathy (section 6.1.5).

CAUTIONS. Angiotensin-II receptor antagonists should be used with caution in renal artery stenosis (see also Renal Effects under ACE Inhibitors, section 2.5.5.1). Monitoring of plasma-potassium concentration is advised, particularly in the elderly and in patients with renal impairment; lower initial doses may be appropriate in these patients. Angiotensin-II receptor antagonists should be used with caution in aortic or mitral valve stenosis and in obstructive hypertrophic cardiomyopathy. Afro-Caribbean patients, particularly those with left ventricular hypertrophy, may not benefit from an angiotensin-II receptor antagonist. **Interactions:** Appendix 1 (angiotensin-II receptor antagonists).

CONTRA-INDICATIONS. Angiotensin-II receptor antagonists, like the ACE inhibitors, should be avoided in pregnancy (see also Appendix 4).

SIDE-EFFECTS. Side-effects are usually mild. Symptomatic hypotension including dizziness may occur, particularly in patients with intravascular volume depletion (e.g. those taking high-dose diuretics). Hyperkalaemia occurs occasionally; angioedema has also been reported with some angiotensin-II receptor antagonists.

CANDESARTAN CILEXETIL

Indications: hypertension; heart failure with impaired left ventricular systolic function (see also notes above)

Cautions: see notes above; hepatic impairment (Appendix 2); renal impairment (Appendix 3)

Contra-indications: see notes above; breast-feeding (Appendix 5); cholestasis

Side-effects: see notes above; also vertigo, headache; *very rarely* nausea, hepatitis, blood disorders, hyponatraemia, back pain, arthralgia, myalgia, rash, urticaria, pruritus

Dose: hypertension, initially 8 mg (hepatic impairment 2 mg, renal impairment or intravascular volume depletion 4 mg) once daily, increased if necessary at intervals of 4 weeks to max. 32 mg once daily; usual maintenance dose 8 mg once daily

Heart failure, initially 4 mg once daily, increased at intervals of at least 2 weeks to 'target' dose of 32 mg once daily or to max. tolerated dose

Amias® (Takeda) PoM

Tablets, candesartan cilexetil 2 mg, net price 7-tab pack = £2.99; 4 mg (scored), 7-tab pack = £3.24, 28-tab pack = £8.15; 8 mg (pink, scored), 28-tab pack = £9.89; 16 mg (pink, scored), 28-tab pack = £12.72; 32 mg (pink), 28-tab pack = £16.13

EPROSARTAN

Indications: hypertension (see also notes above)

Cautions: see notes above; also renal impairment (Appendix 3); breast-feeding (Appendix 5)

Contra-indications: see notes above; also severe hepatic impairment (Appendix 2)

Side-effects: see notes above; also flatulence, arthralgia, rhinitis; hypertriglyceridaemia, rarely anaemia

Dose: 600 mg once daily (elderly over 75 years, mild to moderate hepatic impairment, renal impairment, initially 300 mg once daily); if necessary increased after 2–3 weeks to 800 mg once daily

Teveten® (Solvay) PoM

Tablets, f/c, eprosartan (as mesilate) 300 mg, net price 28-tab pack = £11.63; 400 mg, 56-tab pack = £15.77; 600 mg, 28-tab pack = £14.31. Label: 21

IRBESARTAN

Indications: hypertension; renal disease in hypertensive type 2 diabetes mellitus (see also notes above)
Cautions: see notes above
Contra-indications: see notes above; breast-feeding (Appendix 5)
Side-effects: see notes above; nausea, vomiting, fatigue, musculoskeletal pain; less commonly diarrhoea, dyspepsia, flushing, tachycardia, cough; sexual dysfunction; rarely rash, urticaria; headache, myalgia, arthralgia, tinnitus, taste disturbance, hepatitis, renal dysfunction also reported
Dose: hypertension, initially 150 mg once daily, increased if necessary to 300 mg once daily. Renal disease in hypertensive type 2 diabetes mellitus, initially 150 mg once daily, increased according to response to 300 mg once daily (in haemodialysis or in elderly over 75 years, initial dose of 75 mg once daily may be used)

Aprovel® (Bristol-Myers Squibb, Sanofi-Synthelabo) PoM
Tablets, f/c, irbesartan 75 mg, net price 28-tab pack = £10.29; 150 mg, 28-tab pack = £12.57; 300 mg, 28-tab pack = £16.91

■ With diuretic
NOTE. For hypertension not adequately controlled on individual components

CoAprovel® (Bristol-Myers Squibb, Sanofi-Synthelabo) PoM
Tablets, f/c, both peach, irbesartan 150 mg, hydrochlorothiazide 12.5 mg, net price 28-tab pack = £12.57; irbesartan 300 mg, hydrochlorothiazide 12.5 mg, 28-tab pack = £16.91

LOSARTAN POTASSIUM

Indications: hypertension, including patients with left ventricular hypertrophy; diabetic nephropathy in type 2 diabetes mellitus (see also notes above)
Cautions: see notes above; hepatic impairment (Appendix 2); renal impairment (Appendix 3)
Contra-indications: see notes above; breast-feeding (Appendix 5)
Side-effects: see notes above; diarrhoea, taste disturbance, cough, myalgia, asthenia, fatigue, migraine, vertigo, urticaria, pruritus, rash; *rarely* hepatitis, anaemia (in severe renal disease or following renal transplant), vasculitis (including Henoch-Schönlein purpura)
Dose: usually 50 mg once daily (elderly over 75 years, moderate to severe renal impairment, intravascular volume depletion, initially 25 mg once daily); if necessary increased after several weeks to 100 mg once daily

Cozaar® (MSD) PoM
Tablets, f/c, losartan potassium 25 mg (Half Strength), net price 28-tab pack = £18.09; 50 mg (scored), 28-tab pack = £18.09; 100 mg, 28-tab pack = £24.20

■ With diuretic
NOTE. For hypertension not adequately controlled on individual components

Cozaar-Comp® (MSD) PoM
Tablets, f/c, yellow, losartan potassium 50 mg, hydrochlorothiazide 12.5 mg. Net price 28-tab pack = £18.09

OLMESARTAN MEDOXOMIL

Indications: hypertension (see also notes above)
Cautions: see notes above
Contra-indications: see notes above; hepatic impairment (Appendix 2); moderate to severe renal impairment (Appendix 3); biliary obstruction; breast-feeding (Appendix 5)
Side-effects: see notes above; also abdominal pain, diarrhoea, dyspepsia, nausea, influenza-like symptoms, cough, pharyngitis, rhinitis, haematuria, urinary-tract infection, peripheral oedema, arthritis, musculoskeletal pain; less commonly angina, vertigo, rash
Dose: initially 10 mg once daily; if necessary increased to 20 mg once daily; max. 40 mg daily (ELDERLY max. 20 mg daily)

Olmetec® (Sankyo) ▼ PoM
Tablets, f/c, olmesartan medoxomil 10 mg, net price 28-tab pack = £10.95; 20 mg, 28-tab pack = £12.95; 40 mg, 28-tab pack = £17.50

TELMISARTAN

Indications: hypertension (see also notes above)
Cautions: see notes above; hepatic impairment—avoid if severe (Appendix 2); renal impairment (Appendix 3)
Contra-indications: see notes above; biliary obstruction; breast-feeding (Appendix 5)
Side-effects: see notes above; also gastro-intestinal disturbances; influenza-like symptoms including pharyngitis and sinusitis; arthralgia, myalgia, back pain, leg cramps; eczema; *less commonly* dry mouth, flatulence, anxiety, vertigo, tendinitis-like symptoms, abnormal vision, increased sweating; *rarely* bradycardia, tachycardia, dyspnoea, insomnia, depression, blood disorders, increase in uric acid, eosinophilia, rash, and pruritus
Dose: usually 40 mg once daily (but 20 mg may be sufficient), increased if necessary after at least 4 weeks, to max. 80 mg once daily

Micardis® (Boehringer Ingelheim) PoM
Tablets, telmisartan 20 mg, net price 28-tab pack = £11.34; 40 mg, 28-tab pack = £11.34; 80 mg, 28-tab pack = £14.18

■ With diuretic
NOTE. For patients with hypertension not adequately controlled by telmisartan alone

Micardis Plus® (Boehringer Ingelheim) ▼ PoM
Tablets 40/12.5, red/white, telmisartan 40 mg, hydrochlorothiazide 12.5 mg, net price 28-tab pack = £11.34
Tablets 80/12.5, red/white, telmisartan 80 mg, hydrochlorothiazide 12.5 mg, net price 28-tab pack = £14.18

VALSARTAN

Indications: hypertension; myocardial infarction with left ventricular failure or left ventricular systolic dysfunction (see also notes above)
Cautions: see notes above; mild to moderate hepatic impairment (Appendix 2); renal impairment (Appendix 3)
Contra-indications: see notes above; severe hepatic impairment (Appendix 2), cirrhosis, biliary obstruction, breast-feeding (Appendix 5)
Side-effects: see notes above; fatigue, rarely diarrhoea, headache, epistaxis; thrombocytopenia,

arthralgia, myalgia, taste disturbance, neutropenia reported

Dose: hypertension, usually 80 mg once daily (elderly over 75 years, mild to moderate hepatic impairment, moderate to severe renal impairment, intravascular volume depletion, initially 40 mg once daily); if necessary increased after at least 4 weeks to 160 mg daily

Myocardial infarction, initially 20 mg twice daily increased over several weeks to 160 mg twice daily if tolerated (consider lower dose in mild to moderate hepatic impairment)

Diovan® (Novartis) PoM

Capsules, valsartan 40 mg (grey), net price 7-cap pack = £3.69; 80 mg (grey/pink), 28-cap pack = £16.44; 160 mg (dark grey/pink), 28-cap pack = £21.66

Tablets, yellow, scored, valsartan 40 mg, net price 7-tab pack = £3.69

■ With diuretic

NOTE. For hypertension not adequately controlled by valsartan alone

Co-Diovan® (Novartis) ▼ PoM

Tablets, f/c, valsartan 80 mg, hydrochlorothiazide 12.5 mg (orange), net price 28-tab pack = £16.44; valsartan 160 mg, hydrochlorothiazide 12.5 mg (red), 28-tab pack = £21.66; valsartan 160 mg, hydrochlorothaizide 25 mg (brown-orange), 28-tab pack = £21.66

2.5.6 Ganglion-blocking drugs

Trimetaphan, a ganglion-blocking drug, was used to reduce blood pressure during surgery. It has been discontinued.

2.5.7 Tyrosine hydroxylase inhibitors

Metirosine (*Demser*®, MSD, available on named-patient basis) inhibits the enzyme tyrosine hydroxylase, and hence the synthesis of catecholamines. It is used in the pre-operative management of phaeochromocytoma, and long term in patients unsuitable for surgery; an alpha-adrenoceptor blocking drug (e.g. phenoxybenzamine, section 2.5.4) may also be required. Metirosine should **not** be used to treat essential hypertension.

2.6 Nitrates, calcium-channel blockers, and potassium-channel activators

Nitrates, calcium-channel blockers and potassium-channel activators have a vasodilating effect. Vasodilators are known to act in heart failure either by arteriolar dilatation which reduces both peripheral vascular resistance and left ventricular pressure at systole and results in improved cardiac output, *or* venous dilatation which results in dilatation of capacitance vessels, increase of venous pooling, and diminution of venous return to the heart (decreasing left ventricular end-diastolic pressure).

Angina

Stable angina usually results from atherosclerotic plaques in the coronary arteries, whereas *unstable angina* is usually due to plaque rupture and may occur either in patients with a history of stable angina or in those with previously silent coronary artery disease. It is important to distinguish unstable from stable angina; unstable angina is usually characterised by new onset severe angina or sudden worsening of previously stable angina.

STABLE ANGINA. Acute attacks of stable angina should be managed with sublingual **glyceryl trinitrate**. If attacks occur more than twice a week, regular drug therapy is required and should be introduced in a stepwise manner according to response. **Aspirin** (section 2.9) should be given to patients with angina; a dose of 75 mg daily is suitable. Revascularisation procedures may also be appropriate.

Patients with mild or moderate stable angina who do not have left ventricular dysfunction, may be managed effectively with sublingual glyceryl trinitrate and regular administration of a **beta-blocker** (section 2.4). If necessary a long-acting **dihydropyridine calcium-channel blocker** (section 2.6.2) and then a **long-acting nitrate** (section 2.6.1) may be added. For those without left ventricular dysfunction and in whom beta-blockers are inappropriate, **diltiazem** or **verapamil** may be given (section 2.6.2) and a long-acting nitrate (section 2.6.1) may be added if symptom control is not adequate. For those intolerant of standard treatment, or where standard treatment has failed, nicorandil may be tried.

For patients with left ventricular dysfunction a long-acting nitrate (section 2.6.1) should be used and a long-acting dihydropyridine calcium-channel blocker (section 2.6.2) may be added if necessary.

A **statin** (section 2.12) should be prescribed for those with an elevated plasma-cholesterol concentration.

UNSTABLE ANGINA. Patients with unstable angina should be admitted to hospital. The aims of management of unstable angina are to provide supportive care and pain relief during the acute attack and to prevent myocardial infarction and death.

Initial management. **Aspirin** (chewed or dispersed in water) is given for its antiplatelet effect at a dose of 300 mg (section 2.9). If aspirin is given before arrival at hospital, a note saying that it has been given should be sent with the patient.

Heparin (section 2.8.1) or the low molecular weight heparins **dalteparin** or **enoxaparin** (section 2.8.1) should also be given.

Nitrates (section 2.6.1) are used to relieve ischaemic pain. If sublingual glyceryl trinitrate is not effective, intravenous or buccal glyceryl trinitrate or intravenous isosorbide dinitrate is given.

Patients without contra-indications should receive intravenous or oral **beta-blockers** (section 2.4). In patients without left ventricular dysfunction and in whom beta-blockers are inappropriate, **diltiazem** or **verapamil** may be given (section 2.6.2).

The glycoprotein IIb/IIIa inhibitors **eptifibatide** and **tirofiban** (section 2.9) are recommended (with aspirin and heparin) for unstable angina in patients with a high risk of developing myocardial infarction.

Abciximab, eptifibatide or tirofiban may also be used with aspirin and heparin in patients undergoing percutaneous coronary intervention, to reduce the immediate risk of vascular occlusion.

Revascularisation procedures are often appropriate for patients with unstable angina.

Long-term management. The importance of life-style changes, especially stopping smoking, should be emphasised. Patients should receive low-dose **aspirin** indefinitely—a dose of 75 mg daily is suitable. A **statin** (section 2.12) should also be prescribed. The need for long-term angina treatment or for coronary angiography should be assessed. If there is continuing ischaemia, standard angina treatment should be continued; if not, antianginal treatment may be withdrawn cautiously at least 2 months after the acute attack.

2.6.1 Nitrates

Nitrates have a useful role in *angina* (for details on the management of stable angina, see section 2.6). Although they are potent coronary vasodilators, their principal benefit follows from a reduction in venous return which reduces left ventricular work. Unwanted effects such as flushing, headache, and postural hypotension may limit therapy, especially when angina is severe or when patients are unusually sensitive to the effects of nitrates.

Sublingual **glyceryl trinitrate** is one of the most effective drugs for providing rapid symptomatic relief of angina, but its effect lasts only for 20 to 30 minutes; the 300-microgram tablet is often appropriate when glyceryl trinitrate is first used. The *aerosol spray* provides an alternative method of rapid relief of symptoms for those who find difficulty in dissolving sublingual preparations. Duration of action may be prolonged by *modified-release* and *transdermal* preparations (but tolerance may develop, see below).

Isosorbide dinitrate is active *sublingually* and is a more stable preparation for those who only require nitrates infrequently. It is also effective by mouth for prophylaxis; although the effect is slower in onset, it may persist for several hours. Duration of action of up to 12 hours is claimed for *modified-release* preparations. The activity of isosorbide dinitrate may depend on the production of active metabolites, the most important of which is isosorbide mononitrate. **Isosorbide mononitrate** itself is also licensed for angina prophylaxis; modified-release formulations (for once daily administration) are available.

Glyceryl trinitrate or isosorbide dinitrate may be tried by *intravenous injection* when the sublingual form is ineffective in patients with chest pain due to myocardial infarction or severe ischaemia. Intravenous injections are also useful in the treatment of acute left ventricular failure.

TOLERANCE. Many patients on long-acting or transdermal nitrates rapidly develop tolerance (with reduced therapeutic effects). Reduction of blood-nitrate concentrations to low levels for 4 to 8 hours each day usually maintains effectiveness in such patients. If tolerance is suspected during the use of transdermal patches they should be left off for several consecutive hours in each 24 hours; in the case of modified-release tablets of isosorbide dinitrate (and conventional formulations of isosorbide mononitrate), the second of the two daily doses can be given after about 8 hours rather than after 12 hours. Conventional formulations of isosorbide mononitrate should not usually be given more than twice daily unless small doses are used; modified-release formulations of isosorbide mononitrate should only be given once daily, and used in this way do not produce tolerance.

GLYCERYL TRINITRATE

Indications: prophylaxis and treatment of angina; left ventricular failure

Cautions: severe hepatic or renal impairment; hypothyroidism, malnutrition, or hypothermia; head trauma, cerebral haemorrhage; recent history of myocardial infarction; metal-containing transdermal systems should be removed before cardioversion or diathermy; tolerance (see notes above); **interactions:** Appendix 1 (glyceryl trinitrate)

Contra-indications: hypersensitivity to nitrates; hypotensive conditions and hypovolaemia; hypertrophic obstructive cardiomyopathy, aortic stenosis, cardiac tamponade, constrictive pericarditis, mitral stenosis; marked anaemia, closed-angle glaucoma

Side-effects: throbbing headache, flushing, dizziness, postural hypotension, tachycardia (but paradoxical bradycardia has occurred)

INJECTION. Specific side-effects following injection (particularly if given too rapidly) include severe hypotension, nausea and retching, diaphoresis, apprehension, restlessness, muscle twitching, retrosternal discomfort, palpitation, abdominal pain, syncope; prolonged administration has been associated with methaemoglobinaemia

Dose: *sublingually*, 0.3–1 mg, repeated as required

By mouth, see under preparations

By intravenous infusion, 10–200 micrograms/minute

■ Short-acting tablets and sprays

Glyceryl Trinitrate (Non-proprietary)

Sublingual tablets, glyceryl trinitrate 300 micrograms, net price 100 = £2.71; 500 micrograms, 100 = £2.36; 600 micrograms, 100 = £3.86. Label: 16

NOTE. Glyceryl trinitrate tablets should be supplied in glass containers of not more than 100 tablets, closed with a foil-lined cap, and containing no cotton wool wadding; they should be discarded after 8 weeks in use

Aerosol spray, glyceryl trinitrate 400 micrograms/metered dose. Net price 200-dose unit = £3.13

Dose: treatment or prophylaxis of angina, spray 1–2 doses under tongue and then close mouth

Coro-Nitro Pump Spray® (Roche)

Aerosol spray, glyceryl trinitrate 400 micrograms/metered dose. Net price 200-dose unit = £3.13

Dose: treatment or prophylaxis of angina, spray 1–2 doses under tongue and then close mouth

Glytrin Spray® (Sanofi-Synthelabo)
Aerosol spray, glyceryl trinitrate 400 micrograms/metered dose. Net price 200-dose unit = £3.49
Dose: treatment or prophylaxis of angina, spray 1–2 doses under tongue and then close mouth
Caution: flammable

GTN 300 mcg (Martindale)
Sublingual tablets, glyceryl trinitrate 300 micrograms. Net price 100 = £2.71. Label: 16

Nitrolingual Pumpspray® (Merck)
Aerosol spray, glyceryl trinitrate 400 micrograms/metered dose. Net price 200-dose unit = £3.65; *Duo Pack* (250-dose unit and 75-dose unit) = £4.98
Dose: treatment or prophylaxis of angina, spray 1–2 doses under tongue and then close mouth

Nitromin® (Egis)
Aerosol spray, glyceryl trinitrate 400 micrograms/metered dose, net price 180-dose unit = £2.63, 200-dose unit = £2.82
Dose: treatment or prophylaxis of angina, spray 1–2 doses under tongue and then close mouth

■ Longer-acting tablets

Suscard® (Forest)
Buccal tablets, m/r, glyceryl trinitrate 2 mg, net price 100-tab pack = £12.70; 3 mg, 100-tab pack = £18.33; 5 mg, 100-tab pack = £24.96. Counselling, see below
Dose: treatment of angina, 2 mg as required, increased to 3 mg if necessary; prophylaxis 2–3 mg 3 times daily; 5 mg in severe angina
Unstable angina (adjunct), up to 5 mg with ECG monitoring
Congestive heart failure, 5 mg 3 times daily, increased to 10 mg 3 times daily in severe cases
Acute heart failure, 5 mg repeated until symptoms abate
COUNSELLING. Tablets have rapid onset of effect; they are placed between upper lip and gum, and left to dissolve; vary site to reduce risk of dental caries

Sustac® (Forest)
Tablets, m/r, all pink, glyceryl trinitrate 2.6 mg, net price 90-tab pack = £4.80; 6.4 mg, 90-tab pack = £6.92. Label: 25
Dose: prophylaxis of angina, 2.6–12.8 mg 3 times daily *or* 10 mg 2–3 times daily

■ Parenteral preparations

NOTE. Glass or polyethylene apparatus is preferable; loss of potency will occur if PVC is used

Glyceryl Trinitrate (Non-proprietary) PoM
Injection, glyceryl trinitrate 5 mg/mL. To be diluted before use. Net price 5-mL amp = £6.49; 10-mL amp = £12.98
Excipients: may include ethanol, propylene glycol (see Excipients, p. 2)

Nitrocine® (Schwarz) PoM
Injection, glyceryl trinitrate 1 mg/mL. To be diluted before use or given undiluted with syringe pump. Net price 10-mL amp = £7.34; 50-mL bottle = £17.21
Excipients: include propylene glycol (see Excipients, p. 2)

Nitronal® (Merck) PoM
Injection, glyceryl trinitrate 1 mg/mL. To be diluted before use or given undiluted with syringe pump. Net price 5-mL vial = £1.92; 50-mL vial = £15.67

■ Transdermal preparations

Deponit® (Schwarz)
Patches, self-adhesive, transparent, glyceryl trinitrate, *'5' patch* (releasing approx. 5 mg/24 hours when in contact with skin), net price 28 = £15.96; *'10' patch* (releasing approx. 10 mg/24 hours), 28 = £17.57
Dose: prophylaxis of angina, apply one '5' or one '10' patch to lateral chest wall, upper arm, or shoulder; replace every 24 hours, siting replacement patch on different area; see also notes above

Minitran® (3M)
Patches, self-adhesive, transparent, glyceryl trinitrate, *'5' patch* (releasing approx. 5 mg/24 hours when in contact with skin), net price 30 = £11.62; *'10' patch* (releasing approx. 10 mg/24 hours), 30 = £12.87; *'15' patch* (releasing approx. 15 mg/24 hours), 30 = £14.19
Dose: prophylaxis of angina, apply one '5' patch to chest or upper arm; replace every 24 hours, siting replacement patch on different area; adjust dose according to response; see also notes above
Maintenance of venous patency ('5' patch only), consult product literature

Nitro-Dur® (Schering-Plough)
Patches, self-adhesive, buff, glyceryl trinitrate, *'0.2 mg/h' patch* (releasing approx. 5 mg/24 hours when in contact with skin), net price 28 = £11.01; *'0.4 mg/h' patch* (releasing approx. 10 mg/24 hours), 28 = £12.18; *'0.6 mg/h' patch* (releasing approx. 15 mg/24 hours), 28 = £13.41
Dose: prophylaxis of angina, apply one '0.2 mg/h' patch to chest or outer upper arm; replace every 24 hours, siting replacement patch on different area: adjust dose according to response; see also notes above

Percutol® (PLIVA)
Ointment, glyceryl trinitrate 2%. Net price 60 g = £9.55. Counselling, see administration below
Excipients: include wool fat
Dose: prophylaxis of angina, usual dose 1–2 inches of ointment measured on to *Applirule*®, and applied (usually to chest, arm, or thigh) without rubbing in and secured with surgical tape, every 3–4 hours as required; to determine dose, ½ inch on first day then increased by ½ inch/day until headache occurs, then reduced by ½ inch
NOTE. Approx. 800 micrograms/hour absorbed from 1 inch of ointment

Transiderm-Nitro® (Novartis)
Patches, self-adhesive, pink, glyceryl trinitrate, *'5' patch* (releasing approx. 5 mg/24 hours when in contact with skin), net price 28 = £21.31; *'10' patch* (releasing approx. 10 mg/24 hours), 28 = £23.43
Dose: prophylaxis of angina, apply one '5' or one '10' patch to lateral chest wall; replace every 24 hours, siting replacement patch on different area; max. two '10' patches daily; see also notes above
Prophylaxis of phlebitis and extravasation ('5' patch only), consult product literature

Trintek® (Goldshield)
Patches, self-adhesive, glyceryl trinitrate, '5' patch (releasing approx. 5 mg/24 hours when in contact with skin), net price 30 = £11.84; '10' patch (releasing approx. 10 mg/24 hours), net price 30 = £13.10; '15' patch (releasing approx. 15 mg/24 hours), net price 30 = £14.42
Dose: prophylaxis of angina, apply one '5' patch to lateral chest wall; replace every 24 hours, siting replacement patch on different area; adjust dose according to response, max one '15' patch daily; see also notes above

ISOSORBIDE DINITRATE

Indications: prophylaxis and treatment of angina; left ventricular failure
Cautions: see under Glyceryl Trinitrate

Contra-indications: see under Glyceryl Trinitrate
Side-effects: see under Glyceryl Trinitrate
Dose: *By mouth*, daily in divided doses, angina 30–120 mg, left ventricular failure 40–160 mg, up to 240 mg if required
By intravenous infusion, 2–10 mg/hour; higher doses up to 20 mg/hour may be required

■ Short-acting tablets and sprays

Isosorbide Dinitrate (Non-proprietary)
Tablets, isosorbide dinitrate 10 mg, net price 20 = 76p; 20 mg, 20 = 92p

Angitak® (LPC)
Aerosol spray, isosorbide dinitrate 1.25 mg/metered dose, net price 200-dose unit = £3.95
Dose: treatment or prophylaxis of angina, spray 1–3 doses under tongue whilst holding breath; allow 30 second interval between each dose

■ Modified-release preparations

Cedocard Retard® (Pharmacia)
Retard-20 tablets, m/r, yellow, scored, isosorbide dinitrate 20 mg. Net price 60-tab pack = £6.85. Label: 25
Dose: prophylaxis of angina, 1 tablet every 12 hours
Retard-40 tablets, m/r, orange-red, scored, isosorbide dinitrate 40 mg. Net price 60-tab pack = £13.31. Label: 25
Dose: prophylaxis of angina, 1–2 tablets every 12 hours

Isoket Retard® (Schwarz)
Retard-20 tablets, m/r, scored, isosorbide dinitrate 20 mg. Net price 56-tab pack = £3.23. Label: 25
Retard-40 tablets, m/r, scored, isosorbide dinitrate 40 mg. Net price 56-tab pack = £7.95. Label: 25
Dose: prophylaxis of angina, 20–40 mg every 12 hours

■ Parenteral preparations

Isoket® (Schwarz) PoM
Injection 0.05%, isosorbide dinitrate 500 micrograms/mL. To be diluted before use or given undiluted with syringe pump. Net price 50-mL bottle = £8.94
Injection 0.1%, isosorbide dinitrate 1 mg/mL. To be diluted before use. Net price 10-mL amp = £3.37; 50-mL bottle = £16.70; 100-mL bottle = £25.98
NOTE. Glass or polyethylene infusion apparatus is preferable; loss of potency if PVC used

ISOSORBIDE MONONITRATE

Indications: prophylaxis of angina; adjunct in congestive heart failure
Cautions: see under Glyceryl Trinitrate
Contra-indications: see under Glyceryl Trinitrate
Side-effects: see under Glyceryl Trinitrate
Dose: initially 20 mg 2–3 times daily *or* 40 mg twice daily (10 mg twice daily in those who have not previously received nitrates); up to 120 mg daily in divided doses if required

Isosorbide Mononitrate (Non-proprietary)
Tablets, isosorbide mononitrate 10 mg, net price 56 = £1.13; 20 mg, 56 = £1.13; 40 mg, 56 = £2.77. Label: 25
Brands include *Angeze*®, *Dynamin*®

Elantan® (Schwarz)
Elantan 10 tablets, scored, isosorbide mononitrate 10 mg. Net price 56 = £3.31; 84 = £4.97. Label: 25
Elantan 20 tablets PoM, scored, isosorbide mononitrate 20 mg. Net price 56 = £4.32; 84 = £6.13. Label: 25
Elantan 40 tablets PoM, scored, isosorbide mononitrate 40 mg. Net price 56 = £7.03; 84 = £10.56. Label: 25

Ismo® (Roche)
Ismo 10 tablets, isosorbide mononitrate 10 mg. Net price 60-tab pack = £3.01. Label: 25
Ismo 20 tablets, scored, isosorbide mononitrate 20 mg. Net price 60-tab pack = £4.42. Label: 25
Ismo 40 tablets, scored, isosorbide mononitrate 40 mg. Net price 60-tab pack = £7.25. Label: 25

■ Modified release

Chemydur® **60XL** (Sovereign) PoM
Tablets, m/r, scored, ivory, isosorbide mononitrate 60 mg, net price 28-tab pack = £5.99. Label: 25
Dose: prophylaxis of angina, 1 tablet in the morning (half a tablet for 2–4 days to minimise possibility of headache), increased if necessary to 2 tablets

Elantan LA® (Schwarz)
Elantan LA 25 capsules, m/r, brown/white, enclosing white micropellets, isosorbide mononitrate 25 mg. Net price 28-cap pack = £6.59. Label: 25
Dose: prophylaxis of angina, 1 capsule in the morning, increased if necessary to 2 capsules
Elantan LA 50 capsules, m/r, brown/pink, enclosing white micropellets, isosorbide mononitrate 50 mg. Net price 28-cap pack = £10.54. Label: 25
Dose: prophylaxis of angina, 1 capsule daily in the morning, increased if necessary to 2 capsules

Imdur® (AstraZeneca)
Durules® (= tablets m/r), yellow, f/c, scored, isosorbide mononitrate 60 mg. Net price 28-tab pack = £11.14. Label: 25
Dose: prophylaxis of angina, 1 tablet in the morning (half a tablet if headache occurs), increased to 2 tablets in the morning if required

Isib 60XL® (Ashbourne)
Tablets, m/r, scored, ivory, isosorbide mononitrate 60 mg. Net price 28-tab pack = £8.19. Label: 25
Dose: prophylaxis of angina, 1 tablet in the morning (half a tablet for 2–4 days if headache occurs), increased if necessary to 2 tablets

Ismo Retard® (Roche)
Tablets, m/r, s/c, isosorbide mononitrate 40 mg, net price 30-tab pack = £9.75. Label: 25
Dose: prophylaxis of angina, 1 tablet daily in morning

Isodur® (Galen)
Isodur 25XL capsules, m/r, brown/white, isosorbide mononitrate 25 mg, net price 28-cap pack = £6.05. Label: 25
Isodur 50XL capsules, m/r, brown/pink, isosorbide mononitrate 50 mg, net price 28-cap pack = £9.75. Label: 25
Dose: prophylaxis of angina, 25–50 mg daily in the morning, increased if necessary to 50–100 mg once daily

Isotard® (Strakan)
Isotard 25XL tablets, m/r, ivory, isosorbide mononitrate 25 mg, net price 28-tab pack = £5.95. Label: 25
Isotard 40XL tablets, m/r, ivory, isosorbide mononitrate 40 mg, net price 28-tab pack = £6.78. Label: 25
Isotard 50XL tablets, m/r, ivory, isosorbide mononitrate 50 mg, net price 28-tab pack = £6.78. Label: 25

Isotard 60XL tablets, m/r, ivory, isosorbide mononitrate 60 mg, net price 28-tab pack = £6.78. Label: 25

Dose: prophylaxis of angina, 25–60 mg daily in the morning (if headache occurs with 60-mg tablet, half a 60-mg tablet may be given for 2–4 days), increased if necessary to 50–120 mg daily

Modisal XL® (Sandoz)

Tablets, m/r, ivory, isosorbide mononitrate 60 mg. Net price 28-tab pack = £10.36. Label: 25

Dose: prophylaxis of angina, 1 tablet daily in the morning (half a tablet for first 2–4 days to minimise possibility of headache), increased if necessary to 2 tablets once daily

Monomax® (Trinity-Chiesi) PoM

Monomax® SR, capsules, m/r, isosorbide mononitrate 40 mg, net price 28-cap pack = £8.31; 60 mg, 28-cap pack = £6.75. Label: 25

Dose: prophylaxis of angina, 40–60 mg daily in the morning, increased if necessary to 120 mg daily

NOTE. Also available as *Angeze SR*®

Monomax® XL tablets, m/r, isosorbide mononitrate 60 mg, net price 28-tab pack = £6.75. Label: 25

Dose: prophylaxis of angina, 1 tablet in the morning (half a tablet for first 2–4 days to minimise possibility of headache), increased if necessary to 2 tablets

Monosorb XL 60® (Dexcel) PoM

Tablets, m/r, f/c, isosorbide mononitrate 60 mg. Net price 28-tab pack = £15.53. Label: 25

Dose: prophylaxis of angina, 1 tablet daily in the morning (half a tablet for first 2–4 days to minimise possibility of headache), increased if necessary to 2 tablets

NOTE. Also available as *Monigen® XL, Trangina® XL, Xismox® XL 60*

Zemon® (Neolab)

Zemon 40XL tablets, m/r, ivory, isosorbide mononitrate 40 mg, net price 28-tab pack = £14.25. Label: 25

Zemon 60XL tablets, scored, m/r, ivory, isosorbide mononitrate 60 mg, net price 28-tab pack = £11.14. Label: 25

Dose: prophylaxis of angina, 40–60 mg daily in the morning (half a 60-mg tablet may be given for 2–4 days to minimise possibility of headache), increased if necessary to 80–120 mg once daily

■ With aspirin

NOTE. For prophylaxis of angina and secondary prevention of myocardial infarction; for cautions, contra-indications and side-effects of aspirin see section 2.9

Imazin® **XL** (Napp)

Tablets, aspirin 75 mg, isosorbide mononitrate 60 mg (m/r), net price 28-tab pack = £8.07. Label: 25, 32

Dose: 1 tablet in the morning, increased to 2 tablets if required

Forte tablets, aspirin 150 mg, isosorbide mononitrate 60 mg (m/r), net price 28-tab pack = £8.07. Label: 25, 32

Dose: 1 tablet in the morning

2.6.2 Calcium-channel blockers

Calcium-channel blockers (less correctly called 'calcium-antagonists') interfere with the inward displacement of calcium ions through the slow channels of active cell membranes. They influence the myocardial cells, the cells within the specialised conducting system of the heart, and the cells of vascular smooth muscle. Thus, myocardial contractility may be reduced, the formation and propagation of electrical impulses within the heart may be depressed, and coronary or systemic vascular tone may be diminished.

Calcium-channel blockers differ in their predilection for the various possible sites of action and, therefore, their therapeutic effects are disparate, with much greater variation than those of beta-blockers. There are important differences between verapamil, diltiazem, and the dihydropyridine calcium-channel blockers (amlodipine, felodipine, isradipine, lacidipine, lercanidipine, nicardipine, nifedipine, nimodipine, and nisoldipine). Verapamil and diltiazem should usually be **avoided** in *heart failure* because they may further depress cardiac function and cause clinically significant deterioration.

Verapamil is used for the treatment of *angina* (section 2.6), *hypertension*, and *arrhythmias* (section 2.3.2). It is a highly negatively inotropic calcium channel-blocker and it reduces cardiac output, slows the heart rate, and may impair atrioventricular conduction. It may precipitate heart failure, exacerbate conduction disorders, and cause hypotension at high doses and should **not** be used with beta-blockers (see p. 113). Constipation is the most common side-effect.

Nifedipine relaxes vascular smooth muscle and dilates coronary and peripheral arteries. It has more influence on vessels and less on the myocardium than does verapamil, and unlike verapamil has no anti-arrhythmic activity. It rarely precipitates heart failure because any negative inotropic effect is offset by a reduction in left ventricular work. Short-acting formulations of nifedipine are not recommended for angina or long-term management of hypertension; their use may be associated with large variations in blood pressure and reflex tachycardia. **Nicardipine** has similar effects to those of nifedipine and may produce less reduction of myocardial contractility. **Amlodipine** and **felodipine** also resemble nifedipine and nicardipine in their effects and do not reduce myocardial contractility and they do not produce clinical deterioration in heart failure. They have a longer duration of action and can be given once daily. Nifedipine, nicardipine, amlodipine, and felodipine are used for the treatment of angina (section 2.6) or hypertension. All are valuable in forms of *angina associated with coronary vasospasm*. Side-effects associated with vasodilatation such as flushing and headache (which become less obtrusive after a few days), and ankle swelling (which may respond only partially to diuretics) are common.

Isradipine, **lacidipine**, **lercanidipine** and **nisoldipine** have similar effects to those of nifedipine and nicardipine; isradipine, lacidipine, and lercanidipine are only indicated for *hypertension* whereas nisoldipine is indicated for angina and hypertension.

Nimodipine is related to nifedipine but the smooth muscle relaxant effect preferentially acts on cerebral arteries. Its use is confined to prevention of *vascular spasm following aneurysmal subarachnoid haemorrhage*.

Diltiazem is effective in most forms of *angina* (section 2.6); the longer-acting formulation is also used for *hypertension*. It may be used in patients for whom beta-blockers are contra-indicated or ineffective. It has a less negative inotropic effect than verapamil and significant myocardial depression occurs rarely. Nevertheless because of the risk of bradycardia it should be used with caution in association with beta-blockers.

UNSTABLE ANGINA. Calcium-channel blockers do not reduce the risk of myocardial infarction in unstable angina. The use of diltiazem or verapamil should be reserved for patients resistant to treatment with beta-blockers.

WITHDRAWAL. There is some evidence that sudden withdrawal of calcium-channel blockers may be associated with an exacerbation of angina.

AMLODIPINE

Indications: hypertension, prophylaxis of angina

Cautions: hepatic impairment (Appendix 2); pregnancy (Appendix 4); **interactions:** Appendix 1 (calcium-channel blockers)

Contra-indications: cardiogenic shock, unstable angina, significant aortic stenosis; breast-feeding (Appendix 5)

Side-effects: abdominal pain, nausea; palpitation, flushing, oedema; headache, dizziness, sleep disturbances, fatigue; *less commonly* gastro-intestinal disturbances, dry mouth, taste disturbances, hypotension, syncope, chest pain, dyspnoea, rhinitis, mood changes, tremor, paraesthesia, urinary disturbances, impotence, gynaecomastia, weight changes, myalgia, visual disturbances, tinnitus, pruritus, rashes (including isolated reports of erythema multiforme), alopecia, purpura, and skin discolouration; *very rarely* gastritis, pancreatitis, hepatitis, jaundice, cholestasis, gingival hyperplasia, myocardial infarction, arrhythmias, vasculitis, coughing, hyperglycaemia, thrombocytopenia, angioedema, and urticaria

Dose: hypertension or angina, initially 5 mg once daily; max. 10 mg once daily

NOTE. Tablets from various suppliers may contain different salts (e.g. amlodipine besilate and amlodipine maleate) but the strength is expressed in terms of amlodipine (base); tablets containing different salts are considered interchangeable

Amlodipine (Non-proprietary) PoM

Tablets, amlodipine (as maleate) 5 mg, net price 28-tab pack = £8.89; 10 mg, 28-tab pack = £12.25

Brands include *Amlostin*®

Istin® (Pfizer) PoM

Tablets, amlodipine (as besilate) 5 mg. Net price 28-tab pack = £13.04; 10 mg, 28-tab pack = £19.47

DILTIAZEM HYDROCHLORIDE

Indications: prophylaxis and treatment of angina; hypertension

Cautions: reduce dose in hepatic and renal impairment; heart failure or significantly impaired left ventricular function, bradycardia (avoid if severe), first degree AV block, or prolonged PR interval; **interactions:** Appendix 1 (calcium-channel blockers)

Contra-indications: severe bradycardia, left ventricular failure with pulmonary congestion, second- or third-degree AV block (unless pacemaker fitted), sick sinus syndrome; pregnancy; breast-feeding (Appendix 5)

Side-effects: bradycardia, sino-atrial block, AV block, palpitation, dizziness, hypotension, malaise, asthenia, headache, hot flushes, gastro-intestinal disturbances, oedema (notably of ankles); rarely rashes (including erythema multiforme and exfoliative dermatitis), photosensitivity; hepatitis, gynaecomastia, gum hyperplasia, extrapyramidal symptoms, depression reported

Dose: angina, 60 mg 3 times daily (elderly initially twice daily); increased if necessary to 360 mg daily

Longer-acting formulations, see under preparations below

■ Standard formulations

NOTE. These formulations are licensed as generics and there is no requirement for brand name dispensing. Although their means of formulation has called for the strict designation 'modified-release' their duration of action corresponds to that of tablets requiring administration 3 times daily

Diltiazem (Non-proprietary) PoM

Tablets, m/r (but see note above), diltiazem hydrochloride 60 mg. Net price 100 = £4.01. Label: 25

Brands include *Optil*®

Tildiem® (Sanofi-Synthelabo) PoM

Tablets, m/r (but see note above), off-white, diltiazem hydrochloride 60 mg. Net price 90-tab pack = £8.28. Label: 25

■ Longer-acting formulations

NOTE. Different versions of modified-release preparations may not have the same clinical effect. To avoid confusion between these different formulations of diltiazem, prescribers should specify the brand to be dispensed

Adizem-SR® (Napp) PoM

Capsules, m/r, diltiazem hydrochloride 90 mg (white), net price 56-cap pack = £8.98; 120 mg (brown/white), 56-cap pack = £9.98; 180 mg (brown/white), 56-cap pack = £14.95. Label: 25

Tablets, m/r, f/c, scored, diltiazem hydrochloride 120 mg. Net price 56-tab pack = £14.72. Label: 25

Dose: mild to moderate hypertension, usually 120 mg twice daily (dose form not appropriate for initial dose titration)

Angina, initially 90 mg twice daily (elderly, dose form not appropriate for initial dose titration); increased to 180 mg twice daily if required

Adizem-XL® (Napp) PoM

Capsules, m/r, diltiazem hydrochloride 120 mg (pink/blue), net price 28-cap pack = £9.66; 180 mg (dark pink/blue), 28-cap pack = £10.96; 200 mg (brown), 28-cap pack = £7.82; 240 mg (red/blue), 28-cap pack = £12.17; 300 mg (maroon/blue), 28-cap pack = £9.66. Label: 25

Dose: angina and mild to moderate hypertension, initially 240 mg once daily, increased if necessary to 300 mg once daily; in elderly and in hepatic or renal impairment, initially 120 mg daily

Angitil SR® (Trinity-Chiesi) PoM

Capsules, m/r, diltiazem hydrochloride 90 mg (white), net price 56-cap pack = £7.86; 120 mg (brown), 56-cap pack = £8.73; 180 mg (brown), 56-cap pack = £14.08. Label: 25

Dose: angina and mild to moderate hypertension, initially 90 mg twice daily; increased if necessary to 120 mg or 180 mg twice daily

NOTE. Also available as *Disogram*® *SR*

Angitil XL® (Trinity-Chiesi) PoM

Capsules, m/r, diltiazem hydrochloride 240 mg (white), net price 28-cap pack = £9.44; 300 mg (yellow), 28-cap pack = £8.57. Label: 25

Dose: angina and mild to moderate hypertension, initially 240 mg once daily (elderly and in hepatic and renal impairment, dose form not appropriate for initial dose titration); increased if necessary to 300 mg once daily

NOTE. Also available as *Disogram*® *SR*

Calcicard CR® (IVAX) PoM
Tablets, m/r, both f/c, diltiazem hydrochloride 90 mg, net price 56-tab pack = £6.33; 120 mg, 56-tab pack = £7.04. Label: 25
Dose: mild to moderate hypertension, initially 90 mg or 120 mg twice daily; up to 360 mg daily may be required: ELDERLY and in hepatic and renal impairment, initially 120 mg once daily; up to 240 mg daily may be required
Angina, initially 90 mg or 120 mg twice daily; up to 480 mg daily in divided doses may be required; ELDERLY and in hepatic and renal impairment, dose form not appropriate for initial dose titration; up to 240 mg daily may be required
NOTE. Also available as *Angiozem CR*®

Dilcardia SR® (Generics) PoM
Capsules, m/r, diltiazem hydrochloride 60 mg (pink/white), net price 56-cap pack = £8.31; 90 mg (pink/yellow), 56-cap pack = £10.33; 120 mg (pink/orange), 56-cap pack = £11.49. Label: 25
Dose: angina and mild to moderate hypertension, initially 90 mg twice daily; increased if necessary to 180 mg twice daily; ELDERLY and in hepatic or renal impairment, initially 60 mg twice daily, max. 90 mg twice daily

Dilzem SR® (Zeneus) PoM
Capsules, m/r, all beige, diltiazem hydrochloride 60 mg, net price 56-cap pack = £6.40; 90 mg, 56-cap pack = £9.59; 120 mg, 56-cap pack = £10.95. Label: 25
Dose: angina and mild to moderate hypertension, initially 90 mg twice daily (elderly 60 mg twice daily); up to 180 mg twice daily may be required

Dilzem XL® (Zeneus) PoM
Capsules, m/r, diltiazem hydrochloride 120 mg, net price 28-cap pack = £6.61; 180 mg, 28-cap pack = £9.81; 240 mg, 28-cap pack = £11.70. Label: 25
Dose: angina and mild to moderate hypertension, initially 180 mg once daily (elderly and in hepatic and renal impairment, 120 mg once daily); if necessary may be increased to 360 mg once daily

Slozem® (Merck) PoM
Capsules, m/r, diltiazem hydrochloride 120 mg (pink/clear), net price 28-cap pack = £7.00; 180 mg (pink/clear), 28-cap pack = £7.80; 240 mg (red/clear), 28-cap pack = £8.20; 300 mg (red/white), 28-cap pack = £8.50. Label: 25
Dose: angina and mild to moderate hypertension, initially 240 mg once daily (elderly and in hepatic and renal impairment, 120 mg once daily); if necessary may be increased to 360 mg once daily

Tildiem LA® (Sanofi-Synthelabo) PoM
Capsules, m/r, diltiazem hydrochloride 200 mg (pink/grey, containing white pellets), net price 28-cap pack = £7.83; 300 mg (white/yellow, containing white pellets), 28-cap pack = £9.39. Label: 25
Dose: angina and mild to moderate hypertension, initially 200 mg once daily before or with food, increased if necessary to 300–400 mg daily, max. 500 mg daily; ELDERLY and in hepatic or renal impairment, initially 200 mg daily, increased if necessary to 300 mg daily

Tildiem Retard® (Sanofi-Synthelabo) PoM
Tablets, m/r, diltiazem hydrochloride 90 mg, net price 56-tab pack = £8.55; 120 mg, 56-tab pack = £9.53. Label: 25
COUNSELLING. Tablet membrane may pass through gastro-intestinal tract unchanged, but being porous has no effect on efficacy
Dose: mild to moderate hypertension, initially 90 mg or 120 mg twice daily; increased if necessary to 360 mg daily in divided doses; ELDERLY and in hepatic or renal impairment, initially 120 mg once daily; increased if necessary to 120 mg twice daily
Angina, initially 90 mg or 120 mg twice daily; increased if necessary to 480 mg daily in divided doses; ELDERLY and in hepatic or renal impairment, dose form not appropriate for initial titration; up to 120 mg twice daily may be required

Viazem XL® (Genus) PoM
Capsules, m/r, diltiazem hydrochloride 120 mg (lavender), net price 28-cap pack = £6.60; 180 mg (white/blue-green), 28-cap pack = £7.36; 240 mg (blue-green/lavender), 28-cap pack = £7.74; 300 mg (white/lavender), 28-cap pack = £8.03; 360 mg (blue-green), 28-cap pack = £14.70. Label: 25
Dose: angina and mild to moderate hypertension, initially 180 mg once daily, adjusted according to response to 240 mg once daily; max. 360 mg once daily; ELDERLY and in hepatic or renal impairment, initially 120 mg once daily, adjusted according to response

Zemtard® (Galen) PoM
Zemtard 120XL capsules, m/r, brown/orange, diltiazem hydrochloride 120 mg, net price 28-cap pack = £6.60. Label: 25
Zemtard 180XL capsules, m/r, grey/pink, diltiazem hydrochloride 180 mg, net price 28-cap pack = £7.36. Label: 25
Zemtard 240XL capsules, m/r, blue, diltiazem hydrochloride 240 mg, net price 28-cap pack = £7.74. Label: 25
Zemtard 300XL capsules, m/r, white/blue, diltiazem hydrochloride 300 mg, net price 28-cap pack = £8.03. Label: 25
Dose: angina and mild to moderate hypertension, 180–300 mg once daily, increased if necessary to 360 mg once daily in hypertension and to 480 mg once daily in angina; ELDERLY and in hepatic or renal impairment, initially 120 mg once daily

FELODIPINE

Indications: hypertension, prophylaxis of angina
Cautions: withdraw if ischaemic pain occurs or existing pain worsens shortly after initiating treatment or if cardiogenic shock develops; severe left ventricular dysfunction; avoid grapefruit juice (may affect metabolism); reduce dose in hepatic impairment; breast-feeding (Appendix 5); **interactions:** Appendix 1 (calcium-channel blockers)
Contra-indications: unstable angina, uncontrolled heart failure; significant aortic stenosis; within 1 month of myocardial infarction; pregnancy (Appendix 4)
Side-effects: flushing, headache, palpitation, dizziness, fatigue, gravitational oedema; rarely rash, pruritus, cutaneous vasculitis, gum hyperplasia, urinary frequency, impotence, fever
Dose: hypertension, initially 5 mg (elderly 2.5 mg) daily in the morning; usual maintenance 5–10 mg once daily; doses above 20 mg daily rarely needed
Angina, initially 5 mg daily in the morning, increased if necessary to 10 mg once daily

Felodipine (Non-proprietary) PoM
Tablets, m/r felodipine 5 mg, net price 28-tab pack = £8.93; 10 mg, 28-tab pack = £12.01, 30-tab pack = £12.87. Label: 25
Brands include *Cardioplen XL*®, *Felogen XL*®, *Felotens XL*®, *Keloc SR*®, *Neofel XL*®, *Vascalpha*®

Plendil® (AstraZeneca) PoM
Tablets, m/r, f/c, felodipine 2.5 mg (yellow), net price 28-tab pack = £6.70; 5 mg (pink), 28-tab pack = £8.93; 10 mg (brown), 28-tab pack = £12.01. Label: 25

ISRADIPINE

Indications: hypertension

Cautions: sick sinus syndrome (if pacemaker not fitted); avoid grapefruit juice (may affect metabolism); reduce dose in hepatic or renal impairment; pregnancy (Appendix 4); **interactions:** Appendix 1 (calcium-channel blockers)

Contra-indications: cardiogenic shock; symptomatic or tight aortic stenosis; within 1 month of myocardial infarction; unstable angina; breast-feeding (Appendix 5)

Side-effects: headache, flushing, dizziness, tachycardia and palpitation, localised peripheral oedema; hypotension uncommon; rarely weight gain, fatigue, abdominal discomfort, rashes

Dose: 2.5 mg twice daily (1.25 mg twice daily in elderly, hepatic or renal impairment); increased if necessary after 3–4 weeks to 5 mg twice daily (exceptionally up to 10 mg twice daily); maintenance 2.5 or 5 mg once daily may be sufficient

Prescal® (Novartis) PoM
Tablets, yellow, scored, isradipine 2.5 mg. Net price 56-tab pack = £15.04

LACIDIPINE

Indications: hypertension

Cautions: cardiac conduction abnormalities; poor cardiac reserve; withdraw if ischaemic pain occurs shortly after initiating treatment or if cardiogenic shock develops; avoid grapefruit juice (may affect metabolism); hepatic impairment (Appendix 2); **interactions:** Appendix 1 (calcium-channel blockers)

Contra-indications: aortic stenosis; avoid within 1 month of myocardial infarction; pregnancy (Appendix 4); breast-feeding (Appendix 5)

Side-effects: headache, flushing, oedema, dizziness, palpitation; also asthenia, rash (including pruritus and erythema), gastro-intestinal disturbances, gum hyperplasia, muscle cramps, polyuria, chest pain (see Cautions); mood disturbances

Dose: initially 2 mg as a single daily dose, preferably in the morning; increased after 3–4 weeks to 4 mg daily, then if necessary to 6 mg daily

Motens® (Boehringer Ingelheim) PoM
Tablets, both f/c, lacidipine 2 mg, net price 28-tab pack = £10.23; 4 mg (scored), 28-tab pack = £15.30

LERCANIDIPINE HYDROCHLORIDE

Indications: mild to moderate hypertension

Cautions: left ventricular dysfunction; sick sinus syndrome (if pacemaker not fitted); avoid grapefruit juice (may affect metabolism); hepatic impairment (Appendix 2); **interactions:** Appendix 1 (calcium-channel blockers)

Contra-indications: aortic stenosis; unstable angina, uncontrolled heart failure; within 1 month of myocardial infarction; renal impairment; pregnancy (Appendix 4); breast-feeding

Side-effects: flushing, peripheral oedema, palpitation, tachycardia, headache, dizziness, asthenia; also gastro-intestinal disturbances, hypotension, drowsiness, myalgia, polyuria, rash

Dose: initially 10 mg once daily; increased, if necessary, after at least 2 weeks to 20 mg daily

Zanidip® (Recordati) PoM
Tablets, yellow, f/c, lercanidipine hydrochloride 10 mg, net price 28-tab pack = £5.80. Label: 22

NICARDIPINE HYDROCHLORIDE

Indications: prophylaxis of angina; mild to moderate hypertension

Cautions: withdraw if ischaemic pain occurs or existing pain worsens within 30 minutes of initiating treatment or increasing dose; congestive heart failure or significantly impaired left ventricular function; elderly; avoid grapefruit juice (may affect metabolism); hepatic impairment (Appendix 2); renal impairment (Appendix 3); pregnancy (Appendix 4); **interactions:** Appendix 1 (calcium-channel blockers)

Contra-indications: cardiogenic shock; advanced aortic stenosis; unstable or acute attacks of angina; avoid within 1 month of myocardial infarction; breast-feeding (Appendix 5)

Side-effects: dizziness, headache, peripheral oedema, flushing, palpitation, nausea; also gastro-intestinal disturbances, drowsiness, insomnia, tinnitus, hypotension, rashes, dyspnoea, paraesthesia, frequency of micturition; thrombocytopenia, depression and impotence reported

Dose: initially 20 mg 3 times daily, increased, after at least three days, to 30 mg 3 times daily (usual range 60–120 mg daily)

Nicardipine (Non-proprietary) PoM
Capsules, nicardipine hydrochloride 20 mg, net price 56-cap pack = £8.92; 30 mg, 56-cap pack = £10.56

Cardene® (Yamanouchi) PoM
Capsules, nicardipine hydrochloride 20 mg (blue/white), net price 56-cap pack = £8.57; 30 mg (blue/pale blue), 56-cap pack = £9.95

■ Modified release

Cardene SR® (Yamanouchi) PoM
Capsules, m/r, nicardipine hydrochloride 30 mg, net price 56-cap pack = £10.21; 45 mg (blue), 56-cap pack = £14.86. Label: 25
Dose: mild to moderate hypertension, initially 30 mg twice daily; usual effective dose 45 mg twice daily (range 30–60 mg twice daily)

NIFEDIPINE

Indications: prophylaxis of angina; hypertension; Raynaud's phenomenon

Cautions: withdraw if ischaemic pain occurs or existing pain worsens shortly after initiating treatment; poor cardiac reserve; heart failure or significantly impaired left ventricular function (heart failure deterioration observed); severe hypotension; reduce dose in hepatic impairment (Appendix 2); diabetes mellitus; may inhibit labour; pregnancy (Appendix 4); breast-feeding (Appendix 5); avoid grapefruit juice (may affect metabolism); **interactions:** Appendix 1 (calcium-channel blockers)

Contra-indications: cardiogenic shock; advanced aortic stenosis; within 1 month of myocardial infarction; unstable or acute attacks of angina; porphyria (section 9.8.2)

Side-effects: headache, flushing, dizziness, lethargy; tachycardia, palpitation; short-acting preparations may induce an exaggerated fall in blood pressure and reflex tachycardia which may lead to myocardial or cerebrovascular ischaemia; gravitational oedema, rash (erythema multiforme reported), pruritus, urticaria, nausea, constipation or diarrhoea, increased frequency of micturition, eye pain, visual disturbances, gum hyperplasia, asthenia, paraesthesia, myalgia, tremor, impotence, gynaecomastia; depression, telangiectasia, cholestasis, jaundice reported

Dose: see preparations below

Nifedipine (Non-proprietary) PoM

Capsules, nifedipine 5 mg, net price 84-cap pack = £3.78; 10 mg, 84-cap pack = £4.64

Dose: angina prophylaxis (but not recommended, see notes above) and Raynaud's phenomenon, initially 5 mg 3 times daily, adjusted according to response to 20 mg 3 times daily

Hypertension, not recommended therefore no dose stated

Adalat® (Bayer) PoM

Capsules, both orange, nifedipine 5 mg, net price 90-cap pack = £6.08; 10 mg, 90-cap pack = £7.74

Dose: angina prophylaxis (but not recommended, see notes above) and Raynaud's phenomenon, initially 5 mg 3 times daily, adjusted according to response to 20 mg 3 times daily

Hypertension, not recommended therefore no dose stated

■ Modified release

NOTE. Different versions of modified-release preparations may not have the same clinical effect. To avoid confusion between these different formulations of nifedipine, prescribers should specify the brand to be dispensed. Modified-release formulations may not be suitable for dose titration in hepatic disease

Adalat® LA (Bayer) PoM

LA 20 tablets, m/r, pink, nifedipine 20 mg, net price 28-tab pack = £5.27. Label: 25

LA 30 tablets, m/r, pink, nifedipine 30 mg, net price 28-tab pack = £7.59. Label: 25

LA 60 tablets, m/r, pink, nifedipine 60 mg, net price 28-tab pack = £9.69. Label: 25

COUNSELLING. Tablet membrane may pass through gastro-intestinal tract unchanged, but being porous has no effect on efficacy

Dose: hypertension, 20–30 mg once daily, increased if necessary; max. 90 mg once daily

Angina prophylaxis, 30 mg once daily, increased if necessary; max. 90 mg once daily

Caution: dose form not appropriate for use in hepatic impairment or where there is a history of oesophageal or gastro-intestinal obstruction, decreased lumen diameter of the gastro-intestinal tract, or inflammatory bowel disease (including Crohn's disease)

Adalat® Retard (Bayer) PoM

Retard 10 tablets, m/r, pink, nifedipine 10 mg. Net price 56-tab pack = £8.50. Label: 25

Retard 20 tablets, m/r, pink, nifedipine 20 mg. Net price 56-tab pack = £10.20. Label: 25

Dose: hypertension and angina prophylaxis, 10 mg twice daily, adjusted according to response to 40 mg twice daily

Adipine® MR (Trinity-Chiesi) PoM

Tablets, m/r, nifedipine 10 mg (apricot), net price 56-tab pack = £5.96; 20 mg (pink), 56-tab pack = £7.43. Label: 21, 25

Dose: hypertension and angina prophylaxis, 20 mg twice daily after food (initial titration 10 mg twice daily); max. 40 mg twice daily

Adipine® XL (Trinity-Chiesi) PoM

Tablets, m/r, both red, nifedipine 30 mg, net price 28-tab pack = £5.95; 60 mg, 28-tab pack = £8.95. Label: 25

Dose: hypertension and angina prophylaxis, 30 mg once daily, increased if necessary; max. 90 mg once daily

Cardilate MR® (IVAX) PoM

Tablets, m/r, nifedipine 10 mg (pink), net price 56-tab pack = £4.97; 20 mg (brown), net price 100-tab pack = £16.62. Label: 25

Dose: hypertension and angina prophylaxis, 20 mg twice daily (initial titration 10 mg twice daily); max. 80 mg daily

Coracten SR® (Celltech) PoM

Capsules, m/r, nifedipine 10 mg (grey/pink, enclosing yellow pellets), net price 60-cap pack = £4.27; 20 mg (pink/brown, enclosing yellow pellets), 60-cap pack = £5.93. Label: 25

Dose: hypertension and angina prophylaxis, one 20-mg capsule every 12 hours, adjusted within range 10–40 mg every 12 hours

Coracten XL® (Celltech) PoM

Capsules, m/r, nifedipine 30 mg (brown), net price 28-cap pack = £5.89; 60 mg (orange), 28-cap pack = £8.84. Label: 25

Dose: hypertension and angina prophylaxis, 30 mg once daily, increased if necessary; max. 90 mg once daily

Fortipine LA 40® (Goldshield) PoM

Tablets, m/r, red, nifedipine 40 mg, net price 30-tab pack = £8.00. Label: 21, 25

Dose: hypertension and angina prophylaxis, 40 mg once daily, increased if necessary to 80 mg daily in 1–2 divided doses

Hypolar® Retard 20 (Sandoz) PoM

Tablets, m/r, red, f/c, nifedipine 20 mg. Net price 56-tab pack = £7.00. Label: 25

Dose: hypertension and angina prophylaxis, 20 mg twice daily, increased if necessary to 40 mg twice daily

Nifedipress® MR (Dexcel) PoM

Tablets, m/r, pink, nifedipine 10 mg, net price 56-tab pack = £9.23. Label: 25

Dose: hypertension and angina prophylaxis, initially 10 mg twice daily adjusted according to response to 40 mg twice daily

Nifopress® Retard (Goldshield) PoM

Tablets, m/r, pink, nifedipine 20 mg, net price 112-tab pack = £10.80. Label: 21, 25

Dose: mild to moderate hypertension, angina prophylaxis and Raynaud's phenomenon, usually 20 mg twice daily, adjusted according to response to 40 mg twice daily

Slofedipine® (Winthrop) PoM

Tablets, m/r, pink, nifedipine 20 mg, net price 56-tab pack = £10.32. Label: 25

Dose: hypertension and angina prophylaxis, initially 20 mg twice daily adjusted according to response to 40 mg twice daily

Slofedipine XL® (Winthrop) PoM

Tablets, m/r, brown, nifedipine 30 mg, net price 28-tab pack = £9.89; 60 mg, 28-tab pack = £14.71. Label: 25

Dose: hypertension and angina prophylaxis, 30 mg once daily, increased if necessary to 90 mg once daily

Caution: dose form not appropriate for use in hepatic impairment or where there is a history of oesophageal or gastro-intestinal obstruction, decreased lumen diameter of the gastro-intestinal tract, or inflammatory bowel disease (including Crohn's disease)

Tensipine MR® (Genus) PoM
Tablets, m/r, both pink, nifedipine 10 mg, net price 56-tab pack = £3.75; 20 mg, 56-tab pack = £5.25. Label: 21, 25
Dose: hypertension and angina prophylaxis, initially 10 mg twice daily adjusted according to response to 40 mg twice daily

■ With atenolol
Section 2.4

NIMODIPINE

Indications: prevention and treatment of ischaemic neurological deficits following aneurysmal subarachnoid haemorrhage

Cautions: cerebral oedema or severely raised intracranial pressure; hypotension; avoid concomitant administration of nimodipine tablets and infusion, other calcium-channel blockers, or beta-blockers; concomitant nephrotoxic drugs; avoid grapefruit juice (may affect metabolism); hepatic impairment (Appendix 2); renal impairment (Appendix 3); pregnancy (Appendix 4); **interactions:** Appendix 1 (calcium-channel blockers, alcohol (infusion only))

Contra-indications: within 1 month of myocardial infarction; unstable angina

Side-effects: hypotension, variation in heart-rate, flushing, headache, gastro-intestinal disorders, nausea, sweating and feeling of warmth; thrombocytopenia and ileus reported

Dose: prevention, *by mouth*, 60 mg every 4 hours, starting within 4 days of aneurysmal subarachnoid haemorrhage and continued for 21 days
Treatment, *by intravenous infusion* via central catheter, initially 1 mg/hour (up to 500 micrograms/hour if body-weight less than 70 kg or if blood pressure unstable), increased after 2 hours to 2 mg/hour if no severe fall in blood pressure; continue for at least 5 days (max. 14 days); if surgical intervention during treatment, continue for at least 5 days after surgery; max. total duration of nimodipine use 21 days

Nimotop® (Bayer) PoM
Tablets, yellow, f/c, nimodipine 30 mg. Net price 100-tab pack = £38.85
Intravenous infusion, nimodipine 200 micrograms/mL; also contains ethanol 20% and macrogol '400' 17%. Net price 50-mL vial (with polyethylene infusion catheter) = £13.24
NOTE. Polyethylene, polypropylene or glass apparatus should be used; PVC should be avoided

NISOLDIPINE

Indications: prophylaxis of angina, mild to moderate hypertension

Cautions: elderly; hypotension; avoid grapefruit juice (may affect metabolism); **interactions:** Appendix 1 (calcium-channel blockers)

Contra-indications: cardiogenic shock, aortic stenosis, unstable or acute attacks of angina; within 1 week of myocardial infarction; hepatic impairment (dose form not appropriate); pregnancy (Appendix 4); breast-feeding (Appendix 5)

Side-effects: gravitational oedema, headache, flushing, tachycardia, palpitation; dizziness, asthenia, gastro-intestinal disturbances (including nausea, constipation); less frequently paraesthesia, myalgia, tremor, hypotension, weakness, dyspnoea, allergic skin reactions, increased frequency of micturition; rarely exacerbation of angina, visual disturbances, gynaecomastia, gum hyperplasia

Dose: initially 10 mg daily, preferably before breakfast; if necessary increase at intervals of at least 1 week (usual maintenance in angina 20–40 mg once daily); max. 40 mg daily

Syscor MR® (Forest) PoM
Tablets, m/r, f/c, yellow, nisoldipine 10 mg, net price 28-tab pack = £8.77. Label: 22, 25

VERAPAMIL HYDROCHLORIDE

Indications: see under Dose and preparations

Cautions: first-degree AV block; acute phase of myocardial infarction (avoid if bradycardia, hypotension, left ventricular failure); patients taking beta-blockers (**important:** see below); hepatic impairment (Appendix 2); children, specialist advice only (section 2.3.2); pregnancy (Appendix 4) and breast-feeding (Appendix 5); avoid grapefruit juice (may affect metabolism); **interactions:** Appendix 1 (calcium-channel blockers)
VERAPAMIL AND BETA-BLOCKERS. **Verapamil** injection should not be given to patients recently treated with beta-blockers because of the risk of hypotension and asystole. The suggestion that when verapamil injection has been given first, an interval of 30 minutes before giving a beta-blocker is sufficient has not been confirmed.
It may also be hazardous to give verapamil and a beta-blocker together by mouth (should only be contemplated if myocardial function well preserved).

Contra-indications: hypotension, bradycardia, second- and third-degree AV block, sick sinus syndrome, cardiogenic shock, sino-atrial block; history of heart failure or significantly impaired left ventricular function, even if controlled by therapy; atrial flutter or fibrillation complicating Wolff-Parkinson-White syndrome; porphyria (section 9.8.2)

Side-effects: constipation; less commonly nausea, vomiting, flushing, headache, dizziness, fatigue, ankle oedema; rarely allergic reactions (erythema, pruritus, urticaria, angioedema, Stevens-Johnson syndrome); myalgia, arthralgia, paraesthesia, erythromelalgia; increased prolactin concentration; rarely gynaecomastia and gingival hyperplasia after long-term treatment; after intravenous administration or high doses, hypotension, heart failure, bradycardia, heart block, and asystole

Dose: *by mouth*, supraventricular arrhythmias (but see also Contra-indications), 40–120 mg 3 times daily
Angina, 80–120 mg 3 times daily
Hypertension, 240–480 mg daily in 2–3 divided doses
By slow intravenous injection over 2 minutes (3 minutes in elderly), 5–10 mg (preferably with ECG monitoring); in paroxysmal tachyarrhythmias a further 5 mg after 5–10 minutes if required

Verapamil (Non-proprietary) PoM
Tablets, coated, verapamil hydrochloride 40 mg, net price 20 = 62p; 80 mg, 20 = 60p; 120 mg, 20 = £1.39; 160 mg, 20 = £2.23
Oral solution, verapamil hydrochloride 40 mg/5 mL, net price 150 mL = £36.90
Brands include *Zolvera*®

Cordilox® (IVAX) PoM
Tablets, all yellow, f/c, verapamil hydrochloride 40 mg, net price 84-tab pack = £1.50; 80 mg, 84-tab pack = £2.05; 120 mg, 28-tab pack = £1.15; 160 mg, 56-tab pack = £2.80
Injection, verapamil hydrochloride 2.5 mg/mL, net price 2-mL amp = £1.11

Securon® (Abbott) PoM
Tablets, f/c, verapamil hydrochloride 40 mg, net price 100 = £4.57; 120 mg (scored), 60-tab pack = £6.29
Injection, verapamil hydrochloride 2.5 mg/mL. Net price 2-mL amp = £1.08

■ Modified release

Half Securon SR® (Abbott) PoM
Tablets, m/r, f/c, verapamil hydrochloride 120 mg. Net price 28-tab pack = £7.50. Label: 25
Dose: see *Securon SR*®

Securon SR® (Abbott) PoM
Tablets, m/r, pale green, f/c, scored, verapamil hydrochloride 240 mg. Net price 28-tab pack = £6.29. Label: 25
Dose: hypertension, 240 mg daily (new patients initially 120 mg), increased if necessary to max. 480 mg daily (doses above 240 mg daily as 2 divided doses)
Angina, 240 mg twice daily (may sometimes be reduced to once daily)
Prophylaxis after myocardial infarction where beta-blockers not appropriate (started at least 1 week after infarction), 360 mg daily in divided doses, given as 240 mg in the morning and 120 mg in the evening *or* 120 mg 3 times daily

Univer® (Zeneus) PoM
Capsules, m/r, verapamil hydrochloride 120 mg (yellow/dark blue), net price 28-cap pack = £7.51; 180 mg (yellow), 56-cap pack = £18.15; 240 mg (yellow/dark blue), 28-cap pack = £12.24. Label: 25
Dose: hypertension, 240 mg daily, max. 480 mg daily (new patients, initial dose 120 mg); angina, 360 mg daily, max. 480 mg daily

Verapress MR® (Dexcel) PoM
Tablets, m/r, pale green, f/c, verapamil hydrochloride 240 mg. Net price 28-tab pack = £9.90. Label: 25
Dose: hypertension, 1 tablet daily, increased to twice daily if necessary; angina, 1 tablet twice daily (may sometimes be reduced to once daily)
NOTE. Also available as *Cordilox*® *MR*

Vertab® **SR 240** (Trinity-Chiesi) PoM
Tablets, m/r, pale green, f/c, scored, verapamil hydrochloride 240 mg, net price 28-tab pack = £8.63. Label: 25
Dose: mild to moderate hypertension, 240 mg daily, increased to twice daily if necessary; angina, 240 mg twice daily (may sometimes be reduced to once daily)

2.6.3 Potassium-channel activators

Nicorandil, a potassium-channel activator with a nitrate component, has both arterial and venous vasodilating properties and is licensed for the prevention and long-term treatment of angina (section 2.6). Nicorandil has similar efficacy to other anti-anginal drugs in controlling symptoms; it may produce additional symptomatic benefit in combination with other antianginal drugs [unlicensed indication].

NICORANDIL

Indications: prophylaxis and treatment of angina
Cautions: hypovolaemia; low systolic blood pressure; acute pulmonary oedema; acute myocardial infarction with acute left ventricular failure and low filling pressures; pregnancy (Appendix 4); **interactions:** Appendix 1 (nicorandil)
DRIVING. Patients should be warned not to drive or operate machinery until it is established that their performance is unimpaired
Contra-indications: cardiogenic shock; left ventricular failure with low filling pressures; hypotension; breast-feeding
Side-effects: headache (especially on initiation, usually transitory); cutaneous vasodilatation with flushing; nausea, vomiting, dizziness, weakness also reported; *rarely* oral ulceration, myalgia, and rash; at high dosage, reduction in blood pressure and/or increase in heart rate; angioedema, hepatic dysfunction, and anal ulceration also reported
Dose: initially 10 mg twice daily (if susceptible to headache 5 mg twice daily); usual dose 10–20 mg twice daily; up to 30 mg twice daily may be used

Ikorel® (Rhône-Poulenc Rorer) PoM
Tablets, both scored, nicorandil 10 mg, net price 60-tab pack = £8.18; 20 mg, 60-tab pack = £15.54

2.6.4 Peripheral vasodilators and related drugs

Most serious peripheral vascular disorders, such as *intermittent claudication*, are due to occlusion of vessels, either by spasm or sclerotic plaques. Life-style changes including smoking cessation and exercise training are the most important measures in the conservative management of intermittent claudication. Low-dose aspirin (75 mg daily) should be given as long-term prophylaxis against cardio-vascular events and a statin (section 2.12) should be considered if serum total cholesterol is raised. **Naftidrofuryl** 200 mg 3 times daily may alleviate symptoms and improve pain-free walking distance in moderate disease, but it is not known whether naftidrofuryl has any effect on the outcome of the disease. Patients receiving naftidrofuryl should be assessed for improvement after 3–6 months. **Cilostazol** is licensed for use in intermittent claudication to improve walking distance in patients without peripheral tissue necrosis and who do not have pain at rest. Inositol nicotinate, pentoxifylline (oxpentifylline) and cinnarizine are not established as being effective.

Management of *Raynaud's syndrome* includes avoidance of exposure to cold and stopping smoking. More severe symptoms may require vasodilator treatment, which is most often successful in primary Raynaud's syndrome. **Nifedipine** (section 2.6.2) is useful for reducing the frequency and severity of vasospastic attacks. Alternatively, **naftidrofuryl** may produce symptomatic improvement; **inositol nicotinate** (a nicotinic acid derivative) may also be considered. Cinnarizine, pentoxifylline, prazosin and moxisylyte (thymoxamine) are not established as being effective.

Vasodilator therapy is not established as being effective for *chilblains* (section 13.14).

CILOSTAZOL

Indications: intermittent claudication in patients without rest pain and no peripheral tissue necrosis

Cautions: atrial or ventricular ectopy, atrial fibrillation, atrial flutter; diabetes mellitus (higher risk of intra-ocular bleeding); **interactions:** Appendix 1 (cilostazol)

Contra-indications: predisposition to bleeding (e.g. active peptic ulcer, haemorrhagic stroke in previous 6 months, surgery in previous 3 months, proliferative diabetic retinopathy, poorly controlled hypertension); history of ventricular tachycardia, of ventricular fibrillation and of multifocal ventricular ectopics, prolongation of QT interval, congestive heart failure; moderate or severe hepatic impairment (Appendix 2); renal impairment (Appendix 3); pregnancy (Appendix 4); breast-feeding (Appendix 5)

Side-effects: diarrhoea, abnormal stools, and headache are very common; nausea, vomiting, dyspepsia, flatulence, abdominal pain; tachycardia, palpitation, angina, arrhythmia, chest pain; rhinitis; dizziness; ecchymosis; rash, pruritus; oedema, asthenia; less commonly, gastritis, myocardial infarction, congestive heart failure, postural hypotension, insomnia, anxiety, abnormal dreams, dyspnoea, pneumonia, cough, hypersensitivity reactions, diabetes mellitus, anaemia, haemorrhage, thrombocythaemia, myalgia, renal impairment

Dose: 100 mg twice daily (30 minutes before or 2 hours after food)

Pletal (Otsuka) ▼ PoM
Tablets, cilostazol 100 mg, net price 56-tab pack = £35.31

CINNARIZINE

Indications: peripheral vascular disease, Raynaud's syndrome

Cautions: see section 3.4.1

Contra-indications: see section 3.4.1

Side-effects: see section 3.4.1; also hypotension with high doses, allergic skin reactions, fatigue; *rarely* extrapyramidal symptoms in elderly on prolonged therapy

Dose: initially, 75 mg 3 times daily; maintenance, 75 mg 2–3 times daily

Stugeron Forte® (Janssen-Cilag)
Capsules, orange/ivory, cinnarizine 75 mg. Net price 100-cap pack = £5.23. Label: 2

Stugeron®
See section 4.6

MOXISYLYTE

(Thymoxamine)

Indications: primary Raynaud's syndrome (short-term treatment)

Cautions: diabetes mellitus

Contra-indications: active liver disease; pregnancy (Appendix 4)

Side-effects: nausea, diarrhoea, flushing, headache, dizziness; hepatic reactions including cholestatic jaundice and hepatitis reported to CSM

Dose: initially 40 mg 4 times daily, increased to 80 mg 4 times daily if poor initial response; discontinue after 2 weeks if no response

Opilon® (Concord) PoM
Tablets, yellow, f/c, moxisylyte 40 mg (as hydrochloride). Net price 112-tab pack = £79.98. Label: 21

NAFTIDROFURYL OXALATE

Indications: see under Dose

Side-effects: nausea, epigastric pain, rash, hepatitis, hepatic failure

Dose: peripheral vascular disease (see notes above), 100–200 mg 3 times daily; cerebral vascular disease, 100 mg 3 times daily

Naftidrofuryl (Non-proprietary) PoM
Capsules, naftidrofuryl oxalate 100 mg. Net price 84-cap pack = £7.86. Label: 25, 27

Praxilene® (Merck) PoM
Capsules, pink, naftidrofuryl oxalate 100 mg. Net price 84-cap pack = £8.60. Label: 25, 27

INOSITOL NICOTINATE

Indications: peripheral vascular disease; hyperlipidaemia (section 2.12)

Cautions: cerebrovascular insufficiency, unstable angina

Contra-indications: recent myocardial infarction, acute phase of a cerebrovascular accident; pregnancy (Appendix 4)

Side-effects: nausea, vomiting, hypotension, flushing, syncope, oedema, headache, dizziness, paraesthesia, rash

Dose: 3 g daily in 2–3 divided doses; max. 4 g daily

Hexopal® (Genus)
Tablets, scored, inositol nicotinate 500 mg. Net price 20 = £4.10
Tablets forte, scored, inositol nicotinate 750 mg. Net price 112-tab pack = £34.02

PENTOXIFYLLINE

(Oxpentifylline)

Indications: peripheral vascular disease; venous leg ulcers [unlicensed indication] (Appendix A8.2.5)

Cautions: hypotension, coronary artery disease; renal impairment (Appendix 3), severe hepatic impairment; avoid in porphyria (section 9.8.2); **interactions:** Appendix 1 (pentoxifylline)

Contra-indications: cerebral haemorrhage, extensive retinal haemorrhage, acute myocardial infarction; pregnancy and breast-feeding

Side-effects: gastro-intestinal disturbances, dizziness, agitation, sleep disturbances, headache; rarely flushing, tachycardia, angina, hypotension, thrombocytopenia, intrahepatic cholestasis, hypersensitivity reactions including rash, pruritus and bronchospasm

Dose: 400 mg 2–3 times daily

Trental® (Aventis Pharma) PoM
Tablets, m/r, pink, s/c, pentoxifylline 400 mg. Net price 90-tab pack = £20.48. Label: 21, 25

Other preparations used in peripheral vascular disease

Rutosides (oxerutins, *Paroven*®) are not vasodilators and are not generally regarded as effective preparations as capillary sealants or for the treatment of cramps; side-effects include headache, flushing, rashes, mild gastro-intestinal disturbances.

Paroven® (Novartis Consumer Health)
Capsules, yellow, oxerutins 250 mg. Net price 120-cap pack = £13.05
Dose: relief of symptoms of oedema associated with chronic venous insufficiency, 500 mg twice daily

2.7 Sympathomimetics

The properties of sympathomimetics vary according to whether they act on alpha or on beta adrenergic receptors. Adrenaline (epinephrine) (section 2.7.3) acts on both alpha and beta receptors and increases both heart rate and contractility ($beta_1$ effects); it can cause peripheral vasodilation (a $beta_2$ effect) or vasoconstriction (an alpha effect).

2.7.1 Inotropic sympathomimetics

The cardiac stimulants **dobutamine** and **dopamine** act on $beta_1$ receptors in cardiac muscle, and increase contractility with little effect on rate.

Dopexamine acts on $beta_2$ receptors in cardiac muscle to produce its positive inotropic effect; and on peripheral dopamine receptors to increase renal perfusion; it is reported not to induce vasoconstriction.

Isoprenaline injection is available on special order only.

SHOCK. Shock is a medical emergency associated with a high mortality. The underlying causes of shock such as haemorrhage, sepsis or myocardial insufficiency should be corrected. The profound hypotension of shock must be treated promptly to prevent tissue hypoxia and organ failure. Volume replacement is essential to correct the hypovolaemia associated with haemorrhage and sepsis but may be detrimental in cardiogenic shock. Depending on haemodynamic status, cardiac output may be improved by the use of sympathomimetic inotropes such as adrenaline (epinephrine), dobutamine or dopamine (see notes above). In septic shock, when fluid replacement and inotropic support fail to maintain blood pressure, the vasoconstrictor noradrenaline (norepinephrine) (section 2.7.2) may be considered. In cardiogenic shock peripheral resistance is frequently high and to raise it further may worsen myocardial performance and exacerbate tissue ischaemia.

The use of sympathomimetic inotropes and vasoconstrictors should preferably be confined to the intensive care setting and undertaken with invasive haemodynamic monitoring.

For advice on the management of anaphylactic shock, see section 3.4.3.

DOBUTAMINE

Indications: inotropic support in infarction, cardiac surgery, cardiomyopathies, septic shock, and cardiogenic shock
Cautions: severe hypotension complicating cardiogenic shock; **interactions:** Appendix 1 (sympathomimetics)
Side-effects: tachycardia and marked increase in systolic blood pressure indicate overdosage; phlebitis; *rarely* thrombocytopenia
Dose: *by intravenous infusion*, 2.5–10 micrograms/kg/minute, adjusted according to response

Dobutamine (Non-proprietary) PoM
Strong sterile solution, dobutamine (as hydrochloride) 12.5 mg/mL. For dilution and use as an intravenous infusion. Net price 20-mL amp = £5.25

DOPAMINE HYDROCHLORIDE

Indications: cardiogenic shock in infarction or cardiac surgery
Cautions: correct hypovolaemia; low dose in shock due to acute myocardial infarction—see notes above; **interactions:** Appendix 1 (sympathomimetics)
Contra-indications: tachyarrhythmia, phaeochromocytoma
Side-effects: nausea and vomiting, peripheral vasoconstriction, hypotension, hypertension, tachycardia
Dose: *by intravenous infusion*, 2–5 micrograms/kg/minute initially (see notes above)

Dopamine (Non-proprietary) PoM
Sterile concentrate, dopamine hydrochloride 40 mg/mL, net price 5-mL amp = £3.88; 160 mg/mL, net price 5-mL amp = £14.75. For dilution and use as an intravenous infusion
Intravenous infusion, dopamine hydrochloride 1.6 mg/mL in glucose 5% intravenous infusion, net price 250-mL container (400 mg) = £11.69; 3.2 mg/mL, 250-mL container (800 mg) = £22.93 (both hosp. only)

Select-A-Jet® **Dopamine** (Celltech) PoM
Strong sterile solution, dopamine hydrochloride 40 mg/mL. Net price 5-mL vial = £4.55; 10-mL vial = £7.32. For dilution and use as an intravenous infusion

DOPEXAMINE HYDROCHLORIDE

Indications: inotropic support and vasodilator in exacerbations of chronic heart failure and in heart failure associated with cardiac surgery
Cautions: myocardial infarction, recent angina, hypokalaemia, hyperglycaemia; correct hypovolaemia before starting, monitor blood pressure, pulse, plasma potassium, blood glucose; avoid abrupt withdrawal; **interactions:** Appendix 1 (sympathomimetics)
Contra-indications: left ventricular outlet obstruction such as hypertrophic cardiomyopathy or aortic stenosis; phaeochromocytoma, thrombocytopenia
Side-effects: tachycardia, other arrhythmias; also reported: nausea, vomiting, anginal pain, tremor, headache

Dose: *by intravenous infusion* into central or large peripheral vein, 500 nanograms/kg/minute, may be increased to 1 microgram/kg/minute and further increased up to 6 micrograms/kg/minute in increments of 0.5–1 microgram/kg/minute at intervals of not less than 15 minutes

Dopacard® (Zeneus) PoM
Strong sterile solution, dopexamine hydrochloride 10 mg/mL (1%). For dilution and use as an intravenous infusion. Net price 5-mL amp = £21.00
NOTE. Contact with metal in infusion apparatus should be minimised

2.7.2 Vasoconstrictor sympathomimetics

Vasoconstrictor sympathomimetics raise blood pressure transiently by acting on alpha-adrenergic receptors to constrict peripheral vessels. They are sometimes used as an emergency method of elevating blood pressure where other measures have failed (see also section 2.7.1).

The danger of vasoconstrictors is that although they raise blood pressure they do so at the expense of perfusion of vital organs such as the kidney.

Spinal and epidural anaesthesia may result in sympathetic block with resultant hypotension. Management may include intravenous fluids (which are usually given prophylactically), oxygen, elevation of the legs, and injection of a pressor drug such as ephedrine. As well as constricting peripheral vessels **ephedrine** also accelerates the heart rate (by acting on beta receptors). Use is made of this dual action of ephedrine to manage associated bradycardia (although intravenous injection of atropine sulphate 400 to 600 micrograms may also be required if bradycardia persists).

EPHEDRINE HYDROCHLORIDE

Indications: see under Dose
Cautions: hyperthyroidism, diabetes mellitus, ischaemic heart disease, hypertension, angle-closure glaucoma, elderly, pregnancy (Appendix 4); may cause acute urine retention in prostatic hypertrophy; **interactions:** Appendix 1 (sympathomimetics)
Contra-indications: breast-feeding (Appendix 5)
Side-effects: nausea, vomiting, anorexia; tachycardia (sometimes bradycardia), arrhythmias, anginal pain, vasoconstriction with hypertension, vasodilation with hypotension, dizziness and flushing; dyspnoea; headache, anxiety, restlessness, confusion, psychoses, insomnia, tremor; difficulty in micturition, urine retention; sweating, hypersalivation; changes in blood-glucose concentration
Dose: reversal of hypotension from spinal or epidural anaesthesia, *by slow intravenous injection* of a solution containing ephedrine hydrochloride 3 mg/mL, 3–6 mg (max. 9 mg) repeated every 3–4 minutes according to response to max. 30 mg

Ephedrine Hydrochloride (Non-proprietary) PoM
Injection, ephedrine hydrochloride 3 mg/mL, net price 10-mL amp = £2.83; 30 mg/mL, net price 1-mL amp = £1.70

METARAMINOL

Indications: acute hypotension (see notes above); priapism (section 7.4.5) [unlicensed indication]
Cautions: see under Noradrenaline Acid Tartrate; longer duration of action than noradrenaline (norepinephrine), see below; cirrhosis; pregnancy (Appendix 4); breast-feeding (Appendix 5)
HYPERTENSIVE RESPONSE. Metaraminol has a longer duration of action than noradrenaline, and an excessive vasopressor response may cause a prolonged rise in blood pressure
Contra-indications: see under Noradrenaline Acid Tartrate
Side-effects: see under Noradrenaline Acid Tartrate; tachycardia; fatal ventricular arrhythmia reported in Laennec's cirrhosis
Dose: *by intravenous infusion*, 15–100 mg, adjusted according to response
In emergency, *by intravenous injection*, 0.5–5 mg then *by intravenous infusion*, 15–100 mg, adjusted according to response

Metaraminol (Non-proprietary) PoM
Injection, metaraminol 10 mg (as tartrate)/mL.
Available from regional hospital manufacturing unit ('special order')

NORADRENALINE ACID TARTRATE/ NOREPINEPHRINE BITARTRATE

Indications: see under dose
Cautions: coronary, mesenteric, or peripheral vascular thrombosis; following myocardial infarction, Prinzmetal's variant angina, hyperthyroidism, diabetes mellitus; hypoxia or hypercapnia; uncorrected hypovolaemia; elderly; extravasation at injection site may cause necrosis; **interactions:** Appendix 1 (sympathomimetics)
Contra-indications: hypertension (monitor blood pressure and rate of flow frequently); pregnancy (Appendix 4)
Side-effects: hypertension, headache, bradycardia, arrhythmias, peripheral ischaemia
Dose: acute hypotension, *by intravenous infusion*, via central venous catheter, of a solution containing noradrenaline acid tartrate 80 micrograms/mL (equivalent to noradrenaline base 40 micrograms/mL) at an initial rate of 0.16–0.33 mL/minute, adjusted according to response
Cardiac arrest, *by rapid intravenous or intracardiac injection*, 0.5–0.75 mL of a solution containing noradrenaline acid tartrate 200 micrograms/mL (equivalent to noradrenaline base 100 micrograms/mL)

Noradrenaline/Norepinephrine (Abbott) PoM
Injection, noradrenaline acid tartrate 2 mg/mL (equivalent to noradrenaline base 1 mg/mL). For dilution before use. Net price 2-mL amp = £1.01, 4-mL amp = £1.50, 20-mL amp = £6.35

PHENYLEPHRINE HYDROCHLORIDE

Indications: acute hypotension (see notes above); priapism (section 7.4.5) [unlicensed indication]
Cautions: see under Noradrenaline Acid Tartrate; longer duration of action than noradrenaline (norepinephrine), see below; coronary disease
HYPERTENSIVE RESPONSE. Phenylephrine has a longer duration of action than noradrenaline, and an excessive vasopressor response may cause a prolonged rise in blood pressure

Contra-indications: see under Noradrenaline Acid Tartrate; severe hyperthyroidism; pregnancy (Appendix 4)
Side-effects: see under Noradrenaline Acid Tartrate; tachycardia or reflex bradycardia
Dose: *by subcutaneous or intramuscular injection*, 2–5 mg, followed if necessary by further doses of 1–10 mg
By slow intravenous injection of a 1 mg/mL solution, 100–500 micrograms repeated as necessary after at least 15 minutes
By intravenous infusion, initial rate up to 180 micrograms/minute reduced to 30–60 micrograms/minute according to response

Phenylephrine (Sovereign) PoM
Injection, phenylephrine hydrochloride 10 mg/mL (1%). Net price 1-mL amp = £5.50

2.7.3 Cardiopulmonary resuscitation

The algorithm for cardiopulmonary resuscitation (see inside back cover) reflects the most recent recommendations of the Resuscitation Council (UK). In cardiac arrest **adrenaline (epinephrine)** 1 in 10 000 (100 micrograms/mL) is recommended in a dose of 10 mL by intravenous injection, preferably through a central line. If injected through a peripheral line, the drug must be flushed with at least 20 mL sodium chloride 0.9% injection (to aid entry into the central circulation). Intravenous injection of **amiodarone** 300 mg (from a prefilled syringe *or* diluted in glucose intravenous infusion 5%) should be considered after adrenaline to treat ventricular fibrillation or pulseless ventricular tachycardia in cardiac arrest refractory to defibrillation. **Atropine** 3 mg by intravenous injection (section 15.1.3) as a single dose is also used in cardiopulmonary resuscitation to block vagal activity.

For the management of acute anaphylaxis see section 3.4.3.

ADRENALINE/EPINEPHRINE

Indications: see notes above
Cautions: heart disease, diabetes mellitus, hyperthyroidism, hypertension, arrhythmias, cerebrovascular disease, angle-closure glaucoma, avoid during second stage of labour; **interactions:** Appendix 1 (sympathomimetics)
Side-effects: anxiety, tremor, tachycardia, headache, cold extremities; in overdosage arrhythmias, cerebral haemorrhage, pulmonary oedema; nausea, vomiting, sweating, weakness, dizziness and hyperglycaemia also reported
Dose: see notes above

Adrenaline/Epinephrine 1 in 10 000, Dilute (Non-proprietary) PoM
Injection, adrenaline (as acid tartrate) 100 micrograms/mL. 10-mL amp.
Brands include *Minijet® Adrenaline*

2.8 Anticoagulants and protamine

The main use of anticoagulants is to prevent thrombus formation or extension of an existing thrombus in the slower-moving venous side of the circulation, where the thrombus consists of a fibrin web enmeshed with platelets and red cells. They are therefore widely used in the prevention and treatment of *deep-vein thrombosis in the legs*.

Anticoagulants are of less use in preventing thrombus formation in arteries, for in faster-flowing vessels thrombi are composed mainly of platelets with little fibrin. They are used to prevent thrombi forming on *prosthetic heart valves*.

2.8.1 Parenteral anticoagulants

Heparin

Heparin initiates anticoagulation rapidly but has a short duration of action. It is now often referred to as being **standard** or **unfractionated heparin** to distinguish it from the **low molecular weight heparins** (see p. 119), which have a longer duration of action. For patients at high risk of bleeding, heparin is more suitable than low molecular weight heparin because its effect can be terminated rapidly by stopping the infusion.

TREATMENT. For the initial treatment of *deep-vein thrombosis and pulmonary embolism* heparin is given as an *intravenous loading dose,* followed by *continuous intravenous infusion* (using an infusion pump) or by *intermittent subcutaneous injection*; the use of *intermittent intravenous injection* is no longer recommended. Alternatively, a low molecular weight heparin is given for initial treatment of deep vein thrombosis and pulmonary embolism. An oral anticoagulant (usually warfarin, section 2.8.2) is started at the same time as the heparin (the heparin needs to be continued for at least 5 days and until the INR has been in the therapeutic range for 2 consecutive days). Laboratory monitoring is essential—preferably on a daily basis, determination of the activated partial thromboplastin time (APTT) being the most widely used technique. Heparin is also used in regimens for the management of *myocardial infarction* (see also section 2.10.1), the management of *unstable angina* (section 2.6), and the management of *acute peripheral arterial occlusion*.

PROPHYLAXIS. In patients undergoing *general surgery*, low-dose heparin by subcutaneous injection is widely advocated to *prevent postoperative deep-vein thrombosis and pulmonary embolism* in 'high risk' patients (i.e. those with obesity, malignant disease, history of deep-vein thrombosis or pulmonary embolism, patients over 40 years, or those with an established thrombophilic disorder or who are undergoing large or complicated surgical procedures); laboratory monitoring is not required with this *standard prophylactic regimen*.

To combat the increased risk in *major orthopaedic surgery* an *adjusted dose regimen* may be used (with monitoring) or *low molecular weight heparin* (see below), or aspirin, or in patients at high risk of thromboembolism, warfarin may be selected.

EXTRACORPOREAL CIRCUITS. Heparin is also used in the maintenance of extracorporeal circuits in *cardiopulmonary bypass* and *haemodialysis*.

HAEMORRHAGE. If haemorrhage occurs it is usually sufficient to withdraw heparin, but if rapid reversal of the effects of heparin is required, protamine sulphate (section 2.8.3) is a specific antidote (but only partially reverses the effects of low molecular weight heparins).

HEPARIN

Indications: see under Dose

Cautions: elderly; hypersensitivity to low molecular weight heparins; hepatic impairment (Appendix 2); renal impairment (Appendix 3); pregnancy (Appendix 4); **interactions:** Appendix 1 (heparin)

THROMBOCYTOPENIA. Clinically important thrombocytopenia is immune-mediated, and does not usually develop until after 6 to 10 days; it may be complicated by thrombosis. Platelet counts are recommended for patients receiving heparin (including low molecular weight heparins) for longer than 5 days (heparin should be stopped immediately, and not repeated, in those who develop thrombocytopenia or a 50% reduction of platelet count). Patients requiring continued anticoagulation should preferably be given lepirudin or a heparinoid such as danaparoid

HYPERKALAEMIA. Inhibition of aldosterone secretion by heparin (including low molecular weight heparins) may result in hyperkalaemia; patients with diabetes mellitus, chronic renal failure, acidosis, raised plasma potassium or those taking potassium-sparing drugs seem to be more susceptible. The risk appears to increase with duration of therapy and the CSM has recommended that plasma potassium should be measured in patients at risk before starting heparin and monitored regularly thereafter, particularly if heparin is to be continued for more than 7 days

Contra-indications: haemophilia and other haemorrhagic disorders, thrombocytopenia (including history of heparin-induced thrombocytopenia), peptic ulcer, recent cerebral haemorrhage, severe hypertension, severe liver disease (including oesophageal varices), after major trauma or recent surgery to eye or nervous system, acute bacterial endocarditis; spinal or epidural anaesthesia with treatment doses of heparin; hypersensitivity to heparin

Side-effects: haemorrhage (see notes above), skin necrosis, thrombocytopenia (see Cautions), hyperkalaemia (see Cautions), hypersensitivity reactions (including urticaria, angioedema, and anaphylaxis); osteoporosis after prolonged use (and rarely alopecia)

Dose: treatment of deep-vein thrombosis and pulmonary embolism, *by intravenous injection*, loading dose of 5000 units (10 000 units in severe pulmonary embolism) followed by continuous *infusion* of 15–25 units/kg/hour *or* treatment of deep-vein thrombosis, *by subcutaneous injection* of 15 000 units every 12 hours (laboratory monitoring essential—preferably on a daily basis, and dose adjusted accordingly)

SMALL ADULT OR CHILD, lower loading dose *then*, 15–25 units/kg/hour *by intravenous infusion, or* 250 units/kg every 12 hours *by subcutaneous injection*

Unstable angina, acute peripheral arterial occlusion, as intravenous regimen for deep-vein thrombosis and pulmonary embolism, above

Prophylaxis in orthopaedic surgery, see notes above

Prophylaxis in general surgery (see notes above), *by subcutaneous injection*, 5000 units 2 hours before surgery, then every 8–12 hours for 7 days or until patient is ambulant (monitoring not needed); during pregnancy (with monitoring), 5000–10 000 units every 12 hours (**important:** not intended to cover prevention of prosthetic heart valve thrombosis in pregnancy which calls for separate specialist management)

MYOCARDIAL INFARCTION. For the prevention of *coronary re-occlusion after thrombolysis* heparin is used in a variety of regimens according to locally agreed protocols

For the prevention of *mural thrombosis* heparin is considered effective when given *by subcutaneous injection* of 12 500 units every 12 hours for at least 10 days

Prevention of clotting in extracorporeal circuits, consult product literature

> *Note.* Doses above reflect the guidelines of the British Society for Haematology; for doses of the low molecular weight heparins, see below

Heparin (Non-proprietary) PoM

Injection, heparin sodium 1000 units/mL, net price 1-mL amp = 19p, 5-mL amp = 85p, 5-mL vial = 47p, 10-mL amp = £1.46, 20-mL amp = £2.40; 5000 units/mL, 1-mL amp = 36p, 5-mL amp = £1.00, 5-mL vial = 92p; 25 000 units/mL, 1-mL amp = £1.01, 5-mL vial = £3.68

Calciparine® (Sanofi-Synthelabo) PoM

Injection (subcutaneous only), heparin calcium 25 000 units/mL. Net price 0.2-mL syringe = 60p; 0.5-mL syringe = £1.46

Monoparin® (CP) PoM

Injection, heparin sodium (mucous) 1000 units/mL, net price 1-mL amp = 19p; 5-mL amp = 52p; 10-mL amp = 69p; 20-mL amp = £1.24; 5000 units/mL, 1-mL amp = 36p; 5-mL amp = £1.00; 25 000 units/mL, 0.2-mL amp = 46p, 1-mL amp = £1.01

Monoparin Calcium® (CP) PoM

Injection, heparin calcium 25 000 units/mL. Net price 0.2-mL amp = 48p

Multiparin® (CP) PoM

Injection, heparin sodium (mucous) 1000 units/mL, net price 5-mL vial = 47p; 5000 units/mL, 5-mL vial = 92p; 25 000 units/mL, 5-mL vial = £3.68

Low molecular weight heparins

Bemiparin, **dalteparin**, **enoxaparin**, **reviparin**, and **tinzaparin** are low molecular weight heparins. Low molecular weight heparins are as effective and as safe as unfractionated heparin in the *prevention* of venous thrombo-embolism; in orthopaedic practice they are probably more effective. They have a longer duration of action than unfractionated heparin; *once-daily subcutaneous* dosage means that they are convenient to use. The standard prophylactic regimen does not require monitoring.

Some low molecular weight heparins are also used in the *treatment* of deep-vein thrombosis, pulmonary embolism, unstable coronary artery disease (section 2.6) and for the prevention of clotting in extracorporeal circuits. Routine monitoring of anticoagulant effect of the treatment regimen is not usually required, but may be necessary in patients at increased risk of bleeding (e.g. in renal impairment and those who are underweight or overweight)

HAEMORRHAGE. See under Heparin.

BEMIPARIN SODIUM

Indications: see notes above and under preparations
Cautions: see under Heparin
Contra-indications: see under Heparin; breast-feeding (Appendix 5)
Side-effects: see under Heparin
Dose: see under preparations below

Zibor® (Amdipharm) ▼ PoM

Injection, bemiparin sodium 12 500 units/mL, net price 0.2-mL (2500-unit) prefilled syringe = £3.39; 17 500 units/mL, 0.2-mL (3500-unit) prefilled syringe = £4.52

Dose: prophylaxis of deep-vein thrombosis, *by subcutaneous injection*, moderate risk, 2500 units 2 hours before or 6 hours after surgery then 2500 units every 24 hours for 7–10 days; high risk, 3500 units 2 hours before or 6 hours after surgery then 3500 units every 24 hours for 7–10 days

Prevention of clotting in extracorporeal circuits, consult product literature

Injection, bemiparin sodium 25 000 units/mL, net price 0.2-mL (5000-unit) prefilled syringe = £6.96, 0.3-mL (7500-unit) prefilled syringe = £8.63, 0.4-mL (10 000-unit) prefilled syringe = £12.60

Dose: treatment of deep-vein thrombosis (with or without pulmonary embolism), *by subcutaneous injection*, 115 units/kg every 24 hours for 5–9 days (and until adequate oral anticoagulation established)

DALTEPARIN SODIUM

Indications: see notes above and under preparations
Cautions: see under Heparin; not known to be harmful in pregnancy
Contra-indications: see under Heparin
Side-effects: see under Heparin
Dose: see under preparations below

Fragmin® (Pharmacia) PoM

Injection (single-dose syringe), dalteparin sodium 12 500 units/mL, net price 0.2-mL (2500-unit) syringe = £1.86; 25 000 units/mL, 0.2-mL (5000-unit) syringe = £2.82, 0.3-mL (7500-unit) syringe = £4.23, 0.4-mL (10 000-unit) syringe = £5.65, 0.5-mL (12 500-unit) syringe = £7.06, 0.6-mL (15 000-unit) syringe = £8.47, 0.72-mL (18 000-unit) syringe = £10.16

Dose: prophylaxis of deep-vein thrombosis, in surgical patients, *by subcutaneous injection*, moderate risk, 2500 units 1–2 hours before surgery then 2500 units every 24 hours for 5–7 days or longer; high risk, 2500 units 1–2 hours before surgery, then 2500 units 8–12 hours later (*or* 5000 units on the evening before surgery, then 5000 units on the following evening), then 5000 units every 24 hours for 5–7 days or longer (5 weeks in hip replacement)

Prophylaxis of deep-vein thrombosis in medical patients, *by subcutaneous injection*, 5000 units every 24 hours

Treatment of deep-vein thrombosis and of pulmonary embolism, *by subcutaneous injection*, as a single daily dose, ADULT body-weight under 46 kg, 7500 units daily; body-weight 46–56 kg, 10 000 units daily; body-weight 57–68 kg, 12 500 units daily; body-weight 69–82 kg, 15 000 units daily; body-weight 83 kg and over, 18 000 units daily, with oral anticoagulant treatment until prothrombin complex concentration in therapeutic range (usually for at least 5 days); monitoring of anti-factor Xa not usually required; for patients at increased risk of haemorrhage, see below

Injection, dalteparin sodium 2500 units/mL (for subcutaneous or intravenous use), net price 4-mL (10 000-unit) amp = £5.12; 10 000-units/mL (for subcutaneous or intravenous use), 1-mL (10 000-unit) amp = £5.12; 25 000 units/mL (for subcutaneous use only), 4-mL (100 000-unit) vial = £48.66

Dose: treatment of deep-vein thrombosis and of pulmonary embolism, *by subcutaneous injection*, 200 units/kg (max. 18 000 units) as a single daily dose (*or* 100 units/kg twice daily if increased risk of haemorrhage) with oral anticoagulant treatment until prothrombin complex concentration in therapeutic range (usually for at least 5 days)

NOTE. For monitoring, blood should be taken 3–4 hours after a dose (recommended plasma concentration of anti-Factor Xa 0.5–1 unit/mL); monitoring not required for once-daily treatment regimen and not generally necessary for twice-daily regimen

Unstable coronary artery disease, *by subcutaneous injection,* 120 units/kg every 12 hours (max. 10 000 units twice daily) for 5–8 days

Prevention of clotting in extracorporeal circuits, consult product literature

Injection (graduated syringe), dalteparin sodium 10 000 units/mL, net price 1-mL (10 000-unit) syringe = £5.65

Dose: unstable coronary artery disease (including non-ST-segment-elevation myocardial infarction), *by subcutaneous injection*, 120 units/kg every 12 hours (max. 10 000 units twice daily) for up to 8 days; beyond 8 days (if awaiting angiography or revascularisation) women body-weight less than 80 kg and men less than 70 kg, 5000 units every 12 hours, women body-weight greater than 80 kg and men greater than 70 kg, 7500 units every 12 hours, until day of procedure (max. 45 days)

ENOXAPARIN SODIUM

Indications: see notes above and under preparations
Cautions: see under Heparin; low body-weight (increased risk of bleeding)
Contra-indications: see under Heparin; breast-feeding (Appendix 5)
Side-effects: see under Heparin
Dose: see under preparation below

Clexane® (Rhône-Poulenc Rorer) PoM

Injection, enoxaparin sodium 100 mg/mL, net price 0.2-mL (20-mg, 2000-units) syringe = £3.15, 0.4-mL (40-mg, 4000-units) syringe = £4.20, 0.6-mL (60-mg, 6000-units) syringe = £4.75, 0.8-mL (80-mg, 8000-units) syringe = £5.40, 1-mL (100-mg, 10 000-units) syringe = £6.69; 150 mg/mL (*Clexane*® *Forte*), 0.8-mL (120-mg, 12 000-units) syringe = £9.77, 1-mL (150-mg, 15 000-units) syringe = £11.10

Dose: prophylaxis of deep-vein thrombosis especially in surgical patients, *by subcutaneous injection, moderate risk*, 20 mg (2000 units) approx. 2 hours before surgery then 20 mg (2000 units) every 24 hours for 7–10 days; *high risk* (e.g. orthopaedic surgery), 40 mg (4000 units) 12 hours before surgery then 40 mg (4000 units) every 24 hours for 7–10 days

Prophylaxis of deep-vein thrombosis in medical patients, *by subcutaneous injection*, 40 mg (4000 units) every 24

hours for at least 6 days until patient ambulant (max. 14 days)
Treatment of deep-vein thrombosis or pulmonary embolism, *by subcutaneous injection*, 1.5 mg/kg (150 units/kg) every 24 hours, usually for at least 5 days (and until adequate oral anticoagulation established)
Unstable angina and non-ST-segment-elevation myocardial infarction, *by subcutaneous injection*, 1 mg/kg (100 units/kg) every 12 hours usually for 2–8 days (minimum 2 days)
Prevention of clotting in extracorporeal circuits, consult product literature

REVIPARIN SODIUM

Indications: see notes above and under preparation
Cautions: see under Heparin; platelet count recommended before treatment, on days 1 and 4 of treatment then twice weekly for first 3 weeks of treatment
Contra-indications: see under Heparin; pregnancy (Appendix 4)
Side-effects: see under Heparin
Dose: see under preparation below

Clivarine® (Valeant) PoM
Injection, reviparin sodium 1432 units/0.25-mL syringe, net price 1 syringe = £3.63
Dose: prophylaxis of deep-vein thrombosis, *by subcutaneous injection*, 1432 units 2 hours before surgery, then 1432 units every 24 hours for 7 days (or until patient is mobile)

TINZAPARIN SODIUM

Indications: see notes above and under preparations
Cautions: see under Heparin
Contra-indications: see under Heparin; breast-feeding (Appendix 5)
Side-effects: see under Heparin
Dose: see under preparations below

Innohep® (Leo) PoM
Injection, tinzaparin sodium 10 000 units/mL, net price 2500-unit (0.25-mL) syringe = £2.13, 3500-unit (0.35-mL) syringe = £2.98, 4500-unit (0.45-mL) syringe = £3.83, 20 000-unit (2-mL) vial = £11.36
Dose: prophylaxis of deep-vein thrombosis, *by subcutaneous injection*, general surgery, 3500 units 2 hours before surgery, then 3500 units every 24 hours for 7–10 days; orthopaedic surgery (high risk), 50 units/kg 2 hours before surgery, then 50 units/kg every 24 hours for 7–10 days *or* 4500 units 12 hours before surgery, then 4500 units every 24 hours for 7–10 days
Prevention of clotting in extracorporeal circuits, consult product literature
Injection, tinzaparin sodium 20 000 units/mL, net price 0.5-mL (10 000-unit) syringe = £9.65, 0.7-mL (14 000-unit) syringe = £13.51, 0.9-mL (18 000-unit) syringe = £17.37, 2-mL (40 000-unit) vial = £36.77
Dose: treatment of deep-vein thrombosis and of pulmonary embolism, *by subcutaneous injection*, 175 units/kg once daily for at least 6 days (and until adequate oral anticoagulation established)
NOTE. This treatment regimen does not require anticoagulation monitoring
ASTHMA. Presence of sulphites in formulation may (especially in patients with asthma) lead to hypersensitivity (with bronchospasm and shock)

Heparinoids

Danaparoid is a heparinoid used for prophylaxis of deep-vein thrombosis in patients undergoing general or orthopaedic surgery. Providing there is no evidence of cross-reactivity, it also has a role in patients who develop thrombocytopenia in association with heparin.

DANAPAROID SODIUM

Indications: prevention of deep-vein thrombosis in general or orthopaedic surgery; thromboembolic disease in patients with history of heparin-induced thrombocytopenia
Cautions: recent bleeding or risk of bleeding; antibodies to heparins (risk of antibody-induced thrombocytopenia); hepatic impairment (Appendix 2); renal impairment (Appendix 3); pregnancy (Appendix 4); breast-feeding (Appendix 5)
Contra-indications: haemophilia and other haemorrhagic disorders, thrombocytopenia (unless patient has heparin-induced thrombocytopenia), recent cerebral haemorrhage, severe hypertension, active peptic ulcer (unless this is the reason for operation), diabetic retinopathy, acute bacterial endocarditis, spinal or epidural anaesthesia with treatment doses of danaparoid
Side-effects: haemorrhage; hypersensitivity reactions (including rash)
Dose: prevention of deep-vein thrombosis, *by subcutaneous injection*, 750 units twice daily for 7–10 days; initiate treatment before operation (with last pre-operative dose 1–4 hours before surgery)
Thromboembolic disease in patients with history of heparin-induced thrombocytopenia, *by intravenous injection*, 2500 units (1250 units if body-weight under 55 kg, 3750 units if over 90 kg), followed by *intravenous infusion* of 400 units/hour for 2 hours, *then* 300 units/hour for 2 hours, *then* 200 units/hour for 5 days; monitor antifactor-Xa activity in renal impairment and in patients over 90 kg (consult product literature)

Orgaran® (Organon) PoM
Injection, danaparoid sodium 1250 units/mL, net price 0.6-mL amp (750 units) = £29.80

Hirudins

Lepirudin, a recombinant hirudin, is licensed for anticoagulation in patients with Type II (immune) heparin-induced thrombocytopenia who require parenteral antithrombotic treatment. The dose of lepirudin is adjusted according to activated partial thromboplastin time (APTT). **Bivalirudin**, a hirudin analogue, is a thrombin inhibitor which is licensed as an anticoagulant for patients undergoing percutaneous coronary intervention. The *Scottish Medicines Consortium* has advised (March 2005) that bivalirudin is accepted for restricted use for patients undergoing percutaneous coronary intervention who would have been considered for treatment with unfractionated heparin combined with a glycoprotein IIb/IIIa inhibitor; it should not be used alone.

BIVALIRUDIN

Indications: anticoagulation for patients undergoing percutaneous coronary intervention
Cautions: exposure to lepirudin (theoretical risk from lepirudin antibodies); brachytherapy procedures; renal impairment (Appendix 3); pregnancy (Appendix 4); breast-feeding (Appendix 5)
Contra-indications: severe hypertension; subacute bacterial endocarditis; active bleeding; bleeding disorders
Side-effects: bleeding (discontinue); *less commonly* nausea, vomiting, tachycardia, bradycardia, hypotension, angina, dyspnoea, allergic reactions (including isolated reports of anaphylaxis), headache, thrombocytopenia, anaemia, back and chest pain, and injection-site reactions; *very rarely* thrombosis
Dose: initially *by intravenous injection*, 750 micrograms/kg, then *by intravenous infusion* of 1.75 mg/kg/hour, for up to 4 hours after procedure complete

Angiox® (Nycomed) ▼ PoM
Injection, powder for reconstitution, bivalirudin, net price 250-mg vial = £310.00

LEPIRUDIN

Indications: thromboembolic disease requiring parenteral anticoagulation in patients with heparin-induced thrombocytopenia type II
Cautions: hepatic impairment (Appendix 2); renal impairment (Appendix 3); recent bleeding or risk of bleeding including recent puncture of large vessels, organ biopsy, recent major surgery, stroke, bleeding disorders, severe hypertension, bacterial endocarditis; determine activated partial thromboplastin time 4 hours after start of treatment (or after infusion rate altered) and at least once daily thereafter
Contra-indications: pregnancy and breast-feeding
Side-effects: bleeding; reduced haemoglobin concentration without obvious source of bleeding; fever, hypersensitivity reactions (including rash); injection-site reactions
Dose: initially *by slow intravenous injection* (of 5 mg/mL solution), 400 micrograms/kg followed by *continuous intravenous infusion* of 150 micrograms/kg/hour (max. 16.5 mg/hour), adjusted according to activated partial thromboplastin time, for 2–10 days (longer if necessary)

Refludan® (Pharmion) PoM
Injection, powder for reconstitution, lepirudin. Net price 50-mg vial = £57.00

Heparin flushes

For maintaining patency of peripheral venous catheters, sodium chloride injection 0.9% is as effective as heparin flushes.

Heparin Sodium (Non-proprietary) PoM
Solution, heparin sodium 10 units/mL, net price 5-mL amp = 25p; 100 units/mL, 2-mL amp = 28p
To maintain patency of catheters, cannulas, etc. 10–200 units flushed through every 4–8 hours. Not for therapeutic use

Canusal® (CP) PoM
Solution, heparin sodium 100 units/mL. Net price 2-mL amp = 28p
To maintain patency of catheters, cannulas, etc., 200 units flushed through every 4 hours or as required. Not for therapeutic use

Hepsal® (CP) PoM
Solution, heparin sodium 10 units/mL. Net price 5-mL amp = 25p
To maintain patency of catheters, cannulas, etc., 50 units flushed through every 4 hours or as required. Not for therapeutic use

Epoprostenol

Epoprostenol (prostacyclin) can be given to inhibit platelet aggregation during renal dialysis either alone or with heparin. It is also licensed for the treatment of primary pulmonary hypertension resistant to other treatment, usually with oral anticoagulation. Since its half-life is only about 3 minutes it must be given by continuous intravenous infusion. It is a potent vasodilator and therefore its side-effects include flushing, headache, and hypotension.

EPOPROSTENOL

Indications: see notes above
Cautions: anticoagulant monitoring required when given with heparin; haemorrhagic diathesis; dose titration for pulmonary hypertension should be in hospital (risk of pulmonary oedema); pregnancy (Appendix 4)
Contra-indications: severe left ventricular dysfunction
Side-effects: see notes above; also bradycardia, tachycardia, pallor, sweating with higher doses; gastro-intestinal disturbances; lassitude, anxiety, agitation; dry mouth, jaw pain, chest pain; also reported, hyperglycaemia and injection-site reactions
Dose: see product literature

Flolan® (GSK) PoM
Infusion, powder for reconstitution, epoprostenol (as sodium salt). Net price 500-microgram vial (with diluent) = £64.57; 1.5-mg vial (with diluent) = £130.07

Fondaparinux

Fondaparinux sodium is a synthetic pentasaccharide that inhibits activated factor X. It is licensed for prophylaxis of venous thromboembolism in medical patients and in patients undergoing major orthopaedic surgery of the legs. It is also licensed for treatment of deep-vein thrombosis and of pulmonary embolism.

FONDAPARINUX SODIUM

Indications: see notes above and under preparations
Cautions: bleeding disorders, active gastro-intestinal ulcer disease; recent intracranial haemorrhage; brain, spinal, or ophthalmic surgery; spinal or epidural anaesthesia (risk of spinal haematoma—avoid if using treatment doses); low body-weight; elderly patients; concomitant use of drugs that increase risk of bleeding; hepatic impairment (Appendix 2); renal impairment (App-

endix 3); pregnancy (Appendix 4); breast-feeding (Appendix 5)

Contra-indications: active bleeding; bacterial endocarditis

Side-effects: oedema; haemorrhage, anaemia, thrombocytopenia; purpura; liver enzyme changes; *less commonly* gastro-intestinal disturbances, hypotension, chest pain, dyspnoea, dizziness, vertigo, headache, thrombocythaemia, rash, pruritus, injection-site reactions

Dose: see under preparation below

Arixtra® (GSK) ▼ PoM

Injection, fondaparinux sodium 5 mg/mL, net price 0.5-mL (2.5-mg) prefilled syringe = £6.66

Dose: prophylaxis of venous thromboembolism in surgery, *by subcutaneous injection*, 2.5 mg 6 hours after surgery then 2.5 mg daily for 5–9 days (longer after hip surgery); CHILD under 17 years not recommended

Prophylaxis of venous thromboembolism in medical patients, *by subcutaneous injection*, 2.5 mg daily usually for 6–14 days; CHILD under 17 years not recommended

Injection, fondaparinux sodium 12.5 mg/mL, net price 0.4-mL (5-mg) prefilled syringe = £12.37, 0.6-mL (7.5-mg) prefilled syringe = £12.37, 0.8-mL (10-mg) prefilled syringe = £12.37

Dose: treatment of deep-vein thrombosis and of pulmonary embolism, *by subcutaneous injection*, ADULT body-weight under 50 kg, 5 mg every 24 hours; body-weight 50–100 kg, 7.5 mg every 24 hours; body-weight over 100 kg, 10 mg every 24 hours; usually for at least 5 days (and until adequate oral anticoagulation established); CHILD under 17 years not recommended

2.8.2 Oral anticoagulants

Oral anticoagulants antagonise the effects of vitamin K, and take at least 48 to 72 hours for the anticoagulant effect to develop fully; if an immediate effect is required, heparin must be given concomitantly.

USES. The main indication for an oral anticoagulant is *deep-vein thrombosis*. Patients with *pulmonary embolism* should also be treated, as should those with *atrial fibrillation who are at risk of embolisation* (see also section 2.3.1), and those with *mechanical prosthetic heart valves* (to prevent emboli developing on the valves); an antiplatelet drug may also be useful in these patients.

Warfarin is the drug of choice; **acenocoumarol** (nicoumalone) and **phenindione** are seldom required.

Oral anticoagulants should not be used in cerebral artery thrombosis or peripheral artery occlusion as first-line therapy; aspirin (section 2.9) is more appropriate for reduction of risk in transient ischaemic attacks.

DOSE. Whenever possible, the base-line prothrombin time should be determined but the initial dose should not be delayed whilst awaiting the result.

The usual adult induction dose of warfarin is 10 mg[1] daily for 2 days (higher doses no longer recommended). The subsequent maintenance dose depends upon the prothrombin time, reported as INR (international normalised ratio). The daily maintenance dose of warfarin is usually 3 to 9 mg (taken at the **same time** each day). The indications and target INRs[2] currently recommended by the British Society for Haematology[3] are:

- INR 2–2.5 for prophylaxis of deep-vein thrombosis including surgery on high-risk patients;
- INR 2.5 for treatment of deep-vein thrombosis and pulmonary embolism (or for recurrence in patients no longer receiving warfarin), atrial fibrillation, cardioversion, dilated cardiomyopathy, mural thrombus following myocardial infarction, and rheumatic mitral valve disease;
- INR 3.5 for recurrent deep-vein thrombosis and pulmonary embolism (in patients currently receiving warfarin with INR above 2) and mechanical prosthetic heart valves.

MONITORING. It is essential that the INR be determined daily or on alternate days in early days of treatment, *then* at longer intervals (depending on response[4]) *then* up to every 12 weeks.

HAEMORRHAGE. The main adverse effect of all oral anticoagulants is haemorrhage. Checking the INR and omitting doses when appropriate is essential; if the anticoagulant is stopped but not reversed, the INR should be measured 2–3 days later to ensure that it is falling. The following recommendations (which take into account the recommendations of the British Society for Haematology[3]) are based on the result of the INR and whether there is major or minor bleeding; the recommendations apply to patients taking warfarin:

- Major bleeding—stop warfarin; give phytomenadione (vitamin K_1) 5 mg by slow intravenous injection; give prothrombin complex concentrate (factors II, VII, IX and X) 30–50 units/kg *or* (if no concentrate available) fresh frozen plasma 15 mL/kg
- INR > 8.0, no bleeding or minor bleeding—stop warfarin, restart when INR < 5.0; if there are other risk factors for bleeding give phytomenadione (vitamin K_1) 500 micrograms by slow intravenous injection or 5 mg by mouth (for partial reversal of anticoagulation give smaller oral doses of phytomenadione e.g. 0.5–2.5 mg using the intravenous preparation orally); repeat dose of phytomenadione if INR still too high after 24 hours
- INR 6.0–8.0, no bleeding or minor bleeding—stop warfarin, restart when INR < 5.0
- INR < 6.0 but more than 0.5 units above tar-

1. First dose less than 10 mg if base-line prothrombin time prolonged, if liver-function tests abnormal, or if patient in cardiac failure, on parenteral feeding, less than average body weight, elderly, or receiving other drugs known to potentiate oral anticoagulants.

2. An INR which is within 0.5 units of the target value is generally satisfactory; larger deviations require dosage adjustment. Target values (rather than ranges) are now recommended (except for prophylaxis of deep-vein thrombosis where a range is still recommended).

3. Guidelines on Oral Anticoagulation: third edition. *Br J Haematol* 1998; **101**: 374–87

4. Change in patient's clinical condition, particularly associated with liver disease, intercurrent illness, or drug administration, necessitates more frequent testing. See also **interactions**, Appendix 1 (warfarin). Major changes in diet (especially involving salads and vegetables) and in alcohol consumption may also affect warfarin control.

get value—reduce dose or stop warfarin, restart when INR < 5.0

- Unexpected bleeding at therapeutic levels—always investigate possibility of underlying cause e.g. unsuspected renal or gastro-intestinal tract pathology

PREGNANCY. Oral anticoagulants are teratogenic and should not be given in the first trimester of pregnancy. Women at risk of pregnancy should be warned of this danger since stopping warfarin before the sixth week of gestation may largely avoid the risk of fetal abnormality. Oral anticoagulants cross the placenta with risk of placental or fetal haemorrhage, especially during the last few weeks of pregnancy and at delivery. Therefore, if at all possible, oral anticoagulants should be avoided in pregnancy, especially in the first and third trimesters. Difficult decisions may have to be made, particularly in women with prosthetic heart valves or with a history of recurrent venous thrombosis or pulmonary embolism.

TREATMENT BOOKLETS. Anticoagulant treatment booklets should be issued to patients, and are available for distribution to local healthcare professionals from Health Authorities and also from:

England and Wales:
Astron
The Causeway
Oldham Broadway
Business Park
Chadderton
Oldham OL9 9XD
(0161) 683 2376

Scotland:
Banner Business Supplies
20 South Gyle Crescent
Edinburgh EH12 9EB
(0131) 479 3279

Northern Ireland:
Central Services Agency
25 Adelaide St
Belfast BT2 8FH
(028) 9053 5652

These booklets include advice for patients on anticoagulant treatment.

WARFARIN SODIUM

Indications: prophylaxis of embolisation in rheumatic heart disease and atrial fibrillation; prophylaxis after insertion of prosthetic heart valve; prophylaxis and treatment of venous thrombosis and pulmonary embolism; transient ischaemic attacks

Cautions: recent surgery; hepatic impairment (Appendix 2); renal impairment (Appendix 3); breast-feeding (Appendix 5); avoid cranberry juice; **interactions:** Appendix 1 (coumarins)

Contra-indications: peptic ulcer, severe hypertension, bacterial endocarditis; pregnancy (see notes above and Appendix 4)

Side-effects: haemorrhage—see notes above; other side-effects reported include hypersensitivity, rash, alopecia, diarrhoea, unexplained drop in haematocrit, 'purple toes', skin necrosis, jaundice, hepatic dysfunction; also nausea, vomiting, and pancreatitis

Dose: see notes above

Warfarin (Non-proprietary) PoM

Tablets, warfarin sodium 0.5 mg (white), net price 28-tab pack = £1.00; 1 mg (brown), 28 = £1.47; 3 mg (blue), 28 = £1.30; 5 mg (pink), 28 = £1.76. Label: 10, anticoagulant card

Brands include *Marevan*®

ACENOCOUMAROL

(Nicoumalone)

Indications: see under Warfarin Sodium

Cautions: see under Warfarin Sodium

Contra-indications: see under Warfarin Sodium

Side-effects: see under Warfarin Sodium

Dose: 8–12 mg on 1st day; 4–8 mg on 2nd day; maintenance dose usually 1–8 mg daily

Sinthrome® (Alliance) PoM

Tablets, acenocoumarol 1 mg. Net price 20 = 92p. Label: 10, anticoagulant card

PHENINDIONE

Indications: prophylaxis of embolisation in rheumatic heart disease and atrial fibrillation; prophylaxis after insertion of prosthetic heart valve; prophylaxis and treatment of venous thrombosis and pulmonary embolism

Cautions: see under Warfarin Sodium; **interactions:** Appendix 1 (phenindione)

Contra-indications: see under Warfarin Sodium; breast-feeding (Appendix 5)

Side-effects: see under Warfarin Sodium; also hypersensitivity reactions including rashes, exfoliative dermatitis, exanthema, fever, leucopenia, agranulocytosis, eosinophilia, diarrhoea, renal and hepatic damage; urine coloured pink or orange

Dose: 200 mg on day 1; 100 mg on day 2; maintenance dose usually 50–150 mg daily

Phenindione (Non-proprietary) PoM

Tablets, phenindione 10 mg, net price 100 = £6.80; 25 mg, 100 = £9.50; 50 mg, 100 = £12.10. Label: 10, anticoagulant card, 14, (urine pink or orange)

2.8.3 Protamine sulphate

Although protamine sulphate is used to counteract overdosage with heparin, if used in excess it has an anticoagulant effect.

PROTAMINE SULPHATE

(Protamine Sulfate)

Indications: see above

Cautions: see above; also if increased risk of allergic reaction to protamine (includes previous treatment with protamine or protamine insulin, allergy to fish, men who are infertile or who have had a vasectomy)

Side-effects: nausea, vomiting, lassitude, flushing, hypotension, bradycardia, dyspnoea; hypersensitivity reactions (including angioedema, anaphylaxis) reported

Dose: *by intravenous injection* over approx. 10 minutes, 1 mg neutralises 80–100 units heparin when given within 15 minutes of heparin; if longer time, less protamine required as heparin rapidly excreted; max. 50 mg

Protamine Sulphate (Non-proprietary) PoM

Injection, protamine sulphate 10 mg /mL, net price 5-mL amp = £1.14, 10-mL amp = £3.96

Prosulf® (CP) PoM
Injection,, protamine sulphate 10 mg/mL. Net price 5-mL amp = 96p (glass), £1.20 (polypropylene)

2.9 Antiplatelet drugs

Antiplatelet drugs decrease platelet aggregation and may inhibit thrombus formation in the arterial circulation, where anticoagulants have little effect.

A low dose of **aspirin** is used for the *secondary prevention* of thrombotic cerebrovascular or cardiovascular disease. A single dose of aspirin 150–300 mg is given as soon as possible after an ischaemic event, preferably dispersed in water or chewed. The initial dose is followed by maintenance treatment with aspirin 75 mg daily.

A low dose of aspirin is also of benefit in the *primary prevention* of vascular events when the estimated 10-year cardiovascular disease risk is 20% or greater and provided that blood pressure is controlled (section 2.5)[1].

A low dose of aspirin (75 mg daily) is also given following coronary bypass surgery. For details on the use of aspirin in atrial fibrillation see section 2.3.1, for stable angina see section 2.6 and for intermittent claudication see section 2.6.4.1.

Clopidogrel is licensed for the prevention of ischaemic events in patients with a history of symptomatic ischaemic disease. Clopidogrel, in combination with low-dose aspirin, is also licensed for acute coronary syndrome without ST-segment elevation; in these circumstances the combination is given for at least 1 month but usually no longer than 9–12 months. However, long-term routine use of clopidogrel with aspirin increases the risk of bleeding and the evidence of benefit of such use is not compelling.

The *Scottish Medicines Consortium* has advised (February 2004) that clopidogrel be accepted for restricted use for the treatment of confirmed acute coronary syndrome (without ST-segment elevation), in combination with aspirin. Clopidogrel should be initiated in hospital inpatients **only**.

Dipyridamole is used by mouth as an adjunct to oral anticoagulation for prophylaxis of thromboembolism associated with prosthetic heart valves. Modified-release preparations are licensed for secondary prevention of ischaemic stroke and transient ischaemic attacks. Dipyridamole is also used in combination with low-dose aspirin; evidence of long-term benefit has not been established.

GLYCOPROTEIN IIb/IIIa INHIBITORS. Glycoprotein IIb/IIIa inhibitors prevent platelet aggregation by blocking the binding of fibrinogen to receptors on platelets. **Abciximab** is a monoclonal antibody which binds to glycoprotein IIb/IIIa receptors and to other related sites; it is licensed as an adjunct to heparin and aspirin for the prevention of ischaemic complications in high-risk patients undergoing percutaneous transluminal coronary intervention. Abciximab should be used once only. **Eptifibatide** and **tirofiban** also inhibit glycoprotein IIb/IIIa receptors; they are licensed for use with heparin and aspirin to prevent early myocardial infarction in patients with unstable angina (section 2.6) or non-ST-segment-elevation myocardial infarction. Abciximab, eptifibatide and tirofiban should be used by specialists only.

For use of epoprostenol, see section 2.8.1.

NICE guidance (glycoprotein IIb/IIIa inhibitors for acute coronary syndromes). NICE has recommended (September 2002) that a glycoprotein IIb/IIIa inhibitor (abciximab, eptifibatide, and tirofiban) should be considered in the management of unstable angina or non-ST-segment-elevation myocardial infarction.

A glycoprotein IIb/IIIa inhibitor is recommended for patients at high risk of myocardial infarction or death when early percutaneous coronary intervention is desirable but does not occur immediately; either eptifibatide or tirofiban is recommended in addition to other appropriate drug treatment.

A glycoprotein IIb/IIIa inhibitor is recommended as an adjunct to percutaneous coronary intervention:

- when early percutaneous coronary intervention is indicated but it is delayed;
- in patients with diabetes;
- if the procedure is complex.

NOTE. Only abciximab is licensed as an adjunct to percutaneous coronary intervention

ABCIXIMAB

Indications: prevention of ischaemic cardiac complications in patients undergoing percutaneous coronary intervention; short-term prevention of myocardial infarction in patients with unstable angina not responding to conventional treatment and who are scheduled for percutaneous coronary intervention (use under specialist supervision)

Cautions: measure baseline prothrombin time, activated clotting time, activated partial thromboplastin time, platelet count, haemoglobin and haematocrit; monitor haemoglobin and haematocrit 12 hours and 24 hours after start of treatment and platelet count 2–4 hours and 24 hours after start of treatment; concomitant use of drugs that increase risk of bleeding; discontinue if uncontrollable serious bleeding occurs or emergency cardiac surgery needed; consult product literature for details of procedures to minimise bleeding; elderly; hepatic impairment (Appendix 2); renal impairment (Appendix 3); pregnancy (Appendix 4)

Contra-indications: active internal bleeding; major surgery, intracranial or intraspinal surgery or trauma within last 2 months; stroke within last 2 years; intracranial neoplasm, arteriovenous malformation or aneurysm, severe hypertension, haemorrhagic diathesis, thrombocytopenia, vasculitis, hypertensive retinopathy; breast-feeding (Appendix 5)

Side-effects: bleeding manifestations; nausea, vomiting, hypotension, bradycardia, chest pain, back pain, headache, fever, puncture site pain, thrombocytopenia; *rarely* cardiac tamponade, adult respiratory distress, hypersensitivity reactions

1. Cardiovascular disease risk may be determined from the chart issued by the British Hypertension Society (*J Hum Hypertens* 2004; **18**: 139–85)—see inside back cover. The Joint British Societies' 'Cardiac Risk Assessor' computer programme may also be used to determine cardiovascular disease risk by adding together the coronary heart disease risk and stroke risk.

Dose: ADULT initially *by intravenous injection* over 1 minute, 250 micrograms/kg, then *by intravenous infusion*, 125 nanograms/kg/minute (max. 10 micrograms/minute); for prevention of ischaemic complications start 10–60 minutes before percutaneous coronary intervention and continue infusion for 12 hours; for unstable angina start up to 24 hours before possible percutaneous coronary intervention and continue infusion for 12 hours after intervention

ReoPro® (Lilly) PoM
Injection, abciximab 2 mg/mL, net price 5-mL vial = £260.40

ASPIRIN (antiplatelet)

(Acetylsalicylic Acid)

Indications: prophylaxis of cerebrovascular disease or myocardial infarction (see section 2.10.1 and notes above)

Cautions: asthma; uncontrolled hypertension; previous peptic ulceration (but manufacturer's package insert may advise avoidance of low-dose aspirin in history of peptic ulceration); hepatic impairment (Appendix 2); renal impairment (Appendix 3); pregnancy (Appendix 4); **interactions:** Appendix 1 (aspirin)

Contra-indications: children under 16 years and in breast-feeding (Reye's syndrome, section 4.7.1; Appendix 5); active peptic ulceration; haemophilia and other bleeding disorders

Side-effects: bronchospasm; gastro-intestinal haemorrhage (occasionally major), also other haemorrhage (e.g. subconjunctival)

Dose: see notes above

[1]**Aspirin** (Non-proprietary) PoM
Dispersible tablets, aspirin 75 mg, net price 20 = 19p; 300 mg, see section 4.7.1. Label: 13, 21, 32
Tablets, e/c, aspirin 75 mg, net price 56-tab pack = £1.62; 300 mg, see section 4.7.1. Label: 5, 25, 32
Brands include *Gencardia*®, *Micropirin*®

Angettes 75® (Bristol-Myers Squibb)
Tablets, aspirin 75 mg. Net price 28-tab pack = 94p. Label: 32

Caprin® (Sinclair) PoM
Tablets, e/c, pink, aspirin 75 mg, net price 28-tab pack = £1.55, 56-tab pack = £3.08, 100-tab pack = £5.24; 300 mg, see section 4.7.1. Label: 5, 25, 32

Nu-Seals® **Aspirin** (Alliance) PoM
Tablets, e/c, aspirin 75 mg, net price 56-tab pack = £2.60; 300 mg, see section 4.7.1. Label: 5, 25, 32
NOTE. Tablets may be chewed at diagnosis for rapid absorption

■ With isosorbide mononitrate
Section 2.6.1

CLOPIDOGREL

Indications: see notes above for *Scottish Medicines Consortium* advice; prevention of atherosclerotic events in peripheral arterial disease, or within 35 days of myocardial infarction, or within 6 months of ischaemic stroke, or (given with aspirin—see notes above) in acute coronary syndrome without ST-segment-elevation

Cautions: patients at risk of increased bleeding from trauma, surgery or other pathological conditions; concomitant use of drugs that increase risk of bleeding; discontinue 7 days before elective surgery if antiplatelet effect not desirable; liver impairment (Appendix 2); renal impairment (Appendix 3); pregnancy (Appendix 4); **interactions:** Appendix 1 (clopidogrel)

Contra-indications: active bleeding, breast-feeding (Appendix 5)

Side-effects: dyspepsia, abdominal pain, diarrhoea; bleeding disorders (including gastro-intestinal and intracranial); *less commonly* nausea, vomiting, gastritis, flatulence, constipation, gastric and duodenal ulcers, headache, dizziness, paraesthesia, leucopenia, decreased platelets (very rarely severe thrombocytopenia), eosinophilia, rash, and pruritus; *rarely* vertigo; *very rarely* colitis, pancreatitis, hepatitis, vasculitis, confusion, hallucinations, taste disturbance, blood disorders (including thrombocytopenic purpura, agranulocytosis and pancytopenia), and hypersensitivity-like reactions (including fever, glomerulonephritis, arthralgia, Stevens-Johnson syndrome, lichen planus)

Dose: 75 mg once daily
Acute coronary syndrome, initially 300 mg then 75 mg daily (with aspirin, but see notes above)

Plavix® (Bristol-Myers Squibb, Sanofi-Synthelabo) PoM
Tablets, pink, f/c, clopidogrel (as hydrogen sulphate) 75 mg, net price 28-tab pack = £35.31

DIPYRIDAMOLE

Indications: see notes above and under Dose

Cautions: rapidly worsening angina, aortic stenosis, recent myocardial infarction, heart failure; may exacerbate migraine; hypotension; myasthenia gravis (risk of exacerbation); breast-feeding (Appendix 5); **interactions:** Appendix 1 (dipyridamole)

Side-effects: gastro-intestinal effects, dizziness, myalgia, throbbing headache, hypotension, hot flushes and tachycardia; worsening symptoms of coronary heart disease; hypersensitivity reactions such as rash, urticaria, severe bronchospasm and angioedema; increased bleeding during or after surgery; thrombocytopenia reported

Dose: *by mouth*, 300–600 mg daily in 3–4 divided doses before food
Modified-release preparations, see under preparation below
By intravenous injection, diagnostic only, consult product literature

Dipyridamole (Non-proprietary) PoM
Tablets, coated, dipyridamole 25 mg, net price 20 = 63p; 100 mg, 20 = £1.20; 84 = £5.05. Label: 22
Oral suspension, dipyridamole 50 mg/5 mL, net price 150 mL = £34.00

Persantin® (Boehringer Ingelheim) PoM
Tablets, both s/c, dipyridamole 25 mg (orange), net price 84-tab pack = £1.57; 100 mg, 84-tab pack = £4.38. Label: 22
Injection, dipyridamole 5 mg/mL. Net price 2-mL amp = 11p

1. Aspirin tablets 75 mg may be sold to the public in packs of up to 100 tablets; for details relating to other strengths see section 4.7.1 and *Medicines, Ethics and Practice*, No. 29, London, Pharmaceutical Press, 2005 (and subsequent editions as available)

■ Modified release

Persantin® Retard (Boehringer Ingelheim) PoM
Capsules, m/r, red/orange containing yellow pellets, dipyridamole 200 mg. Net price 60-cap pack = £8.78. Label: 21, 25
Dose: secondary prevention of ischaemic stroke and transient ischaemic attacks (used alone or with aspirin), adjunct to oral anticoagulation for prophylaxis of thromboembolism associated with prosthetic heart valves, 200 mg twice daily preferably with food
NOTE. Dispense in original container (pack contains a desiccant) and discard any capsules remaining 6 weeks after opening

■ With aspirin

For cautions, contra-indications and side-effects of aspirin, see under Aspirin, above

Asasantin® Retard (Boehringer Ingelheim) PoM
Capsules, red/ivory, aspirin 25 mg, dipyridamole 200 mg (m/r), net price 60-cap pack = £7.80. Label: 21, 25
Dose: secondary prevention of ischaemic stroke and transient ischaemic attacks, 1 capsule twice daily
Note: Dispense in original container (pack contains a desiccant) and discard any capsules remaining 6 weeks after opening

EPTIFIBATIDE

Indications: prevention of early myocardial infarction in patients with unstable angina or non-ST-segment-elevation myocardial infarction and with last episode of chest pain within 24 hours (use under specialist supervision)

Cautions: risk of bleeding, concomitant drugs that increase risk of bleeding—discontinue immediately if uncontrolled serious bleeding; measure baseline prothrombin time, activated partial thromboplastin time, platelet count, haemoglobin, haematocrit and serum creatinine; monitor haemoglobin, haematocrit and platelets within 6 hours after start of treatment then at least once daily; discontinue if thrombolytic therapy, intra-aortic balloon pump or emergency cardiac surgery necessary; hepatic impairment (Appendix 2); renal impairment (Appendix 3); pregnancy (Appendix 4); breast-feeding (Appendix 5)

Contra-indications: abnormal bleeding within 30 days, major surgery or severe trauma within 6 weeks, stroke within last 30 days or any history of haemorrhagic stroke, intracranial disease (aneurysm, neoplasm or arteriovenous malformation), severe hypertension, haemorrhagic diathesis, increased prothrombin time or INR, thrombocytopenia, significant hepatic impairment; breast-feeding

Side-effects: bleeding manifestations; *very rarely* anaphylaxis and rash

Dose: initially *by intravenous injection*, 180 micrograms/kg, then *by intravenous infusion*, 2 micrograms/kg/minute for up to 72 hours (up to 96 hours if percutaneous coronary intervention during treatment)

Integrilin® (GSK) PoM
Injection, eptifibatide 2 mg/mL, net price 10-mL (20-mg) vial = £14.45
Infusion, eptifibatide 750 micrograms/mL, net price 100-mL (75-mg) vial = £45.42

TIROFIBAN

Indications: prevention of early myocardial infarction in patients with unstable angina or non-ST-segment-elevation myocardial infarction and with last episode of chest pain within 12 hours (use under specialist supervision)

Cautions: hepatic impairment (avoid if severe; Appendix 2); renal impairment (Appendix 3); major surgery or severe trauma within 3 months (avoid if within 6 weeks); traumatic or protracted cardiopulmonary resuscitation, organ biopsy or lithotripsy within last 2 weeks; risk of bleeding including active peptic ulcer within 3 months; acute pericarditis, aortic dissection, haemorrhagic retinopathy, vasculitis, haematuria, faecal occult blood; severe heart failure, cardiogenic shock, anaemia; puncture of non-compressible vessel within 24 hours; concomitant drugs that increase risk of bleeding (including within 48 hours after thrombolytic); monitor platelet count, haemoglobin and haematocrit before treatment, 2–6 hours after start of treatment and then at least once daily; discontinue if thrombolytic therapy, intra-aortic balloon pump or emergency cardiac surgery necessary; discontinue immediately if serious bleeding uncontrolled by pressure occurs; pregnancy (Appendix 4)

Contra-indications: abnormal bleeding within 30 days, stroke within 30 days or any history of haemorrhagic stroke, intracranial disease (aneurysm, neoplasm or arteriovenous malformation), severe hypertension, haemorrhagic diathesis, increased prothrombin time or INR, thrombocytopenia; breast-feeding (Appendix 5)

Side-effects: bleeding manifestations; reversible thrombocytopenia

Dose: *by intravenous infusion*, initially 400 nanograms/kg/minute for 30 minutes, then 100 nanograms/kg/minute for at least 48 hours (continue during and for 12–24 hours after percutaneous coronary intervention); max. duration of treatment 108 hours

Aggrastat® (MSD) PoM
Concentrate for intravenous infusion, tirofiban (as hydrochloride) 250 micrograms/mL. For dilution before use, net price 50-mL (12.5-mg) vial = £146.11
Intravenous infusion, tirofiban (as hydrochloride) 50 micrograms/mL, net price 250-mL *Intravia®* bag = £160.72

2.10 Myocardial infarction and fibrinolysis

2.10.1 Management of myocardial infarction

Local guidelines for the management of myocardial infarction should be followed where they exist

These notes give an overview of the initial and long-term management of myocardial infarction. The aims of management are to provide supportive care and pain relief, to promote revascularisation and to reduce mortality. Oxygen, diamorphine and nitrates provide initial support and pain relief; aspirin and percutaneous coronary intervention or thrombolytics promote revascularisation; long-term use of aspirin, beta-blockers, ACE inhibitors and statins help to reduce mortality further.

INITIAL MANAGEMENT. **Oxygen** (section 3.6) is administered unless the patient has severe chronic obstructive pulmonary disease.

The pain (and anxiety) of myocardial infarction is managed with slow intravenous injection of **diamorphine** (section 4.7.2); an antiemetic such as metoclopramide (or, if left ventricular function is not compromised, cyclizine) by intravenous injection should also be given (section 4.6).

Aspirin (chewed or dispersed in water) is given for its antiplatelet effect (section 2.9); a dose of 150–300 mg is suitable. If aspirin is given before arrival at hospital, a note saying that it has been given should be sent with the patient.

Patency of the occluded artery can be restored by percutaneous coronary intervention or by giving a **thrombolytic drug** (section 2.10.2), unless contra-indicated. Alteplase, reteplase and streptokinase need to be given within 12 hours of a myocardial infarction, ideally within 1 hour; use after 12 hours requires specialist advice. Tenecteplase should be given within 6 hours of a myocardial infarction. Antibodies to streptokinase appear after 4 days and it should not therefore be used again after this time. **Heparin** is used as adjunctive therapy with alteplase, reteplase, and tenecteplase to prevent re-thrombosis; heparin treatment should be continued for at least 24 hours (consult product literature).

Nitrates (section 2.6.1) are used to relieve ischaemic pain. If sublingual glyceryl trinitrate is not effective, intravenous glyceryl trinitrate or isosorbide dinitrate is given.

Early intravenous administration of some **beta-blockers** (section 2.4) has been shown to be of benefit and patients without contra-indications should receive **atenolol** by intravenous injection at a dose of 5 mg over 5 minutes, and the dose repeated once after 10–15 minutes; **metoprolol** by intravenous injection is an alternative.

ACE inhibitors (section 2.5.5.1) are also of benefit to patients who have no contra-indications; in hypertensive and normotensive patients treatment with an ACE inhibitor can be started within 24 hours of the myocardial infarction and continued for at least 5–6 weeks (see below for long-term treatment).

All patients should be closely monitored for hyperglycaemia; those with diabetes or raised blood-glucose concentration should receive **insulin**.

LONG-TERM MANAGEMENT. Long-term management involves the use of several drugs which should ideally be started before the patient is discharged from hospital.

Aspirin (section 2.9) should be given to all patients, unless contra-indicated, at a dose of 75 mg daily. **Warfarin** (with or without aspirin) may confer greater benefit than aspirin alone, but the risk of bleeding is increased.

Beta-blockers (section 2.4) should be given to all patients in whom they are not contra-indicated and continued for at least 2–3 years. Acebutolol, metoprolol, propranolol and timolol are suitable; for patients with left ventricular dysfunction, carvedilol, bisoprolol or long-acting metoprolol may be appropriate (section 2.5.5).

Verapamil (section 2.6.2) may be useful if a beta-blocker cannot be used; however, other calcium-channel blockers have no place in routine long-term management after a myocardial infarction.

An **ACE inhibitor** (section 2.5.5.1) should be considered for all patients, especially those with evidence of left ventricular dysfunction. If an ACE inhibitor cannot be used, an angiotensin-II receptor antagonist may be used for patients with heart failure; a relatively high dose of the angiotensin-II receptor antagonist may be required to produce benefit.

Nitrates (section 2.6.1) are used for patients with angina.

Statins are beneficial in preventing recurrent coronary events (section 2.12).

2.10.2 Fibrinolytic drugs

Fibrinolytic drugs act as thrombolytics by activating plasminogen to form plasmin, which degrades fibrin and so breaks up thrombi.

The value of thrombolytic drugs for the treatment of *myocardial infarction* has been established (section 2.10.1). **Streptokinase** and **alteplase** have been shown to reduce mortality. **Reteplase** and **tenecteplase** are also licensed for acute myocardial infarction; they are given by intravenous injection (tenecteplase is given as a bolus injection). Thrombolytic drugs are indicated for any patient with acute myocardial infarction for whom the benefit is likely to outweigh the risk of treatment. Trials have shown that the benefit is greatest in those with ECG changes that include ST segment elevation (especially in those with anterior infarction) and in patients with bundle branch block. Patients should not be denied thrombolytic treatment on account of age alone because mortality in this group is high and the reduction in mortality is the same as in younger patients.

Streptokinase is used in the treatment of *life-threatening venous thrombosis*, and in *pulmonary embolism*, but treatment must be started promptly.

CAUTIONS. Risk of bleeding including that from venepuncture or invasive procedures, external chest compression, pregnancy (Appendix 4), abdominal aneurysm or conditions in which thrombolysis might give rise to embolic complications such as enlarged left atrium with atrial fibrillation (risk of dissolution of clot and subsequent embolisation), diabetic retinopathy (very small risk of retinal bleeding), recent or concurrent anticoagulant therapy.

CONTRA-INDICATIONS. Recent haemorrhage, trauma, or surgery (including dental extraction), coagulation defects, bleeding diatheses, aortic dissection, coma, history of cerebrovascular disease especially recent events or with any residual disability, recent symptoms of possible peptic ulceration, heavy vaginal bleeding, severe hypertension, active pulmonary disease with cavitation, acute pancreatitis, severe liver disease, oesophageal varices; also in the case of streptokinase, previous allergic reactions to either streptokinase or anistreplase (no longer available).

Prolonged persistence of antibodies to streptokinase and anistreplase (no longer available) may reduce the effectiveness of subsequent treatment; therefore, streptokinase should not be used again beyond 4 days of first administration of either streptokinase or anistreplase. Antibodies may also appear after topical use of streptokinase on wounds.

SIDE-EFFECTS. Side-effects of thrombolytics are mainly nausea and vomiting and bleeding. When thrombolytics are used in myocardial infarction, reperfusion arrhythmias may occur. Hypotension may also occur and can usually be controlled by elevating the patient's legs, or by reducing the rate of infusion or stopping it temporarily. Back pain has been reported. Bleeding is usually limited to the site of injection, but intracerebral haemorrhage or bleeding from other sites may occur. Serious bleeding calls for discontinuation of the thrombolytic and may require administration of coagulation factors and antifibrinolytic drugs (aprotinin or tranexamic acid). Streptokinase may cause allergic reactions (including rash, flushing and uveitis) and anaphylaxis has been reported (for details of management see Allergic Emergencies, section 3.4.3). Guillain-Barré syndrome has been reported rarely after streptokinase treatment.

ALTEPLASE

(rt-PA, tissue-type plasminogen activator)

Indications: acute myocardial infarction (see notes above and section 2.10.1); pulmonary embolism; acute ischaemic stroke (treatment under specialist neurology physician **only**)

Cautions: see notes above; *in acute stroke*, monitor for intracranial haemorrhage, monitor blood pressure (antihypertensive recommended if systolic above 180 mmHg or diastolic above 105 mmHg); renal impairment (Appendix 3)

Contra-indications: see notes above; *in acute stroke*, convulsion accompanying stroke, severe stroke, history of stroke in patients with diabetes, stroke in last 3 months, hypoglycaemia, hyperglycaemia

Side-effects: see notes above; also risk of cerebral bleeding increased in acute stroke

Dose: myocardial infarction, accelerated regimen (initiated within 6 hours), 15 mg *by intravenous injection*, followed *by intravenous infusion* of 50 mg over 30 minutes, then 35 mg over 60 minutes (total dose 100 mg over 90 minutes); lower doses in patients less than 65 kg

Myocardial infarction, initiated within 6–12 hours, 10 mg *by intravenous injection*, followed *by intravenous infusion* of 50 mg over 60 minutes, then 4 *infusions* each of 10 mg over 30 minutes (total dose 100 mg over 3 hours; max. 1.5 mg/kg in patients less than 65 kg)

Pulmonary embolism, 10 mg *by intravenous injection* over 1–2 minutes, followed *by intravenous infusion* of 90 mg over 2 hours; max. 1.5 mg/kg in patients less than 65 kg

Acute stroke (treatment **must** begin within 3 hours), *by intravenous administration* over 60 minutes, 900 micrograms/kg (max. 90 mg); initial 10% of dose by intravenous injection, remainder by intravenous infusion; ELDERLY over 80 years not recommended

Actilyse® (Boehringer Ingelheim) PoM

Injection, powder for reconstitution, alteplase 10 mg (5.8 million units)/vial, net price per vial (with diluent) = £135.00; 20 mg (11.6 million units)/vial (with diluent and transfer device) = £180.00; 50 mg (29 million units)/vial (with diluent, transfer device, and infusion bag) = £300.00

RETEPLASE

Indications: acute myocardial infarction (see notes above and section 2.10.1)

Cautions: see notes above; breast-feeding (Appendix 5)

Contra-indications: see notes above

Side-effects: see notes above

Dose: *by intravenous injection,* 10 units over not more than 2 minutes, followed after 30 minutes by a further 10 units

Rapilysin® (Roche) PoM

Injection, powder for reconstitution, reteplase 10 units/vial, net price pack of 2 vials (with 2 prefilled syringes of diluent and transfer device) = £666.11

STREPTOKINASE

Indications: acute myocardial infarction (see notes above and section 2.10.1); deep-vein thrombosis, pulmonary embolism, acute arterial thromboembolism, and central retinal venous or arterial thrombosis; topical use (section 13.11.7)

Cautions: see notes above

Contra-indications: see notes above

Side-effects: see notes above

Dose: myocardial infarction, 1 500 000 units over 60 minutes

Deep-vein thrombosis, pulmonary embolism, acute arterial thromboembolism, central retinal venous or arterial thrombosis, *by intravenous infusion*, 250 000 units over 30 minutes, then 100 000 units every hour for up to 12–72 hours according to condition with monitoring of clotting parameters (consult product literature)

Streptokinase (Non-proprietary) PoM

Injection, powder for reconstitution, streptokinase, net price 100 000-unit vial = £10.00; 250 000-unit vial = £14.33; 750 000-unit vial = £38.20; 1.5 million-unit vial = £81.18

Streptase® (ZLB Behring) PoM

Injection, powder for reconstitution, streptokinase, net price 250 000-unit vial = £17.11; 750 000-unit vial = £44.86; 1.5 million-unit vial = £89.72 (hosp. only)

TENECTEPLASE

Indications: acute myocardial infarction (see notes above and section 2.10.1)

Cautions: see notes above; breast-feeding (Appendix 5)

Contra-indications: see notes above

Side-effects: see notes above; also fever

Dose: *by intravenous injection* over 10 seconds, 30–50 mg according to body-weight (500–600 micrograms/kg)—consult product literature; max. 50 mg

Metalyse® (Boehringer Ingelheim) PoM
Injection, powder for reconstitution, tenecteplase, net price 40-mg (8000-unit) vial = £665.00; 50-mg (10 000-unit) vial = £735.00 (both with prefilled syringe of water for injection)

2.11 Antifibrinolytic drugs and haemostatics

Fibrin dissolution can be impaired by the administration of **tranexamic acid**, which inhibits fibrinolysis. It may be useful to prevent bleeding (e.g. in prostatectomy and dental extraction in haemophilia) and can be particularly useful in menorrhagia. Tranexamic acid may also be used in hereditary angioedema, epistaxis and in thrombolytic overdose.

Desmopressin (section 6.5.2) is used in the management of mild to moderate haemophilia.

Aprotinin is a proteolytic enzyme inhibitor acting on plasmin and kallidinogenase (kallikrein). It is indicated for patients at high risk of major blood loss during and after open heart surgery with extracorporeal circulation and for patients in whom optimal blood conservation during open heart surgery is an absolute priority; it is also indicated for the treatment of life-threatening haemorrhage due to hyperplasminaemia (occasionally observed during the mobilisation and dissection of malignant tumours, in acute promyelocytic leukaemia, and following thrombolytic therapy). Aprotinin is also used in liver transplantation [unlicensed].

Etamsylate (ethamsylate) reduces capillary bleeding in the presence of a normal number of platelets. It does not act by fibrin stabilisation, but probably by correcting abnormal adhesion.

APROTININ

Indications: see notes above
Cautions: pregnancy (Appendix 4)
Side-effects: occasionally hypersensitivity reactions and localised thrombophlebitis
Dose: *by slow intravenous injection or infusion*, test dose, 10 000 units (1 mL) at least 10 minutes before remainder of dose (to detect allergy)
Open heart surgery, loading dose, *by slow intravenous injection or infusion* over 20 minutes, 2 000 000 units (200 mL) after induction of anaesthesia and before sternotomy; maintenance dose, *by intravenous infusion* 500 000 units (50 mL) every hour until end of operation (or early postoperative period in septic endocarditis); pump prime, 2 000 000 units (200 mL) in priming volume of extracorporeal circuit (3 000 000 units (300 mL) in septic endocarditis); usual max. 7 000 000 units (700 mL) per treatment course
Hyperplasminaemia, *by slow intravenous injection or infusion*, initially 500 000–1 000 000 units (50–100 mL) at max. rate 10 mL/minute; followed if necessary by 200 000 units (20 mL) every hour until bleeding stops

Trasylol® (Bayer) PoM
Injection, aprotinin 10 000 kallikrein inactivator units/mL. Net price 50-mL vial = £20.53
NOTE. A non-proprietary aprotinin injection containing 10 000 kallikrein inactivator units/mL is also available

ETAMSYLATE

(Ethamsylate)
Indications: blood loss in menorrhagia
Contra-indications: porphyria (see section 9.8.2)
Side-effects: nausea, headache, rashes
Dose: 500 mg 4 times daily during menstruation

Dicynene® (Sanofi-Synthelabo) PoM
Tablets, scored, etamsylate 500 mg, net price 100-tab pack = £8.78

TRANEXAMIC ACID

Indications: see notes above
Cautions: renal impairment (avoid if severe—Appendix 3); massive haematuria (avoid if risk of ureteric obstruction); not for use in disseminated intravascular coagulation; pregnancy (Appendix 4); regular eye examinations and liver function tests in long-term treatment of hereditary angioedema
NOTE. Requirement for regular eye examinations during long-term treatment is based on unsatisfactory evidence
Contra-indications: severe renal impairment, thromboembolic disease
Side-effects: nausea, vomiting, diarrhoea (reduce dose); disturbances in colour vision (discontinue) and thromboembolic events reported rarely; giddiness on rapid intravenous injection
Dose: *by mouth*, local fibrinolysis, 15–25 mg/kg 2–3 times daily
Menorrhagia (initiated when menstruation has started), 1 g 3 times daily for up to 4 days; max. 4 g daily
Hereditary angioedema, 1–1.5 g 2–3 times daily
By slow intravenous injection, local fibrinolysis, 0.5–1 g 3 times daily

Tranexamic acid (Non-proprietary) PoM
Tablets, tranexamic acid 500 mg, net price 60-tab pack = £14.16

Cyklokapron® (Meda) PoM
Tablets, f/c, scored, tranexamic acid 500 mg. Net price 60-tab pack = £14.30
Injection, tranexamic acid 100 mg/mL. Net price 5-mL amp = £1.55

Blood products

NICE guidance (drotrecogin alfa (activated) for severe sepsis). NICE has recommended (September 2004) that drotrecogin alfa (activated) should be considered for adults with severe sepsis that has resulted in the failure of two or more major organs and who are receiving optimum intensive care support. Drotrecogin alfa (activated) should be initiated and supervised only by a specialist consultant with intensive care skills and experience in the care of patients with sepsis.

ANTITHROMBIN III CONCENTRATE

Dried antithrombin III is prepared from human plasma
Indications: congenital deficiency of antithrombin III
Side-effects: nausea, flushing, headache; rarely, allergic reactions and fever
Available from BPL (Dried Antithrombin III)

DROTRECOGIN ALFA (ACTIVATED)

Recombinant activated protein C

Indications: adjunctive treatment of severe sepsis with multiple organ failure

Cautions: increased risk of bleeding, concomitant use of drugs that increase risk of bleeding; pregnancy (Appendix 4); breast-feeding (Appendix 5); **interactions:** Appendix 1 (drotrecogin alfa)

Contra-indications: internal bleeding; intracranial neoplasm or cerebral herniation; chronic severe hepatic disease; thrombocytopenia; not recommended for use in children

Side-effects: bleeding; headache; ecchymosis; pain

Available from Lilly (*Xigris*®▼)

FACTOR VIIa (RECOMBINANT)

Recombinant factor VIIa is used in patients with inhibitors to factors VIII and IX

Available from Novo Nordisk (*NovoSeven*®)

FACTOR VIII FRACTION, DRIED

(Human Antihaemophilic Fraction, Dried)

Dried factor VIII fraction is prepared from human plasma by a suitable fractionation technique

Indications: treatment and prophylaxis of haemorrhage in haemophilia A

Cautions: intravascular haemolysis after large or frequently repeated doses in patients with blood groups A, B, or AB—less likely with high potency concentrates

Side-effects: allergic reactions including chills, fever; hyperfibrinogenaemia occurred after massive doses with earlier products but less likely since fibrinogen content has now been substantially reduced

Available from ZLB Behring (*Beriate*® *P*; *Haemate*® *P*), Baxter (*Hemofil M*®), BPL (*Optivate*®, High Purity Factor VIII and von Willebrand factor concentrate; *Replenate*®; *8Y*®), Grifols (*Alphanate*®; *Fanhdi*®), SNBTS (*Liberate*®, High Potency Factor VIII Concentrate)

NOTE. Preparation of recombinant human antihaemophilic factor VIII (octocog alfa) available from ZLB Behring (*Helixate*® *NexGen*), Baxter Bioscience (*Advate*®▼; *Recombinate*®), Bayer (*Kogenate Bayer*®), Wyeth (*ReFacto*®)

FACTOR VIII INHIBITOR BYPASSING FRACTION

Preparations with factor VIII inhibitor bypassing activity are prepared from human plasma

Human Factor VIII Inhibitor Bypassing Fraction (*FEIBA*®, Baxter Bioscience) is used in patients with factor VIII inhibitors

NOTE. A porcine preparation of antihaemophilic factor for patients with inhibitors to human factor VIII is available from Ipsen (*Hyate C*®)

FACTOR IX FRACTION, DRIED

Dried factor IX fraction is prepared from human plasma by a suitable fractionation technique; it may also contain clotting factors II, VII, and X

Indications: congenital factor IX deficiency (haemophilia B)

Cautions: risk of thrombosis—principally with former low purity products

Contra-indications: disseminated intravascular coagulation

Side-effects: allergic reactions, including chills, fever

Available from ZLB Behring (*Mononine*®), BPL (*Replenine*®*-VF*, Dried Factor IX Fraction), Grifols (*AlphaNine*®), SNBTS (*HT Defix*®, Human Factor IX Concentrate, Heat Treated; *Hipfix*®▼, High Purity Factor IX Concentrate)

NOTE. Preparation of recombinant coagulation factor IX (nonacog alfa) available from Baxter Bioscience (*BeneFIX*®)

FACTOR XIII FRACTION, DRIED

(Human Fibrin-stabilising Factor, Dried)

Indications: congenital factor XIII deficiency

Side-effects: rarely, allergic reactions and fever

Available from ZLB Behring (*Fibrogammin*® *P*)

FRESH FROZEN PLASMA

Fresh frozen plasma is prepared from the supernatant liquid obtained by centrifugation of one donation of whole blood

Indications: to replace coagulation factors or other plasma proteins where their concentration or functional activity is critically reduced, e.g. to reverse warfarin effect

Cautions: avoid in circulatory overload; need for compatibility

Side-effects: allergic reactions including chills, fever, bronchospasm; adult respiratory distress syndrome

Available from Regional Blood Transfusion Services and BPL

NOTE. A preparation of solvent/detergent treated human plasma (frozen) is available from Octapharma (*Octaplas*®)

PROTEIN C CONCENTRATE

Protein C is prepared from human plasma

Indications: congenital protein C deficiency

Cautions: hypersensitivity to heparin

Side-effects: fever, arrhythmia, bleeding and thrombosis reported; rarely allergic reactions

Available from Baxter (*Ceprotin*®▼)

2.12 Lipid-regulating drugs

Lowering the concentration of low density lipoprotein (LDL) cholesterol and raising high density lipoprotein (HDL) cholesterol reduces the progression of coronary atherosclerosis and may even induce regression.

There is evidence that lowering total cholesterol by 20–25% (or lowering the LDL-cholesterol by about 30%) is effective in both the primary and secondary prevention of clinical manifestations of atherosclerotic cardiovascular disease. Therefore, treatment with a lipid-regulating drug should be considered in patients with cardiovascular disease and in those at high risk of developing it because of multiple risk factors (including smoking, hypertension, diabetes mellitus, and a family history of premature cardiovascular disease). Treatment with statins (see Statins, below) has been shown to reduce myocardial infarction, coronary deaths and overall mortality rate and they are the drugs of choice in patients with a high risk of cardiovascular disease. Lipid-regulating drug therapy must be combined with advice on diet and lifestyle measures to reduce cardiovascular disease risk including, if appropriate, reduction of blood pressure (section 2.5) and use of aspirin (section 2.9).

A number of conditions, some familial, are characterised by very high plasma concentrations of cholesterol, or triglycerides, or both. Statins are drugs of first choice for treating hypercholesterolaemia and fibrates for treating hypertriglyceridaemia; statins or fibrates can be used, either alone or together, to treat mixed hyperlipidaemia.

Severe hyperlipidaemia not adequately controlled with maximal dose of a statin, may require use of an additional lipid-regulating drug such as ezetimibe or a fibrate; such treatment should generally be under specialist supervision. Combinations of a statin with nicotinic acid or a fibrate carry an increased risk of side-effects (including rhabdomyolysis) and should be used with caution. In particular, concomitant administration of gemfibrozil with a statin may increase the risk of rhabdomyolysis considerably (see also below); gemfibrozil and statins should therefore **not** be used concomitantly.

Patients wth hypothyroidism should receive adequate thyroid replacement therapy before assessing their requirement for lipid-regulating treatment because correction of hypothyroidism itself may resolve the lipid abnormality. Untreated hypothyroidism increases the risk of myositis with lipid-regulating drugs.

CSM advice (muscle effects). The CSM has advised that rhabdomyolysis associated with lipid-regulating drugs such as the fibrates and statins appears to be rare (approx. 1 case in every 100 000 treatment years) but may be increased in those with renal impairment and possibly in those with hypothyroidism (see also notes above). Concomitant treatment with drugs that increase plasma-statin concentration increase the risk of muscle toxicity; concomitant treatment with a fibrate and a statin may also be associated with an increased risk of serious muscle toxicity.

Anion-exchange resins

Colestyramine (cholestyramine) and **colestipol** are anion-exchange resins used in the management of hypercholesterolaemia. They act by binding bile acids, preventing their reabsorption; this promotes hepatic conversion of cholesterol into bile acids; the resultant increased LDL-receptor activity of liver cells increases the clearance of LDL-cholesterol. Thus both compounds effectively reduce LDL-cholesterol but can aggravate hypertriglyceridaemia.

CAUTIONS. Anion-exchange resins interfere with the absorption of fat-soluble vitamins; supplements of vitamins A, D and K may be required when treatment is prolonged. **Interactions:** Appendix 1 (colestyramine and colestipol).

SIDE-EFFECTS. As colestyramine and colestipol are not absorbed, gastro-intestinal side-effects predominate. Constipation is common, but diarrhoea has occurred, as have nausea, vomiting, and gastro-intestinal discomfort. Hypertriglyceridaemia may be aggravated. An increased bleeding tendency has been reported due to hypoprothrombinaemia associated with vitamin K deficiency.

COUNSELLING. Other drugs should be taken at least 1 hour (in the case of ezetimibe, at least 2 hours) before or 4–6 hours after colestyramine or colestipol to reduce possible interference with absorption.

COLESTYRAMINE

(Cholestyramine)

Indications: hyperlipidaemias, particularly type IIa, in patients who have not responded adequately to diet and other appropriate measures; primary prevention of coronary heart disease in men aged 35–59 years with primary hypercholesterolaemia who have not responded to diet and other appropriate measures; pruritus associated with partial biliary obstruction and primary biliary cirrhosis (section 1.9.2); diarrhoeal disorders (section 1.9.2)

Cautions: see notes above; hepatic impairment (Appendix 2); pregnancy and breast-feeding; **interactions**: Appendix 1 (colestyramine)

Contra-indications: complete biliary obstruction (not likely to be effective)

Side-effects: see notes above; hyperchloraemic acidosis reported on prolonged use

Dose: lipid reduction (after initial introduction over 3–4 weeks) 12–24 g daily in water (or other suitable liquid) in single or up to 4 divided doses; up to 36 g daily if necessary

Pruritus, see section 1.9.2

Diarrhoeal disorders, see section 1.9.2

CHILD 6–12 years, see product literature

Colestyramine (Non-proprietary) PoM

Powder, colestyramine (anhydrous) 4 g/sachet, net price 50-sachet pack = £17.55. Label: 13, counselling, avoid other drugs at same time (see notes above)

Excipients: include aspartame (section 9.4.1)

Questran® (Bristol-Myers Squibb) PoM

Powder, colestyramine (anhydrous) 4 g/sachet. Net price 50-sachet pack = £17.55. Label: 13, counselling, avoid other drugs at same time (see notes above)

Excipients: include sucrose 3.79g/sachet

Questran Light® (Bristol-Myers Squibb) PoM

Powder, sugar-free, colestyramine (anhydrous) 4 g/sachet, net price 50-sachet pack = £18.43. Label: 13, counselling, avoid other drugs at same time (see notes above)

Excipients: include aspartame (section 9.4.1)

COLESTIPOL HYDROCHLORIDE

Indications: hyperlipidaemias, particularly type IIa, in patients who have not responded adequately to diet and other appropriate measures

Cautions: see notes above; pregnancy

Side-effects: see notes above

Dose: 5 g 1–2 times daily in liquid increased if necessary at intervals of 1–2 months to max. of 30 g daily (in single or 2 divided doses)

Colestid® (Pharmacia) PoM

Granules, yellow, colestipol hydrochloride 5 g/sachet. Net price 30 sachets = £15.05. Label: 13, counselling, avoid other drugs at same time (see notes above)

Colestid Orange, granules, yellow/orange, colestipol hydrochloride 5 g/sachet, with aspartame. Net price 30 sachets = £15.05. Label: 13, counselling, avoid other drugs at same time (see notes above)

Ezetimibe

Ezetimibe inhibits the intestinal absorption of cholesterol. It is licensed as adjunctive therapy to dietary manipulation in patients with hypercholesterolaemia in combination with a statin or alone (if a statin is inappropriate), in patients with homozygous familial hypercholesterolaemia in combination with a statin, and in patients with homozygous familial sitosterolaemia (phytosterolaemia).

EZETIMIBE

Indications: adjunct to dietary measures and statin in primary and homozygous familial hypercholesterolaemia (statin omitted in primary hypercholesterolaemia if inappropriate or not tolerated); adjunct to dietary measures in homozygous sitosterolaemia

Cautions: liver impairment (avoid if moderate or severe; Appendix 2); **interactions:** Appendix 1 (ezetimibe)

Contra-indications: breast-feeding (Appendix 5)

Side-effects: gastro-intestinal disturbances; headache, fatigue; myalgia; *rarely* hypersensitivity reactions including rash and angioedema; *very rarely* pancreatitis, cholelithiasis, cholecystitis, thrombocytopenia, and raised creatine kinase

Dose: 10 mg once daily; CHILD under 10 years not recommended

Ezetrol (MSD, Schering-Plough) ▼ PoM
Tablets, ezetimibe 10 mg, net price 28–tab pack = £26.31

■ With simvastatin
See under Simvastatin

Fibrates

Bezafibrate, **ciprofibrate**, **fenofibrate**, and **gemfibrozil** act mainly by decreasing serum triglycerides; they have variable effects on LDL-cholesterol. Although a fibrate may reduce the risk of coronary heart disease events in those with low HDL-cholesterol or with raised triglycerides a statin should be used first.

All can cause a myositis-like syndrome, especially in patients with impaired renal function. Also, combination of a fibrate with a statin increases the risk of muscle effects (especially rhabdomyolysis) and should be used with caution (see CSM advice on p. 132).

BEZAFIBRATE

Indications: hyperlipidaemias of types IIa, IIb, III, IV and V in patients who have not responded adequately to diet and other appropriate measures

Cautions: correct hypothyroidism before initiating treatment (see p. 132); hepatic impairment (Appendix 2); renal impairment (Appendix 3—see also under Myotoxicity below); **interactions:** Appendix 1 (fibrates)

MYOTOXICITY. Special care needed in patients with renal disease, as progressive increases in serum creatinine concentration or failure to follow dosage guidelines may result in myotoxicity (rhabdomyolysis); discontinue if myotoxicity suspected or creatine kinase concentration increases significantly

Contra-indications: severe hepatic and renal impairment, hypoalbuminaemia, primary biliary cirrhosis, gall bladder disease, nephrotic syndrome, pregnancy (Appendix 4); breast-feeding (Appendix 5)

Side-effects: gastro-intestinal disturbances; rash, pruritus; *less commonly*, headache, fatigue, dizziness, insomnia; *rarely* gallstones, hepatomegaly, cholestasis, hypoglycaemia, impotence, anaemia, leucopenia, thrombocytopenia, increased risk of bleeding, alopecia, photosensitivity reactions, raised serum creatinine (unrelated to renal impairment), and myotoxicity (with myasthenia or myalgia)—special risk in renal impairment (see Cautions)

Dose: see preparations below

Bezafibrate (Non-proprietary) PoM
Tablets, bezafibrate 200 mg, net price 100-tab pack = £9.35. Label: 21
Dose: 200 mg 3 times daily

Bezalip® (Roche) PoM
Tablets, f/c, bezafibrate 200 mg. Net price 100-tab pack = £9.15. Label: 21
Dose: 200 mg 3 times daily

■ Modified release

Bezalip® **Mono** (Roche) PoM
Tablets, m/r, f/c, bezafibrate 400 mg. Net price 30-tab pack = £8.09. Label: 21, 25
Dose: 1 tablet daily (dose form not appropriate in renal impairment)
NOTE. Modified-release tablets containing bezafibrate 400 mg also available; brands include *Zimbacol*® *XL*

CIPROFIBRATE

Indications: hyperlipidaemias of types IIa, IIb, III, and IV in patients who have not responded adequately to diet

Cautions: see under Bezafibrate

Contra-indications: see under Bezafibrate

Side-effects: see under Bezafibrate

Dose: 100 mg daily

Modalim® (Sanofi-Synthelabo) PoM
Tablets, scored, ciprofibrate 100 mg. Net price 28-tab pack = £14.72

FENOFIBRATE

Indications: hyperlipidaemias of types IIa, IIb, III, IV, and V in patients who have not responded adequately to diet and other appropriate measures

Cautions: see under Bezafibrate; liver function tests recommended every 3 months for first year (discontinue treatment if significantly raised); renal impairment (avoid if severe; Appendix 3)

Contra-indications: gall bladder disease; photosensitivity to ketoprofen; severe hepatic impairment (Appendix 2); pregnancy (Appendix 4); breast-feeding (Appendix 5)

Side-effects: see under Bezafibrate; also *very rarely* hepatitis, pancreatitis, and interstitial pneumopathies

Dose: see preparations below

Fenofibrate (Non-proprietary) PoM
Capsules, fenofibrate 200 mg, net price 30-cap pack = £14.75. Label: 21
Dose: 1 capsule daily (dose form not appropriate for children or in renal impairment)
Brands include *Fenogal*®

Lipantil® (Fournier) PoM

Lipantil® Micro 67 capsules, yellow, fenofibrate (micronised) 67 mg, net price 90-cap pack = £23.30. Label: 21

Dose: initially 3 capsules daily in divided doses; usual range 2–4 capsules daily; CHILD 4–15 years 1 capsule/20 kg daily

Lipantil® Micro 200 capsules, orange, fenofibrate (micronised) 200 mg, net price 28-cap pack = £17.95. Label: 21

Dose: initially 1 capsule daily (dose form not appropriate for children or in renal impairment)

Lipantil® Micro 267 capsules, orange/cream, fenofibrate (micronised) 267 mg, net price 28-cap pack = £21.75. Label: 21

Dose: severe hyperlipidaemia, 1 capsule daily (dose form not appropriate for children or in renal impairment)

NOTE. For an equivalent therapeutic effect, 100 mg previously available non-micronised fenofibrate ≡ 67 mg micronised fenofibrate

Supralip® **160** (Fournier) PoM

Tablets, f/c, fenofibrate 160 mg, net price 28-tab pack = £14.75. Label: 21, 25

Dose: 160 mg daily (dose form not appropriate for children or in renal impairment)

GEMFIBROZIL

Indications: hyperlipidaemias of types IIa, IIb, III, IV and V in patients who have not responded adequately to diet and other appropriate measures; primary prevention of cardiovascular disease in men with hyperlipidaemias that have not responded to diet and other appropriate measures

Cautions: lipid profile, blood counts, and liver-function tests before initiating long-term treatment; preferably avoid use with statins (high risk of rhabdomyolysis); correct hypothyroidism before initiating treatment (see p. 132); elderly; renal impairment (Appendix 3); **interactions:** Appendix 1 (fibrates)

Contra-indications: alcoholism, biliary-tract disease including gallstones; photosensitivity to fibrates; hepatic impairment (Appendix 2); pregnancy (Appendix 4); breast-feeding (Appendix 5)

Side-effects: gastro-intestinal disturbances; headache, fatigue, vertigo; eczema, rash; *less commonly* atrial fibrillation; *rarely* pancreatitis, appendicitis, disturbances in liver function including hepatitis and cholestatic jaundice, dizziness, paraesthesia, sexual dysfunction, thrombocytopenia, anaemia, leucopenia, eosinophilia, bone-marrow suppression, myalgia, myopathy, myasthenia, myositis accompanied by increase in creatine kinase (discontinue if raised significantly), blurred vision, exfoliative dermatitis, alopecia, and photosensitivity)

Dose: 1.2 g daily, usually in 2 divided doses; range 0.9–1.2 g daily; CHILD not recommended

Gemfibrozil (Non-proprietary) PoM

Capsules, gemfibrozil 300 mg, net price 112-cap pack = £28.26. Label: 22

Tablets, gemfibrozil 600 mg, net price 30-tab pack = £14.49. Label: 22

Lopid® (Pfizer) PoM

'300' capsules, white/maroon, gemfibrozil 300 mg. Net price 112-cap pack = £35.57. Label: 22

'600' tablets, f/c, gemfibrozil 600 mg. Net price 56-tab pack = £35.57. Label: 22

Statins

The statins (**atorvastatin**, **fluvastatin**, **pravastatin**, **rosuvastatin**, and **simvastatin**) competitively inhibit 3-hydroxy-3-methylglutaryl coenzyme A (HMG CoA) reductase, an enzyme involved in cholesterol synthesis, especially in the liver. They are more effective than other classes of drugs in lowering LDL-cholesterol but less effective than the fibrates in reducing triglycerides.

Statins reduce all atherosclerotic cardiovascular disease events, and total mortality. They should be considered for all patients, including the elderly, at risk of cardiovascular disease such as those with coronary heart disease (including history of angina or acute myocardial infarction), occlusive arterial disease (including peripheral vascular disease, non-haemorrhagic stroke or transient ischaemic attacks), or diabetes mellitus.

Statins are also used for the *secondary prevention* of cardiovascular disease events in patients with coronary heart disease (including history of angina or acute myocardial infarction), peripheral artery disease, or a history of stroke. Although statins produce these benefits irrespective of the initial cholesterol concentration, patients with a total serum-cholesterol concentration of 5 mmol/litre or greater are likely to benefit most. Statins also reduce the incidence of non-haemorrhagic stroke when used for secondary prevention in cardiovascular disease.

Statins are also used for the *primary prevention* of cardiovascular disease events in patients at increased risk. Risk of cardiovascular disease events is not accurately predicted from cholesterol concentrations alone and methods that take into account factors such as smoking, hypertension and age should be used to estimate risk. Patients with a 10-year cardiovascular disease risk of ≥ 20%[1] stand to benefit from primary prevention irrespective of the cholesterol concentration, in association with lifestyle measures and other appropriate interventions.

For primary and secondary prevention of cardiovascular disease, statin treatment should be adjusted to achieve a target total cholesterol concentration of less than 5 mmol/litre (or a reduction of 25% if that produces a lower concentration); in terms of LDL-cholesterol, the target should be below 3 mmol/litre (or a reduction of about 30% if that produces a lower concentration).

CAUTIONS. Statins should be used with caution in those with a history of liver disease or with a high alcohol intake (use should be avoided in active liver disease). Hypothyroidism should be managed adequately before starting treatment with a statin (see p. 132). Liver-function tests should be carried out before and within 1–3 months of starting treatment and thereafter at intervals of 6 months for 1 year, unless indicated sooner by signs or symptoms suggestive of hepatotoxicity. Treatment should be discontinued if serum transaminase concentration rises to, and persists at, 3 times the upper limit of the

1. Cardiovascular disease risk may be determined from the chart issued by the British Hypertension Society (*J Hum Hypertens* 2004; **18**: 139–85)—see inside back cover. The Joint British Societies' 'Cardiac Risk Assessor' computer programme may also be used to determine cardiovascular disease risk by adding together the coronary heart disease risk and stroke risk.

reference range. Statins should be used with caution in those with risk factors for myopathy or rhabdomyolysis; patients should be advised to report unexplained muscle pain (see Muscle Effects below). Statins should be avoided in porphyria (section 9.8.2) but rosuvastatin thought to be safe. **Interactions:** Appendix 1 (statins).

CONTRA-INDICATIONS. Statins are contra-indicated in active liver disease (or persistently abnormal liver function tests), in pregnancy (adequate contraception required during treatment and for 1 month afterwards) and breast-feeding (see Appendix 4 and Appendix 5).

SIDE-EFFECTS. Reversible myositis is a rare but significant side-effect of the statins (see also Muscle Effects, p. 132 and below). The statins also cause headache, altered liver-function tests (rarely, hepatitis), paraesthesia, and gastro-intestinal effects including abdominal pain, flatulence, constipation, diarrhoea, nausea and vomiting. Rash and hypersensitivity reactions (including angioedema and anaphylaxis) have been reported rarely.

MUSCLE EFFECTS. Myalgia, myositis and myopathy have been reported with the statins; if myopathy is suspected and creatine kinase is markedly elevated (more than 5 times upper limit of normal), or muscular symptoms are severe, treatment should be discontinued; in patients at high risk of muscle effects, a statin should not be started if creatine kinase is elevated. There is an increased incidence of myopathy if the statins are given at high doses or given with a fibrate (see also CSM advice on p. 132), with lipid-lowering doses of nicotinic acid, or with immunosuppressants such as ciclosporin; close monitoring of liver function and, if symptomatic, of creatine kinase is required in patients receiving these drugs. Rhabdomyolysis with acute renal impairment secondary to myoglobinuria has also been reported.

COUNSELLING. Advise patient to report promptly unexplained muscle pain, tenderness, weakness.

ATORVASTATIN

Indications: primary hypercholesterolaemia, heterozygous familial hypercholesterolaemia, homozygous familial hypercholesterolaemia or combined (mixed) hyperlipidaemia in patients who have not responded adequately to diet and other appropriate measures

Cautions: see notes above

Contra-indications: see notes above

Side-effects: see notes above; also chest pain, angina; insomnia, dizziness, hypoaesthesia, arthralgia; back pain; *less commonly* anorexia, malaise, weight gain, amnesia, impotence, thrombocytopenia, tinnitus, and alopecia; *rarely* pancreatitis, peripheral neuropathy, and peripheral oedema; *very rarely* cholestatic jaundice, hypoglycaemia, hyperglycaemia, and Stevens-Johnson syndrome

Dose: primary hypercholesterolaemia and combined hyperlipidaemia, usually 10 mg once daily; if necessary, may be increased at intervals of at least 4 weeks to max. 80 mg once daily; CHILD 10–17 years usually 10 mg once daily (limited experience with doses above 20 mg daily)

Familial hypercholesterolaemia, initially 10 mg daily, increased at intervals of at least 4 weeks to 40 mg once daily; if necessary, further increased to max. 80 mg once daily (or 40 mg once daily combined with anion-exchange resin in heterozygous familial hypercholesterolaemia); CHILD 10–17 years up to 20 mg once daily (limited experience with higher doses)

Lipitor® (Pfizer) PoM

Tablets, all f/c, atorvastatin (as calcium trihydrate) 10 mg, net price 28-tab pack = £18.03; 20 mg, 28-tab pack = £24.64; 40 mg 28-tab pack = £28.21; 80 mg, 28-tab pack = £28.21. Counselling, muscle effects, see notes above

FLUVASTATIN

NOTE. The *Scottish Medicines Consortium* has advised (February 2004) that fluvastatin is accepted for restricted use for the secondary prevention of coronary events after percutaneous coronary angioplasty; if the patient has previously been receiving another statin, then there is no need to change the statin

Indications: adjunct to diet in primary hypercholesterolaemia or combined (mixed) hyperlipidaemia (types IIa and IIb); adjunct to diet to slow progression of coronary atherosclerosis in primary hypercholesterolaemia and concomitant coronary heart disease; prevention of coronary events after percutaneous coronary intervention

Cautions: see notes above

Contra-indications: see notes above

Side-effects: see notes above; also insomnia; *very rarely* dysaesthesia, hypoesthesia, peripheral neuropathy, thrombocytopenia, vasculitis, eczema, dermatitis, bullous exanthema, and lupus erythematosus-like syndrome

Dose: hypercholesterolaemia or combined hyperlipidaemia, initially 20–40 mg daily in the evening, adjusted at intervals of at least 4 weeks; up to 80 mg daily may be required; CHILD and ADOLESCENT under 18 years, not recommended

Prevention of progression of coronary atherosclerosis, 40 mg daily in the evening

Following percutaneous coronary intervention, 80 mg daily

Lescol® (Novartis) PoM

Capsules, fluvastatin (as sodium salt) 20 mg (brown/yellow), net price 28-cap pack = £12.72; 40 mg (brown/orange), 28-cap pack = £12.72, 56-cap pack = £25.44. Counselling, muscle effects, see notes above

■ Modified release

Lescol® **XL** (Novartis) PoM

Tablets, m/r, yellow, fluvastatin (as sodium salt) 80 mg, net price 28-tab pack = £16.00. Label: 25, counselling, muscle effects, see notes above

Dose: 80 mg once daily (dose form not appropriate for initial dose titration in hypercholesterolaemia or combined hyperlipidaemia)

PRAVASTATIN SODIUM

Indications: adjunct to diet for primary hypercholesterolaemia or combined (mixed) hyperlipidaemias in patients who have not responded adequately to dietary control; adjunct to diet to prevent cardiovascular events in patients with hypercholesterolaemia; prevention of cardiovascular events in patients with previous myocardial infarction or unstable angina; reduction of hyperlipidaemia in patients receiving immunosuppressive therapy following solid-organ transplantation

Cautions: see notes above; renal impairment (Appendix 3)

Contra-indications: see notes above

Side-effects: see notes above; *less commonly* fatigue, dizziness, sleep disturbances, abnormal urination (including dysuria, nocturia and frequency), sexual dysfunction, visual disturbances, alopecia, *very rarely* pancreatitis, jaundice, fulminant hepatic necrosis, peripheral neuropathy, lupus erythematosus-like syndrome

Dose: hypercholesterolaemia or combined hyperlipidaemias, 10–40 mg once daily at night, adjusted at intervals of not less than 4 weeks

Familial hypercholesterolaemia, CHILD 8–13 years 10–20 mg once daily at night, 14–18 years 10–40 mg once daily at night

Prevention of cardiovascular events, 40 mg once daily at night

Post-transplantation hyperlipidaemia, initially 20 mg once daily at night, increased if necessary (under close medical supervision) to max. 40 mg

Pravastatin (Non-proprietary) PoM

Tablets, pravastatin sodium 10 mg, net price 28-tab pack = £3.42; 20 mg, 28-tab pack = £5.89; 40 mg, 28-tab pack = £6.55. Counselling, muscle effects, see notes above

Lipostat® (Squibb) PoM

Tablets, all yellow, pravastatin sodium 10 mg, net price 28-tab pack = £15.05; 20 mg, 28-tab pack = £27.61; 40 mg, 28-tab pack = £27.61. Counselling, muscle effects, see notes above

ROSUVASTATIN

Indications: primary hypercholesterolaemia (type IIa including heterozygous familial hypercholesterolaemia), mixed dyslipidaemia (type IIb), or homozygous familial hypercholesterolaemia in patients who have not responded adequately to diet and other appropriate measures

Cautions: see notes above; patients of Asian origin (see under Dose); max. dose 20 mg in patients with risk factors for myopathy or rhabdomyolysis (including personal or family history of muscular disorders or toxicity)

Contra-indications: see notes above; renal impairment (Appendix 3)

Side-effects: see notes above; also dizziness and asthenia; proteinuria; *rarely* jaundice, arthralgia, and polyneuropathy

Dose: 10 mg once daily increased if necessary after not less than 4 weeks to 20 mg once daily; increased after a further 4 weeks to 40 mg only in severe hypercholesterolaemia with high cardiovascular risk and under specialist supervision; patient of Asian origin, max. 20 mg daily

NOTE. Max. 20 mg daily with concomitant ciclosporin or fibrate

Crestor® (AstraZeneca) ▼ PoM

Tablets, all pink, f/c, rosuvastatin (as calcium salt) 10 mg, net price 28-tab pack = £18.03; 20 mg, 28-tab pack = £29.69; 40 mg, 28-tab pack = £29.69. Counselling, muscle effects, see notes above

SIMVASTATIN

Indications: primary hypercholesterolaemia, homozygous familial hypercholesterolaemia or combined (mixed) hyperlipidaemia in patients who have not responded adequately to diet and other appropriate measures; prevention of cardiovascular events in patients with atherosclerotic cardiovascular disease or diabetes mellitus

Cautions: see notes above; renal impairment (Appendix 3)

Contra-indications: see notes above; also porphyria (see section 9.8.2)

Side-effects: see notes above; also alopecia, anaemia, dizziness, peripheral neuropathy, hepatitis, jaundice, pancreatitis

Dose: primary hypercholesterolaemia, combined hyperlipidaemia, 10–20 mg daily at night, adjusted at intervals of at least 4 weeks; usual range 10–80 mg once daily at night

Homozygous familial hypercholesterolaemia, 40 mg daily at night *or* 80 mg daily in 3 divided doses (with largest dose at night)

Prevention of cardiovascular events, initially 20–40 mg once daily at night, adjusted at intervals of at least 4 weeks; max. 80 mg once daily at night

NOTE. Max. 10 mg daily with concomitant ciclosporin, fibrate or lipid-lowering dose of nicotinic acid. Max. 20 mg daily with concomitant amiodarone or verapamil. Max. 40 mg daily with diltiazem

[1]**Simvastatin** (Non-proprietary) PoM

Tablets, simvastatin 10 mg, net price 28-tab pack = £2.12, 20 mg, 28-tab pack = £2.26; 40 mg, 28-tab pack = £4.87; 80 mg, 28-tab pack = £26.79. Counselling, muscle effects, see notes above

Brands include *Simvador*®, *Simzal*®

[1]**Zocor**® (MSD) PoM

Tablets, all f/c, simvastatin 10 mg (peach), net price 28-tab pack = £18.03; 20 mg (tan), 28-tab pack = £29.69; 40 mg (red), 28-tab pack = £29.69; 80 mg (red), 28-tab pack = £29.69. Counselling, muscle effects, see notes above

■ With ezetimibe

NOTE. For hypercholesterolaemia in patients stabilised on the individual components in the same proportions, or for patients not adequately controlled by statin alone. The *Scottish Medicines Consortium* has advised (June 2005) that Inegy® is accepted for restricted use for patients not adequately controlled with a maximal dose of a statin. For cautions, contra-indications, and side-effects of ezetimibe, see Ezetimibe

Inegy® (MSD, Schering-Plough) ▼ PoM

Tablets, simvastatin 20 mg, ezetimibe 10 mg, net price 28-tab pack = £33.42; simvastatin 40 mg, ezetimibe 10 mg, 28-tab pack = £38.98; simvastatin 80 mg, ezetimibe 10 mg, 28-tab pack = £41.21. Counselling, muscle effects, see notes above

Nicotinic acid group

The value of **nicotinic acid** is limited by its side-effects, especially vasodilatation. In doses of 1.5 to 3 g daily it lowers both cholesterol and triglyceride concentrations by inhibiting synthesis; it also increases HDL-cholesterol. Nicotinic acid is licensed for use with a statin if the statin alone cannot adequately control dyslipidaemia (raised LDL-cholesterol, triglyceridaemia, and low HDL-choles-

1. Simvastatin 10 mg tablets can be sold to the public to reduce risk of first coronary event in individuals at moderate risk of coronary heart disease (approx. 10–15% risk of major event in 10 years), max. daily dose 10 mg and pack size of 28 tablets; treatment should form part of a programme to reduce risk of coronary heart disease; a proprietary brand *Zocor Heart-Pro*® is on sale to the public

terol); it can be used alone if the patient is intolerant of statins (for advice on treatment of dyslipidaemia, including use of combination treatment, see p. 131). The *Scottish Medicines Consortium* has advised (April 2004) that *Niaspan®* is not recommended for the treatment of hypercholesterolaemia and mixed dyslipidaemia; this is because of a lack of appropriate studies comparing *Niaspan®* with other lipid-regulating drugs.

Acipimox seems to have fewer side-effects than nicotinic acid but may be less effective in its lipid-modulating capabilities.

ACIPIMOX

Indications: hyperlipidaemias of types IIa, IIb, and IV in patients who have not responded adequately to diet and other appropriate measures

Cautions: renal impairment (Appendix 3)

Contra-indications: peptic ulcer; pregnancy (Appendix 4); breast-feeding (Appendix 5)

Side-effects: vasodilatation, flushing, itching, rashes, urticaria, erythema; heartburn, epigastric pain, nausea, diarrhoea, headache, malaise, dry eyes; rarely angioedema, bronchospasm, anaphylaxis

Dose: usually 500–750 mg daily in divided doses

Olbetam® (Pharmacia) PoM

Capsules, brown/pink, acipimox 250 mg. Net price 90-cap pack = £46.33. Label: 21

NICOTINIC ACID

Indications: adjunct to statin in dyslipidaemia or used alone if statin not tolerated (see also p. 131)

Cautions: unstable angina, acute myocardial infarction, diabetes mellitus, gout, history of peptic ulceration; hepatic impairment (Appendix 2); renal impairment; pregnancy (Appendix 4); **interactions:** Appendix 1 (nicotinic acid)

Contra-indications: arterial bleeding; active peptic ulcer disease; breast-feeding

Side-effects: diarrhoea, nausea, vomiting, abdominal pain, dyspepsia; flushing; pruritus, rash; *less commonly* tachycardia, palpitation, shortness of breath, peripheral oedema, headache, dizziness, increase in uric acid, hypophosphataemia, prolonged prothrombin time, and reduced platelet count; *rarely* hypotension, syncope, rhinitis, insomnia, reduced glucose tolerance, myalgia, myopathy, and myasthenia; *very rarely* anorexia, rhabdomyolysis

NOTE. Prostaglandin-mediated symptoms (such as flushing) can be reduced by low initial doses taken with meals

Dose: initially 100–200 mg 3 times daily (see above), gradually increased over 2–4 weeks to 1–2 g 3 times daily

NOTE. Doses of standard-release and modified-release formulations are **not** equivalent; when switching formulation initiate treatment with low dose and increase gradually as recommended

Nicotinic Acid[1] (Non-proprietary) PoM

Tablets, nicotinic acid 50 mg, net price 100 = £9.25. Label: 21

1. May be sold to the public unless max. daily dose exceeds 600 mg or if intended for treatment of hyperlipidaemia

■ Modified release

Niaspan (Merck) PoM

Tablets, m/r, nicotinic acid 500 mg, net price 56-tab pack = £17.25; 750 mg, 56-tab pack = £26.25; 1 g, 56-tab pack = £29.50; 21-day starter pack of 7 × 375-mg tab with 7 × 500-mg tab and 7 × 750-mg tab = £14.00. Label: 21, 25

Dose: 375 mg once daily at night (after a low-fat snack) for 1 week, then 500 mg once daily at night for 1 week, then 750 mg once daily at night for 1 week, then 1 g once daily at night for 4 weeks, increased if necessary in steps of 500 mg at intervals of at least 4 weeks to max. 2 g daily; usual maintenance dose 1–2 g once daily at night

Fish oils

A fish-oil preparation (*Maxepa®*), rich in **omega-3-marine triglycerides**, is useful in the treatment of severe hypertriglyceridaemia; however, it can sometimes aggravate hypercholesterolaemia.

The preparation *Omacor®*, which contains **omega-3-acid ethyl esters**, is licensed for hypertriglyceridaemia and secondary prevention after myocardial infarction. However, its capacity to reduce cardiovascular events or mortality is unknown. The *Scottish Medicines Consortium* has advised (November 2002) that *Omacor®* is not recommended for the treatment of hypertriglyceridaemia.

OMEGA-3-ACID ETHYL ESTERS

Indications: adjunct to diet and statin in type IIb or III hypertriglyceridaemia; adjunct to diet in type IV hypertriglyceridaemia; adjunct in secondary prevention after myocardial infarction

Cautions: haemorrhagic disorders, anticoagulant treatment (bleeding time increased); hepatic impairment (Appendix 2); pregnancy (Appendix 4)

Contra-indications: breast-feeding (Appendix 5)

Side-effects: gastro-intestinal disturbances; *less commonly* taste disturbances, dizziness, and hypersensitivity reactions; *rarely* hepatic disorders, headache, hyperglycaemia, acne, and rash; *very rarely* hypotension, nasal dryness, urticaria, and increased white cell count

Dose: see under preparation below

Omacor® (Solvay)

Capsules, 1 g of 90% omega-3-acid ethyl esters containing eicosapentaenoic acid 46% and docosahexaenoic acid 38%, alpha-tocopherol 4 mg, net price 28-cap pack = £13.89, 100-cap pack = £49.60. Label: 21

Dose: hypertriglyceridaemia, initially 2 capsules daily with food, increased if necessary to 4 capsules daily

Secondary prevention after myocardial infarction, 1 capsule daily with food

OMEGA-3-MARINE TRIGLYCERIDES

Indications: adjunct in the reduction of plasma triglycerides in patients with severe hypertriglyceridaemia judged to be at special risk of ischaemic heart disease or pancreatitis

Cautions: haemorrhagic disorders, anticoagulant treatment; aspirin-sensitive asthma; diabetes mellitus

Side-effects: occasional nausea and belching

Dose: see under preparations below

Maxepa® (Seven Seas)

Capsules, 1 g (approx. 1.1 mL) concentrated fish oils containing eicosapentaenoic acid 170 mg, docosahexaenoic acid 115 mg. Vitamin A content less than 100 units/g, vitamin D content less than 10 units/g, net price 200-cap pack = £27.28. Label: 21

Dose: 5 capsules twice daily with food

Liquid, golden-coloured, concentrated fish oils containing eicosapentaenoic acid 170 mg, docosahexaenoic acid 115 mg/g (1.1 mL). Vitamin A content less than 100 units/g, vitamin D content less than 10 units/g, net price 150 mL = £20.46. Label: 21

Dose: 5 mL twice daily with food

2.13 Local sclerosants

Ethanolamine oleate and sodium tetradecyl sulphate are used in sclerotherapy of varicose veins, and phenol is used in haemorrhoids (section 1.7.3).

ETHANOLAMINE OLEATE

(Monoethanolamine Oleate)

Indications: sclerotherapy of varicose veins

Cautions: extravasation may cause necrosis of tissues

Contra-indications: inability to walk, acute phlebitis, oral contraceptive use, obese legs

Side-effects: allergic reactions (including anaphylaxis)

Ethanolamine Oleate PoM

Injection, ethanolamine oleate 5%, net price 2-mL amp = £2.62, 5-mL amp = £2.27

Dose: by slow injection into empty isolated segment of vein, 2–5 mL divided between 3–4 sites; repeated at weekly intervals

SODIUM TETRADECYL SULPHATE

Indications: sclerotherapy of varicose veins

Cautions: see under Ethanolamine Oleate

Contra-indications: see under Ethanolamine Oleate

Side-effects: see under Ethanolamine Oleate

Fibro-Vein® (STD Pharmaceutical) PoM

Injection, sodium tetradecyl sulphate 0.2%, net price 5-mL amp = £5.00; 0.5%, 2-mL amp = £2.60; 1%, 2-mL amp = £3.00; 3%, 2-mL amp = £3.70, 5-mL vial = £9.30

Dose: by slow injection into empty isolated segment of vein, 0.1–1 mL according to site and condition being treated (consult product literature)

3: Respiratory system

3.1 Bronchodilators

Asthma

Drugs used in the management of asthma include $beta_2$ agonists (section 3.1.1), antimuscarinic bronchodilators (section 3.1.2), theophylline (section 3.1.3), corticosteroids (section 3.2), cromoglicate and nedocromil (section 3.3.1), and leukotriene receptor antagonists (section 3.3.2).

For tables outlining the management of chronic asthma and acute severe asthma see p. 140 and p. 141. For advice on the management of medical emergencies in dental practice, see p. 21.

Administration of drugs for asthma

INHALATION. This route delivers the drug directly to the airways; the dose is smaller than that for the drug given by mouth and side-effects are reduced. *Pressurised metered-dose inhalers* are an effective and convenient method of administering many drugs used for asthma. A spacer device (section 3.1.5) may improve drug delivery, particularly for young children and those who have difficulty using a pressurised metered-dose inhaler; spacers also reduce local adverse effects from inhaled corticosteroids. Breath-actuated devices including dry powder inhalers are also available.

Solutions for nebulisation are available for use in acute severe asthma. They are administered over 5–10 minutes from a nebuliser, usually driven by oxygen in hospital. Electric compressors are best suited to domiciliary use.

ORAL. The oral route is used when administration by inhalation is not possible. Systemic side-effects occur more frequently when a drug is given orally rather than by inhalation. Drugs given by mouth for the treatment of asthma include $beta_2$ agonists, corticosteroids, theophylline and leukotriene receptor antagonists.

PARENTERAL. Drugs such as $beta_2$ agonists, corticosteroids, and aminophylline may be given by injection in acute severe asthma when administration by nebulisation is inadequate or inappropriate. If the patient is being treated in the community, urgent transfer to hospital should be arranged.

Pregnancy and breast-feeding

It is particularly important that asthma should be well controlled during pregnancy; where this is achieved

MANAGEMENT OF CHRONIC ASTHMA IN ADULTS AND CHILDREN

Start at **step most appropriate** to initial severity

Chronic asthma: adults and schoolchildren

Step 1: occasional relief bronchodilators

Inhaled short-acting $beta_2$ agonist as required (up to once daily)

NOTE. Move to step 2 if needed 3 times a week or more, or if night-time symptoms more than once a week or if exacerbation in the last 2 years requiring systemic corticosteroid or nebulised bronchodilator; check compliance and inhaler technique

Step 2: regular inhaled preventer therapy

Inhaled short-acting $beta_2$ agonist as required

plus

Regular standard-dose[1] inhaled corticosteroid (alternatives[2] are considerably less effective)

Step 3: inhaled corticosteroids + long-acting inhaled $beta_2$ agonist

Inhaled short-acting $beta_2$ agonist as required

plus

Regular standard-dose[1] inhaled corticosteroid

plus

Regular inhaled long-acting $beta_2$ agonist (salmeterol *or* formoterol) but discontinue long-acting $beta_2$ agonist in the absence of response

If asthma not controlled

Increase dose of inhaled corticosteroid to upper end of standard dose[1]

If asthma still not controlled

Add one of

- Leukotriene receptor antagonist
- Modified-release oral theophylline
- Modified-release oral $beta_2$ agonist

Step 4: high-dose inhaled corticosteroids + regular bronchodilators

Inhaled short-acting $beta_2$ agonist as required

with

Regular high-dose[3] inhaled corticosteroid

plus

Inhaled long-acting $beta_2$ agonist

plus

In adults 6-week sequential therapeutic trial of one or more of

- Leukotriene receptor antagonist
- Modified-release oral theophylline
- Modified-release oral $beta_2$ agonist

Step 5: regular corticosteroid tablets

Inhaled short-acting $beta_2$ agonist as required

with

Regular high-dose[3] inhaled corticosteroid

and

one or more long-acting bronchodilators (see step 4)

plus

Regular prednisolone tablets (as single daily dose)

NOTE. In addition to regular prednisolone, continue high-dose inhaled corticosteroid (in exceptional cases may exceed licensed doses); these patients should normally be referred to an asthma clinic

Stepping down

Review treatment every 3 months; if control achieved stepwise reduction may be possible; use lowest possible dose of corticosteroid; reduce dose of *inhaled* corticosteroid slowly (consider reduction every 3 months, decreasing dose by up to 50% each time) to the lowest dose which controls asthma

Chronic asthma: children under 5 years[4]

Step 1: occasional relief bronchodilators

Short-acting $beta_2$ agonist as required (not more than once daily)

NOTE. Whenever possible inhaled (less effective and more side-effects when given by mouth); check compliance, technique and that inhaler device is appropriate

Move to step 2 if needed 3 times a week or more, or if night-time symptoms more than once a week or if exacerbation in last 2 years

Step 2: regular preventer therapy

Inhaled short-acting $beta_2$ agonist as required

plus

Either regular standard-dose[1] inhaled corticosteroid

Or (if inhaled corticosteroid cannot be used) leukotriene receptor antagonist (alternatives[2] are considerably less effective)

Step 3: add-on therapy

Children 2–5 years:

Inhaled short-acting $beta_2$ agonist as required

plus

Regular inhaled corticosteroid in standard dose[1]

plus

Leukotriene receptor antagonist

Children under 2 years:

Refer to respiratory paediatrician

Step 4: persistent poor control

Refer to respiratory paediatrician

Stepping down

Regularly review need for treatment

1. Standard-dose inhaled corticosteroids (given through metered dose inhaler) are beclometasone dipropionate or budesonide 100–400 micrograms (CHILD 100–200 micrograms) twice daily *or* fluticasone propionate 50–200 micrograms (CHILD 50–100 micrograms) twice daily *or* mometasone furoate (given through dry powder inhaler) 200 micrograms twice daily; initial dose according to severity of asthma; use large-volume spacer in children under 5 years
2. Alternatives to inhaled corticosteroid are leukotriene receptor antagonist, theophylline, and in adults, regular cromoglicate, and in children over 5 years, regular nedocromil
3. High-dose inhaled corticosteroids (given through metered dose inhaler) are beclometasone dipropionate or budesonide 0.8–2 mg daily (in divided doses) *or* fluticasone propionate 0.4–1 mg daily (in divided doses) *or* mometasone furoate (given through dry powder inhaler) up to 800 micrograms daily (in 2 divided doses); CHILD 5–12 years, beclometasone dipropionate or budesonide up to 400 micrograms twice daily *or* fluticasone propionate up to 200 micrograms twice daily; use a large-volume spacer
4. Lung-function measurements cannot be used to guide management in those under 5 years

Advice on the management of chronic asthma is based on the recommendations of the British Thoracic Society and Scottish Intercollegiate Guidelines Network (updated on 20 April 2004)

MANAGEMENT OF ACUTE SEVERE ASTHMA IN GENERAL PRACTICE

MANAGEMENT OF ACUTE SEVERE ASTHMA IN GENERAL PRACTICE

Moderate asthma exacerbation

— Peak flow >50–75% of predicted or best
— No features of acute severe asthma
— Increasing symptoms

Treat at home but response to treatment **must** be assessed before doctor leaves

Treatment:

High-flow oxygen if available
Salbutamol or terbutaline via large-volume spacer (4–6 puffs each inhaled separately; dose repeated every 10–20 minutes if necessary) or nebuliser
Monitor response 15–30 minutes after nebulisation
Give oral prednisolone 40–50 mg daily for at least 5 days and step up usual treatment

Follow up

Monitor symptoms and peak flow
Set up asthma action plan
Review in surgery within 48 hours
Modify treatment at review according to guidelines for chronic asthma (see Management of Chronic Asthma in Adults and Children)

Important: regard each emergency consultation as being for **acute severe asthma** until shown otherwise.

Important: failure to respond adequately **at any time** requires immediate referral to hospital.

Acute severe asthma in adults

— Cannot complete sentences in one breath
— Pulse ≥ 110 beats/minute
— Respiration ≥ 25 breaths/minute
— Peak flow 33–50% of predicted or best

Seriously consider hospital admission if more than one of above features present

Treatment:

High-flow oxygen if available
Salbutamol or terbutaline via large-volume spacer (4–6 puffs each inhaled separately; dose repeated every 10–20 minutes if necessary) or nebuliser (oxygen driven if available)
Oral prednisolone 40–50 mg daily for at least 5 days (or i/v hydrocortisone 400 mg daily in 4 divided doses)
Monitor response 15–30 minutes after nebulisation

If any signs of acute asthma persist:

Arrange hospital admission
While awaiting ambulance repeat nebulised $beta_2$ agonist and give with nebulised ipratropium 500 micrograms

Alternatively if symptoms have improved, respiration and pulse settling, and peak flow >50% of predicted or best:

Step up usual treatment *and* continue prednisolone for at least 5 days

Follow up

Monitor symptoms and peak flow, set up asthma action plan, review in surgery within 24 hours, modify treatment at review (see Management of Chronic Asthma)

Life-threatening asthma in adults

— Silent chest
— Cyanosis
— Feeble respiratory effort
— Bradycardia, exhaustion, arrhythmia, hypotension, confusion, or coma
— Peak flow <33% of predicted or best
— Arterial oxygen saturation <92%

Arrange **immediate** hospital admission

Treatment:

Oral prednisolone 40–50mg daily for at least 5 days (or i/v hydrocortisone 400 mg daily in 4 divided doses) (immediately)
Oxygen-driven nebuliser in ambulance
Nebulised[1] $beta_2$ agonist with nebulised ipratropium
Stay with patient until ambulance arrives

1. If nebuliser not available give 1 puff of $beta_2$ agonist using large-volume spacer and repeat 10–20 times

Important: patients with severe or life-threatening attacks may not be distressed and may not have all these abnormalities; the presence of any should alert doctor.

Acute episodes or exacerbations of asthma in young children in primary care

Mild/moderate episode in young children
– short-acting $beta_2$ agonist from metered dose inhaler *via* large-volume spacer (and face mask in very young), up to 10 puffs; alternatively give by nebuliser
– if favourable response (respiratory rate reduced, reduced use of accessory muscles, improved 'behaviour' pattern), repeat inhaled $beta_2$ agonist as needed
– start short course of oral prednisolone for 3 days (under 2 years 10 mg; 2–5 years 20 mg; over 5 years 30–40 mg daily; those already on prednisolone tablets 2 mg/kg up to max. 60 mg)
– consider i/v hydrocortisone in those who are unable to retain oral prednisolone

If unresponsive or relapse within 3–4 hours:
– immediately refer to hospital
– give nebulised $beta_2$ agonist with nebulised ipratropium 250 micrograms every 20–30 minutes
– give high-flow oxygen *via* face mask

Signs of acute asthma in children

Acute severe asthma:
– too breathless to talk
– too breathless to feed
– respiration >50 breaths/minute (> 30/minute in children over 5 years)
– pulse >130 beats/minute (>120 beats/minute in children over 5 years)
– in younger children, use of accessory muscles of breathing
– in older children, peak flow ≤50% of predicted or best

Life-threatening features:
– cyanosis, silent chest, or poor respiratory effort
– exhaustion
– agitation, hypotension, confusion, reduced level of consciousness, or coma
– in older children, peak flow <33% of predicted or best

Advice on the management of acute asthma is based on the recommendations of the British Thoracic Society and Scottish Intercollegiate Guidelines Network (updated on 20 April 2004)

asthma has no important effects on pregnancy, labour, or on the fetus. Drugs for asthma should preferably be administered by inhalation to minimise exposure of the fetus.

Severe exacerbations of asthma can have an adverse effect on pregnancy and should be treated promptly with conventional therapy, including oral or parenteral administration of a corticosteroid and nebulisation of a beta$_2$ agonist; prednisolone is the preferred corticosteroid for oral administration since very little of the drug reaches the fetus. Oxygen should be given immediately to maintain arterial oxygen saturation above 95% and prevent maternal and fetal hypoxia. Inhaled drugs, theophylline, and prednisolone can be taken as normal during breast-feeding.

Acute severe asthma

Severe asthma can be fatal and **must** be treated promptly and energetically. It is characterised by persistent dyspnoea poorly relieved by bronchodilators, exhaustion, a high pulse rate (usually over 110/minute), and a very low peak expiratory flow. As asthma becomes more severe, wheezing may be absent. Such patients should be given **oxygen** (if available) and **salbutamol** or **terbutaline** by nebuliser. This should be followed by a large dose of a **corticosteroid** (section 6.3.2)—for adults, prednisolone 30–60 mg by mouth or hydrocortisone 200 mg (preferably as sodium succinate) intravenously; for children, prednisolone 1–2 mg/kg by mouth (1–4 years max. 20 mg, 5–15 years max. 40 mg) or hydrocortisone 100 mg (preferably as sodium succinate) intravenously; if vomiting occurs, the parenteral route may be preferred for the first dose. For a table outlining the management of acute severe asthma, see p. 141.

If there is little response **ipratropium** by nebuliser (section 3.1.2) should be considered. Most patients do not require and do not benefit from the addition of intravenous aminophylline or of a beta$_2$ agonist; both cause more adverse effects than nebulised beta$_2$ agonists. Nevertheless, an occasional patient who has not been taking theophylline, may benefit from a slow intravenous infusion of aminophylline. Patients with severe asthma may be helped by **magnesium sulphate** [unlicensed indication] but evidence of benefit is limited; it may be given by intravenous infusion of magnesium sulphate 1.2–2 g over 20 minutes or by nebulisation of 2.5 mL isotonic magnesium sulphate (60 mg/mL) in 2.5 mL salbutamol nebuliser solution (1 mg/mL).

Treatment of these patients is safer in hospital where resuscitation facilities are immediately available. Treatment should **never** be delayed for investigations, patients should **never** be sedated, and the possibility of a pneumothorax should be considered.

If the patient deteriorates despite appropriate pharmacological treatment, intermittent positive pressure ventilation may be needed.

Chronic obstructive pulmonary disease

Smoking cessation (section 4.10) reduces the progressive decline in lung function in chronic obstructive pulmonary disease (COPD, chronic bronchitis, or emphysema). Infection can complicate chronic obstructive pulmonary disease and may be prevented by vaccination (pneumococcal vaccine and influenza vaccine, section 14.4).

A trial of a high-dose inhaled corticosteroid *or* an oral corticosteroid is recommended for patients with moderate airflow obstruction to ensure that asthma has not been overlooked.

Chronic obstructive pulmonary disease may be helped by an inhaled **short-acting beta$_2$ agonist** (section 3.1.1.1) or a **short-acting antimuscarinic bronchodilator** (section 3.1.2) used as required.

When the airways obstruction is more severe, a regular inhaled **antimuscarinic bronchodilator** (section 3.1.2) should be added. In those who remain symptomatic or have two or more exacerbations in a year, a **long-acting beta$_2$ agonist** should be added. If symptoms persist despite a trial of short-acting bronchodilators or a long-acting beta$_2$ agonist or a **long-acting antimuscarinic bronchodilator** or if the patient is unable to use inhaled therapy, theophylline (section 3.1.3) can be used.

In moderate or severe chronic obstructive pulmonary disease, a combination of a long-acting beta$_2$ agonist and an inhaled corticosteroid (section 3.2) should be tried. Combination treatment should be discontinued if there is no benefit after 4 weeks.

Long-term **oxygen** therapy (section 3.6) prolongs survival in patients with severe chronic obstructive pulmonary disease and hypoxaemia.

In an exacerbation of chronic obstructive pulmonary disease, bronchodilator therapy can be administered through a nebuliser if necessary and oxygen given if appropriate. A short course of oral corticosteroid (section 3.2) should be given if increased breathlessness interferes with daily activities. Antibacterial treatment (Table 1, section 5.1) is required when the sputum becomes purulent or if there are other signs of infection.

Croup

Mild croup requires no specific treatment and can be managed in the community. More severe croup (or mild croup that might cause complications) calls for hospital admission; a single dose of a corticosteroid (e.g. dexamethasone 150 micrograms/kg by mouth, section 6.3.2) may be administered before transfer to hospital. In hospital, dexamethasone 150 micrograms/kg (by mouth or by injection) or budesonide 2 mg (by nebulisation, section 3.2) will often reduce symptoms; the dose may need to be repeated after 12 hours if necessary. For severe croup not effectively controlled with corticosteroid treatment, nebulised adrenaline solution 1 in 1000 (1 mg/mL) may be given with close clinical monitoring in a dose of 400 micrograms/kg (max. 5 mg) repeated after 30 minutes if necessary; the effects of nebulised adrenaline last 2–3 hours and the child needs to be monitored carefully for recurrence of the obstruction.

3.1.1 Adrenoceptor agonists
(Sympathomimetics)

The selective beta$_2$ agonists (selective beta$_2$-adrenoceptor agonists, selective beta$_2$ stimulants) (section

3.1.1.1) such as salbutamol or terbutaline are the safest and most effective short-acting beta$_2$ agonists for asthma. Less selective beta$_2$ agonists such as orciprenaline (section 3.1.1.2) should be avoided whenever possible.

Adrenaline (epinephrine) (which has both alpha- and beta-adrenoceptor agonist properties) is used in the emergency management of allergic and anaphylactic reactions (section 3.4.3) and in the management of croup (see above).

3.1.1.1 Selective beta$_2$ agonists

Mild to moderate symptoms of asthma respond rapidly to the inhalation of a selective short-acting beta$_2$ agonist such as **salbutamol** or **terbutaline**. If beta$_2$ agonist inhalation is needed more often than once daily, prophylactic treatment should be considered, using a stepped approach as outlined on p. 140.

Salmeterol and **formoterol** (eformoterol) are longer-acting beta$_2$ agonists which are administered by inhalation. They should not be used for the relief of an acute asthma attack. Salmeterol and formoterol should be added to existing corticosteroid therapy and not replace it. They can be useful in nocturnal asthma. Patients with asthma who use salmeterol must also use an inhaled corticosteroid (see Chronic Asthma table, p. 140) because salmeterol may increase life-threatening attacks when given without an inhaled corticosteroid. Formoterol is also licensed for short-term symptom relief.

REGULAR TREATMENT. Short-acting beta$_2$ agonists should not be prescribed for use on a regular basis in patients with mild or moderate asthma since regular treatment provides no clinical benefit. However, regular use of the longer acting beta$_2$ agonists, salmeterol and formoterol, is of benefit.

Chronic Asthma table, see p. 140
Acute Severe Asthma table, see p. 141

INHALATION. *Pressurised-metered dose inhalers* are an effective and convenient method of drug administration in mild to moderate asthma. A spacer device (section 3.1.5) may improve drug delivery. At recommended inhaled doses the duration of action of salbutamol, terbutaline and fenoterol is about 3 to 5 hours and for salmeterol and formoterol 12 hours. The **dose**, the frequency, and the maximum number of inhalations in 24 hours of the beta$_2$ agonist should be **stated explicitly** to the patient. The patient should be advised to seek medical advice when the prescribed dose of beta$_2$ agonist fails to provide the usual degree of symptomatic relief because this usually indicates a worsening of the asthma and the patient may require a prophylactic drug such as an inhaled corticosteroid (see Chronic Asthma table, p. 140).

Nebuliser (or respirator) solutions of salbutamol and terbutaline are used for the treatment of acute asthma in hospital or in general practice. Patients with a severe attack of asthma should preferably have oxygen during nebulisation since beta$_2$ agonists can increase arterial hypoxaemia. For the use of nebulisers in chronic obstructive pulmonary disease, see section 3.1.5. The dose given by nebuliser is substantially higher than that given by inhaler. Patients should therefore be warned that it is dangerous to exceed the prescribed dose and they should seek medical advice if they fail to respond to the usual dose of the respirator solution. See also guidelines in section 3.1.5.

CFC-FREE INHALERS. Chlorofluorocarbon (CFC) propellants in pressurised metered-dose inhalers are being replaced by hydrofluoroalkane (HFA) propellants. Patients receiving CFC-free inhalers should be reassured about the efficacy of the new inhalers and counselled that the aerosol may feel and taste different; any difficulty with the new inhaler should be discussed with the doctor or pharmacist.

ORAL. Oral preparations of beta$_2$ agonists may be used by patients who cannot manage the inhaled route. They are sometimes used for children, but inhaled beta$_2$ agonists are more effective and have fewer side-effects. The longer-acting oral preparations including bambuterol may be of value in nocturnal asthma but they have a limited role and inhaled long-acting beta$_2$ agonists are usually preferred.

PARENTERAL. Salbutamol or terbutaline are given by intravenous infusion for severe asthma. The regular use of beta$_2$ agonists by the subcutaneous route is not recommended since the evidence of benefit is uncertain and it may be difficult to withdraw such treatment once started. Patients supplied with a selective beta$_2$ agonist injection for severe attacks should be advised to attend hospital immediately after using the injection, for further assessment. Beta$_2$ agonists may also be given by intramuscular injection.

CHILDREN. Selective beta$_2$ agonists are useful even in children under the age of 18 months. They are most effective by the inhaled route; a pressurised metered-dose inhaler should be used with a spacer device in children under 5 years (see NICE guidance, section 3.1.5). A beta$_2$ agonist may also be given by mouth but administration by inhalation is preferred; a long-acting inhaled beta$_2$ agonist may be used where appropriate (see Chronic Asthma table, p. 140). In severe attacks nebulisation using a selective beta$_2$ agonist or ipratropium is advisable (see also Asthma tables, p. 140 and p. 141).

CAUTIONS. Beta$_2$ agonists should be used with caution in hyperthyroidism, cardiovascular disease, arrhythmias, susceptibility to QT-interval prolongation, and hypertension. If high doses are needed during pregnancy they should be given by inhalation because a parenteral beta$_2$ agonist can affect the myometrium (section 7.1.3) and possibly cause cardiac problems; see also Pregnancy and Breast-feeding, section 3.1. Beta$_2$ agonists should be used with caution in diabetes—monitor blood glucose (risk of ketoacidosis, especially when beta$_2$ agonist given intravenously). **Interactions:** Appendix 1 (sympathomimetics, beta$_2$)

HYPOKALAEMIA. The CSM has advised that potentially serious hypokalaemia may result from beta$_2$ agonist therapy. Particular caution is required in severe asthma, because this effect may be potentiated by concomitant treatment with theophylline and its derivatives, corticosteroids, and diuretics, and by hypoxia. Plasma-potassium concentration should therefore be monitored in severe asthma

SIDE-EFFECTS. Side-effects of the beta$_2$ agonists include fine tremor (particularly in the hands), nervous tension, headache, muscle cramps, and palpitations. Other side-effects include tachycardia and arrhythmias and disturbances of sleep and behaviour in children. Paradoxical bronchospasm, urticaria, and angioedema have also been reported. $Beta_2$ agonists are associated with hypokalaemia after high doses (for CSM advice see under Cautions). Pain may occur on intramuscular injection.

SALBUTAMOL

Indications: asthma and other conditions associated with reversible airways obstruction; premature labour (section 7.1.3)

Cautions: see notes above

Side-effects: see notes above

Dose: *by mouth*, 4 mg (elderly and sensitive patients initially 2 mg) 3–4 times daily; max. single dose 8 mg (but unlikely to provide much extra benefit or to be tolerated); CHILD under 2 years 100 micrograms/kg 4 times daily [unlicensed]; 2–6 years 1–2 mg 3–4 times daily, 6–12 years 2 mg 3–4 times daily

By subcutaneous or intramuscular injection, 500 micrograms, repeated every 4 hours if necessary

By slow intravenous injection, 250 micrograms, repeated if necessary

By intravenous infusion, initially 5 micrograms/minute, adjusted according to response and heart-rate usually in range 3–20 micrograms/minute, or more if necessary; CHILD 1 month–12 years 0.1–1 microgram/kg/minute [unlicensed]

By aerosol inhalation, 100–200 micrograms (1–2 puffs); for persistent symptoms up to 4 times daily (but see also Chronic Asthma table); CHILD 100 micrograms (1 puff), increased to 200 micrograms (2 puffs) if necessary; for persistent symptoms up to 4 times daily (but see also Chronic Asthma table)

Prophylaxis in exercise-induced bronchospasm, 200 micrograms (2 puffs); CHILD 100 micrograms (1 puff), increased to 200 micrograms (2 puffs) if necessary

By inhalation of powder (for *Ventolin Accuhaler*® and *Asmasal*® dose see under preparation), 200–400 micrograms; for persistent symptoms up to 4 times daily (but see also Chronic Asthma table); CHILD 200 micrograms

Prophylaxis in exercise-induced bronchospasm (*powder*), 400 micrograms; CHILD 200 micrograms

NOTE. Bioavailability appears to be lower, so recommended doses for dry powder inhalers are twice those in a metered inhaler

By inhalation of nebulised solution, chronic bronchospasm unresponsive to conventional therapy and severe acute asthma, ADULT and CHILD over 18 months 2.5 mg, repeated up to 4 times daily; may be increased to 5 mg if necessary, but medical assessment should be considered since alternative therapy may be indicated; CHILD under 18 months, [unlicensed] (transient hypoxaemia may occur—consider supplemental oxygen), 1.25–2.5 mg up to 4 times daily but more frequent administration may be needed in severe cases

■ Oral

Salbutamol (Non-proprietary) PoM

Tablets, salbutamol (as sulphate) 2 mg, net price 20 = £1.54; 4 mg, 20 = £1.46

Oral solution, salbutamol (as sulphate) 2 mg/5 mL, net price 150 mL = £1.41

Brands include *Salapin*® (sugar-free)

Ventmax® SR (Trinity) PoM

Capsules, m/r, salbutamol (as sulphate) 4 mg (green/grey), net price 56-cap pack = £8.57; 8 mg (white), 56-cap pack = £10.28. Label: 25

Dose: 8 mg twice daily; CHILD 3–12 years 4 mg twice daily

Ventolin® (A&H) PoM

Syrup, sugar-free, salbutamol (as sulphate) 2 mg/5 mL, net price 150 mL = 60p

Volmax® (A&H) PoM

Tablets, m/r, salbutamol (as sulphate) 4 mg, net price 56-tab pack = £9.81; 8 mg, 56-tab pack = £11.77. Label: 25

Dose: 8 mg twice daily; CHILD 3–12 years 4 mg twice daily

■ Parenteral

Ventolin® (A&H) PoM

Injection, salbutamol (as sulphate) 500 micrograms/mL, net price 1-mL amp = 40p

Solution for intravenous infusion, salbutamol (as sulphate) 1 mg/mL. Dilute before use. Net price 5-mL amp = £2.58

■ Inhalation

COUNSELLING. Advise patients not to exceed prescribed dose and to follow manufacturer's directions; if a previously effective dose of inhaled salbutamol fails to provide at least 3 hours relief, a doctor's advice should be obtained as soon as possible.

Patients receiving CFC-free inhalers should be reassured about their efficacy and counselled that aerosol may feel and taste different

Salbutamol (Non-proprietary) PoM

Aerosol inhalation, salbutamol 100 micrograms/metered inhalation, net price 200-dose unit = £2.99. Counselling, dose

Excipients: include CFC propellants

Aerosol inhalation, salbutamol (as sulphate) 100 micrograms/metered inhalation, net price 200-dose unit = £2.99. Counselling, dose, change to CFC-free inhaler

Excipients: include HFA-134a (a non-CFC propellant), alcohol

Brands include *Salamol*®

NOTE. Can be supplied against a generic prescription but if CFC-free not specified will be reimbursed at price for CFC-containing inhaler

Dry powder for inhalation, salbutamol 100 micrograms/metered inhalation, net price 200-dose unit = £3.46; 200 micrograms/metered inhalation, 100-dose unit = £5.05, 200-dose unit = £6.92. Counselling, dose

Brands include *Easyhaler® Salbutamol*, *Pulvinal® Salbutamol*

Inhalation powder, hard capsule (for use with *Cyclohaler*® device), salbutamol 200 micrograms, net price 120-cap pack = £4.78; 400 micrograms, 120-cap pack = £8.08

Brands include *Salbutamol Cyclocaps*®

Nebuliser solution, salbutamol (as sulphate) 1 mg/mL, net price 20 × 2.5 mL (2.5 mg) = £1.99; 2 mg/mL, 20 × 2.5 mL (5 mg) = £3.98. May be diluted with sterile sodium chloride 0.9%

Brands include *Salamol Steri-Neb*®

Airomir® (IVAX) PoM
Aerosol inhalation, salbutamol (as sulphate) 100 micrograms/metered inhalation, net price 200-dose unit = £1.97. Counselling, dose, change to CFC-free inhaler
Excipients: include HFA-134a (a non-CFC propellant), alcohol
Also available as *Salbulin*® (3M)
NOTE. Can be supplied against a generic prescription but if 'CFC-free' not specified will be reimbursed at price for CFC-containing inhaler
Autohaler (breath-actuated aerosol inhalation), salbutamol (as sulphate) 100 micrograms/metered inhalation, net price 200-dose unit = £6.02. Counselling, dose, change to CFC-free inhaler
Excipients: include HFA-134a (a non-CFC propellant), alcohol

Asmasal Clickhaler® (Celltech) PoM
Dry powder for inhalation, salbutamol (as sulphate) 95 micrograms/metered inhalation, net price 200-dose unit = £5.88. Counselling, dose
Dose: acute bronchospasm 1–2 puffs
Persistent symptoms, 2 puffs 3–4 times daily
Prophylaxis in exercise-induced bronchospasm, 2 puffs

Salamol Easi-Breathe® (IVAX) PoM
Aerosol inhalation, salbutamol 100 micrograms/metered inhalation, net price 200-dose breath-actuated unit = £1.58 Counselling, dose
Excipients: include alcohol, HFA-134a (a non-CFC propellant)

Ventodisks® (A&H) PoM
Dry powder for inhalation, disks containing 8 blisters of salbutamol (as sulphate) 200 micrograms/blister, net price 15 disks with *Diskhaler*® device = £6.98, 15-disk refill = £6.45; 400 micrograms/blister, 15 disks with *Diskhaler*® device = £11.83, 15-disk refill = £11.29. Counselling, dose

Ventolin® (A&H) PoM
Accuhaler® (dry powder for inhalation), disk containing 60 blisters of salbutamol (as sulphate) 200 micrograms/blister with *Accuhaler*® device, net price = £5.12. Counselling, dose
Dose: by inhalation of powder, 200 micrograms; for persistent symptoms up to 4 times daily (but see also Chronic Asthma table); CHILD 200 micrograms
Prophylaxis in allergen- or exercise-induced bronchospasm, 200 micrograms
Evohaler® *aerosol inhalation*, salbutamol (as sulphate) 100 micrograms/metered inhalation, net price 200-dose unit = £1.50. Counselling, dose, change to CFC-free inhaler
Excipients: include HFA-134a (a non-CFC propellant)
NOTE. Can be supplied against a generic prescription but if CFC-free not specified will be reimbursed at price for CFC-containing inhaler
Nebules® (for use with nebuliser), salbutamol (as sulphate) 1 mg/mL, net price 20 × 2.5 mL (2.5 mg) = £1.75; 2 mg/mL, 20 × 2.5 mL (5 mg) = £2.95. May be diluted with sterile sodium chloride 0.9% if administration time in excess of 10 minutes is required
Respirator solution (for use with a nebuliser or ventilator), salbutamol (as sulphate) 5 mg/mL. Net price 20 mL = £2.27 (hosp. only). May be diluted with sterile sodium chloride 0.9%

■ Compound preparations
For some **compound preparations** containing salbutamol, see section 3.1.4

Chronic Asthma table, see p. 140
Acute Severe Asthma table, see p. 141

TERBUTALINE SULPHATE

Indications: asthma and other conditions associated with reversible airways obstruction; premature labour (section 7.1.3)
Cautions: see notes above
Side-effects: see notes above
Dose: *by mouth*, initially 2.5 mg 3 times daily for 1–2 weeks, then up to 5 mg 3 times daily
CHILD 75 micrograms/kg 3 times daily; 7–15 years 2.5 mg 2–3 times daily
By subcutaneous, intramuscular, or slow intravenous injection, 250–500 micrograms up to 4 times daily; CHILD 2–15 years 10 micrograms/kg to a max. of 300 micrograms
By continuous intravenous infusion as a solution containing 3–5 micrograms/mL, 1.5–5 micrograms/minute for 8–10 hours; reduce dose for children
By aerosol inhalation, ADULT and CHILD 250–500 micrograms (1–2 puffs); for persistent symptoms up to 3–4 times daily (but see also Chronic Asthma table)
By inhalation of powder (*Turbohaler*®), 500 micrograms (1 inhalation); for persistent symptoms up to 4 times daily (but see also Chronic Asthma table)
By inhalation of nebulised solution, 5–10 mg 2–4 times daily; additional doses may be necessary in severe acute asthma; CHILD, up to 3 years 2 mg, 3–6 years 3 mg; 6–8 years 4 mg, over 8 years 5 mg, 2–4 times daily

■ Oral and parenteral

Bricanyl® (AstraZeneca) PoM
Tablets, scored, terbutaline sulphate 5 mg. Net price 20 = 82p
Syrup, sugar-free, terbutaline sulphate 1.5 mg/5 mL. Net price 300 mL = £2.60
Injection, terbutaline sulphate 500 micrograms/mL. Net price 1-mL amp = 30p; 5-mL amp = £1.40

Bricanyl SA® (AstraZeneca) PoM
Tablets, m/r, terbutaline sulphate 7.5 mg. Net price 20 = £1.71. Label: 25
Dose: 7.5 mg twice daily

Monovent® (Sandoz) PoM
Syrup, sugar-free, terbutaline sulphate 1.5 mg/5 mL. Net price 300 mL = £2.15

■ Inhalation
COUNSELLING. Advise patients not to exceed prescribed dose and to follow manufacturer's directions; if a previously effective dose of inhaled terbutaline fails to provide at least 3 hours relief, a doctor's advice should be obtained as soon as possible

Bricanyl® (AstraZeneca) PoM
Aerosol inhalation, terbutaline sulphate 250 micrograms/metered inhalation. Net price 400-dose unit = £5.84. Counselling, dose
Excipients: include CFC propellants
Turbohaler® (= dry powder inhaler), terbutaline sulphate 500 micrograms/metered inhalation. Net price 100-dose unit = £6.92. Counselling, dose
Respules® (= single-dose units for nebulisation), terbutaline sulphate 2.5 mg/mL. Net price 20 × 2-mL units (5-mg) = £4.04
Respirator solution (for use with a nebuliser or ventilator), terbutaline sulphate 10 mg/mL. Net price 20 mL = £2.91. Before use dilute with sterile sodium chloride 0.9%

BAMBUTEROL HYDROCHLORIDE

NOTE. Bambuterol is a pro-drug of terbutaline

Indications: asthma and other conditions associated with reversible airways obstruction

Cautions: see notes above; renal impairment (Appendix 3); hepatic impairment (avoid if severe); manufacturer advises avoid in pregnancy

Side-effects: see notes above

Dose: 20 mg once daily at bedtime if patient has previously tolerated $beta_2$ agonists; other patients, initially 10 mg once daily at bedtime, increased if necessary after 1–2 weeks to 20 mg once daily; CHILD not recommended

Bambec® (AstraZeneca) PoM

Tablets, both scored, bambuterol hydrochloride 10 mg, net price 28-tab pack = £12.05; 20 mg, 28-tab pack = £13.14

FENOTEROL HYDROBROMIDE

Indications: reversible airways obstruction

Cautions: see notes above

Side-effects: see notes above

■ Compound preparations

For **compound preparation** containing fenoterol, see section 3.1.4

FORMOTEROL FUMARATE

(Eformoterol fumarate)

Indications: reversible airways obstruction (including nocturnal asthma and prevention of exercise-induced bronchospasm) in patients requiring long-term regular bronchodilator therapy, see also Chronic Asthma table, p. 140; chronic obstructive pulmonary disease

Cautions: see notes above; severe liver cirrhosis (Appendix 2); pregnancy (Appendix 4 and notes above); breast-feeding (Appendix 5)

Side-effects: see notes above; oropharyngeal irritation, taste disturbances, rash, insomnia, nausea and pruritus also reported; **important:** potential for paradoxical bronchospasm (calling for discontinuation and alternative therapy)

Dose: see under preparations below

COUNSELLING. Advise patients not to exceed prescribed dose, and to follow manufacturer's directions; if a previously effective dose of inhaled formoterol fails to provide adequate relief, a doctor's advice should be obtained as soon as possible

Foradil® (Novartis) PoM

Dry powder for inhalation, formoterol fumarate 12 micrograms/capsule, net price 60-dose unit (with inhaler device) = £26.57. Counselling, dose

Dose: by inhalation of powder, asthma, ADULT and CHILD over 5 years, 12 micrograms twice daily, increased to 24 micrograms twice daily in more severe airways obstruction

Chronic obstructive pulmonary disease, 12 micrograms twice daily

Oxis® (AstraZeneca) PoM

Turbohaler® (= dry powder inhaler), formoterol fumarate 4.5 micrograms/metered inhalation, net price 60-dose unit = £24.80; 9 micrograms/metered inhalation, 60-dose unit = £24.80. Counselling, dose

Dose: by inhalation of powder, asthma, 4.5–9 micrograms 1–2 times daily, increased to 18 micrograms twice daily in more severe airways obstruction; for short-term symptom relief (but not acute asthma) additional doses may be taken to max. 54 micrograms daily (max. single dose 27 micrograms); reassess treatment if additional doses required on more than 2 days a week

CHILD over 6 years, 9 micrograms 1–2 times daily, max. 18 micrograms daily

Prevention of exercise-induced bronchospasm ADULT and CHILD over 6 years, 9 micrograms before exercise

Chronic obstructive pulmonary disease, 9 micrograms 1–2 times daily; max. 36 micrograms daily (max. single dose 18 micrograms)

NOTE. Each metered inhalation of *Oxis*® *6 Turbohaler*® delivers 4.5 micrograms formoterol fumarate; each metered inhalation of *Oxis*® *12 Turbohaler*® delivers 9 micrograms formoterol fumarate

SALMETEROL

Indications: reversible airways obstruction (including nocturnal asthma and prevention of exercise-induced bronchospasm) in patients requiring long-term regular bronchodilator therapy, see also Chronic Asthma table, p. 140; chronic obstructive pulmonary disease

NOTE. Not for immediate relief of acute asthma attacks; existing corticosteroid therapy should not be reduced or withdrawn

Cautions: see notes above

Side-effects: see notes above; **important:** potential for paradoxical bronchospasm (calling for discontinuation and alternative therapy)

Dose: *by inhalation*, asthma, 50 micrograms (2 puffs or 1 blister) twice daily; up to 100 micrograms (4 puffs or 2 blisters) twice daily in more severe airways obstruction; CHILD over 4 years, 50 micrograms (2 puffs or 1 blister) twice daily

Chronic obstructive pulmonary disease 50 micrograms (2 puffs or 1 blister) twice daily

COUNSELLING. Advise patients that salmeterol should **not** be used for relief of acute attacks, not to exceed prescribed dose, and to follow manufacturer's directions; if a previously effective dose of inhaled salmeterol fails to provide adequate relief, a doctor's advice should be obtained as soon as possible

Serevent® (A&H) PoM

Accuhaler® (dry powder for inhalation), disk containing 60 blisters of salmeterol (as xinafoate) 50 micrograms/blister with *Accuhaler*® device, net price = £29.26. Counselling, dose

Aerosol inhalation, salmeterol (as xinafoate) 25 micrograms/metered inhalation, net price 120-dose unit = £29.26. Counselling, dose

Excipients: include CFC propellants

Diskhaler® (dry powder for inhalation), disks containing 4 blisters of salmeterol (as xinafoate) 50 micrograms/blister, net price 15 disks with *Diskhaler*® device = £35.79, 15-disk refill = £35.15. Counselling, dose

3.1.1.2 Other adrenoceptor agonists

Ephedrine and the partially selective beta agonist, orciprenaline, are less suitable and less safe for use as bronchodilators than the selective $beta_2$ agonists, because they are more likely to cause arrhythmias and other side-effects. They should be avoided whenever possible.

Adrenaline (epinephrine) injection (1 in 1000) is used in the emergency treatment of acute allergic and anaphylactic reactions (section 3.4.3). Adrenaline solution (1 in 1000) is used by nebulisation in the management of severe croup (section 3.1).

EPHEDRINE HYDROCHLORIDE

Indications: reversible airways obstruction, but see notes above

Cautions: hyperthyroidism, diabetes mellitus, ischaemic heart disease, hypertension, renal impairment, elderly; prostatic hypertrophy (risk of acute retention); interaction with MAOIs a disadvantage; **interactions:** Appendix 1 (sympathomimetics)

Side-effects: tachycardia, anxiety, restlessness, insomnia common; also tremor, arrhythmias, dry mouth, cold extremities

Dose: 15–60 mg 3 times daily; CHILD up to 1 year 7.5 mg 3 times daily, 1–5 years 15 mg 3 times daily, 6–12 years 30 mg 3 times daily

[1]**Ephedrine Hydrochloride** (Non-proprietary) PoM

Tablets, ephedrine hydrochloride 15 mg, net price 28 = £1.70; 30 mg, 28 = £1.76

1. For exemptions see *Medicines, Ethics and Practice*, No. 29, London, Pharmaceutical Press, 2005 (and subsequent editions as available)

■ Preparations on sale to the public

For a list of **cough and decongestant preparations on sale to the public**, including those containing ephedrine, see section 3.9.2

ORCIPRENALINE SULPHATE

Indications: reversible airways obstruction, but see notes above

Cautions: see section 3.1.1.1 and notes above; **interactions:** Appendix 1 (sympathomimetics)

Side-effects: see section 3.1.1.1 and notes above

Dose: 20 mg 4 times daily; CHILD up to 1 year 5–10 mg 3 times daily, 1–3 years 5–10 mg 4 times daily, 3–12 years 40–60 mg daily in divided doses

Alupent® (Boehringer Ingelheim) PoM

Syrup, sugar-free, orciprenaline sulphate 10 mg/5 mL, net price 300 mL = £6.75

3.1.2 Antimuscarinic bronchodilators

Ipratropium can provide short-term relief in chronic asthma, but short-acting beta$_2$ agonists act more quickly and are preferred. Ipratropium by nebulisation may be added to other standard treatment in life-threatening asthma or where acute asthma fails to improve with standard therapy (see Acute Severe Asthma table, p. 141).

Antimuscarinic bronchodilators are effective in chronic obstructive pulmonary disease. The aerosol inhalation of ipratropium has a maximum effect 30–60 minutes after use; its duration of action is 3 to 6 hours and bronchodilation can usually be maintained with treatment 3 times a day.

Tiotropium, a long-acting antimuscarinic bronchodilator, is licensed for maintenance treatment of chronic obstructive pulmonary disease; it is not suitable for the relief of acute bronchospasm.

CAUTIONS. Antimuscarinic bronchodilators should be used with caution in glaucoma (see below), prostatic hyperplasia and bladder outflow obstruction; **interactions:** Appendix 1 (antimuscarinics)

GLAUCOMA. *Acute angle-closure glaucoma* reported with nebulised ipratropium, particularly when given with nebulised salbutamol (and possibly other beta$_2$ agonists); care needed to protect patient's eyes from nebulised drug or from drug powder

SIDE-EFFECTS. The side-effects of antimuscarinic bronchodilators include dry mouth, nausea, constipation, and headache. Tachycardia and atrial fibrillation have also been reported.

IPRATROPIUM BROMIDE

Indications: reversible airways obstruction, particularly in chronic obstructive pulmonary disease

Cautions: see notes above; also *first dose* of nebulised solution should be inhaled under medical supervision (risk of paradoxical bronchospasm)

Side-effects: see notes above

Dose: *by aerosol inhalation*, 20–40 micrograms, 3–4 times daily; CHILD up to 6 years 20 micrograms 3 times daily, 6–12 years 20–40 micrograms 3 times daily

By inhalation of powder, 40 micrograms 3–4 times daily (may be doubled in less responsive patients); CHILD under 12 years, not recommended

By inhalation of nebulised solution, reversible airways obstruction in chronic obstructive pulmonary disease, 250–500 micrograms 3–4 times daily

Acute bronchospasm (see also Acute Asthma table, p. 141), 500 micrograms repeated as necessary; CHILD under 5 years 125–250 micrograms, max. 1 mg daily; 6–12 years 250 micrograms, max. 1 mg daily

COUNSELLING. Advise patient not to exceed prescribed dose and to follow manufacturer's directions

Ipratropium Bromide (Non-proprietary) PoM

Nebuliser solution, ipratropium bromide 250 micrograms/mL, net price 20 × 1-mL (250-microgram) unit-dose vials = £6.75, 60 × 1-mL = £21.78; 20 × 2-mL (500-microgram) = £7.43, 60 × 2-mL = £26.97. If dilution is necessary use only sterile sodium chloride 0.9%

Atrovent® (Boehringer Ingelheim) PoM

Aerocaps® (dry powder for inhalation; for use with *Atrovent Aerohaler*®), green, ipratropium bromide 40 micrograms, net price pack of 100 caps with *Aerohaler*® = £14.53; 100 caps = £10.53. Counselling, dose

Aerosol inhalation▼, ipratropium bromide 20 micrograms/metered inhalation, net price 200-dose unit = £4.21. Counselling, dose, change to CFC-free inhaler

Excipients: include HFA-134a (a non-CFC propellant), alcohol

Nebuliser solution, isotonic, ipratropium bromide 250 micrograms/mL, net price 20 × 1-mL unit-dose vials = £5.18, 60 × 1-mL vials = £15.55; 20 × 2-mL vials = £6.08, 60 × 2-mL vials = £18.24. If dilution is necessary use only sterile sodium chloride 0.9%

NOTE. One *Atrovent Aerocap*® is equivalent to 2 puffs of *Atrovent*® metered aerosol inhalation

Ipratropium Steri-Neb® (IVAX) PoM
Nebuliser solution, isotonic, ipratropium bromide 250 micrograms/mL, net price 20 × 1-mL (250-microgram) unit-dose vials = £8.72; 20 × 2-mL (500-microgram) = £9.94. If dilution is necessary use only sterile sodium chloride 0.9%

Respontin® (A&H) PoM
Nebuliser solution, isotonic, ipratropium bromide 250 micrograms/mL, net price 20 × 1-mL (250-microgram) unit-dose vials = £5.07; 20 × 2-mL (500-microgram) = £5.95. If dilution is necessary use only sterile sodium chloride 0.9%

■ Compound ipratropium preparations
Section 3.1.4

TIOTROPIUM

Indications: maintenance treatment of chronic obstructive pulmonary disease
Cautions: see notes above; renal impairment (Appendix 3); pregnancy (Appendix 4)
Side-effects: see notes above; also pharyngitis, sinusitis, candidiasis; rarely difficulty in micturition (urinary retention reported in elderly men with prostatic hyperplasia)
Dose: *by inhalation of powder*, 18 micrograms once daily, CHILD and ADOLESCENT under 18 years, not recommended

Spiriva® (Boehringer Ingelheim) ▼ PoM
Inhalation powder, hard capsule (for use with *HandiHaler*® device), tiotropium (as tiotropium bromide monohydrate) 18 micrograms, net price 30-cap pack with *HandiHaler*® device = £37.62, 30-cap refill = £36.60

3.1.3 Theophylline

Theophylline is a bronchodilator used for *asthma* and stable *chronic obstructive pulmonary disease*; it is not generally effective in exacerbations of chronic obstructive pulmonary disease. It may have an additive effect when used in conjunction with small doses of $beta_2$ agonists; the combination may increase the risk of side-effects, including hypokalaemia (for CSM advice see p. 143).

Theophylline is metabolised in the liver; there is considerable variation in plasma-theophylline concentration particularly in smokers, in patients with hepatic impairment or heart failure, or if certain drugs are taken concurrently. The plasma-theophylline concentration is *increased* in heart failure, cirrhosis, viral infections, in the elderly, and by drugs that inhibit its metabolism. The plasma-theophylline concentration is *decreased* in smokers and in chronic alcoholism and by drugs that induce liver metabolism. For other interactions of theophylline see Appendix 1.

These differences in theophylline half-life are important because its toxic dose is close to the therapeutic dose. In most individuals a plasma-theophylline concentration of between 10–20 mg/litre is required for satisfactory bronchodilation, although a plasma-theophylline concentration of 10 mg/litre (or less) may be effective. Adverse effects can occur within the range 10–20 mg/litre and both the frequency and severity increase at concentrations above 20 mg/litre.

Theophylline is given by injection as **aminophylline**, a mixture of theophylline with ethylenediamine, which is 20 times more soluble than theophylline alone. Aminophylline injection is needed rarely for severe attacks of asthma. It must be given by **very slow** intravenous injection (over at least 20 minutes); it is too irritant for intramuscular use. Measurement of plasma theophylline concentration may be helpful, and is **essential** if aminophylline is to be given to patients who have been taking theophylline, because serious side-effects such as convulsions and arrhythmias can occasionally precede other symptoms of toxicity.

THEOPHYLLINE

Indications: reversible airways obstruction, acute severe asthma; for guidelines see also Asthma tables (p. 140 and p. 141)
Cautions: cardiac disease, hypertension, hyperthyroidism, peptic ulcer, epilepsy, elderly, fever, hepatic impairment (Appendix 2); pregnancy (Appendix 4) and breast-feeding (Appendix 5); **CSM** advice on hypokalaemia risk, p. 143; avoid in porphyria (section 9.8.2); **interactions:** Appendix 1 (theophylline) and notes above
Side-effects: tachycardia, palpitations, nausea and other gastro-intestinal disturbances, headache, CNS stimulation, insomnia, arrhythmias, and convulsions especially if given rapidly by intravenous injection; **overdosage:** see Emergency Treatment of Poisoning, p. 33
Dose: see below

NOTE. Plasma theophylline concentration for optimum response 10–20 mg/litre (55–110 micromol/litre); narrow margin between therapeutic and toxic dose, see also notes above

■ Modified release

NOTE. The Council of the Royal Pharmaceutical Society of Great Britain advises pharmacists that if a general practitioner prescribes a modified-release oral theophylline preparation without specifying a brand name, the pharmacist should contact the prescriber and agree the brand to be dispensed. Additionally, it is essential that a patient discharged from hospital should be maintained on the brand on which that patient was stabilised as an in-patient.

Nuelin SA® (3M)
SA tablets, m/r, theophylline 175 mg. Net price 60-tab pack = £3.19. Label: 25
Dose: 175–350 mg every 12 hours; CHILD over 6 years 175 mg every 12 hours
SA 250 tablets, m/r, scored, theophylline 250 mg. Net price 60-tab pack = £4.46. Label: 25
Dose: 250–500 mg every 12 hours; CHILD over 6 years 125–250 mg every 12 hours

Slo-Phyllin® (Merck)
Capsules, all m/r, theophylline 60 mg (white/clear, enclosing white pellets), net price 56-cap pack = £2.30; 125 mg (brown/clear, enclosing white pellets), 56-cap pack = £2.90; 250 mg (blue/clear, enclosing white pellets), 56-cap pack = £3.62. Label: 25, or counselling, see below
Dose: 250–500 mg every 12 hours; CHILD, every 12 hours, 2–6 years 60–120 mg, 7–12 years 125–250 mg
COUNSELLING. Swallow whole with fluid *or* swallow enclosed granules with soft food (e.g. yoghurt)

Uniphyllin Continus® (Napp)
Tablets, m/r, all scored, theophylline 200 mg, net price 56-tab pack = £3.13; 300 mg, 56-tab pack = £4.77; 400 mg, 56-tab pack = £5.65. Label: 25
Dose: 200 mg every 12 hours increased according to response to 400 mg every 12 hours
May be appropriate to give larger evening or morning dose to achieve optimum therapeutic effect when symptoms most severe; in patients whose night or daytime symptoms persist despite other therapy, who are not currently receiving theophylline, total daily requirement may be added as single evening or morning dose
CHILD 9 mg/kg twice daily; some children with chronic asthma may require 10–16 mg/kg every 12 hours

For a list of **cough and decongestant preparations on sale to the public**, including those containing theophylline, see section 3.9.2

AMINOPHYLLINE

NOTE. Aminophylline is a stable mixture or combination of theophylline and ethylenediamine; the ethylenediamine confers greater solubility in water

Indications: reversible airways obstruction, acute severe asthma

Cautions: see under Theophylline

Side-effects: see under Theophylline; also allergy to ethylenediamine can cause urticaria, erythema, and exfoliative dermatitis

Dose: see under preparations, below
NOTE. Plasma theophylline concentration for optimum response 10–20 mg/litre (55–110 micromol/litre); narrow margin between therapeutic and toxic dose, see also notes above

Aminophylline (Non-proprietary) PoM
Injection, aminophylline 25 mg/mL, net price 10-mL amp = 68p
Brands include *Minijet*® *Aminophylline*
Dose: deteriorating acute severe asthma **not** previously treated with theophylline, *by slow intravenous injection* over at least 20 minutes (with close monitoring), 250–500 mg (5 mg/kg), then as for acute severe asthma; CHILD 5 mg/kg, then as for acute severe asthma
Acute severe asthma, *by intravenous infusion* (with close monitoring), 500 micrograms/kg/hour, adjusted according to plasma-theophylline concentration; CHILD 6 months–9 years 1 mg/kg/hour, 10–16 years 800 micrograms/kg/hour, adjusted according to plasma-theophylline concentration
NOTE. Patients taking oral theophylline or aminophylline should not normally receive intravenous aminophylline unless plasma-theophylline concentration is available to guide dosage

■ Modified release

NOTE. Advice about modified-release theophylline preparations on p. 148 also applies to modified-release aminophylline preparations

Phyllocontin Continus® (Napp)
Tablets, m/r, yellow, f/c, aminophylline hydrate 225 mg. Net price 56-tab pack = £2.54. Label: 25
Dose: 1 tablet twice daily initially, increased after 1 week to 2 tablets twice daily
NOTE. Brands of modified-release tablets containing aminophylline 225 mg include *Amnivent*® *225 SR*, *Norphyllin*® *SR*
Forte tablets, m/r, yellow, f/c, aminophylline hydrate 350 mg. Net price 56-tab pack = £4.22. Label: 25
NOTE. *Forte* tablets are for smokers and other patients with decreased theophylline half-life (see notes above)
Paediatric tablets, m/r, peach, aminophylline hydrate 100 mg. Net price 56-tab pack = £1.63. Label: 25
Dose: CHILD over 3 years, 6 mg/kg twice daily initially, increased after 1 week to 12 mg/kg twice daily; some children with chronic asthma may require 13–20 mg/kg every 12 hours

3.1.4 Compound bronchodilator preparations

In general, patients are best treated with single-ingredient preparations, such as a selective beta$_2$ agonist (section 3.1.1.1) or ipratropium bromide (section 3.1.2), so that the dose of each drug can be adjusted. This flexibility is lost with combinations. However, a combination product may be appropriate for patients stabilised on individual components in the same proportion.

For **cautions, contra-indications** and **side-effects** see under individual drugs.

Combivent® (Boehringer Ingelheim) PoM
Aerosol inhalation, ipratropium bromide 20 micrograms, salbutamol (as sulphate) 100 micrograms/metered inhalation. Net price 200-dose unit = £6.45. Counselling, dose
Excipients: include CFC propellants
Dose: bronchospasm associated with chronic obstructive pulmonary disease, 2 puffs 4 times daily; CHILD under 12 years not recommended
Nebuliser solution, isotonic, ipratropium bromide 500 micrograms, salbutamol (as sulphate) 2.5 mg/2.5-mL vial, net price 60 unit-dose vials = £25.08
Dose: bronchospasm in chronic obstructive pulmonary disease, *by inhalation of nebulised solution*, 1 vial 3–4 times daily; CHILD under 12 years not recommended
GLAUCOMA. In addition to other potential side-effects acute angle-closure glaucoma has been reported with nebulised ipratropium—for details, see p. 147

Duovent® (Boehringer Ingelheim) PoM
Nebuliser solution, isotonic, fenoterol hydrobromide 1.25 mg, ipratropium bromide 500 micrograms/4-mL vial, net price 20 unit-dose vials = £11.00
Dose: acute severe asthma or acute exacerbation of chronic asthma, *by inhalation of nebulised solution*, 1 vial (4 mL); may be repeated up to max. 4 vials in 24 hours; CHILD under 14 years, not recommended
GLAUCOMA. In addition to other potential side-effects acute angle-closure glaucoma has been reported with nebulised ipratropium—for details, see p. 147

3.1.5 Peak flow meters, inhaler devices and nebulisers

Peak flow meters

Measurement of peak flow is particularly helpful for patients who are 'poor perceivers' and hence slow to detect deterioration in their asthma, and for those with moderate or severe asthma.

Standard-range peak flow meters are suitable for both adults and children; low-range peak flow meters are appropriate for severely restricted airflow in adults and children. Patients must be given clear guidelines as to the action they should take if their peak flow falls below a certain level. Patients can be encouraged to adjust some of their own treatment (within specified limits) according to changes in peak flow rate.

Standard Range Peak Flow Meter

Conforms to standard EN 13826

MicroPeak®, range 60–800 litres/minute, net price = £6.50, replacement mouthpiece = 38p (Micro Medical)

Mini-Wright®, range 60–800 litres/minute, net price = £6.86, replacement mouthpiece = 38p (Clement Clarke)

Pocketpeak®, range 60–800 litres/minute, net price = £6.53, replacement mouthpiece = 38p (Ferraris)

Vitalograph, range 50–800 litres/minute, net price = £5.95 (coloured children's version also available), replacement mouthpiece = 40p (Vitalograph)

NOTE. Readings from new peak flow meters are often lower than those obtained from old Wright-scale peak flow meters and the correct chart should be used

Low Range Peak Flow Meter

Compliant to standard EN 13826 except for reduced measurement range

Mini-Wright®, range 30–400 litres/minute, net price = £6.90, replacement mouthpiece = 38p (Clement Clarke)

Pocketpeak®, range 50–400 litres/minute, net price = £6.53, replacement mouthpiece = 38p (Ferraris)

Vitalograph, range 50–400 litres/minute, net price = £5.95, replacement mouthpiece = 40p (Vitalograph)

NOTE. Readings from new peak flow meters are often lower than those obtained from old Wright-scale peak flow meters and the correct chart should be used

Drug delivery devices

INHALER DEVICES. These include *pressurised metered-dose inhalers*, *breath-actuated inhalers* and *dry powder inhalers*. Many patients can be taught to use a pressurised metered-dose inhaler effectively but some patients, particularly the elderly and small children, find it difficult to use them. *Spacer devices* (see below) can help such patients because they remove the need to co-ordinate actuation with inhalation and are effective even for children under 5 years. Alternatively, breath-actuated inhalers or dry powder inhalers (which are activated by patient's inhalation) may be used but they are less suitable for young children. On changing from a pressurised metered-dose inhaler to a dry powder inhaler patients may notice a lack of sensation in the mouth and throat previously associated with each actuation. Coughing may also occur.

The patient should be instructed carefully on the use of the inhaler and it is important to check that the inhaler continues to be used correctly because inadequate inhalation technique may be mistaken for a lack of response to the drug.

NICE guidance (inhaler devices for children with chronic asthma)

The National Institute for Health and Clinical Excellence has advised that the child's needs, ability to develop and maintain effective technique, and likelihood of good compliance should govern the choice of inhaler and spacer device; only then should cost be considered

For children aged under 5 years:

- corticosteroid and bronchodilator therapy should be delivered by pressurised metered-dose inhaler and spacer device, with a facemask if necessary;
- if this is not effective, and depending on the child's condition, nebulised therapy may be considered and, in children over 3 years, a dry powder inhaler may also be considered [but see notes above];

For children aged 5–15 years:

- corticosteroid therapy should be routinely delivered by a pressurised metered-dose inhaler and spacer device
- children and their carers should be trained in the use of the chosen device; suitability of the device should be reviewed at least annually. Inhaler technique and compliance should be monitored

SPACER DEVICES. Spacer devices remove the need for co-ordination between actuation of a pressurised metered-dose inhaler and inhalation. The spacer device reduces the velocity of the aerosol and subsequent impaction on the oropharynx. In addition the device allows more time for evaporation of the propellant so that a larger proportion of the particles can be inhaled and deposited in the lungs. The size of the spacer is important, the larger spacers with a one-way valve (*Nebuhaler*®, *Volumatic*®) being most effective. Spacer devices are particularly useful for patients with poor inhalation technique, for children, for patients requiring higher doses, for nocturnal asthma, and for patients prone to candidiasis with inhaled corticosteroids. It is important to prescribe a spacer device that is compatible with the metered-dose inhaler.

USE AND CARE OF SPACER DEVICES. Patients should inhale from the spacer device as soon as possible after actuation because the drug aerosol is very short-lived; single-dose actuation is recommended. The device should be cleansed once a month by washing in mild detergent, rinsed and then allowing to dry in air (wiping or more frequent cleaning should be avoided since any electrostatic charge may affect drug delivery). Spacer devices should be replaced every 6–12 months.

Able Spacer® (Clement Clarke)

Spacer device, small-volume device. For use with pressurised (aerosol) inhalers, net price standard device = £4.20; with infant, child or adult mask = £6.86

AeroChamber® **Plus** (GSK)

Spacer device, medium-volume device. For use with *Airomir*®, *Alvesco*®, *Atrovent*®, *Atrovent*® *Forte*, *Combivent*®, *Duovent*®, *Salbulin*®, and *Qvar*® inhalers, net price standard device (blue) = £4.36, with mask (blue) = £7.27; infant device (orange) with mask = £4.36; child device (yellow) with mask = £7.27

Babyhaler® (A&H) NHS

Spacer device for paediatric use with *Becotide*®*-50* and *Ventolin*® inhalers. Net price = £11.34

E-Z Spacer® (Vitalograph) NHS
Spacer device, large-volume, collapsible device. For use with pressurised (aerosol) inhalers, price (direct from manufacturer) = £23.00

Haleraid® (A&H) NHS
Device to place over standard inhalers to aid when strength in hands is impaired (e.g. in arthritis). Available as *Haleraid®-120* for 120-dose inhalers and *Haleraid®-200* for 200-dose inhalers. Net price = 80p

Nebuhaler® (AstraZeneca)
Spacer device, large-volume device. For use with *Bricanyl*® and *Pulmicort*® inhalers, net price = £4.28; with paediatric mask = £4.28

PARI Vortex Spacer® (Pari) NHS
Spacer device, small-volume device. For use with a pressurised (aerosol) inhaler, net price with mouthpiece = £6.07; with mask for infant or child = £7.91; with adult mask = £9.97

Pocket Chamber® (Ferraris)
Spacer device, small-volume device. For use with a pressurised (aerosol) inhaler, net price = £4.18; with infant, small, medium, or large mask = £9.75

Spinhaler® (Rhône-Poulenc Rorer)
Breath-actuated device for use with *Intal Spincaps*®. Net price = £1.92

Nebulisers

In England and Wales nebulisers and compressors are not available on the NHS (but they are free of VAT); some nebulisers (but not compressors) are available on form GP10A in Scotland (for details consult Scottish Drug Tariff).

A nebuliser converts a solution of a drug into an aerosol for inhalation. It is used to deliver higher doses of drug to the airways than is usual with standard inhalers. The main indications for use of a nebuliser are:

- to deliver a $beta_2$ agonist or ipratropium to a patient with an *acute exacerbation* of asthma or of chronic obstructive pulmonary disease;
- to deliver a $beta_2$ agonist or ipratropium on a *regular basis* to a patient with severe asthma or reversible airways obstruction who has been shown to benefit from regular treatment with higher doses;
- to deliver *prophylactic medication* such as a corticosteroid to a patient unable to use other inhalational devices (particularly to a young child);
- to deliver an antibiotic (such as colistin) to a patient with chronic purulent infection (as in cystic fibrosis or bronchiectasis);
- to deliver pentamidine for the prophylaxis and treatment of pneumocystis pneumonia.

The proportion of a nebuliser solution that reaches the lungs depends on the type of nebuliser and although it can be as high as 30%, it is more frequently close to 10% and sometimes below 10%. The remaining solution is left in the nebuliser as residual volume or it is deposited in the mouthpiece and tubing. The extent to which the nebulised solution is deposited in the airways or alveoli depends on particle size. Particles with a mass median diameter of 1–5 microns are deposited in the airways and are therefore appropriate for asthma whereas a particle size of 1–2 microns is needed for alveolar deposition of pentamidine to combat pneumocystis infection. The type of nebuliser is therefore chosen according to the deposition required and according to the viscosity of the solution (antibiotic solutions usually being more viscous).

Some jet nebulisers are able to increase drug output during inspiration and hence increase efficiency.

The patient should be aware that the dose of a bronchodilator given by nebulisation is usually **much higher** than that from an aerosol inhaler.

The British Thoracic Society has advised that nebulised bronchodilators may be given to patients with chronic persistent asthma or those with sudden catastrophic severe asthma (brittle asthma). In chronic asthma, nebulised bronchodilators should only be used to relieve persistent daily wheeze (see Chronic Asthma table p. 140). The British Thoracic Society has recommended that the use of nebulisers in chronic persistent asthma should only be considered:

- after a review of the diagnosis;
- if the airflow obstruction is significantly reversible by bronchodilators without unacceptable side-effects;
- after the patient has been using the usual hand-held inhaler correctly;
- after a larger dose of bronchodilator from a hand-held inhaler (with a spacer if necessary) has been tried for at least 2 weeks;
- if the patient is complying with the prescribed dose and frequency of anti-inflammatory treatment including regular use of high-dose inhaled corticosteroid.

Before prescribing a nebuliser, a home trial should preferably be undertaken to monitor peak flow for up to 2 weeks on standard treatment and up to 2 weeks on nebulised treatment. If prescribed, patients must:

- have clear instructions from doctor, specialist nurse or pharmacist on the use of the nebuliser and on peak-flow monitoring;
- be instructed not to treat acute attacks at home without also seeking help;
- receive an education program;
- have regular follow up including peak-flow monitoring and be seen by doctor, specialist nurse or physiotherapist.

Jet nebulisers

Jet nebulisers are more widely used than ultrasonic nebulisers. Most jet nebulisers require an optimum gas flow rate of 6–8 litres/minute and in hospital can be driven by piped air or oxygen. Domiciliary oxygen cylinders do not provide an adequate flow rate therefore an electrical compressor is required for domiciliary use.

For patients with *chronic obstructive pulmonary disease and hypercapnia*, oxygen can be dangerous and the nebuliser should be driven by air (see also p. 143). In exacerbations of chronic obstructive pulmonary disease, the nebuliser should be driven by compressed air in hypercapnia or acidosis. If oxygen is required, it should be given simultaneously by nasal cannula.

Important: the Department of Health has reminded users of the need to use the correct grade of tubing when connecting a nebuliser to a medical gas supply or compressor.

Medix Lifecare Nebuliser Chamber® (Medix) NHS
Jet nebuliser, disposable; for use with bronchodilators, antimuscarinics, corticosteroids, and antibacterials, replacement recommended every 2–3 months if used 4 times a day. Compatible with *AC 2000 Hi Flo®* NHS, *World Traveller Hi Flo®* NHS, and *Econoneb®* NHS, net price = £1.00

Medix Lifecare Nebuliser System® (Medix) NHS
Jet nebuliser, consisting of mouthpiece, tubing, and nebuliser chamber, net price = £2.00; mask kits with tubing and nebuliser chamber also available, net price (adult) = £2.00; (child) = £2.10

PARI LC PLUS FILTER® (Pari) NHS
Jet nebuliser, closed system, non-disposable, for hospital or home use; for use with bronchodilators, antibacterials and corticosteroids; replacement recommended yearly if used 4 times a day. Compatible with *PARI Turbo BOY'N'®* NHS, *PARI Junior BOY'N'®* NHS and *PARI UNI light mobil®* NHS compressors, net price = £24.80, replacement filters 100 = £35.70

PARI LC PLUS® (Pari) NHS
Jet nebuliser, non-disposable, for hospital or home use; for use with bronchodilators, antibacterials, and corticosteroids, replacement recommended yearly if used 4 times a day. Compatible with *PARI Turbo BOY'N'®* NHS, *PARI Junior BOY'N'®* NHS, *PARI UNI light mobil®* NHS and *PARI WALK BOY®* NHS compressors, net price = £15.45

PARI BABY® (Pari) NHS
Jet nebuliser, non-disposable, for hospital or home use; for use with bronchodilators, antibacterials and corticosteroids; replacement recommended yearly if used 4 times a day. Compatible with *PARI Turbo BOY'N'®* NHS, *PARI Junior BOY'N'®* NHS, *PARI UNI light mobil®* NHS, *PARI WALK BOY®* NHS compressors. Available separately for children aged less than 1 year, 1–4 years or 4–7 years, net price (with mask and connection tube) = £31.40

Sidestream Durable® (Profile Respiratory) NHS
Jet nebuliser, non-disposable, for home use; for use with bronchodilators; yearly replacement recommended if 4 six-minute treatments used per day. Compatible with *Freeway Freedom®* NHS and *Porta-Neb®* NHS, net price year pack = £20.40 (*Porta-Neb®*), £29.00 (*Freeway Freedom®*). *Disposable Sidestream®* NHS nebuliser also available

Ventstream® (Profile Respiratory) NHS
Jet nebuliser, closed-system, for use with low flow compressors, compatible with *Porta-Neb®* NHS, and *Freeway Freedom®* NHS compressors; for use with antibacterials, bronchodilators, and corticosteroids, replacement recommended yearly if used 3 times a day, net price year pack with filter = £39.00 (*Porta-Neb®*), £41.00 (*Freeway Freedom®*)

Home compressors with nebulisers

AC 2000 HI FLO® (Medix) NHS
Home and hospital use, containing 1 *Jet Nebuliser®* NHS set with mouthpiece, 1 adult and 1 child mask,1 spare inlet filter, filter spanner. Mains operated. Nebulises bronchodilators, corticosteroids, and antibacterials, net price = £117.00; carrying case available

AC 4000® (Medix) NHS
Home and hospital use, containing 1 *Jet Nebuliser®* NHS set with mouthpiece, 1 adult and 1 child face mask, 1 spare inlet filter, filter spanner. Mains operated. Nebulises bronchodilators, corticosteroids, and antibacterials, net price = £80.10

Aquilon® (Henleys) NHS
Portable, home use, with 1 adult or 1 child mask and tubing. Mains operated; for use with bronchodilators, corticosteroids and antibacterials, net price = £82.50

Econoneb® (Medix) NHS
Home, clinic and hospital use, used with 1 *Jet Nebuliser®* NHS set with mouthpiece, 1 adult and 1 child mask, 1 spare inlet filter, filter spanner. Nebulises bronchodilators, corticosteroids, and antibacterials. Mains operated, net price = £99.00

Freeway Freedom® (Profile Respiratory) NHS
Portable, containing *Sidestream Durable®* NHS nebuliser, 1 adult mask, 1 child mask, 1 angled mouthpiece, 1 coiled *Duratube®*, 4 inlet filters, charger and power lead, net price = £203.20; with *Ventstream®* NHS nebuliser, 1 straight mouthpiece, 1 coiled *Duratube®*, 4 inlet filters, 1 aerosol hose, charger and power lead, net price = £203.20

PARI Junior BOY'N'® (Pari) NHS
Portable, for hospital or home use, containing *PARI LC PLUS Junior* NHS nebuliser with child mouthpiece, mask, connection tube, and mains cable. Filter replacement recommended every 12 months. Compatible with *PARI LC PLUS®* NHS, *PARI LC PLUS Filter®* NHS, and *PARI Baby®* NHS nebulisers, net price = £70.00

PARI Turbo BOY'N'® (Pari) NHS
Portable, for hospital or home use, containing *PARI LC PLUS* NHS nebuliser with adult mouthpiece, mask, connection tube and mains cable. Filter replacement recommended every 12 months. Compatible with *PARI LC PLUS®* NHS, *PARI LC PLUS FILTER®* NHS, and *PARI BABY®* NHS nebulisers, net price = £65.00

PARI UNI light mobil® (Pari) NHS
Portable, containing *PARI LC PLUS®* NHS nebuliser with connection tube, mains cable, rechargeable battery, car battery adaptor, and carrying case. Compatible with *PARI BABY®* NHS, and *PARI LC PLUS FILTER®* NHS nebulisers. Nebulises bronchodilators, corticosteroids, and antibacterials, net price = £180.00

Porta-Neb® (Profile Respiratory) NHS
Portable, containing *Sidestream Durable®* NHS nebuliser, 1 adult mask, 1 child mask, 1 angled mouthpiece, 1 coiled *Duratube®*, 4 inlet filters. Mains operated, net price = £94.00; with *Ventstream®* NHS nebuliser, 1 straight mouthpiece, 1 coiled *Duratube®*, 4 inlet filters, aerosol hose. Mains operated, net price = £104.80

De Vilbiss 5650® (De Vilbiss) NHS
Home, clinic use, containing disposable nebuliser set, mouthpiece, mask, mains lead, tubing, thumb-valve. For use with bronchodilators, net price = £142.14

De Vilbiss 4650® (De Vilbiss) NHS
Home, clinic and hospital use, with mouthpiece. Mains operated, net price = £93.95

Tourer® (Henleys) NHS
Portable, home use. Mains/car battery operated; for use with bronchodilators, corticosteroids and antibacterials, net price = £101.25

Ultima® (Henleys) NHS
Portable, home use. Rechargable or mains/car battery operated. Nebulises bronchodilators and corticosteroids, net price = £156.00 (includes case)

World Traveller HI FLO® (Medix) NHS
Portable, containing 1 *Jet Nebuliser®* NHS set with mouthpiece, 1 adult and 1 child mask, 1 spare inlet filter, filter spanner. Battery, car, and mains operated; rechargeable battery pack available. Nebulises bronchodilators, corticosteroids, and antibacterials, net price excluding battery = £166.00; with battery = £216.00; carrying case available

Compressors

Omron CX3® (Omron) NHS
Home and hospital use. Mains operated, net price = £48.75

Omron compAIR CX^Pro® (Omron) NHS
Home and hospital use. Mains operated, net price = £56.78 (includes 1 adult mask, child mask, 5 spare filters, and carrying case)

System 22 CR60® (Profile Respiratory) NHS
Hospital use, high flow compressor. Mains operated, net price = £199.90. Also compatible with *System 22 Antibiotic Tee®* NHS for nebulisation of high viscosity drugs such as antibacterials

Turboneb® (Medix) NHS
Hospital use, high flow compressor. Nebulises bronchodilators, corticosteroids, antibacterials, and pentamidine. Mains operated, net price = £125.00

■ Ultrasonic nebulisers

Ultrasonic nebulisers produce an aerosol by ultrasonic vibration of the drug solution and therefore do not require a gas flow

F16 Wave® (Parkside) NHS

Portable, adjustable delivery rate. Mains/car battery operated or rechargeable battery pack (supplied), net price = £130.00

Liberty® (Medix) NHS

Portable, home and clinic use, containing disposable mouthpiece and chamber cover. Mains and car battery operated. Nebulises bronchodilators and antibacterials, net price £112.49

Omron MicroAIR® (Omron) NHS

Portable, battery operated, net price = £149.96 (includes 1 adult mask, 1 child mask, and carrying case; mains adaptor also available)

Omron NE-U17® (Omron) NHS

Clinic and hospital use, mains operated, net price = £650.17

Ultra Neb 2000® (De Vilbiss) NHS

Hospital, clinic and home use, delivery rate adjustable. Supplied with stand, net price = £1205.00

Nebuliser diluent

Nebulisation may be carried out using an undiluted nebuliser solution or it may require dilution beforehand. The usual diluent is sterile sodium chloride 0.9% (physiological saline).

Sodium Chloride (Non-proprietary) PoM

Nebuliser solution, sodium chloride 0.9%, net price 20 × 2.5 mL = £5.49

Brands include *Saline Steripoule*®, *Saline Steri-Neb*®

3.2 Corticosteroids

Corticosteroids are very effective in *asthma*; they reduce airway inflammation (and hence reduce oedema and secretion of mucus into the airway).

In *chronic obstructive pulmonary disease* inhaled corticosteroid treatment may reduce exacerbations. An inhaled corticosteroid [unlicensed indication] should be considered (in addition to bronchodilator treatment) if the peak flow is worse than 50% of the predicted value and if the patient has had 2 or more exacerbations in a year which require antibacterial treatment or an oral corticosteroid. A trial of an inhaled corticosteroid for about 3 weeks can distinguish patients who have asthma from those who have chronic obstructive pulmonary disease.

INHALATION. Inhaled corticosteroids are recommended for prophylactic treatment of asthma when patients are using a beta$_2$ agonist more than 3 times a week or if symptoms disturb sleep more than once a week or if the patient has suffered exacerbations in the last 2 years requiring a systemic corticosteroid or a nebulised bronchodilator (see Chronic Asthma table, p. 140). *Regular use* of inhaled corticosteroids reduces the risk of exacerbation of asthma.

Corticosteroid inhalers must be used regularly for maximum benefit; alleviation of symptoms usually occurs 3 to 7 days after initiation. **Beclometasone dipropionate** (beclomethasone dipropionate), **budesonide** and **fluticasone propionate** appear to be equally effective. Preparations that combine a corticosteroid with a long-acting beta$_2$ agonist may be helpful for patients stabilised on the individual components in the same proportion.

Doses for CFC-free corticosteroid inhalers may be different from those that contain CFCs.

CFC-FREE INHALERS. Chlorofluorocarbon (CFC) propellants in pressurised aerosol inhalers are being replaced by hydrofluoroalkane (HFA) propellants. Patients receiving CFC-free inhalers should be reassured about the efficacy of the new inhalers and counselled that the aerosol may feel and taste different; any difficulty with the new inhaler should be discussed with the doctor or pharmacist.

If the inhaled corticosteroid causes coughing, the use of a beta$_2$ agonist beforehand may help.

Patients taking long-term oral corticosteroids for asthma can often be transferred to an inhaled corticosteroid but the transfer must be slow, with gradual reduction in the dose of the oral corticosteroid, and at a time when the asthma is well controlled.

High-dose corticosteroid inhalers are suitable for patients who respond only partially to standard-dose inhalers and long-acting beta$_2$ agonists or other long-acting bronchodilators (see Chronic Asthma, table, p. 140). High doses should be continued only if there is clear benefit over the lower dose. The recommended maximum dose of an inhaled corticosteroid should not generally be exceeded. However, if higher doses are required (e.g. fluticasone in a dose above 500 micrograms twice daily in an adult or 200 micrograms twice daily in a child aged 4–16 years), then they should be initiated by specialists.

Systemic corticosteroid therapy may be necessary during episodes of infection or if the asthma is worsening, when higher doses are needed and access of inhaled drug to small airways may be reduced; patients may need a reserve supply of tablets.

CAUTIONS OF INHALED CORTICOSTEROIDS. An inhaled corticosteroid should be used cautiously in active or quiescent tuberculosis; systemic therapy may be required during periods of stress or when either airways obstruction or mucus prevent drug access to smaller airways; **interactions:** Appendix 1 (corticosteroids)

PARADOXICAL BRONCHOSPASM. The potential for paradoxical bronchospasm (calling for discontinuation and alternative therapy) should be borne in mind—mild bronchospasm may be prevented by inhalation of a short-acting beta$_2$ agonist (or by transfer from an aerosol inhalation to a dry powder inhalation).

SIDE-EFFECTS OF INHALED CORTICOSTEROIDS. Inhaled corticosteroids have considerably fewer systemic effects than oral corticosteroids, but adverse effects have been reported.

Higher doses of inhaled corticosteroids have the potential to induce adrenal suppression (section 6.3.2) and patients on high doses should be given a 'steroid card'; such patients may need corticosteroid cover during an episode of stress (e.g. an operation). Inhaled corticosteroids in children have been associated with adrenal crisis and coma; excessive doses should be **avoided**, particularly of fluticasone, which should be given in a dose of 50–100 micrograms twice daily and the dose should not exceed 200 micrograms twice daily.

Bone mineral density may be reduced following long-term inhalation of higher doses of corticosteroids, predisposing patients to osteoporosis (section 6.6). It is therefore sensible to ensure that the dose of an inhaled corticosteroid is no higher than necessary to keep a patient's asthma under good control. Treatment with an inhaled corticosteroid can usually be stopped after a mild exacerbation as long as the patient knows that it is necessary to reinstate it should the asthma deteriorate or the peak flow rate fall.

In children, growth retardation associated with oral corticosteroid therapy does not seem to be a significant problem with recommended doses of inhaled therapy; although initial growth velocity may be reduced, there appears to be no effect on achieving normal adult height. However, the CSM recommends that the height of children receiving prolonged treatment is monitored; if growth is slowed, referral to a paediatrician should be considered. Large-volume spacer devices should be used for administering inhaled corticosteroids in children under 5 years (see NICE guidance, section 3.1.5); they are also useful in older children and adults, particularly if high doses are required. Spacer devices increase airway deposition and reduce oropharyngeal deposition.

A small increased risk of glaucoma with prolonged high doses of inhaled corticosteroids has been reported; cataracts have also been reported with inhaled corticosteroids. Hoarseness and candidiasis of the mouth or throat have been reported, usually only with large doses (see also below). Hypersensitivity reactions (including rash and angioedema) have been reported rarely.

CANDIDIASIS. Candidiasis can be reduced by using spacer, see notes above, and it responds to antifungal lozenges (section 12.3.2) without discontinuation of therapy—rinsing the mouth with water (or cleaning child's teeth) after inhalation of a dose may also be helpful.

ORAL. An acute attack of asthma should be treated with a short course of an oral corticosteroid starting with a high dose, e.g. prednisolone 40–50 mg daily for a few days. Patients whose asthma has deteriorated rapidly usually respond quickly to corticosteroids. The dose can usually be stopped abruptly in a mild exacerbation of asthma (see also Withdrawal of Corticosteroids, section 6.3.2) but it should be reduced gradually in those with poorer asthma control, to reduce the possibility of serious relapse. For use of corticosteroids in the emergency treatment of acute severe asthma see table on p. 141.

In chronic continuing asthma, when the response to other drugs has been inadequate, longer term administration of an oral corticosteroid may be necessary; in such cases high doses of an inhaled corticosteroid should be continued to minimise oral corticosteroid requirements. In chronic obstructive pulmonary disease prednisolone 30 mg daily should be given for 7–14 days; treatment can be stopped abruptly. Prolonged treatment with oral prednisolone is of no benefit and maintenance treatment is not normally recommended.

An oral corticosteroid should normally be taken as a single dose in the morning to reduce the disturbance to circadian cortisol secretion. Dosage should always be titrated to the lowest dose that controls symptoms. Regular peak flow measurements help to optimise the dose.

Alternate-day administration has not been very successful in the management of asthma in adults because control can deteriorate during the second 24 hours. If alternate-day administration is introduced, pulmonary function should be monitored carefully over the 48 hours.

PARENTERAL. For the use of hydrocortisone injection in the emergency treatment of acute severe asthma, see Acute Severe Asthma table, p. 141.

BECLOMETASONE DIPROPIONATE

(Beclomethasone Dipropionate)

Indications: prophylaxis of asthma (see also Chronic Asthma table, p. 140)

Cautions: see notes above

Side-effects: see notes above; *very rarely* anxiety, sleep disorders, and behavioural changes

Dose: Standard-dose inhalers

By aerosol inhalation (for *Qvar*® dose see under preparation), 200 micrograms twice daily *or* 100 micrograms 3–4 times daily (in more severe cases initially 600–800 micrograms daily); CHILD 50–100 micrograms 2–4 times daily

By inhalation of powder (for *Asmabec*® dose see under preparation), 400 micrograms twice daily *or* 200 micrograms 3–4 times daily; CHILD 100 micrograms 2–4 times daily *or* 200 micrograms twice daily

High-dose inhalers

By aerosol inhalation (for *Qvar*® dose see under preparation), 500 micrograms twice daily *or* 250 micrograms 4 times daily; if necessary may be increased to 500 micrograms 4 times daily; CHILD not recommended

By inhalation of powder (for *Asmabec*® dose see under preparation), 400 micrograms twice daily; if necessary may be increased to 800 micrograms twice daily; CHILD not recommended

■ Standard-dose inhalers

Beclometasone (Non-proprietary) PoM

Aerosol inhalation, beclometasone dipropionate 50 micrograms/metered inhalation, net price 200-dose unit = £4.62; 100 micrograms/metered inhalation, 200-dose unit = £8.24; 200 micrograms/metered inhalation, 200-dose unit = £8.14. Label: 8, counselling, dose

Excipients: include CFC propellants

Brands include *Beclazone*®, *Filair*®

Dry powder for inhalation, beclometasone dipropionate 100 micrograms/metered inhalation, net price 100-dose unit = £5.58; 200 micrograms/metered inhalation, 100-dose unit = £10.29. Label: 8, counselling, dose

Brands include *Pulvinal*® *Beclometasone Dipropionate*

Inhalation powder, hard capsule (for use with *Cyclohaler*® device), beclometasone dipropionate 100 micrograms, net price 120-cap pack = £7.59; 200 micrograms, 120-cap pack = £14.41. Label: 8, counselling, dose

Brands include *Beclometasone Cyclocaps*®

AeroBec® (3M) PoM

AeroBec 50 Autohaler® (breath-actuated aerosol inhalation), beclometasone dipropionate 50 micrograms/metered inhalation, net price 200-dose unit = £4.04. Label: 8, counselling, dose

Excipients: include CFC propellants

AeroBec 100 Autohaler® (breath-actuated aerosol inhalation), beclometasone dipropionate 100 micrograms/metered inhalation, net price 200-dose unit = £7.66. Label: 8, counselling, dose

Excipients: include CFC propellants

Asmabec Clickhaler® (Celltech) PoM
Dry powder for inhalation, beclometasone dipropionate 50 micrograms/metered inhalation, net price 200-dose unit = £6.68; 100 micrograms/metered inhalation, 200-dose unit = £9.81. Label: 8, counselling, dose

Dose: by inhalation of powder, 200–400 micrograms daily, in 2–4 divided doses (in more severe cases initially 0.8–1.6 mg daily, in 2–4 divided doses—see also High-dose inhalers); CHILD 50–100 micrograms 2–4 times daily

Beclazone Easi-Breathe® (IVAX) PoM
Aerosol inhalation, beclometasone dipropionate 50 micrograms/metered inhalation, net price 200-dose breath-actuated unit = £3.26; 100 micrograms/metered inhalation, 200-dose breath-actuated unit = £6.18. Label: 8, counselling, dose

Excipients: include CFC propellants

Becodisks® (A&H) PoM
Dry powder for inhalation, disks containing 8 blisters of beclometasone dipropionate 100 micrograms/blister, net price 15 disks with *Diskhaler*® device = £12.00, 15-disk refill = £11.42; 200 micrograms/blister, 15 disks with *Diskhaler*® device = £22.87, 15-disk refill = £22.28. Label: 8, counselling, dose

Becotide® (A&H) PoM
Becotide®-50 aerosol inhalation, beclometasone dipropionate 50 micrograms/metered inhalation. Net price 200-dose unit = £1.79. Label: 8, counselling, dose

Excipients: include CFC propellants

Becotide®-100 aerosol inhalation, beclometasone dipropionate 100 micrograms/metered inhalation. Net price 200-dose unit = £2.79. Label: 8, counselling, dose

Excipients: include CFC propellants

Becotide®-200 aerosol inhalation, beclometasone dipropionate 200 micrograms/metered inhalation. Net price 200-dose unit = £8.14. Label: 8, counselling, dose, 10, steroid card

Excipients: include CFC propellants

NOTE. *Becotide®-200* not indicated for children

Qvar® (IVAX) PoM
Qvar® 50 aerosol inhalation, beclometasone dipropionate 50 micrograms/metered inhalation, net price 200-dose unit = £7.87. Label: 8, counselling, dose

Qvar® 100 aerosol inhalation, beclometasone dipropionate 100 micrograms/metered inhalation, net price 200-dose unit = £17.21. Label: 8, counselling, dose, 10, steroid card

Qvar 50 Autohaler® (breath-actuated aerosol inhalation), beclometasone dipropionate 50 micrograms/metered inhalation, net price 200-dose unit = £7.87. Label: 8, counselling, dose

Qvar 100 Autohaler® (breath-actuated aerosol inhalation), beclometasone dipropionate 100 micrograms/metered inhalation, net price 200-dose unit = £17.21. Label: 8, counselling, dose, 10, steroid card

Excipients: include HFA-134a (a non-CFC propellant), ethanol

Qvar Easi-Breathe® (breath-actuated aerosol inhalation), beclometasone dipropionate 50 micrograms/metered inhalation, net price 200-dose = £8.24; 100 micrograms/metered inhalation, 200-dose = £18.02. Label: 8, counselling, dose, 10, steroid card

Excipients: include HFA-134a (a non-CFC propellant), ethanol

Dose: by aerosol inhalation, 50–200 micrograms twice daily, if necessary may be increased to max. 400 micrograms twice daily; CHILD not recommended

NOTE. When transferring a patient from a CFC-containing inhaler (asthma well controlled), initially a 100-microgram metered dose of *Qvar*® should be substituted for:

- 200–250 micrograms of beclometasone dipropionate or budesonide
- 100 micrograms of fluticasone propionate

When transferring a patient from a CFC-containing inhaler (asthma poorly controlled), initially a 100-microgram metered dose of *Qvar*® should be substituted for 100 micrograms of beclometasone dipropionate, budesonide or fluticasone propionate

■ High-dose inhalers

NOTE. High-dose inhalers not indicated for children

Chronic Asthma table, see p. 140
Acute Severe Asthma table, see p. 141

Beclometasone (Non-proprietary) PoM
Aerosol inhalation, beclometasone dipropionate 250 micrograms/metered inhalation, net price 200-dose unit = £16.37. Label: 8, counselling, dose, 10, steroid card

Excipients: include CFC propellants

Brands include *Beclazone*®, *Filair Forte*®

Dry powder for inhalation, beclometasone dipropionate 400 micrograms/metered inhalation, net price 100-dose unit = £20.41. Label: 8, counselling, dose, 10, steroid card

Brands include *Pulvinal® Beclometasone Dipropionate*

Inhalation powder, hard capsule (for use with *Cyclohaler*® device), beclometasone dipropionate 400 micrograms, net price 120-cap pack = £27.38. Label: 8, counselling, dose, 10, steroid card

Brands include *Beclometasone 400 Cyclocaps*®

AeroBec Forte® (3M) PoM
Aerosol inhalation, beclometasone dipropionate 250 micrograms/metered inhalation, net price 200-inhalation breath-actuated unit (*Autohaler*®) = £16.76. Label: 8, counselling, dose, 10, steroid card

Excipients: include CFC propellants

Asmabec Clickhaler® (Celltech) PoM
Dry powder for inhalation, beclometasone dipropionate 250 micrograms/metered inhalation, net price 100-dose unit = £12.31. Label: 8, counselling, dose, 10, steroid card

Dose: by inhalation of powder, 500 micrograms twice daily *or* 250 micrograms 4 times daily; if necessary may be increased to 500 micrograms 4 times daily; CHILD not recommended

Beclazone Easi-Breathe® (IVAX) PoM
Aerosol inhalation, beclometasone dipropionate 250 micrograms/metered inhalation, net price 200-dose breath-actuated unit = £13.52. Label: 8, counselling, dose, 10, steroid card

Excipients: include CFC propellants

Becloforte® (A&H) PoM
Aerosol inhalation, beclometasone dipropionate 250 micrograms/metered inhalation. Net price 200-dose unit = £6.99. Label: 8, counselling, dose, 10, steroid card

Excipients: include CFC propellants

Becodisks® (A&H) PoM
Dry powder for inhalation, disks containing 8 blisters of beclometasone dipropionate 400 micrograms/blister, 15 disks with *Diskhaler*® device = £45.14, 15-disk refill = £44.57. Label: 8, counselling, dose, 10, steroid card

Qvar® (IVAX) PoM
See under Standard-dose inhalers above

BUDESONIDE

Indications: prophylaxis of asthma (see also Chronic Asthma table, p. 140)
Cautions: see notes above
Side-effects: see notes above
Dose: see preparations below

Budesonide (Non-proprietary) PoM
Dry powder for inhalation, budesonide 200 micrograms, net price 100-dose unit = £18.50, 100-dose refill = £9.59
Brands include *Novolizer*®▼
Inhalation powder, hard capsule (for use with *Cyclohaler*® device), budesonide 200 micrograms, net price 100-cap pack = £15.48; 400 micrograms, 50-cap pack = £15.48. Label: 8, counselling, dose, 10, steroid card
Brands include *Budesonide Cyclocaps*®
Dose: 0.2–1.6 mg daily in divided doses adjusted as necessary; CHILD over 6 years 200–400 micrograms daily in divided doses adjusted as necessary (max. 800 micrograms daily)

Pulmicort® (AstraZeneca) PoM
LS aerosol inhalation, budesonide 50 micrograms/metered inhalation. Net price 200-dose unit = £7.33. Label: 8, counselling, dose
Excipients: include CFC propellants
Aerosol inhalation, budesonide 200 micrograms/metered inhalation. Net price 200-dose unit with or without *NebuChamber*® = £20.90; 100-dose unit = £7.60 (hosp. only; may be difficult to obtain). Label: 8, counselling, dose, 10, steroid card
Excipients: include CFC propellants
Dose: by aerosol inhalation, 200 micrograms twice daily; may be reduced in well-controlled asthma to not less than 200 micrograms daily; in severe asthma dose may be increased to 1.6 mg daily; CHILD 50–400 micrograms twice daily; in severe asthma may be increased to 800 micrograms daily
Turbohaler® (= dry powder inhaler), budesonide 100 micrograms/metered inhalation, net price 200-dose unit = £18.50; 200 micrograms/metered inhalation, 100-dose unit = £18.50; 400 micrograms/metered inhalation, 50-dose unit = £18.50. Label: 8, counselling, dose, 10, steroid card
Dose: by inhalation of powder, when starting treatment, during periods of severe asthma, and while reducing or discontinuing oral corticosteroid, 0.2–1.6 mg daily in 2 divided doses; in less severe cases 200–400 micrograms once daily (each evening); patients already controlled on inhaled beclometasone dipropionate or budesonide administered twice daily may be transferred to once-daily dosing (each evening) at the same equivalent total daily dose (up to 800 micrograms once daily); CHILD under 12 years 200–800 micrograms daily in 2 divided doses (800 micrograms daily in severe asthma) *or* 200–400 micrograms once daily (each evening)
Respules® (= single-dose units for nebulisation), budesonide 250 micrograms/mL, net price 20 × 2-mL (500-microgram) unit = £32.00; 500 micrograms/mL, 20 × 2-mL (1-mg) unit = £44.64. May be diluted with sterile sodium chloride 0.9%. Label: 8, counselling, dose, 10, steroid card
Dose: by inhalation of nebulised suspension, when starting treatment, during periods of severe asthma, and while reducing or discontinuing oral corticosteroids, 1–2 mg twice daily (may be increased further in very severe asthma); CHILD 3 months–12 years, 0.5–1 mg twice daily
Maintenance, usually half above doses
Croup, 2 mg as a single dose (*or* as two 1-mg doses separated by 30 minutes)

■ Compound preparations

Symbicort® (AstraZeneca) PoM
Symbicort 100/6 Turbohaler® (= dry powder inhaler), budesonide 80 micrograms, formoterol fumarate 4.5 micrograms/metered inhalation, net price 120-dose unit = £33.00. Label: 8, counselling, dose, 10, steroid card
NOTE. Each metered inhalation of *Symbicort*® *100/6* delivers the same quantity of budesonide as a 100-microgram metered inhalation of *Pulmicort Turbohaler*® and of formoterol fumarate as a 4.5-microgram metered inhalation of *Oxis*® *6 Turbohaler*®
Dose: by inhalation of powder, asthma, 1–2 puffs twice daily increased if necessary to max. 4 puffs twice daily, reduced to 1 puff once daily if control maintained; ADOLESCENT 12–17 years 1–2 puffs twice daily reduced to 1 puff once daily if control maintained; CHILD over 6 years, 2 puffs twice daily reduced to 1 puff once daily if control maintained
Symbicort 200/6 Turbohaler® (=dry powder inhaler), budesonide 160 micrograms, formoterol fumarate 4.5 micrograms/metered inhalation, net price 120-dose unit = £38.00. Label: 8, counselling, dose, 10, steroid card
NOTE. Each metered inhalation of *Symbicort*® *200/6* delivers the same quantity of budesonide as a 200-microgram metered inhalation of *Pulmicort Turbohaler*® and of formoterol fumarate as a 4.5-microgram metered inhalation of *Oxis*® *6 Turbohaler*®
Dose: by inhalation of powder, asthma, 1–2 puffs twice daily increased if necessary to max. 4 puffs twice daily, reduced to 1 puff once daily if control maintained; ADOLESCENT 12–17 years 1–2 puffs twice daily reduced to 1 puff once daily if control maintained; CHILD under 12 years not recommended
Chronic obstructive pulmonary disease, 2 puffs twice daily; CHILD not recommended
Symbicort 400/12 Turbohaler® (=dry powder inhaler), budesonide 320 micrograms, formoterol fumarate 9 micrograms/metered inhalation, net price 60-dose unit = £38.00. Label: 8, counselling, dose, 10, steroid card
NOTE. Each metered inhalation of *Symbicort*® *400/12* delivers the same quantity of budesonide as a 400-microgram metered inhalation of *Pulmicort Turbohaler*® and of formoterol fumarate as a 9-microgram metered inhalation of *Oxis*® *12 Turbohaler*®
Dose: by inhalation of powder, asthma, 1 puff twice daily increased if necessary to max. 2 puffs twice daily, reduced to 1 puff once daily if control maintained; ADOLESCENT 12–17 years 1 puff twice daily reduced to 1 puff once daily if control maintained; CHILD under 12 years not recommended
Chronic obstructive pulmonary disease, 1 puff twice daily; CHILD not recommended

CICLESONIDE

Indications: prophylaxis of asthma
Cautions: see notes above
Side-effects: see notes above
Dose: *by aerosol inhalation*, 160 micrograms daily as a single dose reduced to 80 micrograms daily if

control maintained; CHILD and ADOLESCENT under 18 years not recommended

Alvesco® (Altana) ▼ PoM
Aerosol inhalation, ciclesonide 80 micrograms/metered inhalation, net price 120-dose unit = £28.56; 160 micrograms/metered inhalation, 120-dose unit = £33.60. Label: 8, counselling, dose
Excipients: include HFA-134a (a non-CFC propellant), ethanol

FLUTICASONE PROPIONATE

Indications: prophylaxis of asthma (see also Chronic Asthma table, p. 140)
Cautions: see notes above
Side-effects: see notes above
Dose: see preparations below

Flixotide® (A&H) PoM
Accuhaler® (dry powder for inhalation), disk containing 60 blisters of fluticasone propionate 50 micrograms/blister with *Accuhaler*® device, net price = £6.38; 100 micrograms/blister with *Accuhaler*® device = £8.93; 250 micrograms/blister with *Accuhaler*® device = £21.26; 500 micrograms/blister with *Accuhaler*® device = £36.14. Label: 8, counselling, dose; 250- and 500-microgram strengths also label 10, steroid card
NOTE. *Flixotide Accuhaler*® 250 micrograms and 500 micrograms are not indicated for children
Dose: by inhalation of powder, ADULT and CHILD over 16 years, 100–250 micrograms twice daily, increased according to severity of asthma to 1 mg twice daily; CHILD 4–16 years, 50–100 micrograms twice daily adjusted as necessary; max. 200 micrograms twice daily
Diskhaler® (dry powder for inhalation), fluticasone propionate 50 micrograms/blister, net price 15 disks of 4 blisters with *Diskhaler*® device = £8.17, 15-disk refill = £7.64; 100 micrograms/blister, 15 disks of 4 blisters with *Diskhaler*® device = £12.71, 15-disk refill = £12.18; 250 micrograms/blister, 15 disks of 4 blisters with *Diskhaler*® device = £24.11, 15-disk refill = £23.58; 500 micrograms/blister, 15 disks of 4 blisters with *Diskhaler*® device = £40.05, 15-disk refill = £39.52. Label: 8, counselling, dose; 250- and 500-microgram strengths also label 10, steroid card
NOTE. *Flixotide Diskhaler*® 250 micrograms and 500 micrograms are not indicated for children
Dose: by inhalation of powder, ADULT and CHILD over 16 years, 100–250 micrograms twice daily, increased according to severity of asthma to 1 mg twice daily; CHILD 4–16 years, 50–100 micrograms twice daily adjusted as necessary; max. 200 micrograms twice daily
Evohaler® *aerosol inhalation*, fluticasone propionate 50 micrograms/metered inhalation, net price 120-dose unit = £5.44; 125 micrograms/metered inhalation, 120-dose unit = £21.26; 250 micrograms/metered inhalation, 120-dose unit = £36.14. Label: 8, counselling, dose, change to CFC-free inhaler; 250-microgram strength also label 10, steroid card
Excipients: include HFA-134a (a non-CFC propellant)
NOTE. *Flixotide Evohaler*® 125 micrograms and 250 micrograms not indicated for children
Dose: by aerosol inhalation, ADULT and CHILD over 16 years, 100–250 micrograms twice daily, increased according to severity of asthma to 1 mg twice daily; CHILD 4–16 years, 50–100 micrograms twice daily adjusted as necessary; max. 200 micrograms twice daily
Nebules® (= single-dose units for nebulisation) fluticasone propionate 250 micrograms/mL, net price 10 × 2-mL (500-microgram) unit = £9.34; 1 mg/mL, 10 × 2-mL (2-mg) unit = £37.35. May be diluted with sterile sodium chloride 0.9%. Label: 8, counselling, dose, 10, steroid card
Dose: by inhalation of nebulised suspension, ADULT and CHILD over 16 years, 0.5–2 mg twice daily; CHILD 4–16 years, 1 mg twice daily

■ Compound preparations

Seretide® (A&H) PoM
Seretide 100 Accuhaler® (dry powder for inhalation), disk containing 60 blisters of fluticasone propionate 100 micrograms, salmeterol (as xinafoate) 50 micrograms/blister with *Accuhaler*® device, net price = £31.19. Label: 8, counselling, dose
Dose: by inhalation of powder, asthma, ADULT and CHILD over 4 years, 1 blister twice daily, reduced to 1 blister once daily if control maintained
Seretide 250 Accuhaler® (dry powder for inhalation), disk containing 60 blisters of fluticasone propionate 250 micrograms, salmeterol (as xinafoate) 50 micrograms/blister with *Accuhaler*® device, net price = £36.65. Label: 8, counselling, dose, 10, steroid card
Dose: by inhalation of powder, asthma, ADULT and CHILD over 12 years, 1 blister twice daily
Seretide 500 Accuhaler® (dry powder for inhalation), disk containing 60 blisters of fluticasone propionate 500 micrograms, salmeterol (as xinafoate) 50 micrograms/blister with *Accuhaler*® device, net price = £40.92. Label: 8, counselling, dose, 10, steroid card
Dose: by inhalation of powder, asthma, ADULT and CHILD over 12 years, 1 blister twice daily
Chronic obstructive pulmonary disease, ADULT 1 blister twice daily
Seretide 50 Evohaler® (aerosol inhalation), fluticasone propionate 50 micrograms, salmeterol (as xinafoate) 25 micrograms/metered inhalation, net price 120-dose unit = £19.50. Label: 8, counselling, dose, change to CFC-free inhaler
Excipients: include HFA-134a (a non-CFC propellant)
Dose: by aerosol inhalation, asthma, ADULT and CHILD over 4 years, 2 puffs twice daily, reduced to 2 puffs once daily if control maintained
Seretide 125 Evohaler® (aerosol inhalation), fluticasone propionate 125 micrograms, salmeterol (as xinafoate) 25 micrograms/metered inhalation, net price 120-dose unit = £39.41. Label: 8, counselling, dose, change to CFC-free inhaler, 10, steroid card
Excipients: include HFA-134a (a non-CFC propellant)
Dose: by aerosol inhalation, asthma, ADULT and CHILD over 12 years, 2 puffs twice daily
Seretide 250 Evohaler® (aerosol inhalation), fluticasone propionate 250 micrograms, salmeterol (as xinafoate) 25 micrograms/metered inhalation, net price 120-dose unit = £66.98. Label: 8, counselling, dose, change to CFC-free inhaler, 10, steroid card
Excipients: include HFA-134a (a non-CFC propellant)
Dose: by aerosol inhalation, asthma, ADULT and CHILD over 12 years, 2 puffs twice daily

MOMETASONE FUROATE

Indications: prophylaxis of asthma (see also Chronic Asthma table, p. 140)
Cautions: see notes above
Side-effects: see notes above; also pharyngitis
Dose: *by inhalation of powder*, 200–400 micrograms as a single dose in the evening or in 2

divided doses; dose increased to 400 micrograms twice daily if necessary; CHILD not recommended

Asmanex® (Schering-Plough) ▼ PoM
Twisthaler (= dry powder inhaler), mometasone furoate 200 micrograms/metered inhalation, net price 30-dose unit = £16.00, 60-dose unit = £24.00; 400 micrograms/metered inhalation, 30-dose unit = £22.20, 60-dose unit = £36.75. Label: 8, counselling, dose, 10, steroid card

3.3 Cromoglicate, related therapy and leukotriene receptor antagonists

3.3.1 Cromoglicate and related therapy

The mode of action of **sodium cromoglicate** and **nedocromil** is not completely understood. They may be of value in asthma with an allergic basis, but, in practice, it is difficult to predict who will benefit; they could probably be given for 4 to 6 weeks to assess response. Dose frequency is adjusted according to response but is usually 3 to 4 times a day initially; this may subsequently be reduced.

In general, *prophylaxis* with sodium cromoglicate is less effective than prophylaxis with corticosteroid inhalations (see Chronic Asthma table, p. 140). There is evidence of efficacy of nedocromil in children aged 5–12 years. Sodium cromoglicate is of no value in the treatment of acute attacks of asthma.

Sodium cromoglicate can prevent exercise-induced asthma. However, exercise-induced asthma may reflect poor overall control and the patient should be assessed.

If inhalation of the dry powder form of sodium cromoglicate causes bronchospasm a selective beta$_2$-adrenoceptor stimulant such as salbutamol or terbutaline should be inhaled a few minutes beforehand. The nebuliser solution is an alternative means of delivery for children who cannot manage the dry powder inhaler or the aerosol.

SODIUM CROMOGLICATE

(Sodium Cromoglycate)

Indications: prophylaxis of asthma; food allergy (section 1.5); allergic conjunctivitis (section 11.4.2); allergic rhinitis (section 12.2.1)

Side-effects: coughing, transient bronchospasm, and throat irritation due to inhalation of powder (see also notes above)

Dose: *by aerosol inhalation*, ADULT and CHILD, 10 mg (2 puffs) 4 times daily, increased in severe cases or during periods of risk to 6–8 times daily; additional doses may also be taken before exercise; maintenance 5 mg (1 puff) 4 times daily

By inhalation of powder (*Spincaps*®), ADULT and CHILD, 20 mg 4 times daily, increased in severe cases to 8 times daily; additional doses may also be taken before exercise

By inhalation of nebulised solution, ADULT and CHILD, 20 mg 4 times daily, increased in severe cases to 6 times daily

COUNSELLING. Regular use is necessary

Sodium Cromoglicate (Non-proprietary) PoM
Aerosol inhalation, sodium cromoglicate 5 mg/metered inhalation. Net price 112-dose unit = £5.92. Label: 8
Excipients: include CFC propellants
Brands include *Cromogen*®

Cromogen Easi-Breathe® (IVAX) PoM
Aerosol inhalation, sodium cromoglicate 5 mg/metered inhalation. Net price 112-dose breath-actuated unit = £13.91. Label: 8
Excipients: include CFC propellants

Intal® (Rhône-Poulenc Rorer) PoM
Aerosol inhalation, sodium cromoglicate 5 mg/metered inhalation. Net price 112-dose unit = £5.92; 2 × 112-dose unit with spacer device (*Syncroner*®) = £35.31; also available with large volume spacer inhaler (*Fisonair*®), complete unit = £20.52. Label: 8
Excipients: include CFC propellants
Spincaps®, yellow/clear, sodium cromoglicate 20 mg. Net price 112-cap pack = £15.44. Label: 8
Spinhaler insufflator® (for use with *Intal Spincaps*). Net price = £1.92
Nebuliser solution sodium cromoglicate 10 mg/mL. Net price 2-mL amp = 32p. For use with power-operated nebuliser

NEDOCROMIL SODIUM

Indications: prophylaxis of asthma

Side-effects: see under Sodium Cromoglicate; also headache, nausea, vomiting, dyspepsia and abdominal pain; bitter taste (masked by mint flavour)

Dose: *by aerosol inhalation*, ADULT and CHILD over 6 years 4 mg (2 puffs) 4 times daily, when control achieved may be possible to reduce to twice daily

COUNSELLING. Regular use is necessary

Tilade® (Sanofi-Aventis) PoM
Aerosol inhalation, mint-flavoured, nedocromil sodium 2 mg/metered inhalation. Net price 2 × 56-dose units = £39.97; 2 × 112-dose units with spacer device (*Syncroner*®) = £79.93. Label: 8
Excipients: include CFC propellants

Related therapy

Antihistamines are of no value in the treatment of bronchial asthma. **Ketotifen** is an antihistamine with an action said to resemble that of sodium cromoglicate, but it has proved ineffective in asthma. Specialists sometimes use it in the management of urticaria [unlicensed indication].

KETOTIFEN

Indications: see notes above

Cautions: previous anti-asthmatic treatment should be continued for a minimum of 2 weeks after initiation of ketotifen treatment; pregnancy (Appendix 4) and breast-feeding (Appendix 5); **interactions:** Appendix 1 (antihistamines)—also, manufacturer advises avoid with oral antidiabetics (fall in thrombocyte count reported)

DRIVING. Drowsiness may affect performance of skilled tasks (e.g. driving); effects of alcohol enhanced

Side-effects: drowsiness, dry mouth, slight dizziness; CNS stimulation, weight gain also reported

Dose: 1 mg twice daily with food increased if necessary to 2 mg twice daily; initial treatment in readily sedated patients 0.5–1 mg at night; CHILD over 2 years 1 mg twice daily

Zaditen® (Novartis) PoM

Tablets, scored, ketotifen (as hydrogen fumarate) 1 mg. Net price 60-tab pack = £9.77. Label: 2, 8, 21

Elixir, ketotifen (as hydrogen fumarate) 1 mg/5 mL. Net price 300 mL = £11.57. Label: 2, 8, 21

3.3.2 Leukotriene receptor antagonists

The leukotriene receptor antagonists, **montelukast** and **zafirlukast**, block the effects of cysteinyl leukotrienes in the airways. They are effective in asthma when used alone or with an inhaled corticosteroid (see Chronic Asthma table, p. 140). Montelukast has not been shown to be more effective than a standard dose of inhaled corticosteroid but the two drugs appear to have an additive effect. The leukotriene receptor antagonists may be of benefit in exercise-induced asthma and in those with concomitant rhinitis but they are less effective in those with severe asthma who are also receiving high doses of other drugs.

Churg-Strauss syndrome has occurred very rarely in association with the use of leukotriene receptor antagonists; in many of the reported cases the reaction followed the reduction or withdrawal of oral corticosteroid therapy. The CSM has advised that prescribers should be alert to the development of eosinophilia, vasculitic rash, worsening pulmonary symptoms, cardiac complications, or peripheral neuropathy.

MONTELUKAST

Indications: prophylaxis of asthma, see notes above and Chronic Asthma table, p. 140

Cautions: pregnancy (Appendix 4) and breast-feeding (Appendix 5); Churg-Strauss syndrome, see notes above; **interactions:** Appendix 1 (leukotriene antagonists)

Side-effects: gastro-intestinal disturbances, dry mouth, thirst; hypersensitivity reactions including anaphylaxis, angioedema and skin reactions; asthenia, dizziness, agitation, restlessness, paraesthesia, headache, sleep disorders (insomnia, drowsiness, abnormal dreams); arthralgia, myalgia and muscle cramps; palpitations, increased bleeding tendency, cholestatic hepatitis, raised serum transaminases, oedema, hallucinations, and seizures also reported

Dose: 10 mg daily in the evening; CHILD 6 months–5 years 4 mg daily in the evening, 6–14 years 5 mg daily in the evening

Singulair® (MSD) PoM

Chewable tablets, both pink, cherry-flavoured, montelukast (as sodium salt) 4 mg, net price 28-tab pack = £25.69; 5 mg, 28-tab pack = £25.69. Label: 24

Excipients: include aspartame equivalent to phenylalanine 674 micrograms/4-mg tablet and 842 micrograms/5-mg tablet (section 9.4.1)

Granules, montelukast (as sodium salt) 4 mg, net price 28-sachet pack = £25.69. Counselling, administration

COUNSELLING. Granules may be swallowed or mixed with cold food (but not fluid) and taken immediately

Tablets, beige, f/c, montelukast (as sodium salt) 10 mg, net price 28-tab pack = £26.97

ZAFIRLUKAST

Indications: prophylaxis of asthma, see notes above and Chronic Asthma table, p. 140

Cautions: elderly, pregnancy (Appendix 4), renal impairment (Appendix 3); Churg-Strauss syndrome, see notes above; **interactions:** Appendix 1 (leukotriene antagonists)

HEPATIC DISORDERS. Patients or their carers should be told how to recognise development of liver disorder and advised to seek medical attention if symptoms or signs such as persistent nausea, vomiting, malaise or jaundice develop

Contra-indications: hepatic impairment; breast-feeding (Appendix 5)

Side-effects: gastro-intestinal disturbances, headache, insomnia, malaise; *rarely* bleeding disorders, hypersensitivity reactions including angioedema and skin reactions, arthralgia, myalgia, hepatitis, hyperbilirubinaemia, thrombocytopenia; *very rarely* agranulocytosis; also respiratory-tract infection in the elderly

Dose: 20 mg twice daily; CHILD under 12 years, not recommended

Accolate® (AstraZeneca) PoM

Tablets, f/c, zafirlukast 20 mg, net price 56-tab pack = £28.26. Label: 23

3.4 Antihistamines, hyposensitisation, and allergic emergencies

3.4.1 Antihistamines

All antihistamines are of potential value in the treatment of nasal allergies, particularly seasonal allergic rhinitis (hay fever), and they may be of some value in vasomotor rhinitis. They reduce rhinorrhoea and sneezing but are usually less effective for nasal congestion. Antihistamines are used topically in the eye (section 11.4.2), in the nose (section 12.2.1), and on the skin (section 13.3).

Oral antihistamines are also of some value in preventing urticaria and are used to treat urticarial rashes, pruritus, and insect bites and stings; they are also used in drug allergies. Injections of chlorphenamine (chlorpheniramine) or promethazine are used as an adjunct to adrenaline (epinephrine) in the emergency treatment of anaphylaxis and angio-edema (section 3.4.3). For the use of antihistamines (including cinnarizine, cyclizine, and promethazine teoclate) in nausea and vomiting, see section 4.6. Buclizine is included as an anti-emetic in a preparation for migraine (section 4.7.4.1). For reference to the use of antihistamines for occasional insomnia, see section 4.1.1.

Antihistamines differ in their duration of action and incidence of drowsiness and antimuscarinic effects. Many older antihistamines are relatively short acting but some (e.g. promethazine) act for up to 12 hours, while most of the newer non-sedating antihistamines are long acting.

All older antihistamines cause sedation but **alimemazine** (trimeprazine) and **promethazine** may be more sedating whereas **chlorphenamine** and **cyclizine** (section 4.6) may be less so. This sedating activity is sometimes used to manage the pruritus associated with some allergies. There is little evidence that any one of the older, 'sedating' antihistamines is superior to another and patients vary widely in their response.

Non-sedating antihistamines such as **acrivastine**, **cetirizine**, **desloratadine** (an active metabolite of loratadine), **fexofenadine** (an active metabolite of terfenadine), **levocetirizine** (an isomer of cetirizine), **loratadine**, **mizolastine**, and **terfenadine** cause less sedation and psychomotor impairment than the older antihistamines because they penetrate the blood brain barrier only to a slight extent. Terfenadine is associated with hazardous arrhythmias.

DENTAL SURGERY. Antihistamines are used widely as anti-emetics (section 4.6) but diazepam is likely to be more effective in patients with an overactive vomiting reflex. See also Anaphylaxis under Medical Emergencies in Dental Practice, p. 20.

CAUTIONS AND CONTRA-INDICATIONS. Sedating antihistamines have significant antimuscarinic activity and they should therefore be used with caution in prostatic hypertrophy, urinary retention, glaucoma and pyloroduodenal obstruction. Antihistamines should be used with caution in hepatic disease (Appendix 2) and dose reduction may be necessary in renal impairment (Appendix 3). Caution may be required in epilepsy. Children and the elderly are more susceptible to side-effects. Many antihistamines should be avoided in porphyria although some (e.g. chlorphenamine and cetirizine) are thought to be safe (section 9.8.2). **Interactions:** Appendix 1 (antihistamines); **important:** see also under Terfenadine.

SIDE-EFFECTS. Drowsiness is a significant side-effect with most of the older antihistamines although paradoxical stimulation may occur rarely, especially with high doses or in children and the elderly. Drowsiness may diminish after a few days of treatment and is considerably less of a problem with the newer antihistamines (see also notes above). Side-effects that are more common with the older antihistamines include headache, psychomotor impairment, and antimuscarinic effects such as urinary retention, dry mouth, blurred vision, and gastro-intestinal disturbances.

Other side-effects of antihistamines include palpitations and arrhythmias (**important:** see especially risks associated with *terfenadine,* below), hypotension, hypersensitivity reactions (including bronchospasm, angioedema, and anaphylaxis, rashes and photosensitivity reactions), extrapyramidal effects, dizziness, confusion, depression, sleep disturbances, tremor, convulsions, blood disorders, and liver dysfunction.

Non-sedating antihistamines

DRIVING. Although drowsiness is rare, nevertheless patients should be advised that it can occur and may affect performance of skilled tasks (e.g. driving); excess alcohol should be avoided.

ACRIVASTINE

Indications: symptomatic relief of allergy such as hay fever, urticaria
Cautions: see notes above; pregnancy (Appendix 4) and breast-feeding (Appendix 5)
Contra-indications: see notes above; also avoid in renal impairment (Appendix 3); hypersensitivity to triprolidine
Side-effects: see notes above; incidence of sedation and antimuscarinic effects low
Dose: 8 mg 3 times daily; CHILD under 12 years, not recommended; ELDERLY not recommended

■ Preparations

Capsules can be sold to the public for the treatment of hay fever and allergic skin conditions in adults and children over 12 years provided packs do not contain over 10 days' supply (*Benadryl® Allergy Relief*)

CETIRIZINE HYDROCHLORIDE

Indications: symptomatic relief of allergy such as hay fever, urticaria
Cautions: see notes above
Contra-indications: see notes above; also pregnancy (Appendix 4) and breast-feeding (Appendix 5)
Side-effects: see notes above; incidence of sedation and antimuscarinic effects low
Dose: ADULT and CHILD over 6 years, 10 mg daily *or* 5 mg twice daily; CHILD 2–6 years, hay fever, 5 mg daily *or* 2.5 mg twice daily

Cetirizine (Non-proprietary)
Tablets, cetirizine hydrochloride 10 mg, net price 30-tab pack = £1.44. Counselling, driving
Oral solution, cetirizine hydrochloride 5 mg/5 mL, net price 200 mL = £8.63. Counselling, driving
Proprietary brands of cetirizine on sale to the public include *AllerTek®*, *Benadryl® One A Day*, *Piriteze® Allergy*, *Zirtek® Allergy*, *Zirtek® Allergy Relief*

DESLORATADINE

NOTE. Desloratadine is a metabolite of loratadine
Indications: symptomatic relief of allergy such as hay fever, urticaria
Cautions: see notes above
Contra-indications: see notes above; also hypersensitivity to loratadine; pregnancy (Appendix 4) and breast-feeding (Appendix 5)
Side-effects: see notes above; also fatigue; incidence of sedation and antimuscarinic effects low

Dose: ADULT and ADOLESCENT over 12 years, 5 mg daily; CHILD 1–5 years 1.25 mg daily, 6–11 years 2.5 mg daily

Neoclarityn® (Schering-Plough) ▼ PoM
Tablets, blue, f/c, desloratadine 5 mg, net price 30-tab pack = £7.04. Counselling, driving
Syrup, desloratadine 2.5 mg/5 mL, net price 100 mL (bubblegum-flavour) = £7.04. Counselling, driving

FEXOFENADINE HYDROCHLORIDE

NOTE. Fexofenadine is a metabolite of terfenadine
Indications: see under Dose
Cautions: see notes above; also pregnancy (Appendix 4)
Contra-indications: see notes above; also breast-feeding (Appendix 5)
Side-effects: see notes above; incidence of sedation and antimuscarinic effects low
Dose: seasonal allergic rhinitis, 120 mg once daily; CHILD 6–11 years, 30 mg twice daily
Chronic idiopathic urticaria, 180 mg once daily; CHILD under 12 years, not recommended

Telfast® (Aventis Pharma) PoM
Tablets, f/c, peach, fexofenadine hydrochloride 30 mg, net price 60-tab pack = £5.68; 120 mg, 30-tab pack = £6.23; 180 mg, 30-tab pack = £7.89. Counselling, driving

LEVOCETIRIZINE HYDROCHLORIDE

NOTE. Levocetirizine is an isomer of cetirizine
Indications: symptomatic relief of allergy such as hay fever, urticaria
Cautions: see notes above; also pregnancy (Appendix 4) and breast-feeding (Appendix 5)
Contra-indications: see notes above; also severe renal impairment
Side-effects: see notes above; incidence of sedation and antimuscarinic effects low
Dose: ADULT and CHILD over 6 years, 5 mg daily

Xyzal® (UCB Pharma) ▼ PoM
Tablets, f/c, levocetirizine hydrochloride 5 mg, net price 30-tab pack = £7.45. Counselling, driving

LORATADINE

Indications: symptomatic relief of allergy such as hay fever, urticaria
Cautions: see notes above
Contra-indications: see notes above; also pregnancy (Appendix 4) and breast-feeding (Appendix 5)
Side-effects: see notes above; incidence of sedation and antimuscarinic effects low
Dose: ADULT and CHILD over 6 years 10 mg daily; CHILD 2–5 years 5 mg daily

Loratadine (Non-proprietary)
Tablets, loratadine 10 mg, net price 30-tab pack = £2.45
Syrup, loratadine 5 mg/5 mL, net price 100 mL = £7.57. Counselling, driving
Proprietary brands of loratadine on sale to the public include *Boots Hayfever and Allergy Relief All Day*®, *Boots Hayfever and Allergy Relief Fast Melting Tablets*®, and *Clarityn Allergy*® NHS

MIZOLASTINE

Indications: symptomatic relief of allergy such as hay fever, urticaria
Cautions: see notes above
Contra-indications: see notes above; also susceptibility to QT-interval prolongation (including cardiac disease and hypokalaemia); significant hepatic impairment; pregnancy (Appendix 4) and breast-feeding (Appendix 5)
Side-effects: see notes above; also may cause weight gain; incidence of sedation and antimuscarinic effects low
Dose: 10 mg daily; CHILD under 12 years, not recommended

Mizollen® (Schwarz) PoM
Tablets, m/r, f/c, scored, mizolastine 10 mg, net price 30-tab pack = £5.77. Label: 25, Counselling, driving

TERFENADINE

Indications: symptomatic relief of allergy such as allergic rhinitis, urticaria
Cautions: see notes above
Contra-indications: see notes above; avoid grapefruit juice (may inhibit metabolism of terfenadine); **important:** see also Arrhythmias, below; also pregnancy (Appendix 4) and breast-feeding (Appendix 5)
ARRHYTHMIAS. Rare hazardous arrhythmias are associated with terfenadine particularly in association with increased terfenadine blood concentration. Recommendations include:

- not to exceed recommended dose
- avoid in significant hepatic impairment
- avoid in hypokalaemia (or other electrolyte imbalance)
- avoid in known or suspected prolonged QT interval
- avoid concomitant administration of drugs that prolong the QT interval or inhibit the metabolism of terfenadine, or those liable to produce electrolyte imbalance or are potentially arrhythmogenic; for details, see **interactions**: Appendix 1 (antihistamines)
- discontinue if syncope occurs and evaluate for potential arrhythmias

Side-effects: see notes above; incidence of sedation and antimuscarinic effects low; erythema multiforme and galactorrhoea reported; **important:** ventricular arrhythmias (including torsades de pointes) have followed excessive dosage, see also Arrhythmias above
Dose: allergic rhinitis and conjunctivitis, ADULT and CHILD over 50 kg, 60 mg daily increased if necessary to 120 mg daily in single or 2 divided doses
Allergic skin disorders, ADULT and CHILD over 50 kg, 120 mg daily in single or 2 divided doses

Terfenadine (Non-proprietary) PoM
Tablets, terfenadine 60 mg, net price 60-tab pack = £2.44. Counselling, driving
NOTE. May be difficult to obtain

Sedating antihistamines

DRIVING. Drowsiness may affect performance of skilled tasks (e.g. driving); sedating effects enhanced by alcohol.

ALIMEMAZINE TARTRATE

(Trimeprazine tartrate)

Indications: urticaria and pruritus, premedication

Cautions: see notes above; also pregnancy (Appendix 4); see also section 4.2.1

Contra-indications: see notes above; also breast-feeding (Appendix 5); see also section 4.2.1

Side-effects: see notes above; see also section 4.2.1

Dose: urticaria and pruritus, 10 mg 2–3 times daily, in severe cases up to max. 100 mg daily has been used; ELDERLY 10 mg 1–2 times daily; CHILD over 2 years 2.5–5 mg 3–4 times daily

Premedication, CHILD 2–7 years up to 2 mg/kg 1–2 hours before operation

Vallergan® (Castlemead) PoM

Tablets, blue, f/c, alimemazine tartrate 10 mg, net price 28-tab pack = £3.01. Label: 2

Syrup, straw-coloured, alimemazine tartrate 7.5 mg /5 mL, net price 100 mL = £3.44. Label: 2

Syrup forte, alimemazine tartrate 30 mg/5 mL, net price 100 mL = £5.32. Label: 2

CHLORPHENAMINE MALEATE

(Chlorpheniramine maleate)

Indications: symptomatic relief of allergy such as hay fever, urticaria; emergency treatment of anaphylactic reactions (section 3.4.3)

Cautions: see notes above; also pregnancy (Appendix 4) and breast-feeding (Appendix 5)

Contra-indications: see notes above

Side-effects: see notes above; also exfoliative dermatitis and tinnitus reported; injections may cause transient hypotension or CNS stimulation and may be irritant

Dose: *by mouth*, 4 mg every 4–6 hours, max. 24 mg daily; INFANT under 1 year not recommended, 1–2 years 1 mg twice daily; CHILD 2–5 years 1 mg every 4–6 hours, max. 6 mg daily; 6–12 years 2 mg every 4–6 hours, max. 12 mg daily

By subcutaneous or intramuscular injection or by intravenous injection over 1 minute, 10–20 mg; max. 40 mg in 24 hours; INFANT 1 month–1 year 250 micrograms/kg; CHILD 1–12 years 200 micrograms/kg *or* 1–5 years 2.5–5 mg, 6–12 years 5–10 mg

Chlorphenamine (Non-proprietary)

Tablets, chlorphenamine maleate 4 mg, net price 28 = £1.48. Label: 2

DENTAL PRESCRIBING ON NHS. Chlorphenamine tablets may be prescribed

Oral solution, chlorphenamine maleate 2 mg/5 mL, net price 150 mL = £2.28. Label: 2

Injection PoM[1], chlorphenamine maleate 10 mg/mL, net price 1-mL amp = £1.62

1. PoM restriction does not apply where administration is for saving life in emergency

Piriton® (GSK Consumer Healthcare)

Tablets, yellow, scored, chlorphenamine maleate 4 mg, net price 20 = 19p. Label: 2

Syrup, chlorphenamine maleate 2 mg/5 mL, net price 150 mL = £2.28. Label: 2

NOTE. In addition to *Piriton Allergy*® NHS, proprietary brands of chlorphenamine maleate tablets on sale to the public include *Allerief*®, *Boots Allergy Relief Antihistamine Tablets*, *Calimal*®

For a list of **cough and decongestant preparations on sale to the public**, including those containing chlorphenamine, see section 3.9.2

CLEMASTINE

Indications: symptomatic relief of allergy such as hay fever, urticaria

Cautions: see notes above; also pregnancy (Appendix 4) and breast-feeding (Appendix 5)

Contra-indications: see notes above

Side-effects: see notes above

Dose: 1 mg twice daily, increased up to 6 mg daily if required; INFANT under 1 year not recommended, CHILD 1–3 years 250–500 micrograms twice daily; 3–6 years 500 micrograms twice daily; 6–12 years 0.5–1 mg twice daily

Tavegil® (Novartis Consumer Health)

Tablets, scored, clemastine (as hydrogen fumarate) 1 mg. Net price 60-tab pack = £2.35. Label: 2

CYPROHEPTADINE HYDROCHLORIDE

Indications: symptomatic relief of allergy such as hay fever, urticaria; migraine (section 4.7.4.2)

Cautions: see notes above; also pregnancy (Appendix 4) and breast-feeding (Appendix 5)

Contra-indications: see notes above

Side-effects: see notes above

Dose: allergy, usual dose 4 mg 3–4 times daily; usual range 4–20 mg daily, max. 32 mg daily; INFANT under 2 years not recommended, CHILD 2–6 years 2 mg 2–3 times daily, max. 12 mg daily; 7–14 years 4 mg 2–3 times daily, max. 16 mg daily

Migraine, 4 mg with a further 4 mg after 30 minutes if necessary; maintenance, 4 mg every 4–6 hours

Periactin® (MSD)

Tablets, scored, cyproheptadine hydrochloride 4 mg. Net price 30 = 86p. Label: 2

DIPHENHYDRAMINE HYDROCHLORIDE

Indications: see under Preparations

Cautions: see notes above

Contra-indications: see notes above

Side-effects: see notes above

■ Preparations

Proprietary brands of diphenhydramine hydrochloride on sale to the public to aid relief of temporary sleep disturbance in adults include:

Dreemon® (diphenhydramine hydrochloride 10 mg/5 mL, diphenhydramine hydrochloride tablets 25 mg), *Medinex*® (diphenhydramine hydrochloride 10 mg/5 mL), *Nightcalm*® (diphenhydramine hydrochloride tablets 25 mg), *Nytol*® NHS (diphenhydramine hydrochloride tablets 25 mg and 50 mg), and *Panadol Night*® (diphenhydramine hydrochloride 25 mg and paracetamol 500 mg, for relief of temporary sleeplessness and night-time pain)

For a list of **cough and decongestant preparations on sale to the public**, including those containing diphenhydramine, see section 3.9.2

DOXYLAMINE

Cautions: see notes above
Contra-indications: see notes above
Side-effects: see notes above

■ Preparations

Ingredient of **cough and decongestant preparations** (section 3.9.2) and of **compound analgesics** (section 4.7.1) on sale to the public

HYDROXYZINE HYDROCHLORIDE

Indications: pruritus, anxiety (short-term) (section 4.1.2)
Cautions: see notes above
Contra-indications: see notes above; also pregnancy (Appendix 4) and breast-feeding (Appendix 5)
Side-effects: see notes above
Dose: pruritus, initially 25 mg at night increased if necessary to 25 mg 3–4 times daily; CHILD 6 months–6 years initially 5–15 mg daily increased if necessary to 50 mg daily in divided doses; over 6 years initially 15–25 mg daily increased if necessary to 50–100 mg daily in divided doses
Anxiety (adults only), 50–100 mg 4 times daily

Atarax® (Pfizer) PoM
Tablets, both s/c, hydroxyzine hydrochloride 10 mg (orange), net price 84-tab pack = £1.82; 25 mg (green), 28-tab pack = £1.22. Label: 2

Ucerax® (UCB Pharma) PoM
Tablets NHS, f/c, scored, hydroxyzine hydrochloride 25 mg, net price 25-tab pack = 85p. Label: 2
Syrup, hydroxyzine hydrochloride 10 mg/5 mL. Net price 200-mL pack = £1.78. Label: 2

PROMETHAZINE HYDROCHLORIDE

Indications: symptomatic relief of allergy such as hay fever, urticaria; premedication; emergency treatment of anaphylactic reactions (section 3.4.3); sedation (section 4.1.1); motion sickness (section 4.6)
Cautions: see notes above; also pregnancy (Appendix 4) and breast-feeding (Appendix 5)
Contra-indications: see notes above
Side-effects: see notes above; intramuscular injection may be painful
Dose: *by mouth*, 25 mg at night increased to 25 mg twice daily if necessary *or* 10–20 mg 2–3 times daily; CHILD under 2 years not recommended, 2–5 years 5–15 mg daily in 1–2 divided doses, 5–10 years 10–25 mg daily in 1–2 divided doses
Premedication, CHILD under 2 years not recommended, 2–5 years 15–20 mg, 5–10 years 20–25 mg
By deep intramuscular injection, 25–50 mg; max. 100 mg; CHILD 5–10 years 6.25–12.5 mg
Premedication, 25–50 mg 1 hour before operation; CHILD 5–10 years, 6.25–12.5 mg
By slow intravenous injection in emergencies, 25–50 mg as a solution containing 2.5 mg/mL in water for injections; max. 100 mg

Phenergan® (Rhône-Poulenc Rorer)
Tablets, both blue, f/c, promethazine hydrochloride 10 mg, net price 56-tab pack = £1.71; 25 mg, 56-tab pack = £2.55. Label: 2
DENTAL PRESCRIBING ON NHS. May be prescribed as Promethazine Hydrochloride Tablets 10 mg or 25 mg
Elixir, sugar-free, golden, promethazine hydrochloride 5 mg/5 mL. Net price 100 mL = £1.49. Label: 2
DENTAL PRESCRIBING ON NHS. May be prescribed as Promethazine Hydrochloride Oral Solution 5 mg/5 mL
Injection PoM[1], promethazine hydrochloride 25 mg/mL. Net price 1-mL amp = 58p
Promethazine hydrochloride injection 25 mg/mL (1-mL and 2-mL ampoules) also available from Antigen
NOTE. Proprietary brands of promethazine hydrochloride on sale to the public include *Phenergan Nightime*® (promethazine hydrochloride tablets 25 mg, for occasional insomnia in adults), *Sominex*® NHS (promethazine hydrochloride tablets 20 mg, for occasional insomnia in adults)

For a list of **cough and decongestant preparations on sale to the public**, including those containing promethazine, see section 3.9.2

1. PoM restriction does not apply where administration is for saving life in emergency

TRIPROLIDINE HYDROCHLORIDE

Cautions: see notes above
Contra-indications: see notes above
Side-effects: see notes above

■ Preparations

For a list of **cough and decongestant preparations on sale to the public**, including those containing triprolidine, see section 3.9.2

3.4.2 Hyposensitisation

Except for wasp and bee sting allergy, specific hyposensitisation with allergen extract vaccines has usually shown little benefit in asthma. Hyposensitisation may be effective in allergic rhinitis if sensitisation to a particular allergen can be proven. However, the benefit of hyposensitisation needs to be balanced against the significant risk of anaphylaxis, particularly in patients with asthma (see CSM advice below).

Diagnostic skin tests alone are unreliable and should only be used in conjunction with a detailed history of allergen exposure.

CSM advice. After re-examination of the efficacy and safety of desensitising vaccines, the CSM has concluded that they should only be used for the following indications:

- Seasonal allergic hay fever (which has not responded to anti-allergy drugs) caused by pollens, using licensed products only—patients with *asthma* should not be treated with desensitising vaccines as they are more likely to develop severe adverse reactions.
- Hypersensitivity to wasp and bee venoms—since reactions can be life-threatening, *asthma* is not an absolute contra-indication.

There is inadequate evidence of benefit from desensitisation to other allergens such as house dust, house dust mite, animal danders and foods and desensitisation is **not** recommended. Desensitising vaccines should be avoided in pregnant women, in children under five years old, and in those taking beta-blockers.

Bronchospasm usually develops within 1 hour and anaphylaxis within 30 minutes of injection. Therefore patients need to be monitored for 1 hour after injection. If symptoms or signs of hypersensitivity develop (e.g. rash, urticaria, bronchospasm, faintness), **even when mild**, the patient should be observed until these have **resolved completely**.

For details of the management of anaphylactic shock, see section 3.4.3.

Each set of allergen extracts usually contains vials for the administration of graded amounts of allergen to patients undergoing hyposensitisation. Maintenance sets containing vials at the highest strength are also available. Product literature must be consulted for details of allergens, vial strengths, and administration

BEE AND WASP ALLERGEN EXTRACTS

Indications: hypersensitivity to wasp or bee venom (see notes above)

Cautions: see notes above including CSM advice and consult product literature

CSM advice. The CSM has advised that facilities for cardiopulmonary resuscitation must be immediately available and patients monitored closely for one hour after each injection, for full details see above.

Contra-indications: see notes above and consult product literature

Side-effects: consult product literature

Dose: *by subcutaneous injection*, consult product literature

Pharmalgen® (ALK-Abelló) PoM

Bee venom extract (*Apis mellifera*) or wasp venom extract (*Vespula* spp.). Net price initial treatment set = £59.77 (bee), £73.28 (wasp); maintenance treatment set = £69.54 (bee), £89.45 (wasp)

GRASS AND TREE POLLEN EXTRACTS

Indications: treatment of seasonal allergic hay fever due to grass or tree pollen in patients who have failed to respond to anti-allergy drugs (see notes above)

Cautions: see notes above including CSM advice and consult product literature

CSM advice. The CSM has advised that facilities for cardiopulmonary resuscitation must be immediately available and patients must be monitored closely for one hour after each injection, for full details see above.

Contra-indications: see notes above and consult product literature

Side-effects: consult product literature

Dose: *by subcutaneous injection*, consult product literature

Pollinex® (Allergy) PoM

Grass or tree pollen extract, net price initial treatment set (3 vials) = £170.00; extension course treatment (1 vial) = £150.00

3.4.3 Allergic emergencies

Adrenaline (**epinephrine**) provides physiological reversal of the immediate symptoms (such as laryngeal oedema, bronchospasm, and hypotension) associated with hypersensitivity reactions such as *anaphylaxis* and *angioedema*. See below for full details of adrenaline administration and for adjunctive treatment.

Anaphylaxis

Anaphylactic shock requires prompt energetic treatment of *laryngeal oedema, bronchospasm*, and *hypotension*. Atopic individuals are particularly susceptible. Insect stings are a recognised risk (in particular wasp and bee stings). Certain foods, including eggs, fish, cow's milk protein, peanuts, and nuts may also precipitate anaphylaxis. Medicinal products particularly associated with anaphylaxis include blood products, vaccines, hyposensitising (allergen) preparations, antibacterials, aspirin and other NSAIDs, heparin, and neuromuscular blocking drugs. In the case of drugs, anaphylaxis is more likely after parenteral administration; resuscitation facilities must always be available for injections associated with special risk. Anaphylactic reactions may also be associated with *additives and excipients* in foods and medicines. Refined arachis (peanut) oil, which may be present in some medicinal products, is unlikely to cause an allergic reaction—nevertheless it is wise to check the full formula of preparations which may contain allergenic fats or oils.

First-line treatment includes securing the airway, restoration of blood pressure (laying the patient flat, raising the feet), and administration of **adrenaline** (epinephrine) injection. This is given **intramuscularly** in a dose of 500 micrograms (0.5 mL adrenaline injection 1 in 1000); a dose of 300 micrograms (0.3 mL adrenaline injection 1 in 1000) may be appropriate for *immediate self-administration*. The dose is repeated if necessary at 5-minute intervals according to blood pressure, pulse and respiratory function (important: possible need for *intravenous route* using *dilute solution*, see below). **Oxygen** administration is also of primary importance. An antihistamine (e.g. **chlorphenamine** (chlorphenir-amine), given by slow intravenous injection in a dose of 10–20 mg, see p. 162) is a useful adjunctive treatment, given after adrenaline injection and continued for 24 to 48 hours to prevent relapse. Patients receiving beta-blockers or those receiving anti-depressants require special consideration (see under Adrenaline, p. 165).

Continuing deterioration requires further treatment including intravenous fluids (section 9.2.2), intravenous aminophylline (see p. 149) or a nebulised $beta_2$ agonist (such as salbutamol or terbutaline, see p. 144 and p. 145); in addition to oxygen, assisted respiration and possibly emergency tracheotomy may be necessary.

An intravenous corticosteroid e.g. **hydrocortisone** (as sodium succinate) in a dose of 100–300 mg (section 6.3.2) is of secondary value in the initial management of anaphylactic shock because the onset of action is delayed for several hours, but should be given to prevent further deterioration in severely affected patients.

When a patient is so ill that there is doubt as to the adequacy of the circulation, the initial injection of adrenaline may need to be given as a *dilute solution by the intravenous route*, for details of cautions, dose and strength, see under Intravenous Adrenaline (Epinephrine), below.

Some patients with severe allergy to insect stings or foods are encouraged to carry prefilled adrenaline syringes for *self-administration* during periods of risk.

For advice on the management of medical emergencies in dental practice, see p. 20.

Angioedema

Angioedema is dangerous if *laryngeal oedema* is present. In this circumstance adrenaline (epinephrine) injection and oxygen should be given as described under Anaphylaxis (see above); antihistamines and corticosteroids should also be given (see again above). Tracheal intubation and other measures may be necessary.

The administration of C_1 esterase inhibitor (in fresh frozen plasma or in partially purified form) may terminate acute attacks of *hereditary angioedema*, but is not practical for long-term prophylaxis. **Tranexamic acid** (section 2.11) and **danazol** (section 6.7.2) [unlicensed indication] are used for long-term prophylaxis of hereditary angiodema.

Intramuscular adrenaline (epinephrine)

The *intramuscular route* is the *first choice route* for the administration of adrenaline (epinephrine) in the management of anaphylactic shock. Adrenaline has a rapid onset of action after intramuscular administration and in the shocked patient its absorption from the intramuscular site is faster and more reliable than from the subcutaneous site (the intravenous route should be reserved for extreme emergency when there is doubt about the adequacy of the circulation; for details of cautions, dose and strength see under Intravenous Adrenaline (Epinephrine), below).

Patients with severe allergy should ideally be instructed in the self-administration of adrenaline by intramuscular injection (for details see under Self-administration of Adrenaline (Epinephrine), below).

Prompt injection of adrenaline is of paramount importance. The following adrenaline doses are based on the revised recommendations of the Project Team of the Resuscitation Council (UK).

Dose of **intramuscular** injection of adrenaline (epinephrine) for anaphylactic shock. Subcutaneous injection **not** generally recommended.

Age	Dose	Volume of adrenaline **1 in 1000** (1 mg/mL)
Under 6 months	50 micrograms	0.05 mL[1]
6 months–6 years	120 micrograms	0.12 mL[1]
6–12 years	250 micrograms	0.25 mL
Adult and adolescent	500 micrograms	0.5 mL

These doses may be repeated several times if necessary at 5-minute intervals according to blood pressure, pulse and respiratory function.

1. Use suitable syringe for measuring small volume

Intravenous adrenaline (epinephrine)

Where the patient is severely ill and there is real doubt about adequacy of the circulation and absorption from the intramuscular injection site, adrenaline (epinephrine) may be given by **slow** *intravenous injection* in a dose of 500 micrograms (5 mL of the dilute 1 in 10 000 adrenaline injection) given at a rate of 100 micrograms (1 mL of the dilute 1 in 10 000 adrenaline injection) per minute, *stopping when a response has been obtained*; children can be given a dose of 10 micrograms/kg (0.1 mL/kg of the dilute 1 in 10 000 adrenaline injection) by **slow** *intravenous injection* over several minutes. Great vigilance is needed to ensure that the *correct strength* is used; anaphylactic shock kits need to make a *very clear distinction* between the 1 in 10 000 strength and the 1 in 1000 strength. It is also important that, where intramuscular injection might still succeed, time should not be wasted seeking intravenous access.

For reference to the use of the intravenous route for *cardiac resuscitation*, see section 2.7.3.

Self-administration of adrenaline (epinephrine)

Individuals at considerable risk of anaphylaxis need to carry adrenaline (epinephrine) at all times and need to be *instructed in advance* how to inject it. In addition, the packs need to be labelled so that in the case of rapid collapse someone else is able to administer the adrenaline. It is important to ensure that an adequate supply is provided to treat symptoms until medical assistance is available.

Some patients may best cope with a pre-assembled syringe fitted with a needle suitable for very rapid administration (if necessary by a bystander). *Anapen*® and *EpiPen*® consist of a fully assembled syringe and needle delivering a dose of 300 micrograms of adrenaline by *intramuscular injection*; 150-microgram versions (*Anapen*® *Junior*, *EpiPen*® *Jr*) are also available for use in children. Other products for the immediate treatment of anaphylaxis are available but are not licensed for use in the UK. *Ana-Guard*® is a prefilled syringe that delivers two 300-microgram doses of adrenaline *by subcutaneous or intramuscular injection*; it can be adjusted to administer smaller doses for children. *Ana-Kit*® includes a prefilled adrenaline syringe, chewable tablets of chlorphenamine maleate (chlorpheniramine maleate) 2 mg, 2 sterile pads impregnated with 70% isopropyl alcohol, and a tourniquet. *Ana-Guard*® and *Ana-Kit*® are available on a named-patient basis from IDIS.

ADRENALINE/EPINEPHRINE

Indications: emergency treatment of acute anaphylaxis; angioedema; cardiopulmonary resuscitation (section 2.7.3); priapism [unlicensed indication] (section 7.4.5)

Cautions: hyperthyroidism, diabetes mellitus, heart disease, hypertension, arrhythmias, cerebrovascular disease, angle-closure glaucoma, second stage of labour, elderly patients

INTERACTIONS. Severe anaphylaxis in patients on non-cardioselective beta-blockers may not respond to adrenaline injection calling for intravenous injection of salbutamol (see p. 144); furthermore, adrenaline may cause severe hypertension in those receiving beta-blockers. Patients on tricyclic antidepressants are considerably more susceptible to arrhythmias, calling for a much reduced dose of adrenaline. Other **interactions**, see Appendix 1 (sympathomimetics).

Side-effects: anxiety, tremor, tachycardia, arrhythmias, headache, cold extremities; also hypertension (risk of cerebral haemorrhage) and pulmonary oedema (on excessive dosage or extreme sensitivity); nausea, vomiting, sweating, weakness, dizziness and hyperglycaemia also reported

Dose: acute anaphylaxis, *by intramuscular injection* (preferably midpoint in anterolateral thigh) (*or by subcutaneous injection*) of 1 in 1000 (1 mg/mL) solution, see notes and table above

Acute anaphylaxis when there is doubt as to the adequacy of the circulation, *by slow intravenous injection* of 1 in 10 000 (100 micrograms/mL) solution (extreme caution), see notes above

IMPORTANT. Intravenous route should be used with **extreme care**, see notes above

■ Intramuscular or subcutaneous

[1]**Adrenaline/Epinephrine 1 in 1000** (Non-proprietary) PoM
Injection, adrenaline (as acid tartrate) 1 mg/mL, net price 0.5-mL amp = 51p; 1-mL amp = 42p
Excipients: include sulphites

[1]**Minijet® Adrenaline** (Celltech) PoM
Injection, adrenaline (as hydrochloride) 1 in 1000 (1 mg/mL). Net price 1 mL (with 25 gauge × 0.25 inch needle for subcutaneous injection) = £8.11, 1 mL (with 21 gauge × 1.5 inch needle for intramuscular injection) = £5.00 (both disposable syringes)
Excipients: include sulphites

■ Intravenous

Extreme caution, see notes above

Adrenaline/Epinephrine 1 in 10 000, Dilute (Non-proprietary) PoM
Injection, adrenaline (as acid tartrate) 100 micrograms/mL, 10-mL amp, 1-mL and 10-mL pre-filled syringe
Excipients: include sulphites
Brands include *Minijet® Adrenaline*

■ Intramuscular injection for self-administration

Anapen® (Celltech) PoM
[1]*Anapen® 0.3 mg solution for injection* (delivering a single dose of adrenaline 300 micrograms), adrenaline 1 mg/mL (1 in 1000), net price 1.05-mL auto-injector device = £30.67
Excipients: include sulphites
NOTE. 0.75 mL of the solution remains in the auto-injector device after use
Dose: by intramuscular injection, ADULT and CHILD over 30 kg, 300 micrograms repeated after 10–15 minutes as necessary

Anapen® Junior 0.15 mg solution for injection (delivering a single dose of adrenaline 150 micrograms), adrenaline 500 micrograms/mL (1 in 2000), net price 1.05-mL auto-injector device = £30.67
Excipients: include sulphites
NOTE. 0.75 mL of the solution remains in the auto-injector device after use
Dose: by intramuscular injection, CHILD 15–30 kg, 150 micrograms repeated after 10–15 minutes as necessary

EpiPen® (ALK-Abelló) PoM
[1]*EpiPen® Auto-injector 0.3 mg* (delivering a single dose of adrenaline 300 micrograms), adrenaline 1 mg/mL (1 in 1000), net price 2-mL auto-injector = £28.05
Excipients: include sulphites
NOTE. 1.7 mL of the solution remains in the *Auto-injector* after use
Dose: by intramuscular injection, ADULT and CHILD over 30 kg, 300 micrograms repeated after 15 minutes as necessary

Epipen® Jr Auto-injector 0.15 mg (delivering a single dose of adrenaline 150 micrograms), adrenaline 500 micrograms/mL (1 in 2000), net price 2-mL auto-injector = £28.05
Excipients: include sulphites
NOTE. 1.7 mL of the solution remains in the *Auto-injector* after use
Dose: by intramuscular injection, CHILD 15–30 kg, 150 micrograms (but on the basis of a dose of 10 micrograms/kg, 300 micrograms may be more appropriate for some children) repeated after 15 minutes as necessary

1. PoM restriction does not apply to adrenaline injection 1 mg/mL where administration is for saving life in emergency

3.5 Respiratory stimulants and pulmonary surfactants

3.5.1 Respiratory stimulants

Respiratory stimulants (analeptic drugs) have a limited place in the treatment of ventilatory failure in patients with chronic obstructive pulmonary disease. They are effective only when given by intravenous injection or infusion and have a short duration of action. Their use has largely been replaced by ventilatory support including nasal intermittent positive pressure ventilation. However, occasionally when ventilatory support is contra-indicated and in patients with hypercapnic respiratory failure who are becoming drowsy or comatose, respiratory stimulants in the short term may arouse patients sufficiently to co-operate and clear their secretions.

Respiratory stimulants can also be harmful in respiratory failure since they stimulate non-respiratory as well as respiratory muscles. They should only be given under **expert supervision** in hospital and must be combined with active physiotherapy. There is at present no oral respiratory stimulant available for long-term use in chronic respiratory failure.

Doxapram is given by continuous intravenous infusion. Frequent arterial blood gas and pH measurements are necessary during treatment to ensure correct dosage.

DOXAPRAM HYDROCHLORIDE

Indications: see under Dose

Cautions: give with oxygen in severe irreversible airways obstruction or severely decreased lung compliance (because of increased work load of breathing); give with $beta_2$ agonist in bronchoconstriction; hypertension (avoid if severe), impaired cardiac reserve; hepatic impairment, pregnancy (compelling reasons only); **interactions:** Appendix 1 (doxapram)

Contra-indications: severe hypertension, status asthmaticus, coronary artery disease, thyrotoxicosis, epilepsy, physical obstruction of respiratory tract

Side-effects: perineal warmth, dizziness, sweating, moderate increase in blood pressure and heart rate; side-effects reported in postoperative period (causal effect not established) include muscle fasciculation, hyperactivity, confusion, hallucinations, cough, dyspnoea, laryngospasm, bronchospasm, sinus tachycardia, bradycardia, extrasystoles, nausea, vomiting and salivation

Dose: postoperative respiratory depression, *by intravenous injection* over at least 30 seconds, 1–1.5 mg/kg repeated if necessary after intervals of 1 hour *or* alternatively *by intravenous infusion*, 2–3 mg/minute adjusted according to response; CHILD not recommended

Acute respiratory failure, *by intravenous infusion*, 1.5–4 mg/minute adjusted according to response (given concurrently with oxygen and whenever possible monitor with frequent measurement of blood gas tensions); CHILD not recommended

Dopram® (Anpharm) PoM

Injection, doxapram hydrochloride 20 mg/mL. Net price 5-mL amp = £2.24

Intravenous infusion, doxapram hydrochloride 2 mg/mL in glucose 5%. Net price 500-mL bottle = £21.33

3.5.2 Pulmonary surfactants

Pulmonary surfactants are used in the management of respiratory distress syndrome (hyaline membrane disease) in neonates and preterm neonates. They may also be given prophylactically to those considered at risk of developing the syndrome.

CAUTIONS. Continuous monitoring is required to avoid hyperoxaemia (due to rapid improvement in arterial oxygen concentration).

SIDE-EFFECTS. Pulmonary haemorrhage, especially in more preterm neonates, is a rare complication of therapy; obstruction of the endotracheal tube by mucous secretions has also been reported.

BERACTANT

Indications: treatment of respiratory distress syndrome in neonates over 700 g; prophylaxis of respiratory distress syndrome in preterm neonates

Cautions: see notes above

Side-effects: see notes above

Dose: *by endotracheal tube*, phospholipid 100 mg/kg equivalent to a volume of 4 mL/kg, preferably within 8 hours of birth; may be repeated within 48 hours at intervals of at least 6 hours for up to 4 doses

Survanta® (Abbott) PoM

Suspension, beractant (bovine lung extract) providing phospholipid 25 mg/mL, with lipids and proteins, net price 8-mL vial = £306.43

PORACTANT ALFA

Indications: treatment of respiratory distress syndrome or hyaline membrane disease in neonates over 700 g; prophylaxis of respiratory distress syndrome in preterm neonates

Cautions: see notes above

Side-effects: see notes above

Dose: *by endotracheal tube*, treatment, 100–200 mg/kg; further doses of 100 mg/kg may be repeated 12 hours later and after further 12 hours if still intubated; max. total dose 300–400 mg/kg; prophylaxis, 100–200 mg/kg soon after birth (preferably within 15 minutes); further doses of 100 mg/kg may be repeated 6–12 hours later and after further 12 hours if still intubated; max. total dose 300–400 mg/kg

Curosurf® (Trinity) PoM

Suspension, poractant alfa (porcine lung phospholipid fraction) 80 mg/mL, net price 1.5-mL vial = £382.00; 3-mL vial = £764.00

3.6 Oxygen

Oxygen should be regarded as a drug. It is prescribed for hypoxaemic patients to increase alveolar oxygen tension and decrease the work of breathing necessary to maintain a given arterial oxygen tension. The concentration depends on the condition being treated; an inappropriate concentration may have serious or even lethal effects.

High concentration oxygen therapy, with concentrations of up to 60%, is safe in conditions such as pneumonia, pulmonary thromboembolism, and fibrosing alveolitis. In such conditions low arterial oxygen (P_aO_2) is usually associated with low or normal arterial carbon dioxide (P_aCO_2), therefore there is little risk of hypoventilation and carbon dioxide retention.

In acute severe asthma, the arterial carbon dioxide (P_aCO_2) is usually subnormal but as asthma deteriorates it may rise steeply (particularly in children). These patients usually require high concentrations of oxygen and if the arterial carbon dioxide (P_aCO_2) remains high despite other treatment intermittent positive pressure ventilation needs to be considered urgently. Where facilities for blood gas measurement are not immediately available, for example while transferring the patient to hospital, 40 to 60% oxygen delivered through a high-flow mask is recommended.

Low concentration oxygen therapy (controlled oxygen therapy) is reserved for patients with ventilatory failure due to chronic obstructive pulmonary disease or other causes. The concentration should not exceed 28% and in some patients a concentration above 24% may be excessive. The aim is to provide the patient with enough oxygen to correct hypoxaemia but without worsening existing carbon dioxide retention and respiratory acidosis. Treatment should be initiated in hospital because repeated blood gas measurements are required to assess the correct concentration.

DOMICILIARY OXYGEN. Oxygen should only be prescribed for patients in the home after careful evaluation in hospital by respiratory experts; it should never be prescribed on a placebo basis.

Patients should be **advised of the fire risks** when receiving oxygen therapy.

AIR TRAVEL. Some patients with arterial hypoxaemia will require supplementary oxygen for air travel. The patient's requirement should be discussed with the airline before travel.

Intermittent oxygen therapy

Oxygen is occasionally prescribed for intermittent use for episodes of hypoxaemia of short duration, for example asthma. It is important, however, that the patient does not rely on oxygen instead of obtaining medical help or taking more specific treatment.

Alternatively, intermittent oxygen may be prescribed for patients with advanced irreversible respiratory disorders to increase mobility and capacity for exercise and to ease discomfort, for example in chronic obstructive pulmonary disease. Appropriate patients may be prescribed portable equipment through the hospital service, refillable from cylinders in the home.

Under the NHS oxygen may be supplied by pharmacy contractors as **oxygen cylinders**. Oxygen flow can be adjusted as the cylinders are equipped with an oxygen flow meter with 'medium' (2 litres/minute) and 'high' (4 litres/minute) settings. The Health Authorities have lists of pharmacy contractors who provide domiciliary oxygen services.

Patients are supplied with either constant or variable performance masks. The *Intersurgical 010 28%* or *Ventimask Mk IV 28%* are constant performance masks and provide a nearly constant supply of oxygen (28%) despite variations in oxygen flow rate and the patient's breathing pattern. The variable performance masks include the *Intersurgical 005 Mask* and the *Venticaire Mask*; the concentration of oxygen supplied to the patient varies with the rate of flow of oxygen and with the patient's breathing pattern. If a mask which provides 24% oxygen is required, it may be ordered from BOC Medical.

Giving oxygen by nasal cannula allows the patient to talk and eat but the concentration is not controlled and the method may not be appropriate for acute respiratory failure. When given through a nasal cannula at a rate of 1–2 litres/minute the inspiratory oxygen concentration is usually low, but it varies with ventilation and can be high if the patient is underventilating.

PORTABLE OXYGEN CYLINDERS. Medigas and BOC supply a portable oxygen cylinder called 'PD oxygen cylinder', which has the same bull-nose fitting as the normal domiciliary headsets (prescriptions must therefore specify 'PD oxygen cylinder'). The PD oxygen cylinder holds 300 litres of oxygen which will last approximately 2 hours at a standard flow rate of 2 litres/minute.

Long-term oxygen therapy

Long-term administration of oxygen (at least 15 hours daily) prolongs survival in some patients with chronic obstructive pulmonary disease.

The Royal College of Physicians has produced guidelines for oxygen therapy (*Domiciliary oxygen therapy services: Clinical guidelines and advice for prescribers*; June 1999). Assessment for long-term oxygen therapy requires measurement of arterial blood gas tensions. Measurements should be taken on 2 occasions at least 3 weeks apart to demonstrate clinical stability, and not sooner than 4 weeks after an acute exacerbation of the disease. The guidelines recommend that long-term oxygen therapy should be considered for patients with:

- chronic obstructive pulmonary disease with $P_aO_2 < 7.3$ kPa when breathing air during a period of clinical stability;
- chronic obstructive pulmonary disease with P_aO_2 7.3–8 kPa in the presence of secondary polycythaemia, nocturnal hypoxaemia, peripheral oedema or evidence of pulmonary hypertension;
- interstitial lung disease with $P_aO_2 < 8$ kPa and in patients with $P_aO_2 > 8$ kPa with disabling dyspnoea;
- cystic fibrosis when $P_aO_2 < 7.3$ kPa *or* if P_aO_2 7.3–8 kPa in the presence of secondary polycythaemia, nocturnal hypoxaemia, pulmonary hypertension or peripheral oedema;
- pulmonary hypertension, without parenchymal lung involvement when $P_aO_2 < 8$ kPa;
- neuromuscular or skeletal disorders, after specialist assessment;
- obstructive sleep apnoea despite continuous positive airways pressure therapy, after specialist assessment;
- pulmonary malignancy or other terminal disease with disabling dyspnoea;
- heart failure with daytime $P_aO_2 < 7.3$ kPa (on air) or with nocturnal hypoxaemia;
- paediatric respiratory disease, after specialist assessment.

Increased respiratory depression is seldom a problem in patients with stable respiratory failure treated with low concentrations of oxygen although it may occur during exacerbations; patients and relatives should be warned to call for medical help if drowsiness or confusion occur.

Oxygen concentrators are more economical for patients requiring oxygen for long periods, and in England and Wales are prescribable on the NHS on a regional tendering basis (see below). A concentrator is recommended for a patient requiring oxygen for more than 8 hours a day (or 21 cylinders per month). Exceptionally, if a higher concentration of oxygen is required the output of 2 oxygen concentrators can be combined using a 'Y' connection.

A nasal cannula is usually preferred for long-term oxygen therapy from an oxygen concentrator. It can, however, produce dermatitis and mucosal drying in sensitive individuals. Nasal cannulas are supplied with oxygen concentrators but they are not prescribable on the NHS.

Prescribing arrangements for oxygen concentrators

Oxygen concentrators and accessories (face mask, nasal cannula, and humidifier) should be prescribed on form FP10 or form WP10 in Wales and the amount of oxygen required (hours per day) and flow rate specified. If required, a back-up oxygen set and cylinder can be prescribed at the same time. The patient should be informed that the supplier will be in contact to make arrangements and that the prescription form is to be given to the person who installs the concentrator.

The prescriber should contact the supplier by telephone (see table below) who will send written confirmation of the order to the prescriber, the patient, and the Primary Care Trust or the Health Authority. The same procedure should be followed for a back-up oxygen set and cylinder if required.

Primary Care Trust or Health Authority regional group	Supplier
South Western London South (includes Kent, Surrey, and Sussex)	BOC Medical *to order*: Dial 0800 136 603
Eastern London North North Western and North Wales West Midlands	De Vilbiss Medequip Ltd *to order*: Dial 0800 020 202
Central and South Wales Northern Yorkshire (South and West) and Humberside	Air Products *to order*: Dial 0800 373 580

In **Scotland** refer the patient for assessment by a respiratory consultant. If the need for a concentrator is confirmed the consultant will arrange for the provision of a concentrator through the Common Services Agency.

3.7 Mucolytics

Mucolytics are sometimes prescribed to facilitate expectoration by reducing sputum viscosity. Mucolytics reduce exacerbations in patients with chronic obstructive pulmonary disease and a chronic productive cough. Steam inhalation with postural drainage is effective in bronchiectasis and in some cases of chronic bronchitis.

Mucolytics should be used with caution in those with a history of peptic ulceration because they may disrupt the gastric mucosal barrier.

For reference to dornase alfa, see below.

CARBOCISTEINE

Indications: reduction of sputum viscosity
Cautions: see notes above
Contra-indications: active peptic ulceration
Side-effects: occasional gastro-intestinal irritation, rashes
Dose: initially 750 mg 3 times daily, then 1.5 g daily in divided doses as condition improves; CHILD 2–5 years 62.5–125 mg 4 times daily, 6–12 years 250 mg 3 times daily

Carbocisteine (Beacon) PoM
Capsules, carbocisteine 375 mg. Net price 30-cap pack = £4.17
Brands include *Mucodyne*®
Oral liquid, carbocisteine 125 mg/5 mL, net price 300 mL = £4.57; 250 mg/5 mL, 300 mL = £5.84
Brands include *Mucodyne*® *Paediatric* 125 mg/5 mL and *Mucodyne*® 250 mg/5 mL

MECYSTEINE HYDROCHLORIDE

(Methyl Cysteine Hydrochloride)
Indications: reduction of sputum viscosity
Cautions: see notes above
Dose: 200 mg 4 times daily for 2 days, then 200 mg 3 times daily for 6 weeks, then 200 mg twice daily; CHILD over 5 years 100 mg 3 times daily

Visclair® (Sinclair)
Tablets, yellow, s/c, e/c, mecysteine hydrochloride 100 mg. Net price 20 = £3.66. Label: 5, 22, 25

Dornase alfa

Dornase alfa is a genetically engineered version of a naturally occurring human enzyme which cleaves extracellular deoxyribonucleic acid (DNA). It is used in cystic fibrosis and is administered by inhalation using a jet nebuliser (section 3.1.5).

DORNASE ALFA

Phosphorylated glycosylated recombinant human deoxyribonuclease 1 (rhDNase)
Indications: management of cystic fibrosis patients with a forced vital capacity (FVC) of greater than 40% of predicted to improve pulmonary function
Cautions: pregnancy (Appendix 4); breast-feeding (Appendix 5)
Side-effects: pharyngitis, voice changes, chest pain; occasionally laryngitis, rashes, urticaria, conjunctivitis
Dose: *by inhalation of nebulised solution* (by jet nebuliser), 2500 units (2.5 mg) once daily (patients over 21 years may benefit from twice daily dosage); CHILD under 5 years not recommended

Pulmozyme® (Roche) PoM
Nebuliser solution, dornase alfa 1000 units (1 mg)/mL. Net price 2.5-mL (2500 units) vial = £18.52
NOTE. For use undiluted with jet nebulisers only; ultrasonic nebulisers are unsuitable

3.8 Aromatic inhalations

Inhalations containing volatile substances such as eucalyptus oil are traditionally used and although the vapour may contain little of the additive it encourages deliberate inspiration of warm moist air which is often comforting in bronchitis; boiling water should not be used owing to the risk of scalding. Inhalations are also used for the relief of nasal obstruction in acute rhinitis or sinusitis. Menthol and eucalyptus inhalation is used to relieve sinusitis affecting the maxillary antrum (section 12.2.2)

CHILDREN. The use of strong aromatic decongestants (applied as rubs or to pillows) is not advised for infants under the age of 3 months. Carers of young infants in whom nasal obstruction with mucus is a problem can readily be taught appropriate techniques of suction aspiration but sodium chloride 0.9% given as nasal drops is preferred.

Benzoin Tincture, Compound, BP
(Friars' Balsam)
Tincture, balsamic acids approx. 4.5%. Label: 15
Dose: add one teaspoonful to a pint of hot, **not** boiling, water and inhale the vapour

Menthol and Eucalyptus Inhalation, BP 1980
Inhalation, racementhol or levomenthol 2 g, eucalyptus oil 10 mL, light magnesium carbonate 7 g, water to 100 mL
Dose: add one teaspoonful to a pint of hot, **not** boiling, water and inhale the vapour
DENTAL PRESCRIBING ON THE NHS. Menthol and Eucalyptus Inhalation BP, 1980 may be prescribed

Karvol® (Crookes) NHS
Inhalation capsules, levomenthol 35.55 mg, with chlorobutanol, pine oils, terpineol, and thymol, net price 10-cap pack = £2.25; 20-cap pack = £4.06
Inhalation solution, levomenthol 7.9%, with chlorobutanol, pine oils, terpineol, and thymol, net price 12-mL dropper bottle = £1.90
Dose: express into handkerchief or add to a pint of hot, **not** boiling, water the contents of 1 capsule or 6 drops of solution; avoid in infants under 3 months

3.9 Cough preparations

3.9.1 Cough suppressants

Cough is usually a symptom of an underlying disorder e.g. asthma (section 3.1.1), gastro-oesophageal reflux disease (section 1.1), and 'post-nasal drip'; where there is no identifiable cause, cough suppressants may be useful, for example if sleep is disturbed. They may cause sputum retention and this may be harmful in patients with chronic bronchitis and bronchiectasis.

Codeine may be effective but it is constipating and can cause dependence; **dextromethorphan** and **pholcodine** have fewer side-effects.

Sedating antihistamines, such as diphenhydramine, are used as the cough suppressant component of many compound cough preparations on sale to the public; all tend to cause drowsiness which may reflect their main mode of action.

CHILDREN. The use of cough suppressants containing codeine or similar opioid analgesics is not generally recommended in children and should be avoided altogether in those under 1 year of age.

CODEINE PHOSPHATE

Indications: dry or painful cough; diarrhoea (section 1.4.2); pain (section 4.7.2)
Cautions: asthma; hepatic and renal impairment; history of drug abuse; see also notes above and section 4.7.2; **interactions:** Appendix 1 (opioid analgesics)
Contra-indications: liver disease, ventilatory failure
Side-effects: constipation, respiratory depression in sensitive patients or if given large doses

[1]**Codeine Linctus, BP** PoM
Linctus (= oral solution), codeine phosphate 15 mg/5 mL. Net price 100 mL = 40p (diabetic, 73p)
Brands include *Galcodine*®
Dose: 5–10 mL 3–4 times daily; CHILD (but not generally recommended) 5–12 years, 2.5–5 mL
NOTE. BP directs that when Diabetic Codeine Linctus is prescribed, Codeine Linctus formulated with a vehicle appropriate for administration to diabetics, whether or not labelled 'Diabetic Codeine Linctus', shall be dispensed or supplied

1. Can be sold to the public provided the maximum single dose does not exceed 5 mL

Codeine Linctus, Paediatric, BP
Linctus (= oral solution), codeine phosphate 3 mg/5 mL. Net price 100 mL = 18p
Brands include *Galcodine® Paediatric* (sugar-free)
Dose: CHILD (but not generally recommended) 1–5 years 5 mL 3–4 times daily
NOTE. BP directs that Paediatric Codeine Linctus may be prepared extemporaneously by diluting Codeine Linctus with a suitable vehicle in accordance with the manufacturer's instructions

For a list of **cough and decongestant preparations on sale to the public**, including those containing codeine, see section 3.9.2

PHOLCODINE

Indications: dry or painful cough
Cautions: see under Codeine Phosphate
Contra-indications: see under Codeine Phosphate
Side-effects: see under Codeine Phosphate

Pholcodine Linctus, BP
Linctus (= oral solution), pholcodine 5 mg/5 mL in a suitable flavoured vehicle, containing citric acid monohydrate 1%. Net price 100 mL = 24p
Brands include *Pavacol-D*® (sugar-free), *Galenphol*® (sugar-free)
Dose: 5–10 mL 3–4 times daily; CHILD (but not generally recommended, see notes above) 5–12 years 2.5–5 mL

Pholcodine Linctus, Strong, BP
Linctus (= oral solution), pholcodine 10 mg/5 mL in a suitable flavoured vehicle, containing citric acid monohydrate 2%. Net price 100 mL = 33p
Dose: 5 mL 3–4 times daily
Brands include *Galenphol*®

Galenphol® (Thornton & Ross)
Paediatric linctus (= oral solution), orange, sugar-free, pholcodine 2 mg/5 mL. Net price 90-mL pack = £1.11
Dose: CHILD (but not generally recommended, see notes above) 1–5 years 5–10 mL 3 times daily; 6–12 years 10 mL 3 times daily

For a list of **cough and decongestant preparations on sale to the public**, including those containing pholcodine, see section 3.9.2

Palliative care

Diamorphine and methadone have been used to control distressing cough in terminal lung cancer although morphine is now preferred (see p. 15). In other circumstances they are contra-indicated because they induce sputum retention and ventilatory failure as well as causing opioid dependence. Methadone linctus should be avoided because it has a long duration of action and tends to accumulate.

METHADONE HYDROCHLORIDE

Indications: cough in terminal disease
Cautions: see notes in section 4.7.2
Contra-indications: see notes in section 4.7.2
Side-effects: see notes in section 4.7.2; longer-acting than morphine therefore effects may be cumulative
Dose: see below

Methadone Linctus CD

Linctus (= oral solution), methadone hydrochloride 2 mg/5 mL in a suitable vehicle with a tolu flavour. Label: 2

Dose: 2.5–5 mL every 4–6 hours, reduced to twice daily on prolonged use

MORPHINE HYDROCHLORIDE

Indications: cough in terminal disease (see also Prescribing in Palliative Care p. 15)
Cautions: see notes in section 4.7.2
Contra-indications: see notes in section 4.7.2
Side-effects: see notes in section 4.7.2
Dose: initially 5 mg every 4 hours

■ Preparation

Section 4.7.2

3.9.2 Expectorant and demulcent cough preparations

Expectorants are claimed to promote expulsion of bronchial secretions but there is no evidence that any drug can specifically facilitate expectoration. The assumption that sub-emetic doses of expectorants, such as ammonium chloride, ipecacuanha, and squill promote expectoration is a myth. However, a simple expectorant mixture may serve a useful placebo function and has the advantage of being inexpensive.

Demulcent cough preparations contain soothing substances such as syrup or glycerol and some patients believe that such preparations relieve a dry irritating cough. Preparations such as **simple linctus** have the advantage of being harmless and inexpensive; **paediatric simple linctus** is particularly useful in children.

Compound preparations are on sale to the public for the treatment of cough and colds; the rationale for some is dubious.

Ammonia and Ipecacuanha Mixture, BP

Mixture, ammonium bicarbonate 200 mg, liquorice liquid extract 0.5 mL, ipecacuanha tincture 0.3 mL, concentrated camphor water 0.1 mL, concentrated anise water 0.05 mL, double-strength chloroform water 5 mL, water to 10 mL. It should be recently prepared

Dose: 10–20 mL 3–4 times daily

Simple Linctus, BP

Linctus (= oral solution), citric acid monohydrate 2.5% in a suitable vehicle with an anise flavour. Net price 100 mL = 18p

Dose: 5 mL 3–4 times daily

A sugar-free version is also available

Simple Linctus, Paediatric, BP

Linctus (= oral solution), citric acid monohydrate 0.625% in a suitable vehicle with an anise flavour. Net price 100 mL = 17p

Dose: CHILD 5–10 mL 3–4 times daily

A sugar-free version is also available

■ Preparations on sale to the public

Systemic cough and decongestant preparations on sale to the public, together with their significant ingredients.

Important: in overdose contact **Poisons Information Services** (p. 27) for full details of the ingredients.

Adult Meltus® **Expectorant with Decongestant** (guaifenesin, pseudoephedrine, menthol), **Advil Cold and Sinus®** (ibuprofen, pseudoephedrine)

Baby Meltus® (dilute acetic acid), **Beechams All-In-One®** (guaifenesin, paracetamol, phenylephrine), **Beechams Flu-Plus Caplets®** (paracetamol, phenylephrine), **Beechams Hot Lemon®**, **Hot Lemon and Honey®**, **Hot Blackcurrant®**, **Beechams Powders Capsules® with Decongestant** (paracetamol, phenylephrine), **Benadryl Plus Capsules®** (acrivastine, pseudoephedrine), **Benylin Chesty Coughs® Original** (diphenhydramine, menthol), **Benylin Children's Chesty Coughs®** (guaifenesin), **Benylin Children's Night Coughs®** (diphenhydramine, menthol), **Benylin Children's Dry Coughs®** (pholcodine), **Benylin Children's Coughs and Colds®** (dextromethorphan, triprolidine), **Benylin with Codeine®** (codeine, diphenhydramine, menthol), **Benylin Cough and Congestion®** (dextromethorphan, diphenhydramine, menthol, pseudoephedrine), **Benylin Dry Cough®** (dextromethorphan, diphenhydramine, menthol), **Benylin Four Flu®** (diphenhydramine, paracetamol, pseudoephedrine), **Benylin Non-drowsy for Chesty Coughs®** (guaifenesin, menthol), **Benylin Non-drowsy for Dry Coughs®** (dextromethorphan), **Benylin Day & Night Tablets®** (*day tablets*, paracetamol, pseudoephedrine, *night tablets*, paracetamol, diphenhydramine), **Boots Bronchial Cough Mixture®** (ammonium carbonate, ammonium chloride, guaifenesin), **Boots Catarrh Cough Syrup®** (codeine, creosote), **Boots Chesty Cough Syrup 1 Year Plus®** (guaifenesin), **Boots Cough and Decongestant Syrup 2 Years Plus®** (guaifenesin, pseudoephedrine), **Boots Cough Syrup 3 Months Plus®** (glycerol), **Boots Cold and Flu Relief Tablets®** (paracetamol, phenylephrine), **Boots Decongestant Tablets®** (pseudoephedrine), **Boots Decongestant Tablets with Paracetamol®** (paracetamol, pseudoephedrine), **Boots Night Time Cough Syrup 1 Year Plus®** (diphenhydramine, pholcodine), **Buttercup Infant Cough Syrup®** (ipecacuanha,), **Buttercup Syrup®** (capsicum, squill), **Buttercup Syrup Honey and Lemon Flavour®** (ipecacuanha, menthol)

Cabdrivers® (dextromethorphan, menthol), **CAM®** (ephedrine), **Contac® Non Drowsy 12 Hour Relief** (pseudoephedrine), **Covonia Bronchial Balsam®** (dextromethorphan, menthol), **Covonia Mentholated Cough Mixture®** (liquorice, menthol, squill), **Covonia Night Time Formula®** (dextromethorphan, diphenhydramine)

Day Nurse® (paracetamol, pholcodine, pseudoephedrine), **Do-Do Chesteze®** (ephedrine, theophylline)

Expulin® (chlorphenamine, menthol, pholcodine, pseudoephedrine),

Famel Original® (codeine, creosote), **Franol®** (ephedrine, theophylline), **Franol Plus®** (ephedrine, theophylline)

Galcodine® (codeine), **Galcodine Paediatric**® (codeine), **Galenphol**® (pholcodine), **Galenphol Paediatric**® (pholcodine), **Galenphol Strong**® (pholcodine), **Galloway's**® (ipecacuanha, squill), **Galsud**® (pseudoephedrine)

Haymine® (chlorphenamine, ephedrine), **Hill's Balsam Adult Expectorant**® (ipecacuanha, pholcodine), **Hill's Balsam Cough Suppressant**® (pholcodine), **Histalix**® (ammonium chloride, diphenhydramine, menthol)

Jackson's All Fours® (guaifenesin), **Jackson's Bronchial Balsam**® (guaifenesin), **Jackson's Little Healers**® (ipecacuanha), **Jackson's Troublesome Coughs**® (ipecacuanha), **Junior Meltus Dry Cough**® (dextromethorphan, pseudoephedrine), **Junior Meltus Expectorant**® (guaifenesin)

Lemsip® **Cold & Flu Breathe Easy** (paracetamol, phenylephrine), **Lemsip**® **Cold & Flu Lemon** or **Blackcurrant** (paracetamol, phenylephrine), **Lemsip**® **Cold & Flu Sinus 12 Hr Ibuprofen + Pseudoephedrine** (ibuprofen, pseudoephedrine), **Lemsip**® **Cough Chesty** (guaifenesin), **Lemsip**® **Flu Lemon** (paracetamol, pseudoephedrine), **Lemsip**® **Max Cold & Flu Capsules** (caffeine, paracetamol, phenylephrine), **Lemsip**® **Max Cold & Flu Direct Lemon** or **Blackcurrant** (paracetamol, phenylephrine), **Lemsip**® **Max Cold & Flu Lemon** (paracetamol, phenylephrine), **Lemsip**® **Max Flu 12 HR Ibuprofen + Pseudoephedrine** (ibuprofen, pseudoephedrine), **Lemsip**® **Max Sinus Capsules** (caffeine, paracetamol, phenylephrine),- **Liqufruta Garlic**® (guaifenesin)

Medised® (paracetamol, promethazine), **Meltus Baby**® (dilute acetic acid), **Meltus Dry Cough**® (dextromethorphan, pseudoephedrine), **Meltus Expectorant**®, **Meltus Honey and Lemon**® (guaifenesin), **Multi-action Actifed Tablets**® (pseudoephedrine, triprolidine), **Multi-action Actifed Dry Coughs**® (dextromethorphan, pseudoephedrine, triprolidine), **Multi-action Actifed Syrup**® (pseudoephedrine, triprolidine), **Multi-action Actifed Chesty Coughs**® (guaifenesin, pseudoephedrine, triprolidine)

Night Nurse® (dextromethorphan, paracetamol, promethazine), **Nirolex for Chesty Coughs with Decongestant**® (guaifenesin, pseudoephedrine), **Nirolex Chesty Cough Linctus**® (guaifenesin), **Nirolex Day Cold Comfort**® (paracetamol, pholcodine, pseudoephedrine), **Nirolex Dry Cough Linctus**® (glycerol), **Nirolex for Dry Coughs with Decongestant**® (dextromethorphan, pseudoephedrine), **Nirolex for Night Time Coughs**® (diphenhydramine, pholcodine), **Non-Drowsy Sinutab**® (paracetamol, pseudoephedrine), **Non-Drowsy Sudafed Congestion Cold and Flu Tablets**® (paracetamol, pseudoephedrine), **Non-Drowsy Sudafed Congestion Relief**® (phenylephrine), **Non-Drowsy Sudafed Decongestant Tablets**® (pseudoephedrine), **Non-Drowsy Sudafed Dual Relief**® (paracetamol, phenylephrine), **Non-Drowsy Sudafed Dual Relief Max**® (ibuprofen, pseudoephedrine), **Non-Drowsy Sudafed Expectorant**® (guaifenesin, pseudoephedrine), **Non-Drowsy Sudafed 12 Hour Relief**® (pseudoephedrine), **Non-Drowsy Sudafed Linctus**® (dextromethorphan, pseudoephedrine), **Non-Drowsy Sudafed Plus Tablets**® (pseudoephedrine, triprolidine), **Numark Cold Relief Powders**® (paracetamol), **Nurofen**® **Cold and Flu** (ibuprofen, pseudoephedrine), **Nurofen**® **Sinus** (ibuprofen, pseudoephedrine),

Otrivine® **Mu-Cron** (paracetamol, pseudoephedrine)

Pavacol D® (pholcodine), **Pulmo Bailly**® (codeine, guaiacol)

Robitussin Chesty Cough® (guaifenesin), **Robitussin Chesty Cough with Congestion**® (guaifenesin, pseudoephedrine), **Robitussin Dry Cough**® (dextromethorphan), **Robitussin Soft Pastilles For Dry Cough**® (dextromethorphan)

Sudafed Plus® (pseudoephedrine, triprolidine)

Tixycolds® (diphenhydramine, pseudoephedrine), **Tixylix Chesty Cough**® (guaifenesin), **Tixylix Cough and Cold**® (chlorphenamine, pholcodine, pseudoephedrine), **Tixylix Daytime**® (pholcodine), **Tixylix Night-time**® (pholcodine, promethazine), **Tixyplus**® **Active Relief for Colds and Flu** (diphenhydramine, paracetamol)

Uniflu with Gregovite C® (caffeine, codeine, diphenhydramine, paracetamol, phenylephrine)

Venos Expectorant® (guaifenesin), **Vicks Medinite**® (dextromethorphan, doxylamine, ephedrine, paracetamol), **Vicks Vaposyrup for Tickly Coughs**® (menthol), **Vicks Vaposyrup Chesty Cough**® (guaifenesin), **Vicks Vaposyrup Dry Cough**® (dextromethorphan)

3.10 Systemic nasal decongestants

Nasal decongestants for administration by mouth may not be as effective as preparations for local application (section 12.2.2) but they do not give rise to rebound nasal congestion on withdrawal. **Pseudoephedrine** is available over-the-counter; it has few sympathomimetic effects.

Systemic decongestants should be used with **caution** in diabetes, hypertension, hyperthyroidism, raised intra-ocular pressure, prostate hypertrophy, hepatic impairment, renal impairment, and ischaemic heart disease and **avoided** in patients taking monoamine oxidase inhibitors; **interactions:** Appendix 1 (sympathomimetics).

Systemic compound preparations containing pseudoephedrine are shown in the list of cough and decongestant preparations on sale to the public (section 3.9.2). Many preparations also contain antihistamines, which may cause drowsiness and affect the ability to drive or operate machinery.

Preparations containing phenylpropanolamine have been discontinued.

PSEUDOEPHEDRINE HYDROCHLORIDE

Indications: see notes above
Cautions: see notes above
Side-effects: tachycardia, anxiety, restlessness, insomnia; rarely hallucinations, rash; urinary retention also reported
Dose: see preparations below

Galpseud® (Thornton & Ross)
Tablets, pseudoephedrine hydrochloride 60 mg. Net price 20 = 91p
Dose: 1 tablet 4 times daily
Linctus, orange, sugar-free, pseudoephedrine hydrochloride 30 mg/5 mL. Net price 100 mL = 69p
Dose: 10 mL 3 times daily; CHILD 2–6 years 2.5 mL, 6–12 years 5 mL

Sudafed® (Warner Lambert)
Tablets, red, f/c, pseudoephedrine hydrochloride 60 mg. Net price 24 = £2.12
Dose: 1 tablet every 4–6 hours (up to 4 times daily)

Elixir, red, pseudoephedrine hydrochloride 30 mg/ 5 mL. Net price 100 mL = £1.48
Dose: 10 mL every 4–6 hours (up to 4 times daily); CHILD 2–5 years 2.5 mL, 6–12 years 5 mL
NOTE. The brand name *Sudafed*® is also used for preparations containing dextromethorphan, guaifenesin, ibuprofen, paracetamol, phenylephrine, triprolidine (p. 171 and p. 222), oxymetazoline, and xylometazoline (p. 551)

■ Preparations on sale to the public

For a list of systemic **cough and decongestant preparations on sale to the public**, including those containing pseudoephedrine, see p. 171

4: Central nervous system

4.1 Hypnotics and anxiolytics

Most anxiolytics ('sedatives') will induce sleep when given at night and most hypnotics will sedate when given during the day. Prescribing of these drugs is widespread but dependence (both physical and psychological) and tolerance occurs. This may lead to difficulty in withdrawing the drug after the patient has been taking it regularly for more than a few weeks (see Dependence and Withdrawal, below). Hypnotics and anxiolytics should therefore be reserved for short courses to alleviate acute conditions after causal factors have been established.

Benzodiazepines are the most commonly used anxiolytics and hypnotics; they act at benzodiazepine receptors which are associated with gamma-aminobutyric acid (GABA) receptors. Older drugs such as meprobamate and barbiturates (section 4.1.3) are **not** recommended—they have more side-effects and interactions than benzodiazepines and are much more dangerous in overdosage.

PARADOXICAL EFFECTS. A paradoxical increase in hostility and aggression may be reported by patients taking benzodiazepines. The effects range from talkativeness and excitement, to aggressive and antisocial acts. Adjustment of the dose (up or down) usually attenuates the impulses. Increased anxiety and perceptual disorders are other paradoxical effects. Increased hostility and aggression after barbiturates and alcohol usually indicates intoxication.

DRIVING. Hypnotics and anxiolytics may impair judgement and increase reaction time, and so affect ability to drive or operate machinery; they increase the effects of alcohol. Moreover the hangover effects of a night dose may impair driving on the following day. See also Drugs and Driving under General Guidance, p. 2.

DEPENDENCE AND WITHDRAWAL. Withdrawal of a benzodiazepine should be gradual because abrupt withdrawal may produce confusion, toxic psychosis, convulsions, or a condition resembling delirium tremens. Abrupt withdrawal of a barbiturate (section 4.1.3) is even more likely to have serious effects.

The benzodiazepine withdrawal syndrome may develop at any time up to 3 weeks after stopping a long-acting benzodiazepine, but may occur within a few hours in the case of a short-acting one. It is characterised by insomnia, anxiety, loss of appetite and of body-weight, tremor, perspiration, tinnitus, and perceptual disturbances. These symptoms may be similar to the original complaint and encourage further prescribing; some symptoms may continue for weeks or months after stopping benzodiazepines.

A benzodiazepine can be withdrawn in steps of about one-eighth (range one-tenth to one-quarter) of the daily dose every fortnight. A suggested withdrawal protocol for patients who have difficulty is as follows:

1. Transfer patient to equivalent daily dose of diazepam[1] preferably taken at night
2. Reduce diazepam dose in fortnightly steps of 2 or 2.5 mg; if withdrawal symptoms occur, maintain this dose until symptoms improve
3. Reduce dose further, if necessary in smaller fortnightly steps[2]; it is better to reduce too slowly rather than too quickly
4. Stop completely; time needed for withdrawal can vary from about 4 weeks to a year or more

Counselling may help; beta-blockers should **only** be tried if other measures fail; antidepressants should be used **only** for clinical depression or for panic disorder; **avoid** antipsychotics (which may aggravate withdrawal symptoms).

CSM advice.

1. Benzodiazepines are indicated for the short-term relief (two to four weeks only) of anxiety that is severe, disabling or subjecting the individual to unacceptable distress, occurring alone or in association with insomnia or short-term psychosomatic, organic or psychotic illness.
2. The use of benzodiazepines to treat short-term 'mild' anxiety is inappropriate and unsuitable.
3. Benzodiazepines should be used to treat insomnia only when it is severe, disabling, or subjecting the individual to extreme distress.

4.1.1 Hypnotics

Before a hypnotic is prescribed the cause of the insomnia should be established and, where possible, underlying factors should be treated. However, it should be noted that some patients have unrealistic sleep expectations, and others understate their alcohol consumption which is often the cause of the insomnia.

Transient insomnia may occur in those who normally sleep well and may be due to extraneous factors such as noise, shift work, and jet lag. If a hypnotic is indicated one that is rapidly eliminated should be chosen, and only one or two doses should be given.

Short-term insomnia is usually related to an emotional problem or serious medical illness. It may last for a few weeks and may recur; a hypnotic can be useful but should not be given for more than three weeks (preferably only one week). Intermittent use is desirable with omission of some doses. A rapidly eliminated drug is generally appropriate.

Chronic insomnia is rarely benefited by hypnotics and is more often due to mild dependence caused by injudicious prescribing. Psychiatric disorders such as anxiety, depression, and abuse of drugs and alcohol are common causes. Sleep disturbance is very common in depressive illness and early wakening is often a useful pointer. The underlying psychiatric complaint should be treated, adapting the drug regimen to alleviate insomnia. For example, amitriptyline or mirtazapine prescribed for depression will also help to promote sleep if taken at night. Other causes of insomnia include daytime catnapping and physical causes such as pain, pruritus, and dyspnoea.

Hypnotics should **not** be prescribed indiscriminately and routine prescribing is undesirable. They should be reserved for short courses in the acutely distressed. Tolerance to their effects develops within 3 to 14 days of continuous use and long-term efficacy cannot be assured. A major drawback of long-term use is that withdrawal causes rebound insomnia and precipitates a withdrawal syndrome (section 4.1).

Where prolonged administration is unavoidable hypnotics should be discontinued as soon as feasible and the patient warned that sleep may be disturbed for a few days before normal rhythm is re-established; broken sleep with vivid dreams and increased REM (rapid eye movement) sleep may persist for several weeks.

CHILDREN. The prescribing of hypnotics to children, except for occasional use such as for night terrors and somnambulism (sleep-walking), is not justified.

ELDERLY. Hypnotics should be avoided in the elderly, who are at risk of becoming ataxic and confused and so liable to fall and injure themselves.

DENTAL PROCEDURES. Some anxious patients may benefit from the use of a hypnotic for 1 to 3 nights before the dental appointment. Hypnotics do not relieve pain, and if pain interferes with sleep an appropriate analgesic should be given. **Diazepam** (section 4.1.2), **nitrazepam** or **temazepam** are used at night for dental patients. Temazepam is preferred when it is important to minimise any residual effect the following day. For information on anxiolytics for dental procedures, see section 15.1.4.1.

Benzodiazepines

Benzodiazepines used as hypnotics include **nitrazepam** and **flurazepam** which have a prolonged action and may give rise to residual effects on the following day; repeated doses tend to be cumulative.

Loprazolam, **lormetazepam**, and **temazepam** act for a shorter time and they have little or no hangover effect. Withdrawal phenomena are more common with the short-acting benzodiazepines.

If insomnia is associated with daytime anxiety then the use of a long-acting benzodiazepine anxiolytic such as **diazepam** given as a single dose at night may effectively treat both symptoms.

For general guidelines on benzodiazepine prescribing see section 4.1.2 and for benzodiazepine withdrawal see section 4.1.

1. Approximate equivalent doses, diazepam 5 mg
≡chlordiazepoxide 15 mg
≡loprazolam 0.5–1 mg
≡lorazepam 500 micrograms
≡lormetazepam 0.5–1 mg
≡nitrazepam 5 mg
≡oxazepam 15 mg
≡temazepam 10 mg

2. Steps may be adjusted according to initial dose and duration of treatment and can range from diazepam 500 micrograms (one-quarter of a 2-mg tablet) to 2.5 mg

NITRAZEPAM

Indications: insomnia (short-term use)

Cautions: respiratory disease, muscle weakness, history of drug or alcohol abuse, marked personality disorder, pregnancy (Appendix 4), breast-feeding (Appendix 5); reduce dose in elderly and debilitated, and in hepatic impairment (avoid if severe; Appendix 2) and renal impairment (Appendix 3); avoid prolonged use (and abrupt withdrawal thereafter); porphyria (section 9.8.2); **interactions:** Appendix 1 (anxiolytics and hypnotics)

DRIVING. Drowsiness may persist the next day and affect performance of skilled tasks (e.g. driving); effects of alcohol enhanced

Contra-indications: respiratory depression; acute pulmonary insufficiency; severe hepatic impairment, myasthenia gravis, sleep apnoea syndrome; not for use alone to treat depression (or anxiety associated with depression) or chronic psychosis

Side-effects: drowsiness and lightheadedness the next day; confusion and ataxia (especially in the elderly); amnesia may occur; dependence; see also under Diazepam (section 4.1.2); **overdosage:** see Emergency Treatment of Poisoning, p. 32

Dose: 5–10 mg at bedtime; ELDERLY (or debilitated) 2.5–5 mg; CHILD not recommended

Nitrazepam (Non-proprietary) PoM

Tablets, nitrazepam 5 mg, net price 20 = £1.16. Label: 19

Brands include *Mogadon*® NHS, *Remnos*® NHS

DENTAL PRESCRIBING ON NHS. Nitrazepam Tablets may be prescribed

Oral suspension, nitrazepam 2.5 mg/5 mL. Net price 150 mL = £5.30. Label: 19

Brands include *Somnite*® NHS

FLURAZEPAM

Indications: insomnia (short-term use)

Cautions: see under Nitrazepam

Contra-indications: see under Nitrazepam

Side-effects: see under Nitrazepam

Dose: 15–30 mg at bedtime; ELDERLY (or debilitated) 15 mg; CHILD not recommended

Dalmane® (Valeant) PoM NHS

Capsules, flurazepam (as hydrochloride), 15 mg (grey/yellow), net price 30-cap pack = £5.44; 30 mg (black/grey), 30-cap pack = £6.98. Label: 19

LOPRAZOLAM

Indications: insomnia (short-term use)

Cautions: see under Nitrazepam

Contra-indications: see under Nitrazepam

Side-effects: see under Nitrazepam; shorter acting

Dose: 1 mg at bedtime, increased to 1.5 or 2 mg if required; ELDERLY (or debilitated) 0.5 or 1 mg; CHILD not recommended

Loprazolam (Non-proprietary) PoM

Tablets, loprazolam 1 mg (as mesilate). Net price 28-tab pack = £4.46. Label: 19

LORMETAZEPAM

Indications: insomnia (short-term use)

Cautions: see under Nitrazepam

Contra-indications: see under Nitrazepam

Side-effects: see under Nitrazepam; shorter acting

Dose: 0.5–1.5 mg at bedtime; ELDERLY (or debilitated) 500 micrograms; CHILD not recommended

Lormetazepam (Non-proprietary) PoM

Tablets, lormetazepam 500 micrograms, net price 28-tab pack = £6.98; 1 mg, 28-tab pack = £8.15. Label: 19

TEMAZEPAM

Indications: insomnia (short-term use); see also section 15.1.4.1 for peri-operative use

Cautions: see under Nitrazepam

Contra-indications: see under Nitrazepam

Side-effects: see under Nitrazepam; shorter acting

Dose: 10–20 mg at bedtime, exceptional circumstances 30–40 mg; ELDERLY (or debilitated) 10 mg at bedtime, exceptional circumstances 20 mg; CHILD not recommended

[1]**Temazepam** (Non-proprietary) CD

Tablets, temazepam 10 mg, net price 28-tab pack = 95p; 20 mg, 28-tab pack = £1.58. Label: 19

Oral solution, temazepam 10 mg/5 mL, net price 300 mL = £9.95. Label: 19

NOTE. Sugar-free versions are available and can be ordered by specifying 'sugar-free' on the prescription

DENTAL PRESCRIBING ON NHS. Temazepam Tablets or Oral Solution may be prescribed

1. See p. 7 for prescribing requirements for temazepam

Zaleplon, zolpidem, and zopiclone

Zaleplon, **zolpidem** and **zopiclone** are non-benzodiazepine hypnotics, but they act at the benzodiazepine receptor. Zolpidem and zopiclone have a short duration of action; zaleplon is very short acting. All three drugs are not licensed for long-term use; dependence has been reported in a small number of patients.

ZALEPLON

Indications: insomnia (short-term use—up to 2 weeks)

Cautions: respiratory insufficiency (avoid if severe); hepatic impairment (avoid if severe; Appendix 2); history of drug or alcohol abuse; avoid prolonged use (and abrupt withdrawal thereafter); pregnancy (Appendix 4); not for use alone to treat depression

Contra-indications: sleep apnoea syndrome, myasthenia gravis; not for use alone to treat psychosis; breast-feeding (Appendix 5)

Side-effects: amnesia, paraesthesia, drowsiness, asthenia; nausea, incoordination, confusion, impaired concentration, dizziness, hallucinations, disturbances of hearing, smell, speech, and vision, photosensitivity; dependence; paradoxical effects (discontinue—see also section 4.1)

Dose: 10 mg at bedtime or after going to bed if difficulty falling asleep; ELDERLY 5 mg; CHILD under 18 years not recommended

NOTE. Patients should be advised not to take a second dose during a single night

Sonata® (Wyeth) PoM

Capsules, zaleplon 5 mg (white/light brown), net price 14-cap pack = £3.12; 10 mg (white), 14-cap pack = £3.76. Label: 2

ZOLPIDEM TARTRATE

Indications: insomnia (short-term use—up to 4 weeks)

Cautions: depression, history of drug or alcohol abuse, hepatic impairment (avoid if severe; Appendix 2); renal impairment; elderly; avoid prolonged use (and abrupt withdrawal thereafter); **interactions:** Appendix 1 (anxiolytics and hypnotics)

DRIVING. Drowsiness may persist the next day and affect performance of skilled tasks (e.g. driving); effects of alcohol enhanced

Contra-indications: obstructive sleep apnoea, acute or severe respiratory depression, myasthenia gravis, severe hepatic impairment, psychotic illness, pregnancy, breast-feeding (Appendix 5)

Side-effects: diarrhoea, nausea, vomiting, vertigo, dizziness, headache, drowsiness, asthenia, amnesia; dependence, memory disturbances, nightmares, nocturnal restlessness, depression, confusion, perceptual disturbances or diplopia, tremor, ataxia, falls, skin reactions, changes in libido; paradoxical effects—see section 4.1

Dose: 10 mg at bedtime; ELDERLY (or debilitated) 5 mg; CHILD not recommended

Zolpidem (Non-proprietary) PoM

Tablets, zolpidem tartrate 5 mg, net price 28-tab pack = £3.17; 10 mg, 28-tab pack = £3.67. Label: 19

Stilnoct® (Sanofi-Synthelabo) PoM

Tablets, both f/c, zolpidem tartrate 5 mg, net price 28-tab pack = £3.08; 10 mg, 28-tab pack = £4.48. Label: 19

ZOPICLONE

Indications: insomnia (short-term use—up to 4 weeks)

Cautions: hepatic impairment (avoid if severe; Appendix 2) and renal impairment (Appendix 3); elderly; history of drug abuse, psychiatric illness; avoid prolonged use (and abrupt withdrawal thereafter); **interactions:** Appendix 1 (anxiolytics and hypnotics)

DRIVING. Drowsiness may persist the next day and affect performance of skilled tasks (e.g. driving); effects of alcohol enhanced

Contra-indications: myasthenia gravis, respiratory failure, severe sleep apnoea syndrome, severe hepatic impairment; pregnancy and breast-feeding (Appendix 5)

Side-effects: bitter or metallic taste; gastro-intestinal disturbances including nausea and vomiting, dry mouth, aggression; irritability, confusion, depressed mood; drowsiness, dizziness, lightheadedness, and incoordination, headache; dependence; hypersensitivity reactions reported (including urticaria and rashes); hallucinations, nightmares, amnesia reported

Dose: 7.5 mg at bedtime; ELDERLY initially 3.75 mg at bedtime increased if necessary; CHILD not recommended

Zopiclone (Non-proprietary) PoM

Tablets, zopiclone 3.75 mg, net price 28-tab pack = £2.87; 7.5 mg, 28-tab pack = £2.56. Label: 19

Brands include *Zileze*®

Zimovane® (Rhône-Poulenc Rorer) PoM

Tablets, f/c, zopiclone 3.75 mg (*Zimovane*® *LS*, blue), net price 28-tab pack = £2.33; 7.5 mg, 28-tab pack = £3.39. Label: 19

Chloral and derivatives

Chloral hydrate and derivatives were formerly popular hypnotics for children (but the use of hypnotics in children is not usually justified). There is no convincing evidence that they are particularly useful in the elderly and their role as hypnotics is now very limited. **Triclofos** causes fewer gastro-intestinal disturbances than chloral hydrate.

CHLORAL HYDRATE

Indications: insomnia (short-term use)

Cautions: respiratory disease, history of drug or alcohol abuse, marked personality disorder; reduce dose in elderly and debilitated; avoid prolonged use (and abrupt withdrawal thereafter); avoid contact with skin and mucous membranes; hepatic impairment (avoid if severe—Appendix 2); **interactions:** Appendix 1 (anxiolytics and hypnotics)

DRIVING. Drowsiness may persist the next day and affect performance of skilled tasks (e.g. driving); effects of alcohol enhanced

Contra-indications: severe cardiac disease, gastritis, severe hepatic impairment, severe renal impairment; pregnancy; breast-feeding (Appendix 5); porphyria (section 9.8.2)

Side-effects: gastric irritation (nausea and vomiting reported), abdominal distention and flatulence; also ataxia, confusion, rashes, headache, light-headedness, ketonuria, excitement, nightmares, delirium (especially on abrupt withdrawal); dependence (may be associated with gastritis and renal damage) on prolonged use

Dose: see under preparations below

Chloral Mixture, BP 2000 PoM

(Chloral Oral Solution)

Mixture, chloral hydrate 500 mg/5 mL in a suitable vehicle. Extemporaneous preparations should be recently prepared according to the following formula: chloral hydrate 1 g, syrup 2 mL, water to 10 mL. Net price 100 mL = 53p. Label: 19, 27

Dose: 5–20 mL; CHILD 1–5 years 2.5–5 mL, 6–12 years 5–10 mL, taken well diluted with water at bedtime

Chloral Elixir, Paediatric, BP 2000 PoM

(Chloral Oral Solution, Paediatric)

Elixir, chloral hydrate 4% in a suitable vehicle with a blackcurrant flavour. Extemporaneous preparations should be recently prepared according to the following formula: chloral hydrate 200 mg, water 0.1 mL, blackcurrant syrup 1 mL, syrup to 5 mL. Net price 100 mL = £1.02. Label: 1, 27

Dose: up to 1 year 5 mL, taken well diluted with water at bedtime

■ Cloral betaine

Welldorm® (Alphashow) PoM

Tablets, blue-purple, f/c, cloral betaine 707 mg (≡ chloral hydrate 414 mg). Net price 30-tab pack = £2.43. Label: 19, 27

Dose: 1–2 tablets with water or milk at bedtime, max. 5 tablets (2 g chloral hydrate) daily

Elixir, red, chloral hydrate 143.3 mg/5 mL. Net price 150-mL pack = £2.05. Label: 19, 27

Dose: 15–45 mL (0.4–1.3 g chloral hydrate) with water or milk, at bedtime, max. 70 mL (2 g chloral hydrate) daily; CHILD 1–1.75 mL/kg (30–50 mg/kg chloral hydrate), max. 35 mL (1 g chloral hydrate) daily

TRICLOFOS SODIUM

Indications: insomnia (short-term use)
Cautions: see Chloral Hydrate
Contra-indications: see Chloral Hydrate
Side-effects: see Chloral Hydrate but less gastric irritation
Dose: see under preparation below

Triclofos Oral Solution, BP PoM
(Triclofos Elixir)
Oral solution, triclofos sodium 500 mg/5 mL. Net price 300 mL = £27.83. Label: 19
Dose: 10–20 mL (1–2 g triclofos sodium) at bedtime; CHILD up to 1 year 25–30 mg/kg, 1–5 years 2.5–5 mL (250–500 mg triclofos sodium), 6–12 years 5–10 mL (0.5–1 g triclofos sodium)

Clomethiazole

Clomethiazole (chlormethiazole) may be a useful hypnotic for elderly patients because of its freedom from hangover but, as with all hypnotics, routine administration is undesirable and dependence occurs. It is licensed for use as a hypnotic only in the elderly (and for *very short-term use* in younger adults to attenuate alcohol withdrawal symptoms, see section 4.10).

CLOMETHIAZOLE

(Chlormethiazole)
Indications: see under Dose; alcohol withdrawal (section 4.10)
Cautions: cardiac and respiratory disease (confusional state may indicate hypoxia); history of drug abuse; marked personality disorder; elderly; excessive sedation may occur (particularly with higher doses); hepatic impairment (especially if severe because sedation can mask hepatic coma; Appendix 2); renal impairment (Appendix 3); avoid prolonged use (and abrupt withdrawal thereafter); **interactions:** Appendix 1 (anxiolytics and hypnotics)
DRIVING. Drowsiness may persist the next day and affect performance of skilled tasks (e.g. driving); effects of alcohol enhanced
Contra-indications: acute pulmonary insufficiency; alcohol-dependent patients who continue to drink
Side-effects: nasal congestion and irritation (increased nasopharyngeal and bronchial secretions), conjunctival irritation, headache; rarely, paradoxical excitement, confusion, dependence, gastro-intestinal disturbances, rash, urticaria, bullous eruption, anaphylaxis, alterations in liver enzymes
Dose: severe insomnia in the elderly (short-term use), 1–2 capsules (*or* 5–10 mL syrup) at bedtime; CHILD not recommended
Restlessness and agitation in the elderly, 1 capsule (*or* 5 mL syrup) 3 times daily
Alcohol withdrawal, initially 2–4 capsules, if necessary repeated after some hours; day 1 (first 24 hours), 9–12 capsules in 3–4 divided doses; day 2, 6–8 capsules in 3–4 divided doses; day 3, 4–6 capsules in 3–4 divided doses; then gradually reduced over days 4–6; total treatment for not more than 9 days
NOTE. For an equivalent therapeutic effect 1 capsule ≡ 5 mL syrup

Heminevrin® (AstraZeneca) PoM
Capsules, grey-brown, clomethiazole base 192 mg in an oily basis. Net price 60-cap pack = £4.78. Label: 19
Syrup, sugar-free, clomethiazole edisilate 250 mg/5 mL. Net price 300-mL pack = £4.00. Label: 19

Antihistamines

Some **antihistamines** such as diphenhydramine (section 3.4.1) and promethazine are on sale to the public for occasional insomnia; their prolonged duration of action may often lead to drowsiness the following day. The sedative effect of antihistamines may diminish after a few days of continued treatment; antihistamines are associated with headache, psychomotor impairment and antimuscarinic effects.

Promethazine is also popular for use in children, but the use of hypnotics in children is not usually justified.

PROMETHAZINE HYDROCHLORIDE

Indications: night sedation and insomnia (short-term use); other indications (section 3.4.1, section 4.6)
Cautions: section 3.4.1
Contra-indications: section 3.4.1
Side-effects: section 3.4.1
Dose: *by mouth*, 25 mg at bedtime increased to 50 mg if necessary; CHILD under 2 years not recommended, 2–5 years 15–20 mg, 5–10 years 20–25 mg, at bedtime

■ Preparations
Section 3.4.1

Alcohol

Alcohol is a poor hypnotic because its diuretic action interferes with sleep during the latter part of the night. With chronic use, alcohol disturbs sleep patterns and causes insomnia; **interactions:** Appendix 1 (alcohol).

4.1.2 Anxiolytics

Benzodiazepine anxiolytics can be effective in alleviating anxiety states. Although these drugs are often prescribed to almost anyone with stress-related symptoms, unhappiness, or minor physical disease, their use in many situations is unjustified. In particular, they are not appropriate for treating depression or chronic psychosis. In bereavement, psychological adjustment may be inhibited by benzodiazepines. In children anxiolytic treatment should be used only to relieve acute anxiety (and related insomnia) caused by fear (e.g. before surgery).

Anxiolytic treatment should be limited to the lowest possible dose for the shortest possible time (see CSM advice, section 4.1). Dependence is particularly likely in patients with a history of alcohol or drug abuse and in patients with marked personality disorders.

Anxiolytics, particularly the benzodiazepines, have been termed 'minor tranquillisers'. This term is misleading because not only do they differ markedly from the antipsychotic drugs ('major tranquillisers') but their use is by no means minor. Antipsychotics, in low doses, are also sometimes used in severe anxiety for their sedative action but long-term use should be avoided in view of a possible risk of tardive dyskinesia (section 4.2.1).

Some antidepressants (section 4.3) are licensed for use in anxiety and related disorders; see section 4.3 for a comment on their role in chronic anxiety, generalised anxiety disorder, and panic disorders. The use of antihistamines (e.g. hydroxyzine, section 3.4.1) for their sedative effect in anxiety is not considered to be appropriate.

Benzodiazepines

Benzodiazepines are indicated for the *short-term relief of severe anxiety* but long-term use should be avoided (see p. 174). Diazepam, alprazolam, chlordiazepoxide, clobazam, and clorazepate have a sustained action. Shorter-acting compounds such as **lorazepam** and **oxazepam** may be preferred in patients with hepatic impairment but they carry a greater risk of withdrawal symptoms.

In *panic disorders* (with or without agoraphobia) resistant to antidepressant therapy (section 4.3), a benzodiazepine (lorazepam 3–5 mg daily or clonazepam 1–2 mg daily (section 4.8.1) [both unlicensed]) may be used; alternatively, a benzodiazepine may be used as short-term adjunctive therapy at the start of antidepressant treatment to prevent the initial worsening of symptoms.

Diazepam or lorazepam are very occasionally administered intravenously for the *control of panic attacks*. This route is the most rapid but the procedure is not without risk (section 4.8.2) and should be used only when alternative measures have failed. The intramuscular route has no advantage over the oral route.

For guidelines on benzodiazepine withdrawal, see p. 174.

DIAZEPAM

Indications: short-term use in anxiety or insomnia, adjunct in acute alcohol withdrawal; status epilepticus (section 4.8.2); febrile convulsions (section 4.8.3); muscle spasm (section 10.2.2); peri-operative use (section 15.1.4.1)

Cautions: respiratory disease, muscle weakness, history of drug or alcohol abuse, marked personality disorder, pregnancy (Appendix 4), breast-feeding (Appendix 5); reduce dose in elderly and debilitated, and in hepatic impairment (avoid if severe; Appendix 2), renal impairment (Appendix 3); avoid prolonged use (and abrupt withdrawal thereafter); special precautions for intravenous injection (section 4.8.2); porphyria (section 9.8.2); **interactions:** Appendix 1 (anxiolytics and hypnotics)

DRIVING. Drowsiness may affect performance of skilled tasks (e.g. driving); effects of alcohol enhanced

Contra-indications: respiratory depression; acute pulmonary insufficiency; sleep apnoea syndrome; severe hepatic impairment; not for chronic psychosis; should not be used alone in depression or in anxiety with depression; avoid injections containing benzyl alcohol in neonates (see under preparations below)

Side-effects: drowsiness and lightheadedness the next day; confusion and ataxia (especially in the elderly); amnesia; dependence; paradoxical increase in aggression (see also section 4.1); muscle weakness; *occasionally:* headache, vertigo, hypotension, salivation changes, gastro-intestinal disturbances, visual disturbances, dysarthria, tremor, changes in libido, incontinence, urinary retention; blood disorders and jaundice reported; skin reactions; on intravenous injection, pain, thrombophlebitis, and rarely apnoea; **overdosage:** see Emergency Treatment of Poisoning, p. 32

Dose: *by mouth*, anxiety, 2 mg 3 times daily increased if necessary to 15–30 mg daily in divided doses; ELDERLY (or debilitated) half adult dose

Insomnia associated with anxiety, 5–15 mg at bedtime

CHILD night terrors and somnambulism, 1–5 mg at bedtime

By intramuscular injection or slow intravenous injection (into a large vein, at a rate of not more than 5 mg/minute), for severe acute anxiety, control of acute panic attacks, and acute alcohol withdrawal, 10 mg, repeated if necessary after not less than 4 hours

NOTE. Only use intramuscular route when oral and intravenous routes not possible; special precautions for intravenous injection see section 4.8.2

By intravenous infusion—section 4.8.2

By rectum as rectal solution, acute anxiety and agitation, 500 micrograms/kg repeated after 12 hours as required; ELDERLY 250 micrograms/kg; CHILD not recommended

CHILD febrile convulsions, see p. 250

By rectum as suppositories, anxiety when oral route not appropriate, 10–30 mg (higher dose divided); dose form not appropriate for less than 10 mg

Diazepam (Non-proprietary) [PoM]

Tablets, diazepam 2 mg, net price 20 = 81p; 5 mg, 20 = 59p; 10 mg, 20 = £1.03. Label: 2 or 19

Brands include *Rimapam*® [NHS], *Tensium*® [NHS]

Oral solution, diazepam 2 mg/5 mL, net price 100 mL = £1.75. Label: 2 or 19

Brands include *Dialar*® [NHS]

Strong oral solution, diazepam 5 mg/5 mL, net price 100-mL pack = £6.38. Label: 2 or 19 [NHS]

Brands include *Dialar*® [NHS]

Injection (solution), diazepam 5 mg/mL. Do not dilute (except for intravenous infusion). Net price 2-mL amp = 32p

Excipients: may include benzyl alcohol (avoid in neonates, see Excipients, p. 2), ethanol, propylene glycol

Injection (emulsion), diazepam 5 mg/mL. For intravenous injection or infusion. Net price 2-mL amp = 84p

Brands include *Diazemuls*®

Rectal tubes (= rectal solution), diazepam 2 mg/mL, net price 1.25-mL (2.5-mg) tube = 90p, 2.5-mL (5-mg) tube = £1.27; 4 mg/mL, 2.5-mL (10-mg) tube = £1.49

Brands include *Diazepam Rectubes*®, *Stesolid*®

Suppositories, diazepam 10 mg, net price 6 = £10.20. Label: 2 or 19

Brands include *Valclair*®

DENTAL PRESCRIBING ON NHS. Diazepam Tablets or Diazepam Oral Solution 2 mg/5 mL may be prescribed

ALPRAZOLAM

Indications: anxiety (short-term use)

Cautions: see under Diazepam

Contra-indications: see under Diazepam
Side-effects: see under Diazepam
Dose: 250–500 micrograms 3 times daily (elderly or debilitated 250 micrograms 2–3 times daily), increased if necessary to a total of 3 mg daily; CHILD not recommended

Xanax® (Pharmacia) PoM NHS
Tablets, both scored, alprazolam 250 micrograms, net price 60-tab pack = £3.18; 500 micrograms (pink), 60-tab pack = £6.09. Label: 2

CHLORDIAZEPOXIDE

Indications: anxiety (short-term use); adjunct in acute alcohol withdrawal (section 4.10)
Cautions: see under Diazepam
Contra-indications: see under Diazepam
Side-effects: see under Diazepam
Dose: anxiety, 10 mg 3 times daily increased if necessary to 60–100 mg daily in divided doses; ELDERLY (or debilitated) half adult dose; CHILD not recommended
NOTE. The doses stated above refer equally to chlordiazepoxide and to its hydrochloride

Chlordiazepoxide (Non-proprietary) PoM
Capsules, chlordiazepoxide hydrochloride 5 mg, net price 20 = 83p; 10 mg, 20 = £1.15. Label: 2
Brands include *Librium*® NHS, *Tropium*® NHS

Chlordiazepoxide Hydrochloride (Non-proprietary) PoM
Tablets, chlordiazepoxide hydrochloride 5 mg, net price 20 = 79p; 10 mg, 20 = £1.09. Label: 2

CLORAZEPATE DIPOTASSIUM

Indications: anxiety (short-term use)
Cautions: see under Diazepam
Contra-indications: see under Diazepam
Side-effects: see under Diazepam
Dose: 7.5–22.5 mg daily in 2–3 divided doses *or* a single dose of 15 mg at bedtime; ELDERLY (or debilitated) half adult dose; CHILD not recommended

Tranxene® (Boehringer Ingelheim) PoM NHS
Capsules, clorazepate dipotassium 7.5 mg (maroon/grey), net price 20-cap pack = £2.66. Label: 2 or 19

LORAZEPAM

Indications: short-term use in anxiety or insomnia; status epilepticus (section 4.8.2); peri-operative (section 15.1.4.1)
Cautions: see under Diazepam; short acting; when given parenterally, facilities for managing respiratory depression with mechanical ventilation must be at hand
Contra-indications: see under Diazepam
Side-effects: see under Diazepam
Dose: *by mouth*, anxiety, 1–4 mg daily in divided doses; ELDERLY (or debilitated) half adult dose
Insomnia associated with anxiety, 1–2 mg at bedtime; CHILD not recommended
By intramuscular or slow intravenous injection (into a large vein), acute panic attacks, 25–30 micrograms/kg (usual range 1.5–2.5 mg), repeated every 6 hours if necessary; CHILD not recommended
NOTE. Only use intramuscular route when oral and intravenous routes not possible

Lorazepam (Non-proprietary) PoM
Tablets, lorazepam 1 mg, net price 20 = £1.54; 2.5 mg, 20 = £2.54. Label: 2 or 19
Injection, lorazepam 4 mg/mL. Net price 1-mL amp = 37p
Excipients: include benzyl alcohol, propylene glycol (see Excipients, p. 2)
Brands include *Ativan*®
NOTE. For intramuscular injection it should be diluted with an equal volume of water for injections or physiological saline (but only use when oral and intravenous routes not possible)

OXAZEPAM

Indications: anxiety (short-term use)
Cautions: see under Diazepam; short acting
Contra-indications: see under Diazepam
Side-effects: see under Diazepam
Dose: anxiety, 15–30 mg (elderly or debilitated 10–20 mg) 3–4 times daily; CHILD not recommended
Insomnia associated with anxiety, 15–25 mg (max. 50 mg) at bedtime; CHILD not recommended

Oxazepam (Non-proprietary) PoM
Tablets, oxazepam 10 mg, net price 20 = 96p; 15 mg, 20 = £1.34; 30 mg, 20 = 49p. Label: 2

Buspirone

Buspirone is thought to act at specific serotonin ($5HT_{1A}$) receptors. Response to treatment may take up to 2 weeks. It does not alleviate the symptoms of benzodiazepine withdrawal. Therefore a patient taking a benzodiazepine still needs to have the benzodiazepine withdrawn gradually; it is advisable to do this before starting buspirone. The dependence and abuse potential of buspirone is low; it is, however, licensed for short-term use only (but specialists occasionally use it for several months).

BUSPIRONE HYDROCHLORIDE

Indications: anxiety (short-term use)
Cautions: does not alleviate benzodiazepine withdrawal (see notes above); **interactions:** Appendix 1 (anxiolytics and hypnotics)
DRIVING. May affect performance of skilled tasks (e.g. driving); effects of alcohol may be enhanced
Contra-indications: epilepsy, severe hepatic impairment (Appendix 2), moderate to severe renal impairment (Appendix 3), pregnancy (Appendix 4) and breast-feeding (Appendix 5)
Side-effects: nausea, dizziness, headache, nervousness, lightheadedness, excitement; rarely tachycardia, palpitations, chest pain, drowsiness, confusion, seizures, dry mouth, fatigue, and sweating
Dose: initially 5 mg 2–3 times daily, increased as necessary every 2–3 days; usual range 15–30 mg daily in divided doses; max. 45 mg daily; CHILD not recommended

Buspirone Hydrochloride (Non-proprietary) PoM
Tablets, buspirone hydrochloride 5 mg, net price 30-tab pack = £10.72; 10 mg, 30-tab pack = £16.59. Counselling, driving

Buspar® (Bristol-Myers Squibb) PoM
Tablets, buspirone hydrochloride 5 mg, net price 90-tab pack = £28.08; 10 mg, 90-tab pack = £42.12. Counselling, driving

Beta-blockers

Beta-blockers (e.g. propranolol, oxprenolol) (section 2.4) do not affect psychological symptoms, such as worry, tension, and fear, but they do reduce autonomic symptoms, such as palpitation and tremor; they do not reduce non-autonomic symptoms, such as muscle tension. Beta-blockers are therefore indicated for patients with predominantly somatic symptoms; this, in turn, may prevent the onset of worry and fear. Patients with predominantly psychological symptoms may obtain no benefit.

Meprobamate

Meprobamate is **less effective** than the benzodiazepines, more hazardous in overdosage, and can also induce dependence. It is **not** recommended.

MEPROBAMATE

Indications: short-term use in anxiety, but see notes above

Cautions: respiratory disease, muscle weakness, epilepsy (may induce seizures), history of drug or alcohol abuse, marked personality disorder, pregnancy (Appendix 4); elderly and debilitated; hepatic impairment (Appendix 2), renal impairment (Appendix 3); avoid prolonged use, abrupt withdrawal may precipitate convulsions; **interactions:** Appendix 1 (anxiolytics and hypnotics)

DRIVING. Drowsiness may affect performance of skilled tasks (e.g. driving); effects of alcohol enhanced

Contra-indications: acute pulmonary insufficiency; respiratory depression; porphyria (section 9.8.2); breast-feeding (Appendix 5)

Side-effects: see under Diazepam, but incidence greater and drowsiness most common side-effect; also gastro-intestinal disturbances, hypotension, paraesthesia, weakness, CNS effects including headache, paradoxical excitement, disturbances of vision; rarely agranulocytosis and rashes

Dose: 400 mg 3–4 times daily; elderly patients half adult dose or less; CHILD not recommended

Meprobamate (Non-proprietary) CD
Tablets, scored, meprobamate 400 mg. Net price 84-tab pack = £19.95. Label: 2

4.1.3 Barbiturates

The intermediate-acting **barbiturates** have a place only in the treatment of severe intractable insomnia in patients **already taking** barbiturates; they should be **avoided** in the elderly. The long-acting barbiturate, phenobarbital is still sometimes of value in epilepsy (section 4.8.1) but its use as a sedative is unjustified. The very short-acting barbiturate thiopental is used in anaesthesia (section 15.1.1).

BARBITURATES

Indications: severe intractable insomnia **only** in patients already taking barbiturates; see also notes above

Cautions: avoid use where possible; dependence and tolerance readily occur; abrupt withdrawal may precipitate serious withdrawal syndrome (rebound insomnia, anxiety, tremor, dizziness, nausea, convulsions, delirium, and death); repeated doses are cumulative and may lead to excessive sedation; respiratory disease; renal impairment (Appendix 3); hepatic impairment; **interactions:** Appendix 1 (barbiturates)

DRIVING. Drowsiness may persist the next day and affect performance of skilled tasks (e.g. driving); effects of alcohol enhanced

Contra-indications: insomnia caused by pain; porphyria (section 9.8.2); severe hepatic impairment; children, young adults, elderly and debilitated patients, also patients with history of drug or alcohol abuse; pregnancy (Appendix 4); breast-feeding (Appendix 5)

Side-effects: include hangover with drowsiness, dizziness, ataxia, respiratory depression, hypersensitivity reactions, headache, particularly in elderly; paradoxical excitement and confusion occasionally precede sleep

Dose: see under preparations below

Amytal® (Flynn) CD
Tablets, amobarbital (amylobarbitone) 50 mg, net price 20 = £1.84. Label: 19
Dose: 100–200 mg at bedtime (**important:** but see also contra-indications)

Sodium Amytal® (Flynn) CD
Capsules, both blue, amobarbital (amylobarbitone) sodium 60 mg, net price 20 = £3.43; 200 mg, 20 = £6.75. Label: 19
Dose: 60–200 mg at bedtime (**important:** but see also contra-indications)

Soneryl® (Concord) CD
Tablets, pink, scored, butobarbital (butobarbitone) 100 mg. Net price 56-tab pack = £10.65. Label: 19
Dose: 100–200 mg at bedtime (**important:** but see also contra-indications)

■ Preparations containing secobarbital (quinalbarbitone)

NOTE. Secobarbital (quinalbarbitone) is in schedule 2 of the Misuse of Drugs Regulations 2001; receipt and supply must therefore be recorded in the CD register.

Seconal Sodium® (Flynn) CD
Capsules, both orange, secobarbital (quinalbarbitone) sodium 50 mg, net price 20 = £5.30; 100 mg, 20 = £6.96. Label: 19
Dose: 100 mg at bedtime (**important:** but see also contra-indications)

Tuinal® (Flynn) CD
Capsules, orange/blue, a mixture of amobarbital (amylobarbitone) sodium 50 mg, secobarbital (quinalbarbitone) sodium 50 mg. Net price 20 = £3.88. Label: 19
Dose: 1–2 capsules at bedtime (**important:** but see also contra-indications)
NOTE. Prescriptions need only specify 'Tuinal capsules'

4.2 Drugs used in psychoses and related disorders

Advice of Royal College of Psychiatrists on doses above BNF upper limit. Unless otherwise stated, doses in the BNF are licensed doses—any higher dose is therefore **unlicensed** (for an explanation of the significance of this, see p. 1).

1. Consider alternative approaches including adjuvant therapy and newer or atypical neuroleptics such as clozapine.
2. Bear in mind risk factors, including obesity—particular caution is indicated in older patients especially those over 70.
3. Consider potential for drug interactions—see **interactions:** Appendix 1 (antipsychotics).
4. Carry out ECG to exclude untoward abnormalities such as prolonged QT interval; repeat ECG periodically and reduce dose if prolonged QT interval or other adverse abnormality develops.
5. Increase dose slowly and not more often than once weekly.
6. Carry out regular pulse, blood pressure, and temperature checks; ensure that patient maintains adequate fluid intake.
7. Consider high-dose therapy to be for limited period and review regularly; abandon if no improvement after 3 months (return to standard dosage).

Important: When prescribing an antipsychotic for administration on an emergency basis, the intramuscular dose should be **lower** than the corresponding oral dose (owing to absence of first-pass effect), particularly if the patient is very active (increased blood flow to muscle considerably increases the rate of absorption). The prescription should specify the dose for **each route** and should **not** imply that the same dose can be given by mouth or by intramuscular injection. The dose of antipsychotic for emergency use should be reviewed at least **daily**.

4.2.1 Antipsychotic drugs

Antipsychotic drugs are also known as 'neuroleptics' and (misleadingly) as 'major tranquillisers'. Antipsychotic drugs generally tranquillise without impairing consciousness and without causing paradoxical excitement but they should not be regarded merely as tranquillisers. For conditions such as schizophrenia the tranquillising effect is of secondary importance.

In the short term they are used to quieten disturbed patients whatever the underlying psychopathology, which may be schizophrenia, brain damage, mania, toxic delirium, or agitated depression. Antipsychotic drugs are used to alleviate severe anxiety but this too should be a short-term measure.

SCHIZOPHRENIA. Antipsychotic drugs relieve florid psychotic symptoms such as thought disorder, hallucinations, and delusions, and prevent relapse. Although they are usually less effective in apathetic withdrawn patients, they sometimes appear to have an activating influence. Patients with acute schizophrenia generally respond better than those with chronic symptoms.

Long-term treatment of a patient with a definite diagnosis of schizophrenia may be necessary even after the first episode of illness in order to prevent the manifest illness from becoming chronic. Withdrawal of drug treatment requires careful surveillance because the patient who appears well on medication may suffer a disastrous relapse if treatment is withdrawn inappropriately. In addition the need for continuation of treatment may not become immediately evident because relapse is often delayed for several weeks after cessation of treatment.

Antipsychotic drugs are considered to act by interfering with dopaminergic transmission in the brain by blocking dopamine D_2 receptors, which may give rise to the extrapyramidal effects described below, and also to hyperprolactinaemia. Antipsychotic drugs may also affect cholinergic, alpha-adrenergic, histaminergic, and serotonergic receptors.

CAUTIONS AND CONTRA-INDICATIONS. Antipsychotics should be used with **caution** in patients with hepatic impairment (Appendix 2), renal impairment (Appendix 3), cardiovascular disease, Parkinson's disease (may be exacerbated by antipsychotics), epilepsy (and conditions predisposing to epilepsy), depression, myasthenia gravis, prostatic hypertrophy, or a personal or family history of angle-closure glaucoma (avoid chlorpromazine, pericyazine and prochlorperazine in these conditions). Caution is also required in severe respiratory disease and in patients with a history of jaundice or who have blood dyscrasias (perform blood counts if unexplained infection or fever develops). Antipsychotics should be used with caution in the elderly, who are particularly susceptible to postural hypotension and to hyper- or hypothermia in very hot or cold weather. Serious consideration should be given before prescribing these drugs for elderly patients. As photosensitisation may occur with higher dosages, patients should avoid direct sunlight.

Antipsychotic drugs may be **contra-indicated** in comatose states, CNS depression, and phaeochromocytoma. Most antipsychotics are best avoided during pregnancy, unless essential (Appendix 4) and it is advisable to discontinue breast-feeding during treatment (Appendix 5); **interactions:** Appendix 1 (antipsychotics)

DRIVING. Drowsiness may affect performance of skilled tasks (e.g. driving or operating machinery), especially at start of treatment; effects of alcohol are enhanced

WITHDRAWAL. Withdrawal of antipsychotic drugs after long-term therapy should always be gradual and closely monitored to avoid the risk of acute withdrawal syndromes or rapid relapse.

SIDE-EFFECTS. Extrapyramidal symptoms are the most troublesome. They occur most frequently with the piperazine phenothiazines (fluphenazine, perphenazine, prochlorperazine, and trifluoperazine), the butyrophenones (benperidol and haloperidol), and the depot preparations. They are easy to recognise but cannot be predicted accurately because they depend on the dose, the type of drug, and on individual susceptibility.

Extrapyramidal symptoms consist of:

- *parkinsonian symptoms* (including tremor), which may occur more commonly in adults or the elderly and may appear gradually;
- *dystonia* (abnormal face and body movements) and *dyskinesia*, which occur more commonly in children or young adults and appear after only a few doses;
- *akathisia* (restlessness), which characteristically occurs after large initial doses and may

resemble an exacerbation of the condition being treated; and

- *tardive dyskinesia* (rhythmic, involuntary movements of tongue, face, and jaw), which usually develops on long-term therapy or with high dosage, but it may develop on short-term treatment with low doses—short-lived tardive dyskinesia may occur after withdrawal of the drug.

Parkinsonian symptoms remit if the drug is withdrawn and may be suppressed by the administration of **antimuscarinic** drugs (section 4.9.2). However, routine administration of such drugs is not justified because not all patients are affected and because they may unmask or worsen tardive dyskinesia.

Tardive dyskinesia is of particular concern because it may be irreversible on withdrawing therapy and treatment is usually ineffective. However, some manufacturers suggest that drug withdrawal at the earliest signs of tardive dyskinesia (fine vermicular movements of the tongue) may halt its full development. Tardive dyskinesia occurs fairly frequently, especially in the elderly, and treatment must be carefully and regularly reviewed.

Hypotension and interference with temperature regulation are dose-related side-effects and are liable to cause dangerous falls and hypothermia or hyperthermia in the elderly.

Neuroleptic malignant syndrome (hyperthermia, fluctuating level of consciousness, muscular rigidity, and autonomic dysfunction with pallor, tachycardia, labile blood pressure, sweating, and urinary incontinence) is a rare but potentially fatal side-effect of some drugs. Discontinuation of the antipsychotic is essential because there is no proven effective treatment, but cooling, bromocriptine, and dantrolene have been used. The syndrome, which usually lasts for 5–7 days after drug discontinuation, may be unduly prolonged if depot preparations have been used.

Other side-effects include: drowsiness; apathy; agitation, excitement and insomnia; convulsions; dizziness; headache; confusion; gastro-intestinal disturbances; nasal congestion; antimuscarinic symptoms (such as dry mouth, constipation, difficulty with micturition, and blurred vision); cardiovascular symptoms (such as hypotension, tachycardia, and arrhythmias); ECG changes (cases of sudden death have occurred); endocrine effects such as menstrual disturbances, galactorrhoea, gynaecomastia, impotence, and weight gain; blood dyscrasias (such as agranulocytosis and leucopenia), photosensitisation, contact sensitisation and rashes, and jaundice (including cholestatic); corneal and lens opacities, and purplish pigmentation of the skin, cornea, conjunctiva, and retina.

Overdosage: for poisoning with phenothiazines and related compounds, see Emergency Treatment of Poisoning, p. 33.

CLASSIFICATION OF ANTIPSYCHOTICS. The **phenothiazine** derivatives can be divided into 3 main groups.

Group 1: chlorpromazine, levomepromazine (methotrimeprazine), and promazine, generally characterised by pronounced sedative effects and moderate antimuscarinic and extrapyramidal side-effects.

Group 2: pericyazine and pipotiazine, generally characterised by moderate sedative effects, marked antimuscarinic effects, but fewer extrapyramidal side-effects than groups 1 or 3.

Group 3: fluphenazine, perphenazine, prochlorperazine, and trifluoperazine, generally characterised by fewer sedative effects, fewer antimuscarinic effects, but more pronounced extrapyramidal side-effects than groups 1 and 2.

Drugs of other chemical groups tend to resemble the phenothiazines of *group 3*. They include the **butyrophenones** (benperidol and haloperidol); **diphenylbutylpiperidines** (pimozide); **thioxanthenes** (flupentixol and zuclopenthixol); and the **substituted benzamides** (sulpiride).

For details of the newer antipsychotic drugs amisulpride, clozapine, olanzapine, quetiapine, risperidone, sertindole, and zotepine, see under Atypical Antipsychotics, p. 188.

CHOICE. As indicated above, the various drugs differ somewhat in predominant actions and side-effects. Selection is influenced by the degree of sedation required and the patient's susceptibility to extrapyramidal side-effects. However, the differences between antipsychotic drugs are less important than the great variability in patient response; moreover, tolerance to secondary effects such as sedation usually develops. The atypical antipsychotics may be appropriate if extrapyramidal side-effects are a particular concern (see under Atypical Antipsychotics, below). Clozapine is used for schizophrenia when other antipsychotics are ineffective or not tolerated.

Prescribing of more than one antipsychotic at the same time is **not** recommended; it may constitute a hazard and there is no significant evidence that side-effects are minimised.

Chlorpromazine is still widely used despite the wide range of adverse effects associated with it. It has a marked sedating effect and is useful for treating violent patients without causing stupor. Agitated states in the elderly can be controlled without confusion, a dose of 10 to 25 mg once or twice daily usually being adequate.

Flupentixol (flupenthixol) and **pimozide** (see CSM advice p. 186) are less sedating than chlorpromazine.

Sulpiride in high doses controls florid positive symptoms, but in lower doses it has an alerting effect on apathetic withdrawn schizophrenics.

Fluphenazine, **haloperidol**, and **trifluoperazine** are also of value but their use is limited by the high incidence of extrapyramidal symptoms. Haloperidol may be preferred for the rapid control of hyperactive psychotic states; it causes less hypotension than chlorpromazine and is therefore also popular for agitation and restlessness in the elderly, despite the high incidence of extrapyramidal side-effects.

Promazine is not sufficiently active by mouth to be used as an antipsychotic drug; it has been used to treat agitation and restlessness in the elderly (see Other uses, below).

OTHER USES. Nausea and vomiting (section 4.6), choreas, motor tics (section 4.9.3), and intractable hiccup (see under Chlorpromazine Hydrochloride and under Haloperidol). **Benperidol** is used in deviant antisocial sexual behaviour but its value is not established; see also section 6.4.2 for the role of cyproterone acetate.

Psychomotor agitation and, in the elderly, agitation and restlessness, should be investigated for an underlying cause; they can be managed with low doses of chlorpromazine or haloperidol used for short periods. The use of promazine for agitation and restlessness in the elderly has declined. **Olanzapine** and **risperidone** may be effective for agitation and restlessness in the elderly [both unlicensed].

Equivalent doses of oral antipsychotics

These equivalences are intended **only** as an approximate guide; individual dosage instructions should **also** be checked; patients should be carefully monitored after **any** change in medication

Antipsychotic	Daily dose
Chlorpromazine	100 mg
Clozapine	50 mg
Haloperidol	2–3 mg
Pimozide	2 mg
Risperidone	0.5–1 mg
Sulpiride	200 mg
Trifluoperazine	5 mg

Important. These equivalences must **not** be extrapolated beyond the max. dose for the drug. Higher doses require careful titration in specialist units and the equivalences shown here may not be appropriate

> **Dosage.** After an initial period of stabilisation, in most patients, the long half-life of antipsychotic drugs allows the total daily oral dose to be given as a single dose. For the advice of The Royal College of Psychiatrists on doses above the BNF upper limit, see p. 181.

BENPERIDOL

Indications: control of deviant antisocial sexual behaviour (but see notes above)

Cautions: see notes above; also manufacturer advises regular blood counts and liver function tests during long-term treatment

Contra-indications: see notes above

Side-effects: see notes above

Dose: 0.25–1.5 mg daily in divided doses, adjusted according to the response; ELDERLY (or debilitated) initially half adult dose; CHILD not recommended

Benquil® (Concord) PoM

Tablets, scored, benperidol 250 micrograms, net price 112-tab pack = £104.00. Label: 2

CHLORPROMAZINE HYDROCHLORIDE

WARNING. Owing to the risk of contact sensitisation, pharmacists, nurses, and other health workers should avoid direct contact with chlorpromazine; tablets should not be crushed and solutions should be handled with care

Indications: see under Dose; antiemetic in palliative care (section 4.6)

Cautions: see notes above; also patients should remain supine and the blood pressure monitored for 30 minutes after intramuscular injection

Contra-indications: see notes above

Side-effects: see notes above; also intramuscular injection may be painful, cause hypotension and tachycardia, and give rise to nodule formation

Dose: *by mouth*, schizophrenia and other psychoses, mania, short-term adjunctive management of severe anxiety, psychomotor agitation, excitement, and violent or dangerously impulsive behaviour initially 25 mg 3 times daily (*or* 75 mg at night), adjusted according to response, to usual maintenance dose of 75–300 mg daily (but up to 1 g daily may be required in psychoses); ELDERLY (or debilitated) third to half adult dose; CHILD (childhood schizophrenia and autism) 1–5 years 500 micrograms/kg every 4–6 hours (max. 40 mg daily); 6–12 years third to half adult dose (max. 75 mg daily)

Intractable hiccup, 25–50 mg 3–4 times daily

By deep intramuscular injection, (for relief of acute symptoms but see also Cautions and Side-effects), 25–50 mg every 6–8 hours; CHILD, 1–5 years 500 micrograms/kg every 6–8 hours (max. 40 mg daily); 6–12 years 500 micrograms/kg every 6–8 hours (max. 75 mg daily)

Induction of hypothermia (to prevent shivering), *by deep intramuscular injection*, 25–50 mg every 6–8 hours; CHILD 1–12 years, initially 0.5–1 mg/kg, followed by maintenance 500 micrograms/kg every 4–6 hours

By rectum in suppositories as chlorpromazine base 100 mg every 6–8 hours [unlicensed]

NOTE. For equivalent therapeutic effect 100 mg chlorpromazine base given *rectally* as a suppository ≡ 20–25 mg chlorpromazine hydrochloride *by intramuscular injection* ≡ 40–50 mg of chlorpromazine base or hydrochloride *by mouth*

Chlorpromazine (Non-proprietary) PoM

Tablets, coated, chlorpromazine hydrochloride 10 mg, net price 56-tab pack = 71p; 25 mg, 28-tab pack = £2.23; 50 mg, 28-tab pack = £1.95; 100 mg, 28-tab pack = £2.37. Label: 2, 11

Brands include *Chloractil*®

Oral solution, chlorpromazine hydrochloride 25 mg/5 mL, net price 150 mL = £1.35, 100 mg/5 mL, 150 mL = £3.57. Label: 2, 11

Injection, chlorpromazine hydrochloride 25 mg/mL, net price 1-mL amp = 60p; 2-mL amp = 63p

Suppositories, chlorpromazine 100 mg. Label: 2, 11

'Special order' [unlicensed] product; contact Martindale or regional hospital manufacturing unit

Largactil® (Hawgreen) PoM

Tablets, all off-white, f/c, chlorpromazine hydrochloride 10 mg. Net price 56-tab pack = 66p; 25 mg, 56-tab pack = 91p; 50 mg, 56-tab pack = £1.91; 100 mg, 56-tab pack = £3.54. Label: 2, 11

Syrup, brown, chlorpromazine hydrochloride 25 mg/5 mL. Net price 100-mL pack = £1.03. Label: 2, 11

Suspension forte, orange, sugar-free, chlorpromazine hydrochloride 100 mg (as embonate)/5 mL. Net price 100-mL pack = £2.38. Label: 2, 11

Injection, chlorpromazine hydrochloride 25 mg/mL. Net price 2-mL amp = 63p

FLUPENTIXOL

(Flupenthixol)

Indications: schizophrenia and other psychoses, particularly with apathy and withdrawal but not mania or psychomotor hyperactivity; depression (section 4.3.4)

Cautions: see notes above; avoid in porphyria (section 9.8.2)

Contra-indications: see notes above; also excitable and overactive patients
Side-effects: see notes above; less sedating but extrapyramidal symptoms frequent
Dose: psychosis, initially 3–9 mg twice daily adjusted according to the response; max. 18 mg daily; ELDERLY (or debilitated) initially quarter to half adult dose; CHILD not recommended

Depixol® (Lundbeck) PoM
Tablets, yellow, s/c, flupentixol 3 mg (as dihydrochloride). Net price 20 = £2.78. Label: 2
Depot injection (flupentixol decanoate): section 4.2.2

FLUPHENAZINE HYDROCHLORIDE

Indications: see under Dose
Cautions: see notes above
Contra-indications: see notes above; also marked cerebral atherosclerosis
Side-effects: see notes above; less sedating and fewer antimuscarinic or hypotensive symptoms, but extrapyramidal symptoms, particularly dystonic reactions and akathisia, more frequent; systemic lupus erythematosus, inappropriate antidiuretic hormone secretion, oedema, also reported
Dose: schizophrenia and other psychoses, mania, initially 2.5–10 mg daily in 2–3 divided doses, adjusted according to response to 20 mg daily; doses above 20 mg daily (10 mg in elderly) only with special caution; CHILD not recommended
Short-term adjunctive management of severe anxiety, psychomotor agitation, excitement, and violent or dangerously impulsive behaviour, initially 1 mg twice daily, increased as necessary to 2 mg twice daily; CHILD not recommended

Moditen® (Sanofi-Synthelabo) PoM
Tablets, both s/c, fluphenazine hydrochloride 1 mg (pink), net price 20 = £1.06; 2.5 mg (yellow), 20 = £1.33. Label: 2

Modecate® PoM
Section 4.2.2

HALOPERIDOL

Indications: see under Dose; motor tics (section 4.9.3)
Cautions: see notes above; also subarachnoid haemorrhage and metabolic disturbances such as hypokalaemia, hypocalcaemia, or hypomagnesaemia
Contra-indications: see notes above
Side-effects: see notes above, but less sedating and fewer antimuscarinic or hypotensive symptoms; pigmentation and photosensitivity reactions rare; extrapyramidal symptoms, particularly dystonic reactions and akathisia especially in thyrotoxic patients; rarely weight loss; hypoglycaemia; inappropriate antidiuretic hormone secretion
Dose: *by mouth*, schizophrenia and other psychoses, mania, short-term adjunctive management of psychomotor agitation, excitement, and violent or dangerously impulsive behaviour, initially 1.5–3 mg 2–3 times daily *or* 3–5 mg 2–3 times daily in severely affected or resistant patients; in resistant schizophrenia up to 30 mg daily may be needed; adjusted according to response to lowest effective maintenance dose (as low as 5–10 mg daily); ELDERLY (or debilitated) initially half adult dose; CHILD initially 25–50 micrograms/kg daily (in 2 divided doses) to max. 10 mg
Agitation and restlessness in the elderly, initially 0.5–1.5 mg once or twice daily
Short-term adjunctive management of severe anxiety, 500 micrograms twice daily; CHILD not recommended
Intractable hiccup, 1.5 mg 3 times daily adjusted according to response; CHILD not recommended
Nausea and vomiting, 1 mg daily (see also Prescribing in Palliative Care, p. 16)
By intramuscular or by intravenous injection, initially 2–10 mg, then every 4–8 hours according to response to total max. 18 mg daily; severely disturbed patients may require initial dose of up to 18 mg; ELDERLY (or debilitated) initially half adult dose; CHILD not recommended
Nausea and vomiting, 0.5–2 mg

Haloperidol (Non-proprietary) PoM
Tablets, haloperidol 500 micrograms, net price 28-tab pack = 91p; 1.5 mg, 20 = £1.92; 5 mg, 20 = £3.77; 10 mg, 20 = £4.26; 20 mg, 20 = £8.70. Label: 2

Dozic® (Rosemont) PoM
Oral liquid, sugar-free, haloperidol 1 mg/mL. Net price 100-mL pack = £6.86. Label: 2

Haldol® (Janssen-Cilag) PoM
Tablets, both scored, haloperidol 5 mg (blue), net price 20 = £1.56; 10 mg (yellow), 20 = £3.05. Label: 2
Oral liquid, sugar-free, haloperidol 2 mg/mL. Net price 100-mL pack (with pipette) = £4.83. Label: 2
Injection, haloperidol 5 mg/mL. Net price 1-mL amp = 31p
Depot injection (haloperidol decanoate): section 4.2.2

Serenace® (IVAX) PoM
Capsules, green, haloperidol 500 micrograms, net price 30-cap pack = 98p. Label: 2
Tablets, haloperidol 1.5 mg, net price 30-tab pack = £1.73; 5 mg (pink), 30-tab pack = £4.90; 10 mg (pale pink), 30-tab pack = £8.81. Label: 2
Oral liquid, sugar-free, haloperidol 2 mg/mL, net price 500-mL pack = £43.83. Label: 2
Injection, haloperidol 5 mg/mL, net price 1-mL amp = 59p; 10 mg/mL, 2-mL amp = £2.03

LEVOMEPROMAZINE

(Methotrimeprazine)
Indications: see under Dose
Cautions: see notes above; patients receiving large initial doses should remain supine
ELDERLY. Risk of postural hypotension; not recommended for ambulant patients over 50 years unless risk of hypotensive reaction assessed
Contra-indications: see notes above
Side-effects: see notes above; occasionally raised erythrocyte sedimentation rate occurs
Dose: *by mouth*, schizophrenia, initially 25–50 mg daily in divided doses increased as necessary; bedpatients initially 100–200 mg daily usually in 3 divided doses, increased if necessary to 1 g daily; ELDERLY, see Cautions
Adjunctive treatment in palliative care (including management of pain and associated restlessness, distress, or vomiting), 12.5–50 mg every 4–8 hours, but see also Prescribing in Palliative Care, p. 15 and p. 16

By intramuscular injection or by intravenous injection (by intravenous injection after dilution with an equal volume of sodium chloride 0.9% injection), adjunct in palliative care, 12.5–25 mg (severe agitation up to 50 mg) every 6–8 hours if necessary

By continuous subcutaneous infusion, adjunct in palliative care (via syringe driver), diluted in a suitable volume of sodium chloride 0.9% injection, see Prescribing in Palliative Care, p. 16; CHILD (experience limited), 0.35–3 mg/kg daily

Nozinan® (Link) PoM

Tablets, scored, levomepromazine maleate 25 mg, net price 84-tab pack = £20.26. Label: 2

Injection, levomepromazine hydrochloride 25 mg/mL, net price 1-mL amp = £2.01

PERICYAZINE

(Periciazine)

Indications: see under Dose

Cautions: see notes above

Contra-indications: see notes above

Side-effects: see notes above; more sedating; hypotension common when treatment initiated; respiratory depression

Dose: schizophrenia and other psychoses, initially 75 mg daily in divided doses increased at weekly intervals by steps of 25 mg according to response; usual max. 300 mg daily (elderly initially 15–30 mg daily)

Short-term adjunctive management of severe anxiety, psychomotor agitation, and violent or dangerously impulsive behaviour, initially 15–30 mg (elderly 5–10 mg) daily divided into 2 doses, taking the larger dose at bedtime, adjusted according to response

CHILD and INFANT over 1 year (severe mental or behavioural disorders only), initially, 500 micrograms daily for 10-kg child, increased by 1 mg for each additional 5 kg to max. total daily dose of 10 mg; dose may be gradually increased according to response but maintenance should not exceed twice initial dose

INFANT under 1 year not recommended

Neulactil® (JHC) PoM

Tablets, all yellow, scored, pericyazine 2.5 mg, net price 84-tab pack = £7.15; 10 mg, 84-tab pack = £19.33. Label: 2

Syrup forte, brown, pericyazine 10 mg/5 mL. Net price 100-mL pack = £9.37. Label: 2

PERPHENAZINE

Indications: see under Dose; anti-emetic (section 4.6)

Cautions: see notes above

Contra-indications: see notes above; also agitation and restlessness in the elderly

Side-effects: see notes above; less sedating; extrapyramidal symptoms, especially dystonia, more frequent, particularly at high dosage; rarely systemic lupus erythematosus

Dose: schizophrenia and other psychoses, mania, short-term adjunctive management of anxiety, severe psychomotor agitation, excitement, and violent or dangerously impulsive behaviour, initially 4 mg 3 times daily adjusted according to the response; max. 24 mg daily; ELDERLY quarter to half adult dose (but see Cautions); CHILD under 14 years not recommended

Fentazin® (Goldshield) PoM

Tablets, both s/c, perphenazine 2 mg, net price 20 = £3.73; 4 mg, 20 = £4.39. Label: 2

PIMOZIDE

Indications: see under Dose

Cautions: see notes above

CSM WARNING. Following reports of sudden unexplained death, the CSM recommends ECG before treatment. The CSM also recommends that patients on pimozide should have an annual ECG (if the QT interval is prolonged, treatment should be reviewed and either withdrawn or dose reduced under close supervision) and that pimozide should **not** be given with other antipsychotic drugs (including depot preparations), tricyclic antidepressants or other drugs which prolong the QT interval, such as certain antimalarials, anti-arrhythmic drugs and certain antihistamines and should **not** be given with drugs which cause electrolyte disturbances (especially diuretics)

Contra-indications: see notes above; history of arrhythmias or congenital QT prolongation

Side-effects: see notes above; less sedating; serious arrhythmias reported; glycosuria and, rarely, hyponatraemia reported

Dose: schizophrenia, initially 2 mg daily, increased according to response in steps of 2–4 mg at intervals of not less than 1 week; usual dose range 2–20 mg daily; ELDERLY half usual starting dose; CHILD not recommended

Monosymptomatic hypochondriacal psychosis, paranoid psychosis, initially 4 mg daily, increased according to response in steps of 2–4 mg at intervals of not less than 1 week; max. 16 mg daily; ELDERLY half usual starting dose; CHILD not recommended

Orap® (Janssen-Cilag) PoM

Tablets, scored, green, pimozide 4 mg, net price 20 = £5.83. Label: 2

PROCHLORPERAZINE

Indications: see under Dose; anti-emetic (section 4.6)

Cautions: see notes above; also hypotension more likely after intramuscular injection

Contra-indications: see notes above; children, but see section 4.6 for use as anti-emetic

Side-effects: see notes above; less sedating; extrapyramidal symptoms, particularly dystonias, more frequent; respiratory depression may occur in susceptible patients

Dose: *by mouth*, schizophrenia and other psychoses, mania, prochlorperazine maleate or mesilate, 12.5 mg twice daily for 7 days adjusted at intervals of 4–7 days to usual dose of 75–100 mg daily according to response; CHILD not recommended

Short-term adjunctive management of severe anxiety, 15–20 mg daily in divided doses; max. 40 mg daily; CHILD not recommended

By deep intramuscular injection, psychoses, mania, prochlorperazine mesilate 12.5–25 mg 2–3 times daily; CHILD not recommended

By rectum in suppositories, psychoses, mania, the equivalent of prochlorperazine maleate 25 mg 2–3 times daily; CHILD not recommended

■ Preparations

Section 4.6

PROMAZINE HYDROCHLORIDE

Indications: see under Dose
Cautions: see notes above; also cerebral arteriosclerosis
Contra-indications: see notes above
Side-effects: see notes above; also haemolytic anaemia
Dose: *by mouth*, short-term adjunctive management of psychomotor agitation, 100–200 mg 4 times daily; CHILD not recommended
Agitation and restlessness in elderly, 25–50 mg 4 times daily
By intramuscular injection, short-term adjunctive management of psychomotor agitation, 50 mg (25 mg in elderly or debilitated), repeated if necessary after 6–8 hours; CHILD not recommended

Promazine (Non-proprietary) PoM
Tablets ▲, coated, promazine hydrochloride 25 mg, net price 20 = 85p; 50 mg, 20 = £1.37. Label: 2
Oral solution ▲, promazine hydrochloride 25 mg/5 mL, net price 150 mL = £3.51; 50 mg/5 mL, 150 mL = £3.51. Label: 2

SULPIRIDE

Indications: schizophrenia
Cautions: see notes above; also excited, agitated, or aggressive patients (even low doses may aggravate symptoms)
Contra-indications: see notes above; also porphyria (section 9.8.2)
Side-effects: see notes above; also hepatitis
Dose: 200–400 mg twice daily; max. 800 mg daily in predominantly negative symptoms, and 2.4 g daily in mainly positive symptoms; ELDERLY, lower initial dose, increased gradually according to response; CHILD under 14 years not recommended

Sulpiride (Non-proprietary) PoM
Tablets, sulpiride 200 mg, net price 100-tab pack = £13.97; 400 mg, 100-tab pack = £36.29. Label: 2

Dolmatil® (Sanofi-Synthelabo) PoM
Tablets, both scored, sulpiride 200 mg, net price 100-tab pack = £13.85; 400 mg (f/c), 100-tab pack = £36.29. Label: 2

Sulpitil® (Pharmacia) PoM
Tablets, scored, sulpiride 200 mg. Net price 28-tab pack = £4.29; 112-tab pack = £12.85. Label: 2

Sulpor® (Rosemont) PoM
Oral solution, sugar-free, lemon- and aniseed-flavoured, sulpiride 200 mg/5 mL, net price 150 mL = £25.38. Label: 2

TRIFLUOPERAZINE

Indications: see under Dose; anti-emetic (section 4.6)
Cautions: see notes above
Contra-indications: see notes above
Side-effects: see notes above; extrapyramidal symptoms more frequent, especially at doses exceeding 6 mg daily; pancytopenia; thrombocytopenia; hyperpyrexia; anorexia
Dose: *by mouth* (reduce initial doses in elderly by at least half)
Schizophrenia and other psychoses, short-term adjunctive management of psychomotor agitation, excitement, and violent or dangerously impulsive behaviour, initially 5 mg twice daily, *or* 10 mg daily in modified-release form, increased by 5 mg after 1 week, then at intervals of 3 days, according to the response; CHILD up to 12 years, initially up to 5 mg daily in divided doses, adjusted according to response, age, and body-weight
Short-term adjunctive management of severe anxiety, 2–4 mg daily in divided doses *or* 2–4 mg daily in modified-release form, increased if necessary to 6 mg daily; CHILD 3–5 years up to 1 mg daily, 6–12 years up to 4 mg daily

Trifluoperazine (Non-proprietary) PoM
Tablets, coated, trifluoperazine (as hydrochloride) 1 mg, net price 20 = 53p; 5 mg, 20 = 87p. Label: 2
Oral solution, trifluoperazine (as hydrochloride) 5 mg/5 mL. Net price 200-mL = £11.07. Label: 2

Stelazine® (Goldshield) PoM
Tablets, both blue, f/c, trifluoperazine (as hydrochloride) 1 mg, net price 20 = 61p; 5 mg, 20 = 87p. Label: 2
Spansules® (= capsules m/r), all clear/yellow, enclosing dark blue, light blue, and white pellets, trifluoperazine (as hydrochloride) 2 mg, net price 60-cap pack = £4.65; 10 mg, 30-cap pack = £2.83; 15 mg, 30-cap pack = £4.27. Label: 2, 25
Syrup, sugar-free, yellow, trifluoperazine (as hydrochloride) 1 mg/5 mL, net price 200-mL pack = £2.95. Label: 2
Oral solution forte, sugar-free, yellow, peach-flavour, trifluoperazine (as hydrochloride) 5 mg/5 mL, net price 200-mL pack = £10.99. Label: 2

ZUCLOPENTHIXOL ACETATE

Indications: short-term management of acute psychosis, mania, or exacerbations of chronic psychosis
Cautions: see notes above; avoid in porphyria (section 9.8.2)
Contra-indications: see notes above
Side-effects: see notes above
Dose: *by deep intramuscular injection* into the gluteal muscle or lateral thigh, 50–150 mg (ELDERLY 50–100 mg), if necessary repeated after 2–3 days (1 additional dose may be needed 1–2 days after the first injection); max. cumulative dose 400 mg per course and max. 4 injections; max. duration of treatment 2 weeks—if maintenance treatment necessary change to an oral antipsychotic 2–3 days after last injection, *or* to a longer acting antipsychotic depot injection given concomitantly with last injection of zuclopenthixol acetate; CHILD not recommended

Clopixol Acuphase® (Lundbeck) PoM
Injection (oily), zuclopenthixol acetate 50 mg/mL. Net price 1-mL amp = £4.84; 2-mL amp = £9.33

ZUCLOPENTHIXOL DIHYDROCHLORIDE

Indications: schizophrenia and other psychoses, particularly when associated with agitated, aggressive, or hostile behaviour
Cautions: see notes above; avoid in porphyria (section 9.8.2)
Contra-indications: see notes above; apathetic or withdrawn states

Side-effects: see notes above; urinary frequency or incontinence; weight loss (less common than weight gain)

Dose: initially 20–30 mg daily in divided doses, increasing to a max. of 150 mg daily if necessary; usual maintenance dose 20–50 mg daily; ELDERLY (or debilitated) initially quarter to half adult dose; CHILD not recommended

Clopixol® (Lundbeck) PoM

Tablets, all f/c, pink, zuclopenthixol (as dihydrochloride) 2 mg, net price 20 = 60p; 10 mg, 20 = £1.61; 25 mg, 20 = £3.22. Label: 2

Depot injection (zuclopenthixol decanoate): section 4.2.2

Atypical antipsychotics

The 'atypical antipsychotics' **amisulpride**, **aripiprazole**, **clozapine**, **olanzapine**, **quetiapine**, **risperidone**, and **zotepine** may be better tolerated than other antipsychotics; extrapyramidal symptoms may be less frequent than with older antipsychotics.

Aripiprazole, clozapine, olanzapine, quetiapine, and sertindole cause little or no elevation of prolactin concentration; when changing from other antipsychotics, a reduction in prolactin may increase fertility.

Clozapine is licensed for the treatment of schizophrenia only in patients unresponsive to, or intolerant of, conventional antipsychotic drugs. It can cause agranulocytosis and its use is restricted to patients registered with a clozapine patient monitoring service (see under preparations, below).

Sertindole has been reintroduced following an earlier suspension of the drug because of concerns about arrhythmias; its use is restricted to patients who are enrolled in clinical studies and who are intolerant of at least one other antipsychotic.

NICE guidance (atypical antipsychotics for schizophrenia). NICE has recommended (June 2002) that:

- the atypical antipsychotics (amisulpride, olanzapine, quetiapine, risperidone, and zotepine) should be considered when choosing first-line treatment of *newly diagnosed schizophrenia*;
- an atypical antipsychotic is considered the treatment option of choice for managing an *acute schizophrenic episode* when discussion with the individual is not possible;
- an atypical antipsychotic should be considered for an individual who is suffering unacceptable side-effects from a conventional antipsychotic;
- an atypical antipsychotic should be considered for an individual in relapse whose symptoms were previously inadequately controlled;
- changing to an atypical antipsychotic is not necessary if a conventional antipsychotic controls symptoms adequately and the individual does not suffer unacceptable side-effects;
- clozapine should be introduced if schizophrenia is inadequately controlled despite the sequential use of two or more antipsychotics (one of which should be an atypical antipsychotic) each for at least 6–8 weeks.

CAUTIONS AND CONTRA-INDICATIONS. While atypical antipsychotics have not generally been associated with clinically significant prolongation of the QT interval, they should be used with care if prescribed with other drugs that increase the QT interval. Atypical antipsychotics should be used with caution in patients with cardiovascular disease, or a history of epilepsy; they should be used with caution in the elderly; **interactions:** Appendix 1 (antipsychotics).

Atypical antipsychotics and stroke. Olanzapine and risperidone are associated with an increased risk of stroke in elderly patients with dementia. The CSM has advised:

- risperidone or olanzapine should **not** be used for treating behavioural symptoms of dementia;
- for acute psychotic conditions in elderly patients with dementia, risperidone should be limited to short-term use under specialist advice; olanzapine is not licensed for acute psychoses;
- the possibility of cerebrovascular events should be considered carefully before treating any patient with a history of stroke or transient ischaemic attack; risk factors for cerebrovascular disease (e.g. hypertension, diabetes, smoking, and atrial fibrillation) should also be considered.

DRIVING. Atypical antipsychotics may affect performance of skilled tasks (e.g. driving); effects of alcohol are enhanced.

WITHDRAWAL. Withdrawal of antipsychotic drugs after long-term therapy should always be gradual and closely monitored to avoid the risk of acute withdrawal syndromes or rapid relapse.

SIDE-EFFECTS. Side-effects of the atypical antipsychotics include weight gain, dizziness, postural hypotension (especially during initial dose titration) which may be associated with syncope or reflex tachycardia in some patients, extrapyramidal symptoms (usually mild and transient and which respond to dose reduction or to an antimuscarinic drug), and occasionally tardive dyskinesia on long-term administration (discontinue drug on appearance of early signs). Hyperglycaemia and sometimes diabetes can occur, particularly with clozapine and olanzapine; monitoring weight and plasma glucose may identify the development of hyperglycaemia. Neuroleptic malignant syndrome has been reported rarely.

AMISULPRIDE

Indications: schizophrenia

Cautions: see notes above; also renal impairment (Appendix 3); Parkinson's disease; elderly (risk of hypotension or sedation)

Contra-indications: see notes above; also pregnancy (Appendix 4) and breast-feeding (Appendix 5), phaeochromocytoma, prolactin-dependent tumours

Side-effects: see notes above; also insomnia, anxiety, agitation, drowsiness, gastro-intestinal disorders such as constipation, nausea, vomiting, and dry mouth; hyperprolactinaemia (with galactorrhoea, amenorrhoea, gynaecomastia, breast pain, sexual dysfunction), occasionally bradycardia

Dose: acute psychotic episode, 400–800 mg daily in divided doses, adjusted according to response; max. 1.2 g daily

Predominantly negative symptoms, 50–300 mg daily; CHILD under 15 years, not recommended

NOTE. Doses up to 300 mg may be administered once daily

Solian® (Sanofi-Synthelabo) PoM

Tablets, scored, amisulpride 50 mg, net price 60-tab pack = £18.36; 100 mg, 60-tab pack = £36.72; 200 mg, 60-tab pack = £61.38, 400 mg, 60-tab pack = £122.76. Label: 2

Solution, 100 mg/mL, net price 60 mL (caramel flavour) = £30.69. Label: 2

ARIPIPRAZOLE

Indications: schizophrenia

Cautions: see notes above; history of convulsions; elderly (reduce initial dose); hepatic impairment (Appendix 2); pregnancy (Appendix 4)

Contra-indications: see notes above; breast-feeding (Appendix 5)

Side-effects: see notes above; nausea, vomiting, dyspepsia, constipation, insomnia, akathisia, somnolence, tremor, headache, asthenia, blurred vision; *less commonly* tachycardia, seizures; *very rarely* increased salivation, pancreatitis, chest pain, agitation, speech disorder, stiffness, rhabdomyolysis

Dose: 15 mg daily; max. 30 mg daily; CHILD and ADOLESCENT not recommended

Abilify® (Bristol-Myers Squibb) ▼ PoM

Tablets, aripiprazole 5 mg (blue), net price 28-tab pack = £101.63; 10 mg (pink), 28-tab pack = £101.63; 15 mg (yellow), 28-tab pack = £101.63; 30 mg (pink), 28-tab pack = £203.26. Counselling, driving

CLOZAPINE

Indications: schizophrenia (including psychosis in Parkinson's disease) in patients unresponsive to, or intolerant of, conventional antipsychotic drugs

Cautions: see notes above; monitor leucocyte and differential blood counts (see Agranulocytosis, below); taper off conventional neuroleptic before starting; hepatic impairment (Appendix 2); renal impairment (Appendix 3); prostatic hypertrophy, angle-closure glaucoma

WITHDRAWAL. On planned withdrawal reduce dose over 1–2 weeks to avoid risk of rebound psychosis. If abrupt withdrawal necessary observe patient carefully

AGRANULOCYTOSIS. Neutropenia and potentially fatal agranulocytosis reported. Leucocyte and differential blood counts must be normal before starting; monitor counts every week for 18 weeks then at least every 2 weeks and if clozapine continued and blood count stable after 1 year at least every 4 weeks (and 4 weeks after discontinuation); if leucocyte count below 3000/mm^3 or if absolute neutrophil count below 1500/mm^3 discontinue permanently and refer to haematologist. Avoid drugs which depress leucopoiesis; patients should report immediately symptoms of infection, especially influenza-like illness

MYOCARDITIS AND CARDIOMYOPATHY. Fatal myocarditis (most commonly in first 2 months) and cardiomyopathy reported. The CSM has advised:

- physical examination and medical history before starting clozapine;
- specialist examination if cardiac abnormalities or history of heart disease found—clozapine initiated only in absence of severe heart disease and if benefit outweighs risk;
- persistent tachycardia especially in first 2 months should prompt observation for other indicators for myocarditis or cardiomyopathy;
- if myocarditis or cardiomyopathy suspected clozapine should be stopped and patient evaluated urgently by cardiologist;
- discontinue permanently in clozapine-induced myocarditis or cardiomyopathy

GASTRO-INTESTINAL OBSTRUCTION. Reactions resembling gastro-intestinal obstruction reported. Clozapine should be used cautiously with drugs which cause constipation (e.g. antimuscarinic drugs) or in history of colonic disease or bowel surgery. Monitor for constipation and prescribe laxative if required

Contra-indications: severe cardiac disorders (e.g. myocarditis; see Myocarditis and Cardiomyopathy, above); active liver disease (Appendix 2), severe renal impairment (Appendix 3); history of neutropenia or agranulocytosis; bone-marrow disorders; paralytic ileus (see Gastro-intestinal Obstruction, above); alcoholic and toxic psychoses; history of circulatory collapse; drug intoxication; coma or severe CNS depression; uncontrolled epilepsy; pregnancy (Appendix 4) and breast-feeding (Appendix 5)

Side-effects: see notes above; also constipation (see Gastro-intestinal Obstruction, above), hypersalivation, nausea, vomiting; tachycardia, ECG changes, hypertension; drowsiness, blurred vision, headache, tremor, rigidity, extrapyramidal symptoms, convulsions, fatigue, impaired temperature regulation, fever; hepatitis, cholestatic jaundice, pancreatitis; urinary incontinence and retention; agranulocytosis (**important:** see Agranulocytosis, above), leucopenia, eosinophilia, leucocytosis; rarely dysphagia, circulatory collapse, arrhythmias, myocarditis (**important:** see Myocarditis and Cardiomyopathy, above), pericarditis, thromboembolism, confusion, delirium, restlessness, agitation, diabetes mellitus; also reported, intestinal obstruction, paralytic ileus (see Gastro-intestinal Obstruction, above), enlarged parotid gland, fulminant hepatic necrosis, thrombocytopenia, thrombocythaemia, hypertriglyceridaemia, hypercholesterolaemia, cardiomyopathy, cardiac arrest, respiratory arrest, interstitial nephritis, priapism, skin reactions

Dose: schizophrenia, ADULT over 16 years (close medical supervision on initiation—risk of collapse due to hypotension) 12.5 mg once or twice on first day then 25–50 mg on second day then increased gradually (if well tolerated) in steps of 25–50 mg daily over 14–21 days up to 300 mg daily in divided doses (larger dose at night, up to 200 mg daily may be taken as a single dose at bedtime); if necessary may be further increased in steps of 50–100 mg once (preferably) or twice weekly; usual dose 200–450 mg daily (max. 900 mg daily)

NOTE. *Restarting* after *interval of more than 2 days*, 12.5 mg once or twice on first day (but may be feasible to increase more quickly than on initiation)—extreme caution if previous respiratory or cardiac arrest with initial dosing

ELDERLY AND SPECIAL RISK GROUPS. In *elderly*, 12.5 mg once on first day—subsequent adjustments restricted to 25 mg daily

Psychosis in Parkinson's disease, ADULT over 16 years, 12.5 mg at bedtime then increased in steps of 12.5 mg up to twice weekly to 50 mg at bedtime; usual dose range 25–37.5 mg at bedtime; exceptionally, dose may be increased further in steps of

12.5 mg weekly to max. 100 mg daily in 1–2 divided doses

Clozaril® (Novartis) PoM
Tablets, both yellow, clozapine 25 mg (scored), net price 28-tab pack = £6.17, 84-tab pack (hosp. only) = £18.49; 100 mg, 28-tab pack = £24.64, 84-tab pack (hosp. only) = £73.92. Label: 2, 10, patient information leaflet
NOTE. Patient, prescriber, and supplying pharmacist must be registered with the Clozaril Patient Monitoring Service—takes several days to do this

Denzapine® (Denfleet) PoM
Tablets, both yellow, scored, clozapine 25 mg, net price 28-tab pack = £6.17, 84-tab pack = £18.49; 100 mg, 28-tab pack = £24.64, 84-tab pack = £73.92. Label: 2, 10, patient information leaflet
NOTE. Patient, prescriber, and supplying pharmacist must be registered with the Denzapine Patient Monitoring Service—takes several days to do this

Zaponex® (IVAX) PoM
Tablets, both yellow, scored, clozapine 25 mg, net price 84-tab pack = £22.17; 100 mg, 84-tab pack = £88.68. Label: 2, 10, patient information leaflet
NOTE. Patient, prescriber, and supplying pharmacist must be registered with the Zaponex Treatment Access System—takes several days to do this

OLANZAPINE

Indications: see under Dose

Cautions: see notes above (including advice on atypical antipsychotics and stroke); also prostatic hypertrophy, paralytic ileus, diabetes mellitus (risk of exacerbation or ketoacidosis), low leucocyte or neutrophil count, bone-marrow depression, hypereosinophilic disorders, myeloproliferative disease, Parkinson's disease; hepatic impairment (Appendix 2); renal impairment (Appendix 3); pregnancy (Appendix 4); **interactions:** Appendix 1 (antipsychotics)
CNS AND RESPIRATORY DEPRESSION. Blood pressure, pulse and respiratory rate should be monitored for at least 4 hours after intramuscular injection, particularly in those also receiving another antipsychotic or benzodiazepine

Contra-indications: angle-closure glaucoma; breast-feeding (Appendix 5); *for injection*, acute myocardial infarction, unstable angina, severe hypotension or bradycardia, sick sinus syndrome, recent heart surgery

Side-effects: see notes above; also mild, transient antimuscarinic effects; drowsiness, speech difficulty, exacerbation of Parkinson's disease, abnormal gait, hallucinations, akathisia, asthenia, increased appetite, increased body temperature, raised triglyceride concentration, oedema, hyperprolactinaemia (but clinical manifestations rare); urinary incontinence; eosinophilia; *less commonly* hypotension, bradycardia, photosensitivity; *rarely* thromboembolism, seizures, urinary retention, priapism, leucopenia, neutropenia, thrombocytopenia, rhabdomyolysis, rash, hepatitis, pancreatitis; *with injection*, injection-site reactions, sinus pause, hypoventilation

Dose: schizophrenia, combination therapy for mania, preventing recurrence in bipolar disorder, *by mouth*, ADULT over 18 years, 10 mg daily adjusted to usual range of 5–20 mg daily; doses greater than 10 mg daily only after reassessment; max. 20 mg daily

Monotherapy for mania, *by mouth*, ADULT over 18 years, 15 mg daily adjusted to usual range of 5–20 mg daily; doses greater than 15 mg only after reassessment; max. 20 mg daily

Control of agitation and disturbed behaviour in schizophrenia or mania, *by intramuscular injection*, ADULT over 18 years, initially 5–10 mg (usual dose 10 mg) as a single dose followed by 5–10 mg after 2 hours if necessary; ELDERLY initially 2.5–5 mg as a single dose followed by 2.5–5 mg after 2 hours if necessary; max. 3 injections daily for 3 days; max. daily combined oral and parenteral dose 20 mg

NOTE. When one or more factors present that might result in slower metabolism (e.g. female gender, elderly, non-smoker) consider lower initial dose and more gradual dose increase

Zyprexa® (Lilly) PoM
Tablets, f/c, olanzapine 2.5 mg, net price 28-tab pack = £33.29; 5 mg, 28-tab pack = £48.78; 7.5 mg, 56-tab pack = £146.34; 10 mg, 28-tab pack = £79.45, 56-tab pack = £158.90; 15 mg (blue), 28-tab pack = £146.34. Label: 2
Orodispersible tablet (*Velotab*®), olanzapine 5 mg, net price 28-tab pack = £56.10; 10 mg, 28-tab pack = £112.19; 15 mg, 28-tab pack = £168.29. Label: 2, counselling, administration
Excipients: include aspartame (section 9.4.1)
COUNSELLING. *Velotab*® may be placed on the tongue and allowed to dissolve or dispersed in water, orange juice, apple juice, milk, or coffee
Injection▼, powder for reconstitution, olanzapine 5 mg/mL, net price 10-mg vial = £3.48

QUETIAPINE

Indications: schizophrenia; treatment of episodes of mania either alone or with mood stabilisers

Cautions: see notes above; also pregnancy (Appendix 4), hepatic impairment (Appendix 2), renal impairment (Appendix 3), cerebrovascular disease

Contra-indications: breast-feeding (Appendix 5)

Side-effects: see notes above; also drowsiness, dyspepsia, constipation, dry mouth, mild asthenia, rhinitis, tachycardia; leucopenia, neutropenia and occasionally eosinophilia reported; elevated plasma-triglyceride and cholesterol concentrations, reduced plasma-thyroid hormone concentrations; possible QT interval prolongation; rarely oedema; very rarely priapism

Dose: schizophrenia 25 mg twice daily on day 1, 50 mg twice daily on day 2, 100 mg twice daily on day 3, 150 mg twice daily on day 4, then adjusted according to response, usual range 300–450 mg daily in 2 divided doses; max. 750 mg daily; ELDERLY initially 25 mg daily as a single dose, increased in steps of 25–50 mg daily in 2 divided doses; CHILD and ADOLESCENT not recommended

Mania, 50 mg twice daily on day 1, 100 mg twice daily on day 2, 150 mg twice daily on day 3, 200 mg twice daily on day 4, then adjusted according to response in steps of up to 200 mg daily to max. 800 mg daily; usual range 400–800 mg daily in 2 divided doses; ELDERLY initially 25 mg daily as a single dose, increased in steps of 25–50 mg daily in 2 divided doses; CHILD and ADOLESCENT not recommended

Seroquel® (AstraZeneca) PoM
Tablets, f/c, quetiapine (as fumarate) 25 mg (peach), net price 60-tab pack = £28.20; 100 mg (yellow),

60-tab pack = £113.10; 150 mg (pale yellow), 60-tab pack = £113.10; 200 mg (white), 60-tab pack = £113.10; 300 mg (white), 60-tab pack = £170.00. Label: 2

RISPERIDONE

Indications: acute and chronic psychoses, mania

Cautions: see notes above (including advice on atypical antipsychotics and stroke); Parkinson's disease; pregnancy (Appendix 4); hepatic impairment (Appendix 2), renal impairment (Appendix 3)

Contra-indications: breast-feeding (Appendix 5)

Side-effects: see notes above; also insomnia, agitation, anxiety, headache; *less commonly* drowsiness, impaired concentration, fatigue, blurred vision, constipation, nausea and vomiting, dyspepsia, abdominal pain, hyperprolactinaemia (with galactorrhoea, menstrual disturbances, gynaecomastia), sexual dysfunction, priapism, urinary incontinence, tachycardia, hypertension, oedema, rash, rhinitis; cerebrovascular accident, neutropenia and thrombocytopenia have been reported; *rarely* seizures, hyponatraemia, abnormal temperature regulation, and epistaxis

Dose: psychoses, 2 mg in 1–2 divided doses on first day *then* 4 mg in 1–2 divided doses on second day (slower titration appropriate in some patients); usual dose range 4–6 mg daily; doses above 10 mg daily only if benefit considered to outweigh risk (max. 16 mg daily); ELDERLY (or in hepatic or renal impairment) initially 500 micrograms twice daily increased in steps of 500 micrograms twice daily to 1–2 mg twice daily; CHILD under 15 years not recommended

Mania, initially 2 mg once daily, increased if necessary in steps of 1 mg daily; usual dose range 1–6 mg daily; ELDERLY (or in hepatic or renal impairment) initially 500 micrograms twice daily increased in steps of 500 micrograms twice daily to 1–2 mg twice daily

Risperdal® (Janssen-Cilag) PoM

Tablets, f/c, scored, risperidone 500 micrograms (brown-red), net price 20-tab pack = £7.06; 1 mg (white), 20-tab pack = £11.61, 60-tab pack = £34.84; 2 mg (orange), 60-tab pack = £68.69; 3 mg (yellow), 60-tab pack = £101.01; 4 mg (green), 60-tab pack = £133.34; 6 mg (yellow), 28-tab pack = £94.28. Label: 2

Orodispersible tablets (*Quicklet®*), all pink, risperidone 500 micrograms, net price 28-tab pack = £11.43; 1 mg, 28-tab pack = £18.39; 2 mg, 28-tab pack = £34.66. Label: 2, counselling, administration

Excipients: include aspartame (section 9.4.1)

COUNSELLING. Tablets should be placed on the tongue, allowed to dissolve and swallowed

Liquid, risperidone 1 mg/mL, net price 100 mL = £56.12. Label: 2

NOTE. Liquid may be diluted with mineral water, orange juice or black coffee (should be taken immediately)

Depot injection: section 4.2.2

SERTINDOLE

Indications: schizophrenia, see also notes above

Cautions: see notes above; hepatic impairment (Appendix 2); diabetes; correct hypokalaemia or hypomagnesaemia before treatment; monitor ECG during treatment; monitor blood pressure during dose titration and early maintenance therapy (risk of postural hypotension)

Contra-indications: see notes above; pregnancy (Appendix 4), breast-feeding (Appendix 5), severe hepatic impairment, QT interval prolongation (ECG required before and during treatment—consult product literature); concomitant administration of drugs which prolong QT interval (see interactions); uncorrected hypokalaemia or hypomagnesaemia

Side-effects: see notes above; prolonged QT interval, peripheral oedema, dry mouth, rhinitis, nasal congestion, dyspnoea, paraesthesia, abnormal ejaculation (decreased volume); rarely seizures, hyperglycaemia

Dose: initially 4 mg daily increased in steps of 4 mg at intervals of 4–5 days to usual maintenance of 12–20 mg as a single daily dose; max. 24 mg daily; ELDERLY consider slower dose titration and lower maintenance dose; CHILD and ADOLESCENT not recommended

Serdolect® (Lundbeck) ▼ PoM

Tablets, f/c, sertindole 4 mg, 30-tab pack; 12 mg 28-tab pack; 16 mg, 28-tab pack; 20 mg 28-tab pack

Available only on named-patient basis (see notes above)

ZOTEPINE

Indications: schizophrenia

Cautions: see notes above; personal or close family history of epilepsy; withdrawal of concomitantly prescribed CNS depressants; QT interval prolongation—ECG required (before treatment and at each dose increase) in patients at risk of arrhythmias; monitor plasma electrolytes particularly before treatment and at each dose increase; hepatic impairment (Appendix 2); renal impairment (Appendix 3); prostatic hypertrophy, urinary retention, angle-closure glaucoma, paralytic ileus, pregnancy (Appendix 4)

Contra-indications: acute intoxication with CNS depressants; high doses of concomitantly prescribed antipsychotics; acute gout (avoid for 3 weeks after episode resolves), history of nephrolithiasis; breast-feeding (Appendix 5)

Side-effects: see notes above; constipation, dyspepsia, dry mouth, tachycardia, QT interval prolongation, rhinitis, agitation, anxiety, depression, asthenia, headache, EEG abnormalities, insomnia, drowsiness, hyperthermia or hypothermia, increased salivation, blood dyscrasias (including leucocytosis, leucopenia), raised erythrocyte sedimentation rate, blurred vision, sweating; less frequently anorexia, diarrhoea, nausea and vomiting, abdominal pain, hypertension, influenza-like syndrome, cough, dyspnoea, confusion, convulsions, decreased libido, speech disorder, vertigo, hyperprolactinaemia, anaemia, thrombocythaemia, increased serum creatinine, hypoglycaemia and hyperglycaemia, hyperlipidaemia, hypouricaemia, oedema, thirst, impotence, urinary incontinence, arthralgia, myalgia, conjunctivitis, acne, dry skin, rash; rarely bradycardia, epistaxis, abdominal enlargement, amnesia, ataxia, coma, delirium, hypaesthesia, myoclonus, thrombocytopenia, abnormal ejaculation, urinary retention, menstrual irregularities, myasthenia, alopecia, photosensitivity

Dose: initially 25 mg 3 times daily increased according to response at intervals of 4 days to max. 100 mg 3 times daily; ELDERLY initially 25 mg twice daily increased according to response to max. 75 mg twice daily; CHILD and ADOLESCENT under 18 years not recommended

Zoleptil® (Orion) PoM
Tablets, s/c, zotepine 25 mg (white), net price 30-tab pack = £14.33, 90-tab pack = £42.98; 50 mg (yellow), 30-tab pack = £19.10, 90-tab pack = £57.30; 100 mg (pink), 30-tab pack = £31.52, 90-tab pack = £94.55. Label: 2

4.2.2 Antipsychotic depot injections

Long-acting depot injections are used for maintenance therapy especially when compliance with oral treatment is unreliable. However, depot injections of conventional antipsychotics may give rise to a higher incidence of extrapyramidal reactions than oral preparations; extrapyramidal reactions occur less frequently with atypical antipsychotics such as risperidone.

ADMINISTRATION. Depot antipsychotics are administered by deep intramuscular injection at intervals of 1 to 4 weeks. When initiating therapy with sustained-release preparations of conventional antipsychotics, patients should first be given a small test-dose as undesirable side-effects are prolonged. In general not more than 2–3 mL of oily injection should be administered at any one site; correct injection technique (including the use of z-track technique) and rotation of injection sites are essential. If the dose needs to be reduced to alleviate side-effects, it is important to recognise that the plasma-drug concentration may not fall for some time after reducing the dose, therefore it may be a month or longer before side-effects subside.

DOSAGE. Individual responses to neuroleptic drugs are very variable and to achieve optimum effect, dosage and dosage interval must be titrated according to the patient's response. For the advice of The Royal College of Psychiatrists on doses above the BNF upper limit, see p. 181 "

Equivalent doses of depot antipsychotics

These equivalences are intended **only** as an approximate guide; individual dosage instructions should **also** be checked; patients should be carefully monitored after **any** change in medication

Antipsychotic	Dose (mg)	Interval
Flupentixol decanoate	40	2 weeks
Fluphenazine decanoate	25	2 weeks
Haloperidol (as decanoate)	100	4 weeks
Pipotiazine palmitate	50	4 weeks
Zuclopenthixol decanoate	200	2 weeks

Important. These equivalences must **not** be extrapolated beyond the max. dose for the drug

CHOICE. There is no clear-cut division in the use of the conventional antipsychotics, but **zuclopenthixol** may be suitable for the treatment of agitated or aggressive patients whereas **flupentixol** can cause over-excitement in such patients. The incidence of extrapyramidal reactions is similar for the conventional antipsychotics.

CAUTIONS. See section 4.2.1. Treatment requires careful monitoring for optimum effect. When transferring from oral to depot therapy, dosage by mouth should be reduced gradually.

CONTRA-INDICATIONS. See section 4.2.1. Do not use in children.

SIDE-EFFECTS. See section 4.2.1. Pain may occur at injection site and occasionally erythema, swelling, and nodules. For side-effects of specific antipsychotics see under the relevant drug.

FLUPENTIXOL DECANOATE

(Flupenthixol Decanoate)

Indications: maintenance in schizophrenia and other psychoses

Cautions: see notes on p. 182 and also under Flupentixol (section 4.2.1) and notes above; an alternative antipsychotic may be necessary if symptoms such as aggression or agitation appear

Contra-indications: see notes on p. 182 and also under Flupentixol (section 4.2.1) and notes above

Side-effects: see notes on p. 182 and also under Flupentixol (section 4.2.1) and notes above, but may have a mood elevating effect

Dose: *by deep intramuscular injection* into the gluteal muscle, test dose 20 mg, then after at least 7 days 20–40 mg repeated at intervals of 2–4 weeks, adjusted according to response; max. 400 mg weekly; usual maintenance dose 50 mg every 4 weeks to 300 mg every 2 weeks; ELDERLY initially quarter to half adult dose; CHILD not recommended

Depixol® (Lundbeck) PoM
Injection (oily), flupentixol decanoate 20 mg/mL. Net price 1-mL amp = £1.52; 2-mL amp = £2.54

Depixol Conc.® (Lundbeck) PoM
Injection (oily), flupentixol decanoate 100 mg/mL. Net price 0.5-mL amp = £3.42; 1-mL amp = £6.25

Depixol Low Volume® (Lundbeck) PoM
Injection (oily), flupentixol decanoate 200 mg/mL. Net price 1-mL amp = £19.52

FLUPHENAZINE DECANOATE

Indications: maintenance in schizophrenia and other psychoses

Cautions: see notes on p. 182 and also notes above

Contra-indications: see notes on p. 182 and also notes above

Side-effects: see notes on p. 182 and also under Fluphenazine Hydrochloride (section 4.2.1) and notes above; also extrapyramidal symptoms usually appear a few hours after injection and continue for about 2 days but may be delayed

Dose: *by deep intramuscular injection* into the gluteal muscle, test dose 12.5 mg (6.25 mg in elderly), then after 4–7 days 12.5–100 mg repeated at intervals of 14–35 days, adjusted according to response; CHILD not recommended

Fluphenazine decanoate (Non-proprietary) PoM
Injection (oily), fluphenazine decanoate 25 mg/mL, net price 1-mL amp = £2.35; 100 mg/mL, 0.5-mL amp = £4.50, 1-mL amp = £8.79
Excipients: include sesame oil

Modecate® (Sanofi-Synthelabo) PoM
Injection (oily), fluphenazine decanoate 25 mg/mL. Net price 0.5-mL amp = £1.35, 1-mL amp = £2.35, 2-mL amp = £4.62
Excipients: include sesame oil

Modecate Concentrate® (Sanofi-Synthelabo) PoM
Injection (oily), fluphenazine decanoate 100 mg/mL. Net price 0.5-mL amp = £4.66, 1-mL amp = £9.10
Excipients: include sesame oil

HALOPERIDOL

Indications: maintenance in schizophrenia and other psychoses
Cautions: see notes on p. 182 and also under Haloperidol (section 4.2.1) and notes above
Contra-indications: see notes on p. 182 and also under Haloperidol (section 4.2.1) and notes above
Side-effects: see notes on p. 182 and also under Haloperidol (section 4.2.1) and notes above
Dose: *by deep intramuscular injection* into the gluteal muscle, initially 50 mg every 4 weeks, if necessary increasing by 50-mg increments to 300 mg every 4 weeks; higher doses may be needed in some patients; ELDERLY, initially 12.5–25 mg every 4 weeks; CHILD not recommended
NOTE. If 2-weekly administration preferred, doses should be halved

Haldol Decanoate® (Janssen-Cilag) PoM
Injection (oily), haloperidol (as decanoate) 50 mg/mL, net price 1-mL amp = £4.13; 100 mg/mL, 1-mL amp = £5.48
Excipients: include sesame oil

PIPOTIAZINE PALMITATE

(Pipothiazine Palmitate)
Indications: maintenance in schizophrenia and other psychoses
Cautions: see notes on p. 182 and notes above
Contra-indications: see notes on p. 182 and notes above
Side-effects: see notes on p. 182 and notes above
Dose: *by deep intramuscular injection* into the gluteal muscle, test dose 25 mg, then a further 25–50 mg after 4–7 days, then adjusted according to response at intervals of 4 weeks; usual maintenance range 50–100 mg (max. 200 mg) every 4 weeks; ELDERLY initially 5–10 mg; CHILD not recommended

Piportil Depot® (JHC) PoM
Injection (oily), pipotiazine palmitate 50 mg/mL. Net price 1-mL amp = £10.52; 2-mL amp = £17.21
Excipients: include sesame oil

RISPERIDONE

Indications: schizophrenia and other psychoses in patients tolerant to risperidone by mouth
Cautions: see under Risperidone (section 4.2.1) and notes above
Contra-indications: see under Risperidone (section 4.2.1)
Side-effects: see under Risperidone (section 4.2.1); also depression, tremor; *less commonly* apathy, weight loss, abnormal vision, pruritus; injection-site reactions also reported
Dose: *by deep intramuscular injection* into the gluteal muscle, patients taking oral risperidone up to 4 mg daily, initially 25 mg every 2 weeks; patients taking oral risperidone over 4 mg daily, initially 37.5 mg every 2 weeks; dose adjusted at intervals of at least 4 weeks in steps of 12.5 mg to max. 50 mg (ELDERLY 25 mg) every 2 weeks; CHILD and ADOLESCENT under 18 years not recommended
NOTE. During initiation risperidone by mouth continued if necessary for max. 3 weeks; risperidone by mouth may also be used during dose adjustment of depot injection

Risperdal Consta® (Janssen-Cilag) ▼ PoM
Injection, powder for reconstitution, risperidone 25-mg vial, net price = £82.92; 37.5-mg vial = £115.84; 50-mg vial = £148.55 (all with diluent)

ZUCLOPENTHIXOL DECANOATE

Indications: maintenance in schizophrenia and other psychoses, particularly with aggression and agitation
Cautions: see notes on p. 182 and notes above; avoid in porphyria (section 9.8.2)
Contra-indications: see notes on p. 182 and notes above
Side-effects: see notes on p. 182 and notes above
Dose: *by deep intramuscular injection* into the gluteal muscle, test dose 100 mg, followed after at least 7 days by 200–500 mg or more, repeated at intervals of 1–4 weeks, adjusted according to response; max. 600 mg weekly; ELDERLY quarter to half usual starting dose; CHILD not recommended

Clopixol® (Lundbeck) PoM
Injection (oily), zuclopenthixol decanoate 200 mg/mL. Net price 1-mL amp = £3.15

Clopixol Conc.® (Lundbeck) PoM
Injection (oily), zuclopenthixol decanoate 500 mg/mL. Net price 1-mL amp = £7.44

4.2.3 Antimanic drugs

Drugs are used in mania both to control acute attacks and also to prevent their recurrence.

Benzodiazepines

Use of benzodiazepines (section 4.1) may be helpful in the initial stages of treatment until lithium achieves its full effect; they should not be used for long periods because of the risk of dependence.

Antipsychotic drugs

In an acute attack of mania, treatment with an antipsychotic drug (section 4.2.1) is usually required because it may take a few days for lithium to exert its antimanic effect. Lithium may be given concurrently with the antipsychotic drug, and treatment with the antipsychotic gradually tailed off as lithium becomes effective. Alternatively, lithium therapy may be commenced once the patient's mood has been stabilised with the antipsychotic. The adjunctive use of atypical antipsychotics such as olanzapine (section 4.2.1) and risperidone [unlicensed indication] with either lithium or valproic acid may also be of benefit.

High doses of haloperidol, fluphenazine, or flupentixol may be hazardous when used with lithium; irreversible toxic encephalopathy has been reported.

Carbamazepine

Carbamazepine (section 4.8.1) may be used for the prophylaxis of bipolar disorder (manic-depressive disorder) in patients unresponsive to lithium; it seems to be particularly effective in patients with rapid cycling manic-depressive illness (4 or more affective episodes per year).

Valproic acid

Valproic acid (as the semisodium salt) is licensed for the treatment of manic episodes associated with bipolar disorder. It may be useful in patients unresponsive to lithium. Sodium valproate (section 4.8.1) has also been used, but it is unlicensed for this indication.

VALPROIC ACID

Indications: treatment of manic episodes associated with bipolar disorder

Cautions: see Sodium Valproate (section 4.8.1); monitor closely if dose greater than 45 mg/kg daily

Contra-indications: see Sodium Valproate (section 4.8.1)

Side-effects: see Sodium Valproate (section 4.8.1)

Dose: initially 750 mg daily in 2–3 divided doses, increased according to response, usual dose 1–2 g daily; CHILD and ADOLESCENT under 18 years not recommended

Depakote® (Sanofi-Synthelabo) PoM

Tablets, e/c, valproic acid (as semisodium valproate) 250 mg, net price 90-tab pack = £43.19; 500 mg, 90-tab pack = £72.19. Label: 25

NOTE. Semisodium valproate comprises equimolar amounts of sodium valproate and valproic acid.

Lithium

Lithium salts are used in the prophylaxis and treatment of mania, in the prophylaxis of bipolar disorder (manic-depressive disorder) and in the prophylaxis of recurrent depression (unipolar illness or unipolar depression). Lithium is unsuitable for children.

The decision to give prophylactic lithium usually requires *specialist advice*, and must be based on careful consideration of the likelihood of recurrence in the individual patient, and the benefit weighed against the risks. In long-term use lithium has been associated with thyroid disorders and mild cognitive and memory impairment. Long-term treatment should therefore be undertaken only with careful assessment of risk and benefit, and with regular monitoring of thyroid function. The need for continued therapy should be assessed regularly and patients should be maintained on lithium after 3–5 years only if benefit persists.

SERUM CONCENTRATIONS. Lithium salts have a narrow therapeutic/toxic ratio and should therefore not be prescribed unless facilities for monitoring serum-lithium concentrations are available. There seem few if any reasons for preferring one or other of the salts of lithium available. Doses are adjusted to achieve serum-lithium concentration of 0.4–1 mmol/litre (lower end of the range for maintenance therapy and elderly patients) on samples taken 12 hours after the preceding dose. It is important to determine the optimum range for each individual patient.

Overdosage, usually with serum-lithium concentration of over 1.5 mmol/litre, may be fatal and toxic effects include tremor, ataxia, dysarthria, nystagmus, renal impairment, and convulsions. If these potentially hazardous signs occur, treatment should be stopped, serum-lithium concentrations redetermined, and steps taken to reverse lithium toxicity. In mild cases withdrawal of lithium and administration of generous amounts of sodium salts and fluid will reverse the toxicity. Serum-lithium concentration in excess of 2 mmol/litre require urgent treatment as indicated under Emergency Treatment of Poisoning, p. 32.

INTERACTIONS. Lithium toxicity is made worse by sodium depletion, therefore concurrent use of diuretics (particularly thiazides) is hazardous and should be avoided. For other **interactions** with lithium, see Appendix 1 (lithium).

WITHDRAWAL. While there is no clear evidence of withdrawal or rebound psychosis, abrupt discontinuation of lithium increases the risk of relapse. If lithium is to be discontinued, the dose should be reduced gradually over a period of a few weeks and patients should be warned of possible relapse if discontinued abruptly.

> **Lithium cards.** A lithium treatment card available from pharmacies tells patients how to take lithium preparations, what to do if a dose is missed, and what side-effects to expect. It also explains why regular blood tests are important and warns that some medicines and illnesses can change serum-lithium concentration
> Cards may be obtained from NPA Services, 38–42 St. Peter's St, St. Albans, Herts AL1 3NP.

LITHIUM CARBONATE

Indications: treatment and prophylaxis of mania, bipolar disorder, and recurrent depression (see also notes above); aggressive or self-mutilating behaviour

Cautions: measure serum-lithium concentration regularly (every 3 months on stabilised regimens), measure thyroid function every 6–12 months on stabilised regimens and advise patient to seek attention if symptoms of hypothyroidism develop (women at greater risk) e.g. lethargy, feeling cold; maintain adequate sodium and fluid intake; test renal function before initiating and if evidence of toxicity, avoid in renal impairment (Appendix 3), cardiac disease, and conditions with sodium imbalance such as Addison's disease; reduce dose or discontinue in diarrhoea, vomiting and intercurrent infection (especially if sweating profusely); psoriasis (risk of exacerbation) pregnancy (Appendix 4), breast-feeding (Appendix 5), elderly (reduce dose), diuretic treatment, myasthenia gravis; surgery (section 15.1); avoid abrupt withdrawal (see notes above); **interactions:** Appendix 1 (lithium)

COUNSELLING. Patients should maintain adequate fluid intake and avoid dietary changes which reduce or increase sodium intake

Side-effects: gastro-intestinal disturbances, fine tremor, renal impairment (particularly impaired urinary concentration and polyuria), polydipsia, leucocytosis; also weight gain and oedema (may respond to dose reduction); hyperparathyroidism and hypercalcaemia reported; signs of intoxication are blurred vision, increasing gastro-intestinal disturbances (anorexia, vomiting, diarrhoea), muscle weakness, increased CNS disturbances (mild drowsiness and sluggishness increasing to giddiness with ataxia, coarse tremor, lack of co-ordination, dysarthria), and require withdrawal of treatment; with severe **overdosage** (serum-lithium concentration above 2 mmol/litre) hyperreflexia and hyperextension of limbs, convulsions, toxic psychoses, syncope, renal failure, circulatory failure, coma, and occasionally, death; goitre, raised antidiuretic hormone concentration, hypothyroidism, hypokalaemia, ECG changes, and kidney changes may also occur; see also Emergency Treatment of Poisoning, p. 32

Dose: see under preparations below, adjusted to achieve a serum-lithium concentration of 0.4–1 mmol/litre 12 hours after a dose on days 4–7 of treatment, then every week until dosage has remained constant for 4 weeks and every 3 months thereafter; doses are initially divided throughout the day, but once daily administration is preferred when serum-lithium concentration stabilised

NOTE. **Preparations vary widely in bioavailability**; changing the preparation requires the same precautions as initiation of treatment

NOTE. Lithium carbonate 200 mg ≡ lithium citrate 509 mg

Camcolit® (Norgine) PoM

Camcolit 250® *tablets*, f/c, scored, lithium carbonate 250 mg (Li^+ 6.8 mmol), net price 20 = 64p. Label: 10, lithium card, counselling, see above

Camcolit 400® *tablets*, m/r, f/c, scored, lithium carbonate 400 mg (Li^+ 10.8 mmol), net price 20 = 86p. Label: 10, lithium card, 25, counselling, see above

Dose: (serum monitoring, see above):
Treatment, initially 1–1.5 g daily; prophylaxis, initially 300–400 mg daily; CHILD not recommended

NOTE. *Camcolit 400*® also available as *Lithonate*® (TEVA UK)

Liskonum® (GSK) PoM

Tablets, m/r, f/c, scored, lithium carbonate 450 mg (Li^+ 12.2 mmol), net price 60-tab pack = £2.88. Label: 10, lithium card, 25, counselling, see above

Dose: (serum monitoring, see above):
Treatment, initially 450–675 mg twice daily (elderly initially 225 mg twice daily); prophylaxis, initially 450 mg twice daily (elderly 225 mg twice daily); CHILD not recommended

Priadel® (Sanofi-Synthelabo) PoM

Tablets, m/r, both scored, lithium carbonate 200 mg (Li^+ 5.4 mmol), net price 20 = 59p; 400 mg (Li^+ 10.8 mmol), 20 = 78p. Label: 10, lithium card, 25, counselling, see above

Dose: (serum monitoring, see above):
Treatment and prophylaxis, initially 0.4–1.2 g daily as a single dose or in 2 divided doses (elderly or patients less than 50 kg, 400 mg daily); CHILD not recommended

Liquid, see under Lithium Citrate below

LITHIUM CITRATE

Indications: see under Lithium Carbonate and notes above

Cautions: see under Lithium Carbonate and notes above

COUNSELLING. Patients should maintain an adequate fluid intake and should avoid dietary changes which might reduce or increase sodium intake; lithium treatment cards are available from pharmacies (see above)

Side-effects: see under Lithium Carbonate and notes above

Dose: see under preparations below, adjusted to achieve serum-lithium concentration of 0.4–1 mmol/litre as described under Lithium Carbonate

NOTE. **Preparations vary widely in bioavailability**; changing the preparation requires the same precautions as initiation of treatment

NOTE. Lithium carbonate 200 mg ≡ lithium citrate 509 mg

Li-Liquid® (Rosemont) PoM

Oral solution, lithium citrate 509 mg/5 mL (Li^+ 5.4 mmol/5 mL), yellow, net price 150-mL pack = £5.79; 1.018 g/5 mL (Li^+ 10.8 mmol/5 mL), orange, 150-mL pack = £11.58. Label: 10, lithium card, counselling, see above

Dose: (plasma monitoring, see above):
Treatment and prophylaxis, initially 1.018–3.054 g daily in 2 divided doses (elderly or patients less than 50 kg, initially 509 mg twice daily); CHILD not recommended

Priadel® (Sanofi-Synthelabo) PoM

Tablets, see under Lithium Carbonate, above

Liquid, sugar-free, lithium citrate 520 mg/5 mL (approx. Li^+ 5.4 mmol/5 mL), net price 150-mL pack = £5.84. Label: 10, lithium card, counselling, see above

Dose: (plasma monitoring, see above):
Treatment and prophylaxis, initially 1.04–3.12 g daily in 2 divided doses (elderly or patients less than 50 kg, 520 mg twice daily); CHILD not recommended

4.3 Antidepressant drugs

Antidepressant drugs are effective in the treatment of major depression of moderate and severe degree including major depression associated with physical illness and that following childbirth; they are also effective for dysthymia (lower grade chronic depression). Antidepressant drugs are not generally effective in milder forms of acute depression but a trial may be considered in cases refractory to psychological treatments.

CHOICE. The major classes of antidepressants include the tricyclics and related antidepressants, the selective serotonin re-uptake inhibitors (SSRIs), and the monoamine oxidase inhibitors (MAOIs). A number of antidepressants cannot be accommodated easily into this classification; these are included in section 4.3.4.

Choice of antidepressant should be based on the individual patient's requirements, including the presence of concomitant disease, existing therapy, suicide risk, and previous response to antidepressant therapy.

Either tricyclic and related antidepressants or SSRIs are generally preferred because MAOIs may be less effective and show dangerous interactions with some foods and drugs.

Tricyclic antidepressants may be suitable for many depressed patients. If the potential side-effects of the older tricyclics are of concern, an SSRI or one of the newer classes of antidepressants may be appropriate. Although SSRIs appear to be better tolerated than older drugs, the difference is too small to justify always choosing an SSRI as first-line treatment.

Compared to older **tricyclics** (e.g. amitriptyline), the **tricyclic-related drugs** (e.g. trazodone) have a lower incidence of antimuscarinic side-effects, such as dry mouth and constipation. The tricyclic-related drugs may also be associated with a lower risk of cardiotoxicity in overdosage, but some have additional side-effects (for further details see section 4.3.1).

The **selective serotonin re-uptake inhibitors** (SSRIs) have fewer antimuscarinic side-effects than the older tricyclics and they are also less cardiotoxic in overdosage. Therefore, although no more effective, they are preferred where there is a significant risk of deliberate overdosing or where concomitant conditions preclude the use of other antidepressants. SSRIs are also preferred to tricyclic antidepressants for depression in patients with diabetes. The SSRIs do, however, have characteristic side-effects of their own; gastro-intestinal side-effects such as nausea and vomiting are common and bleeding disorders have been reported.

For severely ill inpatients and those in whom maximising efficacy is of overriding importance, a tricyclic may be more effective than an SSRI or an MAOI. Venlafaxine, at a dose of 150 mg or greater, may also be more effective than SSRIs for major depression of at least moderate severity. Where the depression is very severe electroconvulsive therapy (ECT) may be indicated.

MAOIs may be more effective than tricyclics in non-hospitalised patients with 'atypical depression'; MAOI treatment should be initiated by those experienced in its use.

Although anxiety is often present in depressive illness (and may be the presenting symptom), the use of an antipsychotic or an anxiolytic may mask the true diagnosis. Anxiolytics (section 4.1.2) or antipsychotics (section 4.2.1) should therefore be used with caution in depression but they are useful adjuncts in agitated patients.

See also section 4.2.3 for references to the management of bipolar disorders.

St John's wort (*Hypericum perforatum*) is a popular unlicensed herbal remedy for treating mild depression. However, preparations of St John's wort can induce drug metabolising enzymes and a number of important interactions with conventional drugs have been identified, see Appendix 1 (St John's wort). The amount of active ingredient can vary between different preparations of St John's wort and switching from one to another can change the degree of enzyme induction. Furthermore, when a patient stops taking St John's wort, concentrations of interacting drugs may increase, leading to toxicity. Antidepressants should **not** be used with St John's wort because of the potential for interaction.

Hyponatraemia and antidepressant therapy. Hyponatraemia (usually in the elderly and possibly due to inappropriate secretion of antidiuretic hormone) has been associated with all types of antidepressants; however, it has been reported more frequently with SSRIs than with other antidepressants. The CSM has advised that hyponatraemia should be considered in all patients who develop drowsiness, confusion, or convulsions while taking an antidepressant.

MANAGEMENT. Patients should be reviewed every 1–2 weeks at the start of antidepressant treatment. Treatment should be continued for at least 4 weeks (6 weeks in the elderly) before considering whether to switch antidepressant due to lack of efficacy. In cases of partial response, continue for a further 2 weeks (elderly patients may take longer to respond).

Following remission, antidepressant treatment should be continued at the same dose for at least 4–6 months (about 12 months in the elderly). Patients with a history of recurrent depression should continue to receive maintenance treatment (for at least 5 years and possibly indefinitely). Lithium (section 4.2.3) is an effective second-line alternative for maintenance treatment.

Combination of two antidepressants can be dangerous and is rarely justified (except under specialist supervision).

FAILURE TO RESPOND. Failure to respond to an initial course of antidepressant, may necessitate an increase in the dose, switching to a different antidepressant class, or in patients with 'atypical' major depression, the use of an MAOI. Failure to respond to a second antidepressant may require the addition of an augmenting drug such as lithium or liothyronine (specialist use), psychotherapy, or ECT. Adjunctive therapy with lithium or an MAOI should only be initiated by doctors with special experience of these combinations.

WITHDRAWAL. Gastro-intestinal symptoms of nausea, vomiting, and anorexia, accompanied by headache, giddiness, 'chills', and insomnia, and sometimes by hypomania, panic-anxiety, and extreme motor restlessness may occur if an antidepressant (particularly an MAOI) is stopped suddenly after regular administration for 8 weeks or more. The dose should preferably be reduced gradually over about 4 weeks, or longer if withdrawal symptoms emerge (6 months in patients who have been on long-term maintenance treatment). SSRIs have been associated with a specific withdrawal syndrome (section 4.3.3).

ANXIETY. Management of *acute anxiety* generally involves the use of a benzodiazepine or buspirone (section 4.1.2). For *chronic anxiety* (of longer than 4 weeks' duration), it may be appropriate to use an antidepressant before a benzodiazepine. *Generalised anxiety disorder* which does not respond to buspirone or to a benzodiazepine is treated with an antidepressant. Antidepressants such as SSRIs and venlafaxine may be effective in specific anxiety disorders.

Compound preparations of an antidepressant and an anxiolytic are not recommended because it is not possible to adjust the dosage of the individual components separately. Whereas antidepressants are given continuously over several months, anxiolytics are prescribed on a short-term basis.

PANIC DISORDERS. Antidepressants are generally used for *panic disorders* and *phobias*; clomipramine (section 4.3.1) is licensed for *obsessional and phobic states*; escitalopram and paroxetine (section 4.3.3) and moclobemide (section 4.3.2) are licensed for the management of social phobia. However, in panic disorders (with or without agoraphobia) resistant to antidepressant therapy, a benzodiazepine may be considered (section 4.1.2).

4.3.1 Tricyclic and related antidepressant drugs

This section covers tricyclic antidepressants and also 1-, 2-, and 4-ring structured drugs with broadly similar properties.

These drugs are most effective for treating moderate to severe *endogenous depression* associated with psychomotor and physiological changes such as loss of appetite and sleep disturbances; improvement in sleep is usually the first benefit of therapy. Since there may be an interval of 2 weeks before the antidepressant action takes place electroconvulsive treatment may be required in severe depression when delay is hazardous or intolerable.

Some tricyclic antidepressants are also effective in the management of *panic disorder*.

For reference to the role of some tricyclic antidepressants in some forms of *neuralgia*, see section 4.7.3, and in *nocturnal enuresis* in children, see section 7.4.2.

DOSAGE. About 10 to 20% of patients fail to respond to tricyclic and related antidepressant drugs and inadequate dosage may account for some of these failures. It is important to use doses that are sufficiently high for effective treatment but not so high as to cause toxic effects. Low doses should be used for initial treatment in the **elderly** (see under Side-effects, below).

In most patients the long half-life of tricyclic antidepressant drugs allows **once-daily** administration, usually at night; the use of modified-release preparations is therefore unnecessary.

CHOICE. Tricyclic and related antidepressant drugs can be roughly divided into those with additional sedative properties and those which are less so. Agitated and anxious patients tend to respond best to the sedative compounds whereas withdrawn and apathetic patients will often obtain most benefit from the less sedating ones. Those with **sedative** properties include amitriptyline, clomipramine, dosulepin (dothiepin), doxepin, maprotiline, mianserin, trazodone, and trimipramine. Those with **less sedative** properties include amoxapine, imipramine, lofepramine, and nortriptyline.

Imipramine is well established and relatively safe and effective, but it has more marked antimuscarinic and cardiac side-effects than compounds such as **doxepin**, **mianserin**, and **trazodone**; this may be important in individual patients. **Amitriptyline** and **dosulepin** (dothiepin) are effective but they are particularly dangerous in overdosage (see Overdosage, below). **Lofepramine** also has a lower incidence of antimuscarinic and sedative side-effects and is less dangerous in overdosage; it is, however, infrequently associated with hepatic toxicity. **Amoxapine** is related to the antipsychotic loxapine and its side-effects include tardive dyskinesia.

For a comparison of tricyclic and related antidepressants with SSRIs and related antidepressants and MAOIs, see section 4.3.

SIDE-EFFECTS. *Arrhythmias* and *heart block* occasionally follow the use of tricyclic antidepressants, particularly amitriptyline, and may be a factor in the sudden death of patients with cardiac disease. They are also sometimes associated with *convulsions* (and should be prescribed with special caution in epilepsy as they lower the convulsive threshold); maprotiline has particularly been associated with convulsions. *Hepatic* and *haematological* reactions may occur and have been particularly associated with mianserin.

Other side-effects of tricyclic and related antidepressants include *drowsiness, dry mouth, blurred vision, constipation,* and *urinary retention* (all attributed to antimuscarinic activity), and sweating. The patient should be encouraged to persist with treatment as some tolerance to these side-effects seems to develop. They are reduced if low doses are given initially and then gradually increased, but this must be balanced against the need to obtain a full therapeutic effect as soon as possible. Gradual introduction of treatment is particularly important in the elderly, who, because of the hypotensive effects of these drugs, are prone to attacks of *dizziness* or even *syncope*. Another side-effect to which the elderly are particularly susceptible is *hyponatraemia* (see CSM advice on p. 196).

Neuroleptic malignant syndrome (section 4.2.1) may, very rarely, arise in the course of antidepressant treatment.

OVERDOSAGE. Limited quantities of tricyclic antidepressants should be prescribed at any one time because their cardiovascular effects are dangerous in overdosage. In particular, overdosage with dosulepin (dothiepin) and amitriptyline is associated with a relatively high rate of fatality. For advice on **overdosage** see Emergency Treatment of Poisoning, p. 31

WITHDRAWAL. If possible tricyclic and related antidepressants should be withdrawn slowly (see also section 4.3).

INTERACTIONS. A tricyclic or related antidepressant (or an SSRI or related antidepressant) should not be started until 2 weeks after stopping an MAOI (3 weeks if starting clomipramine or imipramine). Conversely, an MAOI should not be started until at least 7–14 days after a tricyclic or related antidepressant (3 weeks in the case of clomipramine or imipramine) has been stopped. For guidance relating to the reversible monoamine oxidase inhibitor, moclobemide, see p. 202. For other tricyclic antidepressant **interactions**, see Appendix 1 (antidepressants, tricyclic and antidepressants, tricyclic (related)).

Tricyclic antidepressants

AMITRIPTYLINE HYDROCHLORIDE

Indications: depressive illness, particularly where sedation is required; nocturnal enuresis in children (section 7.4.2)

Cautions: cardiac disease (particularly with arrhythmias, see Contra-indications below), history of epilepsy, pregnancy (Appendix 4), breast-feeding (Appendix 5), elderly, hepatic impairment (avoid if severe; Appendix 2), thyroid disease, phaeochromocytoma, history of mania, psychoses (may aggravate psychotic symptoms), angle-closure glaucoma, history of urinary retention, concurrent electroconvulsive therapy; if possible avoid abrupt withdrawal; anaesthesia (increased risk of arrhythmias and hypotension, see surgery section 15.1); porphyria (section 9.8.2); see section 7.4.2 for additional nocturnal enuresis warnings; **interactions:** Appendix 1 (antidepressants, tricyclic)

DRIVING. Drowsiness may affect performance of skilled tasks (e.g. driving); effects of alcohol enhanced

Contra-indications: recent myocardial infarction, arrhythmias (particularly heart block), not indicated in manic phase, severe liver disease

Side-effects: dry mouth, sedation, blurred vision (disturbance of accommodation, increased intra-ocular pressure), constipation, nausea, difficulty with micturition; cardiovascular side-effects (such as ECG changes, arrhythmias, postural hypotension, tachycardia, syncope, particularly with high doses); sweating, tremor, rashes and hypersensitivity reactions (including urticaria, photosensitivity), behavioural disturbances (particularly children), hypomania or mania, confusion or delirium (particularly elderly), headache, interference with sexual function, blood sugar changes; increased appetite and weight gain (occasionally weight loss); endocrine side-effects such as testicular enlargement, gynaecomastia, galactorrhoea; also convulsions (see also Cautions), movement disorders and dyskinesias, dysarthria, paraesthesia, taste disturbances, tinnitus, fever, agranulocytosis, leucopenia, eosinophilia, purpura, thrombocytopenia, hyponatraemia (may be due to inappropriate antidiuretic hormone secretion) see CSM advice, p. 196, abnormal liver function tests (jaundice); for a general outline of side-effects see also notes above; **overdosage:** see Emergency Treatment of Poisoning, p. 31 (high rate of fatality—see notes above)

Dose: depression, initially 75 mg (elderly and adolescents 30–75 mg) daily in divided doses *or* as a single dose at bedtime increased gradually as necessary to 150–200 mg; CHILD under 16 years not recommended for depression

Nocturnal enuresis, CHILD 7–10 years 10–20 mg, 11–16 years 25–50 mg at night; max. period of treatment (including gradual withdrawal) 3 months—full physical examination before further course

Amitriptyline (Non-proprietary) PoM
Tablets, coated, amitriptyline hydrochloride 10 mg, net price 20 = 71p; 25 mg, 20 = £1.22; 50 mg, 20 = £1.14. Label: 2

Oral solution, amitriptyline (as hydrochloride) 25 mg/5 mL, net price 200 mL = £16.53; 50 mg/5 mL, 200 mL = £18.00. Label: 2

■ Compound preparations

Triptafen® (Goldshield) PoM
Tablets, pink, s/c, amitriptyline hydrochloride 25 mg, perphenazine 2 mg. Net price 20 = £4.25. Label: 2

Triptafen-M® (Goldshield) PoM
Tablets, pink, s/c, amitriptyline hydrochloride 10 mg, perphenazine 2 mg. Net price 20 = £3.80. Label: 2

AMOXAPINE

Indications: depressive illness

Cautions: see under Amitriptyline Hydrochloride

Contra-indications: see under Amitriptyline Hydrochloride

Side-effects: see under Amitriptyline Hydrochloride; tardive dyskinesia reported; menstrual irregularities, breast enlargement

Dose: initially 100–150 mg daily in divided doses *or* as a single dose at bedtime increased as necessary to max. 300 mg daily; ELDERLY initially 25 mg twice daily increased as necessary after 5–7 days to max. 50 mg 3 times daily; CHILD under 16 years not recommended

Asendis® (Goldshield) PoM
Tablets, amoxapine 50 mg (orange, scored), net price 84-tab pack = £16.78; 100 mg (blue, scored), 56-tab pack = £18.65. Label: 2

CLOMIPRAMINE HYDROCHLORIDE

Indications: depressive illness, phobic and obsessional states; adjunctive treatment of cataplexy associated with narcolepsy

Cautions: see under Amitriptyline Hydrochloride

Contra-indications: see under Amitriptyline Hydrochloride

Side-effects: see under Amitriptyline Hydrochloride; also diarrhoea; hair loss reported

Dose: depressive illness, initially 10 mg daily, increased gradually as necessary to 30–150 mg daily in divided doses *or* as a single dose at bedtime; max. 250 mg daily; ELDERLY initially 10 mg daily increased carefully over approx. 10 days to 30–75 mg daily; CHILD not recommended

Phobic and obsessional states, initially 25 mg daily (ELDERLY 10 mg daily) increased over 2 weeks to 100–150 mg daily; CHILD not recommended

Adjunctive treatment of cataplexy associated with narcolepsy, initially 10 mg daily, gradually increased until satisfactory response (range 10–75 mg daily)

Clomipramine (Non-proprietary) PoM
Capsules, clomipramine hydrochloride 10 mg, net price 28-cap pack = £1.58; 25 mg, 28-cap pack = £1.97; 50 mg, 28-cap pack = £3.86. Label: 2

Anafranil® (Cephalon) PoM
Capsules, clomipramine hydrochloride 10 mg (yellow/caramel), net price 84-cap pack = £3.23; 25 mg (orange/caramel), 84-cap pack = £6.35; 50 mg (grey/caramel), 56-cap pack = £8.06. Label: 2

Anafranil SR® (Cephalon) PoM 
Tablets, m/r, grey-red, f/c, clomipramine hydrochloride 75 mg. Net price 28-tab pack = £8.83. Label: 2, 25

DOSULEPIN HYDROCHLORIDE

(Dothiepin hydrochloride)

Indications: depressive illness, particularly where sedation is required

Cautions: see under Amitriptyline Hydrochloride

Contra-indications: see under Amitriptyline Hydrochloride

Side-effects: see under Amitriptyline Hydrochloride (high rate of fatality—see notes above)

Dose: initially 75 mg (ELDERLY 50–75 mg) daily in divided doses *or* as a single dose at bedtime, increased gradually as necessary to 150 mg daily (ELDERLY 75 mg may be sufficient); up to 225 mg daily in some circumstances (e.g. hospital use); CHILD not recommended

Dosulepin (Non-proprietary) PoM
Capsules, dosulepin hydrochloride 25 mg, net price 20 = 92p. Label: 2
Brands include *Dothapax*®, *Prepadine*®
Tablets, dosulepin hydrochloride 75 mg, net price 28-tab pack = £2.08. Label: 2
Brands include *Dothapax*®, *Prepadine*®

Prothiaden® (Abbott) PoM
Capsules, red/red-brown, dosulepin hydrochloride 25 mg. Net price 20 = £1.11. Label: 2
Tablets, red, s/c, dosulepin hydrochloride 75 mg. Net price 28-tab pack = £2.97. Label: 2

DOXEPIN

Indications: depressive illness, particularly where sedation is required; skin (section 13.3)

Cautions: see under Amitriptyline Hydrochloride

Contra-indications: see under Amitriptyline Hydrochloride; breast-feeding (Appendix 5)

Side-effects: see under Amitriptyline Hydrochloride

Dose: initially 75 mg daily in divided doses *or* as a single dose at bedtime, increased as necessary to max. 300 mg daily in 3 divided doses (up to 100 mg may be given as a single dose); ELDERLY initially 10–50 mg daily, range of 30–50 mg daily may be adequate; CHILD not recommended

Sinequan® (Pfizer) PoM
Capsules, doxepin (as hydrochloride) 10 mg (orange), net price 56-cap pack = £1.33; 25 mg (orange/blue), 28-cap pack = 96p; 50 mg (blue), 28-cap pack = £1.57; 75 mg (yellow/blue), 28-cap pack = £2.49. Label: 2

IMIPRAMINE HYDROCHLORIDE

Indications: depressive illness; nocturnal enuresis in children (see section 7.4.2)

Cautions: see under Amitriptyline Hydrochloride

Contra-indications: see under Amitriptyline Hydrochloride

Side-effects: see under Amitriptyline Hydrochloride, but less sedating

Dose: depression, initially up to 75 mg daily in divided doses increased gradually to 150–200 mg (up to 300 mg in hospital patients); up to 150 mg may be given as a single dose at bedtime; ELDERLY initially 10 mg daily, increased gradually to 30–50 mg daily; CHILD not recommended for depression
Nocturnal enuresis, CHILD 7 years 25 mg, 8–11 years 25–50 mg, over 11 years 50–75 mg at bedtime; max. period of treatment (including gradual withdrawal) 3 months—full physical examination before further course

Imipramine (Non-proprietary) PoM
Tablets, coated, imipramine hydrochloride 10 mg, net price 20 = £1.19; 25 mg, 20 = £1.26. Label: 2

Tofranil® (Novartis) PoM
Tablets, red-brown, s/c, imipramine hydrochloride 25 mg, net price 84-tab pack = £3.66. Label: 2

LOFEPRAMINE

Indications: depressive illness

Cautions: see under Amitriptyline Hydrochloride

Contra-indications: see under Amitriptyline Hydrochloride; hepatic and severe renal impairment

Side-effects: see under Amitriptyline Hydrochloride, but less sedating, lower incidence of antimuscarinic effects and less dangerous in overdosage; hepatic disorders reported

Dose: 140–210 mg daily in divided doses; ELDERLY may respond to lower doses; CHILD not recommended

Lofepramine (Non-proprietary) PoM
Tablets, lofepramine 70 mg (as hydrochloride). Net price 56-tab pack = £14.87. Label: 2
Brands include *Feprapax*®
Oral suspension, lofepramine 70 mg/5 mL (as hydrochloride). Net price 150 mL = £22.22. Label: 2
Brands include *Lomont*® (sugar-free)

Gamanil® (Merck) PoM
Tablets, f/c, brown-violet, lofepramine 70 mg (as hydrochloride). Net price 56-tab pack = £9.84. Label: 2

NORTRIPTYLINE

Indications: depressive illness; nocturnal enuresis in children (section 7.4.2)

Cautions: see under Amitriptyline Hydrochloride; manufacturer advises plasma-nortriptyline concentration monitoring if dose above 100 mg daily, but evidence of practical value uncertain

Contra-indications: see under Amitriptyline Hydrochloride

Side-effects: see under Amitriptyline Hydrochloride, but less sedating

Dose: depression, low dose initially increased as necessary to 75–100 mg daily in divided doses *or* as a single dose (max. 150 mg daily); ADOLESCENT and ELDERLY 30–50 mg daily in divided doses; CHILD not recommended for depression
Nocturnal enuresis, CHILD 7 years 10 mg, 8–11 years 10–20 mg, over 11 years 25–35 mg, at night; max period of treatment (including gradual withdrawal) 3 months—full physical examination and ECG before further course

Allegron® (King) PoM
Tablets, nortriptyline (as hydrochloride) 10 mg, net price 20 = £2.48; 25 mg (orange, scored), 20 = £4.90. Label: 2

■ Compound preparations

Motival® (Sanofi-Synthelabo) PoM
Tablets, pink, s/c, fluphenazine hydrochloride 500 micrograms, nortriptyline 10 mg (as hydrochloride). Net price 20 = 67p. Label: 2

TRIMIPRAMINE

Indications: depressive illness, particularly where sedation required

Cautions: see under Amitriptyline Hydrochloride

Contra-indications: see under Amitriptyline Hydrochloride

Side-effects: see under Amitriptyline Hydrochloride

Dose: initially 50–75 mg daily in divided doses *or* as a single dose at bedtime, increased as necessary to 150–300 mg daily; ELDERLY initially 10–25 mg 3 times daily, maintenance half adult dose may be sufficient; CHILD not recommended

Surmontil® (Aventis Pharma) PoM
Capsules, green/white, trimipramine 50 mg (as maleate). Net price 28-cap pack = £7.91. Label: 2
Tablets, trimipramine (as maleate) 10 mg, net price 28-tab pack = £3.57, 84-tab pack = £10.69; 25 mg, 28-tab pack = £4.71, 84-tab pack = £14.10. Label: 2

Related antidepressants

MAPROTILINE HYDROCHLORIDE

Indications: depressive illness, particularly where sedation is required

Cautions: see under Amitriptyline Hydrochloride; **interactions:** Appendix 1 (antidepressants, tricyclic (related))

Contra-indications: see under Amitriptyline Hydrochloride; history of epilepsy

Side-effects: see under Amitriptyline Hydrochloride, antimuscarinic effects may occur less frequently but rashes common and increased risk of convulsions at higher dosage

Dose: initially 25–75 mg (elderly 30 mg) daily in 3 divided doses *or* as a single dose at bedtime, increased gradually as necessary to max. 150 mg daily; CHILD not recommended

Ludiomil® (Novartis) PoM
Tablets, all f/c, maprotiline hydrochloride 25 mg (greyish-red), net price 28-tab pack = £2.53; 50 mg (light orange), 28-tab pack = £5.02; 75 mg (brownish-orange), 28-tab pack = £7.46. Label: 2
Excipients: include gluten

MIANSERIN HYDROCHLORIDE

Indications: depressive illness, particularly where sedation is required

Cautions: see under Amitriptyline Hydrochloride; **interactions:** Appendix 1 (antidepressants, tricyclic (related))

BLOOD COUNTS. A full **blood count** is recommended every 4 weeks during the first 3 months of treatment; clinical monitoring should continue subsequently and treatment should be stopped and a full blood count obtained if *fever, sore throat, stomatitis*, or other signs of infection develop.

Contra-indications: see under Amitriptyline Hydrochloride

Side-effects: see under Amitriptyline Hydrochloride, fewer and milder antimuscarinic and cardiovascular effects; leucopenia, agranulocytosis and aplastic anaemia (particularly in the elderly); jaundice; arthritis, arthralgia

Dose: initially 30–40 mg (elderly 30 mg) daily in divided doses *or* as a single dose at bedtime, increased gradually as necessary; usual dose range 30–90 mg; CHILD not recommended

Mianserin (Non-proprietary) PoM
Tablets, mianserin hydrochloride 10 mg, net price 20 = £3.66; 20 mg, 20 = £2.96; 30 mg, 20 = £6.24. Label: 2, 25

TRAZODONE HYDROCHLORIDE

Indications: depressive illness, particularly where sedation is required; anxiety

Cautions: see under Amitriptyline Hydrochloride; **interactions:** Appendix 1 (antidepressants, tricyclic (related))

Contra-indications: see under Amitriptyline Hydrochloride

Side-effects: see under Amitriptyline Hydrochloride but fewer antimuscarinic and cardiovascular effects; rarely priapism (discontinue immediately)

Dose: depression, initially 150 mg (elderly 100 mg) daily in divided doses after food *or* as a single dose at bedtime; may be increased to 300 mg daily; hospital patients up to max. 600 mg daily in divided doses

Anxiety, 75 mg daily, increasing if necessary to 300 mg daily

CHILD not recommended

Trazodone (Non-proprietary) PoM
Capsules, trazodone hydrochloride 50 mg, net price 84-cap pack = £26.04; 100 mg, 56-cap pack = £28.55. Label: 2, 21
Tablets, trazodone hydrochloride 150 mg, net price 28-tab pack = £17.03. Label: 2, 21

Molipaxin® (Hoechst Marion Roussel) PoM
Capsules, trazodone hydrochloride 50 mg (violet/green), net price 84-cap pack = £20.74; 100 mg (violet/fawn), 56-cap pack = £24.40. Label: 2, 21
Tablets, pink, f/c, trazodone hydrochloride 150 mg. Net price 28-tab pack = £13.94. Label: 2, 21
Liquid, sugar-free, trazodone hydrochloride 50 mg/5 mL, net price 120 mL = £9.28. Label: 2, 21

4.3.2 Monoamine-oxidase inhibitors (MAOIs)

Monoamine-oxidase inhibitors are used much less frequently than tricyclic and related antidepressants, or SSRIs and related antidepressants because of the dangers of dietary and drug interactions and the fact that it is easier to prescribe MAOIs when tricyclic antidepressants have been unsuccessful than vice versa. **Tranylcypromine** is the most **hazardous** of the MAOIs because of its stimulant action. The drugs of choice are **phenelzine** or **isocarboxazid** which are less stimulant and therefore safer.

Phobic patients and depressed patients with atypical, hypochondriacal, or hysterical features are said to respond best to MAOIs. However, MAOIs should be tried in any patients who are refractory to treatment with other antidepressants as there is occasionally a dramatic response. Response to treatment may be delayed for 3 weeks or more and may take an additional 1 or 2 weeks to become maximal.

WITHDRAWAL. If possible MAOIs should be withdrawn slowly (see also section 4.3).

INTERACTIONS. MAOIs inhibit monoamine oxidase, thereby causing an accumulation of amine neurotransmitters. The metabolism of some amine drugs such as *indirect-acting sympathomimetics* (present in many cough and decongestant preparations, see section 3.10) is also inhibited and their pressor action may be potentiated; the pressor effect of tyramine (in some foods, such as mature cheese, pickled herring, broad bean pods, and *Bovril*®, *Oxo*®, *Marmite*® or any similar meat or yeast extract or fermented soya bean extract) may also be dangerously potentiated. These interactions may cause a dangerous rise in blood pressure. An early warning symptom may be a throbbing headache. Patients should be advised to eat only fresh foods and avoid food that is suspected of being stale or 'going off'. This is especially important with meat, fish, poultry or offal; game should be avoided. The danger of interaction persists for up to 2 weeks after treatment with MAOIs is discontinued. Patients should also avoid alcoholic drinks or de-alcoholised (low alcohol) drinks.

Other antidepressants should **not** be started for 2 weeks after treatment with MAOIs has been stopped (3 weeks if starting clomipramine or imipramine). Some psychiatrists use selected tricyclics in conjunction with MAOIs but this is hazardous, indeed potentially lethal, except in experienced hands and there is no evidence that the combination is more effective than when either constituent is used alone. The combination of tranylcypromine with clomipramine is particularly **dangerous**.

Conversely, an MAOI should not be started until at least 7–14 days after a tricyclic or related antidepressant (3 weeks in the case of clomipramine or imipramine) has been stopped.

In addition, an MAOI should not be started for at least 2 weeks after a previous MAOI has been stopped (then started at a reduced dose).

For other interactions with MAOIs including those with opioid analgesics (notably pethidine), see Appendix 1 (MAOIs). For guidance on interactions relating to the reversible monoamine oxidase inhibitor, moclobemide, see p. 202; for guidance on interactions relating to SSRIs, see p. 202.

PHENELZINE

Indications: depressive illness

Cautions: diabetes mellitus, cardiovascular disease, epilepsy, blood disorders, concurrent electroconvulsive therapy; elderly (great caution); monitor blood pressure (risk of postural hypotension and hypertensive responses—discontinue if palpitations or frequent headaches); if possible avoid abrupt withdrawal; severe hypertensive reactions to certain drugs and foods; avoid in agitated patients; porphyria (section 9.8.2); pregnancy (Appendix 4) and breast-feeding; surgery (section 15.1); **interactions:** Appendix 1 (MAOIs)

DRIVING. Drowsiness may affect performance of skilled tasks (e.g. driving)

Contra-indications: hepatic impairment or abnormal liver function tests (Appendix 2), cerebrovascular disease, phaeochromocytoma; not indicated in manic phase

Side-effects: commonly postural hypotension (especially in elderly) and dizziness; less common side-effects include drowsiness, insomnia, headache, weakness and fatigue, dry mouth, constipation and other gastro-intestinal disturbances, oedema, myoclonic movement, hyperreflexia, elevated liver enzymes; agitation and tremors, nervousness, euphoria, arrhythmias, blurred vision, nystagmus, difficulty in micturition, sweating, convulsions, rashes, purpura, leucopenia, sexual disturbances, and weight gain with inappropriate appetite may also occur; psychotic episodes with hypomanic behaviour, confusion, and hallucinations may be induced in susceptible persons; jaundice has been reported and, on rare occasions, fatal progressive hepatocellular necrosis; paraesthesia, peripheral neuritis, peripheral neuropathy may be due to pyridoxine deficiency; for CSM advice on possible hyponatraemia, see p. 196

Dose: 15 mg 3 times daily, increased if necessary to 4 times daily after 2 weeks (hospital patients, max. 30 mg 3 times daily), then reduced gradually to lowest possible maintenance dose (15 mg on alternate days may be adequate); CHILD not recommended

Nardil® (Concord) PoM
Tablets, orange, f/c, phenelzine (as sulphate) 15 mg, net price 20 = £3.99. Label: 3, 10, patient information leaflet

ISOCARBOXAZID

Indications: depressive illness

Cautions: see under Phenelzine

Contra-indications: see under Phenelzine

Side-effects: see under Phenelzine

Dose: initially 30 mg daily in single or divided doses until improvement occurs (increased after 4 weeks if necessary to max. 60 mg daily for 4–6 weeks under close supervision), then reduced to usual maintenance dose 10–20 mg daily (but up to 40 mg daily may be required); ELDERLY 5–10 mg daily; CHILD not recommended

Isocarboxazid (Non-proprietary) PoM
Tablets, pink, scored, isocarboxazid 10 mg. Net price 50 = £27.79. Label: 3, 10, patient information leaflet

TRANYLCYPROMINE

Indications: depressive illness

Cautions: see under Phenelzine

Contra-indications: see under Phenelzine; hyperthyroidism

Side-effects: see under Phenelzine; insomnia if given in evening; hypertensive crises with throbbing headache requiring discontinuation of treatment more frequent than with other MAOIs; liver damage less frequent than with phenelzine

Dose: initially 10 mg twice daily not later than 3 p.m., increasing the second daily dose to 20 mg after 1 week if necessary; doses above 30 mg daily under close supervision only; usual maintenance dose 10 mg daily; CHILD not recommended

Tranylcypromine (Non-proprietary) PoM
Tablets, tranylcypromine (as sulphate) 10 mg. Net price 28-tab pack = £5.08. Label: 3, 10, patient information leaflet

Reversible MAOIs

Moclobemide is indicated for major depression and social phobia; it is reported to act by reversible inhibition of monoamine oxidase type A (it is therefore termed a RIMA). It should be reserved as a second-line treatment.

INTERACTIONS. Moclobemide is claimed to cause less potentiation of the pressor effect of tyramine than the traditional (irreversible) MAOIs, but patients should avoid consuming large amounts of tyramine-rich food (such as mature cheese, yeast extracts and fermented soya bean products).

The risk of drug interactions is also claimed to be less but patients still need to avoid sympathomimetics such as ephedrine and pseudoephedrine. In addition, moclobemide should not be given with another antidepressant. Owing to its short duration of action no treatment-free period is required after it has been stopped but it should not be started until at least a week after a tricyclic or related antidepressant or an SSRI or related antidepressant has been stopped (2 weeks in the case of sertraline, and at least 5 weeks in the case of fluoxetine), or for at least a week after an MAOI has been stopped. For other interactions, see Appendix 1 (moclobemide).

MOCLOBEMIDE

Indications: depressive illness; social phobia

Cautions: avoid in agitated or excited patients (or give with sedative for up to 2–3 weeks), thyrotoxicosis, hepatic impairment (Appendix 2), may provoke manic episodes in bipolar disorders, pregnancy (Appendix 4) and breast-feeding (Appendix 5—patient information leaflet advises avoid); **interactions:** see notes above and Appendix 1 (moclobemide)

Contra-indications: acute confusional states, phaeochromocytoma

Side-effects: sleep disturbances, dizziness, gastro-intestinal disorders, headache, restlessness, agitation; paraesthesia, dry mouth, visual disturbances, oedema, skin reactions, confusional states reported; rarely raised liver enzymes, galactorrhoea; for CSM advice on possible hyponatraemia, see p. 196

Dose: depression, initially 300 mg daily usually in divided doses after food, adjusted according to response; usual range 150–600 mg daily; CHILD not recommended

Social phobia, initially 300 mg daily increased on fourth day to 600 mg daily in 2 divided doses, continued for 8–12 weeks to assess efficacy; CHILD not recommended

Moclobemide (Non-proprietary) PoM
Tablets, moclobemide 150 mg, net price 30-tab pack = £6.51; 300 mg, 30-tab pack = £12.55. Label: 10, patient information leaflet, 21

Manerix® (Roche) PoM
Tablets, yellow, f/c, scored, moclobemide 150 mg, net price 30-tab pack = £9.33; 300 mg, 30-tab pack = £13.99. Label: 10, patient information leaflet, 21

4.3.3 Selective serotonin re-uptake inhibitors

Citalopram, **escitalopram**, **fluoxetine**, **fluvoxamine, paroxetine**, and **sertraline** selectively inhibit the re-uptake of serotonin (5-hydroxytryptamine, 5-HT); they are termed selective serotonin re-uptake inhibitors (SSRIs). For a general comment on the management of depression and on the comparison between *tricyclic and related antidepressants* and the *SSRIs and related antidepressants*, see section 4.3.

CSM advice (depressive illness in children and adolescents). The CSM has advised that the balance of risks and benefits for the treatment of depressive illness in individuals under 18 years is considered unfavourable for the SSRIs citalopram, escitalopram, paroxetine, and sertraline, and for mirtazapine and venlafaxine. Clinical trials have failed to show efficacy and have shown an increase in harmful outcomes. However, it is recognised that specialists may sometimes decide to use these drugs in response to individual clinical need; children and adolescents should be monitored carefully for suicidal behaviour, self-harm or hostility, particularly at the beginning of treatment.
Only fluoxetine has been shown in clinical trials to be effective for treating depressive illness in children and adolescents. However, it is possible that, in common with the other SSRIs, it is associatd with a small risk of self-harm and suicidal thoughts. Overall, the balance of risks and benefits for fluoxetine in the treatment of depressive illness in individuals under 18 years is considered favourable, but children and adolescents must be carefully monitored as above.

CAUTIONS. SSRIs should be used with caution in patients with epilepsy (avoid if poorly controlled, discontinue if convulsions develop), concurrent electroconvulsive therapy (prolonged seizures reported with fluoxetine), history of mania, cardiac disease, diabetes mellitus, angle-closure glaucoma, concomitant use of drugs that increase risk of bleeding, history of bleeding disorders (especially gastro-intestinal bleeding), hepatic impairment (Appendix 2), renal impairment (Appendix 3), pregnancy (Appendix 4), and breast-feeding (Appendix 5). The risk of suicidal behaviour is possibly higher in young adults, calling for close monitoring of those receiving SSRIs (see also CSM advice above). SSRIs may also impair performance of skilled tasks (e.g. driving). **Interactions:** see below and Appendix 1 (antidepressants, SSRI).

WITHDRAWAL. Gastro-intestinal disturbances, headache, anxiety, dizziness, paraesthesia, sleep disturbances, fatigue, influenza-like symptoms, and sweating are the most common features of abrupt withdrawal of an SSRI or marked reduction of the dose; the dose should be tapered over a few weeks to avoid these effects.

INTERACTIONS. An SSRI or related antidepressant should not be started until 2 weeks after stopping an MAOI. Conversely, an MAOI should not be started until at least a week after an SSRI or related antidepressant has been stopped (2 weeks in the case of sertraline, at least 5 weeks in the case of fluoxetine). For guidance relating to the reversible monoamine oxidase inhibitor, moclobemide, see above. For other SSRI antidepressant interactions, see Appendix 1 (antidepressants, SSRI).

CONTRA-INDICATIONS. SSRIs should not be used if the patient enters a manic phase.

SIDE-EFFECTS. SSRIs are less sedating and have fewer antimuscarinic and cardiotoxic effects than tricyclic antidepressants (section 4.3). Side-effects of the SSRIs include gastro-intestinal effects (dose-related and fairly common—include nausea, vomiting, dyspepsia, abdominal pain, diarrhoea, constipation), anorexia with weight loss (increased appetite and weight gain also reported) and hypersensitivity reactions including rash (consider discontinuation—may be sign of impending serious systemic reaction, possibly associated with vasculitis), urticaria, angioedema, anaphylaxis, arthralgia, myalgia and photosensitivity; other side-effects include dry mouth, nervousness, anxiety, headache, insomnia, tremor, dizziness, asthenia, hallucinations, drowsiness, convulsions (see Cautions above), galactorrhoea, sexual dysfunction, urinary retention, sweating, hypomania or mania (see Cautions above), movement disorders and dyskinesias, visual disturbances, hyponatraemia (may be due to inappropriate antidiuretic hormone secretion—see CSM warning, section 4.3), and cutaneous bleeding disorders including ecchymoses and purpura. Suicidal ideation has been linked with SSRIs but causality has not been established.

CITALOPRAM

Indications: depressive illness, panic disorder
Cautions: see notes above
Contra-indications: see notes above
Side-effects: see notes above; also palpitation, tachycardia, postural hypotension, coughing, yawning, confusion, impaired concentration, malaise, amnesia, migraine, paraesthesia, abnormal dreams, taste disturbance, increased salivation, rhinitis, tinnitus, polyuria, micturition disorders, euphoria
Dose: see preparations below

Citalopram (Non-proprietary) PoM
Tablets, citalopram (as hydrobromide) 10 mg, net price 28-tab pack = £7.04; 20 mg, 28-tab pack = £12.63; 40 mg, 28-tab pack = £20.82. Counselling, driving

Cipramil® (Lundbeck) PoM
Tablets, f/c, citalopram (as hydrobromide) 10 mg, net price 28-tab pack = £8.97; 20 mg (scored), 28-tab pack = £14.91; 40 mg, 28-tab pack = £25.20. Counselling, driving
Dose: depressive illness, 20 mg daily as a single dose in the morning or evening increased if necessary to max. 60 mg daily (ELDERLY max. 40 mg daily); CHILD and ADOLESCENT under 18 years not recommended (see CSM advice p. 202)
Panic disorder, initially 10 mg daily increased to 20 mg after 7 days, usual dose 20–30 mg daily; max. 60 mg daily (ELDERLY max. 40 mg daily); CHILD and ADOLESCENT under 18 years not recommended
Oral drops, sugar-free, citalopram (as hydrochloride) 40 mg/mL, net price 15 mL = £20.16. Counselling, driving, administration
Dose: depressive illness, 16 mg daily as a single dose in the morning or evening increased if necessary to max. 48 mg daily (ELDERLY max. 32 mg daily); CHILD and ADOLESCENT under 18 years not recommended (see CSM advice p. 202)
Panic disorder, initially 8 mg daily as a single dose increased to 16 mg daily after 7 days, usual dose 16–24 mg daily; max. 48 mg daily; (ELDERLY max. 32 mg daily); CHILD and ADOLESCENT under 18 years not recommended
Excipients: include alcohol
NOTE. 8 mg (4 drops) Cipramil® oral drops may be considered to be equivalent in therapeutic effect to 10-mg Cipramil® tablet
Mix with water, orange juice, or apple juice before taking

ESCITALOPRAM

NOTE. Escitalopram is an isomer of citalopram
Indications: see under Dose
Cautions: see notes above
Contra-indications: see notes above
Side-effects: see notes above; also postural hypotension, sinusitis, yawning, pyrexia, taste disturbance reported
Dose: depressive illness, 10 mg once daily increased if necessary to max. 20 mg daily; ELDERLY initially half adult dose, lower maintenance dose may be sufficient; CHILD and ADOLESCENT under 18 years not recommended (see CSM advice p. 202)
Panic disorder, initially 5 mg daily increased to 10 mg daily after 7 days; max. 20 mg daily; ELDERLY initially half adult dose, lower maintenance dose may be sufficient; CHILD and ADOLESCENT under 18 years not recommended
Social anxiety disorder, initially 10 mg daily adjusted after 2–4 weeks; usual dose 5–20 mg daily; CHILD and ADOLESCENT under 18 years not recommended

Cipralex® (Lundbeck) ▼ PoM
Tablets, f/c, scored, escitalopram (as oxalate) 5 mg, net price 28-tab pack = £8.97; 10 mg, 28-tab pack = £14.91; 20 mg, 28-tab pack = £25.20. Counselling, driving

FLUOXETINE

Indications: see under Dose
Cautions: see notes above
Contra-indications: see notes above
Side-effects: see notes above; also possible changes in blood sugar, fever, neuroleptic malignant syndrome-like event; also reported (no causal relationship established): abnormal bleeding, aplastic anaemia, cerebrovascular accident, ecchymoses, gastro-intestinal haemorrhage, haemolytic anaemia, pancreatitis, pancytopenia, thrombocytopenia, thrombocytopenic purpura, vaginal bleeding on withdrawal, violent behaviour; hair loss also reported
Dose: depressive illness, 20 mg once daily increased after 3 weeks if necessary, usual dose 20–60 mg (ELDERLY 20–40 mg) once daily; max. 80 mg (ELDERLY max. 60 mg) once daily; CHILD and ADOLESCENT under 18 years not recommended
Bulimia nervosa, 60 mg once daily; max. 80 mg once daily; CHILD and ADOLESCENT under 18 years not recommended
Obsessive-compulsive disorder, initially 20 mg once daily increased after two weeks if necessary, usual dose 20–60 mg (ELDERLY 20–40 mg) once daily; max. 80 mg (ELDERLY max. 60 mg) once daily; discontinue if no improvement within 10 weeks; CHILD and ADOLESCENT under 18 years not recommended
LONG DURATION OF ACTION. Consider the long half-life of fluoxetine when adjusting dosage (or in overdosage)

Fluoxetine (Non-proprietary) PoM
Capsules, fluoxetine (as hydrochloride) 20 mg, net price 30-cap pack = £1.56; 60 mg, 30-cap pack = £47.61. Counselling, driving
Brands include *Oxactin*®
Liquid, fluoxetine (as hydrochloride) 20 mg/5 mL, net price 70 mL = £11.87. Counselling, driving

Prozac® (Dista) PoM
Capsules, fluoxetine (as hydrochloride) 20 mg (green/yellow), net price 30-cap pack = £14.21; 60 mg (yellow), 30-cap pack = £47.61. Counselling, driving
Liquid, fluoxetine (as hydrochloride) 20 mg/5 mL. Net price 70 mL = £13.26. Counselling, driving

FLUVOXAMINE MALEATE

Indications: depressive illness, obsessive-compulsive disorder

Cautions: see notes above

CSM ADVICE. The CSM has advised that concomitant use of fluvoxamine and theophylline or aminophylline should usually be avoided; see also **interactions:** Appendix 1 (antidepressants, SSRIs)

Contra-indications: see notes above

Side-effects: see notes above; palpitation, tachycardia (may also cause bradycardia); *rarely* postural hypotension, confusion, ataxia, paraesthesia, malaise, taste disturbance, neuroleptic malignant syndome-like event, abnormal liver function tests, usually symptomatic (discontinue treatment)

Dose: depression, initially 50–100 mg daily in the evening, increased gradually if necessary to max. 300 mg daily (over 150 mg in divided doses); usual maintenance dose 100 mg daily; CHILD and ADOLESCENT under 18 years not recommended

Obsessive-compulsive disorder, initially 50 mg in the evening increased gradually if necessary after some weeks to max. 300 mg daily (over 150 mg in divided doses); usual maintenance dose 100–300 mg daily; CHILD over 8 years initially 25 mg daily increased if necessary in steps of 25 mg every 4–7 days to max. 200 mg daily (over 50 mg in divided doses)

NOTE. If no improvement in obsessive-compulsive disorder within 10 weeks, treatment should be reconsidered

Fluvoxamine (Non-proprietary) PoM
Tablets, fluvoxamine maleate 50 mg, net price 60-tab pack = £10.98; 100 mg, 30-tab pack = £11.98. Counselling, driving

Faverin® (Solvay) PoM
Tablets, f/c, scored, fluvoxamine maleate 50 mg, net price 60-tab pack = £17.10; 100 mg, 30-tab pack = £17.10. Counselling, driving

PAROXETINE

Indications: major depression, obsessive-compulsive disorder, panic disorder; social phobia; post-traumatic stress disorder; generalised anxiety disorder

Cautions: see notes above

IMPORTANT. During initial treatment of panic disorder, there is potential for worsening of panic symptoms

CSM ADVICE. Extrapyramidal reactions (including orofacial dystonias) and withdrawal syndrome are reported to the CSM more commonly with paroxetine than with other SSRIs

Contra-indications: see notes above

Side-effects: see notes above; also yawning; *less commonly* arrhythmias, transient changes in blood pressure, confusion; *rarely* panic attacks, depersonalisation, and neuroleptic malignant syndrome-like event; *very rarely* peripheral oedema, acute glaucoma, hepatic disorders (e.g. hepatitis)

Dose: major depression, social anxiety disorder, post-traumatic stress disorder, generalised anxiety disorder, usually 20 mg each morning, increased gradually in steps of 10 mg to max. 50 mg daily (ELDERLY 40 mg daily) but doses higher than 20 mg not necessary, see CSM advice below; CHILD and ADOLESCENT under 18 years not recommended (see CSM advice p. 202)

Obsessive compulsive disorder, initially 20 mg each morning, increased gradually in steps of 10 mg to usual dose of 40 mg daily; max. 60 mg daily (ELDERLY 40 mg daily) but doses higher than 40 mg not necessary, see CSM advice below; CHILD and ADOLESCENT under 18 years not recommended

Panic disorder, initially 10 mg each morning, increased gradually in steps of 10 mg to usual dose of 40 mg daily; max. 60 mg daily (ELDERLY 40 mg daily) but doses higher than 40 mg not necessary, see CSM advice below; CHILD and ADOLESCENT under 18 years not recommended

CSM ADVICE. The recommended dose for the treatment of depression, social anxiety disorder, generalised anxiety disorder, and post-traumatic stress disorder is 20 mg daily and for obsessive-compulsive disorder and panic disorder it is 40 mg daily. There is no evidence that higher doses are more effective.

Paroxetine (Non-proprietary) PoM
Tablets, paroxetine (as hydrochloride) 20 mg, net price 30-tab pack = £6.86. Label: 21, counselling, driving

Seroxat® (GSK) PoM
Tablets, both f/c, scored, paroxetine (as hydrochloride) 20 mg, net price 30-tab pack = £13.21; 30 mg (blue), 30-tab pack = £23.18. Label: 21, counselling, driving
Liquid, orange, sugar-free, paroxetine (as hydrochloride) 10 mg/5 mL. Net price 150-mL pack = £9.49. Label: 21, counselling, driving

SERTRALINE

Indications: depressive illness, obsessive-compulsive disorder (under specialist supervision in children), post-traumatic stress disorder in women

Cautions: see notes above

Contra-indications: see notes above

Side-effects: see notes above; tachycardia, confusion, amnesia, aggressive behaviour, psychosis, pancreatitis, hepatitis, jaundice, liver failure, menstrual irregularities, paraesthesia; thrombocytopenia also reported (causal relationship not established)

Dose: depressive illness, initially 50 mg daily, increased if necessary by increments of 50 mg over several weeks to max. 200 mg daily; usual maintenance dose 50 mg daily; CHILD and ADOLESCENT under 18 years not recommended (see CSM advice p. 202)

Obsessive-compulsive disorder, ADULT and ADOLESCENT over 13 years initially 50 mg daily, increased if necessary in steps of

50 mg over several weeks; usual dose range 50–200 mg daily; CHILD 6–12 years initially 25 mg daily, increased to 50 mg daily after 1 week, further increased if necessary in steps of 50 mg at intervals of at least 1 week (max. 200 mg daily); CHILD under 6 years not recommended

Post-traumatic stress disorder, initially 25 mg daily, increased after 1 week to 50 mg daily; if response is partial and if drug tolerated, dose increased in steps of 50 mg over several weeks to max. 200 mg daily; CHILD and ADOLESCENT under 18 years not recommended

Lustral® (Pfizer) PoM
Tablets, both f/c, sertraline (as hydrochloride) 50 mg (scored), net price 28-tab pack = £17.82; 100 mg, 28-tab pack = £29.16. Counselling, driving

4.3.4 Other antidepressant drugs

Duloxetine inhibits the re-uptake of both serotonin and noradrenaline and is licensed to treat major depressive disorder.

The thioxanthene **flupentixol** (*Fluanxol*®) has antidepressant properties, and low doses (1 to 3 mg daily) are given by mouth for this purpose. Flupentixol is also used for the treatment of psychoses (section 4.2.1 and section 4.2.2)

Mirtazapine, a presynaptic α_2-antagonist, increases central noradrenergic and serotonergic neurotransmission. It has few antimuscarinic effects, but causes sedation during initial treatment.

Reboxetine, a selective inhibitor of noradrenaline re-uptake, has been introduced for the treatment of depressive illness.

Tryptophan is licensed as adjunctive therapy for depression resistant to standard antidepressants; it has been associated with the eosinophilia-myalgia syndrome. Tryptophan should be initiated under specialist supervision.

Venlafaxine is a serotonin and noradrenaline re-uptake inhibitor (SNRI); it lacks the sedative and antimuscarinic effects of the tricyclic antidepressants. The CSM has recommended that because of concerns about toxicity in overdose, treatment with venlafaxine should be initiated and maintained under specialist supervision only. The CSM has advised that venlafaxine should not be used in patients with heart disease, electrolyte imbalance and hypertension.

DULOXETINE

Indications: major depressive disorder; stress urinary incontinence (section 7.4.2)

Cautions: see section 7.4.2; pregnancy (Appendix 4); **interactions:** Appendix 1 (duloxetine)

Contra-indications: hepatic impairment; renal impairment (Appendix 3); breast-feeding (Appendix 5)

Side-effects: see section 7.4.2

Dose: 60 mg once daily; CHILD and ADOLESCENT under 18 years not recommended

Cymbalta® (Lilly) ▼ PoM
Capsules, duloxetine (as hydrochloride) 30 mg (white/blue), net price 28-cap pack = £22.40; 60 mg (green/blue), 28-cap pack = £27.72, 84-cap pack = £83.16. Label: 2

Yentreve® (Lilly) ▼ PoM
Section 7.4.2 (stress urinary incontinence)

FLUPENTIXOL

(Flupenthixol)

Indications: depressive illness; psychoses (section 4.2.1)

Cautions: cardiovascular disease (including cardiac disorders and cerebral arteriosclerosis), senile confusional states, parkinsonism, hepatic impairment (Appendix 2), renal impairment (Appendix 3); avoid in excitable and overactive patients; porphyria (section 9.8.2); see also section 4.2.1; **interactions**: Appendix 1 (antipsychotics)

Side-effects: restlessness, insomnia; hypomania reported; rarely dizziness, tremor, visual disturbances, headache, hyperprolactinaemia, extrapyramidal symptoms

Dose: initially 1 mg (elderly 500 micrograms) in the morning, increased after 1 week to 2 mg (elderly 1 mg) if necessary; max. 3 mg (elderly 2 mg) daily, doses above 2 mg (elderly 1 mg) being divided in 2 portions, second dose not after 4 p.m. Discontinue if no response after 1 week at max. dosage; CHILD and ADOLESCENT under 18 years not recommended

COUNSELLING. Although drowsiness may occur, can also have an alerting effect so should not be taken in the evening

Fluanxol® (Lundbeck) PoM
Tablets, both red, s/c, flupentixol (as dihydrochloride) 500 micrograms, net price 60-tab pack = £2.88; 1 mg, 60-tab pack = £4.86. Label: 2, counselling, administration

MIRTAZAPINE

Indications: depressive illness

Cautions: epilepsy, hepatic or renal impairment, cardiac disorders, hypotension, history of urinary retention, angle-closure glaucoma, diabetes mellitus, psychoses (may aggravate psychotic symptoms), history of bipolar depression, avoid abrupt withdrawal; manufacturer advises avoid in pregnancy and in breast-feeding (Appendix 5); **interactions:** Appendix 1 (mirtazapine)

BLOOD DISORDERS. Patients should be advised to report any fever, sore throat, stomatitis or other signs of infection during treatment. Blood count should be performed and the drug stopped immediately if blood dyscrasia suspected

Side-effects: increased appetite and weight gain, oedema, sedation; less commonly dizziness, headache; rarely postural hypotension, abnormal dreams, mania, convulsions, tremor, myoclonus, paraesthesia, arthralgia, myalgia, restless legs, exanthema, reversible agranulocytosis (see Cautions above)

Dose: initially 15 mg daily at bedtime increased according to response up to 45 mg daily as a single dose at bedtime or in 2 divided doses; CHILD and ADOLESCENT under 18 years not recommended (see CSM advice, p. 202)

Mirtazapine (Non-proprietary) PoM
Tablets, mirtazapine 30 mg, net price 28-tab pack = £22.99. Label: 2, 25
Oral solution, mirtazapine 15 mg/mL, net price 66 mL = £47.00. Label: 2

Zispin SolTab® (Organon) PoM
Orodispersible tablets, mirtazapine 15 mg, net price 6-tab pack = £3.84, 30-tab pack = £19.19; 30 mg, 30-tab pack = £19.19; 45 mg, 30-tab pack = £19.19. Label: 2, counselling, administration
Excipients: include aspartame
COUNSELLING. *Zispin SolTab*® should be placed on the tongue, allowed to disperse and swallowed

REBOXETINE

Indications: depressive illness
Cautions: severe renal impairment (Appendix 3), hepatic impairment (Appendix 2), history of cardiovascular disease and epilepsy, bipolar disorders, urinary retention, prostatic hypertrophy, glaucoma; **interactions:** Appendix 1 (reboxetine)
Contra-indications: pregnancy (Appendix 4) and breast-feeding (Appendix 5)
Side-effects: insomnia, sweating, dizziness, postural hypotension, vertigo, paraesthesia, impotence, dysuria, urinary retention (mainly in men), dry mouth, constipation, tachycardia; lowering of plasma-potassium concentration on prolonged administration in the elderly
Dose: 4 mg twice daily increased if necessary after 3–4 weeks to 10 mg daily in divided doses, max. 12 mg daily; CHILD and ELDERLY not recommended

Edronax® (Pharmacia) PoM
Tablets, scored, reboxetine (as mesilate) 4 mg. Net price 60-tab pack = £18.91. Counselling, driving

TRYPTOPHAN

(L-Tryptophan)
Indications: see notes above
Cautions: eosinophilia-myalgia syndrome has been reported—close monitoring required (withhold treatment if increased eosinophil count, myalgia, arthralgia, fever, dyspnoea, neuropathy, oedema or skin lesions develop until possibility of eosinophilia-myalgia syndrome excluded); pregnancy and breast-feeding; **interactions:** Appendix 1 (tryptophan)
Contra-indications: history of eosinophilia-myalgia syndrome following use of tryptophan
Side-effects: drowsiness, nausea, headache, light-headedness; eosinophilia-myalgia syndrome, see Cautions
Dose: 1 g 3 times daily; max. 6 g daily; ELDERLY lower dose may be appropriate especially where renal or hepatic impairment; CHILD not recommended

Optimax® (Merck) PoM
Tablets, scored, tryptophan 500 mg. Net price 84-tab pack = £19.56. Label: 3

VENLAFAXINE

Indications: moderate to severe depressive illness, generalised anxiety disorder (under specialist supervision, see CSM advice p. 205)
Cautions: ECG required before treatment, measure blood pressure before and periodically during treatment; history of epilepsy, angle-closure glaucoma; concomitant use of drugs that increase risk of bleeding, history of bleeding disorders; hepatic impairment (Appendix 2); renal impairment (Appendix 3); **interactions:** Appendix 1 (venlafaxine)
DRIVING. May affect performance of skilled tasks (e.g. driving)
WITHDRAWAL. Gastro-intestinal disturbances, headache, anxiety, dizziness, paraesthesia, tremor, sleep disturbances, and sweating are most common features of withdrawal if treatment stopped abruptly or if dose reduced markedly; dose should be reduced over several weeks
Contra-indications: see CSM advice, p. 202 and p. 205; heart disease, electrolyte disturbance, hypertension; severe hepatic or renal impairment; pregnancy (Appendix 4) and breast-feeding (Appendix 5)
Side-effects: constipation, nausea; dizziness, dry mouth, insomnia, nervousness, drowsiness, asthenia, headache; sexual dysfunction; sweating; commonly anorexia, weight changes, diarrhoea, dyspepsia, vomiting, abdominal pain; hypertension, palpitation, vasodilatation, changes in serum cholesterol; chills, pyrexia, dyspnoea, yawning; abnormal dreams, agitation, anxiety, confusion, hypertonia, paraesthesia, tremor; urinary frequency, menstrual disturbances; arthralgia, myalgia; visual disturbances, mydriasis; tinnitus; pruritus, rash; *less commonly* apathy, bruxism, taste disturbances, hypotension and postural hypotension, arrhythmias, syndrome of inappropriate anti-diuretic hormone secretion (see advice on Hyponatraemia, p. 196), hallucinations, myoclonus, urinary retention, bleeding disorders (including ecchymosis and rarely haemorrhage), alopecia, hypersensitivity reactions including angioedema, urticaria, photosensitivity; *rarely* prolonged QT interval, ataxia, incoordination, speech disorder, extrapyramidal effects, suicidal ideation, mania and hypomania, aggression, seizures, serotonin syndrome and neuroleptic malignant syndrome, increased prolactin concentration, blood dyscrasias, rhabdomyolysis, erythema multiforme, Stevens-Johnson syndrome; hepatitis and pancreatitis reported
Dose: depression, initially 75 mg daily in 2 divided doses increased if necessary after at least 3–4 weeks to 150 mg daily in 2 divided doses; severely depressed or hospitalised patients, increased further if necessary in steps of up to 75 mg every 2–3 days to max. 375 mg daily then gradually reduced; CHILD and ADOLESCENT under 18 years not recommended (see CSM advice p. 202)
Generalised anxiety disorder, see under preparations below

Efexor® (Wyeth) PoM
Tablets, all peach, venlafaxine (as hydrochloride) 37.5 mg, net price 56-tab pack = £23.41; 75 mg, 56-tab pack = £39.03. Label: 3, 21, counselling, driving

■ Modified release

Efexor® **XL** (Wyeth) PoM
Capsules, m/r, venlafaxine (as hydrochloride) 75 mg (peach), net price 28-cap pack = £23.41,

150 mg (orange), 28-cap pack = £39.03. Label: 3, 21, 25, counselling, driving

Dose: depression, 75 mg daily as a single dose, increased if necessary after at least 2 weeks to 150 mg once daily; max. 225 mg once daily; ADOLESCENT and CHILD under 18 years not recommended (see CSM advice, p. 202), Generalised anxiety disorder, 75 mg daily as a single dose; discontinue if no response after 8 weeks; ADOLESCENT and CHILD under 18 years not recommended

4.4 CNS stimulants and other drugs used for attention deficit hyperactivity disorder

Central nervous system stimulants include the **amphetamines** (notably dexamfetamine) **and related drugs** (e.g. methylphenidate). They have very few indications and in particular, should **not** be used to treat depression, obesity, senility, debility, or for relief of fatigue.

Caffeine is a weak stimulant present in tea and coffee. It is included in many analgesic preparations (section 4.7.1) but does not contribute to their analgesic or anti-inflammatory effect. Over-indulgence may lead to a state of anxiety.

The **amphetamines** have a limited field of usefulness and their use should be **discouraged** as they may cause dependence and psychotic states. They have **no place** in the management of **depression** or **obesity**.

Patients with *narcolepsy* may derive benefit from treatment with dexamfetamine.

Methylphenidate is used for the management of *attention deficit hyperactivity disorder* (ADHD) in children and adolescents as part of a comprehensive treatment programme. Growth is not generally affected but it is advisable to monitor growth during treatment. **Dexamfetamine** (dexamphetamine) is an alternative in children who do not respond to other drugs. **Atomoxetine** is licensed for the management of attention deficit hyperactivity disorder in children. Drug treatment of attention deficit hyperactivity disorder should be initiated by a specialist in ADHD but may be continued by general practitioners, under a shared-care arrangement.

Modafinil is used for the treatment of daytime sleepiness associated with narcolepsy or obstructive sleep apnoea syndrome; dependence with long-term use cannot be excluded and it should therefore be used with caution.

ATOMOXETINE

Indications: attention deficit hyperactivity disorder (initiated by a specialist physician experienced in managing the condition)

Cautions: cardiovascular disease including hypertension, tachycardia, and postural hypotension; monitor growth in children; hepatic impairment (see Hepatic Disorders below; Appendix 2); pregnancy (Appendix 4); breast-feeding (Appendix 5); **interactions:** Appendix 1 (atomoxetine)

HEPATIC DISORDERS. Following rare reports of hepatic disorders, the CSM has advised that patients and carers should be advised of the risk and be told how to recognise symptoms; prompt medical attention should be sought in case of abdominal pain, unexplained nausea, malaise, darkening of the urine or jaundice

Contra-indications: angle-closure glaucoma

Side-effects: anorexia, dry mouth, nausea, vomiting, abdominal pain, constipation, dyspepsia, flatulence; palpitation, tachycardia, increased blood pressure, postural hypotension, hot flushes; sleep disturbance, dizziness, headache, fatigue, lethargy, depression, anxiety, tremor, rigors; urinary retention, enuresis, prostatitis, sexual dysfunction, menstrual disturbances; mydriasis, conjunctivitis; dermatitis, pruritus, rash, sweating, weight changes; *less commonly* cold extremities; *rarely* hepatic disorders (see Hepatic Disorders above)

Dose: ADOLESCENT body-weight over 70 kg, initially 40 mg daily for 7 days then increased according to response to usual maintenance dose 80 mg daily; max. 100 mg daily; CHILD over 6 years and ADOLESCENT body-weight up to 70 kg, initially 500 micrograms/kg daily for 7 days then increased according to response to usual maintenance dose 1.2 mg/kg daily

NOTE. Total daily dose may be given *either* as a single dose in the morning *or* in 2 divided doses with last dose no later than early evening

Strattera® (Lilly) ▼ PoM

Capsules, atomoxetine (as hydrochloride) 10 mg (white), net price 7-cap pack = £13.65, 28-cap pack = £54.60; 18 mg (gold/white), 7-cap pack = £13.65, 28-cap pack = £54.60; 25 mg (blue/white), 7-cap pack = £13.65, 28-cap pack = £54.60; 40 mg (blue), 7-cap pack = £13.65, 28-cap pack = £54.60; 60 mg (blue/gold), 28-cap pack = £54.60. Label: 3

DEXAMFETAMINE SULPHATE

(Dexamphetamine sulphate)

Indications: narcolepsy, adjunct in the management of refractory hyperkinetic states in children (under specialist supervision)

Cautions: mild hypertension (contra-indicated if moderate or severe)—monitor blood pressure; history of epilepsy (discontinue if convulsions occur); tics and Tourette syndrome (use with caution)—discontinue if tics occur; monitor growth in children (see also below); avoid abrupt withdrawal; data on safety and efficacy of long-term use not complete; porphyria (see section 9.8.2); **interactions:** Appendix 1 (sympathomimetics)

SPECIAL CAUTIONS IN CHILDREN. Monitor height and weight as growth retardation may occur during prolonged therapy (drug free periods may allow catch-up in growth but withdraw slowly to avoid inducing depression or renewed hyperactivity). In psychotic children may exacerbate behavioural disturbances and thought disorder

DRIVING. May affect performance of skilled tasks (e.g. driving); effects of alcohol unpredictable

Contra-indications: cardiovascular disease including moderate to severe hypertension, hyperexcitability or agitated states, hyperthyroidism, history of drug or alcohol abuse, glaucoma, pregnancy (Appendix 4) and breast-feeding (Appendix 5)

Side-effects: insomnia, restlessness, irritability and excitability, nervousness, night terrors, euphoria, tremor, dizziness, headache; convulsions (see also Cautions); dependence and tolerance, sometimes psychosis; anorexia, gastro-intestinal symptoms, growth retardation in children (see also under Cautions); dry mouth, sweating, tachycardia (and anginal pain), palpitation, increased blood pressure; visual disturbances; cardiomyopathy reported with chronic use; central stimulants have provoked choreoathetoid movements, tics and Tourette syndrome in predisposed individuals (see also Cautions above); **overdosage:** see Emergency Treatment of Poisoning, p. 33

Dose: narcolepsy, 10 mg (ELDERLY, 5 mg) daily in divided doses increased by 10 mg (ELDERLY, 5 mg) daily at intervals of 1 week to a max. of 60 mg daily

Hyperkinesia, CHILD over 6 years 5–10 mg daily, increased if necessary by 5 mg at intervals of 1 week to usual max. 20 mg daily (older children have received max. 40 mg daily); under 6 years not recommended

Dexedrine® (Celltech) CD
Tablets, scored, dexamfetamine sulphate 5 mg. Net price 28-tab pack = £3.00. Counselling, driving

METHYLPHENIDATE HYDROCHLORIDE

Indications: part of a comprehensive treatment programme for attention-deficit hyperactivity disorder when remedial measures alone prove insufficient (under specialist supervision)

Cautions: monitor growth (if prolonged treatment), blood pressure and full blood count; history of drug or alcohol dependence; psychosis; epilepsy (discontinue if increased seizure frequency); avoid abrupt withdrawal; pregnancy (Appendix 4); **interactions:** Appendix 1 (sympathomimetics)

Contra-indications: anxiety or agitation; tics or a family history of Tourette syndrome; hyperthyroidism, severe angina, cardiac arrythmias, glaucoma; breast-feeding (Appendix 5)

Side-effects: abdominal pain, nausea, vomiting, dry mouth; tachycardia, palpitation, arrythmias, changes in blood pressure; insomnia, nervousness, anorexia, headache, drowsiness, dizziness, movement disorders; arthralgia; rash, pruritus, alopecia; *rarely* cerebral arteritis, angina, hyperactivity, convulsions, psychosis, tics including Tourette syndrome, neuroleptic malignant syndrome, tolerance and dependence, growth retardation, reduced weight gain, blood disorders including leucopenia and thrombocytopenia, muscle cramps, visual disturbances, exfoliative dermatitis, erythema multiforme

Dose: CHILD over 6 years, initially 5 mg 1–2 times daily, increased if necessary at weekly intervals by 5–10 mg daily to max. 60 mg daily in divided doses; discontinue if no response after 1 month, also suspend periodically to assess child's condition (usually finally discontinued during or after puberty); under 6 years not recommended

EVENING DOSE. If effect wears off in evening (with rebound hyperactivity) a dose at bedtime may be appropriate (establish need with trial bedtime dose)

Methylphenidate Hydrochloride (Non-proprietary) CD
Tablets, methylphenidate hydrochloride 5 mg, net price 30-tab pack = £2.78; 10 mg, 30-tab pack = £5.27; 20 mg, 30-tab pack = £9.98
Brands include *Equasym*®

Ritalin® (Cephalon) CD
Tablets, scored, methylphenidate hydrochloride 10 mg, net price 30-tab pack = £5.57

■ Modified release

Concerta® **XL** (Janssen-Cilag) ▼ CD
Tablets, m/r, methylphenidate hydrochloride 18 mg (yellow), net price 30-tab pack = £27.00; 36 mg (white), 30-tab pack = £36.75. Label: 25
COUNSELLING. Tablet membrane may pass through gastro-intestinal tract unchanged
Cautions: dose form not appropriate for use in dysphagia or where gastro-intestinal lumen restricted
Dose: CHILD over 6 years, initially 18 mg once daily (in the morning), increased if necessary in weekly steps of 18 mg according to response, max. 54 mg once daily; discontinue if no response after 1 month; suspend periodically to assess condition (usually finally discontinued during or after puberty); CHILD under 6 years not recommended
NOTE. Total daily dose of 15 mg of standard-release formulation is considered equivalent to *Concerta*® *XL* 18 mg once daily

Equasym XL® (UCB Pharma) CD
Capsules, m/r, methylphenidate hydrochloride 10 mg (white/green), net price 30-cap pack = £25.00; 20 mg (white/blue), 30-cap pack = £30.00; 30 mg (white/brown), 30-cap pack = £35.00. Label: 25
Dose: CHILD over 6 years, initially 10 mg once daily in the morning before breakfast, increased gradually if necessary to max. 60 mg daily; discontinue if no response after 1 month; suspend periodically to assess condition (usually finally discontinued during or after puberty); CHILD under 6 years not recommended

MODAFINIL

Indications: daytime sleepiness associated with chronic pathological conditions including narcolepsy, obstructive sleep apnoea syndrome, and chronic shift work

Cautions: hepatic impairment (Appendix 2); renal impairment (Appendix 3); monitor blood pressure and heart rate in hypertensive patients (but see below); possibility of dependence; **interactions:** Appendix 1 (modafinil)

Contra-indications: pregnancy (Appendix 4) and breast-feeding (Appendix 5); moderate to severe hypertension; history of left ventricular hypertrophy, cor pulmonale, or of clinically significant signs of CNS stimulant-induced mitral valve prolapse (including ischaemic ECG changes, chest pain and arrhythmias)

Side-effects: dry mouth, appetite changes, gastro-intestinal disturbances (including nausea, diarrhoea, constipation, and dyspepsia), abdominal pain; tachycardia, vasodilation, chest pain, dyspnoea; headache (uncommonly migraine), anxiety, insomnia, dizziness, depression, confusion, abnormal thinking, paraesthesia, incoordination, hypertonia, asthenia; visual disturbances; less commonly, mouth ulcers, dysphagia, taste disturbances; hypertension, hypotension, arrhythmia, peripheral oedema, hypercholesterolaemia; rhinitis; dyskinesia, amnesia, emotional lability, abnormal dreams, agitation, tremor, vertigo, decreased libido, weight changes, hyperglycaemia; urinary frequency, myasthenia, muscle cramps, menstrual disturbances; eosinophilia, leucopenia; glossitis, pharyngitis, sinusitis, epistaxis; myalgia, arthralgia; acne, sweating, rash, pruritus, dry eye

Dose: narcolepsy and obstructive sleep apnoea syndrome, initially 200 mg daily, *either* in 2 divided doses morning and at noon *or* as a single

dose in the morning, dose adjusted according to response to 200–400 mg daily in 2 divided doses or as a single dose; ELDERLY initiate at 100 mg daily; CHILD not recommended
Chronic shift work sleep disorder, 200 mg taken 1 hour before the start of the work shift

Provigil® (Cephalon) ▼ PoM
Tablets, modafinil 100 mg, net price 30-tab pack = £60.00; 200 mg, 30 tab-pack = £120.00

Cocaine

Cocaine is a drug of addiction which causes central nervous stimulation. Its clinical use is mainly as a topical local anaesthetic (section 15.2). It has been included in analgesic elixirs for the relief of pain in palliative care but this use is obsolete. For management of cocaine poisoning, see p. 33.

4.5 Drugs used in the treatment of obesity

Obesity is associated with many health problems including cardiovascular disease, diabetes mellitus, gallstones and osteoarthritis. Factors that aggravate obesity may include depression, other psychosocial problems, and some drugs.

The main treatment of the obese individual is a suitable diet, carefully explained to the individual, with appropriate support and encouragement; the individual should also be advised to increase physical activity. Smoking cessation (while maintaining body weight) may be worthwhile before attempting supervised weight loss since cigarette smoking may be more harmful than obesity. Attendance at groups (e.g. 'weight-watchers') helps some individuals.

Severe obesity should be managed in an appropriate setting by staff who have been trained in the management of obesity; the individual should receive advice on diet and lifestyle modification and be monitored for changes in weight as well as in blood pressure, blood lipids and other associated conditions.

An anti-obesity drug should be considered only for those with a body mass index (BMI, individual's body-weight divided by the square of the individual's height) of 30 kg/m^2 or greater in whom at least 3 months of managed care involving supervised diet, exercise and behaviour modification fails to achieve a realistic reduction in weight. In the presence of risk factors (such as diabetes, coronary heart disease, hypertension, and obstructive sleep apnoea), it may be appropriate to prescribe a drug to individuals with a BMI of 27 kg/m^2 or greater, provided that such use is permitted by the drug's marketing authorisation. Drugs should **never** be used as the sole element of treatment. The individual should be monitored on a regular basis; drug treatment should be discontinued if weight loss is less than 5% after the first 12 weeks or if the individual regains weight at any time whilst receiving drug treatment.

Drugs specifically licensed for the treatment of obesity are **orlistat** (section 4.5.1) and **sibutramine** (section 4.5.2). There is little evidence to guide selection between the two drugs, but it may be appropriate to choose orlistat for those who have a high intake of fats whereas sibutramine may be chosen for those who cannot control their eating; the cautions, contra-indications and side-effects of the two drugs should also be considered.

Combination therapy involving more than one anti-obesity drug is **contra-indicated** until further information about efficacy and long-term safety is available.

Thyroid hormones have **no** place in the treatment of obesity except in biochemically proven hypothyroid patients. The use of diuretics, chorionic gonadotrophin, or amphetamines is **not** appropriate for weight reduction.

4.5.1 Anti-obesity drugs acting on the gastro-intestinal tract

Orlistat, a lipase inhibitor, reduces the absorption of dietary fat. It is used in conjunction with a mildly hypocaloric diet in individuals with a body mass index (BMI) of 30 kg/m^2 or more *or* in individuals with a BMI of 28 kg/m^2 in the presence of other risk factors such as type 2 diabetes, hypertension, or hypercholesterolaemia.

Orlistat should be used in conjunction with other measures to manage obesity (section 4.5). NICE has recommended (March 2001) that treatment with orlistat should be continued beyond 6 months only if at least 10% weight has been lost since the start of treatment.

Some of the weight loss in those taking orlistat probably results from individuals reducing their fat intake to avoid severe gastro-intestinal effects including steatorrhoea. Vitamin supplementation (especially of vitamin D) may be considered if there is concern about deficiency of fat-soluble vitamins. On stopping orlistat, there may be a gradual reversal of weight loss.

The most commonly used bulk-forming drug is **methylcellulose** (section 1.6.1). It is claimed to reduce intake by producing a feeling of satiety but there is little evidence to support its use in the management of obesity.

ORLISTAT

Indications: adjunct in obesity (see notes above)
Cautions: diabetes mellitus; may impair absorption of fat-soluble vitamins; **interactions:** Appendix 1 (orlistat)
MULTIVITAMINS. If a multivitamin supplement is required, it should be taken at least 2 hours after orlistat dose or at bedtime
Contra-indications: chronic malabsorption syndrome; cholestasis; pregnancy (Appendix 4) and breast-feeding (Appendix 5)
Side-effects: oily leakage from rectum, flatulence, faecal urgency, liquid or oily stools, faecal incontinence, abdominal distension and pain (gastro-intestinal effects minimised by reduced fat intake), tooth and gingival disorders; respiratory infec-

tions; anxiety, headache; menstrual disturbances, urinary-tract infection; fatigue; also reported diverticulitis, cholelithiasis, hepatitis, hypersensitivity reactions, and bullous eruptions

Dose: 120 mg taken immediately before, during, or up to 1 hour after each main meal (up to max. 360 mg daily); continue treatment beyond 12 weeks only if weight loss since start of treatment exceeds 5% (see also notes above); CHILD not recommended

NOTE. If a meal is missed or contains no fat, the dose of orlistat should be omitted

Xenical® (Roche) PoM

Capsules, turquoise, orlistat 120 mg, net price 84-cap pack = £39.51

4.5.2 Centrally acting appetite suppressants

Sibutramine inhibits the re-uptake of noradrenaline and serotonin. It is used in the adjunctive management of obesity in individuals with a body mass index (BMI) of 30 kg/m^2 or more (and no associated co-morbidity) or in individuals with a BMI of 27 kg/m^2 or more in the presence of other risk factors such as type 2 diabetes or hypercholesterolaemia. Sibutramine is not licensed for use longer than 1 year; on stopping it, there may be a reversal of weight loss.

Dexfenfluramine, fenfluramine, and phentermine have been associated with valvular heart disease and the rare but serious risk of pulmonary hypertension.

NICE guidance (sibutramine). NICE has recommended that sibutramine should be prescribed in accordance with the summary of product characteristics and under the following conditions:

- it should be prescribed only for individuals who have attempted seriously to lose weight by diet, exercise, and other behavioural modification;
- arrangements should exist for appropriate healthcare professionals to offer specific advice, support, and counselling on diet, physical activity, and behavioural strategies to those receiving sibutramine.

SIBUTRAMINE HYDROCHLORIDE

Indications: adjunct in obesity (see notes above)

Cautions: monitor blood pressure and pulse rate (every 2 weeks for first 3 months *then* monthly for 3 months *then* at least every 3 months)—discontinue if blood pressure exceeds 145/90 mmHg or if systolic or diastolic pressure raised by more than 10 mmHg or if pulse rate raised by 10 beats per minute at 2 consecutive visits; sleep apnoea syndrome (increased risk of hypertension); epilepsy; hepatic impairment (avoid if severe; Appendix 2); renal impairment (avoid if severe; Appendix 3); open angle glaucoma, history of ocular hypertension; monitor for pulmonary hypertension; family history of motor or vocal tics, history of depression; predisposition to bleeding, concomitant use of drugs that increase risk of bleeding; **interactions:** Appendix 1 (sibutramine)

DISCONTINUATION OF TREATMENT. Discontinue treatment if:

- weight loss after 3 months less than 5% of initial body-weight;
- weight loss stabilises at less than 5% of initial body-weight;
- individuals regain 3 kg or more after previous weight loss

In individuals with co-morbid conditions, treatment should be continued only if weight loss is associated with other clinical benefits

Contra-indications: history of major eating disorders; psychiatric illness, Tourette syndrome; history of coronary artery disease, congestive heart failure, tachycardia, peripheral arterial occlusive disease, arrhythmias, and of cerebrovascular disease; uncontrolled hypertension; hyperthyroidism; prostatic hypertrophy; phaeochromocytoma; angle closure glaucoma; history of drug or alcohol abuse; pregnancy (Appendix 4); breast-feeding (Appendix 5)

Side-effects: constipation, dry mouth, nausea, taste disturbances, diarrhoea, vomiting; tachycardia, palpitations, hypertension, flushing, insomnia, lightheadedness, paraesthesia, headache, anxiety, depression, seizures; sexual dysfunction, menstrual disturbances, urinary retention; thrombocytopenia; blurred vision, sweating, hypersensitivity reactions including Henoch-Shönlein purpura, rash, urticaria, angioedema and anaphylaxis; interstitial nephritis, glomerulonephritis

Dose: initially 10 mg daily in the morning, increased if weight loss less than 2 kg after 4 weeks to 15 mg daily; discontinue if weight loss less than 2 kg after 4 weeks at higher dose (see also Discontinuation of Treatment above); max. period of treatment 1 year; CHILD, ADOLESCENT under 18 years, and ELDERLY over 65 years not recommended

Reductil® (Abbott) PoM

Capsules, sibutramine hydrochloride 10 mg (blue/yellow), net price 28-cap pack = £41.29; 15 mg (blue/white), 28-cap pack = £45.14

4.6 Drugs used in nausea and vertigo

Anti-emetics should be prescribed only when the cause of vomiting is known because otherwise they may delay diagnosis, particularly in children. Anti-emetics are unnecessary and sometimes harmful when the cause can be treated, such as in diabetic ketoacidosis, or in digoxin or antiepileptic overdose.

If anti-emetic drug treatment is indicated, the drug is chosen according to the aetiology of vomiting.

Antihistamines are effective against nausea and vomiting resulting from many underlying conditions. There is no evidence that any one antihistamine is superior to another but their duration of action and incidence of adverse effects (drowsiness and antimuscarinic effects) differ.

The **phenothiazines** are dopamine antagonists and act centrally by blocking the chemoreceptor trigger zone. They are of considerable value for the prophylaxis and treatment of nausea and vomiting associated with diffuse neoplastic disease, radiation sickness, and the emesis caused by drugs such as opioids, general anaesthetics, and cytotoxics. **Prochlorperazine**, **perphenazine**, and **trifluoperazine** are less sedating than **chlorpromazine**; severe dystonic reactions sometimes occur with phenothiazines, especially in children. Other antipsychotic drugs including **haloperidol** and **levomepromazine** (**methotrimeprazine**) (section 4.2.1) are also used for the relief of nausea. Some phenothiazines are available as rectal suppositories, which can be useful in patients with persistent vomiting or with severe nausea; prochlorperazine can also be administered as a buccal tablet which is placed between the upper lip and the gum.

Metoclopramide is an effective anti-emetic and its activity closely resembles that of the phenothiazines. Metoclopramide also acts directly on the gastro-intestinal tract and it may be superior to the phenothiazines for emesis associated with gastroduodenal, hepatic, and biliary disease. In postoperative nausea and vomiting, metoclopramide in a dose of 10 mg has limited efficacy. High-dose metoclopramide injection is now less commonly used for cytotoxic-induced nausea and vomiting. As with the phenothiazines, metoclopramide can induce acute dystonic reactions involving facial and skeletal muscle spasms and oculogyric crises. These dystonic effects are more common in the young (especially girls and young women) and the very old; they usually occur shortly after starting treatment with metoclopramide and subside within 24 hours of stopping it. Injection of an antiparkinsonian drug such as procyclidine (section 4.9.2) will abort dystonic attacks.

Domperidone acts at the chemoreceptor trigger zone; it is used for the relief of nausea and vomiting, especially when associated with cytotoxic therapy. It has the advantage over metoclopramide and the phenothiazines of being less likely to cause central effects such as sedation and dystonic reactions because it does not readily cross the blood-brain barrier. In Parkinson's disease, it is used to prevent nausea and vomiting during treatment with apomorphine and also to treat nausea caused by other dopaminergic drugs (section 4.9.1). Domperidone is also used to treat vomiting due to emergency hormonal contraception (section 7.3.1).

Dolasetron, **granisetron**, **ondansetron**, and **tropisetron** are specific $5HT_3$ antagonists which block $5HT_3$ receptors in the gastro-intestinal tract and in the CNS. They are of value in the management of nausea and vomiting in patients receiving cytotoxics and in postoperative nausea and vomiting. **Palonosetron** is licensed for prevention of nausea and vomiting associated with moderately or highly emetogenic cytotoxic chemotherapy.

Dexamethasone (section 6.3.2) has anti-emetic effects and it is used in vomiting associated with cancer chemotherapy. It can be used alone or with metoclopramide, prochlorperazine, lorazepam, or a $5HT_3$ antagonist (see also section 8.1).

Aprepitant, a neurokinin 1 receptor antagonist, is licensed for the prevention of acute and delayed nausea and vomiting associated with cisplatin-based cytotoxic chemotherapy; it is given with dexamethasone and a $5HT_3$ antagonist.

Nabilone is a synthetic cannabinoid with anti-emetic properties. It may be used for nausea and vomiting caused by cytotoxic chemotherapy that is unresponsive to conventional anti-emetics. Side-effects such as drowsiness and dizziness occur frequently with standard doses.

Vomiting of pregnancy

Nausea in the first trimester of pregnancy is generally mild and does not require drug therapy. On rare occasions if vomiting is severe, short-term treatment with an antihistamine, such as **promethazine**, may be required. **Prochlorperazine** or **metoclopramide** may be considered as second-line treatments. If symptoms do not settle in 24 to 48 hours then specialist opinion should be sought. Hyperemesis gravidarum is a more serious condition, which requires intravenous fluid and electrolyte replacement and sometimes nutritional support. Supplementation with thiamine must be considered in order to reduce the risk of Wernicke's encephalopathy.

Postoperative nausea and vomiting

The incidence of postoperative nausea and vomiting depends on many factors including the anaesthetic used, the type and duration of surgery, and the patient's sex. The aim is to prevent postoperative nausea and vomiting from occurring. Drugs used include some **phenothiazines** (e.g. prochlorperazine), **metoclopramide** (but 10-mg dose has limited efficacy and higher parenteral doses associated with greater side-effects), **$5HT_3$ antagonists**, **antihistamines** (such as cyclizine), and **dexamethasone**. A combination of two anti-emetic drugs acting at different sites may be needed in resistant postoperative nausea and vomiting.

Motion sickness

Anti-emetics should be given to prevent motion sickness rather than after nausea or vomiting develop. The most effective drug for the prevention of motion sickness is **hyoscine**. A transdermal hyoscine patch provides prolonged activity but it needs to be applied several hours before travelling. The sedating antihistamines are slightly less effective against motion sickness, but are generally better tolerated than hyoscine. If a sedative effect is desired **promethazine** is useful, but generally a slightly less sedating antihistamine such as **cyclizine** or **cinnarizine** is preferred. The $5HT_3$ antagonists, domperidone, metoclopramide, and the phenothiazines (except the antihistamine phenothiazine promethazine) are **ineffective** in motion sickness.

Other vestibular disorders

Management of vestibular diseases is aimed at treating the underlying cause as well as treating symptoms of the balance disturbance and associated nausea and vomiting. Vertigo and nausea associated with Ménière's disease and middle-ear surgery can be difficult to treat.

Betahistine is an analogue of histamine and is claimed to reduce endolymphatic pressure by improving the microcirculation. Betahistine is licensed for vertigo, tinnitus, and hearing loss associated with Ménière's disease.

A **diuretic** alone or combined with salt restriction may provide some benefit in vertigo associated with Ménière's disease. **Antihistamines** (such as cinnarizine), and **phenothiazines** (such as prochlorperazine) are effective for prophylaxis and treatment.

For advice to avoid the inappropriate prescribing of drugs (notably phenothiazines) for dizziness in the elderly, see Prescribing for the Elderly, p. 18

Cytotoxic chemotherapy

For the management of nausea and vomiting induced by cytotoxic chemotherapy, see section 8.1.

Palliative care

For the management of nausea and vomiting in palliative care, see p. 16

Migraine

For the management of nausea and vomiting associated with migraine, see p. 235

Antihistamines

CINNARIZINE

Indications: vestibular disorders, such as vertigo, tinnitus, nausea, and vomiting in Ménière's disease; motion sickness; vascular disease (section 2.6.4)

Cautions: see section 3.4.1; risk of hypotension with high doses

Contra-indications: see section 3.4.1

Side-effects: see section 3.4.1

Dose: vestibular disorders, 30 mg 3 times daily; CHILD 5–12 years half adult dose

Motion sickness, 30 mg 2 hours before travel then 15 mg every 8 hours during journey if necessary; CHILD 5–12 years half adult dose

Cinnarizine (Non-proprietary)
Tablets, cinnarizine 15 mg. Net price 20 = £1.61. Label: 2
Brands include *Cinazière*®

Stugeron® (Janssen-Cilag)
Tablets, scored, cinnarizine 15 mg. Net price 20 = 71p. Label: 2

Stugeron Forte®
See section 2.6.4

CYCLIZINE

Indications: nausea, vomiting, vertigo, motion sickness, labyrinthine disorders

Cautions: see section 3.4.1; severe heart failure; may counteract haemodynamic benefits of opioids; **interactions:** Appendix 1 (antihistamines)

Contra-indications: see section 3.4.1

Side-effects: see section 3.4.1

Dose: *by mouth*, cyclizine hydrochloride 50 mg up to 3 times daily; CHILD 6–12 years 25 mg up to 3 times daily

By intramuscular or intravenous injection, cyclizine lactate 50 mg 3 times daily

Valoid® (Amdipharm)
Tablets, scored, cyclizine hydrochloride 50 mg. Net price 20 = £1.44. Label: 2
Injection [PoM], cyclizine lactate 50 mg/mL. Net price 1-mL amp = 70p

MECLOZINE HYDROCHLORIDE

Indications: see under preparations

Cautions: see section 3.4.1; **interactions:** Appendix 1 (antihistamines)

DRIVING. Drowsiness may affect performance of skilled tasks (e.g. driving); effects of alcohol enhanced

Contra-indications: see section 3.4.1

Side-effects: see section 3.4.1

■ Preparations

A proprietary brand of meclozine hydrochloride tablets 12.5 mg (*Sea-legs*®) is on sale to the public for motion sickness

PROMETHAZINE HYDROCHLORIDE

Indications: nausea, vomiting, vertigo, labyrinthine disorders, motion sickness; other indications (section 3.4.1, section 4.1.1, section 15.1.4.1)

Cautions: see section 3.4.1; also pregnancy (Appendix 4) and breast-feeding (Appendix 5)

Contra-indications: see section 3.4.1

Side-effects: see section 3.4.1 but more sedating; intramuscular injection may be painful

Dose: motion sickness prevention, 20–25 mg at bedtime on night before travel, repeat following morning if necessary; CHILD under 2 years not recommended, 2–5 years 5 mg at night and following morning if necessary, 5–10 years 10 mg at night and following morning if necessary

■ Preparations

Section 3.4.1

PROMETHAZINE TEOCLATE

Indications: nausea, vertigo, labyrinthine disorders, motion sickness (acts longer than the hydrochloride)

Cautions: see section 3.4.1; also pregnancy (Appendix 4) and breast-feeding (Appendix 5)

Contra-indications: see section 3.4.1

Side-effects: see section 3.4.1

Dose: 25–75 mg, max. 100 mg, daily; CHILD 5–10 years, 12.5–37.5 mg daily

Motion sickness prevention, 25 mg at bedtime on night before travel *or* 25 mg 1–2 hours before travel; CHILD 5–10 years half adult dose

Severe vomiting in pregnancy, 25 mg at bedtime, increased if necessary to max. 100 mg daily (but see also Vomiting of Pregnancy in notes above)

Avomine® (Manx)
Tablets, scored, promethazine teoclate 25 mg. Net price 10-tab pack = £1.13; 28-tab pack = £3.13. Label: 2

Phenothiazines and related drugs

CHLORPROMAZINE HYDROCHLORIDE

Indications: nausea and vomiting of terminal illness (where other drugs have failed or are not available); other indications (section 4.2.1 and section 15.1.4.1)

Cautions: see Chlorpromazine Hydrochloride, section 4.2.1

Contra-indications: see Chlorpromazine Hydrochloride, section 4.2.1

Side-effects: see Chlorpromazine Hydrochloride, section 4.2.1

Dose: *by mouth*, 10–25 mg every 4–6 hours; CHILD 500 micrograms/kg every 4–6 hours (1–5 years max. 40 mg daily, 6–12 years max. 75 mg daily)

By deep intramuscular injection initially 25 mg then 25–50 mg every 3–4 hours until vomiting stops; CHILD 500 micrograms/kg every 6–8 hours (1–5 years max. 40 mg daily, 6–12 years max. 75 mg daily)

By rectum in suppositories, chlorpromazine 100 mg every 6–8 hours [unlicensed]

■ Preparations
Section 4.2.1

PERPHENAZINE

Indications: severe nausea, vomiting (see notes above); other indications (section 4.2.1)

Cautions: see Perphenazine (section 4.2.1)

Contra-indications: see Perphenazine (section 4.2.1)

Side-effects: see Perphenazine (section 4.2.1); extrapyramidal symptoms particularly in young adults, elderly, and debilitated

Dose: 4 mg 3 times daily, adjusted according to response; max. 24 mg daily (chemotherapy-induced); ELDERLY quarter to half adult dose; CHILD under 14 years not recommended

■ Preparations
Section 4.2.1

PROCHLORPERAZINE

Indications: severe nausea, vomiting, vertigo, labyrinthine disorders (see notes above); other indications section 4.2.1

Cautions: see under Prochlorperazine (section 4.2.1); oral route only for children (avoid if under 10 kg); elderly (see notes above)

Contra-indications: see under Prochlorperazine (section 4.2.1)

Side-effects: see under Prochlorperazine (section 4.2.1); extrapyramidal symptoms, particularly in children, elderly, and debilitated

Dose: doses are expressed as prochlorperazine maleate or mesilate; 1 mg prochlorperazine maleate ≡ 1 mg prochlorperazine mesilate

By mouth, nausea and vomiting, acute attack, 20 mg initially then 10 mg after 2 hours; prevention 5–10 mg 2–3 times daily; CHILD (over 10 kg only) 250 micrograms/kg 2–3 times daily

Labyrinthine disorders, 5 mg 3 times daily, gradually increased if necessary to 30 mg daily in divided doses, then reduced after several weeks to 5–10 mg daily; CHILD not recommended

By deep intramuscular injection, nausea and vomiting, 12.5 mg when required followed if necessary after 6 hours by an oral dose, as above; CHILD not recommended

By rectum in suppositories, nausea and vomiting, 25 mg followed if necessary after 6 hours by oral dose, as above; *or* due to migraine, 5 mg 3 times daily; CHILD not recommended

Prochlorperazine (Non-proprietary) PoM

Tablets, prochlorperazine maleate 5 mg, net price 20 = £1.01. Label: 2

Brands include *Prozière*®

Stemetil® (Castlemead) PoM

Tablets, prochlorperazine maleate 5 mg (off-white), net price 84-tab pack = £6.18; 25 mg (scored), 56-tab pack = £10.91. Label: 2

Syrup, straw-coloured, prochlorperazine mesilate 5 mg/5 mL. Net price 100-mL pack = £3.48. Label: 2

Eff (= effervescent granules), sugar-free, prochlorperazine mesilate 5 mg/sachet. Net price 21-sachet pack = £6.46. Label: 2, 13

Excipients: include aspartame (section 9.4.1)

Injection, prochlorperazine mesilate 12.5 mg/mL. Net price 1-mL amp = 54p

Suppositories, prochlorperazine maleate (as prochlorperazine), 5 mg, net price 10 = £8.74; 25 mg, 10 = £11.46. Label: 2

■ Buccal preparation

[1]**Buccastem**® (R&C) PoM

Tablets (buccal), pale yellow, prochlorperazine maleate 3 mg. Net price 5 × 10-tab pack = £5.75. Label: 2, counselling, administration, see under Dose below

Dose: 1–2 tablets twice daily; tablets are placed high between upper lip and gum and left to dissolve; CHILD not recommended

1. Prochlorperazine maleate can be sold to the public for adults over 18 years (provided packs do not contain more than 24 mg) for the treatment of nausea and vomiting in previously diagnosed migraine only (max. daily dose 12 mg); a proprietary brand (*Buccastem*® *M*) is on sale to the public

TRIFLUOPERAZINE

Indications: severe nausea and vomiting (see notes above); other indications (section 4.2.1)

Cautions: see section 4.2.1

Contra-indications: see section 4.2.1

Side-effects: see section 4.2.1; extrapyramidal symptoms, particularly in children, elderly, and debilitated

Dose: 2–4 mg daily in divided doses *or* as a single dose of a modified-release preparation; max. 6 mg daily; CHILD 3–5 years up to 1 mg daily, 6–12 years up to 4 mg daily

■ Preparations
Section 4.2.1

Domperidone and metoclopramide

DOMPERIDONE

Indications: nausea and vomiting, dyspepsia, gastro-oesophageal reflux

Cautions: renal impairment (Appendix 3); pregnancy (Appendix 4) and breast-feeding (Appendix 5); not recommended for routine prophylaxis of post-operative vomiting or for chronic administration; **interactions:** Appendix 1 (domperidone)

Contra-indications: prolactinoma, hepatic impairment; where increased gastro-intestinal motility harmful

Side-effects: rarely gastro-intestinal disturbances (including cramps), raised prolactin concentration; extrapyramidal effects and rashes reported

Dose: *by mouth*, ADULT and ADOLESCENT body-weight over 35 kg, 10–20 mg 3–4 times daily; max. 80 mg daily; CHILD body-weight up to 34 kg, 250–500 micrograms/kg 3–4 times daily; max. 2.4 mg/kg in 24 hours

By rectum in suppositories, ADULT and ADOLESCENT body-weight over 35 kg, 60 mg twice daily; CHILD 15–34 kg, 30 mg twice daily; CHILD body-weight under 15 kg, not recommended

[1]**Domperidone** (Non-proprietary) PoM
Tablets, 10 mg (as maleate), net price 30-tab pack = £2.11; 100-tab pack = £4.86

1. Domperidone can be sold to the public (provided packs do not contain more than 200 mg) for the relief of postprandial symptoms of excessive fullness, nausea, epigastric bloating and belching occasionally accompanied by epigastric discomfort and heartburn (max. single dose 10 mg, max. daily dose 40 mg); a proprietary brand (*Motilium® 10*) is on sale to the public

Motilium® (Sanofi-Synthelabo) PoM
Tablets, f/c, domperidone 10 mg (as maleate). Net price 30-tab pack = £2.35; 100-tab pack = £7.84
Suspension, sugar-free, domperidone 5 mg/5 mL. Net price 200-mL pack = £1.80
Suppositories domperidone 30 mg. Net price 10 = £2.65

■ Compound preparations (for migraine)
section 4.7.4.1

METOCLOPRAMIDE HYDROCHLORIDE

Indications: adults, nausea and vomiting, particularly in gastro-intestinal disorders (section 1.2) and treatment with cytotoxics or radiotherapy; migraine (section 4.7.4.1)

PATIENTS UNDER 20 YEARS. Use restricted to severe intractable vomiting of known cause, vomiting of radiotherapy and cytotoxics, aid to gastro-intestinal intubation, pre-medication; also, dose should be determined on the basis of body-weight

Cautions: hepatic impairment (Appendix 2), renal impairment (Appendix 3); elderly, young adults, and children (measure dose accurately, preferably with a pipette); may mask underlying disorders such as cerebral irritation; epilepsy; pregnancy (Appendix 4); porphyria (section 9.8.2); **interactions:** Appendix 1 (metoclopramide)

Contra-indications: gastro-intestinal obstruction, perforation or haemorrhage; 3–4 days after gastro-intestinal surgery; phaeochromocytoma; breast-feeding (Appendix 5)

Side-effects: extrapyramidal effects (especially in children and young adults—see notes above), hyperprolactinaemia, occasionally tardive dyskinesia on prolonged administration; also reported, drowsiness, restlessness, diarrhoea, depression, neuroleptic malignant syndrome, rashes, pruritus, oedema; cardiac conduction abnormalities reported following intravenous administration; rarely methaemoglobinaemia (more severe in G6PD deficiency)

Dose: *by mouth, or by intramuscular injection or by intravenous injection* over 1–2 minutes, 10 mg (5 mg in young adults 15–19 years under 60 kg) 3 times daily; CHILD up to 1 year (up to 10 kg) 1 mg twice daily, 1–3 years (10–14 kg) 1 mg 2–3 times daily, 3–5 years (15–19 kg) 2 mg 2–3 times daily, 5–9 years (20–29 kg) 2 mg 3 times daily, 9–14 years (30 kg and over) 5 mg 3 times daily

NOTE. Daily dose of metoclopramide should not normally exceed 500 micrograms/kg, particularly for children and young adults (restricted use, see above)

For diagnostic procedures, as a single dose 5–10 minutes before examination, 10–20 mg (10 mg in young adults 15–19 years); CHILD under 3 years 1 mg, 3–9 years 2 mg, 9–14 years 5 mg

Metoclopramide (Non-proprietary) PoM
Tablets, metoclopramide hydrochloride 10 mg, net price 28-tab pack = £1.32
Oral solution, metoclopramide hydrochloride 5 mg/5 mL, net price 100-mL pack = £2.55
NOTE. Sugar-free versions are available and can be ordered by specifying 'sugar-free' on the prescription
Injection, metoclopramide hydrochloride 5 mg/mL, net price 2-mL amp = 26p

Maxolon® (Shire) PoM
Tablets, scored, metoclopramide hydrochloride 10 mg, net price 84-tab pack = £5.24
Syrup, sugar-free, metoclopramide hydrochloride 5 mg/5 mL. Net price 200-mL pack = £3.83
Paediatric liquid, sugar-free, metoclopramide hydrochloride 1 mg/mL. Net price 15-mL pack with pipette = £1.51. Counselling, use of pipette
Injection, metoclopramide hydrochloride 5 mg/mL. Net price 2-mL amp = 27p

■ High-dose (with cytotoxic chemotherapy only)

Maxolon High Dose® (Shire) PoM
Injection, metoclopramide hydrochloride 5 mg/mL. Net price 20-mL amp = £2.67.
For dilution and use as an intravenous infusion in nausea and vomiting associated with cytotoxic chemotherapy only
Dose: by continuous intravenous infusion (preferred method), initially (before starting chemotherapy), 2–4 mg/kg over 15–20 minutes, then 3–5 mg/kg over 8–12 hours; max. in 24 hours, 10 mg/kg
By intermittent intravenous infusion, initially (before starting chemotherapy), up to 2 mg/kg over at least 15 minutes then up to 2 mg/kg over at least 15 minutes every 2 hours; max. in 24 hours, 10 mg/kg

■ Modified-release preparations
NOTE. All unsuitable for patients under 20 years

Gastrobid Continus® (Napp) PoM
Tablets, m/r, metoclopramide hydrochloride 15 mg. Net price 56-tab pack = £7.75. Label: 25
Dose: patients over 20 years, 1 tablet twice daily

Maxolon SR® (Shire) PoM
Capsules, m/r, clear, enclosing white granules, metoclopramide hydrochloride 15 mg. Net price 56-cap pack = £7.01. Label: 25
Dose: patients over 20 years, 1 capsule twice daily

■ Compound preparations (for migraine)
Section 4.7.4.1

5HT$_3$ antagonists

DOLASETRON MESILATE

Indications: see under Dose

Cautions: prolonged QT interval, cardiac conduction disorders, concomitant administration of drugs that prolong QT interval, congestive cardiac failure; pregnancy and breast-feeding; **interactions:** Appendix 1 (dolasetron)

Side-effects: diarrhoea, constipation, dyspepsia, abdominal pain, flatulence, taste disturbances; tachycardia, bradycardia, ECG changes, flushing; fever, shivering; headache, sleep disorder, fatigue, dizziness, drowsiness, anorexia; hypersensitivity reactions including rash, pruritus, urticaria, angioedema and anaphylaxis; rarely intestinal obstruction, pancreatitis, jaundice, seizures, cardiac arrhythmia, injection-site reactions; very rarely severe hypotension and bradycardia following intravenous injection

Dose: prevention of nausea and vomiting induced by cytotoxic chemotherapy, *by mouth*, 200 mg one hour before treatment *or by intravenous injection* (over 30 seconds) *or by intravenous infusion*, 100 mg 30 minutes before treatment

Prevention of delayed nausea and vomiting after chemotherapy cycle, *by mouth*, 200 mg once daily

NOTE. Dolasetron can be used for a maximum of 4 consecutive days in relation to any one chemotherapy cycle

Prevention of postoperative nausea and vomiting, *by mouth*, 50 mg before induction of anaesthesia *or by intravenous injection* (over 30 seconds) *or by intravenous infusion*, 12.5 mg at cessation of anaesthesia

Treatment of postoperative nausea and vomiting, *by intravenous injection* (over 30 seconds) *or by intravenous infusion*, 12.5 mg

CHILD not recommended

Anzemet® (Amdipharm) ▼ PoM

Tablets, f/c, pink, dolasetron mesilate 50 mg, net price 3-tab pack = £13.50; 200 mg, 3-tab pack = £42.00, 6-tab pack = £84.00

Injection, dolasetron mesilate 20 mg/mL, net price 0.625-mL (12.5-mg) amp = £4.00, 5-mL (100-mg) amp = £13.00

GRANISETRON

Indications: see under Dose

Cautions: pregnancy (Appendix 4) and breast-feeding (Appendix 5)

Side-effects: constipation, headache, rash; transient increases in liver enzymes; hypersensitivity reactions reported

Dose: nausea and vomiting induced by cytotoxic chemotherapy or radiotherapy, *by mouth*, 1–2 mg within 1 hour before start of treatment, then 2 mg daily in 1–2 divided doses during treatment; when intravenous infusion also used, max. combined total 9 mg in 24 hours; CHILD 20 micrograms/kg (max. 1 mg) within 1 hour before start of treatment, then 20 micrograms/kg (max. 1 mg) twice daily for up to 5 days during treatment

By intravenous injection (diluted in 15 mL sodium chloride 0.9% and given over not less than 30 seconds) *or by intravenous infusion* (over 5 minutes, see Appendix 6), prevention, 3 mg before start of cytotoxic therapy (up to 2 additional 3-mg doses may be given within 24 hours); treatment, as for prevention (the two additional doses must not be given less than 10 minutes apart); max. 9 mg in 24 hours; CHILD, *by intravenous infusion*, (over 5 minutes), prevention, 40 micrograms/kg (max. 3 mg) before start of cytotoxic therapy; treatment, as for prevention—one additional dose of 40 micrograms/kg (max. 3 mg) may be given within 24 hours (not less than 10 minutes after initial dose)

Postoperative nausea and vomiting, *by intravenous injection* (diluted to 5 mL and given over 30 seconds), prevention, 1 mg before induction of anaesthesia; treatment, 1 mg, given as for prevention; max. 2 mg in one day; CHILD not recommended

Kytril® (Roche) PoM

Tablets, f/c, granisetron (as hydrochloride) 1 mg, net price 10-tab pack = £65.49; 2 mg, 5-tab pack = £65.49

Paediatric liquid, sugar-free, granisetron (as hydrochloride) 1 mg/5 mL, net price 30 mL = £39.29

Sterile solution, granisetron (as hydrochloride) 1 mg/mL, for dilution and use as injection or infusion, net price 1-mL amp = £8.60, 3-mL amp = £25.79

ONDANSETRON

Indications: see under Dose

Cautions: pregnancy (Appendix 4) and breast-feeding (Appendix 5); moderate or severe hepatic impairment (Appendix 2); **interactions:** Appendix 1 (ondansetron)

Side-effects: constipation; headache, sensation of warmth or flushing, hiccups; occasional alterations in liver enzymes; hypersensitivity reactions reported; occasional transient visual disturbances and dizziness following intravenous administration; involuntary movements, seizures, chest pain, arrhythmias, hypotension and bradycardia also reported; suppositories may cause rectal irritation

Dose: moderately emetogenic chemotherapy or radiotherapy, *by mouth*, 8 mg 1–2 hours before treatment *or by rectum*, 16 mg 1–2 hours before treatment *or by intramuscular injection or slow intravenous injection*, 8 mg immediately before treatment

then by mouth, 8 mg every 12 hours for up to 5 days *or by rectum*, 16 mg daily for up to 5 days

Severely emetogenic chemotherapy, *by intramuscular injection or slow intravenous injection*, 8 mg immediately before treatment, where necessary followed by 8 mg at intervals of 2–4 hours for 2 further doses (*or* followed by 1 mg/hour *by continuous intravenous infusion* for up to 24 hours)

then by mouth, 8 mg every 12 hours for up to 5 days *or by rectum*, 16 mg daily for up to 5 days

alternatively, by intravenous infusion over at least 15 minutes, 32 mg immediately before treatment *or by rectum*, 16 mg 1–2 hours before treatment

then by mouth, 8 mg every 12 hours for up to 5 days *or by rectum*, 16 mg daily for up to 5 days

CHILD, *by slow intravenous injection or by intravenous infusion* over 15 minutes, 5 mg/m^2 immediately before chemotherapy then, 4 mg *by mouth* every 12 hours for up to 5 days

Prevention of postoperative nausea and vomiting, *by*

mouth, 16 mg 1 hour before anaesthesia *or* 8 mg 1 hour before anaesthesia followed by 8 mg at intervals of 8 hours for 2 further doses
alternatively, by intramuscular or slow intravenous injection, 4 mg at induction of anaesthesia; CHILD over 2 years, *by slow intravenous injection*, 100 micrograms/kg (max. 4 mg) before, during, or after induction of anaesthesia
Treatment of postoperative nausea and vomiting, *by intramuscular or slow intravenous injection*, 4 mg; CHILD over 2 years, *by slow intravenous injection*, 100 micrograms/kg (max. 4 mg)

Zofran® (GSK) PoM
Tablets, both yellow, f/c, ondansetron (as hydrochloride) 4 mg, net price 30-tab pack = £107.91; 8 mg, 10-tab pack = £71.94
Oral lyophilisates (*Zofran Melt*®), ondansetron 4 mg, net price 10-tab pack = £35.97; 8 mg, 10-tab pack = £71.94. Counselling, administration
COUNSELLING. Tablets should be placed on the tongue, allowed to disperse and swallowed
Excipients: include aspartame (section 9.4.1)
Syrup, sugar-free, ondansetron (as hydrochloride) 4 mg/5 mL. Net price 50-mL pack = £35.97
Injection, ondansetron (as hydrochloride) 2 mg/mL, net price 2-mL amp = £5.99; 4-mL amp = £11.99
Suppositories, ondansetron 16 mg. Net price 1 = £14.39

PALONOSETRON

Indications: prevention of nausea and vomiting induced by moderately and severely emetogenic chemotherapy
Cautions: history of constipation; intestinal obstruction; concomitant administration of drugs that prolong QT interval; pregnancy (Appendix 4); breast-feeding (Appendix 5)
DRIVING. Dizziness or drowsiness may affect performance of skilled tasks (e.g. driving)
Side-effects: diarrhoea, constipation; headache, dizziness; *less commonly* dyspepsia, abdominal pain, dry mouth, flatulence, changes in blood pressure, tachycardia, bradycardia, arrhythmia, myocardial ischaemia, hiccups, drowsiness, asthenia, insomnia, anxiety, euphoria, paraesthesia, peripheral neuropathy, anorexia, motion sickness, influenza-like symptoms, urinary retention, glycosuria, hyperglycaemia, electrolyte disturbance, arthralgia, eye irritation, amblyopia, tinnitus, rash, pruritus
Dose: *by intravenous injection* (over 30 seconds), 250 micrograms as a single dose 30 minutes before treatment; do not repeat dose within 7 days; CHILD and ADOLESCENT under 18 years not recommended

Aloxi® (Cambridge) ▼ PoM
Injection, palonosetron (as hydrochloride) 50 micrograms/mL, net price 5-mL amp = £55.89

TROPISETRON

Indications: see under Dose
Cautions: uncontrolled hypertension (has been aggravated by doses higher than recommended); cardiac conduction disorders; arrhythmias, concomitant administration of drugs that prolong QT interval; pregnancy (Appendix 4), breast-feeding; **interactions:** Appendix 1 (tropisetron)
DRIVING. Dizziness or drowsiness may affect performance of skilled tasks (e.g. driving)
Side-effects: constipation, diarrhoea, abdominal pain; headache, dizziness, fatigue; hypersensitivity reactions reported (including facial flushing, urticaria, chest tightness, dyspnoea, bronchospasm and hypotension); collapse, syncope, bradycardia, cardiovascular collapse also reported (causal relationship not established)
Dose: prevention of nausea and vomiting induced by cytotoxic chemotherapy, *by slow intravenous injection or by intravenous infusion*, 5 mg shortly before chemotherapy, then 5 mg *by mouth* every morning at least 1 hour before food for 5 days; CHILD over 2 years, *by intravenous injection* over at least 1 minute or *by intravenous infusion*, 200 micrograms/kg (max. 5 mg) shortly before chemotherapy, then 200 micrograms/kg daily for 4 days; CHILD 25 kg and over, *by intravenous injection* over at least 1 minute or *by intravenous infusion*, 5 mg shortly before chemotherapy, then *by mouth* (preferably) or *by intravenous injection* over at least 1 minute or *by intravenous infusion*, 5 mg daily for 5 days
Postoperative nausea and vomiting, *by slow intravenous injection* or *by intravenous infusion*, prevention, 2 mg shortly before induction of anaesthesia; treatment, 2 mg within 2 hours of the end of anaesthesia

Navoban® (Novartis) PoM
Capsules, white/yellow, tropisetron (as hydrochloride) 5 mg, net price 5-cap pack = £53.86; 50-cap pack = £538.60. Label: 23
Injection, tropisetron (as hydrochloride), 1 mg/mL, net price 2-mL amp = £4.86, 5-mL amp = £12.16

Neurokinin receptor antagonist

APREPITANT

Indications: adjunct to dexamethasone and a $5HT_3$ antagonist in preventing nausea and vomiting associated with moderately and highly emetogenic chemotherapy
Cautions: hepatic impairment (Appendix 2); pregnancy (Appendix 4); **interactions:** Appendix 1 (aprepitant)
Contra-indications: breast-feeding (Appendix 5)
Side-effects: hiccups, dyspepsia, diarrhoea, constipation, anorexia, asthenia, headache, dizziness; *less commonly* weight changes, dry mouth, colitis, flatulence, stomatitis, abdominal pain, gastro-oesophageal reflux, duodenal ulcer, oedema, bradycardia, cough, disorientation, euphoria, anxiety, confusion, thirst, abnormal dreams, hyperglycaemia, polyuria, anaemia, dysuria, haematuria, myalgia, conjunctivitis, pharyngitis, sneezing, tinnitus, sweating, oily skin, pruritus, rash, acne, photosensitivity, flushing, hyponatraemia
Dose: 125 mg 1 hour before chemotherapy, then 80 mg daily as a single dose for the next 2 days; consult product literature for dose of concomitant corticosteroid and $5HT_3$ antagonist; CHILD and ADOLESCENT under 18 years not recommended

Emend® (MSD) ▼ PoM
Capsules, aprepitant 80 mg, net price 2-cap pack = £31.61; 125 mg (white/pink), 5-cap pack = £79.03; 3-day pack of one 125-mg capsule and two 80-mg capsules = £47.42

Cannabinoid

NABILONE

Indications: nausea and vomiting caused by cytotoxic chemotherapy, unresponsive to conventional anti-emetics (under close observation, preferably in hospital setting)

Cautions: history of psychiatric disorder; elderly; hypertension; heart disease; adverse effects on mental state can persist for 48–72 hours after stopping; pregnancy (Appendix 4); **interactions:** Appendix 1 (nabilone)

DRIVING. Drowsiness may affect performance of skilled tasks (e.g. driving); effects of alcohol enhanced

Contra-indications: severe hepatic impairment; pregnancy and breast-feeding (Appendix 5)

Side-effects: drowsiness, vertigo, euphoria, dry mouth, ataxia, visual disturbance, concentration difficulties, sleep disturbance, dysphoria, hypotension, headache and nausea; also confusion, disorientation, hallucinations, psychosis, depression, decreased coordination, tremors, tachycardia, decreased appetite, and abdominal pain

BEHAVIOURAL EFFECTS. Patients should be made aware of possible changes of mood and other adverse behavioural effects

Dose: initially 1 mg twice daily, increased if necessary to 2 mg twice daily, throughout each cycle of cytotoxic therapy and, if necessary, for 48 hours after the last dose of each cycle; max. 6 mg daily given in 3 divided doses. The first dose should be taken the night before initiation of cytotoxic treatment and the second dose 1–3 hours before the first dose of cytotoxic drug; ADOLESCENT and CHILD under 18 years not recommended

Nabilone (Cambridge) PoM
Capsules, blue/white, nabilone 1 mg. Net price 20-cap pack = £125.84. Label: 2, counselling, behavioural effects

Hyoscine

HYOSCINE HYDROBROMIDE

(Scopolamine Hydrobromide)

Indications: motion sickness; premedication (section 15.1.3)

Cautions: elderly, urinary retention, cardiovascular disease, gastro-intestinal obstruction, hepatic or renal impairment; porphyria (section 9.8.2); pregnancy (Appendix 4) and breast-feeding (Appendix 5); **interactions:** Appendix 1 (antimuscarinics)

DRIVING. Drowsiness may affect performance of skilled tasks (e.g. driving) and may persist for up to 24 hours or longer after removal of patch: effects of alcohol enhanced

Contra-indications: closed-angle glaucoma

Side-effects: drowsiness, dry mouth, dizziness, blurred vision, difficulty with micturition

Dose: motion sickness, *by mouth*, 300 micrograms 30 minutes before start of journey followed by 300 micrograms every 6 hours if required; max. 3 doses in 24 hours; CHILD 4–10 years 75–150 micrograms, over 10 years 150–300 micrograms

NOTE. Proprietary brands of hyoscine hydrobromide tablets (*Joy-rides*®, *Kwells*®) are on sale to the public for motion sickness

Injection, see section 15.1.3

Scopoderm TTS® (Novartis Consumer Health) PoM
Patch, self-adhesive, pink, releasing hyoscine approx. 1 mg/72 hours when in contact with skin. Net price 2 = £4.30. Label: 19, counselling, see below

Dose: motion sickness prevention, apply 1 patch to hairless area of skin behind ear 5–6 hours before journey; replace if necessary after 72 hours, siting replacement patch behind other ear; CHILD under 10 years not recommended

COUNSELLING. Explain accompanying instructions to patient and in particular emphasise advice to wash hands after handling and to wash application site after removing, and to use one patch at a time

NOTE. The brand name *Scopoderm*® is used for a hyoscine patch that is available for sale to the public

Other drugs for Ménière's disease

Betahistine has been promoted as a specific treatment for Ménière's disease.

BETAHISTINE DIHYDROCHLORIDE

Indications: vertigo, tinnitus and hearing loss associated with Ménière's disease

Cautions: asthma, history of peptic ulcer; pregnancy and breast-feeding; **interactions:** Appendix 1 (betahistine)

Contra-indications: phaeochromocytoma

Side-effects: gastro-intestinal disturbances; headache, rashes and pruritus reported

Dose: initially 16 mg 3 times daily, preferably with food; maintenance 24–48 mg daily; CHILD not recommended

Betahistine Dihydrochloride (Non-proprietary) PoM
Tablets, betahistine dihydrochloride 8 mg, net price 120-tab pack = £3.34; 16 mg, 84-tab pack = £3.99. Label: 21

Serc® (Solvay) PoM
Tablets, betahistine dihydrochloride 8 mg (*Serc*®*-8*), net price 120-tab pack = £9.04; 16 mg (*Serc*®*-16*), 84-tab pack = £12.65 Label: 21

4.7 Analgesics

The non-opioid drugs (section 4.7.1), paracetamol and aspirin (and other NSAIDs), are particularly suitable for pain in musculoskeletal conditions, whereas the opioid analgesics (section 4.7.2) are more suitable for moderate to severe pain, particularly of visceral origin.

PAIN IN PALLIATIVE CARE. For advice on pain relief in palliative care see p. 14.

PAIN IN SICKLE-CELL DISEASE. The pain of mild sickle-cell crises is managed with paracetamol, an NSAID, codeine, or dihydrocodeine. Severe crises may require the use of morphine or diamorphine; concomitant use of an NSAID may potentiate analgesia and allow lower doses of the opioid to be used. Pethidine should be avoided if possible because accumulation of a neurotoxic metabolite can precipitate seizures; the relatively short half-life of pethidine necessitates frequent injections.

DENTAL AND OROFACIAL PAIN. Analgesics should be used judiciously in dental care as a **temporary** measure until the cause of the pain has been dealt with.

Dental pain of inflammatory origin, such as that associated with pulpitis, apical infection, localised osteitis (dry socket) or pericoronitis is usually best managed by treating the infection, providing drainage, restorative procedures, and other local measures. Analgesics provide temporary relief of pain (usually for about 1 to 7 days) until the causative factors have been brought under control. In the case of pulpitis, intra-osseous infection or abscess, reliance on analgesics alone is usually inappropriate.

Similarly the pain and discomfort associated with acute problems of the oral mucosa (e.g. acute herpetic gingivostomatitis, erythema multiforme) may be relieved by **benzydamine** mouthwash or spray (see p. 553) until the cause of the mucosal disorder has been dealt with. However, where a patient is febrile, the antipyretic action of **paracetamol** (see p. 220) or **ibuprofen** (see p. 503) is often helpful.

The *choice* of an analgesic for dental purposes should be based on its suitability for the patient. Most dental pain is relieved effectively by non-steroidal anti-inflammatory drugs (NSAIDs). NSAIDs that are used for dental pain include **ibuprofen**, **aspirin**, and **diflunisal**; for further details see section 4.7.1 and section 10.1.1. **Paracetamol** has analgesic and antipyretic effects but no anti-inflammatory effect.

Opioid analgesics (section 4.7.2) such as **dihydrocodeine** and **pethidine** act on the central nervous system and are traditionally used for *moderate to severe pain*. However, opioid analgesics are relatively ineffective in dental pain and their side-effects can be unpleasant. Paracetamol, ibuprofen, aspirin, or diflunisal are adequate for most cases of dental pain and an opioid is rarely required.

Combining a non-opioid with an opioid analgesic can provide greater relief of pain than a non-opioid analgesic given alone. However, this applies only when an appropriate dose combination is used. Most combination analgesic preparations have not been shown to provide greater relief of pain than an adequate dose of the non-opioid component given alone. Moreover, combination preparations have the disadvantage of an increased number of side-effects.

Any analgesic given before a dental procedure should have a low risk of increasing postoperative bleeding. In the case of pain after the dental procedure, taking an analgesic before the effect of the local anaesthetic has worn off can improve control. Postoperative analgesia with ibuprofen or aspirin is usually continued for about 24 to 72 hours.

Temporomandibular joint pain dysfunction syndrome can be related to anxiety in some patients who may clench or grind their teeth (bruxism) during the day or night. The muscle spasm (which appears to be the main source of pain) may be treated empirically with an overlay appliance which provides a free sliding occlusion and may also interfere with grinding. In addition, **diazepam** (section 4.1.2), which has muscle relaxant as well as anxiolytic properties, may be helpful but it should only be prescribed on a short-term basis during the acute phase. Analgesics such as aspirin (section 4.7.1) or ibuprofen (section 10.1.1) may also be required.

For the management of neuropathic and functional pain (including atypical facial pain and trigeminal neuralgia), see section 4.7.3.

DYSMENORRHOEA. Use of an oral contraceptive prevents the pain of dysmenorrhoea which is generally associated with ovulatory cycles. If treatment is necessary paracetamol or an NSAID (section 10.1.1) will generally provide adequate relief of pain. The vomiting and severe pain associated with dysmenorrhoea in women with endometriosis may call for an antiemetic (in addition to an analgesic). Antispasmodics (such as alverine citrate, section 1.2) have been advocated for dysmenorrhoea but the antispasmodic action does not generally provide significant relief.

4.7.1 Non-opioid analgesics

Aspirin is indicated for headache, transient musculoskeletal pain, dysmenorrhoea and pyrexia. In inflammatory conditions, most physicians prefer anti-inflammatory treatment with another NSAID which may be better tolerated and more convenient for the patient. Aspirin is used increasingly for its antiplatelet properties (section 2.9). Aspirin tablets or dispersible aspirin tablets are adequate for most purposes as they act rapidly.

Gastric irritation may be a problem; it is minimised by taking the dose after food. Enteric-coated preparations are available, but have a slow onset of action and are therefore unsuitable for single-dose analgesic use (though their prolonged action may be useful for night pain).

Aspirin interacts significantly with a number of other drugs and its interaction with warfarin is a **special hazard**, see **interactions:** Appendix 1 (aspirin).

Paracetamol is similar in efficacy to aspirin, but has no demonstrable anti-inflammatory activity; it is less irritant to the stomach and for that reason is now generally preferred to aspirin, particularly in the elderly. **Overdosage** with paracetamol is particularly dangerous as it may cause hepatic damage which is sometimes not apparent for 4 to 6 days (see Emergency Treatment of Poisoning, p. 29).

Nefopam may have a place in the relief of persistent pain unresponsive to other non-opioid analgesics. It causes little or no respiratory depression, but sympathomimetic and antimuscarinic side-effects may be troublesome.

Non-steroidal anti-inflammatory analgesics (NSAIDs, section 10.1.1) are particularly useful for the treatment of patients with chronic disease accompanied by pain and inflammation. Some of them are also used in the short-term treatment of mild to moderate pain including transient musculoskeletal pain but paracetamol is now often preferred, particularly in the elderly (see also p. 19). They are also suitable for the relief of pain in *dysmenorrhoea* and to treat pain caused by *secondary bone tumours*, many of which produce lysis of bone and release prostaglandins (see Prescribing in Palliative Care, p. 14). Selective inhibitors of cyclo-oxygenase-2 may be used in preference to non-selective NSAIDs for patients at high risk of developing serious gastro-intestinal side-effects. NSAIDs including ketorolac are also used for peri-operative analgesia (section 15.1.4.2).

DENTAL AND OROFACIAL PAIN. Most dental pain is relieved effectively by NSAIDs (section 10.1.1). **Aspirin** is effective against mild to moderate dental pain; dispersible tablets provide a rapidly absorbed form of aspirin suitable for most purposes.

The analgesic effect of **paracetamol** in mild to moderate dental pain is probably less than that of aspirin, but it does not affect bleeding time or interact significantly with warfarin. Moreover, it is less irritant to the stomach. Paracetamol is a suitable analgesic for children; sugar-free versions can be requested by specifying 'sugar-free' on the prescription.

For further information on the management of dental and orofacial pain, see p. 218.

Compound analgesic preparations

Compound analgesic preparations that contain a simple analgesic (such as aspirin or paracetamol) with an opioid component reduce the scope for effective titration of the individual components in the management of pain of varying intensity.

Compound analgesic preparations containing paracetamol or aspirin with a *low dose* of an opioid analgesic (e.g. 8 mg of codeine phosphate per compound tablet) are commonly used, but the advantages have not been substantiated. The low dose of the opioid may be enough to cause opioid side-effects (in particular, constipation) and can complicate the treatment of **overdosage** (see p. 31) yet may not provide significant additional relief of pain.

Co-proxamol (dextropropoxyphene in combination with paracetamol) (p. 222) has little more analgesic effect than paracetamol alone. An important disadvantage of co-proxamol is that overdosage (which may be combined with alcohol) is complicated by respiratory depression and acute heart failure due to the dextropropoxyphene and by hepatotoxicity due to the paracetamol. Rapid treatment is essential (see Emergency Treatment of Poisoning, p. 31). Co-proxamol is to be withdrawn from the market and the CSM has advised that co-proxamol treatment should **no longer** be prescribed; patients who are already receiving it should have their treatment reviewed and another analgesic considered.

A *full dose* of the opioid component (e.g. 60 mg codeine phosphate) in compound analgesic preparations effectively augments the analgesic activity but is associated with the full range of opioid side-effects (including nausea, vomiting, severe constipation, drowsiness, respiratory depression, and risk of dependence on long-term administration). For details of the **side-effects**, **cautions** and **contra-indications** of opioid analgesics, see p. 223 (**important:** the elderly are particularly susceptible to opioid side-effects and should receive lower doses).

In general, when assessing pain, it is necessary to weigh up carefully whether there is a need for a non-opioid and an opioid analgesic to be taken simultaneously.

For information on the use of combination analgesic preparations in dental and orofacial pain, see p. 218

Caffeine is a weak stimulant that is often included, in small doses, in analgesic preparations. It is claimed that the addition of caffeine may enhance the analgesic effect, but the alerting effect, mild habit-forming effect and possible provocation of headache may not always be desirable. Moreover, in excessive dosage or on withdrawal caffeine may itself induce headache.

ASPIRIN

(Acetylsalicylic Acid)

Indications: mild to moderate pain, pyrexia; see also section 10.1.1; antiplatelet (section 2.9)

Cautions: asthma, allergic disease, hepatic impairment (Appendix 2), renal impairment (Appendix 3), dehydration; preferably avoid during fever or viral infection in adolescents (risk of Reye's syndrome, see below); pregnancy (Appendix 4); elderly; G6PD-deficiency (section 9.1.5); **interactions:** Appendix 1 (aspirin)

Contra-indications: children and adolescents under 16 years and in breast-feeding (Reye's syndrome, see below; Appendix 5); previous or active peptic ulceration, haemophilia; not for treatment of gout

HYPERSENSITIVITY. Aspirin and other NSAIDs are **contra-indicated** in patients with a history of hypersensitivity to aspirin or any other NSAID—*which includes those* in whom attacks of *asthma, angioedema, urticaria or rhinitis* have been precipitated by aspirin or any other NSAID

REYE'S SYNDROME. Owing to an association with Reye's syndrome, the CSM has advised that aspirin-containing preparations should not be given to children and adolescents under 16 years, unless specifically indicated, e.g. for Kawasaki syndrome.

Side-effects: generally mild and infrequent but high incidence of gastro-intestinal irritation with slight asymptomatic blood loss, increased bleeding time, bronchospasm and skin reactions in hypersensitive patients. Prolonged administration, see section 10.1.1. **Overdosage:** see Emergency Treatment of Poisoning, p. 29

Dose: 300–900 mg every 4–6 hours when necessary; max. 4 g daily; CHILD and ADOLESCENT not recommended (see Reye's syndrome above)
Rectal route, see below

Aspirin (Non-proprietary)
Tablets PoM[1], aspirin 300 mg. Net price 20 = 21p. Label: 21, 32

1. May be sold to the public provided packs contain no more than 32 capsules or tablets; pharmacists can sell multiple packs up to a total quantity of 100 capsules or tablets in justifiable circumstances; for details see *Medicines, Ethics and Practice*, No. 29, London, Pharmaceutical Press, 2005 (and subsequent editions as available)

Tablets [PoM][1], e/c, aspirin 300 mg, net price 100-tab pack = £4.89; 75 mg, see section 2.9. Label: 5, 25, 32

Dispersible tablets [PoM][1], aspirin 300 mg, net price 20 = 22p; 75 mg, see section 2.9. Label: 13, 21, 32

NOTE. BP directs that when no strength is stated the 300-mg strength should be dispensed, and that when soluble aspirin tablets are prescribed, dispersible aspirin tablets shall be dispensed.

DENTAL PRESCRIBING ON NHS. Aspirin Dispersible Tablets 300 mg may be prescribed

Caprin® (Pinewood)

Tablets [PoM][1], e/c, f/c, pink, aspirin 300 mg, net price 100-tab pack = £4.89; 75 mg, see section 2.9. Label: 5, 25, 32

Nu-Seals® **Aspirin** (Alliance)

Tablets [PoM][1], e/c, aspirin 300 mg, net price 100-tab pack = £3.46; 75 mg, see section 2.9. Label: 5, 25, 32

■ With codeine phosphate 8 mg

[1]**Co-codaprin** (Non-proprietary) [PoM] [CD]

Dispersible tablets, co-codaprin 8/400 (codeine phosphate 8 mg, aspirin 400 mg). Net price 20 = £1.26. Label: 13, 21, 32

Dose: 1–2 tablets in water every 4–6 hours; max. 8 tablets daily

When co-codaprin tablets or dispersible tablets are prescribed and no strength is stated, tablets or dispersible tablets, respectively, containing codeine phosphate 8 mg and aspirin 400 mg should be dispensed

■ Other compound preparations

Aspav® (Alpharma) [PoM] [CD]

Dispersible tablets, aspirin 500 mg, papaveretum 7.71 mg (providing the equivalent of 5 mg of anhydrous morphine). Net price 30-tab pack = £5.98. Label: 2, 13, 21, 32

Dose: 1–2 tablets in water every 4–6 hours if necessary; max. 8 tablets daily

■ Preparations on sale to the public

For a list of **preparations** containing aspirin and paracetamol **on sale to the public**, see p. 222.

PARACETAMOL

(Acetaminophen)

Indications: mild to moderate pain, pyrexia

Cautions: hepatic impairment (Appendix 2); renal impairment (Appendix 3), alcohol dependence; **interactions:** Appendix 1 (paracetamol)

Side-effects: side-effects rare, but rashes, blood disorders (including thrombocytopenia, leucopenia, neutropenia) reported; hypotension also reported on infusion; **important:** liver damage (and less frequently renal damage) following **overdosage**, see Emergency Treatment of Poisoning, p. 29

Dose: *by mouth*, 0.5–1 g every 4–6 hours to a max. of 4 g daily; CHILD 2 months 60 mg for post-immunisation pyrexia; otherwise under 3 months (on doctor's advice only), 10 mg/kg (5 mg/kg if jaundiced); 3 months–1 year 60–120 mg, 1–5 years 120–250 mg, 6–12 years 250–500 mg; these doses may be repeated every 4–6 hours when necessary (max. of 4 doses in 24 hours)

By intravenous infusion over 15 minutes, ADULT and CHILD over 50 kg, 1 g every 4–6 hours; max. 4 g daily; ADULT and CHILD 10–50 kg, 15 mg/kg every 4–6 hours; max. 60 mg/kg daily

For full Joint Committee on Vaccination and Immunisation recommendation on post-immunisation pyrexia, see section 14.1

Rectal route, see below

Paracetamol (Non-proprietary)

Tablets [PoM][1], paracetamol 500 mg. Net price 20 = 21p. Label: 29, 30

Brands include *Panadol*® [NHS]

Soluble Tablets (= Dispersible tablets) [PoM][2], paracetamol 500 mg. Net price 60-tab pack = £5.43. Label: 13, 29, 30

Brands include *Panadol Soluble*® [NHS]

Paediatric Soluble Tablets (= Paediatric dispersible tablets), paracetamol 120 mg. Net price 16-tab pack = 91p. Label: 13, 30

Brands include *Disprol*® *Soluble Paracetamol* [NHS]

Oral Suspension 120 mg/5 mL (= Paediatric Mixture), paracetamol 120 mg/5 mL. Net price 100 mL = 42p. Label: 30

NOTE. BP directs that when Paediatric Paracetamol Oral Suspension or Paediatric Paracetamol Mixture is prescribed Paracetamol Oral Suspension 120 mg/5 mL should be dispensed; sugar-free versions can be ordered by specifying 'sugar-free'on the prescription

Brands include *Calpol*® *Paediatric*, *Calpol*® *Paediatric* sugar-free, *Disprol*® *Paediatric*, *Medinol*® *Paediatric* sugar-free, *Paldesic*®, *Panadol*® sugar-free

Oral Suspension 250 mg/5 mL (= Mixture), paracetamol 250 mg/5 mL. Net price 100 mL = 73p. Label: 30

Brands include *Calpol*®*6 Plus* [NHS], *Medinol*® *Over 6* [NHS], *Paldesic*®

Suppositories, paracetamol 60 mg, net price 10 = £9.96; 125 mg, 10 = £11.50; 250 mg, 10 = £23.00; 500 mg, 10 = £9.90. Label: 30

Dose: by rectum, ADULT and CHILD over 12 years 0.5–1 g up to 4 times daily, CHILD 1–5 years 125–250 mg, 6–12 years 250–500 mg

Brands include *Alvedon*®

DENTAL PRESCRIBING ON NHS. Paracetamol Tablets, Paracetamol Soluble Tablets 500 mg, and Paracetamol Oral Suspension may be prescribed

Perfalgan® (Bristol-Myers Squibb) ▼ [PoM]

Intravenous infusion, paracetamol 10 mg/mL, net price 100-mL vial = £1.50

■ Co-codamol 8/500

When co-codamol tablets, dispersible (or effervescent) tablets, or capsules are prescribed and **no strength is stated**, tablets, dispersible (or effervescent) tablets, or capsules, respectively, containing codeine phosphate **8 mg** and paracetamol **500 mg** should be dispensed.

Co-codamol 8/500[2] (Non-proprietary) [PoM] [CD]

Tablets, co-codamol 8/500 (codeine phosphate 8 mg, paracetamol 500 mg) Net price 20 = 23p. Label: 29, 30

Brands include *Panadeine*® [NHS]

Dose: 1–2 tablets every 4–6 hours; max. 8 tablets daily; CHILD 6–12 years ½–1 tablet

1. May be sold to the public provided packs contain no more than 32 capsules or tablets; pharmacists can sell multiple packs up to a total quantity of 100 capsules or tablets in justifiable circumstances; for details see *Medicines, Ethics and Practice*, No. 29, London, Pharmaceutical Press, 2005 (and subsequent editions as available)

2. May be sold to the public under certain circumstances; for exemptions see *Medicines, Ethics and Practice*, No. 29, London, Pharmaceutical Press, 2005 (and subsequent editions as available)

Effervescent or *dispersible tablets*, co-codamol 8/500 (codeine phosphate 8 mg, paracetamol 500 mg). Net price 20 = £1.34. Label: 13, 29, 30
Brands include *Paracodol*® NHS

Dose: 1–2 tablets in water every 4–6 hours, max. 8 tablets daily; CHILD 6–12 years ½–1 tablet, max. 4 daily
NOTE. The Drug Tariff allows tablets of co-codamol labelled 'dispersible' to be dispensed against an order for 'effervescent' and *vice versa*

Capsules, co-codamol 8/500 (codeine phosphate 8 mg, paracetamol 500 mg). Net price 10-cap pack = £1.10, 20-cap pack = £1.66. Label: 29, 30
Brands include *Paracodol*® NHS

Dose: 1–2 capsules every 4 hours; max. 8 capsules daily

■ Co-codamol 15/500

When co-codamol tablets, dispersible (or effervescent) tablets, or capsules are prescribed and **no strength is stated**, tablets, dispersible (or effervescent) tablets, or capsules, respectively, containing codeine phosphate **8 mg** and paracetamol **500 mg** should be dispensed (see preparations above).

See warnings and notes on p. 219 (**important:** special care in elderly—reduce dose)

Codipar (Goldshield) PoM

Caplets (= tablets), co-codamol 15/500 (codeine phosphate 15 mg, paracetamol 500 mg). Net price 100-tab pack = £7.50. Label: 2, 29, 30

Dose: 1–2 tablets every 4 hours; max. 8 daily; CHILD not recommended

■ Co-codamol 30/500

When co-codamol tablets, dispersible (or effervescent) tablets, or capsules are prescribed and **no strength is stated**, tablets, dispersible (or effervescent) tablets, or capsules, respectively, containing codeine phosphate **8 mg** and on paracetamol **500 mg** should be dispensed (see preparations above).

See warnings and notes on p. 219 (**important:** special care in elderly—reduce dose)

Co-codamol 30/500 (Non-proprietary) PoM

Tablets, co-codamol 30/500 (codeine phosphate 30 mg, paracetamol 500 mg), net price 100-tab pack = £6.88. Label: 2, 29, 30

Dose: 1–2 tablets every 4 hours; max. 8 tablets daily; CHILD not recommended

Capsules, co-codamol 30/500 (codeine phosphate 30 mg, paracetamol 500 mg), net price 100-cap pack = £8.01. Label: 2, 29, 30
Brands include *Medocodene*®, *Zapain*®

Dose: 1–2 capsules every 4 hours; max. 8 capsules daily; CHILD not recommended

Kapake® (Galen) PoM

Tablets, scored, co-codamol 30/500 (codeine phosphate 30 mg, paracetamol 500 mg). Net price 30-tab pack = £2.26 (hosp. only), 100-tab pack = £7.10. Label: 2, 29, 30

Dose: 1–2 tablets every 4 hours; max. 8 tablets daily; CHILD not recommended

Capsules, co-codamol 30/500 (codeine phosphate 30 mg, paracetamol 500 mg), net price 100-cap pack = £7.10. Label: 2, 29, 30

Dose: 1–2 capsules every 4 hours; max. 8 capsules daily; CHILD not recommended

Effervescent tablets, co-codamol 30/500 (codeine phosphate 30 mg, paracetamol 500 mg). Contains Na^+ 16.9 mmol/tablet; avoid in *renal impairment*, net price 100-tab pack = £8.30. Label: 2, 13, 29, 30

Dose: 2 tablets in water every 4 hours; max. 8 daily; CHILD not recommended

Solpadol® (Sanofi-Synthelabo) PoM

Caplets(= tablets), co-codamol 30/500 (codeine phosphate 30 mg, paracetamol 500 mg). Net price 100-tab pack = £7.54. Label: 2, 29, 30

Dose: 2 tablets every 4 hours; max. 8 daily; CHILD not recommended

Capsules, grey/purple, co-codamol 30/500 (codeine phosphate 30 mg, paracetamol 500 mg). Net price 100-cap pack = £7.54. Label: 2, 29, 30

Dose: 1–2 capsules every 4 hours; max. 8 capsules daily; CHILD not recommended
NOTE. May be difficult to obtain

Effervescent tablets, co-codamol 30/500 (codeine phosphate 30 mg, paracetamol 500 mg). Contains Na^+ 16.9 mmol/tablet; avoid in *renal impairment*. Net price 100-tab pack = £9.05. Label: 2, 13, 29, 30

Dose: 2 tablets in water every 4 hours; max. 8 daily; CHILD not recommended

Tylex® (Schwarz) PoM

Capsules, co-codamol 30/500 (codeine phosphate 30 mg, paracetamol 500 mg). Net price 100-cap pack = £8.01. Label: 2, 29, 30

Dose: 1–2 capsules every 4 hours; max. 8 capsules daily; CHILD not recommended

Effervescent tablets, co-codamol 30/500 (codeine phosphate 30 mg, paracetamol 500 mg). Contains Na^+ 13.6 mmol/tablet; avoid in *renal impairment*. Net price 90-tab pack = £7.94. Label: 2, 13, 29, 30
Excipients: include aspartame 25 mg/tablet (see section 9.4.1)

Dose: 1–2 tablets in water every 4 hours; max. 8 tablets daily; CHILD not recommended

■ With methionine (co-methiamol)

A mixture of methionine and paracetamol; methionine has no analgesic activity but may prevent paracetamol-induced liver toxicity if overdose taken

Paradote® (Penn)

Tablets, f/c, co-methiamol 100/500 (DL-methionine 100 mg, paracetamol 500 mg). Net price 24-tab pack = £1.05, 96-tab pack = £2.77. Label: 29, 30

Dose: 2 tablets every 4 hours; max. 8 tablets daily; CHILD 12 years and under, not recommended

■ With dihydrocodeine tartrate 10 mg

See notes on p. 219

Co-dydramol (Non-proprietary) PoM

Tablets, scored, co-dydramol 10/500 (dihydrocodeine tartrate 10 mg, paracetamol 500 mg). Net price 20 = 49p. Label: 21, 29, 30

Dose: 1–2 tablets every 4–6 hours; max. 8 tablets daily; CHILD not recommended
When co-dydramol tablets are prescribed and no strength is stated tablets containing dihydrocodeine tartrate 10 mg and paracetamol 500 mg should be dispensed.
NOTE. Tablets containing paracetamol 500 mg and dihydrocodeine 7.46 mg (*Paramol*® NHS) are on sale to the public. The name *Paramol*® was formerly applied to a brand of co-dydramol tablets

■ With dihydrocodeine tartrate 20 or 30 mg

See warnings and notes on p. 219 (**important:** special care in elderly—reduce dose)

Remedeine® (Napp) PoM

Tablets, paracetamol 500 mg, dihydrocodeine tartrate 20 mg. Net price 112-tab pack = £10.21. Label: 2, 21, 29, 30

Dose: 1–2 tablets every 4–6 hours; max. 8 tablets daily; CHILD not recommended

Forte tablets, paracetamol 500 mg, dihydrocodeine tartrate 30 mg. Net price 56-tab pack = £6.31. Label: 2, 21, 29, 30

Dose: 1–2 tablets every 4–6 hours; max. 8 tablets daily; CHILD not recommended

■ Other compound preparations

Patients should not be initiated on co-proxamol therapy; see also notes on p. 219

Co-proxamol (Non-proprietary) PoM

Tablets, co-proxamol 32.5/325 (dextropropoxyphene hydrochloride 32.5 mg, paracetamol 325 mg). Net price 20 = 30p. Label: 2, 10, patient information leaflet (if available), 29, 30

Brands include *Cosalgesic*® NHS, *Distalgesic*® NHS

Dose: patients already receiving co-proxamol, 2 tablets 3–4 times daily; max. 8 tablets daily; ADOLESCENT and CHILD under 18 years, not recommended

When co-proxamol tablets are prescribed and no strength is stated tablets containing dextropropoxyphene hydrochloride 32.5 mg and paracetamol 325 mg should be dispensed.

■ Preparations on Sale to the Public

The following is a list of preparations on sale to the public that contain **aspirin** or **paracetamol**, **alone** or with **other ingredients**. Other significant ingredients (such as codeine and caffeine) are listed. For details of preparations containing ibuprofen on sale to the public, see section 10.1.1.

Important: in overdose contact **Poisons Information Services** (p. 27) for full details of the ingredients

Alka-Seltzer® (aspirin), **Alka-Seltzer XS**® (aspirin, caffeine, paracetamol), **Anadin**® (aspirin, caffeine), **Anadin Cold Control**® (paracetamol, caffeine, phenylephrine), **Anadin Extra**®, **Anadin Extra Soluble**® (both aspirin, caffeine, paracetamol), **Anadin Paracetamol**® (paracetamol), **Angettes 75**® (aspirin), **Askit**® (aspirin, aloxiprin = polymeric product of aspirin, caffeine), **Aspro Clear**® (aspirin),

Beechams-All-In-One® (paracetamol, guaifenesin, phenylephrine), **Beechams Cold & Flu**®, **Beechams Flu-Plus Hot Berry Fruits**®, **Beechams Flu-Plus Powder**®, **Beechams Hot Lemon**®, **Hot Lemon and Honey**®, **Hot Blackcurrant**® (all paracetamol, phenylephrine), **Beechams Flu-Plus Caplets**® (paracetamol, caffeine, phenylephrine), **Beechams Lemon Tablets**® (aspirin), **Beechams Powders**® (aspirin, caffeine), **Beechams Powders Capsules**® (paracetamol, caffeine, phenylephrine), **Benylin 4 Flu**® (paracetamol, diphenhydramine, pseudoephedrine), **Benylin Day and Night**® (*day tablets*, paracetamol, pseudoephedrine, *night tablets*, paracetamol, diphenhydramine), **Boots Cold & Flu Relief Tablets**® (paracetamol, caffeine, phenylephrine), **Boots Pain Relief Paracetamol Suspension 3 Months Plus**® (paracetamol), **Boots Cold Relief Hot Blackcurrant**®, **Hot Lemon**® (paracetamol), **Boots Migraine Relief**® (paracetamol, codeine), **Boots Seltzer**® (aspirin), **Boots Tension Headache Relief**® (paracetamol, caffeine, codeine, doxylamine)

Calpol Fast Melts®, **Calpol Infant**®, **Calpol 6 Plus**® (all paracetamol), **Caprin**® (aspirin), **Codis 500**® (aspirin, codeine), **Mrs. Cullen's**® (aspirin, caffeine)

Day Nurse® (paracetamol, dextromethorphan, pseudoephedrine), **De Witt's Analgesic Pills**® (paracetamol, caffeine), **Disprin**®, **Disprin Direct**® (all aspirin), **Disprin Extra**® (aspirin, paracetamol), **Disprol**® (paracetamol), **Doans Backache Pills**® (paracetamol, sodium salicylate), **Dolvan**® (paracetamol, diphenhydramine, ephedrine, caffeine), **Dozol**® (paracetamol, diphenhydramine)

Feminax® (paracetamol, caffeine, codeine, hyoscine), **Fennings Children's Cooling Powders**® (paracetamol)

Galpamol® (paracetamol)

Hedex® (paracetamol), **Hedex Extra**® (paracetamol, caffeine)

Infadrops® (paracetamol)

Lemsip Cold & Flu Breathe Easy® (paracetamol, phenylephrine), **Lemsip Cold & Flu Combined Relief Capsules**® (paracetamol, caffeine, phenylephrine), **Lemsip Cold & Flu Max Strength**® (paracetamol, phenylephrine), **Lemsip Lemon**® or **Blackcurrant**®, **Lemsip Max Strength**® (all paracetamol, phenylephrine)

Mandanol® (paracetamol), **Maximum Strength Aspro Clear**® (aspirin), **Medinol**® (paracetamol), **Medised**® (paracetamol, promethazine), **Midrid**® (paracetamol, isometheptene mucate), **Migraleve**® (*pink tablets*, paracetamol, codeine, buclizine, *yellow tablets*, paracetamol, codeine)

Night Nurse® (paracetamol, dextromethorphan, promethazine), **Nirolex Day Cold Comfort**® (paracetamol, pholcodine, pseudoephedrine), **Nirolex Night Cold Comfort**® (paracetamol, pseudoephedrine, diphenhydramine, pholcodeine), **Non-Drowsy Sinutab**® (paracetamol, pseudoephedrine), **Nurse Sykes' Powders**® (aspirin, caffeine, paracetamol)

Panadol® (paracetamol), **Panadol Extra**® (paracetamol, caffeine), **Panadol Night**® (paracetamol, diphenhydramine), **Panadol Soluble**® (paracetamol), **Panadol Ultra**® (paracetamol, codeine), **Paracets**® (paracetamol), **Paracets Plus**® (paracetamol, caffeine, phenylephrine), **Paracodol**® (paracetamol, codeine), **Paradote**® (co-methiamol (paracetamol, DL-methionine)), **Paramol**® (paracetamol, dihydrocodeine), **Phensic**® (aspirin, caffeine), **Propain**® (paracetamol, caffeine, codeine, diphenhydramine), **Propain Plus**® (paracetamol, caffeine, codeine, doxylamine)

Resolve® (paracetamol)

Solpadeine® **Headache** (caffeine, paracetamol), **Solpadeine**® **Max** (codeine, paracetamol), **Solpadeine**® **Plus** (codeine, caffeine, paracetamol), **Sudafed-Co**® (paracetamol, pseudoephedrine), **Syndol**® (paracetamol, caffeine, codeine, doxylamine)

Ultramol Soluble® (paracetamol, codeine, caffeine), **Uniflu with Gregovite C**® (paracetamol, caffeine, codeine, diphenhydramine, phenylephrine)

Veganin® (caffeine, codeine, paracetamol), **Vicks Medinite**® (paracetamol, dextromethorphan, doxylamine, ephedrine)

NEFOPAM HYDROCHLORIDE

Indications: moderate pain

Cautions: hepatic or renal disease, elderly, urinary retention; pregnancy (Appendix 4) and breastfeeding; **interactions:** Appendix 1 (nefopam)

Contra-indications: convulsive disorders; not indicated for myocardial infarction

Side-effects: nausea, nervousness, urinary retention, dry mouth, lightheadedness; less frequently vomiting, blurred vision, drowsiness, sweating, insomnia, tachycardia, headache; confusion and hallucinations also reported; may colour urine (pink)

Dose: *by mouth*, initially 60 mg (elderly, 30 mg) 3 times daily, adjusted according to response; usual range 30–90 mg 3 times daily; CHILD not recommended

By intramuscular injection, 20 mg every 6 hours; CHILD not recommended

NOTE. Nefopam hydrochloride 20 mg by injection ≡ 60 mg by mouth

Acupan® (3M) PoM

Tablets, f/c, nefopam hydrochloride 30 mg. Net price 90-tab pack = £11.18. Label: 2, 14

Injection, nefopam hydrochloride 20 mg/mL. Net price 1-mL amp = 69p

4.7.2 Opioid analgesics

Opioid analgesics are usually used to relieve moderate to severe pain particularly of visceral origin. Repeated administration may cause dependence and tolerance, but this is no deterrent in the control of pain in terminal illness, for guidelines see Prescribing in Palliative Care, p. 14. Regular use of a potent opioid may be appropriate for certain cases of chronic non-malignant pain; treatment should be supervised by a specialist and the patient should be assessed at regular intervals.

SIDE-EFFECTS. Opioid analgesics share many side-effects though qualitative and quantitative differences exist. The most common include nausea, vomiting, constipation, and drowsiness. Larger doses produce respiratory depression and hypotension. **Overdosage**, see Emergency Treatment of Poisoning, p. 31.

INTERACTIONS. See Appendix 1 (opioid analgesics) (**important:** special hazard with *pethidine and possibly other opioids* and MAOIs).

DRIVING. Drowsiness may affect performance of skilled tasks (e.g. driving); effects of alcohol enhanced.

CHOICE. **Morphine** remains the most valuable opioid analgesic for severe pain although it frequently causes nausea and vomiting. It is the standard against which other opioid analgesics are compared. In addition to relief of pain, morphine also confers a state of euphoria and mental detachment.

Morphine is the opioid of choice for the oral treatment of *severe pain in palliative care*. It is given regularly every 4 hours (or every 12 or 24 hours as modified-release preparations). For guidelines on dosage adjustment in palliative care, see p. 14.

Buprenorphine has both opioid agonist and antagonist properties and may precipitate withdrawal symptoms, including pain, in patients dependent on other opioids. It has abuse potential and may itself cause dependence. It has a much longer duration of action than morphine and sublingually is an effective analgesic for 6 to 8 hours. Vomiting may be a problem. Unlike most opioid analgesics, the effects of buprenorphine are only partially reversed by naloxone.

Codeine is effective for the relief of mild to moderate pain but is too constipating for long-term use.

Diphenoxylate (in combination with atropine, as co-phenotrope) is used in acute diarrhoea (see section 1.4.2).

Dipipanone used alone is less sedating than morphine but the only preparation available contains an anti-emetic and is therefore not suitable for regular regimens in palliative care.

Diamorphine (heroin) is a powerful opioid analgesic. It may cause less nausea and hypotension than morphine. In *palliative care* the greater solubility of diamorphine allows effective doses to be injected in smaller volumes and this is important in the emaciated patient.

Dihydrocodeine has an analgesic efficacy similar to that of codeine. The dose of dihydrocodeine by mouth is usually 30 mg every 4 hours; doubling the dose to 60 mg may provide some additional pain relief but this may be at the cost of more nausea and vomiting. A 40-mg tablet is now also available.

Alfentanil, **fentanyl** and **remifentanil** are used by injection for intra-operative analgesia (section 15.1.4.3); fentanyl is available in a transdermal drug delivery system as a self-adhesive patch which is changed every 72 hours.

Meptazinol is claimed to have a low incidence of respiratory depression. It has a reported length of action of 2 to 7 hours with onset within 15 minutes.

Methadone is less sedating than morphine and acts for longer periods. In prolonged use, methadone should not be administered more often than twice daily to avoid the risk of accumulation and opioid overdosage. Methadone may be used instead of morphine in the occasional patient who experiences excitation (or exacerbation of pain) with morphine.

Oxycodone has an efficacy and side-effect profile similar to that of morphine. It is used primarily for control of *pain in palliative care*. It is used as the pectinate in suppositories (special order from BCM Specials).

Pentazocine has both agonist and antagonist properties and precipitates withdrawal symptoms, including pain in patients dependent on other opioids. By injection it is more potent than dihydrocodeine or codeine, but hallucinations and thought disturbances may occur. It is not recommended and, in particular, should be avoided after myocardial infarction as it may increase pulmonary and aortic blood pressure as well as cardiac work.

Pethidine produces prompt but short-lasting analgesia; it is less constipating than morphine, but even in high doses is a less potent analgesic. It is not suitable for severe continuing pain. It is used for analgesia in labour; however, other opioids, such as morphine or diamorphine, are often preferred for obstetric pain.

Tramadol produces analgesia by two mechanisms: an opioid effect and an enhancement of serotonergic and adrenergic pathways. It has fewer of the typical opioid side-effects (notably, less respiratory depression, less constipation and less addiction potential); psychiatric reactions have been reported.

DOSE. The dose of opioids in the BNF may need to be **adjusted individually** according to the degree of analgesia and side-effects; patients' response to opioids varies widely.

POSTOPERATIVE ANALGESIA. The use of intra-operative opioids affects the prescribing of postoperative analgesics and in many cases delays the need for a postoperative analgesic. A postoperative opioid analgesic should be given with care since it may potentiate any residual respiratory depression (for the treatment of opioid-induced respiratory depression, see section 15.1.7). Non-opioid analgesics are also used for postoperative pain (section 15.1.4.2).

Morphine and **papaveretum** are used most widely. **Tramadol** is not as effective in severe pain as other opioid analgesics. **Buprenorphine** may antagonise the analgesic effect of previously administered opioids and is generally not recommended. **Pethidine** is metabolised to norpethidine which may accumulate, particularly in renal impairment; norpethidine stimulates the central nervous system and may cause convulsions. **Meptazinol** is rarely used.

Opioids are also given epidurally [unlicensed route] in the postoperative period but are associated with side-effects such as pruritus, urinary retention, nausea and vomiting; respiratory depression can be delayed, particularly with morphine.

For details of patient-controlled analgesia (PCA) to relieve postoperative pain, consult hospital protocols. Formulations specifically designed for PCA are available (*Pharma-Ject® Morphine Sulphate*).

DENTAL AND OROFACIAL PAIN. Opioid analgesics are **relatively ineffective** in dental pain. Like other opioids, **dihydrocodeine** often causes nausea and vomiting which limits its value in dental pain; if taken for more than a few doses it is also liable to cause constipation. Dihydrocodeine is not very effective in postoperative dental pain.

Pethidine can be taken by mouth, but for optimal effect, it needs to be given by injection. Its efficacy in postoperative dental pain is not proven and its use in dentistry is likely to be minimal. The side-effects of pethidine are similar to those of dihydrocodeine and, apart from constipation, pethidine is also more likely to cause them. Dependence is unlikely if very few tablets are prescribed on very few occasions; nevertheless, dental surgeons need to be aware of the possibility that addicts may seek to acquire supplies.

For the management of dental and orofacial pain, see p. 218.

ADDICTS. Although caution is necessary, addicts (and ex-addicts) may be treated with analgesics in the same way as other people when there is a real clinical need. Doctors do not require a special licence to prescribe opioid analgesics for addicts for relief of pain due to organic disease or injury.

MORPHINE SALTS

Indications: see notes above and under Dose; acute diarrhoea (section 1.4.2); cough in terminal care (section 3.9.1)

Cautions: hypotension, hypothyroidism, asthma (avoid during attack) and decreased respiratory reserve, prostatic hypertrophy; pregnancy (Appendix 4), breast-feeding (Appendix 5); may precipitate coma in hepatic impairment (reduce dose or avoid but many such patients tolerate morphine well); reduce dose or avoid in renal impairment (see also Appendix 3), elderly and debilitated (reduce dose); convulsive disorders, dependence (severe withdrawal symptoms if withdrawn abruptly); use of cough suppressants containing opioid analgesics not generally recommended in children and should be avoided altogether in those under at least 1 year; **interactions:** Appendix 1 (opioid analgesics)

PALLIATIVE CARE. In the control of pain in terminal illness these cautions should not necessarily be a deterrent to the use of opioid analgesics

Contra-indications: avoid in acute respiratory depression, acute alcoholism and where risk of paralytic ileus; also avoid in raised intracranial pressure or head injury (affects pupillary responses vital for neurological assessment); avoid injection in phaeochromocytoma (risk of pressor response to histamine release)

Side-effects: nausea and vomiting (particularly in initial stages), constipation, and drowsiness; larger doses produce respiratory depression, hypotension, and muscle rigidity; other side-effects include difficulty with micturition, ureteric or biliary spasm, dry mouth, sweating, headache, facial flushing, vertigo, bradycardia, tachycardia, palpitation, postural hypotension, hypothermia, hallucinations, dysphoria, mood changes, dependence, miosis, decreased libido or potency, rashes, urticaria and pruritus; **overdosage:** see Emergency Treatment of Poisoning, p. 31; for reversal of opioid-induced respiratory depression, see section 15.1.7.

Dose: acute pain, *by subcutaneous injection* (not suitable for oedematous patients) *or by intramuscular injection*, 10 mg every 4 hours if necessary (15 mg for heavier well-muscled patients); NEONATE up to 1 month 150 micrograms/kg; INFANT 1–12 months 200 micrograms/kg; CHILD 1–5 years 2.5–5 mg; CHILD 6–12 years 5–10 mg

By slow intravenous injection, quarter to half corresponding intramuscular dose

Premedication, *by subcutaneous or intramuscular injection*, up to 10 mg 60–90 minutes before operation; CHILD, *by intramuscular injection*, 150 micrograms/kg

Postoperative pain, *by subcutaneous or intramuscular injection*, 10 mg every 2–4 hours if necessary (15 mg for heavier well-muscled patients); NEONATE up to 1 month 150 micrograms/kg; INFANT 1–12 months 200 micrograms/kg; CHILD 1–5 years 2.5–5 mg; CHILD 6–12 years 5–10 mg

NOTE. In the postoperative period, the patient should be closely monitored for pain relief as well as for side-effects especially respiratory depression

Patient controlled analgesia (PCA), consult hospital protocols

Myocardial infarction, *by slow intravenous injection* (2 mg/minute), 10 mg followed by a further 5–10 mg if necessary; elderly or frail patients, reduce dose by half

Acute pulmonary oedema, *by slow intravenous injection* (2 mg/minute) 5–10 mg

Chronic pain, *by mouth or by subcutaneous injection* (not suitable for oedematous patients) *or by intramuscular injection*, 5–20 mg regularly every 4 hours; dose may be increased according to needs; oral dose should be approx. double corresponding intramuscular dose and approximately triple corresponding intramuscular *diamorphine* dose (see also Prescribing in Palliative Care, p. 14); *by rectum*, as suppositories, 15–30 mg regularly every 4 hours

NOTE. The doses stated above refer equally to morphine hydrochloride, sulphate, and tartrate; see below for doses of **modified-release** preparations.

■ Oral solutions

NOTE. For advice on transfer from oral solutions of morphine to modified-release preparations of morphine, see Prescribing in Palliative Care, p. 14

Morphine Oral Solutions

PoM or CD

Oral solutions of morphine can be prescribed by writing the formula:

Morphine hydrochloride 5 mg

Chloroform water to 5 mL

NOTE. The proportion of morphine hydrochloride may be altered when specified by the prescriber; if above 13 mg per 5 mL the solution becomes **CD**. For sample prescription see Controlled Drugs and Drug Dependence, p. 7. It is usual to adjust the strength so that the dose volume is 5 or 10 mL.

Oramorph® (Boehringer Ingelheim)
Oramorph® oral solution PoM, morphine sulphate 10 mg/5 mL. Net price 100-mL pack = £1.87; 300-mL pack = £5.21; 500-mL pack = £7.86. Label: 2
Oramorph® Unit Dose Vials 10 mg PoM (oral vials), sugar-free, morphine sulphate 10 mg/5-mL vial, net price 20 vials = £2.65. Label: 2
Oramorph® Unit Dose Vials 30 mg CD (oral vials), sugar-free, morphine sulphate 30 mg/5-mL vial, net price 20 vials = £7.44. Label: 2
Oramorph® concentrated oral solution CD, sugar-free, morphine sulphate 100 mg/5 mL. Net price 30-mL pack = £5.24; 120-mL pack = £19.57 (both with calibrated dropper). Label: 2
Oramorph® Unit Dose Vials 100 mg CD (oral vials), sugar-free, morphine sulphate 100 mg/5-mL vial, net price 20 vials = £24.80. Label: 2

■ Tablets

Sevredol® (Napp) CD
Tablets, f/c, scored, morphine sulphate 10 mg (blue), net price 56-tab pack = £5.61; 20 mg (pink), 56-tab pack = £11.21; 50 mg (pale green), 56-tab pack = £28.02. Label: 2
Dose: severe pain uncontrolled by weaker opioid, 10–50 mg every 4 hours (dose adjusted according to response); CHILD 3–5 years, 5 mg every 4 hours; 6–12 years, 5–10 mg

■ Modified-release oral preparations

Morcap® SR (Mayne) CD
Capsules, m/r, clear enclosing ivory and brown pellets, morphine sulphate 20 mg, net price 60-cap pack = £10.80; 50 mg, 60-cap pack = £26.40; 100 mg, 60-cap pack = £50.10. Label: 2, counselling, see below
Dose: every 12 or 24 hours, dose adjusted according to daily morphine requirements, for further advice on determining dose, see Prescribing in Palliative Care, p. 14; dosage requirements should be reviewed if the brand is altered
COUNSELLING. Swallow whole or open capsule and sprinkle contents on soft food
NOTE. Prescription must also specify 'capsules' (i.e. 'Morcap SR capsules')

Morphgesic® SR (Amdipharm) CD
Tablets, m/r, f/c, morphine sulphate 10 mg (buff), net price 60-tab pack = £4.09; 30 mg (violet), 60-tab pack = £9.81; 60 mg (orange), 60-tab pack = £19.15; 100 mg (grey), 60-tab pack = £30.30. Label: 2, 25
Dose: every 12 hours, dose adjusted according to daily morphine requirements, for further advice on determining dose, see Prescribing in Palliative Care, p. 14; dosage requirements should be reviewed if the brand is altered
NOTE. Prescriptions must also specify 'tablets' (i.e. Morphgesic SR tablets)

MST Continus® (Napp) CD
Tablets, m/r, f/c, morphine sulphate 5 mg (white), net price 60-tab pack = £3.29; 10 mg (brown), 60-tab pack = £5.48; 15 mg (green), 60-tab pack = £9.61; 30 mg (purple), 60-tab pack = £13.17; 60 mg (orange), 60-tab pack = £25.69; 100 mg (grey), 60-tab pack = £40.66; 200 mg (green), 60-tab pack = £81.34. Label: 2, 25
Suspension (= sachet of granules to mix with water), m/r, pink, morphine sulphate 20 mg/sachet, net price 30-sachet pack = £24.58; 30 mg/sachet, 30-sachet pack = £25.54; 60 mg/sachet, 30-sachet pack = £51.09; 100 mg/sachet, 30-sachet pack = £85.15; 200 mg/sachet pack, 30-sachet pack = £170.30. Label: 2, 13
Dose: every 12 hours, dose adjusted according to daily morphine requirements, for further advice on determining dose, see Prescribing in Palliative Care, p. 14; dosage requirements should be reviewed if the brand is altered
NOTE. Prescriptions must also specify 'tablets' or 'suspension' (i.e. 'MST Continus tablets' or 'MST Continus suspension')

MXL® (Napp) CD
Capsules, m/r, morphine sulphate 30 mg (light blue), net price 28-cap pack = £10.91; 60 mg (brown), 28-cap pack = £14.95; 90 mg (pink), 28-cap pack = £22.04; 120 mg (green), 28-cap pack = £29.15; 150 mg (blue), 28-cap pack = £36.43; 200 mg (red-brown), 28-cap pack = £46.15. Label: 2, counselling, see below
Dose: every 24 hours, dose adjusted according to daily morphine requirements, for further advice on determining dose, see Prescribing in Palliative Care, p. 14; dosage requirements should be reviewed if the brand is altered
COUNSELLING. Swallow whole or open capsule and sprinkle contents on soft food
NOTE. Prescriptions must also specify 'capsules' (i.e. 'MXL capsules')

Zomorph® (Link) CD
Capsules, m/r, morphine sulphate 10 mg (yellow/clear enclosing pale yellow pellets), net price 60-cap pack = £4.08; 30 mg (pink/clear enclosing pale yellow pellets), 60-cap pack = £9.77; 60 mg (orange/clear enclosing pale yellow pellets), 60-cap pack = £19.06; 100 mg (white/clear enclosing pale yellow pellets), 60-cap pack = £30.18; 200 mg (clear enclosing pale yellow pellets), 60-cap pack = £60.35. Label: 2, counselling, see below
Dose: every 12 hours, dose adjusted according to daily morphine requirements, for further advice on determining doses, see Prescribing in Palliative Care, p. 14; dosage requirements should be reviewed if the brand is altered
COUNSELLING. Swallow whole or open capsule and sprinkle contents on soft food
NOTE. Prescriptions must also specify 'capsules' (i.e. 'Zomorph capsules')

■ Suppositories

Morphine (Non-proprietary) CD
Suppositories, morphine hydrochloride or sulphate 10 mg, net price 12 = £7.24; 15 mg, 12 = £7.14; 20 mg, 12 = £8.92; 30 mg, 12 = £10.41. Label: 2
Available from Aurum, Martindale
NOTE. Both the strength of the suppositories and the morphine salt contained in them must be specified by the prescriber

■ Injections

Morphine Sulphate (Non-proprietary) CD
Injection, morphine sulphate 10, 15, 20, and 30 mg/mL, net price 1- and 2-mL amp (all) = 72p–£1.09; 10 mg/mL, 1-mL prefilled syringe = £5.00
Intravenous infusion, morphine sulphate 1 mg/mL, net price 50-mL vial = £5.00; 2 mg/mL, 50-mL vial = £5.10

Minijet® Morphine Sulphate (Celltech) CD
Injection, morphine sulphate 1 mg/mL, net price 10-mL disposable syringe = £7.36

■ Injection with anti-emetic

CAUTION. In myocardial infarction cyclizine may aggravate severe heart failure and counteract the haemodynamic benefits of opioids, see section 4.6. **Not recommended** in palliative care, see Nausea and Vomiting, p. 16

Cyclimorph® (Amdipharm) CD

Cyclimorph-10® Injection, morphine tartrate 10 mg, cyclizine tartrate 50 mg/mL. Net price 1-mL amp = £1.34

Dose: moderate to severe pain (short-term use only) by subcutaneous, intramuscular, or intravenous injection, 1 mL, repeated not more often than every 4 hours, with not more than 3 doses in any 24-hour period

Cyclimorph-15® Injection, morphine tartrate 15 mg, cyclizine tartrate 50 mg/mL. Net price 1-mL amp = £1.39

Dose: moderate to severe pain (short-term use only) by subcutaneous, intramuscular, or intravenous injection, 1 mL, repeated not more often than every 4 hours, with not more than 3 doses in any 24-hour period

BUPRENORPHINE

Indications: moderate to severe pain; peri-operative analgesia; opioid dependence (section 4.10)

Cautions: see under Morphine Salts and notes above; effects only partially reversed by naloxone; **interactions:** Appendix 1 (opioid analgesics)

FEVER OR EXTERNAL HEAT. Monitor patients using patches for increased side-effects if fever present (increased absorption possible); avoid exposing application site to external heat (may also increase absorption)

Contra-indications: see under Morphine Salts and notes above

Side-effects: see under Morphine Salts and notes above; can give rise to mild withdrawal symptoms in patients dependent on opioids; hiccups, dyspnoea; with patches, local reactions such as erythema and pruritus; delayed local allergic reactions with severe inflammation—discontinue treatment

Dose: moderate to severe pain, *by sublingual administration*, initially 200–400 micrograms every 8 hours, increasing if necessary to 200–400 micrograms every 6–8 hours; CHILD over 6 years, 16–25 kg, 100 micrograms every 6–8 hours; 25–37.5 kg, 100–200 micrograms every 6–8 hours; 37.5–50 kg, 200–300 micrograms every 6–8 hours

By intramuscular or slow intravenous injection, 300–600 micrograms every 6–8 hours; CHILD over 6 months 3–6 micrograms/kg every 6–8 hours (max. 9 micrograms/kg)

Premedication, *by sublingual administration*, 400 micrograms

By intramuscular injection, 300 micrograms

Intra-operative analgesia, *by slow intravenous injection*, 300–450 micrograms

Temgesic® (Schering-Plough) CD

Tablets (sublingual), buprenorphine (as hydrochloride), 200 micrograms, net price 50-tab pack = £5.33; 400 micrograms, 50-tab pack = £10.66. Label: 2, 26

Injection, buprenorphine (as hydrochloride) 300 micrograms/mL, net price 1-mL amp = 49p

Transtec® (Napp) ▼ CD

Patches, self-adhesive, skin-coloured, buprenorphine, '35' patch (releasing 35 micrograms/hour for 72 hours), net price 5 = £28.97; '52.5' patch (releasing 52.5 micrograms/hour for 72 hours), 5 = £43.46; '70' patch (releasing 70 micrograms/hour for 72 hours), 5 = £57.94. Label: 2

Dose: moderate to severe pain unresponsive to non-opioid analgesics, ADULT over 18 years, apply to dry, non-irritated, non-hairy skin on upper torso, removing after 72 hours and siting replacement patch on a different area (avoid same area for at least 6 days). Patients who have not previously received strong opioid analgesic, initially, one '35 micrograms/hour' patch replaced after 72 hours; patients who have received strong opioid analgesic, initial dose based on previous 24-hour opioid requirement, consult product literature

DOSE ADJUSTMENT. When starting, analgesic effect should **not** be evaluated until the system has been worn for **24 hours** (to allow for gradual increase in plasma-buprenorphine concentration)—if necessary, dose should be adjusted at 72-hour intervals using a patch of the next strength *or* using 2 patches of the same strength (applied at *same time* to avoid confusion). Max. 2 patches can be used at any one time. For breakthrough pain, consider 200–400 micrograms buprenorphine sublingually. **Important:** it may take approx. 30 hours for the plasma-buprenorphine concentration to decrease by 50% after patch is removed

LONG DURATION OF ACTION. In view of the long duration of action, patients who have severe side-effects should be monitored for up to 30 hours after removing patch

CODEINE PHOSPHATE

Indications: mild to moderate pain; diarrhoea (section 1.4.2); cough suppression (section 3.9.1)

Cautions: see under Morphine Salts and notes above; use of cough suppressants containing codeine or similar opioid analgesics not generally recommended in children and should be avoided altogether in those under 1 year; **interactions:** Appendix 1 (opioid analgesics)

Contra-indications: see under Morphine Salts and notes above

Side-effects: see under Morphine Salts and notes above

Dose: *by mouth*, 30–60 mg every 4 hours when necessary, to a max. of 240 mg daily; CHILD 1–12 years, 3 mg/kg daily in divided doses

By intramuscular injection, 30–60 mg every 4 hours when necessary

Codeine Phosphate (Non-proprietary)

Tablets PoM, codeine phosphate 15 mg, net price 20 = 91p; 30 mg, 20 = £1.64; 60 mg, 20 = £2.09. Label: 2

NOTE. As for schedule 2 controlled drugs, travellers needing to take codeine phosphate preparations abroad may require a doctor's letter explaining why they are necessary

Syrup PoM, codeine phosphate 25 mg/5 mL. Net price 100 mL = 90p. Label: 2

Injection CD, codeine phosphate 60 mg/mL. Net price 1-mL amp = £2.37

Codeine Linctuses Section 3.9.1

NOTE. Codeine is an ingredient of some compound analgesic preparations, section 4.7.1 and section 10.1.1 (*Codafen Continus®*)

DIAMORPHINE HYDROCHLORIDE

(Heroin Hydrochloride)

Indications: see notes above; acute pulmonary oedema

Cautions: see under Morphine Salts and notes above; **interactions:** Appendix 1 (opioid analgesics)

Contra-indications: see under Morphine Salts and notes above

Side-effects: see under Morphine Salts and notes above

Dose: acute pain, *by subcutaneous or intramuscular injection*, 5 mg repeated every 4 hours if necessary (up to 10 mg for heavier well-muscled patients)

By slow intravenous injection, quarter to half corresponding intramuscular dose

Myocardial infarction, *by slow intravenous injection* (1 mg/minute), 5 mg followed by a further 2.5–5 mg if necessary; elderly or frail patients, reduce dose by half

Acute pulmonary oedema, *by slow intravenous injection* (1 mg/minute) 2.5–5 mg

Chronic pain, *by mouth or by subcutaneous or intramuscular injection*, 5–10 mg regularly every 4 hours; dose may be increased according to needs; intramuscular dose should be approx. half corresponding oral dose, and approx. one third corresponding oral *morphine* dose—see also Prescribing in Palliative Care, p. 14; *by subcutaneous infusion* (using syringe driver), see Prescribing in Palliative Care, p. 17

Diamorphine (Non-proprietary) CD

Tablets, diamorphine hydrochloride 10 mg. Net price 100-tab pack = £12.30. Label: 2

Injection, powder for reconstitution, diamorphine hydrochloride. Net price 5-mg amp = £1.18, 10-mg amp = £1.36, 30-mg amp = £1.62, 100-mg amp = £4.50, 500-mg amp = £20.68

DIHYDROCODEINE TARTRATE

Indications: moderate to severe pain

Cautions: see under Morphine Salts and notes above; **interactions:** Appendix 1 (opioid analgesics)

Contra-indications: see under Morphine Salts and notes above

Side-effects: see under Morphine Salts and notes above

Dose: *by mouth*, 30 mg every 4–6 hours when necessary (see also notes above); CHILD over 4 years 0.5–1 mg/kg every 4–6 hours

By deep subcutaneous or intramuscular injection, up to 50 mg repeated every 4–6 hours if necessary; CHILD over 4 years 0.5–1 mg/kg every 4–6 hours

Dihydrocodeine (Non-proprietary)

Tablets PoM, dihydrocodeine tartrate 30 mg. Net price 20 = 99p. Label: 2, 21

DENTAL PRESCRIBING ON NHS. Dihydrocodeine Tablets 30 mg may be prescribed

Oral solution PoM, dihydrocodeine tartrate 10 mg/5 mL. Net price 150 mL = £3.08. Label: 2, 21

Injection CD, dihydrocodeine tartrate 50 mg/mL. Net price 1-mL amp = £2.29

DF 118 Forte® (Martindale) PoM

Tablets, dihydrocodeine tartrate 40 mg. Net price 100-tab pack = £11.51. Label: 2, 21

Dose: severe pain, 40–80 mg 3 times daily; max. 240 mg daily; CHILD not recommended

■ Modified release

DHC Continus® (Napp) PoM

Tablets, m/r, dihydrocodeine tartrate 60 mg, net price 56-tab pack = £5.50; 90 mg, 56-tab pack = £8.66; 120 mg, 56-tab pack = £11.57. Label: 2, 25

Dose: chronic severe pain, 60–120 mg every 12 hours; CHILD not recommended

NOTE. Dihydrocodeine is an ingredient of some compound analgesic preparations, see section 4.7.1

DIPIPANONE HYDROCHLORIDE

Indications: moderate to severe pain

Cautions: see under Morphine Salts and notes above; **interactions:** Appendix 1 (opioid analgesics)

Contra-indications: see under Morphine Salts and notes above

Side-effects: see under Morphine Salts and notes above

Dose: see preparation below

Diconal® (Amdipharm) CD

Tablets, pink, scored, dipipanone hydrochloride 10 mg, cyclizine hydrochloride 30 mg. Net price 50-tab pack = £8.57. Label: 2

Dose: acute pain, 1 tablet gradually increased to 3 tablets every 6 hours; CHILD not recommended

CAUTION. **Not recommended** in palliative care, see Nausea and vomiting p. 16

FENTANYL

Indications: breakthrough pain in patients already receiving opioid therapy for chronic cancer pain (lozenges); chronic intractable pain (patches), other indications (section 15.1.4.3)

Cautions: see under Morphine Salts and notes above; **interactions:** Appendix 1 (opioid analgesics)

FEVER OR EXTERNAL HEAT. Monitor patients using patches for increased side-effects if fever present (increased absorption possible); avoid exposing application site to external heat (may also increase absorption)

Contra-indications: see under Morphine Salts and notes above

Side-effects: see under Morphine Salts and notes above; with patches, local reactions such as rash, erythema and itching reported

Dose: see under preparation, below

CONVERSION. (from oral morphine to transdermal fentanyl), see Prescribing in Palliative Care, p. 15

Actiq® (Cephalon) CD

Lozenge, (with oromucosal applicator), fentanyl (as citrate) 200 micrograms, net price 3 = £18.58, 30 = £185.80; 400 micrograms, 3 = £18.58, 30 = £185.80; 600 micrograms, 3 = £18.58, 30 = £185.80; 800 micrograms, 3 = £18.58, 30 = £185.80; 1.2 mg, 3 = £18.58, 30 = £185.80; 1.6 mg, 3 = £18.58, 30 = £185.80. Label: 2

Dose: initially 200 micrograms (over 15 minutes) repeated if necessary 15 minutes after first dose (no more than 2 dose units for each pain episode); adjust dose according to response; max. 4 dose units daily

NOTE. If more than 4 episodes of breakthrough pain each day, adjust dose of background analgesic

Durogesic® DTrans® (Janssen-Cilag) CD

Patches, self-adhesive, transparent, fentanyl, '25' patch (releasing approx. 25 micrograms/hour for 72 hours), net price 5 = £27.52; '50' patch (releasing approx. 50 micrograms/hour for 72 hours), 5 = £51.40; '75' patch (releasing approx. 75 micrograms/hour for 72 hours), 5 = £71.66; '100' patch (releasing approx. 100 micrograms/hour for 72 hours), 5 = £88.32. Label: 2

NOTE. Prescriptions must also specify 'patches' (i.e. 'Durogesic DTrans patches')

Dose: apply to dry, non-irritated, non-irradiated, non-hairy skin on torso or upper arm, removing after 72 hours and siting replacement patch on a different area (avoid using the same area for several days). Patients who have not previously received a strong opioid analgesic, initial dose, one '25 micrograms/hour' patch replaced after 72 hours; patients who have received a strong opioid analgesic, initial dose based on previous 24-hour opioid requirement (oral morphine sulphate 90 mg over 24 hours is approximately equivalent to one '25 micrograms/hour' patch, consult product literature for details); CHILD not recommended

DOSE ADJUSTMENT. When starting, evaluation of the analgesic effect should **not** be made before the system has been worn for **24 hours** (to allow for the gradual increase in plasma-fentanyl concentration)—previous analgesic therapy should be phased out gradually from time of first patch application; if necessary dose should be adjusted at 72-hour intervals in steps of '25 micrograms/hour'. More than one patch may be used at a time for doses greater than '100 micrograms/hour'(but applied at *same time* to avoid confusion)—consider additional or alternative analgesic therapy if dose required exceeds 300 micrograms/hour (**important:** it may take 17 hours or longer for the plasma-fentanyl concentration to decrease by 50%, therefore replacement opioid therapy should be initiated at a low dose, increasing gradually).

LONG DURATION OF ACTION. In view of the long duration of action, patients who have had severe side-effects should be monitored for up to 24 hours after patch removal

NOTE. Prescriptions for fentanyl patches can be written to show the strength in terms of the release rate and it is acceptable to write '*Fentanyl 25 patches*' to prescribe patches that release fentanyl 25 micrograms per hour. The dosage should be expressed in terms of the interval between applying a patch and replacing it with a new one, e.g. '*one patch to be applied every 72 hours*'. The total quantity of patches should be written in words and figures.

HYDROMORPHONE HYDROCHLORIDE

Indications: severe pain in cancer

Cautions: see Morphine Salts and notes above; **interactions:** Appendix 1 (opioid analgesics)

Contra-indications: see Morphine Salts and notes above

Side-effects: see Morphine Salts and notes above

Dose: see under preparations below

Palladone® (Napp) CD

Capsules, hydromorphone hydrochloride 1.3 mg (orange/clear), net price 56-cap pack = £8.82; 2.6 mg (red/clear), 56-cap pack = £17.64. Label: 2, counselling, see below

Dose: 1.3 mg every 4 hours, increased if necessary according to severity of pain; CHILD under 12 years not recommended

COUNSELLING. Swallow whole or open capsule and sprinkle contents on soft food

■ Modified release

Palladone® **SR** (Napp) CD

Capsules, m/r, hydromorphone hydrochloride 2 mg (yellow/clear), net price 56-cap pack = £20.98; 4 mg (pale blue/clear), 56-cap pack = £28.75; 8 mg (pink/clear), 56-cap pack = £56.08; 16 mg (brown/clear), 56-cap pack = £106.53; 24 mg (dark blue/clear), 56-cap pack = £159.82. Label: 2, counselling, see below

Dose: 4 mg every 12 hours, increased if necessary according to severity of pain; CHILD under 12 years not recommended

COUNSELLING. Swallow whole or open capsule and sprinkle contents on soft food

MEPTAZINOL

Indications: moderate to severe pain, including postoperative and obstetric pain and renal colic; peri-operative analgesia, see section 15.1.4.3

Cautions: see under Morphine Salts and notes above; effects only partially reversed by naloxone; **interactions:** Appendix 1 (opioid analgesics)

Contra-indications: see under Morphine Salts and notes above

Side-effects: see under Morphine Salts and notes above

Dose: *by mouth*, 200 mg every 3–6 hours as required; CHILD not recommended

By intramuscular injection, 75–100 mg every 2–4 hours if necessary; obstetric analgesia, 100–150 mg according to patient's weight (2 mg/kg); CHILD not recommended

By slow intravenous injection, 50–100 mg every 2–4 hours if necessary; CHILD not recommended

Meptid® (Shire) PoM

Tablets, orange, f/c, meptazinol 200 mg, net price 112-tab pack = £22.11. Label: 2

Injection, meptazinol 100 mg (as hydrochloride)/mL, net price 1-mL amp = £1.92

METHADONE HYDROCHLORIDE

Indications: severe pain, see notes above; cough in terminal disease (section 3.9.1); adjunct in treatment of opioid dependence (section 4.10)

Cautions: see under Morphine Salts and notes above; **interactions:** Appendix 1 (opioid analgesics)

Contra-indications: see under Morphine Salts and notes above

Side-effects: see under Morphine Salts and notes above

Dose: *by mouth or by subcutaneous or intramuscular injection*, 5–10 mg every 6–8 hours, adjusted according to response; on prolonged use not to be given more frequenly than every 12 hours; CHILD not recommended

Methadone (Non-proprietary) CD

Tablets, methadone hydrochloride 5 mg. Net price 50 = £2.97. Label: 2

Brands include *Physeptone*®

Injection▼, methadone hydrochloride, 10 mg/mL, net price 1-mL amp = 86p, 2-mL amp = £1.45, 3.5-mL amp = £1.78, 5-mL amp = £1.92

Brands include *Physeptone*®, *Synastone*®

OXYCODONE HYDROCHLORIDE

Indications: moderate to severe pain in patients with cancer; postoperative pain; severe pain

Cautions: see under Morphine Salts and notes above; avoid in porphyria (section 9.8.2); **interactions:** Appendix 1 (opioid analgesics)

Contra-indications: see under Morphine Salts and notes above; moderate to severe hepatic impairment; severe renal impairment

Side-effects: see under Morphine Salts and notes above

Dose: *by mouth*, initially, 5 mg every 4–6 hours, increased if necessary according to severity of pain, usual max. 400 mg daily, but some patients may require higher doses; CHILD under 18 years not recommended

By slow intravenous injection, 1–10 mg every 4 hours when necessary
By subcutaneous injection, initially 5 mg every 4 hours when necessary
By subcutaneous infusion, initially 7.5 mg/24 hours adjusted according to response
Patient controlled analgesia (PCA), consult hospital protocols
NOTE. 2 mg oral oxycodone is approximately equivalent to 1 mg parenteral oxycodone

OxyNorm® (Napp) CD
Capsules, oxycodone hydrochloride 5 mg (orange/beige), net price 56-cap pack = £11.09; 10 mg (white/beige), 56-cap pack = £22.18; 20 mg (pink/beige), 56-cap pack = £44.35. Label: 2
Liquid (= oral solution), sugar-free, oxycodone hydrochloride 5 mg/5 mL, net price 250 mL = £9.43. Label: 2
Concentrate (= concentrated oral solution), sugar-free, oxycodone hydrochloride 10 mg/mL, net price 120 mL = £45.25. Label: 2
Injection ▼, oxycodone hydrochloride 10 mg/mL, net price 1-mL amp = £1.47, 2-mL amp = £2.94
NOTE. The *Scottish Medicines Consortium* has advised (October 2004) that *OxyNorm*® injection is used only in patients with cancer who have difficulty in tolerating morphine or diamorphine

■ Modified release

OxyContin® (Napp) CD
Tablets, f/c, m/r, oxycodone hydrochloride 5 mg (blue), net price 28-tab pack = £12.16; 10 mg (white), 56-tab pack = £24.30; 20 mg (pink), 56-tab pack = £48.60; 40 mg (yellow), 56-tab pack = £97.22; 80 mg (green), 56-tab pack = £194.44. Label: 2, 25
Dose: initially, 10 mg every 12 hours, increased if necessary according to severity of pain, usual max. 200 mg every 12 hours, but some patients may require higher doses; CHILD under 18 years not recommended

PAPAVERETUM

IMPORTANT. Do **not** confuse with papaverine (section 7.4.5)
A mixture of 253 parts of morphine hydrochloride, 23 parts of papaverine hydrochloride and 20 parts of codeine hydrochloride
The CSM has advised that to avoid confusion the figures of 7.7 mg/ml or 15.4 mg/ml should be used for prescribing purposes

Indications: premedication; enhancement of anaesthesia (but see section 15.1.4.3); postoperative analgesia; severe chronic pain
Cautions: see Morphine Salts and notes above
Contra-indications: see Morphine Salts and notes above
Side-effects: see Morphine Salts and notes above
Dose: *by subcutaneous, intramuscular, or intravenous injection*, 7.7–15.4 mg repeated every 4 hours if necessary (ELDERLY initially 7.7 mg); CHILD up to 1 month 115 micrograms/kg, 1–12 months 154 micrograms/kg, 1–5 years 1.93–3.85 mg, 6–12 years, 3.85–7.7 mg
INTRAVENOUS DOSE. In general the intravenous dose should be 25–50% of the corresponding subcutaneous or intramuscular dose

Papaveretum (Non-proprietary) CD
Injection, papaveretum 15.4 mg/mL (providing the equivalent of 10 mg of anhydrous morphine/mL), net price 1-mL amp = £1.36
NOTE. The name *Omnopon*® was formerly used for papaveretum preparations

■ With hyoscine

Papaveretum and Hyoscine Injection (Non-proprietary) CD
Injection, papaveretum 15.4 mg (providing the equivalent of 10 mg of anhydrous morphine), hyoscine hydrobromide 400 micrograms/mL. Net price 1-mL amp = £2.98
Dose: premedication, by subcutaneous or intramuscular injection, 0.5–1 mL

■ With aspirin

Section 4.7.1

PENTAZOCINE ◢

Indications: moderate to severe pain, but see notes above
Cautions: see under Morphine Salts and notes above; avoid in porphyria (section 9.8.2); **interactions:** Appendix 1 (opioid analgesics)
Contra-indications: see under Morphine Salts and notes above; patients dependent on opioids; arterial or pulmonary hypertension, heart failure
Side-effects: see under Morphine Salts and notes above; occasional hallucinations
Dose: *by mouth*, pentazocine hydrochloride 50 mg every 3–4 hours preferably after food (range 25–100 mg); max. 600 mg daily; CHILD 6–12 years 25 mg
By subcutaneous, intramuscular, or intravenous injection, moderate pain, pentazocine 30 mg, severe pain 45–60 mg every 3–4 hours when necessary; CHILD over 1 year, *by subcutaneous or intramuscular injection*, up to 1 mg/kg, *by intravenous injection* up to 500 micrograms/kg
By rectum in suppositories, pentazocine 50 mg up to 4 times daily; CHILD not recommended

Pentazocine (Non-proprietary) CD ◢
Capsules, pentazocine hydrochloride 50 mg. Net price 28-cap pack = £4.46. Label: 2, 21
Brands include *Fortral*® NHS
Tablets, pentazocine hydrochloride 25 mg. Net price 20-tab pack = £1.43. Label: 2, 21
Brands include *Fortral*® NHS
Injection, pentazocine 30 mg (as lactate)/mL. Net price 1-mL amp = £1.67; 2-mL amp = £3.21
Brands include *Fortral*® NHS
Suppositories, pentazocine 50 mg (as lactate). Net price 20 = £19.93. Label: 2
Brands include *Fortral*® NHS

PETHIDINE HYDROCHLORIDE

Indications: moderate to severe pain, obstetric analgesia; peri-operative analgesia
Cautions: see under Morphine Salts and notes above; not suitable for severe continuing pain; **interactions:** Appendix 1 (opioid analgesics)
Contra-indications: see under Morphine Salts and notes above; severe renal impairment
Side-effects: see under Morphine Salts and notes above; convulsions reported in **overdosage**
Dose: acute pain, *by mouth*, 50–150 mg every 4 hours; CHILD 0.5–2 mg/kg
By subcutaneous or intramuscular injection, 25–100 mg, repeated after 4 hours; CHILD, *by intramuscular injection*, 0.5–2 mg/kg
By slow intravenous injection, 25–50 mg, repeated after 4 hours

Obstetric analgesia, *by subcutaneous or intramuscular injection*, 50–100 mg, repeated 1–3 hours later if necessary; max. 400 mg in 24 hours

Premedication, *by intramuscular injection*, 25–100 mg 1 hour before operation; CHILD 0.5–2 mg/kg

Postoperative pain, *by subcutaneous or intramuscular injection*, 25–100 mg, every 2–3 hours if necessary; CHILD, *by intramuscular injection*, 0.5–2 mg/kg

NOTE. In the postoperative period, the patient should be closely monitored for pain relief as well as for side-effects especially respiratory depression

Pethidine (Non-proprietary) CD

Tablets, pethidine hydrochloride 50 mg, net price 20 = £1.97. Label: 2

DENTAL PRESCRIBING ON NHS. Pethidine Tablets may be prescribed

Injection, pethidine hydrochloride 50 mg/mL, net price 1-mL amp = 53p, 2-mL amp = 56p; 10 mg/mL, 5-mL amp = £2.06, 10-mL amp = £2.18

Pamergan P100® (Martindale) CD

Injection, pethidine hydrochloride 50 mg, promethazine hydrochloride 25 mg/mL. Net price 2-mL amp = 70p

Dose: *by intramuscular injection*, premedication, 2 mL 60–90 minutes before operation; CHILD 8–12 years 0.75 mL, 13–16 years 1 mL

Obstetric analgesia, 1–2 mL every 4 hours if necessary

Severe pain, 1–2 mL every 4–6 hours if necessary

NOTE. Although usually given intramuscularly, may be given intravenously after dilution to at least 10 mL with water for injections

TRAMADOL HYDROCHLORIDE

Indications: moderate to severe pain

Cautions: see under Morphine Salts and notes above; history of epilepsy (convulsions reported, usually after rapid intravenous injection); manufacturer advises avoid in pregnancy (Appendix 4) and breast-feeding (Appendix 5); not suitable as substitute in opioid-dependent patients; **interactions:** Appendix 1 (opioid analgesics)

GENERAL ANAESTHESIA. Not recommended for analgesia during potentially very light planes of general anaesthesia (possibly increased operative recall reported)

Contra-indications: see under Morphine Salts and notes above

Side-effects: see under Morphine Salts and notes above; also abdominal discomfort, diarrhoea, hypotension and occasionally hypertension; paraesthesia, anaphylaxis, and confusion reported

Dose: *by mouth*, 50–100 mg not more often than every 4 hours; total of more than 400 mg daily by mouth not usually required; CHILD not recommended

By intramuscular injection or by intravenous injection (over 2–3 minutes) *or by intravenous infusion*, 50–100 mg every 4–6 hours

Postoperative pain, 100 mg initially then 50 mg every 10–20 minutes if necessary during first hour to total max. 250 mg (including initial dose) in first hour, *then* 50–100 mg every 4–6 hours; max. 600 mg daily; CHILD not recommended

Tramadol Hydrochloride (Non-proprietary) PoM

Capsules, tramadol hydrochloride 50 mg. Net price 30-cap pack = £3.22, 100-cap pack = £4.91. Label: 2

Brands include *Tramake*®

Injection, tramadol hydrochloride 50 mg/mL. Net price 2-mL amp = £1.15

Tramake Insts® (Galen) PoM

Sachets, effervescent powder, sugar-free, lemon-flavoured, tramadol hydrochloride 50 mg (contains Na^+ 9.7 mmol/sachet), net price 60-sachet pack = £8.75; 100 mg (contains Na^+ 14.6 mmol/sachet), 60-sachet pack = £17.00. Label: 2, 13

Excipients: include aspartame (section 9.4.1)

Zamadol® (Viatris) PoM

Capsules, tramadol hydrochloride 50 mg, net price 100-cap pack = £8.00. Label: 2

Orodispersible tablets (*Zamadol Melt*®), tramadol hydrochloride 50 mg, net price 60-tab pack = £7.12, 100-tab pack = £11.88. Label: 2, counselling, administration

Excipients: include aspartame

COUNSELLING. *Zamadol Melt*® should be sucked and then swallowed. May also be dispersed in water

Injection, tramadol hydrochloride 50 mg/mL, net price 2-mL amp = £1.10

Zydol® (Grünenthal) PoM

Capsules, green/yellow, tramadol hydrochloride 50 mg. Net price 100-cap pack = £16.91. Label: 2

Soluble tablets, tramadol hydrochloride 50 mg, net price 20-tab pack = £3.05, 100-tab pack = £15.23. Label: 2, 13

Injection, tramadol hydrochloride 50 mg/mL. Net price 2-mL amp = £1.24

■ Modified release

Dromadol® **SR** (IVAX) PoM

Tablets, m/r, tramadol hydrochloride 100 mg (white), net price 60-tab pack = £16.00; 150 mg (beige), 60-tab pack = £24.00; 200 mg (orange), 60-tab pack = £32.00. Label: 2, 25

Dose: initially 100 mg twice daily increased if necessary; usual max. 200 mg twice daily; CHILD under 12 years not recommended

Larapam® **SR** (Sandoz) PoM

Tablets, m/r, tramadol hydrochloride 100 mg, net price 60-tab pack = £18.25; 150 mg, 60-tab pack = £27.35; 200 mg, 60-tab pack = £36.50. Label: 2, 25

Dose: initially 100 mg twice daily increased if necessary; usual max. 200 mg twice daily; CHILD under 12 years not recommended

Zamadol® **SR** (Viatris) PoM

Capsules, m/r, tramadol hydrochloride 50 mg (green), net price 60-cap pack = £7.64; 100 mg, net price 60-cap pack = £15.28; 150 mg (dark green), 60-cap pack = £22.92; 200 mg (yellow), 60-cap pack = £30.55. Label: 2

Dose: 50–100 mg twice daily increased if necessary to 150–200 mg twice daily; total of more than 400 mg daily not usually required; CHILD under 12 years not recommended

COUNSELLING. Swallow whole or open capsule and swallow contents immediately without chewing

Zydol SR® (Grünenthal) PoM

Tablets, m/r, f/c, tramadol hydrochloride 100 mg, net price 60-tab pack = £18.26; 150 mg (beige), 60-tab pack = £27.39; 200 mg (orange), 60-tab pack = £36.52. Label: 2, 25

Dose: 100 mg twice daily increased if necessary to 150–200 mg twice daily; total of more than 400 mg daily not usually required; CHILD not recommended

Zydol XL® (Grünenthal) PoM

Tablets, m/r, f/c, tramadol hydrochloride 150 mg, net price 30-tab pack = £15.22; 200 mg, 30-tab pack = £20.29; 300 mg, 30-tab pack = £30.44; 400 mg, 30-tab pack = £40.59. Label: 2, 25

Dose: 150 mg daily increased if necessary; more than 400 mg once daily not usually required; CHILD not recommended

■ With paracetamol

Tramacet® (Janssen-Cilag) ▼ PoM

Tablets, f/c, yellow, tramadol hydrochloride 37.5 mg, paracetamol 325 mg, net price 60-tab pack = £10.07. Label: 2, 25, 29, 30

Dose: 2 tablets not more than every 6 hours; max. 8 tablets daily; CHILD under 12 years not recommended

4.7.3 Neuropathic and functional pain

Neuropathic pain, which occurs as a result of damage to neural tissue, includes *postherpetic neuralgia, phantom limb pain, complex regional pain syndrome* (reflex sympathetic dystrophy, causalgia) *compression neuropathies, peripheral neuropathies* (e.g. due to diabetes, haematological malignancies, rheumatoid arthritis, alcoholism, drug misuse), *trauma, central pain* (e.g. pain following stroke, spinal cord injury and syringomyelia) and *idiopathic neuropathy*. The pain occurs in an area of sensory deficit and may be described as burning, shooting or scalding and is often accompanied by pain that is evoked by a non-noxious stimulus (allodynia).

Trigeminal neuralgia is also caused by dysfunction of neural tissue, but its management is distinct from other forms of neuropathic pain.

Neuropathic pain is generally managed with a tricyclic antidepressant and certain antiepileptic drugs. Neuropathic pain may respond only partially to opioid analgesics. Of the opioids, methadone, tramadol, and oxycodone are probably the most effective for neuropathic pain and they may be considered when other measures fail. Nerve blocks, transcutaneous electrical nerve stimulation (TENS) and, in selected cases, central electrical stimulation may help. Many patients with chronic neuropathic pain require multidisciplinary management, including physiotherapy and psychological support.

Amitriptyline is prescribed most frequently [unlicensed indication], initially at 10–25 mg each night. The dose may be increased gradually to about 75 mg daily if required (higher doses under specialist supervision); **nortriptyline**, a metabolite of amitriptyline, also given at an initial dose of 10–25 mg at night may produce fewer side-effects. **Gabapentin** and **pregabalin** (section 4.8.1) are licensed for the treatment of neuropathic pain.

Capsaicin (section 10.3.2) is licensed for neuropathic pain (but the intense burning sensation during initial treatment may limit use). Drugs, that are now generally reserved for use under specialist supervision include **sodium valproate** and occasionally **phenytoin**. **Ketamine** (section 15.1.1), an NMDA antagonist, or **lidocaine (lignocaine)** by intravenous infusion may also be useful in some forms of neuropathic pain [both unlicensed indication; specialist use only].

A **corticosteroid** may help to relieve pressure in compression neuropathy and thereby reduce pain. The management of trigeminal neuralgia and postherpetic neuralgia are outlined below; for the management of neuropathic pain in *palliative care* see p. 15; for the management of diabetic neuropathy, see section 6.1.5.

Trigeminal neuralgia

Surgery may be the treatment of choice in many patients; a neurological assessment will identify those who stand to benefit. **Carbamazepine** (section 4.8.1) taken during the acute stages of trigeminal neuralgia, reduces the frequency and severity of attacks. It is very effective for the severe pain associated with trigeminal neuralgia and (less commonly) glossopharyngeal neuralgia. Plasma-carbamazepine concentration should be monitored when high doses are given. Small doses should be used initially to reduce the incidence of side-effects e.g. dizziness. **Oxcarbazepine** [unlicensed indication] is an alternative to carbamazepine. **Gabapentin** and **lamotrigine** [unlicensed indication] are also used in trigeminal neuralgia. Some cases respond to **phenytoin** (section 4.8.1); the drug may be given by intravenous infusion (possibly as fosphenytoin) in a crisis (specialist use only).

Postherpetic neuralgia

Postherpetic neuralgia follows acute herpes zoster infection (shingles), particularly in the elderly. If **amitriptyline** fails to manage the pain adequately, **gabapentin** may improve control. A topical analgesic preparation containing **capsaicin** 0.075% (section 10.3.2) is licensed for use in postherpetic neuralgia. Application of topical local anaesthetic preparations may be helpful in some patients.

Functional facial pain

Chronic oral and facial pain (e.g. atypical facial pain, oral dysaesthesia or temporomandibular joint pain dysfunction syndrome) may call for prolonged use of analgesics or for other drugs. Tricyclic antidepressants (section 4.3.1) may be useful for facial pain [unlicensed indication], but are not on the Dental Practitioners' List. Long-term prescribing for disorders of this type should follow a full investigation and usually involves specialists. Patients on long-term therapy need to be monitored both for progress and for side-effects.

4.7.4 Antimigraine drugs

4.7.4.1 Treatment of the acute migraine attack

Treatment of a migraine attack should be guided by response to previous treatment and the severity of the attacks. A **simple analgesic** such as aspirin, paracetamol (preferably in a soluble or dispersible form) or an NSAID is often effective; concomitant **antiemetic** treatment may be required. If treatment with an analgesic is inadequate, an attack may be treated with a specific antimigraine compound such as a **$5HT_1$ agonist** ('triptan'). **Ergot alkaloids** are rarely required now; oral and rectal preparations are associated with many side-effects and they should be avoided in cerebrovascular or cardiovascular disease.

Frequent and prolonged use of analgesics for migraine (opioid and non-opioid analgesics, $5HT_1$ agonists, and ergotamine) is associated with analgesic-induced headaches; therefore, increasing consumption of these medicines needs careful management.

Analgesics

Most migraine headaches respond to analgesics such as **aspirin** or **paracetamol** (section 4.7.1) but because peristalsis is often reduced during migraine attacks the medication may not be sufficiently well absorbed to be effective; dispersible or effervescent preparations are therefore preferred.

The NSAID **tolfenamic acid** is licensed specifically for the treatment of an acute attack of migraine; **diclofenac potassium**, **flurbiprofen**, **ibuprofen**, and **naproxen sodium** (section 10.1.1) are also licensed for use in migraine.

ANALGESICS

■ Aspirin
Section 4.7.1

■ Paracetamol
Section 4.7.1

■ Non-steroidal anti-inflammatory drugs (NSAIDs)
Section 10.1.1

■ With anti-emetics

Domperamol® (Servier) PoM
Tablets, f/c, paracetamol 500 mg, domperidone (as maleate) 10 mg, net price 16-tab pack = £6.51. Label: 17, 30
Dose: 2 tablets at onset of attack then up to every 4 hours; max. 8 tablets daily; CHILD not recommended

Migraleve® (Pfizer Consumer)
Tablets, all f/c, *pink tablets*, buclizine hydrochloride 6.25 mg, paracetamol 500 mg, codeine phosphate 8 mg; *yellow tablets*, paracetamol 500 mg, codeine phosphate 8 mg. Net price 48-tab *Migraleve* PoM (32 pink + 16 yellow) = £5.10; 48 pink (*Migraleve Pink*) = £5.56; 48 yellow (*Migraleve Yellow*) = £4.70. Label: 2, (*Migraleve Pink*), 17, 30
Dose: 2 pink tablets at onset of attack, or if it is imminent, then 2 yellow tablets every 4 hours if necessary; max. in 24 hours 2 pink and 6 yellow; CHILD under 10 years, only under close medical supervision; 10–14 years, half adult dose

MigraMax® (Zeneus) PoM
Oral powder, aspirin (as lysine acetylsalicylate) 900 mg, metoclopramide hydrochloride 10 mg/sachet, net price 6-sachet pack = £7.00, 20-sachet pack = £23.33. Label: 13, 21, 32
Dose: ADULT over 20 years 1 sachet in water at onset of attack, repeated after 2 hours if necessary (max. 3 sachets in 24 hours); YOUNG ADULT (under 20 years) and CHILD not recommended
IMPORTANT. Metoclopramide can cause **severe extrapyramidal effects**, particularly in children and young adults (for further details, see p. 211)
Excipients: include aspartame (section 9.4.1)

Paramax® (Sanofi-Synthelabo) PoM
Tablets, scored, paracetamol 500 mg, metoclopramide hydrochloride 5 mg. Net price 42-tab pack = £6.69. Label: 17, 30
Sachets, effervescent powder, sugar-free, the contents of 1 sachet = 1 tablet; to be dissolved in ¼ tumblerful of liquid before administration. Net price 42-sachet pack = £8.69. Label: 13, 17, 30
Dose: (tablets or sachets): 2 at onset of attack then every 4 hours when necessary to max. of 6 in 24 hours; YOUNG ADULT 12–19 years, 1 at onset of attack then 1 every 4 hours when necessary to max. of 3 in 24 hours (max. dose of metoclopramide 500 micrograms/kg daily)
IMPORTANT. Metoclopramide can cause **severe extrapyramidal effects**, particularly in children and young adults (for further details, see p. 211)

TOLFENAMIC ACID

Indications: treatment of acute migraine attacks
Cautions: see NSAIDs, section 10.1.1
Contra-indications: see NSAIDs, section 10.1.1
Side-effects: see NSAIDs, section 10.1.1; also dysuria (most commonly in men), tremor, euphoria, and fatigue reported
Dose: 200 mg at onset repeated once after 1–2 hours if necessary

Clotam® (Provalis) PoM
Rapid Tablets, tolfenamic acid 200 mg. Net price 10-tab pack = £15.00

$5HT_1$ agonists

A $5HT_1$ agonist is of considerable value in the treatment of an acute migraine attack. The $5HT_1$ agonists ('triptans') act on the 5HT (serotonin) 1B/1D receptors and they are therefore sometimes referred to as $5HT_{1B/1D}$-receptor agonists. A $5HT_1$ agonist may be used during the established headache phase of an attack and is the preferred treatment in those who fail to respond to conventional analgesics.

The $5HT_1$ agonists available for treating migraine are **almotriptan**, **eletriptan**, **frovatriptan**, **naratriptan**, **rizatriptan**, **sumatriptan**, and **zolmitriptan**. Sumatriptan is also of value in cluster headache (section 4.7.4.3).

CAUTIONS. $5HT_1$ agonists should be used with caution in conditions which predispose to coronary artery disease (pre-existing cardiac disease, see Contra-indications below); hepatic impairment (see Appendix 2); pregnancy (see Appendix 4) and breast-feeding (see Appendix 5). $5HT_1$ agonists are recommended as monotherapy and should not be taken concurrently with other therapies for acute migraine; see also **interactions**: Appendix 1 ($5HT_1$ agonists). Little information is available on the use of these drugs in the elderly (over 65 years).

CONTRA-INDICATIONS. $5HT_1$ agonists should not be used for prophylaxis and they are contra-indicated in ischaemic heart disease, previous myocardial infarction, coronary vasospasm (including Prinzmetal's angina), and uncontrolled or severe hypertension.

SIDE-EFFECTS. Side-effects of the $5HT_1$ agonists include sensations of tingling, heat, heaviness, pressure, or tightness of any part of the body (including throat and chest—discontinue if intense, may be due to coronary vasoconstriction or to anaphylaxis; see also CSM advice under Sumatriptan); flushing, dizziness, feeling of weakness; fatigue; nausea and vomiting also reported.

ALMOTRIPTAN

Indications: treatment of acute migraine attacks

Cautions: see under $5HT_1$ agonists above; hepatic impairment (avoid if severe—Appendix 2); severe renal impairment (Appendix 3); sensitivity to sulphonamides; **interactions:** Appendix 1 ($5HT_1$ agonists)

Contra-indications: see under $5HT_1$ agonists above; previous cerebrovascular accident or transient ischaemic attack; peripheral vascular disease

Side-effects: see under $5HT_1$ agonists above; transient increase in blood pressure, drowsiness; also paraesthesia, diarrhoea, dyspepsia, dry mouth, myalgia, headache, tinnitus

Dose: 12.5 mg as soon as possible after onset repeated after 2 hours if migraine recurs (patient not responding should not take second dose for same attack); max. 25 mg in 24 hours; CHILD and ADOLESCENT under 18 years not recommended

Almogran® (Organon) ▼ PoM

Tablets, f/c, almotriptan (as hydrogen malate) 12.5 mg, net price 3-tab pack = £9.07; 6-tab pack = £18.14; 9-tab pack = £27.20. Label: 3

ELETRIPTAN

Indications: treatment of acute migraine attacks

Cautions: see under $5HT_1$ agonists above; hepatic impairment (avoid if severe); renal impairment (avoid if severe—Appendix 3); **interactions**: Appendix 1 ($5HT_1$ agonists)

Contra-indications: see under $5HT_1$ agonists above; previous cerebrovascular accident or transient ischaemic attack; peripheral vascular disease

Side-effects: see under $5HT_1$ agonists above; also dry mouth, dyspepsia, abdominal pain, tachycardia, asthenia, drowsiness, ataxia, speech impairment, myasthenia, myalgia, pharyngitis, sweating; less commonly diarrhoea, anorexia, glossitis, thirst, oedema, increased urinary frequency, transient increase in blood pressure, insomnia, depression, confusion, tremor, agitation, euphoria, malaise, arthralgia, dyspnoea, rhinitis, rash, pruritus, visual disturbances, taste disturbance, tinnitus; rarely bradycardia

Dose: 40 mg as soon as possible after onset repeated after 2 hours if migraine recurs (patient not responding should not take second dose for same attack); increase to 80 mg for subsequent attacks if 40-mg dose inadequate; max. 80 mg in 24 hours; CHILD and ADOLESCENT under 18 years not recommended

Relpax® (Pfizer) ▼ PoM

Tablets, f/c, orange, eletriptan (as hydrobromide) 20 mg, net price 6-tab pack = £22.50; 40 mg, 6-tab pack = £22.50. Label: 3

FROVATRIPTAN

Indications: treatment of acute migraine attacks

Cautions: see under $5HT_1$ agonists above; **interactions:** Appendix 1 ($5HT_1$ agonists)

Contra-indications: see under $5HT_1$ agonists above; severe hepatic impairment; previous cerebrovascular attack or transient ischaemic attack; peripheral vascular disease

Side-effects: see under $5HT_1$ agonists above; dry mouth, gastro-intestinal disturbances, palpitation, paraesthesia, drowsiness, sweating; taste disturbances, tachycardia (rarely bradycardia), hypertension, rhinitis, pharyngitis, sinusitis, laryngitis, tremor, muscle spasm, anxiety, insomnia, confusion, nervousness, agitation, impaired concentration, mood disturbances, thirst, micturition disorders, pruritus, tinnitus; rarely bilirubinaemia, stomatitis, hyperventilation, amnesia, abnormal dreams, syncope, hypocalcaemia, hypoglycaemia, urticaria

Dose: 2.5 mg as soon as possible after onset repeated after 2 hours if migraine recurs (patient not responding should not take second dose for same attack); max. 5 mg in 24 hours; CHILD and ADOLESCENT under 18 years not recommended; ELDERLY over 65 years not recommended

Migard® (Menarini) ▼ PoM

Tablets, f/c, frovatriptan (as succinate) 2.5 mg, net price 6-tab pack = £16.67. Label: 3

NARATRIPTAN

Indications: treatment of acute migraine attacks

Cautions: see under $5HT_1$ agonists above; renal impairment (Appendix 3); sensitivity to sulphonamides; **interactions:** Appendix 1 ($5HT_1$ agonists)

DRIVING. Drowsiness may affect performance of skilled tasks (e.g. driving)

Contra-indications: see under $5HT_1$ agonists above; previous cerebrovascular accident or transient ischaemic attack; peripheral vascular disease

Side-effects: see under $5HT_1$ agonists above, bradycardia or tachycardia; visual disturbances; ischaemic colitis reported

Dose: 2.5 mg as soon as possible after onset; if migraine recurs after initial response, dose may be repeated after 4 hours (patient not responding should not take second dose for same attack); max. 5 mg in 24 hours; CHILD and ADOLESCENT under 18 years not recommended

Naramig® (GSK) PoM

Tablets, f/c, green, naratriptan (as hydrochloride) 2.5 mg, net price 6-tab pack = £24.55, 12-tab pack = £49.10. Label: 3

RIZATRIPTAN

Indications: treatment of acute migraine attacks

Cautions: see under $5HT_1$ agonists above; renal impairment (Appendix 3); **interactions:** Appendix 1 ($5HT_1$ agonists)

DRIVING. Drowsiness may affect performance of skilled tasks (e.g. driving)

Contra-indications: see under $5HT_1$ agonists above; previous cerebrovascular accident or transient ischaemic attack; peripheral vascular disease

Side-effects: see under $5HT_1$ agonists above; drowsiness, palpitation, tachycardia, dry mouth, diarrhoea, dyspepsia, thirst, pharyngeal discomfort, dyspnoea, headache, paraesthesia, decreased alertness, insomnia, tremor, ataxia, nervousness, vertigo, confusion, myalgia and muscle weakness, sweating, urticaria, pruritus, blurred vision; rarely syncope, hypertension; hypersensitivity reactions (including rash, angioedema, and toxic epidermal necrolysis) and taste disturbance reported

Dose: 10 mg as soon as possible after onset repeated after 2 hours if migraine recurs (patient not responding should not take second dose for same attack); max. 20 mg in 24 hours; CHILD and ADOLESCENT under 18 years not recommended

NOTE. Halve dose in patients taking propranolol; not to be taken within 2 hours of taking propranolol

Maxalt® (MSD) PoM

Tablets, pink, rizatriptan (as benzoate) 5 mg, net price 6-tab pack = £26.74; 10 mg, 3-tab pack = £13.37, 6-tab pack = £26.74. Label: 3

Wafers (*Maxalt*® *Melt*), rizatriptan (as benzoate) 10 mg, net price 3-wafer pack = £13.37, 6-wafer pack = £26.74. Label: 3, counselling, administration

COUNSELLING. *Maxalt*® *Melt* wafers should be placed on the tongue and allowed to dissolve

Excipients: include aspartame equivalent to phenylalanine 2.1 mg (section 9.4.1)

SUMATRIPTAN

Indications: treatment of acute migraine attacks; cluster headache (subcutaneous injection only)

Cautions: see under $5HT_1$ agonists above; history of seizures; renal impairment; sensitivity to sulphonamides; **interactions:** Appendix 1 ($5HT_1$ agonists)

DRIVING. Drowsiness may affect performance of skilled tasks (e.g. driving)

Contra-indications: see under $5HT_1$ agonists above; previous cerebrovascular accident or transient ischaemic attack; peripheral vascular disease; moderate and severe hypertension

Side-effects: see under $5HT_1$ agonists above; drowsiness, transient increase in blood pressure, hypotension, bradycardia or tachycardia, visual disturbances, ischaemic colitis, Raynaud's syndrome, seizures reported; erythema at injection site; nasal irritation and taste disturbance with nasal spray

CSM advice. Following reports of chest pain and tightness (coronary vasoconstriction) CSM has emphasised that sumatriptan should **not** be used in ischaemic heart disease or Prinzmetal's angina, and that use with ergotamine should be **avoided** (see also Cautions).

Dose: *by mouth*, 50 mg (some patients may require 100 mg) as soon as possible after onset (patient not responding should not take second dose for same attack); dose may be repeated after not less than 2 hours if migraine recurs; max. 300 mg in 24 hours; CHILD and ADOLESCENT under 18 years not recommended

By subcutaneous injection using auto-injector, 6 mg as soon as possible after onset (patients not responding should not take second dose for same attack); dose may be repeated once after not less than 1 hour if migraine recurs; max. 12 mg in 24 hours; CHILD and ADOLESCENT under 18 years not recommended

IMPORTANT. **Not** for intravenous injection which may cause coronary vasospasm and angina

Intranasally, 10–20 mg (ADOLESCENT 12–17 years 10 mg) into one nostril as soon as possible after onset (patient not responding should not take a second dose for same attack); dose may be repeated once after not less than 2 hours if migraine recurs; max. 40 mg (ADOLESCENT 12–17 years 20 mg) in 24 hours; CHILD under 12 years not recommended

Imigran® (GSK) PoM

Tablets, f/c, sumatriptan (as succinate) 50 mg, net price 6-tab pack = £27.62, 12-tab pack = £52.48; 100 mg, 6-tab pack = £44.64, 12-tab pack = £89.28. Label: 3, 10, patient information leaflet

Injection, sumatriptan (as succinate) 12 mg/mL (= 6 mg/0.5-mL syringe), net price, treatment pack (2 × 0.5-mL prefilled syringes and auto-injector) = £44.19; refill pack 2 × 0.5-mL prefilled cartridges = £42.05; 6 × 0.5-mL prefilled cartridges = £126.13. Label: 3, 10, patient information leaflet

Nasal spray, sumatriptan 10 mg/0.1-mL actuation, net price 2 unit-dose spray device = £12.28; 20 mg/0.1-mL actuation, 2 unit-dose spray device = £12.28, 6 unit-dose spray device = £36.83. Label: 3, 10, patient information leaflet

Imigran® **RADIS** (GSK) PoM

Tablets, f/c, sumatriptan (as succinate) 50 mg (pink), net price 6-tab pack = £24.87, 12-tab pack = £49.77; 100 mg (white), 6-tab pack = £44.64, 12-tab pack = £89.28. Label: 3, 10, patient information leaflet

ZOLMITRIPTAN

Indications: treatment of acute migraine attacks

Cautions: see under $5HT_1$ agonists above; should not be taken within 12 hours of any other $5HT_1$ agonist; **interactions:** Appendix 1 ($5HT_1$ agonists)

Contra-indications: see under $5HT_1$ agonists above; Wolff-Parkinson-White syndrome or arrhythmias associated with accessory cardiac conduction pathways; previous cerebrovascular accident or transient ischaemic attack

Side-effects: see under $5HT_1$ agonists above; drowsiness, transient increase in blood pressure, dry mouth, myalgia, muscle weakness, dysaesthesia; rarely, gastro-intestinal ischaemia, angina, myocardial infarction, tachycardia, palpitations, headache, polyuria, splenic infarction; taste disturbance and nasal discomfort with nasal spray

Dose: *by mouth*, 2.5 mg as soon as possible after onset repeated after not less than 2 hours if migraine persists or recurs (increase to 5 mg for subsequent attacks in patients not achieving satisfactory relief with 2.5-mg dose); max. 10 mg in 24 hours; CHILD not recommended

Intranasally, 5 mg (1 spray) into one nostril as soon as possible after onset repeated after not less than 2 hours if migraine persists or recurs; max. 10 mg in 24 hours; CHILD not recommended

Zomig® (AstraZeneca) PoM

Tablets, f/c, yellow, zolmitriptan 2.5 mg, net price 6-tab pack = £24.00, 12-tab pack = £48.00

Orodispersible tablets (*Zomig Rapimelt*®), zolmitriptan 2.5 mg, net-price 6-tab pack = £24.00; 5 mg, 6-tab pack = £26.16 Counselling, administration

COUNSELLING. *Zomig Rapimelt*® should be placed on the tongue, allowed to disperse and swallowed

Excipients: include aspartame equivalent to phenylalanine 2.81 mg/tablet (section 9.4.1)

Nasal spray▼, zolmitriptan 5 mg/0.1-mL unit-dose spray device, net price 6 unit-dose sprays = £40.50

Ergot alkaloids

The value of **ergotamine** for migraine is limited by difficulties in absorption and by its side-effects, particularly nausea, vomiting, abdominal pain, and *muscular cramps*; it is best avoided. The recommended doses of ergotamine preparations should **not** be exceeded and treatment should **not** be repeated at intervals of less than 4 days.

To avoid habituation the frequency of administration of ergotamine should be limited to **no more than** twice a month. It should **never** be prescribed prophylactically but in the management of cluster headache a low dose (e.g. ergotamine 1 mg at night for 6 nights in 7) is occasionally given for 1 to 2 weeks [unlicensed indication].

ERGOTAMINE TARTRATE

Indications: treatment of acute migraine attacks and migraine variants unresponsive to analgesics

Cautions: risk of peripheral vasospasm (see advice below); elderly; dependence (see Ergot alkaloids above), should not be used for migraine prophylaxis; **interactions:** Appendix 1 (ergot alkaloids) and under Sumatriptan (Cautions), below

PERIPHERAL VASOSPASM. Warn patient to stop treatment immediately if numbness or tingling of extremities develops and to contact doctor.

Contra-indications: peripheral vascular disease, coronary heart disease, obliterative vascular disease and Raynaud's syndrome, temporal arteritis, hepatic impairment (Appendix 2), renal impairment (Appendix 3), sepsis, severe or inadequately controlled hypertension, hyperthyroidism, pregnancy (Appendix 4), breast-feeding (Appendix 5), porphyria (section 9.8.2)

Side-effects: nausea, vomiting, vertigo, abdominal pain, diarrhoea, muscle cramps, and occasionally headache provoked (usually because of prolonged excessive dosage or abrupt withdrawal); precordial pain, myocardial and intestinal ischaemia, rarely myocardial infarction; repeated high dosage may cause ergotism with gangrene and confusion; pleural, peritoneal and heart-valve fibrosis may occur with excessive use; rectal or anal stricture or ulceration and rectovaginal fistula reported with prolonged use of suppositories

Dose: see under preparations below

Cafergot® (Alliance) PoM

Tablets, ergotamine tartrate 1 mg, caffeine 100 mg. Net price 30-tab pack = £5.02. Label: 18, counselling, dosage

Dose: 1–2 tablets at onset; max. 4 tablets in 24 hours; not to be repeated at intervals of less than 4 days; max. 8 tablets in one week (but see also notes above); CHILD not recommended

Suppositories, ergotamine tartrate 2 mg, caffeine 100 mg. Net price 30 = £10.13. Label: 18, counselling, dosage

Dose: 1 suppository at onset; max. 2 in 24 hours; not to be repeated at intervals of less than 4 days; max. 4 suppositories in one week (but see also notes above); CHILD not recommended

Migril® (CP) PoM

Tablets, scored, ergotamine tartrate 2 mg, cyclizine hydrochloride 50 mg, caffeine hydrate 100 mg. Net price 20 = £11.67. Label: 2, 18, counselling, dosage

Dose: 1 tablet at onset, followed after 30 minutes by ½–1 tablet, repeated every 30 minutes if necessary; max. 4 tablets per attack and 6 tablets in one week (but see also notes above); CHILD not recommended

Anti-emetics

Anti-emetics (section 4.6), such as **metoclopramide** or **domperidone**, or phenothiazine and antihistamine anti-emetics, relieve the nausea associated with migraine attacks. Anti-emetics may be given by intramuscular injection or rectally if vomiting is a problem. Metoclopramide and domperidone have the added advantage of promoting gastric emptying and normal peristalsis; a single dose should be given at the onset of symptoms. Oral analgesic preparations containing metoclopramide or domperidone are a convenient alternative (**important:** for warnings relating to extrapyramidal effects of metoclopramide particularly in children and young adults, see p. 211).

Other drugs for migraine

Isometheptene mucate (in combination with paracetamol) is licensed for the treatment of acute attacks of migraine; other more effective treatments are available.

ISOMETHEPTENE MUCATE

Indications: treatment of acute migraine attacks

Cautions: cardiovascular disease, hepatic and renal impairment, diabetes mellitus, hyperthyroidism; **interactions:** Appendix 1 (sympathomimetics)

Contra-indications: glaucoma, severe cardiac, hepatic and renal impairment, severe hypertension, pregnancy and breast-feeding; porphyria (section 9.8.2)

Side-effects: dizziness, circulatory disturbances, rashes, blood disorders also reported

[1]**Midrid**® (Manx) PoM

Capsules, red, isometheptene mucate 65 mg, paracetamol 325 mg. Net price 30-cap pack = £5.50. Label: 30, counselling, dosage

Dose: migraine, 2 capsules at onset of attack, followed by 1 capsule every hour if necessary; max. 5 capsules in 12 hours; CHILD not recommended

1. A pack containing 15 capsules may be sold to the public

4.7.4.2 Prophylaxis of migraine

Where migraine attacks are frequent, possible provoking factors such as stress, irregular life-style (e.g. lack of sleep), or chemical triggers (e.g. alcohol and nitrates) should be sought; combined oral contraceptives may also provoke migraine, see section 7.3.1 for advice.

Preventative treatment for migraine should be considered for patients who:

- suffer at least two attacks a month;
- suffer an increasing frequency of headaches;
- suffer significant disability despite suitable treatment for migraine attacks;
- cannot take suitable treatment for migraine attacks.

Prophylaxis is also necessary in some rare migraine subtypes and those at risk of migrainous infarction.

Pizotifen is an antihistamine and serotonin antagonist structurally related to the tricyclic antidepressants. It affords good prophylaxis but may cause weight gain. To avoid undue drowsiness treatment may be started at 500 micrograms at night and gradually increased to 3 mg; it is rarely necessary to exceed this dose.

The **beta-blockers** propranolol, metoprolol, nadolol, and timolol (section 2.4) are all effective. Propranolol is the most commonly used in an initial dose of 40 mg 2 to 3 times daily by mouth. Beta-blockers may also be given as a single daily dose of a long-acting preparation. The value of beta-blockers is limited by their contra-indications (section 2.4) and also by their interactions (see Appendix 1, beta-blockers).

Amitriptyline (section 4.3.1) [unlicensed indication] may usefully be prescribed in a dose of 10 mg at night, increasing to a maintenance dose of 50–75 mg at night.

Sodium valproate (section 4.8.1) may be effective for migraine prophylaxis [unlicensed indication] in a starting dose of 300 mg twice daily, increased if necessary to 1.2 g daily in divided doses. **Valproic acid** (as semisodium valproate) (section 4.2.3) is similarly effective [unlicensed indication] in a starting dose of 250 mg twice daily, increased if necessary to 1 g daily in divided doses. Alternatively, **topiramate** (section 4.8.1) started at a dose of 25 mg daily increased gradually to 100–200 mg daily in divided doses may be effective [unlicensed indication].

Cyproheptadine (section 3.4.1), an antihistamine with serotonin-antagonist and calcium channel-blocking properties, may also be tried in refractory cases.

Clonidine (*Dixarit*®) is **not** recommended and may aggravate depression or produce insomnia. **Methysergide**, a semi-synthetic ergot alkaloid, has dangerous side-effects (retroperitoneal fibrosis and fibrosis of the heart valves and pleura); **important:** it should only be administered under hospital supervision.

PIZOTIFEN

Indications: prevention of vascular headache including classical migraine, common migraine, and cluster headache

Cautions: urinary retention; angle-closure glaucoma, renal impairment; pregnancy and breast-feeding (Appendix 5); **interactions:** Appendix 1 (pizotifen)

DRIVING. Drowsiness may affect performance of skilled tasks (e.g. driving); effects of alcohol enhanced

Side-effects: antimuscarinic effects, drowsiness, increased appetite and weight gain; occasionally nausea, dizziness; rarely anxiety, aggression, and depression; CNS stimulation may occur in children

Dose: 1.5 mg at night *or* 500 micrograms 3 times daily (but see also notes above), adjusted according to response; max. single dose 3 mg, max. daily dose 4.5 mg; CHILD over 2 years, up to 1.5 mg daily in divided doses; max. single dose at night 1 mg

Pizotifen (Non-proprietary) PoM

Tablets, pizotifen (as hydrogen malate), 500 micrograms, net price 28-tab pack = £2.28; 1.5 mg, 28-tab pack = £4.99. Label: 2

Sanomigran® (Novartis) PoM

Tablets, both ivory-yellow, s/c, pizotifen (as hydrogen malate), 500 micrograms, net price 60-tab pack = £2.57; 1.5 mg, 28-tab pack = £4.28. Label: 2

Elixir, pizotifen (as hydrogen malate) 250 micrograms/5 mL, net price 300 mL = £4.51. Label: 2

CLONIDINE HYDROCHLORIDE

Indications: prevention of recurrent migraine (but see notes above), vascular headache, menopausal flushing; hypertension (section 2.5.2)

Cautions: depressive illness, concurrent antihypertensive therapy; porphyria (section 9.8.2); **interactions:** Appendix 1 (alpha$_2$-adrenoceptor stimulant)

Side-effects: dry mouth, sedation, dizziness, nausea, nocturnal restlessness; occasionally rashes

Dose: 50 micrograms twice daily, increased after 2 weeks to 75 micrograms twice daily if necessary; CHILD not recommended

Clonidine (Non-proprietary) PoM

Tablets, clonidine hydrochloride 25 micrograms. Net price 112-tab pack = £10.54

Dixarit® (Boehringer Ingelheim) PoM

Tablets, blue, s/c, clonidine hydrochloride 25 micrograms. Net price 112-tab pack = £7.11

Catapres® PoM

Section 2.5.2 (hypertension)

METHYSERGIDE

Indications: prevention of severe recurrent migraine, cluster headache and other vascular headaches in patients who are refractory to other treatment and whose lives are seriously disrupted (**important:** hospital supervision only, see notes above); diarrhoea associated with carcinoid syndrome

Cautions: history of peptic ulceration; avoid abrupt withdrawal of treatment; after 6 months withdraw (gradually over 2 to 3 weeks) for reassessment for at least 1 month (see also notes above); **interactions:** Appendix 1 (ergot alkaloids)

Contra-indications: renal, hepatic, pulmonary, and cardiovascular disease, severe hypertension, collagen disease, cellulitis, urinary-tract disorders, cachectic or septic conditions, pregnancy, breast-feeding

Side-effects: nausea, vomiting, heartburn, abdominal discomfort, drowsiness, and dizziness occur frequently in initial treatment; mental and behavioural disturbances, insomnia, oedema, weight gain, rashes, loss of scalp hair, cramps, arterial spasm (including coronary artery spasm with angina and possible myocardial infarction), paraesthesias of extremities, postural hypotension, and tachycardia also occur; retroperitoneal and other abnormal fibrotic reactions may occur on prolonged administration, requiring immediate withdrawal of treatment

Dose: initially 1 mg at bedtime, increased gradually over about 2 weeks to 1–2 mg 3 times daily with food (see notes above); CHILD not recommended

Diarrhoea associated with carcinoid syndrome, usual range, 12–20 mg daily (hospital supervision); CHILD not recommended

Deseril® (Alliance) PoM

Tablets, s/c, methysergide (as maleate) 1 mg, net price 60-tab pack = £13.46. Label: 2, 21

4.7.4.3 Cluster headache

Cluster headache rarely responds to standard analgesics. **Sumatriptan** given by subcutaneous injection is the drug of choice for the *treatment* of cluster headache. Alternatively, 100% **oxygen** at a rate of 7–12 litres/minute is useful in aborting an attack.

Prophylaxis of cluster headache is considered if the attacks are frequent, or last over 3 weeks, or if the attacks cannot be treated effectively. **Verapamil** or **lithium** [both unlicensed use] are used for prophylaxis. **Ergotamine**, used on an intermittent basis is an alternative for patients with short bouts, but it should **not** be used for prolonged periods. **Methysergide** is effective but must be used with extreme caution (see section 4.7.4.2) and only if other drugs cannot be used or if they are not effective.

4.8 Antiepileptics

4.8.1 Control of epilepsy

The object of treatment is to prevent the occurrence of seizures by maintaining an effective dose of one or more antiepileptic drugs. Careful adjustment of doses is necessary, starting with low doses and increasing gradually until seizures are controlled or there are overdose effects.

The frequency of administration is often determined by the plasma half-life, and should be kept as low as possible to encourage better patient compliance. Most antiepileptics, when used in average dosage, may be given twice daily. Phenobarbital and sometimes phenytoin, which have long half-lives, may often be given as a daily dose at bedtime. However, with large doses, some antiepileptics may need to be administered 3 times daily to avoid adverse effects associated with high peak plasma concentrations. Young children metabolise antiepileptics more rapidly than adults and therefore require more frequent doses and a higher amount per kilogram body-weight.

COMBINATION THERAPY. Therapy with two or more antiepileptic drugs concurrently may be necessary; it should preferably only be used when monotherapy with several alternative drugs has proved ineffective. Combination therapy enhances toxicity and drug interactions may occur between antiepileptics (see below).

INTERACTIONS. Interactions between antiepileptics are complex and may enhance toxicity without a corresponding increase in antiepileptic effect. Interactions are usually caused by *hepatic enzyme induction* or *hepatic enzyme inhibition*; *displacement from protein binding sites* is not usually a problem. These interactions are highly variable and unpredictable. Plasma monitoring is therefore often advisable with combination therapy.

Significant interactions that occur **between antiepileptics** themselves are as follows:

> NOTE. Check under each drug for possible interactions when two or more antiepileptic drugs are used

Carbamazepine
- *often lowers* plasma concentration of *clobazam, clonazepam, lamotrigine, an active metabolite of oxcarbazepine*, and of *phenytoin* (but may also raise phenytoin concentration), *tiagabine, topiramate, valproate*, and *zonisamide*
- *sometimes lowers* plasma concentration of *ethosuximide, and primidone* (but tendency for corresponding increase in phenobarbital level)

Ethosuximide
- *sometimes raises* plasma concentration of *phenytoin*

Gabapentin
- no interactions with gabapentin reported

Lamotrigine
- *sometimes raises* plasma concentration of *an active metabolite of carbamazepine* (but evidence is conflicting)

Levetiracetam
- no interactions with levetiracetam reported

Oxcarbazepine
- *sometimes lowers* plasma concentration of *carbamazepine* (but may raise concentration of *an active metabolite of carbamazepine*)
- *sometimes raises* plasma concentration of *phenytoin*
- *often raises* plasma concentration of *phenobarbital*

Phenobarbital *or* Primidone
- *often lowers* plasma concentration of *carbamazepine, clonazepam, lamotrigine, an active metabolite of oxcarbazepine*, and of *phenytoin* (but may also raise phenytoin concentration), *tiagabine, valproate*, and *zonisamide*
- *sometimes lowers* plasma concentration of *ethosuximide*

Phenytoin
- *often lowers* plasma concentration of *clonazepam, carbamazepine, lamotrigine, an active metabolite of oxcarbazepine*, and of *tiagabine, topiramate, valproate*, and *zonisamide*
- *often raises* plasma concentration of *phenobarbital*
- *sometimes lowers* plasma concentration of *ethosuximide, and primidone* (by increasing conversion to phenobarbital)

Pregabalin
- no interactions with pregabalin reported

Topiramate
- *sometimes raises* plasma concentration of *phenytoin*

Valproate
- *sometimes lowers* plasma concentration of *an active metabolite of oxcarbazepine*
- *often raises* plasma concentration of *an active metabolite of carbamazepine*, and of *lamotrigine, primidone, phenobarbital, and phenytoin* (but may also lower)
- *sometimes raises* plasma concentration of *ethosuximide, and primidone* (and tendency for significant increase in phenobarbital level)

Vigabatrin
often lowers plasma concentration of *phenytoin*
sometimes lowers plasma concentration of *phenobarbital, and primidone*

Zonisamide
sometimes increases plasma concentration of *carbamazepine* (but may also lower carbamazepine concentration)

For other important interactions see **Appendix 1**, and for FPA guidelines on enzyme-inducing antiepileptics and **oral contraceptives**, see section 7.3.1.

WITHDRAWAL. Abrupt withdrawal of antiepileptics, particularly the barbiturates and benzodiazepines, should be avoided, as this may precipitate severe rebound seizures. Reduction in dosage should be carried out in stages and, in the case of the barbiturates, the withdrawal process may take months. The changeover from one antiepileptic drug regimen to another should be made cautiously, withdrawing the first drug only when the new regimen has been largely established.

The decision to withdraw all antiepileptics from a seizure-free patient, and its timing, is often difficult and may depend on individual patient factors. Even in patients who have been seizure-free for several years, there is a significant risk of seizure recurrence on drug withdrawal.

In patients receiving several antiepileptic drugs, only one drug should be withdrawn at a time.

DRIVING. Patients suffering from epilepsy may drive a motor vehicle (but not a heavy goods or public service vehicle) provided that they have had a seizure-free period of one year or, if subject to attacks only while asleep, have established a 3-year period of asleep attacks without awake attacks. Patients affected by drowsiness should not drive or operate machinery.

Guidance issued by the Drivers Medical Unit of the Driver and Vehicle Licensing Agency (DVLA) recommends that patients should be advised not to drive during withdrawal of antiepileptic drugs, or for 6 months afterwards (see also Drugs and Driving under General Guidance, p. 2).

PREGNANCY AND BREAST-FEEDING. During pregnancy, total plasma concentrations of antiepileptics (particularly of phenytoin) may fall, particularly in the later stages but free plasma concentrations may remain the same (or even rise). There is an increased risk of teratogenicity associated with the use of antiepileptic drugs (reduced if treatment is limited to a single drug). In view of the increased risk of neural tube and other defects associated, in particular, with **carbamazepine**, **oxcarbazepine**, **phenytoin** and **valproate** women taking antiepileptic drugs who *may become pregnant* should be **informed of the possible consequences**. Those who *wish to become pregnant* should be referred to an appropriate specialist for advice. Women who become pregnant should be **counselled** and offered **antenatal screening** (alpha-fetoprotein measurement and a second trimester ultrasound scan).

To counteract the risk of neural tube defects adequate folate supplements are advised for women before and during pregnancy; to prevent recurrence of neural tube defects, women should receive folic acid 5 mg daily (section 9.1.2)—this dose may also be appropriate for women receiving antiepileptic drugs.

In view of the risk of neonatal bleeding associated with carbamazepine, phenobarbital and phenytoin, prophylactic vitamin K_1 (section 9.6.6) is recommended for the mother before delivery (as well as for the neonate).

Breast-feeding is acceptable with all antiepileptic drugs, taken in normal doses, with the possible exception of the barbiturates, and also some of the more recently introduced ones, see Appendix 5.

Partial seizures with or without secondary generalisation

Carbamazepine, **lamotrigine**, **sodium valproate** and **phenytoin** can be used in monotherapy for secondarily generalised tonic-clonic seizures and for partial (focal) seizures; alternatively, **oxcarbazepine** monotherapy can be used. **Phenobarbital** (phenobarbitone) and **primidone** are also effective but they are more sedating and are not used as first-line drugs.

Where a single drug has failed to control the seizures, combination therapy can be tried with the above drugs or with additional drugs, such as gabapentin, tiagabine, topiramate, or vigabatrin; alternatives include acetazolamide, clobazam, and clonazepam.

Generalised seizures

TONIC-CLONIC SEIZURES (GRAND MAL). The drugs of choice for tonic-clonic seizures are **carbamazepine**, **lamotrigine**, **phenytoin**, and **sodium valproate**. For those patients who have tonic-clonic seizures as part of the syndrome of primary generalised epilepsy, **sodium valproate** is the drug of choice. **Phenobarbital** and **primidone** are also effective but may be more sedating.

ABSENCE SEIZURES (PETIT MAL). **Ethosuximide** and **sodium valproate** are the drugs of choice in simple absence seizures. Sodium valproate is also highly effective in treating the tonic-clonic seizures which may co-exist with absence seizures in primary generalised epilepsy. **Lamotrigine** may also be effective [unlicensed indication].

MYOCLONIC SEIZURES. Myoclonic seizures (myoclonic jerks) occur in a variety of syndromes, and response to treatment varies considerably. **Sodium valproate** is the drug of choice and **clonazepam**, **ethosuximide**, or **lamotrigine** may be used. For reference to the adjunctive use of piracetam, see section 4.9.3.

ATYPICAL ABSENCE, ATONIC, AND TONIC SEIZURES. These seizure types are usually seen in childhood, in specific epileptic syndromes, or associated with cerebral damage or mental retardation. They may respond poorly to the traditional drugs. **Phenytoin**, **sodium valproate**, **lamotrigine**, **clonazepam**, **ethosuximide**, and **phenobarbital** may be tried. Second-line antiepileptic drugs that are occasionally helpful, include **acetazolamide** and **corticosteroids**.

Carbamazepine and oxcarbazepine

Carbamazepine is a drug of choice for simple and complex partial seizures and for tonic-clonic seizures secondary to a focal discharge. It has a wider therapeutic index than phenytoin and the relationship between dose and plasma-carbamazepine concentration is linear, but monitoring of plasma-carbamazepine concentrations may be helpful in determining optimum dosage. It has generally fewer side-effects than phenytoin or the barbiturates, but reversible blurring of vision, dizziness, and unsteadiness are dose-related, and may be dose-limiting. These side-effects may be reduced by altering the timing of medication; use of modified-release tablets also significantly lessens the incidence of dose-related side-effects. It is essential to initiate carbamazepine therapy at a low dose and build this up slowly with increments of 100–200 mg every two weeks.

Oxcarbazepine is licensed for the treatment of partial seizures with or without secondarily generalised tonic-clonic seizures. Oxcarbazepine induces hepatic enzymes to a lesser extent than carbamazepine.

CARBAMAZEPINE

Indications: partial and secondary generalised tonic-clonic seizures, some primary generalised seizures; trigeminal neuralgia; prophylaxis of bipolar disorder unresponsive to lithium

Cautions: hepatic impairment (Appendix 2) or renal impairment; cardiac disease (see also Contra-indications), skin reactions (see also Blood, hepatic or skin disorders below and under Side-effects), history of haematological reactions to other drugs; manufacturer recommends blood counts and hepatic and renal function tests (but evidence of practical value unsatisfactory); glaucoma; pregnancy (**important:** see p. 238 and Appendix 4 (neural tube screening)), breast-feeding (see p. 238 and Appendix 5); avoid abrupt withdrawal; **interactions:** see p. 237 and Appendix 1 (carbamazepine)

BLOOD, HEPATIC OR SKIN DISORDERS. Patients or their carers should be told how to recognise signs of blood, liver, or skin disorders, and advised to seek immediate medical attention if symptoms such as fever, sore throat, rash, mouth ulcers, bruising, or bleeding develop. Leucopenia which is severe, progressive or associated with clinical symptoms requires withdrawal (if necessary under cover of suitable alternative).

Contra-indications: AV conduction abnormalities (unless paced); history of bone marrow depression, porphyria (section 9.8.2)

Side-effects: nausea and vomiting, dizziness, drowsiness, headache, ataxia, confusion and agitation (elderly), visual disturbances (especially double vision and often associated with peak plasma concentrations); constipation or diarrhoea, anorexia; mild transient generalised erythematous rash may occur in a large number of patients (withdraw if worsens or is accompanied by other symptoms); leucopenia and other blood disorders (including thrombocytopenia, agranulocytosis and aplastic anaemia); other side-effects include cholestatic jaundice, hepatitis and acute renal failure, Stevens-Johnson syndrome, toxic epidermal necrolysis, alopecia, thromboembolism, arthralgia, fever, proteinuria, lymph node enlargement, cardiac conduction disturbances (sometimes arrhythmias), dyskinesias, paraesthesia, depression, impotence (and impaired fertility), gynaecomastia, galactorrhoea, aggression, activation of psychosis; photosensitivity, pulmonary hypersensitivity (with dyspnoea and pneumonitis), hyponatraemia, oedema, and disturbances of bone metabolism (with osteomalacia) also reported; suppositories may cause occasional rectal irritation

Dose: *by mouth*, epilepsy, initially, 100–200 mg 1–2 times daily, increased slowly (see notes above) to usual dose of 0.8–1.2 g daily in divided doses; in some cases 1.6–2 g daily may be needed; ELDERLY reduce initial dose; CHILD daily in divided doses, up to 1 year 100–200 mg, 1–5 years 200–400 mg, 5–10 years 400–600 mg, 10–15 years 0.6–1 g

Trigeminal neuralgia, initially 100 mg 1–2 times daily (but some patients may require higher initial dose), increased gradually according to response; usual dose 200 mg 3–4 times daily, up to 1.6 g daily in some patients

Prophylaxis of bipolar disorder unresponsive to lithium (see also section 4.2.3), initially 400 mg daily in divided doses increased until symptoms controlled; usual range 400–600 mg daily; max. 1.6 g daily

By rectum, as suppositories, see below

NOTE. Plasma concentration for optimum response 4–12 mg/litre (20–50 micromol/litre)

Carbamazepine (Non-proprietary) [PoM]

Tablets, carbamazepine 100 mg, net price 20 = 58p; 200 mg, 20 = £1.07; 400 mg, 20 = £2.11. Label: 3, 8, counselling, blood, hepatic or skin disorder symptoms (see above), driving (see notes above)

Brands include *Carbagen*®, *Epimaz*®

NOTE. Different preparations may vary in bioavailability; to avoid reduced effect or excessive side-effects, it may be prudent to avoid changing the formulation (see also notes above on how side-effects may be reduced)

DENTAL PRESCRIBING ON NHS. Carbamazepine Tablets may be prescribed

Tegretol® (Cephalon) [PoM]

Tablets, all scored, carbamazepine 100 mg, net price 84-tab pack = £2.43; 200 mg, 84-tab pack = £4.50; 400 mg, 56-tab pack = £5.90. Label: 3, 8, counselling, blood, hepatic or skin disorder symptoms (see above), driving (see notes above)

Chewtabs, orange, carbamazepine 100 mg, net price 56-tab pack = £3.54; 200 mg, 56-tab pack = £6.59. Label: 3, 8, 21, 24, counselling, blood, hepatic or skin disorder symptoms (see above), driving (see notes above)

Liquid, sugar-free, carbamazepine 100 mg/5 mL. Net price 300-mL pack = £6.86. Label: 3, 8, counselling, blood, hepatic or skin disorder symptoms (see above), driving (see notes above)

Suppositories, carbamazepine 125 mg, net price 5 = £9.00; 250 mg, 5 = £12.00. Label: 3, 8, counselling, blood, hepatic or skin disorder symptoms (see above), driving (see notes above)

Dose: epilepsy, for short-term use (max. 7 days) when oral therapy temporarily not possible; suppositories of 125 mg may be considered to be approximately equivalent in therapeutic effect to tablets of 100 mg but final adjustment should always depend on clinical response (plasma concentration monitoring recommended); max. by rectum 1 g daily in 4 divided doses

■ Modified release

Carbagen SR (Generics) [PoM]

Tablets, m/r, f/c, both scored, carbamazepine 200 mg, net price 56-tab pack = £4.88; 400 mg, 56-

tab pack = £9.63. Label: 3, 8, 25, counselling, blood, hepatic or skin disorder symptoms (see above), driving (see notes above)

Dose: epilepsy (ADULT and CHILD over 5 years), as above; trigeminal neuralgia, as above; total daily dose given in 1–2 divided doses; bipolar disorder, as above

Tegretol® Retard (Cephalon) PoM

Tablets, m/r, both scored, carbamazepine 200 mg (beige-orange), net price 56-tab pack = £5.26; 400 mg (brown-orange), 56-tab pack = £10.34. Label: 3, 8, 25, counselling, blood, hepatic or skin disorder symptoms (see above), driving (see notes above)

Dose: epilepsy (ADULT and CHILD over 5 years), as above; trigeminal neuralgia, as above; total daily dose given in 2 divided doses

OXCARBAZEPINE

Indications: monotherapy and adjunctive treatment of partial seizures with or without secondarily generalised tonic-clonic seizures

Cautions: hypersensitivity to carbamazepine; avoid abrupt withdrawal; elderly, hyponatraemia (monitor plasma-sodium concentration in patients at risk), heart failure (monitor body-weight), cardiac conduction disorders; avoid in porphyria (section 9.8.2); hepatic impairment (Appendix 2); renal impairment (Appendix 3); pregnancy (see p. 238 and Appendix 4); breast-feeding (Appendix 5); **interactions:** Appendix 1 (oxcarbazepine)

BLOOD, HEPATIC OR SKIN DISORDERS. Patients or their carers should be told how to recognise signs of blood, liver, or skin disorders, and advised to seek immediate medical attention if symptoms such as lethargy, confusion, muscular twitching, fever, sore throat, rash, blistering, mouth ulcers, bruising, or bleeding develop

Side-effects: nausea, vomiting, constipation, diarrhoea, abdominal pain; dizziness, headache, drowsiness, agitation, amnesia, asthenia, ataxia, confusion, impaired concentration, depression, tremor; hyponatraemia; acne, alopecia, rash; vertigo, nystagmus, visual disorders including diplopia; *less commonly* urticaria, leucopenia; *rarely* arrhythmias, Stevens-Johnson syndrome, systemic lupus erythematosus, hepatitis, pancreatitis, thrombocytopenia, angioedema, hypersensitivity reactions

Dose: initially 300 mg twice daily increased according to response in steps of up to 600 mg daily at weekly intervals; usual dose range 0.6–2.4 g daily in divided doses; CHILD over 6 years, 8–10 mg/kg daily in 2 divided doses increased according to response in steps of up to 10 mg/kg daily at weekly intervals (in adjunctive therapy, maintenance dose approx. 30 mg/kg daily); max. 46 mg/kg daily in divided doses

NOTE. In adjunctive therapy, the dose of concomitant antiepileptics may need to be reduced when using high doses of oxcarbazepine

Trileptal® (Novartis) PoM

Tablets, f/c, scored, all yellow, oxcarbazepine 150 mg, net price 50-tab pack = £10.00; 300 mg, 50-tab pack = £20.00; 600 mg, 50-tab pack = £40.00. Label: 3, 8, counselling, blood, hepatic or skin disorders (see above), driving (see notes above)

Oral suspension, sugar-free, oxcarbazepine 300 mg/5 mL, net price 250 mL (with oral syringe) = £40.00. Label: 3, 8, counselling, blood, hepatic or skin disorders (see above), driving (see notes above)

Excipients: include propylene glycol

Ethosuximide

Ethosuximide is sometimes used in simple absence seizures; it may also be used in myoclonic seizures and in atypical absence, atonic, and tonic seizures.

ETHOSUXIMIDE

Indications: absence seizures

Cautions: see notes above; hepatic and renal impairment; manufacturer recommends blood counts and hepatic and renal function tests (but evidence of practical value unsatisfactory); pregnancy (see p. 238 and Appendix 4) and breast-feeding (Appendix 5); avoid sudden withdrawal; porphyria (see section 9.8.2); **interactions:** Appendix 1 (ethosuximide)

BLOOD DISORDERS. Patients or their carers should be told how to recognise signs of blood disorders, and advised to seek immediate medical attention if symptoms such as fever, sore throat, mouth ulcers, bruising or bleeding develop

Side-effects: gastro-intestinal disturbances, weight loss, drowsiness, dizziness, ataxia, dyskinesia, hiccup, photophobia, headache, depression, and mild euphoria. Psychotic states, rashes, hepatic and renal changes (see Cautions), and haematological disorders such as agranulocytosis and aplastic anaemia occur rarely (blood counts required if signs or symptoms of infection); systemic lupus erythematosus and erythema multiforme (Stevens-Johnson syndrome) reported; other side-effects reported include gum hypertrophy, swelling of tongue, irritability, hyperactivity, sleep disturbances, night terrors, inability to concentrate, aggressiveness, increased libido, myopia, vaginal bleeding

Dose: ADULT and CHILD over 6 years initially, 500 mg daily, increased by 250 mg at intervals of 4–7 days to usual dose of 1–1.5 g daily; occasionally up to 2 g daily may be needed; CHILD up to 6 years initially 250 mg daily, increased gradually to usual dose of 20 mg/kg daily

NOTE. Plasma concentration for optimum response 40–100 mg/litre (300–700 micromol/litre)

Emeside® (LAB) PoM

Capsules, orange, ethosuximide 250 mg. Net price 112-cap pack = £12.27. Label: 8, counselling, blood disorders (see above), driving (see notes above)

Syrup, blackcurrant, ethosuximide 250 mg/5 mL. Net price 200-mL pack = £6.60. Label: 8, counselling, blood disorders (see above), driving (see notes above)

Zarontin® (Parke-Davis) PoM

Capsules, yellow, ethosuximide 250 mg. Net price 56-cap pack = £5.41. Label: 8, counselling, blood disorders (see above), driving (see notes above)

Syrup, yellow, ethosuximide 250 mg/5 mL. Net price 200-mL pack = £4.48. Label: 8, counselling, blood disorders (see above), driving (see notes above)

Gabapentin and pregabalin

Gabapentin and **pregabalin** can be given as adjunctive therapy in partial epilepsy with or without secondary generalisation. They are also licensed for the treatment of neuropathic pain (section 4.7.3).

GABAPENTIN

Indications: adjunctive treatment of partial seizures with or without secondary generalisation not satisfactorily controlled with other antiepileptics; neuropathic pain (section 4.7.3)

Cautions: avoid sudden withdrawal (may cause anxiety, insomnia, nausea, pain and sweating—taper off over at least 1 week); history of psychotic illness, elderly (may need to reduce dose), renal impairment (Appendix 3), diabetes mellitus, false positive readings with some urinary protein tests; pregnancy (see p. 238 and Appendix 4) and breast-feeding (see p. 238 and Appendix 5); **interactions:** Appendix 1 (gabapentin)

Side-effects: diarrhoea, dry mouth, dyspepsia, nausea and vomiting; peripheral oedema; dizziness, drowsiness, anxiety, abnormal gait, amnesia, ataxia, fatigue, nystagmus, tremor, asthenia, paraesthesia, abnormal thinking, emotional lability, hyperkinesia; infections (including urinary tract and upper respiratory tract); weight gain; dysarthria, arthralgia; diplopia, amblyopia; rash; *less commonly* constipation, flatulence, dyspnoea, impotence, leucopenia; *rarely* depression, hallucinations and psychosis, headache, pancreatitis, urinary incontinence; alopecia, allergic reactions (including urticaria, angioedema, and Stevens-Johnson Syndrome); chest pain, palpitations, movement disorders, thrombocytopenia, tinnitus, and acute renal failure also reported

Dose: epilepsy, 300 mg on day 1, then 300 mg twice daily on day 2, then 300 mg 3 times daily (approx. every 8 hours) on day 3, then increased according to response in steps of 300 mg daily (in 3 divided doses) to max. 2.4 g daily, usual range 0.9–1.2 g daily; CHILD 6–12 years (specialist use only) 10 mg/kg on day 1, then 20 mg/kg on day 2, then 25–35 mg/kg daily (in 3 divided doses approx. every 8 hours), maintenance 900 mg daily (body-weight 26–36 kg) or 1.2 g daily (body-weight 37–50 kg)

Neuropathic pain, 300 mg on day 1, then 300 mg twice daily on day 2, then 300 mg 3 times daily on day 3, then increased according to response in steps of 300 mg daily (in 3 divided doses) to max. 1.8 g daily

Gabapentin (Non-proprietary) PoM

Capsules, gabapentin 100 mg, net price 100-cap pack = £25.61; 300 mg, 100-cap pack = £57.39; 400 mg, 100-cap pack = 64.36. Label: 3, 5, 8, counselling, driving (see notes above)

Tablets, gabapentin 600 mg, net price 100-tab pack = £106.00; 800 mg, 100-tab pack = £133.31. Label: 3, 5, 8, counselling, driving (see notes above)

Neurontin® (Parke-Davis) PoM

Capsules, gabapentin 100 mg (white), net price 100-cap pack = £22.86; 300 mg (yellow), 100-cap pack = £53.00; 400 mg (orange), 100-cap pack = £61.33; titration pack of 40 × 300-mg (yellow) capsules with 10 × 600-mg tablets = £31.80. Label: 3, 5, 8, counselling, driving (see notes above)

Tablets, gabapentin 600 mg, net price 100-tab pack = £106.00; 800 mg, 100-tab pack = £122.66. Label: 3, 5, 8, counselling, driving (see notes above)

PREGABALIN

Indications: peripheral neuropathic pain; adjunctive therapy for partial seizures with or without secondary generalisation

Cautions: avoid abrupt withdrawal (taper-off over at least 1 week); renal impairment (Appendix 3); pregnancy (Appendix 4)

Contra-indications: breast-feeding (Appendix 5)

Side-effects: dry mouth, constipation, vomiting, flatulence; oedema; dizziness, drowsiness, attention disturbance, disturbances in muscle control and movement, memory impairment, speech disorder, paraesthesia, euphoria, confusion, fatigue, appetite changes, weight gain; changes in sexual function; visual disturbances and ocular disorders (including blurred vision, diplopia, eye strain and eye irritation); less commonly abdominal distension, increased salivation, gastro-oesophageal reflux disease, taste disturbance, thirst, hot flushes, tachycardia, syncope, dyspnoea, chest tightness, nasal dryness, stupor, depersonalisation, depression, insomnia, hallucinations, agitation, mood swings, panic attacks, apathy, dysuria, urinary incontinence, thrombocytopenia, joint swelling, muscle cramp, myalgia, arthralgia, sweating, and rash; rarely ascites, dysphagia, pancreatitis, hypotension, hypertension, cold extremities, first-degree AV block, arrhythmia, bradycardia, nasopharyngitis, cough, epistaxis, rhinitis, parosmia, pyrexia, rigors, disinhibition, weight loss, hypoglycaemia or hyperglycaemia, renal failure, menstrual disturbances, breast pain, breast discharge, breast hypertrophy, neutropenia, rhabdomyolysis, hyperacusis, hypokalaemia, and leucocytosis

Dose: neuropathic pain, initially 150 mg daily in 2–3 divided doses, increased if necessary after 3–7 days to 300 mg daily in 2–3 divided doses, increased further if necessary after 7 days to max. 600 mg daily in 2–3 divided doses; CHILD and ADOLESCENT not recommended

Epilepsy, initially 150 mg daily in 2–3 divided doses, increased if necessary after 7 days to 300 mg daily in 2–3 divided doses, increased further if necessary after 7 days to max. 600 mg daily in 2–3 divided doses; CHILD and ADOLESCENT not recommended

Lyrica® (Pfizer) ▼ PoM

Capsules, pregabalin 25 mg (white), net price 56-cap pack = £64.40, 84-cap pack = £96.60; 50 mg (white), 84-cap pack = £96.60; 75 mg (white/orange), 56-cap pack = £64.40; 100 mg (orange), 84-cap pack = £96.60; 150 mg (white), 56-cap pack = £64.40; 200 mg (orange), 84-cap pack = £96.60; 300 mg (white/orange), 56-cap pack = £64.40. Label: 3, 8, counselling, driving (see notes above)

Lamotrigine

Lamotrigine is an antiepileptic for partial seizures and primary and secondarily generalised tonic-clonic seizures. It is also used for myoclonic seizures and may be tried for atypical absence, atonic, and tonic seizures in the Lennox-Gastaut syndrome. Lamotrigine may cause serious skin rash especially in children; dose recommendations should be adhered to closely.

Lamotrigine is used either as sole treatment or as an adjunct to treatment with other antiepileptic drugs. Valproate increases plasma-lamotrigine concentration whereas the enzyme inducing antiepileptics reduce it; care is therefore required in choosing the appropriate initial dose and subsequent titration. Where the potential for interaction is not known, treatment should be initiated with lower doses such as those used with valproate.

LAMOTRIGINE

Indications: monotherapy and adjunctive treatment of partial seizures and primary and secondarily generalised tonic-clonic seizures; seizures associated with Lennox-Gastaut syndrome

Cautions: closely monitor (including hepatic, renal and clotting parameters) and consider withdrawal if rash, fever, influenza-like symptoms, drowsiness, or worsening of seizure control develops (although causal relationship not established, lamotrigine given with other antiepileptics has been associated with rapidly progressive illness with status epilepticus, multi-organ dysfunction, disseminated intravascular coagulation and death); avoid abrupt withdrawal (taper off over 2 weeks or longer) unless serious skin reaction occurs; hepatic impairment (Appendix 2); renal impairment (Appendix 3); elderly; pregnancy (Appendix 4) and breast-feeding (Appendix 5); monitor bodyweight in children and review dose if necessary; **interactions:** see p. 237 and Appendix 1 (lamotrigine)

BLOOD DISORDERS. The CSM has advised prescribers to be alert for symptoms and signs suggestive of bone-marrow failure such as anaemia, bruising, or infection. Aplastic anaemia, bone-marrow depression and pancytopenia have been associated rarely with lamotrigine.

Side-effects: commonly rashes (see also below)—fever, malaise, influenza-like symptoms, drowsiness and rarely hepatic dysfunction, lymphadenopathy, leucopenia, and thrombocytopenia reported in conjunction with rash; angioedema, and photosensitivity also reported; diplopia, blurred vision, conjunctivitis, dizziness, drowsiness, insomnia, headache, ataxia, tiredness, gastro-intestinal disturbances (including vomiting), irritability, aggression, tremor, agitation, confusion; headache, nausea, dizziness, diplopia and ataxia in patients also taking carbamazepine usually resolve when dose of either drug reduced

SKIN REACTIONS. Serious skin reactions including Stevens-Johnson syndrome and toxic epidermal necrolysis (rarely with fatalities) have developed especially in children; most rashes occur in the first 8 weeks. The CSM has advised that factors associated with increased risk of serious skin reactions include concomitant use of valproate, initial lamotrigine dosing higher than recommended, and more rapid dose escalation than recommended.

COUNSELLING. Warn patients to see their doctor immediately if rash or influenza-like symptoms associated with hypersensitivity develop

Dose: IMPORTANT. Do not confuse the different combinations; see also notes above

Monotherapy, initially 25 mg daily for 14 days, increased to 50 mg daily for further 14 days, then increased by max. of 50–100 mg every 7–14 days; usual maintenance as monotherapy, 100–200 mg daily in 1–2 divided doses (up to 500 mg daily has been required)

Adjunctive therapy *with valproate*, initially 25 mg every other day for 14 days then 25 mg daily for further 14 days, thereafter increased by max. of 25–50 mg every 7–14 days; usual maintenance, 100–200 mg daily in 1–2 divided doses

Adjunctive therapy (with enzyme inducing drugs) *without valproate*, initially 50 mg daily for 14 days then 50 mg twice daily for further 14 days, thereafter increased by max. of 100 mg every 7–14 days; usual maintenance 200–400 mg daily in 2 divided doses (up to 700 mg daily has been required)

CHILD under 12 years, *monotherapy*, not recommended

CHILD 2–12 years, adjunctive therapy *with valproate*, initially 150 micrograms/kg daily for 14 days (those weighing 17–33 kg may receive 5 mg on alternate days for first 14 days) then 300 micrograms/kg daily for further 14 days, thereafter increased by 300 micrograms/kg every 7–14 days; usual maintenance 1–5 mg/kg daily in 1–2 divided doses

CHILD 2–12 years adjunctive therapy (with enzyme inducing drugs) *without valproate*, initially 600 micrograms/kg daily in 2 divided doses for 14 days then 1.2 mg/kg daily in 2 divided doses for further 14 days, thereafter increased by 1.2 mg/kg every 7–14 days; usual maintenance 5–15 mg/kg daily in 2 divided doses

Lamotrigine (Non-proprietary) PoM

Tablets, lamotrigine 25 mg, net price 56-tab pack = £17.35; 50 mg, 56-tab pack = £29.50; 100 mg, 56-tab pack = £50.88; 200 mg, 30-tab pack = £46.34, 56-tab pack = £86.50. Label: 8, counselling, driving (see notes above)

Dispersible tablets, lamotrigine 5 mg, net price 28-tab pack = £8.04; 25 mg, 56-tab pack = £20.31; 100 mg, 56-tab pack = £59.76. Label: 8, 13, counselling, driving (see notes above)

Lamictal® (GSK) PoM

Tablets, all yellow, lamotrigine 25 mg, net price 21-tab pack (*'Valproate Add-on therapy' Starter Pack*) = £7.65, 42-tab pack (*'Monotherapy' Starter Pack*) = £15.30, 56-tab pack = £20.41; 50 mg, 42-tab pack (*'Non-valproate Add-on therapy' Starter Pack*) = £26.02, 56-tab pack = £34.70; 100 mg, 56-tab pack = £59.86; 200 mg, 56-tab pack = £101.76. Label: 8, counselling, driving (see notes above)

Dispersible tablets, chewable, lamotrigine 2 mg, net price 30-tab pack = £ 8.71; 5 mg, 28-tab pack = £8.14; 25 mg, 56-tab pack = £20.41; 100 mg, 56-tab pack = £59.86. Label: 8, 13, counselling, driving (see notes above)

Levetiracetam

Levetiracetam is licensed for the adjunctive treatment of partial seizures.

LEVETIRACETAM

Indications: adjunctive treatment of partial seizures with or without secondary generalisation

Cautions: hepatic impairment (Appendix 2); renal impairment (Appendix 3); pregnancy (see p. 238 and Appendix 4); breast-feeding (Appendix 5); avoid sudden withdrawal

Side-effects: drowsiness, asthenia, dizziness; less commonly, anorexia, diarrhoea, dyspepsia, nausea, amnesia, ataxia, depression, emotional lability, aggression, insomnia, nervousness, tremor, vertigo, headache, diplopia, rash; also

reported anxiety, psychosis, leucopenia, pancytopenia, thrombocytopenia
Dose: initially 1 g daily in 2 divided doses, adjusted in increments of 1 g every 2 to 4 weeks; max. 3 g daily in 2 divided doses; CHILD under 16 years not recommended

Keppra® (UCB Pharma) ▼ PoM
Tablets, f/c, levetiracetam 250 mg (blue), net price 60-tab pack = £29.70; 500 mg (yellow), 60-tab pack = £52.30; 750 mg (orange) 60-tab pack = £89.10; 1 g (white), 60-tab pack = £101.10. Label: 8
Oral solution, sugar-free, levetiracetam 100 mg/mL, net price 300 mL = £71.00. Label: 8

Phenobarbital and other barbiturates

Phenobarbital (phenobarbitone) is effective for tonic-clonic and partial seizures but may be sedative in adults and cause behavioural disturbances and hyperkinesia in children. It may be tried for atypical absence, atonic, and tonic seizures. Rebound seizures may be a problem on withdrawal. Monitoring plasma concentrations is less useful than with other drugs because tolerance occurs.

Primidone is largely converted to phenobarbital and this is probably responsible for its antiepileptic action. A small starting dose of primidone (125 mg) is essential, and the drug should be introduced over several weeks.

PHENOBARBITAL

(Phenobarbitone)
Indications: all forms of epilepsy except absence seizures; status epilepticus (section 4.8.2)
Cautions: elderly, debilitated, children, hepatic impairment (Appendix 2), renal impairment (Appendix 3), respiratory depression (avoid if severe), pregnancy (Appendix 4) and breast-feeding (Appendix 5) (see notes above); avoid sudden withdrawal; see also notes above; avoid in porphyria (see section 9.8.2); **interactions:** see p. 237 and Appendix 1 (barbiturates)
Side-effects: drowsiness, lethargy, mental depression, ataxia and allergic skin reactions; paradoxical excitement, restlessness and confusion in the elderly and hyperkinesia in children; megaloblastic anaemia (may be treated with folic acid)
Dose: *by mouth*, 60–180 mg at night; CHILD 5–8 mg/kg daily
Control of acute seizures, *by intramuscular injection*, 200 mg, repeated after 6 hours if necessary; CHILD 15 mg/kg as a single dose
Status epilepticus, *by intravenous injection* (dilute injection 1 in 10 with water for injections), 10 mg/kg at a rate of not more than 100 mg/minute; max. 1 g
NOTE. For therapeutic purposes phenobarbital and phenobarbital sodium may be considered equivalent in effect. Plasma concentration for optimum response 15–40 mg/litre (60–180 micromol/litre)

[1]**Phenobarbital** (Non-proprietary) CD
Tablets, phenobarbital 15 mg, net price 28-tab pack = 63p; 30 mg, 28-tab pack = 66p; 60 mg, 28-tab pack = 72p. Label: 2, 8, counselling, driving (see notes above)
Elixir, phenobarbital 15 mg/5 mL in a suitable flavoured vehicle, containing alcohol 38%, net price 100 mL = 77p. Label: 2, 8, counselling, driving (see notes above)
NOTE. Some hospitals supply **alcohol-free** formulations of varying phenobarbital strengths
Injection, phenobarbital sodium 200 mg/mL in propylene glycol 90% and water for injections 10%, net price 1-mL amp = £1.82
NOTE. Must be diluted before intravenous administration (see under Dose)

1. See p. 7 for prescribing requirements for phenobarbital

PRIMIDONE

Indications: all forms of epilepsy except absence seizures; essential tremor (also section 4.9.3)
Cautions: see under Phenobarbital; **interactions:** see p. 237 and Appendix 1 (primidone)
Side-effects: see under Phenobarbital; drowsiness, ataxia, nausea, visual disturbances, and rashes, particularly at first, usually reversible on continued administration
Dose: epilepsy, ADULT and CHILD over 9 years, initially, 125 mg daily at bedtime, increased by 125 mg every 3 days to 500 mg daily in 2 divided doses then increased by 250 mg every 3 days to max. 1.5 g daily in divided doses; CHILD under 2 years, 250–500 mg daily in 2 divided doses; 2–5 years, 500–750 mg daily in 2 divided doses; 6–9 years 0.75–1 g daily in 2 divided doses
Essential tremor, initially 50 mg daily increased gradually over 2–3 weeks according to response; max. 750 mg daily
NOTE. Monitor plasma concentrations of derived phenobarbital. Optimum range as for phenobarbital

Mysoline® (Acorus) PoM
Tablets, scored, primidone 250 mg. Net price 100-tab pack = £12.60. Label: 2, 8, counselling, driving (see notes above)

Phenytoin

Phenytoin is effective in tonic-clonic and partial seizures. It has a narrow therapeutic index and the relationship between dose and plasma concentration is non-linear; small dosage increases in some patients may produce large rises in plasma concentrations with acute toxic side-effects. Monitoring of plasma concentration greatly assists dosage adjustment. A few missed doses or a small change in drug absorption may result in a marked change in plasma concentration.

Phenytoin may cause coarse facies, acne, hirsutism, and gingival hyperplasia and so may be particularly undesirable in adolescent patients.

When only parenteral administration is possible, **fosphenytoin** (section 4.8.2), a pro-drug of phenytoin, may be convenient to give. Whereas phenytoin can be given intravenously only, fosphenytoin may also be given by intramuscular injection.

PHENYTOIN

Indications: all forms of epilepsy except absence seizures; trigeminal neuralgia if carbamazepine inappropriate (see also section 4.7.3)
Cautions: hepatic impairment (reduce dose), pregnancy (**important:** see notes above and Appendix 4), breast-feeding (see notes above and Appendix 5); avoid sudden withdrawal; manufacturer recommends blood counts (but evidence of

practical value unsatisfactory); avoid in porphyria (section 9.8.2); see also notes above; **interactions:** see p. 237 and Appendix 1 (phenytoin)

BLOOD OR SKIN DISORDERS. Patients or their carers should be told how to recognise signs of blood or skin disorders, and advised to seek immediate medical attention if symptoms such as fever, sore throat, rash, mouth ulcers, bruising, or bleeding develop. Leucopenia which is severe, progressive or associated with clinical symptoms requires withdrawal (if necessary under cover of suitable alternative)

Side-effects: nausea, vomiting, mental confusion, dizziness, headache, tremor, transient nervousness, insomnia occur commonly; rarely dyskinesias, peripheral neuropathy; ataxia, slurred speech, nystagmus and blurred vision are signs of overdosage; rashes (discontinue; if mild re-introduce cautiously but discontinue immediately if recurrence), gingival hypertrophy and tenderness, coarse facies, acne and hirsutism, fever and hepatitis; lupus erythematosus, Stevens-Johnson syndrome, toxic epidermal necrolysis, polyarteritis nodosa; lymphadenopathy; rarely haematological effects, including megaloblastic anaemia (may be treated with folic acid), leucopenia, thrombocytopenia, agranulocytosis, and aplastic anaemia; plasma-calcium concentration may be lowered (rickets and osteomalacia)

Dose: *by mouth*, initially 3–4 mg/kg daily *or* 150–300 mg daily (as a single dose *or* in 2 divided doses) increased gradually as necessary (with plasma-phenytoin concentration monitoring); usual dose 200–500 mg daily (exceptionally, higher doses may be used); CHILD initially 5 mg/kg daily in 2 divided doses, usual dose range 4–8 mg/kg daily (max. 300 mg)

By intravenous injection—section 4.8.2

NOTE. Plasma concentration for optimum response 10–20 mg/litre (40–80 micromol/litre)

COUNSELLING. Take preferably with or after food

Phenytoin (Non-proprietary) PoM

Tablets, coated, phenytoin sodium 100 mg, net price 28-tab pack = £3.87. Label: 8, counselling, administration, blood or skin disorder symptoms (see above), driving (see notes above)

NOTE. On the basis of single dose tests there are no clinically relevant differences in bioavailability between available phenytoin sodium tablets and capsules but there may be a pharmacokinetic basis for maintaining the same brand of phenytoin in some patients

Epanutin® (Pfizer) PoM

Capsules, phenytoin sodium 25 mg (white/purple), net price 28-cap pack = 66p; 50 mg (white/pink), 28-cap pack = 67p; 100 mg (white/orange), 20-cap pack = 67p; 300 mg (white/green), 20-cap pack = £2.02. Label: 8, counselling, administration, blood or skin disorder symptoms (see above), driving (see notes above)

Infatabs® (= chewable tablets), yellow, scored, phenytoin 50 mg. Net price 20 = £1.32. Label: 8, 24, counselling, blood or skin disorder symptoms (see above), driving (see notes above)

NOTE. Contain phenytoin 50 mg (as against phenytoin sodium) therefore care is needed on changing to capsules or tablets containing phenytoin sodium

Suspension, red, phenytoin 30 mg/5 mL. Net price 100 mL = 85p. Label: 8, counselling, administration, blood or skin disorder symptoms (see above), driving (see notes above)

NOTE. Suspension of phenytoin 90 mg in 15 mL may be considered to be approximately equivalent in therapeutic effect to capsules or tablets containing phenytoin sodium 100 mg, but nevertheless care is needed in making changes

Tiagabine

Tiagabine is used as adjunctive treatment for partial seizures, with or without secondary generalisation.

TIAGABINE

Indications: adjunctive treatment for partial seizures with or without secondary generalisation not satisfactorily controlled with other antiepileptics

Cautions: avoid in porphyria (section 9.8.2); hepatic impairment (Appendix 2); avoid abrupt withdrawal; **interactions:** Appendix 1 (tiagabine)

DRIVING. May impair performance of skilled tasks (e.g. driving)

Side-effects: diarrhoea, dizziness, tiredness, nervousness, tremor, concentration difficulties, emotional lability, speech impairment; rarely, confusion, depression, drowsiness, psychosis; leucopenia reported

Dose: adjunctive therapy, with *enzyme-inducing* drugs, 5 mg twice daily for 1 week, then increased at weekly intervals in steps of 5–10 mg daily; usual maintenance dose 30–45 mg daily (doses above 30 mg given in 3 divided doses); in patients receiving *non-enzyme-inducing* drugs, initial maintenance dose should be 15–30 mg daily; CHILD under 12 years not recommended

Gabitril® (Cephalon) PoM

Tablets, f/c, scored, tiagabine (as hydrochloride) 5 mg, net price 100-tab pack = £43.37; 10 mg, 100-tab pack = £86.74; 15 mg, 100-tab pack = £130.11. Label: 21

Topiramate

Topiramate can be given alone or as adjunctive treatment in generalised tonic-clonic seizures or partial seizures with or without secondary generalisation. It can also be used as adjunctive treatment for seizures associated with Lennox-Gastaut syndrome.

TOPIRAMATE

Indications: monotherapy and adjunctive treatment of generalised tonic-clonic seizures or partial seizures with or without secondary generalisation; adjunctive treatment of seizures in Lennox-Gastaut syndrome

Cautions: avoid abrupt withdrawal; ensure adequate hydration (especially if predisposition to nephrolithiasis or in strenuous activity or warm environment); avoid in porphyria (section 9.8.2); pregnancy (see notes above and Appendix 4); hepatic impairment (Appendix 2); renal impairment (Appendix 3); **interactions:** see p. 237 and Appendix 1 (topiramate)

CSM ADVICE. Topiramate has been associated with acute myopia with secondary angle-closure glaucoma, typically occurring within 1 month of starting treatment. Choroidal effusions resulting in anterior displacement of the lens and iris have also been reported. The CSM advises that if raised intra-ocular pressure occurs:

- seek specialist ophthalmological advice;
- use appropriate measures to reduce intra-ocular pressure;
- stop topiramate as rapidly as feasible

Contra-indications: breast-feeding

Side-effects: nausea, abdominal pain, weight loss, anorexia; paraesthesia; hypoaesthesia, headache, fatigue, dizziness, somnolence, insomnia, impaired memory and concentration, anxiety, depression, nervousness, mood instability; rarely reduced sweating mainly in children, metabolic acidosis

ADJUNCTIVE THERAPY. Commonly agitation, ataxia, asthenia, confusion, cognitive impairment, speech disorders, visual disturbances; also increased salivation, hyperkinesia and personality disorder in children; less commonly taste disturbances; abnormal gait, incoordination, psychotic reactions including hallucinations; leucopenia

Dose: monotherapy, initially 25 mg daily at night for 1 week *then* increased in steps of 25–50 mg daily at intervals of 1–2 weeks taken in 2 divided doses; usual dose 100 mg daily in 2 divided doses; max. 400 mg daily; CHILD 6–16 years, initially 0.5–1 mg/kg daily at night for 1 week *then* increased in steps of 0.5–1 mg/kg daily at intervals of 1–2 weeks taken in 2 divided doses; usual dose 3–6 mg/kg daily in 2 divided doses; max. 16 mg/kg daily

Adjunctive therapy, initially 25 mg daily for 1 week *then* increased in steps of 25–50 mg daily at intervals of 1–2 weeks; usual dose 200–400 mg daily in 2 divided doses; max. 800 mg daily; CHILD 2–16 years, initially 25 mg daily at night for one week *then* increased in steps of 1–3 mg/kg daily at intervals of 1–2 weeks taken in 2 divided doses; recommended dose range 5–9 mg/kg daily in 2 divided doses; max. 30 mg/kg daily

NOTE. If patient cannot tolerate titration regimen recommended above then smaller steps or longer interval between steps may be used

Topamax® (Janssen-Cilag) PoM

Tablets, f/c, topiramate 25 mg, net price 60-tab pack = £20.92; 50 mg (light yellow), 60-tab pack = £34.36; 100 mg (yellow), 60-tab pack = £61.56; 200 mg (salmon), 60-tab pack = £119.54. Label: 3, 8, counselling, driving (see notes above)

Sprinkle capsules, topiramate 15 mg, net price 60-cap pack = £16.04; 25 mg, 60-cap pack = £24.05; 50 mg, 60-cap pack = £39.52. Label: 3, 8, counselling, administration, driving (see notes above)

COUNSELLING. Swallow whole or open capsule and sprinkle contents on soft food

Valproate

Sodium valproate is effective in controlling tonic-clonic seizures, particularly in primary generalised epilepsy. It is a drug of choice in primary generalised epilepsy, generalised absences and myoclonic seizures, and may be tried in atypical absence, atonic, and tonic seizures. Controlled trials in partial epilepsy suggest that it has similar efficacy to that of carbamazepine and phenytoin. Plasma-valproate concentrations are not a useful index of efficacy, therefore routine monitoring is unhelpful. The drug has widespread metabolic effects, and may have dose-related side-effects.

Valproic acid (as semisodium valproate) (section 4.2.3) is licensed for acute mania associated with bipolar disorder.

SODIUM VALPROATE

Indications: all forms of epilepsy

Cautions: monitor liver function before therapy and during first 6 months especially in patients most at risk (see also below), ensure no undue potential for bleeding before starting and before surgery; renal impairment (Appendix 3); pregnancy (**important** see notes above and Appendix 4 (neural tube screening)); breast-feeding (Appendix 5); systemic lupus erythematosus; false-positive urine tests for ketones; avoid sudden withdrawal; see also notes above; **interactions:** see p. 237 and Appendix 1 (valproate)

LIVER TOXICITY. Liver dysfunction (including fatal hepatic failure) has occurred in association with valproate (especially in children under 3 years of age and those with metabolic or degenerative disorders, organic brain disease or severe seizure disorders associated with mental retardation) usually in the first 6 months of therapy and usually involving multiple antiepileptic therapy (monotherapy preferred). Raised liver enzymes are not uncommon during valproate treatment and are usually transient but patients should be reassessed clinically and liver function (including prothrombin time) monitored until return to normal—an abnormally prolonged prothrombin time (particularly in association with other relevant abnormalities) requires discontinuation of treatment. Any concomitant use of salicylates should be stopped.

BLOOD OR HEPATIC DISORDERS. Patients or their carers should be told how to recognise signs of blood or liver disorders, and advised to seek immediate medical attention if symptoms develop (advice is given on patient information leaflet).

PANCREATITIS. Patients or their carers should be told how to recognise signs of pancreatitis, and advised to seek immediate medical attention if symptoms such as abdominal pain, nausea and vomiting develop; discontinue sodium valproate if pancreatitis is diagnosed

Contra-indications: active liver disease, family history of severe hepatic dysfunction, porphyria (section 9.8.2)

Side-effects: gastric irritation, nausea, ataxia and tremor; hyperammonaemia, increased appetite and weight gain; transient hair loss (regrowth may be curly), oedema, thrombocytopenia, and inhibition of platelet aggregation; impaired hepatic function leading rarely to fatal hepatic failure (see also under Cautions—withdraw treatment immediately if vomiting, anorexia, jaundice, drowsiness, or loss of seizure control occurs); rashes; sedation reported (rarely lethargy and confusion associated with too high an initial dose) and also increased alertness (occasionally aggression, hyperactivity and behavioural disturbances); rarely pancreatitis (measure plasma amylase in acute abdominal pain; see also Pancreatitis under Cautions above), extrapyramidal symptoms, dementia, leucopenia, pancytopenia, red cell hypoplasia, fibrinogen reduction; irregular periods, amenorrhoea, gynaecomastia, hearing loss, Fanconi's syndrome, toxic epidermal necrolysis, Stevens-Johnson syndrome, vasculitis, hirsutism and acne also reported

Dose: *by mouth*, initially, 600 mg daily given in 2 divided doses, preferably after food, increasing by 200 mg/day at 3-day intervals to a max. of 2.5 g daily in divided doses, usual maintenance 1–2 g daily (20–30 mg/kg daily); CHILD up to 20 kg, initially 20 mg/kg daily in divided doses, may be increased provided plasma concentrations monitored (above 40 mg/kg daily also monitor clinical chemistry and haematological parameters); over 20 kg, initially 400 mg daily in divided doses increased until control (usually in range of 20–30 mg/kg daily); max. 35 mg/kg daily

By intravenous injection (over 3–5 minutes) or *by intravenous infusion*, continuation of valproate treatment when oral therapy not possible, same as current dose by oral route

Initiation of valproate therapy (when oral valproate not possible), *by intravenous injection* (over 3–5 minutes), 400–800 mg (up to 10 mg/kg) followed by *intravenous infusion* up to max. 2.5 g daily; CHILD, usually 20–30 mg/kg daily, may be increased provided plasma concentrations monitored (above 40 mg/kg daily also monitor clinical chemistry and haematological parameters)

Sodium Valproate (Non-proprietary) PoM

Tablets (crushable), scored, sodium valproate 100 mg. Net price 20 = 78p. Label: 8, counselling, blood or hepatic disorder symptoms (see above), driving (see notes above)

Tablets, e/c, sodium valproate 200 mg, net price 20 = £1.44; 500 mg, 20 = £3.58. Label: 5, 8, 25, counselling, blood or hepatic disorder symptoms (see above), driving (see notes above)

Brands include *Orlept*®

Oral solution, sodium valproate 200 mg/5 mL. Net price 100 mL = £2.25. Label: 8, counselling, blood or hepatic disorder symptoms (see above), driving (see notes above)

Brands include *Orlept*® sugar-free

Epilim® (Sanofi-Synthelabo) PoM

Tablets (crushable), scored, sodium valproate 100 mg. Net price 20 = 78p. Label: 8, counselling, blood or hepatic disorder symptoms (see above), driving (see notes above)

Tablets, both e/c, lilac, sodium valproate 200 mg, net price 20 = £1.28; 500 mg, 20 = £3.21. Label: 5, 8, 25, counselling, blood or hepatic disorder symptoms (see above), driving (see notes above)

Liquid, red, sugar-free, sodium valproate 200 mg/5 mL. Net price 300-mL pack = £6.48. Label: 8, counselling, blood or hepatic disorder symptoms (see above), driving (see notes above)

Syrup, red, sodium valproate 200 mg/5 mL. Net price 300-mL pack = £6.48. Label: 8, counselling, blood or hepatic disorder symptoms (see above), driving (see notes above)

Epilim Chrono® (Sanofi-Synthelabo) PoM

Tablets, m/r, all lilac, sodium valproate 200 mg (as sodium valproate and valproic acid), net price 100-tab pack = £8.09; 300 mg, 100-tab pack = £12.13; 500 mg, 100-tab pack = £20.21. Label: 8, 25, counselling, blood or hepatic disorder symptoms (see above), driving (see notes above)

Dose: ADULT and CHILD over 20 kg, as above, total daily dose given in 1–2 divided doses

Epilim® **Intravenous** (Sanofi-Synthelabo) PoM

Injection, powder for reconstitution, sodium valproate. Net price 400-mg vial (with 4-mL amp water for injections) = £9.65

■ Valproic acid

Convulex® (Pharmacia) PoM

Capsules, e/c, valproic acid 150 mg, net price 100-cap pack = £3.68; 300 mg, 100-cap pack = £7.35; 500 mg, 100-cap pack = £12.25. Label: 8, 25, counselling, blood or hepatic disorder symptoms (see above), driving (see notes above)

Dose: ADULT and CHILD as for sodium valproate, in 2–4 divided doses

EQUIVALENCE TO SODIUM VALPROATE. Manufacturer advises that *Convulex*® has a 1:1 dose relationship with products containing sodium valproate, but nevertheless care is needed in making changes.

Vigabatrin

For partial epilepsy with or without secondary generalisation, **vigabatrin** is given in combination with other antiepileptic treatment; its use is restricted to patients in whom all other combinations are inadequate or are not tolerated. It can be used as sole therapy in the management of infantile spasms in West's syndrome.

About one-third of patients treated with vigabatrin have suffered visual field defects; counselling and **careful monitoring** for this side-effect are required (see also Visual Field Defects under Cautions below). Vigabatrin has prominent behavioural side-effects in some patients.

VIGABATRIN

Indications: initiated and supervised by appropriate specialist, adjunctive treatment of partial seizures with or without secondary generalisation not satisfactorily controlled with other antiepileptics; monotherapy for management of infantile spasms (West's syndrome)

Cautions: renal impairment (Appendix 3); elderly; closely monitor neurological function; avoid sudden withdrawal (taper off over 2–4 weeks); history of psychosis, depression or behavioural problems; pregnancy (see p. 238 and Appendix 4) and breast-feeding (Appendix 5); absence seizures (may be exacerbated); **interactions:** see p. 237 and Appendix 1 (vigabatrin)

VISUAL FIELD DEFECTS. Vigabatrin is associated with visual field defects. The CSM has advised that onset of symptoms varies from 1 month to several years after starting. In most cases, visual field defects have persisted despite discontinuation. Product literature advises visual field testing before treatment and at 6-month intervals; a procedure for testing visual fields in those with a developmental age of less than 9 years is available from the manufacturers. Patients should be warned to report any new visual symptoms that develop and those with symptoms should be referred for an urgent ophthalmological opinion. Gradual withdrawal of vigabatrin should be considered.

Contra-indications: visual field defects

Side-effects: drowsiness (rarely, encephalopathic symptoms consisting of marked sedation, stupor, and confusion with non-specific slow wave EEG—reduce dose or withdraw), fatigue, visual field defects (see also under Cautions), dizziness, nervousness, irritability, behavioural effects such as excitation and agitation especially in children; depression, abnormal thinking, headache, nystagmus, ataxia, tremor, paraesthesia, impaired concentration; less commonly confusion, aggression, psychosis, mania, memory disturbance, visual disturbance (e.g. diplopia); also weight gain, oedema, gastro-intestinal disturbances, alopecia, rash; less commonly, urticaria, occasional increase in seizure frequency (especially if myoclonic), decrease in liver enzymes, slight decrease in haemoglobin; photophobia and retinal disorders (e.g. peripheral retinal atrophy); optic neuritis, optic atrophy, hallucinations also reported

Dose: with current antiepileptic therapy, initially 1 g daily in single or 2 divided doses then increased according to response in steps of 500 mg at weekly intervals; usual range 2–3 g daily (max. 3 g daily); CHILD initially 40 mg/kg daily in single or 2 divided doses then adjusted according to body-weight 10–15 kg, 0.5–1 g daily; body-weight 15–30 kg, 1–1.5 g daily; body-weight 30–50 kg, 1.5–3 g daily; body-weight over 50 kg, 2–3 g daily

Infantile spasms (West's syndrome), *monotherapy*, 50 mg/kg daily, adjusted according to response over 7 days; up to 150 mg/kg daily used with good tolerability

Sabril® (Aventis Pharma) PoM

Tablets, f/c, scored, vigabatrin 500 mg, net price 100-tab pack = £30.84. Label: 3, 8, counselling, driving (see notes above)

Powder, sugar-free, vigabatrin 500 mg/sachet. Net price 50-sachet pack = £17.08. Label: 3, 8, 13, counselling, driving (see notes above)

NOTE. The contents of a sachet should be dissolved in water or a soft drink immediately before taking

Zonisamide

Zonisamide is used as adjunctive treatment for partial seizures with or without secondary generalisation.

ZONISAMIDE

Indications: adjunctive therapy for partial seizures with or without secondary generalisation

Cautions: elderly; ensure adequate hydration (especially if predisposition to nephrolithiasis or in strenuous activity or warm environment); concomitant use of drugs that increase risk of hyperthermia or nephrolithiasis; avoid abrupt withdrawal; hepatic impairment (avoid if severe—Appendix 2); renal impairment (Appendix 3); pregnancy (Appendix 4); **interactions:** see p. 237 and Appendix 1 (zonisamide)

Contra-indications: hypersensitivity to sulphonamides; breast-feeding (Appendix 5)

Side-effects: nausea, diarrhoea, gastro-intestinal pain; drowsiness, dizziness, confusion, agitation, irritability, depression, ataxia, speech disorder, impaired memory and attention, anorexia and weight loss, pyrexia; diplopia; rash (consider withdrawal); *less commonly* vomiting, cholelithiasis, cholecystitis, convulsions, psychosis, urinary calculus, hypokalaemia; *very rarely* dyspnoea, hallucinations, insomnia, suicidal ideation, amnesia, coma, myasthenic syndrome, neuroleptic malignant syndrome, heat stroke, hydronephrosis, renal impairment, metabolic acidosis, blood disorders, rhabdomyolysis, impaired sweating, pruritus, Stevens-Johnson syndrome, hepatitis, pancreatitis

Dose: initially 50 mg daily in 2 divided doses, increased after 7 days to 100 mg daily in 2 divided doses; then increase if necessary by 100 mg every 7 days; usual maintenance 300–500 mg daily in 1–2 divided doses; CHILD and ADOLESCENT under 18 years not recommended

Zonegran® (Eisai) ▼ PoM

Capsules, zonisamide 25 mg (white), net price 14-cap pack = £8.82; 50 mg (white/grey), 56-cap pack = £47.04; 100 mg (white/red), 56-cap pack = £62.72. Label: 3

Benzodiazepines

Clonazepam is occasionally used in tonic-clonic or partial seizures, but its sedative side-effects may be prominent. **Clobazam** may be used as adjunctive therapy in the treatment of epilepsy (section 4.1.2), but the effectiveness of these and other **benzodiazepines** may wane considerably after weeks or months of continuous therapy.

CLOBAZAM

Indications: adjunct in epilepsy; anxiety (short-term use)

Cautions: see under Diazepam (section 4.1.2)

Contra-indications: see under Diazepam (section 4.1.2)

Side-effects: see under Diazepam (section 4.1.2)

Dose: epilepsy, 20–30 mg daily; max. 60 mg daily; CHILD over 3 years, not more than half adult dose

Anxiety, 20–30 mg daily in divided doses or as a single dose at bedtime, increased in severe anxiety (in hospital patients) to a max. of 60 mg daily in divided doses; ELDERLY (or debilitated) 10–20 mg daily

[1]**Clobazam** (Non-proprietary) PoM NHS

Tablets, clobazam 10 mg. Net price 30-tab pack = £9.74. Label: 2 or 19, 8, counselling, driving (see notes above)

Brands include *Frisium*® NHS

1. NHS except for epilepsy and endorsed 'SLS'

CLONAZEPAM

Indications: all forms of epilepsy; myoclonus; status epilepticus (section 4.8.2)

Cautions: see notes above; elderly and debilitated, respiratory disease, spinal or cerebellar ataxia; history of alcohol or drug abuse, depression or suicidal ideation; avoid sudden withdrawal; porphyria (section 9.8.2); hepatic impairment (avoid if severe; Appendix 2); renal impairment; pregnancy (see notes above and Appendix 4); breast-feeding (see notes above and Appendix 5); **interactions:** Appendix 1 (anxiolytics and hypnotics)

DRIVING. Drowsiness may affect performance of skilled tasks (e.g. driving); effects of alcohol enhanced

Contra-indications: respiratory depression; acute pulmonary insufficiency; sleep apnoea syndrome

Side-effects: drowsiness, fatigue, dizziness; muscle hypotonia, co-ordination disturbances; also poor concentration, restlessness, confusion, amnesia, dependence and withdrawal; salivary or bronchial hypersecretion in infants and small children; *rarely* gastro-intestinal symptoms, respiratory depression, headache, paradoxical effects including aggression and anxiety, sexual dysfunction, urinary incontinence, urticaria, pruritus, reversible hair loss, skin pigmentation changes; dysarthria, ataxia, and visual disturbances on long-term treatment; blood disorders reported; **overdosage:** see Emergency Treatment of Poisoning, p. 32

Dose: 1 mg (elderly, 500 micrograms), initially at night for 4 nights, increased over 2–4 weeks to a usual maintenance dose of 4–8 mg daily in divided doses; CHILD up to 1 year 250 micrograms increased as above to 0.5–1 mg, 1–5 years 250 micrograms increased to 1–3 mg, 5–12 years 500 micrograms increased to 3–6 mg

Rivotril® (Roche) PoM
Tablets, both scored, clonazepam 500 micrograms (beige), net price 100 = £3.92; 2 mg (white), 100 = £5.23. Label: 2, 8, counselling, driving (see notes above)
Injection, section 4.8.2

Other drugs

Acetazolamide (section 11.6), a carbonic anhydrase inhibitor, is a second-line drug for both tonic-clonic and partial seizures. It is occasionally helpful in atypical absence, atonic, and tonic seizures.

Piracetam (section 4.9.3) is used as adjunctive treatment for cortical myoclonus.

4.8.2 Drugs used in status epilepticus

Initial management of status epilepticus includes positioning the patient to avoid injury, supporting respiration including the provision of oxygen, maintaining blood pressure, and the correction of any hypoglycaemia. The use of parenteral **thiamine** should be considered if alcohol abuse is suspected; **pyridoxine** should be administered if the status epilepticus is caused by pyridoxine deficiency.

Major status epilepticus should be treated initially with intravenous **lorazepam**. Intravenous **diazepam** may also be used, but lorazepam has a longer duration of antiepileptic action. Diazepam is associated with a high risk of venous thrombophlebitis which is reduced by using an emulsion (*Diazemuls*®). Alternatively, in prolonged or recurrent seizures, a single dose of **midazolam** (section 15.1.4.1) can be given [unlicensed use] by the buccal route (in a dose of 10 mg) or intranasally (200 micrograms/kg).

Where facilities for resuscitation are not immediately available, small doses of lorazepam or diazepam can be given intravenously, or diazepam can be administered as a rectal solution. Absorption from intramuscular injection or from suppositories is too slow for treatment of status epilepticus.

Clonazepam can also be used as an alternative.

If seizures recur or fail to respond after 30 minutes, phenytoin sodium, fosphenytoin, or phenobarbital sodium should be used.

Phenytoin sodium may be given by slow intravenous injection, with ECG monitoring, followed by the maintenance dosage. Intramuscular use of phenytoin is not recommended (absorption is slow and erratic).

Alternatively, **fosphenytoin**, a pro-drug of phenytoin, can be given more rapidly and when given intravenously causes fewer injection site reactions compared to phenytoin. Intravenous administration requires ECG monitoring. Although it can also be given intramuscularly, absorption is too slow by this route for treatment of status epilepticus. Doses of fosphenytoin should be expressed in terms of phenytoin sodium.

Alternatively, **phenobarbital sodium** can be given by intravenous injection (section 4.8.1).

Paraldehyde also remains a valuable drug. Given rectally it causes little respiratory depression and is therefore useful where facilities for resuscitation are poor.

If the above measures fail to control seizures, anaesthesia with thiopental (section 15.1.1) or in adults, a non-barbiturate anaesthetic such as propofol [unlicensed indication] (section 15.1.1), should be instituted with full intensive care support.

For advice on the management of medical emergencies in dental practice, see p. 20

DIAZEPAM

Indications: status epilepticus; convulsions due to poisoning (see Emergency Treatment of Poisoning); other indications (section 4.1.2, section 10.2.2, and section 15.1.4.1)

Cautions: see section 4.1.2; when given intravenously facilities for reversing respiratory depression with mechanical ventilation must be at hand (but see also notes above)

SPECIAL CAUTIONS FOR INTRAVENOUS INFUSION. Intravenous infusion of diazepam is potentially hazardous (especially if prolonged), calling for close and constant observation and best carried out in specialist centres with intensive care facilities. Prolonged infusion may lead to accumulation and delay recovery

Contra-indications: see section 4.1.2

Side-effects: see section 4.1.2; hypotension and apnoea

Dose: *by intravenous injection*, 10–20 mg at a rate of 0.5 mL (2.5 mg) per 30 seconds, repeated if necessary after 30–60 minutes; may be followed by *intravenous infusion* to max. 3 mg/kg over 24 hours; CHILD 200–300 micrograms/kg *or* 1 mg per year of age

By rectum as rectal solution, ADULT and CHILD over 10 kg 500 micrograms/kg, up to max. 30 mg (ELDERLY 250 micrograms/kg, up to max. 15 mg); repeated after 12 hours if necessary

Diazepam (Non-proprietary) PoM
Injection (solution), diazepam 5 mg/mL. See Appendix 6. Net price 2-mL amp = 32p
Excipients: may include benzyl alcohol (avoid in neonates, see Excipients, p. 2), ethanol, propylene glycol
Injection (emulsion), diazepam 5 mg/mL (0.5%). See Appendix 6. Net price 2-mL amp = 84p
Brands include *Diazemuls*®
Rectal tubes (= rectal solution), diazepam 2 mg/mL, net price 1.25-mL (2.5-mg) tube = 90p, 2.5-mL (5-mg) tube = £1.27; 4 mg/mL, 2.5-mL (10-mg) tube = £1.49
Brands include *Diazepam Rectubes*®, *Stesolid*®

■ Oral preparations
Section 4.1.2

CLONAZEPAM

Indications: status epilepticus; other forms of epilepsy, and myoclonus (section 4.8.1)

Cautions: see section 4.8.1; facilities for reversing respiratory depression with mechanical ventilation must be at hand (but see also notes above)

INTRAVENOUS INFUSION. Intravenous infusion of clonazepam is potentially hazardous (especially if prolonged), calling for close and constant observation and best carried out in specialist centres with intensive care facilities. Prolonged infusion may lead to accumulation and delay recovery

Contra-indications: see section 4.8.1; avoid injections containing benzyl alcohol in neonates (see under preparations below)
Side-effects: see section 4.8.1; hypotension and apnoea
Dose: *by intravenous injection* into a large vein (over at least 2 minutes) *or by intravenous infusion*, 1 mg, repeated if necessary; CHILD all ages, 500 micrograms

Rivotril® (Roche) PoM
Injection, clonazepam 1 mg/mL in solvent, for dilution with 1 mL water for injections immediately before injection or as described in Appendix 6. Net price 1-mL amp (with 1 mL water for injections) = 63p
Excipients: include benzyl alcohol (avoid in neonates, see Excipients, p. 2), ethanol, propylene glycol

■ Oral preparations
Section 4.8.1

FOSPHENYTOIN SODIUM

NOTE. Fosphenytoin is a pro-drug of phenytoin
Indications: status epilepticus; seizures associated with neurosurgery or head injury; when phenytoin by mouth not possible
Cautions: see Phenytoin Sodium; liver impairment (Appendix 2); renal impairment (Appendix 3); resuscitation facilities must be available; **interactions:** see p. 237 and Appendix 1 (phenytoin)
Contra-indications: see Phenytoin Sodium
Side-effects: see Phenytoin Sodium
CSM ADVICE. Intravenous infusion of fosphenytoin has been associated with severe cardiovascular reactions including asystole, ventricular fibrillation, and cardiac arrest. Hypotension, bradycardia, and heart block have also been reported. The CSM advises:

- monitor heart rate, blood pressure, and respiratory function for duration of infusion
- observe patient for at least 30 minutes after infusion
- if hypotension occurs, reduce infusion rate or discontinue
- reduce dose or infusion rate in elderly, and in renal or hepatic impairment.

Dose: expressed as **phenytoin sodium equivalent** (PE); fosphenytoin sodium 1.5 mg ≡ phenytoin sodium 1 mg
Status epilepticus, *by intravenous infusion* (at a rate of 100–150 mg(PE)/minute), initially 15 mg(PE)/kg then *by intramuscular injection* or *by intravenous infusion* (at a rate of 50–100 mg(PE)/minute), 4–5 mg(PE)/kg daily in 1–2 divided doses, dose adjusted according to response and trough plasma-phenytoin concentration
CHILD 5 years and over, *by intravenous infusion* (at a rate of 2–3 mg(PE)/kg/minute), initially 15 mg(PE)/kg then *by intravenous infusion* (at a rate of 1–2 mg(PE)/kg/minute), 4–5 mg(PE)/kg daily in 1–4 divided doses, dose adjusted according to response and trough plasma-phenytoin concentration
Prophylaxis or treatment of seizures associated with neurosurgery or head injury, *by intramuscular injection* or *by intravenous infusion* (at a rate of 50–100 mg(PE)/minute), initially 10–15 mg(PE)/kg then *by intramuscular injection* or *by intravenous infusion* (at a rate of 50–100 mg(PE)/minute), 4–5 mg(PE)/kg daily (in 1–2 divided doses), dose adjusted according to response and trough plasma-phenytoin concentration
CHILD 5 years and over, *by intravenous infusion* (at a rate of 1–2 mg(PE)/kg/minute), initially 10–15 mg(PE)/kg then 4–5 mg(PE)/kg daily in 1–4 divided doses, dose adjusted according to response and trough plasma-phenytoin concentration
Temporary substitution for oral phenytoin, *by intramuscular injection* or *by intravenous infusion* (at a rate of 50–100 mg(PE)/minute), same dose and dosing frequency as oral phenytoin therapy; CHILD 5 years and over, *by intravenous infusion* (at a rate of 1–2 mg(PE)/kg/minute), same dose and dosing frequency as oral phenytoin therapy
ELDERLY consider 10–25% reduction in dose or infusion rate

NOTE. Prescriptions for fosphenytoin sodium should state the dose in terms of phenytoin sodium equivalent (PE)

Pro-Epanutin® (Pfizer) PoM
Injection, fosphenytoin sodium 75 mg/mL (equivalent to phenytoin sodium 50 mg/mL), net price 10-mL vial = £40.00
Electrolytes: phosphate 3.7 micromol/mg fosphenytoin sodium (phosphate 5.6 micromol/mg phenytoin sodium)

LORAZEPAM

Indications: status epilepticus; other indications (section 4.1.2)
Cautions: see section 4.1.2
Contra-indications: see under Diazepam (section 4.1.2)
Side-effects: see under Diazepam (section 4.1.2)
Dose: *by intravenous injection* (into large vein), 4 mg; CHILD 2 mg

■ Preparations
Section 4.1.2

PARALDEHYDE

Indications: status epilepticus
Cautions: bronchopulmonary disease, hepatic impairment; pregnancy (Appendix 4) and breast-feeding (Appendix 5); **interactions:** Appendix 1 (paraldehyde)
Contra-indications: gastric disorders; rectal administration in colitis
Side-effects: rashes; rectal irritation after enema
Dose: *by rectum*, usually 10–20 mL; CHILD up to 3 months 0.5 mL, 3–6 months 1 mL, 6–12 months 1.5 mL, 1–2 years 2 mL, 3–5 years 3–4 mL, 6–12 years 5–6 mL
ADMINISTRATION. Administer as an enema containing 1 part paraldehyde diluted with 9 parts physiological saline (some centres mix paraldehyde with an equal volume of arachis (peanut) oil instead)
NOTE. Do not use paraldehyde if it has a brownish colour or an odour of acetic acid. Avoid contact with rubber and plastics.

Paraldehyde (Non-proprietary) PoM
Injection, sterile paraldehyde, net price 5-mL amp = £9.49

PHENYTOIN SODIUM

Indications: status epilepticus; seizures in neurosurgery; arrhythmias, but now obsolete (section 2.3.2)
Cautions: hypotension and heart failure; resuscitation facilities must be available; injection solutions alkaline (irritant to tissues); see also p. 243;

interactions: see p. 237 and Appendix 1 (phenytoin)

Contra-indications: sinus bradycardia, sino-atrial block, and second- and third-degree heart block; Stokes-Adams syndrome; porphyria (section 9.8.2)

Side-effects: intravenous injection may cause cardiovascular and CNS depression (particularly if injection too rapid) with arrhythmias, hypotension, and cardiovascular collapse; alterations in respiratory function (including respiratory arrest); see also p. 243

Dose: *by slow intravenous injection or infusion* (with blood pressure and ECG monitoring), status epilepticus, 15 mg/kg at a rate not exceeding 50 mg per minute, as a loading dose (see also notes above); maintenance doses of about 100 mg should be given thereafter at intervals of every 6–8 hours, monitored by measurement of plasma concentrations; rate and dose reduced according to weight; CHILD 15 mg/kg as a loading dose (neonate 15–20 mg/kg at rate of 1–3 mg/kg/minute)

Ventricular arrhythmias (but use now obsolete), *by intravenous injection* via caval catheter, 3.5–5 mg/kg at a rate not exceeding 50 mg/minute, with blood pressure and ECG monitoring; repeat once if necessary

NOTE. Phenytoin is licensed for administration by intravenous infusion (at the same rate of administration as the injection—not exceeding 50 mg/minute, for further details of the infusion, see Appendix 6). To avoid local venous irritation each injection or infusion should be preceded and followed by an injection of sterile physiological saline through the same needle or catheter

By intramuscular injection, not recommended (see notes above)

Phenytoin (Non-proprietary) PoM

Injection, phenytoin sodium 50 mg/mL with propylene glycol 40% and alcohol 10% in water for injections, net price 5-mL amp = £3.40

Epanutin® Ready-Mixed Parenteral (Pfizer) PoM

Injection, phenytoin sodium 50 mg/mL with propylene glycol 40% and alcohol 10% in water for injections. Net price 5-mL amp = £4.88

■ Oral preparations

Section 4.8.1

4.8.3 Febrile convulsions

Brief febrile convulsions need only simple treatment such as tepid sponging or bathing, or antipyretic medication, e.g. **paracetamol** (section 4.7.1). *Prolonged febrile convulsions* (those lasting 15 minutes or longer), *recurrent convulsions*, or those occurring in a child at known risk must be treated more actively, as there is the possibility of resulting brain damage. **Diazepam** is the drug of choice given either by slow intravenous injection in a dose of 250 micrograms/kg (section 4.8.2) or preferably rectally in solution (section 4.8.2) in a dose of 500 micrograms/kg (max. 10 mg), repeated if necessary. The rectal route is preferred as satisfactory absorption is achieved within minutes and administration is much easier. Suppositories are not suitable because absorption is too slow.

Intermittent prophylaxis (i.e. the anticonvulsant administered at the onset of fever) is possible in only a small proportion of children. Again **diazepam** is the treatment of choice, orally or rectally.

The exact role of continuous prophylaxis in children at risk from prolonged or complex febrile convulsions is controversial. It is probably indicated in only a small proportion of children, including those whose first seizure occurred at under 14 months or who have pre-existing neurological abnormalities or who have had previous prolonged or focal convulsions. Thus long-term anticonvulsant prophylaxis is rarely indicated.

4.9 Drugs used in parkinsonism and related disorders

In idiopathic Parkinson's disease, the progressive degeneration of pigmented neurones in the substantia nigra leads to a deficiency of the neurotransmitter dopamine. The resulting neurochemical imbalance in the basal ganglia causes the characteristic signs and symptoms of the illness. Drug therapy does not prevent disease progression, but it improves most patients' quality of life.

When initiating treatment, patients should be advised about its limitations and possible side-effects. About 5–10% of patients with Parkinson's disease respond poorly to treatment.

Symptoms resembling Parkinson's disease can occur in diseases such as progressive supranuclear palsy and multiple system atrophy, but they do not normally respond to the drugs used in the treatment of idiopathic Parkinson's disease.

ELDERLY. Antiparkinsonian drugs can cause confusion in the elderly. It is particularly important to initiate treatment with low doses and to increase the dose gradually.

4.9.1 Dopaminergic drugs used in parkinsonism

Treatment for Parkinson's disease should be initiated under the supervision of a physician specialising in Parkinson's disease. Treatment is usually not started until symptoms cause significant disruption of daily activities.

The dopamine receptor agonists, **bromocriptine**, **cabergoline**, **lisuride** (lysuride), **pergolide**, **pramipexole**, and **ropinirole**, have a direct action on dopamine receptors. The treatment of new patients is often started with dopamine receptor agonists. They are also used with levodopa in more advanced disease.

When used alone, dopamine receptor agonists cause fewer motor complications in long-term treatment compared with levodopa treatment but their improvement on overall motor performance is slightly less. The dopamine receptor agonists are associated with more neuropsychiatric side-effects than levodopa. The ergot-derived dopamine receptor agonists, bromocriptine, cabergoline, lisuride, and pergolide have been associated with fibrotic reactions (see notes below).

Doses of dopamine receptor agonists should be increased slowly according to response and tolerability. They should also be withdrawn gradually.

Apomorphine is a dopamine receptor agonist that is used in advanced disease (see below).

Fibrotic reactions. The CSM has advised that ergot-derived dopamine receptor agonists, bromocriptine, cabergoline, lisuride, and pergolide have been associated with pulmonary, retroperitoneal, and pericardial fibrotic reactions. Before starting treatment with these ergot derivatives it may be appropriate to measure the erythrocyte sedimentation rate and serum creatinine and to obtain a chest X-ray. Patients should be monitored for dyspnoea, persistent cough, chest pain, cardiac failure, and abdominal pain or tenderness. If long-term treatment is expected, then lung-function tests may also be helpful.

Levodopa, the amino-acid precursor of dopamine, acts by replenishing depleted striatal dopamine; it is given with an extracerebral **dopa-decarboxylase inhibitor** that reduces the peripheral conversion of levodopa to dopamine, thereby limiting side-effects such as nausea, vomiting and cardiovascular effects. Additionally, effective brain-dopamine concentrations can be achieved with lower doses of levodopa. The extracerebral dopa-decarboxylase inhibitors used with levodopa are benserazide (in **co-beneldopa**) and carbidopa (in **co-careldopa**).

Levodopa, in combination with a dopa-decarboxylase inhibitor, is useful in the elderly or frail, in patients with other significant illnesses, and in those with more severe symptoms. It is effective and well tolerated in the majority of patients.

Levodopa therapy should be initiated at a low dose and increased in small steps; the final dose should be as low as possible. Intervals between doses should be chosen to suit the needs of the individual patient.

NOTE. When co-careldopa is used, the total daily dose of carbidopa should be at least 70 mg. A lower dose may not achieve full inhibition of extracerebral dopa-decarboxylase, with a resultant increase in side-effects.

Nausea and vomiting with co-beneldopa or co-careldopa are rarely dose-limiting but domperidone (section 4.6) may be useful in controlling these effects.

Levodopa treatment is associated with the development of potentially troublesome motor complications including response fluctuations and dyskinesias. Response fluctuations are characterised by large variations in motor performance, with normal function during the 'on' period, and weakness and restricted mobility during the 'off' period. 'End-of-dose' deterioration also occurs, where the duration of benefit after each dose becomes progressively shorter. Modified-release preparations may help with 'end-of-dose' deterioration or nocturnal immobility and rigidity. Motor complications are particularly problematic in young patients treated with levodopa.

Selegiline is a monoamine-oxidase-B inhibitor used in conjunction with levodopa to reduce 'end-of-dose' deterioration in advanced Parkinson's disease. Early treatment with selegiline alone may delay the need for levodopa therapy for some months but other more effective drugs are preferred. When combined with levodopa, selegiline should be avoided or used with great caution in postural hypotension.

Entacapone and **tolcapone** prevent the peripheral breakdown of levodopa, allowing more levodopa to reach the brain. They are licensed for use as an adjunct to co-beneldopa or co-careldopa for patients with Parkinson's disease who experience 'end-of-dose' deterioration and cannot be stabilised on these combinations. Due to the risk of hepatotoxicity, tolcapone should be prescribed under specialist supervision only, when other combinations have proved ineffective.

Amantadine has modest antiparkinsonian effects. It improves mild bradykinetic disabilities as well as tremor and rigidity. It may also be useful for dyskinesias in more advanced disease. Tolerance to its effects may develop and confusion and hallucinations may occasionally occur. Withdrawal of amantadine should be gradual irrespective of the patient's response to treatment.

Apomorphine is a potent dopamine agonist that is sometimes helpful in advanced disease for patients experiencing unpredictable 'off' periods with levodopa treatment. For the treatment of Parkinson's disease it is only available for parenteral administration. Apomorphine is highly emetogenic; patients must receive domperidone for at least 2 days before starting treatment. Specialist supervision is advisable throughout apomorphine treatment.

Sudden onset of sleep. Excessive daytime sleepiness and sudden onset of sleep can occur with co-careldopa, co-beneldopa, and the dopamine receptor agonists.

Patients starting treatment with these drugs should be warned of the possibility of these effects and of the need to exercise caution when driving or operating machinery.

Patients who have suffered excessive sedation or sudden onset of sleep, should refrain from driving or operating machines, until those effects have stopped recurring.

LEVODOPA

Indications: parkinsonism (but not drug-induced extrapyramidal symptoms), see notes above

Cautions: pulmonary disease, peptic ulceration, cardiovascular disease, diabetes mellitus, osteomalacia, open-angle glaucoma, history of skin melanoma (risk of activation), psychiatric illness (avoid if severe); warn patients about excessive drowsiness (see notes above); in prolonged therapy, psychiatric, hepatic, haematological, renal, and cardiovascular surveillance is advisable; warn patients to resume normal activities gradually; avoid abrupt withdrawal; **interactions:** Appendix 1 (levodopa)

Contra-indications: closed-angle glaucoma; pregnancy (Appendix 4) and breast-feeding (Appendix 5)

Side-effects: anorexia, nausea and vomiting, insomnia, agitation, postural hypotension (rarely labile hypertension), dizziness, tachycardia, arrhythmias, reddish discoloration of urine and other body fluids, rarely hypersensitivity; abnormal involuntary movements and psychiatric symptoms which include hypomania and psychosis may be dose-limiting; depression, drowsiness, headache, flushing, sweating, gastro-intestinal bleeding, peripheral neuropathy, taste disturbance, pruritus, rash, and liver enzyme changes also reported; syndrome resembling neuroleptic malignant syndrome reported on withdrawal

Dose: initially 125–500 mg daily in divided doses after meals, increased according to response (but rarely used alone, see notes above)

Levodopa (Non-proprietary) PoM 
Tablets—product discontinued

CO-BENELDOPA

A mixture of benserazide hydrochloride and levodopa in mass proportions corresponding to 1 part of benserazide and 4 parts of levodopa

Indications: see under Levodopa and notes above
Cautions: see under Levodopa and notes above
Contra-indications: see under Levodopa
Side-effects: see under Levodopa and notes above
Dose: expressed as levodopa, initially 50 mg 3–4 times daily (100 mg 3 times daily in advanced disease), increased by 100 mg once or twice weekly according to response; usual maintenance dose 400–800 mg daily in divided doses after meals; ELDERLY initially 50 mg once or twice daily, increased by 50 mg every 3–4 days according to response

NOTE. When transferring patients from other levodopa preparations, it is recommended that the previous preparation should be discontinued 12 hours beforehand (although interval can be shorter); 3 capsules co-beneldopa 25/100 (*Madopar 125*®) should be substituted for 2 g levodopa; if transferring from another levodopa/dopa-decarboxylase inhibitor preparation, initial dose, expressed as levodopa, should be 50 mg 3–4 times daily

Madopar® (Roche) PoM
Capsules 62.5, blue/grey, co-beneldopa 12.5/50 (benserazide 12.5 mg (as hydrochloride), levodopa 50 mg). Net price 100-cap pack = £6.20. Label: 14, counselling, driving, see notes above
Capsules 125, blue/pink, co-beneldopa 25/100 (benserazide 25 mg (as hydrochloride), levodopa 100 mg). Net price 100-cap pack = £8.64. Label: 14, counselling, driving, see notes above
Capsules 250, blue/caramel, co-beneldopa 50/200 (benserazide 50 mg (as hydrochloride), levodopa 200 mg). Net price 100-cap pack = £14.73. Label: 14, counselling, driving, see notes above
Dispersible tablets 62.5, scored, co-beneldopa 12.5/50 (benserazide 12.5 mg (as hydrochloride), levodopa 50 mg). Net price 100-tab pack = £7.37. Label: 14, counselling, administration, see below, driving see notes above
Dispersible tablets 125, scored, co-beneldopa 25/100 (benserazide 25 mg (as hydrochloride) levodopa 100 mg). Net price 100-tab pack = £13.06. Label: 14, counselling, administration, see below, driving see notes above

NOTE. The tablets may be dispersed in water or orange squash (not orange juice) or swallowed whole

■ Modified release

Madopar® **CR** (Roche) PoM
Capsules 125, m/r, dark green/light blue, co-beneldopa 25/100 (benserazide 25 mg (as hydrochloride), levodopa 100 mg). Net price 100-cap pack = £15.96. Label: 5, 14, 25, counselling, driving, see notes above

Dose: Patients not receiving levodopa therapy, initially 1 capsule 3 times daily (max. initial dose 6 capsules daily)
Fluctuations in response related to plasma-levodopa concentration or to timing of dose, initially 1 capsule substituted for every 100 mg of levodopa and given at same dosage frequency, subsequently increased every 2–3 days according to response; average increase of 50% needed over previous levodopa dose and titration may take up to 4 weeks
Supplementary dose of conventional *Madopar*® may be needed with first morning dose; if response still poor to total daily dose of *Madopar*® *CR* plus *Madopar*® corresponding to 1.2 g levodopa, consider alternative therapy

CO-CARELDOPA

A mixture of carbidopa and levodopa; the proportions are expressed in the form *x/y* where *x* and *y* are the strengths in milligrams of carbidopa and levodopa respectively

Indications: see under Levodopa and notes above
Cautions: see under Levodopa and notes above
Contra-indications: see under Levodopa
Side-effects: see under Levodopa and notes above
Dose: see preparations

NOTE. Carbidopa 70–100 mg daily is necessary to achieve full inhibition of peripheral dopa-decarboxylase

Sinemet® (Bristol-Myers Squibb) PoM
Sinemet-62.5® *tablets*, yellow, scored, co-careldopa 12.5/50 (carbidopa 12.5 mg (as monohydrate), levodopa 50 mg), net price 90-tab pack = £7.03. Label: 14, counselling, driving, see notes above

NOTE. 2 tablets *Sinemet-62.5*® ≡ 1 tablet *Sinemet Plus*®; *Sinemet-62.5*® previously known as *Sinemet LS*®

Sinemet-110® *tablets*, blue, scored, co-careldopa 10/100 (carbidopa 10 mg (as monohydrate), levodopa 100 mg), net price 90-tab pack = £6.84. Label: 14, counselling, driving, see notes above
Sinemet-Plus® *tablets*, yellow, scored, co-careldopa 25/100 (carbidopa 25 mg (as monohydrate), levodopa 100 mg), net price 90-tab pack = £10.05. Label: 14, counselling, driving, see notes above

NOTE. The daily dose of carbidopa required to achieve full inhibition of extracerebral dopa-decarboxylase is 75 mg; co-careldopa 25/100 provides an adequate dose of carbidopa when low doses of levodopa are needed

Sinemet-275® *tablets*, blue, scored, co-careldopa 25/250 (carbidopa 25 mg (as monohydrate), levodopa 250 mg), net price 90-tab pack = £14.28. Label: 14, counselling, driving, see notes above

Dose: expressed as levodopa, initially 100 mg (with carbidopa 25 mg, as *Sinemet-Plus*®) 3 times daily, increased by 50–100 mg (with carbidopa 12.5–25 mg, as *Sinemet-62.5*® or *Sinemet-Plus*®) daily or on alternate days according to response, up to 800 mg (with carbidopa 200 mg) daily in divided doses
Alternatively, initially 50–100 mg (with carbidopa 10–12.5 mg, as *Sinemet-62.5*® or *Sinemet-110*®) 3–4 times daily, increased by 50–100 mg daily or on alternate days according to response, up to 800 mg (with carbidopa 80–100 mg) daily in divided doses
Alternatively, initially 125 mg (with carbidopa 12.5 mg, as ½ tablet of *Sinemet-275*®) 1–2 times daily, increased by 125 mg (with carbidopa 12.5 mg) daily or on alternate days according to response

NOTE. When transferring patients from levodopa, 1 tablet co-careldopa 25/250 (*Sinemet-275*®) 3–4 times daily should be substituted for patients receiving more than 1.5 g levodopa daily; 1 tablet co-careldopa 25/100 (*Sinemet-Plus*®) 3–4 times daily should be substituted for patients receiving less than 1.5 g levodopa daily; levodopa should be discontinued 12 hours beforehand

■ Modified release

Half Sinemet® CR (Bristol-Myers Squibb) PoM
Tablets, m/r, pink, co-careldopa 25/100 (carbidopa 25 mg (as monohydrate), levodopa 100 mg), net price 60-tab pack = £12.07. Label: 14, 25, counselling, driving, see notes above
Dose: for fine adjustment of *Sinemet® CR* dose (see below)

Sinemet® CR (Bristol-Myers Squibb) PoM
Tablets, m/r, peach, co-careldopa 50/200 (carbidopa 50 mg (as monohydrate), levodopa 200 mg), net price 60-tab pack = £12.07. Label: 14, 25, counselling, driving, see notes above
Dose: initial treatment or fluctuations in response to conventional levodopa therapy, 1 *Sinemet® CR* tablet twice daily; both dose and interval then adjusted according to response at intervals of not less than 3 days; if transferring from existing levodopa therapy withdraw 8 hours beforehand; 1 tablet *Sinemet® CR* twice daily can be substituted for a daily dose of levodopa 300–400 mg in conventional *Sinemet®* tablets

Tilolec® (Tillomed) PoM
Tilolec® 100/25 tablets, m/r, orange-brown, co-careldopa 25/100 (carbidopa 25 mg (as monohydrate), levodopa 100 mg), net price 60-tab pack = £18.90. Label: 14, 25, counselling, driving, see notes above
Tilolec® 200/50 tablets, m/r, orange-brown, co-careldopa 50/200 (carbidopa 50 mg (as monohydrate), levodopa 200 mg), net price 60-tab pack = £22.15. Label: 14, 25, counselling, driving, see notes above
Dose: initiation of treatment, 1 tablet *Tilolec® 100/25* twice daily or 1 tablet *Tilolec® 200/50* twice daily (initial max. 3 tablets *Tilolec® 200/50* daily in 2–3 divided doses) adjusting dose and frequency according to response at intervals of at least 2 days; max. 8 tablets *Tilolec® 200/50* daily in divided doses
Switching from immediate-release co-careldopa, withdraw existing treatment 12 hours beforehand then substitute *Tilolec® 100/25* 1 tablet twice daily for levodopa 100–200 mg daily or *Tilolec® 200/50* 1 tablet twice daily for levodopa 300–400 mg daily, then adjust dose and frequency according to response at intervals of at least 3 days; max. 8 tablets *Tilolec® 200/50* daily in divided doses

■ With entacapone
NOTE. For Parkinson's disease and end-of-dose motor fluctuations not adequately controlled with levodopa and dopa-decarboxylase inhibitor treatment

Stalevo® (Orion) ▼ PoM
Stalevo 50 mg/12.5 mg/200 mg tablets, f/c, brown, levodopa 50 mg, carbidopa 12.5 mg, entacapone 200 mg, net price 30-tab pack = £21.72, 100-tab pack = £72.40. Label: 14 (urine reddish-brown), 25, counselling, driving, see notes above
Stalevo 100 mg/25 mg/200 mg tablets, f/c, brown, levodopa 100 mg, carbidopa 25 mg, entacapone 200 mg, net price 30-tab pack = £21.72, 100-tab pack = £72.40. Label: 14 (urine reddish-brown), 25, counselling, driving, see notes above
Stalevo 150 mg/37.5 mg/200 mg tablets, f/c, brown, levodopa 150 mg, carbidopa 37.5 mg, entacapone 200 mg, net price 30-tab pack = £21.72, 100-tab pack = £72.40. Label: 14 (urine reddish-brown), 25, counselling, driving, see notes above
Dose: only 1 tablet of *Stalevo®* to be taken for each dose
Patients receiving standard-release co-careldopa or co-beneldopa alone, initiate *Stalevo®* at a dose that provides similar (or slightly lower) amount of levodopa
Patients with dyskinesia or receiving more than 800 mg levodopa daily, introduce entacapone before transferring to *Stalevo®* (levodopa dose may need to be reduced by 10–30% initially)
Patients receiving entacapone and standard-release co-careldopa or co-beneldopa, initiate *Stalevo®* at a dose that provides similar (or slightly higher) amount of levodopa

AMANTADINE HYDROCHLORIDE

Indications: Parkinson's disease (but not drug-induced extrapyramidal symptoms); antiviral (section 5.3.4)

Cautions: hepatic, or renal impairment (Appendix 3), congestive heart disease (may exacerbate oedema), confused or hallucinatory states, elderly; avoid abrupt discontinuation in Parkinson's disease; **interactions:** Appendix 1 (amantadine)
DRIVING. May affect performance of skilled tasks (e.g. driving)

Contra-indications: epilepsy, history of gastric ulceration, severe renal impairment; pregnancy (Appendix 4), breast-feeding (Appendix 5)

Side-effects: anorexia, nausea, nervousness, inability to concentrate, insomnia, dizziness, convulsions, hallucinations or feelings of detachment, blurred vision, gastro-intestinal disturbances, livedo reticularis and peripheral oedema; rarely leucopenia, rashes

Dose: Parkinson's disease, 100 mg daily increased after one week to 100 mg twice daily, usually in conjunction with other treatment; some patients may require higher doses, max. 400 mg daily; ELDERLY 65 years and over, 100 mg daily adjusted according to response
Post-herpetic neuralgia, 100 mg twice daily for 14 days, continued for a further 14 days if necessary

Symmetrel® (Alliance) PoM
Capsules, red-brown, amantadine hydrochloride 100 mg. Net price 56-cap pack = £16.88. Counselling, driving
Syrup, amantadine hydrochloride 50 mg/5 mL. Net price 150-mL pack = £5.55. Counselling, driving

Lysovir® (Alliance) PoM
See p. 327

APOMORPHINE HYDROCHLORIDE

Indications: refractory motor fluctuations in Parkinson's disease ('off' episodes) inadequately controlled by levodopa or other dopaminergics (for capable and motivated patients under specialist supervision); erectile dysfunction (section 7.4.5)

Cautions: tendency to nausea and vomiting; pulmonary, cardiovascular or endocrine disease, renal impairment; elderly and debilitated, history of postural hypotension (special care on initiation); hepatic, haemopoietic, renal, and cardiovascular monitoring; *on administration with levodopa* test initially and every 6 months for haemolytic anaemia (development calls for specialist haematological care with dose reduction and possible discontinuation); **interactions:** Appendix 1 (apomorphine)

Contra-indications: respiratory or CNS depression, hepatic impairment, hypersensitivity to opioids; neuropsychiatric problems or dementia; not suitable if 'on' response to levodopa marred by severe dyskinesia, hypotonia or psychiatric effects; pregnancy and breast-feeding; not for intravenous administration

Side-effects: nausea and vomiting (see below under Dose), dyskinesias during 'on' periods (may require discontinuation); postural instability and falls (impaired speech and balance may not improve), increasing cognitive impairment, and personality change during 'on' phase; confusion and hallucinations (if continued, specialist observation required with possible gradual dose reduction), sedation, postural hypotension; also euphoria, light-headedness, restlessness, tremors; haemolytic anaemia with levodopa (see Cautions) and rarely eosinophilia; local reactions common (include nodule formation and possible ulceration)—rotate injection sites, dilute with sodium chloride 0.9%, consider ultrasound, ensure no infection

Dose: *by subcutaneous injection*, usual range (after initiation as below) 3–30 mg daily in divided doses; subcutaneous infusion may be preferable in those requiring division of injections into more than 10 doses daily; max. single dose 10 mg; ADOLESCENT (under 18 years) and CHILD not recommended

By continuous subcutaneous infusion (those requiring division into more than 10 injections daily) initially 1 mg/hour daily increased according to response (not more often than every 4 hours) in max. steps of 500 micrograms/hour, to usual rate of 1–4 mg/hour (14–60 micrograms/kg/hour); change infusion site every 12 hours and give during waking hours only (24-hour infusions not advised unless severe night-time symptoms)—intermittent bolus boosts also usually needed; CHILD and ADOLESCENT under 18 years not recommended

Total daily dose by either route (or combined routes) max. 100 mg

REQUIREMENTS FOR INITIATION. *Hospital admission* and at least 2 days of pretreatment with domperidone for nausea and vomiting, *after at least 3 days* withhold existing antiparkinsonian medication overnight to provoke 'off' episode, *determine* threshold dose, *re-establish* other antiparkinsonian drugs, *determine* effective apomorphine regimen, *teach* to administer by subcutaneous injection into lower abdomen or outer thigh at first sign of 'off' episode, *discharge* from hospital, *monitor* frequently and *adjust* dosage regimen as appropriate (domperidone may normally be withdrawn over several weeks or longer)—for full details of initiation requirements, consult product literature

APO-go® (Britannia) PoM

Injection, apomorphine hydrochloride 10 mg/mL, net price 2-mL amp = £7.59, 5-mL amp = £14.62

Injection (APO-go® Pen), apomorphine hydrochloride 10 mg/mL, net price 3-mL pen injector = £24.78

Injection (APO-go® PFS), apomorphine hydrochloride 5 mg/mL, net price 10-mL prefilled syringe = £14.62

BROMOCRIPTINE

Indications: parkinsonism (but not drug-induced extrapyramidal symptoms); endocrine disorders, section 6.7.1

Cautions: section 6.7.1; fibrotic reactions—see CSM advice in notes above

HYPOTENSIVE REACTIONS. Hypotensive reactions in some patients may be disturbing during the first few days of treatment and particular care should be exercised when driving or operating machinery; tolerance may be reduced by alcohol

Contra-indications: section 6.7.1

Side-effects: section 6.7.1

Dose: first week 1–1.25 mg at night, second week 2–2.5 mg at night, third week 2.5 mg twice daily, fourth week 2.5 mg 3 times daily then increasing by 2.5 mg every 3–14 days according to response to a usual range of 10–40 mg daily; taken with food

■ Preparations

Section 6.7.1

CABERGOLINE

Indications: adjunct to levodopa (with dopa-decarboxylase inhibitor) in Parkinson's disease; endocrine disorders (section 6.7.1)

Cautions: section 6.7.1; fibrotic reactions—see CSM advice in notes above

HYPOTENSIVE REACTIONS. Hypotensive reactions in some patients may be disturbing during the first few days of treatment; tolerance may be reduced by alcohol

Contra-indications: section 6.7.1

Side-effects: section 6.7.1

Dose: initially 1 mg daily, increased by increments of 0.5–1 mg at 7 or 14 day intervals; usual range 2–6 mg daily

NOTE. Concurrent dose of levodopa may be decreased gradually while dose of cabergoline is increased

Cabaser® (Pharmacia) PoM

Tablets, all scored, cabergoline 1 mg, net price 20-tab pack = £83.00; 2 mg, 20-tab pack = £83.00; 4 mg, 16-tab pack = £75.84. Label: 21, counselling, hypotensive reactions, driving, see notes above

NOTE. Dispense in original container (contains desiccant)

ENTACAPONE

Indications: adjunct to levodopa with dopa-decarboxylase inhibitor in Parkinson's disease and 'end-of-dose' motor fluctuations

Cautions: concurrent levodopa dose may need to be reduced by about 10–30%; **interactions:** Appendix 1 (entacapone)

Contra-indications: pregnancy (Appendix 4) and breast-feeding (Appendix 5); hepatic impairment; phaeochromocytoma; history of neuroleptic malignant syndrome or non-traumatic rhabdomyolysis

Side-effects: nausea, vomiting, abdominal pain, constipation, diarrhoea, urine may be coloured reddish-brown, dry mouth, dyskinesias; dizziness; rarely hepatitis

Dose: 200 mg with each dose of levodopa with dopa-decarboxylase inhibitor; max. 2 g daily

Comtess® (Orion) PoM

Tablets, f/c, brown/orange, entacapone 200 mg, net price 30-tab pack = £18.00, 100-tab pack = £60.00. Label: 14, (urine reddish-brown), counselling, driving, see notes above

LISURIDE MALEATE

(Lysuride maleate)

Indications: Parkinson's disease, used alone or as an adjunct to levodopa

Cautions: history of pituitary tumour; history of psychotic disturbance; pregnancy; porphyria (section 9.8.2); fibrotic reactions—see CSM advice in notes above; **interactions:** Appendix 1 (lisuride)
HYPOTENSIVE REACTIONS. Hypotensive reactions in some patients may be disturbing during the first few days of treatment and particular care should be exercised when driving or operating machinery

Contra-indications: severe disturbances of peripheral circulation; coronary insufficiency

Side-effects: see notes above; nausea and vomiting; dizziness; headache, lethargy, malaise, drowsiness, psychotic reactions (including hallucinations); occasionally severe hypotension, rashes; rarely abdominal pain and constipation; Raynaud's phenomenon reported

Dose: initially 200 micrograms at bedtime with food increased as necessary at weekly intervals to 200 micrograms twice daily (midday and bedtime) then to 200 micrograms 3 times daily (morning, midday, and bedtime); further increases made by adding 200 micrograms each week first to the bedtime dose, then to the midday dose and finally to the morning dose; max. 5 mg daily in 3 divided doses after food

Lisuride Maleate (Non-proprietary) PoM
Tablets, scored, lisuride maleate 200 micrograms. Net price 100-tab pack = £45.27. Label: 21, counselling, hypotensive reactions

PERGOLIDE

Indications: alone or as adjunct to levodopa in Parkinson's disease where dopamine receptor agonists other than ergot derivative not appropriate

Cautions: arrhythmias or underlying cardiac disease; before treatment assess for asymptomatic valvular disease (see notes above—Fibrotic Reactions); history of confusion or hallucinations, dyskinesia (may exacerbate); increase dose gradually and avoid abrupt withdrawal; porphyria (section 9.8.2); pregnancy (Appendix 4); breast-feeding (Appendix 5); **interactions:** Appendix 1 (pergolide)
HYPOTENSIVE REACTIONS. Hypotensive reactions in some patients may be disturbing during the first few days of treatment and particular care should be exercised when driving or operating machinery

Contra-indications: history of fibrotic disorders; cardiac valve disease

Side-effects: see notes above; hallucinations, confusion, dizziness, dyskinesia, drowsiness, abdominal pain, nausea, vomiting, dyspepsia, diplopia, rhinitis, dyspnoea, pleuritis, pleural effusion, pleural fibrosis, pericarditis, pericardial effusion, cardiac valvulopathy, and retroperitoneal fibrosis, insomnia, constipation or diarrhoea, hypotension, syncope, tachycardia and atrial premature contractions, rash, fever, Raynaud's phenomenon reported; neuroleptic malignant syndrome also reported

Dose: monotherapy, 50 micrograms at night on day 1, then 50 micrograms twice daily on days 2–4, then increased by 100–250 micrograms daily every 3–4 days (given in 3 divided doses) up to a daily dose of 1.5 mg at day 28; after day 30, further increases of up to 250 micrograms twice a week; usual maintenance dose approx. 2–2.5 mg daily; max. 5 mg daily

Adjunctive therapy with levodopa, 50 micrograms daily for 2 days, increased gradually by 100–150 micrograms every 3 days over next 12 days, usually given in 3 divided doses; further increases of 250 micrograms every 3 days; usual maintenance dose 3 mg daily; max. 5 mg daily; during pergolide titration levodopa dose may be reduced cautiously

Pergolide (Non-proprietary) PoM
Tablets, pergolide (as mesilate) 50 micrograms, net price 100-tab pack = £31.38; 250 micrograms, 100-tab pack = £35.66; 1 mg, 100-tab pack = £84.16. Counselling, hypotensive reactions, driving, see notes above

Celance® (Lilly) PoM
Tablets, all scored, pergolide (as mesilate) 50 micrograms (ivory), net price 100-tab pack = £32.44; 250 micrograms (green), 100-tab pack = £48.92; 1 mg (pink), 100-tab pack = £176.58. Counselling, hypotensive reactions, driving, see notes above

PRAMIPEXOLE

Indications: Parkinson's disease, used alone or as adjunct to levodopa

Cautions: psychotic disorders; ophthalmological testing recommended (risk of visual disorders); severe cardiovascular disease; avoid abrupt withdrawal (risk of neuroleptic malignant syndrome); renal impairment (Appendix 3); pregnancy (Appendix 4); **interactions:** Appendix 1 (pramipexole)
HYPOTENSIVE REACTIONS. Hypotensive reactions may be disturbing in some patients during the first few days of treatment

Contra-indications: breast-feeding (Appendix 5)

Side-effects: see notes above; also nausea, constipation, confusion, drowsiness (including sudden onset of sleep) and insomnia, dizziness, hallucinations (mostly visual), dyskinesia during initial dose titration (more frequent in women—reduce levodopa dose), peripheral oedema; changes in libido also reported

Dose: initially, 264 micrograms daily in 3 divided doses, doubling the dose every 5–7 days to 1.08 mg daily in 3 divided doses; further increased if necessary by 540 micrograms daily at weekly intervals; max. 3.3 mg daily in 3 divided doses
NOTE. During pramipexole dose titration and maintenance, levodopa dose may be reduced
IMPORTANT. Doses and strengths are stated in terms of pramipexole (base); equivalent strengths in terms of pramipexole dihydrochloride monohydrate (salt) are as follows: 88 micrograms base ≡ 125 micrograms salt; 180 micrograms base ≡ 250 micrograms salt; 700 micrograms base ≡ 1 mg salt

Mirapexin® (Boehringer Ingelheim) PoM
Tablets, pramipexole (as hydrochloride) 88 micrograms, net price 30-tab pack = £9.25; 180 micrograms (scored), 30-tab pack = £18.50, 100-tab pack = £61.67; 700 micrograms (scored), 30-tab pack = £58.89, 100-tab pack = £196.32. Counselling, hypotensive reactions, driving, see notes above

ROPINIROLE

Indications: Parkinson's disease, either used alone or as an adjunct to levodopa; see also notes above

Cautions: hepatic impairment (Appendix 2); renal impairment (Appendix 3); severe cardiovascular disease, major psychotic disorders, avoid abrupt withdrawal; **interactions:** Appendix 1 (ropinirole)

Contra-indications: pregnancy and breast-feeding

Side-effects: see notes above; nausea, drowsiness (including sudden onset of sleep), leg oedema, abdominal pain, vomiting and syncope; dyskinesia, hallucinations and confusion reported in adjunctive therapy; occasionally severe hypotension and bradycardia

Dose: initially 750 micrograms daily in 3 divided doses, increased by increments of 750 micrograms at weekly intervals to 3 mg daily; further increased by increments of up to 3 mg at weekly intervals according to response; usual range 3–9 mg daily (but higher doses may be required if used with levodopa); max. 24 mg daily

NOTE. When administered as adjunct to levodopa, concurrent dose of levodopa may be reduced by approx. 20%

Requip® (GSK) PoM

Tablets, f/c, ropinirole (as hydrochloride) 1 mg (green), net price 84-tab pack = £47.26; 2 mg (pink), 84-tab pack = £94.53; 5 mg (blue), 84-tab pack = £163.27; 28-day starter pack of 42 × 250-microgram (white) tablets, 42 × 500-microgram (yellow) tablets, and 21 × 1-mg (green) tablets = £40.10; 28-day follow-on pack of 42 × 500-microgram (yellow) tablets, 42 × 1-mg (green) tablets, and 63 × 2-mg (pink) tablets = £74.40. Label: 21, counselling, driving, see notes above

SELEGILINE HYDROCHLORIDE

Indications: Parkinson's disease, used alone or as adjunct to levodopa

Cautions: gastric and duodenal ulceration (avoid in active ulceration), uncontrolled hypertension, arrhythmias, angina, psychosis, side-effects of levodopa may be increased, concurrent levodopa dosage may need to be reduced by 10–50%; **interactions:** Appendix 1 (selegiline)

Contra-indications: pregnancy (Appendix 4), breast-feeding (Appendix 5)

Side-effects: nausea, dry mouth; postural hypotension; dyskinesia, vertigo, sleeping disorders, confusion, hallucinations; rarely arrhythmias, agitation, headache, micturition difficulties, skin reactions

Dose: 10 mg in the morning, or 5 mg at breakfast and midday; ELDERLY see below

ELDERLY. To avoid initial confusion and agitation, it may be appropriate to start treatment with a dose of 2.5 mg daily, particularly in the elderly

Selegiline Hydrochloride (Non-proprietary) PoM

Tablets, selegiline hydrochloride 5 mg, net price 56-tab pack = £5.15; 10 mg, 30-tab pack = £5.32

Eldepryl® (Orion) PoM

Tablets, both scored, selegiline hydrochloride 5 mg, net price 60-tab pack = £10.35; 10 mg, 30-tab pack = £10.10

Oral liquid, selegiline hydrochloride 10 mg/5 mL, net price 200 mL = £18.72

■ Oral lyophilisate

Zelapar® (Zeneus) PoM

Oral lyophilisates (= freeze-dried tablets), yellow, selegiline hydrochloride 1.25 mg, net price 30-tab pack = £59.95. Counselling, administration

Dose: initially 1.25 mg daily before breakfast

COUNSELLING. Tablets should be placed on the tongue and allowed to dissolve. Advise patient not to drink, rinse, or wash mouth out for 5 minutes after taking the tablet

Excipients: include aspartame (section 9.4.1)

NOTE. Patients receiving 10 mg conventional selegiline hydrochloride tablets can be switched to *Zelapar*® 1.25 mg

TOLCAPONE

Indications: adjunct to levodopa with dopa-decarboxylase inhibitor in Parkinson's disease and 'end-of-dose' motor fluctuations if another inhibitor of peripheral levodopa breakdown inappropriate (under specialist supervision)

Cautions: most patients receiving more than 600 mg levodopa daily require reduction of levodopa dose; pregnancy (Appendix 4); **interactions:** Appendix 1 (tolcapone)

HEPATOTOXICITY. Potentially life-threatening hepatotoxicity including fulminant hepatitis reported usually in first 6 months; monitor liver function before treatment, every 2 weeks for first year, every 4 weeks for next 6 months and every 8 weeks thereafter (restart monitoring schedule if dose increased); discontinue if abnormal liver function tests or symptoms of liver disorder (counselling, see below); do not re-introduce tolcapone once discontinued

COUNSELLING. Patients should be told how to recognise signs of liver disorder and advised to seek immediate medical attention if symptoms such as anorexia, nausea, vomiting, fatigue, abdominal pain, dark urine, or pruritus develop

Contra-indications: hepatic impairment or raised liver enzymes (see Hepatotoxicity above), severe dyskinesia, phaeochromocytoma, previous history of neuroleptic malignant syndrome, rhabdomyolysis, or hyperthermia; breast-feeding (Appendix 5)

Side-effects: diarrhoea, constipation, dyspepsia, abdominal pain, xerostomia, hepatotoxicity (see above); chest pain; confusion; intensification of urine colour; increase in levodopa-related side-effects; neuroleptic malignant syndrome reported on dose reduction or withdrawal

Dose: 100 mg 3 times daily, leave 6 hours between each dose; max. 200 mg 3 times daily in exceptional circumstances; first daily dose should be taken at the same time as levodopa with dopa-decarboxylase inhibitor

NOTE. Continue beyond 3 weeks **only** if substantial improvement

Tasmar® (Valeant) ▼ PoM

Tablets, f/c, yellow, tolcapone 100 mg, net price 100-tab pack = £95.20. Label: 14, 25

4.9.2 Antimuscarinic drugs used in parkinsonism

Antimuscarinic drugs exert their antiparkinsonian action by reducing the effects of the central cholinergic excess that occurs as a result of dopamine deficiency. Antimuscarinic drugs are useful in drug-induced parkinsonism, but they are generally not used in idiopathic Parkinson's disease because they are less effective than dopaminergic drugs and they are associated with cognitive impairment.

The antimuscarinic drugs, **benzatropine**, **orphenadrine**, **procyclidine**, and **trihexyphenidyl** (benzhexol), reduce the symptoms of parkinsonism induced by antipsychotic drugs, but there is no justification for giving them routinely in the absence of parkinsonian side-effects. Tardive dyskinesia is not improved by antimuscarinic drugs and may be made worse.

In idiopathic Parkinson's disease, antimuscarinic drugs reduce tremor and rigidity but they have little effect on bradykinesia. They may be useful in reducing sialorrhoea.

No important differences exist between the antimuscarinic drugs, but some patients tolerate one better than another.

Benzatropine may be given parenterally and it is effective emergency treatment for acute drug-induced dystonic reactions which may be severe.

BENZATROPINE MESILATE

(Benztropine mesylate)

Indications: see Trihexyphenidyl Hydrochloride

Cautions: see Trihexyphenidyl Hydrochloride

Contra-indications: see Trihexyphenidyl Hydrochloride; avoid in children under 3 years

Side-effects: see Trihexyphenidyl Hydrochloride, but causes sedation rather than stimulation

Dose: *by mouth*, 0.5–1 mg daily usually at bedtime, gradually increased; max. 6 mg daily; usual maintenance dose 1–4 mg daily in single or divided doses; ELDERLY preferably lower end of range

By intramuscular or intravenous injection, 1–2 mg, repeated if symptoms reappear; ELDERLY preferably lower end of range

Cogentin® (MSD) PoM

Injection, benzatropine mesilate 1 mg/mL. Net price 2-mL amp = 92p

ORPHENADRINE HYDROCHLORIDE

Indications: see Trihexyphenidyl Hydrochloride

Cautions: see Trihexyphenidyl Hydrochloride

Contra-indications: see Trihexyphenidyl Hydrochloride; porphyria (section 9.8.2)

Side-effects: see Trihexyphenidyl Hydrochloride; may cause insomnia

Dose: 150 mg daily in divided doses, increased gradually; max. 400 mg daily; ELDERLY preferably lower end of range

Orphenadrine Hydrochloride (Non-proprietary) PoM

Tablets, orphenadrine hydrochloride 50 mg, net price 20 = £1.15. Counselling, driving

Oral solution, orphenadrine hydrochloride 50 mg/5 mL. Net price 200 mL = £9.47. Counselling, driving

Biorphen® (Alliance) PoM

Elixir, sugar-free, orphenadrine hydrochloride 25 mg/5 mL. Net price 200 mL = £7.07. Counselling, driving

Disipal® (Yamanouchi) PoM

Tablets, yellow, s/c, orphenadrine hydrochloride 50 mg. Net price 20 = 69p. Counselling, driving

Excipients: include tartrazine

PROCYCLIDINE HYDROCHLORIDE

Indications: see Trihexyphenidyl Hydrochloride

Cautions: see Trihexyphenidyl Hydrochloride

Contra-indications: see Trihexyphenidyl Hydrochloride

Side-effects: see Trihexyphenidyl Hydrochloride

Dose: *by mouth*, 2.5 mg 3 times daily, increased gradually if necessary; usual max. 30 mg daily (60 mg daily in exceptional circumstances); ELDERLY preferably lower end of range

Acute dystonia, *by intramuscular or intravenous injection*, 5–10 mg (occasionally more than 10 mg), usually effective in 5–10 minutes but may need 30 minutes for relief

Procyclidine (Non-proprietary) PoM

Tablets, procyclidine hydrochloride 5 mg. Net price 20 = £1.53. Counselling, driving

Arpicolin® (Rosemont) PoM

Syrup, sugar-free, procyclidine hydrochloride 2.5 mg/5 mL, net price 150 mL = £4.22; 5 mg/5 mL, 150 mL pack = £7.54. Counselling, driving

Kemadrin® (GSK) PoM

Tablets, scored, procyclidine hydrochloride 5 mg. Net price 20 = 94p. Counselling, driving

Kemadrin® (Auden Mckenzie) PoM

Injection, procyclidine hydrochloride 5 mg/mL, net price 2-mL amp = £1.49

TRIHEXYPHENIDYL HYDROCHLORIDE

(Benzhexol hydrochloride)

Indications: parkinsonism; drug-induced extrapyramidal symptoms (but not tardive dyskinesia, see notes above)

Cautions: cardiovascular disease, glaucoma, gastro-intestinal obstruction, prostatic hypertrophy; elderly; avoid abrupt withdrawal; liable to abuse; hepatic impairment; renal impairment; pregnancy; breast-feeding; **interactions:** Appendix 1 (antimuscarinics)

DRIVING. May affect performance of skilled tasks (e.g. driving)

Side-effects: constipation, dry mouth; blurred vision; *less commonly* nausea, vomiting, agitation, confusion, hallucinations, euphoria, insomnia, restlessness, urinary retention; paranoid delusions and impaired memory also reported

Dose: 1 mg daily, increased gradually; usual maintenance dose 5–15 mg daily in 3–4 divided doses (max. 20 mg daily); ELDERLY preferably lower end of range

CHILD not recommended

Trihexyphenidyl (Non-proprietary) PoM

Tablets, trihexyphenidyl hydrochloride 2 mg, net price 20 = 69p; 5 mg, 20 = 85p. Counselling, before or after food (see notes above), driving

Broflex® (Alliance) PoM

Syrup, pink, trihexyphenidyl hydrochloride 5 mg/5 mL. Net price 200 mL = £6.20. Counselling, before or after food (see notes above), driving

4.9.3 Drugs used in essential tremor, chorea, tics, and related disorders

Tetrabenazine is mainly used to control movement disorders in Huntington's chorea and related disorders. It may act by depleting nerve endings of dopamine. It has useful action in only a proportion of patients and its use may be limited by the development of depression.

Haloperidol may be useful in improving motor tics and symptoms of Gilles de la Tourette syndrome and related choreas. **Pimozide** (see section 4.2.1 for CSM warning), **clonidine** (section 4.7.4.2) and **sulpiride** (section 4.2.1) are also used in Gilles de la Tourette syndrome. **Trihexyphenidyl (benzhexol)** (section 4.9.2) at high dosage may also improve some movement disorders; it is sometimes necessary to build the dose up over many weeks, to 20 to 30 mg daily or higher. **Chlorpromazine** and **haloperidol** are used to relieve intractable hiccup (section 4.2.1).

Propranolol or another beta-adrenoceptor blocking drug (section 2.4) may be useful in treating essential tremor or tremors associated with anxiety or thyrotoxicosis. Propranolol is given in a dosage of 40 mg 2 or 3 times daily, increased if necessary; 80 to 160 mg daily is usually required for maintenance.

Primidone (section 4.8.1) in some cases provides relief from benign essential tremor; the dose is increased slowly to reduce side-effects.

Piracetam is used as an adjunctive treatment for myoclonus of cortical origin.

Riluzole is used to extend life or the time to mechanical ventilation in patients with motor neurone disease who have amyotrophic lateral sclerosis.

NICE guidance (riluzole). NICE has recommended (January 2001) riluzole to treat individuals with the amyotrophic lateral sclerosis (ALS) form of motor neurone disease (MND). Treatment should be initiated by a specialist in MND but it can then be supervised under a shared-care arrangement involving the general practitioner.

HALOPERIDOL

Indications: motor tics, adjunctive treatment in choreas and Gilles de la Tourette syndrome; other indications, section 4.2.1

Cautions: section 4.2.1

Contra-indications: section 4.2.1

Side-effects: section 4.2.1

Dose: *by mouth*, 0.5–1.5 mg 3 times daily adjusted according to the response; 10 mg daily or more may occasionally be necessary in Gilles de la Tourette syndrome; CHILD, Gilles de la Tourette syndrome up to 10 mg daily

■ Preparations

Section 4.2.1

PIRACETAM

Indications: adjunctive treatment of cortical myoclonus

Cautions: avoid abrupt withdrawal; elderly; renal impairment (avoid if severe; Appendix 3)

Contra-indications: hepatic and severe renal impairment; pregnancy and breast-feeding

Side-effects: diarrhoea, weight gain; somnolence, insomnia, nervousness, depression; hyperkinesia; rash

Dose: initially 7.2 g daily in 2–3 divided doses, increased according to response by 4.8 g daily every 3–4 days to max. 20 g daily (subsequently, attempts should be made to reduce dose of concurrent therapy); CHILD under 16 years not recommended

ORAL SOLUTION. Follow the oral solution with a glass of water (or soft drink) to reduce bitter taste.

Nootropil® (UCB Pharma) PoM

Tablets, f/c, scored, piracetam 800 mg, net price 90-tab pack = £14.69; 1.2 g, 56-tab pack = £13.71. Label: 3

Oral solution, piracetam, 333.3 mg/mL, net price 300-mL pack = £20.39. Label: 3

RILUZOLE

Indications: to extend life or the time to mechanical ventilation for patients with amyotrophic lateral sclerosis, initiated by specialists experienced in the management of motor neurone disease

Cautions: history of abnormal hepatic function (consult product literature for details)

BLOOD DISORDERS. Patients or their carers should be told how to recognise signs of neutropenia and advised to seek immediate medical attention if symptoms such as fever occur; white blood cell counts should be determined in febrile illness; neutropenia requires discontinuation of riluzole

DRIVING. Dizziness or vertigo may affect performance of skilled tasks (e.g. driving)

Contra-indications: hepatic and renal impairment (Appendix 3); pregnancy (Appendix 4) and breast-feeding (Appendix 5)

Side-effects: nausea, vomiting, asthenia, tachycardia, somnolence, headache, dizziness, vertigo, abdominal pain, circumoral paraesthesia, alterations in liver function tests

Dose: 50 mg twice daily; CHILD not recommended

Rilutek® (Aventis Pharma) PoM

Tablets, f/c, riluzole 50 mg. Net price 56-tab pack = £179.37. Counselling, blood disorders, driving

TETRABENAZINE

Indications: see under Dose

Cautions: pregnancy (Appendix 4); avoid in breast-feeding; **interactions:** Appendix 1 (tetrabenazine)

DRIVING. May affect performance of skilled tasks (e.g. driving)

Side-effects: drowsiness, gastro-intestinal disturbances, depression, extrapyramidal dysfunction, hypotension; rarely parkinsonism; neuroleptic malignant syndrome reported

Dose: movement disorders due to Huntington's chorea, hemiballismus, senile chorea, and related neurological conditions, initially 12.5 mg twice daily (elderly 12.5 mg daily) gradually increased to 12.5–25 mg 3 times daily; max. 200 mg daily

Moderate to severe tardive dyskinesia, initially 12.5 mg daily, gradually increased according to response

Xenazine® **25** (Cambridge) PoM

Tablets, pale yellow-buff, scored, tetrabenazine 25 mg. Net price 112-tab pack = £100.00. Label: 2

Torsion dystonias and other involuntary movements

BOTULINUM A TOXIN

Indications: focal spasticity, including arm symptoms in conjunction with physiotherapy, dynamic equinus foot deformity caused by spasticity in ambulant paediatric cerebral palsy patients over 2 years, and hand and wrist disability associated with stroke; blepharospasm; hemifacial spasm; spasmodic torticollis; severe hyperhidrosis of axillae (all specialist use only)

Cautions: potential for anaphylaxis; history of dysphagia

SPECIFIC CAUTIONS FOR BLEPHAROSPASM OR HEMIFACIAL SPASM. Avoid deep or misplaced injections—relevant anatomy (and any alterations due to previous surgery) must be understood before injecting; caution if risk of angle closure glaucoma; reduced blinking can lead to corneal exposure, persistent epithelial defect and corneal ulceration (especially in those with VIIth nerve disorders)—careful testing of corneal sensation in previously operated eyes, avoidance of injection in lower lid area to avoid ectropion and vigorous treatment of epithelial defect needed

SPECIFIC CAUTIONS FOR TORTICOLLIS. Patients with defective neuromuscular transmission (risk of excessive muscle weakness)

COUNSELLING. All patients should be alerted to possible side-effects

Contra-indications: generalised disorders of muscle activity (e.g. myasthenia gravis); pregnancy (Appendix 4), breast-feeding (Appendix 5)

Side-effects: increased electrophysiologic jitter in some distant muscles; misplaced injections may paralyse nearby muscle groups and excessive doses may paralyse distant muscles; influenza-like syndrome, rarely hypersensitivity reactions including rash, pruritus and anaphylaxis; antibody formation (substantial deterioration in response); arrhythmia and myocardial infarction; injection site reactions

SPECIFIC SIDE-EFFECTS IN BLEPHAROSPASM OR HEMIFACIAL SPASM. Ptosis; less frequently keratitis, lagophthalmos, dry eye, irritation, photophobia, lacrimation; ectropion, entropion, diplopia, dizziness, skin rash, facial weakness (including drooping), tiredness, visual disturbance, blurring of vision; rarely eyelid bruising and swelling (minimised by applying gentle pressure at injection site immediately after injection); angle closure glaucoma, corneal ulceration.

SPECIFIC SIDE-EFFECTS IN PAEDIATRIC CEREBRAL PALSY. Myalgia, urinary incontinence, somnolence, malaise, paraesthesia

SPECIFIC SIDE-EFFECTS IN TORTICOLLIS. Dysphagia and pooling of saliva (occurs most frequently after injection into sternomastoid muscle); nausea, dry mouth, rhinitis, drowsiness, headache, dizziness, hypertonia, malaise, stiffness; less frequently dyspnoea, fever, voice alteration, diplopia, and ptosis; rarely respiratory difficulties (associated with high doses); CSM has warned of persistent dysphagia and sequelae (including death)—**important**

Dose: consult product literature (**important:** specific to **each individual preparation** and **not interchangeable**)

Botox® (Allergan) PoM
Injection, powder for reconstitution, botulinum A neurotoxin complex, net price 100-unit vial = £128.93

Dysport® (Ipsen) PoM
Injection, powder for reconstitution, botulinum A toxin-haemagglutinin complex, net price 500-unit vial = £153.21

BOTULINUM B TOXIN

Indications: spasmodic torticollis (cervical dystonia)—specialist use only

Cautions: inadvertent injection into a blood vessel; tolerance may occur

Contra-indications: neuromuscular or neuromuscular junctional disorders; pregnancy (Appendix 4) and breast-feeding (Appendix 5)

Side-effects: increased electrophysiologic jitter in some distant muscles; dry mouth, dysphagia; also dyspepsia, worsening torticollis, neck pain, myasthenia, voice changes, taste disturbances

Dose: *by intramuscular injection*, initially 5000–10 000 units divided between 2–4 most affected muscles; adjust dose and frequency according to response; **important: not** interchangeable with other botulinum toxin preparations

NeuroBloc® (Zeneus) PoM
Injection, botulinum B toxin 5000 units/mL, net price 0.5-mL vial = £111.20; 1-mL vial = £148.27; 2-mL vial = £197.69

NOTE. May be diluted with sodium chloride 0.9%

4.10 Drugs used in substance dependence

This section includes drugs used in alcohol dependence, cigarette smoking, and opioid dependence.

The health departments of the UK have produced a report, *Drug Misuse and Dependence* which contains guidelines on clinical management.

Drug Misuse and Dependence, London, The Stationery Office, 1999 can be obtained from:

The Publications Centre
PO Box 276, London SW8 5DT
Telephone orders (087) 0600 5522
Fax (087) 0600 5533

or from The Stationery Office bookshops and through all good booksellers.

It is **important** to be aware that *people who misuse drugs* may be at risk not only from the intrinsic toxicity of the drug itself but also from the practice of injecting preparations intended for administration by mouth. Excipients used in the production of oral dose forms are usually insoluble and may lead to *abscess formation at the site of injection*, or even to *necrosis and gangrene*; moreover, deposits in the heart or lungs may lead to *severe cardiac or pulmonary toxicity*. Additional hazards include *infection* following the use of a dirty needle or an unsterilised diluent.

Alcohol dependence

Disulfiram is used as an adjunct to the treatment of alcohol dependence. It gives rise to extremely unpleasant systemic reactions after the ingestion of even a small amount of alcohol because it leads to accumulation of acetaldehyde in the body. Reactions include flushing of the face, throbbing headache, palpitation, tachycardia, nausea, vomiting, and, with large doses of alcohol, arrhythmias, hypotension, and collapse. Small amounts of alcohol included in many oral medicines may be sufficient to precipitate a reaction (even toiletries and mouthwashes that contain alcohol should be avoided). It may be advisable for patients to carry a card warning of the danger of administration of alcohol.

Long-acting **benzodiazepines** (section 4.1) are used to attenuate withdrawal symptoms but they also have a dependence potential. To minimise the risk of dependence, administration should be for a limited period only (e.g. **chlordiazepoxide** 10–50 mg 4 times daily, gradually reducing over 7–14 days). Benzodiazepines should not be prescribed if the patient is likely to continue drinking alcohol.

Clomethiazole (chlormethiazole) (section 4.1.1) should be used for the management of withdrawal in an **in-patient setting only**. It is associated with a risk of dependence and should not be prescribed if the patient is likely to continue drinking alcohol.

Acamprosate, in combination with counselling, may be helpful in maintaining abstinence in alcohol-dependent patients. It should be initiated as soon as possible *after* abstinence has been achieved and should be maintained if the patient relapses. Continued alcohol abuse, however, negates the therapeutic benefit of acamprosate.

ACAMPROSATE CALCIUM

Indications: maintenance of abstinence in alcohol dependence

Cautions: continued alcohol abuse (risk of treatment failure)

Contra-indications: renal and severe hepatic impairment; pregnancy and breast-feeding

Side-effects: diarrhoea, nausea, vomiting, abdominal pain, pruritus, occasionally maculopapular rash, rarely bullous skin reactions; fluctuation in libido

Dose: ADULT 18–65 years, 60 kg and over, 666 mg 3 times daily; less than 60 kg, 666 mg at breakfast, 333 mg at midday and 333 mg at night

TREATMENT COURSE. Treatment should be initiated as soon as possible after alcohol withdrawal period and maintained if patient relapses; recommended treatment period 1 year

Campral EC® (Merck) PoM
Tablet, e/c, acamprosate calcium 333 mg. Net price 168-tab pack = £28.92. Label: 21, 25
Electrolytes: Ca^{2+} 0.8 mmol/tablet

DISULFIRAM

Indications: adjunct in the treatment of chronic alcohol dependence (under specialist supervision)

Cautions: ensure that alcohol not consumed for at least 24 hours before initiating treatment; see also notes above; alcohol challenge **not** recommended on routine basis (if considered essential—specialist units only with resuscitation facilities); hepatic or renal impairment, respiratory disease, diabetes mellitus, epilepsy; **interactions:** Appendix 1 (disulfiram)

ALCOHOL REACTION. Patients should be warned of unpredictable and occasionally severe nature of disulfiram-alcohol interactions. Reactions can occur within 10 minutes and last several hours (may require intensive supportive therapy—oxygen should be available). Patients should not ingest alcohol at all and should be warned of possible presence of alcohol in liquid medicines, remedies, tonics, foods and even in toiletries (alcohol should also be avoided for at least 1 week after stopping)

Contra-indications: cardiac failure, coronary artery disease, history of cerebrovascular accident, hypertension, psychosis, severe personality disorder, suicide risk, pregnancy (Appendix 4), breast-feeding (Appendix 5)

Side-effects: initially drowsiness and fatigue; nausea, vomiting, halitosis, reduced libido; rarely psychotic reactions (depression, paranoia, schizophrenia, mania), allergic dermatitis, peripheral neuritis, hepatic cell damage

Dose: 800 mg as a single dose on first day, reducing over 5 days to 100–200 mg daily; should not be continued for longer than 6 months without review; CHILD not recommended

Antabuse® (Alpharma) PoM
Tablets, scored, disulfiram 200 mg. Net price 50-tab pack = £26.28. Label: 2, counselling, alcohol reaction

Cigarette smoking

Smoking cessation interventions are a cost-effective way of reducing ill health and prolonging life. Smokers should be advised to stop and offered help if interested in doing so, with follow-up where appropriate.

Where possible, smokers should have access to a smoking cessation clinic for behavioural support. **Nicotine replacement therapy** and **bupropion** are effective aids to smoking cessation for those smoking more than 10 cigarettes a day. Bupropion has been used as an antidepressant but its mode of action in smoking cessation is not clear and may involve an effect on noradrenaline and dopamine neurotransmission. Nicotine replacement therapy is regarded as the pharmacological treatment of choice in the management of smoking cessation.

NICE guidance (nicotine replacement therapy and bupropion for smoking cessation)

NICE has recommended (March 2002) that nicotine replacement therapy or bupropion should be prescribed only for a smoker who commits to a target stop date. The smoker should be offered advice and encouragement to aid smoking cessation.

Therapy to aid smoking cessation is chosen according to the smoker's likely compliance, availability of counselling and support, previous experience of smoking-cessation aids, contra-indications and adverse effects of the products, and the smoker's preferences.

Initial supply of the prescribed smoking-cessation therapy should be sufficient to last only 2 weeks after the target stop date; normally this will be 2 weeks of nicotine replacement therapy or 3–4 weeks of bupropion. A second prescription should be issued only if the smoker demonstrates a continuing attempt to stop smoking.

If an attempt to stop smoking is unsuccessful, the NHS should not normally fund a further attempt within 6 months.

There is currently insufficient evidence to recommend the combined use of nicotine replacement therapy and bupropion.

> **CSM advice (bupropion).** The CSM has issued a reminder that bupropion is contra-indicated in patients with a history of seizures or of eating disorders, a CNS tumour, or who are experiencing acute symptoms of alcohol or benzodiazepine withdrawal. Bupropion should not be prescribed to patients with other risk factors for seizures unless the potential benefit of smoking cessation clearly outweighs the risk. Factors that increase the risk of seizures include concomitant administration of drugs that can lower the seizure threshold (e.g. antidepressants, antimalarials [such as mefloquine and chloroquine], antipsychotics, quinolones, sedating antihistamines, systemic corticosteroids, theophylline, tramadol), alcohol abuse, history of head trauma, diabetes, and use of stimulants and anorectics.

BUPROPION

(Amfebutamone)

Indications: adjunct to smoking cessation in combination with motivational support

Cautions: elderly; hepatic impairment (Appendix 2, avoid in severe hepatic cirrhosis), renal impairment (Appendix 3); predisposition to seizures (see CSM advice above); measure blood pressure before and during treatment (monitor weekly if used with nicotine products); **interactions**: Appendix 1 (bupropion)

DRIVING. May impair performance of skilled tasks (e.g. driving)

Contra-indications: history of seizures, of eating disorders (see CSM advice above) and of bipolar disorder; pregnancy (Appendix 4); breast-feeding (Appendix 5)

Side-effects: dry mouth, gastro-intestinal disturbances, insomnia (reduced by avoiding dose at bedtime), tremor, impaired concentration, headache, dizziness, depression, agitation, anxiety, rash, pruritus, sweating, hypersensitivity reactions (may resemble serum sickness), fever, taste disturbances; less commonly chest pain, asthenia, tachycardia, hypertension, flushing, anorexia, tinnitus, visual disturbances; rarely palpitations, postural hypotension, vasodilation, hallucinations, depersonalisation, seizures, abnormal dreams, memory impairment, paraesthesia, incoordination, urinary retention, urinary frequency, Stevens-Johnson syndrome, jaundice, hepatitis, blood-glucose disturbances, exacerbation of psoriasis

Dose: start 1–2 weeks before target stop date, initially 150 mg daily for 6 days then 150 mg twice daily (max. single dose 150 mg, max. daily dose 300 mg; minimum 8 hours between doses); max. period of treatment 7–9 weeks; discontinue if abstinence not achieved at 7 weeks; consider max. 150 mg daily in patients with risk factors for seizures (see CSM advice above); ELDERLY max. 150 mg daily; CHILD and ADOLESCENT under 18 years not recommended

Zyban® (GSK) ▼ PoM

Tablets, m/r, f/c, bupropion (as hydrochloride) 150 mg, net price 60-tab pack = £39.85. Label: 25

NICOTINE

Indications: adjunct to smoking cessation

Cautions: cardiovascular disease (avoid if severe); peripheral vascular disease; hyperthyroidism; diabetes mellitus; phaeochromocytoma, renal impairment (Appendix 3) and hepatic impairment; history of gastritis and peptic ulcers; should not smoke or use nicotine replacement products in combination; pregnancy (Appendix 4); breast-feeding (Appendix 5); *patches*, exercise may increase absorption and side-effects, skin disorders (patches should not be placed on broken skin)

Contra-indications: severe cardiovascular disease (including severe arrhythmias or immediate post-myocardial infarction period); recent cerebrovascular accident (including transient ischaemic attacks)

Side-effects: nausea, dizziness, headache and cold and influenza-like symptoms, palpitations, dyspepsia and other gastro-intestinal disturbances, hiccups, insomnia, vivid dreams, myalgia; other side-effects reported include chest pain, blood pressure changes, anxiety and irritability, somnolence and impaired concentration, abnormal hunger, dysmenorrhoea, rash; *with patches*, skin reactions (discontinue if severe)—vasculitis also reported; *with spray*, nasal irritation, nose bleeds, watering eyes, ear sensations; *with gum, lozenges, sublingual tablets* or *inhalator*, aphthous ulceration (sometimes with swelling of tongue); *with spray, inhalator, lozenges, sublingual tablets* or *gum*, throat irritation; *with inhalator*, cough, rhinitis, pharyngitis, stomatitis, sinusitis, dry mouth; *with lozenges* or *sublingual tablets*, unpleasant taste

Dose: see under preparations, below

NOTE. Proprietary brands of nicotine products on sale to the public include *Boots Nicotine Gum* 2 mg, 4 mg, *Boots Nicotine Inhalator* 10 mg, and *Boots NRT Patch* 7 mg/24 hours, 14 mg/24 hours, 21 mg/24 hours

Nicorette® (Pharmacia)

Nicorette Microtab (sublingual), nicotine (as a cyclodextrin complex) 2 mg, net price starter pack of 2 × 15-tablet discs with dispenser = £3.57; refill pack of 7 × 15-tablet discs = £9.84. Label: 26

Dose: individuals smoking 20 cigarettes or less daily, *sublingually*, 2 mg each hour; for patients who fail to stop smoking or have significant withdrawal symptoms, consider increasing to 4 mg each hour

Individuals smoking more than 20 cigarettes daily, 4 mg each hour

Max. 80 mg daily; treatment should be continued for at least 3 months followed by a gradual reduction in dosage; max. period of treatment should not exceed 6 months

Nicorette chewing gum, sugar-free, nicotine (as resin) 2 mg, net price pack of 15 = £1.71, pack of 30 = £3.25, pack of 105 = £8.89; 4 mg, net price pack of 15 = £2.11, pack of 30 = £3.99, pack of 105 = £10.83

NOTE. Also available in mint and freshmint flavours

Dose: individuals smoking 20 cigarettes or fewer daily, initially one 2-mg piece chewed slowly for approx. 30 minutes, when urge to smoke occurs; individuals smoking more than 20 cigarettes daily or needing more than 15 pieces of 2-mg gum daily may need the 4-mg strength; max. 15 pieces of 4-mg strength daily; withdraw gradually after 3 months

Nicorette patches, self-adhesive, all beige, nicotine, *'5 mg' patch* (releasing approx. 5 mg/16 hours), net price 7 = £9.07; *'10 mg' patch* (releasing approx. 10 mg/16 hours), 7 = £9.07; *'15 mg' patch* (releasing approx. 15 mg/16 hours), 2 = £2.85, 7 = £9.07

Dose: apply on waking to dry, non-hairy skin on hip, chest or upper arm, removing after approx. 16 hours, usually when retiring to bed; site next patch on different area (avoid using same area on consecutive days); initially '15-mg' patch for 16 hours daily for 8 weeks then if abstinence achieved '10-mg' patch for 16 hours daily for 2 weeks then '5-mg' patch for 16 hours daily for 2 weeks; review treatment if abstinence not achieved in 3 months—further courses may be given if considered beneficial

Nicorette nasal spray, nicotine 500 micrograms/metered spray. Net price 200-spray unit = £10.99

Dose: apply 1 spray into each nostril as required to max. twice an hour for 16 hours daily (max. 64 sprays daily) for 8 weeks, then reduce gradually over next 4 weeks (reduce by half at end of first 2 weeks, stop altogether at end of next 2 weeks); max. treatment length 3 months

Nicorette inhalator (nicotine-impregnated plug for use in inhalator mouthpiece), nicotine 10 mg/cartridge. Net price 6-cartridge (starter) pack = £3.39, 42-cartridge (refill) pack = £11.37

Dose: inhale when urge to smoke occurs; initially use between 6 and 12 cartridges daily for up to 8 weeks, then reduce number of cartridges used by half over next 2 weeks and then stop altogether at end of further 2 weeks; review treatment if abstinence not achieved in 3 months

Nicotinell® (Novartis Consumer Health)

Chewing gum, sugar-free, nicotine 2 mg, net price pack of 12 = £1.59, pack of 24 = £3.01, pack of 96 = £8.26; 4 mg, pack of 12 = £1.70, pack of 24 = £3.30, pack of 96 = £10.26

NOTE. Also available in fruit, liquorice and mint flavours

Dose: initially one 2-mg or 4-mg piece chewed slowly for approx. 30 minutes, when urge to smoke occurs; max. 60 mg daily; withdraw gradually after 3 months

Nicotinell mint lozenge, sugar-free, nicotine (as bitartrate) 1 mg, net price pack of 12 = £1.71, pack of 36 = £4.27, pack of 96 = £9.12; 2 mg, net price pack of 12 = £1.99, pack of 36 = £4.95, pack of 96 = £10.60. Label: 24

Excipients: include aspartame (section 9.4.1)

Dose: initially 1 lozenge every 1–2 hours, when urge to smoke occurs; max. 30 mg daily; withdraw gradually after 3 months; max. period of treatment should not usually exceed 6 months

TTS Patches, self-adhesive, all yellowish-ochre, nicotine, *'10' patch* (releasing approx. 7 mg/24 hours), net price 7 = £9.12; *'20' patch* (releasing approx. 14 mg/24 hours), net price 2 = £2.57, 7 = £9.40; *'30' patch* (releasing approx. 21 mg/24 hours), net price 2 = £2.85, 7 = £9.97, 21 = £24.51

Dose: apply to dry, non-hairy skin on trunk or upper arm, removing after 24 hours and siting replacement patch on a different area (avoid using the same area for several days); individuals smoking 20 cigarettes daily or fewer, initially '20' patch daily; individuals smoking more than 20 cigarettes daily, initially '30' patch daily; withdraw gradually, reducing dose every 3–4 weeks; review treatment if abstinence not achieved in 3 months

NiQuitin CQ® (GSK Consumer Healthcare)

Chewing gum, sugar-free, mint-flavour, nicotine 2 mg, net price pack of 12 = £1.71, pack of 24 = £2.85, pack of 96 = £8.55; 4 mg, net price pack of 12 = £1.71, pack of 24 = £2.85, pack of 96 = £8.55

Dose: initially 1 piece chewed slowly for approx. 30 minutes, when urge to smoke occurs; max. 15 pieces daily; withdraw gradually after 3 months

Lozenges, sugar-free, nicotine (as polacrilex) 2 mg, net price pack of 36 = £5.12, pack of 72 = £9.97; 4 mg, pack of 36 = £5.12, pack of 72 = £9.97. Contains 0.65 mmol Na^+/lozenge

Excipients: include aspartame (section 9.4.1)

Dose: initially 1 lozenge every 1–2 hours (when urge to smoke occurs) (max. 15 lozenges daily) for 6 weeks, then 1 lozenge every 2–4 hours for 3 weeks, then 1 lozenge every 4–8 hours for 3 weeks; withdraw gradually after 3 months; max. period of treatment should not exceed 6 months

Patches, self-adhesive, pink/beige, nicotine *'7 mg' patch* (releasing approx. 7 mg/24 hours), net price 7 = £9.97; *'14 mg' patch* (releasing approx. 14 mg/24 hours), 7 = £9.97; *'21 mg' patch* (releasing approx. 21 mg/24 hours), 7 = £9.97, 14 = £18.79

NOTE. Also available as a clear patch

Dose: apply on waking to dry, non-hairy skin site, removing after 24 hours and siting replacement patch on different area (avoid using same area for 7 days); individuals smoking 10 or more cigarettes daily, initially '21-mg' patch daily for 6 weeks then '14-mg' patch daily for 2 weeks then '7-mg' patch daily for 2 weeks; review treatment if abstinence not achieved in 10 weeks

Individuals smoking less than 10 cigarettes daily, initially '14-mg' patch daily for 6 weeks then '7-mg' patch daily for 2 weeks

NOTE. Patients using the '21-mg' patch who experience excessive side-effects, which do not resolve within a few days, should change to '14-mg' patch for the remainder of the initial 6 weeks before switching to the '7-mg' patch for the final 2 weeks

Opioid dependence

The management of opioid dependence requires medical, social, and psychological treatment; access to a multidisciplinary team is valuable. Treatment with opioid substitutes or with naltrexone is best initiated under the supervision of an appropriately qualified physician.

Methadone, an opioid *agonist*, can be substituted for opioids such as diamorphine, preventing the onset of withdrawal symptoms; it is itself addictive and should only be prescribed for those who are physically dependent on opioids. It is administered in a single daily dose usually as methadone oral solution 1 mg/mL. The dose is adjusted according to the degree of dependence.

Buprenorphine is an opioid partial agonist. Because of its abuse and dependence potential it should be prescribed only for those who are already physically dependent on opioids. It can be used as substitution therapy for patients with moderate opioid dependence. In patients dependent on high doses of opioids, buprenorphine may precipitate withdrawal due to its partial antagonist properties; in these patients, the daily opioid dose should be reduced gradually before initiating therapy with buprenorphine.

Naltrexone, an opioid *antagonist*, blocks the action of opioids and precipitates withdrawal symptoms in opioid-dependent subjects. Because the euphoric action of opioid agonists is blocked by naltrexone it is given to former addicts as an aid to prevent relapse.

Lofexidine is used for the alleviation of symptoms in individuals whose opioid use is well controlled and are undergoing opioid withdrawal. Like clonidine it is an alpha-adrenergic agonist and appears to act centrally to produce a reduction in sympathetic tone, but reduction in blood pressure is less marked.

BUPRENORPHINE

Indications: adjunct in the treatment of opioid dependence; premedication, peri-operative analgesia, analgesia in other situations (section 4.7.2)

Cautions: see section 4.7.2 and notes above; effects only partially reversed by naloxone
Contra-indications: see section 4.7.2; breast-feeding (Appendix 5)
Side-effects: see section 4.7.2
Dose: *by sublingual administration*, initially, 0.8–4 mg as a single daily dose, adjusted according to response; max. 32 mg daily; withdraw gradually; CHILD under 16 years not recommended

NOTE. In those who have not undergone opioid withdrawal, buprenorphine should be administered at least 4 hours after last use of opioid or when signs of craving appear

For those receiving methadone, dose of methadone should be reduced to max. 30 mg daily before starting buprenorphine

Subutex® (Schering-Plough) CD
Tablets (sublingual), buprenorphine (as hydrochloride) 400 micrograms, net price 7-tab pack = £1.60; 2 mg, 7-tab pack = £6.72; 8 mg, 7-tab pack = £20.16. Label: 2, 26

LOFEXIDINE HYDROCHLORIDE

Indications: management of symptoms of opioid withdrawal
Cautions: severe coronary insufficiency, recent myocardial infarction, cerebrovascular disease, marked bradycardia (monitor pulse rate frequently); history of QT prolongation; concomitant administration of drugs that prolong QT interval; renal impairment; history of depression (on longer treatment); pregnancy and breast-feeding; withdraw gradually over 2–4 days (or longer) to minimise risk of rebound hypertension and associated symptoms; **interactions:** Appendix 1 (lofexidine)
Side-effects: drowsiness, dry mucous membranes (particularly dry mouth, throat and nose), hypotension, bradycardia, rebound hypertension on withdrawal (see Cautions); sedation and coma in overdosage
Dose: initially, 200 micrograms twice daily, increased as necessary in steps of 200–400 micrograms daily to max. 2.4 mg daily; recommended duration of treatment 7–10 days if no opioid use (but longer may be required); withdraw gradually over 2–4 days or longer; CHILD not recommended

BritLofex® (Britannia) PoM
Tablets, peach, f/c, lofexidine hydrochloride 200 micrograms. Net price 60-tab pack = £61.79. Label: 2

METHADONE HYDROCHLORIDE

Indications: adjunct in treatment of opioid dependence, see notes above; analgesia (section 4.7.2); cough in terminal disease (section 3.9.1)
Cautions: section 4.7.2
Contra-indications: section 4.7.2
Side-effects: section 4.7.2; **overdosage:** see Emergency Treatment of Poisoning, p. 31

IMPORTANT. Methadone, even in low doses is a **special hazard** for children; non-dependent adults are also at risk of toxicity; dependent adults are at risk if tolerance is incorrectly assessed during induction

INCOMPATIBILITY. Syrup preserved with hydroxybenzoate (parabens) esters may be incompatible with methadone hydrochloride.

Dose: initially 10–40 mg daily, increased by up to 10 mg daily (max. weekly increase 30 mg) until no signs of withdrawal or intoxication; usual dose range 60–120 mg daily; CHILD not recommended (see also important note above)

NOTE. Methadone hydrochloride doses in the BNF may differ from those in the product literature

Methadone (Non-proprietary) CD
Oral solution 1 mg/mL, methadone hydrochloride 1 mg/mL, net price 30 mL = 44p, 50 mL = 73p, 100 mL = £1.35, 500 mL = £7.59. Label: 2

Brands include *Metharose*® (sugar-free), *Physeptone* (also as sugar-free)

IMPORTANT. This preparation is 2½ times the strength of Methadone Linctus; many preparations of this strength are licensed for opioid drug addiction only but some are also licensed for analgesia in severe pain

Injection ▼, methadone hydrochloride 25 mg/mL, net price 2-mL amp = £2.05; 50 mg/mL, 1-mL amp = £2.05

Brands include *Synastone*®

Methadose® (Rosemont) CD
Oral concentrate, methadone hydrochloride 10 mg/mL (blue), net price 150 mL = £12.01; 20 mg/mL (brown), 150 mL = £24.02. Label: 2

NOTE. The final strength of the methadone mixture to be dispensed to the patient must be specified on the prescription

IMPORTANT. Care is required in prescribing and dispensing the **correct strength** since any confusion could lead to an overdose; this preparation should be dispensed only **after dilution** as appropriate with *Methadose*® *Diluent* (life of diluted solution 3 months) and is for drug dependent persons (see also p. 7)

NALTREXONE HYDROCHLORIDE

Indications: adjunct to prevent relapse in detoxified formerly opioid-dependent patients (who have remained opioid-free for at least 7–10 days)
Cautions: hepatic and renal impairment; liver function tests needed before and during treatment; test for opioid dependence with naloxone; avoid concomitant use of opioids but increased dose of opioid analgesic may be required for pain (monitor for opioid intoxication); pregnancy, breast-feeding

WARNING FOR PATIENTS. Patients need to be warned that an attempt to overcome the block could result in acute opioid intoxication

Contra-indications: patients currently dependent on opioids; acute hepatitis or liver failure
Side-effects: nausea, vomiting, abdominal pain; anxiety, nervousness, sleeping difficulty, headache, reduced energy; joint and muscle pain; less frequently, loss of appetite, diarrhoea, constipation, increased thirst; chest pain; increased sweating and lacrimation; increased energy, 'feeling down', irritability, dizziness, chills; delayed ejaculation, decreased potency; rash; occasionally, liver function abnormalities; reversible idiopathic thrombocytopenia reported
Dose: (initiate in specialist clinics only) 25 mg initially then 50 mg daily; the total weekly dose may be divided and given on 3 days of the week for improved compliance (e.g. 100 mg on Monday and Wednesday, and 150 mg on Friday); CHILD not recommended

Nalorex® (Bristol-Myers Squibb) PoM
Tablets, yellow, f/c, scored, naltrexone hydrochloride 50 mg. Net price 28-tab pack = £42.51

4.11 Drugs for dementia

Acetylcholinesterase inhibiting drugs are used in the treatment of Alzheimer's disease, specifically for mild to moderate disease. The evidence to support the use of these drugs relates to their cognitive enhancement.

Treatment with drugs for dementia should be initiated and supervised only by a specialist experienced in the management of dementia.

Benefit is assessed by repeating the cognitive assessment at around 3 months. Such assessment cannot demonstrate how the disease may have progressed in the absence of treatment but it can give a good guide to response. Up to half the patients given these drugs will show a slower rate of cognitive decline. The drug should be discontinued in those thought not to be responding. Many specialists repeat the cognitive assessment 4 to 6 weeks after discontinuation to assess deterioration; if significant deterioration occurs during this short period, consideration should be given to restarting therapy.

Donepezil is a reversible inhibitor of acetylcholinesterase that can be given once daily. **Galantamine** is a reversible inhibitor of acetylcholinesterase and it also has nicotinic receptor agonist properties. It is given twice daily. **Rivastigmine** is a reversible non-competitive inhibitor of acetylcholinesterases, which is given twice daily.

Acetylcholinesterase inhibitors can cause unwanted dose-related cholinergic effects and should be started at a low dose and the dose increased according to response and tolerability.

Memantine is a NMDA-receptor antagonist that affects glutamate transmission; it is licensed for treating moderate to severe Alzheimer's disease.

NICE guidance (Alzheimer's disease). NICE has recommended (January 2001) that, for the adjunctive treatment of mild and moderate Alzheimer's disease in those whose mini mental-state examination (MMSE) score is above 12 points, donepezil, galantamine, and rivastigmine should be available under the following conditions:

- Alzheimer's disease must be diagnosed in a specialist clinic; the clinic should also assess cognitive, global and behavioural functioning, activities of daily living, and the likelihood of compliance with treatment;
- treatment should be initiated by specialists but may be continued by general practitioners under a shared-care protocol;
- the carers' views of the condition should be sought before and during drug treatment;
- the patient should be assessed 2–4 months after maintenance dose is established; drug treatment should continue only if MMSE score has improved or has not deteriorated *and* if behavioural or functional assessment shows improvement;
- the patient should be assessed every 6 months and drug treatment should normally continue only if MMSE score remains above 12 points and if treatment is considered to have a worthwhile effect on the global, functional and behavioural condition.

DONEPEZIL HYDROCHLORIDE

Indications: mild to moderate dementia in Alzheimer's disease

Cautions: sick sinus syndrome or other supraventricular conduction abnormalities; susceptibility to peptic ulcers; asthma, chronic obstructive pulmonary disease; may exacerbate extrapyramidal symptoms; hepatic impairment; **interactions:** Appendix 1 (parasympathomimetics)

Contra-indications: pregnancy and breast-feeding

Side-effects: nausea, vomiting, anorexia, diarrhoea, fatigue, insomnia, headache, dizziness, syncope, psychiatric disturbances, muscle cramps, urinary incontinence, rash, pruritus; less frequently, bradycardia, convulsions, gastric and duodenal ulcers, gastro-intestinal haemorrhage; rarely, sino-atrial block, AV block, hepatitis reported; potential for bladder outflow obstruction

Dose: 5 mg once daily at bedtime, increased if necessary after one month to 10 mg daily; max. 10 mg daily

Aricept® (Pfizer, Eisai) PoM

Tablets, f/c, donepezil hydrochloride 5 mg, net price 28-tab pack = £63.54; 10 mg (yellow), 28-tab pack = £89.06.

GALANTAMINE

Indications: mild to moderate dementia in Alzheimer's disease

Cautions: sick sinus syndrome or other supraventricular conduction abnormalities; susceptibility to peptic ulcers; asthma, chronic obstructive pulmonary disease; avoid in urinary retention and gastro-intestinal obstruction; hepatic impairment (Appendix 2—avoid if severe); pregnancy (Appendix 4); **interactions:** Appendix 1 (parasympathomimetics)

Contra-indications: severe renal impairment; breast-feeding (Appendix 5)

Side-effects: nausea, vomiting, diarrhoea, abdominal pain, dyspepsia; rhinitis; drowsiness, dizziness, insomnia, confusion, depression, headache, fatigue, anorexia; weight loss; *rarely* bradycardia, syncope, convulsions, hallucinations, agitation, aggression, exacerbation of Parkinson's disease, hypokalaemia, rash; *very rarely* gastrointestinal bleeding, dysphagia, dehydration, hypotension, AV block, tremor, sweating

Dose: initially 4 mg twice daily for 4 weeks increased to 8 mg twice daily for 4 weeks; maintenance 8–12 mg twice daily

Reminyl® (Shire) PoM

Tablets, all f/c, galantamine (as hydrobromide) 4 mg (white), net price 56-tab pack = £54.60; 8 mg (pink), 56-tab pack = £68.32; 12 mg (orange-brown), 56-tab pack = £84.00 Label: 3, 21

Oral solution, galantamine (as hydrobromide) 4 mg/mL, net price 100 mL with pipette = £120.00. Label: 3, 21

■ Modified release

Reminyl® **XL** (Shire) PoM

Capsules, m/r, galantamine (as hydrobromide) 8 mg (white), net price 28-cap pack = £54.60; 16 mg (pink), 28-cap pack = £68.32; 24 mg (beige), 28-cap pack = £84.00. Label: 3, 21, 25

Dose: initially 8 mg daily for 4 weeks increased to 16 mg daily for 4 weeks; maintenance 16–24 mg daily

MEMANTINE HYDROCHLORIDE

Indications: moderate to severe dementia in Alzheimer's disease

Cautions: renal impairment (avoid if severe—Appendix 3); history of convulsions; pregnancy (Appendix 4); **interactions:** Appendix 1 (memantine)

Contra-indications: breast-feeding

Side-effects: dizziness, confusion, headache, hallucinations, tiredness; less commonly, vomiting, anxiety, hypertonia, cystitis, increased libido; seizures reported

Dose: initially, 5 mg in the morning, increased in steps of 5 mg at intervals of 1 week up to max. 10 mg twice daily

Ebixa® (Lundbeck) ▼ PoM

Tablets, f/c, scored, memantine hydrochloride 10 mg, net price 28-tab pack = £34.50, 56-tab pack = £69.01, 112-tab pack = £138.01

Oral drops, memantine hydrochloride 10 mg/g, net price 50 g = £61.61, 100 g = £123.23

NOTE. 5 mg ≡ 10 drops of memantine hydrochloride oral drops

RIVASTIGMINE

Indications: mild to moderate dementia in Alzheimer's disease

Cautions: renal impairment, mild to moderate hepatic impairment (Appendix 2); sick sinus syndrome, conduction abnormalities; gastric or duodenal ulcers (and those at risk of developing ulcers); history of asthma or chronic obstructive pulmonary disease; history of seizures, bladder outflow obstruction, pregnancy (Appendix 4); may exacerbate extrapyramidal symptoms (including worsening of Parkinson's disease); monitor body-weight; **interactions:** Appendix 1 (parasympathomimetics)

NOTE. If treatment interrupted for more than several days, re–introduce with initial dose and increase gradually (see Dose)

Contra-indications: breast-feeding (Appendix 5)

Side-effects: nausea, vomiting, diarrhoea, dyspepsia, anorexia, abdominal pain; dizziness, headache, drowsiness, tremor, asthenia, malaise, agitation, confusion; sweating; less commonly, syncope, depression, insomnia; rarely gastric or duodenal ulceration, gastro-intestinal haemorrhage, pancreatitis, angina pectoris, arrhythmias, bradycardia, hypertension, convulsions, hallucinations, urinary infection, rash

NOTE. Gastro-intestinal side-effects may occur more commonly in women

Dose: initially 1.5 mg twice daily, increased in steps of 1.5 mg twice daily at intervals of at least 2 weeks according to response and tolerance; usual range 3–6 mg twice daily; max. 6 mg twice daily

Exelon® (Novartis) PoM

Capsules, rivastigmine (as hydrogen tartrate) 1.5 mg (yellow), net price 28-cap pack = £34.02, 56-cap pack = £68.04; 3 mg (orange), 28-cap pack = £34.02, 56-cap pack = £68.04; 4.5 mg (red), 28-cap pack = £34.02, 56-cap pack = £68.04; 6 mg (red/orange), 28-cap pack = £34.02, 56-cap pack = £68.04. Label: 21, 25

Oral solution, rivastigmine (as hydrogen tartrate) 2 mg/mL, net price 120 mL (with oral syringe) = £116.64. Label: 21

5: Infections

Notifiable diseases

Doctors must notify the Proper Officer of the local authority (usually the consultant in communicable disease control) when attending a patient suspected of suffering from any of the diseases listed below; a form is available from the Proper Officer.

Anthrax	Ophthalmia neonatorum
Cholera	Paratyphoid fever
Diphtheria	Plague
Dysentery (amoebic or bacillary)	Poliomyelitis, acute
Encephalitis, acute	Rabies
Food poisoning	Relapsing fever
Haemorrhagic fever (viral)	Rubella
Hepatitis, viral	Scarlet fever
Leprosy	Smallpox
Leptospirosis	Tetanus
Malaria	Tuberculosis
Measles	Typhoid fever
Meningitis	Typhus
Meningococcal septicaemia (without meningitis)	Whooping cough
Mumps	Yellow fever

NOTE. It is good practice for doctors to also inform the consultant in communicable disease control of instances of other infections (e.g. psittacosis) where there could be a public health risk.

5.1 Antibacterial drugs

CHOICE OF A SUITABLE DRUG. Before selecting an antibacterial the clinician must first consider two factors—the patient and the known or likely causative organism. Factors related to the patient which must be considered include history of allergy, renal and hepatic function, susceptibility to infection (i.e. whether immunocompromised), ability to tolerate drugs by mouth, severity of illness, ethnic origin, age, whether taking other medication and, if female, whether pregnant, breast-feeding or taking an oral contraceptive.

The known or likely organism and its antibacterial sensitivity, in association with the above factors, will suggest one or more antibacterials, the final choice depending on the microbiological, pharmacological, and toxicological properties.

An example of a rational approach to the selection of an antibacterial is treatment of a urinary-tract infection in a patient complaining of nausea in early pregnancy. The organism is reported as being resistant to ampicillin but sensitive to nitrofurantoin (can cause nausea), gentamicin (can be given only by injection and best avoided in pregnancy), tetracycline (causes dental discoloration) and trimethoprim (folate antagonist therefore theoretical teratogenic risk), and cefalexin. The safest antibiotics in pregnancy are the penicillins and cephalosporins; therefore, cefalexin would be indicated for this patient.

The principles involved in selection of an antibacterial must allow for a number of variables including changing renal and hepatic function, increasing bacterial resistance, and new information on side-effects. Duration of therapy, dosage, and route of administration depend on site, type and severity of infection and response.

ANTIBACTERIAL POLICIES. Local policies often limit the antibacterials that may be used to achieve reasonable economy consistent with adequate cover, and to reduce the development of resistant organisms. A policy may indicate a range of drugs for general use, and permit other drugs only on the advice of the microbiologist or physician responsible for the control of infectious diseases.

BEFORE STARTING THERAPY. The following precepts should be considered before starting:

- Viral infections should not be treated with antibacterials. However, antibacterials are occasionally helpful in controlling secondary bacterial infection (e.g. acute necrotising ulcerative gingivitis secondary to herpes simplex infection);
- Samples should be taken for culture and sensitivity testing; **'blind'** antibacterial prescribing for unexplained pyrexia usually leads to further difficulty in establishing the diagnosis;
- Knowledge of **prevalent organisms** and their current sensitivity is of great help in choosing an antibacterial before bacteriological confirmation is available;
- The **dose** of an antibacterial varies according to a number of factors including age, weight, hepatic function, renal function, and severity of infection. The prescribing of the so-called 'standard' dose in serious infections may result in failure of treatment or even death of the patient; therefore it is important to prescribe a dose appropriate to the condition. An inadequate dose may also increase the likelihood of antibacterial resistance. On the other hand, for an antibacterial with a narrow margin between the toxic and therapeutic dose (e.g. an aminoglycoside) it is also important to avoid an excessive dose and the concentration of the drug in the plasma may need to be monitored;
- The **route** of administration of an antibacterial often depends on the severity of the infection. Life-threatening infections require intravenous therapy. Whenever possible painful intramuscular injections should be avoided in children;
- **Duration** of therapy depends on the nature of the infection and the response to treatment. Courses should not be unduly prolonged because they encourage resistance, they may lead to side-effects and they are costly. However, in certain infections such as tuberculosis or chronic osteomyelitis it is necessary to treat for prolonged periods. Conversely a single dose of an antibacterial may cure uncomplicated urinary-tract infections.

ORAL BACTERIAL INFECTIONS. Antibacterial drugs should only be prescribed for the *treatment* of oral infections on the basis of defined need. They may be used in conjunction with (but not as an alternative to) other appropriate measures, such as providing drainage or extracting a tooth.

The 'blind' prescribing of an antibacterial for unexplained pyrexia, cervical lymphadenopathy, or facial swelling can lead to difficulty in establishing the diagnosis. Bacteriological sampling should always be carried out in severe oral infections.

Oral infections which call for antibacterial treatment include acute suppurative pulpitis, acute periapical or periodontal abscess, cellulitis, oral-antral fistula (and acute sinusitis), severe pericoronitis, localised osteitis, acute necrotising ulcerative gingivitis, and destructive forms of chronic periodontal disease. Most of these infections are readily resolved by the early establishment of drainage and removal of the cause (typically an infected necrotic pulp). Antibacterials may be indicated if treatment has to be delayed and they are essential in immunocompromised patients or in those with conditions such as diabetes or Paget's disease. Certain rarer infections including bacterial sialadenitis, osteomyelitis, actinomycosis, and infections involving fascial spaces such as Ludwig's angina, require antibiotics and specialist hospital care.

Antibacterial drugs may also be useful after dental surgery in some cases of spreading infection. Infection may spread to involve local lymph nodes, to fascial spaces (where it can cause airway obstruction), or into the bloodstream (where it can lead to cavernous sinus thrombosis and other serious complications). Extension of an infection can also lead to maxillary sinusitis; osteomyelitis is a complication, which usually arises when host resistance is reduced.

If the oral infection fails to respond to antibacterial treatment within 48 hours the antibacterial should be changed, preferably on the basis of bacteriological investigation. Failure to respond may also suggest an incorrect diagnosis, lack of essential additional measures (such as drainage), poor host resistance, or poor patient compliance.

Combination of a penicillin (or erythromycin) with metronidazole may sometimes be helpful for the treatment of severe or resistant oral infections.

See also **Penicillins** (section 5.1.1), **Cephalosporins** (section 5.1.2), **Tetracyclines** (section 5.1.3), **Macrolides** (section 5.1.5), **Clindamycin** (section 5.1.6), **Metronidazole** (section 5.1.11), **Fusidic acid** (section 13.10.1.2).

SUPERINFECTION. In general, broad-spectrum antibacterial drugs such as the cephalosporins are more likely to be associated with adverse reactions related to the selection of resistant organisms e.g. *fungal infections* or *antibiotic-associated colitis* (pseudomembranous colitis); other problems associated with superinfection include vaginitis and pruritus ani.

THERAPY. Suggested treatment is shown in table 1. When the pathogen has been isolated treatment may be changed to a more appropriate antibacterial if necessary. If no bacterium is cultured the antibacterial can be continued or stopped on clinical grounds. Infections for which prophylaxis is useful are listed in table 2.

Table 1. Summary of antibacterial therapy

If treating a patient suspected of suffering from a notifiable disease, the consultant in communicable disease control should be informed (see p. 266)

Gastro-intestinal system

Gastro-enteritis

Antibacterial not usually indicated

Frequently self-limiting and may not be bacterial

Campylobacter enteritis

Ciprofloxacin *or* erythromycin

Invasive salmonellosis

Ciprofloxacin *or* cefotaxime

Includes severe infections which may be invasive

Shigellosis

Ciprofloxacin *or* trimethoprim

Antibacterial not indicated for mild cases. Ciprofloxacin should be used for trimethoprim-resistant strains

Typhoid fever

Ciprofloxacin *or* cefotaxime *or* chloramphenicol

Infections from Indian subcontinent, Middle-East, and South-East Asia may be multiple-antibacterial-resistant and sensitivity should be tested; azithromycin [unlicensed indication] may be an option in mild or moderate disease caused by multiple antibacterial-resistant organisms

Antibiotic-associated colitis (pseudomembranous colitis)

Oral metronidazole *or* oral vancomycin

Give metronidazole by intravenous infusion if oral treatment inappropriate

Biliary-tract infection

A cephalosporin *or* gentamicin

Peritonitis

A cephalosporin (*or* gentamicin) + metronidazole (*or* clindamycin)

Peritoneal dialysis-associated peritonitis

Either vancomycin[1] + ceftazidime added to dialysis fluid *or* vancomycin added to dialysis fluid + ciprofloxacin by mouth

Treat for 14 days or longer

Cardiovascular system

Endocarditis: initial 'blind' therapy

Flucloxacillin (*or* benzylpenicillin if symptoms less severe) + gentamicin

Substitute flucloxacillin (or benzylpenicillin) with vancomycin + rifampicin if cardiac prostheses present, or if penicillin-allergic, or if methicillin-resistant *Staphylococcus aureus* suspected

Endocarditis caused by staphylococci

Flucloxacillin (*or* vancomycin + rifampicin if penicillin-allergic or if methicillin-resistant *Staphylococcus aureus*)

Treat for at least 4 weeks; treat prosthetic valve endocarditis for at least 6 weeks and if using flucloxacillin add rifampicin for at least 2 weeks

Endocarditis caused by streptococci (e.g. viridans streptococci)

Benzylpenicillin (*or* vancomycin[1] if penicillin-allergic or highly penicillin-resistant) + gentamicin

Treat endocarditis caused by fully sensitive streptococci with benzylpenicillin or vancomycin alone for 4 weeks *or* (if no cardiac or embolic complications) with benzylpenicillin + gentamicin for 2 weeks; treat more resistant organisms for 4–6 weeks (stopping gentamicin after 2 weeks for organisms moderately sensitive to penicillin); if aminoglycoside cannot be used and if streptococci moderately sensitive to penicillin, treat with benzylpenicillin alone for 4 weeks; treat prosthetic valve endocarditis for at least 6 weeks (stopping gentamicin after 2 weeks if organisms fully sensitive to penicillin)

Endocarditis caused by enterococci (e.g. *Enterococcus faecalis*)

Amoxicillin[2] (*or* vancomycin[1] if penicillin-allergic or penicillin-resistant) + gentamicin

Treat for at least 4 weeks (at least 6 weeks for prosthetic valve endocarditis); if gentamicin-resistant, substitute gentamicin with streptomycin

Endocarditis caused by haemophilus, actinobacillus, cardiobacterium, eikenella, and kingella species ('HACEK' organisms)

Amoxicillin[2] (*or* ceftriaxone if amoxicillin-resistant) + low-dose gentamicin

Treat for 4 weeks (6 weeks for prosthetic valve endocarditis); stop gentamicin after 2 weeks

Respiratory system

***Haemophilus influenzae* epiglottitis**

Cefotaxime *or* chloramphenicol

Give intravenously

Exacerbations of chronic bronchitis

Amoxicillin[2] *or* tetracycline (*or* erythromycin[3])

Some pneumococci and *Haemophilus influenzae* strains tetracycline-resistant; 15% *H. influenzae* strains amoxicillin-resistant

Uncomplicated community-acquired pneumonia

Amoxicillin[2] (*or* benzylpenicillin if previously healthy chest *or* erythromycin[3] if penicillin-allergic)

Add flucloxacillin if staphylococci suspected, e.g. in influenza or measles; treat for 7 days (14–21 days for infections caused by staphylococci); pneumococci with decreased penicillin sensitivity being isolated but not yet common in UK; add erythromycin[3] if atypical pathogens suspected

Severe community-acquired pneumonia of unknown aetiology

Cefuroxime (or cefotaxime) + erythromycin[3]

Add flucloxacillin if staphylococci suspected; treat for 10 days (14–21 days if staphylococci, legionella, or Gram-negative enteric bacilli suspected)

Pneumonia possibly caused by atypical pathogens

Erythromycin[3]

Severe Legionella infections may require addition of rifampicin; tetracycline is an alternative for chlamydial and mycoplasma infections; treat for at least 14 days (14–21 days for legionella)

Hospital-acquired pneumonia

A broad-spectrum cephalosporin (e.g. cefotaxime or ceftazidime) *or* an antipseudomonal penicillin or another antipseudomonal beta-lactam

An aminoglycoside may be added in severe illness

1. Where vancomycin is suggested teicoplanin may be used.

2. Where amoxicillin is suggested ampicillin may be used.

3. Where erythromycin is suggested another macrolide (e.g. azithromycin or clarithromycin) may be used.

Central nervous system

Meningitis: initial 'blind' therapy

- Transfer patient urgently to hospital.
- If bacterial meningitis and especially if *meningococcal disease* suspected, general practitioners should give benzylpenicillin (see p. 274 for dose) before urgent transfer to hospital; cefotaxime (section 5.1.2) may be an alternative in penicillin allergy; chloramphenicol (section 5.1.7) may be used if history of anaphylaxis to penicillin or to cephalosporins
- Consider adjunctive treatment with dexamethasone (particularly if pneumococcal meningitis suspected in adults) starting before or with first dose of antibacterial; avoid dexamethasone in septic shock, or if immunocompromised, or in meningitis following surgery

Meningitis caused by meningococci

Benzylpenicillin *or* cefotaxime

Treat for at least 5 days; substitute chloramphenicol if history of anaphylaxis to penicillin or to cephalosporins; to eliminate nasopharyngeal carriage give rifampicin for 2 days to patients treated with benzylpenicillin or chloramphenicol

Meningitis caused by pneumococci

Cefotaxime

Treat for 10–14 days; substitute benzylpenicillin if organism penicillin-sensitive; if organism highly penicillin- and cephalosporin-resistant, add vancomycin and if necessary rifampicin; consider early adjunctive treatment with dexamethasone (but may reduce penetration of vancomycin into cerebrospinal fluid; section 6.3.2)

Meningitis caused by *Haemophilus influenzae*

Cefotaxime

Treat for at least 10 days; substitute chloramphenicol if history of anaphylaxis to penicillin or to cephalosporins or if organism resistant to cefotaxime; consider early adjunctive treatment with dexamethasone (section 6.3.2); for *H. influenzae* type b give rifampicin for 4 days before hospital discharge

Meningitis caused by Listeria

Amoxicillin[1] + gentamicin

Treat for 10–14 days

Urinary tract

Acute pyelonephritis

A broad-spectrum cephalosporin *or* a quinolone

Treat for 14 days; longer treatment may be necessary in complicated pyelonephritis

Acute prostatitis

A quinolone *or* trimethoprim

Treat for 28 days; in severe infection, start treatment with a high dose broad-spectrum cephalosporin (e.g. cefuroxime or cefotaxime) + gentamicin

'Lower' urinary-tract infection

Trimethoprim *or* amoxicillin[1] *or* nitrofurantoin *or* oral cephalosporin

Treat for 7 days but a short course (e.g. 3 days) of trimethoprim or amoxicillin is usually adequate for uncomplicated urinary-tract infections in women

Genital system

Syphilis

Procaine benzylpenicillin [unlicensed] *or* doxycycline *or* erythromycin

Treat early syphilis for 14 days (10 days with procaine benzylpenicillin); treat late latent syphilis (asymptomatic infection of more than 2 years) with procaine benzylpenicillin for 17 days (or with doxycycline for 28 days); treat asymptomatic contacts of patients with infectious syphilis with doxycycline for 14 days; contact tracing recommended

Uncomplicated gonorrhoea

Cefixime [unlicensed indication] *or* ciprofloxacin

Single-dose treatment in uncomplicated infection; choice depends on locality where infection acquired; pharyngeal infection requires treatment with ceftriaxone; use ciprofloxacin only if organism sensitive; contact-tracing recommended; remember chlamydia

Uncomplicated genital chlamydial infection, non-gonococcal urethritis and non-specific genital infection

Doxycycline *or* azithromycin

Treat with doxycycline for 7 days or with azithromycin as a single dose; alternatively, treat with erythromycin for 14 days; contact tracing recommended

Pelvic inflammatory disease

Ofloxacin + metronidazole

Treat for at least 14 days; in severely ill patients substitute initial treatment with doxycycline + ceftriaxone + metronidazole, then switch to oral treatment with doxycycline + metronidazole to complete 14 days' treatment; contact tracing recommended; remember gonorrhoea

Blood

Community-acquired septicaemia

A broad-spectrum antipseudomonal penicillin (e.g. *Tazocin*®, *Timentin*®) *or* a broad-spectrum cephalosporin (e.g. ceftazidime, cefotaxime)

Add aminoglycoside if pseudomonas suspected, or if severe sepsis, or if patient recently discharged from hospital; add vancomycin[2] if methicillin-resistant *Staphylococcus aureus* suspected; add metronidazole to broad-spectrum cephalosporin if anaerobic infection suspected

Hospital-acquired septicaemia

A broad-spectrum antipseudomonal beta-lactam antibacterial (e.g. ceftazidime, *Tazocin*®, *Timentin*®, imipenem (with cilastatin as *Primaxin*®) *or* meropenem)

Add aminoglycoside if pseudomonas suspected, or if multiple-resistant organisms suspected, or if severe sepsis; add vancomycin[2] if methicillin-resistant *Staphylococcus aureus* suspected; add metronidazole to broad-spectrum cephalosporin if anaerobic infection suspected

Septicaemia related to vascular catheter

Vancomycin[2]

Add an aminoglycoside + a broad-spectrum antipseudomonal beta-lactam if Gram-negative sepsis suspected, especially in the immunocompromised; consider removing vascular catheter, particularly if infection caused by *Staphylococcus aureus*, pseudomonas, or candida

Meningococcal septicaemia

Benzylpenicillin *or* cefotaxime

If meningococcal disease suspected, general practitioners advised to give a single dose of benzylpenicillin (see p. 274 for dose) before urgent transfer to hospital; cefotaxime (section 5.1.2) may be an alternative in penicillin allergy; chloramphenicol may be used if history of anaphylaxis to penicillin or to cephalosporins; give rifampicin for 2 days to patients treated with benzylpenicillin or chloramphenicol

Musculoskeletal system

Osteomyelitis

Flucloxacillin *or* clindamycin if penicillin-allergic (*or* vancomycin[2] if resistant *Staphylococcus epidermidis* or methicillin-resistant *Staph. aureus*)

Treat acute infection for 4–6 weeks and chronic infection for at least 12 weeks; combine vancomycin[2] with either fusidic acid or rifampicin if prostheses present or if life-threatening condition

Septic arthritis

Flucloxacillin + fusidic acid *or* clindamycin alone if penicillin-allergic (*or* vancomycin[2] if resistant *Staphylococcus epidermidis* or methicillin-resistant *Staph. aureus*)

Treat for 6–12 weeks; combine vancomycin[2] with either fusidic acid or rifampicin if prostheses present or if life-threatening condition

---

1. Where amoxicillin is suggested ampicillin may be used.

2. Where vancomycin is suggested teicoplanin may be used.

Eye

Purulent conjunctivitis

Chloramphenicol *or* gentamicin eye-drops

Ear, nose, and oropharynx

Pericoronitis

Metronidazole *or* amoxicillin

Antibacterial required only in presence of systemic features of infection or of trismus or persistent swelling despite local treatment; treat for 3 days or until symptoms resolve

Acute necrotising ulcerative gingivitis

Metronidazole *or* amoxicillin

Antibacterial required only if systemic features of infection; treat for 3 days or until symptoms resolve

Periapical or periodontal abscess

Amoxicillin *or* metronidazole

Antibacterial required only in severe disease with cellulitis or if systemic features of infection; treat for 5 days

Periodontitis

Metronidazole *or* doxycycline

Antibacterial required for severe disease or disease unresponsive to local treatment

Throat infections

Phenoxymethylpenicillin (*or* erythromycin[1] if penicillin-allergic)

Most throat infections are caused by viruses and many do not require antibiotic therapy; prescribe antibacterial for beta-haemolytic streptococcal pharyngitis (treat for 10 days), if history of valvular heart disease, if marked systemic upset, if peritonsillar cellulitis or if at increased risk from acute infection (e.g. in immunosuppression, diabetes); **avoid** amoxicillin if possibility of glandular fever, see section 5.1.1.3; initial parenteral therapy (in severe infection) with benzylpenicillin, then oral therapy with phenoxymethylpenicillin *or* amoxicillin[2]

Sinusitis

Amoxicillin[2] *or* doxycycline *or* erythromycin[1]

Antibacterial should usually be used only for persistent symptoms and purulent discharge lasting at least 7 days or if severe symptoms; treat for 7–10 days

Otitis externa

Flucloxacillin (*or* erythromycin[1] if penicillin-allergic)

Use ciprofloxacin (or an aminoglycoside) if pseudomonas suspected, see section 12.1.1

Otitis media

Amoxicillin[2] (*or* erythromycin[1] if penicillin-allergic)

Many infections caused by viruses; most uncomplicated cases resolve without antibacterial treatment; in children without systemic features, antibacterial treatment may be started after 72 hours if no improvement, or earlier if deterioration; treat for 5 days (longer if severely ill); initial parenteral therapy in severe infections; consider co-amoxiclav or ceftriaxone if no improvement after 24–48 hours

Skin

Impetigo

Topical fusidic acid (*or* mupirocin if methicillin-resistant *Staphylococcus aureus*); oral flucloxacillin *or* erythromycin[1] if widespread

Topical treatment for 7 days usually adequate; max. duration of topical treatment 10 days; seek local microbiology advice before using topical treatment in hospital; oral treatment for 7 days; add phenoxymethylpenicillin to flucloxacillin if streptococcal infection suspected

1. Where erythromycin is suggested another macrolide (e.g. azithromycin or clarithromycin) may be used.

2. Where amoxicillin is suggested ampicillin may be used.

Erysipelas

Phenoxymethylpenicillin (*or* erythromycin[1] if penicillin-allergic)

Add flucloxacillin to phenoxymethylpenicillin if staphylococcus suspected; substitute benzylpenicillin for phenoxymethylpenicillin if parenteral treatment required

Cellulitis

Benzylpenicillin + flucloxacillin (*or* erythromycin[1] alone if penicillin-allergic)

Substitute phenoxymethylpenicillin for benzylpenicillin if oral treatment appropriate; discontinue flucloxacillin if streptococcal infection confirmed

Animal and human bites

Co-amoxiclav alone (*or* doxycycline + metronidazole if penicillin-allergic)

Cleanse wound thoroughly; for tetanus-prone wound, give human tetanus immunoglobulin (with a tetanus-containing vaccine if necessary, according to immunisation history and risk of infection), see under Tetanus Vaccines, section 14.4; consider rabies prophylaxis (section 14.4) for bites from animals in endemic countries; assess risk of blood-borne viruses

Acne

See section 13.6

Table 2. Summary of antibacterial prophylaxis

Prevention of recurrence of rheumatic fever

Phenoxymethylpenicillin 250 mg twice daily *or* sulfadiazine 1 g daily (500 mg daily for patients under 30 kg)

Prevention of secondary case of meningococcal meningitis[3]

Rifampicin 600 mg every 12 hours for 2 days; CHILD 10 mg/kg (under 1 year, 5 mg/kg) every 12 hours for 2 days

or ciprofloxacin [not licensed for this indication] 500 mg as a single dose; CHILD 5–12 years 250 mg

or i/m ceftriaxone [not licensed for this indication] 250 mg as a single dose; CHILD under 12 years 125 mg

Prevention of secondary case of *Haemophilus influenzae* type b disease[3]

Rifampicin 600 mg once daily for 4 days (regimen of choice for adults); CHILD 1–3 months 10 mg/kg once daily for 4 days, over 3 months 20 mg/kg once daily for 4 days (max. 600 mg daily)

Prevention of secondary case of diphtheria in non-immune patient

Erythromycin 500 mg every 6 hours for 7 days; CHILD up to 2 years 125 mg every 6 hours, 2–8 years 250 mg every 6 hours

Treat for further 10 days if nasopharyngeal swabs positive after first 7 days' treatment

3. For details of those who should receive chemoprophylaxis contact a consultant in communicable disease control (or a consultant in infectious diseases or the local Health Protection Agency laboratory). Unless there has been mouth-to-mouth contact (or direct exposure to infectious droplets from a patient with meningococcal disease), healthcare workers do not generally require chemoprophylaxis.

Prevention of endocarditis[1] in patients with heart-valve lesion, septal defect, patent ductus, prosthetic valve, or history of endocarditis

Dental procedures[2] *under local or no anaesthesia*, patients who have not received more than a single dose of a penicillin[3] in the previous month, including those with a prosthetic valve (but not those who have had endocarditis), oral amoxicillin 3 g 1 hour before procedure; CHILD under 5 years quarter adult dose; 5–10 years half adult dose

patients who are penicillin-allergic or have received more than a single dose of a penicillin[3] in the previous month, oral clindamycin[4] 600 mg 1 hour before procedure; CHILD under 5 years clindamycin[4] 150 mg *or* azithromycin[5] 200 mg; 5–10 years clindamycin[4] 300 mg *or* azithromycin[5] 300 mg

patients who have had endocarditis, amoxicillin + gentamicin, as under general anaesthesia

Dental procedures[2] *under general anaesthesia*, *no special risk* (including patients who have not received more than a single dose of a penicillin in the previous month),
either i/v amoxicillin 1 g at induction, then oral amoxicillin 500 mg 6 hours later; CHILD under 5 years quarter adult dose; 5–10 years half adult dose
or oral amoxicillin 3 g 4 hours before induction then oral amoxicillin 3 g as soon as possible after procedure; CHILD under 5 years quarter adult dose; 5–10 years half adult dose

special risk (patients with a prosthetic valve or who have had endocarditis), i/v amoxicillin 1 g + i/v gentamicin 120 mg at induction, then oral amoxicillin 500 mg 6 hours later; CHILD under 5 years amoxicillin quarter adult dose, gentamicin 2 mg/kg; 5–10 years amoxicillin half adult dose, gentamicin 2 mg/kg

patients who are penicillin-allergic or who have received more than a single dose of a penicillin in the previous month,
either i/v vancomycin 1 g over at least 100 minutes then i/v gentamicin 120 mg at induction or 15 minutes before procedure; CHILD under 10 years vancomycin 20 mg/kg, gentamicin 2 mg/kg
or i/v teicoplanin 400 mg + gentamicin 120 mg at induction or 15 minutes before procedure; CHILD under 14 years teicoplanin 6 mg/kg, gentamicin 2 mg/kg
or i/v clindamycin[4] 300 mg over at least 10 minutes at induction or 15 minutes before procedure then oral or i/v clindamycin 150 mg 6 hours later; CHILD under 5 years quarter adult dose; 5–10 years half adult dose

Upper respiratory-tract procedures, as for dental procedures; post-operative dose may be given parenterally if swallowing is painful

Genito-urinary procedures, as for *special risk* patients undergoing dental procedures under general anaesthesia except that clindamycin is not given, see above; if urine infected, prophylaxis should also cover infective organism

Obstetric, gynaecological and gastro-intestinal procedures (prophylaxis required for patients with prosthetic valves or those who have had endocarditis only), as for genito-urinary procedures

Joint prostheses and dental treatment. Advice of a Working Party of the British Society for Antimicrobial Chemotherapy is that patients with prosthetic joint implants (including total hip replacements) do not require antibiotic prophylaxis for dental treatment. The Working Party considers that it is unacceptable to expose patients to the adverse effects of antibiotics when there is no evidence that such prophylaxis is of any benefit, but that those who develop any intercurrent infection require prompt treatment with antibiotics to which the infecting organisms are sensitive.
The Working Party has commented that joint infections have rarely been shown to follow dental procedures and are even more rarely caused by oral streptococci.

Dermatological procedures. Advice of a Working Party of the British Society for Antimicrobial Chemotherapy is that patients who undergo dermatological procedures[6] do not require antibacterial prophylaxis against endocarditis.

Immunosuppression and indwelling intraperitoneal catheters. Advice of a Working Party of the British Society for Antimicrobial Chemotherapy is that patients who are immunosuppressed (including transplant patients) and patients with indwelling intraperitoneal catheters do not require antibiotic prophylaxis for dental treatment provided there is no other indication for prophylaxis.
The Working Party has commented that there is little evidence that dental treatment is followed by infection in immunosuppressed and immunodeficient patients nor is there evidence that dental treatment is followed by infection in patients with indwelling intraperitoneal catheters.

---

1. Advice on the prevention of endocarditis reflects the recommendations of a Working Party of the British Society for Antimicrobial Chemotherapy, *Lancet*, 1982, **2**, 1323–26; *idem*, 1986, **1**, 1267; *idem*, 1990, **335**, 88–9; *idem*, 1992, **339**, 1292–93; *idem*, 1997, **350**, 1100; also *J Antimicrob Chemother*, 1993; **31**, 437–8

2. Dental procedures that require antibacterial prophylaxis are, *extractions*, *scaling*, and *surgery involving gingival tissues* (see also p. 23). Antibiotic prophylaxis for dental procedures may be supplemented with *chlorhexidine gluconate gel 1%* or *chlorhexidine gluconate mouthwash 0.2%*, used 5 minutes before procedure. Oral antibacterial should be taken in the presence of a dental surgeon or a dental nurse

3. For multistage procedures a max. of 2 single doses of a penicillin may be given in a month; alternative drugs should be used for further treatment and the penicillin should not be used again for 3–4 months

4. If **clindamycin** is used, periodontal or other multistage procedures should not be repeated at intervals of less than 2 weeks; clindamycin is not licensed for use in endocarditis prophylaxis but it is recommended by the Endocarditis Working Party

5. Azithromycin is not licensed for use in endocarditis prophylaxis but it is recommended by the Endocarditis Working Party

6. The British Association of Dermatologists Therapy Guidelines and Audit Subcommittee advise that such dermatological procedures include skin biopsies and excision of moles or of malignant lesions

Prevention of secondary case of pertussis in non-immune patient or partially immune patient

Erythromycin[1] ADULT and CHILD over 8 years, 250–500 mg every 6 hours for 7 days; CHILD under 2 years 125 mg every 6 hours, 2–8 years 250 mg every 6 hours

Prevention of pneumococcal infection in asplenia or in patients with sickle cell disease

Phenoxymethylpenicillin 500 mg every 12 hours; CHILD under 5 years 125 mg every 12 hours, 6–12 years 250 mg every 12 hours—if cover also needed for *H. influenzae* in CHILD give amoxicillin instead (under 5 years 125 mg every 12 hours, over 5 years 250 mg every 12 hours)

NOTE. Antibiotic prophylaxis is not fully reliable; for vaccines in asplenia see p. 605

Prevention of gas-gangrene in high lower-limb amputations or following major trauma

Benzylpenicillin 300–600 mg every 6 hours for 5 days *or* if penicillin-allergic metronidazole 400–500 mg every 8 hours

Prevention of tuberculosis in susceptible close contacts or those who have become tuberculin positive[2]

Isoniazid 300 mg daily for 6 months; CHILD 5–10 mg/kg daily (max. 300 mg daily)
or isoniazid 300 mg daily + rifampicin 600 mg daily (450 mg if less than 50 kg) for 3 months; CHILD isoniazid 5–10 mg/kg daily (max. 300 mg daily) + rifampicin 10 mg/kg daily (max. 600 mg daily)

Prevention of infection in gastro-intestinal procedures

Operations on stomach or oesophagus for carcinoma
Single dose[3] of i/v gentamicin *or* i/v cefuroxime

Open biliary surgery
Single dose[3] of i/v cefuroxime + i/v metronidazole[4] *or* i/v gentamicin + i/v metronidazole[4]

Resections of colon and rectum for carcinoma, and resections in inflammatory bowel disease, and appendicectomy
Single dose[3] of i/v gentamicin + i/v metronidazole[4] *or* i/v cefuroxime + i/v metronidazole[4] *or* i/v co-amoxiclav alone

Endoscopic retrograde cholangiopancreatography
Single dose of i/v gentamicin *or* oral or i/v ciprofloxacin
Prophylaxis particularly recommended if bile stasis, pancreatic pseudocyst, previous cholangitis or neutropenia

Prevention of infection in orthopaedic surgery

Joint replacement including hip and knee and management of fractures
Single dose[3] of i/v cefuroxime or i/v flucloxacillin
Substitute i/v vancomycin if history of allergy to penicillins or to cephalosporins; use cefuroxime + metronidazole for complex open fractures with extensive soft-tissue damage; prophylaxis continued for 24 hours in open fractures (longer if complex open fractures)

Prevention of infection in urological procedures

Transrectal prostate biopsy
Single dose[3] of i/v cefuroxime + i/v metronidazole[4] *or* i/v gentamicin + i/v metronidazole[4]

Transurethral resection of prostate
Single dose[3] of oral ciprofloxacin *or* i/v gentamicin *or* i/v cefuroxime

Prevention of infection in obstetric and gynaecological surgery

Caesarean section
Single dose[3] of i/v cefuroxime
Administer immediately after umbilical cord is clamped; substitute i/v clindamycin if history of allergy to penicillins or cephalosporins

Hysterectomy
Single dose[3] of i/v cefuroxime + i/v metronidazole[4] *or* i/v gentamicin + i/v metronidazole[4] *or* i/v co-amoxiclav alone

Termination of pregnancy
Single dose[3] of oral metronidazole
If genital chlamydial infection cannot be ruled out, give doxycycline (section 5.1.3) postoperatively

Prevention of infection in vascular surgery

Reconstructive arterial surgery of abdomen, pelvis or legs
Single dose[3] of i/v cefuroxime *or* i/v gentamicin
Add i/v metronidazole for patients at risk from anaerobic infections including those with diabetes, gangrene, or undergoing amputation; substitute i/v vancomycin for cefuroxime or gentamicin if high risk of methicillin-resistant *Staphylococcus aureus*

---

1. Where erythromycin is suggested another macrolide (e.g. azithromycin or clarithromycin) may be used.

2. The Joint Tuberculosis Committee recommends chemoprophylaxis for patients with documented recent tuberculin conversion, for some tuberculin-positive children identified in BCG schools programme, for children under 2 years in close contact with smear-positive tuberculosis (including those previously vaccinated with BCG but now showing strongly positive tuberculin test), for children under 16 years showing a positive tuberculin test at new immigrant or contact screening; chemoprophylaxis should be considered in immigrant adults 16–34 years without a BCG scar but with strongly positive tuberculin test. See also section 5.1.9, for advice on immunocompromised patients and on prevention of tuberculosis

3. Additional intra-operative or postoperative doses of antibacterial may be given for prolonged procedures or if there is major blood loss

4. Metronidazole may alternatively be given by suppository but to allow adequate absorption, it should be given 2 hours before surgery

5.1.1 Penicillins

The penicillins are bactericidal and act by interfering with bacterial cell wall synthesis. They diffuse well into body tissues and fluids, but penetration into the cerebrospinal fluid is poor except when the meninges are inflamed. They are excreted in the urine in therapeutic concentrations.

The most important side-effect of the penicillins is hypersensitivity which causes rashes and anaphylaxis and can be fatal. Allergic reactions to penicillins occur in 1–10% of exposed individuals; anaphylactic reactions occur in fewer than 0.05% of treated patients. Patients with a history of atopic allergy (e.g. asthma, eczema, hay fever) are more likely to be allergic to penicillins. Individuals with a history of anaphylaxis, urticaria, or rash immediately after penicillin administration are at risk of immediate hypersensitivity to a penicillin; these individuals should not receive a penicillin, a cephalosporin or another beta-lactam antibiotic. Patients who are allergic to one penicillin will be allergic to all because the hypersensitivity is related to the basic penicillin structure. Individuals with a history of a minor rash (i.e. non-confluent rash restricted to a small area of the body) or a rash that occurs more than 72 hours after penicillin administration are probably not allergic to penicillin and in these individuals a penicillin should not be withheld unnecessarily for serious infections; the possibility of an allergic reaction should, however, be borne in mind.

A rare but serious toxic effect of the penicillins is encephalopathy due to cerebral irritation. This may result from excessively high doses or in patients with severe renal failure. The penicillins should **not** be given by intrathecal injection because they can cause encephalopathy which may be fatal.

Another problem relating to high doses of penicillin, or normal doses given to patients with renal failure, is the accumulation of electrolyte since most injectable penicillins contain either sodium or potassium.

Diarrhoea frequently occurs during oral penicillin therapy. It is most common with broad-spectrum penicillins, which can also cause antibiotic-associated colitis.

5.1.1.1 Benzylpenicillin and phenoxymethylpenicillin

Benzylpenicillin (Penicillin G) remains an important and useful antibiotic but is inactivated by bacterial beta-lactamases. It is effective for many streptococcal (including pneumococcal), gonococcal, and meningococcal infections and also for anthrax (section 5.1.12), diphtheria, gas-gangrene, leptospirosis, and treatment of Lyme disease (section 5.1.1.3) in children. Pneumococci, meningococci, and gonococci which have decreased sensitivity to penicillin have been isolated; benzylpenicillin is no longer the drug of first choice for pneumococcal meningitis. Although benzylpenicillin is effective in the treatment of tetanus, metronidazole (section 5.1.11) is preferred. Benzylpenicillin is inactivated by gastric acid and absorption from the gut is low; therefore it is best given by injection.

Procaine benzylpenicillin (procaine penicillin) (available on a named-patient basis from IDIS) is used for the treatment of early syphilis and late latent syphilis; it is given in a dose of 600 mg daily by intramuscular injection.

Phenoxymethylpenicillin (Penicillin V) has a similar antibacterial spectrum to benzylpenicillin, but is less active. It is gastric acid-stable, so is suitable for oral administration. It should not be used for serious infections because absorption can be unpredictable and plasma concentrations variable. It is indicated principally for respiratory-tract infections in children, for streptococcal tonsillitis, and for continuing treatment after one or more injections of benzylpenicillin when clinical response has begun. It should not be used for meningococcal or gonococcal infections. Phenoxymethylpenicillin is used for prophylaxis against streptococcal infections following rheumatic fever and against pneumococcal infections following splenectomy or in sickle-cell disease.

ORAL INFECTIONS. Phenoxymethylpenicillin is effective for dentoalveolar abscess.

BENZYLPENICILLIN

(Penicillin G)

Indications: throat infections, otitis media, endocarditis, meningococcal disease, pneumonia, cellulitis (Table 1, section 5.1); anthrax; prophylaxis in limb amputation (Table 2, section 5.1); see also notes above

Cautions: history of allergy; false-positive urinary glucose (if tested for reducing substances); renal impairment (Appendix 3); **interactions:** Appendix 1 (penicillins)

Contra-indications: penicillin hypersensitivity

Side-effects: hypersensitivity reactions including urticaria, fever, joint pains, rashes, angioedema, anaphylaxis, serum sickness-like reaction; *rarely* CNS toxicity including convulsions (especially with high doses or in severe renal impairment), interstitial nephritis, haemolytic anaemia, leucopenia, thrombocytopenia, and coagulation disorders; also reported diarrhoea (including antibiotic-associated colitis)

Dose: *by intramuscular or by slow intravenous injection or by infusion*, 2.4–4.8 g daily in 4 divided doses, increased if necessary in more serious infections (single doses over 1.2 g intravenous route only; see also below); PRETERM NEONATE and NEONATE under 1 week, 50 mg/kg daily in 2 divided doses; NEONATE 1–4 weeks, 75 mg/kg daily in 3 divided doses; CHILD 1 month–12 years, 100 mg/kg daily in 4 divided doses (higher doses may be required, see also below); intravenous route recommended in neonates and infants

Endocarditis (in combination with another antibacterial if necessary, see Table 1, section 5.1), *by slow intravenous injection or by infusion*, 7.2 g daily in 6 divided doses, increased if necessary (e.g. in enterococcal endocarditis or if benzylpenicillin used alone) to 14.4 g daily in 6 divided doses

Anthrax (in combination with other antibacterials, see also section 5.1.12), *by slow intravenous injection* or *by infusion*, 2.4 g every 4 hours; CHILD 150 mg/kg daily in 4 divided doses

Intrapartum prophylaxis against group B streptococcal infection, *by slow intravenous injection or by infusion*, initially 3 g then 1.5 g every 4 hours until delivery

Meningococcal disease, *by slow intravenous injection or by infusion*, 2.4 g every 4 hours; PRETERM NEONATE and NEONATE under 1 week, 100 mg/kg daily in 2 divided doses; NEONATE 1–4 weeks, 150 mg/kg daily in 3 divided doses; CHILD 1 month–12 years, 180–300 mg/kg daily in 4–6 divided doses

Important. If bacterial meningitis and especially if meningococcal disease is suspected general practitioners are advised to give a single injection of benzylpenicillin by intravenous injection (or by intramuscular injection) before transferring the patient urgently to hospital. Suitable doses are: ADULT 1.2 g; INFANT under 1 year 300 mg; CHILD 1–9 years 600 mg, 10 years and over as for adult. In **penicillin allergy**, cefotaxime (section 5.1.2) may be an alternative; chloramphenicol may be used if there is a history of anaphylaxis to penicillins

By intrathecal injection, **not** recommended

NOTE. Benzylpenicillin doses in BNF may differ from those in product literature

Crystapen® (Britannia) PoM

Injection, powder for reconstitution, benzylpenicillin sodium (unbuffered), net price 600-mg vial = 43p, 2-vial 'GP pack' = £1.90; 1.2-g vial = 87p

Electrolytes: Na^+ 1.68 mmol/600-mg vial; 3.36 mmol/1.2-g vial

PHENOXYMETHYLPENICILLIN

(Penicillin V)

Indications: oral infections (see notes above); tonsillitis, otitis media, erysipelas, cellulitis; rheumatic fever and pneumococcal infection prophylaxis (Table 2, section 5.1)

Cautions: see under Benzylpenicillin; **interactions:** Appendix 1 (penicillins)

Contra-indications: see under Benzylpenicillin

Side-effects: see under Benzylpenicillin

Dose: 500 mg every 6 hours increased up to 1 g every 6 hours in severe infections; CHILD up to 1 year 62.5 mg every 6 hours, increased up to 12.5 mg/kg every 6 hours in severe infections; 1–5 years, 125 mg every 6 hours, increased up to 12.5 mg/kg every 6 hours in severe infections; 6–12 years, 250 mg every 6 hours, increased up to 12.5 mg/kg every 6 hours in severe infections

NOTE. Phenoxymethylpenicillin doses in the BNF may differ from those in product literature

Phenoxymethylpenicillin (Non-proprietary) PoM

Tablets, phenoxymethylpenicillin (as potassium salt) 250 mg, net price 28-tab pack = £1.71. Label: 9, 23

Oral solution, phenoxymethylpenicillin (as potassium salt) for reconstitution with water, net price 125 mg/5 mL, 100 mL = £1.62; 250 mg/5 mL, 100 mL = £2.26. Label: 9, 23

DENTAL PRESCRIBING ON NHS. Phenoxymethylpenicillin Tablets and Oral Solution may be prescribed

5.1.1.2 Penicillinase-resistant penicillins

Most staphylococci are now resistant to benzylpenicillin because they produce penicillinases. **Flucloxacillin**, however, is not inactivated by these enzymes and is thus effective in infections caused by penicillin-resistant staphylococci, which is the sole indication for its use. Flucloxacillin is acid-stable and can, therefore, be given by mouth as well as by injection.

Flucloxacillin is well absorbed from the gut. For CSM warning on hepatic disorders see under Flucloxacillin.

MRSA. *Staphylococcus aureus* strains resistant to methicillin [now discontinued] (methicillin-resistant *Staph. aureus*, MRSA) and to flucloxacillin have emerged; some of these organisms may be sensitive to vancomycin or teicoplanin (section 5.1.7). Strains may be susceptible to rifampicin, sodium fusidate, tetracyclines, aminoglycosides, macrolides, and clindamycin. Rifampicin or sodium fusidate should not be used alone because resistance may develop rapidly. Trimethoprim alone may be used for urinary-tract infections caused by some MRSA strains. Linezolid (section 5.1.7) and the combination of the streptogramin antibiotics quinupristin and dalfopristin (section 5.1.7) are active against MRSA but these antibacterial drugs should be reserved for organisms resistant to treatment with other antibacterials or for patients who cannot tolerate other antibacterial drugs. Treatment is guided by the sensitivity of the infecting strain. For eradication of nasal carriage of MRSA see section 12.2.3.

FLUCLOXACILLIN

Indications: infections due to beta-lactamase-producing staphylococci including otitis externa; adjunct in pneumonia, impetigo, cellulitis, osteomyelitis and in staphylococcal endocarditis (Table 1, section 5.1)

Cautions: see under Benzylpenicillin (section 5.1.1.1); also hepatic impairment (see CSM advice below); risk of kernicterus in jaundiced neonates when high doses given parenterally

CSM advice (hepatic disorders). CSM has advised that very rarely cholestatic jaundice and hepatitis may occur up to several weeks after treatment with flucloxacillin has been stopped. Administration for more than 2 weeks and increasing age are risk factors. CSM has reminded that:

- flucloxacillin should not be used in patients with a history of hepatic dysfunction associated with flucloxacillin;
- flucloxacillin should be used with caution in patients with hepatic impairment;
- careful enquiry should be made about hypersensitivity reactions to beta-lactam antibacterials.

Contra-indications: see under Benzylpenicillin (section 5.1.1.1)

Side-effects: see under Benzylpenicillin (section 5.1.1.1); also gastro-intestinal disturbances; *very rarely* hepatitis and cholestatic jaundice (see also CSM advice above)

Dose: *by mouth*, 250–500 mg every 6 hours, at least 30 minutes before food; CHILD under 2 years quarter adult dose; 2–10 years half adult dose
By intramuscular injection, 250–500 mg every 6 hours; CHILD under 2 years quarter adult dose; 2–10 years half adult dose
By slow intravenous injection or by intravenous infusion, 0.25–2 g every 6 hours; CHILD under 2 years quarter adult dose; 2–10 years half adult dose
Endocarditis (in combination with another antibacterial, see Table 1, section 5.1), body-weight under 85 kg, 8 g daily in 4 divided doses; body-weight over 85 kg, 12 g daily in 6 divided doses
Osteomyelitis (see Table 1, section 5.1), up to 8 g daily in 3–4 divided doses

NOTE. Flucloxacillin doses in BNF may differ from those in product literature

Flucloxacillin (Non-proprietary) PoM
Capsules, flucloxacillin (as sodium salt) 250 mg, net price 20 = £2.29; 500 mg, 20 = £4.45. Label: 9, 23
Brands include *Fluclomix*®, *Galfloxin*®, *Ladropen*®
Oral solution (= elixir or syrup), flucloxacillin (as sodium salt) for reconstitution with water, 125 mg/5 mL, net price 100 mL = £4.43; 250 mg/5 mL, 100 mL = £6.97. Label: 9, 23
Brands include *Ladropen*®
Injection, powder for reconstitution, flucloxacillin (as sodium salt). Net price 250-mg vial = 91p; 500-mg vial = £1.81; 1-g vial = £3.63

Floxapen® (GSK) PoM
Capsules, both black/caramel, flucloxacillin (as sodium salt) 250 mg, net price 28-cap pack = £6.31; 500 mg, 28-cap pack = £12.66. Label: 9, 23
Syrup, tutti-frutti-and menthol-flavoured, flucloxacillin (as magnesium salt) for reconstitution with water, 125 mg/5 mL, net price 100 mL = £3.25; 250 mg/5 mL, 100 mL = £6.48. Label: 9, 23
Excipients: include sucrose
Injection, powder for reconstitution, flucloxacillin (as sodium salt). Net price 250-mg vial = 91p; 500-mg vial = £1.81; 1-g vial = £3.63
Electrolytes: Na^+ 0.57 mmol/250-mg vial, 1.13 mmol/500-mg vial, 2.26 mmol/1-g vial

5.1.1.3 Broad-spectrum penicillins

Ampicillin is active against certain Gram-positive and Gram-negative organisms but is inactivated by penicillinases including those produced by *Staphylococcus aureus* and by common Gram-negative bacilli such as *Escherichia coli*. Almost all staphylococci, 50% of *E. coli* strains and 15% of *Haemophilus influenzae* strains are now resistant. The likelihood of resistance should therefore be considered before using ampicillin for the 'blind' treatment of infections; in particular, it should not be used for hospital patients without checking sensitivity.

Ampicillin is well excreted in the bile and urine. It is principally indicated for the treatment of exacerbations of chronic bronchitis and middle ear infections, both of which may be due to *Streptococcus pneumoniae* and *H. influenzae*, and for urinary-tract infections (section 5.1.13).

Ampicillin can be given by mouth but less than half the dose is absorbed, and absorption is further decreased by the presence of food in the gut.

Maculopapular rashes commonly occur with ampicillin (and amoxicillin) but are not usually related to true penicillin allergy. They almost always occur in patients with glandular fever; broad-spectrum penicillins should not therefore be used for 'blind' treatment of a sore throat. Rashes are also common in patients with acute or chronic lymphocytic leukaemia or in cytomegalovirus infection.

Amoxicillin (amoxycillin) is a derivative of ampicillin and has a similar antibacterial spectrum. It is better absorbed than ampicillin when given by mouth, producing higher plasma and tissue concentrations; unlike ampicillin, absorption is not affected by the presence of food in the stomach. Amoxicillin is used for endocarditis prophylaxis (section 5.1, table 2); it may also be used for the treatment of Lyme disease [not licensed], see below.

Co-amoxiclav consists of amoxicillin with the beta-lactamase inhibitor clavulanic acid. Clavulanic acid itself has no significant antibacterial activity but, by inactivating beta-lactamases, it makes the combination active against beta-lactamase-producing bacteria that are resistant to amoxicillin. These include resistant strains of *Staph. aureus*, *E. coli*, and *H. influenzae*, as well as many *Bacteroides* and *Klebsiella* spp. Co-amoxiclav should be reserved for infections likely, or known, to be caused by amoxicillin-resistant beta-lactamase-producing strains; for CSM warning on cholestatic jaundice see under Co-amoxiclav.

A combination of ampicillin with flucloxacillin (as co-fluampicil) is available to treat infections involving either streptococci or staphylococci (e.g. cellulitis).

LYME DISEASE. Lyme disease should generally be treated by those experienced in its management. **Doxycycline** is the antibacterial of choice for *early Lyme disease*. **Amoxicillin** [unlicensed indication], **cefuroxime axetil**, or **azithromycin** [unlicensed indication] are alternatives if doxycycline is contra-indicated. Intravenous administration of **cefotaxime**, **ceftriaxone**, or **benzylpenicillin** is recommended for Lyme disease associated with moderate to severe *cardiac* or neurological abnormalities, *late Lyme disease*, and *Lyme arthritis*. The duration of treatment is generally 2–4 weeks; Lyme arthritis requires longer treatment with oral antibacterial drugs.

ORAL INFECTIONS. Amoxicillin or ampicillin are as effective as phenoxymethylpenicillin (section 5.1.1.1) but they are better absorbed; however, they may encourage emergence of resistant organisms. Like phenoxymethylpenicillin, amoxicillin and ampicillin are ineffective against bacteria that produce beta-lactamases. Amoxicillin may be useful for short-course oral regimens. Amoxicillin is also used for prophylaxis of endocarditis (Table 2, section 5.1).

AMOXICILLIN

(Amoxycillin)

Indications: see under Ampicillin; oral infections (see notes above); also endocarditis prophylaxis (Table 2, section 5.1) and treatment (Table 1, section 5.1); anthrax (section 5.1.12); adjunct in listerial meningitis (Table 1, section 5.1); *Helicobacter pylori* eradication (section 1.3)
Cautions: see under Ampicillin; maintain adequate hydration with high doses (particularly during parenteral therapy)
Contra-indications: see under Ampicillin

Side-effects: see under Ampicillin

Dose: *by mouth*, 250 mg every 8 hours, doubled in severe infections; CHILD up to 10 years, 125 mg every 8 hours, doubled in severe infections

Otitis media, 1 g every 8 hours; CHILD 40 mg/kg daily in 3 divided doses (max. 3 g daily)

Pneumonia, 0.5–1 g every 8 hours

Anthrax (treatment and post-exposure prophylaxis—see also section 5.1.12), 500 mg every 8 hours; CHILD body-weight under 20 kg, 80 mg/kg daily in 3 divided doses, body-weight over 20 kg, adult dose

Short-course oral therapy

Dental abscess, 3 g repeated after 8 hours

Urinary-tract infections, 3 g repeated after 10–12 hours

By intramuscular injection, 500 mg every 8 hours; CHILD, 50–100 mg/kg daily in divided doses

By intravenous injection or infusion, 500 mg every 8 hours increased to 1 g every 6 hours in severe infections; CHILD, 50–100 mg/kg daily in divided doses

Listerial meningitis (in combination with another antibiotic, see Table 1, section 5.1), *by intravenous infusion*, 2 g every 4 hours for 10–14 days

Endocarditis (in combination with another antibiotic if necessary, see Table 1, section 5.1), *by intravenous infusion*, 2 g every 6 hours, increased to 2 g every 4 hours e.g. in enterococcal endocarditis or if amoxicillin used alone

NOTE. Amoxicillin doses in BNF may differ from those in product literature

Amoxicillin (Non-proprietary) PoM

Capsules, amoxicillin (as trihydrate) 250 mg, net price 21 = £1.27; 500 mg, 21 = £2.22. Label: 9

Brands include *Amix*®, *Amoram*®, *Amoxident*®, *Galenamox*®, *Rimoxallin*®

Oral suspension, amoxicillin (as trihydrate) for reconstitution with water, 125 mg/5 mL, net price 100 mL = £1.17; 250 mg/5 mL, 100 mL = £1.78. Label: 9

NOTE. Sugar-free versions are available and can be ordered by specifying 'sugar-free' on the prescription

Brands include *Amix*®, *Amoram*®, *Galenamox*®, *Rimoxallin*®

Sachets, sugar-free, amoxicillin (as trihydrate) 3 g/sachet, net price 2-sachet pack = £6.23, 14-sachet pack = £31.94. Label: 9, 13

Injection, powder for reconstitution, amoxicillin (as sodium salt), net price 250-mg vial = 32p; 500-mg vial = 58p; 1-g vial = £1.16

DENTAL PRESCRIBING ON NHS. Amoxicillin Capsules and Oral Suspension may be prescribed. Amoxicillin Sachets may be prescribed as Amoxicillin Oral Powder

Amoxil® (GSK) PoM

Capsules, both maroon/gold, amoxicillin (as trihydrate), 250 mg, net price 21-cap pack = £3.59; 500 mg, 21-cap pack = £7.19. Label: 9

Syrup SF, both sugar-free, peach- strawberry- and lemon-flavoured, amoxicillin (as trihydrate) for reconstitution with water, 125 mg/5 mL, net price 100 mL = 59p; 250 mg/5 mL, 100 mL = 59p. Label: 9

Paediatric suspension, amoxicillin 125 mg (as trihydrate)/1.25 mL when reconstituted with water, net price 20 mL (peach- strawberry- and lemon-flavoured) = £3.38. Label: 9, counselling , use of pipette

Excipients: include sucrose 600 mg/1.25 mL

Sachets SF, powder, sugar-free, amoxicillin (as trihydrate) 3 g/sachet, 2-sachet pack (peach-strawberry- and lemon-flavoured) = £2.99. Label: 9, 13

Injection, powder for reconstitution, amoxicillin (as sodium salt), net price 500-mg vial = 58p; 1-g vial = £1.16

Electrolytes: Na^+ 3.3 mmol/g

AMPICILLIN

Indications: urinary-tract infections, otitis media, sinusitis, oral infections (see notes above), bronchitis, uncomplicated community-acquired pneumonia (Table 1, section 5.1), *Haemophilus influenzae* infections, invasive salmonellosis; listerial meningitis (Table 1, section 5.1)

Cautions: history of allergy; renal impairment (Appendix 3); erythematous rashes common in glandular fever, cytomegalovirus infection, and acute or chronic lymphocytic leukaemia (see notes above); **interactions:** Appendix 1 (penicillins)

Contra-indications: penicillin hypersensitivity

Side-effects: nausea, vomiting, diarrhoea; rashes (discontinue treatment); rarely, antibiotic-associated colitis; see also under Benzylpenicillin (section 5.1.1.1)

Dose: *by mouth*, 0.25–1 g every 6 hours, at least 30 minutes before food; CHILD under 10 years, half adult dose

Urinary-tract infections, 500 mg every 8 hours; CHILD under 10 years, half adult dose

By intramuscular injection or intravenous injection or infusion, 500 mg every 4–6 hours; CHILD under 10 years, half adult dose

Endocarditis (in combination with another antibiotic if necessary), *by intravenous infusion*, 2 g every 6 hours, increased to 2 g every 4 hours e.g. in enterococcal endocarditis or if ampicillin used alone

Listerial meningitis (in combination with another antibiotic), *by intravenous infusion*, 2 g every 4 hours for 10–14 days; NEONATE 50 mg/kg every 6 hours; INFANT 1–3 months, 50–100 mg/kg every 6 hours; CHILD 3 months–12 years, 100 mg/kg every 6 hours (max. 12 g daily)

NOTE. Ampicillin doses in BNF may differ from those in product literature

Ampicillin (Non-proprietary) PoM

Capsules, ampicillin 250 mg, net price 20 = 62p; 500 mg, 20 = £2.16. Label: 9, 23

Brands include *Rimacillin*®

Oral suspension, ampicillin 125 mg/5 mL when reconstituted with water, net price 100 mL = £3.04; 250 mg/5 mL, 100 mL = £5.20. Label: 9, 23

Brands include *Rimacillin*®

Injection, powder for reconstitution, ampicillin (as sodium salt), net price 500-mg vial = 68p

DENTAL PRESCRIBING ON NHS. Ampicillin Capsules and Oral Suspension may be prescribed

Penbritin® (Chemidex) PoM

Capsules, both black/red, ampicillin (as trihydrate) 250 mg, net price 28-cap pack = £2.10. Label: 9, 23

■ With flucloxacillin

See Co-fluampicil

CO-AMOXICLAV

A mixture of amoxicillin (as the trihydrate or as the sodium salt) and clavulanic acid (as potassium clavulanate); the proportions are expressed in the form *x/y* where *x* and *y* are the strengths in milligrams of amoxicillin and clavulanic acid respectively

Indications: infections due to beta-lactamase-producing strains (where amoxicillin alone not appropriate) including respiratory-tract infections, genito-urinary and abdominal infections, cellulitis, animal bites, severe dental infection with spreading cellulitis

Cautions: see under Ampicillin and notes above; also caution in hepatic impairment (monitor hepatic function), pregnancy; maintain adequate hydration with high doses (particularly during parenteral therapy)

CHOLESTATIC JAUNDICE. CSM has advised that cholestatic jaundice can occur either during or shortly after the use of co-amoxiclav. An epidemiological study has shown that the risk of acute liver toxicity was about 6 times greater with co-amoxiclav than with amoxicillin. Cholestatic jaundice is more common in patients above the age of 65 years and in men; these reactions have only rarely been reported in children. Jaundice is usually self-limiting and very rarely fatal. The duration of treatment should be appropriate to the indication and should not usually exceed 14 days

Contra-indications: penicillin hypersensitivity, history of co-amoxiclav-associated or penicillin-associated jaundice or hepatic dysfunction

Side-effects: see under Ampicillin; hepatitis, cholestatic jaundice (see above); Stevens-Johnson syndrome, toxic epidermal necrolysis, exfoliative dermatitis, vasculitis reported; rarely prolongation of bleeding time, dizziness, headache, convulsions (particularly with high doses or in renal impairment); superficial staining of teeth with suspension, phlebitis at injection site

Dose: *by mouth*, expressed as amoxicillin, 250 mg every 8 hours, dose doubled in severe infections; CHILD see under preparations below (under 6 years *Augmentin® '125/31 SF'* suspension; 6–12 years *Augmentin® '250/62 SF'* suspension *or* for short-term treatment with twice daily dosage in CHILD 2 months–12 years *Augmentin-Duo® 400/57* suspension)

Severe dental infections (but not generally first-line, see notes above), expressed as amoxicillin, 250 mg every 8 hours for 5 days

By intravenous injection over 3–4 minutes *or by intravenous infusion*, expressed as amoxicillin, 1 g every 8 hours increased to 1 g every 6 hours in more serious infections; INFANTS up to 3 months 25 mg/kg every 8 hours (every 12 hours in the perinatal period and in premature infants); CHILD 3 months–12 years, 25 mg/kg every 8 hours increased to 25 mg/kg every 6 hours in more serious infections

Surgical prophylaxis, expressed as amoxicillin, 1 g at induction; for high risk procedures (e.g. colorectal surgery) up to 2–3 further doses of 1 g may be given every 8 hours

Co-amoxiclav (Non-proprietary) PoM

Tablets, co-amoxiclav 250/125 (amoxicillin 250 mg as trihydrate, clavulanic acid 125 mg as potassium salt), net price 21-tab pack = £5.77. Label: 9

Brands include *Amiclav®*

Tablets, co-amoxiclav 500/125 (amoxicillin 500 mg as trihydrate, clavulanic acid 125 mg as potassium salt), net price 21-tab pack = £14.24. Label: 9

Oral suspension, co-amoxiclav 125/31 (amoxicillin 125 mg as trihydrate, clavulanic acid 31.25 mg as potassium salt)/5 mL when reconstituted with water, net price 100 mL = £4.57. Label: 9

Oral suspension, co-amoxiclav 250/62 (amoxicillin 250 mg as trihydrate, clavulanic acid 62.5 mg as potassium salt)/5 mL when reconstituted with water, net price 100 mL = £6.42. Label: 9

Injection 500/100, powder for reconstitution, co-amoxiclav 500/100 (amoxicillin 500 mg as sodium salt, clavulanic acid 100 mg as potassium salt), net price per vial = £1.49

Injection 1000/200, powder for reconstitution, co-amoxiclav 1000/200 (amoxicillin 1 g as sodium salt, clavulanic acid 200 mg as potassium salt), net price per vial = £2.97

Augmentin® (GSK) PoM

Tablets 375 mg, f/c, co-amoxiclav 250/125 (amoxicillin 250 mg as trihydrate, clavulanic acid 125 mg as potassium salt), net price 21-tab pack = £4.45. Label: 9

Tablets 625 mg, f/c, co-amoxiclav 500/125 (amoxicillin 500 mg as trihydrate, clavulanic acid 125 mg as potassium salt). Net price 21-tab pack = £8.49. Label: 9

Dispersible tablets, sugar-free, co-amoxiclav 250/125 (amoxicillin 250 mg as trihydrate, clavulanic acid 125 mg as potassium salt). Net price 21-tab pack = £10.22. Label: 9, 13

Suspension '125/31 SF', sugar-free, co-amoxiclav 125/31 (amoxicillin 125 mg as trihydrate, clavulanic acid 31 mg as potassium salt)/5 mL when reconstituted with water. Net price 100 mL (raspberry-and orange-flavoured) = £4.25. Label: 9

Excipients: include aspartame 12.5 mg/5 mL (section 9.4.1)

Dose: CHILD 1–6 years (10–18 kg) 5 mL every 8 hours *or* INFANT and CHILD up to 6 years 0.8 mL/kg daily in 3 divided doses; in severe infections dose increased to 1.6 mL/kg daily in 3 divided doses

Suspension '250/62 SF', sugar-free, co-amoxiclav 250/62 (amoxicillin 250 mg as trihydrate, clavulanic acid 62 mg as potassium salt)/5 mL when reconstituted with water. Net price 100 mL (raspberry-and orange-flavoured) = £5.97. Label: 9

Excipients: include aspartame 12.5 mg/5 mL (section 9.4.1)

Dose: CHILD 6–12 years (18–40 kg) 5 mL every 8 hours *or* 0.4 mL/kg daily in 3 divided doses; in severe infections dose increased to 0.8 mL/kg daily in 3 divided doses

Injection 600 mg, powder for reconstitution, co-amoxiclav 500/100 (amoxicillin 500 mg as sodium salt, clavulanic acid 100 mg as potassium salt). Net price per vial = £1.38

Electrolytes: Na^+ 1.35 mmol, K^+ 0.5 mmol/600-mg vial

Injection 1.2 g, powder for reconstitution, co-amoxiclav 1000/200 (amoxicillin 1 g as sodium salt, clavulanic acid 200 mg as potassium salt). Net price per vial = £2.76

Electrolytes: Na^+ 2.7 mmol, K^+ 1 mmol/1.2-g vial

Augmentin-Duo® (GSK) PoM

Suspension '400/57', sugar-free, strawberry-flavoured, co-amoxiclav 400/57 (amoxicillin 400 mg as trihydrate, clavulanic acid 57 mg as potassium salt)/5 mL when reconstituted with water. Net price 35 mL = £4.38, 70 mL = £6.15. Label: 9

Excipients: include aspartame 12.5 mg/5 mL (section 9.4.1)

Dose: CHILD 2 months–2 years 0.15 mL/kg twice daily, 2–6 years (13–21 kg) 2.5 mL twice daily, 7–12 years (22–40 kg) 5 mL twice daily, doubled in severe infections

CO-FLUAMPICIL

A mixture of equal parts by mass of flucloxacillin and ampicillin

Indications: mixed infections involving beta-lactamase-producing staphylococci

Cautions: see under Ampicillin and Flucloxacillin

Contra-indications: see under Ampicillin and Flucloxacillin

Side-effects: see under Ampicillin and Flucloxacillin

Dose: *by mouth*, co-fluampicil, 250/250 every 6 hours, dose doubled in severe infections; CHILD under 10 years half adult dose, dose doubled in severe infections

By intramuscular or slow intravenous injection or by intravenous infusion, co-fluampicil 250/250 every 6 hours, dose doubled in severe infections; CHILD under 2 years quarter adult dose, 2–10 years half adult dose, dose doubled in severe infections

Co-fluampicil (Non-proprietary) PoM

Capsules, co-fluampicil 250/250 (flucloxacillin 250 mg as sodium salt, ampicillin 250 mg as trihydrate), net price 28-cap pack = £8.86. Label: 9, 22

Brands include *Flu-Amp*®

Magnapen® (CP) PoM

Capsules, black/turquoise, co-fluampicil 250/250 (flucloxacillin 250 mg as sodium salt, ampicillin 250 mg as trihydrate), net price 20-cap pack = £6.15. Label: 9, 22

Syrup, co-fluampicil 125/125 (flucloxacillin 125 mg as magnesium salt, ampicillin 125 mg as trihydrate)/5 mL when reconstituted with water, net price 100 mL = £4.99. Label: 9, 22

Excipients: include sucrose 3.14 g/5 mL

Injection 500 mg, powder for reconstitution, co-fluampicil 250/250 (flucloxacillin 250 mg as sodium salt, ampicillin 250 mg as sodium salt), net price per vial = £1.33

Electrolytes: Na^+ 1.3 mmol/vial

5.1.1.4 Antipseudomonal penicillins

The carboxypenicillin, **ticarcillin**, is principally indicated for serious infections caused by *Pseudomonas aeruginosa* although it also has activity against certain other Gram-negative bacilli including *Proteus* spp. and *Bacteroides fragilis*.

Ticarcillin is now available only in combination with clavulanic acid (section 5.1.1.3); the combination (*Timentin*®) is active against beta-lactamase-producing bacteria resistant to ticarcillin.

Tazocin® contains the ureidopenicillin ***piperacillin*** with the beta-lactamase inhibitor tazobactam. Piperacillin is more active than ticarcillin against *Ps. aeruginosa*. The spectrum of activity of *Tazocin*® is comparable to that of the carbapenems, imipenem and meropenem (section 5.1.2).

For pseudomonas septicaemias (especially in neutropenia or endocarditis) these antipseudomonal penicillins should be given with an aminoglycoside (e.g. gentamicin or netilmicin, section 5.1.4) since they have a synergistic effect. Penicillins and aminoglycosides must not, however, be mixed in the same syringe or infusion.

Owing to the sodium content of many of these antibiotics, high doses may lead to hypernatraemia.

PIPERACILLIN

Indications: see preparations

Cautions: see under Benzylpenicillin (section 5.1.1.1); renal impairment (Appendix 3); pregnancy (Appendix 4); breast-feeding (Appendix 5)

Contra-indications: see under Benzylpenicillin (section 5.1.1.1)

Side-effects: see under Benzylpenicillin (section 5.1.1.1); also nausea, vomiting, diarrhoea; *less commonly* stomatitis, dyspepsia, constipation, jaundice, hypotension, headache, insomnia, and injection-site reactions; *rarely* abdominal pain, hepatitis, oedema, fatigue, and eosinophilia; *very rarely* hypoglycaemia, hypokalaemia, pancytopenia, Stevens-Johnson syndrome, and toxic epidermal necrolysis

Dose: see preparations

■ With tazobactam

Tazocin® (Lederle) PoM

Injection 2.25 g, powder for reconstitution, piperacillin 2 g (as sodium salt), tazobactam 250 mg (as sodium salt). Net price per vial = £7.96

Electrolytes: Na^+ 4.69 mmol/2.25-g vial

Injection 4.5 g, powder for reconstitution, piperacillin 4 g (as sodium salt), tazobactam 500 mg (as sodium salt). Net price per vial = £15.79

Electrolytes: Na^+ 9.37 mmol/4.5-g vial

Dose: lower respiratory-tract, urinary-tract, intra-abdominal and skin infections, and septicaemia, ADULT and CHILD over 12 years, *by intravenous injection* over 3–5 minutes *or by intravenous infusion*, 2.25–4.5 g every 6–8 hours, usually 4.5 g every 8 hours

Complicated appendicitis, *by intravenous injection* over 3–5 minutes or by *intravenous infusion*, CHILD 2–12 years, 112.5 mg/kg every 8 hours (max. 4.5 g every 8 hours) for 5–14 days; CHILD under 2 years, not recommended

Infections in neutropenic patients (in combination with an aminoglycoside), *by intravenous injection* over 3–5 minutes *or by intravenous infusion*, ADULT and CHILD over 50 kg, 4.5 g every 6 hours; CHILD less than 50 kg, 90 mg/kg every 6 hours

TICARCILLIN

Indications: infections due to *Pseudomonas* and *Proteus* spp, see notes above

Cautions: see under Benzylpenicillin (section 5.1.1.1)

Contra-indications: see under Benzylpenicillin (section 5.1.1.1)

Side-effects: see under Benzylpenicillin (section 5.1.1.1); also nausea, vomiting, coagulation disorders, haemorrhagic cystitis (more frequent in children), injection-site reactions, Stevens-Johnson syndrome, toxic epidermal necrolysis, hypokalaemia, eosinophilia

Dose: see under preparation

■ With clavulanic acid

NOTE. For a CSM warning on cholestatic jaundice possibly associated with clavulanic acid, see under Co-amoxiclav p. 277.

Timentin (GSK) PoM

Injection 3.2 g, powder for reconstitution, ticarcillin 3 g (as sodium salt), clavulanic acid 200 mg (as potassium salt). Net price per vial = £5.66

Electrolytes: Na^+ 16 mmol, K^+ 1 mmol /3.2-g vial

Dose: *by intravenous infusion*, 3.2 g every 6–8 hours increased to every 4 hours in more severe infections; CHILD 80 mg/kg every 6–8 hours (every 12 hours in neonates)

5.1.1.5 Mecillinams

Pivmecillinam has significant activity against many Gram-negative bacteria including *Escherichia coli*, klebsiella, enterobacter, and salmonellae. It is not active against *Pseudomonas aeruginosa* or enterococci. Pivmecillinam is hydrolysed to mecillinam, which is the active drug.

PIVMECILLINAM HYDROCHLORIDE

Indications: see under Dose below

Cautions: see under Benzylpenicillin (section 5.1.1.1); also liver and renal function tests required in long-term use; avoid in porphyria (section 9.8.2); pregnancy; **interactions:** Appendix 1 (penicillins)

Contra-indications: see under Benzylpenicillin (section 5.1.1.1); also carnitine deficiency, oesophageal strictures, gastro-intestinal obstruction, infants under 3 months

Side-effects: see under Benzylpenicillin (section 5.1.1.1); nausea, vomiting, dyspepsia; also reduced serum and total body carnitine (especially with long-term or repeated use)

Dose: acute uncomplicated cystitis, ADULT and CHILD over 40 kg, initially 400 mg then 200 mg every 8 hours for 3 days

Chronic or recurrent bacteriuria, ADULT and CHILD over 40 kg, 400 mg every 6–8 hours

Urinary-tract infections, CHILD under 40 kg, 20–40 mg/kg daily in 3–4 divided doses

Salmonellosis, not recommended therefore no dose stated

COUNSELLING. Tablets should be swallowed whole with plenty of fluid during meals while sitting or standing

Selexid® (Leo) PoM

Tablets, f/c, pivmecillinam hydrochloride 200 mg, net price 10-tab pack = £4.50. Label 9, 21, 27, counselling, posture (see Dose above)

5.1.2 Cephalosporins and other beta-lactams

Antibiotics in this section include the **cephalosporins**, such as cefotaxime, ceftazidime, cefuroxime, cefalexin and cefradine, the **monobactam**, aztreonam, and the **carbapenems**, imipenem (a thienamycin derivative) and meropenem.

Cephalosporins

The cephalosporins are broad-spectrum antibiotics which are used for the treatment of septicaemia, pneumonia, meningitis, biliary-tract infections, peritonitis, and urinary-tract infections. The pharmacology of the cephalosporins is similar to that of the penicillins, excretion being principally renal. Cephalosporins penetrate the cerebrospinal fluid poorly unless the meninges are inflamed; cefotaxime is a suitable cephalosporin for infections of the CNS (e.g meningitis).

The principal side-effect of the cephalosporins is hypersensitivity and about 10% of penicillin-sensitive patients will also be allergic to the cephalosporins.

Cefradine (cephradine) has generally been replaced by the newer cephalosporins.

Cefuroxime is a 'second generation' cephalosporin that is less susceptible than the earlier cephalosporins to inactivation by beta-lactamases. It is, therefore, active against certain bacteria which are resistant to the other drugs and has greater activity against *Haemophilus influenzae* and *Neisseria gonorrhoeae*.

Cefotaxime, **ceftazidime** and **ceftriaxone** are 'third generation' cephalosporins with greater activity than the 'second generation' cephalosporins against certain Gram-negative bacteria. However, they are less active than cefuroxime against Gram-positive bacteria, most notably *Staphylococcus aureus*. Their broad antibacterial spectrum may encourage superinfection with resistant bacteria or fungi.

Ceftazidime has good activity against pseudomonas. It is also active against other Gram-negative bacteria.

Ceftriaxone has a longer half-life and therefore needs to be given only once daily. Indications include serious infections such as septicaemia, pneumonia, and meningitis. The calcium salt of ceftriaxone forms a precipitate in the gall bladder which may rarely cause symptoms but these usually resolve when the antibiotic is stopped.

Cefpirome is licensed for urinary-tract, lower respiratory-tract and skin infections, bacteraemia, and infections associated with neutropenia.

ORALLY ACTIVE CEPHALOSPORINS. The orally active 'first generation' cephalosporins, **cefalexin** (cephalexin), **cefradine**, and **cefadroxil** and the 'second generation' cephalosporins, **cefaclor** and **cefprozil**, have a similar antimicrobial spectrum. They are useful for urinary-tract infections which do not respond to other drugs or which occur in pregnancy, respiratory-tract infections, otitis media, sinusitis, and skin and soft-tissue infections. Cefaclor has good activity against *H. influenzae*, but it is associated with protracted skin reactions especially in children. Cefadroxil has a long duration of action and can be given twice daily; it has poor activity against *H. influenzae*. **Cefuroxime axetil**, an ester of the 'second generation' cephalosporin cefuroxime, has the same antibacterial spectrum as the parent compound; it is poorly absorbed.

Cefixime has a longer duration of action than the other cephalosporins that are active by mouth. It is only licensed for acute infections.

Cefpodoxime proxetil is more active than the other oral cephalosporins against respiratory bacterial pathogens and it is licensed for upper and lower respiratory-tract infections.

For treatment of Lyme disease, see section 5.1.1.3.

ORAL INFECTIONS. The cephalosporins offer little advantage over the penicillins in dental infections, often being less active against anaerobes. Infections due to oral streptococci (often termed viridans streptococci) which become resistant to penicillin are usually also resistant to cephalosporins. This is of importance in the case of patients who have had rheumatic fever and are on long-term penicillin therapy. Cefalexin and cefradine have been used in the treatment of oral infections.

CEFACLOR

Indications: infections due to sensitive Gram-positive and Gram-negative bacteria, but see notes above

Cautions: sensitivity to beta-lactam antibacterials (avoid if history of immediate hypersensitivity reaction); renal impairment (Appendix 3); pregnancy and breast-feeding (but appropriate to use); false positive urinary glucose (if tested for reducing substances) and false positive Coombs' test; **interactions:** Appendix 1 (cephalosporins)

Contra-indications: cephalosporin hypersensitivity

Side-effects: diarrhoea and rarely antibiotic-associated colitis (CSM has warned both more likely with higher doses), nausea and vomiting, abdominal discomfort, headache; allergic reactions including rashes, pruritus, urticaria, serum sickness-like reactions with rashes, fever and arthralgia, and anaphylaxis; erythema multiforme, toxic epidermal necrolysis reported; disturbances in liver enzymes, transient hepatitis and cholestatic jaundice; other side-effects reported include eosinophilia and blood disorders (including thrombocytopenia, leucopenia, agranulocytosis, aplastic anaemia and haemolytic anaemia); reversible interstitial nephritis, hyperactivity, nervousness, sleep disturbances, hallucinations, confusion, hypertonia, and dizziness

Dose: 250 mg every 8 hours, doubled for severe infections; max. 4 g daily; CHILD over 1 month, 20 mg/kg daily in 3 divided doses, doubled for severe infections, max. 1 g daily; *or* 1 month–1 year, 62.5 mg every 8 hours; 1–5 years, 125 mg; over 5 years, 250 mg; doses doubled for severe infections

Cefaclor (Non-proprietary) PoM

Capsules, cefaclor (as monohydrate) 250 mg, net price 21-cap pack = £8.99; 500 mg 50-cap pack = £33.66. Label: 9

Brands include *Keftid*®

Suspension, cefaclor (as monohydrate) for reconstitution with water, 125 mg/5 mL, net price 100 mL = £4.23; 250 mg/5 mL, 100 mL = £7.38. Label: 9

NOTE. Sugar-free versions are available and can be ordered by specifying 'sugar-free' on the prescription

Brands include *Keftid*®

Distaclor® (Flynn) PoM

Capsules, cefaclor (as monohydrate) 500 mg (violet/grey), net price 20 = £17.33. Label: 9

Suspension, both pink, cefaclor (as monohydrate) for reconstitution with water, 125 mg/5 mL, net price 100 mL = £4.13; 250 mg/5 mL, 100 mL = £8.26. Label: 9

Distaclor MR® (Flynn) PoM

Tablets, m/r, both blue, cefaclor (as monohydrate) 375 mg. Net price 14-tab pack = £6.93. Label: 9, 21, 25

Dose: 375 mg every 12 hours with food, dose doubled for pneumonia

Lower urinary-tract infections, 375 mg every 12 hours with food

CEFADROXIL

Indications: see under Cefaclor; see also notes above

Cautions: see under Cefaclor

Contra-indications: see under Cefaclor

Side-effects: see under Cefaclor

Dose: patients over 40 kg, 0.5–1 g twice daily; skin, soft tissue, and simple urinary-tract infections, 1 g daily; CHILD under 1 year, 25 mg/kg daily in divided doses; 1–6 years, 250 mg twice daily; over 6 years, 500 mg twice daily

Cefadroxil (Non-proprietary) PoM

Capsules, cefadroxil (as monohydrate) 500 mg, net price 20-cap pack = £5.64. Label: 9

Baxan® (Bristol-Myers Squibb) PoM

Capsules, cefadroxil (as monohydrate) 500 mg, net price 20-cap pack = £5.64. Label: 9

Suspension, cefadroxil (as monohydrate) for reconstitution with water, 125 mg/5 mL, net price 60 mL = £1.75; 250 mg/5 mL, 60 mL = £3.48; 500 mg/5 mL, 60 mL = £5.21. Label: 9

CEFALEXIN

(Cephalexin)

Indications: see under Cefaclor

Cautions: see under Cefaclor

Contra-indications: see under Cefaclor

Side-effects: see under Cefaclor

Dose: 250 mg every 6 hours *or* 500 mg every 8–12 hours increased to 1–1.5 g every 6–8 hours for severe infections; CHILD 25 mg/kg daily in divided doses, doubled for severe infections, max. 100 mg/kg daily; *or* under 1 year 125 mg every 12 hours, 1–5 years 125 mg every 8 hours, 6–12 years 250 mg every 8 hours

Prophylaxis of recurrent urinary-tract infection, ADULT 125 mg at night

Cefalexin (Non-proprietary) PoM

Capsules, cefalexin 250 mg, net price 28-cap pack = £3.39; 500 mg, 21-cap pack = £3.61. Label: 9

Tablets, cefalexin 250 mg, net price 28-tab pack = £2.42; 500 mg, 21-tab pack = £4.83. Label: 9

Oral suspension, cefalexin for reconstitution with water, 125 mg/5 mL, net price 100 mL = £1.31; 250 mg/5 mL, 100 mL = £3.26. Label: 9

DENTAL PRESCRIBING ON NHS. Cefalexin Capsules, Tablets, and Oral Suspension may be prescribed

Ceporex® (Galen) PoM

Capsules, both caramel/grey, cefalexin 250 mg, net price 28-cap pack = £4.02; 500 mg, 28-cap pack = £7.85. Label: 9

Tablets, all pink, f/c, cefalexin 250 mg, net price 28-tab pack = £4.02; 500 mg, 28-tab pack = £7.85. Label: 9

Syrup, all orange, cefalexin for reconstitution with water, 125 mg/5 mL, net price 100 mL = £1.43; 250 mg/5 mL, 100 mL = £2.87; 500 mg/5 mL, 100 mL = £5.57. Label: 9

Keflex® (Flynn) PoM

Capsules, cefalexin 250 mg (green/white), net price 28-cap pack = £1.76; 500 mg (pale green/dark green), 21-cap pack = £2.66. Label: 9

Tablets, both peach, cefalexin 250 mg, net price 28-tab pack = £2.09; 500 mg (scored), 21-tab pack = £2.47. Label: 9

Suspension, cefalexin for reconstitution with water, 125 mg/5 mL, net price 100 mL = 88p; 250 mg/5 mL, 100 mL = £1.51. Label: 9

CEFIXIME

Indications: see under Cefaclor (acute infections only); gonorrhoea [unlicensed indication] (Table 1, section 5.1)
Cautions: see under Cefaclor
Contra-indications: see under Cefaclor
Side-effects: see under Cefaclor
Dose: ADULT and CHILD over 10 years, 200–400 mg daily in 1–2 divided doses; CHILD over 6 months 8 mg/kg daily in 1–2 divided doses *or* 6 months–1 year 75 mg daily; 1–4 years 100 mg daily; 5–10 years 200 mg daily
Gonorrhoea [unlicensed indication], 400 mg as a single dose

Suprax® (Rhône-Poulenc Rorer) PoM
Tablets, f/c, scored, cefixime 200 mg. Net price 7-tab pack = £13.23. Label: 9
Paediatric oral suspension, cefixime 100 mg/5 mL when reconstituted with water, net price 50 mL (with double-ended spoon for measuring 3.75 mL or 5 mL since dilution not recommended) = £10.53, 100 mL = £18.91. Label: 9

CEFOTAXIME

Indications: see under Cefaclor; gonorrhoea; surgical prophylaxis; Haemophilus epiglottitis and meningitis (Table 1, section 5.1); see also notes above
Cautions: see under Cefaclor
Contra-indications: see under Cefaclor
Side-effects: see under Cefaclor; rarely arrhythmias following rapid injection reported
Dose: *by intramuscular or intravenous injection or by intravenous infusion*, 1 g every 12 hours increased in severe infections (e.g. meningitis) to 8 g daily in 4 divided doses; higher doses (up to 12 g daily in 3–4 divided doses) may be required; NEONATE 50 mg/kg daily in 2–4 divided doses increased to 150–200 mg/kg daily in severe infections; CHILD 100–150 mg/kg daily in 2–4 divided doses increased up to 200 mg/kg daily in very severe infections
Gonorrhoea, 500 mg as a single dose
Important. If bacterial meningitis and especially if meningococcal disease is suspected the patient should be transferred urgently to hospital. If benzylpenicillin cannot be given (e.g. because of an allergy), a single dose of cefotaxime may be given (if available) before urgent transfer to hospital. Suitable doses of cefotaxime by intravenous injection (or by intramuscular injection) are ADULT and CHILD over 12 years 1 g; CHILD under 12 years 50 mg/kg; chloramphenicol (section 5.1.7) may be used if there is a history of anaphylaxis to penicillins or cephalosporins

Cefotaxime (Non-proprietary) PoM
Injection, powder for reconstitution, cefotaxime (as sodium salt), net price 500-mg vial = £2.14; 1-g vial = £4.31; 2-g vial = £8.57

Claforan® (Aventis Pharma) PoM
Injection, powder for reconstitution, cefotaxime (as sodium salt), net price 500-mg vial = £2.14; 1-g vial (with or without infusion connector) = £4.31; 2-g vial (with or without infusion connector) = £8.57
Electrolytes: Na^+ 2.09 mmol/g

CEFPIROME

Indications: see under Cefaclor and notes above
Cautions: see under Cefaclor; interference with creatinine assays using picrate method
Contra-indications: see under Cefaclor
Side-effects: see under Cefaclor; taste disturbance shortly after injection reported
Dose: *by intravenous injection or infusion*, complicated upper and lower urinary-tract, skin and soft-tissue infections, 1 g every 12 hours increased to 2 g every 12 hours in very severe infections
Lower respiratory-tract infections, 1–2 g every 12 hours
Severe infections including bacteraemia and septicaemia and infections in neutropenic patients, 2 g every 12 hours
CHILD under 12 years not recommended

Cefrom® (Hoechst Marion Roussel) PoM
Injection, powder for reconstitution, cefpirome (as sulphate), net price 1-g vial = £10.75; 2-g vial = £21.50

CEFPODOXIME

Indications: see under Dose
Cautions: see under Cefaclor
Contra-indications: see under Cefaclor
Side-effects: see under Cefaclor
Dose: upper respiratory-tract infections (but in pharyngitis and tonsillitis reserved for infections which are recurrent, chronic, or resistant to other antibacterials), 100 mg twice daily (200 mg twice daily in sinusitis)
Lower respiratory-tract infections (including bronchitis and pneumonia), 100–200 mg twice daily
Skin and soft tissue infections, 200 mg twice daily
Uncomplicated urinary-tract infections, 100 mg twice daily (200 mg twice daily in uncomplicated upper urinary-tract infections)
Uncomplicated gonorrhoea, 200 mg as a single dose
CHILD 15 days–6 months 4 mg/kg every 12 hours, 6 months–2 years 40 mg every 12 hours, 3–8 years 80 mg every 12 hours, over 9 years 100 mg every 12 hours

Orelox® (Hoechst Marion Roussel) PoM
Tablets, f/c, cefpodoxime 100 mg (as proxetil), net price 10-tab pack = £10.18. Label: 5, 9, 21
Oral suspension, cefpodoxime (as proxetil) for reconstitution with water, 40 mg/5 mL, net price 100 mL = £11.97. Label: 5, 9, 21
Excipients: include aspartame (section 9.4.1)

CEFPROZIL

Indications: see under Dose
Cautions: see under Cefaclor
Contra-indications: see under Cefaclor
Side-effects: see under Cefaclor
Dose: upper respiratory-tract infections and skin and soft tissue infections, 500 mg once daily usually for 10 days; CHILD 6 months–12 years, 20 mg/kg (max. 500 mg) once daily
Acute exacerbation of chronic bronchitis, 500 mg every 12 hours usually for 10 days
Otitis media, CHILD 6 months–12 years, 20 mg/kg (max. 500 mg) every 12 hours

Cefzil® (Bristol-Myers Squibb) PoM
Tablets, cefprozil, 250 mg (orange), net price 20-tab pack = £14.95; 500 mg, 10-tab pack = £14.95. Label: 9
Suspension, cefprozil, 250 mg/5 mL when reconstituted with water, net price 100 mL = £15.22. Label: 9
Excipients: include aspartame equivalent to phenylalanine 28 mg/5 mL (section 9.4.1)

CEFRADINE

(Cephradine)

Indications: see under Cefaclor; surgical prophylaxis

Cautions: see under Cefaclor

Contra-indications: see under Cefaclor

Side-effects: see under Cefaclor

Dose: *by mouth*, 250–500 mg every 6 hours *or* 0.5–1 g every 12 hours; up to 1 g every 6 hours in severe infections; CHILD, 25–50 mg/kg daily in 2–4 divided doses

By deep intramuscular injection or by intravenous injection over 3–5 minutes *or by intravenous infusion*, 0.5–1 g every 6 hours, increased to 8 g daily in severe infections; CHILD 50–100 mg/kg daily in 4 divided doses

Surgical prophylaxis, *by deep intramuscular injection or by intravenous injection* over 3–5 minutes, 1–2 g at induction

Cefradine (Non-proprietary) PoM
Capsules, cefradine 250 mg, net price 20-cap pack = £5.20; 500 mg, 20-cap pack = £10.28 Label: 9
Brands include *Nicef*®
DENTAL PRESCRIBING ON NHS. Cefradine Capsules may be prescribed

Velosef® (Squibb) PoM
Capsules, cefradine 250 mg (orange/blue), net price 20-cap pack = £3.55; 500 mg (blue), 20-cap pack = £7.00. Label: 9
Syrup, cefradine 250 mg/5 mL when reconstituted with water. Net price 100 mL = £4.22. Label: 9
DENTAL PRESCRIBING ON NHS. *Velosef*® syrup may be prescribed as Cefradine Oral Solution
Injection, powder for reconstitution, cefradine. Net price 500-mg vial = 99p; 1-g vial = £1.95

CEFTAZIDIME

Indications: see under Cefaclor; see also notes above

Cautions: see under Cefaclor

Contra-indications: see under Cefaclor

Side-effects: see under Cefaclor

Dose: *by deep intramuscular injection or intravenous injection or infusion*, 1 g every 8 hours *or* 2 g every 12 hours; 2 g every 8–12 hours *or* 3 g every 12 hours in severe infections; single doses over 1 g intravenous route only; ELDERLY usual max. 3 g daily; CHILD, up to 2 months 25–60 mg/kg daily in 2 divided doses, over 2 months 30–100 mg/kg daily in 2–3 divided doses; up to 150 mg/kg daily (max. 6 g daily) in 3 divided doses if immunocompromised or meningitis; intravenous route recommended for children

Urinary-tract and less serious infections, 0.5–1 g every 12 hours

Pseudomonal lung infection in cystic fibrosis, ADULT 100–150 mg/kg daily in 3 divided doses; CHILD up to 150 mg/kg daily (max. 6 g daily) in 3 divided doses; intravenous route recommended for children

Surgical prophylaxis, prostatic surgery, 1 g at induction of anaesthesia repeated if necessary when catheter removed

Fortum® (GSK) PoM
Injection, powder for reconstitution, ceftazidime (as pentahydrate), with sodium carbonate, net price 250-mg vial = £2.20, 500-mg vial = £4.40, 1-g vial = £8.79, 2-g vial (for injection and for infusion, both) = £17.59, 3-g vial (for injection or infusion) = £25.76; *Monovial*, 2 g vial (with transfer needle) = £17.59
Electrolytes: Na^+ 2.3 mmol/g

Kefadim® (Flynn) PoM
Injection, powder for reconstitution, ceftazidime (as pentahydrate), with sodium carbonate, net price 1-g vial = £7.92; 2-g vial = £15.84
Electrolytes: Na^+ 2.3 mmol/g

CEFTRIAXONE

Indications: see under Cefaclor and notes above; surgical prophylaxis; prophylaxis of meningococcal meningitis [unlicensed indication] (Table 2, section 5.1)

Cautions: see under Cefaclor; severe renal impairment (Appendix 3); hepatic impairment if accompanied by renal impairment (Appendix 2); premature neonates; may displace bilirubin from serum albumin, administer over 60 minutes in neonates (see also Contra-indications); treatment longer than 14 days, renal failure, dehydration, or concomitant total parenteral nutrition—risk of ceftriaxone precipitation in gall bladder

Contra-indications: see under Cefaclor; neonates with jaundice, hypoalbuminaemia, acidosis or impaired bilirubin binding

Side-effects: see under Cefaclor; calcium ceftriaxone precipitates in urine (particularly in very young, dehydrated or those who are immobilised) or in gall bladder—consider discontinuation if symptomatic; rarely prolongation of prothrombin time, pancreatitis

Dose: *by deep intramuscular injection, or by intravenous injection* over at least 2–4 minutes, *or by intravenous infusion*, 1 g daily; 2–4 g daily in severe infections; intramuscular doses over 1 g divided between more than one site

NEONATE *by intravenous infusion* over 60 minutes, 20–50 mg/kg daily (max. 50 mg/kg daily) INFANT and CHILD under 50 kg, *by deep intramuscular injection, or by intravenous injection* over 2–4 minutes, *or by intravenous infusion*, 20–50 mg/kg daily; up to 80 mg/kg daily in severe infections; doses of 50 mg/kg and over by intravenous infusion only; 50 kg and over, adult dose

Endocarditis caused by haemophilus, actinobacillus, cardiobacterium, eikenella, and kingella species ('HACEK organisms') (in combination with another antibacterial if necessary, see Table 1, section 5.1; [unlicensed indication]), *by intravenous injection* over 2–4 minutes *or by intravenous infusion*, 2–4 g daily as a single dose

Uncomplicated gonorrhoea, *by deep intramuscular injection*, 250 mg as a single dose

Surgical prophylaxis, *by deep intramuscular injection or by intravenous injection* over at least 2–4 minutes, 1 g at induction; colorectal surgery, *by deep intramuscular injection or by intravenous injection* over at least 2–4 minutes *or by intravenous infusion*, 2 g at induction; intramuscular doses over 1 g divided between more than one site

Ceftriaxone (Non-proprietary) PoM
Injection, powder for reconstitution, ceftriaxone (as sodium salt), net price 1-g vial = £10.17; 2-g vial = £20.36

Rocephin® (Roche) PoM
Injection, powder for reconstitution, ceftriaxone (as sodium salt), net price 250-mg vial = £2.55; 1-g vial = £10.17; 2-g vial = £20.36
Electrolytes: Na^+ 3.6 mmol /g

CEFUROXIME

Indications: see under Cefaclor; surgical prophylaxis; more active against *Haemophilus influenzae* and *Neisseria gonorrhoeae*; Lyme disease
Cautions: see under Cefaclor
Contra-indications: see under Cefaclor
Side-effects: see under Cefaclor
Dose: *by mouth* (as cefuroxime axetil), 250 mg twice daily in most infections including mild to moderate lower respiratory-tract infections (e.g. bronchitis); doubled for more severe lower respiratory-tract infections or if pneumonia suspected
Urinary-tract infection, 125 mg twice daily, doubled in pyelonephritis
Gonorrhoea, 1 g as a single dose
CHILD over 3 months, 125 mg twice daily, if necessary doubled in child over 2 years with otitis media
Lyme disease, ADULT and CHILD over 12 years, 500 mg twice daily for 20 days
By intramuscular injection or intravenous injection or infusion, 750 mg every 6–8 hours; 1.5 g every 6–8 hours in severe infections; single doses over 750 mg intravenous route only
CHILD usual dose 60 mg/kg daily (range 30–100 mg/kg daily) in 3–4 divided doses (2–3 divided doses in neonates)
Gonorrhoea, 1.5 g as a single dose *by intramuscular injection* (divided between 2 sites)
Surgical prophylaxis, 1.5 g *by intravenous injection* at induction; up to 3 further doses of 750 mg may be given *by intramuscular or intravenous* injection every 8 hours for high-risk procedures
Meningitis, 3 g intravenously every 8 hours; CHILD, 200–240 mg/kg daily (in 3–4 divided doses) reduced to 100 mg/kg daily after 3 days or on clinical improvement; NEONATE, 100 mg/kg daily reduced to 50 mg/kg daily

Zinacef® (GSK) PoM
Injection, powder for reconstitution, cefuroxime (as sodium salt). Net price 250-mg vial = 94p; 750-mg vial = £2.34; 1.5-g vial = £4.70
Electrolytes: Na^+ 1.8 mmol/750-mg vial

Zinnat® (GSK) PoM
Tablets, both f/c, cefuroxime (as axetil) 125 mg, net price 14-tab pack = £4.84; 250 mg, 14-tab pack = £9.67. Label: 9, 21, 25
Suspension, cefuroxime (as axetil) 125 mg/5 mL when reconstituted with water, net price 70 mL = £5.52. Label: 9, 21
Excipients: include aspartame (section 9.4.1)

Other beta-lactam antibiotics

Aztreonam is a monocyclic beta-lactam ('monobactam') antibiotic with an antibacterial spectrum limited to Gram-negative aerobic bacteria including *Pseudomonas aeruginosa*, *Neisseria meningitidis*, and *Haemophilus influenzae*; it should not be used alone for 'blind' treatment since it is not active against Gram-positive organisms. Aztreonam is also effective against *Neisseria gonorrhoeae* (but not against concurrent chlamydial infection). Side-effects are similar to those of the other beta-lactams although aztreonam may be less likely to cause hypersensitivity in penicillin-sensitive patients.

Imipenem, a carbapenem, has a broad spectrum of activity which includes many aerobic and anaerobic Gram-positive and Gram-negative bacteria. Imipenem is partially inactivated in the kidney by enzymatic activity and is therefore administered in combination with **cilastatin**, a specific enzyme inhibitor, which blocks its renal metabolism. Side-effects are similar to those of other beta-lactam antibiotics; neurotoxicity has been observed at very high dosage or in renal failure.

Meropenem is similar to imipenem but is stable to the renal enzyme which inactivates imipenem and therefore can be given without cilastatin. Meropenem has less seizure-inducing potential and can be used to treat central nervous system infection.

Ertapenem has a broad spectrum of activity that covers Gram-positive and Gram-negative organisms and anaerobes. It is licensed for treating abdominal and gynaecological infections and for community-acquired pneumonia, but it is not active against atypical respiratory pathogens and it has limited activity against penicillin-resistant pneumococci. Unlike imipenem and meropenem, ertapenem is not active against *Pseudomonas* or against *Acinetobacter* spp.

AZTREONAM

Indications: Gram-negative infections including *Pseudomonas aeruginosa*, *Haemophilus influenzae*, and *Neisseria meningitidis*
Cautions: hypersensitivity to beta-lactam antibiotics; hepatic impairment; renal impairment (Appendix 3); breast-feeding (Appendix 5); **interactions:** Appendix 1 (aztreonam)
Contra-indications: aztreonam hypersensitivity; pregnancy (Appendix 4)
Side-effects: nausea, vomiting, diarrhoea, abdominal cramps; mouth ulcers, altered taste; jaundice and hepatitis; flushing; hypersensitivity reactions; blood disorders (including thrombocytopenia and neutropenia); rashes, injection-site reactions; rarely hypotension, seizures, asthenia, confusion, dizziness, headache, halitosis, and breast tenderness; very rarely antibiotic-associated colitis, gastro-intestinal bleeding, and toxic epidermal necrolysis
Dose: *by deep intramuscular injection or by intravenous injection* over 3–5 minutes *or by intravenous infusion,* 1 g every 8 hours *or* 2 g every 12 hours; 2 g every 6–8 hours for severe infections (including systemic *Pseudomonas aeruginosa* and lung infections in cystic fibrosis); single doses over 1 g intravenous route only
CHILD over 1 week, *by intravenous injection or infusion*, 30 mg/kg every 6–8 hours increased in

severe infections for child of 2 years or older to 50 mg/kg every 6–8 hours; max. 8 g daily
Urinary-tract infections, 0.5–1 g every 8–12 hours
Gonorrhoea, cystitis, *by intramuscular injection*, 1 g as a single dose

Azactam® (Squibb) PoM
Injection, powder for reconstitution, aztreonam. Net price 500-mg vial = £4.48; 1-g vial = £8.95; 2-g vial = £17.90

ERTAPENEM

Indications: abdominal infections; acute gynaecological infections; community-acquired pneumonia
Cautions: renal impairment (Appendix 3); pregnancy (Appendix 4); **interactions:** Appendix 1 (ertapenem)
Contra-indications: hypersensitivity to beta-lactam antibiotics; breast-feeding (Appendix 5)
Side-effects: diarrhoea, nausea, vomiting, headache, injection-site reactions, rash, pruritus, raised platelet count; less commonly dry mouth, taste disturbances, dyspepsia, abdominal pain, anorexia, constipation, antibiotic-associated colitis, hypotension, chest pain, oedema, pharyngeal discomfort, dyspnoea, dizziness, sleep disturbances, confusion, asthenia, seizures, vaginitis, raised glucose; rarely dysphagia, cholecystitis, liver disorder (including jaundice), arrhythmia, increase in blood pressure, syncope, nasal congestion, cough, wheezing, hypersensitivity reactions, anxiety, depression, agitation, tremor, pelvic peritonitis, renal impairment, muscle cramp, scleral disorder, blood disorders (including neutropenia, thrombocytopenia, haemorrhage), hypoglycaemia, electrolyte disturbances; very rarely hallucinations
Dose: *by intravenous infusion*, ADULT over 18 years, 1 g once daily

Invanz® (MSD) ▼ PoM
Intravenous infusion, powder for reconstitution, ertapenem (as sodium salt), net price 1-g vial = £31.65
Electrolytes: Na^+ 6 mmol/1-g vial

IMIPENEM WITH CILASTATIN

Indications: aerobic and anaerobic Gram-positive and Gram-negative infections; surgical prophylaxis; hospital-acquired septicaemia (Table 1, section 5.1); not indicated for CNS infections
Cautions: sensitivity to beta-lactam antibacterials (avoid if history of immediate hypersensitivity reaction); renal impairment (Appendix 3); CNS disorders (e.g. epilepsy); pregnancy (Appendix 4); breast-feeding (Appendix 5); **interactions:** Appendix 1 (imipenem with cilastatin)
Side-effects: nausea, vomiting, diarrhoea (antibiotic-associated colitis reported), taste disturbances, tooth or tongue discoloration, hearing loss; blood disorders, positive Coombs' test; allergic reactions (with rash, pruritus, urticaria, Stevens-Johnson syndrome, fever, anaphylactic reactions, rarely toxic epidermal necrolysis, exfoliative dermatitis); myoclonic activity, convulsions, confusion and mental disturbances reported; slight increases in liver enzymes and bilirubin reported, rarely hepatitis; increases in serum creatinine and blood urea; red coloration of urine in children reported; local reactions: erythema, pain and induration, and thrombophlebitis
Dose: *by deep intramuscular injection*, mild to moderate infections, in terms of imipenem, 500–750 mg every 12 hours
By intravenous infusion, in terms of imipenem, 1–2 g daily (in 3–4 divided doses); less sensitive organisms, up to 50 mg/kg daily (max. 4 g daily) in 3–4 divided doses; CHILD 3 months and older, 60 mg/kg (up to max. of 2 g) daily in 4 divided doses; over 40 kg, adult dose
Surgical prophylaxis, *by intravenous infusion*, 1 g at induction repeated after 3 hours, supplemented in high risk (e.g. colorectal) surgery by doses of 500 mg 8 and 16 hours after induction

Primaxin® (MSD) PoM
Intramuscular injection, powder for reconstitution, imipenem (as monohydrate) 500 mg with cilastatin (as sodium salt) 500 mg, net price per vial = £12.00
Electrolytes: Na^+ 1.47 mmol/vial
Intravenous infusion, powder for reconstitution, imipenem (as monohydrate) 500 mg with cilastatin (as sodium salt) 500 mg, net price per vial = £12.00; *Monovial* (vial with transfer needle) = £12.00
Electrolytes: Na^+ 1.72 mmol/vial

MEROPENEM

Indications: aerobic and anaerobic Gram-positive and Gram-negative infections
Cautions: sensitivity to beta-lactam antibacterials (avoid if history of immediate hypersensitivity reaction); hepatic impairment (monitor liver function; Appendix 2); renal impairment (Appendix 3); pregnancy (Appendix 4); breast-feeding (Appendix 5); **interactions:** Appendix 1 (meropenem)
Side-effects: nausea, vomiting, diarrhoea (antibiotic-associated colitis reported), abdominal pain; disturbances in liver function tests; thrombocytopenia (reduction in partial thromboplastin time reported), positive Coombs' test, eosinophilia, leucopenia, neutropenia; headache, paraesthesia; hypersensitivity reactions including rash, pruritus, urticaria, angioedema, and anaphylaxis; also reported, convulsions, Stevens-Johnson syndrome and toxic epidermal necrolysis; local reactions including pain and thrombophlebitis at injection site
Dose: *by intravenous injection* over 5 minutes *or by intravenous infusion*, 500 mg every 8 hours, dose doubled in hospital-acquired pneumonia, peritonitis, septicaemia and infections in neutropenic patients; CHILD 3 months–12 years [not licensed for infection in neutropenia] 10–20 mg/kg every 8 hours, over 50 kg body weight adult dose
Meningitis, 2 g every 8 hours; CHILD 3 months–12 years 40 mg/kg every 8 hours, over 50 kg body weight adult dose
Exacerbations of chronic lower respiratory-tract infection in cystic fibrosis, up to 2 g every 8 hours; CHILD 4–18 years 25–40 mg/kg every 8 hours

Meronem® (AstraZeneca) PoM
Injection, powder for reconstitution, meropenem (as trihydrate), net price 500-mg vial = £14.33; 1-g vial = £28.65
Electrolytes: Na^+ 3.9 mmol/g

5.1.3 Tetracyclines

The tetracyclines are broad-spectrum antibiotics whose value has decreased owing to increasing bacterial resistance. They remain, however, the treatment of choice for infections caused by chlamydia (trachoma, psittacosis, salpingitis, urethritis, and lymphogranuloma venereum), rickettsia (including Q-fever), brucella (doxycycline with either streptomycin or rifampicin), and the spirochaete, *Borrelia burgdorferi* (Lyme disease—see section 5.1.1.3). They are also used in respiratory and genital mycoplasma infections, in acne, in destructive (refractory) periodontal disease, in exacerbations of chronic bronchitis (because of their activity against *Haemophilus influenzae*), and for leptospirosis in penicillin hypersensitivity (as an alternative to erythromycin).

Microbiologically, there is little to choose between the various tetracyclines, the only exception being **minocycline** which has a broader spectrum; it is active against *Neisseria meningitidis* and has been used for meningococcal prophylaxis but is no longer recommended because of side-effects including dizziness and vertigo (see section 5.1, table 2 for current recommendations). *Deteclo*® (a combination of tetracycline, chlortetracycline and demeclocycline) does not have any advantages over preparations containing a single tetracycline.

ORAL INFECTIONS. In adults, tetracyclines can be effective against oral anaerobes but the development of resistance (especially by oral streptococci) has reduced their usefulness for the treatment of acute oral infections; they may still have a role in the treatment of destructive (refractory) forms of periodontal disease. Doxycycline has a longer duration of action than tetracycline or oxytetracycline and need only be given once daily; it is reported to be more active against anaerobes than some other tetracyclines.

For the use of doxycycline in the treatment of recurrent aphthous ulceration, oral herpes, or as an adjunct to gingival scaling and root planing for periodontitis, see section 12.3.1 and section 12.3.2.

CAUTIONS. Tetracyclines should be used with caution in patients with hepatic impairment (Appendix 2) or those receiving potentially hepatotoxic drugs. Tetracyclines may increase muscle weakness in patients with myasthenia gravis, and exacerbate systemic lupus erythematosus. Antacids, and aluminium, calcium, iron, magnesium and zinc salts decrease the absorption of tetracyclines; milk also reduces the absorption of demeclocycline, oxytetracycline, and tetracycline. Other **interactions:** Appendix 1 (tetracyclines).

CONTRA-INDICATIONS. Deposition of tetracyclines in growing bone and teeth (by binding to calcium) causes staining and occasionally dental hypoplasia, and they should **not** be given to children under 12 years, or to pregnant (Appendixes 4) or breast-feeding women (Appendix 5). However, doxycycline may be used in children for treatment and post-exposure prophylaxis of anthrax when an alternative antibacterial cannot be given [unlicensed indication]. With the exception of **doxycycline** and **minocycline**, the tetracyclines may exacerbate renal failure and should **not** be given to patients with kidney disease (Appendix 3).

SIDE-EFFECTS. Side-effects of the tetracyclines include nausea, vomiting, diarrhoea (antibiotic-associated colitis reported occasionally), dysphagia, and oesophageal irritation. Other rare side-effects include hepatotoxicity, pancreatitis, blood disorders, photosensitivity (particularly with demeclocycline), and hypersensitivity reactions (including rash, exfoliative dermatitis, Stevens-Johnson syndrome, urticaria, angioedema, anaphylaxis, pericarditis). Headache and visual disturbances may indicate benign intracranial hypertension (discontinue treatment); bulging fontanelles have been reported in infants.

TETRACYCLINE

Indications: see notes above; acne vulgaris, rosacea (section 13.6)
Cautions: see notes above
Contra-indications: see notes above
Side-effects: see notes above; also acute renal failure, skin discoloration
Dose: *by mouth*, 250 mg every 6 hours, increased in severe infections to 500 mg every 6–8 hours
Acne, see section 13.6.2
Non-gonococcal urethritis, 500 mg every 6 hours for 7–14 days (21 days if failure or relapse after first course)
COUNSELLING. Tablets should be swallowed whole with plenty of fluid while sitting or standing

Tetracycline (Non-proprietary) PoM
Tablets, coated, tetracycline hydrochloride 250 mg, net price 28-tab pack = £2.17. Label: 7, 9, 23, counselling, posture
DENTAL PRESCRIBING ON NHS. Tetracycline Tablets may be prescribed

■ Compound preparations

Deteclo® (Goldshield) PoM
Tablets, blue, f/c, tetracycline hydrochloride 115.4 mg, chlortetracycline hydrochloride 115.4 mg, demeclocycline hydrochloride 69.2 mg, net price 14-tab pack = £1.83. Label: 7, 9, 11, 23, counselling, posture
Dose: 1 tablet every 12 hours; 3–4 tablets daily in more severe infections

DEMECLOCYCLINE HYDROCHLORIDE

Indications: see notes above; also inappropriate secretion of antidiuretic hormone, section 6.5.2
Cautions: see notes above, but photosensitivity more common (avoid exposure to sunlight or sun lamps)
Contra-indications: see notes above
Side-effects: see notes above; also reversible nephrogenic diabetes insipidus, acute renal failure
Dose: 150 mg every 6 hours *or* 300 mg every 12 hours

Ledermycin® (Goldshield) PoM
Capsules, red, demeclocycline hydrochloride 150 mg, net price 28-cap pack = £6.94. Label: 7, 9, 11, 23

DOXYCYCLINE

Indications: see notes above; chronic prostatitis; sinusitis, syphilis, pelvic inflammatory disease (Table 1, section 5.1); treatment and prophylaxis of anthrax [unlicensed indication]; malaria treatment and prophylaxis (section 5.4.1); recurrent aphthous ulceration, adjunct to gingival scaling and root planing for periodontitis (section 12.3.1); oral herpes simplex (section 12.3.2); rosacea [unlicensed indication], acne vulgaris (section 13.6)

Cautions: see notes above, but may be used in renal impairment; alcohol dependence; photosensitivity reported (avoid exposure to sunlight or sun lamps); avoid in porphyria (section 9.8.2)

Contra-indications: see notes above

Side-effects: see notes above; also anorexia, flushing, and tinnitus

Dose: 200 mg on first day, then 100 mg daily; severe infections (including refractory urinary-tract infections), 200 mg daily

Early syphilis, 100 mg twice daily for 14 days; late latent syphilis 200 mg twice daily for 28 days

Uncomplicated genital chlamydia, non-gonococcal urethritis, 100 mg twice daily for 7 days (14 days in pelvic inflammatory disease, see also Table 1, section 5.1)

Anthrax (treatment or post-exposure prophylaxis; see also section 5.1.12), 100 mg twice daily; CHILD (only if alternative antibacterial cannot be given) [unlicensed dose] 5 mg/kg daily in 2 divided doses (max. 200 mg daily)

COUNSELLING. Capsules should be swallowed whole with plenty of fluid during meals while sitting or standing

NOTE. Doxycycline doses in BNF may differ from those in product literature

Doxycycline (Non-proprietary) PoM

Capsules, doxycycline (as hyclate) 50 mg, net price 28-cap pack = £4.14; 100 mg, 8-cap pack = £2.34. Label: 6, 9, 11, 27, counselling, posture

Brands include *Doxylar*®

DENTAL PRESCRIBING ON NHS. Doxycycline Capsules 100 mg may be prescribed

Vibramycin® (Pfizer) PoM

Capsules, doxycycline (as hyclate) 50 mg (green/ivory), net price 28-cap pack = £7.74; 100 mg (green), 8-cap pack = £4.18. Label: 6, 9, 11, 27, counselling, posture

Vibramycin-D® (Pfizer) PoM

Dispersible tablets, yellow, scored, doxycycline 100 mg, net price 8-tab pack = £4.91. Label: 6, 9, 11, 13

LYMECYCLINE

Indications: see notes above

Cautions: see notes above

Contra-indications: see notes above

Side-effects: see notes above

Dose: 408 mg every 12 hours, increased to 1.224–1.632 g daily in severe infections

Acne, 408 mg daily for at least 8 weeks

Tetralysal 300® (Galderma) PoM

Capsules, red/yellow, lymecycline 408 mg (= tetracycline 300 mg). Net price 28-cap pack = £7.16. Label: 6, 9

MINOCYCLINE

Indications: see notes above; meningococcal carrier state; acne vulgaris (section 13.6.2)

Cautions: see notes above, but may be used in renal impairment; if treatment continued for longer than 6 months, monitor every 3 months for hepatotoxicity, pigmentation and for systemic lupus erythematosus—discontinue if these develop or if pre-existing systemic lupus erythematosus worsens

Contra-indications: see notes above

Side-effects: see notes above; also anorexia, dizziness, tinnitus and vertigo (more common in women), acute renal failure; pigmentation (sometimes irreversible), discoloration of conjunctiva, tears and sweat, systemic lupus erythematosus

Dose: 100 mg twice daily

Acne, see section 13.6.2

Prophylaxis of asymptomatic meningococcal carrier state (but no longer recommended, see notes above), 100 mg twice daily for 5 days usually followed by rifampicin

COUNSELLING. Tablets or capsules should be swallowed whole with plenty of fluid while sitting or standing

Minocycline (Non-proprietary) PoM

Capsules, minocycline (as hydrochloride) 50 mg, net price 56-cap pack = £17.20; 100 mg, 28-cap pack = £14.74. Label: 6, 9, counselling, posture

Brands include *Aknemin*®

Tablets, minocycline (as hydrochloride) 50 mg, net price 28-tab pack = £8.46, 84-tab pack = £16.20 100 mg, 28-tab pack = £13.85. Label: 6, 9, counselling, posture

Brands include *Blemix*®

Minocin MR® (Lederle) PoM

Capsules, m/r, orange/brown (enclosing yellow and white pellets), minocycline (as hydrochloride) 100 mg. Net price 56-cap pack = £21.14. Label: 6, 25

Dose: acne, 1 capsule daily

Sebomin MR® (Alpharma) PoM

Capsules, m/r, orange, minocycline (as hydrochloride) 100 mg, net price 56-cap pack = £21.14. Label: 6, 25

Dose: acne, 1 capsule daily

OXYTETRACYCLINE

Indications: see notes above; acne vulgaris, rosacea (section 13.6)

Cautions: see notes above; porphyria (section 9.8.2)

Contra-indications: see notes above

Side-effects: see notes above

Dose: 250–500 mg every 6 hours

Acne, see section 13.6.2

Oxytetracycline (Non-proprietary) PoM

Tablets, coated, oxytetracycline dihydrate 250 mg, net price 28-tab pack = 81p. Label: 7, 9, 23

Brands include *Oxymycin*®, *Oxytetramix*®

DENTAL PRESCRIBING ON NHS. Oxtetracycline Tablets may be prescribed

5.1.4 Aminoglycosides

These include amikacin, gentamicin, neomycin, netilmicin, streptomycin, and tobramycin. All are bactericidal and active against some Gram-positive and many Gram-negative organisms. Amikacin, gentamicin, and tobramycin are also active against

Pseudomonas aeruginosa; streptomycin is active against *Mycobacterium tuberculosis* and is now almost entirely reserved for tuberculosis (section 5.1.9).

The aminoglycosides are not absorbed from the gut (although there is a risk of absorption in inflammatory bowel disease and liver failure) and must therefore be given by injection for systemic infections.

Excretion is principally via the kidney and accumulation occurs in renal impairment.

Most side-effects of this group of antibiotics are dose-related therefore care must be taken with dosage and whenever possible treatment should not exceed 7 days. The important side-effects are ototoxicity, and nephrotoxicity; they occur most commonly in the elderly and in patients with renal failure.

If there is impairment of renal function (or high pre-dose serum concentrations) the interval between doses must be increased; if the renal impairment is severe the dose itself should be reduced as well.

Aminoglycosides may impair neuromuscular transmission and should not be given to patients with myasthenia gravis; large doses given during surgery have been responsible for a transient myasthenic syndrome in patients with normal neuromuscular function.

Aminoglycosides should preferably not be given with potentially ototoxic diuretics (e.g. furosemide (frusemide)); if concurrent use is unavoidable administration of the aminoglycoside and of the diuretic should be separated by as long a period as practicable.

SERUM CONCENTRATIONS. Serum concentration monitoring avoids both excessive and subtherapeutic concentrations thus preventing toxicity and ensuring efficacy. In patients with normal renal function, aminoglycoside concentrations should be measured after 3 or 4 doses; patients with renal impairment may require earlier and more frequent measurement of aminoglycoside concentration.

Blood samples should be taken approximately 1 hour after intramuscular or intravenous administration ('peak' concentration) and also just before the next dose ('trough' concentration).

Serum aminoglycoside concentrations should be measured in all patients and **must** be determined in infants, in the elderly, in obesity, and in cystic fibrosis, *or* if high doses are being given, *or* if there is renal impairment.

ONCE DAILY DOSAGE. Although aminoglycosides are generally given in 2–3 divided doses during the 24 hours, *once daily administration* is more convenient (while ensuring adequate serum concentration) but **expert advice** about dosage and serum concentrations should be obtained.

ENDOCARDITIS. **Gentamicin** is used in combination with other antibiotics for the treatment of bacterial endocarditis (Table 1, section 5.1). Serum-gentamicin concentration should be determined twice each week (more often in renal impairment). **Streptomycin** may be used as an alternative in gentamicin-resistant enterococcal endocarditis.

Gentamicin is the aminoglycoside of choice in the UK and is used widely for the treatment of serious infections. It has a broad spectrum but is inactive against anaerobes and has poor activity against haemolytic streptococci and pneumococci. When used for the 'blind' therapy of undiagnosed serious infections it is usually given in conjunction with a penicillin or metronidazole (or both). Gentamicin is used together with another antibiotic for the treatment of endocarditis (see above and Table 1, section 5.1).

Loading and maintenance doses of gentamicin may be calculated on the basis of the patient's weight and renal function (e.g. using a nomogram); adjustments are then made according to serum-gentamicin concentrations. High doses are occasionally indicated for serious infections, especially in the neonate or the immunocompromised patient. Whenever possible treatment should not exceed 7 days.

Amikacin is more stable than gentamicin to enzyme inactivation. Amikacin is used in the treatment of serious infections caused by gentamicin-resistant Gram-negative bacilli.

Netilmicin has similar activity to gentamicin, but may cause less ototoxicity in those needing treatment for longer than 10 days. Netilmicin is active against a number of gentamicin-resistant Gram-negative bacilli but is less active against *Ps. aeruginosa* than gentamicin or tobramycin.

Tobramycin has similar activity to gentamicin. It is slightly more active against *Ps. aeruginosa* but shows less activity against certain other Gram-negative bacteria. Tobramycin may be administered by nebuliser on a cyclical basis (28 days of tobramycin followed by a 28–day tobramycin-free interval) for the treatment of chronic pulmonary *Ps. aeruginosa* infection in cystic fibrosis; however, resistance may develop and some patients do not respond to treatment.

Neomycin is too toxic for parenteral administration and can only be used for infections of the skin or mucous membranes or to reduce the bacterial population of the colon prior to bowel surgery or in hepatic failure. Oral administration may lead to malabsorption. Small amounts of neomycin may be absorbed from the gut in patients with hepatic failure and, as these patients may also be uraemic, cumulation may occur with resultant ototoxicity.

GENTAMICIN

Indications: septicaemia and neonatal sepsis; meningitis and other CNS infections; biliary-tract infection, acute pyelonephritis or prostatitis, endocarditis (see notes above); pneumonia in hospital patients, adjunct in listerial meningitis (Table 1, section 5.1); eye (section 11.3.1); ear (section 12.1.1)

Cautions: pregnancy (Appendix 4), renal impairment, neonates, infants and elderly (adjust dose and monitor renal, auditory and vestibular function together with serum gentamicin concentrations); avoid prolonged use; conditions characterised by muscular weakness; obesity (use ideal body-weight to calculate dose and monitor serum-gentamicin concentration closely); see also notes above; **interactions:** Appendix 1 (aminoglycosides)

Contra-indications: myasthenia gravis

Side-effects: vestibular and auditory damage, nephrotoxicity; rarely, hypomagnesaemia on prolonged therapy, antibiotic-associated colitis, stomatitis; also reported, nausea, vomiting, rash, blood disorders; see also notes above

Dose: *by intramuscular or by slow intravenous injection* over at least 3 minutes *or by intravenous infusion*, 3–5 mg/kg daily (in divided doses every 8 hours), see also notes above

NEONATE up to 2 weeks, 3 mg/kg every 12 hours; CHILD 2 weeks–12 years, 2 mg/kg every 8 hours

Endocarditis (in combination with other antibacterials, see Table 1, section 5.1), ADULT 1 mg/kg every 8 hours

Endocarditis prophylaxis, Table 2, section 5.1

By intrathecal injection, seek specialist advice, 1 mg daily (increased if necessary to 5 mg daily)

NOTE. One-hour ('peak') serum concentration should be 5–10 mg/litre (3–5 mg/litre for endocarditis); pre-dose ('trough') concentration should be less than 2 mg/litre (less than 1 mg/litre for endocarditis)

Gentamicin (Non-proprietary) PoM
Injection, gentamicin (as sulphate), net price 40 mg/mL, 1-mL amp = £1.40, 2-mL amp = £1.54, 2-mL vial = £1.48
Paediatric injection, gentamicin (as sulphate) 10 mg/mL, net price 2-mL vial = £1.80
Intrathecal injection, gentamicin (as sulphate) 5 mg/mL, net price 1-mL amp = 74p

Cidomycin® (Beacon) PoM
Injection, gentamicin (as sulphate) 40 mg/mL. Net price 2-mL amp or vial = £1.48

Genticin® (Roche) PoM
Injection, gentamicin (as sulphate) 40 mg/mL. Net price 2-mL amp = £1.40

Isotonic Gentamicin Injection (Baxter) PoM
Intravenous infusion, gentamicin (as sulphate) 800 micrograms/mL in sodium chloride intravenous infusion 0.9%. Net price 100-mL (80-mg) *Viaflex®* bag = £1.61
Electrolytes: Na^+ 15.4 mmol/100-mL bag

AMIKACIN

Indications: serious Gram-negative infections resistant to gentamicin

Cautions: see under Gentamicin

Contra-indications: see under Gentamicin

Side-effects: see under Gentamicin

Dose: *by intramuscular or by slow intravenous injection or by infusion*, 15 mg/kg daily in 2 divided doses, increased to 22.5 mg/kg daily in 3 divided doses in severe infections; max. 1.5 g daily for up to 10 days (max. cumulative dose 15 g); CHILD 15 mg/kg daily in 2 divided doses; NEONATE loading dose of 10 mg/kg then 15 mg/kg daily in 2 divided doses

NOTE. One-hour ('peak') serum concentration should not exceed 30 mg/litre; pre-dose ('trough') concentration should be less than 10 mg/litre

Amikacin (Non-proprietary) PoM
Injection, amikacin (as sulphate) 250 mg/mL. Net price 2-mL vial = £10.14
Electrolytes: Na^+ 0.56 mmol/500-mg vial

Amikin® (Bristol-Myers Squibb) PoM
Injection, amikacin (as sulphate) 250 mg/mL. Net price 2-mL vial = £10.14
Electrolytes: $Na^+ < 0.5$ mmol/vial
Paediatric injection, amikacin (as sulphate) 50 mg/mL. Net price 2-mL vial = £2.36
Electrolytes: $Na^+ < 0.5$ mmol/vial

NEOMYCIN SULPHATE

Indications: bowel sterilisation before surgery, see also notes above

Cautions: see under Gentamicin but too toxic for systemic use, see notes above

Contra-indications: see under Gentamicin; intestinal obstruction

Side-effects: see under Gentamicin but poorly absorbed on oral administration; increased salivation, stomatitis, impaired intestinal absorption with steatorrhoea and diarrhoea

Dose: *by mouth*, pre-operative bowel sterilisation, 1 g every hour for 4 hours, then 1 g every 4 hours for 2–3 days

Hepatic coma, up to 4 g daily in divided doses usually for max. 14 days

Neomycin (Non-proprietary) PoM
Tablets, neomycin sulphate 500 mg. Net price 20 = £3.44
Brands include *Nivemycin®*

NETILMICIN

Indications: serious Gram-negative infections resistant to gentamicin

Cautions: see under Gentamicin

Contra-indications: see under Gentamicin

Side-effects: see under Gentamicin

Dose: *by intramuscular injection or by intravenous injection over 3–5 minutes or by intravenous infusion*, 4–6 mg/kg daily, as a single daily dose or in divided doses every 8 or 12 hours; in severe infections, up to 7.5 mg/kg daily in divided doses every 8 hours (reduced as soon as clinically indicated, usually within 48 hours); PRETERM NEONATE and NEONATE up to 1 week, 3 mg/kg every 12 hours; INFANT 1 week–1 year, 2.5–3 mg/kg every 8 hours; CHILD over 1 year, 2–2.5 mg/kg every 8 hours

Urinary-tract infection, 150 mg as a single daily dose for 5 days

Gonorrhoea, 300 mg as a single dose

NOTE. For divided daily dose regimens, one-hour ('peak') serum concentration should not exceed 12 mg/litre; pre-dose ('trough') concentration should be less than 2 mg/litre

Netillin® (Schering-Plough) PoM
Injection, netilmicin (as sulphate) 10 mg/mL, net price 1.5-mL (15-mg) amp = £1.42; 50 mg/mL, 1-mL (50-mg) amp = £2.11; 100 mg/mL, 1-mL (100-mg) amp = £2.75; 1.5-mL (150-mg) amp = £3.92, 2-mL (200-mg) amp = £5.09

TOBRAMYCIN

Indications: see under Gentamicin and notes above

Cautions: see under Gentamicin

SPECIFIC CAUTIONS FOR INHALED TREATMENT. Other inhaled drugs should be administered before tobramycin; monitor for bronchospasm with initial dose, measure peak flow before and after nebulisation—if bronchospasm occurs, repeat test using bronchodilator; monitor renal function before treatment and then annually; severe haemoptysis

Contra-indications: see under Gentamicin

Side-effects: see under Gentamicin; *on inhalation*, mouth ulcers, voice alteration, cough, bronchospasm (see Cautions)

Dose: *by intramuscular injection or by slow intravenous injection or by intravenous infusion*, 3 mg/kg daily in divided doses every 8 hours, see also notes above; in severe infections up to 5 mg/kg daily in divided doses every 6–8 hours (reduced to

3 mg/kg as soon as clinically indicated); NEONATE 2 mg/kg every 12 hours; CHILD over 1 week 2–2.5 mg/kg every 8 hours

Urinary-tract infection, *by intramuscular injection*, 2–3 mg/kg daily as a single dose

NOTE. One-hour ('peak') serum concentration should not exceed 10 mg/litre; pre-dose ('trough') concentration should be less than 2 mg/litre

Tobramycin (Non-proprietary) PoM

Injection, tobramycin (as sulphate) 40 mg/mL, net price 1-mL (40-mg) vial = £2.73, 2-mL (80-mg) vial = £4.16, 6-mL (240-mg) vial = £12.47

Nebcin® (King) PoM

Injection, tobramycin (as sulphate) 10 mg/mL, net price 2-mL (20-mg) vial = £2.21; 40 mg/mL, 2-mL (80-mg) vial = £5.37

Tobi® (Chiron) PoM

Nebuliser solution, tobramycin 60 mg/mL, net price 56 × 5-mL (300-mg) unit = £1540.00

Dose: chronic pulmonary *Pseudomonas aeruginosa* infection in cystic fibrosis patients, *by inhalation of nebulised solution*, ADULT and CHILD over 6 years, 300 mg every 12 hours for 28 days, courses repeated after 28-day interval

5.1.5 Macrolides

Erythromycin has an antibacterial spectrum that is similar but not identical to that of penicillin; it is thus an alternative in penicillin-allergic patients.

Indications for erythromycin include respiratory infections, whooping cough, legionnaires' disease, and campylobacter enteritis. It is active against many penicillin-resistant staphylococci but some are now also resistant to erythromycin; it has poor activity against *Haemophilus influenzae*. Erythromycin is also active against chlamydia and mycoplasmas.

Erythromycin causes nausea, vomiting, and diarrhoea in some patients; in mild to moderate infections this can be avoided by giving a lower dose (250 mg 4 times daily) but if a more serious infection, such as Legionella pneumonia, is suspected higher doses are needed.

Azithromycin is a macrolide with slightly less activity than erythromycin against Gram-positive bacteria but enhanced activity against some Gram-negative organisms including *H. influenzae*. Plasma concentrations are very low but tissue concentrations are much higher. It has a long tissue half-life and once daily dosage is recommended. For treatment of Lyme disease, see section 5.1.1.3. Azithromycin is also used in the treatment of trachoma [unlicensed indication] (section 11.3.1).

Clarithromycin is an erythromycin derivative with slightly greater activity than the parent compound. Tissue concentrations are higher than with erythromycin. It is given twice daily.

Azithromycin and clarithromycin cause fewer gastro-intestinal side-effects than erythromycin.

Spiramycin is also a macrolide (section 5.4.7).

The ketolide **telithromycin** is a derivative of erythromycin. The antibacterial spectrum of telithromycin is similar to that of macrolides and it is also active against penicillin- and erythromycin-resistant *Streptococcus pneumoniae*.

ORAL INFECTIONS. Erythromycin is an alternative for oral infections in penicillin-allergic patients or where a beta-lactamase producing organism is involved. However, many organisms are now resistant to erythromycin or rapidly develop resistance; its use should therefore be limited to short courses. Metronidazole (section 5.1.11) may be preferred as an alternative to a penicillin.

For prophylaxis of infective endocarditis in patients allergic to penicillin, a single-dose of oral clindamycin is used; see Table 2, section 5.1. Single-dose azithromycin is used for prophylaxis of endocarditis in those unable to take clindamycin [unlicensed indication].

ERYTHROMYCIN

Indications: alternative to penicillin in hypersensitive patients; oral infections (see notes above); campylobacter enteritis, syphilis, non-gonococcal urethritis, respiratory-tract infections (including legionnaires' disease), skin infections (Table 1, section 5.1); chronic prostatitis; diphtheria and whooping cough prophylaxis (Table 2, section 5.1); acne vulgaris and rosacea (section 13.6)

Cautions: hepatic impairment (Appendix 2); renal impairment (Appendix 3); predisposition to QT interval prolongation (including electrolyte disturbances, concomitant use of drugs that prolong QT interval); avoid in porphyria (section 9.8.2); pregnancy (not known to be harmful) and breast-feeding (only small amounts in milk); **interactions:** Appendix 1 (macrolides)

ARRHYTHMIAS. Avoid concomitant administration with pimozide or terfenadine [other interactions, Appendix 1]

Side-effects: nausea, vomiting, abdominal discomfort, diarrhoea (antibiotic-associated colitis reported); less frequently urticaria, rashes and other allergic reactions; reversible hearing loss reported after large doses; cholestatic jaundice, infantile hypertrophic pyloric stenosis, cardiac effects (including chest pain and arrhythmias), myasthenia-like syndrome, Stevens-Johnson syndrome, and toxic epidermal necrolysis also reported

Dose: *by mouth*, ADULT and CHILD over 8 years, 250–500 mg every 6 hours *or* 0.5–1 g every 12 hours (see notes above); up to 4 g daily in severe infections; CHILD up to 2 years 125 mg every 6 hours, 2–8 years 250 mg every 6 hours, doses doubled for severe infections

Early syphilis, 500 mg 4 times daily for 14 days

Uncomplicated genital chlamydia, non-gonococcal urethritis, 500 mg twice daily for 14 days

By intravenous infusion, ADULT and CHILD severe infections, 50 mg/kg daily by continuous infusion *or* in divided doses every 6 hours; mild infections (oral treatment not possible), 25 mg/kg daily; NEONATE 30–45 mg/kg daily in 3 divided doses

Erythromycin (Non-proprietary) PoM

Capsules, enclosing e/c microgranules, erythromycin 250 mg, net price 28-cap pack = £5.95. Label: 5, 9, 25

Brands include *Tiloryth*®

Tablets, e/c, erythromycin 250 mg, net price 20 = £1.15. Label: 5, 9, 25

Brands include *Rommix*®

DENTAL PRESCRIBING ON NHS. Erythromycin Tablets e/c may be prescribed

Erythromycin Ethyl Succinate (Non-proprietary) PoM

Oral suspension, erythromycin (as ethyl succinate) for reconstitution with water 125 mg/5 mL, net price 100 mL = £2.37; 250 mg/5 mL, 100 mL = £3.32; 500 mg/5 mL, 100 mL = £4.84. Label: 9

NOTE. Sugar-free versions are available and can be ordered by specifying 'sugar-free' on the prescription

Brands include *Primacine*®

DENTAL PRESCRIBING ON NHS. Erythromycin Ethyl Succinate Oral Suspension may be prescribed

Erythromycin Lactobionate (Non-proprietary) PoM

Intravenous infusion, powder for reconstitution, erythromycin (as lactobionate), net price 1-g vial = £9.98

Erymax® (Zeneus) PoM

Capsules, opaque orange/clear orange, enclosing orange and white e/c pellets, erythromycin 250 mg, net price 28-cap pack = £5.95, 112-cap pack = £23.80. Label: 5, 9, 25

Dose: 1 capsule every 6 hours *or* 2 capsules every 12 hours; acne, 1 capsule twice daily for 1 month then 1 capsule daily

Erythrocin® (Abbott) PoM

Tablets, both f/c, erythromycin (as stearate), 250 mg, net price 20 = £2.92; 500 mg, 20 = £6.01. Label: 9

DENTAL PRESCRIBING ON NHS. May be prescribed as Erythromycin Stearate Tablets

Erythroped® (Abbott) PoM

Suspension SF, sugar-free, banana-flavoured, erythromycin (as ethyl succinate) for reconstitution with water, 125 mg/5 mL (*Suspension PI SF*), net price 140 mL = £3.18; 250 mg/5 mL, 140 mL = £6.20; 500 mg/5 mL (*Suspension SF Forte*), 140 mL = £10.99. Label: 9

Erythroped A® (Abbott) PoM

Tablets, yellow, f/c, erythromycin 500 mg (as ethyl succinate). Net price 28-tab pack = £8.29. Label: 9

DENTAL PRESCRIBING ON NHS. May be prescribed as Erythromycin Ethyl Succinate Tablets

AZITHROMYCIN

Indications: respiratory-tract infections; otitis media; skin and soft-tissue infections; uncomplicated genital chlamydial infections and non-gonococcal urethritis (Table 1, section 5.1); mild or moderate typhoid due to multiple-antibacterial-resistant organisms [unlicensed indication]; prophylaxis of endocarditis in children [unlicensed indication] (Table 2, section 5.1)

Cautions: see under Erythromycin; pregnancy (Appendix 4) and breast-feeding (Appendix 5); **interactions:** Appendix 1 (macrolides)

Contra-indications: hepatic impairment

Side-effects: see under Erythromycin; also anorexia, dyspepsia, flatulence, constipation, pancreatitis, hepatitis, syncope, dizziness, headache, drowsiness, agitation, anxiety, hyperactivity, asthenia, paraesthesia, convulsions, mild neutropenia, thrombocytopenia, interstitial nephritis, acute renal failure, arthralgia, photosensitivity; *rarely* taste disturbances, tongue discoloration, and hepatic failure

Dose: 500 mg once daily for 3 days; CHILD over 6 months 10 mg/kg once daily for 3 days; *or* body-weight 15–25 kg, 200 mg once daily for 3 days; body-weight 26–35 kg, 300 mg once daily for 3 days; body-weight 36–45 kg, 400 mg once daily for 3 days

Uncomplicated genital chlamydial infections and non-gonococcal urethritis, 1 g as a single dose

Typhoid [unlicensed indication], 500 mg once daily for 7 days

Zithromax® (Pfizer) PoM

Capsules, azithromycin (as dihydrate) 250 mg, net price 4-cap pack = £8.95, 6-cap pack = £13.43. Label: 5, 9, 23

Oral suspension, cherry/banana-flavoured, azithromycin (as dihydrate) 200 mg/5 mL when reconstituted with water. Net price 15-mL pack = £5.08, 22.5-mL pack = £7.62, 30-mL pack = £13.80. Label: 5, 9

DENTAL PRESCRIBING ON NHS. May be prescribed as Azithromycin Oral Suspension 200 mg/5 mL

CLARITHROMYCIN

Indications: respiratory-tract infections, mild to moderate skin and soft tissue infections, otitis media; *Helicobacter pylori* eradication (section 1.3)

Cautions: see under Erythromycin; renal impairment (Appendix 3); pregnancy (Appendix 4); breast-feeding (Appendix 5); **interactions:** Appendix 1 (macrolides)

ARRHYTHMIAS. Avoid concomitant administration with pimozide or terfenadine [other interactions, Appendix 1]

Side-effects: see under Erythromycin; also reported, dyspepsia, headache, smell and taste disturbances, tooth and tongue discoloration, stomatitis, glossitis, pancreatitis, arthralgia, myalgia, dizziness, vertigo, tinnitus, anxiety, insomnia, nightmares, confusion, psychosis, convulsions, paraesthesia, hypoglycaemia, hepatitis, renal failure, leucopenia, and thrombocytopenia; on intravenous infusion, local tenderness, phlebitis

Dose: *by mouth*, 250 mg every 12 hours for 7 days, increased in severe infections to 500 mg every 12 hours for up to 14 days; CHILD body-weight under 8 kg, 7.5 mg/kg twice daily; 8–11 kg (1–2 years), 62.5 mg twice daily; 12–19 kg (3–6 years), 125 mg twice daily; 20–29 kg (7–9 years), 187.5 mg twice daily; 30–40 kg (10–12 years), 250 mg twice daily

By intravenous infusion into larger proximal vein, 500 mg twice daily; CHILD not recommended

Clarithromycin (Non-proprietary) PoM

Tablets, clarithromycin 250 mg, net price 14-tab pack = £10.94; 500 mg, 14-tab pack = £21.90. Label: 9

Klaricid® (Abbott) PoM

Tablets, both yellow, f/c, clarithromycin 250 mg, net price 14-tab pack = £10.94; 500 mg, 14-tab pack = £21.90, 20-tab pack = £31.29. Label: 9

Paediatric suspension, clarithromycin for reconstitution with water 125 mg/5 mL, net price 70 mL = £5.58, 100 mL = £9.60; 250 mg/5 mL, 70 mL = £11.16. Label: 9

Granules, clarithromycin 250 mg/sachet, net price 14-sachet pack = £11.68. Label: 9, 13

Intravenous infusion, powder for reconstitution, clarithromycin. Net price 500-mg vial = £11.46

Electrolytes: Na^+ < 0.5 mmol/500-mg vial

Klaricid XL® (Abbott) PoM

Tablets, m/r, yellow, clarithromycin 500 mg, net price 7-tab pack = £9.90, 14-tab pack = £19.81. Label: 9, 21, 25

Dose: 500 mg once daily (doubled in severe infections) for 7–14 days

TELITHROMYCIN

Indications: community-acquired pneumonia; exacerbation of chronic bronchitis; sinusitis; beta-haemolytic streptococcal pharyngitis or tonsillitis when beta-lactam antibiotics are inappropriate

Cautions: hepatic impairment; renal impairment (Appendix 3); pregnancy (Appendix 4); coronary heart disease, ventricular arrhythmias, bradycardia, hypokalaemia, hypomagnesaemia—risk of QT interval prolongation; concomitant administration of drugs that prolong QT-interval; myasthenia gravis (risk of exacerbation—use only if no other alternative); **interactions:** Appendix 1 (telithromycin)

Contra-indications: breast-feeding (Appendix 5); prolongation of QT interval; congenital or family history of QT interval prolongation (if not excluded by ECG)

ARRHYTHMIAS. Avoid concomitant administration with pimozide or terfenadine [other interactions, Appendix 1]

Side-effects: diarrhoea, nausea, vomiting, flatulence, abdominal pain, taste disturbances; dizziness, headache; *less commonly* constipation, stomatitis, anorexia, flushing, palpitations, drowsiness, insomnia, nervousness, eosinophilia, blurred vision, rash, urticaria, and pruritus; *rarely* cholestatic jaundice, arrhythmias, hypotension, paraesthesia, and diplopia; *very rarely* antibiotic-associated colitis, hepatitis, altered sense of smell, muscle cramp, erythema multiforme

Dose: 800 mg once daily for 5 days for sinusitis or exacerbation of chronic bronchitis *or* for 7–10 days in community-acquired pneumonia; CHILD under 18 years safety and efficacy not established

Beta-haemolytic streptococcal pharyngitis or tonsillitis, ADULT and CHILD over 12 years, 800 mg once daily for 5 days

Ketek® (Aventis Pharma) ▼ PoM

Tablets, orange, f/c, telithromycin 400 mg, net price 10-tab pack = £19.31.Label: 9

5.1.6 Clindamycin

Clindamycin has only a limited use because of serious side-effects. Its most serious toxic effect is antibiotic-associated colitis (section 1.5) which may be fatal and is most common in middle-aged and elderly women, especially following operation. Although antibiotic-associated colitis can occur with most antibacterials it occurs more frequently with clindamycin. Patients should therefore discontinue treatment immediately if diarrhoea develops.

Clindamycin is active against Gram-positive cocci, including penicillin-resistant staphylococci and also against many anaerobes, especially *Bacteroides fragilis*. It is well concentrated in bone and excreted in bile and urine.

Clindamycin is recommended for staphylococcal joint and bone infections such as osteomyelitis, and intra-abdominal sepsis.

Clindamycin is used for prophylaxis of endocarditis in patients allergic to penicillin [unlicensed indication], see Table 2, section 5.1.

ORAL INFECTIONS. Clindamycin should not be used routinely for the treatment of oral infections because it may be no more effective than penicillins against anaerobes and there may be cross-resistance with erythromycin-resistant bacteria.

CLINDAMYCIN

Indications: see notes above; staphylococcal bone and joint infections, peritonitis; endocarditis prophylaxis [unlicensed indication], table 2, section 5.1

Cautions: discontinue immediately if diarrhoea or colitis develops; hepatic impairment (Appendix 2); renal impairment; monitor liver and renal function on prolonged therapy and in neonates and infants; pregnancy (Appendix 4); breast-feeding (Appendix 5); avoid rapid intravenous administration; avoid in porphyria (section 9.8.2); **interactions:** Appendix 1 (clindamycin)

Contra-indications: diarrhoeal states; avoid injections containing benzyl alcohol in neonates (see under preparations below)

Side-effects: diarrhoea (discontinue treatment), abdominal discomfort, oesophagitis, nausea, vomiting, antibiotic-associated colitis; jaundice and altered liver function tests; neutropenia, eosinophilia, agranulocytosis and thrombocytopenia reported; rash, pruritus, urticaria, anaphylactoid reactions, Stevens-Johnson syndrome, exfoliative and vesiculobullous dermatitis reported; pain, induration, and abscess after intramuscular injection; thrombophlebitis after intravenous injection

Dose: *by mouth*, 150–300 mg every 6 hours; up to 450 mg every 6 hours in severe infections; CHILD, 3–6 mg/kg every 6 hours

COUNSELLING. Patients should discontinue immediately and contact doctor if diarrhoea develops; capsules should be swallowed with a glass of water.

By deep intramuscular injection or by intravenous infusion, 0.6–2.7 g daily (in 2–4 divided doses); life-threatening infection, up to 4.8 g daily; single doses above 600 mg by intravenous infusion only; single doses by intravenous infusion not to exceed 1.2 g

CHILD over 1 month, 15–40 mg/kg daily in 3–4 divided doses; severe infections, at least 300 mg daily regardless of weight

Clindamycin (Non-proprietary) PoM

Capsules, clindamycin (as hydrochloride) 150 mg, net price 24-cap pack = £13.72. Label: 9, 27, counselling, see above (diarrhoea)

DENTAL PRESCRIBING ON NHS. Clindamycin Capsules may be prescribed

Dalacin C® (Pharmacia) PoM

Capsules, clindamycin (as hydrochloride) 75 mg (lavender), net price 24-cap pack = £7.45; 150 mg, (lavender/maroon), 24-cap pack = £13.72. Label: 9, 27, counselling, see above (diarrhoea)

DENTAL PRESCRIBING ON NHS. May be prescribed as Clindamycin Capsules

Injection, clindamycin (as phosphate) 150 mg/mL, net price 2-mL amp = £6.20; 4-mL amp = £12.35

Excipients: include benzyl alcohol (avoid in neonates, see Excipients, p. 2)

5.1.7 Some other antibacterials

Antibacterials discussed in this section include chloramphenicol, fusidic acid, glycopeptide antibiotics (vancomycin and teicoplanin), linezolid, the streptogramins (quinupristin and dalfopristin) and the polymyxin, colistin.

Chloramphenicol

Chloramphenicol is a potent broad-spectrum antibiotic; however, it is associated with serious haematological side-effects when given systemically and should therefore be reserved for the treatment of life-threatening infections, particularly those caused by *Haemophilus influenzae*, and also for typhoid fever.

Chloramphenicol eye drops (section 11.3.1) and chloramphenicol ear drops (section 12.1.1) are also available.

CHLORAMPHENICOL

Indications: see notes above

Cautions: avoid repeated courses and prolonged treatment; reduce doses in hepatic impairment (Appendix 2); renal impairment (Appendix 3); blood counts required before and periodically during treatment; monitor plasma-chloramphenicol concentration in neonates (see below); **interactions:** Appendix 1 (chloramphenicol)

Contra-indications: pregnancy (Appendix 4), breast-feeding (Appendix 5), porphyria (section 9.8.2)

Side-effects: blood disorders including reversible and irreversible aplastic anaemia (with reports of resulting leukaemia), peripheral neuritis, optic neuritis, headache, depression, urticaria, erythema multiforme, nausea, vomiting, diarrhoea, stomatitis, glossitis, dry mouth; nocturnal haemoglobinuria reported; grey syndrome (abdominal distension, pallid cyanosis, circulatory collapse) may follow excessive doses in neonates with immature hepatic metabolism

Dose: *by mouth or by intravenous injection or infusion*, 50 mg/kg daily in 4 divided doses (exceptionally, can be doubled for severe infections such as septicaemia and meningitis, providing high doses reduced as soon as clinically indicated); CHILD, haemophilus epiglottitis and pyogenic meningitis, 50–100 mg/kg daily in divided doses (high dosages decreased as soon as clinically indicated); NEONATE under 2 weeks 25 mg/kg daily (in 4 divided doses); INFANT 2 weeks–1 year 50 mg/kg daily (in 4 divided doses)

NOTE. Plasma concentration monitoring required in neonates and preferred in those under 4 years of age, in the elderly, and in hepatic impairment; recommended peak plasma concentration (approx. 1 hour after intravenous injection or infusion) 15–25 mg/litre; pre-dose ('trough') concentration should not exceed 15 mg/litre

Chloramphenicol (Non-proprietary) PoM

Capsules, chloramphenicol 250 mg. Net price 60 = £20.74

Kemicetine® (Pharmacia) PoM

Injection, powder for reconstitution, chloramphenicol (as sodium succinate). Net price 1-g vial = £1.39

Electrolytes: Na^+ 3.14 mmol/g

Fusidic acid

Fusidic acid and its salts are narrow-spectrum antibiotics. The only indication for their use is in infections caused by penicillin-resistant staphylococci, especially osteomyelitis, as they are well concentrated in bone; they are also used for staphylococcal endocarditis. A second antistaphylococcal antibiotic is usually required to prevent emergence of resistance.

SODIUM FUSIDATE

Indications: penicillin-resistant staphylococcal infection including osteomyelitis; staphylococcal endocarditis in combination with other antibacterials (Table 1, section 5.1)

Cautions: monitor liver function with high doses, on prolonged therapy or in hepatic impairment (Appendix 2); elimination may be reduced in hepatic impairment or biliary disease or biliary obstruction; pregnancy (Appendix 4); breast-feeding (Appendix 5); **interactions:** Appendix 1 (fusidic acid)

Side-effects: nausea, vomiting, reversible jaundice, especially after high dosage or rapid infusion (withdraw therapy if persistent); rarely hypersensitivity reactions, acute renal failure (usually with jaundice), blood disorders

Dose: see under Preparations, below

Sodium fusidate (Leo) PoM

Intravenous infusion, powder for reconstitution, sodium fusidate 500 mg (= fusidic acid 480 mg), with buffer, net price per vial (with diluent) = £7.78

Electrolytes: Na^+ 3.1 mmol/vial when reconstituted with buffer

Dose: as sodium fusidate, by intravenous infusion, ADULT over 50 kg, 500 mg 3 times daily; ADULT under 50 kg and CHILD, 6–7 mg/kg 3 times daily

Fucidin® (Leo) PoM

Tablets, f/c, sodium fusidate 250 mg, net price 10-tab pack = £6.02. Label: 9

Dose: as sodium fusidate, 500 mg every 8 hours, doubled for severe infections

Skin infection, as sodium fusidate, 250 mg every 12 hours for 5–10 days

Suspension, off-white, banana- and orange-flavoured, fusidic acid 250 mg/5 mL, net price 50 mL = £6.73. Label: 9, 21

Dose: as fusidic acid, ADULT 750 mg every 8 hours; CHILD up to 1 year 50 mg/kg daily (in 3 divided doses), 1–5 years 250 mg every 8 hours, 5–12 years 500 mg every 8 hours

NOTE. Fusidic acid is incompletely absorbed and doses recommended for suspension are proportionately higher than those for sodium fusidate tablets

Vancomycin and teicoplanin

The glycopeptide antibiotics vancomycin and teicoplanin have bactericidal activity against aerobic and anaerobic Gram-positive bacteria including multi-resistant staphylococci. However, there are reports of *Staphylococcus aureus* with reduced susceptibility to glycopeptides. There are increasing reports of glycopeptide-resistant enterococci.

Vancomycin is used *by the intravenous route* in the prophylaxis and treatment of endocarditis and other serious infections caused by Gram-positive cocci. It has a relatively long duration of action and can therefore be given every 12 hours. Vancomycin (added to dialysis fluid) is also used in the treatment of peritonitis associated with peritoneal dialysis [unlicensed route] (Table 1 section 5.1).

Vancomycin given *by mouth* is effective in the treatment of antibiotic-associated colitis (pseudomembranous colitis, see also section 1.5); a dose of 125 mg every 6 hours for 7 to 10 days is considered adequate (higher dose may be considered if the infection fails to respond or if it is severe). Vancomycin should **not** be given by mouth for systemic infections since it is not significantly absorbed.

Teicoplanin is very similar to vancomycin but has a significantly longer duration of action allowing once-daily administration. Unlike vancomycin, teicoplanin can be given by intramuscular as well as by intravenous injection; it is not given by mouth.

VANCOMYCIN

Indications: see notes above

Cautions: avoid rapid infusion (risk of anaphylactoid reactions, see Side-effects); rotate infusion sites; renal impairment (Appendix 3); elderly; avoid if history of deafness; all patients require plasma-vancomycin measurement (after 3 or 4 doses if renal function normal, earlier if renal impairment), blood counts, urinalysis, and renal function tests; monitor auditory function in elderly or if renal impairment; pregnancy (Appendix 4) and breast-feeding (Appendix 5); systemic absorption may follow oral administration especially in inflammatory bowel disorders or following multiple doses; **interactions:** Appendix 1 (vancomycin)

Side-effects: after parenteral administration: nephrotoxicity including renal failure and interstitial nephritis; ototoxicity (discontinue if tinnitus occurs); blood disorders including neutropenia (usually after 1 week or cumulative dose of 25 g), rarely agranulocytosis and thrombocytopenia; nausea; chills, fever; eosinophilia, anaphylaxis, rashes (including exfoliative dermatitis, Stevens-Johnson syndrome, toxic epidermal necrolysis, and vasculitis); phlebitis (irritant to tissue); on rapid infusion, severe hypotension (including shock and cardiac arrest), wheezing, dyspnoea, urticaria, pruritus, flushing of the upper body ('red man' syndrome), pain and muscle spasm of back and chest

Dose: *by mouth*, antibiotic-associated colitis, 125 mg every 6 hours for 7–10 days, see notes above; CHILD 5 mg/kg every 6 hours, over 5 years, half adult dose

NOTE. Oral paediatric dose is lower than that on product literature but is adequate

By intravenous infusion, 500 mg every 6 hours *or* 1 g every 12 hours; ELDERLY over 65 years, 500 mg every 12 hours *or* 1 g once daily; NEONATE up to 1 week, 15 mg/kg initially then 10 mg/kg every 12 hours; 1–4 weeks, 15 mg/kg initially then 10 mg/kg every 8 hours; CHILD over 1 month, 10 mg/kg every 6 hours

Endocarditis prophylaxis, section 5.1, table 2

NOTE. Plasma concentration monitoring required; pre-dose ('trough') concentration should be 5–10 mg/litre (10–15 mg/litre in endocarditis); vancomycin doses in BNF may differ from those in product literature

Vancomycin (Non-proprietary) PoM

Capsules, vancomycin (as hydrochloride) 125 mg, net price 28-cap pack = £66.23; 250 mg, 28-cap pack = £132.47. Label: 9

Injection, powder for reconstitution, vancomycin (as hydrochloride), for use as an infusion, net price 500-mg vial = £8.05; 1-g vial = £16.11

NOTE. Can be used to prepare solution for oral administration

Vancocin® (Flynn) PoM

Injection, powder for reconstitution, vancomycin (as hydrochloride), for use as an infusion, net price 500-mg vial = £8.05; 1-g vial = £16.11

NOTE. Can be used to prepare solution for oral administration

TEICOPLANIN

Indications: potentially serious Gram-positive infections including endocarditis, dialysis-associated peritonitis, and serious infections due to *Staphylococcus aureus*; prophylaxis in endocarditis [unlicensed indication] and in orthopaedic surgery at risk of infection with Gram-positive organisms

Cautions: vancomycin sensitivity; blood counts and liver and kidney function tests required; renal impairment (Appendix 3)—monitor renal and auditory function on prolonged administration or if other nephrotoxic or neurotoxic drugs given; pregnancy (Appendix 4) and breast-feeding; **interactions:** Appendix 1 (teicoplanin)

Side-effects: nausea, vomiting, diarrhoea; rash, pruritus, fever, bronchospasm, rigors, urticaria, angioedema, anaphylaxis; dizziness, headache; blood disorders including eosinophilia, leucopenia, neutropenia, and thrombocytopenia; disturbances in liver enzymes, transient increase of serum creatinine, renal failure; tinnitus, mild hearing loss, and vestibular disorders also reported; rarely exfoliative dermatitis, Stevens-Johnson syndrome, toxic epidermal necrolysis; local reactions include erythema, pain, thrombophlebitis, injection site abscess and rarely flushing with infusion

Dose: *by intramuscular injection or by intravenous injection or infusion*, initially 400 mg (for severe infections, *by intravenous injection or infusion*, initially 400 mg every 12 hours for 3 doses), then 200 mg daily (400 mg daily for severe infections); higher doses may be required in patients of over 85 kg and in severe burns or endocarditis (consult product literature)

CHILD over 2 months *by intravenous injection or infusion*, initially 10 mg/kg every 12 hours for 3 doses, subsequently 6 mg/kg daily (severe infections or in neutropenia, 10 mg/kg daily); subsequent doses can be given *by intramuscular injection* (but intravenous administration preferred in children); NEONATE *by intravenous infusion*, initially a single dose of 16 mg/kg, subsequently 8 mg/kg daily

Orthopaedic surgery prophylaxis, *by intravenous injection*, 400 mg at induction of anaesthesia

Endocarditis prophylaxis [unlicensed indication], section 5.1, table 2

Targocid® (Aventis Pharma) PoM
Injection, powder for reconstitution, teicoplanin, net price 200-mg vial (with diluent) = £17.58; 400-mg vial (with diluent) = £35.62
Electrolytes: Na^+ < 0.5 mmol/200- and 400-mg vial

Linezolid

Linezolid, an oxazolidinone antibacterial, is active against Gram-positive bacteria including methicillin-resistant *Staphylococcus aureus* (MRSA), and vancomycin-resistant enterococci. Resistance to linezolid can develop with prolonged treatment or if the dose is less than that recommended. Linezolid should be reserved for infections resistant to other antibacterials or when other antibacterials are not tolerated. Linezolid is not sufficiently active against common Gram-negative organisms.

LINEZOLID

Indications: pneumonia, complicated skin and soft-tissue infections caused by Gram-positive bacteria (initiated under expert supervision)

Cautions: monitor full blood count (including platelet count) weekly (see also CSM Advice below); unless close observation and blood-pressure monitoring possible, avoid in uncontrolled hypertension, phaeochromocytoma, carcinoid tumour, thyrotoxicosis, bipolar depression, schizophrenia, or acute confusional states; hepatic impairment (Appendix 2); renal impairment (Appendix 3); pregnancy (Appendix 4); **interactions:** Appendix 1 (MAOIs)

CSM advice. Haematopoietic disorders (including thrombocytopenia, anaemia, leucopenia, and pancytopenia) have been reported in patients receiving linezolid. It is recommended that full blood counts are monitored weekly. Close monitoring is recommended in patients who:

- receive treatment for more than 10–14 days;
- have pre-existing myelosuppression;
- are receiving drugs that may have adverse effects on haemoglobin, blood counts, or platelet function;
- have severe renal impairment.

If significant myelosuppression occurs, treatment should be stopped unless it is considered essential, in which case intensive monitoring of blood counts and appropriate management should be implemented.

MONOAMINE OXIDASE INHIBITION. Linezolid is a reversible, non-selective monoamine oxidase inhibitor (MAOI). Patients should avoid consuming large amounts of tyramine-rich foods (such as mature cheese, yeast extracts, undistilled alcoholic beverages, and fermented soya bean products). In addition, linezolid should not be given with another MAOI or within 2 weeks of stopping another MAOI. Unless close observation and blood-pressure monitoring is possible, avoid in those receiving SSRIs, $5HT_1$ agonists ('triptans'), tricyclic antidepressants, sympathomimetics, dopaminergics, buspirone, pethidine and possibly other opioid analgesics. For other interactions see Appendix 1 (MAOIs)

Contra-indications: breast-feeding (Appendix 5); see also Monoamine oxidase inhibition above

Side-effects: diarrhoea (antibiotic-associated colitis reported), nausea, vomiting, taste disturbances; headache; *less commonly* thirst, dry mouth, glossitis, stomatitis, tongue discoloration, abdominal pain, dyspepsia, gastritis, constipation, pancreatitis, hypertension, fever, fatigue, dizziness, insomnia, neuropathy, tinnitus, polyuria, anaemia, leucopenia, thrombocytopenia, eosinophilia, electrolyte disturbances, blurred vision, rash, pruritus, diaphoresis, and injection-site reactions; *very rarely* transient ischaemic attacks, renal failure, pancytopenia and Stevens-Johnson syndrome

Dose: *by mouth*, ADULT over 18 years, 600 mg every 12 hours for 10–14 days

By intravenous infusion over 30–120 minutes, ADULT over 18 years, 600 mg every 12 hours

Zyvox (Pharmacia) ▼ PoM
Tablets, f/c, linezolid 600 mg, net price 10-tab pack = £445.00. Label: 9, 10, patient information leaflet
Suspension, yellow, orange-flavoured, linezolid 100 mg/5 mL when reconstituted with water, net price 150 mL = £222.50. Label: 9, 10 patient information leaflet
Excipients: include aspartame 20 mg/5 mL (section 9.4.1); Na^+ < 0.5 mmol/5 mL
Intravenous infusion, linezolid 2 mg/mL, net price 300-mL *Excel*® bag = £44.50
Excipients: include Na^+ 5 mmol/300-mL bag, glucose 13.71 g/300-mL bag

Quinupristin and dalfopristin

A combination of the streptogramin antibiotics, **quinupristin** and **dalfopristin** (as *Synercid*®) is licensed for infections due to Gram-positive bacteria. The combination should be reserved for treating infections which have failed to respond to other antibacterials (e.g. methicillin-resistant *Staphylococcus aureus*, MRSA) or for patients who cannot be treated with other antibacterials. Quinupristin and dalfopristin are not active against *Enterococcus faecalis* and they need to be given in combination with other antibacterials for mixed infections which also involve Gram-negative organisms.

QUINUPRISTIN WITH DALFOPRISTIN

A mixture of quinupristin and dalfopristin (both as mesilate salts) in the proportions 3 parts to 7 parts

Indications: serious Gram-positive infections where no alternative antibacterial is suitable including hospital-acquired pneumonia, skin and soft-tissue infections, infections due to vancomycin-resistant *Enterococcus faecium*

Cautions: hepatic impairment (avoid if severe; Appendix 2); pregnancy (Appendix 4); predisposition to cardiac arrhythmias (including congenital QT syndrome, concomitant use of drugs that prolong QT interval, cardiac hypertrophy, dilated cardiomyopathy, hypokalaemia, hypomagnesaemia, bradycardia); **interactions**: Appendix 1 (quinupristin with dalfopristin)

Contra-indications: plasma-bilirubin concentration greater than 3 times upper limit of reference range; breast-feeding (Appendix 5)

Side-effects: nausea, vomiting, diarrhoea, headache, arthralgia, myalgia, asthenia, rash, pruritus, anaemia, leucopenia, eosinophilia, raised urea and creatinine; injection-site reactions on peripheral venous administration; less frequently oral candidiasis, stomatitis, constipation, abdominal pain, antibiotic-associated colitis, anorexia, peripheral oedema, hypotension, chest pain, arrhythmias, dyspnoea, hypersensitivity reactions (including anaphylaxis and urticaria), insomnia, anxiety, confusion, dizziness, paraesthesia, hypertonia, hepatitis, jaundice, pancreatitis, gout; also reported, thrombocytopenia, pancytopenia, electrolyte disturbances

Dose: expressed as a combination of quinupristin and dalfopristin (in a ratio of 3:7)

ADULT over 18 years, by *intravenous infusion* into central vein, 7.5 mg/kg every 8 hours for 7 days in skin and soft-tissue infections; for 10 days in hospital-acquired pneumonia; duration of treatment in *E. faecium* infection depends on site of infection

NOTE. In emergency, first dose may be administered *via* peripheral line until central venous catheter in place

Synercid® (Aventis Pharma) PoM

Intravenous infusion, powder for reconstitution, quinupristin (as mesilate) 150 mg, dalfopristin (as mesilate) 350 mg, net price 500-mg vial = £37.00

Electrolytes: Na^+ approx. 16 mmol/500-mg vial

Polymyxins

The polymyxin antibiotic, **colistin**, is active against Gram-negative organisms, including *Pseudomonas aeruginosa*. It is **not** absorbed by mouth and thus needs to be given by injection to obtain a systemic effect; however, it is toxic and has few, if any, indications for systemic use.

Colistin is used by mouth in bowel sterilisation regimens in neutropenic patients (usually with nystatin); it is **not** recommended for gastro-intestinal infections. It is also given by inhalation of a nebulised solution as an adjunct to standard antibacterial therapy in patients with cystic fibrosis.

Both colistin and polymyxin B are included in some preparations for topical application.

COLISTIN

Indications: see notes above

Cautions: renal impairment (Appendix 3); porphyria (section 9.8.2); risk of bronchospasm on inhalation—may be prevented or treated with a selective $beta_2$ agonist; **interactions:** Appendix 1 (polymyxins)

Contra-indications: myasthenia gravis; pregnancy (Appendix 4); breast-feeding (Appendix 5)

Side-effects: neurotoxicity reported especially with excessive doses (including apnoea, perioral and peripheral paraesthesia, vertigo; rarely vasomotor instability, slurred speech, confusion, psychosis, visual disturbances); nephrotoxicity; hypersensitivity reactions including rash; injection-site reactions; inhalation may cause sore throat, sore mouth, cough, bronchospasm

Dose: *by mouth*, bowel sterilisation, 1.5–3 million-units every 8 hours

By intravenous injection into a totally implantable venous access device, *or by intravenous infusion* (but see notes above), ADULT and CHILD body-weight under 60 kg, 50 000–75 000 units/kg daily in 3 divided doses; body-weight over 60 kg, 1–2 million units every 8 hours

NOTE. Plasma concentration monitoring required in neonates, renal impairment, and in cystic fibrosis; recommended 'peak' plasma-colistin concentration (approx. 30 minutes after intravenous injection or infusion) 10–15 mg/litre (125–200 units/mL)

By inhalation of nebulised solution, ADULT and CHILD over 2 years, 1–2 million units every 12 hours; CHILD under 2 years, 0.5–1 million units every 12 hours

Colomycin® (Forest) PoM

Tablets, scored, colistin sulphate 1.5 million units. Net price 50 = £58.28

Syrup, colistin sulphate 250 000 units/5 mL when reconstituted with water. Net price 80 mL = £3.48

Injection, powder for reconstitution, colistimethate sodium (colistin sulphomethate sodium). Net price 500 000-unit vial = £1.14; 1 million-unit vial = £1.68; 2 million-unit vial = £3.09

Electrolytes: (before reconstitution) $Na^+ < 0.5$ mmol/500 000-unit, 1 million-unit, and 2 million-unit vial

NOTE. *Colomycin*® Injection (dissolved in physiological saline) may be used for nebulisation

Promixin (Profile) PoM

Powder for nebuliser solution, colistimethate sodium (colistin sulphomethate sodium), net price 1 million-unit vial = £4.60. For use with *Prodose*® NHS nebuliser

Injection, powder for reconstitution, colistimethate sodium (colistin sulphomethate sodium), net price 1 million unit-vial = £2.30

Electrolytes: (before reconstitution) $Na^+ < 0.5$ mmol/1 million-unit vial

5.1.8 Sulphonamides and trimethoprim

The importance of the sulphonamides has decreased as a result of increasing bacterial resistance and their replacement by antibacterials which are generally more active and less toxic.

Sulfamethoxazole (sulphamethoxazole) and trimethoprim are used in combination (as **co-trimoxazole**) because of their synergistic activity. However, co-trimoxazole is associated with rare but serious side-effects (e.g. Stevens-Johnson syndrome and blood dyscrasias, notably bone marrow depression and agranulocytosis) especially in the elderly (see CSM recommendations below).

CSM recommendations. Co-trimoxazole should be limited to the role of drug of choice in *Pneumocystis carinii* (*Pneumocystis jiroveci*) pneumonia; it is also indicated for *toxoplasmosis* and *nocardiasis*. It should now only be considered for use in *acute exacerbations of chronic bronchitis* and *infections of the urinary tract* when there is good bacteriological evidence of sensitivity to co-trimoxazole and good reason to prefer this combination to a single antibacterial; similarly it should only be used in *acute otitis media in children* when there is good reason to prefer it.

Trimethoprim can be used alone for urinary- and respiratory-tract infections and for prostatitis, shigellosis, and invasive salmonella infections. Trimethoprim has side-effects similar to co-trimoxazole but they are less severe and occur less frequently.

For *topical preparations* of sulphonamides used in the treatment of burns see section 13.10.1.1.

CO-TRIMOXAZOLE

A mixture of trimethoprim and sulfamethoxazole in the proportions of 1 part to 5 parts

Indications: see CSM recommendations above

Cautions: maintain adequate fluid intake; avoid in blood disorders (unless under specialist supervision); monitor blood counts on prolonged treatment; discontinue immediately if blood disorders or rash develop; predisposition to folate deficiency or hyperkalaemia; elderly (see CSM recommendations above); asthma; G6PD deficiency (section 9.1.5); avoid in infants under 6 weeks (except for treatment or prophylaxis of pneumocystis pneumonia); hepatic impairment (avoid if severe); renal impairment (avoid if severe; Appendix 3); pregnancy (Appendix 4); breast-feeding (Appendix 5); **interactions:** Appendix 1 (trimethoprim, sulfamethoxazole)

Contra-indications: porphyria (section 9.8.2)

Side-effects: nausea, diarrhoea; headache; rash (very rarely including Stevens-Johnson syndrome, toxic epidermal necrolysis, photosensitivity)—discontinue immediately; *less commonly* vomiting; *very rarely* glossitis, stomatitis, anorexia, liver damage (including jaundice and hepatic necrosis), pancreatitis, antibiotic-associated colitis, myocarditis, cough and shortness of breath, pulmonary infiltrates, aseptic meningitis, depression, convulsions, peripheral neuropathy, ataxia, tinnitus, vertigo, hallucinations, hypoglycaemia, blood disorders (including leucopenia, thrombocytopenia, megaloblastic anaemia, eosinophilia), hyperkalaemia, hyponatraemia, renal disorders including interstitial nephritis, arthralgia, myalgia, vasculitis, and systemic lupus erythematosus

Dose: *by mouth*, 960 mg every 12 hours; CHILD, every 12 hours, 6 weeks–5 months, 120 mg; 6 months–5 years, 240 mg; 6–12 years, 480 mg

By intravenous infusion, 960 mg every 12 hours increased to 1.44 g every 12 hours in severe infections; CHILD 36 mg/kg daily in 2 divided doses increased to 54 mg/kg daily in severe infections

Treatment of *Pneumocystis carinii* (*Pneumocystis jiroveci*) infections (undertaken where facilities for appropriate monitoring available—consult microbiologist and product literature), *by mouth or by intravenous infusion*, ADULT and CHILD over 4 weeks 120 mg/kg daily in 2–4 divided doses for 14 days

Prophylaxis of *Pneumocystis carinii* (*Pneumocystis jiroveci*) infections, *by mouth*, 960 mg once daily (may be reduced to 480 mg once daily to improve tolerance) *or* 960 mg on alternate days (3 times a week) *or* 960 mg twice daily on alternate days (3 times a week); CHILD 6 weeks–5 months 120 mg twice daily on 3 consecutive days per week *or* 7 days per week; 6 months–5 years 240 mg; 6–12 years 480 mg

NOTE. 480 mg of co-trimoxazole consists of sulfamethoxazole 400 mg and trimethoprim 80 mg

Co-trimoxazole (Non-proprietary) PoM

Tablets, co-trimoxazole 480 mg, net price 28-tab pack = £5.19, 960 mg, 20 = £4.69. Label: 9

Brands include *Fectrim*®, *Fectrim*® *Forte*

Paediatric oral suspension, co-trimoxazole 240 mg/5 mL, net price 100 mL = £1.12. Label: 9

Oral suspension, co-trimoxazole 480 mg/5 mL. Net price 100 mL = £4.41. Label: 9

Strong sterile solution, co-trimoxazole 96 mg/mL. For dilution and use as an intravenous infusion. Net price 5-mL amp = £1.58, 10-mL amp = £3.06

Septrin® (GSK) PoM

Tablets, co-trimoxazole 480 mg. Net price 20 = £3.10. Label: 9

Forte tablets, scored, co-trimoxazole 960 mg. Net price 20 = £4.69. Label: 9

Adult suspension, co-trimoxazole 480 mg/5 mL. Net price 100 mL (vanilla-flavoured) = £4.41. Label: 9

Paediatric suspension, sugar-free, co-trimoxazole 240 mg/5 mL. Net price 100 mL (banana- and vanilla-flavoured) = £2.45. Label: 9

Intravenous infusion, co-trimoxazole 96 mg/mL. To be diluted before use. Net price 5-mL amp = £1.48

Excipients: include propylene glycol, sulphites

SULFADIAZINE

(Sulphadiazine)

Indications: prevention of rheumatic fever recurrence, toxoplasmosis [unlicensed]—see section 5.4.7

Cautions: see under Co-trimoxazole; renal impairment (avoid if severe; Appendix 3); pregnancy (Appendix 4); breast-feeding (Appendix 5); **interactions:** Appendix 1 (sulphonamides)

Contra-indications: see under Co-trimoxazole

Side-effects: see under Co-trimoxazole

Dose: prevention of rheumatic fever, *by mouth*, 1 g daily (500 mg daily for patients less than 30kg)

Sulfadiazine (Non-proprietary) PoM

Tablets, sulfadiazine 500 mg, net price 56-tab pack = £17.60. Label: 9, 27

Injection, sulfadiazine (as sodium salt) 250 mg/mL, net price 4-mL amp = £4.97

TRIMETHOPRIM

Indications: urinary-tract infections, acute and chronic bronchitis

Cautions: renal impairment (Appendix 3); pregnancy (Appendix 4); breast-feeding (Appendix 5); predisposition to folate deficiency; elderly; manufacturer recommends blood counts on long-term therapy (but evidence of practical value unsatisfactory); neonates (specialist supervision required); porphyria (section 9.8.2); **interactions:** Appendix 1 (trimethoprim)

BLOOD DISORDERS. On long-term treatment, patients and their carers should be told how to recognise signs of blood disorders and advised to seek immediate medical attention if symptoms such as fever, sore throat, rash, mouth ulcers, purpura, bruising or bleeding develop

Contra-indications: blood dyscrasias

Side-effects: gastro-intestinal disturbances including nausea and vomiting, pruritus, rashes, hyperkalaemia, depression of haematopoiesis; rarely erythema multiforme, toxic epidermal necrolysis, photosensitivity and other allergic reactions including angioedema and anaphylaxis; aseptic meningitis reported

Dose: acute infections, 200 mg every 12 hours; CHILD, every 12 hours, 6 weeks–5 months 25 mg, 6 months–5 years 50 mg, 6–12 years 100 mg

Chronic infections and prophylaxis, 100 mg at night; CHILD 1–2 mg/kg at night

Trimethoprim (Non-proprietary) PoM
Tablets, trimethoprim 100 mg, net price 20 = 74p; 200 mg, 20 = £2.00. Label: 9
Brands include *Trimopan*®
Suspension, trimethoprim 50 mg/5 mL, net price 100 mL = £1.77. Label: 9

Monotrim® (Solvay) PoM
Suspension, sugar-free, trimethoprim 50 mg/5 mL. Net price 100 mL = £1.77. Label: 9

5.1.9 Antituberculous drugs

Tuberculosis is treated in two phases—an *initial phase* using at least three drugs and a *continuation phase* using two drugs in fully sensitive cases. Treatment requires specialised knowledge, particularly where the disease involves resistant organisms or non-respiratory organs.

The regimens given below are based on the Joint Tuberculosis Committee of the British Thoracic Society guidelines for the treatment of tuberculosis in the UK; variations occur in other countries. Either the unsupervised regimen or the supervised regimen described below should be used; the two regimens should **not** be used concurrently.

INITIAL PHASE. The concurrent use of at least three drugs during the initial phase is designed to reduce the bacterial population as rapidly as possible and to prevent the emergence of drug-resistant bacteria. The drugs are best given as combination preparations unless one of the components cannot be given because of resistance or intolerance. The treatment of choice for the initial phase is the daily use of isoniazid, rifampicin, pyrazinamide and ethambutol; ethambutol can be omitted from the regimen if the risk of resistance to isoniazid is low (e.g. those who have not been treated previously for tuberculosis, those who are not immunosuppressed, and those who have not been in contact with organisms likely to be drug resistant). Streptomycin is rarely used in the UK but it may be used in the initial phase of treatment if resistance to isoniazid has been established before therapy is commenced. The initial phase drugs should be continued for 2 months. Where a positive culture for *M. tuberculosis* has been obtained, but susceptibility results are not available after 2 months, treatment with pyrazinamide (and ethambutol if appropriate) should be continued until full susceptibility is confirmed, even if this is for longer than 2 months.

CONTINUATION PHASE. After the initial phase, treatment is continued for a further 4 months with isoniazid and rifampicin (preferably given as a combination preparation). Longer treatment is necessary for meningitis and for resistant organisms which may also require modification of the regimen.

UNSUPERVISED TREATMENT. The following regimen should be used for patients who are likely to take antituberculous drugs reliably **without supervision**. Patients who are unlikely to comply with daily administration of antituberculous drugs should be treated with the regimen described under Supervised Treatment.

Recommended dosage for standard unsupervised 6-month treatment

Rifater® [rifampicin, isoniazid, and pyrazinamide] (for 2-month initial phase only)
ADULT under 40 kg 3 tablets daily, 40–49 kg 4 tablets daily, 50–64 kg 5 tablets daily, over 65 kg 6 tablets daily

[1]**Ethambutol** (for 2-month initial phase only)
ADULT AND CHILD 15 mg/kg daily

Rifinah® or ***Rimactazid***® [rifampicin and isoniazid] (for 4-month continuation phase following initial treatment with *Rifater*®)
ADULT under 50 kg 3 tablets daily of *Rifinah*®*-150*, 50 kg and over, 2 tablets daily of *Rifinah*®*-300* or *Rimactazid*®*-300*

or (if combination preparations not appropriate):

Isoniazid (for 2-month initial and 4-month continuation phases)
ADULT 300 mg daily; CHILD 5–10 mg/kg (max. 300 mg) daily

Rifampicin (for 2-month initial and 4-month continuation phases)
ADULT under 50 kg 450 mg daily, 50 kg and over 600 mg daily; CHILD 10 mg/kg (max. 600 mg) daily

Pyrazinamide (for 2-month initial phase only)
ADULT under 50 kg 1.5 g daily, 50 kg and over 2 g daily; CHILD 35 mg/kg daily

[1]**Ethambutol** (for 2-month initial phase only)
ADULT AND CHILD 15 mg/kg daily

PREGNANCY AND BREAST-FEEDING. The standard regimen (above) may be used during pregnancy and breast-feeding. Streptomycin should not be given in pregnancy.

CHILDREN. Children are given isoniazid, rifampicin, and pyrazinamide for the first 2 months followed by isoniazid and rifampicin during the next 4 months. Ethambutol should be included in the first 2 months in children with a high risk of resistant infection (see Initial Phase, above). However, care is needed in young children because of the difficulty in testing eyesight and in obtaining reports of visual symptoms (see below).

SUPERVISED TREATMENT. Drug administration needs to be **fully supervised** (directly observed therapy, DOT) in patients who cannot comply reliably with the treatment regimen. These patients are given isoniazid, rifampicin, pyrazinamide and ethambutol (or streptomycin) 3 times a week under supervision for the first 2 months followed by isoniazid and rifampicin 3 times a week for a further 4 months.

Recommended dosage for intermittent supervised 6-month treatment

Isoniazid (for 2-month initial and 4-month continuation phases)
ADULT AND CHILD 15 mg/kg (max. 900 mg) 3 times a week

Rifampicin (for 2-month initial and 4-month continuation phases)
ADULT 600–900 mg 3 times a week; CHILD 15 mg/kg (max. 900 mg) 3 times a week

Pyrazinamide (for 2-month initial phase only)
ADULT under 50 kg 2 g 3 times a week, 50 kg and over 2.5 g 3 times a week; CHILD 50 mg/kg 3 times a week

[1]**Ethambutol** (for 2-month initial phase only)
ADULT AND CHILD 30 mg/kg 3 times a week

---

1. Ethambutol may be omitted from the regimen if the risk of isoniazid resistance is low

IMMUNOCOMPROMISED PATIENTS. Multi-resistant *Mycobacterium tuberculosis* may be present in immunocompromised patients. The organism should always be cultured to confirm its type and drug sensitivity. Confirmed *M. tuberculosis* infection sensitive to first-line drugs should be treated with a standard 6-month regimen; after completing treatment, patients should be closely monitored. The regimen may need to be modified if infection is caused by resistant organisms, and specialist advice is needed.

Specialist advice should be sought about tuberculosis treatment or chemoprophylaxis in a HIV-positive individual; care is required in choosing the regimen and in avoiding potentially hazardous interactions.

Infection may also be caused by other mycobacteria e.g. *M. avium* complex in which case specialist advice on management is needed.

PREVENTION OF TUBERCULOSIS. Some individuals may develop tuberculosis owing to reactivation of previously latent disease. Chemoprophylaxis may be required in those who have evidence of latent tuberculosis and are receiving treatment with immunosuppressants (including cytotoxics and possibly long-term treatment with systemic corticosteroids). In these cases, isoniazid chemoprophylaxis may be given for 6 months; longer chemoprophylaxis is not recommended.

For prevention of tuberculosis in susceptible close contacts or those who have become tuberculin-positive, see Table 2, section 5.1. For advice on immunisation against tuberculosis, see section 14.4

MONITORING. Since isoniazid, rifampicin and pyrazinamide are associated with liver toxicity (see Appendix 2), *hepatic function* should be checked before treatment with these drugs. Those with pre-existing liver disease or alcohol dependence should have frequent checks particularly in the first 2 months. If there is no evidence of liver disease (and pre-treatment liver function is normal), further checks are only necessary if the patient develops fever, malaise, vomiting, jaundice or unexplained deterioration during treatment. In view of the need to comply fully with antituberculous treatment on the one hand and to guard against serious liver damage on the other, patients and their carers should be informed carefully how to recognise signs of liver disorders and advised to discontinue treatment and seek **immediate** medical attention should symptoms of liver disease occur.

Renal function should be checked before treatment with antituberculous drugs and appropriate dosage adjustments made. Streptomycin or ethambutol should preferably be avoided in patients with renal impairment, but if used, the dose should be reduced and the plasma-drug concentration monitored.

Visual acuity should be tested before ethambutol is used (see below).

> Major causes of treatment failure are incorrect prescribing by the physician and inadequate compliance by the patient. Monthly tablet counts and urine examination (rifampicin imparts an orange-red coloration) may be useful indicators of compliance with treatment. Avoid both excessive and inadequate dosage. Treatment should be supervised by a specialist physician.

Isoniazid is cheap and highly effective. Like rifampicin it should always be included in any antituberculous regimen unless there is a specific contra-indication. Its only common side-effect is peripheral neuropathy which is more likely to occur where there are pre-existing risk factors such as diabetes, alcohol dependence, chronic renal failure, malnutrition and HIV infection. In these circumstances pyridoxine 10 mg daily (or 20 mg daily if suitable product not available) (section 9.6.2) should be given prophylactically from the start of treatment. Other side-effects such as hepatitis (important: see Monitoring above) and psychosis are rare.

Rifampicin, a rifamycin, is a key component of any antituberculous regimen. Like isoniazid it should always be included unless there is a specific contra-indication.

During the first two months ('initial phase') of rifampicin administration transient disturbance of liver function with elevated serum transaminases is common but generally does not require interruption of treatment. Occasionally more serious liver toxicity requires a change of treatment particularly in those with pre-existing liver disease (important: see Monitoring above).

On intermittent treatment six toxicity syndromes have been recognised—influenza-like, abdominal, and respiratory symptoms, shock, renal failure, and thrombocytopenic purpura—and can occur in 20 to 30% of patients.

Rifampicin induces hepatic enzymes which accelerate the metabolism of several drugs including oestrogens, corticosteroids, phenytoin, sulphonylureas, and anticoagulants; **interactions:** Appendix 1 (rifamycins). **Important:** the effectiveness of hormonal contraceptives is reduced and alternative family planning advice should be offered (section 7.3.1).

Rifabutin, a newly introduced rifamycin, is indicated for *prophylaxis* against *M. avium* complex infections in patients with a low CD4 count; it is also licensed for the *treatment* of non-tuberculous mycobacterial disease and pulmonary tuberculosis. **Important:** as with rifampicin it induces hepatic enzymes and the effectiveness of hormonal contraceptives is reduced requiring alternative family planning methods.

Pyrazinamide [unlicensed] is a bactericidal drug only active against intracellular dividing forms of *Mycobacterium tuberculosis*; it exerts its main effect only in the first two or three months. It is particularly useful in tuberculous meningitis because of good meningeal penetration. It is not active against *M. bovis*. Serious liver toxicity may occasionally occur (important: see Monitoring above).

Ethambutol is included in a treatment regimen if isoniazid resistance is suspected; it can be omitted if the risk of resistance is low.

Side-effects of ethambutol are largely confined to visual disturbances in the form of loss of acuity, colour blindness, and restriction of visual fields. These toxic effects are more common where excessive dosage is used or if the patient's renal function is impaired. The earliest features of ocular toxicity are subjective and patients should be advised to discontinue therapy immediately if they develop deterioration in vision and promptly seek further advice. Early discontinuation of the drug is almost always followed by recovery of eyesight. Patients who cannot understand warnings about visual side-effects should, if possible, be given an alternative drug. In particular, ethambutol should be used with caution in children until they are at least 5 years old and capable of reporting symptomatic visual changes accurately.

Visual acuity should be tested by Snellen chart before treatment with ethambutol.

Streptomycin [unlicensed] is now rarely used in the UK except for resistant organisms. It is given intramuscularly in a dose of 15 mg/kg (max. 1 g) daily; the dose is reduced in those under 50 kg, those over 40 years or those with renal impairment. Plasma-drug concentration should be measured in patients with impaired renal function in whom streptomycin must be used with great care. Side-effects increase after a cumulative dose of 100 g, which should only be exceeded in exceptional circumstances.

Drug-resistant tuberculosis should be treated by a specialist physician with experience in such cases, and where appropriate facilities for infection-control exist. Second-line drugs available for infections caused by resistant organisms, or when first-line drugs cause unacceptable side-effects, include amikacin, capreomycin, cycloserine, newer macrolides (e.g. azithromycin and clarithromycin), quinolones (e.g. moxifloxacin and levofloxacin) and protionamide (prothionamide) (no longer on UK market).

CAPREOMYCIN

Indications: in combination with other drugs, tuberculosis resistant to first-line drugs

Cautions: hepatic impairment; renal impairment (Appendix 3); auditory impairment; monitor renal, hepatic, auditory, and vestibular function and electrolytes; pregnancy (teratogenic in *animals*; Appendix 4) and breast-feeding (Appendix 5); **interactions:** Appendix 1 (capreomycin)

Side-effects: hypersensitivity reactions including urticaria and rashes; leucocytosis or leucopenia, rarely thrombocytopenia; changes in liver function tests; nephrotoxicity, electrolyte disturbances; hearing loss with tinnitus and vertigo; neuromuscular block after large doses, pain and induration at injection site

Dose: *by deep intramuscular injection*, 1 g daily (not more than 20 mg/kg) for 2–4 months, then 1 g 2–3 times each week

Capastat® (King) PoM

Injection, powder for reconstitution, capreomycin sulphate 1 million units (= capreomycin approx. 1 g). Net price per vial = £16.01

CYCLOSERINE

Indications: in combination with other drugs, tuberculosis resistant to first-line drugs

Cautions: reduce dose in renal impairment (avoid if severe); monitor haematological, renal, and hepatic function; pregnancy (Appendix 4); breast-feeding (Appendix 5); **interactions:** Appendix 1 (cycloserine)

Contra-indications: severe renal impairment, epilepsy, depression, severe anxiety, psychotic states, alcohol dependence, porphyria (section 9.8.2)

Side-effects: mainly neurological, including headache, dizziness, vertigo, drowsiness, tremor, convulsions, confusion, psychosis, depression (discontinue or reduce dose if symptoms of CNS toxicity); rashes, allergic dermatitis (discontinue or reduce dose); megaloblastic anaemia; changes in liver function tests; heart failure at high doses reported

Dose: initially 250 mg every 12 hours for 2 weeks increased according to blood concentration and response to max. 500 mg every 12 hours; CHILD initially 10 mg/kg daily adjusted according to blood concentration and response

NOTE. Blood concentration monitoring required especially in renal impairment or if dose exceeds 500 mg daily or if signs of toxicity; blood concentration should not exceed 30 mg/litre

Cycloserine (King) PoM

Capsules, red/grey cycloserine 250 mg, net price 100-cap pack = £220.69. Label: 2, 8

ETHAMBUTOL HYDROCHLORIDE

Indications: tuberculosis, in combination with other drugs

Cautions: reduce dose in renal impairment and if creatinine clearance less than 30 mL/minute, also monitor plasma-ethambutol concentration (Appendix 3); elderly; pregnancy; test visual acuity before treatment and warn patients to report visual changes—see notes above; young children (see notes above)—routine ophthalmological monitoring recommended

Contra-indications: optic neuritis, poor vision

Side-effects: optic neuritis, red/green colour blindness, peripheral neuritis, rarely rash, pruritus, urticaria, thrombocytopenia

Dose: see notes above

NOTE. 'Peak' concentration (2–2.5 hours after dose) should be 2–6 mg/litre (7–22 micromol/litre); 'trough' (pre-dose) concentration should be less than 1 mg/litre (4 micromol/litre); for advice on laboratory assay of ethambutol contact the Poisons Unit at New Cross Hospital (Tel (020) 7771 5360)

Ethambutol (Non-proprietary) PoM

Tablets, ethambutol hydrochloride 100 mg (yellow), net price 56-tab pack = £11.50; 400 mg (grey), 56-tab pack = £42.73. Label: 8

ISONIAZID

Indications: tuberculosis, in combination with other drugs; prophylaxis—Table 2, section 5.1

Cautions: hepatic impairment (Appendix 2; see also below); renal impairment (Appendix 3); slow acetylator status (increased risk of side-effects); epilepsy; history of psychosis; alcohol dependence, malnutrition, diabetes mellitus, HIV infection (risk of peripheral neuritis); pregnancy (Appendix 4) and breast-feeding (Appendix 5); porphyria (section 9.8.2); **interactions:** Appendix 1 (isoniazid)

HEPATIC DISORDERS. Patients or their carers should be told how to recognise signs of liver disorder, and advised to discontinue treatment and seek immediate medical attention if symptoms such as persistent nausea, vomiting, malaise or jaundice develop

Contra-indications: drug-induced liver disease

Side-effects: nausea, vomiting, constipation, dry mouth; peripheral neuritis with high doses (pyridoxine prophylaxis, see notes above), optic neuritis, convulsions, psychotic episodes, vertigo; hypersensitivity reactions including fever, erythema multiforme, purpura; blood disorders including agranulocytosis, haemolytic anaemia, aplastic anaemia; hepatitis (especially over age of 35 years); systemic lupus erythematosus-like syndrome, pellagra, hyperreflexia, difficulty with micturition, hyperglycaemia, and gynaecomastia reported

Dose: *by mouth or by intramuscular or intravenous injection*, see notes above

Isoniazid (Non-proprietary) PoM

Tablets, isoniazid 50 mg, net price 56-tab pack = £5.78; 100 mg, 28-tab pack = £5.77. Label: 8, 22

Elixir (BPC), isoniazid 50 mg, citric acid monohydrate 12.5 mg, sodium citrate 60 mg, concentrated anise water 0.05 mL, compound tartrazine solution 0.05 mL, glycerol 1 mL, double-strength chloroform water 2 mL, water to 5 mL. Label: 8, 22

'Special order' [unlicensed] product; contact Martindale, Rosemont, or regional hospital manufacturing unit

Injection, isoniazid 25 mg/mL, net price 2-mL amp = £7.39

PYRAZINAMIDE

Indications: tuberculosis in combination with other drugs

Cautions: pregnancy (Appendix 4); hepatic impairment (monitor hepatic function, see also below and Appendix 2); diabetes; gout (avoid in acute attack); **interactions:** Appendix 1 (pyrazinamide)

HEPATIC DISORDERS. Patients or their carers should be told how to recognise signs of liver disorder, and advised to discontinue treatment and seek immediate medical attention if symptoms such as persistent nausea, vomiting, malaise or jaundice develop

Contra-indications: porphyria (section 9.8.2)

Side-effects: hepatotoxicity including fever, anorexia, hepatomegaly, splenomegaly, jaundice, liver failure; nausea, vomiting, flushing, dysuria, arthralgia, sideroblastic anaemia, rash and occasionally photosensitivity

Dose: see notes above

Pyrazinamide (Non-proprietary) PoM

Tablets, scored, pyrazinamide 500 mg. Label: 8

Available on named-patient basis from IDIS

RIFABUTIN

Indications: see under Dose

Cautions: see under Rifampicin; hepatic impairment (Appendix 2); renal impairment (Appendix 3); pregnancy (Appendix 4); breast-feeding (Appendix 5); porphyria (section 9.8.2)

Side-effects: nausea, vomiting; leucopenia, thrombocytopenia, anaemia, rarely haemolysis; raised liver enzymes, jaundice, rarely hepatitis; uveitis following high doses or administration with drugs which raise plasma concentration—see also **interactions:** Appendix 1 (rifamycins); arthralgia, myalgia, influenza-like syndrome, dyspnoea; also hypersensitivity reactions including fever, rash, eosinophilia, bronchospasm, shock; skin, urine, saliva and other body secretions coloured orange-red; asymptomatic corneal opacities reported with long-term use

Dose: prophylaxis of *Mycobacterium avium* complex infections in immunosuppressed patients with low CD4 count (see product literature), 300 mg daily as a single dose

Treatment of non-tuberculous mycobacterial disease, in combination with other drugs, 450–600 mg daily as a single dose for up to 6 months after cultures negative

Treatment of pulmonary tuberculosis, in combination with other drugs, 150–450 mg daily as a single dose for at least 6 months

CHILD not recommended

Mycobutin® (Pharmacia) PoM

Capsules, red-brown, rifabutin 150 mg. Net price 30-cap pack = £90.38. Label: 8, 14, counselling, lenses, see under Rifampicin

RIFAMPICIN

Indications: see under Dose

Cautions: hepatic impairment (Appendix 2; liver function tests and blood counts in hepatic disorders, alcohol dependence, and on prolonged therapy, see also below); renal impairment (if above 600 mg daily); pregnancy and breast-feeding (see notes above and Appendix 4 and Appendix 5); porphyria (section 9.8.2); **important:** advise patients on hormonal contraceptives to use additional means (see also section 7.3.1); discolours soft contact lenses; see also notes above; **interactions:** Appendix 1 (rifamycins)

NOTE. If treatment interrupted re-introduce with low dosage and increase gradually; discontinue permanently if serious side-effects develop

HEPATIC DISORDERS. Patients or their carers should be told how to recognise signs of liver disorder, and advised to discontinue treatment and seek immediate medical attention if symptoms such as persistent nausea, vomiting, malaise or jaundice develop

Contra-indications: jaundice

Side-effects: gastro-intestinal symptoms including anorexia, nausea, vomiting, diarrhoea (antibiotic-associated colitis reported); headache, drowsiness; those occurring mainly on intermittent therapy include influenza-like symptoms (with chills, fever, dizziness, bone pain), respiratory symptoms (including shortness of breath), collapse and shock, haemolytic anaemia, acute renal failure, and thrombocytopenic purpura; alterations of liver function, jaundice; flushing, urticaria, and rashes; other side-effects reported include oedema, muscular weakness and myopathy, exfoliative dermatitis, toxic epidermal necrolysis, pemphigoid reactions, leucopenia, eosinophilia, menstrual disturbances; urine, saliva, and other body secretions coloured orange-red; thrombophlebitis reported if infusion used for prolonged period

Dose: brucellosis, legionnaires' disease, endocarditis and serious staphylococcal infections, in combination with other drugs, *by mouth or by intravenous infusion*, 0.6–1.2 g daily (in 2–4 divided doses)

Tuberculosis, in combination with other drugs, see notes above

Leprosy, section 5.1.10

Prophylaxis of meningococcal meningitis and *Haemophilus influenzae* (type b) infection, section 5.1, table 2

Rifampicin (Non-proprietary) PoM

Capsules, rifampicin 150 mg, net price 20 = £6.02.; 300 mg, 20 = £12.00. Label: 8, 14, 22, counselling, see lenses above

Rifadin® (Aventis Pharma) PoM

Capsules, rifampicin 150 mg (blue/red), net price 20 = £3.81; 300 mg (red), 20 = £7.62. Label: 8, 14, 22, counselling, see lenses above

Syrup, red, rifampicin 100 mg/5 mL (raspberry-flavoured). Net price 120 mL = £3.70. Label: 8, 14, 22, counselling, see lenses above
Intravenous infusion, powder for reconstitution, rifampicin. Net price 600-mg vial (with solvent) = £7.98
Electrolytes: Na^+ < 0.5 mmol/vial

Rimactane® (Sandoz) PoM
Capsules, rifampicin 150 mg (red), net price 60-cap pack = £11.35; 300 mg (red/brown), 60-cap pack = £22.69. Label: 8, 14, 22, counselling, see lenses above

■ Combined preparations

Rifater® (Aventis Pharma) PoM
Tablets, pink, s/c, rifampicin 120 mg, isoniazid 50 mg, pyrazinamide 300 mg. Net price 20 = £4.39. Label: 8, 14, 22, counselling, see lenses above
Dose: initial treatment of pulmonary tuberculosis, patients up to 40 kg 3 tablets daily preferably before breakfast, 40–49 kg 4 tablets daily, 50–64 kg 5 tablets daily, 65 kg or more, 6 tablets daily; not suitable for use in children

Rifinah 150® (Aventis Pharma) PoM
Tablets, pink, s/c, rifampicin 150 mg, isoniazid 100 mg, net price 84-tab pack = £16.55. Label: 8, 14, 22, counselling, see lenses above
Dose: ADULT under 50 kg, 3 tablets daily, preferably before breakfast

Rifinah 300® (Aventis Pharma) PoM
Tablets, orange, s/c, rifampicin 300 mg, isoniazid 150 mg, net price 56-tab pack = £21.87. Label: 8, 14, 22, counselling, see lenses above
Dose: ADULT 50 kg and over, 2 tablets daily, preferably before breakfast

Rimactazid 300® (Sandoz) PoM
Tablets, orange, s/c, rifampicin 300 mg, isoniazid 150 mg, net price 60-tab pack = £38.77. Label: 8, 14, 22, counselling, see lenses above
Dose: ADULT 50 kg and over, 2 tablets daily, preferably before breakfast

STREPTOMYCIN

Indications: tuberculosis, in combination with other drugs; adjunct to doxycycline in brucellosis; enterococcal endocarditis (Table 1, section 5.1)
Cautions: see under Aminoglycosides, section 5.1.4; **interactions:** Appendix 1 (aminoglycosides)
Contra-indications: see under Aminoglycosides, section 5.1.4
Side-effects: see under Aminoglycosides, section 5.1.4; also hypersensitivity reactions, paraesthesia of mouth
Dose: *by deep intramuscular injection*, tuberculosis, see notes above; brucellosis, expert advice essential
NOTE. One-hour ('peak') concentration should be 15–40 mg/litre; pre-dose ('trough') concentration should be less than 5 mg/litre (less than 1 mg/litre in renal impairment or in those over 50 years)

Streptomycin Sulphate (Non-proprietary) PoM
Injection, powder for reconstitution, streptomycin (as sulphate), net price 1-g vial = £8.25
Available on named-patient basis from Celltech

5.1.10 Antileprotic drugs

Advice from a member of the Panel of Leprosy Opinion is essential for the treatment of leprosy (Hansen's disease). Details of the Panel can be obtained from the Department of Health telephone (020) 7972 4480.

The World Health Organization has made recommendations to overcome the problem of dapsone resistance and to prevent the emergence of resistance to other antileprotic drugs. Drugs recommended are **dapsone**, **rifampicin** (section 5.1.9), and **clofazimine**. Other drugs with significant activity against *Mycobacterium leprae* include ofloxacin, minocycline and clarithromycin, but none of these are as active as rifampicin; at present they should be reserved as second-line drugs for leprosy.

A three-drug regimen is recommended for *multibacillary leprosy* (lepromatous, borderline-lepromatous, and borderline leprosy) and a two-drug regimen for *paucibacillary leprosy* (borderline-tuberculoid, tuberculoid, and indeterminate). The following regimens are widely used throughout the world (with minor local variations):

Multibacillary leprosy (3-drug regimen)

Rifampicin	600 mg once-monthly, supervised (450 mg for adults weighing less than 35 kg)
Dapsone	100 mg daily, self-administered (50 mg daily or 1–2 mg/kg daily for adults weighing less than 35 kg)
Clofazimine	300 mg once-monthly, supervised, *and* 50 mg daily (or 100 mg on alternate days), self-administered

Multibacillary leprosy should be treated for at least 2 years. Treatment should be continued unchanged during both type I (reversal) or type II (erythema nodosum leprosum) reactions. During reversal reactions neuritic pain or weakness can herald the rapid onset of permanent nerve damage. Treatment with prednisolone (initially 40–60 mg daily) should be instituted at once. Mild type II reactions may respond to aspirin or chloroquine. Severe type II reactions may require corticosteroids; thalidomide [unlicensed] is also useful in men and post-menopausal women who have become corticosteroid dependent, but it should be used under **specialist supervision** and it should **never** be used in women of child-bearing potential (significant teratogenic risk—for CSM guidance on prescribing, see *Current Problems in Pharmacovigilance* 1994; **20**, 8). Increased doses of clofazimine 100 mg 3 times daily for the first month with subsequent reductions, are also useful but may take 4–6 weeks to attain full effect.

Paucibacillary leprosy (2-drug regimen)

Rifampicin	600 mg once-monthly, supervised (450 mg for those weighing less than 35 kg)
Dapsone	100 mg daily, self-administered (50 mg daily or 1–2 mg/kg daily for adults weighing less than 35 kg)

Paucibacillary leprosy should be treated for 6 months. If treatment is interrupted the regimen should be recommenced where it was left off to complete the full course.

Neither the multibacillary nor the paucibacillary antileprosy regimen is sufficient to treat tuberculosis.

DAPSONE

Indications: leprosy, dermatitis herpetiformis; *Pneumocystis carinii* pneumonia (section 5.4.8)

Cautions: cardiac or pulmonary disease; anaemia (treat severe anaemia before starting); susceptibility to haemolysis including G6PD deficiency (section 9.1.5)—susceptible breast-feeding infants also at risk (Appendix 5); pregnancy (Appendix 4); avoid in porphyria (section 9.8.2); **interactions:** Appendix 1 (dapsone)

BLOOD DISORDERS. On long-term treatment, patients and their carers should be told how to recognise signs of blood disorders and advised to seek immediate medical attention if symptoms such as fever, sore throat, rash, mouth ulcers, purpura, bruising or bleeding develop

Side-effects: (dose-related and uncommon at doses used for leprosy), haemolysis, methaemoglobinaemia, neuropathy, allergic dermatitis (rarely including toxic epidermal necrolysis and Stevens-Johnson syndrome), anorexia, nausea, vomiting, tachycardia, headache, insomnia, psychosis, hepatitis, agranulocytosis; dapsone syndrome (rash with fever and eosinophilia)—discontinue immediately (may progress to exfoliative dermatitis, hepatitis, hypoalbuminaemia, psychosis and death)

Dose: leprosy, 1–2 mg/kg daily, see notes above

Dermatitis herpetiformis, see specialist literature

Dapsone (Non-proprietary) PoM

Tablets, dapsone 50 mg, net price 28-tab pack = £4.06; 100 mg, 28-tab pack = £5.31. Label: 8

CLOFAZIMINE

Indications: leprosy

Cautions: hepatic and renal impairment; pregnancy and breast-feeding; may discolour soft contact lenses; avoid if persistent abdominal pain and diarrhoea

Side-effects: nausea, vomiting (hospitalise if persistent), abdominal pain; headache, tiredness; brownish-black discoloration of lesions and skin including areas exposed to light; reversible hair discoloration; dry skin; red discoloration of faeces, urine and other body fluids; also rash, pruritus, photosensitivity, acne-like eruptions, anorexia, eosinophilic enteropathy, bowel obstruction, dry eyes, dimmed vision, macular and subepithelial corneal pigmentation; elevation of blood sugar, weight loss, splenic infarction, lymphadenopathy

Dose: leprosy, see notes above

Lepromatous lepra reactions, dosage increased to 300 mg daily for max. of 3 months

Clofazimine (Non-proprietary) PoM

Capsules, clofazimine 100 mg. Label: 8, 14, 21

Available on named-patient basis

5.1.11 Metronidazole and tinidazole

Metronidazole is an antimicrobial drug with high activity against anaerobic bacteria and protozoa; indications include trichomonal vaginitis (section 5.4.3), bacterial vaginosis (notably *Gardnerella vaginalis* infections), and *Entamoeba histolytica* and *Giardia lamblia* infections (section 5.4.2). It is also used for surgical and gynaecological sepsis in which its activity against colonic anaerobes, especially *Bacteroides fragilis*, is important. Metronidazole is also effective in the treatment of antibiotic-associated colitis (pseudomembranous colitis, see also section 1.5). Metronidazole by the rectal route is an effective alternative to the intravenous route when oral administration is not possible. Intravenous metronidazole is used for the treatment of established cases of tetanus; diazepam (section 10.2.2) and tetanus immunoglobulin (section 14.5) are also used.

Topical metronidazole (section 13.10.1.2) reduces the odour produced by anaerobic bacteria in fungating tumours; it is also used in the management of rosacea (section 13.6).

Tinidazole is similar to metronidazole but has a longer duration of action.

ORAL INFECTIONS. Metronidazole is an alternative to a penicillin for the treatment of many oral infections where the patient is allergic to penicillin or the infection is due to beta-lactamase-producing anaerobes (Table 1, section 5.1). It is the drug of first choice for the treatment of acute necrotising ulcerative gingivitis (Vincent's infection) and pericoronitis; suitable alternatives are amoxicillin (section 5.1.1.3) and erythromycin (section 5.1.5). For these purposes metronidazole in a dose of 200 mg 3 times daily for 3 days is sufficient, but the duration of treatment may need to be longer in pericoronitis. Tinidazole is licensed for the treatment of acute ulcerative gingivitis.

METRONIDAZOLE

Indications: anaerobic infections (including dental), see under Dose below; protozoal infections (section 5.4.2); *Helicobacter pylori* eradication (section 1.3); skin (section 13.10.1.2)

Cautions: disulfiram-like reaction with alcohol, hepatic impairment and hepatic encephalopathy (Appendix 2); pregnancy (Appendix 4) and breast-feeding (Appendix 5); avoid in porphyria (section 9.8.2); clinical and laboratory monitoring advised if treatment exceeds 10 days; **interactions:** Appendix 1 (metronidazole)

Side-effects: nausea, vomiting, unpleasant taste, furred tongue, and gastro-intestinal disturbances; rashes; rarely drowsiness, headache, dizziness, ataxia, darkening of urine, erythema multiforme, pruritus, urticaria, angioedema, and anaphylaxis; also reported abnormal liver function tests, hepatitis, jaundice, thrombocytopenia, aplastic anaemia, myalgia, arthralgia; on prolonged or intensive therapy peripheral neuropathy, transient epileptiform seizures, and leucopenia

Dose: anaerobic infections (usually treated for 7 days and for 10 days in antibiotic-associated colitis), *by mouth*, *either* 800 mg initially then 400 mg every 8 hours *or* 500 mg every 8 hours, CHILD 7.5 mg/kg every 8 hours; *by rectum*, 1 g every 8 hours for 3 days, then 1 g every 12 hours, CHILD every 8 hours for 3 days, then every 12 hours, age up to 1 year 125 mg, 1–5 years 250 mg, 5–10 years 500 mg, over 10 years, adult dose; *by intravenous infusion* over 20 minutes, 500 mg every 8 hours; CHILD 7.5 mg/kg every 8 hours

Leg ulcers and pressure sores, *by mouth*, 400 mg every 8 hours for 7 days

Bacterial vaginosis, *by mouth*, 400–500 mg twice daily for 5–7 days *or* 2 g as a single dose

Pelvic inflammatory disease (see also Table 1, section 5.1), *by mouth*, 400 mg twice daily for 14 days
Acute ulcerative gingivitis, *by mouth*, 200–250 mg every 8 hours for 3 days; CHILD 1–3 years 50 mg every 8 hours for 3 days; 3–7 years 100 mg every 12 hours; 7–10 years 100 mg every 8 hours
Acute oral infections, *by mouth*, 200 mg every 8 hours for 3–7 days (see also notes above); CHILD 1–3 years 50 mg every 8 hours for 3–7 days; 3–7 years 100 mg every 12 hours; 7–10 years 100 mg every 8 hours
Surgical prophylaxis, *by mouth*, 400–500 mg 2 hours before surgery; up to 3 further doses of 400–500 mg may be given every 8 hours for high-risk procedures; CHILD 7.5 mg/kg 2 hours before surgery; up to 3 further doses of 7.5 mg/kg may be given every 8 hours for high-risk procedures
By rectum, 1 g 2 hours before surgery; up to 3 further doses of 1 g may be given every 8 hours for high-risk procedures; CHILD 5–10 years 500 mg 2 hours before surgery; up to 3 further doses of 500 mg may be given every 8 hours for high-risk procedures
By intravenous infusion (if rectal administration inappropriate), 500 mg at induction; up to 3 further doses of 500 mg may be given every 8 hours for high-risk procedures; CHILD 7.5 mg/kg at induction; up to 3 further doses of 7.5 mg/kg may be given every 8 hours for high-risk procedures

NOTE. Metronidazole doses in BNF may differ from those in product literature

Metronidazole (Non-proprietary) PoM
Tablets, metronidazole 200 mg, net price 20 = £1.47; 400 mg, 20 = £1.06. Label: 4, 9, 21, 25, 27
Brands include *Vaginyl*®
Tablets, metronidazole 500 mg, net price 21-tab pack = £6.13. Label: 4, 9, 21, 25, 27
Suspension, metronidazole (as benzoate) 200 mg/5 mL. Net price 100 mL = £7.70. Label: 4, 9, 23
Brands include *Norzol*®
Intravenous infusion, metronidazole 5 mg/mL. Net price 20-mL amp = £1.53, 100-mL container = £3.41

DENTAL PRESCRIBING ON NHS. Metronidazole Tablets and Oral Suspension may be prescribed

Flagyl® (Hawgreen) PoM
Tablets, both f/c, ivory, metronidazole 200 mg, net price 21-tab pack = £3.62; 400 mg, 14-tab pack = £5.12. Label: 4, 9, 21, 25, 27
Suppositories, metronidazole 500 mg, net price 10 = £12.25; 1 g, 10 = £18.60. Label: 4, 9

Flagyl® (Aventis Pharma) PoM
Intravenous infusion, metronidazole 5 mg/mL, net price 100-mL *Viaflex*® bag = £3.41
Electrolytes: Na^+ 13.6 mmol/100-mL bag

Flagyl S® (Hawgreen) PoM
Suspension, orange- and lemon-flavoured, metronidazole (as benzoate) 200 mg/5 mL. Net price 100 mL = £9.01. Label: 4, 9, 23

Metrolyl® (Sandoz) PoM
Intravenous infusion, metronidazole 5 mg/mL, net price 100-mL Steriflex® bag = £1.22
Electrolytes: Na^+ 14.53 mmol/100-mL bag
Suppositories, metronidazole 500 mg, net price 10 = £12.34; 1 g, 10 = £18.34. Label: 4, 9

TINIDAZOLE

Indications: anaerobic infections, see under Dose below; protozoal infections (section 5.4.2); *Helicobacter pylori* eradication (section 1.3)
Cautions: see under Metronidazole; pregnancy (manufacturer advises avoid in first trimester); avoid in porphyria (section 9.8.2); **interactions:** Appendix 1 (tinidazole)
Side-effects: see under Metronidazole
Dose: anaerobic infections *by mouth*, 2 g initially, followed by 1 g daily *or* 500 mg twice daily, usually for 5–6 days
Bacterial vaginosis and acute ulcerative gingivitis, a single 2-g dose
Abdominal surgery prophylaxis, a single 2-g dose approximately 12 hours before surgery

Fasigyn® (Pfizer) PoM
Tablets, f/c, tinidazole 500 mg. Net price 20-tab pack = £13.80. Label: 4, 9, 21, 25

5.1.12 Quinolones

Nalidixic acid and **norfloxacin** are effective in uncomplicated urinary-tract infections.

Ciprofloxacin is active against both Gram-positive and Gram-negative bacteria. It is particularly active against Gram-negative bacteria, including salmonella, shigella, campylobacter, neisseria, and pseudomonas. Ciprofloxacin has only moderate activity against Gram-positive bacteria such as *Streptococcus pneumoniae* and *Enterococcus faecalis*; it should not be used for pneumococcal pneumonia. It is active against chlamydia and some mycobacteria. Most anaerobic organisms are not susceptible. Uses for ciprofloxacin include infections of the respiratory tract (but not for pneumococcal pneumonia) and of the urinary tract, and of the gastro-intestinal system (including typhoid fever), and gonorrhoea and septicaemia caused by sensitive organisms.

Ofloxacin is used for urinary-tract infections, lower respiratory-tract infections, gonorrhoea, and non-gonococcal urethritis and cervicitis.

Levofloxacin is active against Gram-positive and Gram-negative organisms. It has greater activity against pneumococci than ciprofloxacin. Levofloxacin is licensed for community-acquired pneumonia but it is considered to be **second-line treatment** for this indication.

Although ciprofloxacin, levofloxacin and ofloxacin are licensed for skin and soft-tissue infections, many staphylococci are resistant to the quinolones and their use should be avoided in MRSA infections.

Moxifloxacin should be used for treating acute exacerbations of chronic bronchitis **only** if conventional treatment has failed or is contra-indicated, and for **second-line treatment** of community-acquired pneumonia. Moxifloxacin is active against Gram-positive and Gram-negative organisms. It has greater activity against Gram-positive organisms including pneumococci than ciprofloxacin. Moxifloxacin is not active against *Pseudomonas aeruginosa* or methicillin-resistant *Staphylococcus aureus* (MRSA).

ANTHRAX. *Inhalation* or *gastro-intestinal anthrax* should be treated initially with either **ciprofloxacin** or **doxycycline** [unlicensed indication] (section 5.1.3) combined with one or two other antibacterials (such as amoxicillin, benzylpenicillin, chloramphenicol, clarithromycin, clindamycin, imipenem with cilastatin, rifampicin [unlicensed indication], and vancomycin). When the condition improves and the sensitivity of the *Bacillus anthracis* strain is known, treatment may be switched to a single antibacterial. Treatment should continue for 60 days because germination may be delayed.

Cutaneous anthrax should be treated with either ciprofloxacin [unlicensed indication] or doxycycline [unlicensed indication] (section 5.1.3) for 7 days. Treatment may be switched to amoxicillin (section 5.1.1.3) if the infecting strain is susceptible. Treatment may need to be extended to 60 days if exposure is due to aerosol. A combination of antibacterials for 14 days is recommended for cutaneous anthrax with systemic features, extensive oedema, or lesions of the head or neck.

Ciprofloxacin or doxycycline may be given for *post-exposure prophylaxis*. If exposure is confirmed, antibacterial prophylaxis should continue for 60 days. Antibacterial prophylaxis may be switched to amoxicillin after 10–14 days if the strain of *B. anthracis* is susceptible. Vaccination against anthrax (section 14.4) may allow the duration of antibacterial prophylaxis to be shortened.

CAUTIONS. Quinolones should be used with caution in patients with a history of epilepsy or conditions that predispose to seizures, in G6PD deficiency (section 9.1.5), myasthenia gravis (risk of exacerbation), in renal impairment (Appendix 3); pregnancy (Appendix 4), during breast-feeding (Appendix 5), and in children or adolescents (arthropathy has developed in weight-bearing joints in young *animals*—see below). Exposure to excessive sunlight should be avoided (discontinue if photosensitivity occurs). The CSM has warned that quinolones may induce **convulsions** in patients with or without a history of convulsions; taking NSAIDs at the same time may also induce them. Other **interactions:** Appendix 1 (quinolones).

USE IN CHILDREN. Quinolones cause arthropathy in the weight-bearing joints of immature *animals* and are therefore generally not recommended in children and growing adolescents. However, the significance of this effect in humans is uncertain and in some specific circumstances short-term use of a quinolone in children may be justified. Nalidixic acid is used for urinary-tract infections in children over 3 months of age. Ciprofloxacin is licensed for pseudomonal infections in cystic fibrosis (for children above 5 years of age), and for treatment and prophylaxis of inhalational anthrax.

CSM advice (tendon damage). Tendon damage (including rupture) has been reported rarely in patients receiving quinolones. Tendon rupture may occur within 48 hours of starting treatment. The CSM has reminded that:

- quinolones are contra-indicated in patients with a history of tendon disorders related to quinolone use;
- elderly patients are more prone to tendinitis;
- the risk of tendon rupture is increased by the concomitant use of corticosteroids;
- if tendinitis is suspected, the quinolone should be discontinued immediately.

SIDE-EFFECTS. Side-effects of the quinolones include nausea, vomiting, dyspepsia, abdominal pain, diarrhoea (rarely antibiotic-associated colitis), headache, dizziness, sleep disorders, rash (rarely Stevens-Johnson syndrome and toxic epidermal necrolysis), and pruritus. Less frequent side-effects include anorexia, increase in blood urea and creatinine; drowsiness, restlessness, asthenia, depression, confusion, hallucinations, convulsions, tremor, paraesthesia, hypoaesthesia; photosensitivity, hypersensitivity reactions including fever, urticaria, angioedema, arthralgia, myalgia, and anaphylaxis; blood disorders (including eosinophilia, leucopenia, thrombocytopenia); disturbances in vision, taste, hearing and smell. Also isolated reports of tendon inflammation and damage (especially in the elderly and in those taking corticosteroids, see also CSM advice above). Other side-effects that have been reported include haemolytic anaemia, renal failure, interstitial nephritis, and hepatic dysfunction (including hepatitis and cholestatic jaundice). The drug should be **discontinued** if psychiatric, neurological or hypersensitivity reactions (including severe rash) occur.

CIPROFLOXACIN

Indications: see notes above and under Dose; eye infections (section 11.3.1)

Cautions: see notes above; avoid excessive alkalinity of urine and ensure adequate fluid intake (risk of crystalluria); **interactions:** Appendix 1 (quinolones)

DRIVING. May impair performance of skilled tasks (e.g. driving); effects enhanced by alcohol

Side-effects: see notes above; also flatulence, dysphagia, pancreatitis, tachycardia, hypotension, oedema, hot flushes, sweating, movement disorders, tinnitus, vasculitis, tenosynovitis, erythema nodosum, haemorrhagic bullae, petechiae and hyperglycaemia; pain and phlebitis at injection site

Dose: *by mouth*, respiratory-tract infections, 250–750 mg twice daily

Urinary-tract infections, 250–500 mg twice daily (100 mg twice daily for 3 days in acute uncomplicated cystitis in women)

Chronic prostatitis, 500 mg twice daily for 28 days

Gonorrhoea, 500 mg as a single dose

Pseudomonal lower respiratory-tract infection in cystic fibrosis, 750 mg twice daily; CHILD 5–17 years (see Cautions above), up to 20 mg/kg twice daily (max. 1.5 g daily)

Most other infections, 500–750 mg twice daily

Surgical prophylaxis, 750 mg 60–90 minutes before procedure

Prophylaxis of meningococcal meningitis [not licensed], Table 2, section 5.1

By intravenous infusion (over 30–60 minutes; 400 mg over 60 minutes), 200–400 mg twice daily

Pseudomonal lower respiratory-tract infection in cystic fibrosis, 400 mg twice daily; CHILD 5–17 years (see Cautions above), up to 10 mg/kg 3 times daily (max. 1.2 g daily)

Urinary-tract infections, 100 mg twice daily

Gonorrhoea, 100 mg as a single dose

CHILD not recommended (see Cautions above) but where benefit outweighs risk, *by mouth*, 10–30 mg/kg daily in 2 divided doses *or by intravenous infusion*, 8–16 mg/kg daily in 2 divided doses

Anthrax (treatment and post-exposure prophylaxis, see notes above), *by mouth*, 500 mg twice daily; CHILD 30 mg/kg daily in 2 divided doses (max. 1 g daily)
By intravenous infusion, 400 mg twice daily; CHILD 20 mg/kg daily in 2 divided doses (max. 800 mg daily)

Ciprofloxacin (Non-proprietary) PoM
Tablets, ciprofloxacin (as hydrochloride) 100 mg, net price 6-tab pack = £1.23; 250 mg, 10-tab pack = £1.85, 20-tab pack = £2.16; 500 mg, 10-tab pack = £2.84, 20-tab pack = £4.76; 750 mg, 10-tab pack = £3.84. Label: 7, 9, 25, counselling, driving

Ciproxin® (Bayer) PoM
Tablets, all f/c, ciprofloxacin (as hydrochloride) 100 mg, net price 6-tab pack = £2.80; 250 mg (scored), 10-tab pack = £7.50, 20-tab pack = £15.00; 500 mg (scored), 10-tab pack = £14.20, 20-tab pack = £28.40; 750 mg, 10-tab pack = £20.00. Label: 7, 9, 25, counselling, driving
Suspension, strawberry-flavoured, ciprofloxacin for reconstitution with diluent provided, 250 mg/5 mL, net price 100 mL = £15.00. Label: 7, 9, 25, counselling, driving
Intravenous infusion, ciprofloxacin (as lactate) 2 mg/mL, in sodium chloride 0.9%, net price 50-mL bottle = £8.65, 100-mL bottle = £16.89, 200-mL bottle = £25.70
Electrolytes: Na^+ 15.4 mmol/100-mL bottle

LEVOFLOXACIN

Indications: see under Dose
Cautions: see notes above; **interactions:** Appendix 1 (quinolones)
DRIVING. May impair performance of skilled tasks (e.g. driving)
Side-effects: see notes above; rarely anxiety, tachycardia, hypotension, hypoglycaemia, pneumonitis, rhabdomyolysis; local reactions and transient hypotension reported with infusion
Dose: *by mouth*, acute sinusitis, 500 mg daily for 10–14 days
Exacerbation of chronic bronchitis, 250–500 mg daily for 7–10 days
Community-acquired pneumonia, 500 mg once or twice daily for 7–14 days
Urinary-tract infections, 250 mg daily for 7–10 days (for 3 days in uncomplicated infection)
Chronic prostatitis, 500 mg once daily for 28 days
Skin and soft tissue infections, 250 mg daily *or* 500 mg once or twice daily for 7–14 days
By intravenous infusion (over at least 60 minutes for 500 mg), community-acquired pneumonia, 500 mg once or twice daily
Complicated urinary-tract infections, 250 mg daily, increased in severe infections
Skin and soft tissue infections, 500 mg twice daily

Tavanic® (Hoechst Marion Roussel) PoM
Tablets, yellow-red, f/c, scored, levofloxacin 250 mg, net price 5-tab pack = £7.23, 10-tab pack = £14.45; 500 mg, 5-tab pack = £12.93, 10-tab pack = £25.85. Label: 6, 9, 25, counselling, driving
Intravenous infusion, levofloxacin 5 mg/mL, net price 100-mL bottle = £26.40
Electrolytes: Na^+ 15.4 mmol/100-mL bottle

MOXIFLOXACIN

Indications: community-acquired pneumonia; exacerbation of chronic bronchitis; sinusitis
Cautions: see notes above; conditions pre-disposing to arrhythmias, including myocardial ischaemia; **interactions:** Appendix 1 (quinolones)
DRIVING. May impair performance of skilled tasks (e.g. driving)
Contra-indications: see notes above; severe hepatic impairment; history of QT-interval prolongation, bradycardia, history of symptomatic arrhythmias, heart failure with reduced left ventricular ejection fraction, electrolyte disturbances, concomitant use with other drugs known to prolong QT-interval
Side-effects: see notes above; also dry mouth, stomatitis, glossitis, flatulence, constipation, arrhythmias, palpitations, peripheral oedema, angina, blood pressure changes, dyspnoea, anxiety, and sweating; *rarely* hypotension, hyperlipidaemia, agitation, abnormal dreams, incoordination, hyperglycaemia, and dry skin
Dose: 400 mg once daily for 10 days in community-acquired pneumonia, for 5–10 days in exacerbation of chronic bronchitis, for 7 days in sinusitis

Avelox (Bayer) ▼ PoM
Tablets, red, f/c, moxifloxacin (as hydrochloride) 400 mg, net price 5-tab pack = £10.95. Label: 6, 9, counselling, driving

NALIDIXIC ACID

Indications: urinary-tract infections
Cautions: see notes above; avoid in porphyria (section 9.8.2); liver disease; false positive urinary glucose (if tested for reducing substances); monitor blood counts, renal and liver function if treatment exceeds 2 weeks; **interactions:** Appendix 1 (quinolones)
Side-effects: see notes above; also reported toxic psychosis, weakness, increased intracranial pressure, cranial nerve palsy, metabolic acidosis
Dose: 1 g every 6 hours for 7 days, reduced in chronic infections to 500 mg every 6 hours; CHILD over 3 months max. 50 mg/kg daily in divided doses; reduced in prolonged therapy to 30 mg/kg daily

Negram® (Sanofi-Synthelabo) PoM
Tablets, beige, nalidixic acid 500 mg. Net price 56-tab pack = £12.83. Label: 9, 11, 23

Uriben® (Rosemont) PoM
Suspension, pink, nalidixic acid 300 mg/5 mL, net price 150 mL = £11.42. Label: 9, 11

NORFLOXACIN

Indications: see under Dose
Cautions: see notes above; **interactions:** Appendix 1 (quinolones)
DRIVING. May impair performance of skilled tasks (e.g. driving)
Side-effects: see notes above; also euphoria, anxiety, tinnitus, polyneuropathy, exfoliative dermatitis, pancreatitis, vasculitis
Dose: urinary-tract infections, 400 mg twice daily for 7–10 days (for 3 days in uncomplicated lower urinary-tract infections)
Chronic relapsing urinary-tract infections, 400 mg twice daily for up to 12 weeks; may be reduced to

400 mg once daily if adequate suppression within first 4 weeks
Chronic prostatitis, 400 mg twice daily for 28 days

Norfloxacin (Non-proprietary) PoM
Tablets, norfloxacin 400 mg, net price 6-tab pack = £3.35, 14-tab pack = £6.81. Label: 7, 9, 23, counselling, driving

Utinor® (MSD) PoM
Tablets, scored, norfloxacin 400 mg. Net price 6-tab pack = £2.19, 14-tab pack = £5.11. Label: 7, 9, 23, counselling, driving

---

OFLOXACIN

Indications: see under Dose

Cautions: see notes above; hepatic impairment (Appendix 2); history of psychiatric illness; **interactions:** Appendix 1 (quinolones)
DRIVING. May affect performance of skilled tasks (e.g. driving); effects enhanced by alcohol

Side-effects: see notes above; also reported, tachycardia, transient hypotension, vasculitic reactions, anxiety, unsteady gait, neuropathy, extrapyramidal symptoms, psychotic reactions (discontinue treatment—see notes above); very rarely changes in blood sugar; isolated cases of pneumonitis; on intravenous infusion, hypotension and local reactions (including thrombophlebitis)

Dose: *by mouth*, urinary-tract infections, 200–400 mg daily preferably in the morning, increased if necessary in upper urinary-tract infections to 400 mg twice daily
Chronic prostatitis, 200 mg twice daily for 28 days
Lower respiratory-tract infections, 400 mg daily preferably in the morning, increased if necessary to 400 mg twice daily
Skin and soft-tissue infections, 400 mg twice daily
Uncomplicated gonorrhoea, 400 mg as a single dose
Uncomplicated genital chlamydial infection, non-gonococcal urethritis, 400 mg daily in single or divided doses for 7 days
Pelvic inflammatory disease (see also section 5.1, table 1), 400 mg twice daily for 14 days
By intravenous infusion (over at least 30 minutes for each 200 mg), complicated urinary-tract infection, 200 mg daily
Lower respiratory-tract infection, 200 mg twice daily
Septicaemia, 200 mg twice daily
Skin and soft-tissue infections, 400 mg twice daily
Severe or complicated infections, dose may be increased to 400 mg twice daily

Ofloxacin (Non-proprietary) PoM
Tablets, ofloxacin 200 mg, net price 10-tab pack = £9.76; 400 mg, 5-tab pack = £8.65, 10-tab pack = £18.03. Label: 6, 9, 11, counselling, driving

Tarivid® (Aventis Pharma) PoM
Tablets, f/c, scored, ofloxacin 200 mg, net price 10-tab pack = £7.84, 20-tab pack = £15.66; 400 mg (yellow), 5-tab pack = £7.82, 10-tab pack = £15.60. Label: 6, 9, 11, counselling, driving
Intravenous infusion, ofloxacin (as hydrochloride) 2 mg/mL, net price 100-mL bottle = £16.82 (hosp. only)

5.1.13 Urinary-tract infections

Urinary-tract infection is more common in women than in men; when it occurs in men there is frequently an underlying abnormality of the renal tract. Recurrent episodes of infection are an indication for radiological investigation especially in children in whom untreated pyelonephritis may lead to permanent kidney damage.

Escherichia coli is the most common cause of urinary-tract infection; *Staphylococcus saprophyticus* is also common in sexually active young women. Less common causes include Proteus and Klebsiella spp. *Pseudomonas aeruginosa* infections usually occur in the hospital setting and may be associated with functional or anatomical abnormalities of the renal tract. *Staphylococcus epidermidis* and *Enterococcus faecalis* infection may complicate catheterisation or instrumentation.

> Whenever possible a specimen of urine should be collected for culture and sensitivity testing before starting antibacterial therapy. The antibacterial chosen should reflect current local bacterial sensitivity to antibacterials.

Uncomplicated lower urinary-tract infections often respond to amoxicillin, nalidixic acid, nitrofurantoin, or trimethoprim given for 7 days (3 days of trimethoprim or amoxicillin may be adequate for infections in women); those caused by fully sensitive bacteria respond to two 3-g doses of amoxicillin (section 5.1.1.3). Widespread bacterial resistance, especially to ampicillin or amoxicillin has increased the importance of urine culture before therapy. Alternatives for resistant organisms include co-amoxiclav (amoxicillin with clavulanic acid), an oral cephalosporin, pivmecillinam, or a quinolone.

Long-term low dose therapy may be required in selected patients to prevent *recurrence of infection*; indications include frequent relapses and significant kidney damage. Trimethoprim, nitrofurantoin and cefalexin have been recommended for long-term therapy.

Methenamine (hexamine) should **not** generally be used because it requires an acidic urine for its antimicrobial activity and it is ineffective for upper urinary-tract infections; it may, however, have a role in chronic bacteriuria particularly in infection caused by highly resistant Gram-negative bacteria or by yeasts.

Acute pyelonephritis can lead to septicaemia and is best treated initially by injection of a broad-spectrum antibacterial such as cefuroxime or a quinolone especially if the patient is severely ill; gentamicin can also be used.

Prostatitis can be difficult to cure and requires treatment for several weeks with an antibacterial which penetrates prostatic tissue such as trimethoprim, or some quinolones.

Where infection is localised and associated with an indwelling *catheter* a bladder instillation is often effective (section 7.4.4).

Patients with *heart-valve lesions* undergoing instrumentation of the urinary tract should be given a parenteral antibiotic to prevent bacteraemia and endocarditis (section 5.1, table 2).

Urinary-tract infection in *pregnancy* may be asymptomatic and requires prompt treatment to prevent progression to acute pyelonephritis. Penicillins and cephalosporins are suitable for treating urinary-tract infection during pregnancy. Nitrofurantoin may also be used but it should be avoided at term. Sulphonamides, quinolones, and tetracyclines should be avoided during pregnancy; trimethoprim should also preferably be avoided particularly in the first trimester.

In *renal failure* antibacterials normally excreted by the kidney accumulate with resultant toxicity unless the dose is reduced. This applies especially to the aminoglycosides which should be used with great caution; tetracyclines, methenamine, and nitrofurantoin should be avoided altogether.

CHILDREN. Urinary-tract infections in children require prompt antibacterial treatment to minimise the risk of renal scarring. For the first infection, treatment may be initiated with trimethoprim or co-amoxiclav and the choice of antibacterial is reviewed when sensitivity results are available; full doses of the antibacterial drug should be given for 5–7 days. Antibacterial prophylaxis with low doses of trimethoprim or nitrofurantoin should then be given until investigations for the infection are complete; long-term prophylaxis may be necessary in some cases (e.g. vesicoureteric reflux or renal scarring).

Children under 3 months or seriously unwell children over 3 months should be transferred to hospital and treated initially with intravenous antibacterial drugs such as ampicillin with gentamicin or cefotaxime alone until the infection responds; full doses of oral antibacterials are then given for a further period. Antibacterial prophylaxis should then be given as above.

NITROFURANTOIN

Indications: urinary-tract infections

Cautions: anaemia; diabetes mellitus; electrolyte imbalance; vitamin B and folate deficiency; pulmonary disease; hepatic impairment; monitor lung and liver function on long-term therapy, especially in the elderly (discontinue if deterioration in lung function); susceptibility to peripheral neuropathy; false positive urinary glucose (if tested for reducing substances); urine may be coloured yellow or brown; **interactions:** Appendix 1 (nitrofurantoin)

Contra-indications: renal impairment (Appendix 3); infants less than 3 months old, G6PD deficiency (including pregnancy at term, and breast-feeding of affected infants, see section 9.1.5 and Appendix 4 and Appendix 5), porphyria (section 9.8.2)

Side-effects: anorexia, nausea, vomiting, and diarrhoea; acute and chronic pulmonary reactions (pulmonary fibrosis reported; possible association with lupus erythematosus-like syndrome); peripheral neuropathy; also reported, hypersensitivity reactions (including angioedema, anaphylaxis, sialadenitis, urticaria, rash and pruritus); rarely, cholestatic jaundice, hepatitis, exfoliative dermatitis, erythema multiforme, pancreatitis, arthralgia, blood disorders (including agranulocytosis, thrombocytopenia, and aplastic anaemia), benign intracranial hypertension, and transient alopecia

Dose: acute uncomplicated infection, 50 mg every 6 hours with food for 7 days; CHILD over 3 months, 3 mg/kg daily in 4 divided doses

Severe chronic recurrent infection, 100 mg every 6 hours with food for 7 days (dose reduced or discontinued if severe nausea)

Prophylaxis (but see Cautions), 50–100 mg at night; CHILD over 3 months, 1 mg/kg at night

Nitrofurantoin (Non-proprietary) PoM

Tablets, nitrofurantoin 50 mg, net price 20 = £1.06; 100 mg, 20 = £3.22. Label: 9, 14, 21

Oral suspension, nitrofurantoin 25 mg/5 mL, net price 300 mL = £65.00. Label: 9, 14, 21

Furadantin® (Goldshield) PoM

Tablets, all yellow, scored, nitrofurantoin 50 mg, net price 20 = £1.96; 100 mg, 20 = £3.62. Label: 9, 14, 21

Macrobid® (Goldshield) PoM

Capsules, m/r, blue/yellow, nitrofurantoin 100 mg (as nitrofurantoin macrocrystals and nitrofurantoin monohydrate). Net price 14-cap pack = £4.89. Label: 9, 14, 21, 25

Dose: uncomplicated urinary-tract infection, 1 capsule twice daily with food

Genito-urinary surgical prophylaxis, 1 capsule twice daily on day of procedure and for 3 days after

Macrodantin® (Goldshield) PoM

Capsules, nitrofurantoin 50 mg (yellow/white), net price 30-cap pack = £3.05; 100 mg (yellow/white), 20 = £3.84. Label: 9, 14, 21

METHENAMINE HIPPURATE

(Hexamine hippurate)

Indications: prophylaxis and long-term treatment of chronic or recurrent lower urinary-tract infections

Cautions: pregnancy; avoid concurrent administration with sulphonamides (risk of crystalluria) or urinary alkalinising agents; **interactions:** Appendix 1 (methenamine)

Contra-indications: hepatic impairment, severe renal impairment, severe dehydration, gout, metabolic acidosis

Side-effects: gastro-intestinal disturbances, bladder irritation, rash

Dose: 1 g every 12 hours (may be increased in patients with catheters to 1 g every 8 hours); CHILD 6–12 years 500 mg every 12 hours

Hiprex® (3M)

Tablets, scored, methenamine hippurate 1 g. Net price 60-tab pack = £6.58. Label: 9

5.2 Antifungal drugs

Treatment of fungal infections

The systemic treatment of common fungal infections is outlined below; specialist treatment is required in most forms of systemic or disseminated fungal infections. For local treatment of fungal infections, see section 7.2.2 (genital), section 7.4.4 (bladder), section 11.3.2 (eye), section 12.1.1 (ear), section 12.3.2 (oropharynx), and section 13.10.2 (skin).

ASPERGILLOSIS. Aspergillosis most commonly affects the respiratory tract but in severely immunocompromised patients, invasive forms can affect the sinuses, heart, brain, and skin. **Amphotericin** by intravenous infusion is the drug of choice but response varies; liposomal amphotericin, **itraconazole**, or **voriconazole** are alternatives in patients in whom initial treatment has failed. Itraconazole is also used as an adjunct in the treatment of allergic bronchopulmonary aspergillosis [unlicensed indication]. **Caspofungin** is licensed for invasive aspergillosis unresponsive to amphotericin or to itraconazole, or in patients who cannot tolerate amphotericin or itraconazole. The *Scottish Medicines Consortium* (March 2003) does not recommend the use of caspofungin because of a lack of robust data on efficacy and safety in the treatment of invasive aspergillosis.

CANDIDIASIS. Many superficial candidal infections are treated locally including infections of the vagina (section 7.2.2) and of the skin (section 13.10.2).

Oropharyngeal candidiasis generally responds to topical therapy (section 12.3.2); an imidazole or triazole antifungal is given by mouth for unresponsive infections. Fluconazole is effective and is reliably absorbed.

For *deep and disseminated candidiasis*, **amphotericin** by intravenous infusion is used alone or with **flucytosine** by intravenous infusion; an alternative is **fluconazole** given alone for *Candida albicans* infection, particularly in AIDS patients (in whom flucytosine is best avoided because of its bone marrow toxicity). **Voriconazole** is licensed for infections caused by fluconazole-resistant *Candida* spp. (including *C. krusei*). The use of **caspofungin** should be restricted to treating fluconazole-resistant Candida infections that have not responded to amphotericin or in patients intolerant of amphotericin.

CRYPTOCOCCOSIS. Cryptococcosis is uncommon but infection in the immunocompromised, especially in AIDS patients, can be life-threatening; cryptococcal meningitis is the most common form of fungal meningitis. The treatment of choice is **amphotericin** by intravenous infusion with or without **flucytosine** by intravenous infusion. **Fluconazole** given alone is an alternative particularly in AIDS patients with no disturbance of consciousness. Following successful treatment, fluconazole can be used for prophylaxis against relapse until immunity recovers.

HISTOPLASMOSIS. Histoplasmosis is rare in temperate climates; it can be life-threatening, particularly in HIV-infected persons. **Itraconazole** can be used for the treatment of immunocompetent patients with indolent non-meningeal infection including chronic pulmonary histoplasmosis; **ketoconazole** is an alternative in immunocompetent patients. **Amphotericin** by intravenous infusion is preferred in patients with fulminant or severe infections. Following successful treatment, itraconazole can be used for prophylaxis against relapse.

SKIN AND NAIL INFECTIONS. Mild localised fungal infections of the skin (including tinea corporis, tinea cruris, and tinea pedis) respond to topical therapy (section 13.10.2). Systemic therapy (itraconazole, fluconazole, or terbinafine) is appropriate if topical therapy fails, if many areas are affected, or if the site of infection is difficult to treat such as in infections of the nails (onychomycosis) and of the scalp (tinea capitis).

Griseofulvin is used for tinea capitis in adults and children; it was used extensively in tinea of various other sites but it has largely been replaced by newer antifungals. Oral imidazole or triazole antifungals (particularly **itraconazole**) and **terbinafine** are used more commonly because they have a broader spectrum of activity and require a shorter duration of treatment; the role of terbinafine in the management of *Microsporum* species (cat or dog ringworm) is uncertain.

Pityriasis versicolor may be treated with **itraconazole** by mouth if topical therapy is ineffective; **fluconazole** by mouth is an alternative. Oral **terbinafine** is **not** effective for pityriasis versicolor.

Terbinafine and **itraconazole** have largely replaced griseofulvin for the systemic treatment of onychomycosis, particularly of the toenail; terbinafine is considered to be the drug of choice. Itraconazole can be administered as intermittent 'pulse' therapy.

IMMUNOCOMPROMISED PATIENTS. Immunocompromised patients are at particular risk of fungal infections and may receive antifungal drugs prophylactically; oral imidazole or triazole antifungals are the drugs of choice for prophylaxis. **Fluconazole** is more reliably absorbed than itraconazole and ketoconazole and is considered less toxic than ketoconazole on long-term use.

Amphotericin by intravenous infusion is used for the empirical *treatment* of serious fungal infections. Fluconazole is used for treating *Candida albicans* infection. Caspofungin is licensed for the empirical treatment of systemic fungal infections (such as those involving *Candida* spp. or *Aspergillus* spp.) in patients with neutropenia.

Drugs used in fungal infections

POLYENE ANTIFUNGALS. The polyene antifungals include amphotericin and nystatin; neither drug is absorbed when given by mouth. They are used for oral, oropharyngeal, and perioral infections by local application in the mouth (section 12.3.2).

Amphotericin by intravenous infusion is used for the treatment of systemic fungal infections and is active against most fungi and yeasts. It is highly protein bound and penetrates poorly into body fluids and tissues. When given parenterally amphotericin is toxic and side-effects are common. Lipid formulations of amphotericin (*Abelcet*®, *AmBisome*®, and *Amphocil*®) are significantly less toxic and are recommended when the conventional formulation of amphotericin is contra-indicated because of toxicity, especially nephrotoxicity or when response to conventional amphotericin is inadequate; lipid formulations are more expensive.

Nystatin is used principally for *Candida albicans* infections of the skin and mucous membranes, including oesophageal and intestinal candidiasis.

IMIDAZOLE ANTIFUNGALS. Clotrimazole, econazole, fenticonazole, sulconazole, and tioconazole are used for the local treatment of vaginal candidiasis (section 7.2.2) and for dermatophyte infections (section 13.10.2).

Ketoconazole is better absorbed by mouth than other imidazoles. It has been associated with fatal hepatotoxicity; the CSM has advised that prescribers should weigh the potential benefits of ketoconazole treatment against the risk of liver damage and should carefully monitor patients both clinically and biochemically. It should not be used by mouth for superficial fungal infections.

Miconazole can be used locally for oral infections; it is also effective in intestinal infections. Systemic absorption may follow use of miconazole oral gel and may result in significant drug interactions.

TRIAZOLE ANTIFUNGALS. **Fluconazole** is very well absorbed after oral administration. It also achieves good penetration into the cerebrospinal fluid to treat fungal meningitis.

Itraconazole is active against a wide range of dermatophytes. Itraconazole capsules require an acid environment in the stomach for optimal absorption.

Itraconazole has been associated with liver damage and should be avoided or used with caution in patients with liver disease; fluconazole is less frequently associated with hepatotoxicity.

Voriconazole is a broad-spectrum antifungal drug which is licensed for use in life-threatening infections.

OTHER ANTIFUNGALS. **Caspofungin** is active against *Aspergillus* spp. and *Candida* spp. It is given by intravenous infusion for invasive infection. **Flucytosine** is often used with amphotericin in a synergistic combination. Bone marrow depression can occur which limits its use, particularly in AIDS patients; weekly blood counts are necessary during prolonged therapy. Resistance to flucytosine can develop during therapy and sensitivity testing is essential before and during treatment.

Griseofulvin is effective for widespread or intractable dermatophyte infections but has been superseded by newer antifungals, particularly for nail infections. It is usually well tolerated and is licensed for use in children. Duration of therapy is dependent on the site of the infection and may be required for a number of months.

Terbinafine is the drug of choice for fungal nail infections and is also used for ringworm infections where oral treatment is considered appropriate.

AMPHOTERICIN

(Amphotericin B)

Indications: See under Dose

Cautions: when given parenterally, toxicity common (close supervision necessary and test dose required); renal impairment (Appendix 3); hepatic and renal-function tests, blood counts, and plasma electrolyte (including plasma-potassium and magnesium concentration) monitoring required; corticosteroids (avoid except to control reactions); pregnancy (Appendix 4); breast-feeding (Appendix 5); avoid rapid infusion (risk of arrhythmias); **interactions:** Appendix 1 (amphotericin)

ANAPHYLAXIS. The CSM has advised that anaphylaxis occurs rarely with any intravenous amphotericin product and a test dose is advisable before the first infusion; the patient should be carefully observed for about 30 minutes after the test dose. Prophylactic antipyretics or hydrocortisone should only be used in patients who have previously experienced acute adverse reactions (in whom continued treatment with amphotericin is essential)

Side-effects: when given parenterally, anorexia, nausea and vomiting, diarrhoea, epigastric pain; febrile reactions, headache, muscle and joint pain; anaemia; disturbances in renal function (including hypokalaemia and hypomagnesaemia) and renal toxicity; also cardiovascular toxicity (including arrhythmias), blood disorders, neurological disorders (including hearing loss, diplopia, convulsions, peripheral neuropathy), abnormal liver function (discontinue treatment), rash, anaphylactoid reactions (see Anaphylaxis, above); pain and thrombophlebitis at injection site

Dose: *by mouth*, intestinal candidiasis, 100–200 mg every 6 hours; INFANT and CHILD, 100 mg 4 times daily

Prophylaxis NEONATE 100 mg once daily

Oral and perioral infections, see section 12.3.2

By intravenous infusion, see under preparations, below

Fungilin® (Squibb) PoM

Tablets, yellow, scored, amphotericin 100 mg, Net price 56-tab pack = £7.74. Label: 9

Suspension, yellow, sugar-free, amphotericin 100 mg/mL, net price 12 mL = £2.15. Label: 9, counselling, use of pipette

Fungizone® (Squibb) PoM

Intravenous infusion, powder for reconstitution, amphotericin (as sodium deoxycholate complex). Net price 50-mg vial = £3.16

Electrolytes: Na^+ < 0.5 mmol/vial

Dose: by intravenous infusion, systemic fungal infections, initial test dose of 1 mg over 20–30 minutes then 250 micrograms/kg daily, gradually increased if tolerated to 1 mg/kg daily; max. (severe infection) 1.5 mg/kg daily or on alternate days

NOTE. Prolonged treatment usually necessary; if interrupted for longer than 7 days recommence at 250 micrograms/kg daily and increase gradually

■ Lipid formulations

Abelcet® (Zeneus) PoM

Intravenous infusion, amphotericin 5 mg/mL as lipid complex with L-α-dimyristoylphosphatidylcholine and L-α-dimyristoylphosphatidylglycerol. Net price 20-mL vial = £82.13 (hosp. only)

Dose: severe invasive candidiasis; severe systemic fungal infections in patients not responding to conventional amphotericin or to other antifungal drugs or where toxicity or renal impairment precludes conventional amphotericin, including invasive aspergillosis, cryptococcal meningitis and disseminated cryptococcosis in HIV patients, by intravenous infusion, ADULT and CHILD, initial test dose 1 mg over 15 minutes then 5 mg/kg daily for at least 14 days

AmBisome® (Gilead) PoM

Intravenous infusion, powder for reconstitution, amphotericin 50 mg encapsulated in liposomes. Net price 50-mg vial = £96.69

Electrolytes: Na^+ < 0.5 mmol/vial

Excipients: include sucrose 900 mg/vial

Dose: severe systemic or deep mycoses where toxicity (particularly nephrotoxicity) precludes use of conventional amphotericin, by intravenous infusion, ADULT and CHILD initial test dose 1 mg over 10 minutes then 1 mg/kg daily as a single dose increased gradually if necessary to 3 mg/kg daily as a single dose; max. 5 mg/kg daily

Infections in febrile neutropenic patients unresponsive to broad-spectrum antibacterials, ADULT and CHILD, initial test dose 1 mg over 10 minutes then 3 mg/kg daily as a single dose until afebrile for 3 consecutive days; max. period of treatment 42 days

Visceral leishmaniasis, see section 5.4.5 and product literature

NOTE. *Ambisome*® doses in BNF may differ from those in product literature

Amphocil® (Cambridge) PoM

Intravenous infusion, powder for reconstitution, amphotericin as a complex with sodium cholesteryl sulphate. Net price 50-mg vial = £96.81, 100-mg vial = £190.05

Electrolytes: Na^+ < 0.5 mmol/vial

Dose: severe systemic or deep mycoses where toxicity or renal failure preclude use of conventional amphotericin, by intravenous infusion, ADULT and CHILD initial test dose 2 mg over 10 minutes then 1 mg/kg daily as a single dose increased gradually if necessary to 3–4 mg/kg daily as a single dose; max.6 mg/kg daily

CASPOFUNGIN

Indications: invasive aspergillosis either unresponsive to amphotericin or itraconazole or in patients intolerant of amphotericin or itraconazole; invasive candidiasis (see notes above); empirical treatment of systemic fungal infections in patients with neutropenia

Cautions: hepatic impairment (Appendix 2); pregnancy (Appendix 4); **interactions:** Appendix 1 (caspofungin)

Contra-indications: breast-feeding (Appendix 5)

Side-effects: nausea, vomiting, abdominal pain, diarrhoea; tachycardia, flushing; dyspnoea; fever, headache; anaemia, decrease in serum potassium, hypomagnesaemia; rash, pruritus, sweating; injection-site reactions; *less commonly* hypercalcaemia; also reported, hepatic dysfunction, oedema, adult respiratory distress syndrome, hypersensitivity reactions (including anaphylaxis)

Dose: *by intravenous infusion*, ADULT over 18 years, 70 mg on first day then 50 mg once daily (70 mg once daily if body-weight over 80 kg)

Cancidas® (MSD) PoM

Intravenous infusion, powder for reconstitution, caspofungin (as acetate), net price 50-mg vial = £327.67; 70-mg vial = £416.78

FLUCONAZOLE

Indications: see under Dose

Cautions: renal impairment (Appendix 3); pregnancy (Appendix 4) and breast-feeding (Appendix 5); monitor liver function—discontinue if signs or symptoms of hepatic disease (risk of hepatic necrosis); susceptibility to QT interval prolongation; **interactions:** Appendix 1 (antifungals, triazole)

Side-effects: nausea, abdominal discomfort, diarrhoea, flatulence, headache, rash (discontinue treatment or monitor closely if infection invasive or systemic); less frequently dyspepsia, vomiting, taste disturbance, hepatic disorders, hypersensitivity reactions, anaphylaxis, dizziness, seizures, alopecia, pruritus, toxic epidermal necrolysis, Stevens-Johnson syndrome (severe cutaneous reactions more likely in AIDS patients), hyperlipidaemia, leucopenia, thrombocytopenia, and hypokalaemia reported

Dose: vaginal candidiasis (see also Recurrent Vulvovaginal Candidiasis, section 7.2.2) and candidal balanitis, *by mouth*, a single dose of 150 mg

Mucosal candidiasis (except genital), *by mouth*, 50 mg daily (100 mg daily in unusually difficult infections) given for 7–14 days in oropharyngeal candidiasis (max. 14 days except in severely immunocompromised patients); for 14 days in atrophic oral candidiasis associated with dentures; for 14–30 days in other mucosal infections (e.g. oesophagitis, candiduria, non-invasive bronchopulmonary infections); CHILD *by mouth or by intravenous infusion*, 3–6 mg/kg on first day then 3 mg/kg daily (every 72 hours in NEONATE up to 2 weeks old, every 48 hours in neonate 2–4 weeks old)

Tinea pedis, corporis, cruris, pityriasis versicolor, and dermal candidiasis, *by mouth*, 50 mg daily for 2–4 weeks (for up to 6 weeks in tinea pedis); max. duration of treatment 6 weeks

Invasive candidal infections (including candidaemia and disseminated candidiasis) and cryptococcal infections (including meningitis), *by mouth or intravenous infusion*, 400 mg initially then 200 mg daily, increased if necessary to 400 mg daily; treatment continued according to response (at least 6–8 weeks for cryptococcal meningitis); CHILD 6–12 mg/kg daily (every 72 hours in NEONATE up to 2 weeks old, every 48 hours in NEONATE 2–4 weeks old); max. 400 mg daily

Prevention of relapse of cryptococcal meningitis in AIDS patients after completion of primary therapy, *by mouth*, 200 mg daily *or by intravenous infusion*, 100–200 mg daily

Prevention of fungal infections in immunocompromised patients, *by mouth or by intravenous infusion*, 50–400 mg daily adjusted according to risk; 400 mg daily if high risk of systemic infections e.g. following bone-marrow transplantation; commence treatment before anticipated onset of neutropenia and continue for 7 days after neutrophil count in desirable range; CHILD according to extent and duration of neutropenia, 3–12 mg/kg daily (every 72 hours in NEONATE up to 2 weeks old, every 48 hours in NEONATE 2–4 weeks old); max. 400 mg daily

Fluconazole (Non-proprietary) PoM

[1]*Capsules*, fluconazole 50 mg, net price 7-cap pack = £4.48; 150 mg, single-capsule pack = £1.47; 200 mg, 7-cap pack = £25.44. Label: 9, (50 and 200 mg)

DENTAL PRESCRIBING ON NHS. Fluconazole Capsules 50 mg may be prescribed

Intravenous infusion, fluconazole 2 mg/mL, net price 25-mL bottle = £7.32; 100-mL bottle = £29.28

Diflucan® (Pfizer) PoM

[1]*Capsules*, fluconazole 50 mg (blue/white), net price 7-cap pack = £16.61; 150 mg (blue), single-capsule pack = £7.12; 200 mg (purple/white), 7-cap pack = £66.42. Label: 9, (50 and 200 mg)

Oral suspension, orange-flavoured, fluconazole for reconstitution with water, 50 mg/5 mL, net price 35 mL = £16.61; 200 mg/5 mL, 35 mL = £66.42. Label: 9

DENTAL PRESCRIBING ON NHS. May be prescribed as Fluconazole Oral Suspension 50 mg/5 mL

Intravenous infusion, fluconazole 2 mg/mL in sodium chloride intravenous infusion 0.9%, net price 25-mL bottle = £7.32; 100-mL bottle = £29.28

Electrolytes: Na^+ 15 mmol/100-mL bottle

1. Capsules can be sold to the public for vaginal candidiasis and associated candidal balanitis in those aged 16–60 years, in a container or packaging containing not more than 150 mg and labelled to show a max. dose of 150 mg; proprietary brands on sale to the public include *Canesten® Oral*, *Diflucan® One*

FLUCYTOSINE

Indications: systemic yeast and fungal infections; adjunct to amphotericin (or fluconazole) in cryptococcal meningitis, adjunct to amphotericin in severe systemic candidiasis and in other severe or long-standing infections

Cautions: renal impairment (Appendix 3); elderly; blood disorders; liver- and kidney-function tests and blood counts required (weekly in renal impairment or blood disorders); pregnancy (Appendix 4), breast-feeding (Appendix 5); **interactions:** Appendix 1 (flucytosine)

Side-effects: nausea, vomiting, diarrhoea, rashes; less frequently confusion, hallucinations, convulsions, headache, sedation, vertigo, alterations in liver function tests (hepatitis and hepatic necrosis reported); blood disorders including thrombocytopenia, leucopenia, and aplastic anaemia reported

Dose: *by intravenous infusion* over 20–40 minutes, ADULT and CHILD, 200 mg/kg daily in 4 divided doses usually for not more than 7 days; extremely sensitive organisms, 100–150 mg/kg daily may be sufficient; treat for at least 4 months in cryptococcal meningitis

NOTE. For plasma concentration monitoring blood should be taken shortly before starting the next infusion; plasma concentration for optimum response 25–50 mg/litre (200–400 micromol/litre)—should not be allowed to exceed 80 mg/litre (620 micromol/litre)

Ancotil® (Valeant) PoM

Intravenous infusion, flucytosine 10 mg/mL. Net price 250-mL infusion bottle = £30.33 (hosp. only)

Electrolytes: Na^+ 34.5 mmol/250-mL bottle

NOTE. Flucytosine tablets may be available on a named-patient basis from Bell and Croyden

GRISEOFULVIN

Indications: dermatophyte infections of the skin, scalp, hair and nails where topical therapy has failed or is inappropriate

Cautions: interactions: Appendix 1 (griseofulvin)

DRIVING. May impair performance of skilled tasks (e.g. driving); effects of alcohol enhanced

Contra-indications: severe liver disease; systemic lupus erythematosus (risk of exacerbation); porphyria (section 9.8.2); pregnancy (**avoid** pregnancy **during** and for **1 month after** treatment (Appendix 4); men should not father children within 6 months of treatment); breast-feeding (Appendix 5)

Side-effects: nausea, vomiting, diarrhoea; headache; less frequently hepatotoxicity, dizziness, confusion, fatigue, sleep disturbances, impaired co-ordination, peripheral neuropathy, leucopenia, systemic lupus erythematosus, rash (including rarely erythema multiforme, toxic epidermal necrolysis), and photosensitivity

Dose: 500 mg daily in divided doses or as a single dose, in severe infection dose may be doubled, reducing when response occurs; CHILD, 10 mg/kg daily in divided doses or as a single dose

Grisovin® (GSK) PoM

Tablets, both f/c, griseofulvin 125 mg, net price 20 = 48p; 500 mg, 20 = £1.79. Label: 9, 21, counselling, driving

ITRACONAZOLE

Indications: see under Dose

Cautions: absorption reduced in AIDS and neutropenia (monitor plasma-itraconazole concentration and increase dose if necessary); susceptibility to congestive heart failure (see also CSM advice, below); renal impairment (Appendix 3); pregnancy (Appendix 4) and breast-feeding (Appendix 5); **interactions:** Appendix 1 (antifungals, triazole)

HEPATOTOXICITY. Potentially life-threatening hepatotoxicity reported very rarely. Monitor liver function—discontinue if signs of hepatitis develop; avoid or use with caution if history of hepatotoxicity with other drugs or in active liver disease (Appendix 2); use with caution in patients receiving other hepatotoxic drugs

COUNSELLING. Patients should be told how to recognise signs of liver disorder and advised to seek immediate medical attention if symptoms such as anorexia, nausea, vomiting, fatigue, abdominal pain or dark urine develop

CSM advice (heart failure). Following rare reports of heart failure, the CSM has advised caution when prescribing itraconazole to patients at high risk of heart failure. Those at risk include:

- patients receiving high doses and longer treatment courses;
- older patients and those with cardiac disease;
- patients receiving treatment with negative inotropic drugs, e.g. calcium channel blockers.

Side-effects: *very rarely* nausea, vomiting, dyspepsia, abdominal pain, diarrhoea, constipation, jaundice, hepatitis (see also Hepatotoxicity above), heart failure (see CSM advice above), pulmonary oedema, headache, dizziness, peripheral neuropathy (discontinue treatment), menstrual disorder, hypokalaemia, rash, pruritus, Stevens-Johnson syndrome, and alopecia; *with intravenous injection, very rarely* hypertension and hyperglycaemia

Dose: *by mouth*, oropharyngeal candidiasis, 100 mg daily (200 mg daily in AIDS or neutropenia) for 15 days; see also under *Sporanox*® oral liquid below

Vulvovaginal candidiasis, 200 mg twice daily for 1 day

Pityriasis versicolor, 200 mg daily for 7 days

Tinea corporis and tinea cruris, *either* 100 mg daily for 15 days *or* 200 mg daily for 7 days

Tinea pedis and tinea manuum, *either* 100 mg daily for 30 days *or* 200 mg twice daily for 7 days

Onychomycosis, *either* 200 mg daily for 3 months *or* course ('pulse') of 200 mg twice daily for 7 days, subsequent courses repeated after 21-day interval; fingernails 2 courses, toenails 3 courses

Histoplasmosis, 200 mg 1–2 times daily

Systemic aspergillosis, candidiasis and cryptococcosis including cryptococcal meningitis where other antifungal drugs inappropriate or ineffective, 200 mg once daily (candidiasis 100–200 mg once daily) increased in invasive or disseminated disease and in cryptococcal meningitis to 200 mg twice daily

Maintenance in AIDS patients to prevent relapse of underlying fungal infection and prophylaxis in neutropenia when standard therapy inappropriate, 200 mg once daily, increased to 200 mg twice daily if low plasma-itraconazole concentration (see Cautions)

Prophylaxis in patients with haematological malignancy or undergoing bone-marrow transplant, see

under *Sporanox*® oral liquid below
CHILD and ELDERLY safety and efficacy not established

By intravenous infusion, systemic aspergillosis, candidiasis and cryptococcosis including cryptococcal meningitis where other antifungal drugs inappropriate or ineffective, histoplasmosis, 200 mg every 12 hours for 2 days, then 200 mg once daily for max. 12 days; CHILD and ELDERLY safety and efficacy not established

Sporanox® (Janssen-Cilag) PoM

Capsules, blue/pink, enclosing coated beads, itraconazole 100 mg, net price 4-cap pack = £3.98; 15-cap pack = £14.93; 28-cap pack (*Sporanox*®*-Pulse*) = £27.88; 60-cap pack = £59.75. Label: 5, 9, 21, 25

Oral liquid, sugar-free, itraconazole 10 mg/mL, net price 150 mL (with 10-mL measuring cup) = £49.67. Label: 9, 23, counselling, administration

Dose: oral or oesophageal candidiasis in HIV-positive or other immunocompromised patients, 20 mL (2 measuring cups) daily in 1–2 divided doses for 1 week (continue for another week if no response)

Fluconazole-resistant oral or oesophageal candidiasis, 10–20 mL (1–2 measuring cups) twice daily for 2 weeks (continue for another 2 weeks if no response; the higher dose should not be used for longer than 2 weeks if no signs of improvement)

Prophylaxis of deep fungal infections (when standard therapy is inappropriate) in patients with haematological malignancy or undergoing bone-marrow transplantation who are expected to become neutropenic, 5 mg/kg daily in 2 divided doses; start 1 week before transplantation or immediately before chemotherapy and continue until neutrophil count recovers; CHILD and ELDERLY safety and efficacy not established

COUNSELLING. Do not take with food; swish around mouth and swallow, do not rinse afterwards

Concentrate for intravenous infusion, itraconazole 10 mg/mL. For dilution before use. Net price 25-mL amp (with infusion bag and filter) = £67.86

Excipients: include propylene glycol

KETOCONAZOLE

Indications: systemic mycoses, serious chronic resistant mucocutaneous candidiasis, serious resistant gastro-intestinal mycoses, chronic resistant vaginal candidiasis, resistant dermatophyte infections of skin or finger nails (not toe nails); prophylaxis of mycoses in immunosuppressed patients

Cautions: monitor liver function clinically and biochemically—for treatment lasting longer than 14 days perform liver function tests before starting, 14 days after starting, then at monthly intervals (for details consult product literature)—for CSM advice see p. 308; avoid in porphyria (section 9.8.2); **interactions:** Appendix 1 (antifungals, imidazole)

Contra-indications: hepatic impairment; pregnancy (Appendix 4) and breast-feeding

Side-effects: nausea, vomiting, abdominal pain; headache; rashes, urticaria, pruritus; rarely angioedema, thrombocytopenia, paraesthesia, photophobia, dizziness, alopecia, gynaecomastia and oligospermia; fatal liver damage—see also under Cautions, risk of developing hepatitis greater if given for longer than 14 days

Dose: 200 mg once daily with food, usually for 14 days; if response inadequate after 14 days continue until at least 1 week after symptoms have cleared and cultures negative; max. 400 mg (ELDERLY 200 mg) daily
CHILD 3 mg/kg daily
Chronic resistant vaginal candidiasis, 400 mg once daily with food for 5 days
Prophylaxis and maintenance treatment in immunosuppressed patients, 200 mg daily

Nizoral® (Janssen-Cilag) PoM

Tablets, scored, ketoconazole 200 mg. Net price 30-tab pack = £14.91. Label: 5, 9, 21

MICONAZOLE

Indications: see under Dose

Cautions: pregnancy (Appendix 4); breast-feeding; avoid in porphyria (section 9.8.2); **interactions:** Appendix 1 (antifungals, imidazole)

Contra-indications: hepatic impairment

Side-effects: nausea and vomiting, diarrhoea (usually on long-term treatment); rarely allergic reactions; isolated reports of hepatitis

Dose: prevention and treatment of oral and intestinal fungal infections, 5–10 mL in the mouth after food 4 times daily; retain near lesions before swallowing; CHILD under 2 years, 2.5 mL twice daily, 2–6 years, 5 mL twice daily, over 6 years, 5 mL 4 times daily

Localised lesions, smear on affected area with clean finger (dental prostheses should be removed at night and brushed with gel); treatment continued for 48 hours after lesions have resolved

NOTE. Not licensed for use in NEONATE

[1]**Daktarin**® (Janssen-Cilag) PoM

Oral gel, sugar-free, orange-flavoured, miconazole 24 mg/mL (20 mg/g). Net price 15-g tube = £2.45, 80-g tube = £4.75. Label: 9, counselling advised, hold in mouth, after food

1. 15-g tube can be sold to public

NYSTATIN

Indications: candidiasis; vaginal infection (section 7.2.2); oral infection (section 12.3.2); skin infection (section 13.10.2)

Side-effects: nausea, vomiting, diarrhoea at high doses; oral irritation and sensitisation; rash (including urticaria) and rarely Stevens-Johnson syndrome reported

Dose: *by mouth*, intestinal candidiasis 500 000 units every 6 hours, doubled in severe infections; CHILD 100 000 units 4 times daily
Prophylaxis, 1 million units once daily; NEONATE 100 000 units once daily

NOTE. Unlicensed for treatment of candidiasis in NEONATE

Nystatin (Non-proprietary) PoM

Oral suspension, nystatin 100 000 units/mL. Net price 30 mL = £2.05. Label: 9, counselling, use of pipette

Brands include *Nystamont*®

Nystan® (Squibb) PoM

Tablets, brown, s/c, nystatin 500 000 units, net price 56-tab pack = £4.70. Label: 9

Suspension, yellow, nystatin 100 000 units/mL, net price 30 mL with pipette = £2.05. Label: 9, counselling, use of pipette

TERBINAFINE

Indications: dermatophyte infections of the nails, ringworm infections (including tinea pedis, cruris, and corporis) where oral therapy appropriate (due to site, severity or extent)

Cautions: hepatic impairment (Appendix 2) and renal impairment (Appendix 3); pregnancy (Appendix 4), breast-feeding (Appendix 5); psoriasis (risk of exacerbation); autoimmune disease (risk of lupus-erythematosus-like effect); **interactions:** Appendix 1 (terbinafine)

Side-effects: abdominal discomfort, anorexia, nausea, diarrhoea; headache; rash and urticaria occasionally with arthralgia or myalgia; *less commonly* taste disturbance; *rarely* liver toxicity (including jaundice, cholestasis and hepatitis)—discontinue treatment, angioedema, dizziness, malaise, paraesthesia, hypoaesthesia, photosensitivity, serious skin reactions (including Stevens-Johnson syndrome and toxic epidermal necrolysis)—discontinue treatment if progressive skin rash; *very rarely* psychiatric disturbances, blood disorders (including leucopenia and thrombocytopenia), lupus erythematosus-like effect, and exacerbation of psoriasis

Dose: 250 mg daily usually for 2–6 weeks in tinea pedis, 2–4 weeks in tinea cruris, 4 weeks in tinea corporis, 6 weeks–3 months in nail infections (occasionally longer in toenail infections); CHILD [unlicensed] usually for 2 weeks, tinea capitis, over 1 year, body-weight 10–20 kg, 62.5 mg once daily; body-weight 20–40 kg, 125 mg once daily; body-weight over 40 kg, 250 mg once daily

Lamisil® (Novartis) PoM

Tablets, off-white, scored, terbinafine 250 mg (as hydrochloride), net price 14-tab pack = £23.16, 28-tab pack = £44.66. Label: 9

VORICONAZOLE

Indications: invasive aspergillosis; serious infections caused by *Scedosporium* spp., *Fusarium* spp., or invasive fluconazole-resistant *Candida* spp. (including *C. krusei*); candidaemia

Cautions: monitor liver function before treatment and during treatment; haematological malignancy (increased risk of hepatic reactions); hepatic impairment (Appendix 2); monitor renal function; renal impairment (Appendix 3); pregnancy (ensure effective contraception during treatment—Appendix 4); electrolyte disturbances, cardiomyopathy, bradycardia, symptomatic arrhythmias, history of QT interval prolongation, concomitant use with other drugs that prolong QT interval; avoid exposure to sunlight; **interactions:** Appendix 1 (antifungals, triazole)

Contra-indications: breast-feeding (Appendix 5)

Side-effects: gastro-intestinal disturbances (including nausea, vomiting, abdominal pain, diarrhoea), jaundice; oedema, hypotension, chest pain; respiratory distress syndrome, sinusitis; headache, dizziness, asthenia, anxiety, depression, confusion, agitation, hallucinations, paraesthesia, tremor; influenza-like symptoms; hypoglycaemia; haematuria; blood disorders (including anaemia, thrombocytopenia, leucopenia, pancytopenia), acute renal failure, hypokalaemia; visual disturbances including altered perception, blurred vision, and photophobia; rash, pruritus, photosensitivity, alopecia, cheilitis; injection-site reactions; *less commonly* taste disturbances, cholecystitis, pancreatitis, hepatitis, constipation, arrhythmias (including QT interval prolongation), syncope, raised serum cholesterol, hypersensitivity reactions (including flushing), ataxia, nystagmus, hypoaesthesia, adrenocortical insufficiency, arthritis, blepharitis, optic neuritis, scleritis, glossitis, gingivitis, psoriasis, and Stevens-Johnson syndrome; *rarely* pseudomembranous colitis, sleep disturbances, tinnitus, hearing disturbances, extrapyramidal effects, hypertonia, hypothyroidism, hyperthyroidism, discoid lupus erythematosus, toxic epidermal necrolysis, retinal haemorrhage, and optic atrophy

Dose: *by mouth*, ADULT and ADOLESCENT over 12 years, body-weight over 40 kg, 400 mg every 12 hours for 2 doses then 200 mg every 12 hours, increased if necessary to 300 mg every 12 hours; body-weight under 40 kg, 200 mg every 12 hours for 2 doses then 100 mg every 12 hours, increased if necessary to 150 mg every 12 hours; CHILD 2–11 years, 6 mg/kg every 12 hours for 2 doses, then 4 mg/kg every 12 hours

By intravenous infusion, ADULT and CHILD over 2 years, 6 mg/kg every 12 hours for 2 doses, then 4 mg/kg every 12 hours (reduced in ADULT and ADOLESCENT over 12 years to 3 mg/kg every 12 hours if not tolerated) for max. 6 months

Vfend® (Pfizer) PoM

Tablets, f/c, voriconazole 50 mg, net price 28-tablet pack = £227.84; 200 mg, 28-tab pack = £911.36. Label: 11, 23

Oral suspension, voriconazole 200 mg/5 mL when reconstituted with water, net price 75 mL (orange-flavoured) = £501.25. Label: 11, 23

Intravenous infusion, powder for reconstitution, voriconazole, net price 200-mg vial = £77.14

Excipients: include sulphobutylether beta cyclodextrin sodium (risk of accumulation in renal impairment)

Electrolytes: Na^+ 9.62 mmol/vial

5.3 Antiviral drugs

The majority of virus infections resolve spontaneously in immunocompetent subjects. A number of specific treatments for viral infections are available, particularly for the immunocompromised. This section includes notes on herpes simplex and varicella-zoster, human immunodeficiency virus, cytomegalovirus, respiratory syncytial virus, viral hepatitis and influenza.

5.3.1 HIV infection

There is no cure for infection caused by the human immunodeficiency virus (HIV) but a number of drugs slow or halt disease progression. Drugs for HIV infection (antiretrovirals) increase life expectancy considerably but they are toxic. Treatment should be undertaken only by those experienced in their use.

PRINCIPLES OF TREATMENT. Treatment is aimed at reducing the plasma viral load as much as possible and for as long as possible; it should be started before the immune system is irreversibly damaged. The need for early drug treatment should, however, be balanced against the development of toxicity. Commitment to treatment and strict adherence over many years are required; the regimen chosen should take into account convenience and patient tolerance. The development of drug resistance is reduced by using a combination of drugs; such combinations should have synergistic or additive activity while ensuring that their toxicity is not additive. Testing for resistance to antiviral drugs particularly in therapeutic failure should be considered.

INITIATION OF TREATMENT. The optimum time for initiation of antiviral treatment will depend primarily on the CD4 cell count; the plasma viral load and clinical symptoms may also help. Initiating treatment with a combination of drugs ('highly active antiretroviral therapy' which includes 2 nucleoside reverse transcriptase inhibitors with *either* a non-nucleoside reverse transcriptase inhibitor *or* 1 or 2 protease inhibitors) is recommended.

SWITCHING THERAPY. Deterioration of the condition (including clinical and virological changes) may require either switching therapy or adding another antiviral drug. The choice of an alternative regimen depends on factors such as the response to previous treatment, tolerance and the possibility of cross-resistance.

PREGNANCY AND BREAST-FEEDING. Treatment of HIV infection in pregnancy aims to reduce the risk of toxicity to the fetus (although the teratogenic potential of most antiretroviral drugs is unknown), to minimise the viral load and disease progression in the mother, and to prevent transmission of infection to the neonate. **All treatment options require careful assessment by a specialist**. Zidovudine monotherapy reduces transmission of infection to the neonate. However, combination antiretroviral therapy maximises the chance of preventing transmission and represents optimal therapy for the mother.

Breast-feeding by HIV-positive mothers may cause HIV infection in the infant and should be avoided.

POST-EXPOSURE PROPHYLAXIS. Prophylaxis with antiretroviral drugs [unlicensed indication] may be appropriate following occupational exposure to HIV-contaminated material. Immediate expert advice should be sought in such cases; national guidelines on post-exposure prophylaxis for healthcare workers have been developed (by the Chief Medical Officer's Expert Advisory Group on AIDS) and local ones may also be available. Antiretrovirals for prophylaxis are chosen on the basis of efficacy and potential for toxicity.

DRUGS USED FOR HIV INFECTION. **Zidovudine**, a nucleoside reverse transcriptase inhibitor (or 'nucleoside analogue'), was the first anti-HIV drug to be introduced. Higher doses of zidovudine alone were used to prevent the AIDS dementia complex but combination therapy including zidovudine at standard doses is now preferred. Other nucleoside reverse transcriptase inhibitors include **abacavir**, **didanosine**, **emtricitabine**, **lamivudine**, **stavudine**, **tenofovir**, and **zalcitabine**.

The protease inhibitors include **amprenavir**, **atazanavir**, **fosamprenavir** (a pro-drug of amprenavir), **indinavir**, **lopinavir**, **nelfinavir**, **ritonavir**, and **saquinavir**. Ritonavir in low doses boosts the activity of amprenavir, indinavir, lopinavir, and saquinavir increasing the persistence of plasma concentrations of these drugs; at such a low dose, ritonavir has no intrinsic antiviral activity. A combination of lopinavir with low-dose ritonavir is available. The protease inhibitors are metabolised by cytochrome P450 enzyme systems and therefore have a significant potential for drug interactions. Protease inhibitors are associated with lipodystrophy and metabolic effects (see below).

The non-nucleoside reverse transcriptase inhibitors **efavirenz** and **nevirapine** may interact with a number of drugs metabolised in the liver. Nevirapine is associated with a high incidence of rash (including Stevens-Johnson syndrome) and occasionally fatal hepatitis. Rash is also associated with efavirenz but it is usually milder. Efavirenz treatment has also been associated with an increased plasma cholesterol concentration.

Enfuvirtide, which inhibits HIV from fusing to the host cell, is licensed for managing infection that has failed to respond to a regimen of other antiretroviral drugs; enfuvirtide should be combined with other potentially active antiretroviral drugs.

Improvement in immune function as a result of antiretroviral treatment may provoke an inflammatory reaction against residual opportunistic organisms.

LIPODYSTROPHY SYNDROME. Metabolic effects associated with antiretroviral treatment include *fat redistribution*, *insulin resistance* and *dyslipidaemia*; collectively these have been termed *lipodystrophy syndrome*.

Fat redistribution (with loss of subcutaneous fat, increased abdominal fat, 'buffalo hump' and breast enlargement) is associated with regimens containing protease inhibitors and nucleoside reverse transcriptase inhibitors.

Dyslipidaemia (with adverse effects on body lipids) is associated with antiretroviral treatment, particularly with protease inhibitors. Protease inhibitors are associated with insulin resistance and hyperglycaemia. Plasma lipids, blood glucose and the usual risk factors for atherosclerotic disease should be taken into account before prescribing regimens containing a protease inhibitor; patients receiving protease inhibitors should be monitored for changes in plasma lipids and blood glucose.

Nucleoside reverse transcriptase inhibitors

CAUTIONS. Nucleoside reverse transcriptase inhibitors should be used with caution in patients with chronic hepatitis B or C (greater risk of hepatic side-effects), in hepatic impairment (see also Lactic Acidosis below and Appendix 2), in renal impairment (Appendix 3), and in pregnancy (see also above and Appendix 4).

LACTIC ACIDOSIS. Life-threatening lactic acidosis associated with hepatomegaly and hepatic steatosis has been reported with nucleoside reverse transcriptase inhibitors. They should be used with caution in patients (particularly obese women) with hepatomegaly, hepatitis (especially hepatitis C treated with interferon alfa and ribavirin), liver-enzyme abnormalities and with other risk factors for liver disease and hepatic steatosis (including alcohol abuse). Treatment with the nucleoside reverse transcriptase inhibitor should be **discontinued** in case of symptomatic hyperlactataemia, lactic acidosis, progressive hepatomegaly or rapid deterioration of liver function.

SIDE-EFFECTS. Side-effects of the nucleoside reverse transcriptase inhibitors include gastro-intestinal disturbances (such as nausea, vomiting, abdominal pain, flatulence and diarrhoea), anorexia, pancreatitis, liver damage (see also Lactic Acidosis, above), dyspnoea, cough, headache, insomnia, dizziness, fatigue, blood disorders (including anaemia, neutropenia, and thrombocytopenia), myalgia, arthralgia, rash, urticaria, and fever. See notes above for metabolic effects and lipodystrophy (Lipodystrophy Syndrome).

ABACAVIR

Indications: HIV infection in combination with other antiretroviral drugs

Cautions: see notes above; **interactions:** Appendix 1 (abacavir)

HYPERSENSITIVITY REACTIONS. Life-threatening hypersensitivity reactions reported—characterised by fever or rash and possibly nausea, vomiting, diarrhoea, abdominal pain, dyspnoea, cough, lethargy, malaise, headache, and myalgia; less frequently mouth ulceration, oedema, hypotension, sore throat, acute respiratory distress syndrome, anaphylaxis, paraesthesia, arthralgia, conjunctivitis, lymphadenopathy, lymphocytopenia and renal failure (CSM has identified hypersensitivity reactions presenting as sore throat, influenza-like illness, cough and breathlessness); rarely myolysis; laboratory abnormalities may include raised liver function tests (see below) and creatine phosphokinase; symptoms usually appear in the first 6 weeks, but may occur at any time; monitor for symptoms every 2 weeks for 2 months; discontinue immediately if any symptom of hypersensitivity develops and do not rechallenge (risk of more severe hypersensitivity reaction); discontinue if hypersensitivity cannot be ruled out, even when other diagnoses possible—if rechallenge necessary it must be carried out in hospital setting; if abacavir is stopped for any reason other than hypersensitivity, exclude hypersensitivity reaction as the cause and rechallenge only if medical assistance is readily available; care needed with concomitant use of drugs which cause skin toxicity

COUNSELLING. Patients should be told the importance of regular dosing (intermittent therapy may increase the risk of sensitisation), how to recognise signs of hypersensitivity, and advised to seek immediate medical attention if symptoms develop or before re-starting treatment; patients should be advised to keep Alert card with them at all times

Contra-indications: breast-feeding (Appendix 5)

Side-effects: see notes above; also hypersensitivity reactions (see above); *very rarely* Stevens-Johnson syndrome and toxic epidermal necrolysis; rash and gastro-intestinal disturbances more common in children

Dose: 600 mg daily in 1–2 divided doses; CHILD 3 months–12 years, 8 mg/kg every 12 hours (max. 600 mg daily)

Ziagen® (GSK) PoM

Tablets, yellow, f/c, abacavir (as sulphate) 300 mg, net price 60-tab pack = £221.81. Counselling, hypersensitivity reactions

Oral solution, sugar-free, banana and strawberry flavoured, abacavir (as sulphate) 20 mg/mL, net price 240-mL = £59.15. Counselling, hypersensitivity reactions

■ With lamivudine

For **cautions**, **contra-indications** and **side-effects** see under individual drugs

Kivexa (GSK) ▼ PoM

Tablets, orange, f/c, abacavir (as sulphate) 600 mg, lamivudine 300 mg, net price 30-tab pack = £373.94. Counselling, hypersensitivity reactions

Dose: ADULT and CHILD over 12 years, body-weight over 40 kg, 1 tablet once daily

■ With lamivudine and zidovudine

NOTE. For patients stabilised (for 6–8 weeks) on the individual components in the same proportions. For **cautions**, **contra-indications** and **side-effects** see under individual drugs

Trizivir® (GSK) PoM

Tablets, blue-green, f/c, abacavir (as sulphate) 300 mg, lamivudine 150 mg, zidovudine 300 mg, net price 60-tab pack = £540.40. Counselling, hypersensitivity reactions

Dose: ADULT over 18 years, 1 tablet twice daily

DIDANOSINE

(ddI, DDI)

Indications: HIV infection in combination with other antiretroviral drugs

Cautions: see notes above; also history of pancreatitis (preferably avoid, otherwise extreme caution, see also below); peripheral neuropathy or hyperuricaemia (see under Side-effects); dilated retinal examinations recommended (especially in children) every 6 months, or if visual changes occur; **interactions:** Appendix 1 (didanosine)

PANCREATITIS. If symptoms of pancreatitis develop or if serum amylase or lipase is raised (even if asymptomatic) suspend treatment until diagnosis of pancreatitis excluded; on return to normal values re-initiate treatment only if essential (using low dose increased gradually if appropriate). Whenever possible avoid concomitant treatment with other drugs known to cause pancreatic toxicity (e.g. intravenous pentamidine isetionate); monitor closely if concomitant therapy unavoidable. Since significant elevations of triglycerides cause pancreatitis monitor closely if elevated

Contra-indications: breast-feeding (Appendix 5)

Side-effects: see notes above; also pancreatitis (see also under cautions), liver failure, anaphylactic reactions, peripheral neuropathy—suspend (reduced dose may be tolerated when symptoms resolve), diabetes mellitus, hypoglycaemia, acute renal failure, rhabdomyolysis, dry eyes, retinal and optic nerve changes (especially in children), dry mouth, parotid gland enlargement, sialadenitis, alopecia, hyperuricaemia (suspend if raised significantly)

Dose: ADULT under 60 kg 250 mg daily in 1–2 divided doses, 60 kg and over 400 mg daily in 1–2 divided doses; CHILD over 3 months (under 6 years *Videx*® tablets only), 240 mg/m^2 daily (180 mg/m^2 daily in combination with zidovudine) in 1–2 divided doses

Videx® (Bristol-Myers Squibb) PoM

Tablets, both with calcium and magnesium antacids, didanosine 25 mg, net price 60-tab pack =

£26.60; 200 mg, 60-tab pack = £163.68. Label: 23, counselling, administration, see below

Excipients: include aspartame equivalent to phenylalanine 36.5 mg per tablet (section 9.4.1)

NOTE. Antacids in formulation may affect absorption of other drugs—see **interactions:** Appendix 1 (antacids)

COUNSELLING. To ensure sufficient antacid, each dose to be taken as 2 tablets (CHILD under 1 year 1 tablet) chewed thoroughly, crushed or dispersed in water; clear apple juice may be added for flavouring; tablets to be taken 2 hours after atazanavir with ritonavir

Videx® EC capsules, enclosing e/c granules, didanosine 125 mg, net price 30-cap pack = £51.15; 200 mg, 30-cap pack = £81.84; 250 mg, 30-cap pack = £102.30; 400 mg, 30-cap pack = £163.68. Label: 25, counselling, administration, see below

COUNSELLING. Capsules to be taken at least 2 hours before or 2 hours after food

EMTRICITABINE

Indications: HIV infection in combination with other antiretroviral drugs

Cautions: see notes above; also on discontinuation, monitor patients with hepatitis B (risk of exacerbation of hepatitis); **interactions:** Appendix 1 (emtricitabine)

Contra-indications: breast-feeding (Appendix 5)

Side-effects: see notes above; also abnormal dreams, pruritus, and hyperpigmentation

Dose: see preparations

Emtriva® (Gilead) ▼ PoM

Capsules, white/blue, emtricitabine 200 mg, net price 30-cap pack = £163.50

Dose: ADULT and CHILD body-weight over 33 kg, 200 mg once daily

Oral solution, orange, emtricitabine 10 mg/mL, net price 170-mL pack = £46.50

Dose: ADULT and CHILD body-weight over 33 kg, 240 mg once daily; CHILD 4 months–18 years, body-weight under 33 kg, 6 mg/kg once daily

NOTE. 240 mg oral solution ≡ 200 mg capsule; where appropriate the capsule may be used instead of the oral solution

■ With tenofovir

See under Tenofovir

LAMIVUDINE

(3TC)

Indications: see preparations below

Cautions: see notes above; **interactions:** Appendix 1 (lamivudine)

CHRONIC HEPATITIS B. Recurrent hepatitis in patients with chronic hepatitis B may occur on discontinuation of lamivudine. When treating chronic hepatitis B with lamivudine, monitor liver function tests at least every 3 months and serological markers of hepatitis B every 6 months, more frequently in patients with advanced liver disease or following transplantation (monitoring to continue after discontinuation)—consult product literature

Contra-indications: breast-feeding (Appendix 5)

Side-effects: see notes above; also peripheral neuropathy, muscle disorders including rhabdomyolysis, nasal symptoms, alopecia

Dose: see preparations below

Epivir® (GSK) PoM

Tablets, f/c, lamivudine 150 mg (white), net price 60-tab pack = £152.14; 300 mg (grey), 30-tab pack = £167.21

Oral solution, banana- and strawberry-flavoured, lamivudine 50 mg/5 mL, net price 240-mL pack = £41.41

Excipients: include sucrose 1 g/5 mL

Dose: HIV infection in combination with other antiretroviral drugs, 150 mg every 12 hours *or* 300 mg once daily; CHILD 3 months–12 years, 4 mg/kg every 12 hours; max. 300 mg daily

Zeffix® (GSK) PoM

Tablets, brown, f/c, lamivudine 100 mg, net price 28-tab pack = £78.09

Oral solution, banana and strawberry flavoured, lamivudine 25 mg/5 mL, net price 240-mL pack = £22.79

Excipients: include sucrose 1 g/5 mL

Dose: chronic hepatitis B infection with *either* compensated liver disease (with evidence of viral replication and histology of active liver inflammation or fibrosis), *or* decompensated liver disease, 100 mg daily; CHILD [unlicensed indication] 2–11 years, 3 mg/kg once daily (max. 100 mg daily); 12–17 years, adult dose; patients receiving lamivudine for concomitant HIV infection should continue to receive lamivudine in a dose appropriate for HIV infection

■ With abacavir

See under Abacavir

■ With zidovudine

See under Zidovudine

■ With abacavir and zidovudine

See under Abacavir

STAVUDINE

(d4T)

Indications: HIV infection in combination with other antiretroviral drugs

Cautions: see notes above; also history of peripheral neuropathy (see below); history of pancreatitis or concomitant use with other drugs associated with pancreatitis; **interactions:** Appendix 1 (stavudine)

PERIPHERAL NEUROPATHY. Suspend if peripheral neuropathy develops—characterised by persistent numbness, tingling or pain in feet or hands; if symptoms resolve satisfactorily on withdrawal and if stavudine needs to be continued, resume treatment at half previous dose

Contra-indications: breast-feeding (Appendix 5)

Side-effects: see notes above; also peripheral neuropathy, abnormal dreams, cognitive dysfunction, drowsiness, depression; *less commonly* anxiety, gynaecomastia

Dose: ADULT under 60 kg, 30 mg every 12 hours preferably at least 1 hour before food; 60 kg and over, 40 mg every 12 hours; CHILD over 3 months, under 30 kg, 1 mg/kg every 12 hours; 30 kg and over, adult dose

Zerit® (Bristol-Myers Squibb) PoM

Capsules, stavudine 15 mg (yellow/red), net price 56-cap pack = £143.10; 20 mg (brown), 56-cap pack = £148.05; 30 mg (light orange/dark orange), 56-cap pack = £155.25; 40 mg (dark orange), 56-cap pack = £159.94 (all hosp. only)

Oral solution, cherry-flavoured, stavudine for reconstitution with water, 1 mg/mL, net price 200 mL = £24.35

TENOFOVIR DISOPROXIL

Indications: HIV infection in combination with other antiretroviral drugs

Cautions: see notes above; also test renal function and serum phosphate before treatment, then every 4 weeks (more frequently if at increased risk of renal impairment) for 1 year and then every 3 months, interrupt treatment if renal function deteriorates or serum phosphate decreases; **interactions:** Appendix 1 (tenofovir)

Contra-indications: breast-feeding (Appendix 5)

Side-effects: see notes above; also hypophosphataemia, reduced bone density, polyuria, and renal failure

Dose: ADULT over 18 years, 245 mg once daily

Viread® (Gilead) ▼ PoM

Tablets, f/c, blue, tenofovir disoproxil (as fumarate) 245 mg, net price 30-tab pack = £255.00. Label: 21, counselling, administration

COUNSELLING. Patients with swallowing difficulties may disperse tablet in half a glass of water, grape juice, or orange juice

■ With emtricitabine

For **cautions**, **contra-indications** and **side-effects** see under individual drugs

Truvada® (Gilead) ▼ PoM

Tablets, blue, f/c, tenofovir disoproxil (as fumarate) 245 mg, emtricitabine 200 mg, net price 30-tab pack = £418.50. Label: 21, counselling, administration

COUNSELLING. Patients with swallowing difficulties may disperse tablet in half a glass of water, orange juice, or grape juice

Dose: ADULT over 18 years, 1 tablet once daily

ZALCITABINE

(ddC, DDC)

Indications: HIV infection in combination with other antiretroviral drugs

Cautions: see notes above; also patients at risk of developing peripheral neuropathy (see below); pancreatitis (see also below)—monitor serum amylase in those with history of elevated serum amylase, pancreatitis, alcohol abuse, or receiving parenteral nutrition; monitor full blood count; cardiomyopathy, history of congestive cardiac failure; **interactions:** Appendix 1 (zalcitabine)

PERIPHERAL NEUROPATHY. Discontinue immediately if peripheral neuropathy develops—characterised by numbness and burning dysaesthesia possibly followed by sharp shooting pains or severe continuous burning and potentially irreversible pain; extreme caution and close monitoring required in those at risk of peripheral neuropathy (especially those with low CD4 cell count for whom risk is greater and those receiving another drug known to cause peripheral neuropathy)

PANCREATITIS. Discontinue permanently if clinical pancreatitis develops; suspend if raised serum amylase associated with dysglycaemia, rising triglyceride, decreasing serum calcium or other signs of impending pancreatitis until pancreatitis excluded; suspend if treatment required with another drug known to cause pancreatic toxicity (e.g. intravenous pentamidine isetionate); caution and close monitoring if history of pancreatitis (or of elevated serum amylase) or if at risk of pancreatitis

Contra-indications: peripheral neuropathy (see also above); breast-feeding (Appendix 5)

Side-effects: see notes above; also oral ulcers, dysphagia, oesophageal ulcers (suspend zalcitabine if no response to treatment for specific organisms), pancreatitis (see also Cautions), rectal ulcers, flushing, hypertension, chest pain, cardiomyopathy, congestive heart failure, tachycardia, palpitation, syncope, pharyngitis, hypersensitivity reactions, peripheral neuropathy (discontinue immediately, see also Cautions), convulsions, tremor, movement disorders, mood changes, anxiety, sleep disturbances, weight loss, hypoglycaemia, hyperglycaemia, acute renal failure, gout, dry mouth, pruritus, sweating, alopecia, electrolyte disturbances, taste, hearing and visual disturbances

Dose: 750 micrograms every 8 hours; CHILD under 13 years safety and efficacy not established

Hivid® (Roche) PoM

Tablets, both f/c, zalcitabine 375 micrograms (beige), net price 100-tab pack = £92.54; 750 micrograms (grey), 100-tab pack = £140.96

ZIDOVUDINE

(Azidothymidine, AZT)

NOTE. The abbreviation AZT which is sometimes used for zidovudine has also been used for another drug

Indications: HIV infection in combination with other antiretroviral drugs; prevention of maternal-fetal HIV transmission (see notes above under Pregnancy and Breast-feeding)

Cautions: see notes above; also haematological toxicity particularly with high dose and advanced disease (blood tests at least every 2 weeks for first 3 months then at least once a month, early disease with good bone marrow reserves may require less frequent tests e.g. every 1–3 months); vitamin B_{12} deficiency (increased risk of neutropenia); reduce dose or interrupt treatment according to product literature if anaemia or myelosuppression; elderly; **interactions:** Appendix 1 (zidovudine)

Contra-indications: abnormally low neutrophil counts or haemoglobin values (consult product literature); neonates with hyperbilirubinaemia requiring treatment other than phototherapy, or with raised transaminase (consult product literature); breast-feeding (Appendix 5)

Side-effects: see notes above; also anaemia (may require transfusion), taste disturbance, chest pain, influenza-like symptoms, paraesthesia, neuropathy, convulsions, dizziness, drowsiness, insomnia, anxiety, depression, loss of mental acuity, myopathy, gynaecomastia, urinary frequency, sweating, pruritus, pigmentation of nails, skin and oral mucosa

Dose: *by mouth*, 500–600 mg daily in 2–3 divided doses; CHILD over 3 months 360–480 mg/m^2 daily in 3–4 divided doses; max. 200 mg every 6 hours

Prevention of maternal-fetal HIV transmission, seek specialist advice (combination therapy preferred)

Patients temporarily unable to take zidovudine by mouth, *by intravenous infusion* over 1 hour, 1–2 mg/kg every 4 hours (approximating to 1.5–3 mg/kg every 4 hours by mouth) usually for not more than 2 weeks; CHILD 80–160 mg/m^2 every 6 hours (120 mg/m^2 every 6 hours approximates to 180 mg/m^2 every 6 hours by mouth)

Retrovir® (GSK) PoM

Capsules, zidovudine 100 mg (white/blue band), net price 100-cap pack = £110.98; 250 mg (blue/white/dark blue band), 40-cap pack = £110.98

Oral solution, sugar-free, strawberry-flavoured, zidovudine 50 mg/5 mL, net price 200-mL pack with 10-mL oral syringe = £22.20

Injection, zidovudine 10 mg/mL. For dilution and use as an intravenous infusion. Net price 20-mL vial = £11.14

■ With lamivudine

For cautions, contra-indications, and side-effects of lamivudine, see Lamivudine

Combivir® (GSK) PoM
Tablets, f/c, zidovudine 300 mg, lamivudine 150 mg, net price 60-tab pack = £318.60
Dose: 1 tablet twice daily

■ With abacavir and lamivudine

See under Abacavir

Protease inhibitors

CAUTIONS. Protease inhibitors are associated with hyperglycaemia and should be used with caution in diabetes (see also notes above under Lipodystrophy Syndrome). Caution is also needed in patients with haemophilia who may be at increased risk of bleeding. Protease inhibitors should be used with caution in hepatic impairment (Appendix 2); the risk of hepatic side-effects is increased in patients with chronic hepatitis B or C. Atazanavir and fosamprenavir may be used at usual doses in patients with renal impairment, but other protease inhibitors should be used with caution in renal impairment (Appendix 3). Protease inhibitors should also be used with caution during pregnancy (Appendix 4).

SIDE-EFFECTS. Side-effects of the protease inhibitors include gastro-intestinal disturbances (including diarrhoea, nausea, vomiting, abdominal pain, flatulence), hepatic dysfunction, pancreatitis; blood disorders including anaemia, neutropenia, and thrombocytopenia; sleep disturbances, fatigue, headache, dizziness, paraesthesia, myalgia, myositis, rhabdomyolysis; taste disturbances; rash, pruritus, Stevens-Johnson syndrome, hypersensitivity reactions including anaphylaxis; see also notes above for lipodystrophy and metabolic effects.

AMPRENAVIR

Indications: HIV infection in combination with other antiretroviral drugs in patients previously treated with other protease inhibitors

Cautions: see notes above; **interactions:** Appendix 1 (amprenavir)

RASH. Rash may occur, usually in the second week of therapy; discontinue permanently if severe rash with systemic or allergic symptoms or, mucosal involvement; if rash mild or moderate, may continue without interruption—rash usually resolves within 2 weeks and may respond to antihistamines

Contra-indications: breast-feeding (Appendix 5)

Side-effects: see notes above; also reported, rash including rarely Stevens-Johnson syndrome (see also above); tremors, oral or perioral paraesthesia, mood disorders including depression

Dose: see preparations below

Agenerase® (GSK) PoM
Capsules, ivory, amprenavir 50 mg, net price 480-cap pack = £139.50. Label: 5
Excipients: include vitamin E 36 units/50 mg amprenavir (avoid vitamin E supplements)
Dose: ADULT and ADOLESCENT over 12 years, body-weight over 50 kg, 1.2 g every 12 hours; ADULT and ADOLESCENT over 12 years, body-weight under 50 kg and CHILD 4–12 years, 20 mg/kg every 12 hours (max. 2.4 g daily)
With low-dose ritonavir, ADULT and ADOLESCENT over 12 years, body-weight over 50 kg, amprenavir 600 mg every 12 hours with ritonavir 100 mg every 12 hours
Oral solution, grape-bubblegum- and peppermint-flavoured, amprenavir 15 mg/mL, net price 240-mL pack = £33.48. Label: 4, 5
Excipients: include vitamin E 46 units/mL (avoid vitamin E supplements), propylene glycol 550 mg/mL (see Excipients, p. 2)
Dose: ADULT and CHILD over 4 years, 17 mg/kg every 8 hours (max. 2.8 g daily); CHILD under 4 years not recommended
NOTE. The bioavailability of *Agenerase*® oral solution is lower than that of capsules; the two formulations are **not** interchangeable on a milligram-for-milligram basis

ATAZANAVIR

Indications: HIV infection in combination with other antiretroviral drugs in patients previously treated with antiretrovirals

Cautions: see notes above; also concomitant use with drugs that prolong PR interval; cardiac conduction disorders; **interactions:** Appendix 1 (atazanavir)

Contra-indications: breast-feeding (Appendix 5)

Side-effects: see notes above; also mouth ulcers, jaundice, hepatosplenomegaly, hypertension, oedema, palpitation, syncope, chest pain, dyspnoea, peripheral neurological symptoms, abnormal dreams, amnesia, depression, anxiety, gynaecomastia, weight changes, increased appetite, nephrolithiasis, urinary frequency, haematuria, proteinuria, arthralgia, alopecia

Dose: with low-dose ritonavir and food, ADULT over 18 years, 300 mg once daily with ritonavir 100 mg once daily

Reyataz® (Bristol-Myers Squibb) ▼ PoM
Capsules, atazanavir (as sulphate) 100 mg (dark blue/white), net price 60-cap pack = £315.69; 150 mg (dark blue/light blue), 60-cap pack = £315.69; 200 mg (dark blue), 60-cap pack = £315.69. Label: 5, 21

FOSAMPRENAVIR

NOTE. Fosamprenavir is a pro-drug of amprenavir

Indications: HIV infection in combination with other antiretroviral drugs

Cautions: see notes above and under Amprenavir

Contra-indications: breast-feeding (Appendix 5)

Side-effects: see notes above and under Amprenavir

Dose: with low-dose ritonavir, ADULT over 18 years, 700 mg twice daily
NOTE. 700 mg fosamprenavir is equivalent to approx. 600 mg amprenavir

Telzir® (GSK) ▼ PoM
Tablets, f/c, pink, fosamprenavir (as calcium) 700 mg, net price 60-tab pack = £274.92
Oral suspension, fosamprenavir (as calcium) 50 mg/mL, net price 225-mL pack (grape-bubblegum-and peppermint-flavoured) (with 10-mL oral syringe) = £73.31. Label: 23

INDINAVIR

Indications: HIV infection in combination with nucleoside reverse transcriptase inhibitors

Cautions: see notes above; also ensure adequate hydration (risk of nephrolithiasis especially in children); patients at risk of nephrolithiasis (monitor for nephrolithiasis); avoid in porphyria (section 9.8.2); **interactions:** Appendix 1 (indinavir)

Contra-indications: breast-feeding (Appendix 5)

Side-effects: see notes above; also reported, dry mouth, hypoaesthesia, dry skin, hyperpigmentation, alopecia, paronychia, interstitial nephritis (with medullary calcification and cortical atrophy in asymptomatic severe leucocyturia), nephrolithiasis (may require interruption or discontinuation; more frequent in children), dysuria, haematuria, crystalluria, proteinuria, pyuria (in children); haemolytic anaemia

Dose: 800 mg every 8 hours; CHILD and ADOLESCENT 4–17 years, 500 mg/m^2 every 8 hours (max. 800 mg every 8 hours); CHILD under 4 years, safety and efficacy not established

Crixivan® (MSD) PoM

Capsules, indinavir (as sulphate), 200 mg, net price 360-cap pack = £226.28; 400 mg, 90-cap pack = £113.15, 180-cap pack = £226.28. Label: 27, counselling, administration

COUNSELLING. Administer 1 hour before or 2 hours after a meal; may be administered with a low-fat light meal; in combination with didanosine tablets, allow 1 hour between each drug (antacids in didanosine tablets reduce absorption of indinavir)

NOTE. Dispense in original container (contains dessicant)

LOPINAVIR WITH RITONAVIR

Indications: HIV infection in combination with other antiretroviral drugs

Cautions: see notes above; concomitant use with drugs that prolong QT interval; pancreatitis (see below); **interactions:** Appendix 1 (lopinavir, ritonavir)

PANCREATITIS. Signs and symptoms suggestive of pancreatitis (including raised serum amylase and lipase) should be evaluated—discontinue if pancreatitis diagnosed

Contra-indications: breast-feeding (Appendix 5, *Kaletra®*)

Side-effects: see notes and Cautions above; also electrolyte disturbances in children; *less commonly* dysphagia, appetite changes, weight changes, cholecystitis, hypertension, myocardial infarction, palpitation, thrombophlebitis, vasculitis, chest pain, oedema, dyspnoea, cough, agitation, anxiety, amnesia, ataxia, hypertonia, confusion, depression, abnormal dreams, extrapyramidal effects, neuropathy, influenza-like syndrome, Cushing's syndrome, hypothyroidism, menorrhagia, sexual dysfunction, breast enlargement, dehydration, hypercalciuria, lactic acidosis, arthralgia, hyperuricaemia, abnormal vision, otitis media, tinnitus, dry mouth, sialadenitis, mouth ulceration, periodontitis, acne, alopecia, dry skin, sweating, skin discoloration, nail disorders, *rarely* prolonged PR interval

Dose: see preparations below

Kaletra® (Abbott) PoM

Capsules, orange, lopinavir 133.3 mg, ritonavir 33.3 mg, net price 180-cap pack = £307.39. Label: 21

Dose: ADULT and CHILD over 2 years with body surface area of 1.4 m^2 or greater, 3 capsules twice daily with food; CHILD over 2 years with body surface area less than 1.4 m^2, oral solution preferred; if oral solution inappropriate and body surface area 0.4–0.75 m^2, 1 capsule twice daily, body surface area 0.8–1.3 m^2, 2 capsules twice daily

Oral solution, lopinavir 400 mg, ritonavir 100 mg/5 mL, net price 5×60-mL packs = £307.39. Label: 21

Excipients: include propylene glycol 153 mg/mL (see Excipients, p. 2), alcohol 42%

Dose: ADULT and ADOLESCENT, 5 mL twice daily with food; CHILD over 2 years 2.9 mL/m^2 twice daily with food, max. 5 mL twice daily; CHILD under 2 years, safety and efficacy not established

NOTE. 5 mL oral solution ≡ 3 capsules; where appropriate, capsules may be used instead of oral solution

NELFINAVIR

Indications: HIV infection in combination with other antiretroviral drugs

Cautions: see notes above; **interactions:** Appendix 1 (nelfinavir)

Contra-indications: breast-feeding (Appendix 5)

Side-effects: see notes above; also reported, fever

Dose: 1.25 g twice daily *or* 750 mg 3 times daily; CHILD 3–13 years, initially 50–55 mg/kg twice daily (max. 1.25 g twice daily) *or* 25–30 mg/kg 3 times daily (max. 750 mg 3 times daily)

Viracept® (Roche) PoM

Tablets, f/c, nelfinavir (as mesilate) 250 mg, net price 300-tab pack = £273.16. Label: 21

Oral powder, nelfinavir (as mesilate) 50 mg/g. Net price 144 g (with 1-g and 5-g scoop) = £28.72. Label: 21, counselling, administration

Excipients: include aspartame (section 9.4.1)

COUNSELLING. Powder may be mixed with water, milk, formula feeds or pudding; it should **not** be mixed with acidic foods or juices owing to its taste

RITONAVIR

Indications: HIV infection in combination with nucleoside reverse transcriptase inhibitors; low doses used to increase effect of some protease inhibitors

Cautions: see notes above; avoid in porphyria (section 9.8.2); pancreatitis (see below); **interactions:** Appendix 1 (ritonavir)

PANCREATITIS. Signs and symptoms suggestive of pancreatitis (including raised serum amylase and lipase) should be evaluated—discontinue if pancreatitis diagnosed

Contra-indications: breast-feeding (Appendix 5)

Side-effects: see notes and Cautions above; also reported, diarrhoea (may impair absorption—close monitoring required), throat irritation, vasodilatation, syncope, hypotension; drowsiness, circumoral and peripheral paraesthesia, hyperaesthesia, seizures, raised uric acid, dry mouth and ulceration, cough, anxiety, fever, decreased blood thyroxine concentration, menorrhagia, sweating, electrolyte disturbances, increased prothrombin time

Dose: initially 300 mg every 12 hours for 3 days, increased in steps of 100 mg every 12 hours over not longer than 14 days to 600 mg every 12 hours; CHILD over 2 years initially 250 mg/m^2 every 12 hours, increased by 50 mg/m^2 at intervals of 2–3 days to 350 mg/m^2 every 12 hours (max. 600 mg every 12 hours)

Low-dose booster to increase effect of other protease inhibitors, 100–200 mg once or twice daily

Norvir® (Abbott) PoM

Capsules, ritonavir 100 mg, net price 336-cap pack = £377.39. Label 21

Excipients: include alcohol 12%

Oral solution, sugar-free, ritonavir 400 mg/5 mL, net price 5 × 90-mL packs (with measuring cup) = £403.20. Label: 21, counselling, administration
COUNSELLING. Oral solution contains 43% alcohol; bitter taste can be masked by mixing with chocolate milk; do not mix with water, measuring cup must be dry

■ With lopinavir
See under Lopinavir with ritonavir

SAQUINAVIR

Indications: HIV infection in combination with other antiretroviral drugs
Cautions: see notes above; concomitant use of garlic (avoid garlic capsules—reduces plasma-saquinavir concentration); **interactions:** Appendix 1 (saquinavir)
Contra-indications: breast-feeding (Appendix 5)
Side-effects: see notes above; also buccal and mucosal ulceration, chest pain, peripheral neuropathy, mood changes, fever, changes in libido, verruca, nephrolithiasis
Dose: with low-dose ritonavir, ADULT and ADOLESCENT over 16 years, 1 g every 12 hours within 2 hours after a meal
NOTE. To avoid confusion between the different formulations of saquinavir, prescribers should specify the brand to be dispensed; absorption from *Fortovase*® is much greater than from *Invirase*®. Treatment should generally be initiated with *Fortovase*®

Fortovase® (Roche) PoM
Capsules (gel-filled), beige, saquinavir 200 mg, net price 180-cap pack = £97.04. Label: 21

Invirase® (Roche) PoM
Capsules, brown/green, saquinavir (as mesilate) 200 mg, net price 270-cap pack = £240.06. Label: 21
Tablets, orange, f/c, saquinavir (as mesilate) 500 mg, net price 120-tab pack = £266.73. Label: 21

Non-nucleoside reverse transcriptase inhibitors

EFAVIRENZ

Indications: HIV infection in combination with other antiretroviral drugs
Cautions: chronic hepatitis B or C (greater risk of hepatic side-effects), hepatic impairment (avoid if severe; Appendix 2); severe renal impairment (Appendix 3); pregnancy (Appendix 4); elderly; history of mental illness or seizures; **interactions:** Appendix 1 (efavirenz)
RASH. Rash, usually in the first 2 weeks, is the most common side-effect; discontinue if severe rash with blistering, desquamation, mucosal involvement or fever; if rash mild or moderate, may continue without interruption—rash usually resolves within 1 month
PSYCHIATRIC DISORDERS. Patients or their carers should be advised to seek immediate medical attention if symptoms such as severe depression, psychosis or suicidal ideation occur
Contra-indications: breast-feeding (Appendix 5)
Side-effects: rash including Stevens-Johnson syndrome (see Rash above); abdominal pain, diarrhoea, nausea, vomiting; anxiety, depression, sleep disturbances, abnormal dreams, dizziness, headache, fatigue, impaired concentration (administration at bedtime especially in first 2–4 weeks reduces CNS effects); pruritus; *less commonly* pancreatitis, hepatitis, psychosis, mania, suicidal ideation, amnesia, ataxia, convulsions, and blurred vision; also reported hepatic failure, raised serum cholesterol, gynaecomastia, photosensitivity
Dose: *see* preparations below

Sustiva (Bristol-Myers Squibb) ▼ PoM
Capsules, efavirenz 50 mg (yellow/white), net price 30-cap pack = £17.41; 100 mg (white), 30-cap pack = £34.77; 200 mg (yellow), 90-cap pack = £208.40
Dose: ADULT and CHILD over 3 years, body-weight 13–14 kg, 200 mg once daily; body-weight 15–19 kg, 250 mg once daily; body-weight 20–24 kg, 300 mg once daily; body-weight 25–32.4 kg, 350 mg once daily; body-weight 32.5–39 kg, 400 mg once daily; body-weight 40 kg and over, 600 mg once daily
Tablets, f/c, yellow, efavirenz 600 mg, net price 30-tab pack = £208.40
Dose: ADULT and ADOLESCENT over 12 years, body-weight over 40 kg, 600 mg once daily
Oral solution, sugar-free, strawberry and mint flavour, efavirenz 30 mg/mL, net price 180-mL pack = £56.02
Dose: ADULT and CHILD over 5 years, body-weight 13–14 kg, 270 mg once daily; body-weight 15–19 kg, 300 mg once daily; body-weight 20–24 kg, 360 mg once daily; body-weight 25–32.4 kg, 450 mg once daily; body-weight 32.5–39 kg, 510 mg once daily; body-weight 40 kg and over, 720 mg once daily; CHILD 3–4 years, body-weight 13–14 kg, 360 mg once daily; body-weight 15–19 kg, 390 mg once daily; body-weight 20–24 kg, 450 mg once daily; body-weight 25–32.4 kg, 510 mg once daily
NOTE. The bioavailability of *Sustiva*® oral solution is lower than that of the capsules and tablets; the oral solution is **not** interchangeable with either capsules or tablets on a milligram-for-milligram basis

NEVIRAPINE

Indications: progressive or advanced HIV infection, in combination with at least two other antiretroviral drugs
Cautions: hepatic impairment (see below and Appendix 2); chronic hepatitis B or C, high CD4 cell count, and women (all at greater risk of hepatic side-effects—manufacturer advises avoid in women with CD4 cell count greater than 250 cells/mm^3 or in men with CD4 cell count greater than 400 cells/mm^3 unless potential benefit outweighs risk); pregnancy (Appendix 4); **interactions:** Appendix 1 (nevirapine)
HEPATIC DISEASE. Potentially life-threatening hepatotoxicity including fatal fulminant hepatitis reported usually in first 6 weeks; close monitoring required during first 18 weeks; monitor liver function before treatment then every 2 weeks for 2 months then after 1 month and then regularly; discontinue permanently if abnormalities in liver function tests accompanied by hypersensitivity reaction (rash, fever, arthralgia, myalgia, lymphadenopathy, hepatitis, renal impairment, eosinophilia, granulocytopenia); suspend if severe abnormalities in liver function tests but no hypersensitivity reaction—discontinue permanently if significant liver function abnormalities recur; monitor patient closely if mild to moderate abnormalities in liver function tests with no hypersensitivity reaction
NOTE. If treatment interrupted for more than 7 days reintroduce with 200 mg daily (CHILD 4 mg/kg daily) and increase dose cautiously
RASH. Rash, usually in first 6 weeks, is most common side-effect; incidence reduced if introduced at low dose and dose increased gradually; monitor closely for skin

reactions during first 18 weeks; discontinue permanently if severe rash or if rash accompanied by blistering, oral lesions, conjunctivitis, facial oedema, general malaise or hypersensitivity reactions; if rash mild or moderate may continue without interruption but dose should not be increased until rash resolves

COUNSELLING. Patients should be told how to recognise hypersensitivity reactions and advised to discontinue treatment and seek immediate medical attention if symptoms of hepatitis, severe skin reaction or hypersensitivity reactions develop

Contra-indications: breast-feeding (Appendix 5); severe hepatic impairment; post-exposure prophylaxis

Side-effects: rash including Stevens-Johnson syndrome and rarely, toxic epidermal necrolysis (see also Cautions above); nausea, hepatitis (see also Hepatic Disease above), headache; less commonly vomiting, abdominal pain, fatigue, fever, and myalgia; rarely diarrhoea, angioedema, anaphylaxis, hypersensitivity reactions (may involve hepatic reactions and rash, see Hepatic Disease above), arthralgia, anaemia, and granulocytopenia (more frequent in children); very rarely neuropsychiatric reactions

Dose: 200 mg once daily for first 14 days then (if no rash present) 200 mg twice daily; CHILD 2 months–8 years, 4 mg/kg once daily for first 14 days then (if no rash present) 7 mg/kg twice daily (max. 400 mg daily); 8–16 years (but under 50 kg), 4 mg/kg once daily for first 14 days then (if no rash present) 4 mg/kg twice daily (max. 400 mg daily); over 50 kg, adult dose

Viramune® (Boehringer Ingelheim) PoM

Tablets, nevirapine 200 mg, net price 60-tab pack = £160.00. Counselling, hypersensitivity reactions

Suspension, nevirapine 50 mg/5 mL, net price 240-mL pack = £50.40. Counselling, hypersensitivity reactions

Other antiretrovirals

ENFUVIRTIDE

Indications: HIV infection in combination with other antiretroviral drugs for resistant infection or for patients intolerant to other antiretroviral regimens

Cautions: chronic hepatitis B or C (possibly greater risk of hepatic side-effects); hepatic impairment (Appendix 2); renal impairment (Appendix 3); pregnancy (Appendix 4)

HYPERSENSITIVITY REACTIONS. Hypersensitivity reactions including rash, fever, nausea, vomiting, chills, rigors, low blood pressure, respiratory distress, glomerulonephritis, and raised liver enzymes reported; discontinue immediately if any signs or symptoms of systemic hypersensitivity develop and do not rechallenge

COUNSELLING. Patients should be told how to recognise signs of hypersensitivity, and advised to discontinue treatment and seek immediate medical attention if symptoms develop

Contra-indications: breast-feeding (Appendix 5)

Side-effects: injection-site reactions; pancreatitis, gastro-oesophageal reflux disease, anorexia, weight loss; hypertriglyceridaemia; peripheral neuropathy, asthenia, tremor, anxiety, nightmares, irritability, impaired concentration, vertigo; pneumonia, sinusitis, influenza-like illness; diabetes mellitus; haematuria; renal calculi, lymphadenopathy; myalgia; conjuctivitis; dry skin, acne, erythema, skin papilloma; *less commonly* hypersensitivity reactions (see Cautions)

Dose: *by subcutaneous injection*, ADULT and ADOLESCENT over 16 years, 90 mg twice daily; CHILD 6–15 years, 2 mg/kg twice daily (max. 90 mg twice daily)

Fuzeon® (Roche) ▼ PoM

Injection, powder for reconstitution, enfuvirtide 108 mg (= enfuvirtide 90 mg/mL when reconstituted with 1.1 mL water for injections), net price 108-mg vial = £19.13 (with solvent, syringe, and alcohol swabs). Counselling, hypersensitivity reactions

5.3.2 Herpesvirus infections

5.3.2.1 Herpes simplex and varicella–zoster infection

The two most important herpesvirus pathogens are herpes simplex virus (herpesvirus hominis) and varicella–zoster virus.

HERPES SIMPLEX INFECTIONS. Herpes infection of the mouth and lips and in the eye is generally associated with herpes simplex virus serotype 1 (HSV-1); other areas of the skin may also be infected, especially in immunodeficiency. Genital infection is most often associated with HSV-2 and also HSV-1.

In individuals with good immune function, mild infection of the eye (ocular herpes, section 11.3.3) and of the lips (herpes labialis or cold sores, section 13.10.3) is treated with a topical antiviral drug. Primary herpetic gingivostomatitis is managed by changes to diet and with analgesics (section 12.3.2). Severe infection, neonatal herpes infection or infection in immunocompromised individuals requires treatment with a systemic antiviral drug. Primary or recurrent genital herpes simplex infection is treated with an antiviral drug given by mouth; specialist advice should be sought for managing the infection in pregnancy.

VARICELLA–ZOSTER INFECTIONS. Regardless of immune function and the use of any immunoglobulins, neonates with *chickenpox* should be treated with a parenteral antiviral to reduce the risk of severe disease. Chickenpox in otherwise healthy children between 1 month and 12 years is usually mild and antiviral treatment is not usually required.

Chickenpox is more severe in adolescents and adults than in children; antiviral treatment started within 24 hours of the onset of rash may reduce the duration and severity of symptoms in otherwise healthy adults and adolescents. Antiviral treatment is generally recommended in immunocompromised patients and those at special risk (e.g. because of severe cardiovascular or respiratory disease or chronic skin disorder); an antiviral is given for 10 days with at least 7 days of parenteral treatment.

Pregnant women who develop severe chickenpox may be at risk of complications, especially varicella pneumonia. Specialist advice should be sought for the treatment of chickenpox during pregnancy.

In *herpes zoster* (shingles) systemic antiviral treatment can reduce the severity and duration of pain, reduce complications, and reduce viral shedding. Treatment with the antiviral should be started within 72 hours of the onset of rash and is usually continued for 7–10 days.

Immunocompromised patients at high risk of disseminated or severe infection should be treated with a parenteral antiviral drug. Chronic pain which persists after the rash has healed (postherpetic neuralgia) requires specific management (section 4.7.3).

Those who have been exposed to chickenpox and are at special risk of complications may require prophylaxis with varicella-zoster immunoglobulin (see under Specific Immunoglobulins, section 14.5).

CHOICE. **Aciclovir** is active against herpesviruses but does not eradicate them. Uses of aciclovir include systemic treatment of varicella–zoster and the systemic and topical treatment of herpes simplex infections of the skin (section 13.10.3) and mucous membranes (section 7.2.2). It is used by mouth for severe herpetic stomatitis (see also p. 556). Aciclovir eye ointment (section 11.3.3) is used for herpes simplex infections of the eye; it is combined with systemic treatment for ophthalmic zoster.

Famciclovir, a prodrug of penciclovir, is similar to aciclovir and is licensed for use in herpes zoster and genital herpes. Penciclovir itself is used as a cream for herpes simplex labialis (section 13.10.3).

Valaciclovir is an ester of aciclovir, licensed for herpes zoster and herpes simplex infections of the skin and mucous membranes (including genital herpes); it is also licensed for preventing cytomegalovirus disease following renal transplantation. Famciclovir or valaciclovir are suitable alternatives to aciclovir for oral lesions associated with herpes zoster. Valaciclovir once daily may reduce the risk of transmitting genital herpes to heterosexual partners—specialist advice should be sought.

Idoxuridine (section 13.10.3) has been used topically for treating herpes simplex infections of the skin and external genitalia with variable results. Its value in the treatment of shingles is unclear.

Inosine pranobex has been used by mouth for herpes simplex infections; its effectiveness remains unproven.

ACICLOVIR

(Acyclovir)

Indications: herpes simplex and varicella–zoster (see also under Dose)

Cautions: maintain adequate hydration (especially with infusion or high doses); renal impairment (Appendix 3); pregnancy (Appendix 4); breast-feeding (Appendix 5); **interactions:** Appendix 1 (aciclovir)

Side-effects: nausea, vomiting, abdominal pain, diarrhoea, headache, fatigue, rash, urticaria, pruritus, photosensitivity; rarely hepatitis, jaundice, dyspnoea, angioedema, anaphylaxis, neurological reactions (including dizziness, confusion, hallucinations and drowsiness), acute renal failure, decreases in haematological indices; on *intravenous infusion*, severe local inflammation (sometimes leading to ulceration), fever, and rarely agitation, tremors, psychosis and convulsions

Dose: *by mouth*, herpes simplex, treatment, 200 mg (400 mg in the immunocompromised or if absorption impaired) 5 times daily, usually for 5 days (longer if new lesions appear during treatment or if healing incomplete); CHILD under 2 years, half adult dose, over 2 years, adult dose

Herpes simplex, prevention of recurrence, 200 mg 4 times daily *or* 400 mg twice daily possibly reduced to 200 mg 2 or 3 times daily and interrupted every 6–12 months

Herpes simplex, prophylaxis in the immunocompromised, 200–400 mg 4 times daily; CHILD under 2 years, half adult dose, over 2 years, adult dose

Varicella and herpes zoster, treatment, 800 mg 5 times daily for 7 days; CHILD, varicella, 20 mg/kg (max. 800 mg) 4 times daily for 5 days *or* under 2 years 200 mg 4 times daily, 2–5 years 400 mg 4 times daily, over 6 years 800 mg 4 times daily

Attenuation of chickenpox (if varicella–zoster immunoglobulin not indicated) [unlicensed use], ADULT and CHILD 40 mg/kg daily in 4 divided doses for 7 days starting 1 week after exposure

By intravenous infusion, treatment of herpes simplex in the immunocompromised, severe initial genital herpes, and varicella–zoster, 5 mg/kg every 8 hours usually for 5 days, doubled to 10 mg/kg every 8 hours in varicella–zoster in the immunocompromised and in simplex encephalitis (usually given for at least 10 days in encephalitis, possibly for 14–21 days); prophylaxis of herpes simplex in the immunocompromised, 5 mg/kg every 8 hours

NOTE. To avoid excessive dosage in obese patients parenteral dose should be calculated on the basis of ideal body-weight

NEONATE and INFANT up to 3 months, with disseminated herpes simplex, 20 mg/kg every 8 hours for 14 days (21 days if CNS involvement); varicella–zoster [unlicensed use] 10–20 mg/kg every 8 hours for at least 7 days; CHILD 3 months–12 years, herpes simplex or varicella–zoster, 250 mg/m^2 every 8 hours usually for 5 days, doubled to 500 mg/m^2 every 8 hours for varicella–zoster in the immunocompromised and in simplex encephalitis (usually given for at least 10 days in encephalitis, possibly for 14–21 days)

By topical application, see sections 13.10.3 (skin) and 11.3.3 (eye)

Aciclovir (Non-proprietary) PoM

Tablets, aciclovir 200 mg, net price 25-tab pack = £4.01; 400 mg, 56-tab pack = £7.31; 800 mg, 35-tab pack = £45.10. Label: 9

Brands include *Virovir*®

DENTAL PRESCRIBING ON NHS. Aciclovir Tablets 200 mg may be prescribed

Dispersible tablets, aciclovir 200 mg, net price 25-tab pack = £3.45; 400 mg, 56-tab pack = £10.85; 800 mg, 35-tab pack = £11.38. Label: 9

Intravenous infusion, powder for reconstitution, aciclovir (as sodium salt). Net price 250-mg vial = £10.91; 500-mg vial = £20.22

Electrolytes: Na^+ 1.1 mmol/250-mg vial

Intravenous infusion, aciclovir (as sodium salt), 25 mg/mL, net price 10-mL (250-mg) vial = £10.37; 20-mL (500-mg) vial = £19.21; 40-mL (1-g) vial = £40.44

Electrolytes: Na^+ 1.16 mmol/250-mg vial

Zovirax® (GSK) PoM

Tablets, all dispersible, f/c, aciclovir 200 mg (blue), net price 25-tab pack = £18.80; 400 mg (pink), 56-tab pack = £68.98; 800 mg (scored, *Shingles Treatment Pack*), 35-tab pack = £69.85. Label: 9

Suspension, both off-white, sugar-free, aciclovir 200 mg/5 mL (banana-flavoured), net price 125 mL = £29.56; 400 mg/5 mL (*Double Strength Suspension*, orange-flavoured) 100 mL = £33.02. Label: 9

DENTAL PRESCRIBING ON NHS. May be prescribed as Aciclovir 200 mg/5 mL oral Suspension

Intravenous infusion, powder for reconstitution, aciclovir (as sodium salt). Net price 250-mg vial = £10.15; 500-mg vial = £18.81

Electrolytes: Na^+ 1.1 mmol/250-mg vial

FAMCICLOVIR

NOTE. Famciclovir is a pro-drug of penciclovir

Indications: treatment of herpes zoster, acute genital herpes simplex and suppression of recurrent genital herpes

Cautions: hepatic impairment (Appendix 2); renal impairment (Appendix 3); pregnancy (Appendix 4) and breast-feeding (Appendix 5); **interactions:** Appendix 1 (famciclovir)

Side-effects: *rarely* nausea, headache, confusion; *very rarely* vomiting, jaundice, dizziness, drowsiness, hallucinations, rash, and pruritus; abdominal pain and fever have been reported in immunocompromised patients

Dose: herpes zoster, 250 mg 3 times daily for 7 days *or* 750 mg once daily for 7 days (in immunocompromised, 500 mg 3 times daily for 10 days)

Genital herpes, first episode, 250 mg 3 times daily for 5 days (longer if new lesions appear during treatment or if healing incomplete); recurrent infection, 125 mg twice daily for 5 days (in immunocompromised, all episodes, 500 mg twice daily for 7 days)

Genital herpes, suppression, 250 mg twice daily (in HIV patients, 500 mg twice daily) interrupted every 6–12 months

CHILD not recommended

Famvir® (Novartis) PoM

Tablets, all f/c, famciclovir 125 mg, net price 10-tab pack = £30.93; 250 mg, 15-tab pack = £92.79, 21-tab pack = £129.89; 56-tab pack = £346.39; 500 mg, 14-tab pack = £173.22, 30-tab pack = £371.07, 56-tab pack = £692.88; 750 mg, 7-tab pack = £123.99. Label: 9

INOSINE PRANOBEX

Indications: see under Dose

Cautions: renal impairment (Appendix 3); history of gout or hyperuricaemia

Contra-indications: pregnancy

Side-effects: reversible increase in serum and urinary uric acid; *less commonly* nausea, vomiting, epigastric discomfort, headache, vertigo, fatigue, arthralgia, rashes and itching; *rarely* diarrhoea, constipation, anxiety, sleep disturbances, and polyuria

Dose: mucocutaneous herpes simplex, 1 g 4 times daily for 7–14 days

Adjunctive treatment of genital warts, 1 g 3 times daily for 14–28 days

Subacute sclerosing panencephalitis, 50–100 mg/kg daily in 6 divided doses

Imunovir® (Ardern) PoM

Tablets, inosine pranobex 500 mg. Net price 100 = £39.50. Label: 9

VALACICLOVIR

NOTE. Valaciclovir is a pro-drug of aciclovir

Indications: treatment of herpes zoster; treatment of initial and suppression of recurrent herpes simplex infections of skin and mucous membranes including initial and recurrent genital herpes; prevention of cytomegalovirus disease following renal transplantation

Cautions: see under Aciclovir; hepatic impairment (Appendix 2); renal impairment (Appendix 3)

Side-effects: see under Aciclovir but neurological reactions more frequent with high doses

Dose: herpes zoster, 1 g 3 times daily for 7 days

Herpes simplex, first episode, 500 mg twice daily for 5 days (longer if new lesions appear during treatment or if healing incomplete); recurrent infection, 500 mg twice daily for 5 days

Herpes simplex, suppression, 500 mg daily in 1–2 divided doses (in immunocompromised, 500 mg twice daily)

Prevention of cytomegalovirus disease following renal transplantation (preferably starting within 72 hours of transplantation), 2 g 4 times daily usually for 90 days

CHILD not recommended

Valtrex® (GSK) PoM

Tablets, f/c, valaciclovir (as hydrochloride) 500 mg, net price 10-tab pack = £21.86, 42-tab pack = £91.61. Label: 9

5.3.2.2 Cytomegalovirus infection

Recommendations for the optimum maintenance therapy of cytomegalovirus (CMV) infections and the duration of treatment are subject to rapid change.

Ganciclovir is related to aciclovir but it is more active against cytomegalovirus; it is also much more toxic than aciclovir and should therefore be prescribed only when the potential benefit outweighs the risks. Ganciclovir is administered by intravenous infusion for the *initial treatment* of CMV retinitis. Ganciclovir causes profound myelosuppression when given with zidovudine; the two should not normally be given together particularly during initial ganciclovir therapy. The likelihood of ganciclovir resistance increases in patients with a high viral load or in those who receive the drug over a long duration; cross-resistance to cidofovir is common.

Valaciclovir (see above) is licensed for prevention of cytomegalovirus disease following renal transplantation.

Valganciclovir is an ester of ganciclovir which is licensed for the *initial treatment* and *maintenance treatment* of CMV retinitis in AIDS patients. Valganciclovir is also licensed for preventing CMV disease following solid organ transplantation from a cytomegalovirus-positive donor.

Foscarnet is also active against cytomegalovirus; it is toxic and can cause renal impairment.

Cidofovir is given in combination with probenecid for CMV retinitis in AIDS patients when ganciclovir and foscarnet are contra-indicated. Cidofovir is nephrotoxic.

For local treatment of CMV retinitis, see section 11.3.3.

CIDOFOVIR

Indications: cytomegalovirus retinitis in AIDS patients for whom other drugs are inappropriate

Cautions: monitor renal function (serum creatinine and urinary protein) and neutrophil count within 24 hours before each dose; co-treatment with probenecid and prior hydration with intravenous fluids necessary to minimise potential nephrotoxicity (see below); diabetes mellitus (increased risk of ocular hypotony); **interactions:** Appendix 1 (cidofovir)

NEPHROTOXICITY. Do not initiate treatment in renal impairment (assess creatinine clearance and proteinuria—consult product literature); discontinue treatment and give intravenous fluids if renal function deteriorates—consult product literature

OCULAR DISORDERS. Regular ophthalmological examinations recommended; iritis and uveitis have been reported which may respond to a topical corticosteroid with or without a cycloplegic drug—discontinue cidofovir if no response to topical corticosteroid or if condition worsens, or if iritis or uveitis recurs after successful treatment

Contra-indications: renal impairment (creatinine clearance 55 mL/minute or less); concomitant administration of potentially nephrotoxic drugs (discontinue potentially nephrotoxic drugs at least 7 days before starting cidofovir); pregnancy (avoid pregnancy during and for 1 month after treatment, men should not father a child during or within 3 months of treatment; Appendix 4), breast-feeding (Appendix 5)

Side-effects: nephrotoxicity (see Cautions above); neutropenia, fever, asthenia, alopecia, nausea, vomiting, hypotony, decreased intra-ocular pressure, iritis, uveitis (see Cautions above)

Dose: *by intravenous infusion* over 1 hour, initial (induction) treatment, 5 mg/kg once weekly for 2 weeks (give probenecid and intravenous fluids with each dose, see below); CHILD not recommended

Maintenance treatment, beginning 2 weeks after completion of induction, *by intravenous infusion* over 1 hour, 5 mg/kg once every 2 weeks (give probenecid and intravenous fluids with each dose, see below)

PROBENECID CO-TREATMENT. *By mouth* (preferably after food), probenecid 2 g 3 hours before cidofovir infusion followed by probenecid 1 g at 2 hours and 1 g at 8 hours after the end of cidofovir infusion (total probenecid 4 g); for cautions, contra-indications and side-effects of probenecid see section 10.1.4

PRIOR HYDRATION. Sodium chloride 0.9%, *by intravenous infusion*, 1 litre over 1 hour immediately before cidofovir infusion (if tolerated an additional 1 litre may be given over 1–3 hours, starting at the same time as the cidofovir infusion or immediately afterwards)

Vistide® (Pharmacia) PoM

Intravenous infusion, cidofovir 75 mg/mL, net price 5-mL vial = £653.22

CAUTION IN HANDLING. Cidofovir is toxic and personnel should be adequately protected during handling and administration; if solution comes into contact with skin or mucosa, wash off immediately with water

GANCICLOVIR

Indications: life-threatening or sight-threatening cytomegalovirus infections in immunocompromised patients only; prevention of cytomegalovirus disease during immunosuppressive therapy following organ transplantation; local treatment of CMV retinitis (section 11.3.3)

Cautions: close monitoring of full blood count (severe deterioration may require correction and possibly treatment interruption); history of cytopenia; low platelet count; potential carcinogen and teratogen; renal impairment (consult product literature); radiotherapy; ensure adequate hydration during intravenous administration; vesicant—infuse into vein with adequate flow preferably using plastic cannula; children (possible risk of long-term carcinogenic or reproductive toxicity—not for neonatal or congenital cytomegalovirus disease); **interactions:** Appendix 1 (ganciclovir)

Contra-indications: pregnancy (ensure effective contraception during treatment and barrier contraception for men during and for at least 90 days after treatment; Appendix 4); breast-feeding; hypersensitivity to ganciclovir or aciclovir; abnormally low haemoglobin, neutrophil, or platelet counts (consult product literature)

Side-effects: diarrhoea, nausea, vomiting, dyspepsia, abdominal pain, constipation, flatulence, dysphagia, hepatic dysfunction; dyspnoea, chest pain, cough; headache, insomnia, convulsions, dizziness, neuropathy, depression, anxiety, confusion, abnormal thinking, fatigue, weight loss, anorexia; infection, fever, night sweats; anaemia, leucopenia, thrombocytopenia, pancytopenia, renal impairment; myalgia, arthralgia; macular oedema, retinal detachment, vitreous floaters, eye pain; ear pain, taste disturbance; dermatitis, pruritus; injection-site reactions; less commonly mouth ulcers, pancreatitis, arrhythmias, hypotension, anaphylactic reactions, psychosis, tremor, male infertility, haematuria, disturbances in hearing and vision, and alopecia

Dose: *by intravenous infusion*, initially (induction) 5 mg/kg every 12 hours for 14–21 days for treatment or for 7–14 days for prevention; maintenance (for patients at risk of relapse of retinitis) 6 mg/kg daily on 5 days per week *or* 5 mg/kg daily until adequate recovery of immunity; if retinitis progresses initial induction treatment may be repeated

Cymevene® (Roche) PoM

Intravenous infusion, powder for reconstitution, ganciclovir (as sodium salt). Net price 500-mg vial = £31.60

Electrolytes: Na^+ 2 mmol/500-mg vial

CAUTION IN HANDLING. Ganciclovir is toxic and personnel should be adequately protected during handling and administration; if solution comes into contact with skin or mucosa, wash off immediately with soap and water

FOSCARNET SODIUM

Indications: cytomegalovirus retinitis in AIDS patients; mucocutaneous herpes simplex virus infections unresponsive to aciclovir in immunocompromised patients

Cautions: renal impairment (reduce dose or avoid if severe); monitor electrolytes, particularly calcium and magnesium; monitor serum creatinine every second day during induction and every week during maintenance; ensure adequate hydration; avoid rapid infusion; **interactions:** Appendix 1 (foscarnet)

Contra-indications: pregnancy; breast-feeding

Side-effects: nausea, vomiting, diarrhoea (occasionally constipation and dyspepsia), abdominal pain, anorexia; changes in blood pressure and ECG; headache, fatigue, mood disturbances (including psychosis), asthenia, paraesthesia, convulsions, tremor, dizziness, and other neurological disorders; rash; impairment of renal function including acute renal failure; hypocalcaemia (sometimes symptomatic) and other electrolyte disturbances; abnormal liver function tests; decreased haemoglobin concentration, leucopenia, granulocytopenia, thrombocytopenia; thrombophlebitis if given undiluted by peripheral vein; genital irritation and ulceration (due to high concentrations excreted in urine); isolated reports of pancreatitis

Dose: CMV retinitis, *by intravenous infusion*, induction 60 mg/kg every 8 hours for 2–3 weeks then maintenance, 60 mg/kg daily, increased to 90–120 mg/kg if tolerated; if retinitis progresses on maintenance dose, repeat induction regimen

Mucocutaneous herpes simplex infection, *by intravenous infusion*, 40 mg/kg every 8 hours for 2–3 weeks or until lesions heal

Foscavir® (AstraZeneca) PoM
Intravenous infusion, foscarnet sodium hexahydrate 24 mg/mL, net price 250-mL bottle = £34.49

VALGANCICLOVIR

NOTE. Valganciclovir is a pro-drug of ganciclovir

Indications: induction and maintenance treatment of cytomegalovirus retinitis in AIDS patients; prevention of cytomegalovirus disease following solid organ transplantation from a cytomegalovirus-positive donor.

Cautions: see under Ganciclovir

Side-effects: see under Ganciclovir

Dose: CMV retinitis, induction, 900 mg twice daily for 21 days then 900 mg once daily; induction regimen may be repeated if retinitis progresses

Prevention of cytomegalovirus disease following solid organ transplantation (starting within 10 days of transplantation), 900 mg once daily for 100 days

CHILD and ADOLESCENT not recommended

NOTE. Oral valganciclovir 900 mg twice daily is equivalent to intravenous ganciclovir 5 mg/kg twice daily

Valcyte® (Roche) ▼ PoM
Tablets, pink, f/c, valganciclovir (as hydrochloride) 450 mg, net price 60-tab pack = £1148.05.
Label: 21

CAUTION IN HANDLING. Valganciclovir is a potential teratogen and carcinogen and caution is advised for handling of broken tablets; if broken tablets come into contact with skin or mucosa, wash off immediately with water

5.3.3 Viral hepatitis

Treatment for viral hepatitis should be initiated by a specialist. The management of uncomplicated acute viral hepatitis is largely symptomatic. Early treatment of acute hepatitis C with interferon alfa [unlicensed indication] may reduce the risk of chronic infection. Hepatitis B and hepatitis C viruses are major causes of chronic hepatitis. For details on immunisation against hepatitis A and B infections, see section 14.4 (active immunisation) and section 14.5 (passive immunisation).

CHRONIC HEPATITIS B. **Interferon alfa** (section 8.2.4) is used in the treatment of chronic hepatitis B but its use is limited by a response rate of less than 50%, and relapse is frequent. If no improvement occurs after 3–4 months of treatment, interferon alfa should be discontinued. Interferon alfa is contra-indicated in patients receiving immunosuppressant treatment (or who have received it recently). The manufacturers of interferon alfa contra-indicate its use in decompensated liver disease but low doses can be used with great caution in these patients.

Lamivudine (see p. 316) is used for the initial treatment of chronic hepatitis B. It can also be used in patients with decompensated liver disease. Treatment should be continued if there is no loss of efficacy and until seroconversion is adequate (consult product literature); it is continued long-term in decompensated liver disease. Hepatitis B viruses with reduced susceptibility to lamivudine have emerged following extended therapy. In patients infected with HIV and hepatitis B, lamivudine should be given only as part of combination antiretroviral therapy and in a dose appropriate for treating HIV; the use of lamivudine alone is likely to result in lamivudine-resistant HIV.

Adefovir dipivoxil is licensed for the treatment of chronic hepatitis B. It is effectve in lamivudine-resistant chronic hepatitis B. Treatment should be continued, if there is no loss in efficacy, until adequate seroconversion has occurred (consult product literature); it is continued long-term in patients with decompensated liver disease or cirrhosis.

CHRONIC HEPATITIS C. Before starting treatment, the genotype of the infecting hepatitis C virus should be determined and the viral load measured as this may affect choice of treatment regimen. A combination of **ribavirin** (see p. 327) and **peginterferon alfa** (section 8.2.4) is used for the treatment of chronic hepatitis C (see NICE guidance, below). The combination of ribavirin and interferon alfa is less effective than the combination of peginterferon alfa and ribavirin. Peginterferon alfa alone should be used if ribavirin is contra-indicated or not tolerated. Ribavirin monotherapy is ineffective.

NICE guidance (peginterferon alfa, interferon alfa, and ribavirin for chronic hepatitis C). NICE has recommended (January 2004) that the combination of peginterferon alfa and ribavirin should be used for treating moderate to severe chronic hepatitis C in patients aged over 18 years:

- not previously treated with interferon alfa or peginterferon alfa;
- treated previously with interferon alfa alone or in combination with ribavirin;
- whose condition did not respond to peginterferon alfa alone or responded but subsequently relapsed.

Peginterferon alfa alone should be used if ribavirin is contra-indicated or not tolerated. Interferon alfa for either monotherapy or combined therapy should be used only if neutropenia and thrombocytopenia are a particular risk. Patients receiving interferon alfa may be switched to peginterferon alfa.
The duration of treatment depends on genotype and viral load (full guidance available at www.nice.org.uk/TA075).

ADEFOVIR DIPIVOXIL

Indications: chronic hepatitis B infection with *either* compensated liver disease with evidence of viral replication, and histologically documented active liver inflammation and fibrosis *or* decompensated liver disease

Cautions: monitor liver function and viral, and serological markers for hepatitis B every 6 months; discontinue if deterioration in liver function, hepatic steatosis, progressive hepatomegaly or unexplained lactic acidosis; recurrent hepatitis may occur on discontinuation; monitor renal function every 3 months, more frequently in renal impairment (Appendix 3) or in patients receiving nephrotoxic drugs; pregnancy (Appendix 4); elderly; HIV infection (particularly if uncontrolled—theoretical risk of HIV resistance)

Contra-indications: breast-feeding (Appendix 5)

Side-effects: nausea, dyspepsia, abdominal pain, flatulence, diarrhoea, asthenia, headache, renal failure

Dose: ADULT over 18 years, 10 mg once daily

Hepsera (Gilead) ▼ PoM
Tablets, adefovir dipivoxil 10 mg, net price 30-tab pack = £315.00

5.3.4 Influenza

For advice on immunisation against influenza, see section 14.4.

Oseltamivir and **zanamivir** reduce replication of influenza A and B viruses by inhibiting viral neuraminidase. They are most effective for the treatment of influenza if started within a few hours of the onset of symptoms; they are licensed for use within 48 hours of the first symptoms. In otherwise healthy individuals they reduce the duration of symptoms by about 1–1.5 days. The effect of oseltamivir or zanamivir on hospitalisation or on mortality is not clear in those at risk of serious complications from influenza. Oseltamivir is also licensed for prophylaxis when used within 48 hours of exposure to influenza and when influenza is circulating in the community; it is also licensed for use in exceptional circumstances (e.g. when vaccination does not cover the infecting strain) to prevent influenza in an epidemic. Where prophylaxis against influenza A or B is required and oseltamivir cannot be used, zanamivir 10 mg once daily by inhalation, is an alternative [unlicensed indication].

Amantadine is licensed for prophylaxis and treatment of influenza A but it is no longer recommended (see NICE guidance).

NICE guidance (oseltamivir, zanamivir, and amantadine for prophylaxis and treatment of influenza). NICE has recommended (February and September 2003) that the drugs described here are not a substitute for vaccination, which remains the most effective way of preventing illness from influenza. When influenza A or influenza B is circulating in the community:

- amantadine is **not** recommended for post-exposure prophylaxis, seasonal prophylaxis, or treatment of influenza;
- oseltamivir and zanamivir are **not** recommended for seasonal prophylaxis against influenza;
- oseltamivir or zanamivir are **not** recommended for post-exposure prophylaxis, or treatment of otherwise healthy individuals with influenza;
- oseltamivir is recommended for post-exposure prophylaxis in at-risk adults and adolescents over 13 years who are not effectively protected by influenza vaccine and who can commence oseltamivir within 48 hours of close contact with someone suffering from influenza-like illness; prophylaxis is also recommended for residents in care establishments (regardless of influenza vaccination) who can commence oseltamivir within 48 hours if influenza-like illness is present in the establishment;
- oseltamivir and zanamivir are recommended (in accordance with UK licensing) to treat at-risk adults who can start treatment within 48 hours of the onset of symptoms; oseltamivir is recommended for at-risk children who can start treatment within 48 hours of the onset of symptoms;

At-risk patients include those aged over 65 years *or* those who have one or more of the following conditions:

- chronic respiratory disease (including chronic obstructive pulmonary disease and asthma) [but see cautions under Zanamivir below];
- significant cardiovascular disease (excluding hypertension);
- chronic renal disease;
- immunosuppression;
- diabetes mellitus.

Community-based virological surveillance schemes including those run by the Health Protection Agency and the Royal College of General Practitioners should be used to indicate when influenza is circulating in the community.

AMANTADINE HYDROCHLORIDE

Indications: see under Dose; parkinsonism (section 4.9.1)

Cautions: see section 4.9.1

Contra-indications: see section 4.9.1

Side-effects: see section 4.9.1

Dose: Influenza A (see also notes above), ADULT and CHILD over 10 years, treatment, 100 mg daily for 4–5 days; prophylaxis, 100 mg daily usually for 6 weeks *or* with influenza vaccination for 2–3 weeks after vaccination
ELDERLY 100 mg daily

Lysovir® (Alliance) PoM
Capsules, white/green, amantadine hydrochloride 100 mg, net price 5-cap pack = £2.40, 14-cap pack = £4.80. Counselling, driving

Symmetrel® (Alliance) PoM
Section 4.9.1

OSELTAMIVIR

Indications: see notes above

Cautions: renal impairment (Appendix 3); pregnancy (Appendix 4); breast-feeding (Appendix 5)

Side-effects: nausea, vomiting, abdominal pain, dyspepsia, diarrhoea; headache, fatigue, insomnia, dizziness; conjunctivitis, epistaxis; rash; *rarely* hypersensitivity reactions; *very rarely* hepatitis, Stevens-Johnson syndrome

Dose: prevention of influenza, ADULT and ADOLESCENT over 13 years, 75 mg once daily for at least 7 days for post-exposure prophylaxis; for up to 6 weeks during an epidemic

Treatment of influenza, 75 mg every 12 hours for 5 days; CHILD over 1 year, body-weight 15 kg or under, 30 mg every 12 hours, body-weight 16–23 kg, 45 mg every 12 hours, body-weight 24–40 kg, 60 mg every 12 hours, body-weight over 40 kg, adult dose

[1]**Tamiflu**® (Roche) ▼ PoM
Capsules, grey/yellow, oseltamivir (as phosphate) 75 mg, net price 10-cap pack = £16.36. Label: 9
Suspension, sugar-free, tutti-frutti-flavoured, oseltamivir (as phosphate) for reconstitution with water, 60 mg/5 mL, net price 75 mL = £16.36. Label: 9
Excipients: include sorbitol 1.71 g/5 mL

1. NHS except for the treatment and prophylaxis of influenza as indicated in the notes above and NICE guidance; endorse prescription 'SLS'

ZANAMIVIR

Indications: see notes above

Cautions: asthma and chronic pulmonary disease (risk of bronchospasm—short-acting bronchodilator should be available; avoid in severe asthma unless close monitoring possible and appropriate facilities available to treat bronchospasm); uncontrolled chronic illness; other inhaled drugs should be administered before zanamivir; pregnancy (Appendix 4)

Contra-indications: breast-feeding (Appendix 5)

Side-effects: gastro-intestinal disturbances; *very rarely*, bronchospasm, respiratory impairment, angioedema, and rash

Dose: *by inhalation of powder*, 10 mg twice daily for 5 days, CHILD under 12 years not recommended

[1]**Relenza**® (GSK) PoM
Dry powder for inhalation disks containing 4 blisters of zanamivir 5 mg/blister, net price 5 disks with *Diskhaler*® device = £24.55

1. NHS except for the treatment of influenza as indicated in the notes above and NICE guidance; endorse prescription 'SLS'

5.3.5 Respiratory syncytial virus

Ribavirin (tribavirin) inhibits a wide range of DNA and RNA viruses. It is licensed for administration by inhalation for the treatment of severe bronchiolitis caused by the respiratory syncytial virus (RSV) in infants, especially when they have other serious diseases. However, there is no clear evidence that ribavirin produces clinically relevant benefit in RSV bronchiolitis. Ribavirin is given by mouth with peginterferon alfa or interferon alfa for the treatment of chronic hepatitis C infection (see Viral Hepatitis, p. 325). Ribavirin is also effective in Lassa fever [unlicensed indication].

Palivizumab is a monoclonal antibody indicated for the prevention of respiratory syncytial virus infection in infants at high risk of infection; it should be prescribed under specialist supervision and on the basis of the likelihood of hospitalisation. It is licensed for monthly use during the RSV season; the first dose should be administered before the start of the RSV season.

PALIVIZUMAB

Indications: see notes above; prevention of serious respiratory syncytial virus during infectious season in infant under 6 months born at less than 35 weeks gestation, *and* in child under 2 years treated in last 6 months for bronchopulmonary dysplasia, *and* in child under 2 years with haemodynamically significant heart disease

Cautions: moderate to severe acute infection or febrile illness; thrombocytopenia; serum-palivizumab concentration may be reduced after cardiac surgery

Contra-indications: hypersensitivity to humanised monoclonal antibodies

Side-effects: fever, injection-site reactions, nervousness; *less commonly* diarrhoea, vomiting, constipation, haemorrhage, rhinitis, cough, wheeze, pain, drowsiness, asthenia, hyperkinesia, leucopenia, and rash; *rarely* apnoea, hypersensitivity reactions (including anaphylaxis)

Dose: *by intramuscular injection* (preferably in anterolateral thigh), 15 mg/kg once a month during season of RSV risk (children undergoing cardiac bypass surgery, 15 mg/kg as soon as stable after surgery, then at monthly intervals during season of risk); injection volume over 1 mL should be divided between more than one site

Synagis® (Abbott) ▼ PoM
Injection, powder for reconstitution, palivizumab, net price 50-mg vial = £360.40; 100-mg vial = £600.10

RIBAVIRIN

(Tribavirin)

Indications: severe respiratory syncytial virus bronchiolitis in infants and children; in combination with peginterferon alfa or interferon alfa for chronic hepatitis C not previously treated in patients without liver decompensation and who have fibrosis or high inflammatory activity or for relapse following previous response to interferon alfa (see also section 5.3.3)

Cautions:
SPECIFIC CAUTIONS FOR INHALED TREATMENT. Maintain standard supportive respiratory and fluid management therapy; monitor electrolytes closely; monitor equipment for precipitation; pregnant women (and those planning pregnancy) should avoid exposure to aerosol
SPECIFIC CAUTIONS FOR ORAL TREATMENT. Exclude pregnancy before treatment; effective contraception essential during treatment and for 6 months after treatment in women and in men; routine monthly pregnancy tests recommended; condoms must be used if partner of male patient is pregnant (ribavirin excreted in semen); renal impairment (Appendix 3); cardiac disease (assessment including ECG recommended before and during treatment—discontinue if deterioration); gout; determine full blood count, platelets, electrolytes, serum creatinine, liver function tests and uric acid before starting treatment and then on weeks 2 and 4 of treatment, then as indicated clinically—adjust dose if adverse reactions or laboratory abnormalities develop (consult product literature)

Interactions: Appendix 1 (Ribavirin)

Contra-indications: pregnancy (**important teratogenic risk**: see Cautions and Appendix 4); breast-feeding
SPECIFIC CONTRA-INDICATIONS FOR ORAL TREATMENT. Severe cardiac disease, including unstable or uncontrolled cardiac disease in previous 6 months; haemoglobinopathies; severe debilitating medical conditions; severe hepatic dysfunction or decompensated cirrhosis (Appendix 2); autoimmune disease (including autoimmune hepatitis); history of severe psychiatric condition

Side-effects:
SPECIFIC SIDE-EFFECTS FOR INHALED TREATMENT. Worsening respiration, bacterial pneumonia, and pneumothorax reported; rarely non-specific anaemia and haemolysis
SPECIFIC SIDE-EFFECTS FOR ORAL TREATMENT. Haemolytic anaemia (anaemia may be improved by epoetin); also reported (in combination with peginterferon alfa or interferon alfa) nausea, vomiting, dry mouth, stomatitis, glossitis, dyspepsia, abdominal pain, gastritis, peptic ulcer, flatulence, diarrhoea, constipation, pancreatitis, anorexia, weight loss; chest pain, tachycardia, palpitation, syncope, peripheral oedema, flushing; dyspnoea, cough, rhinitis, pharyngitis, interstitial pneumonitis; sleep disturbances, asthenia, impaired concentration and memory, irritability, aggression, anxiety, depression, dizziness, tremor, hypertonia, myalgia, arthralgia, paraesthesia, peripheral neuropathy, influenza-like symptoms, headache; thyroid disorders, menstrual disturbances, reduced libido, impotence; rash, pruritus, urticaria, photosensitivity, alopecia, dry skin; taste disturbance, eye changes including blurred vision, tinnitus; neutropenia, thrombocytopenia, aplastic anaemia, lymphadenopathy, hyperuricaemia

Dose: see preparations below

Copegus (Roche) ▼ PoM
Tablets, f/c, pink, ribavirin 200 mg, net price 42-tab pack = £115.62, 112-tab pack = £308.31, 168-tab pack = £462.47. Label: 21
Dose: chronic hepatitis C (in combination with interferon alfa or peginterferon alfa), ADULT over 18 years, body-weight under 75 kg, 400 mg in the morning and 600 mg in the evening; body-weight 75 kg and over, 600 mg twice daily
NOTE. Chronic hepatitis C genotype 2 or 3 requires a lower dose of *Copegus*® (in combination with peginterferon alfa), usual dose 400 mg twice daily

Rebetol® (Schering-Plough) ▼ PoM
Capsules, ribavirin 200 mg, net price 84-cap pack = £275.65, 140-cap pack = £459.42, 168-cap pack = £551.30. Label: 21
Dose: chronic hepatitis C (in combination with interferon alfa or peginterferon alfa), ADULT over 18 years, body-weight under 65 kg, 400 mg twice daily; body-weight 65–85 kg, 400 mg in the morning and 600 mg in the evening; body-weight over 85 kg, 600 mg twice daily

Virazole® (Valeant) PoM
Inhalation, ribavirin 6 g for reconstitution with 300 mL water for injections. Net price 3 × 6-g vials = £349.00
Dose: bronchiolitis, *by aerosol inhalation or nebulisation* (via small particle aerosol generator) of solution containing 20 mg/mL for 12–18 hours for at least 3 days; max. 7 days

5.4 Antiprotozoal drugs

Advice on specific problems available from:

Advice for healthcare professionals

HPA (Health Protection Agency) Malaria Reference Laboratory	(020) 7636 3924 (prophylaxis only)
National Travel Health Network and Centre	(020) 7380 9234
Scottish Centre for Infection and Environmental Health (registered users of Travax only) www.travax.scot.nhs.uk (for registered users of the NHS Travax website only)	(0141) 300 1130 (weekdays 2–4 p.m. only)
Birmingham	(0121) 424 0357
Liverpool	(0151) 708 9393
London	(020) 7387 9300 (treatment)
Oxford	(01865) 225 430

Advice for travellers

HPA Malaria Reference Laboratory

Recorded advice for Travellers (£1.00/minute standard rate)	09065 508 908
Hospital for Tropical Diseases Travel Healthline (50p/minute)	09061 337 733

www.fitfortravel.scot.nhs.uk

WHO advice on international travel and health www.who.int/ith

5.4.1 Antimalarials

Recommendations on the prophylaxis and treatment of malaria reflect guidelines agreed by UK malaria specialists.

The centres listed above should be consulted for advice on special problems.

Treatment of malaria

If the infective species is **not known**, or if the infection is **mixed**, initial treatment should be as for *falciparum malaria* with quinine, *Malarone*® (proguanil with atovaquone), or *Riamet®* (artemether with lumefantrine). Falciparum malaria can progress rapidly in unprotected individuals and antimalarial treatment should be considered in those with features of severe malaria and possible exposure, even if the initial blood tests for the organism are negative.

Falciparum malaria (treatment)

Falciparum malaria (malignant malaria) is caused by *Plasmodium falciparum*. In most parts of the world *P. falciparum* is now resistant to chloroquine which should not therefore be given for treatment.[1]

Quinine, ***Malarone®*** (proguanil with atovaquone), or ***Riamet®*** (artemether with lumefantrine) can be given *by mouth* if the patient can swallow and retain tablets and there are no serious manifestations (e.g. impaired consciousness); quinine should be given *by intravenous infusion* (see below) if the patient is seriously ill or unable to take tablets. Mefloquine is now rarely used for treatment because of concerns about resistance. Specialist advice should be sought in difficult cases since other drugs such as **artesunate** (given intravenously) and intramuscular **artemether** may be available for 'named-patient use'.

Oral. The adult dosage regimen for **quinine** *by mouth* is:
600 mg (of quinine salt[2]) every 8 hours for 5–7 days *and* (if quinine resistance known or suspected) *followed by*
either **doxycycline** 200 mg daily (as a single dose or in 2 divided doses) for at least 7 days
or **clindamycin** 300 mg 4 times daily for 5 days.
If the parasite is likely to be sensitive, *Fansidar®* 3 tablets as a single dose may be given after a course of quinine.

Alternatively, ***Malarone®*** or ***Riamet®*** may be given instead of quinine; mefloquine is also an alternative but resistance to it has been reported in several regions including south-east Asia. It is not necessary to give doxycycline, clindamycin or *Fansidar®* after *Malarone®*, *Riamet®*, or mefloquine treatment.

The adult dose of ***Malarone®*** *by mouth* is:
4 ('standard') tablets once daily for 3 days.

The dose of ***Riamet®*** *by mouth* for adult with body-weight of over 35 kg is:
4 tablets initially, followed by 5 further doses of 4 tablets each given at 8, 24, 36, 48, and 60 hours (total 24 tablets over 60 hours).

1. For chloroquine-sensitive strains of falciparum malaria chloroquine is effective *by mouth* in the dosage schedule outlined under benign malarias but it should **not** be used unless there is an **unambiguous exposure history** in one of the few remaining areas of chloroquine sensitivity.

If the patient with a *chloroquine-sensitive infection* is seriously ill, chloroquine is given *by continuous intravenous infusion*. The dosage (for adults and children) is chloroquine 10 mg/kg (of base) infused over 8 hours, followed by three 8-hour infusions of 5 mg/kg (of base) each. *Oral therapy* is started as soon as possible to complete the course; the total cumulative dose for the course should be 25 mg/kg of base.

2. Valid for quinine hydrochloride, dihydrochloride, and sulphate; not valid for quinine bisulphate which contains a correspondingly smaller amount of quinine.

The adult dosage regimen for **mefloquine** (resistance reported) *by mouth* is:
20–25 mg/kg (of mefloquine base) as a single dose (up to maximum 1.5 g) *or preferably* as 2 divided doses 6–8 hours apart.

Parenteral. If the patient is seriously ill, **quinine** should be given *by intravenous infusion*. The adult dosage regimen for quinine *by infusion* is:
loading dose[3] of 20 mg/kg[4] (up to maximum 1.4 g) of quinine salt[2] infused over 4 hours *then after 8 hours* maintenance dose of 10 mg/kg[5] (up to maximum 700 mg) of quinine salt[2] infused over 4 hours every 8 hours (until patient can swallow tablets to complete the 7-day course) *followed by either Fansidar® or* doxycycline as above. Alternatively, after at least 2–3 days' treatment with a parenteral quinine salt, treatment may be completed with mefloquine by mouth started at least 12 hours after parenteral quinine salt has been administered.

CHILDREN.

Oral. **Quinine** is well tolerated by children although the salts are bitter. The dosage regimen for quinine *by mouth* for children is:
10 mg/kg (of quinine salt[2]) every 8 hours for 7 days *then* (if quinine resistance known or suspected) *either*
Fansidar® as a single dose: up to 4 years ½ tablet, 5–6 years 1 tablet, 7–9 years 1½ tablets, 10–14 years 2 tablets
or clindamycin 20–40 mg/kg daily in 3 divided doses for 5 days [unlicensed indication]

Alternatively ***Malarone®*** or ***Riamet®*** (or mefloquine, but resistance reported) may be given instead of quinine; it is not necessary to give clindamycin or *Fansidar®* after mefloquine, *Malarone®*, or *Riamet®* treatment. The dose regimen for mefloquine *by mouth* for children is calculated on a mg/kg basis as for adults (see above). The dose regimen for *Malarone® by mouth* for children over 40 kg is the same as for adults (see above); the dose regimen for *Malarone®* for smaller children is reduced as follows:

weight under 11 kg, no suitable dose form
weight 11–20 kg, 1 ('standard') tablet daily for 3 days; weight 21–30 kg, 2 ('standard') tablets daily for 3 days; weight 31–40 kg, 3 ('standard') tablets daily for 3 days.

The dose regimen of *Riamet® by mouth* for children over 12 years and body-weight over 35 kg is the same as for adults (see above).

Parenteral. The dose regimen for quinine *by intravenous infusion* for children is calculated on a mg/kg basis as for adults (see above).

3. In intensive care units the loading dose can alternatively be given as quinine salt[2] 7 mg/kg infused over 30 minutes followed immediately by 10 mg/kg over 4 hours then (after 8 hours) maintenance dose as described.

4. **Important:** the loading dose of 20 mg/kg should **not** be used if the patient has received quinine (or quinidine) or mefloquine during the previous 24 hours

5. Maintenance dose should be reduced to 5–7 mg/kg of salt in patients with renal impairment or if parenteral treatment is required for more than 48 hours.

PREGNANCY. Falciparum malaria is particularly dangerous in pregnancy, especially in the last trimester. The adult treatment doses of oral and intravenous quinine given above (including the loading dose) can safely be given to pregnant women. Alternatively, clindamycin, 300 mg every 6 hours for 5 days [unlicensed indication] can be given in combination with quinine. Doxycycline should be avoided in pregnancy (affects teeth and skeletal development); *Fansidar*®, *Malarone*® and *Riamet*® are also best avoided until more information is available.

Benign malarias (treatment)

Benign malaria is usually caused by *Plasmodium vivax* and less commonly by *P. ovale* and *P. malariae*. **Chloroquine**[1] is the drug of choice for the treatment of benign malarias (but chloroquine-resistant *P. vivax* infection has been reported from New Guinea and some adjacent islands).

The adult dosage regimen for **chloroquine** *by mouth* is:

initial dose of 600 mg (of base) *then*
a single dose of 300 mg after 6 to 8 hours *then*
a single dose of 300 mg daily for 2 days
(approximate total cumulative dose of 25 mg/kg of base)

Chloroquine alone is adequate for *P. malariae* infections but in the case of *P. vivax* and *P. ovale*, a *radical cure* (to destroy parasites in the liver and thus prevent relapses) is required. This is achieved with **primaquine**[2] given after chloroquine; in *P. vivax* infection primaquine is given in an adult dosage of 30 mg daily for 14 days and for *P. ovale* infection it is given in an adult dosage of 15 mg daily for 14 days.

CHILDREN. The dosage regimen of chloroquine for benign malaria in children is:
initial dose of 10 mg/kg (of base) *then*
a single dose of 5 mg/kg after 6–8 hours *then*
a single dose of 5 mg/kg daily for 2 days

For a *radical cure* children are then given primaquine[2] in a dose of 250 micrograms/kg daily.

PREGNANCY. The adult treatment doses of chloroquine can be given for benign malaria. In the case of *P. vivax* or *P. ovale*, however, the radical cure with primaquine should be **postponed** until the pregnancy is over; instead chloroquine should be continued at a dose of 600 mg each week during the pregnancy.

Prophylaxis against malaria

The recommendations on prophylaxis reflect guidelines agreed by UK malaria specialists; the advice is aimed at residents of the UK who travel to endemic areas. The choice of drug for a particular individual should take into account:

risk of exposure to malaria;
extent of drug resistance;
efficacy of the recommended drugs;
side-effects of the drugs;
patient-related factors (e.g. age, pregnancy, renal or hepatic impairment).

PROTECTION AGAINST BITES. **Prophylaxis is not absolute**, and breakthrough infection can occur with any of the drugs recommended. Personal protection against being bitten is very important. Mosquito nets impregnated with permethrin provide the most effective barrier protection against insects; coils, mats and vaporised insecticides are also useful. Diethyltoluamide (DEET) in lotions, sprays or roll-on formulations is safe and effective when applied to the skin but the protective effect only lasts for a few hours. Long sleeves and trousers worn after dusk also provide protection.

LENGTH OF PROPHYLAXIS. In order to determine tolerance and to establish habit, prophylaxis should generally be started one week (preferably 2½ weeks in the case of mefloquine) before travel into an endemic area (or if not possible at earliest opportunity up to 1 or 2 days before travel); *Malarone*® prophylaxis should be started 1–2 days before travel. Prophylaxis should be continued for **4 weeks after leaving** (except for *Malarone*® prophylaxis which should be stopped 1 week after leaving).

In those requiring long-term prophylaxis, chloroquine and proguanil may be used for periods of over 5 years. Mefloquine is licensed for up to 1 year (although it has been used for up to 3 years without undue problems). Doxycycline can be used for up to 2 years while *Malarone*® is licensed for up to 28 days but can be used safely for up to 3 months (and possibly 6 months or longer). Specialist advice should be sought for long-term prophylaxis.

RETURN FROM MALARIAL REGION. It is important to be aware that **any illness** that occurs within 1 year and **especially within 3 months of return might be malaria** even if all recommended precautions against malaria were taken. Travellers should be **warned** of this and told that if they develop any illness **particularly within 3 months** of their return they should go **immediately** to a doctor and specifically mention their exposure to malaria.

CHILDREN. Prophylactic doses are based on guidelines agreed by UK malaria experts and may differ from advice in product literature. Weight is a better guide than age. If in doubt telephone centres listed on p. 328.

EPILEPSY. Both chloroquine and mefloquine are unsuitable for malaria prophylaxis in individuals with a history of epilepsy. In areas *without chloroquine resistance* proguanil 200 mg daily alone is recommended; in areas *with chloroquine resistance*, doxycycline or *Malarone*® may be considered; the metabolism of doxycycline may be influenced by antiepileptics (see **interactions:** Appendix 1 (tetracyclines)).

1. Alternatives to chloroquine for the treatment of benign malaria are *Malarone*® [unlicensed indication], quinine, mefloquine, or *Riamet*® [unlicensed indication]; as with chloroquine, primaquine should be given for radical cure.

2. Before starting primaquine blood should be tested for glucose-6-phosphate dehydrogenase (G6PD) activity since the drug can cause haemolysis in G6PD-deficient patients. In G6PD deficiency primaquine, in a dose for adults of 30 mg once a week (children 500–750 micrograms/kg once a week) for 8 weeks, has been found useful and without undue harmful effects.

ASPLENIA. Asplenic individuals (or those with severe splenic dysfunction) are at particular risk of severe malaria. If travel to malarious areas is unavoidable, rigorous precautions are required against contracting the disease.

RENAL IMPAIRMENT. Avoidance (or dosage reduction) of proguanil is recommended since it is excreted by the kidneys. *Malarone*® should not be used for prophylaxis in patients with creatinine clearance less than 30 mL/minute. Chloroquine is only partially excreted by the kidneys and reduction of the dose for prophylaxis is not required except in severe impairment. Mefloquine is considered to be appropriate to use in renal impairment and does not require dosage reduction. Doxycycline is also considered to be appropriate.

PREGNANCY. Travel to malarious areas should be avoided during pregnancy; if travel is unavoidable, effective prophylaxis must be used. Chloroquine and proguanil may be given in usual doses in areas where *P. falciparum* strains are sensitive; in the case of proguanil, folic acid 5 mg daily should be given. The manufacturer advises that prophylaxis with mefloquine should be avoided as a matter of principle but studies of mefloquine in pregnancy (including use in the first trimester) indicate that it can be considered for travel to chloroquine-resistant areas. Doxycycline is contra-indicated during pregnancy. *Malarone*® should be avoided during pregnancy unless there is no suitable alternative. The centres listed on p. 328 should be consulted for advice on prophylaxis in resistant areas.

BREAST-FEEDING. Prophylaxis is required in **breast-fed infants**; although antimalarials are present in milk, the amounts are too variable to give reliable protection.

Specific recommendations

Where a journey requires two regimens, the regimen for the higher risk area should be used for the whole journey. Those travelling to remote or little-visited areas may require expert advice.

> Risk may vary in different parts of a country—check under all risk levels

> WARNING. Settled immigrants (or long-term visitors) to the UK may be unaware that they will have **lost some of their immunity** and also that the areas where they previously lived **may now be malarious**

North Africa, the Middle East, and Central Asia

VERY LOW RISK. Risk *very low* in Algeria, Egypt (tourist areas malaria-free), Georgia (south-east, July–October), Kyrgystan (but *Low Risk* in south-west, see below), Libya, rural Morocco, most tourist areas of Turkey, Uzbekistan (extreme south-east only):

> chemoprophylaxis not recommended but avoid mosquito bites and consider malaria if fever presents

LOW RISK. Risk *low* in Armenia (June–October), Azerbaijan (southern border areas, June–September), Egypt (El Fayoum only, June–October), rural north Iraq and Basrah Province (May–November), Kyrgystan (south-west, May–October), north border of Syria (May–October), Turkey (plain around Adana, Side, south-east Anatolia, March–November), Turkmenistan (south-east only, June–October): **preferably**

> chloroquine *or* (if chloroquine not appropriate) proguanil hydrochloride

RISK. Risk *present* and *chloroquine resistance present* in Afghanistan (below 2000 m, May–November), Iran, Oman (remote rural areas only), Saudi Arabia (except northern, eastern and central provinces, Asir plateau, and western border cities where very little risk, no risk in Mecca), Tajikistan (June–October), Yemen (no risk in Sana'a):

> chloroquine + proguanil hydrochloride *or* (if chloroquine + proguanil not appropriate) doxycyline

Sub-Saharan Africa

No chemoprophylaxis recommended for Cape Verde and non-rural areas of Mauritius (but avoid mosquito bites and consider malaria if fever presents); *chloroquine prophylaxis* appropriate for rural areas of **Mauritius**

SEASONAL RISK. Risk *present* (in parts of country) and *some chloroquine resistance* in Mauritania (all year in south; July–November in north):

> chloroquine + proguanil hydrochloride *or* (if chloroquine + proguanil not appropriate) mefloquine *or* doxycycline *or Malarone*®

VERY HIGH RISK. Risk *very high* (or *locally very high*) and *chloroquine resistance very widespread* in Angola, Benin, Botswana (northern half, November–June), Burkina Faso, Burundi, Cameroon, Central African Republic, Chad, Comoros, Congo, Democratic Republic of the Congo (formely Zaïre), Djibouti, Equatorial Guinea, Eritrea, Ethiopia (below 2200 m; no risk in Addis Ababa), Gabon, Gambia, Ghana, Guinea, Guinea-Bissau, Ivory Coast, Kenya, Liberia, Madagascar, Malawi, Mali, Mozambique, Namibia (all year along Kavango and Kunene rivers; November–June in northern third), Niger, Nigeria, Principe, Rwanda, São Tomé, Senegal, Sierra Leone, Somalia, South Africa (Kruger Park, north-east, low-altitude areas of Northern Province and Mpumalanga, and north-east KwaZulu-Natal as far south as Tugela river), Sudan, Swaziland, Tanzania, Togo, Uganda, Zambia, Zimbabwe (all year in Zambezi valley; November–June in other areas below 1200 m; risk negligible in Harare and Bulawayo):

mefloquine *or* doxycycline *or* *Malarone*®

NOTE. In Zimbabwe and neighbouring countries, pyrimethamine with dapsone (also known as *Deltaprim*®) prophylaxis is used by local residents (sometimes with chloroquine).

South Asia

VARIABLE RISK. Risk *variable* and *chloroquine resistance usually moderate* in Bangladesh (except in Chittagong Hill Tracts, see below; no risk in Dhaka city), southern districts of Bhutan, India (no risk in parts of mountain states of north; *High Risk* in Assam), Nepal (below 1500 m, especially Terai districts; no risk in Kathmandu), Pakistan (below 2000 m), Sri Lanka (no risk in and just south of Colombo):

chloroquine + proguanil hydrochloride

HIGH RISK. Risk *high* and *chloroquine resistance high* in Bangladesh (only in Chittagong Hill Tracts), India (Assam only):

mefloquine *or* doxycycline *or* *Malarone*®

South-East Asia

VERY LOW RISK. Risk *very low* in Bali, main tourist areas of China (but *substantial risk* in Yunnan and Hainan, see below; *chloroquine prophylaxis* appropriate for other remote areas), Hong Kong, Korea (both Democratic People's Republic and Republic), Malaysia (but *substantial risk* in Sabah, and *variable risk* in deep forests, see below), Sarawak (but *variable risk* in deep forests, see below), Thailand (Bangkok, main tourist centres—**important:** regional risk exists, see under *Great risk*, below):

chemoprophylaxis not recommended but avoid mosquito bites and consider malaria if fever presents

VARIABLE RISK. Risk *variable* and *some chloroquine resistance* in Indonesia (very low risk in Bali, and cities but *substantial risk* in Irian Jaya [West Papua] and Lombok, see below), rural Philippines below 600 m (no risk in cities, Cebu, Bohol, and Catanduanes), deep forests of peninsular Malaysia and Sarawak (but *substantial risk* in Sabah, see below):

chloroquine + proguanil hydrochloride *or* (if chloroquine + proguanil not appropriate) mefloquine *or* *Malarone*®

SUBSTANTIAL RISK. Risk *substantial* and *drug resistance common* in Cambodia (no risk in Phnom Penh; for western provinces, see below), China (Yunnan and Hainan; *chloroquine prophylaxis* appropriate for other remote areas), East Timor, Irian Jaya [West Papua], Laos (no risk in Vientiane), Lombok, Malaysia (Sabah; see also *Very low risk* and *Variable risk* above), Myanmar (formerly Burma; see also *Great risk* below), Vietnam (no risk in cities, Red River delta area, coastal plain north of Nha Trang):

mefloquine *or* doxycycline *or* *Malarone*®

GREAT RISK AND DRUG RESISTANCE PRESENT. Risk *great and mefloquine resistance present* in western provinces of Cambodia, borders of Thailand with Cambodia and Myanmar, and Ko Chang, Myanmar (eastern Shan State):

doxycycline *or* *Malarone*®

Oceania

RISK. Risk *high* and *chloroquine resistance high* in Papua New Guinea (below 1800 m), Solomon Islands, Vanuatu:

doxycycline *or* mefloquine *or* *Malarone*®

Central and South America and the Caribbean

VARIABLE TO LOW RISK. Risk *variable to low* in Argentina (rural areas along northern borders only), rural Belize (except Belize district), rural Costa Rica (below 500 m), Dominican Republic, El Salvador (Santa Ana province in west), Guatemala (below 1500 m), Haiti, Honduras, some rural areas of Mexico (not regularly visited by tourists), Nicaragua, Panama (west of Panama Canal but *variable to high risk* east of Panama Canal, see below), rural Paraguay:

chloroquine *or* (if chloroquine not appropriate) proguanil hydrochloride

VARIABLE TO HIGH RISK. Risk *variable to high* and *chloroquine resistance present* in rural areas of Bolivia (below 2500 m), Ecuador (below 1500 m; no malaria in Galapagos Islands and Guayaquil; see below for Esmeraldas Province), Panama (east of Panama Canal), rural areas of Peru (below 1500 m; see below for Amazon basin area), rural areas of Venezuela (except on coast, Caracas free of malaria):

chloroquine + proguanil hydrochloride *or* (if chloroquine + proguanil not appropriate) mefloquine *or* doxycycline *or* *Malarone*®

HIGH RISK. Risk *high* and *marked chloroquine resistance* in Bolivia (Amazon basin area), Brazil (throughout 'Legal Amazon' area which includes the Amazon basin area, Mato Grosso and Maranhao only; elsewhere *very low risk*—no chemoprophylaxis), Colombia (most areas below 800 m), Ecuador

(Esmeraldas Province), French Guiana, all interior regions of Guyana, Peru (Amazon basin area), Surinam (except Paramaribo and coast), Venezuela (Amazon basin area):

mefloquine *or* doxycycline *or Malarone®*

Standby treatment

> Adults travelling for prolonged periods to areas of chloroquine-resistance who are unlikely to have easy access to medical care should carry a standby treatment course. Self-medication should be **avoided** if medical help is accessible; prophylaxis should be continued during and after the attack.
>
> In order to avoid excessive self-medication, the traveller should be provided with **written instructions** that urgent medical attention should be sought if fever (38°C or more) develops 7 days (or more) after arriving in a malarious area and that self-treatment is indicated if medical help is not immediately available or the condition is worsening.
>
> In view of the continuing emergence of resistant strains and of the different regimens required for different areas expert advice should be sought on the best treatment course for an individual traveller. A drug used for chemoprophylaxis should not be considered for standby treatment for the same traveller.

Artemether with lumefantrine

Artemether with lumefantrine is licensed for the *treatment of acute uncomplicated falciparum malaria.*

ARTEMETHER WITH LUMEFANTRINE

Indications: treatment of acute uncomplicated falciparum malaria; treatment of benign malaria [unlicensed indication]

Cautions: electrolyte disturbances, concomitant use with other drugs known to cause QT-interval prolongation; hepatic impairment (Appendix 2); renal impairment (Appendix 3); pregnancy (Appendix 4); monitor patients unable to take food (greater risk of recrudescence); **interactions:** Appendix 1 (artemether with lumefantrine)

DRIVING. Dizziness may affect performance of skilled tasks (e.g. driving)

Contra-indications: history of arrhythmias, of clinically relevant bradycardia, and of congestive heart failure accompanied by reduced left ventricular ejection fraction; family history of sudden death or of congenital QT interval prolongation; breast-feeding (Appendix 5)

Side-effects: abdominal pain, anorexia, diarrhoea, vomiting, nausea, palpitation, cough, headache, dizziness, sleep disturbances, asthenia, arthralgia, myalgia, pruritus and rash

Dose: see notes above

Riamet® (Novartis) ▼ PoM
Tablets, yellow, artemether 20 mg, lumefantrine 120 mg, net price 24-tab pack = £22.50. Label: 21, counselling, driving

Chloroquine

Chloroquine is used for the *prophylaxis of malaria* in areas of the world where the *risk of chloroquine-resistant falciparum malaria is still low.* It is also used with proguanil when chloroquine-resistant falciparum malaria is present but this regimen may not give optimal protection (see specific recommendations by country, p. 331).

Chloroquine is **no longer recommended** for the *treatment of falciparum malaria* owing to widespread resistance, nor is it recommended if the infective species is *not known* or if the infection is *mixed*; in these cases treatment should be with quinine, *Malarone®*, or *Riamet®* (for details, see p. 328). It is still recommended for the *treatment of benign malarias* (for details, see p. 330).

CHLOROQUINE

Indications: chemoprophylaxis and treatment of malaria, see notes above; rheumatoid arthritis and lupus erythematosus (section 10.1.3)

Cautions: renal impairment (see notes above), pregnancy (but for malaria benefit outweighs risk, see Appendix 4, Antimalarials), may exacerbate psoriasis, neurological disorders (avoid for prophylaxis if history of epilepsy, see notes above), may aggravate myasthenia gravis, severe gastro-intestinal disorders, G6PD deficiency (see section 9.1.5); ophthalmic examination and long-term therapy, see under Chloroquine, section 10.1.3; avoid concurrent therapy with hepatotoxic drugs—other **interactions:** Appendix 1 (chloroquine and hydroxychloroquine)

Side-effects: gastro-intestinal disturbances, headache; also convulsions, visual disturbances, depigmentation or loss of hair, skin reactions (rashes, pruritus); rarely, bone-marrow suppression, hypersensitivity reactions such as urticaria and angioedema; other side-effects (not usually associated with malaria prophylaxis or treatment), see under Chloroquine, section 10.1.3; very toxic in **overdosage**—immediate advice from poisons centres essential (see also p. 32)

Dose: expressed as chloroquine base

Prophylaxis of malaria, preferably started 1 week before entering endemic area and continued for 4 weeks after leaving (see notes above), 300 mg once weekly; INFANT up to 12 weeks body-weight under 6 kg, 37.5 mg once weekly; 12 weeks–11 months body-weight 6–10 kg, 75 mg once weekly; CHILD 1–3 years body-weight 10–16 kg, 112.5 mg once weekly; 4–7 years body-weight 16–25 kg, 150 mg once weekly; 8–12 years body-weight 25–45 kg, 225 mg once weekly; over 13 years body-weight over 45 kg, adult dose

Treatment of malaria, see notes above

COUNSELLING. Warn travellers about **importance** of avoiding mosquito bites, **importance** of taking prophylaxis regularly, and **importance** of immediate visit to doctor if ill within 1 year and **especially** within 3 months of return. For details, see notes above

NOTE. Chloroquine doses in BNF may differ from those in product literature

Chloroquine sulphate (Beacon) PoM
Injection, chloroquine sulphate 54.5 mg/mL (≡ chloroquine base 40 mg/mL), net price 5-mL amp = 79p

[1]**Avloclor**® (AstraZeneca) PoM
Tablets, scored, chloroquine phosphate 250 mg (≡ chloroquine base 155 mg). Net price 20-tab pack = £1.22. Label: 5, counselling, prophylaxis, see above

Malarivon® (Wallace Mfg) PoM
Syrup, chloroquine phosphate 80 mg/5 mL (≡ chloroquine base 50 mg/5 mL), net price 75 mL = £3.35. Label: 5, counselling, prophylaxis, see above

[1]**Nivaquine**® (Beacon)
Tablets, f/c, yellow, chloroquine sulphate 200 mg (≡ chloroquine base 150 mg), net price 28-tab pack = £2.16. Label: 5, counselling, prophylaxis, see above
Syrup, golden, chloroquine sulphate 68 mg/5 mL (≡ chloroquine base 50 mg/5 mL), net price 100 mL = £5.15. Label: 5, counselling, prophylaxis, see above

■ With proguanil
For cautions and side-effects of proguanil see Proguanil; for dose see notes above

Paludrine/Avloclor® (AstraZeneca)
Tablets, travel pack of 14 tablets of chloroquine phosphate 250 mg (≡ chloroquine base 155 mg) and 98 tablets of proguanil hydrochloride 100 mg, net price 112-tab pack = £8.79. Label: 5, 21, counselling, prophylaxis, see above

Mefloquine

Mefloquine is used for the *prophylaxis of malaria* in areas of the world where there is a *high risk of chloroquine-resistant falciparum malaria* (for details, see specific recommendations by country, p. 331).

Mefloquine is now rarely used for the *treatment of falciparum malaria* because of increased resistance (for details, see p. 329). It is effective for the *treatment of benign malarias*, but is not required as chloroquine is usually effective. Mefloquine should not be used for treatment if it has been used for prophylaxis.

The CSM has advised that travellers should be informed about adverse reactions of mefloquine and, if they occur, medical advice should be sought on alternative antimalarials before the next dose is due; the patient information leaflet, which describes adverse reactions should always be provided when dispensing mefloquine.

MEFLOQUINE

Indications: chemoprophylaxis of malaria, treatment of uncomplicated mefloquine-sensitive falciparum malaria (but resistance reported) and chloroquine-resistant vivax malaria, see notes above

Cautions: pregnancy (see notes under Prophylaxis against malaria; Appendix 4)—manufacturer advises **avoid** pregnancy during and for 3 months after; breast-feeding (Appendix 5); avoid for chemoprophylaxis in severe hepatic impairment; cardiac conduction disorders; epilepsy (avoid for prophylaxis); not recommended in infants under 3 months (5 kg); **interactions:** Appendix 1 (mefloquine)

DRIVING. Dizziness or a disturbed sense of balance may affect performance of skilled tasks (e.g. driving); effects may persist for up to 3 weeks

Contra-indications: history of neuropsychiatric disorders, including depression, or convulsions; hypersensitivity to quinine

Side-effects: nausea, vomiting, diarrhoea, abdominal pain; dizziness, loss of balance, headache, sleep disorders (insomnia, drowsiness, abnormal dreams); also neuropsychiatric reactions (including sensory and motor neuropathies, tremor, ataxia, anxiety, depression, suicidal ideation, panic attacks, agitation, hallucinations, psychosis, convulsions), tinnitus and vestibular disorders, visual disturbances, circulatory disorders (hypotension and hypertension), chest pain, tachycardia, bradycardia, cardiac conduction disorders, dyspnoea, muscle weakness, myalgia, arthralgia, rash, urticaria, pruritus, alopecia, asthenia, malaise, fatigue, fever, loss of appetite, leucopenia or leucocytosis, thrombocytopenia; rarely Stevens-Johnson syndrome, AV block, encephalopathy and anaphylaxis

Dose: prophylaxis of malaria, preferably started 2½ weeks before entering endemic area and continued for 4 weeks after leaving (see notes above), ADULT and CHILD body-weight over 45 kg, 250 mg once weekly; body-weight 6–16 kg, 62.5 mg once weekly; body-weight 16–25 kg, 125 mg once weekly; body-weight 25–45 kg, 187.5 mg once weekly

Treatment of malaria, see notes above

COUNSELLING. See CSM advice in notes above. Also warn travellers about **importance** of avoiding mosquito bites, **importance** of taking prophylaxis regularly, and **importance** of immediate visit to doctor if ill within 1 year and **especially** within 3 months of return. For details, see notes above

NOTE. Mefloquine doses in BNF may differ from those in product literature

[2]**Lariam**® (Roche) PoM
Tablets, scored, mefloquine (as hydrochloride) 250 mg. Net price 8-tab pack = £14.53. Label: 21, 25, 27, counselling, driving, prophylaxis, see above

Primaquine

Primaquine is used to eliminate the liver stages of *P. vivax or P. ovale following chloroquine treatment* (for details, see p. 330).

PRIMAQUINE

Indications: adjunct in the treatment of *Plasmodium vivax* and *P. ovale* malaria (eradication of liver stages)

Cautions: G6PD deficiency (test blood, see under Benign Malarias (treatment) above); systemic diseases associated with granulocytopenia (e.g. rheumatoid arthritis, lupus erythematosus);

1. Can be sold to the public provided it is licensed and labelled for the prophylaxis of malaria. Drugs for malaria prophylaxis not prescribable on the NHS; health authorities may investigate circumstances under which antimalarials are prescribed

2. Drugs for malaria prophylaxis not prescribable on the NHS; health authorities may investigate circumstances under which antimalarials prescribed

pregnancy (Appendix 4) and breast-feeding; **interactions:** Appendix 1 (primaquine)

Side-effects: nausea, vomiting, anorexia, abdominal pain; less commonly methaemoglobinaemia, haemolytic anaemia especially in G6PD deficiency, leucopenia

Dose: see notes above

Primaquine (Non-proprietary)
Tablets, primaquine (as phosphate) 7.5 mg or 15 mg
Available on a named-patient basis from Durbin, IDIS

Proguanil

Proguanil is used (usually *with chloroquine*, but occasionally *alone*) for the *prophylaxis of malaria*, (for details, see specific recommendations by country, p. 331).

Proguanil used alone is not suitable for the *treatment of malaria*; *Malarone*® (a combination of atovaquone with proguanil) is, however, licensed for the treatment of acute uncomplicated falciparum malaria. *Malarone*® is also used for the *prophylaxis of falciparum malaria* in areas of *widespread mefloquine or chloroquine resistance*. *Malarone*® is also used as an alternative to mefloquine or doxycycline. *Malarone*® is particularly suitable for short trips to highly chloroquine-resistant areas because it needs to be taken only for 7 days after leaving an endemic area.

PROGUANIL HYDROCHLORIDE

Indications: chemoprophylaxis of malaria

Cautions: renal impairment (see notes under Prophylaxis against malaria and Appendix 3); pregnancy (folate supplements needed); **interactions:** Appendix 1 (proguanil)

Side-effects: mild gastric intolerance, diarrhoea and constipation; occasionally mouth ulcers and stomatitis; *very rarely* cholestasis, vasculitis, skin reactions and hair loss

Dose: prophylaxis of malaria, preferably started 1 week before entering endemic area and continued for 4 weeks after leaving (see notes above), 200 mg once daily; INFANT up to 12 weeks body-weight under 6 kg, 25 mg once daily; 12 weeks–11 months body-weight 6–10 kg, 50 mg once daily; CHILD 1–3 years body-weight 10–16 kg, 75 mg once daily; 4–7 years body-weight 16–25 kg, 100 mg once daily; 8–12 years, body-weight 25–45 kg, 150 mg once daily; over 13 years body-weight over 45 kg, adult dose

COUNSELLING. Warn travellers about **importance** of avoiding mosquito bites, **importance** of taking prophylaxis regularly, and **importance** of immediate visit to doctor if ill within 1 year and **especially** within 3 months of return. For details, see notes above

NOTE. Proguanil doses in BNF may differ from those in product literature

[1]**Paludrine**® (AstraZeneca)
Tablets, scored, proguanil hydrochloride 100 mg. Net price 98-tab pack = £7.43. Label: 21, counselling, prophylaxis, see above

■ With chloroquine
See under Chloroquine

1. Drugs for malaria prophylaxis not prescribable on the NHS; health authorities may investigate circumstances under which antimalarials prescribed

PROGUANIL HYDROCHLORIDE WITH ATOVAQUONE

Indications: treatment of acute uncomplicated falciparum malaria and prophylaxis of falciparum malaria, particularly where resistance to other antimalarial drugs suspected; treatment of benign malaria [unlicensed indication]

Cautions: renal impairment (Appendix 3), diarrhoea or vomiting (reduced absorption of atovaquone), pregnancy (Appendix 4) and breast-feeding (Appendix 5); efficacy not evaluated in cerebral or complicated malaria (including hyperparasitaemia, pulmonary oedema or renal failure); **interactions:** see Appendix 1 (proguanil, atovaquone)

Side-effects: nausea, vomiting, mouth ulcers and stomatitis, diarrhoea, abdominal pain, anorexia, fever; headache, dizziness, abnormal dreams, insomnia, cough, visual disturbances, pruritus, rash, blood disorders, hyponatraemia, and hair loss reported

Dose: see under preparation

COUNSELLING. Warn travellers about **importance** of avoiding mosquito bites, **importance** of taking prophylaxis regularly, and **importance** of immediate visit to doctor if ill within 1 year and **especially** within 3 months of return. For details, see notes above

[1]**Malarone**® (GSK) PoM
Tablets ('standard'), pink, f/c, proguanil hydrochloride 100 mg, atovaquone 250 mg. Net price 12-tab pack = £22.92. Label: 21, counselling, prophylaxis, see below
Dose: prophylaxis of malaria, started 1–2 days before entering endemic area and continued for 1 week after leaving, ADULT and CHILD over 40 kg, 1 tablet daily
Treatment of malaria, ADULT and CHILD body-weight over 40 kg, 4 tablets once daily for 3 days; CHILD body-weight 11–20 kg 1 tablet daily for 3 days; body-weight 21–30 kg 2 tablets once daily for 3 days; body-weight 31–40 kg 3 tablets once daily for 3 days

[1]**Malarone**® **Paediatric** (GSK) ▼ PoM
Paediatric tablets, pink, f/c proguanil hydrochloride 25 mg, atovaquone 62.5 mg, net price 12-tab pack = £7.64. Label: 21, counselling, prophylaxis, see above
Dose: prophylaxis of malaria, started 1–2 days before entering endemic area and continued for 1 week after leaving, CHILD body-weight 11–20 kg, 1 tablet once daily; body-weight 21–30 kg, 2 tablets once daily; body-weight 31–40 kg, 3 tablets once daily; body-weight over 40 kg use *Malarone*® ('standard') tablets, see p. 331
Treatment of malaria, see above

Pyrimethamine

Pyrimethamine should not be used alone, but is used with sulfadoxine (in *Fansidar*®).

Fansidar® is not recommended for the *prophylaxis of malaria*, but it is used in the treatment of *falciparum malaria* and can be used *with (or following) quinine*.

PYRIMETHAMINE

Indications: malaria (but used only in combined preparations incorporating sulfadoxine); toxoplasmosis—section 5.4.7

Cautions: hepatic or renal impairment, pregnancy (Appendix 4); breast-feeding (Appendix 5); blood counts required with prolonged treatment; history of seizures—avoid large loading doses; **interactions:** Appendix 1 (pyrimethamine)

Side-effects: depression of haematopoiesis with high doses, rashes, insomnia

Dose: malaria, no dose stated because not recommended alone

Toxoplasmosis, section 5.4.7

Daraprim® (GSK) PoM
Tablets, scored, pyrimethamine 25 mg. Net price 30-tab pack = £2.17

PYRIMETHAMINE WITH SULFADOXINE

Indications: adjunct to quinine in treatment of *Plasmodium falciparum* malaria (see notes above); **not** recommended for prophylaxis

Cautions: see under Pyrimethamine and under Co-trimoxazole (section 5.1.8); pregnancy (Appendix 4); breast-feeding (Appendix 5); not recommended for prophylaxis (severe side-effects on long-term use); **interactions:** Appendix 1 (pyrimethamine, sulphonamides)

Contra-indications: see under Pyrimethamine and under Co-trimoxazole (section 5.1.8); sulphonamide allergy

Side-effects: see under Pyrimethamine and under Co-trimoxazole (section 5.1.8); pulmonary infiltrates (e.g. eosinophilic or allergic alveolitis) reported—discontinue if cough or shortness of breath

Dose: treatment, see notes above

Prophylaxis, not recommended by UK malaria experts

Fansidar® (Roche) PoM
Tablets, scored, pyrimethamine 25 mg, sulfadoxine 500 mg, net price 3-tab pack = 74p

Quinine

Quinine is not suitable for the *prophylaxis of malaria*.

Quinine is used for the *treatment of falciparum malaria* or if the infective species is *not known* or if the infection is *mixed* (for details see p. 328).

QUININE

Indications: falciparum malaria; nocturnal leg cramps, see section 10.2.2

Cautions: atrial fibrillation, conduction defects, heart block, pregnancy (but appropriate for treatment of malaria; Appendix 4); monitor blood glucose and electrolyte concentration during parenteral treatment; G6PD deficiency (see section 9.1.5); **interactions:** Appendix 1 (quinine)

Contra-indications: haemoglobinuria, myasthenia gravis, optic neuritis

Side-effects: cinchonism, including tinnitus, headache, hot and flushed skin, nausea, abdominal pain, rashes, visual disturbances (including temporary blindness), confusion; hypersensitivity reactions including angioedema, blood disorders (including thrombocytopenia and intravascular coagulation), and acute renal failure; hypoglycaemia (especially after parenteral administration); cardiovascular effects (see Cautions); very toxic in **overdosage**—immediate advice from poisons centres essential (see also p. 32)

Dose: see notes above

NOTE. Quinine (anhydrous base) 100 mg ≡ quinine bisulphate 169 mg ≡ quinine dihydrochloride 122 mg ≡ quinine hydrochloride 122 mg ≡ quinine sulphate 121 mg. Quinine bisulphate 300-mg tablets are available but provide less quinine than 300 mg of the dihydrochloride, hydrochloride, or sulphate

Quinine Sulphate (Non-proprietary) PoM
Tablets, coated, quinine sulphate 200 mg, net price 28-tab pack = £2.07; 300 mg, 28-tab pack = £2.72

Quinine Dihydrochloride (Non-proprietary) PoM
Injection, quinine dihydrochloride 300 mg/mL. For dilution and use as an infusion. 1- and 2-mL amps
'Special order' product; contact Martindale or specialist centres (see p. 328)
NOTE. Intravenous injection of quinine is so hazardous that it has been superseded by infusion

Tetracyclines

Doxycycline (section 5.1.3) is used for the *prophylaxis of malaria* in areas of *widespread mefloquine or chloroquine resistance*. Doxycycline is also used as an alternative to mefloquine or *Malarone*® (for details, see specific recommendations by country, p. 331).

Doxycycline is also used as an *adjunct to quinine in the treatment of falciparum malaria* (for details see p. 329).

DOXYCYCLINE

Indications: prophylaxis of malaria; adjunct to quinine in treatment of *Plasmodium falciparum* malaria; see also section 5.1.3

Cautions: section 5.1.3

Contra-indications: section 5.1.3

Side-effects: section 5.1.3

Dose: prophylaxis of malaria, preferably started 1 week before entering endemic area and continued for 4 weeks after leaving (see notes above), 100 mg once daily

Treatment of falciparum malaria, see notes above

■ Preparations
Section 5.1.3

5.4.2 Amoebicides

Metronidazole is the drug of choice for *acute invasive amoebic dysentery* since it is very effective against vegetative forms of *Entamoeba histolytica* in ulcers; it is given in an adult dose of 800 mg three times daily for 5 days. **Tinidazole** is also effective. Metronidazole and tinidazole are also active against amoebae which may have migrated to the liver. Treatment with metronidazole (or tinidazole) is followed by a 10-day course of diloxanide furoate.

Diloxanide furoate is the drug of choice for asymptomatic patients with *E. histolytica* cysts in the faeces; metronidazole and tinidazole are relatively ineffective. Diloxanide furoate is relatively free from toxic effects and the usual course is of 10 days, given alone for chronic infections or following metronidazole or tinidazole treatment.

For *amoebic abscesses* of the liver **metronidazole** is effective in doses of 400 mg 3 times daily for 5–10 days; tinidazole is an alternative. The course may be repeated after 2 weeks if necessary. Aspiration of the abscess is indicated where it is suspected that it may rupture or where there is no improvement after 72 hours of metronidazole; the aspiration may need to be repeated. Aspiration aids penetration of metronidazole and, for abscesses with more than 100 mL of pus, if carried out in conjunction with drug therapy, may reduce the period of disability.

Diloxanide furoate is not effective against hepatic amoebiasis, but a 10-day course should be given at the completion of metronidazole or tinidazole treatment to destroy any amoebae in the gut.

DILOXANIDE FUROATE

Indications: see notes above; chronic amoebiasis and as adjunct to metronidazole or tinidazole in acute amoebiasis

Contra-indications: pregnancy (Appendix 4), breast-feeding (Appendix 5)

Side-effects: flatulence, vomiting, urticaria, pruritus

Dose: 500 mg every 8 hours for 10 days; CHILD over 25 kg, 20 mg/kg daily in 3 divided doses for 10 days

See also notes above

Diloxanide (Sovereign) PoM

Tablets, diloxanide furoate 500 mg, net price 30-tab pack = £32.95. Label: 9

METRONIDAZOLE

Indications: see under Dose below; anaerobic infections, section 5.1.11

Cautions: section 5.1.11

Side-effects: section 5.1.11

Dose: *by mouth*, invasive intestinal amoebiasis, 800 mg every 8 hours for 5 days; CHILD 1–3 years 200 mg every 8 hours; 3–7 years 200 mg every 6 hours; 7–10 years 400 mg every 8 hours

Extra-intestinal amoebiasis (including liver abscess) and symptomless amoebic cyst passers, 400–800 mg every 8 hours for 5–10 days; CHILD 1–3 years 100–200 mg every 8 hours; 3–7 years 100–200 mg every 6 hours; 7–10 years 200–400 mg every 8 hours

Urogenital trichomoniasis, 200 mg every 8 hours for 7 days *or* 400–500 mg every 12 hours for 5–7 days, *or* 2 g as a single dose; CHILD 1–3 years 50 mg every 8 hours for 7 days; 3–7 years 100 mg every 12 hours; 7–10 years 100 mg every 8 hours

Giardiasis, 2 g daily for 3 days *or* 400 mg 3 times daily for 5 days *or* 500 mg twice daily for 7–10 days; CHILD 1–3 years 500 mg daily for 3 days; 3–7 years 600–800 mg daily; 7–10 years 1 g daily

■ Preparations

Section 5.1.11

TINIDAZOLE

Indications: see under Dose below; anaerobic infections, section 5.1.11

Cautions: section 5.1.11

Side-effects: section 5.1.11

Dose: intestinal amoebiasis, 2 g daily for 2–3 days; CHILD 50–60 mg/kg daily for 3 days

Amoebic involvement of liver, 1.5–2 g daily for 3–6 days; CHILD 50–60 mg/kg daily for 5 days

Urogenital trichomoniasis and giardiasis, single 2 g dose; CHILD single dose of 50–75 mg/kg (repeated once if necessary)

■ Preparations

Section 5.1.11

5.4.3 Trichomonacides

Metronidazole (section 5.4.2) is the treatment of choice for *Trichomonas vaginalis* infection. Contact tracing is recommended and sexual contacts should be treated simultaneously.

If metronidazole is ineffective, **tinidazole** may be tried; it is usually given as a single 2-g dose, with food. A further 2-g dose may be given if there is no clinical improvement.

5.4.4 Antigiardial drugs

Metronidazole (section 5.4.2) is the treatment of choice for *Giardia lamblia* infections, given by mouth in a dosage of 2 g daily for 3 days or 400 mg every 8 hours for 5 days.

Alternative treatments are **tinidazole** (section 5.4.2) 2 g as a single dose or **mepacrine hydrochloride** 100 mg every 8 hours for 5–7 days [unlicensed indication].

MEPACRINE HYDROCHLORIDE

Indications: giardiasis; discoid lupus erythematosus (Antimalarials, section 10.1.3)

Cautions: hepatic impairment, elderly, history of psychosis; avoid in psoriasis; **interactions:** Appendix 1 (mepacrine)

Side-effects: gastro-intestinal disturbances; dizziness, headache; with large doses nausea, vomiting and occasionally transient acute toxic psychosis and CNS stimulation; on prolonged treatment yellow discoloration of skin and urine, chronic dermatoses (including severe exfoliative dermatitis), hepatitis, aplastic anaemia; also reported blue/black discoloration of palate and nails and corneal deposits with visual disturbances

Dose: giardiasis, 100 mg every 8 hours for 5–7 days; CHILD 2 mg/kg every 8 hours

Mepacrine Hydrochloride

Tablets, mepacrine hydrochloride 100 mg. Label: 4, 9, 14, 21

Available from BCM Specials [unlicensed—special order]

5.4.5 Leishmaniacides

Cutaneous leishmaniasis frequently heals spontaneously but if skin lesions are extensive or unsightly, treatment is indicated, as it is in visceral leishmaniasis (kala-azar).

Sodium stibogluconate, an organic pentavalent antimony compound, is the treatment of choice for visceral leishmaniasis. The dose is 20 mg/kg daily (max. 850 mg) for at least 20 days by intramuscular or intravenous injection; the dosage varies with different geographical regions and expert advice should be obtained. Skin lesions are treated for 10 days.

Amphotericin is used with or after an antimony compound for visceral leishmaniasis unresponsive to the antimonial alone; side-effects may be reduced by using liposomal amphotericin (*AmBisome*®—section 5.2) at a dose of 1–3 mg/kg daily for 10–21 days to a cumulative dose of 21–30 mg/kg. Other lipid formulations of amphotericin (*Abelcet*® and *Amphocil*®) are also likely to be effective but less information is available.

Pentamidine isetionate (pentamidine isethionate) (section 5.4.8) has been used in antimony-resistant visceral leishmaniasis, but although the initial response is often good, the relapse rate is high; it is associated with serious side-effects. Other treatments include paromomycin (available on named-patient basis from IDIS).

SODIUM STIBOGLUCONATE

Indications: leishmaniasis

Cautions: hepatic impairment; pregnancy; intravenous injections must be given slowly over 5 minutes (to reduce risk of local thrombosis) and stopped if coughing or substernal pain; mucocutaneous disease (see below); monitor ECG before and during treatment; heart disease (withdraw if conduction disturbances occur); treat intercurrent infection (e.g. pneumonia)

MUCOCUTANEOUS DISEASE. Successful treatment of mucocutaneous leishmaniasis may induce severe inflammation around the lesions (may be life-threatening if pharyngeal or tracheal involvement)—may require corticosteroid

Contra-indications: significant renal impairment; breast-feeding

Side-effects: anorexia, nausea, vomiting, abdominal pain, diarrhoea; ECG changes; coughing (see Cautions); headache, lethargy; arthralgia, myalgia; *rarely* jaundice, flushing, bleeding from nose or gum, substernal pain (see Cautions), vertigo, fever, sweating, and rash; also reported pancreatitis and anaphylaxis; pain and thrombosis on intravenous administration, intramuscular injection also painful

Dose: see notes above

Pentostam® (GSK) PoM

Injection, sodium stibogluconate equivalent to pentavalent antimony 100 mg/mL. Net price 100-mL bottle = £66.43

5.4.6 Trypanocides

The prophylaxis and treatment of trypanosomiasis is difficult and differs according to the strain of organism. Expert advice should therefore be obtained.

5.4.7 Drugs for toxoplasmosis

Most infections caused by *Toxoplasma gondii* are self-limiting, and treatment is not necessary. Exceptions are patients with eye involvement (toxoplasma choroidoretinitis), and those who are immunosuppressed. Toxoplasmic encephalitis is a common complication of AIDS. The treatment of choice is a combination of pyrimethamine and sulfadiazine (sulphadiazine), given for several weeks (expert advice **essential**). Pyrimethamine is a folate antagonist, and adverse reactions to this combination are relatively common (folinic acid supplements and weekly blood counts needed). Alternative regimens use combinations of pyrimethamine with clindamycin or clarithromycin or azithromycin. Long-term secondary prophylaxis is required after treatment of toxoplasmosis in AIDS.

If toxoplasmosis is acquired in pregnancy, transplacental infection may lead to severe disease in the fetus. Spiramycin (available on named-patient basis from IDIS) may reduce the risk of transmission of maternal infection to the fetus.

5.4.8 Drugs for pneumocystis pneumonia

Pneumonia caused by *Pneumocystis carinii* occurs in immunosuppressed patients; it is a common cause of pneumonia in AIDS. Pneumocystis pneumonia should generally be treated by those experienced in its management. Blood gas measurement is used to assess disease severity.

Treatment

MILD TO MODERATE DISEASE. **Co-trimoxazole** (section 5.1.8) in high dosage is the drug of choice for the treatment of mild to moderate pneumocystis pneumonia.

Atovaquone is licensed for the treatment of mild to moderate pneumocystis infection in patients who cannot tolerate co-trimoxazole. A combination of **dapsone** 100 mg daily (section 5.1.10) with **trimethoprim** 5 mg/kg every 6–8 hours (section 5.1.8) is given by mouth for the treatment of mild to moderate disease [unlicensed indication].

A combination of **clindamycin** 600 mg by mouth every 8 hours (section 5.1.6) and **primaquine** 30 mg daily by mouth (section 5.4.1) is used in the treatment of mild to moderate disease [unlicensed indication]; this combination is associated with considerable toxicity.

Inhaled **pentamidine isetionate** is sometimes used for mild disease. It is better tolerated than parenteral pentamidine but systemic absorption may still occur.

SEVERE DISEASE. **Co-trimoxazole** (section 5.1.8) in high dosage, given by mouth or by intravenous infusion, is the drug of choice for the treatment of severe pneumocystis pneumonia. **Pentamidine isetionate** given by intravenous infusion is an alternative for patients who cannot tolerate co-trimoxazole, or who have not responded to it. Pentamidine isetionate is a potentially toxic drug that can cause severe hypotension during or immediately after infusion.

Corticosteroid treatment can be lifesaving in those with severe pneumocystis pneumonia (see Adjunctive Therapy below).

ADJUNCTIVE THERAPY. In moderate to severe infections associated with HIV infection, prednisolone 50–80 mg daily is given by mouth for 5 days (alternatively, hydrocortisone may be given parenterally); the dose is then reduced to complete 21 days of treatment. Corticosteroid treatment should ideally be started at the same time as the anti-pneumocystis therapy and certainly no later than 24–72 hours afterwards. The corticosteroid should be withdrawn before anti-pneumocystis treatment is complete.

Prophylaxis

Prophylaxis against pneumocystis pneumonia should be given to all patients with a history of the infection. Prophylaxis against pneumocystis pneumonia should also be considered for severely immunocompromised patients. Prophylaxis should continue until immunity recovers sufficiently. It should not be discontinued if the patient has oral candidiasis, continues to lose weight, or is receiving cytotoxic therapy or long-term immunosuppressant therapy.

Co-trimoxazole by mouth is the drug of choice for prophylaxis against pneumocystis pneumonia. It is given in a dose of 960 mg daily or 960 mg on alternate days (3 times a week); the dose may be reduced to co-trimoxazole 480 mg daily to improve tolerance.

Intermittent inhalation of **pentamidine isetionate** is used for prophylaxis against penumocystis pneumonia in patients unable to tolerate co-trimoxazole. It is effective but patients may be prone to extrapulmonary infection. Alternatively, **dapsone** 100 mg daily (section 5.1.10) can be used. **Atovaquone** 750 mg twice daily has also been used for prophylaxis [unlicensed indication].

ATOVAQUONE

Indications: treatment of mild to moderate *Pneumocystis carinii* pneumonia in patients intolerant of co-trimoxazole

Cautions: initial diarrhoea and difficulty in taking with food may reduce absorption (and require alternative therapy); other causes of pulmonary disease should be sought and treated; elderly; hepatic impairment (Appendix 2); renal impairment (Appendix 3); pregnancy (Appendix 4); avoid breast-feeding (Appendix 5); **interactions:** Appendix 1 (atovaquone)

Side-effects: nausea, rash; commonly diarrhoea, vomiting, headache, insomnia; fever, anaemia, neutropenia, hyponatraemia

Dose: 750 mg twice daily with food (particularly high fat) for 21 days; CHILD not recommended

Wellvone® (GSK) PoM

Suspension, sugar-free, fruit-flavoured, atovaquone 750 mg/5 mL, net price 210 mL = £405.31. Label: 21

■ With proguanil hydrochloride

See section 5.4.1

PENTAMIDINE ISETIONATE

Indications: see under Dose (should only be given by specialists)

Cautions: risk of severe hypotension following administration (establish baseline blood pressure and administer with patient lying down; monitor blood pressure closely during administration, and at regular intervals, until treatment concluded); hepatic impairment; renal impairment (Appendix 3); hypertension or hypotension; hyperglycaemia or hypoglycaemia; leucopenia, thrombocytopenia, or anaemia; pregnancy (Appendix 4); breast-feeding (Appendix 5); carry out laboratory monitoring according to product literature; care required to protect personnel during handling and administration; **interactions:** Appendix 1 (pentamidine isetionate)

Side-effects: severe reactions, sometimes fatal, due to hypotension, hypoglycaemia, pancreatitis, and arrhythmias; also leucopenia, thrombocytopenia, acute renal failure, hypocalcaemia; also reported: azotaemia, abnormal liver-function tests, anaemia, hyperkalaemia, nausea and vomiting, dizziness, syncope, flushing, hyperglycaemia, rash, and taste disturbances; Stevens-Johnson syndrome reported; on inhalation, bronchoconstriction (may be prevented by prior use of bronchodilators), cough, shortness of breath, and wheezing; discomfort, pain, induration, abscess formation, and muscle necrosis at injection site

Dose: *Pneumocystis carinii* pneumonia, *by intravenous infusion*, 4 mg/kg daily for at least 14 days (reduced according to product literature in renal impairment)

By inhalation of nebulised solution (using suitable equipment—consult product literature) 600 mg pentamidine isetionate daily for 3 weeks; secondary prevention, 300 mg every 4 weeks *or* 150 mg every 2 weeks

Visceral leishmaniasis (kala-azar, section 5.4.5), *by deep intramuscular injection*, 3–4 mg/kg on alternate days to max. total of 10 injections; course may be repeated if necessary

Cutaneous leishmaniasis, *by deep intramuscular injection*, 3–4 mg/kg once or twice weekly until condition resolves (but see also section 5.4.5)

Trypanosomiasis, *by deep intramuscular injection or intravenous infusion*, 4 mg/kg daily or on alternate days to total of 7–10 injections

NOTE. Direct bolus intravenous injection should be avoided whenever possible and **never** given rapidly; intramuscular injections should be deep and preferably given into the buttock

Pentacarinat® (JHC) PoM

Injection, powder for reconstitution, pentamidine isetionate, net price 300-mg vial = £30.45

Nebuliser solution, pentamidine isetionate, net price 300-mg bottle = £32.15

CAUTION IN HANDLING. Pentamidine isetionate is toxic and personnel should be adequately protected during handling and administration—consult product literature

5.5 Anthelmintics

Advice on prophylaxis and treatment of helminth infections is available from:

Birmingham	(0121) 424 0357
Scottish Centre for Infection and Environmental Health (registered users of Travax only)	(0141) 300 1130 (weekdays 2–4 p.m. only)
Liverpool	(0151) 708 9393
London	(020) 7387 9300 (treatment)

5.5.1 Drugs for threadworms
(pinworms, *Enterobius vermicularis*)

Anthelmintics are effective in threadworm infections, but their use needs to be combined with hygienic measures to break the cycle of auto-infection. All members of the family require treatment.

Adult threadworms do not live for longer than 6 weeks and for development of fresh worms, ova must be swallowed and exposed to the action of digestive juices in the upper intestinal tract. Direct multiplication of worms does not take place in the large bowel. Adult female worms lay ova on the perianal skin which causes pruritus; scratching the area then leads to ova being transmitted on fingers to the mouth, often via food eaten with unwashed hands. Washing hands and scrubbing nails before each meal and after each visit to the toilet is essential. A bath taken immediately after rising will remove ova laid during the night.

Mebendazole is the drug of choice for treating threadworm infection in patients of all ages over 2 years. It is given as a single dose; as reinfection is very common, a second dose may be given after 2 weeks.

Piperazine is available in combination with sennosides as a single-dose preparation.

MEBENDAZOLE

Indications: threadworm, roundworm, whipworm, and hookworm infections

Cautions: pregnancy (toxicity in *rats*); breast-feeding (Appendix 5); **interactions:** Appendix 1 (mebendazole)

NOTE. The package insert in the *Vermox*® pack includes the statement that it is not suitable for women known to be pregnant or children under 2 years

Side-effects: rarely abdominal pain, diarrhoea; hypersensitivity reactions (including exanthema, rash, urticaria, and angioedema) reported

Dose: threadworms, ADULT and CHILD over 2 years, 100 mg as a single dose; if reinfection occurs second dose may be needed after 2 weeks; CHILD under 2 years, not yet recommended

Whipworms, ADULT and CHILD over 2 years, 100 mg twice daily for 3 days; CHILD under 2 years, not yet recommended

Roundworms—section 5.5.2

Hookworms—section 5.5.4

[1]**Mebendazole** (Non-proprietary) PoM

Tablets, chewable, mebendazole 100 mg

1. Can be sold to the public if supplied for oral use in the treatment of enterobiasis in adults and children over 2 years provided its container or package is labelled to show a max. single dose of 100 mg and it is supplied in a container or package containing not more than 800 mg; proprietary brands on sale to the public include *Boots Threadworm Tablets 2 Years Plus*®, *Ovex*® and *Pripsen*® *Mebendazole*

Vermox® (Janssen-Cilag) PoM

Tablets, orange, scored, chewable, mebendazole 100 mg. Net price 6-tab pack = £1.45

Suspension, mebendazole 100 mg/5 mL. Net price 30 mL = £1.68

PIPERAZINE

Indications: threadworm and roundworm infections

Cautions: liver impairment (Appendix 2); renal impairment (Appendix 3); epilepsy; pregnancy (Appendix 4); packs on sale to the general public carry a warning to avoid in epilepsy, or in liver or kidney disease, and to seek medical advice in pregnancy; breast-feeding (Appendix 5)

Side-effects: nausea, vomiting, colic, diarrhoea, allergic reactions including urticaria, bronchospasm, and rare reports of arthralgia, fever, Stevens-Johnson syndrome and angioedema; rarely dizziness, muscular incoordination ('worm wobble'); drowsiness, nystagmus, vertigo, blurred vision, confusion and clonic contractions in patients with neurological or renal abnormalities

Dose: see under Preparation, below

Piperazine Citrate (Non-proprietary)

Syrup, piperazine hydrate 750 mg/5 mL (as citrate)
Brands include *Ascalix*®
Dose: consult product literature

Syrup, piperazine hydrate 4 g/30 mL (as citrate)
Brands include *Ascalix*®
Dose: consult product literature

■ With sennosides

For cautions, contra-indications, side-effects of senna see section 1.6.2

Pripsen® (Thornton & Ross)

Oral powder, piperazine phosphate 4 g, total sennosides (calculated as sennoside B) 15.3 mg/sachet. Net price two-dose sachet pack = £1.36. Label: 13

Dose: threadworms, stirred into milk or water, ADULT and CHILD over 6 years, content of 1 sachet as a single dose (bedtime in adults or morning in children), repeated after 14 days; INFANT 3 months–1 year, 1 level 2.5-mL spoonful in the morning, repeated after 14 days; CHILD 1–6 years, 1 level 5-mL spoonful in the morning, repeated after 14 days

Roundworms, first dose as for threadworms; repeat at monthly intervals for up to 3 months if reinfection risk

5.5.2 Ascaricides
(common roundworm infections)

Levamisole (available on named-patient basis from IDIS) is very effective against *Ascaris lumbricoides* and is generally considered to be the drug of choice. It is very well tolerated; mild nausea or vomiting has been reported in about 1% of treated patients; it is given as a single dose of 120–150 mg in adults.

Mebendazole (section 5.5.1) is also active against ascaris; the usual dose is 100 mg twice daily for 3 days. **Piperazine** may be given in a single adult dose, see Piperazine, above.

5.5.3 Drugs for tapeworm infections

Taenicides

Niclosamide (available on named-patient basis from IDIS) is the most widely used drug for tapeworm infections and side-effects are limited to occasional gastro-intestinal upset, lightheadedness, and pruritus; it is not effective against larval worms. Fears of developing cysticercosis in *Taenia solium* infections have proved unfounded. All the same, it is wise to anticipate this possibility by using an anti-emetic on wakening.

Praziquantel (available on named-patient basis from Merck (*Cysticide*®)) is as effective as niclosamide and is given as a single dose of 10–20 mg/kg after a light breakfast (a single dose of 25 mg/kg for *Hymenolepis nana*).

Hydatid disease

Cysts caused by *Echinococcus granulosus* grow slowly and asymptomatic patients do not always require treatment. Surgical treatment remains the method of choice in many situations. **Albendazole** (available on named-patient basis from IDIS (*Zentel*®)) is used in conjunction with surgery to reduce the risk of recurrence or as primary treatment in inoperable cases. Alveolar echinococcosis due to *E. multilocularis* is usually fatal if untreated. Surgical removal with albendazole cover is the treatment of choice, but where effective surgery is impossible, repeated cycles of albendazole (for a year or more) may help. Careful monitoring of liver function is particularly important during drug treatment.

5.5.4 Drugs for hookworms
(ancylostomiasis, necatoriasis)

Hookworms live in the upper small intestine and draw blood from the point of their attachment to their host. An iron-deficiency anaemia may thereby be produced and, if present, effective treatment of the infection requires not only expulsion of the worms but treatment of the anaemia.

Mebendazole (section 5.5.1) has a useful broad-spectrum activity, and is effective against hookworms; the usual dose is 100 mg twice daily for 3 days.

5.5.5 Schistosomicides
(bilharziasis)

Adult *Schistosoma haematobium* worms live in the genito-urinary veins and adult *S. mansoni* in those of the colon and mesentery. *S. japonicum* is more widely distributed in veins of the alimentary tract and portal system.

Praziquantel (available on named-patient basis from Merck (*Cysticide*®)) is effective against all human schistosomes. The dose is 40 mg/kg in 2 divided doses 4–6 hours apart on one day (60 mg/kg in 3 divided doses on one day for *S. japonicum* infections). No serious toxic effects have been reported. Of all the available schistosomicides, it has the most attractive combination of effectiveness, broad-spectrum activity, and low toxicity.

Hycanthone, lucanthone, niridazole, oxamniquine, and sodium stibocaptate have now been superseded.

5.5.6 Filaricides

Diethylcarbamazine (not on UK market) is effective against microfilariae and adults of *Loa loa*, *Wuchereria bancrofti*, and *Brugia malayi*. To minimise reactions treatment is commenced with a dose of diethylcarbamazine citrate 1 mg/kg on the first day and increased gradually over 3 days to 6 mg/kg daily in divided doses; this dosage is maintained for 21 days and usually gives a radical cure for these infections. Close medical supervision is necessary particularly in the early phase of treatment.

In heavy infections there may be a febrile reaction, and in heavy *Loa loa* infection there is a small risk of encephalopathy. In such cases treatment must be given under careful in-patient supervision and stopped at the first sign of cerebral involvement (and specialist advice sought).

Ivermectin (available on named-patient basis from IDIS) is very effective in *onchocerciasis* and it is now the drug of choice. A single dose of 150 micrograms/kg by mouth produces a prolonged reduction in microfilarial levels. Retreatment at intervals of 6 to 12 months depending on symptoms must be given until the adult worms die out. Reactions are usually slight and most commonly take the form of temporary aggravation of itching and rash. Diethylcarbamazine or suramin should no longer be used for onchocerciasis because of their toxicity.

5.5.7 Drugs for cutaneous larva migrans
(creeping eruption)

Dog and cat hookworm larvae may enter human skin where they produce slowly extending itching tracks usually on the foot. Single tracks can be treated with topical tiabendazole (no commercial preparation available). Multiple infections respond to **ivermectin** (available on named-patient basis from IDIS), **albendazole** (available on named-patient basis from IDIS (*Zentel*®)) or **tiabendazole** (thiabendazole) (available on a named-patient basis from IDIS (*Mintezol*®, *Triasox*®)) by mouth.

5.5.8 Drugs for strongyloidiasis

Adult *Strongyloides stercoralis* live in the gut and produce larvae which penetrate the gut wall and invade the tissues, setting up a cycle of auto-infection. **Tiabendazole** (thiabendazole) (available on a named-patient basis from IDIS (*Mintezol*®, *Triasox*®)) is the drug of choice for adults (but side-effects are much more marked in the elderly); it is given at a dosage of 25 mg/kg (max. 1.5 g) every 12 hours for 3 days. **Albendazole** is an alternative (available on named-patient basis from IDIS (*Zentel*®)) with fewer side-effects; it is given in a dose of 400 mg twice daily for 3 days, repeated after 3 weeks if necessary. **Ivermectin** (available on named-patient basis from IDIS) in a dose of 200 micrograms/kg daily for 2 days may be the most effective drug for chronic *Strongyloides* infection.

6: Endocrine system

6.1 Drugs used in diabetes

Diabetes mellitus occurs because of a lack of insulin or resistance to its action. Diabetes is clinically defined by measurement of fasting or random blood-glucose concentration (and occasionally by glucose tolerance test). There are two principal classes of diabetes (and many subtypes not listed here):

TYPE 1 DIABETES. Type 1 diabetes, also referred to as insulin-dependent diabetes mellitus (IDDM), is due to a deficiency of insulin following autoimmune destruction of pancreatic beta cells. Patients with type 1 diabetes require administration of insulin.

TYPE 2 DIABETES. Type 2 diabetes, also referred to as non-insulin-dependent diabetes (NIDDM), is due to reduced secretion of insulin or to peripheral resistance to the action of insulin. Although patients may be controlled on diet alone, many require oral antidiabetic drugs or insulin to maintain satisfactory control. In overweight individuals, type 2 diabetes may be prevented by losing weight and increasing physical activity; use of drugs such as orlistat (section 4.5.1) may be considered in obese patients.

Treatment should be aimed at alleviating symptoms and minimising the risk of long-term complications by appropriate control of diabetes. Other risk factors for cardiovascular disease such as smoking (section 4.10), hypertension (section 2.5), obesity (section 4.5), and hyperlipidaemia (section 2.12) should be addressed.

Diabetes is a strong risk factor for cardiovascular disease. The use of an ACE inhibitor (section 2.5.5.1), of low-dose aspirin (section 2.9) and of a lipid-regulating drug (section 2.12) can be beneficial in patients with diabetes and a high cardiovascular risk. For reference to the use of an ACE inhibitor or an angiotensin-II receptor antagonist in the management of diabetic nephropathy, see section 6.1.5.

PREVENTION OF DIABETIC COMPLICATIONS. Optimal glycaemic control in both type 1 diabetes and type 2 diabetes reduces, in the long term, the risk of microvascular complications including retinopathy, development of proteinuria and to some extent neuropathy. However, a temporary deterioration in established diabetic retinopathy may occur when normalising blood-glucose concentration.

A measure of the total glycated (or glycosylated) haemoglobin (HbA_1) or a specific fraction (HbA_{1c}) provides a good indication of long-term glycaemic control. The ideal HbA_{1c} concentration is between 6.5 and 7.5% but this cannot always be achieved, and for those on insulin there are significantly increased risks of severe hypoglycaemia. Tight control of blood pressure in hypertensive patients with type 2 diabetes reduces mortality significantly and protects visual acuity (by reducing considerably the risks of maculopathy and retinal photocoagulation) (see also section 2.5).

6.1.1 Insulins

6.1.1.1 Short-acting insulins
6.1.1.2 Intermediate- and long-acting insulins
6.1.1.3 Hypodermic equipment

Insulin plays a key role in the regulation of carbohydrate, fat, and protein metabolism. It is a polypeptide hormone of complex structure. There are differences in the amino-acid sequence of animal insulins, human insulins and the human insulin analogues. Insulin may be extracted from pork pancreas and purified by crystallisation; it may also be extracted from beef pancreas, but beef insulins are now rarely used. Human sequence insulin may be produced semisynthetically by enzymatic modification of porcine insulin (emp) or biosynthetically by recombinant DNA technology using bacteria (crb, prb) or yeast (pyr).

All insulin preparations are to a greater or lesser extent immunogenic in man but immunological resistance to insulin action is uncommon. Preparations of human sequence insulin should theoretically be less immunogenic, but no real advantage has been shown in trials.

Insulin is inactivated by gastro-intestinal enzymes, and must therefore be given by injection; the subcutaneous route is ideal in most circumstances. It is usually injected into the upper arms, thighs, buttocks, or abdomen; there may be increased absorption from a limb site if the limb is used in strenuous exercise following the injection. Generally subcutaneous insulin injections cause few problems; fat hypertrophy does however occur but can be minimised by rotating the injection sites. Local allergic reactions are now rare.

Insulin is needed by all patients with ketoacidosis, and it is likely to be needed by most patients with:

- rapid onset of symptoms;
- substantial loss of weight;
- weakness;
- ketonuria.

If the condition worsens, vomiting can occur and patients may rapidly develop ketoacidosis. Insulin is required by almost all children with diabetes. It is also needed for type 2 diabetes when other methods have failed to achieve good control, and temporarily in the presence of intercurrent illness or perioperatively. Pregnant women with type 2 diabetes should be treated with insulin when diet alone fails. The majority of those who are obese can be managed by dietary changes or, if diet alone fails to achieve adequate control, by also administering oral hypoglycaemic drugs (section 6.1.2).

MANAGEMENT OF DIABETES WITH INSULIN. The aim of treatment is to achieve the best possible control of blood-glucose concentration without making the patient obsessional and to avoid disabling hypoglycaemia; close co-operation is needed between the patient and the medical team since good control reduces the risk of complications. Mixtures of insulin preparations may be required and appropriate combinations have to be determined for the individual patient. For patients with acute-onset diabetes, treatment should be started with soluble insulin given 3 times daily with medium-acting insulin at bedtime. For those less severely ill, treatment is usually started with a mixture of premixed short- and medium-acting insulins (most commonly in a proportion of 30% soluble insulin and 70% isophane insulin) given twice daily; 8 units twice daily is a suitable initial dose for most ambulant patients. The proportion of the short-acting soluble component can be increased in those with excessive postprandial hyperglycaemia.

The dose of insulin is adjusted on an individual basis, by gradually increasing the dose but avoiding troublesome hypoglycaemic reactions.

There are 3 main types of insulin preparations:

- those of **short** duration which have a relatively rapid onset of action, namely soluble insulin, insulin lispro and insulin aspart;
- those with an **intermediate** action, e.g. isophane insulin and insulin zinc suspension; and
- those whose action is slower in onset and lasts for **long** periods, e.g. crystalline insulin zinc suspension.

The duration of action of a particular type of insulin varies considerably from one patient to another, and needs to be assessed individually.

EXAMPLES OF RECOMMENDED INSULIN REGIMENS.

- Short-acting insulin mixed with intermediate-acting insulin: twice daily (before meals)
- Short-acting insulin mixed with intermediate-acting insulin: before breakfast
  Short-acting insulin: before evening meal
  Intermediate-acting insulin: at bedtime
- Short-acting insulin: three times daily (before breakfast, midday, and evening meal)
  Intermediate-acting insulin: at bedtime
- Intermediate-acting insulin with or without short-acting insulin: once daily either before breakfast or at bedtime suffices for some patients with type 2 diabetes who need insulin, sometimes in combination with oral hypoglycaemic drugs

Insulin requirements may be increased by infection, stress, accidental or surgical trauma, puberty, and during the second and third trimesters of pregnancy. Requirements may be decreased in patients with renal impairment (Appendix 3) or hepatic impairment and in those with some endocrine disorders (e.g. Addison's disease, hypopituitarism) or coeliac disease. In pregnancy insulin requirements should be assessed frequently by an experienced diabetes physician.

INSULIN ADMINISTRATION. Insulin is generally given by *subcutaneous injection*. Injection devices ('pens') (section 6.1.1.3) which hold the insulin in a cartridge and meter the required dose are convenient to use. The conventional syringe and needle is still the preferred method of insulin administration by many and is also required for insulins not available in cartridge form.

For intensive insulin regimens multiple subcutaneous injections (3 to 4 times daily) are usually recommended.

Short-acting insulins (soluble insulin, insulin aspart and insulin lispro) can also be given by *continuous subcutaneous infusion* using a portable infusion pump. This device delivers a continuous basal insulin infusion and patient-activated bolus doses at meal times. This technique is appropriate only for patients who suffer recurrent hypoglycaemia or marked morning rise in blood-glucose concentration despite optimised multiple-injection regimens. NICE (February 2003) has also recommended continuous subcutaneous infusion as an option in those who suffer repeated or unpredictable hypoglycaemia despite optimal multiple-injection regimens (including the use of insulin glargine where appropriate). Patients on subcutaneous insulin infusion must be highly motivated, able to monitor their blood-glucose concentration, and have expert training, advice and supervision from an experienced healthcare team.

Soluble insulin by the *intravenous route* is reserved for urgent treatment, and for fine control in serious illness and in the perioperative period (see under Diabetes and Surgery, below).

UNITS. The word 'unit' should **not** be abbreviated.

MONITORING. Many patients now monitor their own blood-glucose concentrations (section 6.1.6). Since blood-glucose concentrations vary substantially throughout the day, 'normoglycaemia' cannot always be achieved throughout a 24-hour period without causing damaging hypoglycaemia. It is therefore best to recommend that patients should maintain a blood-glucose concentration of between 4 and 9 mmol/litre for most of the time (4–7 mmol/litre before meals and less than 9 mmol/litre after meals), while accepting that on occasions, for brief periods, it will be above these values; strenuous efforts should be made to prevent the blood-glucose concentration from falling below 4 mmol/litre. Patients should be advised to look for 'peaks' and 'troughs' of blood glucose, and to adjust their insulin dosage only once or twice weekly. Overall it is ideal to aim for an HbA_{1c} (glycosylated haemoglobin) concentration of 6.5–7.5% or less (reference range 4–6%) but this is not always possible without causing disabling hypoglycaemia; in those at risk of arterial disease, the aim should be to maintain the HbA_{1c} concentration at 6.5% or less. HbA_{1c} should be measured every 3–6 months. Fructosamine can also be used for assessment of control; this is simpler and cheaper but the measurement of HbA_{1c} is generally a more reliable method.

The intake of energy and of simple and complex carbohydrates should be adequate to allow normal growth and development but obesity must be avoided. The carbohydrate intake needs to be regulated and should be distributed throughout the day. Fine control of plasma glucose can be achieved by moving portions of carbohydrate from one meal to another without altering the total intake.

HYPOGLYCAEMIA. Hypoglycaemia is a potential problem for all patients receiving insulin and careful instruction to the patient must be directed towards avoiding it.

Loss of warning of hypoglycaemia is common among insulin-treated patients and can be a serious hazard, especially for drivers and those in dangerous occupations. Very tight control of diabetes lowers the blood-glucose concentration needed to trigger hypoglycaemic symptoms; increase in the frequency of hypoglycaemic episodes reduces the warning symptoms experienced by the patient. Beta-blockers can also blunt hypoglycaemic awareness (and also delay recovery).

To restore the warning signs, episodes of hypoglycaemia must be reduced to a minimum; this involves appropriate adjustment of insulin type, dose and frequency together with suitable timing and quantity of meals and snacks.

Some patients have reported loss of hypoglycaemia warning after transfer to human insulin. Clinical studies do not confirm that human insulin decreases hypoglycaemia awareness. If a patient believes that human insulin is responsible for the loss of warning it is reasonable to revert to animal insulin and essential to educate the patient about avoiding hypoglycaemia. Great care should be taken to specify whether a human or an animal preparation is required.

Few patients are now treated with beef insulins; when undertaking conversion from beef to human insulin, the total dose should be reduced by about 10% with careful monitoring for the first few days. When changing between pork and human sequence insulins, a dose change is not usually needed, but careful monitoring is still advised.

DRIVING. Drivers treated with insulin or oral antidiabetic drugs are required to notify the Driver and Vehicle Licensing Agency of their condition, as are drivers of Group 2 vehicles (heavy goods vehicles or public service vehicles) whose diabetes is controlled by diet alone; the Agency's Drivers Medical Unit provides guidance on eligibility to drive. Driving is not permitted when hypoglycaemic awareness is impaired.

Drivers need to be particularly careful to avoid hypoglycaemia (see also above) and should be warned of the problems. Drivers treated with insulin should normally check their blood-glucose concentration before driving and, on long journeys, at 2-hour intervals; these precautions may also be necessary for drivers taking oral antidiabetic drugs who are at particular risk of hypoglycaemia. Drivers treated with insulin should ensure that a supply of sugar is always available in the vehicle and they should avoid driving if they are late for a meal. If hypoglycaemia occurs, or warning signs develop, the driver should:

- stop the vehicle in a safe place;
- switch off the ignition;
- eat or drink a suitable source of sugar;
- wait until recovery is complete before continuing journey; recovery may take 15 minutes or longer and should preferably be confirmed by checking blood-glucose concentration.

DIABETES AND SURGERY. The following regimen is suitable when surgery in a patient with type 1 diabetes requires intravenous infusion of insulin for 12 hours or longer.

- Give an injection of the patient's usual insulin on the night before the operation.
- Early on the day of the operation, start an intravenous infusion of glucose 5% or 10% containing potassium chloride 10 mmol/litre (provided that the patient is not hyperkalaemic) and

infuse at a constant rate appropriate to the patient's fluid requirements (usually 125 mL per hour); make up a solution of soluble insulin 1 unit/mL in sodium chloride 0.9% and infuse intravenously using a syringe pump piggy-backed to the intravenous infusion.

- The rate of the insulin infusion should normally be:
  Blood glucose < 4 mmol/litre, give 0.5 units/hour
  Blood glucose 4–15 mmol/litre, give 2 units/hour
  Blood glucose 15–20 mmol/litre, give 4 units/hour
  Blood glucose > 20 mmol/litre, review.

In resistant cases (such as patients who are in shock or severely ill or those receiving corticosteroids or sympathomimetics) 2–4 times these rates or even more may be needed.

If a syringe pump is not available soluble insulin 16 units/litre should be added to the intravenous infusion of glucose 5% or 10% containing potassium chloride 10 mmol per litre (provided the patient is not hyperkalaemic) and the infusion run at the rate appropriate to the patient's fluid requirements (usually 125 mL per hour) with the insulin dose adjusted as follows:

Blood glucose < 4 mmol/litre, give 8 units/litre
Blood glucose 4–15 mmol/litre, give 16 units/litre
Blood glucose 15–20 mmol/litre, give 32 units/litre
Blood glucose > 20 mmol/litre, review.

The rate of intravenous infusion depends on the volume depletion, cardiac function, age, and other factors. Blood-glucose concentration should be measured pre-operatively and then hourly until stable, thereafter every 2 hours. The duration of action of intravenous insulin is only a few minutes and the infusion must not be stopped unless the patient becomes overtly hypoglycaemic (blood glucose < 3 mmol/litre) in which case it should be stopped for up to 30 minutes. The amount of potassium chloride required in the infusion needs to be assessed by regular measurement of plasma electrolytes. Sodium chloride 0.9% infusion should replace glucose 5% or 10% if the blood glucose is persistently above 15 mmol/litre.

Once the patient starts to eat and drink, give subcutaneous insulin before breakfast and stop intravenous insulin 30 minutes later; the dose may need to be 10–20% more than usual if the patient is still in bed or unwell. If the patient was not previously receiving insulin, an appropriate initial dose is 30–40 units daily in four divided doses using soluble insulin before meals and intermediate-acting insulin at bedtime and the dose adjusted from day to day. Patients with hyperglycaemia often relapse after conversion back to subcutaneous insulin calling for one of the following approaches:

- additional doses of soluble insulin at any of the four injection times (before meals or bedtime) *or*
- temporary addition of intravenous insulin infusion (while continuing the subcutaneous regimen) until blood-glucose concentration is satisfactory *or*
- complete reversion to the intravenous regimen (especially if the patient is unwell).

6.1.1.1 Short-acting insulins

Soluble insulin is a short-acting form of insulin. For maintenance regimens it is usual to inject it 15 to 30 minutes before meals.

Soluble insulin is the most appropriate form of insulin for use in diabetic emergencies and at the time of surgery. It can be given intravenously and intramuscularly, as well as subcutaneously.

When injected subcutaneously, soluble insulin has a rapid onset of action (30 to 60 minutes), a peak action between 2 and 4 hours, and a duration of action of up to 8 hours.

When injected intravenously, soluble insulin has a very short half-life of only about 5 minutes and its effect disappears within 30 minutes.

The human insulin analogues, **insulin lispro** and **insulin aspart**, have a faster onset and shorter duration of action than soluble insulin; as a result, compared to soluble insulin, fasting and preprandial blood-glucose concentration is a little higher, post-prandial blood-glucose concentration is a little lower, and hypoglycaemia occurs slightly less frequently. Subcutaneous injection of insulin lispro or of insulin aspart may be convenient for those who wish to inject shortly before or, when necessary, shortly after a meal. They may also help those prone to pre-lunch hypoglycaemia and those who eat late in the evening and are prone to nocturnal hypoglycaemia. Insulin aspart and insulin lispro may also be administered by subcutaneous infusion.

SOLUBLE INSULIN

(Insulin Injection; Neutral Insulin)

A sterile solution of insulin (i.e. bovine or porcine) or of human insulin; pH 6.6–8.0

Indications: diabetes mellitus; diabetic ketoacidosis (section 6.1.3)

Cautions: see notes above; reduce dose in renal impairment (Appendix 3); **interactions:** Appendix 1 (antidiabetics)

Side-effects: see notes above; transient oedema; local reactions and fat hypertrophy at injection site; rarely hypersensitivity reactions including urticaria, rash; overdose causes hypoglycaemia

Dose: *by subcutaneous, intramuscular, or intravenous injection or intravenous infusion*, according to requirements

COUNSELLING. Show container to patient and confirm that patient is expecting the version dispensed

■ Highly purified animal

Hypurin® Bovine Neutral (CP) PoM
Injection, soluble insulin (bovine, highly purified) 100 units/mL. Net price 10-mL vial = £18.48; cartridges (for *Autopen®* devices) 5 × 1.5 mL = £13.86, 5 × 3 mL = £27.72

Hypurin® Porcine Neutral (CP) PoM
Injection, soluble insulin (porcine, highly purified) 100 units/mL. Net price 10-mL vial = £16.80; cartridges (for *Autopen®* devices) 5 × 1.5 mL = £12.60, 5 × 3 mL = £25.20

Pork Actrapid® (Novo Nordisk) PoM
Injection, soluble insulin (porcine, highly purified) 100 units/mL. Net price 10-mL vial = £4.00

NOTE. Not recommended for use in subcutaneous insulin infusion pumps—may precipitate in catheter or needle

■ Human sequence

Actrapid® (Novo Nordisk) PoM
Injection, soluble insulin (human, pyr) 100 units/mL. Net price 10-mL vial = £7.48; *Actrapid Penfill*® cartridge (for *Innovo*® and *NovoPen*® devices) 5 × 3 mL = £20.08; 5 × 3-mL *Actrapid Novolet* ® prefilled disposable injection devices (range 2–78 units, allowing 2-unit dosage adjustment) = £19.87
NOTE. Not recommended for use in subcutaneous insulin infusion pumps—may precipitate in catheter or needle

Velosulin® (Novo Nordisk) PoM
Injection, soluble insulin (human, pyr) 100 units/mL. Net price 10-mL vial = £7.48

Humulin S® (Lilly) PoM
Injection, soluble insulin (human, prb) 100 units/mL. Net price 10-mL vial = £15.00; 5 × 3-mL cartridge (for *Autopen*® *3 mL* or *HumaPen*®) = £25.56; 5 × 3-mL *Humaject S*® prefilled disposable injection devices (range 2–96 units, allowing 2-unit dosage adjustment) = £24.95

Insuman® **Rapid** (Aventis Pharma) ▼ PoM
Injection, soluble insulin (human, crb) 100 units/mL, net price 5 × 3-mL cartridge (for *OptiPen*® *Pro* NHS) = £23.43; 5 × 3-mL *Insuman*® *Rapid OptiSet*® prefilled disposable injection devices (range 2–40 units, allowing 2-unit dosage adjustment) = £27.90
NOTE. Not recommended for use in subcutaneous insulin infusion pumps

■ Mixed preparations
See Biphasic Isophane Insulin (section 6.1.1.2)

INSULIN ASPART

(Recombinant human insulin analogue)
Indications: diabetes mellitus
Cautions: see under Soluble Insulin; children (use only if benefit likely compared to soluble insulin)
Side-effects: see under Soluble Insulin
Dose: *by subcutaneous injection*, immediately before meals or when necessary shortly after meals, according to requirements
By subcutaneous infusion, intravenous injection or intravenous infusion, according to requirements
COUNSELLING. Show container to patient and confirm that patient is expecting the version dispensed

NovoRapid® (Novo Nordisk) PoM
Injection, insulin aspart (recombinant human insulin analogue) 100 units/mL, net price 10-mL vial = £17.27; *Penfill*® cartridge (for *Innovo*® and *NovoPen*® devices) 5 × 3-mL = £29.43; 5 × 3-mL *FlexPen*® prefilled disposable injection devices (range 1–60 units, allowing 1-unit dosage adjustment) = £32.00

INSULIN LISPRO

(Recombinant human insulin analogue)
Indications: diabetes mellitus
Cautions: see under Soluble Insulin; children (use only if benefit likely compared to soluble insulin)
Side-effects: see under Soluble Insulin
Dose: *by subcutaneous injection* shortly before meals or when necessary shortly after meals, according to requirements
By subcutaneous infusion, or intravenous injection, or intravenous infusion, according to requirements
COUNSELLING. Show container to patient and confirm that patient is expecting the version dispensed

Humalog® (Lilly) PoM
Injection, insulin lispro (recombinant human insulin analogue) 100 units/mL. Net price 10-mL vial = £17.28; 5 × 3-mL cartridge (for *Autopen*® *3 mL* or *HumaPen*®) = £29.46; 5 × 3-mL *Humalog*®*-Pen* prefilled disposable injection devices (range 1–60 units, allowing 1-unit dosage adjustment) = £29.46

6.1.1.2 Intermediate- and long-acting insulins

When given by subcutaneous injection, intermediate- and long-acting insulins have an onset of action of approximately 1–2 hours, a maximal effect at 4–12 hours, and a duration of 16–35 hours. Some are given twice daily in conjunction with short-acting (soluble) insulin, and others are given once daily, particularly in elderly patients. Soluble insulin can be mixed with intermediate and long-acting insulins (except insulin detemir and insulin glargine) in the syringe, essentially retaining the properties of the two components, although there may be some blunting of the initial effect of the soluble insulin component (especially on mixing with protamine zinc insulin, see below).

Isophane insulin is a suspension of insulin with protamine which is of particular value for initiation of twice-daily insulin regimens. Patients usually mix isophane with soluble insulin but ready-mixed preparations may be appropriate (**biphasic isophane insulin**, **biphasic insulin aspart**, or **biphasic insulin lispro**).

Insulin zinc suspension (crystalline) has a more prolonged duration of action; it may be used independently or in **insulin zinc suspension** (30% amorphous, 70% crystalline).

Protamine zinc insulin is usually given once daily with short-acting (soluble) insulin. It has the drawback of binding with the soluble insulin when mixed in the same syringe, and is now rarely used.

Insulin glargine and **insulin detemir** are both human insulin analogues with a prolonged duration of action; insulin glargine is given once daily and insulin detemir is given once or twice daily.

NICE guidance (insulin glargine). NICE has recommended (December 2002) that insulin glargine should be available as an option for patients with type 1 diabetes.
Insulin glargine is **not** recommended for routine use in patients with type 2 diabetes who require insulin, but it may be considered in type 2 diabetes for those:
- who require assistance with injecting their insulin; *or*
- whose lifestyle is significantly restricted by recurrent symptomatic hypoglycaemia; *or*
- who would otherwise need twice-daily basal insulin injections in combination with oral antidiabetic drugs

INSULIN DETEMIR

(Recombinant human insulin analogue—long acting)

Indications: diabetes mellitus

Cautions: see under Soluble Insulin (section 6.1.1.1); pregnancy (Appendix 4)

Side-effects: see under Soluble Insulin (section 6.1.1.1)

Dose: *by subcutaneous injection*, ADULT and CHILD over 6 years, according to requirements

COUNSELLING. Show container to patient and confirm that patient is expecting the version dispensed

Levemir® (Novo Nordisk) ▼ PoM

Injection, insulin detemir (recombinant human insulin analogue) 100 units/mL, net price 5 × 3-mL cartridge (for *NovoPen*® devices) = £39.00; 5 × 3-mL *FlexPen*® prefilled disposable injection device (range 1–60 units, allowing 1-unit dosage adjustment) = £39.00.

INSULIN GLARGINE

(Recombinant human insulin analogue—long acting)

Indications: diabetes mellitus

Cautions: see under Soluble Insulin (section 6.1.1.1); pregnancy (Appendix 4)

Side-effects: see under Soluble Insulin (section 6.1.1.1)

Dose: *by subcutaneous injection*, ADULT and CHILD over 6 years, according to requirements

COUNSELLING. Show container to patient and confirm that patient is expecting the version dispensed

Lantus® (Aventis Pharma) ▼ PoM

Injection, insulin glargine (recombinant human insulin analogue) 100 units/mL, net price 10-mL vial = £26.00; 5 × 3-mL cartridge (for *OptiPen*® *Pro* NHS) = £39.00; 5 × 3-mL *Lantus*® *OptiSet*® prefilled disposable injection devices (range 2–40 units, allowing 2-unit dosage adjustment) = £39.00

INSULIN ZINC SUSPENSION

(Insulin Zinc Suspension (Mixed); I. Z. S.—long acting)

A sterile neutral suspension of bovine and/or porcine insulin or of human insulin in the form of a complex obtained by the addition of a suitable zinc salt; consists of rhombohedral crystals (10–40 microns) and of particles of no uniform shape (not exceeding 2 microns)

Indications: diabetes mellitus

Cautions: see under Soluble Insulin (section 6.1.1.1)

Side-effects: see under Soluble Insulin (section 6.1.1.1)

Dose: *by subcutaneous injection*, according to requirements

COUNSELLING. Show container to patient and confirm that patient is expecting the version dispensed

■ Highly purified animal

Hypurin® **Bovine Lente** (CP) PoM

Injection, insulin zinc suspension (bovine, highly purified) 100 units/mL. Net price 10-mL vial = £18.48

■ Human sequence

Monotard® (Novo Nordisk) PoM

Injection, insulin zinc suspension (human, pyr) 100 units/mL. Net price 10-mL vial = £7.48

INSULIN ZINC SUSPENSION (CRYSTALLINE)

(Cryst. I. Z. S.—long acting)

A sterile neutral suspension of bovine insulin or of human insulin in the form of a complex obtained by the addition of a suitable zinc salt; consists of rhombohedral crystals (10–40 microns)

Indications: diabetes mellitus

Cautions: see under Soluble Insulin (section 6.1.1.1)

Side-effects: see under Soluble Insulin (section 6.1.1.1)

Dose: *by subcutaneous injection*, according to requirements

COUNSELLING. Show container to patient and confirm that patient is expecting the version dispensed

■ Human sequence

Ultratard® (Novo Nordisk) PoM

Injection, insulin zinc suspension, crystalline (human, pyr) 100 units/mL. Net price 10-mL vial = £7.48

ISOPHANE INSULIN

(Isophane Insulin Injection; Isophane Protamine Insulin Injection; Isophane Insulin (NPH)—intermediate acting)

A sterile suspension of bovine or porcine insulin or of human insulin in the form of a complex obtained by the addition of protamine sulphate or another suitable protamine

Indications: diabetes mellitus

Cautions: see under Soluble Insulin (section 6.1.1.1)

Side-effects: see under Soluble Insulin (section 6.1.1.1); protamine may cause allergic reactions

Dose: *by subcutaneous injection*, according to requirements

COUNSELLING. Show container to patient and confirm that patient is expecting the version dispensed

■ Highly purified animal

Hypurin® **Bovine Isophane** (CP) PoM

Injection, isophane insulin (bovine, highly purified) 100 units/mL. Net price 10-mL vial = £18.48; cartridges (for *Autopen*® devices) 5 × 1.5 mL = £13.86, 5 × 3 mL = £27.72

Hypurin® **Porcine Isophane** (CP) PoM

Injection, isophane insulin (porcine, highly purified) 100 units/mL. Net price 10-mL vial = £16.80; cartridges (for *Autopen*® devices) 5 × 1.5 mL = £12.60, 5 × 3 mL = £25.20

Pork Insulatard® (Novo Nordisk) PoM

Injection, isophane insulin (porcine, highly purified) 100 units/mL. Net price 10-mL vial = £4.00

■ Human sequence

Insulatard® (Novo Nordisk) PoM

Injection, isophane insulin (human, pyr) 100 units/mL. Net price 10-mL vial = £7.48; *Insulatard Penfill*® cartridge (for *Innovo*®, or *Novopen*® devices) 5 × 3 mL = £20.08; 5 × 3-mL *Insulatard FlexPen*® prefilled disposable injection devices (range 1–60 units, allowing 1-unit dosage adjustment) = £22.86; 5 × 3-mL *Insulatard Novolet*® prefilled disposable injection devices (range 2–78 units, allowing 2-unit dosage adjustment) = £19.87; 5 × 3-mL *Insulatard InnoLet*® prefilled disposable injection devices (range 1–50 units, allowing 1-unit dosage adjustment) = £20.40

Humulin I® (Lilly) PoM
Injection, isophane insulin (human, prb) 100 units/mL. Net price 10-mL vial = £15.00; 5 × 3-mL cartridge (for *Autopen*® *3 mL* or *HumaPen*®) = £27.22; 5 × 3-mL *Humulin I-Pen*® prefilled disposable injection devices (range 1–60 units, allowing 1-unit dosage adjustment) = £27.22

Insuman® **Basal** (Aventis Pharma) ▼ PoM
Injection, isophane insulin (human, crb) 100 units/mL, net price 5-mL vial = £5.84; 5 × 3-mL cartridge (for *OptiPen*® *Pro* NHS) = £23.43; 5 × 3-mL *Insuman*® *Basal OptiSet*® prefilled disposable injection devices (range 2–40 units, allowing 2-unit dosage adjustment) = £27.90

■ Mixed preparations
See Biphasic Isophane Insulin (below)

PROTAMINE ZINC INSULIN

(Protamine Zinc Insulin Injection—long acting)
A sterile suspension of insulin in the form of a complex obtained by the addition of a suitable protamine and zinc chloride; this preparation was included in BP 1980 but is not included in BP 1988

Indications: diabetes mellitus

Cautions: see under Soluble Insulin (section 6.1.1.1); see also notes above

Side-effects: see under Soluble Insulin (section 6.1.1.1); protamine may cause allergic reactions

Dose: *by subcutaneous injection*, according to requirements

COUNSELLING. Show container to patient and confirm that patient is expecting the version dispensed

Hypurin® **Bovine Protamine Zinc** (CP) PoM
Injection, protamine zinc insulin (bovine, highly purified) 100 units/mL. Net price 10-mL vial = £18.48

Biphasic insulins

BIPHASIC INSULIN ASPART

(Intermediate-acting insulin)

Indications: diabetes mellitus

Cautions: see under Soluble Insulin and Insulin Aspart (section 6.1.1.1)

Side-effects: see under Soluble Insulin (section 6.1.1.1); protamine may cause allergic reactions

Dose: *by subcutaneous injection*, up to 10 minutes before or soon after a meal, according to requirements

COUNSELLING. Show container to patient and confirm that patient is expecting the version dispensed; the proportions of the two components should be checked **carefully** (the order in which the proportions are stated may not be the same in other countries)

NovoMix® **30** (Novo Nordisk) PoM
Injection, biphasic insulin aspart (recombinant human insulin analogue), 30% insulin aspart, 70% insulin aspart protamine, 100 units/mL, net price 5 × 3-mL *Penfill*® cartridges (for *Innovo*® and *NovoPen*® devices) = £29.43; 5 × 3-mL *FlexPen*® prefilled disposable injection devices (range 1–60 units, allowing 1-unit dosage adjustment) = £32.00

BIPHASIC INSULIN LISPRO

(Intermediate-acting insulin)

Indications: diabetes mellitus

Cautions: see under Soluble Insulin and Insulin Lispro (section 6.1.1.1)

Side-effects: see under Soluble Insulin (section 6.1.1.1); protamine may cause allergic reactions

Dose: *by subcutaneous injection*, up to 15 minutes before or soon after a meal, according to requirements

COUNSELLING. Show container to patient and confirm that patient is expecting the version dispensed; the proportions of the two components should be checked **carefully** (the order in which the proportions are stated may not be the same in other countries)

Humalog® **Mix25** (Lilly) PoM
Injection, biphasic insulin lispro (recombinant human insulin analogue), 25% insulin lispro, 75% insulin lispro protamine, 100 units/mL, net price 5 × 3-mL cartridge (for *Autopen*® *3 mL* or *HumaPen*®) = £29.46; 5 × 3-mL prefilled disposable injection devices (range 1–60 units, allowing 1-unit dosage adjustment) = £30.98

Humalog® **Mix50** (Lilly) PoM
Injection, biphasic insulin lispro (recombinant human insulin analogue), 50% insulin lispro, 50% insulin lispro protamine, 100 units/mL, net price 5 × 3-mL prefilled disposable injection devices (range 1–60 units, allowing 1-unit dosage adjustment) = £30.98

BIPHASIC ISOPHANE INSULIN

(Biphasic Isophane Insulin Injection—intermediate acting)
A sterile buffered suspension of either porcine or human insulin complexed with protamine sulphate (or another suitable protamine) in a solution of insulin of the same species

Indications: diabetes mellitus

Cautions: see under Soluble Insulin (section 6.1.1.1)

Side-effects: see under Soluble Insulin (section 6.1.1.1); protamine may cause allergic reactions

Dose: *by subcutaneous injection*, according to requirements

COUNSELLING. Show container to patient and confirm that patient is expecting the version dispensed; the proportions of the two components should be checked **carefully** (the order in which the proportions are stated may not be the same in other countries)

■ Highly purified animal

Hypurin® **Porcine 30/70 Mix** (CP) PoM
Injection, biphasic isophane insulin (porcine, highly purified), 30% soluble, 70% isophane, 100 units/mL. Net price 10-mL vial = £16.80; cartridges (for *Autopen*® devices) 5 × 1.5 ml = £12.60, 5 × 3 mL = £25.20

Pork Mixtard 30® (Novo Nordisk) PoM
Injection, biphasic isophane insulin (porcine, highly purified), 30% soluble, 70% isophane, 100 units/mL. Net price 10-mL vial = £4.00

■ Human sequence

Mixtard® **10** (Novo Nordisk) PoM
Injection, biphasic isophane insulin (human, pyr), 10% soluble, 90% isophane, 100 units/mL. Net

price *Mixtard 10 Penfill*® cartridge (for *Innovo*® or *Novopen*® devices) 5 × 3 mL = £20.08; 5 × 3-mL *Mixtard 10 Novolet*® prefilled disposable injection devices (range 2–78 units, allowing 2-unit dosage adjustment) = £19.87

Mixtard® 20 (Novo Nordisk) PoM
Injection, biphasic isophane insulin (human, pyr), 20% soluble, 80% isophane, 100 units/mL. Net price *Mixtard 20 Penfill*® cartridge (for *Innovo*® or *Novopen*® devices) 5 × 3 mL = £20.08; 5 × 3-mL *Mixtard 20 Novolet*® prefilled disposable injection devices (range 2–78 units, allowing 2-unit dosage adjustment) = £19.87

Mixtard® 30 (Novo Nordisk) PoM
Injection, biphasic isophane insulin (human, pyr), 30% soluble, 70% isophane, 100 units/mL. Net price 10-mL vial = £7.48; *Mixtard 30 Penfill*® cartridge (for *Innovo*® or *Novopen*® devices) 5 × 3 mL = £20.08; 5 × 3-mL *Mixtard 30 Novolet*® prefilled disposable injection devices (range 2–78 units, allowing 2-unit dosage adjustment) = £19.87; 5 × 3-mL *Mixtard 30 InnoLet*® prefilled disposable injection devices (range 1–50 units allowing 1-unit dosage adjustment) = £19.87

Mixtard® 40 (Novo Nordisk) PoM
Injection, biphasic isophane insulin (human, pyr), 40% soluble, 60% isophane, 100 units/mL. Net price *Mixtard 40 Penfill*® cartridge (for *Innovo*® or *Novopen*® devices) 5 × 3 mL = £20.08; 5 × 3-mL *Mixtard 40 Novolet*® prefilled disposable injection devices (range 2–78 units, allowing 2-unit dosage adjustment) = £19.87

Mixtard® 50 (Novo Nordisk) PoM
Injection, biphasic isophane insulin (human, pyr), 50% soluble, 50% isophane, 100 units/mL. Net price *Mixtard 50 Penfill*® cartridge (for *Innovo*® or *Novopen*® devices) 5 × 3 mL = £20.08; 5 × 3-mL *Mixtard 50 Novolet*® prefilled disposable injection devices (range 2–78 units, allowing 2-unit dosage adjustment) = £19.87

Humulin M3® (Lilly) PoM
Injection, biphasic isophane insulin (human, prb), 30% soluble, 70% isophane, 100 units/mL. Net price 10-mL vial = £15.00; 5 × 3-mL cartridge (for *Autopen*® *3 mL* or *HumaPen*®) = £25.56; 5 × 3-mL *Humaject M3*® prefilled disposable injection devices (range 2–96 units, allowing 2-unit dosage adjustment) = £24.95

Insuman® Comb 15 (Aventis Pharma) ▼ PoM
Injection, biphasic isophane insulin (human, crb), 15% soluble, 85% isophane, 100 units/mL, net price 5-mL vial = £5.31; 5 × 3-mL cartridge (for *OptiPen*® *Pro* NHS) = £21.30; 5 × 3-mL *Insuman*® *Comb 15 OptiSet*® prefilled disposable injection devices (range 2–40 units, allowing 2-unit dosage adjustment) = £27.90

Insuman® Comb 25 (Aventis Pharma) ▼ PoM
Injection, biphasic isophane insulin (human, crb), 25% soluble, 75% isophane, 100 units/mL, net price 5-mL vial = £5.84; 5 × 3-mL cartridge (for *OptiPen*® *Pro* NHS) = £23.43; 5 × 3-mL *Insuman*® *Comb 25 OptiSet*® prefilled disposable injection devices (range 2–40 units, allowing 2-unit dosage adjustment) = £27.90

Insuman® Comb 50 (Aventis Pharma) ▼ PoM
Injection, biphasic isophane insulin (human, crb), 50% soluble, 50% isophane, 100 units/mL, net price 5-mL vial = £5.31; 5 × 3-mL cartridge (for *OptiPen*® *Pro* NHS) = £23.43; 5 × 3-mL *Insuman*® *Comb 50 OptiSet*® prefilled disposable injection devices (range 2–40 units, allowing 2-unit dosage adjustment) = £27.90

6.1.1.3 Hypodermic equipment

Patients should be advised on the safe disposal of lancets, single-use syringes, and needles. Suitable arrangements for the safe disposal of contaminated waste must be made before these products are prescribed for patients who are carriers of infectious diseases.

■ Injection devices

Autopen® (Owen Mumford)
Injection device; *Autopen*® *1.5 mL* (for use with CP and Lilly 1.5-mL insulin cartridges), allows adjustment of dosage in multiples of 1 unit, max. 16 units (single-unit version) *or* 2 units, max. 32 units (2-unit version), net price (both) = £14.66; *Autopen*® *24* (for use with Aventis 3-mL insulin cartridges), allows adjustments of dosage in multiples of 1 unit, max. 16 units (single-unit version) *or* 2 units, max. 32 units (2 unit version), net price (both) = £14.44; *Autopen*® *3 mL*, *Autopen*® *Special Edition*, and *Autopen*® *Junior* (for use with Lilly 3-mL insulin cartridges), all allow adjustment of dosage in multiples of 1 unit, max. 21 units (single-unit version) *or* 2 units, max. 42 units (2-unit version), net price (both) = £14.92

HumaPen® Ergo (Lilly)
Injection device, for use with *Humulin*® and *Humalog*® 3-mL cartridges; allows adjustment of dosage in multiples of 1 unit, max. 60 units, net price = £22.39 (available in burgundy and teal)

Innovo® (Novo Nordisk)
Injection device, for use with 3-mL *Penfill*® insulin cartridges; allows adjustment of dosage in multiples of 1 unit, max. 70 units, net price = £26.36 (available in green or orange)

mhi-500® (Medical House)
Needle-free insulin delivery device for use with any 10-mL vial *or* any 3-mL cartridge of insulin (except the Novo Nordisk 3 mL penfills), allows adjustment of dosage in multiples of 0.5 units, max. 50 units, net price *starter pack* for 10-mL adaptor (*mhi-500*® device, 5 nozzles, 2 insulin vial adaptors) = £122.12, for 3-mL adaptor = (*mhi-500*® device, 5 nozzles, 2 insulin cartridge adaptors) = £120.00; *3-month consumables pack* for 10-mL adaptor (13 nozzles, 5 insulin vial adaptors) = £22.54, for 3-mL adaptor (13 nozzles, 5 insulin cartridge adaptors) = £34.45; *vial adaptor pack* (6 insulin vial adaptors) = £7.51, *cartridge adaptor pack* (6 insulin cartridge adaptors) = £7.38; *nozzle pack* (6 nozzles) = £7.51

NovoPen® (Novo Nordisk)
Injection device; for use with *Penfill*® insulin cartridges; *NovoPen*® *Junior* (for 3-mL cartridges), allows adjustment of dosage in multiples of 0.5 units, max. 35 units, net price = £23.21; *NovoPen*® *3 Demi* (for 3-mL cartridges), allows adjustment of dosage in multiples of 0.5 units, max. 35 units, net price = £23.61; *NovoPen*® *3 Classic* or *Fun* (for 3-mL cartridges), allows adjustment of dosage in multiples of 1 unit, max. 70 units, net price = £23.61

OptiPen® Pro 1 (Aventis Pharma)
Injection device, for use with *Insuman*® insulin cartridges; allows adjustment of dosage in multiples of 1 unit, max. 60 units, net price = £22.00

■ Lancets

Lancets—sterile, single use (Drug Tariff)
Ascensia Microlet® 100 = £3.55, 200 = £6.76; *BD Micro-Fine*®+ 100 = £3.16, 200 = £6.13; *Cleanlet Fine*® 100 = £3.19, 200 = £6.13; *Finepoint*® 100 = £3.48; *FreeStyle*® 200 = £6.50; *GlucoMen*® Fine 100 = £3.42, 200 = £6.61; *Hypoguard Supreme*® 100 = £2.75; *MediSense Thin*® 200 = £6.63; *Milward Steri-Let*®, 23 gauge, 100 = £3.00, 200 = £5.70, 28 gauge, 100 = £3.00, 200 = £5.70; *Monolet*® 100 = £3.28, 200 = £6.24; *Monolet Extra* 100 = £3.28; *One Touch UltraSoft*® 100 = £3.49; [1]*Softclix*® 200 = £6.79; [1]*Softclix XL*® 50 = £1.70; [2]*Unilet ComforTouch*® 100 = £3.40, 200 = £6.44; [2]*Unilet General Purpose*® 100 = £3.47, 200 = £6.59; [2]*Unilet General Purpose Superlite*® 100 = £3.46, 200 = £6.56; [3]*Unilet Superlite*® 100 = £3.46, 200 = £6.56; *Vitrex Soft*®, 23-gauge, 100 = £3.00, 200 = £5.70; *Vitrex Gentle*® 28-gauge, 100 = £3.19, 200 = £6.13

Compatible finger-pricking devices (unless indicated otherwise, see footnotes), all NHS: *B-D Lancer*®, *Glucolet*®, *Monojector*®, *Penlet II*®, *Soft Touch*®

1. Use NHS *Softclix*® finger-pricking device
2. NHS *Autolet*® and NHS *Autolet Impression*® are also compatible finger-pricking devices
3. Use NHS *Autolet*®, or NHS *Glucolet*® finger-pricking devices

■ Needles

Hypodermic Needle, Sterile single use (Drug Tariff)
For use with reusable glass syringe, sizes 0.5 mm (25G), 0.45 mm (26G), 0.4 mm (27G). Net price 100-needle pack = £2.53
Brands include *Microlance*®, *Monoject*®

Needles for Prefilled and Reusable Pen Injectors (Drug Tariff)
Screw on, needle length 6.1 mm or less, net price 100-needle pack = £12.08; 6.2–9.9 mm, 100-needle pack = £8.57; 10 mm or more, 100-needle pack = £8.57
Brands include *BD Micro-Fine*®+, *NovoFine*®, *Unifine*® *Pentips*
Snap on, needle length 6.1 mm or less, net price 100-needle pack = £11.82; 6.2–9.9 mm, 100-needle pack = £8.38; 10 mm or more, 100-needle pack = £8.38
Brands include *Penfine*®

■ Syringes

Hypodermic Syringe (Drug Tariff)
Calibrated glass with Luer taper conical fitting, for use with U100 insulin. Net price 0.5 mL and 1 mL = £15.18
Brands include *Abcare*®

Pre-Set U100 Insulin Syringe (Drug Tariff)
Calibrated glass with Luer taper conical fitting, supplied with dosage chart and strong box, for blind patients. Net price 1 mL = £21.99

U100 Insulin Syringe with Needle (Drug Tariff)
Disposable with fixed or separate needle for single use or single patient-use, colour coded orange. Needle length 8 mm, diameters 0.33 mm (29G), 0.3 mm (30G), net price 10 (with needle), 0.3 mL = £1.27, 0.5 mL = £1.23; needle length 12 mm, diameters 0.45 mm (26G), 0.4 mm (27G), 0.36 mm (28G), 0.33 mm (29G), net price 10 (with needle), 0.3 mL = £1.37; 0.5 mL = £1.32; 1 mL = £1.33
Brands include *BD Micro-Fine*®+, *Clinipak*®, *Insupak*®, *Monoject*® *Ultra*, *Omnikan*®, *Plastipak*®, *Unifine*®

■ Accessories

Needle Clipping (Chopping) Device (Drug Tariff)
Consisting of a clipper to remove needle from its hub and container from which cut-off needles cannot be retrieved; designed to hold 1200 needles, not suitable for use with lancets. Net price = £1.24
Brands include *BD Safe-Clip*®

Sharpsbin (Drug Tariff)
Net price 1-litre sharpsbin = 85p

6.1.2 Oral antidiabetic drugs

6.1.2.1 Sulphonylureas
6.1.2.2 Biguanides
6.1.2.3 Other antidiabetics

Oral antidiabetic drugs are used for the treatment of type 2 (non-insulin-dependent) diabetes mellitus. They should be prescribed only if the patient fails to respond adequately to at least 3 months' restriction of energy and carbohydrate intake and an increase in physical activity. They should be used to augment the effect of diet and exercise, and not to replace them.

For patients not adequately controlled by diet and oral hypoglycaemic drugs, insulin may be added to the treatment regimen or substituted for oral therapy. When insulin is added to oral therapy, it is generally given at bedtime as isophane insulin, and when insulin replaces an oral regimen it is generally given as twice-daily injections of a biphasic insulin (or isophane insulin mixed with soluble insulin). Weight gain and hypoglycaemia may be complications of insulin therapy but weight gain may be reduced if the insulin is given in combination with metformin.

6.1.2.1 Sulphonylureas

The sulphonylureas act mainly by augmenting insulin secretion and consequently are effective only when some residual pancreatic beta-cell activity is present; during long-term administration they also have an extrapancreatic action. All may cause hypoglycaemia but this is uncommon and usually indicates excessive dosage. Sulphonylurea-induced hypoglycaemia may persist for many hours and must always be treated in hospital.

Sulphonylureas are considered for patients who are not overweight, or in whom metformin is contra-indicated or not tolerated. Several sulphonylureas are available and choice is determined by side-effects and the duration of action as well as the patient's age and renal function. The long-acting sulphonylureas **chlorpropamide** and **glibenclamide** are associated with a greater risk of hypoglycaemia; for this reason they should be avoided in the elderly and shorter-acting alternatives, such as **gliclazide** or **tolbutamide**, should be used instead. Chlorpropamide also has more side-effects than the other sulphonylureas (see below) and therefore it is no longer recommended.

When the combination of strict diet and sulphonylurea treatment fails other options include:

- combining with metformin (section 6.1.2.2) (reports of increased hazard with this combination remain unconfirmed);
- combining with acarbose (section 6.1.2.3), which may have a small beneficial effect, but flatulence can be a problem;
- combining with pioglitazone or rosiglitazone, but see section 6.1.2.3;
- combining with bedtime isophane insulin (section 6.1.1) but weight gain and hypoglycaemia can occur.

Insulin therapy should be instituted temporarily during intercurrent illness (such as myocardial infarction, coma, infection, and trauma). Sulphonylureas should be omitted on the morning of surgery; insulin is often required because of the ensuing hyperglycaemia in these circumstances.

CAUTIONS. Sulphonylureas can encourage weight gain and should be prescribed only if poor control and symptoms persist despite adequate attempts at dieting; metformin (section 6.1.2.2) is considered the drug of choice in obese patients. Caution is needed in the elderly and in those with mild to moderate hepatic (Appendix 2) and renal impairment (Appendix 3) because of the hazard of hypoglycaemia. The short-acting tolbutamide may be used in renal impairment, as may gliquidone and gliclazide which are principally metabolised in the liver, but careful monitoring of blood-glucose concentration is essential; care is required to choose the smallest possible dose that produces adequate control of blood glucose.

CONTRA-INDICATIONS. Sulphonylureas should be avoided where possible in severe hepatic (Appendix 2) and renal (Appendix 3) impairment and in porphyria (section 9.8.2). They should not be used while breast-feeding and insulin therapy should be substituted during pregnancy (see also Appendix 4). Sulphonylureas are contra-indicated in the presence of ketoacidosis.

SIDE-EFFECTS. Side-effects of sulphonylureas are generally mild and infrequent and include gastro-intestinal disturbances such as nausea, vomiting, diarrhoea and constipation.

Chlorpropamide has appreciably more side-effects, mainly because of its very prolonged duration of action and the consequent hazard of hypoglycaemia and it should no longer be used. It may also cause facial flushing after drinking alcohol; this effect does not normally occur with other sulphonylureas. Chlorpropamide may also enhance antidiuretic hormone secretion and very rarely cause hyponatraemia (hyponatraemia is also reported with glimepiride and glipizide).

Sulphonylureas can occasionally cause a disturbance in liver function, which may rarely lead to cholestatic jaundice, hepatitis and hepatic failure. Hypersensitivity reactions can occur, usually in the first 6–8 weeks of therapy, they consist mainly of allergic skin reactions which progress rarely to erythema multiforme and exfoliative dermatitis, fever and jaundice; photosensitivity has rarely been reported with chlorpropamide and glipizide. Blood disorders are also rare but may include leucopenia, thrombocytopenia, agranulocytosis, pancytopenia, haemolytic anaemia, and aplastic anaemia.

CHLORPROPAMIDE ◢

Indications: type 2 diabetes mellitus (for use in diabetes insipidus, see section 6.5.2)
Cautions: see notes above; **interactions:** Appendix 1 (antidiabetics)
Contra-indications: see notes above
Side-effects: see notes above
Dose: initially 250 mg daily with breakfast (ELDERLY 100–125 mg but avoid—see notes above), adjusted according to response; max. 500 mg daily

Chlorpropamide (Non-proprietary) PoM ◢
Tablets, chlorpropamide 100 mg, net price 20 = £1.70; 250 mg, 20 = £2.00. Label: 4

GLIBENCLAMIDE

Indications: type 2 diabetes mellitus
Cautions: see notes above; **interactions:** Appendix 1 (antidiabetics)
Contra-indications: see notes above
Side-effects: see notes above
Dose: initially 5 mg daily with or immediately after breakfast (ELDERLY 2.5 mg, but avoid—see notes above), adjusted according to response; max. 15 mg daily

Glibenclamide (Non-proprietary) PoM
Tablets, glibenclamide 2.5 mg, net price 28-tab pack = £1.06; 5 mg, 28-tab pack = 96p

Daonil® (Hoechst Marion Roussel) PoM
Tablets, scored, glibenclamide 5 mg. Net price 28-tab pack = £2.69

Semi-Daonil® (Hoechst Marion Roussel) PoM
Tablets, scored, glibenclamide 2.5 mg. Net price 28-tab pack = £1.73

Euglucon® (Aventis Pharma) PoM
Tablets, glibenclamide 2.5 mg, net price 28-tab pack = £1.72; 5 mg (scored), 28-tab pack = £2.69

GLICLAZIDE

Indications: type 2 diabetes mellitus
Cautions: see notes above; **interactions:** Appendix 1 (antidiabetics)
Contra-indications: see notes above
Side-effects: see notes above
Dose: initially, 40–80 mg daily, adjusted according to response; up to 160 mg as a single dose, with breakfast; higher doses divided; max. 320 mg daily

Gliclazide (Non-proprietary) PoM
Tablets, scored, gliclazide 80 mg, net price 28-tab pack = £1.52, 60-tab pack = £2.47
Brands include *DIAGLYK*®

Diamicron® (Servier) PoM
Tablets, scored, gliclazide 80 mg, net price 60-tab pack = £6.51

■ Modified release

Diamicron® **MR** (Servier) PoM
Tablets, m/r, gliclazide 30 mg, net price 28-tab pack = £4.40, 56-tab pack = £8.80. Label: 25
Dose: initially 30 mg daily with breakfast, adjusted according to response every 4 weeks (after 2 weeks if no decrease in blood glucose); max. 120 mg daily
NOTE. *Diamicron*® *MR* 30 mg may be considered to be approximately equivalent in therapeutic effect to standard formulation *Diamicron*® 80 mg

GLIMEPIRIDE

Indications: type 2 diabetes mellitus
Cautions: see notes above; manufacturer recommends regular hepatic and haematological monitoring but limited evidence of clinical value; **interactions**: Appendix 1 (antidiabetics)
Contra-indications: see notes above
Side-effects: see notes above
Dose: initially 1 mg daily, adjusted according to response in 1-mg steps at 1–2 week intervals; usual

max. 4 mg daily (exceptionally, up to 6 mg daily may be used); taken shortly before or with first main meal

Amaryl® (Hoechst Marion Roussel) PoM
Tablets, all scored, glimepiride 1 mg (pink), net price 30-tab pack = £4.51; 2 mg (green), 30-tab pack = £7.42; 3 mg (yellow), 30-tab pack = £11.19; 4 mg (blue), 30-tab pack = £14.82

GLIPIZIDE

Indications: type 2 diabetes mellitus
Cautions: see notes above; **interactions:** Appendix 1 (antidiabetics)
Contra-indications: see notes above
Side-effects: see notes above; also dizziness, drowsiness
Dose: initially 2.5–5 mg daily shortly before breakfast or lunch, adjusted according to response; max. 20 mg daily; up to 15 mg may be given as a single dose; higher doses divided

Glipizide (Non-proprietary) PoM
Tablets, glipizide 5 mg, 56-tab pack = £4.58

Glibenese® (Pfizer) PoM
Tablets, scored, glipizide 5 mg. Net price 56-tab pack = £4.36

Minodiab® (Pharmacia) PoM
Tablets, glipizide 2.5 mg, net price 28-tab pack = £1.48; 5 mg (scored), 28-tab pack = £1.26

GLIQUIDONE

Indications: type 2 diabetes mellitus
Cautions: see notes above; **interactions:** Appendix 1 (antidiabetics)
Contra-indications: see notes above
Side-effects: see notes above
Dose: initially 15 mg daily before breakfast, adjusted to 45–60 mg daily in 2 or 3 divided doses; max. single dose 60 mg, max. daily dose 180 mg

Glurenorm® (Sanofi-Synthelabo) PoM
Tablets, scored, gliquidone 30 mg. Net price 100-tab pack = £17.54

TOLBUTAMIDE

Indications: type 2 diabetes mellitus
Cautions: see notes above; **interactions:** Appendix 1 (antidiabetics)
Contra-indications: see notes above
Side-effects: see notes above; also headache, tinnitus
Dose: 0.5–1.5 g (max. 2 g) daily in divided doses (see notes above); with or immediately after breakfast

Tolbutamide (Non-proprietary) PoM
Tablets, tolbutamide 500 mg. Net price 28-tab pack = £2.39

6.1.2.2 Biguanides

Metformin, the only available biguanide, has a different mode of action from the sulphonylureas, and is not interchangeable with them. It exerts its effect mainly by decreasing gluconeogenesis and by increasing peripheral utilisation of glucose; since it acts only in the presence of endogenous insulin it is effective only if there are some residual functioning pancreatic islet cells.

Metformin is the drug of first choice in overweight patients in whom strict dieting has failed to control diabetes, if appropriate it may also be considered as an option in patients who are not overweight. It is also used when diabetes is inadequately controlled with sulphonylurea treatment. When the combination of strict diet and metformin treatment fails, other options include:

- combining with acarbose (section 6.1.2.3), which may have a small beneficial effect, but flatulence can be a problem;
- combining with insulin (section 6.1.1) but weight gain and hypoglycaemia can be problems (weight gain minimised if insulin given at night);
- combining with a sulphonylurea (section 6.1.2.1) (reports of increased hazard with this combination remain unconfirmed);
- combining with pioglitazone or rosiglitazone (section 6.1.2.3);
- combining with repaglinide or nateglinide (section 6.1.2.3).

Insulin treatment is almost always required in medical and surgical emergencies; insulin should also be substituted before elective surgery (omit metformin the evening before surgery and give insulin if required).

Hypoglycaemia does not usually occur with metformin; other advantages are the lower incidence of weight gain and lower plasma-insulin concentration. It does not exert a hypoglycaemic action in non-diabetic subjects unless given in overdose.

Gastro-intestinal side-effects are initially common with metformin, and may persist in some patients, particularly when very high doses such as 3 g daily are given.

Metformin may provoke lactic acidosis which is most likely to occur in patients with renal impairment; it should not be used in patients with even mild renal impairment.

METFORMIN HYDROCHLORIDE

Indications: diabetes mellitus (see notes above); polycystic ovary syndrome [unlicensed indication]
Cautions: see notes above; determine renal function (using an appropriately sensitive method) before treatment and once or twice annually (more frequently in the elderly or if deterioration suspected); **interactions:** Appendix 1 (antidiabetics)
Contra-indications: renal impairment (Appendix 3), ketoacidosis, withdraw if tissue hypoxia likely (e.g. sepsis, respiratory failure, recent myocardial infarction, hepatic impairment (Appendix 2)), use of iodine-containing X-ray contrast media (do not restart metformin until renal function returns to normal) and use of general anaesthesia (suspend metformin 2 days beforehand and restart when renal function returns to normal), pregnancy (Appendix 4) and breast-feeding (Appendix 5)
Side-effects: anorexia, nausea, vomiting, diarrhoea (usually transient), abdominal pain, metallic taste; *rarely* lactic acidosis (withdraw treatment), decreased vitamin-B_{12} absorption, erythema, pruritus and urticaria; hepatitis also reported
Dose: diabetes mellitus, ADULT and CHILD over 10 years initially 500 mg with breakfast for at least 1 week then 500 mg with breakfast and evening meal for at least 1 week then 500 mg with breakfast, lunch and evening meal; usual max. 2 g daily in divided doses

Polycystic ovary syndrome [unlicensed], initially 500 mg with breakfast for 1 week, then 500 mg with breakfast and evening meal for 1 week, then 1.5–1.7 g daily in 2–3 divided doses

NOTE. Metformin doses in the BNF may differ from those in the product literature

Metformin (Non-proprietary) PoM

Tablets, coated, metformin hydrochloride 500 mg, net price 28-tab pack = £1.41, 84-tab pack= £2.09; 850 mg, 56-tab pack = £1.88. Label: 21

Glucophage® (Merck) PoM

Tablets, f/c, metformin hydrochloride 500 mg, net price 84-tab pack = £2.40; 850 mg, 56-tab pack = £2.67. Label: 21

■ Modified release

Glucophage® SR (Merck) PoM

Tablets, m/r, metformin hydrochloride 500 mg, net price 28 tab-pack = £2.67, 56 tab-pack = £5.34. Label: 21, 25

Dose: initially 500 mg once daily, increased every 10–15 days, max. 2 g once daily with evening meal; if control not achieved use 1 g twice daily with meals and if control still not achieved change to standard-release tablets

NOTE. Patients taking less than 2 g daily of the standard-release metformin may start with the same daily dose of *Glucophage® SR*; not suitable if dose of standard release tablets more than 2 g daily

■ With rosiglitazone

See section 6.1.2.3

6.1.2.3 Other antidiabetics

Acarbose, an inhibitor of intestinal alpha glucosidases, delays the digestion and absorption of starch and sucrose. It has a small but significant effect in lowering blood glucose and is used either on its own or as an adjunct to metformin or to sulphonylureas when they prove inadequate. Postprandial hyperglycaemia in type 1 (insulin-dependent) diabetes can be reduced by acarbose, but it has been little used for this purpose. Flatulence deters some from using acarbose although this side-effect tends to decrease with time.

Nateglinide and **repaglinide** stimulate insulin release. Both drugs have a rapid onset of action and short duration of activity, and should be administered shortly before each main meal. Repaglinide may be given as monotherapy for patients who are not overweight or for those in whom metformin is contra-indicated or not tolerated, or it may be given in combination with metformin. Nateglinide is licensed only for use with metformin.

The thiazolidinediones, **pioglitazone** and **rosiglitazone**, reduce peripheral insulin resistance, leading to a reduction of blood-glucose concentration. Either drug may be used alone or in combination with metformin or with a sulphonylurea (if metformin inappropriate); the combination of a thiazolidinedione plus metformin is preferred to a thiazolidinedione plus sulphonylurea, particularly for obese patients. Inadequate response to a combination of metformin and sulphonylurea may indicate failing insulin release; the introduction of pioglitazone or rosiglitazone has a limited role in these circumstances and insulin treatment should not be delayed. Blood-glucose control may deteriorate temporarily when a thiazolidinedione is substituted for an oral antidiabetic drug that is being used in combination with another. Long-term benefits of the thiazolidinediones have not yet been demonstrated.

NICE guidance (pioglitazone and rosiglitazone for type 2 diabetes mellitus). NICE has advised (August 2003) that the use of a thiazolidinedione (pioglitazone or rosiglitazone) as second-line therapy added to either metformin or a sulphonylurea is **not** recommended [see also notes above], except for:

- patients who are unable to tolerate metformin and sulphonylurea in combination therapy, *or*
- patients in whom either metformin or a sulphonylurea is contra-indicated.

In such cases, the thiazolidinedione should replace whichever drug in the combination is poorly tolerated or contra-indicated.

ACARBOSE

Indications: diabetes mellitus inadequately controlled by diet or by diet with oral antidiabetic drugs

Cautions: monitor liver function; may enhance hypoglycaemic effects of insulin and sulphonylureas (hypoglycaemic episodes may be treated with oral glucose but not with sucrose); **interactions:** Appendix 1 (antidiabetics)

Contra-indications: pregnancy (Appendix 4); breast-feeding (Appendix 5); inflammatory bowel disease (e.g. ulcerative colitis, Crohn's disease), partial intestinal obstruction (or predisposition); hepatic impairment, severe renal impairment; hernia, history of abdominal surgery

Side-effects: flatulence, soft stools, diarrhoea (may need to reduce dose or withdraw), abdominal distention and pain; rarely nausea, abnormal liver function tests and skin reactions; ileus, oedema, jaundice and hepatitis reported

NOTE. Antacids not recommended for treating side-effects (unlikely to be beneficial)

Dose: 50 mg daily initially (to minimise side-effects) increased to 50 mg 3 times daily, then increased if necessary after 6–8 weeks to 100 mg 3 times daily; max. 200 mg 3 times daily; CHILD under 12 years not recommended

COUNSELLING. Tablets should be chewed with first mouthful of food or swallowed whole with a little liquid immediately before food. To counteract possible hypoglycaemia, patients receiving insulin or a sulphonylurea as well as acarbose need to carry glucose (not sucrose—acarbose interferes with sucrose absorption)

Glucobay® (Bayer) PoM

Tablets, acarbose 50 mg, net price 90-tab pack = £6.60; 100 mg (scored), 90-tab pack = £12.51. Counselling, administration

NATEGLINIDE

Indications: type 2 diabetes mellitus in combination with metformin when metformin alone inadequate

Cautions: substitute insulin during intercurrent illness (such as myocardial infarction, coma, infection, and trauma) and during surgery; debilitated and malnourished patients; moderate hepatic impairment (avoid if severe—Appendix 2); **interactions:** Appendix 1 (antidiabetics)

Contra-indications: ketoacidosis; pregnancy (Appendix 4) and breast-feeding (Appendix 5)

Side-effects: hypoglycaemia; hypersensitivity reactions including pruritus, rashes and urticaria

Dose: initially 60 mg 3 times daily within 30 minutes before main meals, adjusted according to response up to max. 180 mg 3 times daily; CHILD and ADOLESCENT under 18 years not recommended

Starlix® (Novartis) PoM
Tablets, f/c, nateglinide 60 mg (pink), net price 84-tab pack = £19.75; 120 mg (yellow), 84-tab pack = £22.50; 180 mg (red), 84-tab pack = £22.50

PIOGLITAZONE

Indications: type 2 diabetes mellitus (alone or combined with metformin or a sulphonylurea—see also notes above)

Cautions: monitor liver function (see below); cardiovascular disease (risk of heart failure); **interactions:** Appendix 1 (antidiabetics)

LIVER TOXICITY. Rare reports of liver dysfunction; monitor liver function before treatment, then every 2 months for 12 months and periodically thereafter; advise patients to seek immediate medical attention if symptoms such as nausea, vomiting, abdominal pain, fatigue and dark urine develop; discontinue if jaundice occurs

Contra-indications: hepatic impairment, history of heart failure, combination with insulin (risk of heart failure), pregnancy (Appendix 4), breast-feeding (Appendix 5)

Side-effects: gastro-intestinal disturbances, weight gain, oedema, anaemia, headache, visual disturbances, dizziness, arthralgia, hypoaesthesia, haematuria, impotence; less commonly hypoglycaemia, fatigue, insomnia, vertigo, sweating, altered blood lipids, proteinuria; see also Liver Toxicity above

Dose: initially 15–30 mg once daily increased to 45 mg once daily according to response

Actos® (Takeda) ▼ PoM
Tablets, pioglitazone (as hydrochloride) 15 mg, net price 28-tab pack = £24.14; 30 mg, 28-tab pack = £33.54; 45 mg, 28-tab pack = £36.96

REPAGLINIDE

Indications: type 2 diabetes mellitus (as monotherapy or in combination with metformin when metformin alone inadequate)

Cautions: substitute insulin during intercurrent illness (such as myocardial infarction, coma, infection, and trauma) and during surgery; debilitated and malnourished patients; renal impairment; **interactions:** Appendix 1 (antidiabetics)

Contra-indications: ketoacidosis; severe hepatic impairment; pregnancy (Appendix 4) and breast-feeding (Appendix 5)

Side-effects: abdominal pain, diarrhoea, constipation, nausea, vomiting; *rarely* hypoglycaemia, hypersensitivity reactions including pruritus, rashes, vasculitis, urticaria, and visual disturbances

Dose: initially 500 micrograms within 30 minutes before main meals (1 mg if transferring from another oral hypoglycaemic), adjusted according to response at intervals of 1–2 weeks; up to 4 mg may be given as a single dose, max. 16 mg daily
CHILD and ADOLESCENT under 18 years and ELDERLY over 75 years, not recommended

NovoNorm® (Novo Nordisk) PoM
Tablets, repaglinide 500 micrograms, net price 30-tab pack = £3.92, 90-tab pack = £11.76; 1 mg (yellow), 30-tab pack = £3.92, 90-tab pack = £11.76; 2 mg (peach), 90-tab pack = £11.76

ROSIGLITAZONE

Indications: type 2 diabetes mellitus (alone *or* combined with metformin *or* with a sulphonylurea *or* with both—see also notes above)

Cautions: monitor liver function (see below); cardiovascular disease (risk of heart failure), renal impairment (Appendix 3); **interactions:** Appendix 1 (antidiabetics)

LIVER TOXICITY. Rare reports of liver dysfunction reported; monitor liver function before treatment and periodically thereafter; advise patients to seek immediate medical attention if symptoms such as nausea, vomiting, abdominal pain, fatigue, anorexia and dark urine develop; discontinue if jaundice occurs or liver enzymes significantly raised

Contra-indications: hepatic impairment, history of heart failure, combination with insulin (risk of heart failure), pregnancy (Appendix 4), breast-feeding (Appendix 5)

Side-effects: gastro-intestinal disturbances, headache, anaemia, altered blood lipids, weight gain, oedema, hypoglycaemia; less commonly increased appetite, heart failure, fatigue, paraesthesia, alopecia, dyspnoea; *rarely* pulmonary oedema; *very rarely* angioedema, urticaria; see also Liver Toxicity above

Dose: initially 4 mg daily; if used alone or in combination with metformin may increase to 8 mg daily (in 1 or 2 divided doses) after 8 weeks according to response; CHILD and ADOLESCENT under 18 years not recommended

Avandia® (GSK) ▼ PoM
Tablets, f/c, rosiglitazone (as maleate) 4 mg (orange), net price 28-tab pack = £24.74, 56-tab pack = £49.48; 8 mg (red/brown), 28-tab pack = £50.78

■ With metformin

For cautions, contra-indications and side-effects of metformin see section 6.1.2.2

Avandamet (GSK) ▼ PoM
Avandamet® *2 mg/500 mg tablets*, f/c, pink, rosiglitazone (as maleate) 2 mg, metformin hydrochloride 500 mg, net price 112-tab pack = £52.45. Label: 21
Avandamet® *2 mg/1 g tablets*, f/c, yellow, rosiglitazone (as maleate) 2 mg, metformin hydrochloride 1 g, net price 56-tab pack = £27.71. Label: 21
Avandamet® *4 mg/1 g tablets*, f/c, pink, rosiglitazone (as maleate) 4 mg, metformin hydrochloride 1 g, net price 56-tab pack = £52.45. Label: 21
Dose: type 2 diabetes mellitus not controlled by metformin alone, initially one *Avandamet*® 2 mg/1 g twice daily, increased after 8 weeks according to response up to two *Avandamet*® 2 mg/500 mg tablets twice daily or one *Avandamet*® 4 mg/1 g tablet twice daily; max. 8 mg rosiglitazone and 2 g metformin hydrochloride daily; CHILD and ADOLESCENT under 18 years not recommended
NOTE. Titration with the individual components (rosiglitazone and metformin) may be desirable before initiation of *Avandamet*®

6.1.3 Diabetic ketoacidosis

Soluble insulin, used intravenously, is the most appropriate form of insulin for the management of diabetic ketoacidotic and hyperosmolar non-ketotic coma. It is preferable to use the type of soluble insulin that the patient has been using previously. It is necessary to achieve and to maintain an adequate plasma-insulin concentration until the metabolic disturbance is brought under control.

Insulin is best given by intravenous infusion, using an infusion pump, and diluted to 1 unit/mL (care in mixing, see Appendix 6). Adequate plasma-insulin concentration can usually be maintained with infusion rates of 6 units/hour for adults and 0.1 units/kg/hour for children. Blood glucose is expected to decrease by about 5 mmol/litre/hour; if the response is inadequate the infusion rate can be doubled or quadrupled. When the blood-glucose concentration has fallen to 10 mmol/litre the infusion rate can be reduced to 3 units/hour for adults (about 0.05 units/kg/hour for children) and continued until the patient is ready to take food by mouth. The insulin infusion should not be stopped before subcutaneous insulin has been started.

No matter how large, a bolus intravenous injection of insulin can provide an adequate plasma concentration for a short time only; therefore if facilities for intravenous infusion are not available the insulin is given by *intramuscular injection*. An initial loading dose of 20 units intramuscularly is followed by 6 units intramuscularly every hour until the blood-glucose concentration falls to 10 mmol/litre; intramuscular injections are then given every 2 hours. Although absorption of insulin is usually rapid after intramuscular injection, it may be impaired in the presence of hypotension and poor tissue perfusion; moreover insulin may accumulate during treatment and late hypoglycaemia should be watched for and treated appropriately.

Intravenous replacement of fluid and electrolytes (section 9.2.2) with **sodium chloride** intravenous infusion is an essential part of the management of ketoacidosis; **potassium chloride** is included in the infusion as appropriate to prevent the hypokalaemia induced by the insulin. **Sodium bicarbonate** infusion (1.26% or 2.74%) is used only in cases of extreme acidosis and shock since the acid-base disturbance is normally corrected by the insulin. When the blood glucose has fallen to approximately 10 mmol/litre **glucose** 5% is infused (maximum 2 litres in 24 hours), but insulin infusion must continue.

6.1.4 Treatment of hypoglycaemia

Initially glucose 10–20 g is given by mouth either in liquid form or as granulated sugar or sugar lumps. Approximately 10 g of glucose is available from 2 teaspoons sugar, 3 sugar lumps, *GlucoGel*® (formerly known as *Hypostop Gel*®; glucose 9.2 g/23-g oral ampoule, available from British BioCell International), milk 200 mL, and non-diet versions of *Lucozade*® *Sparkling Glucose Drink* 50–55 mL, *Coca-Cola*® 90 mL, *Ribena*® *Original* 15 mL (to be diluted). If necessary this may be repeated in 10–15 minutes.

Hypoglycaemia which causes unconsciousness is an emergency. **Glucagon**, a polypeptide hormone produced by the alpha cells of the islets of Langerhans, increases plasma-glucose concentration by mobilising glycogen stored in the liver. In hypoglycaemia, if sugar cannot be given by mouth, glucagon can be given by injection. Carbohydrates should be given as soon as possible to restore liver glycogen; glucagon is not appropriate for chronic hypoglycaemia. It may be issued to close relatives of insulin-treated patients for emergency use in hypoglycaemic attacks. It is often advisable to prescribe on an 'if necessary' basis to hospitalised insulin-treated patients, so that it may be given rapidly by the nurses during an hypoglycaemic emergency. If not effective in 10 minutes intravenous glucose should be given.

Alternatively, 50 mL of **glucose intravenous infusion 20%** (section 9.2.2) may be given intravenously into a large vein through a large-gauge needle; care is required since this concentration is irritant especially if extravasation occurs. Alternatively, 25 mL of glucose intravenous infusion 50% may be given, but this higher concentration is more irritant and viscous making administration difficult. Glucose intravenous infusion 10% may also be used but larger volumes are needed. Close monitoring is necessary in the case of an overdose with a long-acting insulin because further administration of glucose may be required. Patients whose hypoglycaemia is caused by an oral antidiabetic drug should be transferred to hospital because the hypoglycaemic effects of these drugs may persist for many hours.

For advice on the management of medical emergencies in dental practice, see p. 22

GLUCAGON

Indications: see notes above and under Dose

Cautions: see notes above, insulinoma, glucagonoma; ineffective in chronic hypoglycaemia, starvation, and adrenal insufficiency

Contra-indications: phaeochromocytoma

Side-effects: nausea, vomiting, abdominal pain, hypokalaemia, hypotension, rarely hypersensitivity reactions

Dose: insulin-induced hypoglycaemia, *by subcutaneous, intramuscular, or intravenous injection*, ADULT and CHILD over 8 years (or body-weight over 25 kg), 1 mg; CHILD under 8 years (or body-weight under 25 kg), 500 micrograms; if no response within 10 minutes intravenous glucose must be given

Diagnostic aid, consult product literature

Beta-blocker poisoning, see p. 32

NOTE. 1 unit of glucagon = 1 mg of glucagon

[1]**GlucaGen**® **HypoKit** (Novo Nordisk) PoM

Injection, powder for reconstitution, glucagon (rys) as hydrochloride with lactose, net price 1-mg vial with prefilled syringe containing water for injection = £11.52

1. PoM restriction does not apply where administration is for saving life in emergency

Chronic hypoglycaemia

Diazoxide, administered by mouth, is useful in the management of patients with chronic hypoglycaemia from excess endogenous insulin secretion, either from an islet cell tumour or islet cell hyperplasia. It has no place in the management of acute hypoglycaemia.

DIAZOXIDE

Indications: chronic intractable hypoglycaemia (for use in hypertensive crisis see section 2.5.1)

Cautions: ischaemic heart disease, pregnancy (Appendix 4), labour, impaired renal function (Appendix 3); haematological examinations and blood pressure monitoring required during prolonged treatment; growth, bone, and developmental checks in children; **interactions:** Appendix 1 (diazoxide)

Side-effects: anorexia, nausea, vomiting, hyperuricaemia, hypotension, oedema, tachycardia, arrhythmias, extrapyramidal effects; hypertrichosis on prolonged treatment

Dose: *by mouth*, ADULT and CHILD, initially 5 mg/kg daily in 2–3 divided doses

Eudemine® (Celltech) PoM
Tablets, diazoxide 50 mg. Net price 20 = £9.29

6.1.5 Treatment of diabetic nephropathy and neuropathy

Diabetic nephropathy

Regular review of diabetic patients should include an annual test for urinary protein (using *Albustix*®) and serum creatinine measurement. If the urinary protein test is negative, the urine should be tested for microalbuminuria (the earliest sign of nephropathy). If reagent strip tests (*Micral-Test II*® NHS or *Microbumintest*® NHS) are used and prove positive, the result should be confirmed by laboratory analysis of a urine sample. Provided there are no contra-indications, all diabetic patients with nephropathy causing proteinuria or with established microalbuminuria (at least 3 positive tests) should be treated with an ACE inhibitor (section 2.5.5.1) or an angiotensin-II receptor antagonist (section 2.5.5.2) even if the blood pressure is normal; in any case, to minimise the risk of renal deterioration, blood pressure should be carefully controlled (section 2.5).

ACE inhibitors may potentiate the hypoglycaemic effect of insulin and oral antidiabetic drugs; this effect is more likely during the first weeks of combined treatment and in patients with renal impairment.

For the treatment of hypertension in diabetes, see section 2.5.

Diabetic neuropathy

Optimal diabetic control is beneficial for the management of *painful neuropathy* in patients with type 1 diabetes (see also section 4.7.3). **Paracetamol** or a **non-steroidal anti-inflammatory drug** such as ibuprofen (section 10.1.1) may relieve *mild to moderate pain.*

The **tricyclic antidepressants** amitriptyline and nortriptyline (section 4.3.1) are the drugs of choice for painful diabetic neuropathy [unlicensed use]; amitriptyline is given in a dose of 25–75 mg daily (higher doses under specialist supervision). Other classes of antidepressants do not appear to be effective. **Gabapentin** (section 4.8.1) is licensed for the treatment of neuropathic pain and is an effective alternative to a tricyclic antidepressant.

Carbamazepine and **phenytoin** [both unlicensed] (section 4.8.1) may be useful for shooting or stabbing pain, but adverse effects are common; carbamazepine 200–800 mg daily in divided doses has been used.

Capsaicin cream 0.075% (section 10.3.2) is licensed for painful diabetic neuropathy and may have some effect, but it produces an intense burning sensation during the initial treatment period.

Neuropathic pain may respond partially to some **opioid analgesics**, such as dextropropoxyphene, methadone, oxycodone and tramadol, and they may have a role when other treatments have failed.

In *autonomic neuropathy* diabetic diarrhoea can often be managed by 2 or 3 doses of **tetracycline** 250 mg [unlicensed use] (section 5.1.3). Otherwise **codeine phosphate** (section 1.4.2) is the best drug, but other antidiarrhoeal preparations can be tried. An **antiemetic** which promotes gastric transit, such as metoclopramide or domperidone (section 4.6), is helpful for gastroparesis. In rare cases when an antiemetic does not help, erythromycin (especially when given intravenously) may be beneficial but this needs confirmation.

For the management of erectile dysfunction, see section 7.4.5.

In *neuropathic postural hypotension* increased salt intake and the use of the **mineralocorticoid** fludrocortisone 100–400 micrograms daily [unlicensed use] (section 6.3.1) help by increasing plasma volume, but uncomfortable oedema is a common side-effect. Fludrocortisone can also be combined with **flurbiprofen** (section 10.1.1) and **ephedrine hydrochloride** (section 3.1.1.2) [both unlicensed]. **Midodrine** [unlicensed], an alpha agonist, may also be useful in postural hypotension.

Gustatory sweating can be treated with an **antimuscarinic** such as propantheline bromide (section 1.2); side-effects are common. For the management of hyperhidrosis, see section 13.12.

In some patients with *neuropathic oedema*, **ephedrine hydrochloride** [unlicensed use] 30–60 mg 3 times daily offers effective relief.

6.1.6 Diagnostic and monitoring agents for diabetes mellitus

Blood glucose monitoring

Blood glucose monitoring gives a direct measure of the glucose concentration at the time of the test and can detect hypoglycaemia as well as hyperglycaemia. Patients should be properly trained in the use of blood glucose monitoring systems and to take appropriate action on the results obtained. Inadequate understanding of the normal fluctuations in blood glucose may lead to confusion and inappropriate action. It is ideal for patients to observe the 'peaks' and 'troughs' of blood glucose over 24 hours and make adjustments of their insulin no more than once or twice weekly. Daily alterations to the insulin dose are highly undesirable (except during illness).

Blood glucose monitoring is best carried out by means of a meter. Visual colour comparison is sometimes used but is much less satisfactory. Meters give a more precise reading and are useful for patients with poor eyesight or who are colour blind.

NOTE. In the UK blood-glucose concentration is expressed in mmol/litre and Diabetes UK advises that these units should be used for self-monitoring of blood glucose. In other European countries units of mg/100 mL (or mg/dL) are commonly used.

It is advisable to check that the meter is pre-set in the correct units.

■ Test strips

Active® (Roche Diagnostics)
Reagent strips, for blood glucose monitoring, range 0.6–33.3 mmol/litre, for use with *Glucotrend*® and *Accu-Chek*® *Active* NHS meters only. Net price 50-strip pack = £15.83

Advantage II® (Roche Diagnostics)
Reagent strips, for blood glucose monitoring, range 0.6–33.3 mmol/litre, for use with *Accu-Chek*® *Advantage* NHS meter only. Net price 50-strip pack = £15.55

Ascensia® **Autodisc** (Bayer Diagnostics)
Sensor discs, for blood glucose monitoring, range 0.6–33.3 mmol/litre, for use with *Ascensia Breeze*® NHS and *Ascensia Esprit*® *2* NHS meters only. Net price 5 × 10-disc pack = £15.67

Ascensia® **Glucodisc** (Bayer Diagnostics) NHS
Sensor discs, for blood glucose monitoring, range 0.6–33.3 mmol/L, for use with *Ascensia Esprit*® 2 NHS meter only. Net price 5 × 10-disc pack = £15.53

Ascensia® **Microfill** (Bayer Diagnostics)
Sensor strips, for blood glucose monitoring, range 0.6–33.3 mmol/litre, for use with *Ascensia*® *Contour* NHS meter only. Net price 50-strip pack = £15.55

BM-Accutest® (Roche Diagnostics)
Reagent strips, for blood glucose monitoring, range 1.1–33.3 mmol/litre, for use with *Accutrend*® NHS meters only. Net price 50-strip pack = £15.34

Compact® (Roche Diagnostics)
Reagent strips, for blood glucose monitoring, range 0.6–33.3 mmol/litre, for use with *Accu-Chek*® *Compact* and *Accu-Chek*® *Compact Plus* NHS meters only. Net price 3 × 17-strip pack = £15.95

FreeStyle® (TheraSense)
Reagent strips, for blood glucose monitoring, range 1.1–27.8 mmol/litre, for use with *FreeStyle*® NHS meter only. Net price 50-strip pack = £15.67

GlucoMen® (Menarini Diagnostics)
Sensor strips, for blood glucose monitoring, range 1.1–33.3 mmol/litre, for use with *GlucoMen*® *Glycó* NHS meter only. Net price 50-strip pack = £14.94

Glucotide® (Bayer Diagnostics)
Reagent strips, for blood glucose monitoring, range 0.6–33.3 mmol/litre, for use with *Glucometer*® *4* NHS meter only. Net price 50-strip pack = £15.33

Hypoguard® **Supreme** (Hypoguard)
Reagent strips, for blood glucose monitoring, range 2.2–27.7 mmol/litre, for use with *Hypoguard*® *Supreme* NHS meters. Net price 50-strip pack = £13.64

Hypoguard® **Supreme Spectrum** (Hypoguard)
Reagent strips, for blood glucose monitoring, visual range 2.2–27.8 mmol/litre. Net price 50-strip pack = £10.34

MediSense G2® (MediSense)
Sensor strips, for blood glucose monitoring, range 1.1–33.3 mmol/litre. for use with *MediSense Card*® NHS or *MediSense Pen*® NHS meters only. Net price 50-strip pack = £14.40

MediSense® **Optium Plus** (MediSense)
Sensor strips, for blood glucose monitoring, range 1.1–27.7 mmol/litre, for use with *MediSense*® *Optium* NHS meter only. Net price 50-strip pack = £15.30

MediSense® **Soft-Sense** (MediSense)
Sensor strips, for blood glucose monitoring, range 1.7–25 mmol/litre, for use with *MediSense*® *Soft-Sense* NHS meter only. Net price 50-strip pack = £15.55

One Touch® (LifeScan)
Reagent strips, for blood glucose monitoring, range 0–33.3 mmol/litre, for use with *One Touch*® *II*, *Profile* and *Basic* NHS meters only. Net price 50-strip pack = £15.41

One Touch® **Ultra** (LifeScan)
Reagent strips, for blood glucose monitoring, range 1.1–33.3 mmol/litre, for use with *One Touch*® *Ultra* NHS meter only. Net price 50-strip pack = £15.57

PocketScan® (LifeScan)
Reagent strips, for blood glucose monitoring, range 1.1–33.3 mmol/litre, for use with *PocketScan*® NHS meter only. Net price 50-strip pack = £15.21

Prestige® **Smart System** (DiagnoSys)
Reagent strips, for blood glucose monitoring, range 1.4–33.3 mmol/litre, for use with *Prestige*® *Smart System* NHS meter only. Net price 50-strip pack = £15.29

■ Meters

Accu-Chek® **Active** (Roche Diagnostics) NHS
Meter, for blood glucose monitoring (for use with *Active*® test strips). *Accu-Chek*® *Active* system = £7.79

Accu-Chek® **Advantage** (Roche Diagnostics) NHS
Meter, for blood glucose monitoring (for use with *Advantage II*® test strips). *Accu-Chek*® *Advantage* system = £4.20

Accu-Chek® **Compact Plus** (Roche Diagnostics) NHS
Meter, for blood glucose monitoring (for use with *Compact*® test strips). *Accu-Chek*® *Compact Plus* system = £7.79

Ascensia Breeze® (Bayer Diagnostics) NHS
Meter, for blood glucose monitoring (for use with *Ascensia*® *Autodisc* test sensor discs)

Ascensia Contour® (Bayer Diagnostics) NHS
Meter, for blood glucose monitoring (for use with *Ascensia*® *Microfill* sensor strips) = £19.97

Ascensia Esprit® **2** (Bayer Diagnostics) NHS
Meter, for blood glucose monitoring (for use with *Ascensia*® *Glucodisc* test sensor discs) = £17.49

FreeStyle® (TheraSense) NHS
Meter for blood glucose monitoring (for use with *FreeStyle*® test strips) = £25.00

GlucoMen® **Glycó** (Menarini Diagnostics) NHS
Meter, for blood glucose monitoring (for use with *GlucoMen*® sensor strips)

GlucoMen® **PC** (Menarini Diagnostics) NHS
Meter, for blood glucose monitoring (for use with *GlucoMen*® sensor strips)

Glucotrend® (Roche Diagnostics) NHS
Meters, for blood glucose monitoring (for use with *Glucotrend*® test strips). *Glucotrend*® *2 Soft Test System* pack NHS = £25.00; *Glucotrend*® *Premium* pack NHS = £36.74

Hypoguard® **Supreme** (Hypoguard) NHS
Meters, for blood glucose monitoring (for use with *Hypoguard*® *Supreme* test strips). *Hypoguard*® *Supreme Plus* meter = £35.00; *Hypoguard*® *Supreme Extra* meter = £45.00

MediSense® (MediSense) NHS
Meters (Sensor), for blood glucose monitoring. *MediSense Card* = £15.31, *MediSense*® card starter pack = £17.50, *MediSense*® Pen = £30.63, *MediSense*® pen starter pack = £39.38, *MediSense*® *Precision QID* starter pack = £12.00 (all for use with *MediSense G2*® test strips); *MediSense*® *Optium* starter pack (for use with *MediSense*® *Optium* test strips) = £17.50; *MediSense*® *Soft-Sense* meter (for use with *MediSense*® *Soft-Sense* test strips)

One Touch® (LifeScan) NHS
Meters, for blood glucose monitoring (for use with *One Touch*® test strips). *One Touch*® *Basic* system pack = £9.38, *One Touch*® *Profile* system pack = £18.38

One Touch® Ultra (LifeScan) NHS
Meter, for blood glucose monitoring (for use with *One Touch® Ultra* test strips) = £10.00

PocketScan® (LifeScan) NHS
Meter, for blood glucose monitoring (for use with *PocketScan®* test strips). *Complete PocketScan® System* = £17.50

Prestige® Smart System (DiagnoSys) NHS
Meter, for blood glucose monitoring (for use with *Prestige® Smart System* test strips) = £5.63

Urinalysis

Urine testing for glucose is useful in patients who find blood glucose monitoring difficult. Tests for glucose range from reagent strips specific to glucose to reagent tablets which detect all reducing sugars. Few patients still use *Clinitest®*; *Clinistix®* is suitable for screening purposes only. Tests for ketones by patients are rarely required unless they become unwell.

Microalbuminuria can be detected with *Micral-Test II®* NHS or *Microbumintest®* NHS but this should be followed by confirmation in the laboratory, since false positive results are common.

■ Glucose

Clinistix® (Bayer Diagnostics)
Reagent strips, for detection of glucose in urine. Net price 50-strip pack = £3.18

Clinitest® (Bayer Diagnostics)
Reagent tablets, for detection of glucose and other reducing substances in urine. Pocket set NHS (test tube, dropper and 36 tablets), net price = £4.02, 36-tab pack = £2.00, 6-test tube pack NHS = £3.70, 6-dropper pack NHS = £3.80

Diabur-Test 5000® (Roche Diagnostics)
Reagent strips, for detection of glucose in urine. Net price 50-strip pack = £2.63

Diastix® (Bayer Diagnostics)
Reagent strips, for detection of glucose in urine. Net price 50-strip pack = £2.71

Medi-Test® Glucose (BHR)
Reagent strips, for detection of glucose in urine. Net price 50-strip pack = £2.17

■ Ketones

Acetest® (Bayer Diagnostics)
Reagent tablets, for detection of ketones in urine. Net price 100-tab pack = £3.53

Ketostix® (Bayer Diagnostics)
Reagent strips, for detection of ketones in urine. Net price 50-strip pack = £2.87

Ketur Test® (Roche Diagnostics)
Reagent strips, for detection of ketones in urine. Net price 50-strip pack = £2.53

■ Protein

Albustix® (Bayer Diagnostics)
Reagent strips, for detection of protein in urine. Net price 50-strip pack = £3.94

Medi-Test® Protein 2 (BHR)
Reagent strips, for detection of protein in urine. Net price 50-strip pack = £3.03

■ Other reagent strips available for urinalysis include:
Combur-3 Test® NHS (glucose and protein—Roche Diagnostics), *Clinitek Microalbumin®* NHS (albumin and creatinine—Bayer Diagnostics), *Ketodiastix®* NHS (glucose and ketones—Bayer Diagnostics), *Medi-Test Combi 2®* NHS (glucose and protein—BHR), *Micral-Test II®* NHS (albumin—Roche Diagnostics), *Microalbustix®* NHS (albumin and creatinine—Bayer Diagnostics), *Microbumintest®* NHS (albumin—Bayer Diagnostics), *Uristix®* NHS (glucose and protein—Bayer Diagnostics)

Glucose tolerance test

The **glucose** tolerance test is now rarely needed for the diagnosis of diabetes when symptoms of hyperglycaemia are present, though it is still required to establish the presence of gestational diabetes. This generally involves giving anhydrous glucose 75 g (equivalent to Glucose BP 82.5 g) by mouth to the fasting patient, and measuring blood-glucose concentrations at intervals.

The appropriate amount of glucose should be given with 200–300 mL fluid. Anhydrous glucose 75 g may alternatively be given as 113 mL *Polycal®* (Nutricia Clinical) with extra fluid to administer a total volume of 200–300 mL.

6.2 Thyroid and antithyroid drugs

6.2.1 Thyroid hormones

Thyroid hormones are used in hypothyroidism (myxoedema), and also in diffuse non-toxic goitre, Hashimoto's thyroiditis (lymphadenoid goitre), and thyroid carcinoma. Neonatal hypothyroidism requires prompt treatment for normal development.

Levothyroxine sodium (thyroxine sodium) is the treatment of choice for *maintenance* therapy. The initial dose should not exceed 100 micrograms daily, preferably before breakfast, or 25 to 50 micrograms in elderly patients or those with cardiac disease, increased by 25 to 50 micrograms at intervals of at least 4 weeks. The usual maintenance dose to relieve hypothyroidism is 100 to 200 micrograms daily which can be administered as a single dose.

In infants and children doses of thyroxine, for congenital hypothyroidism and juvenile myxoedema, should be titrated according to clinical response, growth assessment, and measurements of plasma thyroxine and thyroid-stimulating hormone.

Liothyronine sodium has a similar action to levothyroxine but is more rapidly metabolised and has a more rapid effect; 20 micrograms is equivalent to 100 micrograms of levothyroxine. Its effects develop after a few hours and disappear within 24 to 48 hours of discontinuing treatment. It may be used in *severe hypothyroid states* when a rapid response is desired.

Liothyronine by intravenous injection is the treatment of choice in *hypothyroid coma*. Adjunctive therapy includes intravenous fluids, hydrocortisone, and treatment of infection; assisted ventilation is often required.

LEVOTHYROXINE SODIUM

(Thyroxine sodium)

Indications: hypothyroidism

Cautions: panhypopituitarism or predisposition to adrenal insufficiency (initiate corticosteroid therapy before starting levothyroxine), elderly, cardiovascular disorders (myocardial insufficiency or myocardial infarction, see Initial Dosage below), long-standing hypothyroidism, diabetes insipidus, diabetes mellitus (dose of antidiabetic drugs including insulin may need to be increased); pregnancy (Appendix 4) and breast-feeding (Appendix 5); **interactions:** Appendix 1 (thyroid hormones)

INITIAL DOSAGE. A pre-therapy ECG is valuable as changes induced by hypothyroidism may be confused with evidence of ischaemia. If metabolism increases too rapidly (causing diarrhoea, nervousness, rapid pulse, insomnia, tremors and sometimes anginal pain where there is latent myocardial ischaemia), reduce dose or withhold for 1–2 days and start again at a lower dose

Contra-indications: thyrotoxicosis

Side-effects: usually at excessive dosage (see Initial Dosage above) include anginal pain, arrhythmias, palpitation, skeletal muscle cramps, tachycardia, diarrhoea, vomiting, tremors, restlessness, excitability, insomnia, headache, flushing, sweating, fever, heat intolerance, excessive loss of weight and muscular weakness

Dose: ADULT, initially 50–100 micrograms (50 micrograms for those over 50 years) daily, preferably before breakfast, adjusted in steps of 50 micrograms every 3–4 weeks until metabolism normalised (usually 100–200 micrograms daily); in cardiac disease, initially 25 micrograms daily *or* 50 micrograms on alternate days, adjusted in steps of 25 micrograms every 4 weeks

Congenital hypothyroidism and juvenile myxoedema, NEONATE up to 1 month initially 5–10 micrograms/kg daily, CHILD over 1 month initially 5 micrograms/kg daily adjusted in steps of 25 micrograms every 2–4 weeks until mild toxic symptoms appear then reduce dose slightly

Levothyroxine (Non-proprietary) PoM

Tablets, levothyroxine sodium 25 micrograms, net price 28-tab pack = 85p; 50 micrograms, 28-tab pack = 57p; 100 micrograms, 28-tab pack = 86p

Brands include *Eltroxin*®

LIOTHYRONINE SODIUM

(L-Tri-iodothyronine sodium)

Indications: see notes above

Cautions: see under Levothyroxine Sodium; (Appendix 4); **interactions:** Appendix 1 (thyroid hormones)

Contra-indications: see under Levothyroxine Sodium

Side-effects: see under Levothyroxine Sodium

Dose: *by mouth,* initially 10–20 micrograms daily gradually increased to 60 micrograms daily in 2–3 divided doses; elderly patients should receive smaller initial doses; CHILD, adult dose reduced in proportion to body-weight

By slow intravenous injection, hypothyroid coma, 5–20 micrograms repeated every 12 hours or as often as every 4 hours if necessary; alternatively 50 micrograms initially then 25 micrograms every 8 hours reducing to 25 micrograms twice daily

Tertroxin® (Goldshield) PoM

Tablets, scored, liothyronine sodium 20 micrograms, net price 100-tab pack = £15.92

Triiodothyronine (Goldshield) PoM

Injection, powder for reconstitution, liothyronine sodium (with dextran). Net price 20-microgram amp = £37.92

6.2.2 Antithyroid drugs

Antithyroid drugs are used for hyperthyroidism either to prepare patients for thyroidectomy or for long-term management. In the UK carbimazole is the most commonly used drug. Propylthiouracil may be used in patients who suffer sensitivity reactions to carbimazole as sensitivity is not necessarily displayed to both drugs. Both drugs act primarily by interfering with the synthesis of thyroid hormones.

CSM warning (neutropenia and agranulocytosis)

Doctors are reminded of the importance of recognising bone marrow suppression induced by carbimazole and the need to stop treatment promptly.

1. Patient should be asked to report symptoms and signs suggestive of infection, especially sore throat.
2. A white blood cell count should be performed if there is any clinical evidence of infection.
3. Carbimazole should be stopped promptly if there is clinical or laboratory evidence of neutropenia.

Carbimazole is given in a dose of 15 to 40 mg daily; occasionally a larger dose may be required. This dose is continued until the patient becomes euthyroid, usually after 4 to 8 weeks and the dose is then gradually reduced to a maintenance dose of 5 to 15 mg. Therapy is usually given for 12 to 18 months. Children may be given carbimazole in an initial dose of 250 micrograms/kg three times daily, adjusted according to response; treatment in children should be undertaken by a specialist. Rashes and pruritus are common but they can be treated with antihistamines without discontinuing therapy; alternatively propylthiouracil may be substituted. All patients should be advised to report any sore throat immediately because of the rare complication of agranulocytosis (see CSM warning, above).

Propylthiouracil is given in a dose of 200 to 400 mg daily in adults and this dose is maintained until the patient becomes euthyroid; the dose may then be gradually reduced to a maintenance dose of 50 to 150 mg daily.

Antithyroid drugs only need to be given once daily because of their prolonged effect on the thyroid. Over-treatment can result in the rapid development of hypothyroidism and should be avoided particularly during pregnancy because it can cause fetal goitre.

A combination of carbimazole, 40 to 60 mg daily with levothyroxine, 50 to 150 micrograms daily, may be used in a *blocking-replacement regimen*; therapy is usually given for 18 months. The blocking-replacement regimen is **not** suitable during pregnancy.

Iodine has been used as an adjunct to antithyroid drugs for 10 to 14 days before partial thyroidectomy; however, there is little evidence of a beneficial effect. Iodine should not be used for long-term treatment because its antithyroid action tends to diminish.

Radioactive sodium iodide (^{131}I) solution is used increasingly for the treatment of thyrotoxicosis at all ages, particularly where medical therapy or compliance is a problem, in patients with cardiac disease, and in patients who relapse after thyroidectomy.

Propranolol is useful for rapid relief of thyrotoxic symptoms and may be used in conjunction with antithyroid drugs or as an adjunct to radioactive iodine. Beta-blockers are also useful in neonatal thyrotoxicosis and in supraventricular arrhythmias due to hyperthyroidism. Propranolol has been used in conjunction with iodine to prepare mildly thyrotoxic patients for surgery but it is preferable to make the patient euthyroid with carbimazole. Laboratory tests of thyroid function are not altered by beta-blockers. Most experience in treating thyrotoxicosis has been gained with propranolol but **nadolol** is also used. For doses and preparations of beta-blockers see section 2.4.

Thyrotoxic crisis ('thyroid storm') requires emergency treatment with intravenous administration of fluids, propranolol (5 mg) and hydrocortisone (100 mg every 6 hours, as sodium succinate), as well as oral iodine solution and carbimazole or propylthiouracil which may need to be administered by nasogastric tube.

PREGNANCY AND BREAST-FEEDING. Radioactive iodine therapy is contra-indicated during pregnancy. Propylthiouracil and carbimazole can be given but the blocking-replacement regimen (see above) is **not** suitable. Both propylthiouracil and carbimazole cross the placenta and in high doses may cause fetal goitre and hypothyroidism—the lowest dose that will control the hyperthyroid state should be used (requirements in Graves' disease tend to fall during pregnancy). Rarely, carbimazole has been associated with aplasia cutis of the neonate.

Carbimazole and propylthiouracil appear in breast milk but this does not preclude breast-feeding as long as neonatal development is closely monitored and the lowest effective dose is used.

CARBIMAZOLE

Indications: hyperthyroidism

Cautions: liver disorders, pregnancy, breast-feeding (see notes above)

Side-effects: nausea, mild gastro-intestinal disturbances, headache, rashes and pruritus, arthralgia; rarely myopathy, alopecia, bone marrow suppression (including pancytopenia and agranulocytosis, see **CSM warning** above), jaundice

Dose: see notes above

COUNSELLING. Warn patient to tell doctor **immediately** if sore throat, mouth ulcers, bruising, fever, malaise, or non-specific illness develops

Neo-Mercazole® (Roche) PoM
Tablets, both pink, carbimazole 5 mg, net price 100-tab pack = £5.05; 20 mg, 100-tab pack = £18.75. Counselling, blood disorder symptoms

IODINE AND IODIDE

Indications: thyrotoxicosis (pre-operative)

Cautions: pregnancy, children; not for long-term treatment

Contra-indications: breast-feeding

Side-effects: hypersensitivity reactions including coryza-like symptoms, headache, lacrimation, conjunctivitis, pain in salivary glands, laryngitis, bronchitis, rashes; on prolonged treatment depression, insomnia, impotence; goitre in infants of mothers taking iodides

Aqueous Iodine Oral Solution
(Lugol's Solution), iodine 5%, potassium iodide 10% in purified water, freshly boiled and cooled, total iodine 130 mg/mL. Net price 100 mL = £1.95. Label: 27
Dose: 0.1–0.3 mL 3 times daily well diluted with milk or water

PROPYLTHIOURACIL

Indications: hyperthyroidism

Cautions: see under Carbimazole; hepatic impairment (Appendix 2), renal impairment (Appendix 3)

Side-effects: see under Carbimazole; leucopenia; rarely cutaneous vasculitis, thrombocytopenia, aplastic anaemia, hypoprothrombinaemia, hepatitis, encephalopathy, hepatic necrosis, nephritis, lupus erythematous-like syndromes

Dose: see notes above

Propylthiouracil (Non-proprietary) PoM
Tablets, propylthiouracil 50 mg. Net price 56-tab pack = £24.90

6.3 Corticosteroids

6.3.1 Replacement therapy

The adrenal cortex normally secretes hydrocortisone (cortisol) which has glucocorticoid activity and weak mineralocorticoid activity. It also secretes the mineralocorticoid aldosterone.

In deficiency states, physiological replacement is best achieved with a combination of **hydrocortisone** (section 6.3.2) and the mineralocorticoid **fludrocortisone**; hydrocortisone alone does not usually provide sufficient mineralocorticoid activity for complete replacement.

In *Addison's disease* or following adrenalectomy, **hydrocortisone** 20 to 30 mg daily by mouth is usually required. This is given in 2 doses, the larger in the morning and the smaller in the evening, mimicking the normal diurnal rhythm of cortisol secretion. The optimum daily dose is determined on the basis of clinical response. Glucocorticoid therapy is supplemented by fludrocortisone 50 to 300 micrograms daily.

In *acute adrenocortical insufficiency*, **hydrocortisone** is given intravenously (preferably as sodium succinate) in doses of 100 mg every 6 to 8 hours in sodium chloride intravenous infusion 0.9%.

In *hypopituitarism* glucocorticoids should be given as in adrenocortical insufficiency, but since the production of aldosterone is also regulated by the renin-angiotensin system a mineralocorticoid is not usually required. Additional replacement therapy with levothyroxine (section 6.2.1) and sex hormones (section 6.4) should be given as indicated by the pattern of hormone deficiency.

FLUDROCORTISONE ACETATE

Indications: mineralocorticoid replacement in adrenocortical insufficiency

Cautions: section 6.3.2; **interactions:** Appendix 1 (corticosteroids)

Contra-indications: section 6.3.2

Side-effects: section 6.3.2
Dose: 50–300 micrograms daily; CHILD 5 micrograms/kg daily

Florinef® (Squibb) PoM
Tablets, pink, scored, fludrocortisone acetate 100 micrograms. Net price 56-tab pack = £2.50. Label: 10, steroid card

6.3.2 Glucocorticoid therapy

In comparing the relative potencies of corticosteroids in terms of their anti-inflammatory (glucocorticoid) effects it should be borne in mind that high glucocorticoid activity in itself is of no advantage unless it is accompanied by relatively low mineralocorticoid activity (see Disadvantages of Corticosteroids below). The mineralocorticoid activity of **fludrocortisone** (section 6.3.1) is so high that its anti-inflammatory activity is of no clinical relevance. The table below shows equivalent anti-inflammatory doses.

Equivalent anti-inflammatory doses of corticosteroids

This table takes no account of mineralocorticoid effects, nor does it take account of variations in duration of action
Prednisolone 5 mg
≡ Betamethasone 750 micrograms
≡ Cortisone acetate 25 mg
≡ Deflazacort 6 mg
≡ Dexamethasone 750 micrograms
≡ Hydrocortisone 20 mg
≡ Methylprednisolone 4 mg
≡ Triamcinolone 4 mg

The relatively high mineralocorticoid activity of **cortisone** and **hydrocortisone**, and the resulting fluid retention, make them unsuitable for disease suppression on a long-term basis. However, they can be used for adrenal replacement therapy (section 6.3.1); hydrocortisone is preferred because cortisone requires conversion in the liver to hydrocortisone. Hydrocortisone is used on a short-term basis by intravenous injection for the emergency management of some conditions. The relatively moderate anti-inflammatory potency of hydrocortisone also makes it a useful topical corticosteroid for the management of inflammatory skin conditions because side-effects (both topical and systemic) are less marked (section 13.4); cortisone is not active topically.

Prednisolone has predominantly glucocorticoid activity and is the corticosteroid most commonly used by mouth for long-term disease suppression.

Betamethasone and **dexamethasone** have very high glucocorticoid activity in conjunction with insignificant mineralocorticoid activity. This makes them particularly suitable for high-dose therapy in conditions where fluid retention would be a disadvantage.

Betamethasone and dexamethasone also have a long duration of action and this, coupled with their lack of mineralocorticoid action makes them particularly suitable for conditions which require suppression of corticotropin (corticotrophin) secretion (e.g. congenital adrenal hyperplasia). Some esters of betamethasone and of **beclometasone** (beclomethasone) exert a considerably more marked topical effect (e.g. on the skin or the lungs) than when given by mouth; use is made of this to obtain topical effects whilst minimising systemic side-effects (e.g. for skin applications and asthma inhalations).

Deflazacort has a high glucocorticoid activity; it is derived from prednisolone.

Disadvantages of corticosteroids

Overdosage or prolonged use may exaggerate some of the normal physiological actions of corticosteroids leading to mineralocorticoid and glucocorticoid side-effects.

Mineralocorticoid side-effects include hypertension, sodium and water retention and potassium loss. They are most marked with fludrocortisone, but are significant with cortisone, hydrocortisone, corticotropin, and tetracosactide (tetracosactrin). Mineralocorticoid actions are negligible with the high potency glucocorticoids, betamethasone and dexamethasone, and occur only slightly with methylprednisolone, prednisolone, and triamcinolone.

Glucocorticoid side-effects include diabetes and osteoporosis (section 6.6), which is a danger, particularly in the elderly, as it may result in osteoporotic fractures for example of the hip or vertebrae; in addition high doses are associated with avascular necrosis of the femoral head. Mental disturbances may occur; a serious paranoid state or depression with risk of suicide may be induced, particularly in patients with a history of mental disorder. Euphoria is frequently observed. Muscle wasting (proximal myopathy) may also occur. Corticosteroid therapy is also weakly linked with peptic ulceration (the potential advantage of soluble or enteric-coated preparations to reduce the risk is speculative only).

High doses of corticosteroids may cause Cushing's syndrome, with moon face, striae, and acne; it is usually reversible on withdrawal of treatment, but this must always be gradually tapered to avoid symptoms of acute adrenal insufficiency (**important:** see also Adrenal Suppression , below).

In children, administration of corticosteroids may result in suppression of growth. For the effect of corticosteroids given in pregnancy, see Pregnancy and Breast-feeding, below.

Adrenal Suppression

During prolonged therapy with corticosteroids, adrenal atrophy develops and may persist for years after stopping. Abrupt withdrawal after a prolonged period may lead to acute adrenal insufficiency, hypotension or death (see Withdrawal of Corticosteroids, below). Withdrawal may also be associated with fever, myalgia, arthralgia, rhinitis, conjunctivitis, painful itchy skin nodules and weight loss.

To compensate for a diminished adrenocortical response caused by prolonged corticosteroid treatment, any significant intercurrent illness, trauma, or surgical procedure requires a temporary increase in corticosteroid dose, or if already stopped, a temporary re-introduction of corticosteroid treatment. Anaesthetists **must** therefore know whether a patient is taking or has been taking a corticosteroid, to avoid a precipitous fall in blood pressure during anaesthesia or in the immediate postoperative period. A suitable regimen for corticosteroid replacement, in patients who have taken more than 10 mg prednisolone daily (or equivalent) within 3 months of surgery, is:

- *Minor surgery under general anaesthesia*—usual oral corticosteroid dose on the morning of surgery or hydrocortisone 25–50 mg (usually the sodium succinate) intravenously at induction; the usual oral corticosteroid dose is recommenced after surgery
- *Moderate or major surgery*—usual oral corticosteroid dose on the morning of surgery and hydrocortisone 25–50 mg intravenously at induction, followed by hydrocortisone 25–50 mg 3 times a day by intravenous injection for 24 hours after moderate surgery or for 48–72 hours after major surgery; the usual pre-operative oral corticosteroid dose is recommenced on stopping hydrocortisone injections

Patients on long-term corticosteroid treatment should carry a Steroid Treatment Card (see below) which gives guidance on minimising risk and provides details of prescriber, drug, dosage and duration of treatment.

Infections

Prolonged courses of corticosteroids increase susceptibility to infections and severity of infections; clinical presentation of infections may also be atypical. Serious infections e.g. *septicaemia* and *tuberculosis* may reach an advanced stage before being recognised, and *amoebiasis* or *strongyloidiasis* may be activated or exacerbated (exclude before initiating a corticosteroid in those at risk or with suggestive symptoms). Fungal or viral *ocular infections* may also be exacerbated (see also section 11.4.1).

CHICKENPOX. Unless they have had chickenpox, patients receiving oral or parenteral corticosteroids for purposes other than replacement should be regarded as being *at risk of severe chickenpox* (see Steroid Treatment Card). Manifestations of fulminant illness include pneumonia, hepatitis and disseminated intravascular coagulation; rash is not necessarily a prominent feature.

Passive immunisation with varicella–zoster immunoglobulin (section 14.5) is needed for exposed non-immune patients receiving systemic corticosteroids or for those who have used them within the previous 3 months; varicella–zoster immunoglobulin should preferably be given within 3 days of exposure and no later than 10 days. Confirmed chickenpox warrants specialist care and urgent treatment (section 5.3.2.1). Corticosteroids should not be stopped and dosage may need to be increased.

Topical, inhaled or rectal corticosteroids are less likely to be associated with an increased risk of severe chickenpox.

MEASLES. Patients taking corticosteroids should be advised to take particular care to avoid exposure to measles and to seek immediate medical advice if exposure occurs. Prophylaxis with intramuscular normal immunoglobulin (section 14.5) may be needed.

> Following concern about severe chickenpox associated with systemic corticosteroids, the CSM has issued a notice that **every** patient prescribed a *systemic* corticosteroid should receive the patient information leaflet supplied by the manufacturer.

> Steroid treatment cards (see below) should also be issued where appropriate. Doctors and pharmacists can obtain supplies of the card from:
>
> *England and Wales*
> NHS Customer Services, Astron
> Causeway Distribution Centre, Oldham Broadway Business Park, Chadderton
> Oldham, OL9 9XD
> Tel: (0161) 683 2376/2382; fax (0161) 683 2396
>
> *Scotland*
> Banner Business Supplies
> 20 South Gyle Crescent
> Edinburgh, EH12 9EB
> Tel: (01506) 448 440; fax (01256) 448 400

For other references to the adverse effects of corticosteroids see section 11.4 (eye) and section 13.4 (skin).

STEROID TREATMENT CARD

I am a patient on STEROID treatment which must not be stopped suddenly

- If you have been taking this medicine for more than three weeks, the dose should be reduced gradually when you stop taking steroids unless your doctor says otherwise.
- Read the patient information leaflet given with the medicine.
- Always carry this card with you and show it to anyone who treats you (for example a doctor, nurse, pharmacist or dentist). For one year after you stop the treatment, you must mention that you have taken steroids.
- If you become ill, or if you come into contact with anyone who has an infectious disease, consult your doctor promptly. If you have never had chickenpox, you should avoid close contact with people who have chickenpox or shingles. If you do come into contact with chickenpox, see your doctor urgently.
- Make sure that the information on the card is kept up to date.

Use of corticosteroids

Dosage of corticosteroids varies widely in different diseases and in different patients. If the use of a corticosteroid can save or prolong life, as in exfoliative dermatitis, pemphigus, acute leukaemia or acute transplant rejection, high doses may need to be given, because the complications of therapy are likely to be less serious than the effects of the disease itself.

When long-term corticosteroid therapy is used in some chronic diseases, the adverse effects of treatment may become greater than the disabilities caused by the disease. To minimise side-effects the maintenance dose should be kept as low as possible.

When potentially less harmful measures are ineffective corticosteroids are used topically for the treatment of inflammatory conditions of the skin (section 13.4). Corticosteroids should be avoided or used only under specialist supervision in psoriasis (section 13.5).

Corticosteroids are used both topically (by rectum) and systemically (by mouth or intravenously) in the management of ulcerative colitis and Crohn's disease (section 1.5 and section 1.7.2).

Use can be made of the mineralocorticoid activity of fludrocortisone to treat postural hypotension in autonomic neuropathy (section 6.1.5).

Although very high doses of corticosteroids have been given by intravenous injection in septic shock, a study of high-dose methylprednisolone sodium succinate did not demonstrate efficacy and, moreover, suggested a higher mortality in some subsets of patients given the high-dose corticosteroid therapy. However, there is evidence that administration of lower doses of hydrocortisone (50 mg intravenously every 6 hours) and fludrocortisone (50 micrograms daily by mouth) is of benefit in patients who have adrenocortical insufficiency as a consequence of septic shock.

Dexamethasone and betamethasone have little if any mineralocorticoid action and their long duration of action makes them particularly suitable for suppressing corticotropin secretion in congenital adrenal hyperplasia where the dose should be tailored to clinical response and by measurement of adrenal androgens and 17-hydroxyprogesterone. In common with all glucocorticoids their suppressive action on the hypothalamic-pituitary-adrenal axis is greatest and most prolonged when they are given at night. In most normal subjects a single dose of 1 mg of dexamethasone at night, depending on weight, is sufficient to inhibit corticotropin secretion for 24 hours. This is the basis of the 'overnight dexamethasone suppression test' for diagnosing Cushing's syndrome.

Betamethasone and dexamethasone are also appropriate for conditions where water retention would be a disadvantage.

A corticosteroid may be used in the management of raised intracranial pressure or cerebral oedema that occurs as a result of malignancy (see also p. 15); high doses of betamethasone or dexamethasone are generally used. However, a corticosteroid should **not** be used for the management of head injury or stroke because it is unlikely to be of benefit and may even be harmful

In acute hypersensitivity reactions such as angioedema of the upper respiratory tract and anaphylactic shock, corticosteroids are indicated as an adjunct to emergency treatment with adrenaline (epinephrine) (section 3.4.3). In such cases hydrocortisone (as sodium succinate) by intravenous injection in a dose of 100 to 300 mg may be required.

Corticosteroids are preferably used by inhalation in the management of asthma (section 3.2) but systemic therapy in association with bronchodilators is required for the emergency treatment of severe acute asthma (section 3.1.1).

Corticosteroids may also be useful in conditions such as auto-immune hepatitis, rheumatoid arthritis and sarcoidosis; they may also lead to remissions of acquired haemolytic anaemia (section 9.1.3), and some cases of the nephrotic syndrome (particularly in children) and thrombocytopenic purpura (section 9.1.4).

Corticosteroids can improve the prognosis of serious conditions such as systemic lupus erythematosus, temporal arteritis, and polyarteritis nodosa; the effects of the disease process may be suppressed and symptoms relieved, but the underlying condition is not cured, although it may ultimately remit. It is usual to begin therapy in these conditions at fairly high dose, such as 40 to 60 mg prednisolone daily, and then to reduce the dose to the lowest commensurate with disease control.

For other references to the use of corticosteroids see Prescribing in Palliative Care, section 8.2.2 (immunosuppresion), section 10.1.2 (rheumatic diseases), section 11.4 (eye), section 12.1.1 (otitis externa), section 12.2.1 (allergic rhinitis), and section 12.3.1 (aphthous ulcers).

Pregnancy and breast-feeding

Following a review of the data on the safety of systemic corticosteroids used in pregnancy and breast-feeding the CSM has concluded:

- corticosteroids vary in their ability to cross the placenta; betamethasone and dexamethasone cross the placenta readily while 88% of prednisolone is inactivated as it crosses the placenta;
- there is no convincing evidence that systemic corticosteroids increase the incidence of congenital abnormalities such as cleft palate or lip;
- when administration is prolonged or repeated during pregnancy, systemic corticosteroids increase the risk of intra-uterine growth restriction; there is no evidence of intra-uterine growth restriction following short-term treatment (e.g. prophylactic treatment for neonatal respiratory distress syndrome);
- any adrenal suppression in the neonate following prenatal exposure usually resolves spontaneously after birth and is rarely clinically important;
- prednisolone appears in small amounts in breast milk but maternal doses of up to 40 mg daily are unlikely to cause systemic effects in the infant; infants should be monitored for adrenal suppression if the mothers are taking a higher dose.

See also Appendix 4.

Administration

Whenever possible *local treatment* with creams, intra-articular injections, inhalations, eye-drops, or enemas should be used in preference to *systemic treatment*. The suppressive action of a corticosteroid on cortisol secretion is least when it is given as a single dose in the morning. In an attempt to reduce pituitary-adrenal suppression further, the total dose for two days can sometimes be taken as a single dose on alternate days; alternate-day administration has not been very successful in the management of asthma (section 3.2). Pituitary-adrenal suppression can also be reduced by means of intermittent therapy with short courses. In some conditions it may be possible to reduce the dose of corticosteroid by adding a small dose of an immunosuppressive drug (section 8.2.1).

Withdrawal of corticosteroids

The CSM has recommended that *gradual* withdrawal of systemic corticosteroids should be considered in those whose disease is unlikely to relapse and have

- recently received repeated courses (particularly if taken for longer than 3 weeks)
- taken a short course within 1 year of stopping long-term therapy
- other possible causes of adrenal suppression
- received more than 40 mg daily prednisolone (or equivalent)
- been given repeat doses in the evening
- received more than 3 weeks' treatment

Systemic corticosteroids may be stopped abruptly in those whose disease is unlikely to relapse *and* who have received treatment for 3 weeks or less *and* who are not included in the patient groups described above.

During corticosteroid withdrawal the dose may be reduced rapidly down to physiological doses (equivalent to prednisolone 7.5 mg daily) and then reduced more slowly. Assessment of the disease may be needed during withdrawal to ensure that relapse does not occur.

PREDNISOLONE

Indications: suppression of inflammatory and allergic disorders; see also notes above; inflammatory bowel disease, section 1.5; asthma, section 3.2; immunosuppression, section 8.2.2; rheumatic disease, section 10.1.2

Cautions: adrenal suppression and infection (see notes above), children and adolescents (growth retardation possibly irreversible), elderly (close supervision required particularly on long-term treatment); frequent monitoring required if history of tuberculosis (or X-ray changes), hypertension, recent myocardial infarction (rupture reported), congestive heart failure, liver failure (Appendix 2), renal impairment, diabetes mellitus including family history, osteoporosis (post-menopausal women at special risk), glaucoma (including family history), corneal perforation, severe affective disorders (particularly if history of steroid-induced psychosis), epilepsy, peptic ulcer, hypothyroidism, history of steroid myopathy; pregnancy (Appendix 4) and breast-feeding (Appendix 5) (see also notes above); **interactions:** Appendix 1 (corticosteroids)

Contra-indications: systemic infection (unless specific antimicrobial therapy given); avoid live virus vaccines in those receiving immunosuppressive doses (serum antibody response diminished)

Side-effects: minimised by using lowest effective dose for minimum period possible;
gastro-intestinal effects include dyspepsia, peptic ulceration (with perforation), abdominal distension, acute pancreatitis, oesophageal ulceration and candidiasis; *musculoskeletal effects* include proximal myopathy, osteoporosis, vertebral and long bone fractures, avascular osteonecrosis, tendon rupture; *endocrine effects* include adrenal suppression, menstrual irregularities and amenorrhoea, Cushing's syndrome (with high doses, usually reversible on withdrawal), hirsutism, weight gain, negative nitrogen and calcium balance, increased appetite; increased susceptibility to and severity of infection; *neuropsychiatric effects* include euphoria, psychological dependence, depression, insomnia, increased intracranial pressure with papilloedema in children (usually after withdrawal), psychosis and aggravation of schizophrenia, aggravation of epilepsy; *ophthalmic effects* include glaucoma, papilloedema, posterior subcapsular cataracts, corneal or scleral thinning and exacerbation of ophthalmic viral or fungal disease; *other side-effects* include impaired healing, skin atrophy, bruising, striae, telangiectasia, acne, myocardial rupture following recent myocardial infarction, fluid and electrolyte disturbance, leucocytosis, hypersensitivity reactions (including anaphylaxis), thromboembolism, nausea, malaise, hiccups

Dose: *by mouth*, initially, up to 10–20 mg daily (severe disease, up to 60 mg daily), preferably taken in the morning after breakfast; can often be reduced within a few days but may need to be continued for several weeks or months
Maintenance, usual range, 2.5–15 mg daily, but higher doses may be needed; cushingoid side-effects increasingly likely with doses above 7.5 mg daily

By intramuscular injection, prednisolone acetate (section 10.1.2.2), 25–100 mg once or twice weekly

Prednisolone (Non-proprietary) PoM

Tablets, prednisolone 1 mg, net price 28-tab pack = £1.42; 5 mg, 28-tab pack = £1.10; 25 mg, 56-tab pack = £9.67. Label: 10, steroid card, 21

Tablets, both e/c, prednisolone 2.5 mg (brown), net price 30-tab pack = 31p; 5 mg (red), 30-tab pack = 51p. Label: 5, 10, steroid card, 25

Brands include *Deltacortril Enteric*®

Soluble tablets, prednisolone 5 mg (as sodium phosphate), net price 30-tab pack = £2.20. Label: 10, steroid card, 13, 21

Injection, see section 10.1.2.2

BETAMETHASONE

Indications: suppression of inflammatory and allergic disorders; congenital adrenal hyperplasia; see also notes above; ear (section 12.1.1); eye (section 11.4.1); nose (section 12.2.1)

Cautions: see notes above and under Prednisolone; transient effect on fetal movements and heart rate

Contra-indications: see notes above and under Prednisolone

Side-effects: see notes above and under Prednisolone

Dose: *by mouth*, usual range 0.5–5 mg daily; see also Administration (above)

By intramuscular injection or slow intravenous injection or infusion, 4–20 mg, repeated up to 4 times in 24 hours; CHILD, *by slow intravenous*

injection, up to 1 year 1 mg, 1–5 years 2 mg, 6–12 years 4 mg

Betnelan® (Celltech) PoM
Tablets, scored, betamethasone 500 micrograms. Net price 100-tab pack = £4.39. Label: 10, steroid card, 21

Betnesol® (Celltech) PoM
Soluble tablets, pink, scored, betamethasone 500 micrograms (as sodium phosphate). Net price 100-tab pack = £5.17. Label: 10, steroid card, 13, 21
Injection, betamethasone 4 mg (as sodium phosphate) /mL. Net price 1-mL amp = £1.22. Label: 10, steroid card

CORTISONE ACETATE

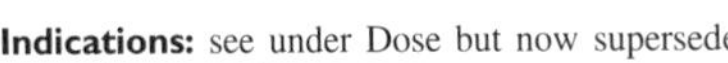

Indications: see under Dose but now superseded, see also notes above
Cautions: see notes above and under Prednisolone
Contra-indications: see notes above and under Prednisolone
Side-effects: see notes above and under Prednisolone
Dose: for replacement therapy, 25–37.5 mg daily in divided doses

Cortisone (Non-proprietary) PoM
Tablets, cortisone acetate 25 mg, net price 56-tab pack = £10.92. Label: 10, steroid card, 21

DEFLAZACORT

Indications: suppression of inflammatory and allergic disorders
Cautions: see notes above and under Prednisolone
Contra-indications: see notes above and under Prednisolone
Side-effects: see notes above and under Prednisolone
Dose: usual maintenance 3–18 mg daily (acute disorders, initially up to 120 mg daily); see also Administration (above)
CHILD 0.25–1.5 mg/kg daily (or on alternate days); see also Administration (above)

Calcort® (Shire) PoM
Tablets, deflazacort 1 mg, net price 100-tab pack = £8.00; 6 mg, 60-tab pack = £16.46; 30 mg, 30-tab pack = £22.80. Label: 5, 10, steroid card

DEXAMETHASONE

Indications: suppression of inflammatory and allergic disorders; diagnosis of Cushing's disease, congenital adrenal hyperplasia; cerebral oedema associated with malignancy; croup (section 3.1); nausea and vomiting with chemotherapy (section 8.1); rheumatic disease (section 10.1.2); eye (section 11.4.1); see also notes above
Cautions: see notes above and under Prednisolone
Contra-indications: see notes above and under Prednisolone
Side-effects: see notes above and under Prednisolone; perineal irritation may follow intravenous administration of the phosphate ester
Dose: *by mouth*, usual range 0.5–10 mg daily; CHILD 10–100 micrograms/kg daily; see also Administration (above)
By intramuscular injection or slow intravenous injection or infusion (as dexamethasone phosphate), initially 0.5–24 mg; CHILD 200–400 micrograms/kg daily
Cerebral oedema (as dexamethasone phosphate), *by intravenous injection*, 10 mg initially, then 4 mg *by intramuscular injection* every 6 hours as required for 2–4 days then gradually reduced and stopped over 5–7 days
Adjunctive treatment of bacterial meningitis, (started with antibacterial treatment, as dexamethasone phosphate) [unlicensed indication], *by intravenous injection*, 10 mg every 6 hours for 4 days; CHILD 150 micrograms/kg every 6 hours for 4 days
NOTE. Dexamethasone 1 mg ≡ dexamethasone phosphate 1.2 mg ≡ dexamethasone sodium phosphate 1.3 mg

Dexamethasone (Non-proprietary) PoM
Tablets, dexamethasone 500 micrograms, net price 20 = 64p; 2 mg, 20 = £1.73. Label: 10, steroid card, 21
Available from Organon
Oral solution, sugar-free, dexamethasone (as dexamethasone sodium phosphate) 2 mg/5 mL, net price 150-mL = £42.30. Label: 10, steroid card, 21
Brands include *Dexsol*®
Injection, dexamethasone phosphate (as dexamethasone sodium phosphate) 4 mg/mL, net price 1-mL amp = £1.00, 2-mL vial = £1.98; 24 mg/mL, 5-mL vial = £16.66. Label: 10, steroid card
Available from Mayne
Injection, dexamethasone (as dexamethasone sodium phosphate) 4 mg/mL, net price 1-mL amp = 83p, 2-mL vial = £1.27. Label: 10, steroid card
Available from Organon

HYDROCORTISONE

Indications: adrenocortical insufficiency (section 6.3.1); shock; see also notes above; hypersensitivity reactions e.g. anaphylactic shock and angioedema (section 3.4.3); inflammatory bowel disease (section 1.5); haemorrhoids (section 1.7.2); rheumatic disease (section 10.1.2); eye (section 11.4.1); skin (section 13.4)
Cautions: see notes above and under Prednisolone
Contra-indications: see notes above and under Prednisolone
Side-effects: see notes above and under Prednisolone; phosphate ester associated with paraesthesia and pain (particularly in the perineal region)
Dose: *by mouth*, replacement therapy, 20–30 mg daily in divided doses—see section 6.3.1; CHILD 10–30 mg
By intramuscular injection or slow intravenous injection or infusion, 100–500 mg, 3–4 times in 24 hours or as required; CHILD *by slow intravenous injection* up to 1 year 25 mg, 1–5 years 50 mg, 6–12 years 100 mg

[1]**Efcortesol**® (Sovereign) PoM
Injection, hydrocortisone 100 mg (as sodium phosphate)/mL, net price 1-mL amp = 75p, 5-mL amp = £3.40. Label: 10, steroid card
NOTE. Paraesthesia and pain (particularly in the perineal region) may follow intravenous injection of the phosphate ester

1. PoM restriction does not apply where administration is for saving life in emergency

Hydrocortone® (MSD) PoM
Tablets, scored, hydrocortisone 10 mg, net price 30-tab pack = 70p; 20 mg, 30-tab pack = £1.07. Label: 10, steroid card, 21

[1]**Solu-Cortef**® (Pharmacia) PoM
Injection, powder for reconstitution, hydrocortisone (as sodium succinate). Net price 100-mg vial = 92p, 100-mg vial with 2-mL amp water for injections = £1.16. Label: 10, steroid card

1. PoM restriction does not apply where administration is for saving life in emergency

METHYLPREDNISOLONE

Indications: suppression of inflammatory and allergic disorders; cerebral oedema associated with malignancy; see also notes above; rheumatic disease (section 10.1.2); skin (section 13.4)
Cautions: see notes above and under Prednisolone; rapid intravenous administration of large doses associated with cardiovascular collapse
Contra-indications: see notes above and under Prednisolone
Side-effects: see notes above and under Prednisolone
Dose: *by mouth*, usual range 2–40 mg daily; see also Administration (above)
By intramuscular injection or slow intravenous injection or infusion, initially 10–500 mg; graft rejection, up to 1 g daily *by intravenous infusion* for up to 3 days

Medrone® (Pharmacia) PoM
Tablets, scored, methylprednisolone 2 mg (pink), net price 30-tab pack = £3.23; 4 mg, 30-tab pack = £6.19; 16 mg, 30-tab pack = £17.17; 100 mg (blue), 20-tab pack = £48.32. Label: 10, steroid card, 21

Solu-Medrone® (Pharmacia) PoM
Injection, powder for reconstitution, methylprednisolone (as sodium succinate) (all with solvent). Net price 40-mg vial = £1.58; 125-mg vial = £4.75; 500-mg vial = £9.60; 1-g vial = £17.30; 2-g vial = £32.86. Label: 10, steroid card

■ Intramuscular depot

Depo-Medrone® (Pharmacia) PoM
Injection (aqueous suspension), methylprednisolone acetate 40 mg/mL. Net price 1-mL vial = £2.87; 2-mL vial = £5.15; 3-mL vial = £7.47. Label: 10, steroid card
Dose: by deep intramuscular injection into gluteal muscle, 40–120 mg, a second injection may be given after 2–3 weeks if required

TRIAMCINOLONE

Indications: suppression of inflammatory and allergic disorders; see also notes above; rheumatic disease, section 10.1.2; mouth, section 12.3.1; skin, section 13.4
Cautions: see notes above and under Prednisolone; high dosage may cause proximal myopathy, avoid in chronic therapy
Contra-indications: see notes above and under Prednisolone
Side-effects: see notes above and under Prednisolone
Dose: *by deep intramuscular injection*, into gluteal muscle, 40 mg of acetonide for depot effect, repeated at intervals according to the patient's response; max. single dose 100 mg

Kenalog® **Intra-articular/Intramuscular** (Squibb) PoM
Injection (aqueous suspension), triamcinolone acetonide 40 mg/mL, net price 1-mL vial = £1.70; 1-mL prefilled syringe = £2.11; 2-mL prefilled syringe = £3.66. Label: 10, steroid card
NOTE. Intramuscular needle with prefilled syringe should be replaced for intra-articular injection

6.4 Sex hormones

6.4.1 Female sex hormones

6.4.1.1 Oestrogens and HRT

Oestrogens are necessary for the development of female secondary sexual characteristics; they also stimulate myometrial hypertrophy with endometrial hyperplasia.

In terms of oestrogenic activity *natural oestrogens* (estradiol (oestradiol), estrone (oestrone), and estriol (oestriol)) have a more appropriate profile for hormone replacement therapy (HRT) than *synthetic oestrogens* (ethinylestradiol (ethinyloestradiol) and mestranol). Tibolone has oestrogenic, progestogenic and weak androgenic activity.

Oestrogen therapy is given cyclically or continuously for a number of gynaecological conditions. If long-term therapy is required a progestogen should normally be added to reduce the risk of cystic hyperplasia of the endometrium (or of endometriotic foci in women who have had a hysterectomy) and possible transformation to cancer.

Oestrogens are no longer used to *suppress lactation* because of their association with thromboembolism.

Hormone replacement therapy

Hormone replacement therapy (HRT) with small doses of an oestrogen (together with a progestogen in women with an intact uterus) is appropriate for alleviating menopausal symptoms such as *vaginal atrophy* or *vasomotor instability*. Oestrogen given systemically in the perimenopausal and postmenopausal period or tibolone given in the postmenopausal period also diminish *postmenopausal osteoporosis* (section 6.6.1) but other drugs (section 6.6) are preferred. Menopausal atrophic vaginitis may respond to a short course of a topical vaginal oestrogen preparation (section 7.2.1) used for a few weeks and repeated if necessary.

Systemic therapy with an oestrogen or drugs with oestrogenic properties alleviates the symptoms of oestrogen deficiency such as *vasomotor symptoms*. Tibolone combines oestrogenic and progestogenic activity with weak androgenic activity; it is given continuously, without cyclical progestogen.

HRT increases the risk of *venous thromboembolism,* of *stroke* and, after some years of use, *endometrial cancer* (reduced by a progestogen) and of *breast cancer* (see below). The CSM advises that the minimum effective dose should be used for the shortest duration. Treatment should be reviewed at least annually and for osteoporosis alternative treatments considered (section 6.6). HRT does not prevent coronary heart disease or protect against a decline in cognitive function and it should **not** be prescribed for these purposes. Experience of treating women over 65 years with HRT is limited.

Clonidine (section 4.7.4.2) may be used to reduce vasomotor symptoms in women who cannot take an oestrogen, but clonidine may cause unacceptable side-effects.

HRT may be used in women with *early natural or surgical menopause (before age 45 years),* since they are at high risk of osteoporosis. For early menopause, HRT can be given until the approximate age of natural menopause (i.e. until age 50 years). Alternatives to HRT should be considered if osteoporosis is the main concern (section 6.6).

In women with an intact uterus, the addition of a progestogen reduces the risk of endometrial cancer but this should be weighed against the increased risk of breast cancer.

The CSM advises that for the treatment of menopausal symptoms the benefits of short-term HRT outweigh the risks in the majority of women, but in healthy women without symptoms the risks outweigh the benefits.

RISK OF BREAST CANCER. The CSM has estimated that using *all* types of HRT, including tibolone, increases the risk of breast cancer within 1–2 years of initiating treatment. The increased risk is related to the duration of HRT use (but not to the age at which HRT is started) and this excess risk disappears within about 5 years of stopping.

About 14 in every 1000 women aged 50–64 years not using HRT have breast cancer diagnosed over 5 years. In those using *oestrogen-only HRT* for 5 years, breast cancer is diagnosed in about 1.5 extra cases in 1000. In those using *combined HRT* for 5 years, breast cancer is diagnosed in about 6 extra cases in 1000. About 31 in every 1000 women aged 50–79 years not using HRT have breast cancer diagnosed over 5 years. In those using oestrogen-only HRT for 5 years no extra cases are diagnosed, but in those using *combined HRT* for 5 years, breast cancer is diagnosed in about 4 extra cases in 1000.

Tibolone increases the risk of breast cancer but to a lesser extent than with *combined HRT.*

RISK OF VENOUS THROMBOEMBOLISM. Women on combined or oestrogen-only HRT are at an increased risk of deep vein thrombosis and of pulmonary embolism especially in the first year.

The CSM has estimated that about 10 in every 1000 *women aged 50–59 years* not using HRT develop venous thromboembolism over 5 years; this figure rises by about 1 extra case in 1000 in those using oestrogen-only HRT and about 4 extra cases in 1000 in those using combined HRT for 5 years. About 20 in every 1000 *women aged 60–69 years* not using HRT develop venous thromboembolism over 5 years; this figure rises by about 4 extra cases in 1000 in those using oestrogen-only HRT and about 9 extra cases in 1000 in those using combined HRT for 5 years. It is not known if tibolone increases the risk of venous thromboembolism.

In *women who have predisposing factors* (such as a personal or family history of deep vein thrombosis or pulmonary embolism, severe varicose veins, obesity, trauma, or prolonged bed-rest) it may be prudent to review the need for HRT as in some cases the risks of HRT may exceed the benefits. See below for advice on surgery.

Travel involving prolonged immobility further increases the risk of deep vein thrombosis, see under Travel in section 7.3.1.

OTHER RISKS. Combined HRT or oestrogen-only HRT slightly increases the risk of *stroke.* The CSM has estimated that about 3 in every 1000 *women aged 50–59 years* not using HRT have a stroke over 5 years; this figure rises by about 2 extra cases in 1000 in those using oestrogen-only HRT and by about 1 extra case in those using combined HRT for 5 years. About 26 in every *1000 women aged 60–69 years* not using HRT have a stroke over 5 years; this figure rises by about 6 extra cases in 1000 in those using oestrogen-only HRT and by about 4 extra cases in those using combined HRT for 5 years.

HRT does not prevent *coronary heart disease* and should not be prescribed for this purpose. HRT possibly increases the risk of coronary heart disease in the first year.

The CSM has estimated that about 3 in every 1000 women aged 50–69 years not using HRT have *endometrial cancer* diagnosed over 5 years; in those using *oestrogen-only HRT* for 5 years endometrial cancer is diagnosed in about 5 extra cases in 1000. The risk of endometrial cancer cannot be reliably estimated in those using combined HRT because the addition of progestogen for at least 12 days per month greatly reduces the additional risk. The risk of endometrial cancer may be different for sequential and continuous combined HRT. The risk of endometrial cancer with tibolone is not known.

The CSM has estimated that about 3 in every 1000 women aged 50–69 years not using HRT have *ovarian cancer* diagnosed over 5 years; this figure rises by about 1 extra case in 1000 in those using *oestrogen-only HRT* for 5 years; the risks in women using combined HRT are unknown.

CHOICE. The choice of HRT for an individual depends on an overall balance of indication, risk, and convenience. A woman with an intact uterus normally requires oestrogen with cyclical progestogen for the last 12 to 14 days of the cycle *or* a preparation which involves continuous administration of an oestrogen and a progestogen (*or* one which provides both oestrogenic and progestogenic activity in a single preparation). Continuous combined preparations or tibolone are **not suitable** for use in the *perimenopause* or within 12 months of the last menstrual period; women who use such preparations may bleed irregularly in the early stages of treatment—if bleeding continues endometrial abnormality should be ruled out and consideration given to changing to cyclical HRT.

An oestrogen alone is suitable for continuous use in women without a uterus. However, in endometriosis, endometrial foci may remain despite hysterectomy and the addition of a progestogen should be considered in these circumstances.

An oestrogen may be given by mouth or it may be given by subcutaneous or transdermal administration, which avoids first-pass metabolism. In the case of subcutaneous implants, recurrence of vasomotor symptoms at supraphysiological plasma concentrations may occur; moreover, there is evidence of prolonged endometrial stimulation after discontinuation (calling for continued cyclical progestogen). For the use of topical HRT preparations see section 7.2.1.

CONTRACEPTION. HRT does **not** provide contraception and a woman is considered potentially fertile for *2 years after her last menstrual period* if she is *under 50 years*, and for *1 year* if she is *over 50 years*. A woman who is under 50 years and free of all risk factors for venous and arterial disease can use a low-oestrogen combined oral contraceptive pill (section 7.3.1) to provide both *relief of menopausal symptoms* and *contraception*; it is recommended that the oral contraceptive be stopped at 50 years of age since there are more suitable alternatives. If any potentially fertile woman needs HRT, *non-hormonal contraceptive measures* (such as condoms, or by this age, contraceptive foam, section 7.3.3) are necessary.

Measurement of follicle-stimulating hormone can help to determine fertility, but high measurements alone (particularly in women aged under 50 years) do not necessarily preclude the possibility of becoming pregnant.

SURGERY. Major surgery under general anaesthesia, including orthopaedic and vascular leg surgery, is a predisposing factor for venous thromboembolism and it may be prudent to stop HRT 4–6 weeks before surgery (see Risk of Venous Thromboembolism, above); it should be restarted only after full mobilisation. If HRT is continued or if discontinuation is not possible (e.g. in non-elective surgery), prophylaxis with heparin and graduated compression hosiery is advised. Oestrogenic activity may persist after removing an estradiol implant (see above).

REASONS TO STOP HRT. For circumstances in which HRT should be stopped, see p. 408.

OESTROGENS FOR HRT

NOTE. Relates only to small amounts of oestrogens given for hormone replacement therapy

Indications: see notes above and under preparations

Cautions: prolonged exposure to unopposed oestrogens may increase risk of developing endometrial cancer (see notes above); migraine (or migraine-like headaches); diabetes (increased risk of heart disease); history of breast nodules or fibrocystic disease—closely monitor breast status (risk of breast cancer, see notes above); risk factors for oestrogen-dependent tumours (e.g. breast cancer in first-degree relative); uterine fibroids may increase in size, symptoms of endometriosis may be exacerbated; factors predisposing to thromboembolism (see notes above); presence of antiphospholipid antibodies (increased risk of thrombotic events); increased risk of gall-bladder disease reported; hypophyseal tumours; porphyria (see section 9.8.2); **interactions:** Appendix 1 (oestrogens)

OTHER CONDITIONS. The product literature advises caution in other conditions including hypertension, renal disease, asthma, epilepsy, sickle-cell disease, melanoma, otosclerosis, multiple sclerosis, and systemic lupus erythematosus (but care required if antiphospholipid antibodies present, see above). Evidence for caution in these conditions is unsatisfactory and many women with these conditions may stand to benefit from HRT.

Contra-indications: pregnancy; oestrogen-dependent cancer, history of breast cancer, active thrombophlebitis, active or recent arterial thromboembolic disease (e.g. angina or myocardial infarction), venous thromboembolism, or history of recurrent venous thromboembolism (unless already on anticoagulant treatment), liver disease (where liver function tests have failed to return to normal), Dubin-Johnson and Rotor syndromes (or monitor closely), untreated endometrial hyperplasia, undiagnosed vaginal bleeding, breast-feeding

Side-effects: see notes above for risks of long-term use; nausea and vomiting, abdominal cramps and bloating, weight changes, breast enlargement and tenderness, premenstrual-like syndrome, sodium and fluid retention, cholestatic jaundice, glucose intolerance, altered blood lipids–may lead to pancreatitis, rashes and chloasma, changes in libido, depression, mood changes, headache, migraine, dizziness, leg cramps (rule out venous thrombosis), vaginal candidiasis, contact lenses may irritate; transdermal delivery systems may cause contact sensitisation (possible severe hypersensitivity reaction on continued exposure), and headache has been reported on vigorous exercise; nasal spray may cause local irritation, rhinorrhoea and epistaxis

WITHDRAWAL BLEEDING. Cyclical HRT (where a progestogen is taken for 12–14 days of each 28-day oestrogen treatment cycle) usually results in *regular withdrawal bleeding* towards the end of the progestogen. The aim of continuous combined HRT (where a combination of oestrogen and progestogen is taken, usually in a single tablet, throughout each 28-day treatment cycle) is to avoid bleeding, but *irregular bleeding* may occur during the early treatment stages (if it continues endometrial abnormality should be excluded and consideration given to cyclical HRT instead)

Dose: see under preparations

COUNSELLING ON PATCHES. Patch should be removed after 3–4 days (or once a week in case of 7-day patch) and replaced with fresh patch on slightly different site; recommended sites: clean, dry, unbroken areas of skin on trunk below waistline; not to be applied on or near breasts or under waistband. If patch falls off in bath allow skin to cool before applying new patch

■ Conjugated oestrogens with progestogen

Premique® (Wyeth) PoM

Premique® *Low Dose tablets*, s/c, ivory, conjugated oestrogen (equine) 300 micrograms and medroxyprogesterone acetate 1.5 mg, net price 3 × 28-tab pack = £29.85

Dose: menopausal symptoms in women with an intact uterus, 1 tablet daily continuously

Premique® *tablets*, s/c, blue, conjugated oestrogen (equine) 625 micrograms and medroxyprogesterone acetate 5 mg. Net price 3 × 28-tab pack = £27.14

Dose: menopausal symptoms and osteoporosis prophylaxis (see section 6.6), in women with intact uterus, 1 tablet daily continuously (starting on day 1 of menstruation if cycles have not ceased)

Premique® *Cycle Calendar pack*, all s/c, 14 white tablets, conjugated oestrogens (equine) 625 micrograms; 14 green tablets, conjugated oestrogens (equine) 625 micrograms and medroxyprogesterone acetate 10 mg, net price 3 × 28-tab pack = £24.87

Dose: menopausal symptoms and osteoporosis prophylaxis (see section 6.6), 1 white tablet daily for 14 days, starting on day 1 of menstruation (or at any time if cycles have ceased or are infrequent) then 1 green tablet daily for 14 days; subsequent courses are repeated without interval

Prempak-C® (Wyeth) PoM

Prempak C® 0.625 Calendar pack, s/c, 28 maroon tablets, conjugated oestrogens (equine) 625 micrograms; 12 light brown tablets, norgestrel 150 micrograms (≡ levonorgestrel 75 micrograms). Net price 3 × 40-tab pack = £17.67

Dose: menopausal symptoms and osteoporosis prophylaxis (see section 6.6), in women with intact uterus, 1 maroon tablet daily continuously, starting on day 1 of menstruation (or at any time if cycles have ceased or are infrequent), and 1 brown tablet daily on days 17–28 of each 28-day treatment cycle; subsequent courses are repeated without interval

Prempak C® 1.25 Calendar pack, s/c, 28 yellow tablets, conjugated oestrogens (equine) 1.25 mg; 12 light brown tablets, norgestrel 150 micrograms (≡ levonorgestrel 75 micrograms). Net price 3 × 40-tab pack = £17.67

Dose: see under 0.625 Calendar pack, but taking 1 yellow tablet daily continuously (instead of 1 maroon tablet) if symptoms not fully controlled with lower strength

■ Estradiol with progestogen

Angeliq® (Schering Health) ▼ PoM

Tablets, f/c, red, estradiol 1mg, drospirenone 2 mg. Net price 3 x 28-tab pack = £25.80

Dose: menopausal symptoms and osteoporosis prophylaxis (see section 6.6), in women with intact uterus, 1 tablet daily continuously (if changing from cyclical HRT begin treatment the day after finishing oestrogen plus progestogen phase)

Cautions: use with care if an increased concentration of potassium might be hazardous; renal impairment (Appendix 3)

NOTE. Unsuitable for use in perimenopausal women or within 12 months of last menstrual period—see choice above

Climagest® (Novartis) PoM

Climagest® 1-mg tablets, 16 grey-blue, estradiol valerate 1 mg; 12 white, estradiol valerate 1 mg and norethisterone 1 mg. Net price 28-tab pack = £4.78; 3 × 28-tab pack = £13.91

Dose: menopausal symptoms, 1 grey-blue tablet daily for 16 days, starting on day 1 of menstruation (or at any time if cycles have ceased or are infrequent) then 1 white tablet for 12 days; subsequent courses are repeated without interval

Climagest® 2-mg tablets, 16 blue, estradiol valerate 2 mg; 12 yellow, estradiol valerate 2 mg and norethisterone 1 mg. Net price 28-tab pack = £4.78; 3 × 28-tab pack = £13.91

Dose: see *Climagest® 1-mg*, but starting with 1 blue tablet daily (instead of 1 grey-blue tablet) if symptoms not controlled with lower strength

Climesse® (Novartis) PoM

Tablets, pink, estradiol valerate 2 mg, norethisterone 700 micrograms. Net price 1 × 28-tab pack = £8.62; 3 × 28-tab pack = £25.86

Dose: menopausal symptoms and osteoporosis prophylaxis (see section 6.6), in women with intact uterus, 1 tablet daily continuously

NOTE. Unsuitable for use in perimenopausal women or within 12 months of last menstrual period—see Choice above

Cyclo-Progynova® (Viatris) PoM

Cyclo-Progynova® 1-mg tablets, all s/c, 11 beige, estradiol valerate 1 mg; 10 brown, estradiol valerate 1 mg and levonorgestrel 250 micrograms. Net price per pack = £3.11

Dose: menopausal symptoms, in women with intact uterus, 1 beige tablet daily for 11 days, starting on day 5 of menstruation (or at any time if cycles have ceased or are infrequent), then 1 brown tablet daily for 10 days, followed by a 7-day interval

Cyclo-Progynova® 2-mg tablets, all s/c, 11 white, estradiol valerate 2 mg; 10 brown, estradiol valerate 2 mg and norgestrel 500 micrograms (≡ levonorgestrel 250 micrograms). Net price per pack = £3.11

Dose: menopausal symptoms and osteoporosis prophylaxis (see section 6.6) as *Cyclo-Progynova® 1-mg*, but starting with 1 white tablet daily for 11 days, then 1 brown tablet daily for 10 days, followed by a 7-day interval

Elleste-Duet® (Pharmacia) PoM

Elleste-Duet® 1-mg tablets, 16 white, estradiol 1 mg; 12 green, estradiol 1 mg and norethisterone acetate 1 mg. Net price 3 × 28-tab pack = £9.72

Dose: menopausal symptoms, 1 white tablet daily for 16 days starting on day 1 of menstruation (or at any time if cycles have ceased or are infrequent), then 1 green tablet daily for 12 days; subsequent courses are repeated without interval

Elleste-Duet® 2-mg tablets, 16 orange, estradiol 2 mg; 12 grey, estradiol 2 mg, norethisterone acetate 1 mg. Net price 3 × 28-tab pack = £9.72

Dose: menopausal symptoms and osteoporosis prophylaxis (see section 6.6), 1 orange tablet daily for 16 days, starting on day 1 of menstruation (or at any time if cycles have ceased or are infrequent) then 1 grey tablet daily for 12 days; subsequent courses are repeated without interval

Elleste-Duet Conti® tablets, f/c, grey, estradiol 2 mg, norethisterone acetate 1 mg. Net price 3 × 28-tab pack = £17.97

Dose: menopausal symptoms and osteoporosis prophylaxis (see section 6.6), in women with intact uterus, 1 tablet daily on a continuous basis (if changing from cyclical HRT begin treatment at the end of scheduled bleed)

NOTE. Unsuitable for use in perimenopausal women or within 12 months of last menstrual period—see Choice above

Estracombi® (Novartis) PoM

Combination pack, self-adhesive patches of *Estraderm TTS® 50* (releasing estradiol approx. 50 micrograms/24 hours) and of *Estragest TTS®* (releasing estradiol approx. 50 micrograms/24 hours and norethisterone acetate 250 micrograms/24 hours); net price 1-month pack (4 of each) = £11.14, 3-month pack (12 of each) = £33.42. Counselling, administration

Dose: menopausal symptoms and osteoporosis prophylaxis (see section 6.6), in women with intact uterus, starting within 5 days of onset of menstruation (or any time if cycles have ceased or are infrequent), 1 *Estraderm TTS® 50* patch to be applied twice weekly for 2 weeks followed by 1 *Estragest TTS®* patch twice weekly for 2 weeks; subsequent courses are repeated without interval

Evorel® (Janssen-Cilag) PoM

Evorel® Conti patches, self-adhesive, (releasing estradiol approx. 50 micrograms/24 hours and norethisterone acetate approx. 170 micrograms/24

hours), net price 8-patch pack = £12.26, 24-patch pack = £36.77. Counselling, administration

Dose: menopausal symptoms and osteoporosis prophylaxis (see section 6.6), in women with intact uterus, 1 patch to be applied twice weekly continuously

Evorel® Pak calendar pack, 8 self-adhesive patches (releasing estradiol approx. 50 micrograms/24 hours) and 12 tablets, norethisterone 1 mg, net price per pack = £8.03. Counselling, administration

Dose: menopausal symptoms and osteoporosis prophylaxis (see section 6.6), in women with intact uterus, apply 1 patch twice weekly continuously (increased if necessary for menopausal symptoms to 2 patches twice weekly after first month) and take 1 tablet daily on days 15–26 of each 28-day treatment cycle

Evorel® Sequi combination pack, 4 self-adhesive patches of *Evorel® 50* (releasing estradiol approx. 50 micrograms/24 hours) and 4 self-adhesive patches of *Evorel® Conti* (releasing estradiol approx. 50 micrograms/24 hours and norethisterone acetate approx. 170 micrograms/24 hours), net price 8-patch pack = £10.45. Counselling, administration

Dose: menopausal symptoms and osteoporosis prophylaxis (see section 6.6), in women with intact uterus, 1 *Evorel® 50* patch to be applied twice weekly for 2 weeks followed by 1 *Evorel® Conti* patch twice weekly for 2 weeks; subsequent courses are repeated without interval

Femapak® (Solvay) PoM

Femapak® 40 combination pack of 8 self-adhesive patches of *Fematrix® 40* (releasing estradiol approx. 40 micrograms/24 hours) and 14 tablets of *Duphaston®* (dydrogesterone 10 mg). Net price per pack = £7.61. Counselling, administration

Dose: see under *Femapak® 80*

Femapak® 80 combination pack of 8 self-adhesive patches of *Fematrix® 80* (releasing estradiol approx. 80 micrograms/24 hours) and 14 tablets of *Duphaston®* (dydrogesterone 10 mg). Net price per pack = £8.06. Counselling, administration

Dose: menopausal symptoms (and osteoporosis prophylaxis (see section 6.6) in case of *Femapak® 80* **only**), in women with intact uterus, starting within 5 days of onset of menstruation (or any time if cycles have ceased or are infrequent), apply 1 patch twice weekly continuously and take 1 tablet daily on days 15–28 of each 28-day treatment cycle; therapy should be initiated with *Femapak® 40* in those with menopausal symptoms, prolonged oestrogen deficiency or anticipated intolerance to higher strengths, subsequently adjusted to lowest effective dose

Femoston® (Solvay) PoM

Femoston® 1/10 tablets, both f/c, 14 white, estradiol 1 mg; 14 grey, estradiol 1 mg, dydrogesterone 10 mg. Net price 3 × 28-tab pack = £13.47

Dose: menopausal symptoms and osteoporosis prophylaxis (see section 6.6), in women with intact uterus, 1 white tablet daily for 14 days, starting within 5 days of onset of menstruation (or any time if cycles have ceased or are infrequent) then 1 grey tablet for 14 days; subsequent courses repeated without interval

Femoston® 2/10 tablets, both f/c, 14 red, estradiol 2 mg; 14 yellow, estradiol 2 mg, dydrogesterone 10 mg. Net price 3 × 28-tab pack = £13.47

Dose: menopausal symptoms and osteoporosis prophylaxis (see section 6.6), in women with intact uterus, 1 red tablet daily for 14 days, starting within 5 days of onset of menstruation (or any time if cycles have ceased or are infrequent) then 1 yellow tablet daily for 14 days; subsequent courses repeated without interval; where therapy required for menopausal symptoms alone, *Femoston® 1/10* given initially and *Femoston® 2/10* substituted if symptoms not controlled

Femoston®-conti tablets, f/c, salmon, estradiol 1 mg, dydrogesterone 5 mg, net price 3 × 28-tab pack = £22.44

Dose: menopausal symptoms and osteoporosis prophylaxis (see section 6.6), in women with intact uterus, 1 tablet daily continuously (if changing from cyclical HRT begin treatment the day after finishing oestrogen plus progestogen phase)

NOTE. Unsuitable for use in perimenopausal women or within 12 months of last menstrual period—see Choice above

FemSeven® Conti (Merck) PoM

Patches, self-adhesive (releasing estradiol approx. 50 micrograms/24 hours and levonorgestrel approx. 7 micrograms/24 hours); net price 4-patch pack = £12.90, 12-patch pack = £ 36.77. Counselling, administration

Dose: menopausal symptoms in women with intact uterus, 1 patch to be applied once a week continuously

NOTE. Unsuitable for use in perimenopausal women or within 12 months of last menstrual period—see Choice above

FemSeven® Sequi (Merck) PoM

Combination pack, self-adhesive patches of *FemSeven® Sequi Phase 1* (releasing estradiol approx. 50 micrograms/24 hours) and of *FemSeven® Sequi Phase 2* (releasing estradiol approx. 50 micrograms/24 hours and levonorgestrel approx. 10 micrograms/24 hours); net price 1-month pack (2 of each) = £10.98, 3-month pack (6 of each) = £31.28. Counselling, administration

Dose: menopausal symptoms in women with intact uterus, 1 *Phase 1* patch applied once a week for 2 weeks followed by 1 *Phase 2* patch once a week for 2 weeks; subsequent courses are repeated without interval

FemTab® Sequi (Merck) PoM

Tablets, both s/c, 16 white, estradiol valerate 2 mg; 12 pink, estradiol valerate 2 mg, levonorgestrel 75 micrograms, net price 3 × 28-tab pack = £15.15

Dose: menopausal symptoms and osteoporosis prophylaxis (see section 6.6), in women with intact uterus, 1 white tablet daily for 16 days, starting on day 5 of menstruation (or any time if cycles have ceased or are infrequent) then 1 pink tablet daily for 12 days; subsequent courses are repeated without interval

Indivina® (Orion) PoM

Indivina® 1 mg/2.5 mg tablets, estradiol valerate 1 mg, medroxyprogesterone acetate 2.5 mg, net price 3 × 28-tab pack = £21.49

Indivina® 1 mg/5 mg tablets, estradiol valerate 1 mg, medroxyprogesterone acetate 5 mg, net price 3 × 28-tab pack = £21.49

Indivina® 2 mg/5 mg tablets, estradiol valerate 2 mg, medroxyprogesterone acetate 5 mg, net price 3 × 28-tab pack = £21.49

Dose: menopausal symptoms and osteoporosis prophylaxis (see section 6.6), in women with intact uterus, 1 tablet daily continuously; initiate therapy with *Indivina® 1 mg/2.5 mg* tablets and adjust according to response; start at end of scheduled bleed if changing from cyclical HRT

NOTE. Less suitable for use in perimenopausal women or within 3 years of last menstrual period—see Choice above

Kliofem® (Novo Nordisk) PoM

Tablets, f/c yellow, estradiol 2 mg, norethisterone acetate 1 mg. Net price 3 × 28-tab pack = £11.43

Dose: menopausal symptoms and osteoporosis prophylaxis (see section 6.6), in women with intact uterus, 1 tablet daily continuously; start at end of scheduled bleed if changing from cyclical HRT

NOTE. Unsuitable for use in perimenopausal women or within 12 months of last menstrual period—see Choice above

Kliovance® (Novo Nordisk) PoM

Tablets, f/c, estradiol 1mg, norethisterone acetate 500 micrograms, net price 3 × 28-tab pack = £14.67

Dose: menopausal symptoms and osteoporosis prophylaxis (see section 6.6), in women with intact uterus, 1 tablet daily continuously; start at end of scheduled bleed if changing from cyclical HRT

NOTE. Unsuitable for use in perimenopausal women or within 12 months of last menstrual period—see Choice above

Novofem (Novo Nordisk) PoM

Tablets, f/c, 16 red, estradiol 1 mg; 12 white, estradiol 1 mg, norethisterone acetate 1 mg, net price 3 × 28-tab pack = £13.50

Dose: menopausal symptoms and osteoporosis prophylaxis (see section 6.6), in women with intact uterus, 1 red tablet daily for 16 days then 1 white tablet daily for 12 days; subsequent courses are repeated without interval; start treatment with red tablet at any time or if changing from cyclical HRT, start treatment the day after finishing oestrogen plus progestogen phase

Nuvelle® (Schering Health) PoM

Nuvelle® tablets, all s/c, 16 white, estradiol valerate 2 mg; 12 pink, estradiol valerate 2 mg and levonorgestrel 75 micrograms. Net price 3 × 28-tab pack = £12.87

Dose: menopausal symptoms and osteoporosis prophylaxis (see section 6.6), in women with intact uterus, 1 white tablet daily for 16 days, starting on day 5 of menstruation (or any time if cycles have ceased or are infrequent) then 1 pink tablet daily for 12 days; subsequent courses are repeated without interval

Nuvelle® Continuous tablets, f/c, pink, estradiol 2 mg, norethisterone acetate 1 mg, net price 3 × 28-tab pack = £16.85

Dose: menopausal symptoms and osteoporosis prophylaxis (see section 6.6), in women with intact uterus, 1 tablet daily continuously; start at end of scheduled bleed if changing from cyclical HRT

NOTE. Unsuitable for use in perimenopausal women or within 12 months of last menstrual period—see Choice above

Tridestra® (Orion) PoM

Tablets, 70 white, estradiol valerate 2 mg; 14 blue, estradiol valerate 2 mg and medroxyprogesterone acetate 20 mg; 7 yellow, inactive. Net price 91-tab pack = £21.40

Dose: menopausal symptoms and osteoporosis prophylaxis (see section 6.6), in women with intact uterus, 1 white tablet daily for 70 days, then 1 blue tablet daily for 14 days, then 1 yellow tablet daily for 7 days; subsequent courses are repeated without interval

Trisequens® (Novo Nordisk) PoM

Tablets, 12 blue, estradiol 2 mg; 10 white, estradiol 2 mg, norethisterone acetate 1 mg; 6 red, estradiol 1 mg, net price 3 × 28-tab pack = £11.10

Dose: menopausal symptoms and osteoporosis prophylaxis (see section 6.6), in women with intact uterus, 1 blue tablet daily, starting on day 5 of menstruation (or at any time if cycles have ceased or are infrequent), then 1 tablet daily in sequence (without interruption)

■ Conjugated oestrogens only

Premarin® (Wyeth) PoM

Tablets, all s/c, conjugated oestrogens (equine) 625 micrograms (maroon), net price 3 × 28-tab pack = £9.72; 1.25 mg (yellow), 3 × 28-tab pack = £13.19

Dose: menopausal symptoms and osteoporosis prophylaxis (see section 6.6), (with progestogen for 12–14 days per cycle in women with intact uterus), 0.625–1.25 mg daily

■ Estradiol only

Estradiol Implants (Organon) PoM

Implant, estradiol 25 mg, net price each = £9.59; 50 mg, each = £19.16; 100 mg, each = £33.40

Dose: by implantation, oestrogen replacement, and osteoporosis prophylaxis (see section 6.6) (with cyclical progestogen for 12–14 days of each cycle in women with intact uterus, see notes above), 25–100 mg as required (usually every 4–8 months) according to oestrogen levels—check before each implant

NOTE. On cessation of treatment or if implants are removed from those with intact uterus, cyclical progesterone should be continued until withdrawal bleed stops

Aerodiol® (Servier) PoM

Nasal spray, estradiol 150 micrograms/metered spray, net price 4.2-mL unit (60 metered sprays) = £7.41

Dose: menopausal symptoms, initially 1 spray into each nostril daily at the same time each day *either* continuously *or* for 21–28 days followed by a 2–7 day treatment-free interval; daily dose adjusted according to response to 1–4 sprays daily in divided doses; with cyclical progestogen for at least 12 days of each cycle in women with intact uterus; not to be used immediately after nasal corticosteroid or nasal vasoconstrictor

NOTE. If patient has a severely blocked nose, *Aerodiol*® may be temporarily administered into the mouth between the cheek and the gum above the upper teeth; in this situation the normal dose should be doubled

Climaval® (Novartis) PoM

Tablets, estradiol valerate 1 mg (grey-blue), net price 1 × 28-tab pack = £2.55, 3 × 28-tab pack = £7.66; 2 mg (blue), 1 × 28-tab pack = £2.55, 3 × 28-tab pack = £7.66

Dose: menopausal symptoms (if patient has had a hysterectomy), 1–2 mg daily

Elleste-Solo® (Pharmacia) PoM

Elleste-Solo® 1-mg tablets, estradiol 1 mg. Net price 3 × 28-tab pack = £5.34

Dose: menopausal symptoms, with cyclical progestogen for 12–14 days of each cycle in women with intact uterus, 1 mg daily starting on day 1 of menstruation (or at any time if cycles have ceased or are infrequent)

Elleste-Solo® 2-mg tablets, orange, estradiol 2 mg. Net price 3 × 28-tab pack = £5.34

Dose: menopausal symptoms not controlled with lower strength and osteoporosis prophylaxis (see section 6.6), with cyclical progestogen for 12–14 days of each cycle in women with intact uterus, 2 mg daily starting on day 1 of menstruation (or at any time if cycles have ceased or are infrequent)

Elleste Solo® **MX** (Pharmacia) PoM

Patches, self-adhesive, estradiol, *MX 40 patch* (releasing approx. 40 micrograms/24 hours), net price 8-patch pack = £5.19; *MX 80 patch* (releasing approx. 80 micrograms/24 hours), 8-patch pack = £5.99. Counselling, administration.

Dose: menopausal symptoms (and osteoporosis prophylaxis in case of *Elleste Solo MX 80*® **only**; see section 6.6), 1 patch to be applied twice weekly continuously starting within 5 days of onset of menstruation (or at any time if cycles have ceased or are infrequent); with cyclical progestogen for 12–14 days of each cycle in women with intact uterus; therapy should be initiated with *MX 40* in those with menopausal symptoms, prolonged oestrogen deficiency or anticipated intolerance to higher strength, dosage may be increased if required, subsequently adjusted to lowest effective dose

Estraderm MX® (Novartis) PoM
Patches, self-adhesive, estradiol, *MX 25 patch* (releasing approx. 25 micrograms/24 hours), net price 8-patch pack = £5.20, 24-patch pack = £15.59; *MX 50 patch* (releasing approx. 50 micrograms/24 hours), 8-patch pack = £5.22, 24-patch pack = £15.65, 20-patch pack (hosp. only) = £13.04; *MX 75 patch* (releasing approx. 75 micrograms/24 hours), 8-patch pack = £6.08, 24-patch pack = £18.25; *MX 100 patch* (releasing approx. 100 micrograms/24 hours), 8-patch pack = £6.31, 24-patch pack = £18.94. Counselling, administration

Dose: menopausal symptoms (and osteoporosis prophylaxis in case of *Estraderm MX*® *50* and *75* **only**; see section 6.6), 1 patch to be applied twice weekly continuously, with cyclical progestogen for 12 days of each cycle in women with intact uterus; therapy should be initiated with *MX 50* for first month, subsequently adjusted to lowest effective dose

Estraderm TTS® (Novartis) PoM
Patches, self-adhesive, estradiol, *TTS 25 patch* (releasing approx. 25 micrograms/24 hours), net price, 8-patch pack = £6.21, 24-patch pack = £18.63; *TTS 50 patch* (releasing approx. 50 micrograms/24 hours), 8-patch pack = £6.23, 24-patch pack = £18.69; *TTS 100 patch* (releasing approx. 100 micrograms/24 hours), 8-patch pack = £7.52, 24-patch pack = £22.63, 20-patch pack (hosp. only) = £16.76. Counselling, administration

Dose: menopausal symptoms (and osteoporosis prophylaxis in case of *Estraderm TTS*® *50* **only**; see section 6.6), 1 patch to be applied twice weekly continuously, with cyclical progestogen for 12 days of each cycle in women with intact uterus; therapy should be initiated with *TTS 50* for first month, subsequently adjusted to lowest effective dose

Estradot® (Novartis) PoM
Patches, self-adhesive, estradiol, *'25' patch* (releasing approx. 25 micrograms/24 hours), net price 8-patch pack = £5.20; *'37.5' patch* (releasing approx. 37.5 micrograms/24 hours), 8-patch pack = £5.21; *'50' patch* (releasing approx. 50 micrograms/24 hours), 8-patch pack = £5.22; *'75' patch* (releasing approx. 75 micrograms/24 hours), 8-patch pack = £6.08; *'100' patch* (releasing approx. 100 micrograms/24 hours), 8-patch pack = £6.31. Counselling, administration

Dose: menopausal symptoms (all strengths) and osteoporosis prophylaxis (*Estradot*® *'50'*, *'75'*, and *'100'* **only**; see section 6.6), 1 patch to be applied twice weekly continuously, with cyclical progestogen for 12 days of each cycle in women with intact uterus; for osteoporosis prophylaxis therapy should be initiated with *'50' patch*

Evorel® (Janssen-Cilag) PoM
Patches, self-adhesive, estradiol, *'25' patch* (releasing approx. 25 micrograms/24 hours), net price 8-patch pack = £2.92; *'50' patch* (releasing approx. 50 micrograms/24 hours), 8-patch pack = £3.31, 24-patch pack = £9.93; *'75' patch* (releasing approx. 75 micrograms/24 hours), 8-patch pack = £3.52; *'100' patch* (releasing approx. 100 micrograms/24 hours), 8-patch pack = £3.65. Counselling, administration

Dose: menopausal symptoms and osteoporosis prophylaxis (except *Evorel*® *25*; see section 6.6), 1 patch to be applied twice weekly continuously, with cyclical progestogen for at least 12 days of each cycle in women with intact uterus; therapy should be initiated with *'50' patch* for first month, subsequently adjusted to lowest effective dose

Fematrix® (Solvay) PoM
Fematrix® *40 patch*, self-adhesive, estradiol, *'40' patch* (releasing approx. 40 micrograms/24 hours). Net price 8-patch pack = £4.95. Counselling, administration

Dose: menopausal symptoms, 1 patch to be applied twice weekly continuously starting within 5 days of onset of menstruation (or at any time if cycles have ceased or are infrequent), with cyclical progestogen for 12–14 days of each cycle in women with intact uterus; *'80' patch* may be used if required (subsequently adjusted to lowest effective dose)

Fematrix® *80 patch*, self-adhesive, estradiol (releasing approx. 80 micrograms/24 hours). Net price 8-patch pack = £5.40. Counselling, administration

Dose: menopausal symptoms and osteoporosis prophylaxis (see section 6.6), as for *Fematrix*® *40*; therapy should be initiated with *Fematrix*® *40* in those with menopausal symptoms, prolonged oestrogen deficiency or anticipated intolerance to higher strength

FemSeven® (Merck) PoM
Patches, self-adhesive, estradiol, *'50' patch* (releasing approx. 50 micrograms/24 hours), net price 4-patch pack = £5.03, 12-patch pack = £15.02; *'75' patch* (releasing approx. 75 micrograms/24 hours), net price 4-patch pack = £5.82; *'100' patch* (releasing approx. 100 micrograms/24 hours), net price 4-patch pack = £6.07. Counselling, administration

Dose: menopausal symptoms and osteoporosis prophylaxis (see section 6.6), 1 patch to be applied once a week continuously, with cyclical progestogen for at least 10 days of each cycle in women with intact uterus; therapy should be initiated with *FemSeven*® *50* patches for the first few months, subsequently adjusted according to response

FemTab® (Merck) PoM
Tablets, s/c, estradiol valerate 1 mg, net price 3 × 28-tab pack = £7.72; 2 mg, 3 × 28-tab pack = £7.72

Dose: menopausal symptoms, 1–2 mg daily continuously; osteoporosis prophylaxis (see section 6.6), 2 mg daily continuously; with cyclical progestogen for 12 days of each cycle in women with intact uterus

Menoring® **50** (Galen) PoM
Vaginal ring, releasing estradiol approx. 50 micrograms/24 hours, net price 1-ring pack = £29.50. Label: 10, patient information leaflet

Dose: for postmenopausal vasomotor and urogenital symptoms in women without a uterus, to be inserted into upper third of vagina and worn continuously; replace after 3 months

Oestrogel® (Hoechst Marion Roussel) PoM
Gel, estradiol 0.06%, net price 64-dose pump pack = £7.39. Counselling, administration

Dose: menopausal symptoms and osteoporosis prophylaxis (see section 6.6), 2 measures (estradiol 1.5 mg) to be applied over an area twice that of the template provided once daily continuously, starting within 5 days of menstruation (or anytime if cycles have ceased or are infrequent), with cyclical progestogen for 12 days of each cycle in women with intact uterus; for menopausal symptoms may be increased if necessary after 1 month to max. 4 measures daily

COUNSELLING. Apply gel to clean, dry, intact skin such as arms, shoulders or inner thighs and allow to dry for 5 minutes before covering with clothing. Not to be applied on or near breasts or on vulval region. Avoid skin contact with another person (particularly male) and avoid other skin products or washing the area for at least 1 hour after application

Progynova® (Schering Health) PoM
Tablets, both s/c, estradiol valerate 1 mg (beige), net price 3 × 28-tab pack = £6.56; 2 mg (blue), 3 × 28-tab pack = £6.56
Dose: menopausal symptoms, 1–2 mg daily continuously; osteoporosis prophylaxis (see section 6.6), 2 mg daily continuously; with cyclical progestogen for 12 days of each cycle in women with intact uterus

Progynova® TS (Schering Health) PoM
Patches, self-adhesive, *Progynova® TS 50* (releasing estradiol approx. 50 micrograms/24 hours), net price 12-patch pack = £16.71; *Progynova® TS 100* (releasing estradiol approx. 100 micrograms/24 hours), 12-patch pack = £18.39. Counselling, administration
Dose: menopausal symptoms, 1 patch to be applied once a week on a continuous or cyclical basis (1 patch per week for three weeks followed by a 7-day patch-free interval); therapy should be initiated with *Progynova® TS 50* and adjusted to lowest effective dose; osteoporosis prophylaxis (see section 6.6), 1 *Progynova® TS 50* patch to be applied once a week on a continuous basis (with cyclical progestogen for 10–14 days of each cycle in women with intact uterus)
NOTE. Women receiving *Progynova® TS 100* patches for menopausal symptoms may continue with this strength for osteoporosis prophylaxis (see section 6.6)

Sandrena® (Organon) PoM
Gel, estradiol (0.1%), 500 microgram/500 mg sachet, net price 28-sachet pack = £5.28, 1 mg/1 g sachet, 28-sachet pack = £6.08. Counselling, administration
Dose: menopausal symptoms, estradiol 1 mg (1 g gel) to be applied once daily over area 1–2 times size of hand; with cyclical progestogen for 12–14 days of each cycle in women with intact uterus; dose may be adjusted after 2–3 cycles to a usual dose of estradiol 0.5–1.5 mg (0.5–1.5 g gel) daily
COUNSELLING. Apply gel to intact areas of skin such as lower trunk or thighs, using right and left sides on alternate days. Wash hands after application. Not to be applied on the breasts or face and avoid contact with eyes. Allow area of application to dry for 5 minutes and do not wash area for at least 1 hour

Zumenon® (Solvay) PoM
Tablets, f/c, estradiol 1 mg, net price 84-tab pack = £6.89; 2 mg (red), 84-tab pack = £6.89
Dose: menopausal symptoms, initially 1 mg daily starting on day 5 of menstruation (or any time if cycles have ceased or are infrequent) adjusted to 1–4 mg daily according to response; osteoporosis prophylaxis (see section 6.6), 2 mg daily; with cyclical progestogen for 10–14 days of each cycle in women with intact uterus

■ Estradiol, estriol and estrone

Hormonin® (Shire) PoM
Tablets, pink, estradiol 600 micrograms, estriol 270 micrograms, estrone 1.4 mg. Net price 84-tab pack = £6.61
Dose: menopausal symptoms and osteoporosis prophylaxis (see section 6.6), 1–2 tablets daily, with cyclical progestogen for 12–14 days of each cycle in women with intact uterus
NOTE. *Hormonin®* tablets can be given continuously or cyclically (21 days out of 28)

■ Estriol only

Ovestin® (Organon) PoM
Tablets, scored, estriol 1 mg. Net price 30-tab pack = £3.91. Label: 25
Dose: genito-urinary symptoms associated with oestrogen-deficiency states, 0.5–3 mg daily, as single dose, for up to 1 month, then 0.5–1 mg daily until restoration of epithelial integrity (short-term use); infertility due to poor cervical penetration, 0.25–1 mg daily on days 6–15 of cycle

■ Estropipate only

Harmogen® (Pharmacia) PoM
Tablets, peach, scored, estropipate 1.5 mg. Net price 28-tab pack = £3.77
Dose: menopausal symptoms and osteoporosis prophylaxis (see section 6.6), 1.5 mg daily continuously (with cyclical progestogen for 10–13 days of each cycle in women with intact uterus); up to 3 mg daily (in single or divided doses) for vasomotor symptoms and menopausal vaginitis

TIBOLONE

Indications: short-term treatment of symptoms of oestrogen deficiency (including women being treated with gonadotrophin releasing hormone analogues); osteoporosis prophylaxis in women at risk of fractures (second-line)

Cautions: see notes above and under Oestrogens for HRT; renal impairment, history of liver disease (Appendix 2), epilepsy, migraine, diabetes mellitus, hypercholesterolaemia; withdraw if signs of thromboembolic disease, abnormal liver function tests or cholestatic jaundice; see also Note below; **interactions:** Appendix 1 (tibolone)

Contra-indications: see notes above and under Oestrogens for HRT; hormone-dependent tumours, history of cardiovascular or cerebrovascular disease (e.g. thrombophlebitis, thromboembolism), uninvestigated vaginal bleeding, severe liver disease, pregnancy, breast-feeding

Side-effects: see notes above; weight changes, oedema, dizziness, nausea, seborrhoeic dermatitis, vaginal bleeding, leucorrhoea, headache, abdominal pain, gastro-intestinal disturbances, increased facial hair; depression, arthralgia, myalgia, migraine, breast cancer (see notes above and section 6.4.1.1), visual disturbances, liver-function changes, rash and pruritus also reported

Dose: 2.5 mg daily
NOTE. Unsuitable for use in the premenopause (unless being treated with gonadotrophin-releasing hormone analogue) and as (or with) an oral contraceptive; also unsuitable for use within 12 months of last menstrual period (may cause irregular bleeding); induce withdrawal bleed with progestogen if transferring from another form of HRT

Livial® (Organon) PoM
Tablets, tibolone 2.5 mg. Net price 28-tab pack = £10.77; 3 × 28-tab pack = £32.29

Ethinylestradiol

Ethinylestradiol (ethinyloestradiol) is licensed for short-term treatment of symptoms of oestrogen deficiency, for osteoporosis prophylaxis if other drugs (section 6.6) cannot be used and for the treatment of female hypogonadism and menstrual disorders.

Ethinylestradiol is occasionally used under **specialist supervision** for the management of *hereditary haemorrhagic telangiectasia* (but evidence of benefit is limited). Side-effects include nausea, fluid retention, and thrombosis. Impotence and gynaecomastia have been reported in men.

For use in prostate cancer, see section 8.3.1.

ETHINYLESTRADIOL

(Ethinyloestradiol)

Indications: see notes above

Cautions: cardiovascular disease (sodium retention with oedema, thromboembolism), hepatic impairment (jaundice), see also under Combined Hormonal Contraceptives (section 7.3.1) and under Oestrogen for HRT (above)

Contra-indications: see under Combined Hormonal Contraceptives (section 7.3.1) and under Oestrogen for HRT (above)

Side-effects: feminising effects in men; see also under Combined Hormonal Contraceptives (section 7.3.1) and under Oestrogen for HRT (above)

Dose: menopausal symptoms and osteoporosis prophylaxis, (with progestogen for 12–14 days per cycle in women with intact uterus), 10–50 micrograms daily for 21 days, repeated after 7-day tablet-free period

Female hypogonadism, 10–50 micrograms daily, usually on cyclical basis; initial oestrogen therapy should be followed by combined oestrogen and progestogen therapy

Menstrual disorders, 20–50 micrograms daily from day 5 to 25 of each cycle, with progestogen added either throughout the cycle or from day 15 to 25

Ethinylestradiol (Non-proprietary) PoM

Tablets, ethinylestradiol 10 micrograms, net price 21-tab pack = £12.86; 50 micrograms, 21-tab pack = £15.16; 1 mg, 28-tab pack = £28.85

Raloxifene

Raloxifene is licensed for the treatment and prevention of *postmenopausal osteoporosis*; unlike hormone replacement therapy, raloxifene does not reduce menopausal vasomotor symptoms.

Raloxifene may reduce the incidence of oestrogen-receptor-positive breast cancer but its role in established breast cancer is not yet clear. The manufacturer advises avoiding its use during treatment for breast cancer.

RALOXIFENE HYDROCHLORIDE

Indications: treatment and prevention of postmenopausal osteoporosis

Cautions: risk factors for venous thromboembolism (discontinue if prolonged immobilisation); breast cancer (see notes above); history of oestrogen-induced hypertriglyceridaemia (monitor serum triglycerides); **interactions:** Appendix 1 (raloxifene)

Contra-indications: history of venous thromboembolism, undiagnosed uterine bleeding, endometrial cancer, hepatic impairment, cholestasis, severe renal impairment; pregnancy and breast-feeding

Side-effects: venous thromboembolism, thrombophlebitis, hot flushes, leg cramps, peripheral oedema, influenza-like symptoms; rarely rashes, gastro-intestinal disturbances, hypertension, headache (including migraine), breast discomfort

Dose: 60 mg once daily

Evista® (Lilly) PoM

Tablets, f/c, raloxifene hydrochloride 60 mg, net price 28-tab pack = £19.86; 84-tab pack = £59.59

6.4.1.2 Progestogens

There are two main groups of progestogen, *progesterone and its analogues* (dydrogesterone and medroxyprogesterone) and *testosterone analogues* (norethisterone and norgestrel). The newer progestogens (desogestrel, norgestimate, and gestodene) are all derivatives of norgestrel; levonorgestrel is the active isomer of norgestrel and has twice its potency. Progesterone and its analogues are less androgenic than the testosterone derivatives and neither progesterone nor dydrogesterone causes virilisation.

Where *endometriosis* requires drug treatment, it may respond to a progestogen, e.g. norethisterone, administered on a continuous basis. Danazol, gestrinone, and gonadorelin analogues are also available (section 6.7.2).

Although oral progestogens have been used widely for *menorrhagia* they are relatively ineffective compared with tranexamic acid (section 2.11) or, particularly where dysmenorrhoea is also a factor, mefenamic acid (section 10.1.1); the levonorgestrel-releasing intra-uterine system (section 7.3.2.3) may be particularly useful for women also requiring contraception. Oral progestogens have also been used for *severe dysmenorrhoea*, but where contraception is also required in younger women the best choice is a combined oral contraceptive (section 7.3.1).

Progestogens have also been advocated for the alleviation of *premenstrual symptoms*, but no convincing physiological basis for such treatment has been shown.

Progestogens have been used for the prevention of spontaneous abortion in women with a history of *recurrent miscarriage* (habitual abortion) but there is no evidence of benefit and they are **not** recommended for this purpose. In pregnant women with antiphospholipid antibody syndrome who have suffered recurrent miscarriage, administration of low-dose aspirin (section 2.9) and a prophylactic dose of a low molecular weight heparin (section 2.8.1) may decrease the risk of fetal loss (use under specialist supervision only).

HORMONE REPLACEMENT THERAPY. In women with a uterus a progestogen needs to be added to *long-term oestrogen therapy for hormone replacement*, to prevent cystic hyperplasia of the endometrium and possible transformation to cancer; it can be added on a cyclical or a continuous basis (see section 6.4.1.1). Combined packs incorporating suitable progestogen tablets are available, see p. 368.

ORAL CONTRACEPTION. Desogestrel, etynodiol (ethynodiol), gestodene, levonorgestrel, norethisterone, and norgestimate are used in *combined oral contraceptives* and in *progestogen-only contraceptives* (section 7.3.1 and section 7.3.2).

CANCER. Progestogens also have a role in *neoplastic disease* (section 8.3.2).

CAUTIONS. Progestogens should be used with caution in conditions that may worsen with fluid retention e.g. epilepsy, hypertension, migraine, asthma, cardiac or renal dysfunction, and in those susceptible to thromboembolism (particular caution with high dose). Care is also required in liver impairment (avoid if severe), and in those with a history of depression. Progestogens can decrease glucose tolerance and diabetes should be monitored closely. For **interactions** see Appendix 1 (progestogens).

CONTRA-INDICATIONS. Progestogens should be avoided in patients with a history of liver tumours, and in severe liver impairment. They are also contra-indicated in those with genital or breast cancer (unless progestogens are being used in the management of these conditions), severe arterial disease, undiagnosed vaginal bleeding and porphyria (section 9.8.2). Progestogens should not be used if there is a history during pregnancy of idiopathic jaundice, severe pruritus, or pemphigoid gestationis.

SIDE-EFFECTS. Side-effects of progestogens include menstrual disturbances, premenstrual-like syndrome (including bloating, fluid retention, breast tenderness), weight gain, nausea, headache, dizziness, insomnia, drowsiness, depression; also skin reactions (including urticaria, pruritus, rash, and acne), hirsutism and alopecia. Jaundice and anaphylactoid reactions have also been reported.

DYDROGESTERONE

Indications: see under Dose and notes above
Cautions: see notes above; breast-feeding (Appendix 5)
Contra-indications: see notes above
Side-effects: see notes above
Dose: endometriosis, 10 mg 2–3 times daily from day 5 to 25 of cycle or continuously
Infertility, irregular cycles, 10 mg twice daily from day 11 to 25 for at least 6 cycles (but not recommended)
Recurrent miscarriage, 10 mg twice daily from day 11 to 25 of cycle until conception, then continuously until week 20 of pregnancy and then gradually reduced (but not recommended, see notes above)
Dysfunctional uterine bleeding, 10 mg twice daily (together with an oestrogen) for 5–7 days to arrest bleeding; 10 mg twice daily (together with an oestrogen) from day 11 to 25 of cycle to prevent bleeding
Dysmenorrhoea (but see notes above), 10 mg twice daily from day 5 to 25 of cycle
Amenorrhoea, 10 mg twice daily from day 11 to 25 of cycle with oestrogen therapy from day 1 to 25 of cycle
Premenstrual syndrome, 10 mg twice daily from day 12 to 26 of cycle increased if necessary (but not recommended, see notes above)
Hormone replacement therapy, with continuous oestrogen therapy, see under *Duphaston® HRT* below

Duphaston® (Solvay) PoM
Tablets, scored, dydrogesterone 10 mg. Net price 60-tab pack = £4.04

Duphaston® HRT (Solvay) PoM
Tablets, scored, dydrogesterone 10 mg. Net price 42-tab pack = £2.83
Dose: 10 mg daily on days 15–28 of each 28-day oestrogen HRT cycle, increased to 10 mg twice daily if withdrawal bleed is early or endometrial biopsy shows inadequate progestational response

MEDROXYPROGESTERONE ACETATE

Indications: see under Dose; contraception (section 7.3.2.2); malignant disease (section 8.3.2)
Cautions: see notes above; breast-feeding (Appendix 5)
Contra-indications: see notes above; pregnancy (Appendix 4)
Side-effects: see notes above; indigestion
Dose: *by mouth*, 2.5–10 mg daily for 5–10 days beginning on day 16 to 21 of cycle, repeated for 2 cycles in dysfunctional uterine bleeding and 3 cycles in secondary amenorrhoea
Mild to moderate endometriosis, 10 mg 3 times daily for 90 consecutive days, beginning on day 1 of cycle
Progestogenic opposition of oestrogen HRT, 10 mg daily for the last 14 days of each 28-day oestrogen HRT cycle

Provera® (Pharmacia) PoM
Tablets, all scored, medroxyprogesterone acetate 2.5 mg (orange), net price 30-tab pack = £1.84; 5 mg (blue), 10-tab pack = £1.23; 10 mg (white), 10-tab pack = £2.47, 90-tab pack = £22.16

■ Combined preparations
Section 6.4.1.1

NORETHISTERONE

Indications: see under Dose; HRT (section 6.4.1.1); contraception (section 7.3.1 and section 7.3.2); malignant disease (section 8.3.2)
Cautions: see notes above; breast-feeding (Appendix 5)
Contra-indications: see notes above; pregnancy (Appendix 4)
Side-effects: see notes above
Dose: endometriosis, 10–15 mg daily for 4–6 months or longer, starting on day 5 of cycle (if spotting occurs increase dose to 20–25 mg daily, reduced once bleeding has stopped)
Dysfunctional uterine bleeding, menorrhagia (but see notes above), 5 mg 3 times daily for 10 days to arrest bleeding; to prevent bleeding 5 mg twice daily from day 19 to 26
Dysmenorrhoea (but see notes above), 5 mg 3 times daily from day 5 to 24 for 3–4 cycles
Premenstrual syndrome, 5 mg 2–3 times daily from day 19 to 26 for several cycles (but not recommended, see notes above)
Postponement of menstruation, 5 mg 3 times daily starting 3 days before anticipated onset (menstruation occurs 2–3 days after stopping)
Progestogenic opposition of menopausal oestrogen HRT, see under *Micronor® HRT*, below

■ Tablets of 5 mg
Norethisterone (Non-proprietary) PoM
Tablets, norethisterone 5 mg, net price 30-tab pack = £2.87; 100-tab pack = £7.17

Primolut N® (Schering Health) PoM
Tablets, norethisterone 5 mg. Net price 30-tab pack = £2.01

Utovlan® (Pharmacia) PoM
Tablets, norethisterone 5 mg, net price 30-tab pack = £1.40, 90-tab pack = £4.21

■ Tablets of 1 mg for HRT

Micronor® HRT (Janssen-Cilag) PoM
Tablets, norethisterone 1 mg. Net price 3 × 12-tab pack = £3.56
Dose: 1 tablet daily on days 15–26 of each 28-day oestrogen HRT cycle

■ Combined preparations
Section 6.4.1.1

PROGESTERONE

Indications: see under preparations

Cautions: see notes above; breast-feeding (Appendix 5)

Contra-indications: see notes above; missed or incomplete abortion

Side-effects: see notes above; injection-site reactions; pain, diarrhoea and flatulence can occur with rectal administration

Crinone® (Serono) PoM
Vaginal gel, progesterone 90 mg/application (8%), 15 = £32.73
Dose: by vagina, infertility due to inadequate luteal phase, insert 1 applicatorful daily starting either after documented ovulation or on day 18–21 of cycle. *In vitro* fertilisation, daily application continued for 30 days after laboratory evidence of pregnancy

Cyclogest® (Alpharma) PoM
Pessaries, progesterone 200 mg, net price 15 = £7.46; 400 mg, 15 = £10.80
Dose: by vagina or rectum, premenstrual syndrome and post-natal depression, 200 mg daily to 400 mg twice daily; for premenstrual syndrome start on day 12–14 and continue until onset of menstruation (but not recommended, see notes above); rectally if barrier methods of contraception are used, in patients who have recently given birth or in those who suffer from vaginal infection or recurrent cystitis

Gestone® (Nordic) PoM
Injection, progesterone 50 mg/mL, 1-mL amp = 57p, 2-mL amp = 75p
Dose: by deep intramuscular injection into buttock, dysfunctional uterine bleeding, 5–10 mg daily for 5–10 days until 2 days before expected onset of menstruation Recurrent miscarriage due to inadequate luteal phase (but not recommended, see notes above) or following *in vitro* fertilisation *or* gamete intra-fallopian transfer, 25–100 mg 2–7 times a week from day 15, or day of embryo *or* gamete transfer, until 8–16 weeks of pregnancy; max. 200 mg daily

6.4.2 Male sex hormones and antagonists

Androgens cause masculinisation; they may be used as replacement therapy in castrated adults and in those who are hypogonadal due to either pituitary or testicular disease. In the normal male they inhibit pituitary gonadotrophin secretion and depress spermatogenesis. Androgens also have an anabolic action which led to the development of anabolic steroids (section 6.4.3).

Androgens are useless as a treatment of impotence and impaired spermatogenesis unless there is associated hypogonadism; they should not be given until the hypogonadism has been properly investigated. Treatment should be under expert supervision.

When given to patients with hypopituitarism they can lead to normal sexual development and potency but not to fertility. If fertility is desired, the usual treatment is with gonadotrophins or pulsatile gonadotrophin-releasing hormone (section 6.5.1) which will stimulate spermatogenesis as well as androgen production.

Caution should be used when androgens or chorionic gonadotrophin are used in treating boys with delayed puberty since the fusion of epiphyses is hastened and may result in short stature.

Intramuscular depot preparations of **testosterone esters** are preferred for replacement therapy. Testosterone enantate, propionate or undecanoate, or alternatively *Sustanon*®, which consists of a mixture of testosterone esters and has a longer duration of action, may be used. Satisfactory replacement therapy can sometimes be obtained with 1 mL of *Sustanon 250*®, given by intramuscular injection once a month, although more frequent dose intervals are often necessary. Implants of testosterone can be used for hypogonadism; the implants are replaced every 4 to 5 months. Menopausal women are also sometimes given implants of testosterone (in a dose of 50–100 mg every 4–8 months) as an adjunct to hormone replacement therapy.

TESTOSTERONE AND ESTERS

Indications: see under preparations

Cautions: cardiac, renal, or hepatic impairment (Appendix 2), elderly, ischaemic heart disease, hypertension, epilepsy, migraine, diabetes mellitus, skeletal metastases (risk of hypercalcaemia), undertake regular examination of the prostate and breast during treatment; pre-pubertal boys (see notes above and under Side-effects); **interactions:** Appendix 1 (testosterone)

Contra-indications: breast cancer in men, prostate cancer, history of primary liver tumours, hypercalcaemia, pregnancy (Appendix 4), breast-feeding (Appendix 5), nephrotic syndrome

Side-effects: prostate abnormalities and prostate cancer, headache, depression, gastro-intestinal bleeding, nausea, cholestatic jaundice, changes in libido, gynaecomastia, polycythaemia, anxiety, asthenia, paraesthesia, hypertension, electrolyte disturbances including sodium retention with oedema and hypercalcaemia, weight gain; increased bone growth; androgenic effects such as hirsutism, male-pattern baldness, seborrhoea, acne, pruritus, excessive frequency and duration of penile erection, precocious sexual development and premature closure of epiphyses in pre-pubertal males, suppression of spermatogenesis in men and virilism in women; *rarely* liver tumours; sleep apnoea also reported; *with patches, buccal tablets, and gel*, local irritation and allergic reactions, bitter taste with *buccal tablets*

■ Oral

Restandol® (Organon) PoM
Capsules, red-brown, testosterone undecanoate 40 mg in oily solution. Net price 28-cap pack = £8.30; 56-cap pack = £16.60. Label: 21, 25
Dose: androgen deficiency, 120–160 mg daily for 2–3 weeks; maintenance 40–120 mg daily

■ Buccal

Striant® SR (Ardana) PoM
Mucoadhesive buccal tablets, m/r, testosterone 30 mg, net price 60-tab pack = £45.84. Counselling, see under Dose below
Dose: hypogonadism, 30 mg every 12 hours; CHILD and ADOLESCENT under 18 years not recommended
COUNSELLING. Place rounded side of tablet on gum above front teeth and hold lip firmly over the gum for 30 seconds. If tablet detaches within 4 hours of next dose, replace with new tablet which is considered the second dose for the day.

■ Intramuscular

Testosterone Enantate (Cambridge) PoM
Injection (oily), testosterone enantate 250 mg/mL. Net price 1-mL amp = £8.33
Dose: by slow intramuscular injection, hypogonadism, initially 250 mg every 2–3 weeks; maintenance 250 mg every 3–6 weeks
Breast cancer, 250 mg every 2–3 weeks

Nebido® (Schering Health) ▼ PoM
Injection (oily), testosterone undecanoate 250 mg/mL. Net price 4-mL amp = £76.70
Dose: by deep intramuscular injection, hypogonadism in men over 18 years, 1 g every 10–14 weeks; if necessary, second dose may be given after 6 weeks to achieve rapid steady state plasma testosterone levels and then every 10–14 weeks

Sustanon 100® (Organon) PoM
Injection (oily), testosterone propionate 20 mg, testosterone phenylpropionate 40 mg, and testosterone isocaproate 40 mg/mL. Net price 1-mL amp = £1.09
Excipients: include arachis (peanut) oil, benzyl alcohol (see Excipients p. 2)
Dose: by deep intramuscular injection, androgen deficiency, 1 mL every 2 weeks

Sustanon 250® (Organon) PoM
Injection (oily), testosterone propionate 30 mg, testosterone phenylpropionate 60 mg, testosterone isocaproate 60 mg, and testosterone decanoate 100 mg/mL. Net price 1-mL amp = £2.55
Excipients: include arachis (peanut) oil, benzyl alcohol (see Excipients p. 2)
Dose: by deep intramuscular injection, androgen deficiency, 1 mL usually every 3 weeks

Virormone® (Nordic) PoM
Injection, testosterone propionate 50 mg/mL. Net price 2-mL amp = 59p
Dose: by intramuscular injection, androgen deficiency, 50 mg 2–3 times weekly
Delayed puberty, 50 mg weekly
Breast cancer in women, 100 mg 2–3 times weekly

■ Implant

Testosterone (Organon) PoM
Implant, testosterone 100 mg, net price = £7.40; 200 mg = £13.79
Dose: by implantation, male hypogonadism, 100–600 mg; 600 mg usually maintains plasma-testosterone concentration within the normal range for 4–5 months
Menopausal women, see notes above

■ Transdermal preparations

Andropatch® (GSK) PoM
Patches, self-adhesive, releasing testosterone approx. 2.5 mg/24 hours, net price 60-patch pack = £49.10; releasing testosterone approx. 5 mg/24 hours, net price 30-patch pack = £49.10. Counselling, administration
Dose: androgen deficiency in men (over 15 years) associated with primary or secondary hypogonadism, apply to clean, dry, unbroken skin on back, abdomen, upper arms or thighs, removing after 24 hours and siting replacement patch on a different area (with an interval of 7 days before using the same site); initially apply patches equivalent to testosterone 5 mg/24 hours (2.5 mg/24 hours in non-virilised patients) at night (approx. 10 p.m.), then adjust to 2.5 mg to 7.5 mg every 24 hours according to plasma-testosterone concentration (those with a body-weight over 130 kg may require 7.5 mg every 24 hours)

Testim® (Ipsen) ▼ PoM
Gel, testosterone 50 mg/5 g tube, net price 30-tube pack = £33.00. Counselling, administration
Excipients: include propylene glycol (see section 13.1.3)
Dose: hypogonadism due to testosterone deficiency in men (over 18 years), 50 mg testosterone (5 g gel) applied once daily; subsequent application adjusted according to response; max. 100 mg (10 g gel) daily
COUNSELLING. Squeeze entire content of tube on to one palm and apply as a thin layer on clean, dry, healthy skin of shoulder or upper arm, preferably in the morning after washing or bathing (if 2 tubes required use 1 per shoulder or upper arm); rub in and allow to dry before putting on clothing to cover site; wash hands with soap after application; avoid washing application site for at least 6 hours
Avoid skin contact with application sites to prevent testosterone transfer to other people, especially pregnant women and children—consult product literature

Testogel® (Schering Health) ▼ PoM
Gel, testosterone 50 mg/5 g sachet, net price 30-sachet pack = £33.00. Counselling, administration
Dose: hypogonadism due to androgen deficiency in men (over 18 years), 50 mg testosterone (5 g gel) to be applied once daily; subsequent application adjusted according to response in 25-mg (2.5 g gel) increments to max. 100 mg (10 g gel) daily
COUNSELLING. Apply thin layer of gel on clean, dry, healthy skin such as shoulders, arms or abdomen, immediately after sachet is opened. Not to be applied on genital area as high alcohol content may cause local irritation. Allow to dry for 3–5 minutes before dressing. Wash hands with soap and water after applying gel, avoid shower or bath for at least 6 hours
Avoid skin contact with gel application sites to prevent testosterone transfer to other people, especially pregnant women and children—consult product literature

MESTEROLONE

Indications: see under Dose
Cautions: see under Testosterone and Esters
Contra-indications: see under Testosterone and Esters
Side-effects: see under Testosterone and Esters but spermatogenesis unimpaired
Dose: androgen deficiency and male infertility associated with hypogonadism, 25 mg 3–4 times daily for several months, reduced to 50–75 mg daily in divided doses for maintenance; CHILD not recommended

Pro-Viron® (Schering Health) PoM
Tablets, scored, mesterolone 25 mg. Net price 30-tab pack = £4.44

Anti-androgens

Cyproterone acetate

Cyproterone acetate is an anti-androgen used in the treatment of severe hypersexuality and sexual deviation in the male. It inhibits spermatogenesis and produces reversible infertility (but is not a male contraceptive); abnormal sperm forms are produced. Fully informed consent is recommended and an initial spermatogram. As hepatic tumours have been produced in *animal* studies, careful consideration should be given to the risk/benefit ratio before treatment. Cyproterone acetate is also used as an adjunct in prostatic cancer (section 8.3.4.2) and in the treatment of acne and hirsutism in women (section 13.6.2).

CYPROTERONE ACETATE

Indications: see notes above; prostate cancer (section 8.3.4.2)

Cautions: ineffective for male hypersexuality in chronic alcoholism (relevance to prostate cancer not known); blood counts initially and throughout treatment; monitor hepatic function regularly (liver function tests should be performed before treatment, see also under Side-effects below); monitor adrenocortical function regularly; diabetes mellitus (see also Contra-indications)

DRIVING. Fatigue and lassitude may impair performance of skilled tasks (e.g. driving)

Contra-indications: (do not apply in prostate cancer) hepatic disease (Appendix 2), severe diabetes (with vascular changes); sickle-cell anaemia, malignant or wasting disease, severe depression, history of thrombo-embolic disorders; youths under 18 years (may arrest bone maturation and testicular development)

Side-effects: fatigue and lassitude, breathlessness, weight changes, reduced sebum production (may clear acne), changes in hair pattern, gynaecomastia (rarely leading to galactorrhoea and benign breast nodules); rarely hypersensitivity reactions, rash and osteoporosis; inhibition of spermatogenesis (see notes above); hepatotoxicity reported (including jaundice, hepatitis and hepatic failure usually in men given 200–300 mg daily for prostatic cancer, see section 8.3.4.2 for details and warnings)

Dose: male hypersexuality, 50 mg twice daily after food

Cyproterone Acetate (Non-proprietary) PoM
Tablets, cyproterone acetate 50 mg, net price 56-tab pack = £31.54. Label 21, counselling, driving

Androcur® (Schering Health) PoM
Tablets, scored, cyproterone acetate 50 mg. Net price 56-tab pack = £25.89. Label: 21, counselling, driving

Dutasteride and finasteride

Dutasteride and **finasteride** are specific inhibitors of the enzyme 5α-reductase, which metabolises testosterone into the more potent androgen, dihydrotestosterone. This inhibition of testosterone metabolism leads to reduction in prostate size, with improvement in urinary flow rate and in obstructive symptoms. Dutasteride and finasteride are alternatives to alpha-blockers (section 7.4.1) particularly in men with a significantly enlarged prostate. Finasteride is also licensed for use with doxazosin in the management of benign prostatic hyperplasia.

A low strength of finasteride is licensed for treating male-pattern baldness in men (section 13.9).

CAUTIONS. Dutasteride and finasteride decrease serum concentration of prostate cancer markers such as prostate-specific antigen; reference values may need adjustment. Both dutasteride and finasteride are excreted in semen and use of a condom is recommended if sexual partner is pregnant or likely to become pregnant. Women of childbearing potential should avoid handling crushed or broken tablets of finasteride and leaking capsules of dutasteride.

CONTRA-INDICATIONS. Dutasteride and finasteride are contra-indicated in women, children, and adolescents.

SIDE-EFFECTS. The side-effects of dutasteride and finasteride include impotence, decreased libido, ejaculation disorders, and breast tenderness and enlargement.

DUTASTERIDE

Indications: benign prostatic hyperplasia

Cautions: see notes above; **interactions:** Appendix 1 (dutasteride)

Contra-indications: see notes above; also severe hepatic impairment

Side-effects: see notes above

Dose: 500 micrograms daily (may require 6 months' treatment before benefit is obtained)

Avodart® (GSK) PoM
Capsules, yellow, dutasteride 500 micrograms, net price 30-cap pack = £24.81. Label: 25

FINASTERIDE

Indications: benign prostatic hyperplasia; male-pattern baldness in men (section 13.9)

Cautions: see notes above; also obstructive uropathy

Side-effects: see notes above; also testicular pain, hypersensitivity reactions (including lip and face swelling, pruritus and rash)

Dose: 5 mg daily, review treatment after 6 months (may require several months' treatment before benefit is obtained)

Proscar® (MSD) PoM
Tablets, blue, f/c, finasteride 5 mg. Net price 28-tab pack = £13.94

6.4.3 Anabolic steroids

Anabolic steroids have some androgenic activity but they cause less virilisation than androgens in women. They are used in the treatment of some *aplastic anaemias* (section 9.1.3). Anabolic steroids have been given for osteoporosis in women but they are no longer advocated for this purpose.

The protein-building properties of anabolic steroids have not proved beneficial in the clinical setting. Their use as body builders or tonics is quite unjustified; some athletes abuse them.

NANDROLONE

Indications: osteoporosis in postmenopausal women (but not recommended, see notes above); aplastic anaemia (section 9.1.3)

Cautions: cardiac and renal impairment, hepatic impairment (Appendix 2), hypertension, diabetes mellitus, epilepsy, migraine; monitor skeletal maturation in young patients; skeletal metastases (risk of hypercalcaemia); **interactions:** Appendix 1 (anabolic steroids)

Contra-indications: severe hepatic impairment, prostate cancer, male breast cancer, pregnancy (Appendix 4) and breast-feeding, porphyria (section 9.8.2)

Side-effects: acne, sodium retention with oedema, virilisation with high doses including voice changes (sometimes irreversible), amenorrhoea, inhibition of spermatogenesis, premature epiphyseal closure; abnormal liver-function tests reported with high doses; liver tumours reported occasionally on prolonged treatment with anabolic steroids

Dose: see below

Deca-Durabolin® (Organon) PoM

Injection (oily), nandrolone decanoate 50 mg/mL, net price 1-mL amp = £3.29

Excipients: include arachis (peanut) oil, benzyl alcohol (see Excipients, p. 2)

Dose: by deep intramuscular injection, 50 mg every 3 weeks

6.5 Hypothalamic and pituitary hormones and anti-oestrogens

Use of preparations in these sections requires detailed prior investigation of the patient and *should be reserved for specialist centres.*

6.5.1 Hypothalamic and anterior pituitary hormones and anti-oestrogens

Anti-oestrogens

The anti-oestrogens **clomifene** (clomiphene) and **tamoxifen** (section 8.3.4.1) are used in the treatment of female infertility due to oligomenorrhoea or secondary amenorrhoea (e.g. associated with polycystic ovarian disease). They induce gonadotrophin release by occupying oestrogen receptors in the hypothalamus, thereby interfering with feedback mechanisms; chorionic gonadotrophin is sometimes used as an adjunct. Patients should be warned that there is a risk of multiple pregnancy (*rarely* more than twins).

CLOMIFENE CITRATE

(Clomiphene Citrate)

Indications: anovulatory infertility—see notes above

Cautions: see notes above; polycystic ovary syndrome (cysts may enlarge during treatment), ovarian hyperstimulation syndrome, uterine fibroids, ectopic pregnancy, incidence of multiple births increased (consider ultrasound monitoring), visual symptoms (discontinue and initiate ophthalmological examination); breast-feeding (Appendix 5)

CSM Advice. The CSM has recommended that clomifene should not normally be used for longer than 6 cycles (possibly increased risk of ovarian cancer)

Contra-indications: hepatic disease (Appendix 2), ovarian cysts, hormone dependent tumours or abnormal uterine bleeding of undetermined cause, pregnancy (exclude before treatment; Appendix 4)

Side-effects: visual disturbances (withdraw), ovarian hyperstimulation (withdraw), hot flushes, abdominal discomfort, occasionally nausea, vomiting, depression, insomnia, breast tenderness, headache, intermenstrual spotting, menorrhagia, endometriosis, convulsions, weight gain, rashes, dizziness, hair loss

Dose: 50 mg daily for 5 days, starting within about 5 days of onset of menstruation (preferably on 2nd day) or at any time (normally preceded by a progestogen-induced withdrawal bleed) if cycles have ceased; second course of 100 mg daily for 5 days may be given in absence of ovulation; most patients who are going to respond will do so to first course; 3 courses should constitute adequate therapeutic trial; long-term cyclical therapy not recommended—see CSM advice, above

Clomifene (Non-proprietary) PoM

Tablets, clomifene citrate 50 mg, net price 30-tab pack = £11.25

Clomid® (Aventis Pharma) PoM

Tablets, yellow, scored, clomifene citrate 50 mg. Net price 30-tab pack = £8.80

Anterior pituitary hormones

Corticotrophins

Tetracosactide (tetracosactrin), an analogue of corticotropin (ACTH), is used to test adrenocortical function; failure of the plasma cortisol concentration to rise after administration of tetracosactide indicates adrenocortical insufficiency.

Both corticotropin and tetracosactide were formerly used as alternatives to corticosteroids in conditions such as Crohn's disease or rheumatoid arthritis; their value was limited by the variable and unpredictable therapeutic response and by the waning of their effect with time.

TETRACOSACTIDE

(Tetracosactrin)

Indications: see notes above

Cautions: as for corticosteroids, section 6.3.2; **important:** risk of anaphylaxis (medical supervision; consult product literature); **interactions:** Appendix 1 (corticosteroids)

Contra-indications: as for corticosteroids, section 6.3.2; avoid injections containing benzyl alcohol in neonates (see under preparations)
Side-effects: as for corticosteroids, section 6.3.2
Dose: see under preparations below

Synacthen® (Alliance) PoM
Injection, tetracosactide 250 micrograms (as acetate)/mL. Net price 1-mL amp = £2.93
Dose: diagnostic (30-minute test), *by intramuscular or intravenous injection*, 250 micrograms as a single dose

Synacthen Depot® (Alliance) PoM
Injection (aqueous suspension), tetracosactide acetate 1 mg/mL, with zinc phosphate complex. Net price 1-mL amp = £4.18
Excipients: include benzyl alcohol (avoid in neonates, see Excipients p. 2)
Dose: diagnostic (5-hour test), *by intramuscular injection*, 1 mg as a single dose
NOTE. Formerly used therapeutically by intramuscular injection, in an initial dose of 1 mg daily (or every 12 hours in acute cases); reduced to 1 mg every 2–3 days, then 1 mg weekly (or 500 micrograms every 2–3 days) but value was limited (see notes above)

Gonadotrophins

Follicle-stimulating hormone (FSH) and luteinising hormone (LH) together (as in **human menopausal gonadotrophin**), follicle-stimulating hormone alone (as in **follitropin**), or chorionic gonadotrophin, are used in the treatment of infertility in women with proven hypopituitarism or who have not responded to clomifene, or in superovulation treatment for assisted conception (such as *in vitro* fertilisation).

The gonadotrophins are also occasionally used in the treatment of hypogonadotrophic hypogonadism and associated oligospermia. There is no justification for their use in primary gonadal failure.

Chorionic gonadotrophin has also been used in delayed puberty in the male to stimulate endogenous testosterone production, but has little advantage over testosterone (section 6.4.2).

CHORIONIC GONADOTROPHIN

(Human Chorionic Gonadotrophin; HCG)
A preparation of a glycoprotein fraction secreted by the placenta and obtained from the urine of pregnant women having the action of the pituitary luteinising hormone
Indications: see notes above
Cautions: cardiac or renal impairment, asthma, epilepsy, migraine; prepubertal boys (risk of premature epiphyseal closure or precocious puberty)
Contra-indications: androgen-dependent tumours
Side-effects: oedema (particularly in males—reduce dose), headache, tiredness, mood changes, gynaecomastia, local reactions; may aggravate ovarian hyperstimulation, multiple pregnancy
Dose: *by subcutaneous or intramuscular injection*, according to patient's response

Choragon® (Ferring) PoM
Injection, powder for reconstitution, chorionic gonadotrophin. Net price 5000-unit amp (with solvent) = £3.26. For intramuscular injection

Pregnyl® (Organon) PoM
Injection, powder for reconstitution, chorionic gonadotrophin. Net price 1500-unit amp = £2.20; 5000-unit amp = £3.27 (both with solvent). For subcutaneous or intramuscular injection

CHORIOGONADOTROPIN ALFA

(Human chorionic gonadotropin)
Indications: see notes above
Cautions: rule out infertility caused by hypothyroidism, adrenocortical deficiency, hyperprolactinaemia, tumours of the pituitary or hypothalamus
Contra-indications: ovarian enlargement or cyst (unless caused by polycystic ovarian disease); ectopic pregnancy in previous 3 months; active thromboembolic disorders; hypothalamus, pituitary, ovarian, uterine or mammary malignancy
Side-effects: nausea, vomiting, abdominal pain; headache, tiredness; injection-site reactions; ovarian hyperstimulation syndrome; rarely diarrhoea, depression, irritability, breast pain; ectopic pregnancy and ovarian torsion reported
Dose: *by subcutaneous injection*, according to patient's response

Ovitrelle® (Serono) ▼ PoM
Injection, choriogonadotropin alfa, net price 6500-unit/0.5 mL (250-micrograms/0.5 mL) prefilled syringe = £33.31

FOLLITROPIN ALFA and BETA

(Recombinant human follicle stimulating hormone)
Indications: see notes above
Cautions: see under Human Menopausal Gonadotrophins
Contra-indications: see under Human Menopausal Gonadotrophins
Side-effects: see under Human Menopausal Gonadotrophins
Dose: *by subcutaneous or intramuscular injection*, according to patient's response

■ Follitropin alfa

Gonal-F® (Serono) PoM
Injection, powder for reconstitution, follitropin alfa. Net price 75-unit amp = £22.31; 450 units/0.75 mL, multidose vial = £133.86; 1050 units/1.75 mL, multidose vial = £312.34 (all with diluent). For subcutaneous injection
Injection, prefilled pen, follitropin alfa 600 units/mL, net price 0.5 mL (300 units) = £97.08, 0.75 mL (450 units) = £145.62, 1.5 mL (900 units) = £291.24. For subcutaneous injection

■ Follitropin beta

Puregon® (Organon) PoM
Injection, follitropin beta 100 units/mL, net price 0.5-mL (50-unit) vial = £18.74; 200 units/mL, 0.5-mL (100-unit) vial = £37.48; 300 units/mL, 0.5-mL (150-unit) vial = £50.62; 400 units/mL, 0.5-mL (200-unit) vial = £67.49; 0.36-mL (300-unit) cartridge = £101.23, 0.72-mL (600-unit) cartridge = £202.47, 1.08-mL (900-unit) cartridge = £303.66, (cartridges for use with *Puregon*® pen). For subcutaneous (cartridges and vials) or intramuscular injection (vials)
Excipients: may include neomycin and streptomycin

HUMAN MENOPAUSAL GONADOTROPHINS

Purified extract of human post-menopausal urine containing follicle-stimulating hormone (FSH) and luteinising hormone (LH); the relative *in vivo* activity is designated as a ratio; the 1:1 ratio is also known as menotrophin

Indications: see notes above

Cautions: rule out infertility caused by adrenal or thyroid disorders, hyperprolactinaemia or tumours of the pituitary or hypothalamus

Contra-indications: ovarian cysts (not caused by polycystic ovarian syndrome); tumours of breast, uterus, ovaries, testes or prostate; vaginal bleeding of unknown cause; pregnancy and breast-feeding

Side-effects: ovarian hyperstimulation, increased risk of multiple pregnancy and miscarriage, hypersensitivity reactions, nausea, vomiting, joint pain, fever, injection site reactions, very rarely thromboembolism; gynaecomastia, acne, and weight gain reported in men

Dose: *by deep intramuscular or subcutaneous injection*, according to patient's response

Menogon® (Ferring) PoM
Injection, powder for reconstitution, menotrophin as follicle-stimulating hormone 75 units, luteinising hormone 75 units, net price per amp (with solvent) = £9.50. For intramuscular injection

Menopur® (Ferring) PoM
Injection, powder for reconstitution, menotrophin as follicle-stimulating hormone 75 units, luteinising hormone 75 units, net price per amp (with solvent) = £13.65. For intramuscular or subcutaneous injection

LUTROPIN ALFA

(Recombinant human luteinising hormone)

Indications: see notes above

Cautions: rule out infertility caused by hypothyroidism, adrenocortical deficiency, hyperprolactinaemia, tumours of the pituitary or hypothalamus

Contra-indications: ovarian enlargement or cyst (unless caused by polycystic ovarian disease); undiagnosed vaginal bleeding; tumours of hypothalamus and pituitary; ovarian, uterine or mammary carcinoma

Side-effects: nausea, vomiting, abdominal and pelvic pain; headache, somnolence; injection-site reactions; ovarian hyperstimulation syndrome, ovarian cyst, breast pain, ectopic pregnancy; thromboembolism, adnexal torsion, and haemoperitoneum

Dose: *by subcutaneous injection*, in conjunction with follicle-stimulating hormone, according to response

Luveris® (Serono) PoM
Injection, powder for reconstitution, lutropin alfa, net price 75-unit vial = £33.31 (with solvent)

Growth hormone

Growth hormone is used to treat deficiency of the hormone in children and in adults (see NICE guidance below). In children it is used in Prader-Willi syndrome, Turner's syndrome and in chronic renal insufficiency; growth hormone has also recently been licensed for use in short children considered small for gestational age at birth.

Growth hormone of human origin (HGH; somatotrophin) has been replaced by a growth hormone of human sequence, **somatropin**, produced using recombinant DNA technology.

NICE guidance (somatropin in children with growth failure). NICE has recommended (May 2002) treatment with somatropin for children with:

- proven growth-hormone deficiency;
- Turner's syndrome;
- Prader-Willi syndrome;
- chronic renal insufficiency before puberty.

Treatment should be initiated and monitored by a paediatrician with expertise in managing growth-hormone disorders; treatment can be continued under a shared-care protocol by a general practitioner.
Treatment should be discontinued if the response is poor (i.e. an increase in growth velocity of less than 50% from baseline) in the first year of therapy.
In children with chronic renal insufficiency, treatment should be stopped after renal transplantation and not restarted for at least a year

NICE guidance (somatropin for adults with growth hormone deficiency). NICE has recommended (August 2003) somatropin in adults **only** if the following 3 criteria are fulfilled:

- Severe growth hormone deficiency, established by an appropriate method,
- Impaired quality of life, measured by means of a specific questionnaire,
- Already receiving treatment for another pituitary hormone deficiency.

Somatropin treatment should be discontinued if the quality of life has not improved sufficiently by 9 months.
Severe growth hormone deficiency developing after linear growth is complete but before the age of 25 years should be treated with growth hormone; treatment should continue until adult peak bone mass has been achieved. Treatment for adult-onset growth hormone deficiency should be stopped only when the patient and the patient's physician consider it appropriate.
Treatment with somatropin should be initiated and managed by a physician with expertise in growth hormone disorders; maintenance treatment can be prescribed in the community under a shared-care protocol.

SOMATROPIN

(Synthetic Human Growth Hormone)

Indications: see under Dose

Cautions: diabetes mellitus (adjustment of antidiabetic therapy may be necessary), papilloedema (see under Side-effects), relative deficiencies of other pituitary hormones (notably hypothyroidism—manufacturers recommend periodic thyroid function tests but limited evidence of clinical value), history of malignant disease, disorders of the epiphysis of the hip (monitor for limping), resolved intracranial hypertension (monitor closely), initiation of treatment close to puberty not recommended in child born small for gestational age; Silver-Russell syndrome; rotate subcutaneous injection sites to prevent lipoatrophy; breast-feeding (Appendix 5); **interactions:** Appendix 1 (somatropin)

Contra-indications: evidence of tumour activity (complete antitumour therapy and ensure intracranial lesions inactive before starting); not to be used after renal transplantation or for growth promotion in children with closed epiphyses (or near closure in Prader-Willi syndrome); severe obesity or severe respiratory impairment in Prader-Willi syndrome; pregnancy (interrupt treatment if pregnancy occurs, Appendix 4)

Side-effects: headache, funduscopy for papilloedema recommended if severe or recurrent headache, visual problems, nausea and vomiting occur—if papilloedema confirmed consider benign intracranial hypertension (rare cases reported); fluid retention (peripheral oedema), arthralgia, myalgia, carpal tunnel syndrome, paraesthesia, antibody formation, hypothyroidism, insulin resistance, hyperglycaemia, hypoglycaemia, reactions at injection site; leukaemia in children with growth hormone deficiency also reported

Dose: Gonadal dysgenesis (Turner's syndrome), *by subcutaneous injection*, 45–50 micrograms/kg daily *or* 1.4 mg/m^2 daily

Deficiency of growth hormone in children, *by subcutaneous or intramuscular injection*, 23–39 micrograms/kg daily *or* 0.7–1 mg/m^2 daily

Growth disturbance in short children born small for gestational age, *by subcutaneous injection*, 35 micrograms/kg daily or 1 mg/m^2 daily

Prader-Willi syndrome, *by subcutaneous injection* in children with growth velocity greater than 1 cm/year, in combination with energy-restricted diet, 35 micrograms/kg daily *or* 1 mg/m^2 daily; max. 2.7 mg daily

Chronic renal insufficiency in children (renal function decreased to less than 50%), *by subcutaneous injection*, 45–50 micrograms/kg daily *or* 1.4 mg/m^2 daily (higher doses may be needed) adjusted if necessary after 6 months

Adult growth hormone deficiency, *by subcutaneous injection*, initially 150–300 micrograms daily, gradually increased if required to max. 1 mg daily; use minimum effective dose (requirements may decrease with age)

NOTE. Dose formerly expressed in units; somatropin 1 mg ≡ 3 units

Genotropin® (Pharmacia) PoM

Injection, two-compartment cartridge containing powder for reconstitution, somatropin (rbe) and diluent, net price 5.3-mg (16-unit) cartridge = £122.87, 12-mg (36-unit) cartridge = £278.20. For use with *Genotropin® Pen* NHS device (available free of charge from clinics). For subcutaneous injection

MiniQuick injection, two-compartment single-dose syringe containing powder for reconstitution, somatropin (rbe) and diluent, net price 0.2-mg (0.6-unit) syringe = £4.64; 0.4-mg (1.2-unit) syringe = £9.27; 0.6-mg (1.8-unit) syringe = £13.91; 0.8-mg (2.4-unit) syringe = £18.55; 1-mg (3-unit) syringe = £23.18; 1.2-mg (3.6-unit) syringe = £27.82; 1.4-mg (4.2-unit) syringe = £32.46; 1.6-mg (4.8-unit) syringe = £37.09; 1.8-mg (5.4-unit) syringe = £41.73; 2-mg (6-unit) syringe = £46.37. For subcutaneous injection

Humatrope® (Lilly) PoM

Injection, powder for reconstitution, somatropin (rbe), net price 6-mg (18-unit) cartridge = £137.25; 12-mg (36-unit) cartridge = £274.50; 24-mg (72-unit) cartridge = £549.00; all supplied with diluent. For subcutaneous or intramuscular injection; cartridges for subcutaneous injection

Norditropin® (Novo Nordisk) PoM

SimpleXx injection, somatropin (epr) 3.3 mg (10 units)/mL, net price 1.5-mL (5-mg, 15-unit) cartridge = £115.90; 6.7 mg (20 units)/mL, 1.5-mL (10-mg, 30-unit) cartridge = £231.80; 10 mg (30 units)/mL, 1.5-mL (15-mg, 45-unit) cartridge = £347.70. For use with appropriate *NordiPen*® NHS device (available free of charge from clinics). For subcutaneous injection

NutropinAq® (Ipsen) PoM

Injection, somatropin (rbe), net price 10 mg (30 units) 2-ml cartridge = £215.57. For use with *NutropinAq® Pen* NHS device (available free of charge from clinics). For subcutaneous injection

Saizen® (Serono) PoM

Injection, powder for reconstitution, somatropin (rmc), net price 1.33-mg (4-unit) vial (with diluent) = £29.28; 3.33-mg (10-unit) vial (with diluent) = £73.20. For subcutaneous or intramuscular injection

Click.easy®, powder for reconstitution, somatropin (rmc), net price 8-mg (24-unit) vial (in *Click.easy*® device with diluent) = £175.68. For use with *One.click*® NHS autoinjector device *or Cool.Click*® NHS needle-free device (both available free of charge from clinics). For subcutaneous injection

Zomacton® (Ferring) PoM

Injection, powder for reconstitution, somatropin (rbe), net price 4-mg (12-unit) vial (with diluent) = £81.32. For use with *ZomaJet® 2* NHS needle-free device or with *Auto-Jector*® NHS (both available free of charge from clinics) or with needles and syringes. For subcutaneous injection

Growth hormone receptor antagonists

Pegvisomant is a genetically modified analogue of human growth hormone and is highly selective growth hormone receptor antagonist. Pegvisomant is licensed for the treatment of acromegaly in patients with inadequate response to surgery, radiation, or both, and to treatment with somatostatin analogues. Pegvisomant should be initiated only by physicians experienced in the treatment of acromegaly.

PEGVISOMANT

Indications: see notes above

Cautions: liver disease (monitor liver enzymes every 4–6 weeks for 6 months or if symptoms of hepatitis develop); diabetes mellitus (adjustment of antidiabetic therapy may be necessary); possible increase in female fertility

Contra-indications: pregnancy and breast-feeding

Side-effects: diarrhoea, constipation, nausea, vomiting, abdominal distension, dyspepsia, flatulence, elevated liver enzymes; hypertension; headache, asthenia, dizziness, drowsiness, tremor, sleep disturbances; influenza-like syndrome, weight gain, hyperglycaemia, hypoglycaemia; arthralgia, myalgia; injection-site reactions, sweating, pruritus, rash; fatigue; hypercholesterolaemia; less commonly thrombocytopenia, leucopenia, leucocytosis, bleeding tendency

Dose: *by subcutaneous injection*, initially 80 mg, then 10 mg daily, increased in steps of 5 mg daily according to response; max. 30 mg daily; CHILD not recommended

Somavert® (Pfizer) ▼ PoM
Injection, powder for reconstitution, pegvisomant, net price 10-mg vial = £50.00; 15-mg vial = £75.00; 20-mg vial = £100.00 (all with solvent)

Thyrotrophin

Thyrotropin alfa is a recombinant form of thyrotrophin (thyroid stimulating hormone). It is licensed for use with or without radioiodine imaging, together with serum thyroglobulin testing, for the detection of thyroid remnants and thyroid cancer in post-thyroidectomy patients.

THYROTROPIN ALFA

(Recombinant human thyroid stimulating hormone, rhTSH)

Indications: detection of thyroid remnants and thyroid cancer in post-thyroidectomy patients

Cautions: presence of thyroglobulin autoantibodies may give false negative results

Contra-indications: pregnancy and breast-feeding; hypersensitivity to bovine or human thyrotrophin

Side-effects: nausea, vomiting; headache, dizziness, asthenia, paraesthesia; pain (including pain at site of metastases), chills, fever, influenza-like symptoms; injection site reactions include urticaria, pruritus and rash

Dose: *by intramuscular injection* into the gluteal muscle, 900 micrograms every 24 hours for 2 doses, consult product literature

Thyrogen® (Genzyme) PoM
Injection, powder for reconstitution, thyrotropin alfa 900 micrograms/vial, net price = £232.50

Hypothalamic hormones

Gonadorelin when injected intravenously in normal subjects leads to a rapid rise in plasma concentrations of both luteinising hormone (LH) and follicle-stimulating hormone (FSH). It has not proved to be very helpful, however, in distinguishing hypothalamic from pituitary lesions. **Gonadorelin analogues** are indicated in endometriosis and infertility (section 6.7.2) and in breast and prostate cancer (section 8.3.4).

Protirelin is a hypothalamic releasing hormone which stimulates the release of thyrotrophin from the pituitary. It is licensed for the diagnosis of mild hyperthyroidism or hypothyroidism, but its use has been superseded by immunoassays for thyroid-stimulating hormone.

Sermorelin, an analogue of growth hormone releasing hormone (somatorelin, GHRH), is licensed as a diagnostic test for secretion of growth hormone.

GONADORELIN

(Gonadotrophin-releasing hormone; GnRH; LH–RH)

Indications: see preparations below

Cautions: pituitary adenoma

Side-effects: rarely, nausea, headache, abdominal pain, increased menstrual bleeding; rarely, hypersensitivity reaction on repeated administration of large doses; irritation at injection site

Dose: see under preparations

HRF® (Intrapharm) PoM
Injection, powder for reconstitution, gonadorelin. Net price 100-microgram vial (with diluent) = £13.72 (hosp. only)
Excipients: include benzyl alcohol (avoid in neonates, see Excipients p. 2)
Dose: for assessment of pituitary function (adults), *by subcutaneous or intravenous injection*, 100 micrograms

PROTIRELIN

(Thyrotrophin-releasing hormone; TRH)

Indications: assessment of thyroid function and thyroid stimulating hormone reserve

Cautions: severe hypopituitarism, myocardial ischaemia, bronchial asthma and obstructive airways disease, pregnancy, breast-feeding (Appendix 5)

Side-effects: after rapid intravenous administration desire to micturate, flushing, dizziness, nausea, strange taste; transient increase in pulse rate and blood pressure; rarely bronchospasm

Dose: *by intravenous injection*, 200 micrograms; CHILD under 12 years 1 microgram/kg

Protirelin (Cambridge) PoM
Injection, protirelin 100 micrograms/mL. Net price 2-mL amp = £9.03

SERMORELIN

Indications: see notes above

Cautions: epilepsy; discontinue growth hormone therapy 1–2 weeks before test; untreated hypothyroidism, antithyroid drugs; obesity, hyperglycaemia, elevated plasma fatty acids; avoid preparations which affect release of growth hormone (includes those affecting release of somatostatin, insulin or glucocorticoids and cyclo-oxygenase inhibitors such as aspirin and indometacin)

Contra-indications: pregnancy and breast-feeding

Side-effects: occasional facial flushing and pain at injection site

Dose: *by intravenous injection*, 1 microgram/kg in the morning after an overnight fast

Geref 50® (Serono) PoM
Injection, powder for reconstitution, sermorelin 50 micrograms (as acetate). Net price per amp (with solvent) = £48.85

6.5.2 Posterior pituitary hormones and antagonists

Posterior pituitary hormones

DIABETES INSIPIDUS. **Vasopressin** (antidiuretic hormone, ADH) is used in the treatment of *pituitary* ('cranial') *diabetes insipidus* as is its analogue **desmopressin**. Dosage is tailored to produce a slight diuresis every 24 hours to avoid water intoxication. Treatment may be required for a limited period only in diabetes insipidus following trauma or pituitary surgery.

Desmopressin is more potent and has a longer duration of action than vasopressin; unlike vasopressin it has no vasoconstrictor effect. It is given by mouth or intranasally for maintenance therapy, and by injection in the postoperative period or in unconscious patients. Desmopressin is also used in the differential diagnosis of diabetes insipidus. Following a dose of 2 micrograms intramuscularly or 20 micrograms intranasally, restoration of the ability to concentrate urine after water deprivation confirms a diagnosis of cranial diabetes insipidus. Failure to respond occurs in nephrogenic diabetes insipidus.

In *nephrogenic* and *partial pituitary diabetes insipidus* benefit may be gained from the paradoxical antidiuretic effect of thiazides (section 2.2.1) e.g. chlortalidone 100 mg twice daily reduced to maintenance dose of 50 mg daily.

Chlorpropamide (section 6.1.2.1) is also useful in partial pituitary diabetes insipidus, and probably acts by sensitising the renal tubules to the action of remaining endogenous vasopressin; it is given in doses of up to 350 mg daily in adults and 200 mg daily in children, care being taken to avoid hypoglycaemia. Carbamazepine (section 4.8.1) is also sometimes useful (in a dose of 200 mg once or twice daily) [unlicensed]; its mode of action may be similar to that of chlorpropamide.

OTHER USES. Desmopressin injection is also used to boost factor VIII concentrations in mild to moderate haemophilia. For a comment on use of desmopressin in nocturnal enuresis see section 7.4.2.

Vasopressin infusion is used to control variceal bleeding in portal hypertension, prior to more definitive treatment and with variable results. Terlipressin, a derivative of vasopressin, is used similarly.

Oxytocin, another posterior pituitary hormone, is indicated in obstetrics (section 7.1.1).

VASOPRESSIN

Indications: pituitary diabetes insipidus; bleeding from oesophageal varices

Cautions: heart failure, hypertension, asthma, epilepsy, migraine or other conditions which might be aggravated by water retention; renal impairment (see also Contra-indications); pregnancy (Appendix 4); avoid fluid overload

Contra-indications: vascular disease (especially disease of coronary arteries) unless extreme caution, chronic nephritis (until reasonable blood nitrogen concentrations attained)

Side-effects: fluid retention, pallor, tremor, sweating, vertigo, headache, nausea, vomiting, belching, abdominal cramps, desire to defaecate, hypersensitivity reactions (including anaphylaxis), constriction of coronary arteries (may cause anginal attacks and myocardial ischaemia), peripheral ischaemia and rarely gangrene

Dose: *by subcutaneous or intramuscular injection*, diabetes insipidus, 5–20 units every four hours

By intravenous infusion, initial control of variceal bleeding, 20 units over 15 minutes

■ Synthetic vasopressin

Pitressin® (Goldshield) PoM

Injection, argipressin (synthetic vasopressin) 20 units/mL. Net price 1-mL amp = £17.14 (hosp. only)

DESMOPRESSIN

Indications: see under Dose

Cautions: see under Vasopressin; less pressor activity, but still considerable caution in renal impairment (Appendix 3), in cardiovascular disease and in hypertension (not indicated for nocturnal enuresis or nocturia in these circumstances); elderly (avoid for nocturnal enuresis and nocturia in those over 65 years); also considerable caution in cystic fibrosis; in nocturia and nocturnal enuresis limit fluid intake to minimum from 1 hour before dose until 8 hours afterwards; in nocturia periodic blood pressure and weight checks needed to monitor for fluid overload; pregnancy (Appendix 4) **interactions:** Appendix 1 (desmopressin)

HYPONATRAEMIC CONVULSIONS. The CSM has advised that patients being treated for primary nocturnal enuresis should be warned to avoid fluid overload (including during swimming) and to stop taking desmopressin during an episode of vomiting or diarrhoea (until fluid balance normal). The risk of hyponatraemic convulsions can also be minimised by keeping to the recommended starting doses and by avoiding concomitant use of drugs which increase secretion of vasopressin (e.g. tricyclic antidepressants)

Contra-indications: cardiac insufficiency and other conditions treated with diuretics; psychogenic polydipsia and polydipsia in alcohol dependence

Side-effects: fluid retention, and hyponatraemia (in more serious cases with convulsions) on administration without restricting fluid intake; stomach pain, headache, nausea, vomiting, allergic reactions, and emotional disturbance in children also reported; epistaxis, nasal congestion, rhinitis with nasal spray

Dose: *by mouth*

Diabetes insipidus, treatment, ADULT and CHILD initially 300 micrograms daily (in 3 divided doses); maintenance, 300–600 micrograms daily in 3 divided doses; range 0.2–1.2 mg daily

Primary nocturnal enuresis (if urine concentrating ability normal), ADULT (under 65 years) and CHILD over 5 years (preferably over 7 years) 200 micrograms at bedtime, only increased to 400 micrograms if lower dose not effective (**important:** see also Cautions); withdraw for at least 1 week for reassessment after 3 months

Postoperative polyuria or polydipsia, adjust dose according to urine osmolality

Intranasally

Diabetes insipidus, diagnosis, ADULT and CHILD 20 micrograms (limit fluid intake to 500 mL from 1 hour before to 8 hours after administration)

Diabetes insipidus, treatment, ADULT 10–40 micrograms daily (in 1–2 divided doses); CHILD 5–20 micrograms daily; infants may require lower doses

Primary nocturnal enuresis (if urine concentrating ability normal), ADULT (under 65 years) and CHILD over 5 years (preferably over 7 years) initially 20 micrograms at bedtime, only increased to 40 micrograms if lower dose not effective (**impor-**

tant: see also Cautions); withdraw for at least 1 week for reassessment after 3 months
Nocturia associated with multiple sclerosis (when other treatments have failed), ADULT (under 65 years) 10–20 micrograms at bedtime (**important:** see also Cautions), dose not to be repeated within 24 hours
Renal function testing (empty bladder at time of administration and limit fluid intake to 500 mL from 1 hour before until 8 hours after administration), ADULT 40 micrograms; INFANT under 1 year 10 micrograms (restrict fluid intake to 50% at next 2 feeds to avoid fluid overload), CHILD 1–15 years 20 micrograms

By injection
Diabetes insipidus, diagnosis (*subcutaneous or intramuscular*), ADULT and CHILD 2 micrograms (limit fluid intake to 500 mL from 1 hour before to 8 hours after administration)
Diabetes insipidus, treatment (*subcutaneous, intramuscular or intravenous*), ADULT 1–4 micrograms daily; INFANT and CHILD 400 nanograms
Renal function testing (empty bladder at time of administration and limit fluid intake to 500 mL from 1 hour before until 8 hours after administration) (*subcutaneous or intramuscular*), ADULT and CHILD 2 micrograms; INFANT 400 nanograms (restrict fluid intake to 50% at next 2 feeds)
Mild to moderate haemophilia and von Willebrand's disease, post lumbar puncture headache, fibrinolytic response testing, consult product literature

Desmopressin acetate (Non-proprietary) PoM
Nasal spray, desmopressin acetate 10 micrograms/metered spray, net price 6-mL unit (60 metered sprays) = £26.04. Counselling, fluid intake, see above
Brands include *Presinex*®
NOTE. Children requiring dose of less than 10 micrograms should be given *DDAVP*® intranasal solution

DDAVP® (Ferring) PoM
Tablets, both scored, desmopressin acetate 100 micrograms, net price 90-tab pack = £45.48; 200 micrograms, 90-tab pack = £90.96. Counselling, fluid intake, see above
Intranasal solution, desmopressin acetate 100 micrograms/mL. Net price 2.5-mL dropper bottle and catheter = £9.72. Counselling, fluid intake, see above
Injection, desmopressin acetate 4 micrograms/mL. Net price 1-mL amp = £1.10

Desmotabs® (Ferring) PoM
Tablets, scored, desmopressin acetate 200 micrograms, net price 30-tab pack = £30.34. Counselling, fluid intake, see above

Desmospray® (Ferring) PoM
Nasal spray, desmopressin acetate 10 micrograms/metered spray. Net price 6-mL unit (60 metered sprays) = £26.04. Counselling, fluid intake, see above
NOTE. Children requiring dose of less than 10 micrograms should be given *DDAVP*® *intranasal solution*

Nocutil® (Norgine) PoM
Nasal spray, desmopressin acetate 10 micrograms/metered spray, net price 5-mL unit (50 metered sprays) = £19.69. Counselling, fluid intake, see above

TERLIPRESSIN

Indications: bleeding from oesophageal varices
Cautions: see under Vasopressin
Contra-indications: see under Vasopressin
Side-effects: see under Vasopressin, but effects milder
Dose: *by intravenous injection*, 2 mg followed by 1 or 2 mg every 4 to 6 hours until bleeding is controlled, for up to 72 hours

Glypressin® (Ferring) PoM
Injection, terlipressin, powder for reconstitution. Net price 1-mg vial with 5 mL diluent = £19.44 (hosp. only)

Antidiuretic hormone antagonists

Demeclocycline (section 5.1.3) may be used in the treatment of hyponatraemia resulting from inappropriate secretion of antidiuretic hormone. It is thought to act by directly blocking the renal tubular effect of antidiuretic hormone. Initially 0.9 to 1.2 g is given daily in divided doses, reduced to 600–900 mg daily for maintenance.

6.6 Drugs affecting bone metabolism

See also calcium (section 9.5.1.1), phosphorus (section 9.5.2), vitamin D (section 9.6.4), and oestrogens in postmenopausal osteoporosis (section 6.4.1.1).

Osteoporosis

Osteoporosis occurs most commonly in postmenopausal women and in those taking long-term oral corticosteroids (glucocorticosteroids). Other risk factors for osteoporosis include low body weight, cigarette smoking, excess alcohol intake, lack of physical activity, family history of osteoporosis, and early menopause.

> Those at risk of osteoporosis should maintain an adequate intake of **calcium and vitamin D** and any deficiency should be corrected by increasing dietary intake or taking supplements.

Elderly patients, especially those who are housebound or live in residential or nursing homes, are at increased risk of calcium and vitamin D deficiency and may benefit from supplements (section 9.5.1.1 and section 9.6.4). Reversible secondary causes of osteoporosis such as hyperthyroidism, hyperparathyroidism, osteomalacia or hypogonadism should be excluded, in both men and women, before treatment for osteoporosis is initiated.

POSTMENOPAUSAL OSTEOPOROSIS. The **bisphosphonates** (alendronic acid, disodium etidronate, and risedronate, section 6.6.2) are effective for preventing postmenopausal osteoporosis. **Hormone replacement therapy** (HRT section 6.4.1.1) is an option where other therapies are contra-indicated, cannot be tolerated, or if there is a lack of response. The CSM has advised that HRT should **not** be considered first-line therapy for long-term prevention of osteoporosis in women over 50 years of age. HRT is of most benefit for the prophylaxis of postmenopausal osteoporosis if started early in menopause and continued for up to 5 years, but bone loss resumes (possibly at an accelerated rate) on stopping HRT. **Calcitonin** (section 6.6.1) may be considered for those at high risk of osteoporosis for whom a bisphosphonate is unsuitable. Women of Afro-Caribbean origin appear to be less susceptible to osteoporosis than those who are white or of Asian origin.

Postmenopausal osteoporosis may be *treated* with a **bisphosphonate** (section 6.6.2). The bisphosphonates (such as alendronate, etidronate, and risedronate) decrease the risk of vertebral fracture; alendronate and risedronate have also been shown to reduce non-vertebral fractures. If bisphosphonates are unsuitable **calcitriol** (section 9.6.4), **calcitonin** or **strontium ranelate** (section 6.6.2) may be considered. Calcitonin [unlicensed indication] may also be useful for pain relief for up to 3 months after a vertebral fracture if other analgesics are ineffective. **Teriparatide** (section 6.6.1) has been introduced for the treatment of postmenopausal oestoporosis.

Raloxifene (section 6.4.1.1) is licensed for the *prophylaxis* and *treatment* of vertebral fractures in postmenopausal women.

> **NICE guidance (bisphosphonates, selective oestrogen receptor modulators and parathyroid hormone for secondary prevention of osteoporotic fragility fractures in postmenopausal women).** NICE has recommended (January 2005) **bisphosphonates** as treatment options for the secondary prevention of osteoporotic fractures in susceptible postmenopausal women. In women who cannot take a bisphosphonate or who have suffered a fragility fracture despite treatment for a year and whose bone mineral density continues to decline, the selective oestrogen receptor modulator **raloxifene** is an alternative. The parathyroid hormone fragment **teriparatide** is recommended for women over 65 years who cannot take a bisphosphonate (or in whom bisphosphonate has failed to prevent a fracture) and have:
>
> - either an extremely low bone mineral density
> - or a very low bone mineral density, suffered more than 2 fractures, and have other risk factors for fractures (e.g. body mass index under 19 kg/m^2, premature menopause, prolonged immobility, history of maternal hip fracture under the age of 75 years).

CORTICOSTEROID-INDUCED OSTEOPOROSIS. To reduce the risk of osteoporosis doses of oral corticosteroids should be as low as possible and courses of treatment as short as possible. The risk of osteoporosis may be related to cumulative dose of corticosteroids; even intermittent courses can therefore increase the risk. The greatest rate of bone loss occurs during the first 6–12 months of corticosteroid use and so early steps to prevent the development of osteoporosis are important. Long-term use of high-dose inhaled corticosteroids may also contribute to corticosteroid-induced osteoporosis(section 3.2).

Patients taking (or who are likely to take) the equivalent of prednisolone 7.5 mg or more each day for 3 months or longer should be assessed and where necessary given prophylactic treatment; those aged over 65 years are at greater risk. Patients taking oral corticosteroids who have sustained a low-trauma fracture should receive treatment for osteoporosis. The therapeutic options for *prophylaxis* and *treatment* of corticosteroid-induced osteoporosis are the same:

- a bisphosphonate such as alendronate, etidronate or risedronate;
- calcitriol.
- hormone replacement (HRT in women, (section 6.4.1) testosterone in men (section 6.4.2))

6.6.1 Calcitonin and teriparatide

Calcitonin is involved with parathyroid hormone in the regulation of bone turnover and hence in the maintenance of calcium balance and homoeostasis. **Calcitonin (salmon) (salcatonin**, synthetic or recombinant salmon calcitonin) is used to lower the plasma-calcium concentration in some patients with hypercalcaemia (notably when associated with malignant disease). Calcitonin is licensed for treatment of Paget's disease of bone. It can also be used in the prevention and treatment of postmenopausal osteoporosis (see section 6.6).

Teriparatide, a recombinant, fragment of parathyroid hormone, has been introduced for the treatment of postmenopausal osteoporosis. *The Scottish Medicines Consortium* has advised (December 2003) that teriparatide should be initiated by specialists experienced in the treatment of osteoporosis.

Cinacalcet (section 9.5.1.2) is licensed for the treatment of hypercalcaemia in parathyroid carcinoma.

CALCITONIN (SALMON)/ SALCATONIN

Indications: see under Dose

Cautions: history of allergy (skin test advised); renal impairment; heart failure; pregnancy (Appendix 4), breast-feeding (Appendix 5)

Contra-indications: hypocalcaemia

Side-effects: nausea, vomiting, diarrhoea, abdominal pain; flushing; dizziness, headache, taste disturbances; musculoskeletal pain; with nasal spray nose and throat irritation, rhinitis, sinusitis and epistaxis; *less commonly* diuresis, oedema, cough, visual disturbances, injection-site reactions, rash, hypersensitivity reactions including pruritus

Dose: hypercalcaemia of malignancy (see also section 9.5.1.2), ADULT over 18 years, *by subcutaneous or intramuscular injection*, 100 units every 6–8 hours adjusted according to response; max. 400 units every 6–8 hours; in severe or emergency cases, *by intravenous infusion*, up to 10 units/kg over at least 6 hours

Paget's disease of bone, ADULT over 18 years, *by subcutaneous or intramuscular injection*, 50 units 3 times weekly to 100 units daily adjusted according to response

Postmenopausal osteoporosis to reduce risk of vertebral fractures, *intranasally*, 200 units (1 spray) into one nostril daily, with dietary calcium and vitamin D supplements (section 9.5.1.1 and section 9.6.4)

Prevention of acute bone loss due to sudden immobility, ADULT over 18 years, *by subcutaneous or intramuscular injection*, 100 units daily in 1–2 divided doses for 2–4 weeks, reduced to 50 units daily at start of mobilisation and continued until fully mobile

Miacalcic® (Novartis) PoM
Nasal spray▼, calcitonin (salmon) 200 units/metered spray, net price 2-mL unit (approx. 14 metered sprays) = £20.99
Injection, calcitonin (salmon) 50 units/mL, net price 1-mL amp = £4.27; 100 units/mL, 1-mL amp = £8.55; 200 units/mL, 2-mL vial = £30.75
For subcutaneous or intramuscular injection and for dilution and use as an intravenous infusion

TERIPARATIDE

Indications: treatment of postmenopausal osteoporosis (initiated by specialist—see notes above)
Cautions: moderate renal impairment (avoid if severe)
Contra-indications: pre-existing hypercalcaemia, metabolic bone diseases, including Paget's disease and hyperparathyroidism, unexplained raised levels of alkaline phosphatase, previous radiation therapy to the skeleton, pregnancy and breast-feeding
Side-effects: gastro-intestinal disorders (including nausea, reflux and haemorrhoids); postural hypotension; dysponea; depression, dizziness, vertigo; urinary disorders, polyuria; muscle cramps, sciatica; increased sweating; injection-site reactions
Dose: *by subcutaneous injection*, 20 micrograms daily; max. duration of treatment 18 months

Forsteo® (Lilly) ▼ PoM
Injection, teriparatide 250 micrograms/mL, net price 3-mL prefilled pen = £271.88
NOTE. 3-ml prefilled pen intended for 28 doses

6.6.2 Bisphosphonates and other drugs affecting bone metabolism

Bisphosphonates are adsorbed onto hydroxyapatite crystals in bone, slowing both their rate of growth and dissolution, and therefore reducing the rate of bone turnover. Bisphosphonates have an important role in the prophylaxis and treatment of osteoporosis and corticosteroid-induced osteoporosis; **alendronic acid** or **risedronate sodium** are considered the drugs of choice for these conditions, but **disodium etidronate** may be considered if these drugs are unsuitable or not tolerated (see also section 6.6).

Bisphosphonates are also used in the treatment of *Paget's disease*, hypercalcaemia of malignancy (section 9.5.1.2). and in bone metastases in breast cancer (section 8.3.4.1). Disodium etidronate can impair bone mineralisation when used continuously or in high doses (such as in the treatment of *Paget's disease*).

Strontium ranelate stimulates bone formation and reduces bone resorption. It is licensed for the treatment of postmenopausal osteoporosis.

ALENDRONIC ACID

Indications: see under Dose
Cautions: upper gastro-intestinal disorders (dysphagia, symptomatic oesophageal disease, gastritis, duodenitis, or ulcers—see also under Contra-indications and Side-effects); history (within 1 year) of ulcers, active gastro-intestinal bleeding, or surgery of the upper gastro-intestinal tract; renal impairment (manufacturer advises avoid if creatinine clearance is less than 35 mL/minute); correct disturbances of calcium and mineral metabolism (e.g. vitamin-D deficiency, hypocalcaemia) before starting and monitor serum calcium during treatment; exclude other causes of osteoporosis; **interactions:** Appendix 1 (bisphosphonates)
Contra-indications: abnormalities of oesophagus and other factors which delay emptying (e.g. stricture or achalasia), hypocalcaemia, pregnancy (Appendix 4) and breast-feeding (Appendix 5)
Side-effects: oesophageal reactions (see below), abdominal pain and distension, dyspepsia, regurgitation, melaena, diarrhoea or constipation, flatulence, musculoskeletal pain, headache; *rarely* rash, pruritus, erythema, photosensitivity, uveitis, scleritis, transient decrease in serum calcium and phosphate; nausea, vomiting, gastritis, peptic ulceration, and hypersensitivity reactions (including urticaria and angioedema) also reported; myalgia, malaise and fever at initiation of treatment; *very rarely* severe skin reactions (including Stevens-Johnson syndrome)
OESOPHAGEAL REACTIONS. Severe oesophageal reactions (oesophagitis, oesophageal ulcers, oesophageal stricture and oesophageal erosions) have been reported; patients should be advised to stop taking the tablets and to seek medical attention if they develop symptoms of oesophageal irritation such as dysphagia, new or worsening heartburn, pain on swallowing or retrosternal pain
Dose: treatment of postmenopausal osteoporosis and osteoporosis in men, 10 mg daily *or* (in postmenopausal osteoporosis) 70 mg once weekly
Prevention of postmenopausal osteoporosis, 5 mg daily
Prevention and treatment of corticosteroid-induced osteoporosis, 5 mg daily (postmenopausal women not receiving hormone replacement therapy, 10 mg daily)
COUNSELLING. Tablets should be swallowed whole with plenty of water while sitting or standing; to be taken on an empty stomach at least 30 minutes before breakfast (or another oral medicine); patient should stand or sit upright for at least 30 minutes after taking tablet

Fosamax® (MSD) PoM
Tablets, alendronic acid (as sodium alendronate) 5 mg, net price 28-tab pack = £25.43; 10 mg, 28-tab pack = £23.12. Counselling, administration

Fosamax® **Once Weekly** (MSD) PoM
Tablets, alendronic acid (as sodium alendronate) 70 mg, net price 4-tab pack = £22.80. Counselling, administration

DISODIUM ETIDRONATE

Indications: see under Dose
Cautions: renal impairment (Appendix 3); **interactions:** Appendix 1 (bisphosphonates)
Contra-indications: moderate to severe renal impairment; pregnancy (Appendix 4) and breast-feeding (Appendix 5); not indicated for osteo-

porosis in presence of hypercalcaemia or hypercalciuria or for osteomalacia

Side-effects: nausea, diarrhoea or constipation, abdominal pain; increased bone pain in Paget's disease, also increased risk of fractures with high doses in Paget's disease (discontinue if fractures occur); rarely exacerbation of asthma, skin reactions (including angioedema, rash, urticaria and pruritus), transient hyperphosphataemia, headache, paraesthesia, peripheral neuropathy reported; blood disorders (including leucopenia, agranulocytosis and pancytopenia) also reported

Dose: Paget's disease of bone, *by mouth*, 5 mg/kg as a single daily dose for up to 6 months; doses above 10 mg/kg daily for up to 3 months may be used with caution but doses above 20 mg/kg daily are not recommended; after interval of not less than 3 months may be repeated where evidence of reactivation—including biochemical indices (avoid premature retreatment)

MONITORING. Serum phosphate, serum alkaline phosphatase and (if possible) urinary hydroxyproline should be measured before starting and at intervals of 3 months—consult product literature for further details

Osteoporosis, see under *Didronel PMO*®

COUNSELLING. Avoid food for at least 2 hours before and after oral treatment, particularly calcium-containing products e.g.milk; also avoid iron and mineral supplements and antacids

Didronel® (Procter & Gamble Pharm.) PoM
Tablets, disodium etidronate 200 mg. Net price 60-tab pack = £34.69. Counselling, food and calcium (see above)

■ With calcium carbonate

For cautions and side-effects of calcium carbonate see section 9.5.1.1

Didronel PMO® (Procter & Gamble Pharm.) PoM
Tablets, 14 white, disodium etidronate 400 mg; 76 pink, effervescent, calcium carbonate 1.25 g (*Cacit*®). Net price per pack = £37.39. Label: 10, patient information leaflet, counselling, food and calcium (see above)

Dose: treatment of osteoporosis, prevention of bone loss in postmenopausal women (particularly if hormone replacement therapy inappropriate), and prevention and treatment of corticosteroid-induced osteoporosis, given in 90-day cycles, 1 *Didronel*® tablet daily for 14 days, then 1 *Cacit*® tablet daily for 76 days

DISODIUM PAMIDRONATE

Disodium pamidronate was formerly called aminohydroxypropylidenediphosphonate disodium (APD)

Indications: see under Dose

Cautions: renal impairment (Appendix 3); assess renal function before each dose; hepatic impairment (Appendix 2); cardiac disease (especially in elderly); previous thyroid surgery (risk of hypocalcaemia); monitor serum electrolytes, calcium and phosphate—possibility of convulsions due to electrolyte changes; avoid concurrent use with other bisphosphonates; **interactions:** Appendix 1 (bisphosphonates)

OSTEONECROSIS OF THE JAW. Osteonecrosis of the jaw reported in cancer patients being treated with bisphosphonate; consider dental examination and preventative treatment before initiating bisphosphonate; avoid invasive dental procedures during treatment

DRIVING. Patients should be warned against driving or operating machinery immediately after treatment (somnolence or dizziness may occur)

Contra-indications: pregnancy (Appendix 4) and breast-feeding (Appendix 5)

Side-effects: hypophosphataemia, fever and influenza-like symptoms (sometimes accompanied by malaise, rigors, fatigue and flushes); nausea, vomiting, anorexia, abdominal pain, diarrhoea, constipation; symptomatic hypocalcaemia (paraesthesia, tetany), hypomagnesaemia, headache, insomnia, drowsiness; hypertension; anaemia, thrombocytopenia, lymphocytopenia; rash; arthralgia, myalgia; rarely muscle cramps, dyspepsia, agitation, confusion, dizziness, lethargy; leucopenia, hypotension, pruritus, hyperkalaemia or hypokalaemia, and hypernatraemia; osteonecrosis (see also Cautions above), isolated cases of seizures, hallucinations, haematuria, acute renal failure, deterioration of renal disease, conjunctivitis and other ocular symptoms; reactivation of herpes simplex and zoster also reported; also injection-site reactions

Dose: *by slow intravenous infusion* (via cannula in a relatively large vein), see also Appendix 6

Hypercalcaemia of malignancy, according to serum calcium concentration 15–60 mg in single infusion or in divided doses over 2–4 days; max. 90 mg per treatment course

Osteolytic lesions and bone pain in bone metastases associated with breast cancer or multiple myeloma, 90 mg every 4 weeks (or every 3 weeks to coincide with chemotherapy in breast cancer)

Paget's disease of bone, 30 mg once a week for 6 weeks (total dose 180 mg) *or* 30 mg in first week then 60 mg every other week (total dose 210 mg); max. total 360 mg (in divided doses of 60 mg) per treatment course; may be repeated every 6 months

CHILD not recommended

CALCIUM AND VITAMIN D SUPPLEMENTS. Oral supplements are advised for those with Paget's disease at risk of calcium or vitamin D deficiency (e.g. through malabsorption or lack of exposure to sunlight) to minimise potential risk of hypocalcaemia

Disodium pamidronate (Non-proprietary) PoM
Concentrate for intravenous infusion, disodium pamidronate 3 mg/mL, net price 5-mL vial = £27.50, 10-mL vial = £55.00; 6 mg/mL, 10-mL vial = £110.00; 9 mg/mL, 10-mL vial = £165.00

Aredia Dry Powder® (Novartis) PoM
Injection, powder for reconstitution, disodium pamidronate, for use as an infusion. Net price 15-mg vial = £29.83; 30-mg vial = £59.66; 90-mg vial = £170.45 (all with diluent)

IBANDRONIC ACID

Indications: see under Dose

Cautions: hepatic impairment (Appendix 2); renal impairment (Appendix 3); monitor renal function and serum calcium, phosphate and magnesium; cardiac disease (avoid fluid overload); breast-feeding (Appendix 5); **interactions:** Appendix 1 (bisphosphonates)

Contra-indications: pregnancy (Appendix 4)

Side-effects: hypocalcaemia, hypophosphataemia, influenza-like symptoms (including fever, chills, and muscle pain), bone pain; oesophageal reactions (see below), diarrhoea, nausea, vomiting, abdominal pain, dyspepsia, pharyngitis; headache, asthenia; rarely anaemia, hypersensitivity reactions (pruritus, bronchospasm and angioedema reported)

OESOPHAGEAL REACTIONS. Severe oesophageal reactions reported with all **oral** bisphosphonates; patients should be advised to stop tablets and seek medical attention for symptoms of oesophageal irritation such as dysphagia, pain on swallowing, retrosternal pain, or heartburn

Dose: reduction of bone damage in bone metastases in breast cancer, *by mouth*, 50 mg daily, *or by intravenous infusion*, 6 mg every 3–4 weeks

Hypercalcaemia of malignancy *by intravenous infusion*, according to serum calcium concentration, 2–4 mg in single infusion

CHILD not recommended

COUNSELLING. Tablets should be swallowed whole with plenty of water while sitting or standing; to be taken on an empty stomach at least 30 minutes before breakfast (or another oral medicine); patient should stand or sit upright for at least 1 hour after taking tablet

Bondronat® (Roche) ▼ PoM

Tablets, f/c, ibandronic acid 50 mg, net price 28-tab pack = £195.00. Counselling, administration

Concentrate for intravenous infusion, ibandronic acid 1 mg/mL, net price 2-mL amp = £94.86, 6-mL vial = £195.00

RISEDRONATE SODIUM

Indications: see under Dose

Cautions: oesophageal abnormalities and other factors which delay transit or emptying (e.g. stricture or achalasia—see also under Side-effects); renal impairment (Appendix 3); correct hypocalcaemia before starting, correct other disturbances of bone and mineral metabolism (e.g. vitamin-D deficiency) at onset of treatment; **interactions:** Appendix 1 (bisphosphonates)

Contra-indications: hypocalcaemia (see Cautions above), pregnancy (Appendix 4) and breast-feeding (Appendix 5)

Side-effects: gastro-intestinal disturbances (including abdominal pain, dyspepsia, nausea, diarrhoea, constipation); dizziness, headache; influenza-like symptoms, musculoskeletal pain; *rarely* oesophageal stricture, oesophagitis, oesphageal ulcer, dysphagia, gastritis, duodenitis, glossitis, peripheral oedema, weight loss, myasthenia, arthralgia, apnoea, bronchitis, sinusitis, rash, nocturia, ambylopia, corneal lesion, dry eye, tinnitus, iritis; *very rarely* hypersensitivity reactions including angioedema

Dose: Paget's disease of bone, 30 mg daily for 2 months; may be repeated if necessary after at least 2 months

Treatment of postmenopausal osteoporosis to reduce risk of vertebral or hip fractures, 5 mg daily *or* 35 mg once weekly

Prevention of osteoporosis (including corticosteroid-induced osteoporosis) in postmenopausal women, 5 mg daily

CHILD not recommended

COUNSELLING. Swallow tablets whole with full glass of water; on rising, take on an empty stomach at least 30 minutes before first food or drink of the day **or**, if taking at any other time of the day, avoid food and drink for at least 2 hours before or after risedronate (particularly avoid calcium-containing products e.g. milk, also avoid iron and mineral supplements and antacids); stand or sit upright for at least 30 minutes; do not take tablets at bedtime or before rising

Actonel® (Procter & Gamble Pharm.) PoM

Tablets, f/c, risedronate sodium 5 mg (yellow), net price 28-tab pack = £19.10; 30 mg (white), 28-tab pack = £152.81. Counselling, administration, food and calcium (see above)

Actonel Once a Week® (Procter & Gamble Pharm.) PoM

Tablets, f/c, risedronate sodium 35 mg (orange), net price 4-tab pack = £20.30. Counselling, administration, food and calcium (see above)

SODIUM CLODRONATE

Indications: see under Dose

Cautions: monitor renal and hepatic function and white cell count; also monitor serum calcium and phosphate periodically; renal dysfunction reported in patients receiving concomitant NSAIDs; maintain adequate fluid intake during treatment; **interactions:** Appendix 1 (bisphosphonates)

Contra-indications: moderate to severe renal impairment; pregnancy (Appendix 4) and breast-feeding (Appendix 5)

Side-effects: nausea, diarrhoea; skin reactions

Dose: osteolytic lesions, hypercalcaemia and bone pain associated with skeletal metastases in patients with breast cancer or multiple myeloma, *by mouth*, 1.6 g daily in single or 2 divided doses increased if necessary to a max. of 3.2 g daily

COUNSELLING. Avoid food for 1 hour before and after treatment, particularly calcium-containing products e.g. milk; also avoid iron and mineral supplements and antacids; maintain adequate fluid intake

Hypercalcaemia of malignancy, *by slow intravenous infusion*, 300 mg daily for max. 7–10 days *or* by single-dose infusion of 1.5 g

Bonefos® (Boehringer Ingelheim) PoM

Capsules, yellow, sodium clodronate 400 mg. Net price 30-cap pack = £34.83, 120-cap pack = £139.33. Counselling, food and calcium

Tablets, f/c, scored, sodium clodronate 800 mg. Net price 10-tab pack = £24.32; 60-tab pack = £145.91. Counselling, food and calcium

Concentrate (= intravenous solution), sodium clodronate 60 mg/mL, for dilution and use as infusion. Net price 5-mL amp = £11.02

Loron® (Roche) PoM

Loron 520® *tablets*, f/c, scored, sodium clodronate 520 mg. Net price 60-tab pack = £161.99.

Label: 10, patient information leaflet, counselling, food and calcium

Dose: 2 tablets daily in single or two divided doses; may be increased to max. 4 tablets daily

STRONTIUM RANELATE

Indications: treatment of postmenopausal osteoporosis to reduce risk of vertebral and hip fractures

Cautions: predisposition to thromboembolism; interferes with colorimetric measurements of calcium in blood and urine; renal impairment (Appendix 3); **interactions**: Appendix 1 (strontium ranelate)

Contra-indications: pregnancy, breast-feeding

Side-effects: nausea, diarrhoea; venous thromboembolism; headache; dermatitis, eczema

Dose: 2 g once daily in water, preferably at bedtime

COUNSELLING. Avoid food for 2 hours before and after taking granules, particularly calcium-containing products e.g. milk; also preferably avoid concomitant antacids containing aluminium and magnesium hydroxides for 2 hours after taking granules

Protelos® (Servier) ▼ PoM
Granules, yellow, strontium ranelate, 2 g/sachet, net price 28-sachets = £25.60. Label: 5, 13, counselling, food and calcium
Excipients: include aspartame (section 9.4.1)

TILUDRONIC ACID

Indications: Paget's disease of bone
Cautions: renal impairment (monitor renal function regularly, see under Contra-indications); correct disturbances of calcium metabolism (e.g. vitamin D deficiency, hypocalcaemia) before starting; avoid concomitant use of indometacin; **interactions:** Appendix 1 (bisphosphonates)
Contra-indications: severe renal impairment, juvenile Paget's disease, pregnancy (Appendix 4) and breast-feeding (Appendix 5)
Side-effects: stomach pain, nausea, diarrhoea; rarely asthenia, dizziness, headache and skin reactions
Dose: 400 mg daily as a single dose for 12 weeks; may be repeated if necessary after 6 months
COUNSELLING. Avoid food for 2 hours before and after treatment, particularly calcium-containing products e.g. milk; also avoid antacids

Skelid® (Sanofi-Synthelabo) PoM
Tablets, tiludronic acid (as tiludronate disodium) 200 mg. Net price 28-tab pack = £99.00. Counselling, food and calcium

ZOLEDRONIC ACID

Indications: see under Dose
Cautions: monitor serum electrolytes, calcium, phosphate and magnesium; assess renal function before each dose; ensure adequate hydration; renal impairment (Appendix 3); severe hepatic impairment (Appendix 2); cardiac disease (avoid fluid overload); **interactions:** Appendix 1 (bisphosphonates)
OSTEONECROSIS OF THE JAW. Osteonecrosis of the jaw reported in cancer patients being treated with bisphosphonate; consider dental examination and preventative treatment before initiating bisphosphonate; avoid invasive dental procedures during treatment
Contra-indications: pregnancy (Appendix 4), breast-feeding (Appendix 5)
Side-effects: hypophosphataemia, anaemia, influenza-like symptoms including bone pain, myalgia, arthralgia, fever and rigors; gastro-intestinal disturbances; headache, conjunctivitis, renal impairment (rarely acute renal failure); *less commonly* taste disturbance, dry mouth, stomatitis, chest pain, hypertension, dyspnoea, cough, dizziness, paraesthesia, tremor, anxiety, sleep disturbance, blurred vision, weight gain, pruritus, rash, sweating, muscle cramps, haematuria, proteinuria, hypersensitivity reactions (including angioedema), asthenia, peripheral oedema, thrombocytopenia, leucopenia, hypomagnesaemia, hypokalaemia, also injection-site reactions; *rarely* bradycardia, confusion, hyperkalaemia, hypernatraemia, pancytopenia, osteonecrosis of the jaw (*see also* Cautions above); *very rarely* uveitis and episcleritis
Dose: reduction of bone damage in advanced malignancies involving bone (with calcium and vitamin D supplement), *by intravenous infusion*, 4 mg every 3–4 weeks
Hypercalcaemia of malignancy, *by intravenous infusion,* 4 mg as a single dose
CHILD not recommended

Zometa® (Novartis) PoM
Concentrate for intravenous infusion, zoledronic acid, 800 micrograms/mL, net price 5-mL (4-mg) vial = £195.00

6.7 Other endocrine drugs

6.7.1 Bromocriptine and other dopaminergic drugs

Bromocriptine is a stimulant of dopamine receptors in the brain; it also inhibits release of prolactin by the pituitary. Bromocriptine is used for the treatment of galactorrhoea and cyclical benign breast disease, and for the treatment of prolactinomas (when it reduces both plasma prolactin concentration and tumour size). Bromocriptine also inhibits the release of growth hormone and is sometimes used in the treatment of acromegaly, but somatostatin analogues (such as octreotide, section 8.3.4.3) are more effective.

Cabergoline has actions and uses similar to those of bromocriptine, but its duration of action is longer. Its side-effects appear to differ from that of bromocriptine and patients intolerant of bromocriptine may be able to tolerate cabergoline (and *vice versa*).

> **Fibrotic reactions.** The CSM has advised that ergot-derived dopamine-receptor agonists, bromocriptine, cabergoline, lisuride, and pergolide have been associated with pulmonary, retroperitoneal, and pericardial fibrotic reactions.
> Before starting treatment with these ergot derivatives it may be appropriate to measure the erythrocyte sedimentation rate and serum creatinine and to obtain a chest X-ray. Patients should be monitored for dyspnoea, persistent cough, chest pain, cardiac failure, and abdominal pain or tenderness. If long-term treatment is expected, then lung-function tests may also be helpful.

Quinagolide has actions and uses similar to those of ergot-derived dopamine agonists, but its side-effects differ slightly.

SUPPRESSION OF LACTATION. Although bromocriptine and cabergoline are licensed to suppress lactation, they are **not** recommended for routine suppression (or for the relief of symptoms of postpartum pain and engorgement) that can be adequately treated with simple analgesics and breast support. If a dopamine-receptor agonist is required, cabergoline is preferred. Quinagolide is not licensed for the suppression of lactation.

Sudden onset of sleep. Excessive daytime sleepiness and sudden onset of sleep can occur with dopaminergic drugs.
Patients starting treatment with these drugs should be warned of the possibility of these effects and of the need to exercise caution when driving or operating machinery.
Patients who have suffered excessive sedation or sudden onset of sleep, should refrain from driving or operating machines, until those effects have stopped recurring.

BROMOCRIPTINE

Indications: see notes above and under Dose; parkinsonism (section 4.9.1)

Cautions: specialist evaluation—monitor for pituitary enlargement, particularly during pregnancy, annual gynaecological assessment (postmenopausal, every 6 months), monitor for peptic ulceration in acromegalic patients; contraceptive advice if appropriate (oral contraceptives may increase prolactin concentration); avoid breast-feeding for about 5 days if lactation prevention fails; history of serious mental disorders (especially psychotic disorders) or cardiovascular disease or Raynaud's syndrome; monitor for retroperitoneal fibrosis (see Fibrotic Reactions in notes above); porphyria (section 9.8.2); hepatic impairment (Appendix 2); **interactions:** Appendix 1 (bromocriptine)

HYPOTENSIVE REACTIONS. Hypotensive reactions may be disturbing in some patients during the first few days of treatment and particular care should be exercised when driving or operating machinery; tolerance may be reduced by alcohol

Contra-indications: hypersensitivity to bromocriptine or other ergot alkaloids; toxaemia of pregnancy and hypertension in postpartum women or in puerperium (see also below)

POSTPARTUM OR PUERPERIUM. Should not be used postpartum or in puerperium in women with high blood pressure, coronary artery disease or symptoms (or history) of serious mental disorder; monitor blood pressure carefully (especially during first few days) in postpartum women. Very rarely hypertension, myocardial infarction, seizures or stroke (both sometimes preceded by severe headache or visual disturbances) and mental disorders have been reported in postpartum women given bromocriptine for lactation suppression—caution with antihypertensive therapy and avoid other ergot alkaloids. Discontinue immediately if hypertension, unremitting headache or signs of CNS toxicity develop

Side-effects: nausea, constipation, headache, drowsiness (see also notes above on Sudden Onset of Sleep), nasal congestion; *less commonly* vomiting, postural hypotension, fatigue, dizziness, dyskinesia, dry mouth, leg cramps; also, particularly with *high doses*, confusion, psychomotor excitation, hallucinations; *rarely* constrictive pericarditis, pericardial effusion, pleural effusion (may necessitate discontinuation), retroperitoneal fibrosis reported (monitoring required)–see Fibrotic Reactions in notes above, hair loss, and allergic skin reactions; *very rarely* gastro-intestinal bleeding, gastric ulcer, vasospasm of fingers and toes particularly in patients with Raynaud's syndrome, and effects like neuroleptic malignant syndrome on withdrawal

Dose: prevention or suppression of lactation (but see notes above and under Cautions), 2.5 mg on day 1 (prevention) or daily for 2–3 days (suppression); then 2.5 mg twice daily for 14 days

Hypogonadism, galactorrhoea, infertility, initially 1–1.25 mg at bedtime, increased gradually; usual dose 7.5 mg daily in divided doses, increased if necessary to max. 30 mg daily, usual dose in infertility without hyperprolactinaemia, 2.5 mg twice daily

Cyclical benign breast disease (see also Breast Pain, section 6.7.2) and cyclical menstrual disorders (particularly breast pain), 1–1.25 mg at bedtime, increased gradually; usual dose 2.5 mg twice daily

Acromegaly, initially 1–1.25 mg at bedtime, increase gradually to 5 mg every 6 hours

Prolactinoma, initially 1–1.25 mg at bedtime; increased gradually to 5 mg every 6 hours (occasional patients may require up to 30 mg daily)

CHILD under 15 years, not recommended

Bromocriptine (Non-proprietary) PoM
Tablets, bromocriptine (as mesilate) 2.5 mg, net price 30-tab pack = £7.03. Label: 21, counselling, hypotensive reactions, driving, see notes above

Parlodel® (Novartis) PoM
Tablets, both scored, bromocriptine (as mesilate) 1 mg, net price 100-tab pack = £9.90; 2.5 mg, 30-tab pack = £5.78. Label: 21, counselling, hypotensive reactions, driving, see notes above
Capsules, bromocriptine (as mesilate) 5 mg (blue/white), net price 100-cap pack = £37.57; 10 mg (white), 100-cap pack = £69.50. Label: 21, counselling, hypotensive reactions, driving, see notes above

CABERGOLINE

Indications: see notes above and under Dose

Cautions: see under Bromocriptine; peptic ulcer, gastro-intestinal bleeding; severe hepatic impairment (Appendix 2); fibrotic lung disease (see Fibrotic Reactions in notes above); monthly pregnancy tests during the amenorrhoeic period; advise non-hormonal contraception if pregnancy not desired (see also Contra-indications); avoid in porphyria (section 9.8.2); **interactions:** Appendix 1 (cabergoline)

HYPOTENSIVE REACTIONS. Hypotensive reactions may be disturbing in some patients during the first few days of treatment and particular care should be exercised when driving or operating machinery; tolerance may be reduced by alcohol

Contra-indications: see under Bromocriptine; exclude pregnancy before starting and discontinue 1 month before intended conception (ovulatory cycles persist for 6 months)—discontinue if pregnancy occurs during treatment (specialist advice needed; Appendix 4); avoid breast-feeding if lactation prevention fails (Appendix 5)

Side-effects: see under Bromocriptine; also dyspepsia, epigastric and abdominal pain, syncope, breast pain, palpitation, angina, epistaxis, peripheral oedema, hemianopia, asthenia, paraesthesia, erythromelalgia, hot flushes, depression

Dose: prevention of lactation (but see notes above and under Contra-indications), during first day postpartum, 1 mg as a single dose; suppression of established lactation (but see notes above) 250 micrograms every 12 hours for 2 days

Hyperprolactinaemic disorders, 500 micrograms weekly (as a single dose *or* as 2 divided doses on separate days) increased at monthly intervals in steps of 500 micrograms until optimal therapeutic response (usually 1 mg weekly, range 0.25–2 mg weekly) with monthly monitoring of serum prolactin levels; reduce initial dose and increase more gradually if patient intolerant; over 1 mg weekly give as divided doses; up to 4.5 mg weekly has been used in hyperprolactinaemic patients

Parkinsonism, section 4.9.1

CHILD under 16 years, not recommended

Dostinex® (Pharmacia) PoM

Tablets, scored, cabergoline 500 micrograms. Net price 8-tab pack = £30.04. Label: 21, counselling, hypotensive reactions, driving, see notes above

QUINAGOLIDE

Indications: see notes above and under Dose

Cautions: see under Bromocriptine; advise non-hormonal contraception if pregnancy not desired; discontinue if pregnancy occurs during treatment (specialist advice needed; Appendix 4); **interactions:** Appendix 1 (quinagolide)

HYPOTENSIVE REACTIONS. Hypotensive reactions may be disturbing in some patients during the first few days of treatment—monitor blood pressure for a few days after starting treatment and following dosage increases; particular care should be exercised when driving or operating machinery; tolerance may be reduced by alcohol

Contra-indications: see under Bromocriptine; hypersensitivity to quinagolide (but not ergot alkaloids); hepatic impairment (Appendix 2); renal impairment (Appendix 3); breast-feeding (Appendix 5)

Side-effects: nausea, vomiting, headache, dizziness, fatigue; less frequently anorexia, abdominal pain, constipation or diarrhoea, oedema, flushing, hypotension, nasal congestion, insomnia; rarely sudden onset of sleep (see notes above), psychosis

Dose: hyperprolactinaemia, 25 micrograms at bedtime for 3 days; increased at intervals of 3 days in steps of 25 micrograms to usual maintenance dose of 75–150 micrograms daily; for doses higher than 300 micrograms daily increase in steps of 75–150 micrograms at intervals of not less than 4 weeks

CHILD not recommended

Norprolac® (Ferring) PoM

Tablets, quinagolide (as hydrochloride) 75 micrograms (white), net price 30-tab pack = £30.00; starter pack of 3 × 25-microgram tabs (pink) with 3 × 50-microgram tabs (blue) = £2.50. Label: 21, counselling, hypotensive reactions

6.7.2 Drugs affecting gonadotrophins

Danazol inhibits pituitary gonadotrophins; it combines androgenic activity with antioestrogenic and antiprogestogenic activity. It is licensed for the treatment of *endometriosis* and for the relief of severe pain and tenderness in *benign fibrocystic breast disease* where other measures have proved unsatisfactory. It may also be effective in the long-term management of *hereditary angioedema* [unlicensed indication].

Gestrinone has general actions similar to those of danazol and is indicated for the treatment of endometriosis.

Cetrorelix and **ganirelix** are luteinising hormone releasing hormone antagonists, which inhibit the release of gonadotrophins (luteinising hormone and follicle-stimulating hormone). They are used in the treatment of infertility by assisted reproductive techniques.

CETRORELIX

Indications: adjunct in the treatment of female infertility (under specialist supervision)

Contra-indications: pregnancy, breast-feeding (Appendix 5), moderate renal impairment (Appendix 3), moderate hepatic impairment (Appendix 2)

Side-effects: nausea, headache, injection site reactions; rarely hypersensitivity reactions

Dose: *by subcutaneous injection* into the lower abdominal wall,

either 250 micrograms in the morning, starting on day 5 or 6 of ovarian stimulation with gonadotrophins (*or* each evening starting on day 5 of ovarian stimulation); continue throughout administration of gonadotrophin including day of ovulation induction (*or* evening before ovulation induction)

or 3 mg on day 7 of ovarian stimulation with gonadotrophins; if ovulation induction not possible on day 5 after 3-mg dose, additional 250 micrograms once daily until day of ovulation induction

Cetrotide® (Serono) PoM

Injection, powder for reconstitution, cetrorelix (as acetate), net price 250-micrograms vial = £24.00; 3-mg vial = £168.00 (both with solvent)

DANAZOL

Indications: see notes above and under Dose

Cautions: cardiac, hepatic, or renal impairment (avoid if severe), elderly, polycythaemia, epilepsy, diabetes mellitus, hypertension, migraine, lipoprotein disorder, history of thrombosis or thromboembolic disease; withdraw if virilisation (may be irreversible on continued use); non-hormonal contraceptive methods should be used, if appropriate; **interactions:** Appendix 1 (danazol)

Contra-indications: pregnancy (Appendix 4), ensure that patients with amenorrhoea are not pregnant; breast-feeding (Appendix 5); severe hepatic, renal or cardiac impairment; thromboembolic disease; undiagnosed genital bleeding; androgen-dependent tumours; porphyria (section 9.8.2)

Side-effects: nausea, dizziness, skin reactions including rashes, photosensitivity and exfoliative dermatitis, fever, backache, nervousness, mood changes, anxiety, changes in libido, vertigo, fatigue, epigastric and pleuritic pain, headache, weight gain; menstrual disturbances, vaginal dryness and irritation, flushing and reduction in breast size; musculo-skeletal spasm, joint pain and swelling, hair loss; androgenic effects including acne, oily skin, oedema, hirsutism, voice changes and rarely clitoral hypertrophy (see also Cautions); temporary alteration in lipoproteins and other metabolic changes, insulin resistance; thrombotic events; leucopenia, thrombocytopenia, eosinophilia, reversible erythrocytosis or polycythaemia reported; headache and visual disturbances may indicate benign intracranial hypertension; rarely cholestatic jaundice, pancreatitis, peliosis hepatis and benign hepatic adenomata

Dose: in women of child-bearing potential, treatment should start during menstruation, preferably on day 1

Endometriosis, 200–800 mg daily in up to 4 divided doses, adjusted to achieve amenorrhoea, usually for 3–6 months

Severe pain and tenderness in benign fibrocystic breast disease not responding to other treatment, 300 mg daily in divided doses usually for 3–6 months

Hereditary angioedema [unlicensed indication], intially 200 mg 2–3 times daily, then reduced according to response

Danazol (Non-proprietary) PoM

Capsules, danazol 100 mg, net price 60-cap pack = £17.04; 200 mg, net price 56-cap pack = £36.02

Danol® (Sanofi-Synthelabo) PoM

Capsules, danazol 100 mg (grey/white), net price 60-cap pack = £17.04; 200 mg (pink/white), 60-cap pack = £33.75

GANIRELIX

Indications: adjunct in the treatment of female infertility (under specialist supervision)

Contra-indications: pregnancy (Appendix 4), breast-feeding (Appendix 5); moderate renal impairment (Appendix 3); moderate hepatic impairment (Appendix 2)

Side-effects: nausea, headache, injection site reactions; dizziness, asthenia and malaise also reported

Dose: *by subcutaneous injection* preferably into the upper leg (rotate injection sites to prevent lipoatrophy), 250 micrograms in the morning (or each afternoon) starting on day 6 of ovarian stimulation with gonadotrophins; continue throughout administration of gonadotrophins including day of ovulation induction (if administering in afternoon, give last dose in afternoon *before* ovulation induction)

Orgalutran® (Organon) PoM

Injection, ganirelix, 500 micrograms/mL, net price 0.5-mL prefilled syringe = £22.32

GESTRINONE

Indications: endometriosis

Cautions: cardiac and renal impairment; **interactions:** Appendix 1 (gestrinone)

Contra-indications: pregnancy (use non-hormonal method of contraception); breast-feeding (Appendix 5); severe cardiac, renal impairment or hepatic impairment; metabolic or vascular disorders associated with previous sex hormone treatment

Side-effects: spotting; acne, oily skin, fluid retention, weight gain, hirsutism, voice change; liver enzyme disturbances; headache; gastro-intestinal disturbances; change in libido, flushing, decrease in breast size; nervousness, depression, change in appetite; muscle cramp

Dose: 2.5 mg twice weekly starting on first day of cycle with second dose 3 days later, repeated on same two days preferably at same time each week; duration of treatment usually 6 months

MISSED DOSES. One missed dose—2.5 mg as soon as possible and maintain original sequence; two or more missed doses—discontinue, re-start on first day of new cycle (following negative pregnancy test)

Dimetriose® (Florizel) PoM

Capsules, gestrinone 2.5 mg, net price 8-cap pack = £103.91

Gonadorelin analogues

Administration of **gonadorelin analogues** produces an initial phase of stimulation; continued administration is followed by down-regulation of gonadotrophin-releasing hormone receptors, thereby reducing the release of gonadotrophins (follicle stimulating hormone and luteinising hormone) which in turn leads to inhibition of androgen and oestrogen production.

Gonadorelin analogues are used in the treatment of endometriosis, precocious puberty, infertility, anaemia due to uterine fibroids (together with iron supplementation), breast cancer (section 8.3.4.1), prostate cancer (section 8.3.4.2) and before intrauterine surgery. Use of leuprorelin and triptorelin for 3 to 4 months before surgery reduces the uterine volume, fibroid size and associated bleeding. For women undergoing hysterectomy or myomectomy, a vaginal procedure is made more feasible following the use of a gonadorelin analogue.

CAUTIONS. Non-hormonal, barrier methods of contraception should be used during entire treatment period with gonadorelin analogues; also use with caution in patients with metabolic bone disease because decrease in bone mineral density can occur.

CONTRA-INDICATIONS. Gonadorelin analogues are contra-indicated for use longer than 6 months (do not repeat), where there is undiagnosed vaginal bleeding, in pregnancy (Appendix 4; exclude pregnancy—also give first injection during menstruation or shortly afterwards *or* use barrier contraception for 1 month beforehand) and in breast-feeding.

SIDE-EFFECTS. Side-effects of the gonadorelin analogues related to the inhibition of oestrogen production include menopausal-like symptoms (e.g. hot flushes, increased sweating, vaginal dryness, dyspareunia and loss of libido) and a decrease in trabecular bone density; these effects can be reduced by hormone replacement (e.g. with an oestrogen and a progestogen or with tibolone). Side-effects of gonadorelin analogues also include headache (rarely migraine) and hypersensitivity reactions including urticaria, pruritus, rash, asthma and anaphylaxis; when treating uterine fibroids bleeding associated with fibroid degeneration can occur; spray formulations can cause irritation of the nasal mucosa including nose bleeds; local reactions at injection site can occur; other side-effects also reported with some gonadorelin analogues include palpitation, hypertension, ovarian cysts (may require withdrawal), changes in breast size, musculoskeletal pain or weakness, visual disturbances, paraesthesia, changes in scalp and body hair, oedema of the face and extremities, weight changes, and mood changes including depression.

BUSERELIN

Indications: see under Dose; prostate cancer (section 8.3.4.2)

Cautions: see notes above; polycystic ovarian disease, depression, hypertension, diabetes

Contra-indications: see notes above; hormone-dependent tumours

Side-effects: see notes above; initially withdrawal bleeding and subsequently breakthrough bleeding, leucorrhoea; nausea, vomiting, constipation, diarrhoea; anxiety, memory and concentration disturbances, sleep disturbances, nervousness, dizziness, drowsiness; breast tenderness, lactation; abdominal pain; fatigue; increased thirst, changes in appetite; acne, dry skin, splitting nails, dry eyes; altered blood lipids, leucopenia, thrombocytopenia; hearing disturbances; reduced glucose tolerance

Dose: endometriosis, *intranasally*, 300 micrograms (one 150-microgram spray in each nostril) 3 times daily (starting on days 1 or 2 of menstruation); max. duration of treatment 6 months (do not repeat)

Pituitary desensitisation before induction of ovulation by gonadotrophins for *in vitro* fertilisation (under specialist supervision), *by subcutaneous injection*, 200–500 micrograms daily given as a single injection (occasionally up to 500 micrograms twice daily may be needed) starting in early follicular phase (day 1) *or*, after exclusion of pregnancy, in midluteal phase (day 21) and continued until down-regulation achieved (usually about 1–3 weeks) then maintained during gonadotrophin administration (stopping gonadotrophin and buserelin on administration of chorionic gonadotrophin at appropriate stage of follicular development)

Intranasally, 150 micrograms (one spray in one nostril) 4 times daily during waking hours (occasionally up to 300 micrograms 4 times daily may be needed) starting in early follicular phase (day 1) *or*, after exclusion of pregnancy, in midluteal phase (day 21) and continued until down-regulation achieved (usually about 2–3 weeks) then maintained during gonadotrophin administration (stopping gonadotrophin and buserelin on administration of chorionic gonadotrophin at appropriate stage of follicular development)

COUNSELLING. Avoid use of nasal decongestants before and for at least 30 minutes after treatment

Suprecur® (Aventis Pharma) PoM

Nasal spray, buserelin (as acetate) 150 micrograms/metered spray. Net price 2 × 100-dose pack (with metered dose pumps) = £75.43. Counselling, nasal decongestants

Injection, buserelin (as acetate) 1mg/mL. Net price 5.5-mL vial = £11.85

GOSERELIN

Indications: see under Dose; prostate cancer (section 8.3.4.2); early and advanced breast cancer (section 8.3.4.1)

Cautions: see notes above; polycystic ovarian disease

Contra-indications: see notes above

Side-effects: see notes above; withdrawal bleeding

Dose: *by subcutaneous injection* into anterior abdominal wall, endometriosis, 3.6 mg every 28 days; max. duration of treatment 6 months (do not repeat); endometrial thinning before intra-uterine surgery, 3.6 mg (may be repeated after 28 days if uterus is large or to allow flexible surgical timing); before surgery in women who have anaemia due to uterine fibroids, 3.6 mg every 28 days (with supplementary iron); max. duration of treatment 3 months

Pituitary desensitisation before induction of ovulation by gonadotrophins for *in vitro* fertilisation (under specialist supervision), after exclusion of pregnancy, 3.6 mg to achieve pituitary down-regulation (usually 1–3 weeks) then gonadotrophin is administered (stopping gonadotrophin on administration of chorionic gonadotrophin at appropriate stage of follicular development)

■ Preparation

Section 8.3.4.2

LEUPRORELIN ACETATE

Indications: see under Dose; prostate cancer (section 8.3.4.2)

Cautions: see notes above; family history of osteoporosis; chronic use of other drugs which reduce bone density including alcohol and tobacco; diabetes

Contra-indications: see notes above

Side-effects: see notes above; breast tenderness; nausea, vomiting, diarrhoea, anorexia; fever, chills; sleep disturbances, dizziness, fatigue, leucopenia, thrombocytopenia, altered blood lipids, pulmonary embolism; spinal fracture, paralysis, hypotension and worsening of depression also reported

Dose: *by subcutaneous or intramuscular injection*, endometriosis, 3.75 mg as a single dose in first 5 days of menstrual cycle then every month for max. 6 months (course not to be repeated)

Endometrial thinning before intra-uterine surgery, 3.75 mg as a single dose (given between days 3 and 5 of menstrual cycle) 5–6 weeks before surgery

Reduction of size of uterine fibroids and of associated bleeding before surgery, 3.75 mg as a single dose every month usually for 3–4 months (max. 6 months)

■ Preparation

Section 8.3.4.2

NAFARELIN

Indications: see under Dose

Cautions: see notes above

Contra-indications: see notes above

Side-effects: see notes above; acne

Dose: women over 18 years, endometriosis, 200 micrograms twice daily as one spray in one nostril in the morning and one spray in the other nostril in the evening (starting on days 2–4 of menstruation), max. duration of treatment 6 months (do not repeat)

Pituitary desensitisation before induction of ovulation by gonadotrophins for *in vitro* fertilisation (under specialist supervision), 400 micrograms (one spray in each nostril) twice daily starting in early follicular phase (day 2) or, after exclusion of pregnancy, in midluteal phase (day 21) and continued until down-regulation achieved (usually within 4 weeks) then maintained (usually for 8–12 days) during gonadotrophin administration (stopping gonadotrophin and nafarelin on administration of chorionic gonadotrophin at follicular maturity); discontinue if down-regulation not achieved within 12 weeks

COUNSELLING. Avoid use of nasal decongestants before and for at least 30 minutes after treatment; repeat dose if sneezing occurs during or immediately after administration

Synarel® (Pharmacia) PoM

Nasal spray, nafarelin (as acetate) 200 micrograms/metered spray. Net price 30-dose unit = £32.28; 60-dose unit = £55.66. Label: 10, patient information leaflet, counselling, see above

---

TRIPTORELIN

Indications: advanced prostate cancer, endometriosis, precocious puberty, reduction in size of uterine fibroids (section 8.3.4.2)

Cautions: see notes above

Contra-indications: see notes above

Side-effects: see notes above; asthenia

Dose: see section 8.3.4.2

■ Preparations

Section 8.3.4.2

Breast pain (mastalgia)

Once any serious underlying cause for breast pain has been ruled out, most women will respond to reassurance and reduction in dietary fat; withdrawal of an oral contraceptive or of hormone replacement therapy may help to resolve the pain.

Mild, non-cyclical breast pain is treated with simple analgesics (section 4.7.1); moderate to severe pain, cyclical pain or symptoms that persist for longer than 6 months may require specific drug treatment. **Bromocriptine** (section 6.7.1) is used in the management of breast pain but is associated with unpleasant side-effects; it acts within 2 months.

Danazol (section 6.7.2) is licensed for the relief of severe pain and tenderness in benign fibrocystic breast disease which has not responded to other treatment.

Tamoxifen (section 8.3.4.1) may be a useful adjunct in the treatment of mastalgia [unlicensed indication] especially when symptoms can definitely be related to cyclic oestrogen production; it may be given on the days of the cycle when symptoms are predicted.

Treatment for breast pain should be reviewed after 6 months and continued if necessary. Symptoms recur in about 50% of women within 2 years of withdrawal of therapy but may be less severe.

6.7.3 Metyrapone and trilostane

Metyrapone is a competitive inhibitor of 11β-hydroxylation in the adrenal cortex; the resulting inhibition of cortisol (and to a lesser extent aldosterone) production leads to an increase in ACTH production which, in turn, leads to increased synthesis and release of cortisol precursors. It may be used as a test of anterior pituitary function.

Although most types of *Cushing's syndrome* are treated surgically, that which occasionally accompanies carcinoma of the bronchus is not usually amenable to surgery. Metyrapone has been found helpful in controlling the symptoms of the disease; it is also used in other forms of Cushing's syndrome to prepare the patient for surgery. The dosages used are either low, and tailored to cortisol production, or high, in which case corticosteroid replacement therapy is also needed.

Trilostane reversibly inhibits 3β-hydroxysteroid dehydrogenase/delta 5-4 isomerase in the adrenal cortex; the resulting inhibition of the synthesis of mineralocorticoids and glucocorticoids may be useful in *Cushing's syndrome* and *primary hyperaldosteronism*. Trilostane appears to be less effective than metyrapone for Cushing's syndrome (where it is tailored to corticosteroid production). It also has a minor role in post-menopausal breast cancer that has relapsed following initial oestrogen antagonist therapy (corticosteroid replacement therapy is also required). **Ketoconazole** (section 5.2) is also used by specialists for the management of *Cushing's syndrome* [unlicensed indication].

See also aminoglutethimide (section 8.3.4)

METYRAPONE

Indications: see notes above and under Dose (specialist supervision in hospital)

Cautions: gross hypopituitarism (risk of precipitating acute adrenal failure); hypertension on long-term administration; hypothyroidism or hepatic impairment (delayed response); many drugs interfere with diagnostic estimation of steroids; avoid in porphyria (section 9.8.2)

DRIVING. Drowsiness may affect the performance of skilled tasks (e.g. driving)

Contra-indications: adrenocortical insufficiency (see Cautions); pregnancy (Appendix 4), breast-feeding (Appendix 5)

Side-effects: occasional nausea, vomiting, dizziness, headache, hypotension, sedation; rarely abdominal pain, allergic skin reactions, hypoadrenalism, hirsutism

Dose: differential diagnosis of ACTH-dependent Cushing's syndrome, 750 mg every 4 hours for 6 doses; CHILD 15 mg/kg (minimum 250 mg) every 4 hours for 6 doses

Management of Cushing's syndrome, range 0.25–6 g daily, tailored to cortisol production; see notes above

Resistant oedema due to increased aldosterone secretion in cirrhosis, nephrotic syndrome, and congestive heart failure (with glucocorticoid replacement therapy) 3 g daily in divided doses

Metopirone® (Alliance) PoM

Capsules, ivory, metyrapone 250 mg. Net price 100-tab pack = £41.44. Label: 21, counselling, driving

---

TRILOSTANE

Indications: see notes above and under Dose (specialist supervision)

Cautions: breast cancer (concurrent corticosteroid replacement therapy needed, see under Dose), adrenal cortical hyperfunction (tailored to cortisol and electrolytes, concurrent corticosteroid therapy may be needed, see under Dose); hepatic and renal impairment; **interactions:** Appendix 1 (trilostane)

Contra-indications: pregnancy (use non-hormonal method of contraception; Appendix 4); breast-feeding; children

Side-effects: flushing, tingling and swelling of mouth, rhinorrhoea, nausea, vomiting, diarrhoea, and rashes reported; rarely granulocytopenia

Dose: adrenal cortical hyperfunction, 240 mg daily in divided doses for at least 3 days then tailored according to response with regular monitoring of plasma electrolytes and circulating corticosteroids (both mineralocorticoid and glucocorticoid replacement therapy may be needed); usual dose: 120–480 mg daily (may be increased to 960 mg)

Postmenopausal breast cancer (with glucocorticoid replacement therapy) following relapse to initial oestrogen receptor antagonist therapy, initially 240 mg daily increased every 3 days in steps of 240 mg to a maintenance dose of 960 mg daily (720 mg daily if not tolerated)

Modrenal® (Bioenvision) PoM

Capsules, trilostane 60 mg (pink/black), net price 100-cap pack = £49.50; 120 mg (pink/yellow), 100-cap pack = £98.50. Label: 21

7: Obstetrics, gynaecology, and urinary-tract disorders

For hormonal therapy of gynaecological disorders see section 6.4.1, section 6.5.1 and section 6.7.2.

7.1 Drugs used in obstetrics

Because of the complexity of dosage regimens in obstetrics, in all cases **detailed specialist literature** should be consulted.

7.1.1 Prostaglandins and oxytocics

Prostaglandins and oxytocics are used to induce abortion or induce or augment labour and to minimise blood loss from the placental site. They include oxytocin, ergometrine, and the prostaglandins. All induce uterine contractions with varying degrees of pain according to the strength of contractions induced.

INDUCTION OF ABORTION. **Gemeprost**, administered vaginally as pessaries is the preferred prostaglandin for the medical induction of late therapeutic abortion. Gemeprost ripens and softens the cervix before surgical abortion, particularly in primigravida. The prostaglandin **misoprostol** is given by mouth or by vaginal administration to induce medical abortion [unlicensed indication]; intravaginal use ripens the cervix before surgical abortion [unlicensed indication]. Extra-amniotic **dinoprostone** is rarely used nowadays.

Pre-treatment with **mifepristone** (section 7.1.2) can facilitate the process of medical abortion. It sensitises the uterus to subsequent administration of a prostaglandin and, therefore, abortion occurs in a shorter time and with a lower dose of prostaglandin.

INDUCTION AND AUGMENTATION OF LABOUR. **Dinoprostone** is available as vaginal tablets, pessaries and vaginal gels for the induction of labour. The intravenous solution is rarely used; it is associated with more side-effects.

Oxytocin (*Syntocinon*®) is administered by slow intravenous infusion, using an infusion pump, to induce or augment labour, usually in conjunction with amniotomy. Uterine activity must be monitored carefully and hyperstimulation avoided. Large doses of oxytocin may result in excessive fluid retention.

Misoprostol is given orally or vaginally for the induction of labour [unlicensed indication].

NICE guidance (induction of labour). NICE has recommended (June 2001) that:

- dinoprostone is preferable to oxytocin for induction of labour in women with intact membranes, regardless of parity or cervical favourability;
- dinoprostone or oxytocin are equally effective for the induction of labour in women with ruptured membranes, regardless of parity or cervical favourability;
- oxytocin should not be started for 6 hours following administration of vaginal prostaglandins;
- when used to induce labour, the recommended dose of oxytocin by intravenous infusion[1] is initially 0.001–0.002 units/minute increased at intervals of at least 30 minutes until a maximum of 3–4 contractions occur every 10 minutes (0.012 units/minute is often adequate); the maximum recommended rate is 0.032 units/minute (licensed max. 0.02 units/minute)

1. Oxytocin should be used in standard dilutions of 10 units/500 mL (infusing 3 mL/hour delivers 0.001 unit/minute) or, for higher doses, 30 units/500 mL (infusing 1 mL/hour delivers 0.001 unit/minute).

PREVENTION AND TREATMENT OF HAEMORRHAGE. Bleeding due to incomplete abortion can be controlled with **ergometrine** and **oxytocin** (*Syntometrine*®) given intramuscularly, the dose is adjusted according to the patient's condition and blood loss. This is commonly used before surgical evacuation of the uterus, particularly when surgery is delayed. Oxytocin and ergometrine combined are more effective in early pregnancy than either drug alone.

For the routine management of the third stage of labour ergometrine 500 micrograms with oxytocin 5 units (*Syntometrine*® 1 mL) is given by intramuscular injection on delivery of the anterior shoulder or, at the latest, immediately after the baby is delivered. If ergometrine is inappropriate (e.g. in pre-eclampsia), oxytocin may be given by intramuscular injection [unlicensed indication].

In excessive uterine bleeding, any placental products remaining in the uterus should be removed. In bleeding caused by uterine atony oxytocic drugs are used in turn as follows:

- oxytocin 5–10 units by intravenous injection
- ergometrine 250–500 micrograms by intravenous injection
- oxytocin 5–30 units in 500 mL infusion fluid given by intravenous infusion at a rate that controls uterine atony

Carboprost has an important role in severe postpartum haemorrhage unresponsive to ergometrine and oxytocin.

Mild secondary postpartum haemorrhage has been treated in domiciliary practice with ergometrine by mouth, but it is rarely used now.

CARBOPROST

Indications: postpartum haemorrhage due to uterine atony in patients unresponsive to ergometrine and oxytocin

Cautions: history of glaucoma or raised intra-ocular pressure, asthma, hypertension, hypotension, anaemia, jaundice, diabetes, epilepsy; uterine scars; excessive dosage may cause uterine rupture; **interactions:** Appendix 1 (prostaglandins)

Contra-indications: untreated pelvic infection; cardiac, renal, pulmonary, or hepatic disease

Side-effects: nausea, vomiting and diarrhoea, hyperthermia and flushing, bronchospasm; less frequent effects include raised blood pressure, dyspnoea, and pulmonary oedema; chills, headache, diaphoresis, dizziness; cardiovascular collapse also reported; erythema and pain at injection site reported

Dose: *by deep intramuscular injection*, 250 micrograms repeated if necessary at intervals of 1½ hours (in severe cases the interval may be reduced but should not be less than 15 minutes); total dose should not exceed 2 mg (8 doses)

Hemabate® (Pharmacia) PoM
Injection, carboprost as trometamol salt (tromethamine salt) 250 micrograms/mL, net price 1-mL amp = £18.20 (hosp. only)

DINOPROSTONE

Indications: see notes above and under preparations below

Cautions: history of asthma, glaucoma and raised intra-ocular pressure; cardiac, hepatic or renal impairment; hypertension; history of epilepsy; uterine scarring; monitor uterine activity and fetal status (particular care if history of uterine hypertony); uterine rupture; see also notes above; effect of oxytocin enhanced (care needed in monitoring uterine activity when used in sequence)—see also under *Propess*® and **interactions:** Appendix 1 (prostaglandins)

Contra-indications: active cardiac, pulmonary, renal or hepatic disease; placenta praevia or unexplained vaginal bleeding during pregnancy, ruptured membranes, major cephalopelvic disproportion or fetal malpresentation, history of caesarean section or major uterine surgery, untreated pelvic infection, fetal distress, grand multiparas and multiple pregnancy, history of difficult or traumatic delivery; avoid extra-amniotic route in cervicitis or vaginitis

Side-effects: nausea, vomiting, diarrhoea; other side-effects include uterine hypertonus, severe uterine contractions, pulmonary or amniotic fluid embolism, abruptio placenta, fetal distress, maternal hypertension, bronchospasm, rapid cervical dilation, fever, backache; uterine hypercontractility with or without fetal bradycardia, low Apgar scores; cardiac arrest, uterine rupture, stillbirth or neonatal death also reported; vaginal symptoms (warmth, irritation, pain); after intravenous administration—flushing, shivering, headache, dizziness, temporary pyrexia and raised white blood cell count; also local tissue reaction and erythema after intravenous administration and possibility of infection after extra-amniotic administration

Dose: see under preparations, below
IMPORTANT. Do not confuse dose of *Prostin E2*® vaginal **gel** with that of *Prostin E2*® vaginal **tablets**—not bioequivalent.

Propess® (Ferring) PoM

Pessaries (within retrieval system), releasing dinoprostone approx. 5 mg over 12 hours. Net price 1-pessary pack = £30.00

Dose: by vagina, cervical ripening and induction of labour at term, 1 pessary inserted high into posterior fornix; if cervical ripening insufficient, remove pessary 8–12 hours later and replace with a second pessary (which should also be removed not more than 12 hours later); max. 2 consecutive pessaries

IMPORTANT. Effect of oxytocin enhanced—particular care needed to monitor uterine activity when oxytocin used in sequence (remove pessary beforehand)

Prostin E2® (Pharmacia) PoM

Intravenous solution ▰, for dilution and use as an infusion, dinoprostone 1 mg/mL, net price 0.75-mL amp = £8.52; 10 mg/mL, 0.5-mL amp = £18.40 (both hosp. only; rarely used, consult product literature for dose and indications)

Extra-amniotic solution ▰, dinoprostone 10 mg/mL. Net price 0.5-mL amp (with diluent) = £18.40 (hosp. only; less commonly used nowadays, consult product literature for dose and indications)

Vaginal gel, dinoprostone 400 micrograms/mL, net price 2.5 mL (1 mg) = £15.25; 800 micrograms/mL, 2.5 mL (2 mg) = £16.80

Dose: by vagina, induction of labour, inserted high into posterior fornix (avoid administration into cervical canal), 1 mg (unfavourable primigravida 2 mg), followed after 6 hours by 1–2 mg if required; max. [gel] 3 mg (unfavourable primigravida 4 mg)

Vaginal tablets, dinoprostone 3 mg. Net price 8-vaginal tab pack = £78.05

Dose: by vagina, induction of labour, inserted high into posterior fornix, 3 mg, followed after 6–8 hours by 3 mg if labour is not established; max. 6 mg [vaginal tablets]

NOTE. *Prostin E2 Vaginal Gel* and *Vaginal Tablets* are **not** bioequivalent

ERGOMETRINE MALEATE

Indications: see notes above

Cautions: cardiac disease, hypertension, hepatic impairment (Appendix 2), and renal impairment (Appendix 3), multiple pregnancy; porphyria (section 9.8.2); **interactions:** Appendix 1 (ergot alkaloids)

Contra-indications: induction of labour, first and second stages of labour, vascular disease, severe cardiac disease, severe hepatic and renal impairment, sepsis, severe hypertension, eclampsia

Side-effects: nausea, vomiting, headache, dizziness, tinnitus, abdominal pain, chest pain, palpitation, dyspnoea, bradycardia, transient hypertension, vasoconstriction; stroke, myocardial infarction and pulmonary oedema also reported

Dose: see notes above

Ergometrine (Non-proprietary) PoM

Tablets ▰, ergometrine maleate 500 micrograms, net price 21-tab pack = £25.00

Injection, ergometrine maleate 500 micrograms/mL. Net price 1-mL amp = 60p

■ With oxytocin

Syntometrine® (Alliance) PoM

Injection, ergometrine maleate 500 micrograms, oxytocin 5 units/mL. Net price 1-mL amp = £1.31

Dose: by intramuscular injection, 1 mL; by intravenous injection, no longer recommended

GEMEPROST

Indications: see under Dose

Cautions: obstructive airways disease, cardiovascular insufficiency, raised intra-ocular pressure, cervicitis or vaginitis; **interactions:** Appendix 1 (prostaglandins)

IMPORTANT. For warnings relating to use of gemeprost in a patient undergoing induction of abortion with mifepristone, see under Mifepristone and Note below

Contra-indications: unexplained vaginal bleeding

Side-effects: vaginal bleeding and uterine pain; nausea, vomiting, or diarrhoea; headache, muscle weakness, dizziness, flushing, chills, backache, dyspnoea, chest pain, palpitation and mild pyrexia; uterine rupture reported (most commonly in multiparas or if history of uterine surgery or if given with intravenous oxytocics); also reported severe hypotension, coronary artery spasm and myocardial infarction

Dose: *by vagina* in pessaries, softening and dilation of the cervix to facilitate transcervical operative procedures in first trimester, inserted into posterior fornix, 1 mg 3 hours before surgery

Second trimester abortion, inserted into posterior fornix, 1 mg every 3 hours for max. of 5 administrations; second course may begin 24 hours after start of treatment (if treatment fails pregnancy should be terminated by another method)

Second trimester intra-uterine death, inserted into posterior fornix, 1 mg every 3 hours for max. of 5 administrations only; monitor for coagulopathy

NOTE. If used in combination with mifepristone, carefully monitor blood pressure and pulse for 6 hours

Gemeprost (Beacon) PoM

Pessaries, gemeprost 1 mg. Net price 5-pessary pack = £215.00

OXYTOCIN

Indications: see under Dose and notes above

Cautions: particular caution needed when given for *induction or enhancement of labour* in presence of borderline cephalopelvic disproportion (avoid if significant), mild or moderate pregnancy-induced hypertension or cardiac disease, women over 35 years or with history of lower-uterine segment caesarean section (see also under Contra-indications below); if fetal death *in utero* or meconium-stained amniotic fluid avoid tumultuous labour (may cause amniotic fluid embolism); water intoxication and hyponatraemia—avoid large infusion volumes and restrict fluid intake by mouth (see also Appendix 6); effects enhanced by concomitant prostaglandins (very careful monitoring), caudal block anaesthesia (may enhance hypertensive effects of sympathomimetic vasopressors), see also **interactions:** Appendix 1 (oxytocin)

Contra-indications: hypertonic uterine contractions, mechanical obstruction to delivery, fetal distress; any condition where spontaneous labour or vaginal delivery inadvisable; avoid prolonged administration in oxytocin-resistant uterine inertia, severe pre-eclamptic toxaemia or severe cardiovascular disease

Side-effects: uterine spasm (may occur at low doses), uterine hyperstimulation (usually with excessive doses—may cause fetal distress, asphyxia and death, or may lead to hypertonicity, tetanic contractions, soft-tissue damage or uterine rupture); water intoxication and hyponatraemia associated with high doses with large infusion volumes of electrolyte-free fluid (see also under Dose below); also nausea, vomiting, arrhythmias; rashes and anaphylactoid reactions (with dyspnoea, hypotension or shock) also reported; placental abruption and amniotic fluid embolism also reported on overdose

Dose: induction of labour for medical reasons or stimulation of labour in hypotonic uterine inertia, *by intravenous infusion*, see NICE guidance above; max. 5 units in 1 day (may be repeated next day starting again at 0.001–0.002 units/minute)

IMPORTANT. Careful monitoring of fetal heart rate and uterine motility essential for dose titration (**avoid** intravenous injection during labour); discontinue immediately in uterine hyperactivity or fetal distress

Caesarean section, *by slow intravenous injection* immediately after delivery, 5 units

Prevention of postpartum haemorrhage, after delivery of placenta, *by slow intravenous injection*, 5 units (if infusion used for induction or enhancement of labour, increase rate during third stage and for next few hours)

NOTE. May be given in a dose of 10 units by intramuscular injection [unlicensed route] instead of oxytocin with ergometrine (*Syntometrine*®), see notes above

Treatment of postpartum haemorrhage, *by slow intravenous injection*, 5–10 units, followed in severe cases *by intravenous infusion* of 5–30 units in 500 mL infusion fluid at a rate sufficient to control uterine atony

IMPORTANT. Avoid rapid intravenous injection (may transiently reduce blood pressure); prolonged administration, see warning below

Incomplete, inevitable or missed abortion, *by slow intravenous injection*, 5 units followed if necessary *by intravenous infusion*, 0.02–0.04 units/minute or faster

IMPORTANT. Prolonged intravenous administration at high doses with large volume of fluid (as possible in inevitable or missed abortion or postpartum haemorrhage) may cause water intoxication with hyponatraemia. To avoid: use electrolyte-containing diluent (i.e. not glucose), increase oxytocin concentration to reduce fluid, restrict fluid intake by mouth; monitor fluid and electrolytes

NOTE. Oxytocin doses in the BNF may differ from those in the product literature

Syntocinon® (Alliance) PoM
Injection, oxytocin, net price 5 units/mL, 1-mL amp = 89p; 10 units/mL, 1-mL amp = £1.01

■ With ergometrine
See Syntometrine®, p. 399

7.1.1.1 Ductus arteriosus

Maintenance of patency

Alprostadil (prostaglandin E_1) is used to maintain patency of the ductus arteriosus in neonates with congenital heart defects, prior to corrective surgery in centres where intensive care is immediately available.

ALPROSTADIL

Indications: congenital heart defects in neonates prior to corrective surgery; erectile dysfunction (section 7.4.5)

Cautions: see notes above; history of haemorrhage, avoid in hyaline membrane disease, monitor arterial pressure; **interactions:** Appendix 1 (prostaglandins)

Side-effects: apnoea (particularly in neonates under 2 kg), flushing, bradycardia, hypotension, tachycardia, cardiac arrest, oedema, diarrhoea, fever, convulsions, disseminated intravascular coagulation, hypokalaemia; cortical proliferation of long bones, weakening of the wall of the ductus arteriosus and pulmonary artery may follow prolonged use; gastric-outlet obstruction reported

Dose: *by intravenous infusion*, initially 50–100 nanograms/kg/minute, then decreased to lowest effective dose

Prostin VR® (Pharmacia) PoM
Intravenous solution, alprostadil 500 micrograms/mL in alcohol. For dilution and use as an infusion. Net price 1-mL amp = £75.19 (hosp. only)

Closure of ductus arteriosus

Indometacin (indomethacin) is used to close a patent ductus arteriosus in premature babies, probably by inhibiting prostaglandin synthesis.

INDOMETACIN

(Indomethacin)

Indications: patent ductus arteriosus in premature babies (under specialist supervision in neonatal intensive care unit); rheumatoid disease (section 10.1.1)

Cautions: may mask symptoms of infection; may reduce urine output by 50% or more (monitor carefully—see also under Anuria or Oliguria, below) and precipitate renal impairment especially if extracellular volume depleted, heart failure, sepsis, or hepatic impairment, or if receiving nephrotoxic drugs; may induce hyponatraemia; monitor renal function and electrolytes; inhibition of platelet aggregation (monitor for bleeding); **interactions:** Appendix 1 (NSAIDs)

ANURIA OR OLIGURIA. If anuria or marked oliguria (urinary output less than 0.6 mL/kg/hour) at time of scheduled second or third dose, delay until renal function returns to normal

Contra-indications: untreated infection, bleeding (especially with active intracranial haemorrhage or gastro-intestinal bleeding); thrombocytopenia, coagulation defects, necrotising enterocolitis, renal impairment

Side-effects: haemorrhagic, renal, gastro-intestinal (including necrotising enterocolitis), metabolic, and coagulation disorders; pulmonary hypertension, intracranial bleeding, fluid retention, and exacerbation of infection

Dose: *by intravenous injection*, over 20–30 minutes (using a suitable syringe driver), 3 doses at intervals of 12–24 hours (provided urine output remains adequate), age less than 48 hours, 200 micrograms/kg then 100 micrograms/kg then 100 micrograms/kg; age 2–7 days, 200 micrograms/kg then 200 micrograms/kg then 200 micrograms/kg; age over 7 days, 200 micrograms/kg then 250 micrograms/kg then 250 micrograms/kg; solution prepared with 1–2 mL sodium chloride 0.9% or water for injections (not glucose and no preservatives)

If ductus arteriosus reopens a second course of 3 injections may be given 48 hours after first course

Indocid PDA® (MSD) PoM
Injection, powder for reconstitution, indometacin (as sodium trihydrate). Net price 3 × 1-mg vials = £22.50 (hosp. only)

7.1.2 Mifepristone

Mifepristone, an antiprogestogenic steroid, sensitises the myometrium to prostaglandin-induced contractions and it softens and dilates the cervix. For the termination of pregnancy, a single dose of mifepristone is followed by vaginal administration of the prostaglandin gemeprost. Although mifepristone is licensed for use in a dose of 600 mg, for medical abortion, a dose of 200 mg is effective for gestation of up to 24 weeks. Guidelines of the Royal College of Obstetricians and Gynaecologists' (September 2004) include the following [unlicensed] regimens for inducing medical abortion:

- For gestation up to 9 weeks, mifepristone 200 mg by mouth followed 1–3 days later by misoprostol 800 micrograms vaginally; in women at more than 7 weeks gestation (49–63 days), if the abortion has not occurred 4 hours after misoprostol, a further dose of misoprostol 400 micrograms may be given vaginally or by mouth
- For gestation between 9 and 13 weeks, mifepristone 200 mg by mouth followed 36–48 hours later by misoprostol 800 micrograms vaginally followed if necessary by a maximum of 4 further doses at 3-hourly intervals of misoprostol 400 micrograms vaginally or by mouth
- For gestation between 13 and 24 weeks, mifepristone 200 mg by mouth followed 36–48 hours later by misoprostol 800 micrograms vaginally then a maximum of 4 further doses at 3-hourly intervals of misoprostol 400 micrograms by mouth

MIFEPRISTONE

Indications: see under dose

Cautions: asthma (avoid if severe); haemorrhagic disorders and anticoagulant therapy; prosthetic heart valve or history of endocarditis (prophylaxis recommended, see section 5.1 table 2); smokers aged over 35 years (increased risk of cardiovascular events); adrenal suppression (may require corticosteroid); not recommended in hepatic or renal impairment; breast-feeding (Appendix 5); avoid aspirin and NSAIDs for analgesia; **interactions**: Appendix 1 (mifepristone)

IMPORTANT. For warnings relating to use of gemeprost in a patient undergoing induction of abortion with mifepristone, see under Gemeprost

Contra-indications: uncontrolled severe asthma; suspected ectopic pregnancy (use other specific means of termination); chronic adrenal failure, porphyria (section 9.8.2)

Side-effects: nausea, vomiting, gastro-intestinal cramps; uterine contractions, vaginal bleeding (sometimes severe) may occur between administration of mifepristone and surgery (and rarely abortion may occur before surgery); *less commonly* hypersensitivity reactions including rash, urticaria, and facial oedema; *rarely* malaise, headache, fever, hot flushes, dizziness, chills

Dose: medical termination of intra-uterine pregnancy of up to 63 days gestation, *by mouth*, mifepristone 600 mg as a single dose under medical supervision, followed 36–48 hours later (unless abortion already complete) by gemeprost 1 mg *by vagina* and observed for at least 6 hours (or until bleeding or pain at acceptable level) with follow-up visit 10–14 days later to verify complete expulsion (if treatment fails essential that pregnancy be terminated by another method)

Softening and dilatation of cervix before mechanical cervical dilatation for termination of pregnancy, 36–48 hours before procedure, *by mouth*, mifepristone 600 mg as a single dose under medical supervision

Termination of pregnancy of 13–24 weeks gestation (in combination with gemeprost), *by mouth*, mifepristone 600 mg as a single dose under medical supervision followed 36–48 hours later by gemeprost 1 mg *by vagina* every 3 hours up to max. 5 mg; if abortion does not occur, 24 hours after start of treatment repeat course of gemeprost 1 mg *by vagina* up to max. 5 mg (if treatment fails pregnancy should be terminated by another method); follow-up visit after appropriate interval to assess vaginal bleeding recommended

NOTE. Careful monitoring essential for 6 hours after administration of gemeprost pessary (risk of profound hypotension)

Labour induction in fetal death *in utero*, *by mouth*, mifepristone 600 mg daily as a single dose for 2 days under medical supervision; if labour not started within 72 hours of first dose, another method should be used

Mifegyne® (Exelgyn) PoM
Tablets, yellow, mifepristone 200 mg. Net price 3-tab pack = £41.83 (supplied to NHS hospitals and premises approved under Abortion Act 1967). Label: 10, patient information leaflet

7.1.3 Myometrial relaxants

Tocolytic drugs postpone *premature labour* and they are used with the aim of reducing harm to the child. However, there is no satisfactory evidence that the use of these drugs reduces mortality. The greatest benefit is gained by using the delay to administer corticosteroid therapy or to implement other measures which improve perinatal health (including transfer to a unit with neonatal intensive care facility).

The oxytocin receptor antagonist, **atosiban**, is licensed for the inhibition of uncomplicated premature labour *between 24 and 33 weeks* of gestation. Atosiban may be preferable to a $beta_2$ agonist because it has fewer side-effects.

The dihydropyridine calcium-channel blocker **nifedipine** (section 2.6.2) also has fewer side-effects than a $beta_2$ agonist. Nifedipine [unlicensed indication] can be given initially in a dose of 20 mg followed by 10–20 mg 3–4 times daily adjusted according to uterine activity.

A $beta_2$ agonist (**ritodrine**, **salbutamol** or **terbutaline**) is used for inhibiting uncomplicated premature labour between 24 and 33 weeks of gestation and it may permit a delay in delivery of at least 48 hours. Prolonged therapy should be avoided since risks to the mother increase after 48 hours and there is a lack of evidence of benefit from further treatment; maintenance treatment is therefore **not recommended**.

Indometacin (indomethacin) (section 10.1.1), a cyclo-oxygenase inhibitor, also inhibits labour [unlicensed indication] and it may be useful in situations where a $beta_2$ agonist is not appropriate; however, there are concerns about neonatal complications such as transient impairment of renal function and premature closure of ductus arteriosus.

ATOSIBAN

Indications: uncomplicated premature labour (see notes above)

Cautions: monitor blood loss after delivery; intra-uterine growth retardation; hepatic impairment (Appendix 2); renal impairment (Appendix 3)

Contra-indications: eclampsia and severe pre-eclampsia, intra-uterine infection, intra-uterine fetal death, antepartum haemorrhage (requiring immediate delivery), placenta praevia, abruptio placenta, intra-uterine growth retardation with abnormal fetal heart rate, premature rupture of membranes after 30 weeks' gestation

Side-effects: nausea, vomiting, tachycardia, hypotension, headache, dizziness, hot flushes, hyperglycaemia, injection site reaction; less commonly pruritus, rash, fever, insomnia

Dose: *by intravenous injection*, initially 6.75 mg over 1 minute, then *by intravenous infusion* 18 mg/hour for 3 hours, then 6 mg/hour for up to 45 hours; max. duration of treatment 48 hours

Tractocile® (Ferring) PoM
Injection, atosiban (as acetate) 7.5 mg/mL, net price 0.9-mL (6.75-mg) vial = £18.60
Concentrate for intravenous infusion, atosiban (as acetate) 7.5 mg/mL, net price 5-mL vial = £53.35

RITODRINE HYDROCHLORIDE

Indications: uncomplicated premature labour (see notes above)

Cautions: suspected cardiac disease (physician experienced in cardiology to assess), hypertension, hyperthyroidism, hypokalaemia (special risk with potassium-depleting diuretics), diabetes mellitus (closely monitor blood glucose during intravenous treatment), mild to moderate pre-eclampsia, monitor blood pressure and pulse rate (should not exceed 140 beats per minute) and avoid over-hydration (Appendix 6); **important:** closely monitor state of hydration (discontinue immediately and institute diuretic therapy if pulmonary oedema occurs); concomitant beta-blocker treatment; drugs likely to enhance sympathomimetic side-effects or induce arrhythmias, see also **interactions**, Appendix 1 (sympathomimetics *and* sympathomimetics, $beta_2$)

Contra-indications: cardiac disease, eclampsia and severe pre-eclampsia, intra-uterine infection, intra-uterine fetal death, antepartum haemorrhage (requires immediate delivery), placenta praevia, cord compression

Side-effects: nausea, vomiting, flushing, sweating, tremor; hypokalaemia, tachycardia, palpitation, and hypotension (left lateral position throughout infusion to minimise risk), uterine bleeding (may be reversed with a non-selective beta-blocker); pulmonary oedema (see below and under Cautions); chest pain or tightness (with or without ECG changes) and arrhythmias reported; salivary gland enlargement also reported; on prolonged administration (several weeks) leucopenia and agranulocytosis reported; liver function abnormalities (including increased transaminases and hepatitis) reported

Dose: *by intravenous infusion* (**important:** minimum fluid volume, see below), initially 50 micrograms/minute, increased gradually according to response by 50 micrograms/minute every 10 minutes until contractions stop or maternal heart rate reaches 140 beats per minute; continue for 12–48 hours after contractions cease (usual rate 150–350 micrograms/minute); max. rate 350 micrograms/minute; or *by intramuscular injection*, 10 mg every 3–8 hours continued for 12–48 hours after contractions have ceased; then *by mouth* (but see notes above), 10 mg 30 minutes before termination of intravenous infusion, repeated every 2 hours for 24 hours, followed by 10–20 mg every 4–6 hours, max. oral dose 120 mg daily

IMPORTANT. Manufacturer states that although *fatal pulmonary oedema* associated with ritodrine infusion is almost certainly multifactorial in origin, evidence suggests that **fluid overload** may be the most important single factor. The volume of infusion should therefore be kept to a minimum; for further guidance see Appendix 6. For specific guidance on infusion rates, consult product literature

Yutopar® (Durbin) PoM
Tablets, yellow, scored, ritodrine hydrochloride 10 mg. Net price 90-tab pack = £25.55
Injection, ritodrine hydrochloride 10 mg/mL. Net price 5-mL amp = £2.98

SALBUTAMOL

Indications: uncomplicated premature labour (see notes above); asthma (section 3.1.1)

Cautions: see under Ritodrine Hydrochloride; **interactions:** Appendix 1 (sympathomimetics, $beta_2$)

Contra-indications: see under Ritodrine Hydrochloride

Side-effects: see under Ritodrine Hydrochloride; headache, rarely muscle cramps; hypersensitivity reactions including bronchospasm, urticaria, and angioedema reported

Dose: *by intravenous infusion*, initially 10 micrograms/minute, rate increased gradually according to response at 10-minute intervals until contractions diminish then increase rate slowly until contractions cease (max. rate 45 micrograms/minute); maintain rate for 1 hour after contractions have stopped, then gradually reduce by 50% every 6 hours; then *by mouth* (but see notes above), 4 mg every 6–8 hours

■ Preparations
Section 3.1.1.1

TERBUTALINE SULPHATE

Indications: uncomplicated premature labour (see notes above); asthma (section 3.1.1)

Cautions: see under Ritodrine Hydrochloride; **interactions:** Appendix 1 (sympathomimetics, $beta_2$)

Contra-indications: see under Ritodrine Hydrochloride
Side-effects: see under Ritodrine Hydrochloride
Dose: *by intravenous infusion*, 5 micrograms/minute for 20 minutes, increased every 20 minutes in steps of 2.5 micrograms/minute until contractions have ceased (more than 10 micrograms/minute should **seldom** be given—20 micrograms/minute should **not** be exceeded), continue for 1 hour then decrease every 20 minutes in steps of 2.5 micrograms/minute to lowest dose that maintains suppression, continue at this level for 12 hours then *by mouth* (but see notes above), 5 mg every 8 hours for as long as is desirable to prolong pregnancy (or alternatively follow the *intravenous infusion* by *subcutaneous injection* 250 micrograms every 6 hours for a few days then *by mouth* as above)

■ Preparations
Section 3.1.1.1

7.2 Treatment of vaginal and vulval conditions

Symptoms are often restricted to the vulva, but infections almost invariably involve the vagina which should also be treated. Applications to the vulva alone are likely to give only symptomatic relief without cure.

Aqueous medicated douches may disturb normal vaginal acidity and bacterial flora.

Topical anaesthetic agents give only symptomatic relief and may cause sensitivity reactions. They are indicated only in cases of pruritus where specific local causes have been excluded.

Systemic drugs are required in the treatment of infections such as gonorrhoea and syphilis (section 5.1).

7.2.1 Preparations for vaginal atrophy

Topical HRT

A cream containing an oestrogen may be applied on a short-term basis to improve the vaginal epithelium in *menopausal atrophic vaginitis*. It is **important** to bear in mind that topical oestrogens should be used in the **smallest effective** amount to minimise systemic effects. Modified-release vaginal tablets and an impregnated vaginal ring are now also available.

The risk of endometrial hyperplasia and carcinoma is increased when *systemic* oestrogens are administered alone for prolonged periods (section 6.4.1.1). The endometrial safety of long-term or repeated use of *topical* vaginal oestrogens is uncertain; treatment should be reviewed at least annually, with special consideration given to any symptoms of endometrial hyperplasia or carcinoma.

Topical oestrogens are also used in postmenopausal women before vaginal surgery for prolapse when there is epithelial atrophy.

For a general comment on hormone replacement therapy, including the role of topical oestrogens, see section 6.4.1.1.

OESTROGENS, TOPICAL

Indications: see notes above
Cautions: see notes above; see also Oestrogens for HRT (section 6.4.1.1); interrupt treatment periodically to assess need for continued treatment
Contra-indications: see notes above; see also Oestrogens for HRT (section 6.4.1.1); pregnancy and breast-feeding
Side-effects: see notes above; see also Oestrogens for HRT (section 6.4.1.1); local irritation

Ortho-Gynest® (Janssen-Cilag) PoM
Intravaginal cream, estriol 0.01%. Net price 80 g with applicator = £2.58
Excipients: include arachis (peanut) oil
Condoms: damages latex condoms and diaphragms
Dose: insert 1 applicatorful daily, preferably in evening; reduced to 1 applicatorful twice a week; attempts to reduce or discontinue should be made at 3–6 month intervals with re-examination
Pessaries, estriol 500 micrograms. Net price 15 pessaries = £5.03
Excipients: include butylated hydroxytoluene
Condoms: damages latex condoms and diaphragms
Dose: insert 1 pessary daily, preferably in the evening, until improvement occurs; maintenance 1 pessary twice a week; attempts to reduce or discontinue should be made at 3–6 month intervals with re-examination

Ovestin® (Organon) PoM
Intravaginal cream, estriol 0.1%. Net price 15 g with applicator = £4.63
Excipients: include cetyl alcohol, polysorbates, stearyl alcohol
Condoms: effect on latex condoms and diaphragms not yet known
Dose: insert 1 applicator-dose daily for 2–3 weeks, then reduce to twice a week (discontinue every 2–3 months for 4 weeks to assess need for further treatment); vaginal surgery, 1 applicator-dose daily for 2 weeks before surgery, resuming 2 weeks after surgery

Premarin® (Wyeth) PoM
Vaginal cream, conjugated oestrogens (equine) 625 micrograms/g. Net price 42.5 g with calibrated applicator = £2.19
Excipients: include cetyl alcohol, propylene glycol
Condoms: effect on latex condoms and diaphragms not yet known
Dose: insert 1–2 g daily starting on day 5 of cycle (or at any time if cycles have ceased) for 3 weeks, repeated after a 1-week interval

Vagifem® (Novo Nordisk) PoM
Vaginal tablets, f/c, m/r, estradiol 25 micrograms in disposable applicators. Net price 15-applicator pack = £7.28
Excipients: none as listed in section 13.1.3
Condoms: no evidence of damage to latex condoms and diaphragms
Dose: insert 1 tablet daily for 2 weeks then reduce to 1 tablet twice weekly; discontinue after 3 months to assess need for further treatment

■ Vaginal ring

Estring® (Pharmacia) PoM
Vaginal ring, releasing estradiol approx. 7.5 micrograms/24 hours. Net price 1-ring pack = £31.42. Label: 10, patient information leaflet
Dose: for postmenopausal urogenital conditions (not suitable for vasomotor symptoms or osteoporosis prophylaxis), to be inserted into upper third of vagina and worn continuously; replace after 3 months; max. duration of continuous treatment 2 years

Non-hormonal preparations

Non-hormonal vaginal preparations include *Replens MD*® which has an acid pH and provides a high moisture content for up to 3 days.

See section 7.2.2 for the pH-modifying preparation *Aci-jel*®.

7.2.2 Vaginal and vulval infections

Effective specific treatments are available for the common vaginal infections.

Fungal infections

Candidal vulvitis can be treated locally with cream but is almost invariably associated with vaginal infection which should also be treated. *Vaginal candidiasis* is treated primarily with antifungal pessaries or cream inserted high into the vagina (including during menstruation). Single-dose preparations offer an advantage when compliance is a problem. Local irritation may occur on application of vaginal antifungal products

Imidazole drugs (clotrimazole, econazole, fenticonazole, and miconazole) are effective in short courses of 3 to 14 days according to the preparation used. Vaginal applications may be supplemented with antifungal cream for vulvitis and to treat other superficial sites of infection.

Nystatin is a well established antifungal drug. One or two pessaries are inserted for 14 to 28 nights; a cream is also used in cases of vulvitis and infection of other superficial sites. Nystatin stains clothing yellow.

Oral treatment of vaginal infection with fluconazole or itraconazole (section 5.2) is also effective; oral ketoconazole has been associated with fatal hepatotoxicity (see section 5.2 for CSM warning).

RECURRENT VULVOVAGINAL CANDIDIASIS. Recurrence is particularly likely if there are predisposing factors such as antibacterial therapy, pregnancy, diabetes mellitus and possibly oral contraceptive use. Possible reservoirs of infection may also lead to recontamination and should be treated; these include other skin sites such as the digits, nail beds, and umbilicus as well as the gastro-intestinal tract and the bladder. The partner may also be the source of re-infection and, if symptomatic, should be treated with cream at the same time.

Treatment against candida may need to be extended for 6 months in recurrent vulvovaginal candidiasis. Some recommended regimens [all unlicensed] include:

- fluconazole (section 5.2) by mouth 100 mg (as a single dose) every week for 6 months
- clotrimazole vaginally 500-mg pessary (as a single dose) every week for 6 months
- itraconazole (section 5.2) by mouth 400 mg (as 2 divided doses on one day) every month for 6 months.

PREPARATIONS FOR VAGINAL AND VULVAL CANDIDIASIS

Side-effects: occasional local irritation

Clotrimazole (Non-proprietary)

Cream (topical), clotrimazole 1%, net price 20 g = £2.12, 50 g = £3.80

Condoms: effect on latex condoms and diaphragms not yet known

Dose: apply to anogenital area 2–3 times daily

Pessary, clotrimazole 500 mg, net price 1 pessary with applicator = £4.29

Dose: insert 1 at night as a single dose

Canesten® (Bayer Consumer Care)

Cream (topical), clotrimazole 1%. Net price 20 g = £2.14; 50 g = £3.80

Excipients: include benzyl alcohol, cetostearyl alcohol, polysorbates

Condoms: damages latex condoms and diaphragms

Dose: apply to anogenital area 2–3 times daily

Thrush Cream (topical), clotrimazole 2%, net price 20 g = £3.42

Excipients: include benzyl alcohol, cetostearyl alcohol, polysorbates

Condoms: damages latex condoms and diaphragms

Dose: apply to anogenital area 2–3 times daily

Vaginal cream (10% VC®*)* PoM, clotrimazole 10%. Net price 5-g applicator pack = £4.50

Excipients: include benzyl alcohol, cetostearyl alcohol, polysorbates

Condoms: damages latex condoms and diaphragms

Dose: insert 5 g at night as a single dose; may be repeated once if necessary

NOTE. Brands for sale to the public include *Canesten*® *Once*

Pessaries, clotrimazole 100 mg, net price 6 pessaries with applicator = £3.30; 200 mg, 3 pessaries with applicator = £3.30

Condoms: damages latex condoms and diaphragms

Dose: insert 200 mg for 3 nights *or* 100 mg for 6 nights

Pessary, clotrimazole 500 mg. Net price 1 with applicator = £3.25

Excipients: none as listed in section 13.1.3

Condoms: damages latex condoms and diaphragms

Dose: insert 1 at night as a single dose

Combi, clotrimazole 500-mg pessary and cream (topical) 2%. Net price 1 pessary and 10 g cream = £4.74

Condoms: damages latex condoms and diaphragms

Ecostatin® (Squibb)

Cream (topical), econazole nitrate 1%. Net price 15 g = £1.49; 30 g = £2.75

Excipients: include butylated hydroxyanisole, fragrance

Condoms: damages latex condoms and diaphragms

Dose: apply to anogenital area twice daily

Pessaries PoM, econazole nitrate 150 mg. Net price 3 with applicator = £3.35

Excipients: none as listed in section 13.1.3

Condoms: damages latex condoms and diaphragms

Dose: insert 1 pessary for 3 nights

Pessary (Ecostatin 1®*)* PoM, econazole nitrate 150 mg, formulated for single-dose therapy. Net price 1 pessary with applicator = £3.35

Excipients: none as listed in section 13.1.3

Condoms: damages latex condoms and diaphragms

Dose: insert 1 pessary at night as a single dose

Twinpack PoM, econazole nitrate 150-mg pessaries and cream 1%. Net price 3 pessaries and 15 g cream = £4.35

Condoms: damages latex condoms and diaphragms

Gyno-Daktarin® (Janssen-Cilag) PoM

Intravaginal cream, miconazole nitrate 2%. Net price 78 g with applicators = £4.70

Excipients: include butylated hydroxyanisole

Condoms: damages latex condoms and diaphragms

Dose: insert 5-g applicatorful once daily for 10–14 days *or* twice daily for 7 days; *topical*, apply to anogenital area twice daily

Pessaries, miconazole nitrate 100 mg. Net price 14 = £3.18
Excipients: none as listed in section 13.1.3
Condoms: damages latex condoms and diaphragms
Dose: insert 1 pessary daily for 14 days or 1 pessary twice daily for 7 days

Combipack, miconazole nitrate 100-mg pessaries and cream (topical) 2%. Net price 14 pessaries and 15 g cream = £4.13
Condoms: damages latex condoms and diaphragms

Ovule (= vaginal capsule) (*Gyno-Daktarin 1*®), miconazole nitrate 1.2 g in a fatty basis. Net price 1 ovule (with finger stall) = £3.18
Excipients: include hydroxybenzoates (parabens)
Condoms: damages latex condoms and diaphragms
Dose: insert 1 ovule at night as a single dose

Gyno-Pevaryl® (Janssen-Cilag) PoM

Cream, econazole nitrate 1%. Net price 15 g = £1.43; 30 g = £3.28
Excipients: none as listed in section 13.1.3
Condoms: damages latex condoms and diaphragms
Dose: insert 5-g applicatorful intravaginally and apply to vulva at night for at least 14 nights

Pessaries, econazole nitrate 150 mg. Net price 3 pessaries = £3.01
Excipients: none as listed in section 13.1.3
Condoms: damages latex condoms and diaphragms
Dose: ADULT and ADOLESCENT over 16 years, insert 1 pessary for 3 nights

Pessary (*Gyno-Pevaryl 1*®), econazole nitrate 150 mg, formulated for single-dose therapy. Net price 1 pessary with applicator = £3.20
Excipients: none as listed in section 13.1.3
Condoms: damages latex condoms and diaphragms
Dose: ADULT and ADOLESCENT over 16 years, insert 1 pessary at night as a single dose

Combipack, econazole nitrate 150-mg pessaries, econazole nitrate 1% cream. Net price 3 pessaries and 15 g cream = £4.13
Condoms: damages latex condoms and diaphragms

CP pack (*Gyno-Pevaryl 1*®), econazole nitrate 150-mg pessary, econazole nitrate 1% cream. Net price 1 pessary and 15 g cream = £4.13
Condoms: damages latex condoms and diaphragms

Nizoral® (Janssen-Cilag) PoM

Cream (topical), ketoconazole 2%. Net price 30 g = £3.62
Excipients: include polysorbates, propylene glycol, stearyl alcohol
Dose: apply to anogenital area once or twice daily

Nystan® (Squibb) PoM

Cream and *Ointment*, see section 13.10.2

Vaginal cream, nystatin 100 000 units/4-g application. Net price 60 g with applicator = £2.77
Excipients: include benzyl alcohol, propylene glycol
Condoms: damages latex condoms and diaphragms
Dose: insert 1–2 applicatorfuls at night for at least 14 nights

Pessaries, yellow, nystatin 100 000 units. Net price 28-pessary pack = £1.96
Excipients: none as listed in section 13.1.3
Condoms: no evidence of damage to latex condoms and diaphragms
Dose: insert 1–2 pessaries at night for at least 14 nights

Pevaryl® (Janssen-Cilag)

Cream, econazole nitrate 1%. Net price 30 g = £2.65
Excipients: include butylated hydroxyanisole, fragrance
Condoms: effect on latex condoms and diaphragms not yet known
Dose: apply to anogenital area twice daily

Other infections

Vaginal preparations intended to restore normal acidity (*Aci-Jel*®) may prevent recurrence of vaginal infections and permit the re-establishment of the normal vaginal flora.

Trichomonal infections commonly involve the lower urinary tract as well as the genital system and need systemic treatment with metronidazole or tinidazole (section 5.1.11).

Bacterial infections with Gram-negative organisms are particularly common in association with gynaecological operations and trauma. Metronidazole is effective against certain Gram-negative organisms, especially *Bacteroides* spp. and may be used prophylactically in gynaecological surgery.

Topical vaginal products containing povidone–iodine can be used to treat vaginitis due to candidal, trichomonal, non-specific or mixed infections; they are also used for the pre-operative preparation of the vagina. Clindamycin cream and metronidazole gel are also indicated for bacterial vaginosis; *Sultrin*® cream is licensed for the treatment of infections due to *Haemophilus vaginalis* only.

The antiviral drugs aciclovir, famciclovir and valaciclovir may be used in the treatment of genital infection due to *herpes simplex virus*, the HSV type 2 being a major cause of genital ulceration. They have a beneficial effect on virus shedding and healing, generally giving relief from pain and other symptoms. See section 5.3.2.1 for systemic preparations, and section 13.10.3 for topical preparations.

PREPARATIONS FOR OTHER VAGINAL INFECTIONS

Aci-Jel® (Janssen-Cilag)

Vaginal jelly, glacial acetic acid 0.94% in a buffered (pH 4) basis. Net price 85 g with applicator = £3.37
Excipients: include hydroxybenzoates (parabens), fragrance
Condoms: effect on latex condoms and diaphragms not yet known
Dose: non-specific infections, insert 1 applicatorful once or twice daily for up to 2 weeks to restore vaginal acidity

Betadine® (Medlock)

Cautions: avoid in pregnancy (Appendix 4) (also if planned) and in breast-feeding (Appendix 5); renal impairment (Appendix 3); avoid regular use in thyroid disorders
Side-effects: rarely sensitivity; may interfere with thyroid function

Vaginal Cleansing Kit, solution, povidone-iodine 10%. Net price 250 mL with measuring bottle and applicator = £2.79
Excipients: include fragrance
Condoms: effect on latex condoms and diaphragms not yet known
Dose: to be diluted and used once daily, preferably in the morning; may be used with *Betadine*® pessaries or vaginal gel

Pessaries, brown, povidone-iodine 200 mg. Net price 28 pessaries with applicator = £6.06
Condoms: effect on latex condoms and diaphragms not yet known

Dalacin® (Pharmacia) PoM

Cream, clindamycin 2% (as phosphate). Net price 40-g pack with 7 applicators = £10.86
Excipients: include benzyl alcohol, cetostearyl alcohol, polysorbates, propylene glycol
Condoms: damages latex condoms and diaphragms
Side-effects: irritation, cervicitis and vaginitis; poorly absorbed into the blood—very low likelihood of systemic effects (section 5.1.6)
Dose: bacterial vaginosis, insert 5-g applicatorful at night for 3–7 nights

Sultrin® (Janssen-Cilag) PoM

Cream, sulfathiazole 3.42%, sulfacetamide 2.86%, sulfabenzamide 3.7%. Net price 80 g with applicator = £3.31

Excipients: include arachis (peanut) oil, cetyl alcohol, hydroxybenzoates (parabens), propylene glycol, wool fat

Condoms: damages latex condoms and diaphragms

Cautions: absorption of sulphonamides may produce systemic effects

Contra-indications: pregnancy and breast-feeding; hypersensitivity to peanuts

Side-effects: sensitivity

Dose: bacterial vaginosis, insert 1 applicatorful of cream twice daily for 10 days, then once daily if necessary (but see also notes above)

Zidoval® (3M) PoM

Vaginal gel, metronidazole 0.75%. Net price 40-g pack with 5 applicators = £4.31

Excipients: include disodium edetate, hydroxybenzoates (parabens), propylene glycol

Cautions: not recommended during menstruation; some absorption may occur, see section 5.1.11 for systemic effects

Side-effects: local effects including irritation, candidiasis, abnormal discharge, pelvic discomfort

Dose: bacterial vaginosis, insert 5-g applicatorful at night for 5 nights

7.3 Contraceptives

Hormonal contraception is the most effective method of fertility control, but has major and minor side-effects, especially for certain groups of women.

Intra-uterine devices are a highly effective method of contraception but may produce undesirable local side-effects. They are most suitable for older parous women, but less appropriate for younger nulliparous women and for those with an increased risk of pelvic inflammatory disease.

Barrier methods alone (condoms, diaphragms, and caps) are less effective but can be very reliable for well-motivated couples if used in conjunction with a **spermicide**. Occasionally sensitivity reactions occur. A female condom (*Femidom*®) is also available; it is prelubricated but does not contain a spermicide.

7.3.1 Combined hormonal contraceptives

Oral contraceptives containing an oestrogen and a progestogen ('combined oral contraceptives') are the most effective preparations for general use. Advantages of combined oral contraceptives include:

- reliable and reversible;
- reduced dysmenorrhoea and menorrhagia;
- reduced incidence of premenstrual tension;
- less symptomatic fibroids and functional ovarian cysts;
- less benign breast disease;
- reduced risk of ovarian and endometrial cancer;
- reduced risk of pelvic inflammatory disease, which may be a risk with intra-uterine devices.

Combined oral contraceptives containing a fixed amount of an oestrogen and a progestogen in each active tablet are termed 'monophasic'; those with varying amounts of the two hormones according to the stage of the cycle are termed 'biphasic' and 'triphasic'. A transdermal patch containing an oestrogen with a progestogen is also available.

CHOICE. The oestrogen content of combined oral contraceptives ranges from 20 to 40 micrograms and generally a preparation with the lowest oestrogen and progestogen content which gives good cycle control and minimal side-effects in the individual woman is chosen.

- *Low strength preparations* (containing ethinylestradiol 20 micrograms) are particularly appropriate for women with risk factors for circulatory disease, provided a combined oral contraceptive is otherwise suitable. It is recommended that the combined oral contraceptive is not continued beyond 50 years of age since more suitable alternatives exist.
- *Standard strength preparations* (containing ethinylestradiol 30 or 35 micrograms or in 30–40 microgram *phased* preparations) are appropriate for standard use—but see Risk of Venous Thromboembolism below. Phased preparations are generally reserved for women who *either* do not have withdrawal bleeding *or* who have breakthrough bleeding with monophasic products.

The progestogens desogestrel, drospirenone, and gestodene (in combination with ethinylestradiol) may be considered for women who have side-effects (such as acne, headache, depression, weight gain, breast symptoms, and breakthrough bleeding) with other progestogens. However, women should be advised that desogestrel and gestodene have also been associated with an increased risk of *venous thromboembolism*. Drospirenone, a derivative of spironolactone, has anti-androgenic and anti-mineralocorticoid activity; it should be used with care if an increased concentration of potassium might be hazardous. The progestogen norelgestromin is combined with ethinylestradiol in a transdermal patch.

RISK OF VENOUS THROMBOEMBOLISM. There is an increased risk of venous thromboembolic disease (particularly during the first year) in users of oral contraceptives but this risk is considerably smaller than that associated with pregnancy (about 60 cases of venous thromboembolic disease per 100 000 pregnancies). In all cases the risk of venous thromboembolism increases with age and in the presence of other risk factors for venous thromboembolism (e.g. obesity). The risk of venous thromboembolism with transdermal patches is not yet known.

The incidence of venous thromboembolism in healthy, non-pregnant women who are not taking an oral contraceptive is about 5 cases per 100 000 women per year. For those using combined oral contraceptives containing second-generation progestogens e.g. levonorgestrel, this incidence is about 15 per 100 000 women per year of use. Some studies have reported a greater risk of venous thromboembolism in women using preparations containing the third-generation progestogens desogestrel and gestodene; the incidence in these women is about 25 per 100 000 women per year of use.

The absolute risk of venous thromboembolism in women using combined oral contraceptives containing these third-generation progestogens remains very small and well below the risk associated with pregnancy. Provided that women are informed of the relative risks of venous thromboembolism and accept them, the choice of oral contraceptive is for the woman together with the prescriber jointly to make in light of her individual medical history and any contra-indications.

TRAVEL. Women taking oral contraceptives, or using the patch are at an increased risk of deep-vein thrombosis during travel involving long periods of immobility (over 5 hours). The risk may be reduced by appropriate exercise during the journey and possibly by wearing elastic hosiery.

MISSED PILL. The critical time for loss of contraceptive protection is when a pill is omitted at the *beginning* or *end* of a cycle (which lengthens the pill-free interval).

If a woman forgets to take a pill, it should be taken as soon as she remembers, and the next one taken at the normal time. If the delay is 24 hours or longer with any pill (especially the first in the packet) the pill may not work. As soon as she remembers, she should continue taking the pill normally. However, she will not be protected for the next 7 days and must either not have sex or she should use another method of contraception such as a condom. If these 7 days run beyond the end of the packet, the next packet should be started at once, omitting the pill-free interval (or in the case of *everyday* (ED) pills, omitting the 7 inactive tablets).

Emergency contraception is recommended if more than 2 combined oral contraceptive tablets are missed from the first 7 tablets in a packet.

DELAYED APPLICATION OR DETACHED PATCH. If a patch is partly detached for less than 24 hours, reapply to the same site or replace with a new patch immediately; no additional contraception is needed and the next patch should be applied on the usual change day. If a patch remains detached for more than 24 hours or if the user is not aware when the patch became detached then stop the current contraceptive cycle and start a new cycle by applying a new patch, giving a new 'Day 1'; an additional non-hormonal contraceptive must be used concurrently for the first 7 days of the new cycle.

If application of a new patch at the start of a new cycle is delayed, contraceptive protection is lost. A new patch should be applied as soon as remembered giving a new 'Day 1'; additional non-hormonal methods of contraception should be used for the first 7 days of the new cycle. If intercourse has occurred during this extended patch-free interval, a possibility of fertilisation should be considered. If application of a patch in the middle of the cycle is delayed (i.e. the patch is not changed on day 8 or day 15):

- for up to 48 hours, apply a new patch immediately; next patch change day remains the same and no additional contraception is required.
- for more than 48 hours, contraceptive protection may have been lost. Stop the current cycle and start a new 4-week cycle immediately by applying a new patch giving a new 'Day 1'; additional non-hormonal contraception should be used for the first 7 days of the new cycle.

If the patch is not removed at the end of the cycle (day 22), remove it as soon as possble and start the next cycle on the usual 'change day', after day 28; no additional contraception is required.

DIARRHOEA AND VOMITING. Vomiting within 2 hours of taking an oral contraceptive *or* very severe diarrhoea can interfere with its absorption. Additional precautions should therefore be used during and for 7 days after recovery (see also under Missed Pill, above). If the vomiting and diarrhoea occurs during the last 7 tablets, the next pill-free interval should be omitted (in the case of ED tablets the inactive ones should be omitted).

INTERACTIONS. The effectiveness of both *combined* and *progestogen-only* oral contraceptives may be considerably reduced by interaction with drugs that induce hepatic enzyme activity (e.g. **carbamazepine**, **griseofulvin**, **modafinil**, **nelfinavir**, **nevirapine**, **oxcarbazepine**, **phenytoin**, **phenobarbital**, **ritonavir**, **topiramate**, and, above all, **rifabutin** and **rifampicin**). A condom with a long-acting method such as injectable contraceptive may be more suitable for patients with HIV infection or at risk of HIV infection and advice on the possibility of interaction with antiretroviral drugs should be sought from HIV specialists.

Family Planning Association (FPA) advice relating to a *short-term course of an enzyme-inducing drug* (for rifampicin and rifabutin, see also below) is that additional contraceptive precautions should be taken whilst taking the enzyme-inducing drug and for at least 7 days after stopping it; if these 7 days run beyond the end of a packet the new packet should be started immediately without a break (in the case of ED tablets the inactive ones should be omitted). It should be noted that **rifampicin** and **rifabutin** are such potent enzyme-inducing drugs that even if a course lasts for less than 7 days the additional contraceptive precautions should be continued for at least 4 weeks after stopping.

FPA advice relating to a *long-term course of an enzyme-inducing drug* (for rifampicin and rifabutin, see also below) in a woman unable to use an alternative method of contraception is to take a combination of oral contraceptives to provide a daily intake of ethinylestradiol 50 micrograms or more [unlicensed use]; 'tricycling' (i.e. taking 3 or 4 packets of monophasic tablets without a break followed by a short tablet-free interval of 4 days) is recommended [but women should be warned of uncertainty about the effectiveness of this regimen]. **Rifampicin** and **rifabutin** are such potent enzyme-inducing drugs that an alternative method of contraception (such as an IUD) is **always** recommended. Since the excretory function of the liver does not return to normal for several weeks after stopping an enzyme-inducing drug, FPA advice relating to *withdrawal* is that appropriate contraceptive measures are required for 4 to 8 weeks after stopping.

The effectiveness of contraceptive patches may also be reduced by drugs that induce hepatic enzyme activity. Additional contraceptive precautions are required whilst taking the enzyme-inducing drug and for 4 weeks after stopping. If concomitant administration runs beyond the 3 weeks of patch treatment, a new treatment cycle should be started immediately without a patch-free break. For women taking long term enzyme-inducing drugs another method of contraception should be considered.

Some **broad-spectrum antibacterials** (e.g. ampicillin, doxycycline) may reduce the efficacy of *combined* oral contraceptives by impairing the bacterial flora responsible for recycling of ethinylestradiol from the large bowel. FPA advice is that additional contraceptive precautions should be taken whilst taking a *short course of a broad-spectrum antibiotic* and for 7 days after stopping. If these 7 days run beyond the end of a packet the next packet should be started immediately without a break (in the case of ED tablets the inactive ones should be omitted). If the antibiotic course *exceeds 3 weeks*, the bacterial flora develops antibiotic resistance and additional precautions become unnecessary; additional precautions are also unnecessary if a woman starting a *combined* oral contraceptive has been on a course of antibiotics for 3 weeks or more.

It is possible that some antibacterials affect the efficacy of contraceptive patches. Additional contraceptive precautions are recommended during concomitant use and for 7 days after discontinuation of the antibacterial (except tetracycline). If concomitant administration runs beyond the 3 weeks of patch treatment, a new treatment cycle should be started immediately without a patch-free break.

SURGERY. Oestrogen-containing contraceptives should preferably be discontinued (and adequate alternative contraceptive arrangements made) 4 weeks before major elective surgery and all surgery to the legs or surgery which involves prolonged immobilisation of a lower limb; they should normally be recommenced at the first menses occurring at least 2 weeks after full mobilisation. A depot injection of a progestogen-only contraceptive may be offered and the oestrogen-containing contraceptive restarted later—if preferred before the next injection would be due. When discontinuation of an oestrogen-containing contraceptive is not possible, e.g. after trauma or if a patient admitted for an elective procedure is still on an oestrogen-containing contraceptive, thromboprophylaxis (with heparin and graduated compression hosiery) is advised. These recommendations do not apply to minor surgery with short duration of anaesthesia, e.g. laparoscopic sterilisation or tooth extraction, or to women using oestrogen-free hormonal contraceptives (whether by mouth or by injection).

REASON TO STOP IMMEDIATELY. Combined hormonal contraceptives or hormone replacement therapy (HRT) should be stopped (pending investigation and treatment), if any of the following occur:

- sudden severe chest pain (even if not radiating to left arm);
- sudden breathlessness (or cough with blood-stained sputum);
- unexplained severe pain in calf of one leg;
- severe stomach pain;
- serious neurological effects including unusual severe, prolonged headache especially if first time or getting progressively worse *or* sudden partial or complete loss of vision *or* sudden disturbance of hearing or other perceptual disorders *or* dysphasia *or* bad fainting attack or collapse *or* first unexplained epileptic seizure *or* weakness, motor disturbances, very marked numbness suddenly affecting one side or one part of body;
- hepatitis, jaundice, liver enlargement;
- blood pressure above systolic 160 mmHg and diastolic 100 mmHg;
- detection of a risk factor see Cautions and Contra-indications under Combined Hormonal Contraceptives;
- prolonged immobility after surgery or leg injury.

COMBINED HORMONAL CONTRACEPTIVES

Indications: contraception; menstrual symptoms (section 6.4.1.2)

Cautions: risk factors for venous thromboembolism (see below and also notes above), arterial disease and migraine, see below; hyperprolactinaemia (seek specialist advice); history of severe depression especially if induced by hormonal contraceptive, sickle-cell disease, inflammatory bowel disease including Crohn's disease; **interactions:** see above and Appendix 1 (oestrogens, progestogens)

RISK FACTORS FOR VENOUS THROMBOEMBOLISM. See also notes above. Use with **caution** if any of following factors present but **avoid** if two or more factors present:

- *family history of venous thromboembolism* in first-degree relative aged under 45 years (avoid contraceptive containing desogestrel or gestodene, *or* if known prothrombotic coagulation abnormality e.g. factor V Leiden or antiphospholipid antibodies (including lupus anticoagulant));
- *obesity*—body mass index above 30 kg/m^2 (avoid if body mass index above 39 kg/m^2);
- *long-term immobilisation* e.g. in a wheelchair (avoid if confined to bed or leg in plaster cast);
- *varicose veins* (avoid during sclerosing treatment or where definite history of thrombosis).

RISK FACTORS FOR ARTERIAL DISEASE. Use with **caution** if any one of following factors present but **avoid** if two or more factors present:

- *family history of arterial disease* in first degree relative aged under 45 years (avoid if atherogenic lipid profile);
- *diabetes mellitus* (avoid if diabetes complications present);
- *hypertension*—blood pressure above *systolic 140 mmHg* and *diastolic 90 mmHg* (avoid if blood pressure above *systolic 160 mmHg* and *diastolic 100 mmHg*);
- *smoking* (avoid if smoking 40 or more cigarettes daily);
- *age* over 35 years (avoid if over 50 years);
- *obesity* (avoid if body mass index above 39 kg/m^2);
- *migraine*—see below.

MIGRAINE. Women should report any increase in headache frequency or onset of focal symptoms (discontinue immediately and refer urgently to neurology expert if focal neurological symptoms not typical of aura persist for more than 1 hour—see also Reason to stop immediately in notes above); **contra-indicated** in

- migraine with typical focal aura,
- severe migraine regularly lasting over 72 hours despite treatment,
- migraine treated with ergot derivatives;

use with **caution** in

- migraine without focal aura,
- migraine controlled with $5HT_1$ agonist (section 4.7.4.1).

Contra-indications: pregnancy (Appendix 4); personal history of venous or arterial thrombosis, severe or multiple risk factors for arterial disease or for venous thromboembolism (see above), heart disease associated with pulmonary hypertension or risk of embolus; migraine (see above), transient cerebral ischaemic attacks without headaches; liver disease including disorders of hepatic excretion (e.g. Dubin-Johnson or Rotor syndromes), infective hepatitis (until liver function returns to normal); systemic lupus erythematosus; porphyria (section 9.8.2); liver adenoma; gallstones; after evacuation of hydatidiform mole (until return to normal of urine and plasma gonadotrophin concentration); history of haemolytic uraemic syndrome or history during pregnancy of pruritus, cholestatic jaundice, chorea or deterioration of otosclerosis, pemphigoid gestationis; breast or genital-tract carcinoma; undiagnosed vaginal bleeding; breast-feeding (until weaning or for 6 months after birth—Appendix 5)

Side-effects: nausea, vomiting, headache, breast tenderness, changes in body weight, fluid retention, thrombosis (more common when factor V Leiden present or in blood groups A, B, and AB; see also notes above), changes in libido, depression, chorea, skin reactions, chloasma, hypertension, contact lenses may irritate, impairment of liver function, hepatic tumours, reduced menstrual loss, 'spotting' in early cycles, absence of withdrawal bleeding; rarely photosensitivity

BREAST CANCER. There is a small increase in the risk of having breast cancer diagnosed in women taking the combined oral contraceptive pill; this relative risk may be due to an earlier diagnosis. In users of combined oral contraceptive pills the cancers are more likely to be localised to the breast. The most important factor for diagnosing breast cancer appears to be the age at which the contraceptive is stopped rather than the duration of use; any increase in the rate of diagnosis diminishes gradually during the 10 years after stopping and disappears by 10 years. The CSM has advised that a possible small increase in the risk of breast cancer should be weighed against the benefits and evidence of the protective effect against cancers of the ovary and endometrium

Dose: *by mouth*, each tablet should be taken at approximately same time each day; if delayed by longer than 12 hours contraceptive protection may be lost

21-day combined (monophasic) preparations, 1 tablet daily for 21 days; subsequent courses repeated after a 7-day interval (during which withdrawal bleeding occurs); first course usually started on day 1 of cycle—if starting on day 4 of cycle or later additional precautions (barrier methods) necessary during first 7 days

Every day (ED) combined (monophasic) preparations, 1 *active* tablet starting on day 1 of cycle (see also under preparations below)—if starting on day 4 of cycle or later additional precautions (barrier methods) necessary during first 7 days; withdrawal bleeding occurs when *inactive* tablets being taken; subsequent courses repeated without interval

Biphasic and triphasic preparations, see under individual preparations below

CHANGING TO COMBINED PREPARATION CONTAINING DIFFERENT PROGESTOGEN. *21-day combined preparations:* continue current pack until last tablet and start first tablet of new brand the next day. If a 7-day break is taken before starting new brand, additional precautions (barrier methods) should be used during first 7 days of taking the new brand. *Every Day (ED) combined preparations:* start the new brand (first tablet of a *21-day preparation* or the first *active* tablet of an *ED preparation*) the day after taking the last *active* tablet of previous brand (omitting the *inactive* tablets).

CHANGING FROM PROGESTOGEN-ONLY TABLET. Start on day 1 of menstruation or any day if amenorrhoea present and pregnancy has been excluded.

SECONDARY AMENORRHOEA (EXCLUDE PREGNANCY). Start any day, additional precautions (barrier methods) necessary during first 7 days.

AFTER CHILDBIRTH (NOT BREAST-FEEDING). Start 3 weeks after birth (increased risk of thrombosis if started earlier); later than 3 weeks postpartum additional precautions (barrier methods) necessary for first 7 days.

Not recommended if woman breast-feeding—oral progestogen-only contraceptive preferred.

AFTER ABORTION OR MISCARRIAGE. Start same day.

By transdermal application, apply first patch on day 1 of cycle, change patch on days 8 and 15; remove third patch on day 22 and apply new patch after 7-day patch-free interval to start subsequent contraceptive cycle

CHANGING FROM COMBINED ORAL CONTRACEPTIVE. Apply patch on the first day of withdrawal bleeding; if no withdrawal bleeding within 5 days of taking last *active* tablet, rule out pregnancy before applying first patch. Unless patch is applied on first day of withdrawal bleeding, additional precautions (barrier methods) should be used concurrently for first 7 days

CHANGING FROM PROGESTOGEN-ONLY METHOD. From an implant, apply first patch on the day implant removed; from an injection, apply first patch when next injection due; from oral progestogen, first patch may be started on any day after stopping pill. For all methods additional precautions (barrier methods) should be used concurrently for first 7 days

AFTER CHILDBIRTH (NOT BREAST-FEEDING). Start 4 weeks after birth; if started later than 4 weeks after birth additional precautions (barrier methods) should be used for first 7 days

AFTER ABORTION OR MISCARRIAGE. Before 20 weeks' gestation start immediately; no additional contraception required if started immediately. After 20 weeks' gestation start on day 21 after abortion or on the first day of first spontaneous menstruation; additional precautions (barrier methods) should be used for first 7 days after applying the patch

Low strength (oral)

■ Ethinylestradiol with Norethisterone

Loestrin 20® (Galen) PoM

Tablets, norethisterone acetate 1 mg, ethinylestradiol 20 micrograms. Net price 3 × 21-tab pack = £2.70

Dose: 1 tablet daily for 21 days; subsequent courses repeated after 7-day tablet-free interval (during which withdrawal bleeding occurs); for starting routines see under Dose above

■ Ethinylestradiol with Desogestrel

See Risk of venous thromboembolism in notes above before prescribing

Mercilon® (Organon) PoM

Tablets, desogestrel 150 micrograms, ethinylestradiol 20 micrograms. Net price 3 × 21-tab pack = £7.97

Dose: 1 tablet daily for 21 days; subsequent courses repeated after 7-day tablet-free interval (during which withdrawal bleeding occurs); for starting routines see under Dose above

■ Ethinylestradiol with Gestodene

See Risk of venous thromboembolism in notes above before prescribing

Femodette® (Schering Health) PoM

Tablets, s/c, gestodene 75 micrograms, ethinylestradiol 20 micrograms, net price 3 × 21-tab pack = £9.00

Dose: 1 tablet daily for 21 days; subsequent courses repeated after 7-day tablet-free interval (during which withdrawal bleeding occurs); for starting routines see under Dose above

Low strength (transdermal)

■ Ethinylestradiol with Norelgestromin

Evra® (Janssen-Cilag) ▼ PoM

Patches, self-adhesive (releasing ethinylestradiol approx. 20 micrograms/24 hours and norelgestromin approx. 150 micrograms/24 hours); net price 9-patch pack = £16.26. Counselling, administration

Dose: 1 patch to be applied once weekly for three weeks, followed by a 7-day patch-free interval; subsequent courses repeated after 7-day patch-free interval (during which withdrawal bleeding occurs); for starting routines see under Dose above

NOTE. Adhesives or bandages should not be used to hold patch in place. If patch no longer sticky do not reapply but use a new patch.

The *Scottish Medicines Consortium* has advised (September 2003) that *Evra*® patches should be restricted for use in women who are likely to comply poorly with combined oral contraceptives

Standard strength

■ Ethinylestradiol with Levonorgestrel

Logynon® (Schering Health) PoM

6 light brown tablets, ethinylestradiol 30 micrograms, levonorgestrel 50 micrograms;

5 white tablets, ethinylestradiol 40 micrograms, levonorgestrel 75 micrograms;

10 ochre tablets, ethinylestradiol 30 micrograms, levonorgestrel 125 micrograms.

Net price 3 × 21-tab pack = £3.92

Dose: 1 tablet daily for 21 days, starting with light brown tablet marked 1 on day 1 of cycle; repeat after 7-day tablet-free interval

Logynon ED® (Schering Health) PoM

6 light brown tablets, ethinylestradiol 30 micrograms, levonorgestrel 50 micrograms;

5 white tablets, ethinylestradiol 40 micrograms, levonorgestrel 75 micrograms;

10 ochre tablets, ethinylestradiol 30 micrograms, levonorgestrel 125 micrograms;

7 white, inactive tablets.

Net price 3 × 28-tab pack = £3.92

Dose: 1 tablet daily for 28 days, starting on day 1 of cycle with active tablet (withdrawal bleeding occurs when inactive tablets being taken); subsequent courses repeated without interval; for starting routines see under Dose above

Microgynon 30® (Schering Health) PoM

Tablets, s/c, levonorgestrel 150 micrograms, ethinylestradiol 30 micrograms. Net price 3 × 21-tab pack = £2.82

Dose: 1 tablet daily for 21 days; subsequent courses repeated after 7-day tablet-free interval (during which withdrawal bleeding occurs); for starting routines see under Dose above

Microgynon 30 ED® (Schering Health) PoM

Tablets, beige, levonorgestrel 150 micrograms, ethinylestradiol 30 micrograms, white inactive tablets. Net price 3 × 28-tab (7 are inactive) pack = £2.56

Dose: 1 tablet daily for 28 days starting on day 1 of cycle with active tablet (withdrawal bleeding occurs when inactive tablets being taken); subsequent courses repeated without interval; for starting routines see also under Dose above

Ovranette® (Wyeth) PoM

Tablets, levonorgestrel 150 micrograms, ethinylestradiol 30 micrograms. Net price 3 × 21-tab pack = £2.29

Dose: 1 tablet daily for 21 days; subsequent courses repeated after 7-day tablet-free interval (during which withdrawal bleeding occurs); for starting routines see under Dose above

Trinordiol® (Wyeth) PoM

6 light brown tablets, ethinylestradiol 30 micrograms, levonorgestrel 50 micrograms;

5 white tablets, ethinylestradiol 40 micrograms, levonorgestrel 75 micrograms;

10 ochre tablets, ethinylestradiol 30 micrograms, levonorgestrel 125 micrograms.

Net price 3 × 21-tab pack = £4.04

Dose: 1 tablet daily for 21 days, starting with light brown tablet marked 1 on day 1 of cycle; repeat after 7-day tablet-free interval

■ Ethinylestradiol with Norethisterone

BiNovum® (Janssen-Cilag) PoM

7 white tablets, ethinylestradiol 35 micrograms, norethisterone 500 micrograms;

14 peach tablets, ethinylestradiol 35 micrograms, norethisterone 1mg.

Net price 3 × 21-tab pack = £2.13

Dose: 1 tablet daily for 21 days, starting with white tablet on day 1 of cycle; repeat after 7-day tablet-free interval

Brevinor® (Pharmacia) PoM

Tablets, blue, norethisterone 500 micrograms, ethinylestradiol 35 micrograms. Net price 3 × 21-tab pack = £1.99

Dose: 1 tablet daily for 21 days; subsequent courses repeated after 7-day tablet-free interval (during which withdrawal bleeding occurs); for starting routines see under Dose above

Loestrin 30® (Galen) PoM

Tablets, norethisterone acetate 1.5 mg, ethinylestradiol 30 micrograms. Net price 3 × 21-tab pack = £3.90

Dose: 1 tablet daily for 21 days; subsequent courses repeated after 7-day tablet-free interval (during which withdrawal bleeding occurs); for starting routines see under Dose above

Norimin® (Pharmacia) PoM

Tablets, norethisterone 1 mg, ethinylestradiol 35 micrograms. Net price 3 × 21-tab pack = £2.28

Dose: 1 tablet daily for 21 days; subsequent courses repeated after 7-day tablet-free interval (during which withdrawal bleeding occurs); for starting routines see under Dose above

Ovysmen® (Janssen-Cilag) PoM

Tablets, norethisterone 500 micrograms, ethinylestradiol 35 micrograms. Net price 3 × 21-tab pack = £1.62

Dose: 1 tablet daily for 21 days; subsequent courses repeated after 7-day tablet-free interval (during which withdrawal bleeding occurs); for starting routines see under Dose above

Synphase® (Pharmacia) PoM
7 blue tablets, ethinylestradiol 35 micrograms, norethisterone 500 micrograms;
9 white tablets, ethinylestradiol 35 micrograms, norethisterone 1 mg;
5 blue tablets, ethinylestradiol 35 micrograms, norethisterone 500 micrograms.
Net price 21-tab pack = £1.20
Dose: 1 tablet daily for 21 days, starting with blue tablet marked 1 on day 1 of cycle; repeat after 7-day tablet-free interval

TriNovum® (Janssen-Cilag) PoM
7 white tablets, ethinylestradiol 35 micrograms, norethisterone 500 micrograms;
7 light peach tablets, ethinylestradiol 35 micrograms, norethisterone 750 micrograms;
7 peach tablets, ethinylestradiol 35 micrograms, norethisterone 1 mg.
Net price 3 × 21-tab pack = £2.95
Dose: 1 tablet daily for 21 days, starting with white tablet on day 1 of cycle; repeat after 7-day tablet-free interval

■ Ethinylestradiol with Norgestimate

Cilest® (Janssen-Cilag) PoM
Tablets, blue, norgestimate 250 micrograms, ethinylestradiol 35 micrograms. Net price 3 × 21-tab pack = £6.10, 6 × 21-tab pack = £12.20
Dose: 1 tablet daily for 21 days; subsequent courses repeated after 7-day tablet-free interval (during which withdrawal bleeding occurs); for starting routines see under Dose above

■ Ethinylestradiol with Desogestrel

See Risk of venous thromboembolism in notes above before prescribing

Marvelon® (Organon) PoM
Tablets, desogestrel 150 micrograms, ethinylestradiol 30 micrograms. Net price 3 × 21-tab pack = £6.70
Dose: 1 tablet daily for 21 days; subsequent courses repeated after 7-day tablet-free interval (during which withdrawal bleeding occurs); for starting routines see under Dose above

■ Ethinylestradiol with Drospirenone

Yasmin® (Schering Health) PoM
Tablets, f/c, yellow, drospirenone 3 mg, ethinylestradiol 30 micrograms. Net price 3 × 21-tab pack = £14.70
Dose: 1 tablet daily for 21 days; subsequent courses repeated after 7-day tablet-free interval (during which withdrawal bleeding occurs); for starting routines see under Dose above
The *Scottish Medicines Consortium* has advised (March 2003) that *Yasmin*® is not recommended

■ Ethinylestradiol with Gestodene

See Risk of venous thromboembolism in notes above before prescribing

Femodene® (Schering Health) PoM
Tablets, s/c, gestodene 75 micrograms, ethinylestradiol 30 micrograms. Net price 3 × 21-tab pack = £6.84
Dose: 1 tablet daily for 21 days; subsequent courses repeated after 7-day tablet-free interval (during which withdrawal bleeding occurs); for starting routines see under Dose above

Femodene® **ED** (Schering Health) PoM
Tablets, s/c, gestodene 75 micrograms, ethinylestradiol 30 micrograms. Net price 3 × 28-tab (7 are inactive) pack = £6.84
Dose: 1 tablet daily for 28 days, starting on day 1 of cycle with active tablet (withdrawal bleeding occurs when inactive tablets being taken); subsequent courses repeated without interval; for starting routines see under Dose above

Minulet® (Wyeth) PoM
Tablets, gestodene 75 micrograms, ethinylestradiol 30 micrograms. Net price 3 × 21-tab pack = £6.36
Dose: 1 tablet daily for 21 days; subsequent courses repeated after 7-day tablet-free interval (during which withdrawal bleeding occurs); for starting routines see under Dose above

Triadene® (Schering Health) PoM
6 beige tablets, ethinylestradiol 30 micrograms, gestodene 50 micrograms;
5 dark brown tablets, ethinylestradiol 40 micrograms, gestodene 70 micrograms;
10 white tablets, ethinylestradiol 30 micrograms, gestodene 100 micrograms.
Net price 3 × 21-tab pack = £9.54
Dose: 1 tablet daily for 21 days, starting with beige tablet marked 'start' on day 1 of cycle; repeat after 7-day tablet-free interval

Tri-Minulet® (Wyeth) PoM
6 beige tablets, ethinylestradiol 30 micrograms, gestodene 50 micrograms;
5 dark brown tablets, ethinylestradiol 40 micrograms, gestodene 70 micrograms;
10 white tablets, ethinylestradiol 30 micrograms, gestodene 100 micrograms.
Net price 3 × 21-tab pack = £8.87
Dose: 1 tablet daily for 21 days, starting with beige tablet marked '1' on day 1 of the cycle; repeat after 7-day tablet-free interval

■ Mestranol with Norethisterone

Norinyl-1® (Pharmacia) PoM
Tablets, norethisterone 1 mg, mestranol 50 micrograms. Net price 3 × 21-tab pack = £2.19
Dose: 1 tablet daily for 21 days; subsequent courses repeated after 7-day tablet-free interval (during which withdrawal bleeding occurs); for starting routines see under Dose above

■ Ethinylestradiol with cyproterone acetate

See co-cyprindiol (section 13.6.2)

Emergency contraception

Hormonal methods

Hormonal emergency contraception involves the use of **levonorgestrel**. It is effective if dose is taken within 72 hours (3 days) of unprotected intercourse; taking the dose as soon as possible increases efficacy. Levonorgestrel may also be used between 72 and 120 hours after unprotected intercourse [unlicensed use] but efficacy decreases with time. Hormonal emergency contraception is less effective than insertion of an intra-uterine device (see below).

If vomiting occurs within 3 hours of taking levonorgestrel, a replacement dose can be given. If an anti-emetic is required domperidone is preferred.

When prescibing hormonal emergency contraception the doctor should explain:

- that the next period may be early or late;
- that a barrier method of contraception needs to be used until the next period;
- the need to return promptly if any lower abdominal pain occurs because this could signify an ectopic pregnancy (and also in 3 to 4 weeks if the subsequent menstrual bleed is abnormally light, heavy or brief, or is absent, or if she is otherwise concerned).

Intra-uterine pregnancy despite treatment: see Appendix 4 (levonorgestrel).

INTERACTIONS. The effectiveness of the hormonal method of emergency contraception is reduced by enzyme-inducing drugs; a copper intra-uterine device may be offered or, otherwise, the dose of levonorgestrel should be increased to a total of 2.25 mg (1.5 mg taken immediately and 750 micrograms taken 12 hours later) [unlicensed dose]. There is no need to increase the dose for emergency contraception if the patient is taking antibacterials that are not enzyme inducers.

LEVONORGESTREL

Indications: emergency contraception

Cautions: see notes above; past ectopic pregnancy, severe malabsorption syndromes, severe liver disease (Appendix 2), pregnancy (see notes above and Appendix 4); breast-feeding (Appendix 5); **interactions:** see notes above and Appendix 1 (progestogens)

Contra-indications: porphyria (section 9.8.2)

Side-effects: menstrual irregularities (see also notes above), nausea, low abdominal pain, fatigue, headache, dizziness, breast tenderness, vomiting

Dose: 1.5 mg as a single dose as soon as possible after coitus (preferably within 12 hours but no later than after 72 hours)

[1]**Levonelle® One Step** (Schering Health)
Tablets, levonorgestrel 1.5 mg, net price 1-tab pack = £13.83

1. Can be sold to women over 16 years when supplying emergency contraception to the public, pharmacists should refer to guidance issued by the Royal Pharmaceutical Society of Great Britain

Levonelle®-2 (Schering Health) PoM
Tablets, levonorgestrel 750 micrograms, net price 2-tab pack = £5.11

Intra-uterine device

Insertion of an intra-uterine device is more effective than the hormonal methods of emergency contraception. A copper intra-uterine contraceptive device (section 7.3.4) can be inserted up to 120 hours (5 days) after unprotected intercourse; sexually transmitted diseases should be tested for and insertion of the device should usually be covered by antibacterial prophylaxis (e,g, azithromycin 1 g as a single dose). If intercourse has occurred more than 5 days previously, the device can still be inserted up to 5 days after the earliest likely calculated ovulation (i.e. within the minimum period before implantation).

7.3.2 Progestogen-only contraceptives

7.3.2.1 Oral progestogen-only contraceptives

Oral progestogen-only preparations may offer a suitable alternative when oestrogens are contra-indicated (including those patients with venous thrombosis or a past history or predisposition to venous thrombosis), but have a higher failure rate than combined preparations. They are suitable for older women, for heavy smokers, and for those with hypertension, valvular heart disease, diabetes mellitus, and migraine. Menstrual irregularities (oligomenorrhoea, menorrhagia) are more common but tend to resolve on long-term treatment.

INTERACTIONS. Effectiveness of oral progestogen-only preparations is not affected by broad-spectrum antibiotics but is reduced by enzyme-inducing drugs and appropriate contraceptive measures are required for at least 4 weeks after stopping the enzyme-inducing drug—see p. 407 and Appendix 1 (progestogens).

SURGERY. All progestogen-only contraceptives (including those given by injection) are suitable for use as an alternative to combined oral contraceptives before major elective surgery, before all surgery to the legs, or before surgery which involves prolonged immobilisation of a lower limb.

STARTING ROUTINE. One tablet daily, on a continuous basis, starting on day 1 of cycle and taken at the same time each day (if delayed by longer than 3 hours contraceptive protection may be lost). Additional contraceptive precautions are not necessary when initiating treatment.

Changing from a combined oral contraceptive: start on the day following completion of the combined oral contraceptive course without a break (or in the case of ED tablets omitting the inactive ones).

After childbirth: start any time after 3 weeks postpartum (increased risk of breakthrough bleeding if started earlier)—lactation is not affected.

MISSED PILL. The following advice is now recommended by family planning organisations:

> 'If you forget a pill, take it as soon as you remember and carry on with the next pill at the right time. If the pill was more than 3 hours (12 hours for *Cerazette*®) overdue you are not protected. Continue normal pill-taking but you must also use another method, such as the condom, for the next 2 days.'

The Faculty of Family Planning and Reproductive Health Care recommends emergency contraception (see p. 411) if one or more progestogen-only contraceptive tablets are missed or taken more than 3 hours late and intercourse has occurred before 2 further tablets have been correctly taken.

DIARRHOEA AND VOMITING. Vomiting within 2 hours after taking an oral contraceptive *or* very severe diarrhoea can interfere with its absorption. Additional precautions should be used during and for 2 days after recovery.

ORAL PROGESTOGEN-ONLY CONTRACEPTIVES

(Progestogen-only pill, 'POP')

Indications: contraception

Cautions: heart disease, sex-steroid dependent cancer, past ectopic pregnancy, malabsorption syndromes, functional ovarian cysts, active liver disease, recurrent cholestatic jaundice, history of jaundice in pregnancy; **interactions:** p. 407 and Appendix 1 (progestogens)

OTHER CONDITIONS. The product literature advises caution in patients with history of thromboembolism, hypertension, diabetes mellitus and migraine; evidence for caution in these conditions is unsatisfactory

Contra-indications: pregnancy, undiagnosed vaginal bleeding; severe arterial disease; liver adenoma, porphyria (section 9.8.2); after evacuation of hydatidiform mole (until return to normal of urine and plasma gonadotrophin values); history of breast cancer but may be used after 5 years if no evidence of current disease

Side-effects: menstrual irregularities (see also notes above); nausea, vomiting, headache, dizziness, breast discomfort, depression, skin disorders, disturbance of appetite, weight changes, changes in libido

BREAST CANCER. There is a small increase in the risk of having breast cancer diagnosed in women using, or who have recently used, a progestogen-only contraceptive pill; this relative risk may be due to an earlier diagnosis. The most important risk factor appears to be the age at which the contraceptive is stopped rather than the duration of use; the risk disappears gradually during the 10 years after stopping and there is no excess risk by 10 years. The CSM has advised that a possible small increase in the risk of breast cancer should be weighed against the benefits

Dose: 1 tablet daily at same time each day, starting on day 1 of cycle then continuously; if administration delayed for 3 hours (12 hours for *Cerazette*®) or more it should be regarded as a 'missed pill', see notes above

Cerazette® (Organon) ▼ PoM

Tablets, f/c, desogestrel 75 micrograms. Net price 3 × 28-tab pack = £8.85

The *Scottish Medicines Consortium* has advised (September 2003) that *Cerazette*® should be restricted for use in women who cannot tolerate oestrogen-containing contraceptives or in whom these preparations are contra-indicated

Femulen® (Pharmacia) PoM

Tablets, etynodiol diacetate 500 micrograms. Net price 3 × 28-tab pack = £3.31

Micronor® (Janssen-Cilag) PoM

Tablets, norethisterone 350 micrograms. Net price 3 × 28-tab pack = £1.80

Microval® (Wyeth) PoM

Tablets, levonorgestrel 30 micrograms. Net price 35-tab pack = 84p

Norgeston® (Schering Health) PoM

Tablets, s/c, levonorgestrel 30 micrograms. Net price 35-tab pack = 98p

Noriday® (Pharmacia) PoM

Tablets, norethisterone 350 micrograms. Net price 3 × 28-tab pack = £2.10

7.3.2.2 Parenteral progestogen-only contraceptives

Medroxyprogesterone acetate (*Depo-Provera*®) is a long-acting progestogen given by intramuscular injection; it is as effective as the combined oral preparations but because of its prolonged action it should never be given without *full counselling backed by the patient information leaflet.* It may be used as a short-term or long-term contraceptive for women who have been counselled about the likelihood of menstrual disturbance and the potential for a delay in return to full fertility. Delayed return of fertility and irregular cycles may occur after discontinuation of treatment but there is no evidence of permanent infertility. Heavy bleeding has been reported in patients given medroxyprogesterone acetate in the immediate puerperium (the first dose is best delayed until 6 weeks after birth). If the woman is not breast-feeding, the first injection may be given within 5 days postpartum (she should be warned that the risk of heavy or prolonged bleeding may be increased).

Reduction in bone mineral density and rare cases of osteoporosis and osteoporotic fractures have also been reported. The reduction in bone mineral density occurs in the first 2–3 years of use and then stabilises. See also CSM advice below.

CSM advice. The CSM has advised that:

- in adolescents, medroxyprogesterone acetate (*Depo-Provera*®) be used only when other methods of contraception are inappropriate;
- in all women, benefits of using medroxyprogesterone acetate beyond 2 years should be evaluated against risks;
- in women with risk factors for osteoporosis an alternative method of contraception instead of medroxyprogesterone acetate should be considered.

Norethisterone enantate (*Noristerat*®) is a long-acting progestogen given as an oily injection which provides contraception for 8 weeks; it is used as short-term interim contraception e.g. before vasectomy becomes effective. The **cautions** and **contra-indications** of oral progestogen-only contraceptives apply except that because the injection also reliably inhibits ovulation, it protects against ectopic pregnancy and functional ovarian cysts.

An **etonogestrel-releasing implant** (*Implanon*®), consisting of a single flexible rod, is also available; the rod is inserted subdermally into the lower surface of the upper arm and it provides effective contraception for up to 3 years. In women with a body mass index greater than 35 kg/m^2, blood etonogestrel concentrations are lower and therefore the implant may not provide effective contraception during the third year; earlier replacement should be considered in such patients. Local reactions such as bruising and itching may occur at the insertion site. The **cautions**, **contra-indications** and **side-effects** of oral preparations apply; the contraceptive effect of *Implanon*® is rapidly reversed on removal of the implant. *The doctor or nurse administering (or removing) the system should be fully trained in the technique and should provide full counselling backed by the patient information leaflet.*

The **levonorgestrel-releasing implant system** (*Norplant*®, Hoechst Marion Roussel) was discontinued in October 1999; any system still in place should have been removed by the end of 2004.

INTERACTIONS. Effectiveness of parenteral progestogen-only contraceptives is not affected by broad-spectrum antibiotics. However, effectiveness of norethisterone and etonogestrel (but not medroxyprogesterone acetate) may be reduced by enzyme-inducing drugs; alternative contraceptive method should be considered or an additional contraceptive method used while the enzyme-inducing drug is being taken.

PARENTERAL PROGESTOGEN-ONLY CONTRACEPTIVES

Indications: contraception, see also notes above and under preparations (roles vary according to preparation)

Cautions: see notes above and under preparations; possible risk of breast cancer, see oral progestogen-only contraceptives (section 7.3.2.1); history during pregnancy of pruritus or of deterioration of otosclerosis, disturbances of lipid metabolism; **interactions:** see notes above and Appendix 1 (progestogens)

COUNSELLING. Full counselling backed by *patient information leaflet* required before administration

Contra-indications: see notes above; history of breast cancer

Side-effects: see notes above; injection-site reactions

Dose: see under preparations

■ Injectable preparations

Depo-Provera® (Pharmacia) PoM

Injection (aqueous suspension), medroxyprogesterone acetate 150 mg/mL, net price 1-mL prefilled syringe = £5.01, 1-mL vial = £5.01. Counselling, see patient information leaflet

Dose: by deep intramuscular injection, 150 mg within first 5 days of cycle or within first 5 days after parturition (delay until 6 weeks after parturition if breast-feeding); for long-term contraception, repeated every 12 weeks (if interval greater than 12 weeks and 5 days, rule out pregnancy before next injection and advise patient to use additional contraceptive measures (e.g. barrier) for 14 days after the injection)

Noristerat® (Schering Health) PoM

Injection (oily), norethisterone enantate 200 mg/mL. Net price 1-mL amp = £3.59. Counselling, see patient information leaflet

Dose: by deep intramuscular injection given very slowly *into gluteal muscle,* short-term contraception, 200 mg within first 5 days of cycle or immediately after parturition (duration 8 weeks); may be repeated once after 8 weeks (withhold breast-feeding for neonates with severe or persistent jaundice requiring medical treatment)

■ Implants

Implanon® (Organon) PoM

Implant, containing etonogestrel 68 mg in each flexible rod, net price = £90.00. Counselling, see patient information leaflet

Dose: by subdermal implantation, no previous hormonal contraceptive, 1 implant inserted during first 5 days of cycle; parturition or abortion in second trimester, 1 implant inserted between days 21–28 after delivery or abortion (if inserted after 28 days additional precautions necessary for next 7 days); abortion in first trimester, 1 implant inserted immediately; changing from an oral contraceptive, consult product literature; remove within 3 years of insertion

7.3.2.3 Intra-uterine progestogen-only device

The progestogen-only intra-uterine system, *Mirena*®, releases **levonorgestrel** directly into the uterine cavity. It is licensed for use as a contraceptive, for the treatment of primary menorrhagia and for the prevention of endometrial hyperplasia during oestrogen replacement therapy. This may therefore be a contraceptive method of choice for women who have excessively heavy menses. The effects of the intra-uterine system are mainly local and hormonal including prevention of endometrial proliferation, thickening of cervical mucus, and suppression of ovulation in some women (in some cycles). In addition to the progestogenic activity, the intra-uterine system itself may contribute slightly to the contraceptive effect. Return of fertility after removal is rapid and appears to be complete. Advantages over copper intra-uterine devices are that there may be an improvement in any dysmenorrhoea and a reduction in blood loss; there is also evidence that the frequency of pelvic inflammatory disease may be reduced (particularly in the youngest age groups who are most at risk).

In primary menorrhagia, menstrual bleeding is reduced significantly within 3–6 months of inserting the levonogestrel intra-uterine system, probably because it prevents endometrial proliferation. Another treatment should be considered if menorrhagia does not improve within this period (section 6.4.1.2).

Generally the **cautions** and **contra-indications** are as for standard intra-uterine devices (section 7.3.4) but the risk of ectopic pregnancy is considerably smaller. Moreover, since the progestogen is released close to the site of the main contraceptive action (on cervical mucus and endometrium) progestogenic side-effects and interactions are less likely to be a problem—in particular, enzyme-inducing drugs are unlikely to significantly reduce the contraceptive effect. Initially changes in the pattern and duration of menstrual bleeding (spotting or prolonged bleeding) are common; endometrial disorders should be ruled out before insertion and the patient should be fully counselled (and provided with a patient information leaflet). Improvement in progestogenic side-effects, such as mastalgia and mood changes, and in the bleeding pattern usually occurs a few months after insertion and bleeding may often become very light or absent. Functional ovarian cysts (usually asymptomatic) may occur and usually resolve spontaneously (ultrasound monitoring recommended).

INTRA-UTERINE PROGESTOGEN-ONLY SYSTEM

Indications: see under Dose

Cautions: see notes above; in case of pregnancy—remove system (teratogenicity cannot be excluded); advanced uterine atrophy; not suitable for emergency contraception; **interactions:** see notes above and Appendix 1 (progestogens)

Contra-indications: see notes above

Side-effects: see notes above; also abdominal pain; peripheral oedema; nervousness; salpingitis and pelvic inflammatory disease; pelvic pain, back pain; *rarely* hirsutism, hair loss, pruritus, migraine, rash

Mirena® (Schering Health) PoM
Intra-uterine system, T-shaped plastic frame (impregnated with barium sulphate and with threads attached to base) with polydimethylsiloxane reservoir releasing levonorgestrel 20 micrograms/24 hours. Net price = £83.16. Counselling, see patient information leaflet

Dose: Contraception and menorrhagia, insert into uterine cavity within 7 days of onset of menstruation (anytime if replacement) or immediately after first-trimester termination by curettage; postpartum insertions should be delayed until 6 weeks after delivery; effective for 5 years.

Prevention of endometrial hyperplasia during oestrogen replacement therapy, insert during last days of menstruation or withdrawal bleeding or anytime if amenorrhoeic; effective for 4 years

7.3.3 Spermicidal contraceptives

Spermicidal contraceptives are useful additional safeguards but do **not** give adequate protection if used alone except where fertility is already significantly diminished (section 6.4.1.1); they are suitable for use with barrier methods. They have two components: a spermicide and a vehicle which itself may have some inhibiting effect on sperm activity.

> **CSM advice.** Products such as petroleum jelly (*Vaseline*®), baby oil and oil-based vaginal and rectal preparations are likely to damage condoms and contraceptive diaphragms made from latex rubber, and may render them less effective as a barrier method of contraception and as a protection from sexually transmitted diseases (including HIV).

Condoms: no evidence of harm to latex condoms and diaphragms with the products listed below

Gynol II® (Janssen-Cilag)
Jelly, nonoxinol '9' 2% in a water-soluble basis. Net price 81 g = £2.61; applicator = 75p
Excipients: include hydroxybenzoates (parabens), propylene glycol, sorbic acid

Ortho-Creme® (Janssen-Cilag)
Cream, nonoxinol '9' 2% in a water-miscible basis. Net price 70 g = £2.44; applicator = 75p
Excipients: include cetyl alcohol, hydroxybenzoates (parabens), propylene glycol, sorbic acid, fragrance

Orthoforms® (Janssen-Cilag)
Pessaries, nonoxinol '9' 5% in a water-soluble basis. Net price 15 pessaries = £2.40
Excipients: none as listed in section 13.1.3

7.3.4 Contraceptive devices

Intra-uterine devices

The intra-uterine device (IUD) is suitable for older parous women and as a second-line contraceptive in young nulliparous women who should be carefully screened because they have an increased background risk of pelvic inflammatory disease.

Smaller devices have been introduced to minimise side-effects; these consist of a plastic carrier wound with copper wire or fitted with copper bands; some also have a central core of silver to prevent fragmentation of the copper. Fertility declines with age and therefore a copper intra-uterine device which is fitted in a woman over the age of 40, may remain in the uterus until menopause. The intra-uterine device *Gyne-T 380*® (Janssen-Cilag) is no longer available, but some women may have the device in place until 2009. The intra-uterine devices *Multiload*® *Cu250* and *Multiload*® *Cu250 Short* (Organon) have been discontinued, but some women may have the devices in place until 2011.

A frameless, copper-bearing intra-uterine device (*GyneFix*®) has been introduced recently. It consists of a knotted, polypropylene thread with 6 copper sleeves; the device is anchored in the uterus by inserting the knot into the uterine fundus. *The healthcare professional inserting (or removing) the device should be fully trained in the technique and should provide full counselling backed by the patient information leaflet.*

The timing and technique of fitting an intra-uterine device are critical for its subsequent performance and call for proper training and experience. Devices should not be fitted during the heavy days of the period; they are best fitted after the end of menstruation and before the calculated time of implantation. The main excess risk of infection occurs in the first 20 days after insertion and is believed to be related to existing carriage of a sexually transmitted disease, therefore pre-screening (at least for chlamydia) should ideally be performed. The woman should be advised to attend *as an emergency* if she experiences sustained pain during the next 20 days.

An intra-uterine device should not be removed in mid-cycle unless an additional contraceptive was used for the previous 7 days. If removal is essential post-coital contraception should be considered.

If an intra-uterine device fails and the woman wishes to continue to full-term the device should be removed in the first trimester if possible.

INTRA-UTERINE CONTRACEPTIVE DEVICES

Indications: see notes above

Cautions: anaemia, menorrhagia (progestogen intra-uterine system might be preferable, section 7.3.2.3), endometriosis, severe primary dysmenorrhoea, history of pelvic inflammatory disease, history of ectopic pregnancy or tubal surgery, diabetes, fertility problems, nulliparity and young age, severely scarred uterus (including after endometrial resection) or severe cervical stenosis; valvular heart disease or history of endocarditis (antibacterial cover needed at insertion—Table 2, section 5.1); drug- or disease-induced immunosuppression (risk of infection—avoid if marked immunosuppression); epilepsy; increased risk of expulsion if inserted before uterine involution; gynaecological examination before insertion, 6–8 weeks after then annually but counsel women to see doctor promptly in case of significant symptoms, especially pain; anticoagulant therapy (avoid if possible); remove if pregnancy occurs; if pregnancy occurs, increased likelihood that it may be ectopic

Contra-indications: pregnancy, severe anaemia, recent sexually transmitted infection (if not fully investigated and treated), unexplained uterine bleeding, distorted or small uterine cavity, genital malignancy, active trophoblastic disease, pelvic inflammatory disease, established or marked immunosuppression; *copper devices:* copper allergy, Wilson's disease, medical diathermy

Side-effects: uterine or cervical perforation, displacement, expulsion; pelvic infection may be exacerbated, menorrhagia, dysmenorrhoea, allergy; *on insertion*: pain (alleviated by NSAID such as ibuprofen 30 minutes before insertion) and bleeding, occasionally epileptic seizure and vasovagal attack

Flexi-T® 300 (FP)
Intra-uterine device, copper wire, surface area approx. 300 mm^2 wound on vertical stem of T-shaped plastic carrier, impregnated with barium sulphate for radio-opacity, monofilament thread attached to base of vertical stem; preloaded in inserter, net price = £8.95
For uterine length over 5 cm; replacement every 5 years (see also notes above)

GyneFix® (FP)
Intra-uterine device, 6 copper sleeves with surface area of 330 mm^2 on polypropylene thread, net price = £25.19
Suitable for all uterine sizes; replacement every 5 years

Multiload® Cu375 (Organon)
Intra-uterine device, as above, with copper surface area approx. 375 mm^2 and vertical stem length 3.5 cm, net price = £9.24
For uterine length 6–9 cm; replacement every 5 years (see notes above)

Nova-T® 380 (Schering Health)
Intra-uterine device, copper wire with silver core, surface area approx. 380 mm^2 wound on vertical stem of T-shaped plastic carrier, impregnated with barium sulphate for radio-opacity, threads attached to base of vertical stem, net price = £13.50
For uterine length 6.5–9 cm; replacement every 5 years (see notes above)

T-Safe® CU 380 A (FP)
Intra-uterine device, copper wire, wound on vertical stem of T-shaped plastic carrier with copper collar on the distal portion of each arm, total surface area approx. 380 mm^2, impregnated with barium sulphate for radio-opacity, threads attached to base of vertical stem, net price = £9.73
For uterine length 6.5–9 cm; replacement every 8 years (see notes above)

Other contraceptive devices

■ Contraceptive caps

Type A contraceptive pessary
Opaque rubber, sizes 1 to 5 (55–75 mm rising in steps of 5 mm), net price = £7.26
Brands include *Dumas Vault Cap®*

Type B contraceptive pessary
Opaque rubber, sizes 22 to 31 mm (rising in steps of 3 mm), net price = £8.46
Brands include *Prentif Cavity Rim Cervical Cap®*

Type C contraceptive pessary
Opaque rubber, sizes 1 to 3 (42, 48 and 54 mm), net price = £7.26
Brands include *Vimule Cap®*

■ Contraceptive diaphragms

Type A Diaphragm with flat metal spring
Transparent rubber with flat metal spring, sizes 55–95 mm (rising in steps of 5 mm), net price = £5.78
Brands include *Reflexions®*

Type B Diaphragm with coiled metal rim
Opaque rubber with coiled metal rim, sizes 60–95 mm (rising in steps of 5 mm), net price = £6.35
Brands include *Ortho®*

Type C Arcing Spring Diaphragm
Opaque rubber with arcing spring, sizes 60–95 mm (rising in steps of 5 mm), net price = £7.23
Brands include *All-Flex®*

■ Fertility thermometer

Fertility (Ovulation) Thermometer (Zeal)
Mercury in glass thermometer, range 35 to 39°C (graduated in 0.1°C), net price = £1.83
For monitoring ovulation for the fertility awareness method of contraception

7.4 Drugs for genito-urinary disorders

For drugs used in the treatment of urinary-tract infections see section 5.1.13.

7.4.1 Drugs for urinary retention

Acute retention is painful and is treated by catheterisation.

Chronic retention is painless and often long-standing. Catheterisation is unnecessary unless there is deterioration of renal function. After the cause has initially been established and treated, drugs may be required to increase detrusor muscle tone.

Benign prostatic hyperplasia is treated either surgically or medically with alpha-blockers (see below) or with the anti-androgen finasteride (section 6.4.2).

Alpha-blockers

The selective alpha-blockers, **alfuzosin**, **doxazosin**, **indoramin**, **prazosin**, **tamsulosin** and **terazosin** relax smooth muscle in benign prostatic hyperplasia producing an increase in urinary flow-rate and an improvement in obstructive symptoms.

CAUTIONS. Since selective alpha-blockers reduce blood pressure, patients receiving antihypertensive treatment may require reduced dosage and specialist supervision. Caution may be required in the elderly and in patients with hepatic impairment (Appendix 2) and severe renal impairment (Appendix 3). For **interactions** see Appendix 1 (alpha-blockers).

CONTRA-INDICATIONS. Alpha-blockers should be avoided in patients with a history of postural hypotension and micturition syncope.

SIDE-EFFECTS. Side-effects of selective alpha-blockers include drowsiness, hypotension (notably postural hypotension), syncope, asthenia, depression, headache, dry mouth, gastro-intestinal disturbances (including nausea, vomiting, diarrhoea, constipation), oedema, blurred vision, rhinitis, erectile disorders (including priapism), tachycardia, and palpitations. Hypersensitivity reactions including rash, pruritus and angioedema have also been reported.

ALFUZOSIN HYDROCHLORIDE

Indications: see notes above
Cautions: see notes above
Contra-indications: see notes above; severe liver impairment
Side-effects: see notes above; flushes, chest pain
Dose: 2.5 mg 3 times daily, max. 10 mg daily; ELDERLY initially 2.5 mg twice daily

FIRST DOSE EFFECT. First dose may cause collapse due to hypotensive effect (therefore should be taken on retiring to bed). Patient should be warned to lie down if symptoms such as dizziness, fatigue or sweating develop, and to remain lying down until they abate completely

Xatral® (Sanofi-Synthelabo) PoM
Tablets, f/c, alfuzosin hydrochloride 2.5 mg, net price 60-tab pack = £21.20. Label: 3, counselling, see dose above

■ Modified release

Xatral® **XL** (Sanofi-Synthelabo) PoM
Tablets, m/r, yellow/white, alfuzosin hydrochloride 10 mg, net price 10-tab pack = £7.37, 30-tab pack = £22.13. Label: 3, 21, 25, counselling, see above
Dose: benign prostatic hyperplasia 10 mg once daily
Acute urinary retention associated with benign prostatic hyperplasia in men over 65 years, 10 mg once daily for 2–3 days during catheterisation and for one day after removal; max. 4 days

DOXAZOSIN

Indications: see notes above and section 2.5.4
Cautions: see notes above and section 2.5.4
Contra-indications: see notes above
Side-effects: see notes above and section 2.5.4
Dose: initially 1 mg daily; dose may be doubled at intervals of 1–2 weeks according to response, up to max. 8 mg daily; usual maintenance 2–4 mg daily

■ Preparations
Section 2.5.4

INDORAMIN

Indications: see notes above and section 2.5.4
Cautions: see notes above and section 2.5.4
Contra-indications: see notes above and section 2.5.4
Side-effects: see notes above and section 2.5.4
Dose: 20 mg twice daily; increased if necessary by 20 mg every 2 weeks to max. 100 mg daily in divided doses; ELDERLY, 20 mg at night may be adequate

Doralese® (GSK) PoM
Tablets, yellow, f/c, indoramin 20 mg, net price 60-tab pack = £11.44. Label: 2

PRAZOSIN HYDROCHLORIDE

Indications: see notes above and section 2.5.4
Cautions: see notes above and section 2.5.4
Contra-indications: see notes above and section 2.5.4
Side-effects: see notes above and section 2.5.4; paraesthesia, arthralgia, epistaxis, nervousness, dyspnoea, hallucinations, alopecia
Dose: initially 500 micrograms twice daily for 3–7 days, subsequently adjusted according to response; usual maintenance (and max.) 2 mg twice daily; ELDERLY initiate with lowest possible dose

FIRST DOSE EFFECT. First dose may cause collapse due to hypotensive effect (therefore should be taken on retiring to bed). Patient should be warned to lie down if symptoms such as dizziness, fatigue or sweating develop, and to remain lying down until they abate completely

■ Preparations
Section 2.5.4

TAMSULOSIN HYDROCHLORIDE

Indications: see notes above
Cautions: see notes above
Contra-indications: see notes above; severe liver impairment
Side-effects: see notes above
Dose: 400 micrograms daily as a single dose after food

Flomax® **MR** (Yamanouchi) PoM
Capsules, m/r, tamsulosin hydrochloride 400 micrograms. Net price 30-cap pack = £20.65. Label: 25

TERAZOSIN

Indications: see notes above and section 2.5.4
Cautions: see notes above and section 2.5.4
Contra-indications: see notes above
Side-effects: see notes above and section 2.5.4; weight gain, paraesthesia, dyspnoea, thrombocytopenia, nervousness, decreased libido, back pain and pain in extremities
Dose: initially 1 mg at bedtime; if necessary dose may be doubled at intervals of 1–2 weeks according to response, up to max. 10 mg once daily; usual maintenance 5–10 mg daily

FIRST DOSE EFFECT. First dose may cause collapse due to hypotensive effect (therefore should be taken on retiring to bed). Patient should be warned to lie down if symptoms such as dizziness, fatigue or sweating develop, and to remain lying down until they abate completely

Terazosin (Non-proprietary) PoM
Tablets, terazosin (as hydrochloride) 2 mg, net price 28-tab pack = £7.06; 5 mg, 28-tab pack = £12.72; 10 mg, 28-tab pack = £25.97 Label.Label: 3, , counselling, see dose above

Hytrin® (Abbott) PoM
Tablets, terazosin (as hydrochloride) 2 mg (yellow) net price, 28-tab pack = £8.07; 5 mg (tan), 28-tab pack = £13.07; 10 mg (blue), 28-tab pack = £26.59; starter pack (for benign prostatic hyperplasia) of

7 × 1-mg tab with 14 × 2-mg tab and 7 × 5-mg tab = £10.97. Label: 3, counselling, see dose above

Parasympathomimetics

The parasympathomimetic **bethanechol** increases detrusor muscle contraction. However, it has only a limited role in the relief of urinary retention; its use has been superseded by catheterisation.

Distigmine inhibits the breakdown of acetylcholine. It may help patients with an upper motor neurone neurogenic bladder.

CAUTIONS and CONTRA-INDICATIONS. Parasympathomimetics should be used with caution or avoided in hyperthyroidism or in cardiac disorders including bradycardia, arrhythmias and recent myocardial infarction. They are contra-indicated in intestinal or urinary obstruction or where increased motility of the gastro-intestinal or urinary tract could be harmful. Parasympathomimetics should also be avoided in gastro-intestinal ulceration, asthma, hypotension, epilepsy, parkinsonism, pregnancy, and breast-feeding. **Interactions**: Appendix 1 (parasympathomimetics)

SIDE-EFFECTS. Parasympathomimetic side-effects such as nausea, vomiting, intestinal colic, bradycardia, blurred vision, and sweating may occur, particularly in the elderly.

BETHANECHOL CHLORIDE 

Indications: urinary retention, but see notes above
Cautions: see notes above
Contra-indications: see notes above
Side-effects: see notes above
Dose: 10–25 mg 3–4 times daily half an hour before food

Myotonine® (Glenwood) PoM
Tablets, both scored, bethanechol chloride 10 mg, net price 20 = £1.01; 25 mg, 20 = £1.30 Label: 22

DISTIGMINE BROMIDE

Indications: postoperative urinary retention (see notes above), neurogenic bladder; myasthenia gravis (section 10.2.1)
Cautions: see notes above; also pregnancy (Appendix 4); breast-feeding
Contra-indications: see notes above; also severe postoperative shock, serious circulatory insufficiency
Side-effects: see notes above, but action slower than bethamecol chloride (therefore side-effects less acute; see also Neostigmine (section 10.2.1); also dyspnoea, muscle twitching, and urinary frequency
Dose: urinary retention, 5 mg daily, half an hour before breakfast
Neurogenic bladder, 5 mg daily or on alternate days, half an hour before breakfast

Ubretid® (Rhône-Poulenc Rorer) PoM
Tablets, scored, distigmine bromide 5 mg. Net price 30-tab pack = £31.26. Label: 22

7.4.2 Drugs for urinary frequency, enuresis, and incontinence

Urinary incontinence

Incontinence in adults which arises from detrusor instability is managed by combining drug therapy with conservative methods for managing urge incontinence such as pelvic floor exercises and bladder training; stress incontinence is generally managed by non-drug methods. **Duloxetine**, an inhibitor of serotonin and noradrenaline re-uptake can be added and is licensed for the treatment of moderate to severe stress incontinence in women; it may be more effective when used as an adjunct to pelvic floor exercises.

Involuntary detrusor contractions cause urgency and urge incontinence, usually with frequency and nocturia. Antimuscarinic drugs reduce these contractions and increase bladder capacity. **Oxybutynin** also has a direct relaxant effect on urinary smooth muscle. Side-effects limit the use of oxybutynin but they may be reduced by starting at a lower dose. A modified-release preparation of oxybutynin is effective and has fewer side-effects; a transdermal patch is also available. The efficacy and side-effects of **tolterodine** are comparable to those of modified-release oxybutynin. **Flavoxate** has less marked side-effects but it is also less effective. **Propiverine**, **solifenacin** and **trospium** are newer antimuscarinic drugs licensed for urinary frequency, urgency, and incontinence. The need for continuing antimuscarinic drug therapy should be reviewed after 6 months.

Propantheline and tricyclic antidepressants were used for urge incontinence but they are little used now because of their side-effects. The use of imipramine is limited by its potential to cause cardiac side-effects.

Purified bovine collagen implant (*Contigen*®, Bard) is indicated for *urinary incontinence* caused by intrinsic sphincter deficiency (poor or non-functioning bladder outlet mechanism). The implant should be inserted only by surgeons or physicians trained in the technique for injection of the implant.

CAUTIONS. Antimuscarinic drugs should be used with caution in the elderly (especially if frail) and in those with autonomic neuropathy. They should also be used with caution in hiatus hernia with reflux oesophagitis, and in hepatic impairment (Appendix 2; avoid propiverine) and renal impairment (Appendix 3). Antimuscarinics may worsen hyperthyroidism, coronary artery disease, congestive heart failure, hypertension, prostatic hypertrophy, arrhythmias and tachycardia. For **interactions** see Appendix 1 (antimuscarinics).

CONTRA-INDICATIONS. Antimuscarinic drugs should be avoided in patients with myasthenia gravis, angle closure glaucoma, significant bladder outflow obstruction or urinary retention, severe ulcerative colitis, toxic megacolon, and in gastro-intestinal obstruction or intestinal atony.

SIDE-EFFECTS. Side-effects of antimuscarinic drugs include dry mouth, gastro-intestinal disturbances including constipation, blurred vision, dry eyes, drowsiness, difficulty in micturition (less commonly urinary retention), palpitation, and skin reactions (including dry skin, rash, and photosensitivity); also headache, diarrhoea, angioedema, arrhythmias and tachycardia. Central nervous system stimulation, such as restlessness, disorientation, hallucination and convulsion may occur; children are at higher risk of these effects. Antimuscarinic drugs may reduce sweating leading to heat sensations and fainting in hot environments or in patients with fever.

DULOXETINE

Indications: moderate to severe stress urinary incontinence in women; major depressive disorder (section 4.3.4)
Cautions: elderly, cardiac disease, hypertension; history of mania; history of seizures; raised intra-ocular pressure, acute narrow-angle glaucoma; bleeding disorders or concomitant use of drugs that increase risk of bleeding; suicidal thoughts or behaviour; avoid abrupt withdrawal; **interactions**: Appendix 1 (duloxetine)
Contra-indications: hepatic impairment; pregnancy (Appendix 4); breast-feeding (Appendix 5)
Side-effects: nausea, vomiting, dyspepsia, constipation, diarrhoea, dry mouth; hot flushes; insomnia or drowsiness, anxiety, headache, dizziness, tremor, nervousness, anorexia; sexual dysfunction; thirst; fatigue, lethargy, weakness; blurred vision; sweating, pruritus; *rarely* urinary retention and hyponatraemia
Dose: 40 mg twice daily, assessed after 2–4 weeks and reduced to 20 mg twice daily if side-effects troublesome; CHILD and ADOLESCENT under 18 years not recommended

Yentreve® (Lilly) ▼ PoM
Capsules, duloxetine (as hydrochloride) 20 mg (blue), net price 56-cap pack = £30.80; 40 mg (orange/blue), 56-cap pack = £30.80. Label: 2

Cymbalta® (Lilly) ▼ PoM
Section 4.3.4 (major depressive episode)

FLAVOXATE HYDROCHLORIDE

Indications: urinary frequency and incontinence, dysuria, urgency; bladder spasms due to catheterisation
Cautions: see notes above; pregnancy (Appendix 4), breast-feeding (Appendix 5)
Contra-indications: see notes above; gastro-intestinal haemorrhage
Side-effects: see notes above; also vertigo, fatigue, eosinophilia
Dose: 200 mg 3 times daily; CHILD under 12 years not recommended

Urispas 200® (Shire) PoM
Tablets, f/c, flavoxate hydrochloride 200 mg, net price 90-tab pack = £11.87

OXYBUTYNIN HYDROCHLORIDE

Indications: urinary frequency, urgency and incontinence, neurogenic bladder instability and nocturnal enuresis
Cautions: see notes above; pregnancy (Appendix 4), porphyria (section 9.8.2)
Contra-indications: see notes above; breast-feeding (Appendix 5)
Side-effects: see notes above; also anorexia, facial flushing (more marked in children) and dizziness; application site reactions with *patches*
Dose: initially 2.5–5 mg 2–3 times daily increased if necessary to max. 5 mg 4 times daily
ELDERLY initially 2.5–3 mg twice daily, increased to 5 mg twice daily according to response and tolerance
CHILD over 5 years, neurogenic bladder instability, 2.5–3 mg twice daily increased to 5 mg twice daily (max. 5 mg 3 times daily); nocturnal enuresis (preferably over 7 years, see notes below), 2.5–3 mg twice daily increased to 5 mg 2–3 times daily (last dose before bedtime)

Oxybutynin Hydrochloride (Non-proprietary) PoM
Tablets, oxybutynin hydrochloride 2.5 mg, net price 56-tab pack = £5.42; 3 mg, 56-tab pack = £9.15; 5 mg, 56-tab pack = £5.87, 84-tab pack = £4.14. Label: 3

Cystrin® (Sanofi-Synthelabo) PoM
Tablets, oxybutynin hydrochloride 3 mg, net price 56-tab pack = £9.15; 5 mg (scored), 84-tab pack = £22.88. Label: 3

Ditropan® (Sanofi-Synthelabo) PoM
Tablets, both blue, scored, oxybutynin hydrochloride 2.5 mg, net price 84-tab pack = £6.86; 5 mg, 84-tab pack = £13.34. Label: 3
Elixir, oxybutynin hydrochloride 2.5 mg/5 mL. Net price 150-mL pack = £4.78. Label: 3

■ Modified release

Lyrinel® **XL** (Janssen-Cilag) PoM
Tablets, m/r, oxybutynin hydrochloride 5 mg (yellow), net price 30-tab pack = £12.34; 10 mg (pink), 30-tab pack = £24.68. Label: 3, 25
Dose: ADULT over 18 years, initially 5 mg daily, adjusted according to response in 5-mg steps at weekly intervals; max. 20 mg daily taken as a single dose
NOTE. Patients taking immediate-release oxybutynin may be transferred to the nearest equivalent daily dose of *Lyrinel*® *XL*

■ Transdermal preparations

Kentera® (UCB Pharma) PoM
Patches, self-adhesive, oxybutynin 36 mg (releasing oxybutynin approx. 3.9 mg/24 hours), net price 8-patch pack = £27.20. Label: 3, counselling, administration
Dose: urinary frequency, urgency and incontinence, apply 1 patch twice weekly to clean, dry, unbroken skin on abdomen, hip or buttocks, remove after every 3–4 days and site replacement patch on a different area (avoid using the same area for 7 days); CHILD and ADOLESCENT not recommended

PROPANTHELINE BROMIDE

Indications: adult enuresis
Cautions: see notes above; ulcerative colitis, pregnancy (Appendix 4) and breast-feeding (Appendix 5)
Contra-indications: see notes above
Side-effects: see notes above; also facial flushing
Dose: initially 15 mg 3 times daily at least one hour before food and 30 mg at bedtime, subsequently adjusted according to response (max. 120 mg daily)

■ Preparations
Section 1.2

PROPIVERINE HYDROCHLORIDE

Indications: urinary frequency, urgency and incontinence; neurogenic bladder instability
Cautions: see notes above
Contra-indications: see notes above; pregnancy (Appendix 4) and breast-feeding (Appendix 5)
Side-effects: see notes above
Dose: 15 mg 1–3 times daily, increased if necessary to max. 15 mg 4 times daily
CHILD not recommended

Detrunorm® (Amdipharm) PoM
Tablets, pink, s/c, propiverine hydrochloride 15 mg, net price 56-tab pack = £24.45. Label: 3

SOLIFENACIN SUCCINATE

Indications: urinary frequency, urgency and urge incontinence
Cautions: see notes above; neurogenic bladder disorder; pregnancy (Appendix 4)
Contra-indications: see notes above; haemodialysis; breast-feeding (Appendix 5)
Side-effects: see notes above; gastro-oesophageal reflux, altered taste; fatigue; oedema
Dose: 5 mg daily, increased if necessary to 10 mg once daily; CHILD not recommended
NOTE. Max. 5 mg daily with concomitant itraconazole, ketoconazole, nelfinavir or ritonavir

Vesicare® (Yamanouchi) ▼ PoM
Tablets, f/c, solifenacin succinate 5 mg (yellow), net price 30-tab pack = £27.62; 10 mg (pink), 30-tab pack = £35.91. Label: 3

TOLTERODINE TARTRATE

Indications: urinary frequency, urgency and incontinence
Cautions: see notes above
Contra-indications: see notes above; pregnancy (Appendix 4) and breast-feeding (Appendix 5)
Side-effects: see notes above; also dyspepsia, fatigue, flatulence, chest pain, dry eyes, peripheral oedema, paraesthesia
Dose: 2 mg twice daily; reduce to 1 mg twice daily if necessary to minimise side-effects
CHILD not recommended

Detrusitol® (Pharmacia) PoM
Tablets, f/c, tolterodine tartrate 1 mg, net price 56-tab pack = £29.03; 2 mg, 56-tab pack = £30.56

■ Modified release

Detrusitol® XL (Pharmacia) PoM
Capsules, blue, m/r, tolterodine tartrate 4 mg, net price 28-cap pack = £29.03. Label: 25
Dose: 4 mg once daily (dose form not appropriate for hepatic and renal impairment)

TROSPIUM CHLORIDE

Indications: urinary frequency, urgency and incontinence
Cautions: see notes above; pregnancy (Appendix 4); breast-feeding (Appendix 5)
Contra-indications: see notes above
Side-effects: see notes above; also flatulence, chest pain, dyspnoea, rash and asthenia
Dose: 20 mg twice daily before food
CHILD not recommended

Regurin® (Galen) PoM
Tablets, brown, f/c, trospium chloride 20 mg, net price 60-tab pack = £26.00. Label 23

Nocturnal enuresis

Nocturnal enuresis is a common occurrence in young children but persists in as many as 5% by 10 years of age. Treatment is not appropriate in children under 5 years and it is usually not needed in those aged under 7 years and in cases where the child and parents are not anxious about the bedwetting; however, children over 10 years usually require prompt treatment. An **enuresis alarm** should be first-line treatment for well-motivated children aged over 7 years because it may achieve a more sustained reduction of enuresis than use of drugs. Use of an alarm may be combined with drug therapy if either method alone is unsuccessful.

Drug therapy is not usually appropriate for children under 7 years of age; it can be used when alternative measures have failed, preferably on a short-term basis, to cover periods away from home for example. The possible side-effects of the various drugs should be borne in mind when they are prescribed.

Desmopressin (section 6.5.2), an analogue of vasopressin, is used for nocturnal enuresis; it is given intranasally or it may be given by mouth as tablets. Particular care is needed to avoid fluid overload and treatment should not be continued for longer than 3 months without stopping for a week for full re-assessment.

Tricyclics (section 4.3.1) such as **amitriptyline**, **imipramine**, and less often **nortriptyline** are also used but behaviour disturbances may occur and relapse is common after withdrawal. Treatment should not normally exceed 3 months unless a full physical examination is given and the child is fully re-assessed; toxicity following overdosage with tricyclics is of particular concern.

7.4.3 Drugs used in urological pain

The acute pain of *ureteric colic* may be relieved with **pethidine** (section 4.7.2). **Diclofenac** by injection or as suppositories (section10.1.1) is also effective and compares favourably with pethidine; other non-steroidal anti-inflammatory drugs are occasionally given by injection.

Lidocaine (lignocaine) gel is a useful topical application in *urethral pain* or to relieve the discomfort of catheterisation (section 15.2).

Alkalinisation of urine

Alkalinisation of urine may be undertaken with **potassium citrate**. The alkalinising action may relieve the discomfort of *cystitis* caused by lower urinary tract infections. **Sodium bicarbonate** is used as a urinary alkalinising agent in some metabolic and renal disorders (section 9.2.1.3).

POTASSIUM CITRATE

Indications: relief of discomfort in mild urinary-tract infections; alkalinisation of urine

Cautions: renal impairment, cardiac disease; elderly; **interactions:** Appendix 1 (potassium salts)
Side-effects: hyperkalaemia on prolonged high dosage, mild diuresis

Potassium Citrate Mixture BP
(Potassium Citrate Oral Solution)
Oral solution, potassium citrate 30%, citric acid monohydrate 5% in a suitable vehicle with a lemon flavour. Extemporaneous preparations should be recently prepared according to the following formula: potassium citrate 3 g, citric acid monohydrate 500 mg, syrup 2.5 mL, quillaia tincture 0.1 mL, lemon spirit 0.05 mL, double-strength chloroform water 3 mL, water to 10 mL. Contains about 28 mmol K^+/10 mL. Label: 27
Dose: 10 mL 3 times daily well diluted with water
NOTE. Concentrates for preparation of Potassium Citrate Mixture BP are available from Hillcross
Proprietary brands of potassium citrate on sale to the public for the relief of discomfort in mild urinary-tract infections include *Cystopurin*® and *Effercitrate*®

SODIUM BICARBONATE

Indications: relief of discomfort in mild urinary-tract infections; alkalinisation of urine
Cautions: hepatic impairment (Appendix 2); renal impairment (Appendix 3), cardiac disease, pregnancy; patients on sodium-restricted diet; elderly; avoid prolonged use; **interactions:** Appendix 1 (antacids)
Side-effects: belching, alkalosis on prolonged use
Dose: 3 g in water every 2 hours until urinary pH exceeds 7; maintenance of alkaline urine 5–10 g daily

■ Preparations
Section 9.2.1.3

SODIUM CITRATE

Indications: relief of discomfort in mild urinary-tract infections
Cautions: renal impairment, cardiac disease, hypertension, pregnancy, patients on a sodium-restricted diet; elderly
Side-effects: mild diuresis
NOTE. Proprietary brands of sodium citrate on sale to the public for the relief of discomfort in mild urinary-tract infections include *Boots Cystitis Relief Sachets* and *Tablets*, *Canesten*® *Oasis* and *Cymalon*®.

Acidification of urine

Urine acidification is difficult; it is very occasionally used in the management of recurrent urinary-tract infections and to prevent renal stone formation, especially in patients with paraplegia or with a neurogenic bladder. Methenamine (section 5.1.13) requires acid urine for its antimicrobial activity.

Ammonium chloride may be used for urinary acidification but tolerance can develop rapidly. Vomiting and, with large doses, hypokalaemia and acidosis can also occur. Ammonium chloride oral solution needs to be prepared extemporaneously and may not be readily available. **Ascorbic acid** is less suitable for urine acidification because it is not always reliable and high doses, which can lead to renal stones in those with hyperoxaluria, are required.

For pH-modifying solutions for the maintenance of indwelling urinary catheters, see section 7.4.4.

Other preparations for urinary disorders

A terpene mixture (*Rowatinex*®) is claimed to be of benefit in *urolithiasis* for the expulsion of calculi.

Rowatinex® (Rowa) PoM
Capsules, yellow, e/c, anethol 4 mg, borneol 10 mg, camphene 15 mg, cineole 3 mg, fenchone 4 mg, pinene 31 mg. Net price 50 = £7.35. Label: 25
Dose: 1–2 capsules 3–4 times daily before food; CHILD not recommended

7.4.4 Bladder instillations and urological surgery

BLADDER INFECTION. Various solutions are available as irrigations or washouts.

Aqueous **chlorhexidine** (section 13.11.2) may be used in the management of common infections of the bladder but it is ineffective against most *Pseudomonas* spp. Solutions containing chlorhexidine 1 in 5000 (0.02%) are used but they may irritate the mucosa and cause burning and haematuria (in which case they should be discontinued); sterile **sodium chloride solution 0.9%** (physiological saline) is usually adequate and is preferred as a mechanical irrigant.

Continuous bladder irrigation with **amphotericin** 50 micrograms/mL (section 5.2) may be of value in mycotic infections.

DISSOLUTION OF BLOOD CLOTS. Clot retention is usually treated by irrigation with sterile **sodium chloride solution 0.9%** but sterile **sodium citrate solution for bladder irrigation 3%** may also be helpful. **Streptokinase-streptodornase** (*Varidase Topical*®, section 13.11.7) is an alternative.

BLADDER CANCER. Bladder instillations of **doxorubicin** (section 8.1.2), **mitomycin** (section 8.1.2), and **thiotepa** (section 8.1.1) are used for recurrent superficial bladder tumours. Such instillations reduce systemic side-effects; adverse effects on the bladder (e.g. micturition disorders and reduction in bladder capacity) may occur.

Instillation of **epirubicin** (section 8.1.2) is used for treatment and prophylaxis of certain forms of superficial bladder cancer; instillation of **doxorubicin** (section 8.1.2) is also used for some papillary tumours.

Instillation of **BCG** (Bacillus Calmette-Guérin), a live attenuated strain derived from *Mycobacterium bovis* (section 8.2.4), is licensed for the treatment of primary or recurrent bladder carcinoma *in-situ* and for the prevention of recurrence following transurethral resection.

INTERSTITIAL CYSTITIS. **Dimethyl sulfoxide** (dimethyl sulphoxide) may be used for symptomatic relief in patients with interstitial cystitis (Hunner's ulcer). 50 mL of a 50% solution (*Rimso-50*®—available on named-patient basis from Britannia) is instilled into the bladder, retained for 15 minutes, and voided by the patient. Treatment is repeated at intervals of 2 weeks. Bladder spasm and hypersensitivity reactions may occur and long-term use requires ophthalmic, renal, and hepatic assessment at intervals of 6 months.

SODIUM CITRATE

Indications: bladder washouts, see notes above

Sterile Sodium Citrate Solution for Bladder Irrigation sodium citrate 3%, dilute hydrochloric acid 0.2%, in purified water, freshly boiled and cooled, and sterilised

Urological surgery

There is a high risk of fluid absorption from the irrigant used in endoscopic surgery within the urinary tract; if this occurs in excess, hypervolaemia, haemolysis, and renal failure may result. **Glycine irrigation solution 1.5%** is the irrigant of choice for transurethral resection of the prostate gland and bladder tumours; **sterile sodium chloride solution 0.9%** (physiological saline) is used for percutaneous renal surgery.

GLYCINE

Indications: bladder irrigation during urological surgery; see notes above
Cautions: see notes above
Side-effects: see notes above

Glycine Irrigation Solution (Non-proprietary)
Irrigation solution, glycine 1.5% in water for injections

Maintenance of indwelling urinary catheters

The deposition which occurs in catheterised patients is usually chiefly composed of phosphate and to minimise this the catheter (if latex) should be changed at least as often as every 6 weeks. If the catheter is to be left for longer periods a silicone catheter should be used together with the appropriate use of catheter maintenance solutions. Repeated blockage usually indicates that the catheter needs to be changed.

CATHETER PATENCY SOLUTIONS

Chlorhexidine 0.02%
Brands include *Uriflex C*®, 100-mL sachet = £2.40; *Uro-Tainer Chlorhexidine*®, 100-mL sachet = £2.60

Sodium chloride 0.9%
Brands include *OptiFlo S*®, 50- and 100-mL sachets = £3.10; *Uriflex S*®, 100-mL sachet = £2.40; *Uriflex SP*®, with integral drug additive port, 100-mL sachet = £2.40; *Uro-Tainer Sodium Chloride*®, 50- and 100-mL sachets = £2.99; *Uro-Tainer M*®, with integral drug additive port, 50- and 100-mL sachets = £2.90

Solution G
Citric acid 3.23%, magnesium oxide 0.38%, sodium bicarbonate 0.7%, disodium edetate 0.01%. Brands include *OptiFlo G*®, 50- and 100-mL sachets = £3.29; *Uriflex G*®, 100-mL sachet = £2.40; *Uro-Tainer® Twin Suby G*, 2 × 30-mL = £4.10

Solution R
Citric acid 6%, gluconolactone 0.6%, magnesium carbonate 2.8%, disodium edetate 0.01%. Brands include *OptiFlo R*®, 50- and 100-mL sachets = £3.29; *Uriflex R*®, 100-mL sachet = £2.40; *Uro-Tainer® Twin Solutio R*, 2 × 30-mL = £4.10

7.4.5 Drugs for erectile dysfunction

Reasons for failure to produce a satisfactory erection include *psychogenic*, *vascular*, *neurogenic*, and *endocrine abnormalities*; impotence can also be drug-induced. Intracavernosal injection or urethral application of vasoactive drugs under careful medical supervision is used for both diagnostic and therapeutic purposes.

Erectile disorders may also be treated with drugs given by mouth which increase the blood flow to the penis. Drugs should be used with caution if the penis is deformed (e.g. in angulation, cavernosal fibrosis, and Peyronie's disease).

PRIAPISM. If priapism occurs with alprostadil, treatment should not be delayed more than 6 hours and is as follows:

Initial therapy by penile aspiration—using aseptic technique a 19–21 gauge butterfly needle inserted into the corpus cavernosum and 20–50 mL of blood aspirated; if necessary the procedure may be repeated on the opposite side.

If initial aspiration is unsuccessful a second 19-21 gauge butterfly needle can be inserted into the opposite corpus cavernosum and sterile physiological saline introduced through the first needle and drained through the second.

If aspiration and lavage of corpora are unsuccessful, *cautious* intracavernosal injection of a sympathomimetic (section 2.7.2) with action on alpha-adrenergic receptors, continuously monitoring blood pressure and pulse (*extreme caution:* coronary heart disease, hypertension, cerebral ischaemia or if taking antidepressant) as follows:

- intracavernosal injections of phenylephrine 100–200 micrograms (0.5–1 mL of a 200 microgram/mL solution) every 5–10 minutes; max. total dose 1 mg [unlicensed indication] [*important:* if suitable strength of phenylephrine injection not available may be specially prepared by diluting 0.1 mL of the phenylephrine 1% (10 mg/mL) injection (section 2.7.2) to 5 mL with sodium chloride 0.9%];
alternatively
- intracavernosal injections of adrenaline 10–20 micrograms (0.5–1mL of a 20 microgram/mL solution) every 5–10 minutes; max. total dose 100 micrograms [unlicensed indication] [*important:* if suitable strength of adrenaline not available may be specially prepared by diluting 0.1 mL of the adrenaline 1 in 1000 (1 mg/mL, section 3.4.3) injection to 5 mL with sodium chloride 0.9%];
alternatively
- intracavernosal injection of metaraminol (*caution: has been associated with fatal hypertensive crises*); metaraminol 1 mg (0.1 mL of 10 mg/mL metaraminol injection, section

2.7.2) is diluted to 50 mL with sodium chloride injection 0.9% and given carefully by slow injection into the corpora in 5-mL injections every 15 minutes [unlicensed indication].

If necessary the sympathomimetic injections can be followed by further aspiration of blood through the same butterfly needle.

If sympathomimetics unsuccessful, urgent surgical referral for management (possibly including shunt procedure).

PRESCRIBING ON THE NHS. Drug treatments for erectile dysfunction may only be prescribed on the NHS under certain circumstances (see individual preparations). The Department of Health (England) has recommended that treatment should also be available from specialist services (commissioned by Health Authorities and Primary Care Groups, and operating under local agreement) when the condition is causing severe distress; specialist centres should use form FP10(HP) or form HBP in Scotland or form WP10HP in Wales and endorse them 'SLS' if the treatment is to be dispensed in the community. The following criteria should be considered when assessing distress:

- significant disruption to normal social and occupational activities;
- a marked effect on mood, behaviour, social and environmental awareness;
- a marked effect on interpersonal relationships.

Alprostadil

Alprostadil (prostaglandin E_1) is given by intracavernosal injection or intraurethral application for the management of erectile dysfunction (after exclusion of treatable medical causes); it is also used as a diagnostic test.

ALPROSTADIL

Indications: erectile dysfunction (including aid to diagnosis); neonatal congenital heart defects (section 7.1.1.1)

Cautions: priapism—patients should be instructed to report any erection lasting 4 hours or longer—for management, see section 7.4.5; anatomical deformations of penis (painful erection more likely)—follow up regularly to detect signs of penile fibrosis (consider discontinuation if angulation, cavernosal fibrosis or Peyronie's disease develop); **interactions:** Appendix 1 (prostaglandins)

Contra-indications: predisposition to prolonged erection (as in sickle cell anaemia, multiple myeloma or leukaemia); not for use with other agents for erectile dysfunction, in patients with penile implants or when sexual activity medically inadvisable; urethral application also contra-indicated in urethral stricture, severe hypospadia, severe curvature, balanitis, urethritis

Side-effects: penile pain, priapism (see section 7.4.5 and under Cautions); reactions at injection site include haematoma, haemosiderin deposits, penile rash, penile oedema, penile fibrosis, haemorrhage, inflammation; other local reactions include urethral burning and bleeding, penile warmth, numbness, penile or urinary-tract infection, irritation, sensitivity, phimosis, pruritus, erythema, venous leak, abnormal ejaculation; systemic effects reported include testicular pain and swelling, scrotal disorders, changes in micturition (including haematuria), nausea, dry mouth, fainting, hypotension (very rarely circulatory collapse) or hypertension, rapid pulse, vasodilatation, chest pain, supraventricular extrasystole, peripheral vascular disorder, dizziness, weakness, localised pain (buttocks, legs, genital, perineal, abdominal), headache, pelvic pain, back pain, influenza-like syndrome, swelling of the leg veins

Dose: see under preparations below

■ Intracavernosal injection

[1]**Caverject**® (Pharmacia) PoM NHS

Injection, powder for reconstitution, alprostadil, net price 5-microgram vial = £7.73; 10-microgram vial = £9.24; 20-microgram vial = £11.94; 40-microgram vial = £21.58 (all with diluent-filled syringe, needles and swabs)

Caverject® Dual Chamber, double-chamber cartridges (containing alprostadil and diluent), net price 10-microgram cartridge (for doses 2.5–10 micrograms) = £7.35; 20-microgram cartridge (for doses 5–20 micrograms) = £9.50 (both with needles)

Dose: by direct intracavernosal injection, erectile dysfunction, first dose 2.5 micrograms, second dose 5 micrograms (if some response to first dose) *or* 7.5 micrograms (if no response to first dose), increasing in steps of 5–10 micrograms to obtain dose suitable for producing erection not lasting more than 1 hour (neurological dysfunction, first dose 1.25 micrograms, second dose 2.5 micrograms, third dose 5 micrograms, increasing in steps of 5 micrograms to obtain suitable dose); if no response to dose then next higher dose can be given within 1 hour, if there is a response the next dose should not be given for at least 24 hours; usual range 5–20 micrograms; max. 60 micrograms (max. frequency of injection not more than once daily and not more than 3 times in any 1 week)

NOTE. The first dose must be given by medically trained personnel; self-administration may only be undertaken after proper training

Aid to diagnosis, 20 micrograms as a single dose (where evidence of neurological dysfunction, initially 5 micrograms and max. 10 micrograms)—consult product literature for details

[1]**Viridal**® **Duo** (Schwarz) PoM NHS

Starter Pack (hosp. only), contents as for *Continuation Pack* below plus *Duoject* applicator, 10-microgram starter pack = £20.13, 20-microgram starter pack = £24.54, 40-microgram starter pack =

1. NHS except to treat erectile dysfunction in men who:

- have diabetes, multiple sclerosis, Parkinson's disease, poliomyelitis, prostate cancer, severe pelvic injury, single gene neurological disease, spina bifida or spinal cord injury;
- are receiving dialysis for renal failure;
- have had radical pelvic surgery, prostatectomy, or kidney transplant;
- were receiving *Caverject*®, *Erecnos*®, *MUSE*®, *Viagra*® or *Viridal*® for erectile dysfunction, at the expense of the NHS, on 14 September 1998;
- are suffering severe distress as a result of impotence (prescribed in specialist centres only, see notes above).

The prescription must be endorsed 'SLS'.

£29.83; *Continuation Pack*, 2 double-chamber cartridges (containing alprostadil and diluent), 2 needles, swabs, 10-microgram continuation pack = £16.55, 20-microgram continuation pack = £21.39, 40-microgram continuation pack = £27.22; *Duoject*® applicator available free of charge from Schwarz

Dose: by direct intracavernosal injection, erectile dysfunction, initially 2.5 micrograms (1.25 micrograms in neurogenic erectile dysfunction) increasing in steps of 2.5–5 micrograms to obtain dose suitable for producing erection not lasting more than 1 hour; usual range 10–20 micrograms; max. 40 micrograms (max. frequency of injection not more than 2–3 times per week with at least 24 hour interval between injections); erection lasting longer than 2 hours—re-titrate dose; patient should report to doctor erection lasting longer than 4 hours

NOTE. The first dose must be given by medically trained personnel; self-administration may only be undertaken after proper training

■ Urethral application

COUNSELLING. If partner pregnant barrier contraception should be used

[1]**MUSE**® (Meda) PoM NHS

Urethral application, alprostadil, net price 125-microgram single-use applicator = £9.89, 250-microgram single-use applicator = £10.76, 500-microgram single-use applicator = £10.76, 1-mg single-use applicator = £11.01 (all strengths also available in packs of 6 applicators)

Condoms: no evidence of harm to latex condoms and diaphragms

Dose: by direct urethral application, erectile dysfunction, initially 250 micrograms adjusted according to response (usual range 0.125–1 mg); max. 2 doses in 24 hours and 7 doses in 7 days)

NOTE. The first dose must be given by medically trained personnel; self-administration may only be undertaken after proper training

Aid to diagnosis, 500 micrograms as a single dose

Apomorphine

Apomorphine is licensed for the treatment of erectile dysfunction; it is given as sublingual tablets. Compared to subcutaneous injection, absorption from the sublingual site is limited.

APOMORPHINE HYDROCHLORIDE

Indications: erectile dysfunction; Parkinson's disease (section 4.9.1)

Cautions: hepatic impairment (Appendix 2), renal impairment (Appendix 3); uncontrolled hypertension, hypotension; elderly; anatomical deformation of penis (e.g. angulation, cavernosal fibrosis, Peyronie's disease); not recommended for use in combination with other treatments for erectile dysfunction; **interactions:** Appendix 1 (apomorphine)

DRIVING. May impair performance of skilled tasks (e.g. driving)

Contra-indications: recent myocardial infarction; severe unstable angina, severe heart failure or hypotension; conditions where sexual activity is medically inadvisable

Side-effects: nausea, dyspepsia, headache, dizziness, yawning, drowsiness, rhinitis, pharyngitis, cough, flushing, taste disturbance, sweating; vasovagal syndrome; less frequently syncope, stomatitis, mouth ulcers; rarely hypersensitivity reactions including angioedema

Dose: *by sublingual administration*, initially 2 mg approx. 20 minutes before sexual activity, subsequent doses may be increased to 3 mg if necessary; minimum of 8 hours between doses

[1]**Uprima**® (Abbott) PoM NHS

Sublingual tablets, both red, apomorphine hydrochloride 2 mg, net price 2-tab pack = £7.47; 3 mg, 4-tab pack = £14.94. Counselling, driving

Phosphodiesterase type-5 inhibitors

Sildenafil, **tadalafil** and **vardenafil** are phosphodiesterase type-5 inhibitors licensed for the treatment of erectile dysfunction; they are not recommended for use with other treatments for erectile dysfunction. The patient should be assessed appropriately before prescribing sildenafil, tadalafil or vardenafil. Since these drugs are given by mouth there is a potential for drug interactions.

CAUTIONS. Sildenafil, tadalafil and vardenafil should be used with caution in cardiovascular disease, anatomical deformation of the penis (e.g. angulation, cavernosal fibrosis, Peyronie's disease), and in those with a predisposition to prolonged erection (e.g. in sickle-cell disease, multiple myeloma, or leukaemia).

CONTRA-INDICATIONS. Sildenafil, tadalafil and vardenafil are contra-indicated in patients receiving nitrates or in patients in whom vasodilation or sexual activity are inadvisable. In the absence of information, manufacturers contra-indicate these drugs in hypotension, recent stroke, unstable angina, and myocardial infarction.

SIDE-EFFECTS. The side-effects of sildenafil, tadalafil and vardenafil include dyspepsia, vomiting, headache, flushing, dizziness, visual disturbances, raised intra-ocular pressure, and nasal congestion. Hypersensitivity reactions (including rash), priapism, and painful red eyes have been reported.

SILDENAFIL

Indications: erectile dysfunction

Cautions: see notes above; also hepatic impairment (Appendix 2—avoid if severe); renal impairment (Appendix 3); bleeding disorders or active peptic ulceration; **interactions:** Appendix 1 (sildenafil)

Contra-indications: see notes above; also hereditary degenerative retinal disorders

---

1. NHS except to treat erectile dysfunction in men who:

- have diabetes, multiple sclerosis, Parkinson's disease, poliomyelitis, prostate cancer, severe pelvic injury, single gene neurological disease, spina bifida or spinal cord injury;
- are receiving dialysis for renal failure;
- have had radical pelvic surgery, prostatectomy, or kidney transplant;
- were receiving *Caverject*®, *Erecnos*®, *MUSE*®, *Viagra*® or *Viridal*® for erectile dysfunction, at the expense of the NHS, on 14 September 1998;
- are suffering severe distress as a result of impotence (prescribed in specialist centres only, see notes above).

The prescription must be endorsed 'SLS'.

Side-effects: see notes above; also serious cardiovascular events reported

Dose: ADULT over 18 years initially 50 mg approx. 1 hour before sexual activity, subsequent doses adjusted according to response to 25–100 mg as a single dose as needed; max. 1 dose in 24 hours (max. single dose 100 mg)

NOTE. Onset of effect may be delayed if taken with food

[1]**Viagra**® (Pfizer) PoM NHS

Tablets, all blue, f/c, sildenafil (as citrate), 25 mg, net price 4-tab pack = £16.59, 8-tab pack = £33.19; 50 mg, 4-tab pack = £19.34, 8-tab pack = £38.67; 100 mg, 4-tab pack = £23.50, 8-tab pack = £46.99

TADALAFIL

Indications: erectile dysfunction

Cautions: see notes above; also hepatic impairment (Appendix 2); renal impairment (Appendix 3); **interactions:** Appendix 1 (tadalafil)

Contra-indications: see notes above; also moderate heart failure, uncontrolled arrhythmias, uncontrolled hypertension

Side-effects: see notes above; also back pain, myalgia

Dose: initially 10 mg at least 30 minutes before sexual activity, subsequent doses adjusted according to response to 20 mg as a single dose; max. 1 dose in 24 hours (but daily use not recommended)

NOTE. Effect may persist for longer than 24 hours

[1]**Cialis**® (Lilly) ▼ PoM NHS

Tablets, f/c, tadalafil 10 mg (light yellow), net price 4-tab pack = £23.40; 20 mg (yellow), 4-tab pack = £23.40; 8-tab pack = £46.79

VARDENAFIL

Indications: erectile dysfunction

Cautions: see notes above; also hepatic impairment (Appendix 2—avoid if severe); renal impairment (Appendix 3); bleeding disorders or active peptic ulceration; susceptibility to prolongation of QT interval (including concomitant use of drugs which prolong QT interval); **interactions:** Appendix 1 (vardenafil)

Contra-indications: see notes above; also hereditary degenerative retinal disorders

Side-effects: see notes above; also *less commonly* drowsiness, hypertension, tachycardia, palpitation, dyspnoea, back pain, myalgia, and facial oedema; *rarely* hypertonia, hypotension, angina, and epistaxis

Dose: initially 10 mg (ELDERLY 5 mg) approx. 25–60 minutes before sexual activity, subsequent doses adjusted according to response up to max. 20 mg as a single dose; max. 1 dose in 24 hours

NOTE. Onset of effect may be delayed if taken with high-fat meal

[1]**Levitra**® (Bayer) ▼ PoM NHS

Tablets, all orange, f/c, vardenafil (as hydrochloride trihydrate) 5 mg, net price 4-tab pack = £16.58, 8-tab pack = £33.19; 10 mg, 4-tab pack = £19.34, 8-tab pack = £38.67; 20 mg, 4-tab pack = £23.50, 8-tab pack = £46.99

Papaverine and phentolamine

Although not licensed the smooth muscle relaxant **papaverine** has also been given by intracavernosal injection for erectile dysfunction. Patients with neurological or psychogenic impotence are more sensitive to the effect of papaverine than those with vascular abnormalities. **Phentolamine** is added if the response is inadequate [unlicensed indication].

Persistence of the erection for longer than 4 hours is an emergency, see advice in section 7.4.5.

1. NHS except to treat erectile dysfunction in men who:

- have diabetes, multiple sclerosis, Parkinson's disease, poliomyelitis, prostate cancer, severe pelvic injury, single gene neurological disease, spina bifida or spinal cord injury;
- are receiving dialysis for renal failure;
- have had radical pelvic surgery, prostatectomy, or kidney transplant;
- were receiving *Caverject*®, *Erecnos*®, *MUSE*®, *Viagra*® or *Viridal*® for erectile dysfunction, at the expense of the NHS, on 14 September 1998;
- are suffering severe distress as a result of impotence (prescribed in specialist centres only, see notes above).

The prescription must be endorsed 'SLS'.

8: Malignant disease and immunosuppression

8.1 Cytotoxic drugs

The chemotherapy of cancer is complex and should be confined to specialists in oncology. Cytotoxic drugs have both anti-cancer activity and the potential to damage normal tissue. Chemotherapy may be given with a curative intent or it may aim to prolong life or to palliate symptoms. In an increasing number of cases chemotherapy may be combined with radiotherapy or surgery or both as either neoadjuvant treatment (initial chemotherapy aimed at shrinking the primary tumour, thereby rendering local therapy less destructive or more effective) or as adjuvant treatment (which follows definitive treatment of the primary disease, when the risk of sub-clinical metastatic disease is known to be high). All chemotherapy drugs cause side-effects and a balance has to be struck between likely benefit and acceptable toxicity.

CRM guidelines on handling cytotoxic drugs:

1. Trained personnel should reconstitute cytotoxics;
2. Reconstitution should be carried out in designated areas;
3. Protective clothing (including gloves) should be worn;
4. The eyes should be protected and means of first aid should be specified;
5. Pregnant staff should not handle cytotoxics;
6. Adequate care should be taken in the disposal of waste material, including syringes, containers, and absorbent material.

Intrathecal chemotherapy. A Health Service Circular (HSC 2003/010) provides guidance on the introduction of safe practice in NHS Trusts where intrathecal chemotherapy is administered. Support for training programmes is also available.
Copies, and further information may be obtained from:
Department of Health
PO Box 777
London SE1 6XH
Fax: 01623 724524
It is also available from the Department of Health website (www.dh.gov.uk)

Combinations of cytotoxic drugs are frequently more toxic than single drugs but have the advantage in certain tumours of enhanced response, reduced development of drug resistance and increased survival. However for some tumours, single-agent chemotherapy remains the treatment of choice.

> Most cytotoxic drugs are teratogenic, and all may cause life-threatening toxicity; administration should, where possible, be confined to those experienced in their use.
> Because of the complexity of dosage regimens in the treatment of malignant disease, dose statements have been omitted from some of the drug entries in this chapter. *In all cases detailed specialist literature should be consulted.*
> Prescriptions should **not** be repeated except on the instructions of a specialist.

Cytotoxic drugs fall naturally into a number of classes, each with characteristic antitumour activity, sites of action, and toxicity. A knowledge of sites of metabolism and excretion is important because impaired drug handling as a result of disease is not uncommon and may result in enhanced toxicity.

Side-effects of cytotoxic drugs

Side-effects commonly encountered with cytotoxic drugs are discussed below whilst side-effects characteristic of a particular drug or class of drugs (e.g. neurotoxicity with vinca alkaloids) are described in the appropriate sections. Manufacturers' product literature should be consulted for full details of side-effects associated with individual drugs.

EXTRAVASATION OF INTRAVENOUS DRUGS. A number of cytotoxic drugs will cause severe local tissue necrosis if leakage into the extravascular compartment occurs. To reduce the risk of extravasation injury it is recommended that cytotoxic drugs are administered by appropriately trained staff. For information on the prevention and management of extravasation injury see section 10.3.

ORAL MUCOSITIS. A sore mouth is a common complication of cancer chemotherapy; it is most often associated with fluorouracil, methotrexate, and the anthracyclines. It is best to prevent the complication. Good mouth care (rinsing the mouth frequently and effective brushing of the teeth with a soft brush 2–3 times daily) is probably effective. For fluorouracil, sucking ice chips during short infusions of the drug is also helpful.

Once a sore mouth has developed, treatment is much less effective. Saline mouthwashes should be used but there is no good evidence to support the use of antiseptic or anti-inflammatory mouthwashes. In general, mucositis is self-limiting but with poor oral hygiene it can be a focus for blood-borne infection.

HYPERURICAEMIA. Hyperuricaemia, which can result in uric acid crystal formation in the urinary tract with associated renal dysfunction is a complication of the treatment of non-Hodgkin's lymphoma and leukaemia. Allopurinol (see section 10.1.4) should be started 24 hours before treating such tumours; patients should be adequately hydrated. The dose of mercaptopurine or azathioprine should be reduced if allopurinol needs to be given concomitantly (see Appendix 1).

Rasburicase (section 10.1.4) is a recombinant urate oxidase, which has been licensed recently for hyperuricaemia in patients with haematological malignancy, for details, see p. 520.

NAUSEA AND VOMITING. Nausea and vomiting cause considerable distress to many patients who receive chemotherapy, and to a lesser extent abdominal radiotherapy, and may lead to refusal of further treatment. Symptoms may be acute (occurring within 24 hours of treatment), delayed (first occurring more than 24 hours after treatment) or anticipatory (occurring prior to subsequent doses). Delayed and anticipatory symptoms are more difficult to control than acute symptoms and require different management.

Patients vary in their susceptibility to drug-induced nausea and vomiting; those affected more often include women, patients under 50 years of age, anxious patients, and those who experience motion sickness. Susceptibility also increases with repeated exposure to the drug.

Drugs may be divided according to their emetogenic potential and some examples are given below, but the symptoms vary according to the dose, to other drugs administered and to individual susceptibility.

Mildly emetogenic treatment—fluorouracil, etoposide, methotrexate (less than 100 mg/m^2), the vinca alkaloids, and abdominal radiotherapy.

Moderately emetogenic treatment—doxorubicin, intermediate and low doses of cyclophosphamide, mitoxantrone (mitozantrone), and high doses of methotrexate (0.1–1.2 g/m^2).

Highly emetogenic treatment—cisplatin, dacarbazine, and high doses of cyclophosphamide.

Prevention of acute symptoms. For patients at *low risk of emesis*, pretreatment with domperidone or, in adults over 20 years, with metoclopramide, continued for up to 24 hours after chemotherapy, is often effective (section 4.6). If metoclopramide or domperidone are not sufficiently effective, additional drugs such as dexamethasone (6–10 mg by mouth) or lorazepam (1–2 mg by mouth) may be used.

For patients at *high risk of emesis* or when other treatment is inadequate, a specific ($5HT_3$) serotonin antagonist (section 4.6), usually given by mouth, is often highly effective, particularly when used with dexamethasone; adding the neurokinin receptor antagonist, aprepitant (section 4.6) can improve control of cisplatin-related nausea and vomiting.

Prevention of delayed symptoms. Dexamethasone, given by mouth, is the drug of choice for preventing delayed symptoms; it is used alone or with metoclopramide or prochlorperazine. The $5HT_3$ antagonists may be less effective for delayed symptoms.

Prevention of anticipatory symptoms. Good symptom control is the best way to prevent anticipatory symptoms. The addition of lorazepam to antiemetic therapy is helpful because of its amnesic, sedative and anxiolytic effects.

BONE-MARROW SUPPRESSION. All cytotoxic drugs except vincristine and bleomycin cause bone-marrow depression. This commonly occurs 7 to 10 days after administration, but is delayed for certain drugs, such as carmustine, lomustine, and melphalan. Peripheral blood counts must be checked before each treatment, and doses should be reduced or therapy delayed if bone-marrow has not recovered.

Fever in a neutropenic patient (neutrophil count less than 1.0×10^9/litre) requires immediate broad-spectrum antibacterial therapy. Patients at low risk (those receiving chemotherapy for solid tumours, lymphoma or chronic leukaemia) can be treated with oral ciprofloxacin with or without co-amoxiclav (initially in hospital). All other patients should receive parenteral broad-spectrum antibacterial therapy. Appropriate bacteriological investigations should be conducted as soon as possible.

In selected patients, the duration and the severity of neutropenia can be reduced by the use of bone marrow growth factors (colony stimulating factors, section 9.1.6).

Symptomatic anaemia is usually treated with red blood cell transfusions. Epoetin administered subcutaneously is also effective but not widely used.

ALOPECIA. Reversible hair loss is a common complication, although it varies in degree between drugs and individual patients. No pharmacological methods of preventing this are available.

REPRODUCTIVE FUNCTION. Most cytotoxic drugs are teratogenic and should not be administered during pregnancy, especially during the first trimester.

Contraceptive advice should be offered where appropriate before cytotoxic therapy begins (and should cover the duration of contraception required after therapy has ended). Regimens that do not contain an alkylating drug may have less effect on fertility, but those with an alkylating drug carry the risk of causing permanent male sterility (there is no effect on potency). Pre-treatment counselling and consideration of sperm storage may be appropriate. Women are less severely affected, though the span of reproductive life may be shortened by the onset of a premature menopause. No increase in fetal abnormalities or abortion-rate has been recorded in patients who remain fertile after cytotoxic chemotherapy.

THROMBOEMBOLISM. Venous thromboembolism can be a complication of cancer itself, but chemotherapy can also increase the risk. Prophylaxis against thromboembolism may be considered for those receiving chemotherapy.

Drugs for cytotoxic-induced side-effects

Methotrexate-induced mucositis and myelosuppression

Folinic acid (given as calcium folinate) is used to counteract the folate-antagonist action of methotrexate and thus speed recovery from methotrexate-induced mucositis or myelosuppression. It is generally given 24 hours after the methotrexate, in a dose of 15 mg by mouth every 6 hours, for 2–8 doses (depending on the dose of methotrexate). It does not counteract the antibacterial activity of folate antagonists such as trimethoprim.

When folinic acid and fluorouracil are used together in metastatic colorectal cancer the response-rate improves compared to that with fluorouracil alone.

The calcium salt of **levofolinic acid**, a single isomer of folinic acid, is also used for rescue therapy following methotrexate administration and for use with fluorouracil for colorectal cancer. The dose of calcium levofolinate is generally half that of calcium folinate.

The disodium salt of folinic acid is also licensed for rescue therapy following methotrexate therapy and for use with fluorouracil for colorectal cancer.

CALCIUM FOLINATE

(Calcium leucovorin)

Indications: see notes above

Cautions: avoid simultaneous administration of methotrexate; **not** indicated for pernicious anaemia or other megaloblastic anaemias due to vitamin B_{12} deficiency; pregnancy (Appendix 4) and breast-feeding (Appendix 5); **interactions:** Appendix 1 (folates)

IMPORTANT. Intrathecal injection **contra-indicated**

Side-effects: hypersensitivity reactions; rarely pyrexia after parenteral use

Dose: expressed in terms of folinic acid

As an antidote to methotrexate (usually started 24 hours after the beginning of methotrexate infusion), usually up to 120 mg in divided doses over 12–24 hours *by intramuscular or intravenous injection or by intravenous infusion*, followed by 12–15 mg *intramuscularly or* 15 mg *by mouth* every 6 hours for the next 48–72 hours

Suspected methotrexate overdosage, immediate administration of folinic acid at a rate not exceeding 160 mg/minute in a dose equal to (or higher than) the dose of methotrexate

Adjunct to fluorouracil in colorectal cancer, consult product literature

Calcium Folinate (Non-proprietary) PoM

Tablets, scored, folinic acid (as calcium salt) 15 mg, net price 10-tab pack = £40.50, 30-tab pack = £85.74

Brands include *Refolinon*®

NOTE. Not all strengths and pack sizes are available from all manufacturers

Injection, folinic acid (as calcium salt) 3 mg/mL, net price 1-mL amp = £2.28, 10-mL amp = £4.62; 7.5 mg/mL, net price 2-mL amp = £7.80; 10 mg/mL, net price 5-mL vial = £19.41, 10-mL vial = £35.09, 30-mL vial = £94.69, 35-mL vial = £90.98

Brands include *Lederfolin*®

NOTE. Not all strengths and pack sizes are available from all manufacturers

Injection, powder for reconstitution, folinic acid (as calcium salt), net price 15-mg vial = £4.46; 30-mg vial = £8.36

CALCIUM LEVOFOLINATE

(Calcium levoleucovorin)

Indications: see notes above

Cautions: see Calcium Folinate

Side-effects: see Calcium Folinate

Dose: expressed in terms of levofolinic acid

As an antidote to methotrexate (usually started 24 hours after the beginning of methotrexate infusion), usually 7.5 mg, *by intramuscular injection, or by intravenous injection or by intravenous infusion* every 6 hours for 10 doses

Suspected methotrexate overdosage, immediate administration of levofolinic acid at a rate not exceeding 160 mg/minute in a dose which is at least 50% of the dose of methotrexate

Adjunct to fluorouracil in colorectal cancer, consult product literature

Isovorin® (Wyeth) ▼ PoM
Injection, levofolinic acid (as calcium salt) 10 mg/mL, net price 2.5-mL vial = £12.09, 5-mL vial = £26.00, 17.5-mL vial = £84.63

DISODIUM FOLINATE

Indications: see notes above
Cautions: see Calcium Folinate
Side-effects: see Calcium Folinate
Dose: as an antidote to methotrexate, see Calcium Folinate
Adjunct to fluorouracil in colorectal cancer, consult product literature

Sodiofolin® (Medac) PoM
Injection, folinic acid (as disodium salt) 50 mg/mL, net price 2-mL vial = £35.09, 8-mL vial = £126.25, 18-mL vial = £284.07

Urothelial toxicity

Haemorrhagic cystitis is a common manifestation of urothelial toxicity which occurs with the oxazaphosphorines, cyclophosphamide and ifosfamide; it is caused by the metabolite acrolein. **Mesna** reacts specifically with this metabolite in the urinary tract, preventing toxicity. Mesna is used routinely (preferably by mouth) in patients receiving ifosfamide, and in patients receiving cyclophosphamide by the intravenous route at a high dose (e.g. more than 2 g) or in those who experienced urothelial toxicity when given cyclophosphamide previously.

MESNA

Indications: see notes above
Contra-indications: hypersensitivity to thiol-containing compounds
Side-effects: nausea, vomiting, colic, diarrhoea, fatigue, headache, limb and joint pains, depression, irritability, rash, hypotension and tachycardia; rarely hypersensitivity reactions (more common in patients with auto-immune disorders)
Dose: calculated according to oxazaphosphorine (cyclophosphamide or ifosfamide) treatment—for details consult product literature; when given *by mouth*, dose is given 2 hours *before* oxazaphosphorine treatment and repeated 2 and 6 hours *after* treatment; when given *by intravenous injection*, dose is given *with* oxazaphosphorine treatment and repeated 4 and 8 hours *after* treatment

Uromitexan® (Baxter) PoM
Tablets, f/c, mesna 400 mg, net price 10-tab pack = £21.10; 600 mg, 10-tab pack = £27.40
Injection, mesna 100 mg/mL. Net price 4-mL amp = £1.95; 10-mL amp = £4.38
NOTE. For oral administration contents of ampoule are taken in a flavoured drink such as orange juice or cola which may be stored in a refrigerator for up to 24 hours in a sealed container

8.1.1 Alkylating drugs

Extensive experience is available with these drugs, which are among the most widely used in cancer chemotherapy. They act by damaging DNA, thus interfering with cell replication. In addition to the side-effects common to many cytotoxic drugs (section 8.1), there are two problems associated with prolonged usage. Firstly, gametogenesis is often severely affected (section 8.1). Secondly, prolonged use of these drugs, particularly when combined with extensive irradiation, is associated with a marked increase in the incidence of acute non-lymphocytic leukaemia.

Cyclophosphamide is widely used in the treatment of chronic lymphocytic leukaemia, the lymphomas, and solid tumours. It is given by mouth or intravenously and is inactive until metabolised by the liver. A urinary metabolite of cyclophosphamide, acrolein, may cause haemorrhagic cystitis; this is a rare but very serious complication. An increased fluid intake, for 24–48 hours after intravenous injection, will help avoid this complication. When high-dose therapy (e.g. more than 2 g intravenously) is used or when the patient is considered to be at high risk of cystitis (e.g. previous pelvic irradiation) mesna (given initially intravenously then by mouth) will also help prevent this—see under Urothelial toxicity (section 8.1).

Ifosfamide is related to cyclophosphamide and is given intravenously; mesna (section 8.1) is routinely given with it to reduce urothelial toxicity.

Chlorambucil is used to treat chronic lymphocytic leukaemia, non-Hodgkin's lymphoma, Hodgkin's disease, and Waldenstrom's macroglobulinaemia. It is given by mouth. Side-effects, apart from bone-marrow suppression, are uncommon. However, patients occasionally develop severe widespread rashes which can progress to Stevens-Johnson syndrome or to toxic epidermal necrolysis. If a rash occurs further chlorambucil is contra-indicated and cyclophosphamide is substituted.

Melphalan is licensed for the treatment of multiple myeloma, advanced ovarian adenocarcinoma, advanced breast cancer, childhood neuroblastoma, and polycythaemia vera. Melphalan is also licensed for regional arterial perfusion in localised malignant melanoma of the extremities and localised soft-tissue sarcoma of the extremities. Interstitial pneumonitis and life-threatening pulmonary fibrosis are associated with melphalan.

Busulfan (busulphan) is given by mouth to treat chronic myeloid leukaemia. Busulphan given intravenously, followed by cyclophosphamide, is also licensed as conditioning treatment before haematopoietic stem-cell transplantation in adults. Frequent blood tests are necessary because excessive myelosuppression may result in irreversible bone-marrow aplasia. Rarely, progressive pulmonary fibrosis is associated with busulfan. Skin hyperpigmentation is a common side-effect of oral therapy.

Lomustine is a lipid-soluble nitrosourea and is given by mouth. It is mainly used to treat Hodgkin's disease and certain solid tumours. Bone marrow toxicity is delayed, and the drug is therefore given at intervals of 4 to 6 weeks. Permanent bone marrow damage may occur with prolonged use. Nausea and vomiting are common and moderately severe.

Carmustine given intravenously has similar activity to lomustine; it is given to patients with multiple myeloma, non-Hodgkin's lymphomas, and brain tumours. Cumulative renal damage and delayed pulmonary fibrosis may occur with intravenous use. Carmustine implants are licensed for intralesional use in adults, for the treatment of recurrent glioblastoma multiforme as an adjunct to surgery. Carmustine implants are also licensed for high-grade malignant glioma as adjunctive treatment to surgery and radiotherapy.

Estramustine is a combination of an oestrogen and chlormethine used predominantly in prostate cancer. It is given by mouth and has both an antimitotic effect and (by reducing testosterone concentration) a hormonal effect.

Treosulfan is given by mouth or intravenously and is used to treat ovarian cancer. Skin pigmentation is a common side-effect and allergic alveolitis, pulmonary fibrosis and haemorrhagic cystitis occur rarely.

Thiotepa is usually used as an intracavitary drug for the treatment of malignant effusions or bladder cancer (section 7.4.4). It is also occasionally used to treat breast cancer, but requires parenteral administration.

Mitobronitol is occasionally used to treat chronic myeloid leukaemia; it is available on a named-patient basis only (as *Myelobromol*®, Durbin).

BUSULFAN

(Busulphan)

Indications: see notes above

Cautions: see section 8.1 and notes above; avoid in porphyria (section 9.8.2); **interactions:** Appendix 1 (busulfan)

Contra-indications: pregnancy (Appendix 4); breast-feeding

Side-effects: see section 8.1 and notes above

Dose: *by mouth*, chronic myeloid leukaemia, induction of remission, 60 micrograms/kg to max. 4 mg daily; maintenance, 0.5–2 mg daily

By intravenous infusion, consult product literature

Busilvex® (Fabre) ▼ PoM

Concentrate for intravenous infusion, busulfan 6 mg/mL, net price 10-mL vial = £201.25

Myleran® (GSK) PoM

Tablets, f/c, busulfan 2 mg, net price 25-tab pack = £5.20

CARMUSTINE

Indications: see notes above

Cautions: see section 8.1 and notes above

Contra-indications: pregnancy (Appendix 4), breast-feeding

Side-effects: see section 8.1 and notes above; irritant to tissues

BiCNU® (Bristol-Myers Squibb) PoM

Injection, powder for reconstitution, carmustine. Net price 100-mg vial (with diluent) = £12.50

Gliadel® (Link) PoM

Implant, carmustine 7.7 mg, net price = £650.38

CHLORAMBUCIL

Indications: see notes above

Cautions: see section 8.1 and notes above; severe hepatic impairment (Appendix 2); avoid in porphyria (section 9.8.2)

Contra-indications: pregnancy (Appendix 4), breast-feeding

Side-effects: see section 8.1 and notes above

Dose: Hodgkin's disease, used alone, 200 micrograms/kg daily for 4–8 weeks

Non-Hodgkin's lymphoma, used alone, initially 100–200 micrograms/kg daily for 4–8 weeks then dose reduced or given intermittently

Chronic lymphocytic leukaemia, initially 150 micrograms/kg daily until leucocyte count sufficiently reduced; maintenance (started 4 weeks after end of first course) 100 micrograms/kg daily

Waldenstrom's macroglobulinaemia, 6–12 mg daily until leucopenia occurs, then reduce to 2–8 mg daily

Leukeran® (GSK) PoM

Tablets, f/c, brown, chlorambucil 2 mg, net price 25-tab pack = £8.36

CYCLOPHOSPHAMIDE

Indications: see notes above; rheumatoid arthritis (section 10.1.3)

Cautions: see section 8.1 and notes above; hepatic and renal impairment (Appendixes 2 and 3); avoid in porphyria (section 9.8.2); **interactions:** Appendix 1 (cyclophosphamide)

Contra-indications: pregnancy (Appendix 4), breast-feeding (Appendix 5)

Side-effects: see section 8.1 and notes above

Cyclophosphamide (Non-proprietary) PoM

Tablets, s/c, cyclophosphamide (anhydrous) 50 mg, net price 20 = £2.12. Label: 27

Injection, powder for reconstitution, cyclophosphamide, net price 500-mg vial = £2.88; 1-g vial = £5.04

Endoxana® (Baxter) PoM

Tablets, s/c, cyclophosphamide 50 mg, net price 100-tab pack = £12.00. Label: 27

Injection, powder for reconstitution, cyclophosphamide. Net price 200-mg vial = £1.86; 500-mg vial = £3.25; 1-g vial = £5.67

ESTRAMUSTINE PHOSPHATE

Indications: prostate cancer

Cautions: see section 8.1; renal impairment (Appendix 3)

Contra-indications: peptic ulceration, severe liver disease (Appendix 2), cardiac disease

Side-effects: see section 8.1; also gynaecomastia, altered liver function, cardiovascular disorders (angina and rare reports of myocardial infarction)

Dose: 0.14–1.4 g daily in divided doses (usual initial dose 560 mg daily)

COUNSELLING. Each dose should be taken not less than 1 hour before or 2 hours after meals and should not be taken with dairy products

Estracyt® (Pharmacia) PoM

Capsules, estramustine phosphate 140 mg (as disodium salt). Net price 100-cap pack = £171.28. Label: 23, counselling, see above

IFOSFAMIDE

Indications: see notes above

Cautions: see section 8.1 and notes above; renal impairment (Appendix 3); **interactions:** Appendix 1 (ifosfamide)

Contra-indications: hepatic impairment; pregnancy (Appendix 4), breast-feeding

Side-effects: see section 8.1 and notes above

Mitoxana® (Baxter) PoM

Injection, powder for reconstitution, ifosfamide. Net price 1-g vial = £24.57; 2-g vial = £45.49 (hosp. only)

LOMUSTINE

Indications: see notes above
Cautions: see section 8.1 and notes above
Side-effects: see section 8.1 and notes above
Dose: used alone, 120–130 mg/m^2 body-surface every 6–8 weeks

Lomustine (Medac) PoM
Capsules, blue/clear, lomustine 40 mg. Net price 20-cap pack = £344.51
NOTE. The brand name *CCNU*® has been used for lomustine capsules

MELPHALAN

Indications: see notes above
Cautions: see section 8.1 and notes above; renal impairment (Appendix 3); **interactions:** Appendix 1 (melphalan)
Contra-indications: pregnancy (Appendix 4); breast-feeding
Side-effects: see section 8.1 and notes above
Dose: *by mouth*, multiple myeloma, dose may vary according to regimen; typical dose 150 micrograms/kg daily for 4 days, repeated every 6 weeks
Ovarian adenocarcinoma, 200 micrograms/kg daily for 5 days, repeated every 4–8 weeks
Advanced breast cancer, 150 micrograms/kg daily for 5 days, repeated every 6 weeks
Polycythaemia vera, initially, 6–10 mg daily reduced after 5–7 days to 2–4 mg daily until satisfactory response then further reduce to 2–6 mg **per week**
By intravenous injection or infusion and regional arterial perfusion, consult product literature

Alkeran® (GSK) PoM
Tablets, melphalan 2 mg, net price 25 = £11.46
Injection, powder for reconstitution, melphalan 50 mg (as hydrochloride). Net price 50-mg vial (with solvent-diluent) = £27.61

THIOTEPA

Indications: see notes above and section 7.4.4
Cautions: see section 8.1; **interactions:** Appendix 1 (thiotepa)
Contra-indications: pregnancy (Appendix 4); breast-feeding
Side-effects: see section 8.1

Thiotepa (Goldshield) PoM
Injection, powder for reconstitution, thiotepa, net price 15-mg vial = £5.20

TREOSULFAN

Indications: see notes above
Cautions: see section 8.1
Contra-indications: pregnancy; breast-feeding
Side-effects: see section 8.1 and notes above
Dose: *by mouth*, courses of 1–2 g daily in 3–4 divided doses to provide total dose of 21–28 g over initial 8 weeks (with treatment-free intervals during this period—consult product literature)
By intravenous injection or by intraperitoneal administration, consult product literature

Treosulfan (Medac) PoM
Capsules, treosulfan 250 mg. Net price 20 = £67.25
Label: 25
Injection, powder for reconstitution, treosulfan. Net price 1 g = £39.44; 5 g = £152.41 (both in infusion bottle with transfer needle)

8.1.2 Cytotoxic antibiotics

Drugs in this group are widely used. Many cytotoxic antibiotics act as radiomimetics and simultaneous use of radiotherapy should be **avoided** as it may result in markedly enhanced toxicity.

Daunorubicin, doxorubicin, epirubicin and idarubicin are anthracycline antibiotics. Mitoxantrone (mitozantrone) is an anthracycline derivative.

Doxorubicin is used to treat the acute leukaemias, lymphomas, and a variety of solid tumours. It is given by injection into a fast-running infusion, commonly at 21-day intervals. Extravasation can cause severe tissue necrosis. Doxorubicin is largely excreted by the biliary tract, and an elevated bilirubin concentration is an indication for reducing the dose. Supraventricular tachycardia related to drug administration is an uncommon complication. Higher cumulative doses are associated with cardiomyopathy and it is usual to limit total cumulative doses to 450 mg/m^2 because symptomatic and potentially fatal heart failure is common above this dose. Patients with cardiac disease, the elderly, and those who have received myocardial irradiation should be treated cautiously. Cardiac monitoring may assist in determining safe dosage. Some evidence suggests that weekly low-dose administration may be less cardiotoxic. Doxorubicin is also given by bladder instillation for the treatment of transitional cell carcinoma, papillary bladder tumours and carcinoma *in-situ*.

Liposomal formulations of doxorubicin for intravenous use are also available. They may reduce the incidence of cardiotoxicity and lower the potential for local necrosis, but infusion reactions, sometimes severe, may occur. Hand-foot syndrome (painful, macular reddening skin eruptions) occurs commonly with liposomal doxorubicin and may be dose limiting. It can occur after 2–3 treatment cycles and may be prevented by cooling hands and feet and avoiding socks, gloves, or tight-fitting footwear for 4–7 days after treatment.

The *Scottish Medicines Consortium* has advised (December 2003) that pegylated liposomal doxorubicin is **not** recommended for metastatic breast cancer.

> **NICE guidance (paclitaxel, pegylated liposomal doxorubicin and topotecan for second-line or subsequent treatment of advanced ovarian cancer).** See p. 441

Epirubicin is structurally related to doxorubicin and clinical trials suggest that it is as effective in the treatment of breast cancer. A maximum cumulative dose of 0.9–1 g/m^2 is recommended to help avoid cardiotoxicity. Like doxorubicin it is given intravenously and by bladder instillation.

Idarubicin has general properties similar to those of doxorubicin. It is given intravenously and it may also be given by mouth.

Daunorubicin also has general properties similar to those of doxorubicin. It should be given by intravenous infusion and is indicated for acute leukaemias. A liposomal formulation for intravenous use is licensed for AIDS-related Kaposi's sarcoma.

> **Use with trastuzumab.** Concomitant use of anthracyclines with trastuzumab (section 8.1.5) is associated with cardiotoxicity; for details, see p. 444.

Mitoxantrone (**mitozantrone**) is structurally related to doxorubicin; it is used for metastatic breast cancer. Mitoxantrone is also licensed for use in the treatment of non-Hodgkin's lymphoma and adult non-lymphocytic leukaemia. It is given intravenously and is well tolerated but myelosuppression and dose-related cardiotoxicity occur; cardiac examinations are recommended after a cumulative dose of 160 mg/m^2.

Bleomycin is given intravenously or intramuscularly to treat metastatic germ cell cancer and, in some regimens, non-Hodgkin's lymphoma. It causes little bone-marrow suppression but dermatological toxicity is common and increased pigmentation particularly affecting the flexures and subcutaneous sclerotic plaques may occur. Mucositis is also relatively common and an association with Raynaud's phenomenon is reported. Hypersensitivity reactions manifest by chills and fevers commonly occur a few hours after drug administration and may be prevented by simultaneous administration of a corticosteroid, for example hydrocortisone intravenously. The principal problem associated with the use of bleomycin is progressive pulmonary fibrosis. This is dose-related, occurring more commonly at cumulative doses greater than 300 000 units (see Bleomycin, below) and in the elderly. Basal lung crepitations or suspicious chest X-ray changes are an indication to stop therapy with this drug. Patients who have received extensive treatment with bleomycin (e.g. cumulative dose more than 100 000 units—see Bleomycin below) may be at risk of developing respiratory failure if a general anaesthetic is given with high inspired oxygen concentrations. Anaesthetists should be warned of this.

Dactinomycin is principally used to treat paediatric cancers; it is given intravenously. Its side-effects are similar to those of doxorubicin, except that cardiac toxicity is not a problem.

Mitomycin is given intravenously to treat upper gastro-intestinal and breast cancers and by bladder instillation for superficial bladder tumours. It causes delayed bone-marrow toxicity and therefore it is usually administered at 6-weekly intervals. Prolonged use may result in permanent bone-marrow damage. It may also cause lung fibrosis and renal damage.

BLEOMYCIN

Indications: squamous cell carcinoma; see also notes above

Cautions: see section 8.1 and notes above; renal impairment (Appendix 3); caution in handling—irritant to tissues

Contra-indications: pregnancy (Appendix 4); breast-feeding

Side-effects: see section 8.1 and notes above

Bleomycin (Non-proprietary) PoM

Injection, powder for reconstitution, bleomycin (as sulphate). Net price 15 000-unit vial = £15.56

NOTE. To conform to the European Pharmacopoeia vials previously labelled as containing '15 units' of bleomycin are now labelled as containing 15 000 units. The amount of bleomycin in the vial has not changed.

Brands include *Bleo-Kyowa*®

DACTINOMYCIN

(Actinomycin D)

Indications: see notes above

Cautions: see section 8.1 and notes above; caution in handling—irritant to tissues

Contra-indications: pregnancy (Appendix 4); breast-feeding

Side-effects: see section 8.1 and notes above

Cosmegen Lyovac® (MSD) PoM

Injection, powder for reconstitution, dactinomycin, net price 500-microgram vial = £1.50

DAUNORUBICIN

Indications: see notes above

Cautions: see section 8.1 and notes above; hepatic impairment (Appendix 2), renal impairment (Appendix 3); caution in handling—irritant to tissues

Contra-indications: pregnancy (Appendix 4); breast-feeding

Side-effects: see section 8.1 and notes above

Daunorubicin (Non-proprietary) PoM

Injection, powder for reconstitution, daunorubicin (as hydrochloride), net price 20-mg vial = £39.26

NOTE. The brand name *Cerubidin*® was formerly used.

■ Lipid formulation

DaunoXome® (Gilead) PoM

Concentrate for intravenous infusion, daunorubicin encapsulated in liposomes. For dilution before use. Net price 50-mg vial = £137.67

For advanced AIDS-related Kaposi's sarcoma

DOXORUBICIN HYDROCHLORIDE

Indications: see notes above and section 7.4.4

Cautions: see section 8.1 and notes above; hepatic impairment (Appendix 2); caution in handling—irritant to tissues; **interactions:** Appendix 1 (doxorubicin)

Contra-indications: pregnancy (Appendix 4); breast-feeding

Side-effects: see section 8.1 and notes above

Doxorubicin Rapid Dissolution (Pharmacia) PoM

Injection, powder for reconstitution, doxorubicin hydrochloride, net price 10-mg vial = £18.72; 50-mg vial = £93.60

NOTE. This preparation has replaced *Adriamycin*®

Doxorubicin Solution for Injection (Pharmacia) PoM

Injection, doxorubicin hydrochloride 2 mg/mL, net price 5-mL vial = £20.60, 25-mL vial = £103.00, 100-mL vial = £412.00

■ Lipid formulation

Caelyx® (Schering-Plough) PoM

Concentrate for intravenous infusion, pegylated doxorubicin hydrochloride 2 mg/mL encapsulated in liposomes. For dilution before use. Net price 10-mL vial = £382.51, 25-mL vial = £813.49

For AIDS-related Kaposi's sarcoma in patients with low CD4 count and extensive mucocutaneous or visceral disease, for advanced ovarian cancer when platinum-based chemotherapy has failed, and as monotherapy for metastatic breast cancer with increased cardiac risk

Myocet® (Zeneus) ▼ PoM

Injection, powder for reconstitution, doxorubicin hydrochloride (as doxorubicin–citrate complex)

encapsulated in liposomes, net price 50-mg vial (with vials of liposomes and buffer) = £464.50
For use with cyclophosphamide for metastatic breast cancer

EPIRUBICIN HYDROCHLORIDE

Indications: see notes above and section 7.4.4
Cautions: see section 8.1 and notes above; hepatic impairment (Appendix 2); caution in handling—irritant to tissues; **interactions:** Appendix 1 (epirubicin)
Contra-indications: pregnancy (Appendix 4); breast-feeding
Side-effects: see section 8.1 and notes above

Pharmorubicin® Rapid Dissolution (Pharmacia) PoM
Injection, powder for reconstitution, epirubicin hydrochloride. Net price 10-mg vial = £19.31; 20-mg vial = £38.62; 50-mg vial = £96.54

Pharmorubicin® Solution for Injection (Pharmacia) PoM
Injection, epirubicin hydrochloride 2 mg/mL, net price 5-mL vial = £19.31, 25-mL vial = £96.54, 100-mL vial = £386.16

IDARUBICIN HYDROCHLORIDE

Indications: advanced breast cancer after failure of first-line chemotherapy (not including anthracyclines); acute leukaemias—see notes above
Cautions: see section 8.1 and notes above; hepatic impairment (Appendix 2); renal impairment (Appendix 3); caution in handling—irritant to tissues
Contra-indications: pregnancy (Appendix 4); breast-feeding
Side-effects: see section 8.1 and notes above
Dose: *by mouth*, acute non-lymphocytic leukaemia, 30 mg/m^2 daily for 3 days alone *or* 15–30 mg/m^2 daily for 3 days in combination therapy
Advanced breast cancer, 45 mg/m^2 alone, as a single dose *or* divided over 3 consecutive days; repeat every 3–4 weeks
Max. cumulative dose *by mouth* (for all indications) 400 mg/m^2
By intravenous administration, consult product literature

Zavedos® (Pharmacia) PoM
Capsules, idarubicin hydrochloride, 5 mg (red), net price 1-cap pack = £34.56; 10 mg (red/white), 1-cap pack = £69.12; 25 mg (white), 1-cap pack = £172.80. Label: 25
Injection, powder for reconstitution, idarubicin hydrochloride, net price 5-mg vial = £87.36; 10-mg vial = £174.72

MITOMYCIN

Indications: see notes above and section 7.4.4
Cautions: see section 8.1 and notes above; caution in handling—irritant to tissues
Contra-indications: pregnancy (Appendix 4); breast-feeding
Side-effects: see section 8.1 and notes above

Mitomycin C Kyowa® (Kyowa Hakko) PoM
Injection, powder for reconstitution, mitomycin. Net price 2-mg vial = £5.88; 10-mg vial = £19.37; 20-mg vial = £36.94; 40-mg vial = £73.88 (hosp. only)

MITOXANTRONE

(Mitozantrone)
Indications: see notes above
Cautions: see section 8.1 and notes above; intrathecal administration not recommended
Contra-indications: pregnancy (Appendix 4); breast-feeding
Side-effects: see section 8.1 and notes above

Mitoxantrone (Non-proprietary) PoM
Concentrate for intravenous infusion, mitoxantrone (as hydrochloride) 2 mg/mL, net price 10-mL vial = £100.00

Novantrone® (Lederle) PoM
Concentrate for intravenous infusion, mitoxantrone (as hydrochloride) 2 mg/mL, net price 10-mL vial = £139.90, 12.5-mL vial = £174.89, 15-mL vial = £209.81

Onkotrone® (Baxter) PoM
Concentrate for intravenous infusion, mitoxantrone (as hydrochloride) 2 mg/mL, net price 10-mL vial = £135.39, 12.5-mL vial = £169.25, 15-mL vial = £203.04

8.1.3 Antimetabolites

Antimetabolites are incorporated into new nuclear material or combine irreversibly with vital cellular enzymes, preventing normal cellular division.

Methotrexate inhibits the enzyme dihydrofolate reductase, essential for the synthesis of purines and pyrimidines. It is given by mouth, intravenously, intramuscularly, or intrathecally.

Methotrexate is used as maintenance therapy for childhood acute lymphoblastic leukaemia. Other uses include choriocarcinoma, non-Hodgkin's lymphoma, and a number of solid tumours. Intrathecal methotrexate is used in the CNS prophylaxis of childhood acute lymphoblastic leukaemia, and as a therapy for established meningeal cancer or lymphoma.

Methotrexate causes myelosuppression, mucositis, and rarely pneumonitis. It is **contra-indicated** in significant renal impairment because it is excreted primarily by the kidney. It is also contra-indicated in patients with severe hepatic impairment. It should also be **avoided** in the presence of significant pleural effusion or ascites because it can accumulate in these fluids, and its subsequent return to the circulation may cause myelosuppression. Systemic toxicity may follow intrathecal administration and blood counts should be carefully monitored.

Folinic acid (section 8.1) following methotrexate administration helps to prevent methotrexate-induced mucositis or myelosuppression.

Capecitabine, which is metabolised to fluorouracil, is given by mouth. It is used as monotherapy for metastatic colorectal cancer; it has been shown to be of similar efficacy as a combination of fluorouracil and folinic acid. Capecitabine is also licensed for adjuvant treatment of advanced colon cancer following surgery. It is also licensed for second-line treatment of locally advanced or metastatic breast cancer either in combination with docetaxel (where previous therapy included an anthracycline) or alone (after failure of a taxane and anthracycline regimen or where further anthracycline treatment is not indicated).

NICE guidance (capecitabine and tegafur with uracil for metastatic colorectal cancer). NICE has recommended (May 2003) capecitabine or tegafur with uracil (in combination with folinic acid) as an option for the first-line treatment of metastatic colorectal cancer.

NICE guidance (capecitabine for locally advanced or metastatic breast cancer). NICE has recommended (May 2003) capecitabine in combination with docetaxel in preference to docetaxel monotherapy for locally advanced or metastatic breast cancer in people for whom anthracycline-containing regimens are unsuitable or have failed.
Capecitabine monotherapy is recommended as an option for people with locally advanced or metastatic breast cancer who have not previously received capecitabine in combination therapy and for whom anthracycline and taxane-containing regimens have failed or further anthracycline therapy is contra-indicated.

Cytarabine acts by interfering with pyrimidine synthesis. It is given subcutaneously, intravenously, or intrathecally. Its predominant use is in the induction of remission of acute myeloblastic leukaemia. It is a potent myelosuppressant and requires careful haematological monitoring. A liposomal formulation of cytarabine for intrathecal use is licensed for lymphomatous meningitis.

Fludarabine is licensed for the initial treatment of advanced B-cell chronic lymphocytic leukaemia (CLL) or after first-line treatment in patients with sufficient bone-marrow reserves; it is given by mouth or by intravenous injection or by intravenous infusion. Fludarabine is generally well tolerated but it does cause myelosuppression, which may be cumulative. Immunosuppression is also common (see panel on cladribine and fludarabine below) and co-trimoxazole is often used to prevent pneumocystis infection. Immune-mediated haemolytic anaemia, thrombocytopenia, and neutropenia are less common side-effects.

NICE guidance (fludarabine). NICE has recommended (September 2001) oral fludarabine as second-line therapy for B-cell chronic lymphocytic leukaemia (CLL) for patients who have either failed, or are intolerant of, first-line chemotherapy.

Cladribine is an effective but potentially toxic drug given by intravenous infusion for the treatment of hairy cell leukaemia. It is also licensed for chronic lymphocytic leukaemia in patients who have failed to respond to standard regimens containing an alkylating agent; it is given by intravenous infusion. Myelosuppression may be severe and serious neurotoxicity has been reported rarely.

Cladribine and **fludarabine** have a potent and prolonged immunosuppressive effect and only irradiated blood products should be administered to prevent potentially fatal graft-versus-host reaction. Prescribers should consult specialist literature when using highly immunosuppressive drugs.

Gemcitabine is used intravenously; it is given alone for palliative treatment or with cisplatin as a first-line treatment for locally advanced or metastatic non-small cell lung cancer. It is also used in the treatment of locally advanced or metastatic pancreatic cancer. Combined with cisplatin, gemcitabine is also licensed for the treatment of advanced bladder cancer. It is generally well tolerated but may cause mild gastro-intestinal side-effects and rashes; renal impairment, pulmonary toxicity and influenza-like symptoms have also been reported. Haemolytic uraemic syndrome has been reported rarely and gemcitabine should be discontinued if signs of microangiopathic haemolytic anaemia occur.

NICE guidance (gemcitabine). NICE has recommended (May 2001) that gemcitabine is an option for first-line chemotherapy for patients with advanced or metastatic adenocarcinoma of the pancreas and a Karnofsky score of at least 50 [Karnofsky score is a measure of the ability to perform ordinary tasks].
Gemcitabine is not recommended for patients who can have potentially curative surgery. There is insufficient evidence about its use for second-line treatment of pancreatic adenocarcinoma.

NICE guidance (docetaxel, paclitaxel, gemcitabine and vinorelbine for non-small cell lung cancer). NICE has recommended (June 2001) that chemotherapy should be considered for non-small cell lung cancer in patients who are unsuitable for curative treatment or who are unlikely to respond to such treatment.
Gemcitabine, paclitaxel, or vinorelbine should be considered as first-line chemotherapy for advanced non-small cell lung cancer. Combination of each of these drugs with platinum-based chemotherapy, where tolerated, is likely to be most effective.
Docetaxel monotherapy should be considered for locally advanced or metastatic non-small cell lung cancer which relapses after previous chemotherapy.

Fluorouracil is usually given intravenously because absorption following oral administration is unpredictable. It is used to treat a number of solid tumours, including gastro-intestinal tract cancers and breast cancer. It is commonly used with folinic acid in advanced colorectal cancer. It may also be used topically for certain malignant and pre-malignant skin lesions. Toxicity is unusual, but may include myelosuppression, mucositis, and rarely a cerebellar syndrome. On prolonged infusion, a desquamative hand–foot syndrome may occur.

Pemetrexed inhibits thymidylate transferase and other folate-dependent enzymes. It is licensed for use with cisplatin for the treatment of unresectable malignant pleural mesothelioma which has not previously been treated with chemotherapy; it is given by intravenous infusion. Pemetrexed used alone is also licensed for the treatment of locally advanced or metastatic non-small cell lung cancer which has previously been treated with chemotherapy. Common adverse effects include myelosuppression, gastro-intestinal toxicity, and skin disorders.

Raltitrexed, a thymidylate synthase inhibitor, is given intravenously for palliation of advanced colorectal cancer when fluorouracil and folinic acid cannot be used. It is probably of similar efficacy to fluorouracil. Raltitrexed is generally well tolerated, but can cause marked myelosuppression and gastro-intestinal side-effects.

NICE guidance (irinotecan, oxaliplatin and raltitrexed for advanced colorectal cancer). See p. 441

Mercaptopurine is used as maintenance therapy for the acute leukaemias and in the management of ulcerative colitis and Crohn's disease (section 1.5). Azathioprine, which is metabolised to mercaptopurine, is generally used as an immunosuppressant (section 8.2.1 and section 10.1.3). The dose of both drugs should be reduced if the patient is receiving allopurinol since it interferes with their metabolism.

Tegafur (in combination with uracil) is given by mouth, together with calcium folinate, in the management of metastatic colorectal cancer. Tegafur is a prodrug of fluorouracil; uracil inhibits the degradation of fluorouracil. Tegafur (with uracil) has been shown to be of similar efficacy as a combination of fluorouracil and folinic acid for metastatic colorectal cancer. For NICE guidance on capecitabine and tegafur with uracil for metastatic colorectal cancer, see above

Tioguanine (thioguanine) is given by mouth to induce remission in acute myeloid leukaemia.

CAPECITABINE

Indications: see notes above

Cautions: see section 8.1; **interactions:** Appendix 1 (fluorouracil)

Contra-indications: hepatic impairment (Appendix 2), renal impairment (Appendix 3); pregnancy (Appendix 4); breast-feeding

Side-effects: see section 8.1 and notes above; hand–foot (desquamative) syndrome

Dose: ADULT over 18 years, 1.25 g/m^2 twice daily for 14 days; subsequent courses repeated after a 7-day interval

Xeloda® (Roche) ▼ PoM

Tablets, f/c, peach, capecitabine 150 mg, net price 60-tab pack = £44.47; 500 mg, 120-tab pack = £295.06. Label: 21

CLADRIBINE

Indications: see notes above

Cautions: see section 8.1 and notes above; use irradiated blood only; hepatic impairment (Appendix 2); renal impairment (Appendix 3)

Contra-indications: pregnancy (Appendix 4); breast-feeding

Side-effects: see section 8.1 and notes above

Leustat® (Janssen-Cilag) PoM

Injection, cladribine 1 mg/mL. For dilution and use as an infusion, net price 10-mL vial = £173.18

CYTARABINE

Indications: see notes above

Cautions: see section 8.1 and notes above; hepatic impairment (Appendix 2); **interactions:** Appendix 1 (cytarabine)

Contra-indications: pregnancy (Appendix 4); breast-feeding

Side-effects: see section 8.1 and notes above

Cytarabine (Non-proprietary) PoM

Injection (for intravenous, subcutaneous or intrathecal use), cytarabine 20 mg/mL, net price 5-mL vial (Mayne) = £4.00

Injection (for intravenous or subcutaneous use), cytarabine 20 mg/mL, net price 5-mL vial (Pharmacia) = £3.90, 25-mL vial (Pharmacia) = £19.50

Injection (for intravenous or subcutaneous use), cytarabine 100 mg/mL, net price 1-mL vial (Mayne) = £4.00; 5-mL vial (Mayne) = £20.00; 10-mL vial (Mayne) = £40.00, (Pharmacia) = £39.00; 20-mL vial (Mayne) = £79.00, (Pharmacia) = £77.50; 20-mL *Onco-vial*® (Mayne) = £79.00

■ Lipid formulation for intrathecal use

DepoCyte® (Napp) ▼ PoM

Intrathecal injection, cytarabine encapsulated in liposomes, net price 50-mg vial = £1250.00

For lymphomatous meningitis

FLUDARABINE PHOSPHATE

Indications: see notes above

Cautions: see section 8.1 and notes above; use irradiated blood only; renal impairment (Appendix 3) **interactions:** Appendix 1 (fludarabine)

Contra-indications: haemolytic anaemia, pregnancy (Appendix 4); breast-feeding

Side-effects: see section 8.1 and notes above

Dose: *by mouth*, ADULT 40 mg/m^2 for 5 days every 28 days usually for 6 cycles

By intravenous injection or infusion, consult product literature

Fludara® (Schering Health) PoM

Tablets▼, f/c, pink, fludarabine phosphate 10 mg, net price 15-tab pack = £279.00, 20-tab pack = £372.00

Injection, powder for reconstitution, fludarabine phosphate. Net price 50-mg vial = £156.00

FLUOROURACIL

Indications: see notes above

Cautions: see section 8.1 and notes above; caution in handling—irritant to tissues; hepatic impairment (Appendix 2); **interactions:** Appendix 1 (fluorouracil)

Contra-indications: pregnancy (Appendix 4); breast-feeding

Side-effects: see section 8.1 and notes above; also local irritation with topical preparation

Dose: *by mouth*, maintenance 15 mg/kg weekly; max. in one day 1 g

By intravenous injection or infusion or by intra-arterial infusion, consult product literature

Fluorouracil (Non-proprietary) PoM

Capsules, fluorouracil 250 mg.

Available from Cambridge on a named-patient basis

Injection, fluorouracil (as sodium salt) 25 mg/mL, net price 10-mL vial = £3.20, 20-mL vial = £6.40, 100-mL vial = £32.00; 50 mg/mL, 10-mL vial = £6.40, 20-mL vial = £12.80, 50-mL vial = £32.00, 100-mL vial = £64.00

■ Topical preparations

Efudix® (Valeant) PoM

Cream, fluorouracil 5%. Net price 20 g = £17.72

Excipients: include hydroxybenzoates (parabens)

Dose: malignant and pre-malignant skin lesions, apply thinly to the affected area once or twice daily; cover with occlusive dressing in malignant conditions; max. area of skin treated at one time, 500 cm^2; usual duration of initial therapy, 3–4 weeks

GEMCITABINE

Indications: see notes above

Cautions: see section 8.1 and notes above; hepatic impairment (Appendix 2); renal impairment (Appendix 3)

Contra-indications: pregnancy (Appendix 4); breast-feeding

Side-effects: see section 8.1 and notes above

Gemzar® (Lilly) PoM
Injection, powder for reconstitution, gemcitabine (as hydrochloride), net price 200-mg vial = £32.55; 1-g vial = £162.76 (both hosp. only)

MERCAPTOPURINE

Indications: acute leukaemias; inflammatory bowel disease [unlicensed indication] (section 1.5)
Cautions: see section 8.1 and notes above; monitor liver function—hepatic impairment (Appendix 2); renal impairment (Appendix 3); **interactions:** Appendix 1 (mercaptopurine)
Contra-indications: pregnancy (Appendix 4); breast-feeding
Side-effects: see section 8.1 and notes above; also hepatotoxicity; rarely pancreatitis
Dose: initially 2.5 mg/kg daily

Puri-Nethol® (GSK) PoM
Tablets, yellow, scored, mercaptopurine 50 mg. Net price 25-tab pack = £18.78

METHOTREXATE

Indications: see notes above and under Dose; rheumatoid arthritis (section 10.1.3); psoriasis (section 13.5.3)
Cautions: see section 8.1, notes above and section 10.1.3; hepatic impairment (Appendix 2); renal impairment (Appendix 3); **interactions:** Appendix 1 (methotrexate)
Contra-indications: pregnancy (Appendix 4); breast-feeding
Side-effects: see section 8.1, notes above and section 10.1.3
Dose: *by mouth*, leukaemia in children (maintenance), 15 mg/m^2 weekly in combination with other drugs

> **Important.** Note that the above dose is a **weekly** dose. The CSM has received reports of prescription and dispensing errors including fatalities. Attention should be paid to the **strength** of methotrexate tablets prescribed and the **frequency** of dosing

By intravenous injection or infusion, by intra-arterial infusion, or by intramuscular injection, or intrathecal administration, consult product literature

Methotrexate (Non-proprietary) PoM
Injection, methotrexate 2.5 mg (as sodium salt)/mL. Net price 2-mL vial (Mayne) = £1.68
Injection, methotrexate 25 mg (as sodium salt)/mL. Net price 2-mL vial (Mayne) = £4.58, (Goldshield) = £2.62; 8-mL vial (Goldshield) = £10.02; 20-mL vial (Mayne) = £39.09, (Goldshield) = £25.07; 40-mL vial (Goldshield) = £44.57; 200-mL vial (Goldshield) = £200.57
Injection, methotrexate 100 mg/mL (not for intrathecal use). Net price 10-mL vial (Mayne) = £78.33; 50-mL vial (Mayne) = £380.07

■ Oral preparations
Section 10.1.3

PEMETREXED

Indications: see notes above
Cautions: see section 8.1 and notes above; prophylactic folic acid and vitamin-B_{12} supplementation required (consult product literature)
Contra-indications: pregnancy (Appendix 4); breast-feeding (Appendix 5)
Side-effects: see section 8.1 and notes above
Dose: consult product literature

Alimta® (Lilly) ▼ PoM
Injection, powder for reconstitution, pemetrexed 500 mg (as disodium), net price 500-mg vial = £800.00

RALTITREXED

Indications: see notes above
Cautions: see section 8.1 and notes above; hepatic impairment (Appendix 2); renal impairment (Appendix 3)
Contra-indications: pregnancy (Appendix 4); breast-feeding
Side-effects: see section 8.1 and notes above

Tomudex® (AstraZeneca) PoM
Injection, powder for reconstitution, raltitrexed. Net price 2-mg vial = £121.86

TEGAFUR WITH URACIL

Indications: see notes above
Cautions: see section 8.1; cardiac disease; renal impairment; hepatic impairment (avoid if severe—Appendix 2); **interactions:** Appendix 1 (fluorouracil)
Contra-indications: pregnancy (Appendix 4); breast-feeding
Side-effects: see section 8.1 and notes above
Dose: ADULT, tegafur 300 mg/m^2 (with uracil 672 mg/m^2) daily in 3 divided doses for 28 days; subsequent courses repeated after 7-day interval; for dose adjustment due to toxicity, consult product literature

Uftoral® (Bristol-Myers Squibb) ▼ PoM
Capsules, tegafur 100 mg, uracil 224 mg, net price 21-cap pack = £79.88, 28-cap pack = £106.51, 35-cap pack = £133.14, 42-cap pack = £159.77. Label: 23

TIOGUANINE

(Thioguanine)
Indications: acute leukaemias; chronic myeloid leukaemia
Cautions: see section 8.1 and notes above; renal impairment (Appendix 3); **interactions:** Appendix 1 (tioguanine)
Contra-indications: pregnancy (Appendix 4); breast-feeding
Side-effects: see section 8.1 and notes above
Dose: induction, 100–200 mg/m^2 in 1–2 divided doses for 5–20 days; maintenance, usually 60–200 mg/m^2 daily

Lanvis® (GSK) PoM
Tablets, yellow, scored, tioguanine 40 mg. Net price 25-tab pack = £45.41

8.1.4 Vinca alkaloids and etoposide

The vinca alkaloids, **vinblastine**, **vincristine**, and **vindesine**, are used to treat the acute leukaemias, lymphomas, and some solid tumours (e.g. breast and lung cancer). **Vinorelbine**, a semi-synthetic vinca alkaloid, is used for advanced breast cancer (see also NICE guidance below) and for advanced non-small cell lung cancer (see also NICE guidance, p. 434).

Neurotoxicity, usually as peripheral or autonomic neuropathy, occurs with all vinca alkaloids and is a limiting side-effect of vincristine; it occurs less often with vindesine, vinblastine, and vinorelbine. Patients with neurotoxicity commonly have peripheral paraesthesia, loss of deep tendon reflexes, abdominal pain, and constipation. If symptoms of neurotoxicity are severe, doses should be reduced. Motor weakness can also occur, and increasing motor weakness calls for discontinuation of these drugs. Recovery from neurotoxic effects is usually slow but complete.

Myelosuppression is the dose-limiting side-effect of vinblastine, vindesine, and vinorelbine; vincristine causes negligible myelosuppression. The vinca alkaloids may cause reversible alopecia. They cause severe local irritation and care must be taken to avoid extravasation.

> Vinblastine, vincristine, vindesine, and vinorelbine are for **intravenous administration only**. Inadvertent intrathecal administration can cause severe neurotoxicity, which is usually fatal.

> **NICE guidance (vinorelbine for advanced breast cancer).** NICE has recommended (December 2002) that vinorelbine be considered as an option for the second-line (or subsequent) treatment of advanced breast cancer where anthracycline-based regimens have failed or are unsuitable.
> Vinorelbine monotherapy is not recommended as first-line treatment for advanced breast cancer.
> Insufficient information is available to recommend the routine use of vinorelbine in combination with other therapies for advanced breast cancer.

Etoposide may be given orally or by slow intravenous infusion, the oral dose being double the intravenous dose. A preparation containing etoposide phosphate can be given by intravenous injection or infusion. Etoposide is usually given daily for 3–5 days and courses should not be repeated more frequently than at intervals of 21 days. It has particularly useful activity in small cell carcinoma of the bronchus, the lymphomas, and testicular cancer. Toxic effects include alopecia, myelosuppression, nausea, and vomiting.

ETOPOSIDE

Indications: see notes above

Cautions: see section 8.1 and notes above; renal impairment (Appendix 3); **interactions:** Appendix 1 (etoposide)

Contra-indications: see section 8.1 and notes above; severe hepatic impairment; pregnancy (Appendix 4); breast-feeding

Side-effects: see section 8.1 and notes above; irritant to tissues

Dose: *by mouth*, 120–240 mg/m^2 daily for 5 days
By intravenous infusion, consult product literature

Etoposide (Non-proprietary) PoM
Concentrate for intravenous infusion, etoposide 20 mg/mL, net price 5-mL vial = £12.15, 10-mL vial = £29.00, 25-mL vial = £60.75
NOTE. Prices from different suppliers can vary
Brands include *Eposin*®

Etopophos® (Bristol-Myers Squibb) PoM
Injection, powder for reconstitution, etoposide (as phosphate), net price 100-mg vial = £29.87 (hosp. only)

Vepesid® (Bristol-Myers Squibb) PoM
Capsules, both pink, etoposide 50 mg, net price 20 = £105.97; 100 mg, 10-cap pack = £92.60 (hosp. only). Label: 23
Concentrate for intravenous infusion, etoposide 20 mg/mL, net price 5-mL vial = £13.56 (hosp. only)
Excipients: include benzyl alcohol (avoid in neonates, see Excipients, p. 2)

VINBLASTINE SULPHATE

Indications: see notes above

Cautions: see section 8.1 and notes above; hepatic impairment (Appendix 2); caution in handling; **interactions:** Appendix 1 (vinblastine)

Contra-indications: see section 8.1 and notes above; pregnancy (Appendix 4); breast-feeding
IMPORTANT. Intrathecal injection **contra-indicated**

Side-effects: see section 8.1 and notes above; irritant to tissues

Vinblastine (Non-proprietary) PoM
Injection, vinblastine sulphate 1 mg/mL. Net price 10-mL vial = £13.09

Velbe® (Clonmel) PoM
Injection, powder for reconstitution, vinblastine sulphate. Net price 10-mg amp = £14.15

VINCRISTINE SULPHATE

Indications: see notes above

Cautions: see section 8.1 and notes above; hepatic impairment (Appendix 2); caution in handling; **interactions:** Appendix 1 (vincristine)

Contra-indications: see section 8.1 and notes above; pregnancy (Appendix 4); breast-feeding
IMPORTANT. Intrathecal injection **contra-indicated**

Side-effects: see section 8.1 and notes above; irritant to tissues

Vincristine (Non-proprietary) PoM
Injection, vincristine sulphate 1 mg/mL. Net price 1-mL vial = £10.92; 2-mL vial = £21.17; 5-mL vial = £44.16

Oncovin® (Clonmel) PoM
Injection, vincristine sulphate 1 mg/mL, net price 1-mL vial = £14.18; 2-mL vial = £28.05

VINDESINE SULPHATE

Indications: see notes above

Cautions: see section 8.1 and notes above; hepatic impairment (Appendix 2); caution in handling

Contra-indications: see section 8.1 and notes above; pregnancy (Appendix 4); breast-feeding
IMPORTANT. Intrathecal injection **contra-indicated**

Side-effects: see section 8.1 and notes above; irritant to tissues

Eldisine® (Clonmel) PoM
Injection, powder for reconstitution, vindesine sulphate, net price 5-mg vial = £78.30 (hosp. only)

VINORELBINE

Indications: see notes above

Cautions: see section 8.1 and notes above; hepatic impairment (Appendix 2); caution in handling

Contra-indications: see section 8.1 and notes above; pregnancy (Appendix 4); breast-feeding

IMPORTANT. Intrathecal injection **contra-indicated**

Side-effects: see section 8.1 and notes above; irritant to tissues

Navelbine® (Fabre) PoM

Injection concentrate, vinorelbine (as tartrate) 10 mg/mL. Net price 1-mL vial = £29.75; 5-mL vial = £139.98

8.1.5 Other antineoplastic drugs

Amsacrine

Amsacrine has an action and toxic effects similar to those of doxorubicin (section 8.1.2) and is given *intravenously*. It is occasionally used in acute myeloid leukaemia. Side-effects include myelosuppression and mucositis; electrolytes should be monitored as fatal arrhythmias have occurred in association with hypokalaemia.

AMSACRINE

Indications: see notes above

Cautions: see section 8.1 and notes above; reduce dose in renal or hepatic impairment; also caution in handling—irritant to skin and tissues

Contra-indications: pregnancy (Appendix 4); breast-feeding

Side-effects: see section 8.1 and notes above

Amsidine® (Goldshield) PoM

Concentrate for intravenous infusion, amsacrine 5 mg (as lactate)/mL, when reconstituted by mixing two solutions. Net price 1.5-mL (75-mg) amp with 13.5-mL diluent vial = £49.17 (hosp. only)

NOTE. Use glass apparatus for reconstitution

Arsenic trioxide

Arsenic trioxide is licensed for acute promyelocytic leukaemia in patients who have relapsed or failed to respond to previous treatment with a retinoid and chemotherapy.

ARSENIC TRIOXIDE

Indications: see notes above

Cautions: see section 8.1; correct electrolyte abnormalities before treatment; ECG required before and during treatment—consult product literature; avoid concomitant administration with drugs causing QT interval prolongation, hypokalaemia, and hypomagnesaemia; previous treatment with anthracyclines (increased risk of QT interval prolongation); renal impairment (Appendix 3)

Contra-indications: pregnancy (Appendix 4); breast-feeding (Appendix 5)

Side-effects: see section 8.1; leucocyte activation syndrome (requires immediate treatment—consult product literature); hyperglycaemia, hypokalaemia, leucocytosis, QT interval prolongation, atrial fibrillation, atrial flutter, haemorrhage, dyspnoea, pleuritic pain, musculoskeletal pain, paraesthesia, fatigue

Trisenox® (Cell Therapeutics) ▼ PoM

Concentrate for intravenous infusion, arsenic trioxide 1 mg/mL, net price 10-mL amp = £250.90

Bevacizumab

Bevacizumab is an inhibitor of vascular endothelial growth factor. It is licensed for treating metastatic colorectal cancer with a combination *either* of fluorouracil and folinic acid *or* of fluorouracil, folinic acid, and irinotecan. Bevacizumab is given by intravenous infusion.

BEVACIZUMAB

Indications: see notes above

Cautions: see section 8.1; intra-abdominal inflammation (risk of gastro-intestinal perforation); withhold for elective surgery and avoid for at least 28 days after major surgery or until wound fully healed; history of hypertension (increased risk of proteinuria—discontinue if nephrotic syndrome); uncontrolled hypertension; monitor blood pressure during treatment; history of arterial thromboembolism; elderly (increased risk of cardiovascular events)

Contra-indications: pregnancy (Appendix 4); breast-feeding (Appendix 5); untreated CNS metastases

Side-effects: see section 8.1; mucocutaneous bleeding; gastro-intestinal perforation; impaired wound healing; arterial thromboembolism; hypertension (see also Cautions); proteinuria

Avastin® (Roche) ▼ PoM

Concentrate for intravenous infusion, bevacizumab 25 mg/mL, net price 100-mg vial = £242.66; 400-mg vial = £924.40

Bexarotene

Bexarotene is an agonist at the retinoid X receptor, which is involved in the regulation of cell differentiation and proliferation. It is generally well tolerated when given by mouth and it is associated with little myelosuppression or immunosuppression. Bexarotene can cause regression of cutaneous T-cell lymphoma. The main adverse effects are hyperlipidaemia, hypothyroidism, leucopenia, headache, rash, and pruritus.

BEXAROTENE

Indications: skin manifestations of cutaneous T-cell lymphoma refractory to previous systemic treatment

Cautions: see section 8.1 and notes above; hyperlipidaemia (avoid if uncontrolled), hypothyroidism (avoid if uncontrolled); hypersensitivity to retinoids; **interactions:** Appendix 1 (bexarotene)

Contra-indications: see section 8.1 and notes above; history of pancreatitis, hypervitaminosis A, hepatic impairment; pregnancy (Appendix 4); breast-feeding

Side-effects: see section 8.1 and notes above

Dose: initially 300 mg/m^2 daily as a single dose with a meal; adjust dose according to response

Targretin® (Zeneus) ▼ PoM
Capsules, bexarotene 75 mg in a liquid suspension, net price 100-cap pack = £937.50

Bortezomib

Bortezomib is a protease inhibitor, which is licensed for multiple myeloma where the disease has progressed despite the use of at least two therapies. It is given by intravenous injection. Peripheral neuropathy, thrombocytopenia, gastro-intestinal disturbances, pyrexia, postural hypotension, and fatigue are among the most common side-effects.

BORTEZOMIB

Indications: see notes above
Cautions: see section 8.1 and notes above; hepatic impairment (avoid if severe; Appendix 2), renal impairment (Appendix 3); monitor blood-glucose concentration in patients on oral antidiabetics
Side-effects: see section 8.1 and notes above

Velcade® (Ortho Biotech) ▼ PoM
Injection, powder for reconstitution, bortezomib (as mannitol boronic ester), net price 3.5-mg vial = £762.38

Cetuximab

Cetuximab is licensed, in combination with irinotecan, for the treatment of metastatic colorectal cancer in patients with tumours expressing epidermal growth factor receptor in whom previous chemotherapy, that has included irinotecan, has failed.

Cetuximab is given by intravenous infusion. Resuscitation facilities should be available and treatment should be initiated by a specialist.

CETUXIMAB

Indications: see notes above and product literature
Cautions: cardiopulmonary disease, pulmonary disease; pregnancy (Appendix 4)
Contra-indications: breast-feeding (Appendix 5)
Side-effects: infusion-related side-effects including chills, fever, hypersensitivity reactions such as rash, urticaria, airway obstruction, dyspnoea (possibly delayed onset), hypotension; skin reactions including acne, nail disorders; conjunctivitis

Erbitux® (Merck) ▼ PoM
Intravenous infusion, cetuximab 2 mg/mL, net price 50-mL vial = £136.50

Crisantaspase

Crisantaspase is the enzyme asparaginase produced by *Erwinia chrysanthemi*. It is given *intramuscularly* or *subcutaneously* almost exclusively in acute lymphoblastic leukaemia. Facilities for the management of anaphylaxis should be available. Side-effects also include nausea, vomiting, CNS depression, and liver function and blood lipid changes; careful monitoring is therefore necessary and the urine is tested for glucose because of a risk of hyperglycaemia.

CRISANTASPASE

Indications: see notes above
Cautions: see notes above
Contra-indications: pregnancy (Appendix 4); breast-feeding
Side-effects: see notes above

Erwinase® (Ipsen) PoM
Injection, powder for reconstitution, crisantaspase. Net price 10 000-unit vial = £39.94
NOTE. Supplies may be temporarily unavailable

Dacarbazine and temozolomide

Dacarbazine is used to treat metastatic melanoma and, in combination therapy, soft tissue sarcomas. It is also a component of a commonly used combination for Hodgkin's disease (ABVD—doxorubicin [previously *Adriamycin*®], bleomycin, vinblastine, and dacarbazine). It is given *intravenously*. The predominant side-effects are myelosuppression and severe nausea and vomiting.

Temozolomide is structurally related to dacarbazine and is licensed for second-line treatment of malignant glioma.

> **NICE guidance (temozolomide).** NICE has recommended (April 2001) that temozolomide may be considered for the treatment of recurrent malignant glioma, which has not responded to first-line chemotherapy.

DACARBAZINE

Indications: see notes above
Cautions: see section 8.1; hepatic impairment (Appendix 2); renal impairment (Appendix 3); caution in handling
Contra-indications: pregnancy (Appendix 4)
Side-effects: see section 8.1 and notes above; rarely liver necrosis due to hepatic vein thrombosis; irritant to skin and tissues

Dacarbazine (Non-proprietary) PoM
Injection, powder for reconstitution, dacarbazine (as citrate), net price 100-mg vial = £5.11 (Medac) or £5.05 (Pliva); 200-mg vial = £7.24 (Medac) or £7.50 (Mayne) or £7.16 (Pliva); 500-mg vial = £16.50 (Medac); 600-mg vial = £22.50 (Mayne); 1-g vial = £31.80 (Medac)

DTIC-Dome® (Bayer) PoM
Injection, powder for reconstitution, dacarbazine. Net price 200-mg vial = £7.40

TEMOZOLOMIDE

Indications: see notes above
Cautions: see section 8.1; severe hepatic impairment and renal impairment; **interactions:** Appendix 1 (temozolomide)
Contra-indications: pregnancy (Appendix 4); breast-feeding
Side-effects: see section 8.1
Dose: 200 mg/m^2 once daily for 5 days of a 28-day cycle; for patients previously treated with chemotherapy—consult product literature; CHILD under 3 years not recommended

Temodal® (Schering-Plough) PoM
Capsules, temozolomide 5 mg, net price 5-cap pack = £17.30; 20 mg, 5-cap pack = £69.20; 100 mg, 5-cap pack = £346.00; 250 mg, 5-cap pack = £865.00. Label: 23, 25

Hydroxycarbamide

Hydroxycarbamide (hydroxyurea) is an orally active drug used mainly in the treatment of chronic myeloid leukaemia. It is occasionally used for polycythaemia (the usual treatment is venesection). Myelosuppression, nausea, and skin reactions are the most common toxic effects.

HYDROXYCARBAMIDE

(Hydroxyurea)

Indications: see notes above

Cautions: see section 8.1 and notes above

Contra-indications: pregnancy (Appendix 4); breast-feeding

Side-effects: see section 8.1 and notes above

Dose: 20–30 mg/kg daily *or* 80 mg/kg every third day

Hydroxycarbamide (Non-proprietary) PoM
Capsules, hydroxycarbamide 500 mg, net price 20 = £17.20

Hydrea® (Squibb) PoM
Capsules, pink/green, hydroxycarbamide 500 mg. Net price 20 = £2.39

Imatinib

Imatinib is a protein–tyrosine kinase inhibitor, which is licensed for the treatment of newly diagnosed chronic myeloid leukaemia where bone marrow transplantation is not considered first-line treatment and for chronic myeloid leukaemia in chronic phase after failure of interferon alfa, or in accelerated phase, or in blast crisis. It is also licensed for Kit-positive unresectable or metastatic malignant gastro-intestinal stromal tumours (GIST). The most frequent side-effects of imatinib are nausea, vomiting, diarrhoea, oedema, abdominal pain, fatigue, myalgia, headache, and rash; gynaecomastia because of reduced testosterone has been reported.

The *Scottish Medicines Consortium* has advised (March 2002) that imatinib should be used for chronic myeloid leukaemia only under specialist supervision in accordance with British Society of Haematology guidelines (November 2001).

> **NICE guidance (imatinib for chronic myeloid leukaemia).** NICE has recommended (October 2003) imatinib as first-line treatment for Philadelphia-chromosome-positive chronic myeloid leukaemia in the chronic phase and as an option for patients presenting in the accelerated phase or with blast crisis, provided that imatinib has not been used previously.
> Where imatinib has failed to stop disease progression from chronic phase to accelerated phase or blast crisis, continued use is recommended only as part of further clinical study.

IMATINIB

Indications: see notes above

Cautions: consult product literature; pregnancy (Appendix 4 and section 8.1); **interactions:** Appendix 1 (imatinib)

Contra-indications: breast-feeding

Side-effects: see section 8.1 and notes above

Dose: consult product literature

Glivec® (Novartis) ▼ PoM
Tablets, f/c, imatinib (as mesilate) 100 mg (yellow-brown, scored), net price 60-tab pack = £778.68; 400 mg, (yellow), 30-tab pack = £1557.36

Pentostatin

Pentostatin is highly active in hairy cell leukaemia. It is given *intravenously* on alternate weeks and is capable of inducing prolonged complete remission. It is potentially toxic, causing myelosuppression, immunosuppression and a number of other side-effects which may be severe. Its use is probably best confined to specialist centres.

PENTOSTATIN

Indications: see notes above

Cautions: see section 8.1 and notes above; **interactions:** Appendix 1 (pentostatin)

Contra-indications: pregnancy (Appendix 4); breast-feeding

Side-effects: see section 8.1 and notes above

Nipent® (Lederle) PoM
Injection, powder for reconstitution, pentostatin. Net price 10-mg vial = £863.78

Platinum compounds

Carboplatin is widely used in the treatment of advanced ovarian cancer and lung cancer (particulary the small cell type). It is given *intravenously*. The dose of carboplatin is determined according to renal function rather than body surface area. Carboplatin can be given on an outpatient basis and is better tolerated than cisplatin; nausea and vomiting are reduced in severity and nephrotoxicity, neurotoxicity, and ototoxicity are much less of a problem than with cisplatin. It is, however, more myelosuppressive than cisplatin.

Cisplatin is used alone or in combination for the treatment of testicular, lung, cervical, bladder, head and neck, and ovarian cancer (but carboplatin is preferred for ovarian cancer). It is given *intravenously*. Cisplatin requires intensive intravenous hydration and treatment may be complicated by severe nausea and vomiting. Cisplatin is toxic, causing nephrotoxicity (monitoring of renal function is essential), ototoxicity, peripheral neuropathy, hypomagnesaemia and myelosuppression. It is, however, increasingly given in a day-care setting.

Oxaliplatin is licensed in combination with fluorouracil and folinic acid, for the treatment of metastatic colorectal cancer and as adjuvant treatment of colon cancer after resection of the primary tumour; it is given by intravenous infusion. Neurotoxic side-effects (including sensory peripheral neuropathy) are dose limiting. Other side-effects include gastro-intestinal disturbances, ototoxicity, and myelosuppression. Manufacturers advise renal function monitoring in moderate impairment.

NICE guidance (irinotecan, oxaliplatin, and raltitrexed for advanced colorectal cancer). NICE has recommended (March 2002) that oxaliplatin, in combination with fluorouracil and folinic acid, should be considered first-line treatment for advanced colorectal cancer **only** in patients with metastases which are confined to the liver and which could be resected following treatment.
Irinotecan monotherapy is recommended in patients who have failed to respond to an established fluorouracil-containing treatment.
A combination of fluorouracil and folinic acid with either irinotecan or oxaliplatin is **not** recommended for *routine* first-line treatment of advanced colorectal cancer.
Raltitrexed is **not** recommended for the treatment of advanced colorectal cancer. Its use should be confined to clinical studies.

NICE guidance (paclitaxel for ovarian cancer). NICE has recommended (January 2003) that *either* paclitaxel in combination with a platinum compound (cisplatin or carboplatin) *or* a platinum compound alone be used for the first-line treatment of ovarian cancer (usually following surgery).

NICE guidance (paclitaxel, pegylated liposomal doxorubicin, and topotecan for second-line or subsequent treatment of advanced ovarian cancer). NICE has recommended (May 2005) that paclitaxel, combined with a platinum compound, is an option for advanced cancer that relapses 6 months or more after completing initial platinum-based chemotherapy. Paclitaxel alone is an option for advanced ovarian cancer that does not respond to, or relapses within 6 months of completing initial platinum-based chemotherapy.
Pegylated liposomal doxorubicin is an option for advanced ovarian cancer that does not respond to, or relapses within 12 months of completing initial platinum-based chemotherapy.
Paclitaxel alone or pegylated liposomal doxorubicin are options for advanced ovarian cancer in patients who are allergic to platinum compounds. Topotecan alone is an option only for advanced ovarian cancer that does not respond to, or relapses within 6 months of completing initial platinum-based chemotherapy or in those allergic to platinum compounds *and* for whom paclitaxel alone or pegylated liposomal doxorubicin are inappropriate.

CARBOPLATIN

Indications: see notes above
Cautions: see section 8.1 and notes above; renal impairment (Appendix 3); **interactions**: Appendix 1 (platinum compounds)
Contra-indications: pregnancy (Appendix 4); breast-feeding
Side-effects: see section 8.1 and notes above

Carboplatin (Non-proprietary) PoM
Injection, carboplatin 10 mg/mL, net price 5-mL vial = £22.04, 15-mL vial = £56.29, 45-mL vial = £168.85, 60-mL vial = £260.00
NOTE. Prices from different suppliers can vary
Brands include *Onco-vial*®

Paraplatin® (Bristol-Myers Squibb) PoM
Concentrate for intravenous infusion, carboplatin 10 mg/mL, net price 5-mL vial = £21.26, 15-mL vial = £61.22, 45-mL vial = £183.66, 60-mL vial = £244.88

CISPLATIN

Indications: see notes above
Cautions: see section 8.1 and notes above; renal impairment (Appendix 3); **interactions:** Appendix 1 (platinum compounds)
Contra-indications: pregnancy (Appendix 4); breast-feeding
Side-effects: see section 8.1 and notes above

Cisplatin (Non-proprietary) PoM
Injection, cisplatin 1 mg/mL, net price 10-mL vial = £5.85, 50-mL vial = £25.37, 100-mL vial = £50.22
NOTE. Prices from different suppliers can vary
Brands include *Platinex*®
Injection, powder for reconstitution, cisplatin, net price 50-mg vial = £17.00

OXALIPLATIN

Indications: metastatic colorectal cancer in combination with fluorouracil and folinic acid; colon cancer—see notes above
Cautions: see section 8.1 and notes above; renal impairment (Appendix 3); **interactions:** Appendix 1 (platinum compounds)
Contra-indications: see section 8.1; peripheral neuropathy with functional impairment; pregnancy (Appendix 4); breast-feeding
Side-effects: see section 8.1 and notes above

Eloxatin® (Sanofi-Synthelabo) PoM
Injection, powder for reconstitution, oxaliplatin, net price 50-mg vial = £165.00, 100-mg vial = £330.00

Porfimer sodium and temoporfin

Porfimer sodium and **temoporfin** are used in the photodynamic treatment of various tumours. The drugs accumulate in malignant tissue and are activated by laser light to produce a cytotoxic effect.

Porfimer sodium is licensed for photodynamic therapy of non-small cell lung cancer and obstructing oesophageal cancer. Temoporfin is licensed for photodynamic therapy of advanced head and neck cancer.

The *Scottish Medicines Consortium* has advised (May 2004) that temoporfin is **not** recommended for the palliative treatment of advanced head and neck cancer.

PORFIMER SODIUM

Indications: non-small cell lung cancer; oesophageal cancer; see notes above
Cautions: see section 8.1; avoid exposure of skin and eyes to direct sunlight or bright indoor light for at least 30 days
Contra-indications: see section 8.1; severe hepatic impairment; tracheo-oesophageal or broncho-oesophageal fistula; porphyria (section 9.8.2); pregnancy (Appendix 4); breast-feeding (Appendix 5)
Side-effects: see section 8.1; photosensitivity (see Cautions above—sunscreens offer no protection), constipation
Dose: *by intravenous injection* over 3 to 5 minutes, 2 mg/kg
NOTE. For further information on administration and light activation, consult product literature

Photofrin (Sinclair) ▼ PoM
Injection, powder for reconstitution, porfimer sodium, net price 15-mg vial = £154.00; 75-mg vial = £770.00

TEMOPORFIN

Indications: advanced head and neck squamous cell carcinoma refractory to, or unsuitable for, other treatments

Cautions: see section 8.1; avoid exposure of skin and eyes to direct sunlight or bright indoor light for at least 15 days after administration; **interactions:** Appendix 1 (temoporfin)

Contra-indications: see section 8.1; porphyria (section 9.8.2) or other diseases exacerbated by light; elective surgery or ophthalmic slit-lamp examination for 30 days after administration; existing photosensitising treatment; pregnancy; breast-feeding

Side-effects: see section 8.1; photosensitivity (see Cautions above—sunscreens offer no protection), constipation, local haemorrhage, facial pain and oedema, scarring, dysphagia

Dose: *by intravenous injection* over at least 6 minutes, ADULT 150 microgram/kg

NOTE. For use undiluted; for further information on administration and light activation, consult product literature

Foscan® (Biolitec) ▼ PoM
Injection, temoporfin 4 mg/mL, net price 5-mL vial = £4400.00

Procarbazine

Procarbazine is most often used in Hodgkin's disease, for example in MOPP (chlormethine (mustine), vincristine [*Oncovin*®], procarbazine, and prednisolone) chemotherapy. It is given *by mouth*. Toxic effects include nausea, myelosuppression, and a hypersensitivity rash preventing further use of this drug. It is a mild monoamine-oxidase inhibitor but dietary restriction is not considered necessary. Alcohol ingestion may cause a disulfiram-like reaction.

PROCARBAZINE

Indications: see notes above

Cautions: see section 8.1 and notes above; hepatic impairment—avoid if severe; renal impairment—avoid if severe; **interactions:** Appendix 1 (procarbazine)

Contra-indications: pregnancy (Appendix 4); breast-feeding

Side-effects: see section 8.1 and notes above

Dose: used alone, initially 50 mg daily, increased by 50 mg daily to 250–300 mg daily in divided doses; maintenance (on remission) 50–150 mg daily to cumulative total of at least 6 g

Procarbazine (Cambridge) PoM
Capsules, ivory, procarbazine (as hydrochloride) 50 mg, net price 50-cap pack = £37.44. Label: 4

Taxanes

Paclitaxel is a member of the taxane group of drugs. It is given by *intravenous infusion*. Paclitaxel given with carboplatin or cisplatin is used for the treatment of ovarian cancer (see NICE guidance p. 441); the combination is also considered appropriate for women whose ovarian cancer is initially considered inoperable. Paclitaxel is also used in the secondary treatment of metastatic breast cancer (see NICE guidance below). There is limited evidence to support its use in non-small cell lung cancer. Routine premedication with a corticosteroid, an antihistamine and a histamine H_2-receptor antagonist is recommended to prevent severe hypersensitivity reactions; hypersensitivity reactions may occur rarely despite premedication, although more commonly only bradycardia or asymptomatic hypotension occur.

Other side-effects of paclitaxel include myelosuppression, peripheral neuropathy, and cardiac conduction defects with arrhythmias (which are nearly always asymptomatic). It also causes alopecia and muscle pain; nausea and vomiting is mild to moderate.

Docetaxel is licensed for use in locally advanced or metastatic breast cancer and non-small cell lung cancer resistant to other cytotoxic drugs (see NICE guidance on breast cancer, below) or for initial chemotherapy in combination with other cytotoxic drugs. It is also licensed for hormone-resistant prostate cancer and for use with other cytotoxic drugs for adjuvant treatment of operable node-positive breast cancer. Its side-effects are similar to those of paclitaxel but persistent fluid retention (commonly as leg oedema that worsens during treatment) can be resistant to treatment; hypersensitivity reactions also occur. Dexamethasone by mouth is recommended for reducing fluid retention and hypersensitivity reactions.

NICE guidance (paclitaxel, pegylated liposomal doxorubicin and topotecan for second-line or subsequent treatment of advanced ovarian cancer). See p. 441

NICE guidance (breast cancer). NICE has recommended (September 2001) that both docetaxel and paclitaxel should be available for the treatment of advanced breast cancer where initial cytotoxic chemotherapy (including an anthracycline) has failed or is inappropriate. The use of taxanes for adjuvant treatment of early breast cancer or for the first-line treatment of advanced breast cancer should be limited to clinical trials [but see notes above].

NICE guidance (docetaxel, paclitaxel, gemcitabine and vinorelbine for non-small cell lung cancer). See p. 434

DOCETAXEL

Indications: adjuvant treatment of operable node-positive breast cancer, in combination with doxorubicin and cyclophosphamide; with doxorubicin for initial chemotherapy of advanced or metastatic breast cancer; alone or with capecitabine for advanced or metastatic breast cancer where cytotoxic chemotherapy with anthracycline or alkylating drug has failed; with trastuzumab for initial chemotherapy of metastatic breast cancer; advanced or metastatic non-small cell lung cancer where first-line chemotherapy has failed; with cisplatin for unresectable, advanced or metastatic non-small cell lung cancer; with prednisolone for hormone-refractory metastatic prostate cancer

Cautions: see section 8.1 and notes above; hepatic impairment (Appendix 2); **interactions:** Appendix 1 (docetaxel)
Contra-indications: pregnancy (Appendix 4); breast-feeding
Side-effects: see section 8.1 and notes above

Taxotere® (Sanofi-Aventis) PoM
Concentrate for intravenous infusion, docetaxel 40 mg/mL. Net price 0.5-mL vial = £162.75, 2-mL vial = £534.75 (both with diluent) (hosp. only)

PACLITAXEL

Indications: ovarian cancer (advanced or residual disease following laparotomy) in combination with cisplatin; metastatic ovarian cancer where platinum-containing therapy has failed; locally advanced or metastatic breast cancer (in combination with other cytotoxics or alone if other cytotoxics have failed or are inappropriate); adjuvant treatment of node-positive breast cancer following treatment with anthracycline and cyclophosphamide; non-small cell lung cancer (in combination with cisplatin) when surgery or radiotherapy not appropriate; advanced AIDS-related Kaposi's sarcoma where liposomal anthracycline therapy has failed
Cautions: see section 8.1 and notes above; **interactions:** Appendix 1 (paclitaxel)
Contra-indications: see section 8.1 and notes above; severe hepatic impairment; pregnancy (Appendix 4); breast-feeding
Side-effects: see section 8.1 and notes above

Paclitaxel (Non-proprietary) PoM
Concentrate for intravenous infusion, paclitaxel 6 mg/mL, net price 5-mL vial = £112.20, 16.7-mL vial = £336.60, 25-mL vial = £561.00, 50-mL vial = £1009.80
Excipients: include polyoxyl castor oil (risk of anaphylaxis, see Excipients, p. 2)

Taxol® (Bristol-Myers Squibb) PoM
Concentrate for intravenous infusion, paclitaxel 6 mg/mL, net price 5-mL vial = £116.05, 16.7-mL vial = £347.82, 25-mL vial = £521.73, 50-mL vial = £1043.46 (hosp. only)
Excipients: include polyoxyl castor oil (risk of anaphylaxis, see Excipients, p. 2)

Topoisomerase I inhibitors

Irinotecan and topotecan inhibit topoisomerase I, an enzyme involved in DNA replication.

Irinotecan is licensed for metastatic colorectal cancer in combination with fluorouracil and folinic acid or as monotherapy when treatment containing fluorouracil has failed; it is given by intravenous infusion.

NICE guidance (irinotecan, oxaliplatin and raltitrexed for advanced colorectal cancer). See p. 441

Topotecan is given by intravenous infusion in metastatic ovarian cancer when first-line or subsequent therapy has failed.

In addition to dose-limiting myelosuppression, side-effects of irinotecan and topotecan include gastro-intestinal effects (delayed diarrhoea requiring prompt treatment may follow irinotecan treatment), asthenia, alopecia, and anorexia.

NICE guidance (paclitaxel, pegylated liposomal doxorubicin and topotecan for second-line or subsequent treatment of advanced ovarian cancer). See p. 441

IRINOTECAN HYDROCHLORIDE

Indications: metastatic colorectal cancer in combination with fluorouracil and folinic acid or where treatment containing fluorouracil has failed
Cautions: see section 8.1 and notes above; raised plasma-bilirubin concentration (see under Contra-indications and Appendix 2)
Contra-indications: see section 8.1 and notes above, also chronic inflammatory bowel disease, bowel obstruction; plasma bilirubin concentration more than 1.5 times the upper limit of reference range; avoid conception for at least 3 months after cessation of treatment (Appendix 4); breast-feeding
Side-effects: see section 8.1 and notes above; also acute cholinergic syndrome (with early diarrhoea) and delayed diarrhoea (consult product literature)

Campto® (Pfizer) PoM
Concentrate for intravenous infusion, irinotecan hydrochloride 20 mg/mL, net price 2-mL vial = £53.00; 5-mL vial = £130.00

TOPOTECAN

Indications: metastatic ovarian cancer where first-line or subsequent therapy has failed
Cautions: see section 8.1 and notes above; renal impairment (avoid if severe—Appendix 3)
Contra-indications: see section 8.1 and notes above; severe hepatic impairment; pregnancy (Appendix 4); breast-feeding
Side-effects: see section 8.1 and notes above

Hycamtin® (Merck) PoM
Intravenous infusion, powder for reconstitution, topotecan (as hydrochloride), net price 1-mg vial = £97.65; 4-mg vial = £290.62

Trastuzumab

Trastuzumab is licensed, in combination with paclitaxel, for metastatic breast cancer in patients with tumours overexpressing the human epidermal growth factor receptor 2 (HER2) who have not received chemotherapy for metastatic breast cancer and in whom anthracycline treatment is inappropriate; trastuzumab is also licensed for use with docetaxel.

Trastuzumab is also licensed as monotherapy for metastatic breast cancer in patients with tumours that overexpress HER2 who have received at least 2 chemotherapy regimens including, where appropriate, an anthracycline and a taxane; women with oestrogen-receptor-positive breast cancer should also have received hormonal therapy.

Trastuzumab is given by intravenous infusion. Resuscitation facilities should be available and treatment should be initiated by a specialist.

NICE guidance (trastuzumab for advanced breast cancer). NICE has recommended (March 2002) that trastuzumab, used in accordance with the licensed indications for *Herceptin*®, is an option in the management of metastatic breast cancer.

USE WITH ANTHRACYCLINES. Concomitant use of trastuzumab with anthracyclines (section 8.1.2) is associated with cardiotoxicity. The EMEA has advised that the use of anthracyclines even after stopping trastuzumab may carry a higher risk of cardiotoxicity and if possible should be avoided for up to 22 weeks. If anthracyclines need to be used, cardiac function should be monitored.

TRASTUZUMAB

Indications: see notes above and product literature

Cautions: see section 8.1 and notes above; symptomatic heart failure, history of hypertension, coronary artery disease; pregnancy (Appendix 4)

CARDIOTOXICITY. Monitor cardiac function of all patients before and during treatment—for details of monitoring and managing cardiotoxity, consult product literature

Contra-indications: see section 8.1 and notes above; severe dyspnoea at rest; breast-feeding (Appendix 5)

Side-effects: infusion-related side-effects including chills, fever, hypersensitivity reactions such as anaphylaxis, urticaria and angioedema, pulmonary events (possibly delayed onset); cardiotoxicity (see also above); gastro-intestinal symptoms, asthenia, headache, chest pains, arthralgia, myalgia, hypotension

Herceptin® (Roche) ▼ PoM
Injection, powder for reconstitution, trastuzumab, net price 150-mg vial = £407.40. For intravenous infusion

Tretinoin

Tretinoin is licensed for the induction of remission in acute promyelocytic leukaemia. It is used in previously untreated patients as well as in those who have relapsed after standard chemotherapy or who are refractory to it.

TRETINOIN

NOTE. Tretinoin is the acid form of vitamin A

Indications: see notes above; acne (section 13.6.1); photodamage (section 13.8.1)

Cautions: exclude pregnancy before starting treatment and avoid pregnancy during and for at least 1 month after treatment; monitor haematological and coagulation profile, liver function, serum calcium and plasma lipids before and during treatment; increased risk of thrombo-embolism during first month of treatment; hepatic impairment (Appendix 2); renal impairment (Appendix 3); **interactions:** Appendix 1 (retinoids)

Contra-indications: pregnancy (**important teratogenic risk:** see Cautions and Appendix 4) and breast-feeding

Side-effects: retinoic acid syndrome (fever, dyspnoea, acute respiratory distress, pulmonary infiltrates, pleural effusion, hyperleukocytosis, hypotension, oedema, weight gain, hepatic, renal and multi-organ failure) requires immediate treatment—consult product literature; gastro-intestinal disturbances, pancreatitis; arrhythmias, flushing, oedema; headache, benign intracranial hypertension (mainly in children—consider dose reduction if intractable headache in children), shivering, dizziness, confusion, anxiety, depression, insomnia, paraesthesia, visual and hearing disturbances; raised liver enzymes, serum creatinine and lipids; bone and chest pain, alopecia, erythema, rash, pruritus, sweating, dry skin and mucous membranes, cheilitis; thromboembolism, hypercalcaemia, and genital ulceration reported

Dose: ADULT and CHILD 45 mg/m^2 daily in 2 divided doses, max. duration of treatment 90 days (consult product literature for details of concomitant chemotherapy)

Vesanoid® (Roche) PoM
Capsules, yellow/brown, tretinoin 10 mg. Net price 100-cap pack = £170.52. Label: 21

8.2 Drugs affecting the immune response

Immunosuppressant therapy

Immunosuppressants are used to suppress rejection in organ transplant recipients and to treat a variety of chronic inflammatory and autoimmune diseases. Solid organ transplant patients are usually maintained on a corticosteroid combined with a calcineurin inhibitor (ciclosporin or tacrolimus), *or* with an antiproliferative drug (azathioprine or mycophenolate mofetil), *or* with both. Specialist management is required and other immunomodulators may be used to initiate treatment or to treat rejection.

IMPAIRED IMMUNE RESPONSIVENESS. Modification of tissue reactions caused by corticosteroids and other immunosuppressants may result in the rapid *spread of infection*. Corticosteroids may suppress clinical signs of infection and allow diseases such as septicaemia or tuberculosis to reach an advanced stage before being recognised—**important:** for advice on measles and chickenpox (varicella) exposure, see Immunoglobulins (section 14.5). For advice on the use of live vaccines in individuals with impaired immune response, see section 14.1. For general comments and warnings relating to corticosteroids and immunosuppressants see section 6.3.2 (under Prednisolone).

PREGNANCY. Transplant patients immunosuppressed with azathioprine should not discontinue it on becoming pregnant; there is no evidence that azathioprine is teratogenic. However, there have been reports of premature birth and low birth-weight following exposure to azathioprine, particularly in combination with corticosteroids. Spontaneous abortion has been reported following maternal or paternal exposure.

There is less experience of ciclosporin in pregnancy but it does not appear to be any more harmful than azathioprine. The use of these drugs during pregnancy needs to be supervised in specialist units.

Manufacturers contra-indicate the use of tacrolimus and mycophenolate in pregnancy (Appendix 4).

8.2.1 Antiproliferative immunosuppressants

Azathioprine is widely used for transplant recipients and it is also used to treat a number of autoimmune conditions, usually when corticosteroid therapy alone provides inadequate control. It is metabolised to mercaptopurine, and doses should be reduced when allopurinol is given concurrently.

Blood tests and monitoring for signs of myelosuppression are essential in long-term treatment with azathioprine. The enzyme thiopurine methyltransferase (TPMT) metabolises azathioprine; the risk of myelosuppression is increased in those with a low activity of the enzyme, particularly in the very few individuals who are homozygous for low TPMT activity.

Mycophenolate mofetil is metabolised to mycophenolic acid which has a more selective mode of action than azathioprine. It is licensed for the prophylaxis of acute rejection in renal or cardiac transplantation when used in combination with ciclosporin and corticosteroids. There is evidence that compared with similar regimens incorporating azathioprine, mycophenolate mofetil reduces the risk of acute rejection episodes; the risk of opportunistic infections (particularly due to tissue-invasive cytomegalovirus) and the occurrence of blood disorders such as leucopenia may be higher.

Cyclophosphamide (section 8.1.1) is less commonly prescribed as an immunosuppressant.

AZATHIOPRINE

Indications: see notes above; also rheumatoid arthritis (section 10.1.3)

Cautions: monitor for toxicity throughout treatment; monitor full blood count weekly (more frequently with higher doses or if hepatic or renal impairment) for first 4 weeks (manufacturer advises weekly monitoring for 8 weeks but evidence of practical value unsatisfactory), thereafter reduce frequency of monitoring to at least every 3 months; hepatic impairment (Appendix 2); renal impairment (Appendix 3); reduce dose in elderly; pregnancy (see section 8.2)—treatment should not generally be initiated during pregnancy; **interactions:** Appendix 1 (azathioprine)

BONE MARROW SUPPRESSION. Patients should be warned to report immediately any signs or symptoms of bone marrow suppression e.g. inexplicable bruising or bleeding, infection

Contra-indications: hypersensitivity to azathioprine or mercaptopurine; breast-feeding

Side-effects: hypersensitivity reactions (including malaise, dizziness, vomiting, diarrhoea, fever, rigors, myalgia, arthralgia, rash, hypotension and interstitial nephritis—calling for immediate withdrawal); dose-related bone marrow suppression (see also Cautions); liver impairment, cholestatic jaundice, hair loss and increased susceptibility to infections and colitis in patients also receiving corticosteroids; nausea; rarely pancreatitis, pneumonitis, hepatic veno-occlusive disease

Dose: *by mouth, or* (if oral administration not possible—intravenous solution very irritant, see below) *by intravenous injection* over at least 1 minute (followed by 50 mL sodium chloride intravenous infusion), *or by intravenous infusion*, autoimmune conditions, 1–3 mg/kg daily, adjusted according to response (consider withdrawal if no improvement in 3 months)

Suppression of transplant rejection, initially up to 5 mg/kg then 1–4 mg/kg daily according to response

NOTE. Intravenous injection is alkaline and very irritant, intravenous route should therefore be used **only** if oral route not feasible, see also Appendix 6

Azathioprine (Non-proprietary) PoM

Tablets, azathioprine 25 mg, net price 28-tab pack = £9.26; 50 mg, 56-tab pack = £9.97. Label: 21

Brands include *Azamune®*, *Immunoprin®*

Imuran® (GSK) PoM

Tablets, both f/c, azathioprine 25 mg (orange), net price 100-tab pack = £10.99; 50 mg (yellow), 100-tab pack = £7.99. Label: 21

Injection, powder for reconstitution, azathioprine (as sodium salt). Net price 50-mg vial = £15.38

MYCOPHENOLATE MOFETIL

Indications: prophylaxis of acute renal, cardiac, or hepatic transplant rejection (in combination with ciclosporin and corticosteroids) under specialist supervision

Cautions: full blood counts every week for 4 weeks then twice a month for 2 months then every month in the first year (possibly interrupt treatment if neutropenia develops); elderly (increased risk of infection, gastro-intestinal haemorrhage and pulmonary oedema); children (higher incidence of side-effects may call for temporary reduction of dose or interruption); active serious gastro-intestinal disease (risk of haemorrhage, ulceration and perforation); delayed graft function; increased susceptibility to skin cancer (avoid exposure to strong sunlight); **interactions:** Appendix 1 (mycophenolate mofetil)

BONE MARROW SUPPRESSION. Patients should be warned to report immediately any signs or symptoms of bone marrow suppression e.g. infection and inexplicable bruising or bleeding

Contra-indications: pregnancy (exclude before starting and avoid for 6 weeks after discontinuation) (Appendix 4); breast-feeding (Appendix 5)

Side-effects: diarrhoea, abdominal discomfort, gastritis, nausea, vomiting, constipation; cough, influenza-like syndrome; headache; infections (viral, bacterial, and fungal); increased blood creatinine; leucopenia, anaemia, thrombocytopenia; *less commonly* gastro-oesophageal reflux, gastro-intestinal ulceration and bleeding, pancreatitis, abnormal liver function tests, hepatitis, tachycardia, blood pressure changes, oedema, dyspnoea, tremor, insomnia, dizziness, hyperglycaemia, increased risk of malignancies, disturbances of electrolytes and blood lipids, renal tubular necrosis, arthralgia, alopecia, acne

Dose: renal transplantation, *by mouth*, 1 g twice daily starting within 72 hours of transplantation *or by intravenous infusion*, 1 g twice daily starting within 24 hours of transplantation for up to max. 14 days (then transfer to oral therapy); CHILD and ADOLESCENT 2–18 years (and body-surface area over 1.25 m^2) 600 mg/m^2 twice daily (max. 2 g daily)

NOTE. Tablets and capsules not appropriate for dose titration in young children

Cardiac transplantation, *by mouth*, 1.5 g twice daily starting within 5 days of transplantation
Hepatic transplantation, *by intravenous infusion*, 1 g twice daily starting within 24 hours of transplantation for 4 days (up to max. 14 days), then *by mouth*, 1.5 g twice daily as soon as is tolerated

CellCept® (Roche) ▼ PoM
Capsules, blue/brown, mycophenolate mofetil 250 mg, net price 100-cap pack = £87.33
Tablets, lavender, mycophenolate mofetil 500 mg, net price 50-tab pack = £87.33
Oral suspension, mycophenolate mofetil 1 g/5 mL when reconstituted with water, net price 175 mL = £122.25
Intravenous infusion, powder for reconstitution, mycophenolate mofetil (as hydrochloride), net price 500-mg vial = £9.69

■ Mycophenolic acid

Myfortic® (Novartis) PoM
Tablets, e/c, mycophenolic acid (as mycophenolate sodium) 180 mg (green), net price 120-tab pack = £122.49; 360 mg (orange), 120-tab pack = £244.97. Label: 25
Dose: renal transplantation, 720 mg twice daily starting within 72 hours of transplantation
EQUIVALENCE TO MYCOPHENOLATE MOFETIL. Mycophenolic acid 720 mg is approximately equivalent to mycophenolate mofetil 1 g but avoid unnecessary switching because of pharmacokinetic differences

8.2.2 Corticosteroids and other immunosuppressants

Prednisolone (section 6.3.2) is widely used in oncology. It has a marked antitumour effect in acute lymphoblastic leukaemia, Hodgkin's disease, and the non-Hodgkin lymphomas. It has a role in the palliation of symptomatic end-stage malignant disease when it may enhance appetite and produce a sense of well-being (see also Prescribing in Palliative Care, p. 15).

The corticosteroids are also powerful immunosuppressants. They are used to prevent organ transplant rejection, and in high dose to treat rejection episodes.

Ciclosporin (cyclosporin), a calcineurin inhibitor, is a potent immunosuppressant which is virtually non-myelotoxic but markedly nephrotoxic. It has an important role in organ and tissue transplantation, for prevention of graft rejection following bone marrow, kidney, liver, pancreas, heart, lung, and heart-lung transplantation, and for prophylaxis and treatment of graft-versus-host disease.

Tacrolimus is also a calcineurin inhibitor. Although not chemically related to ciclosporin it has a similar mode of action and side-effects, but the incidence of neurotoxicity and nephrotoxicity appears to be greater; cardiomyopathy has also been reported. Disturbance of glucose metabolism also appears to be significant; hypertrichosis appears to be less of a problem than with ciclosporin.

Sirolimus is a potent non-calcineurin inhibiting immunosuppressant introduced recently for renal transplantation. It can cause hyperlipidaemia.

Basiliximab and **daclizumab** are monoclonal antibodies that prevent T-lymphocyte proliferation; they are used for prophylaxis of acute rejection in allogenic renal transplantation. They are given with ciclosporin and corticosteroid immunosuppression regimens; their use should be confined to specialist centres.

Thalidomide [unlicensed drug] should **always** be given under specialist supervision because of its teratogenic potential. It has immunomodulatory and anti-inflammatory activity; it is used in the treatment of refractory myeloma and can delay progression of early disease. It is used alone or in combination with a corticosteroid and an alkylating drug. Thalidomide can cause drowsiness, constipation, and on prolonged use, peripheral neuropathy. It should **never** be given to women of child-bearing potential.

NICE guidance (immunosuppressive therapy for adult renal transplantation). NICE has recommended (September 2004) that for induction therapy in the prophylaxis of organ rejection, either basiliximab or daclizumab are options for combining with a calcineurin inhibitor. For each individual, ciclosporin or tacrolimus is chosen as the calcineurin inhibitor on the basis of side-effects.
Mycophenolate mofetil [mycophenolic acid now also available, see p. 445] is recommended as part of an immunosuppressive regimen only if:

- the calcineurin inhibitor is not tolerated, particularly if nephrotoxicity endangers the transplanted kidney; *or*
- there is very high risk of nephrotoxicity from the calcineurin inhibitor, requiring a reduction in the dose of the calcineurin inhibitor or its avoidance.

Sirolimus is recommended as a component of immunosuppressive regimen **only if** intolerance necessitates the withdrawal of a calcineurin inhibitor.
These recommendations may not be consistent with the marketing authorisations of some of the products.

BASILIXIMAB

Indications: see notes above
Contra-indications: pregnancy (Appendix 4) and breast-feeding
Side-effects: severe hypersensitivity reactions reported rarely; for side-effects of regimen see under Ciclosporin (below) and Prednisolone (section 6.3.2)
Dose: *by intravenous injection or by intravenous infusion*, 20 mg within 2 hours before transplant surgery and 20 mg 4 days after surgery; CHILD and ADOLESCENT under 35 kg, 10 mg within 2 hours before transplant surgery and 10 mg 4 days after surgery; withhold second dose if severe hypersensitivity or graft loss occurs

Simulect® (Novartis) PoM
Injection, powder for reconstitution, basiliximab, net price 10-mg vial = £758.69, 20-mg vial = £842.38 (both with water for injections) . For intravenous infusion

CICLOSPORIN

(Cyclosporin)
Indications: see notes above, and under Dose; atopic dermatitis and psoriasis (section 13.5.3); rheumatoid arthritis (section 10.1.3)
Cautions: monitor kidney function—dose dependent increase in serum creatinine and urea during first few weeks may necessitate dose reduction in transplant patients (exclude rejection if kidney

transplant) or discontinuation in non-transplant patients; monitor liver function (dosage adjustment based on bilirubin and liver enzymes may be needed); monitor blood pressure—discontinue if hypertension develops that cannot be controlled by antihypertensives; hyperuricaemia; monitor serum potassium especially in renal dysfunction (risk of hyperkalaemia); monitor serum magnesium; measure blood lipids before treatment and thereafter as appropriate; pregnancy (see p. 444) and breast-feeding (Appendix 5); porphyria (section 9.8.2); use with tacrolimus specifically contra-indicated and apart from specialist use in transplant patients preferably avoid other immunosuppressants with the exception of corticosteroids (increased risk of infection and lymphoma); **interactions:** Appendix 1 (ciclosporin)

ADDITIONAL CAUTIONS IN NEPHROTIC SYNDROME. ***Contra-indicated*** in uncontrolled hypertension, uncontrolled infections, and malignancy; reduce dose by 25–50% if serum creatinine more than 30% above baseline on more than one measurement; in renal impairment initially 2.5 mg/kg daily; in long-term management, perform renal biopsies at yearly intervals

ADDITIONAL CAUTIONS. Atopic Dermatitis and Psoriasis, section 13.5.3; Rheumatoid Arthritis, section 10.1.3

Side-effects: dose-dependent increase in serum creatinine and urea during first few weeks (see also under Cautions); less commonly renal structural changes on long-term administration; also hypertrichosis, headache, tremor, hypertension (especially in heart transplant patients), hepatic dysfunction, fatigue, gingival hypertrophy, gastro-intestinal disturbances, burning sensation in hands and feet (usually during first week); *occasionally* rash (possibly allergic), mild anaemia, hyperkalaemia, hyperuricaemia, gout, hypomagnesaemia, hypercholesterolaemia, hyperglycaemia, weight increase, oedema, pancreatitis, neuropathy, confusion, paraesthesia, convulsions, benign intracranial hypertension (discontinue), dysmenorrhoea or amenorrhoea; myalgia, muscle weakness, cramps, myopathy, gynaecomastia (in patients receiving concomitant spironolactone), colitis and cortical blindness also reported; thrombocytopenia (sometimes with haemolytic uraemic syndrome) also reported; incidence of malignancies and lymphoproliferative disorders similar to that with other immunosuppressive therapy

Dose: organ transplantation, used alone, ADULT and CHILD over 3 months 10–15 mg/kg *by mouth* 4–12 hours before transplantation followed by 10–15 mg/kg daily for 1–2 weeks postoperatively then reduced gradually to 2–6 mg/kg daily for maintenance (dose should be adjusted according to blood-ciclosporin concentration and renal function); dose lower if given concomitantly with other immunosuppressant therapy (e.g. corticosteroids); if necessary one-third corresponding oral dose can be given *by intravenous infusion* over 2–6 hours

Bone-marrow transplantation, prevention and treatment of graft-versus-host disease, ADULT and CHILD over 3 months 3–5 mg/kg daily *by intravenous infusion* over 2–6 hours from day before transplantation to 2 weeks postoperatively (or 12.5–15 mg/kg daily *by mouth*) then 12.5 mg/kg daily *by mouth* for 3–6 months then tailed off (may take up to a year after transplantation)

Nephrotic syndrome, *by mouth*, 5 mg/kg daily in 2 divided doses; CHILD 6 mg/kg daily in 2 divided doses; maintenance treatment reduce to lowest effective dose according to proteinuria and serum creatinine measurements; discontinue after 3 months if no improvement in glomerulonephritis or glomerulosclerosis (after 6 months in membranous glomerulonephritis)

CONVERSION. Any conversion between brands should be undertaken very carefully and the manufacturer contacted for further information. Currently only *Neoral®* remains available for oral use; *Sandimmun®* capsules and oral solution and *SangCya®* oral solution are available on named-patient basis only for patients who cannot be transferred to another brand of oral ciclosporin

> Because of differences in bioavailability, the brand of ciclosporin to be dispensed should be specified by the prescriber

Neoral® (Novartis) PoM

Capsules, ciclosporin 10 mg (yellow/white), net price 60-cap pack = £16.44; 25 mg (blue/grey), 30-cap pack = £12.00; 50 mg (yellow/white), 30-cap pack = £26.50; 100 mg (blue/grey), 30-cap pack = £50.00. Counselling, administration

Oral solution, yellow, sugar-free, ciclosporin 100 mg/mL, net price 50 mL = £82.00. Counselling, administration

COUNSELLING. Total daily dose should be taken in 2 divided doses. Avoid grapefruit or grapefruit juice for 1 hour before dose

Mix solution with orange juice (or squash) or apple juice (to improve taste) or with water immediately before taking (and rinse with more to ensure total dose). Do not mix with grapefruit juice. Keep medicine measure away from other liquids (including water)

Sandimmun® (Novartis) PoM

Concentrate for intravenous infusion (oily), ciclosporin 50 mg/mL. To be diluted before use. Net price 1-mL amp = £1.94; 5-mL amp = £9.17

Excipients: include polyoxyl castor oil (risk of anaphylaxis, see Excipients, p. 2)

NOTE. Observe for at least 30 minutes after starting infusion and at frequent intervals thereafter

DACLIZUMAB

Indications: see notes above

Contra-indications: pregnancy and breast-feeding

Side-effects: severe hypersensitivity reactions reported rarely; for side-effects of regimen see under Ciclosporin (above) and Prednisolone (section 6.3.2)

Dose: *by intravenous infusion*, ADULT and CHILD, 1 mg/kg within the 24-hour period before transplantation, then 1 mg/kg every 14 days for a total of 5 doses

Zenapax® (Roche) ▼ PoM

Concentrate for intravenous infusion, daclizumab 5 mg/mL, net price 5-mL = £223.68

SIROLIMUS

Indications: prophylaxis of organ rejection in kidney allograft recipients (initially in combination with ciclosporin and corticosteroid, then with corticosteroid only); see also under Dose

Cautions: monitor kidney function when given with ciclosporin; Afro-Caribbean patients may require higher doses; hepatic impairment (Appendix 2; renal impairment (Appendix 3); food may affect absorption (administer at the same time with respect to food); **interactions:** Appendix 1 (sirolimus)

Contra-indications: pregnancy (Appendix 4); breast-feeding (Appendix 5)

Side-effects: lymphocele, oedema, abdominal pain, diarrhoea, tachycardia, anaemia, fever, thrombocytopenia, neutropenia, leucopenia, thrombotic thrombocytopenic purpura, hyperlipidaemias (including hypercholesterolaemia, hypertriglyceridaemia), increase in serum creatinine in patients also receiving ciclosporin, hypokalaemia, arthralgia, acne; less commonly, venous thromboembolism, epistaxis, interstitial lung disease, impaired healing, increased susceptibility to infection, stomatitis, haemolytic uraemia, bone necrosis, rash, pyelonephritis; rarely, pancreatitis, susceptibility to lymphoma and other malignancies particularly of the skin, pancytopenia, hepatic necrosis, hypersensitivity reactions including anaphylaxis

Dose: initially 6 mg, after surgery, then 2 mg once daily (dose adjusted according to blood-sirolimus concentration) in combination with ciclosporin and corticosteroid for 2–3 months (sirolimus given 4 hours after ciclosporin); ciclosporin should then be withdrawn over 4–8 weeks (if not possible, sirolimus should be discontinued and an alternate immunosuppressive regimen used)

NOTE. Pre-dose ('trough') blood-sirolimus concentration (using chromatographic assay) when used with ciclosporin should be 4–12 micrograms/litre; after withdrawal of ciclosporin pre-dose blood-sirolimus concentration should be 12–20 micrograms/litre; close monitoring of blood-sirolimus concentration required in hepatic impairment, during treatment with potent inducers or inhibitors of metabolism and after discontinuing them

When changing between oral solution and tablets, measurement of serum 'trough' blood-sirolimus concentration after 1–2 weeks is recommended

Rapamune (Wyeth) ▼ PoM

Tablets, coated, sirolimus 1 mg, net price 30-tab pack = £90.00; 2 mg, 30-tab pack = £180.00

Oral solution, sirolimus 1 mg/mL, net price 60 mL = £169.00. Counselling, administration

COUNSELLING. Mix solution with at least 60 mL water or orange juice in a glass or plastic container immediately before taking; refill container with at least 120 mL and drink immediately (to ensure total dose). Do not mix with any other liquids

TACROLIMUS

Indications: primary immunosuppression in liver and kidney allograft recipients and allograft rejection resistant to conventional immunosuppressive regimens, see also notes above; moderate to severe atopic eczema (section 13.5.3)

Cautions: see under Ciclosporin; also monitor ECG (**important:** also echocardiography, see CSM warning below), visual status, blood glucose, haematological and neurological parameters; **interactions:** Appendix 1 (tacrolimus)

DRIVING. May affect performance of skilled tasks (e.g. driving)

Contra-indications: hypersensitivity to macrolides; pregnancy (exclude before starting—if contraception needed non-hormonal methods should be used, Appendix 4); breast-feeding (Appendix 5); avoid concurrent administration with ciclosporin (care if patient has previously received ciclosporin)

Side-effects: include gastro-intestinal disturbances including dyspepsia, and inflammatory and ulcerative disorders; hepatic dysfunction, jaundice, bile-duct and gall-bladder abnormalities; hypertension (less frequently hypotension), tachycardia, angina, arrhythmias, thromboembolic and ischaemic events, rarely myocardial hypertrophy, cardiomyopathy (**important:** see CSM warning below); dyspnoea, pleural effusion, tremor, headache, insomnia, paraesthesia, confusion, depression, dizziness, anxiety, convulsions, incoordination, encephalopathy, psychosis; visual and hearing abnormalities; haematological effects including anaemia, leucocytosis, leucopenia, thrombocytopenia, coagulation disorders; altered acid-base balance and glucose metabolism, electrolyte disturbances including hyperkalaemia (less frequently hypokalaemia); altered renal function including increased serum creatinine; hypophosphataemia, hypercalcaemia, hyperuricaemia; muscle cramps, arthralgia; pruritus, alopecia, rash, sweating, acne, photosensitivity; susceptibility to lymphoma and other malignancies particularly of the skin; less commonly ascites, pancreatitis, atelectasis, kidney damage and renal failure, myasthenia, hirsutism, rarely Stevens-Johnson syndrome

CSM WARNING. Cardiomyopathy has been reported in children given tacrolimus after transplantation. Patients should be monitored carefully by echocardiography for hypertrophic changes; dose reduction or discontinuation should be considered if these occur

Dose: liver transplantation, starting 6 hours after transplantation, *by mouth*, 100–200 micrograms/kg daily in 2 divided doses *or by intravenous infusion* over 24 hours, 10–50 micrograms/kg; CHILD *by mouth*, 300 micrograms/kg daily in 2 divided doses *or by intravenous infusion* over 24 hours, 50 micrograms/kg

Renal transplantation, starting within 24 hours of transplantation, *by mouth*, 150–300 micrograms/kg daily in 2 divided doses *or by intravenous infusion* over 24 hours, 50–100 micrograms/kg; CHILD *by mouth*, 300 micrograms/kg daily in 2 divided doses *or by intravenous infusion* over 24 hours, 100 micrograms/kg

Maintenance treatment, dose adjusted according to response

Prograf® (Fujisawa) PoM

Capsules, tacrolimus 500 micrograms (yellow), net price 50-cap pack = £65.69; 1 mg (white), 50-cap pack = £85.22, 100-cap pack = £170.43; 5 mg (greyish-red), 50-cap pack = £314.84. Label: 23, counselling, driving

Concentrate for intravenous infusion, tacrolimus 5 mg/mL. To be diluted before use. Net price 1-mL amp = £62.05

Excipients: include polyoxyl castor oil (risk of anaphylaxis, see Excipients, p. 2)

8.2.3 Rituximab and alemtuzumab

Rituximab, a monoclonal antibody which causes lysis of B lymphocytes, is licensed for the treatment of chemotherapy-resistant advanced follicular lymphoma (see NICE guidance below) and for diffuse large B-cell non-Hodgkin's lymphoma in combination with other chemotherapy (see NICE guidance below). Rituximab has recently been licensed for the treatment of previously untreated advanced follicular lymphoma in combination with other chemotherapy. Full resuscitation facilities should be at hand and as with other cytotoxics, treatment should be undertaken under the close supervision of a specialist.

Rituximab should be used with caution in patients receiving cardiotoxic chemotherapy or with a history of cardiovascular disease because exacerbation of angina, arrhythmia, and heart failure have been reported. Transient hypotension occurs frequently during infusion and antihypertensives may need to be withheld for 12 hours before infusion.

Infusion-related side-effects (including cytokine release syndrome) are reported commonly with rituximab and occur predominantly during the first infusion; they include fever and chills, nausea and vomiting, allergic reactions (such as rash, pruritus, angioedema, bronchospasm and dyspnoea), flushing and tumour pain. Patients should be given an analgesic and an antihistamine before each dose of rituximab to reduce these effects. Premedication with a corticosteroid should also be considered. The infusion may have to be stopped temporarily and the infusion-related effects treated—consult product literature for appropriate management. Evidence of pulmonary infiltration and features of tumour lysis syndrome should be sought if infusion-related effects occur.

Fatalities following **severe** cytokine release syndrome (characterised by severe dyspnoea) and associated with features of tumour lysis syndrome have occurred 1–2 hours after infusion of rituximab. Patients with a high tumour burden as well as those with pulmonary insufficiency or infiltration are at increased risk and should be monitored **very closely** (and a slower rate of infusion considered).

NICE guidance (rituximab for follicular non-Hodgkin's lymphoma). NICE has recommended (March 2002) that for stage III or IV follicular lymphoma, rituximab is used only if the disease is resistant to other chemotherapy or if the patient cannot tolerate such treatment. In these circumstances rituximab should be used as part of a prospective study.

NICE guidance (rituximab for aggressive non-Hodgkin's lymphoma). NICE has recommended (September 2003) rituximab, in combination with cyclophosphamide, doxorubicin, vincristine and prednisolone, for first-line treatment of CD20-positive diffuse large-B-cell lymphoma at clinical stage II, III or IV.

The use of rituximab for localised (stage I) disease should be limited to clinical trials.

Alemtuzumab, another monoclonal antibody that causes lysis of B lymphocytes, is licensed for use in patients with chronic lymphocytic leukaemia which has failed to respond to treatment with an alkylating drug, or which has remitted for only a short period (less than 6 months) following fludarabine treatment. In common with rituximab, it causes infusion-related side-effects including cytokine release syndrome (see above) and premedication with an analgesic, an antihistamine, and a corticosteroid is recommended.

ALEMTUZUMAB

Indications: see notes above

Cautions: see notes above—for full details (including monitoring) consult product literature

Contra-indications: pregnancy (Appendix 4) and breast-feeding (Appendix 5); for full details consult product literature

Side-effects: see notes above—for full details (including monitoring and management of side-effects) consult product literature

Dose: consult product literature

MabCampath® (Schering Health) ▼ PoM
Concentrate for intravenous infusion, alemtuzumab 30 mg/mL, net price 1-mL vial = £274.83

RITUXIMAB

Indications: see notes above

Cautions: see notes above—for full details (including monitoring) consult product literature; pregnancy (Appendix 4)

Contra-indications: breast-feeding

Side-effects: see notes above—but for full details (including monitoring and management of side-effects) consult product literature

MabThera® (Roche) PoM
Concentrate for intravenous infusion, rituximab 10 mg/mL, net price 10-mL vial = £174.63, 50-mL vial = £873.15

8.2.4 Other immunomodulating drugs

Interferon alfa

Interferon alfa has shown some antitumour effect in certain lymphomas and solid tumours. Interferon alfa preparations are also used in the treatment of chronic hepatitis B, and chronic hepatitis C ideally in combination with ribavirin (section 5.3.3). Side-effects are dose-related, but commonly include anorexia, nausea, influenza-like symptoms, and lethargy. Ocular side-effects and depression (including suicidal behaviour) have also been reported. Myelosuppression may occur, particularly affecting granulocyte counts. Cardiovascular problems (hypotension, hypertension, and arrhythmias), nephrotoxicity and hepatotoxicity have been reported. Hypertriglyceridaemia, sometimes severe, has been observed; monitoring of lipid concentration is recommended. Other side-effects include hypersensitivity reactions, thyroid abnormalities, hyperglycaemia, alopecia, psoriasiform rash, confusion, coma and seizures (usually with high doses in the elderly).

Polyethylene glycol-conjugated ('pegylated') derivatives of interferon alfa (**peginterferon alfa-2a** and **peginterferon alfa-2b**) are available; pegylation increases the persistence of the interferon in the blood. The peginterferons are licensed for the treatment of chronic hepatitis C, ideally in combination with ribavirin (see section 5.3.3).

INTERFERON ALFA

Indications: see under preparations

Cautions: consult product literature; **interactions:** Appendix 1 (interferons)

Contra-indications: consult product literature; avoid injections containing benzyl alcohol in neonates (see under preparations below)

Side-effects: see notes above and consult product literature

Dose: consult product literature

IntronA® (Schering-Plough) PoM

Injection, interferon alfa-2b (rbe) 10 million units/mL, net price 2.5-mL vial = £108.00. For subcutaneous or intravenous injection

Injection, powder for reconstitution, interferon alfa-2b (rbe), net price 10-million unit vial (with injection equipment and water for injections) = £43.17. For subcutaneous or intravenous injection

Injection pen, interferon alfa-2b (rbe), net price 15 million units/mL, 1.5-mL cartridge = £77.76; 25 million units/mL, 1.5-mL cartridge = £129.60; 50 million units/mL, 1.5-mL cartridge = £259.20. For subcutaneous injection

NOTE. Each 1.5-mL multidose cartridge delivers 6 doses of 0.2 mL i.e. a total of 1.2 mL

For chronic myelogenous leukaemia (as monotherapy or in combination with cytarabine), hairy cell leukaemia, follicular lymphoma, lymph or liver metastases of carcinoid tumour, chronic hepatitis B, chronic hepatitis C, adjunct to surgery in malignant melanoma and maintenance of remission in multiple myeloma

Roferon-A® (Roche) PoM

Injection, interferon alfa-2a (rbe). Net price 6 million units/mL, 0.5-mL (3 million-unit) prefilled syringe = £15.07; 9 million units/mL, 0.5-mL (4.5 million-unit) prefilled syringe = £22.60; 12 million units/mL, 0.5-mL (6 million-unit) prefilled syringe = £30.12; 18 million units/mL, 0.5-mL (9 million-unit) prefilled syringe = £45.19 36 million units/mL, 0.5-mL (18 million-unit) prefilled syringe = £90.39; 30 million units/mL, 0.6-mL (18 million-unit) cartridge = £90.39, for use with *Roferon* pen device. For subcutaneous injection (cartridges, vials, and prefilled syringes) and intramuscular injection (cartridges and vials)

Excipients: include benzyl alcohol (avoid in neonates, see Excipients, p. 2)

For AIDS-related Kaposi's sarcoma, hairy cell leukaemia, chronic myelogenous leukaemia, recurrent or metastatic renal cell carcinoma, progressive cutaneous T-cell lymphoma, chronic hepatitis B and chronic hepatitis C, follicular non-Hodgkin's lymphoma, adjunct to surgery in malignant melanoma

Viraferon® (Schering-Plough) PoM

Injection, interferon alfa-2b (rbe) 6 million units/mL, net price 3-mL vial = £90.40. For subcutaneous injection

Injection pen, interferon alfa-2b (rbe), net price 15 million units/mL, 1.5-mL cartridge = £90.40. For subcutaneous injection

NOTE. 1.5-mL multidose cartridge delivers 6 doses of 0.2 mL each

For chronic hepatitis B and chronic hepatitis C

PEGINTERFERON ALFA

Indications: combined with ribavirin for chronic hepatitis C; as monotherapy if ribavirin not tolerated or contra-indicated (see section 5.3.3)

Cautions: consult product literature; **interactions:** Appendix 1 (interferons)

Contra-indications: consult product literature

Side-effects: see notes above and consult product literature

Dose: consult product literature

Pegasys® (Roche) ▼ PoM

Injection, peginterferon alfa-2a, net price 135-microgram prefilled syringe = £114.39, 180-microgram prefilled syringe = £132.06. For subcutaneous injection

PegIntron® (Schering-Plough) ▼ PoM

Injection, powder for reconstitution, peginterferon alfa-2b (rbe), net price 50-microgram vial = £62.78, 80-microgram vial = £108.00, 100-microgram vial = £125.55, 120-microgram vial = £162.00, 150-microgram vial = £202.50 (all with injection equipment and water for injections). For subcutaneous injection

ViraferonPeg® (Schering-Plough) ▼ PoM

Injection, powder for reconstitution, peginterferon alfa-2b (rbe), net price 50-microgram vial = £62.78, 80-microgram vial = £100.44, 100-microgram vial = £125.55, 120-microgram vial = £150.66, 150-microgram vial = £188.33 (all with injection equipment and water for injections). For subcutaneous injection

Injection, prefilled pen, powder for reconstitution, peginterferon alfa-2b (rbe), net price 50-microgram pen = £69.05, 80-microgram pen = £118.80, 100-microgram pen = £138.11, 120-microgram pen = £165.73, 150-microgram pen = £207.16 (all with needles and swabs). For subcutaneous injection

Interferon beta

Interferon beta is licensed for use in patients with *relapsing, remitting multiple sclerosis* (characterised by at least two attacks of neurological dysfunction over the previous 2 or 3 years, followed by complete or incomplete recovery) who are able to walk unaided. Not all patients respond and a deterioration in the bouts has been observed in some. Interferon beta-1b is also licensed for use in patients with *secondary progressive multiple sclerosis* but its role in this condition has not been confirmed.

Interferon beta should not be used in those with a history of severe depressive illness (or of suicidal ideation), in those with inadequately controlled epilepsy, or in decompensated hepatic impairment; caution is advised in those with a history of these conditions or with cardiac disorders or myelosuppression. Side-effects reported most frequently include irritation at injection site (including inflammation, hypersensitivity, necrosis) and influenza-like symptoms (fever, chills, myalgia, or malaise) but these decrease over time; nausea and vomiting occur occasionally. Other side-effects include hypersensitivity reactions (including anaphylaxis and urticaria), blood disorders, menstrual disorders, mood and personality changes, suicide attempts, confusion and convulsions; alopecia, hepatitis, and thyroid dysfunction have been reported rarely with interferon beta-1b.

NICE guidance (interferon beta and glatiramer for multiple sclerosis). NICE does not recommend (January 2002) either interferon beta or glatiramer acetate for the treatment of multiple sclerosis in the NHS in England and Wales.
Patients who are currently receiving interferon beta or glatiramer acetate for multiple sclerosis, whether as routine therapy or as part of a clinical trial, should have the option to continue treatment until they and their consultant consider it appropriate to stop, having regard to the established criteria for withdrawal from treatment.

Provision of disease-modifying therapies for multiple sclerosis. The Department of Health, the National Assembly for Wales, the Scottish Executive, the Northern Ireland Department of Health, Social Services & Public Safety, and the manufacturers have reached agreement on a risk-sharing scheme for the NHS supply of interferon beta and glatiramer acetate for multiple sclerosis. Health Service Circular (HSC 2002/004) explains how patients can participate in the scheme. It is available on the Department of Health website (www.dh.gov.uk)

INTERFERON BETA

Indications: see notes above
Cautions: see notes above and consult product literature
Contra-indications: consult product literature; pregnancy (Appendix 4—advise contraceptive measures if appropriate), breast-feeding (Appendix 5)
Side-effects: see notes above and consult product literature
Dose: consult product literature

■ Interferon beta-1a

Avonex® (Biogen) PoM
Injection, interferon beta-1a 60 micrograms (12 million units)/mL, net price 0.5-mL (30-microgram, 6 million-unit) prefilled syringe = £163.50. For intramuscular injection

Rebif® (Serono) PoM
Injection, interferon beta-1a, net price 22-microgram (6 million-unit) prefilled syringe = £54.18; 44-microgram (12 million-unit) prefilled syringe = £71.94. For subcutaneous injection

■ Interferon beta-1b

Betaferon® (Schering Health) PoM
Injection, powder for reconstitution, interferon beta-1b. Net price 300-microgram (9.6 million-unit) vial with diluent = £39.78. For subcutaneous injection
NOTE. An autoinjector device (*Betaject® Light*) is available from Schering Health

Aldesleukin

Aldesleukin (recombinant interleukin-2) is licensed for metastatic renal cell carcinoma; it is usually given by subcutaneous injection. It is now rarely given by intravenous infusion because of an association with a capillary leak syndrome, which can cause pulmonary oedema and hypotension. Aldesleukin produces tumour shrinkage in a small proportion of patients, but it has not been shown to increase survival. Bone-marrow, hepatic, renal, thyroid, and CNS toxicity is common. It is for use in **specialist units only**.
Interactions: Appendix 1 (aldesleukin)

Proleukin® (Chiron) PoM
Injection, powder for reconstitution, aldesleukin. Net price 18-million unit vial = £112.00. For subcutaneous injection
Injection, powder for reconstitution, aldesleukin. Net price 18-million unit vial = £112.00. For intravenous infusion but see notes above
For metastatic renal cell carcinoma, **excluding** patients in whom all three of the following prognostic factors are present: performance status of Eastern Co-operative Oncology Group of 1 or greater, more than one organ with metastatic disease sites, and a period of less than 24 months between initial diagnosis of primary tumour and date of evaluation of treatment.

BCG bladder instillation

BCG (**Bacillus Calmette-Guérin**) is a live attenuated strain derived from *Mycobacterium bovis*. It is licensed as a bladder instillation for the treatment of primary or recurrent bladder carcinoma and for the prevention of recurrence following transurethral resection.

BACILLUS CALMETTE-GUÉRIN

Indications: see notes above; BCG immunisation (section 14.4)
Cautions: screen for active tuberculosis (contra-indicated if tuberculosis confirmed); traumatic catheterisation or urethral or bladder injury (delay administration until mucosal damage healed)
Contra-indications: impaired immune response, HIV infection, urinary-tract infection, severe haematuria, tuberculosis, fever of unknown origin; pregnancy and breast-feeding
Side-effects: cystitis, dysuria, urinary frequency, haematuria, malaise, fever, influenza-like syndrome; also systemic BCG infection (with fatalities)—consult product literature; rarely hypersensitivity reactions (such as arthralgia and rash), orchitis, transient urethral obstruction, bladder contracture, renal abscess; ocular symptoms reported
Dose: consult product literature

ImmuCyst® (Cambridge) PoM
Bladder instillation, freeze-dried powder containing attenuated *Mycobacterium bovis* prepared from the Connaught strain of bacillus of Calmette and Guérin, net price 81-mg vial = £89.00

OncoTICE® (Organon) PoM
Bladder instillation, freeze-dried powder containing attenuated *Mycobacterium bovis* prepared from the TICE strain of bacillus of Calmette and Guérin, net price 12.5-mg vial = £80.00

Glatiramer acetate

Glatiramer is an immunomodulating drug comprising synthetic polypeptides. It is licensed for reducing the frequency of relapses in ambulatory patients with relapsing-remitting multiple sclerosis who have had at least 2 clinical relapses in the past 2 years. Initiation of treatment with glatiramer should be supervised by a specialist.

NICE guidance (interferon beta and glatiramer for multiple sclerosis). See above

Provision of disease-modifying therapies for multiple sclerosis. See above

GLATIRAMER ACETATE

Indications: see notes above
Cautions: cardiac disorders; renal impairment (Appendix 3); breast-feeding (Appendix 5)
Contra-indications: pregnancy (Appendix 4)
Side-effects: flushing, chest pain, palpitations, tachycardia, and dyspnoea may occur within minutes of injection; injection site reactions; nausea, peripheral and face oedema, syncope, asthenia, headache, tremor, sweating, lymphadenopathy, hypertonia, arthralgia, rash; convulsions, hypersensitivity reactions including anaphylaxis, bronchospasm and urticaria reported rarely
Dose: *by subcutaneous injection*, ADULT over 18 years, 20 mg daily

Copaxone® (Teva) PoM
Injection, glatiramer acetate 20 mg/mL, net price 1-mL prefilled syringe = £19.49

8.3 Sex hormones and hormone antagonists in malignant disease

Hormonal manipulation has an important role in the treatment of breast, prostate, and endometrial cancer, and a more marginal role in the treatment of hypernephroma. These treatments are not curative, but may provide excellent palliation of symptoms in selected patients, sometimes for a period of years. Tumour response, and treatment toxicity should be carefully monitored and treatment changed if progression occurs or side-effects exceed benefit.

8.3.1 Oestrogens

Diethylstilbestrol (stilboestrol) is rarely used to treat prostate cancer because of its side-effects. It is occasionally used in postmenopausal women with breast cancer. Toxicity is common and dose-related side-effects include nausea, fluid retention, and venous and arterial thrombosis. Impotence and gynaecomastia always occur in men, and withdrawal bleeding may be a problem in women. Hypercalcaemia and bone pain may also occur in breast cancer.

Ethinylestradiol (ethinyloestradiol) is the most potent oestrogen available; unlike other oestrogens it is only slowly metabolised in the liver. Ethinylestradiol is licensed for the palliative treatment of prostate cancer.

DIETHYLSTILBESTROL

(Stilboestrol)
Indications: see notes above
Cautions: cardiovascular disease
Contra-indications: hepatic impairment (Appendix 2)
Side-effects: sodium retention with oedema, thromboembolism, jaundice, feminising effects in men; see also notes above
Dose: breast cancer, 10–20 mg daily
Prostate cancer, 1–3 mg daily

Diethylstilbestrol (Non-proprietary) PoM
Tablets, diethylstilbestrol 1 mg, net price 28 = £26.40; 5 mg, 28 = £36.64

ETHINYLESTRADIOL

(Ethinyloestradiol)
Indications: see notes above; other indications (section 6.4.1.1)
Cautions: see section 6.4.1.1; **interactions:** Appendix 1 (oestrogens)
Contra-indications: see section 6.4.1.1
Side-effects: see section 6.4.1.1
Dose: prostate cancer (palliative), 0.15–1.5 mg daily

■ Preparations
Section 6.4.1.1

8.3.2 Progestogens

Progestogens have a role in the treatment of endometrial cancer; their use in breast cancer and renal cell cancer has declined. Progestogens are now rarely used to treat prostate cancer. **Medroxyprogesterone** or **megestrol** are usually chosen and can be given orally; high-dose or parenteral treatment cannot be recommended. Side-effects are mild but may include nausea, fluid retention, and weight gain.

MEDROXYPROGESTERONE ACETATE

Indications: see notes above; contraception (section 7.3.2.2); other indications (section 6.4.1.2)
Cautions: see section 6.4.1.2 and notes above; **interactions:** Appendix 1 (progestogens)
Contra-indications: see section 6.4.1.2 and notes above
Side-effects: see section 6.4.1.2 and notes above; glucocorticoid effects at high dose may lead to a cushingoid syndrome
Dose: see preparations below

Farlutal® (Pharmacia) PoM
Injection, medroxyprogesterone acetate 200 mg/mL. Net price 2.5-mL vial = £13.26
Dose: By deep intramuscular injection into the gluteal muscle, breast carcinoma, initially 0.5–1 g daily for 4 weeks; maintenance, 500 mg twice a week
Endometrial carcinoma, initially 500 mg twice weekly for 3 months; maintenance, 500 mg once weekly
Renal adenocarcinoma, initially 500 mg on alternate days for 30 days; maintenance, 500 mg twice weekly until day 60, then 250 mg once weekly
Prostatic adenocarcinoma, initially 500 mg twice weekly; maintenance, 500 mg once weekly

Provera® (Pharmacia) PoM
Tablets, medroxyprogesterone acetate 100 mg (scored), net price 60-tab pack = £29.98, 100-tab pack = £49.94; 200 mg (scored), 30-tab pack = £29.65, 400 mg, 30-tab pack = £58.67
Dose: endometrial and renal cell cancer, 200–400 mg daily; breast cancer, 400–800 mg daily
Tablets, medroxyprogesterone acetate 2.5 mg, 5 mg and 10 mg, see section 6.4.1.2

MEGESTROL ACETATE

Indications: see notes above

Cautions: see under Medroxyprogesterone acetate (section 6.4.1.2) and notes above; **interactions:** Appendix 1 (progestogens)

Contra-indications: see under Medroxyprogesterone acetate (section 6.4.1.2) and notes above

Side-effects: see under Medroxyprogesterone acetate (section 6.4.1.2) and notes above

Dose: breast cancer, 160 mg daily in single or divided doses; endometrial cancer, 40–320 mg daily in divided doses

Megace® (Bristol-Myers Squibb) PoM

Tablets, both scored, megestrol acetate 40 mg, net price 20 = £5.08; 160 mg (off-white), 30-tab pack = £29.30

NORETHISTERONE

Indications: see notes above; other indications (section 6.4.1.2)

Cautions: see section 6.4.1.2 and notes above; **interactions:** Appendix 1 (progestogens)

Contra-indications: see section 6.4.1.2 and notes above

Side-effects: see section 6.4.1.2 and notes above

Dose: breast cancer, 40 mg daily, increased to 60 mg daily if required

■ Preparations

Section 6.4.1.2

8.3.3 Androgens

Testosterone esters (section 6.4.2) have largely been superseded by other drugs for breast cancer.

8.3.4 Hormone antagonists

8.3.4.1 Breast cancer

The management of patients with breast cancer involves surgery, radiotherapy, drug therapy, or a combination of these.

EARLY BREAST CANCER. All women should be considered for adjuvant therapy following surgical removal of the tumour. Adjuvant therapy is used to eradicate the micrometastases that cause relapses. Choice of adjuvant treatment is determined by the risk of recurrence, oestrogen-receptor status of the primary tumour, and menopausal status.

Tamoxifen is an oestrogen-receptor antagonist and is the adjuvant hormonal treatment of choice in all women with oestrogen-receptor-positive breast cancer; it is supplemented in selected cases by cytotoxic chemotherapy. Premenopausal women may also benefit from treatment with a gonadorelin analogue or ovarian ablation.

Treatment with tamoxifen delays the growth of metastases and increases survival; if tolerated it should be continued for 5 years. Tamoxifen also reduces risk of developing cancer in the other breast.

Anastrozole is licensed for the adjuvant treatment of oestrogen-receptor-positive early breast cancer in postmenopausal women. **Letrozole** is licensed for use after tamoxifen in postmenopausal women who have early invasive breast cancer.

Cytotoxic chemotherapy is preferred for both premenopausal and postmenopausal women with oestrogen-receptor-negative breast cancer.

ADVANCED BREAST CANCER. Tamoxifen is used in postmenopausal women with oestrogen-receptor-positive tumours, long disease-free interval following treatment for early breast cancer, and disease limited to bone or soft tissues. However, aromatase inhibitors, such as anastrozole or letrozole, may be more effective and are regarded as preferred treatment in postmenopausal women. Ovarian ablation or a gonadorelin analogue (section 8.3.4.2) should be considered in premenopausal women.

Progestogens such as medroxyprogesterone acetate continue to have a role in postmenopausal women with advanced breast cancer. They are as effective as tamoxifen, but they are not as well tolerated; they are less effective than the aromatase inhibitors.

Cytotoxic chemotherapy is preferred for advanced oestrogen-receptor-negative tumours and for aggressive disease, particularly where metastases involve visceral sites (e.g. the liver) or where the disease-free interval following treatment for early breast cancer is short.

CHEMOPREVENTION. Recent evidence suggests that tamoxifen prophylaxis can reduce breast cancer in women at high risk of the disease. However, the adverse effects of tamoxifen preclude its routine use in most women.

CYTOTOXIC DRUGS USED IN BREAST CANCER. The most common cytotoxic chemotherapy regimen for both adjuvant use and metastatic disease has been cyclophosphamide (section 8.1.1), methotrexate and fluorouracil (both section 8.1.3). However, anthracycline-containing regimens are now increasingly used and should be regarded as standard therapy unless contra-indicated (e.g. in cardiac disease).

Metastatic disease. The choice of chemotherapy regimen will be influenced by whether the patient has previously received adjuvant treatment and the presence of any co-morbidity.

For women who have not previously received chemotherapy, *either* cyclophosphamide, methotrexate and fluorouracil *or* an anthracycline-containing regimen is the standard initial therapy for metastatic breast disease.

Patients with anthracycline-refractory or resistant disease should be considered for treatment with a taxane (section 8.1.5) either alone or in combination with trastuzumab if they have tumours that over-express HER2 (human epidermal growth factor-2). Other cytotoxic drugs with activity against breast cancer include capecitabine (section 8.1.3), mitoxantrone, mitomycin (both section 8.1.2), and vinorelbine (section 8.1.4). In cancers that overexpress HER2, trastuzumab (section 8.1.5) is an option for chemotherapy-resistant disease.

OESTROGEN-RECEPTOR ANTAGONISTS. **Tamoxifen** is an oestrogen-receptor antagonist that is licensed for breast and anovulatory infertility (section 6.5.1).

Fulvestrant is licensed for the treatment of oestrogen-receptor-positive metastatic or locally advanced breast cancer in postmenopausal women in whom disease progresses or relapses while on or after other anti-oestrogen therapy.

Toremifene is licensed for hormone-dependent metastatic breast cancer in postmenopausal women, but it is not often used.

AROMATASE INHIBITORS. Aromatase inhibitors act predominantly by blocking the conversion of androgens to oestrogens in the peripheral tissues. They do not inhibit ovarian oestrogen synthesis and should not be used in premenopausal women.

Anastrozole and **letrozole** are non-steroidal aromatase inhibitors; **exemestane** is a steroidal aromatase inhibitor. Anastrozole and letrozole are at least as effective as tamoxifen for first-line treatment of metastatic breast cancer in postmenopausal women. However, it is not yet known whether the benefits of aromatase inhibitors persist over the long term.

Aminoglutethimide has largely been replaced by the newer, more selective aromatase inhibitors, which are better tolerated. Aminoglutethimide causes adrenal hypofunction and corticosteroid replacement therapy is needed.

GONADORELIN ANALOGUES. **Goserelin** (section 8.3.4.2), a gonadorelin analogue is licensed for the management of advanced breast cancer in premenopausal women.

OTHER DRUGS USED IN BREAST CANCER. **Trilostane** (section 6.7.3) is licensed for postmenopausal breast cancer. It is quite well tolerated but diarrhoea and abdominal discomfort may be a problem. Trilostane causes adrenal hypofunction and corticosteroid replacement therapy is needed.

The use of **bisphosphonates** (section 6.6.2) in patients with metastatic breast cancer may prevent skeletal complications of bone metastases.

TAMOXIFEN

Indications: see under Dose and notes above; mastalgia [unlicensed indication] (section 6.7.2)

Cautions: occasional cystic ovarian swellings in premenopausal women; increased risk of thromboembolic events when used with cytotoxics (see also below); breast-feeding (Appendix 5); endometrial changes (**important:** see below); porphyria (section 9.8.2); **interactions:** Appendix 1 (tamoxifen)

ENDOMETRIAL CHANGES. Increased endometrial changes, including hyperplasia, polyps, cancer, and uterine sarcoma reported; prompt investigation required if abnormal vaginal bleeding including menstrual irregularities, vaginal discharge, and pelvic pain or pressure in those receiving (or who have received) tamoxifen.

Contra-indications: pregnancy (exclude before commencing and advise non-hormonal contraception if appropriate—Appendix 4)

Side-effects: hot flushes, vaginal bleeding and vaginal discharge (**important:** see also Endometrial Changes under Cautions), suppression of menstruation in some premenopausal women, pruritus vulvae, gastro-intestinal disturbances, headache, light-headedness, tumour flare, decreased platelet counts; occasionally oedema, hypercalcaemia if bony metastases, alopecia, rashes, uterine fibroids; also visual disturbances (including corneal changes, cataracts, retinopathy); leucopenia (sometimes with anaemia and thrombocytopenia), rarely neutropenia; hypertriglyceridaemia reported (sometimes with pancreatitis); thromboembolic events reported (see below); liver enzyme changes (rarely fatty liver, cholestasis, hepatitis); rarely interstitial pneumonitis, hypersensitivity reactions including angioedema, Stevens-Johnson syndrome, bullous pemphigoid; see also notes above

RISK OF THROMBOEMBOLISM. Tamoxifen can increase the risk of thromboembolism particularly during and immediately after major surgery or periods of immobility. Patients should be made aware of the symptoms of thromboembolism and advised to report sudden breathlessness and any pain in the calf of one leg

Dose: breast cancer, 20 mg daily

CSM ADVICE. The CSM has advised that tamoxifen in a dose of 20 mg daily substantially increases survival in early breast cancer, and that no further benefit has been demonstrated with higher doses. Patients should be told of the small risk of endometrial cancer (see under Cautions above) and encouraged to report relevant symptoms early. They can, however, be reassured that the benefits of treatment far outweigh the risks

Anovulatory infertility, 20 mg daily on days 2, 3, 4 and 5 of cycle; if necessary the daily dose may be increased to 40 mg then 80 mg for subsequent courses; if cycles irregular, start initial course on any day, with subsequent course starting 45 days later *or* on day 2 of cycle if menstruation occurs

Tamoxifen (Non-proprietary) PoM

Tablets, tamoxifen (as citrate) 10 mg, net price 30-tab pack = £1.97; 20 mg, 30-tab pack = £2.24; 40 mg, 30-tab pack = £8.42

Oral solution, tamoxifen (as citrate) 10 mg/5 mL, net price 150 mL = £29.61

Brands include *Soltamox*®

Nolvadex-D® (AstraZeneca) PoM

Tablets, tamoxifen (as citrate) 20 mg, net-price 30-tab pack = £8.71

AMINOGLUTETHIMIDE

Indications: see notes above and under Dose

Cautions: see notes above; adrenal hypofunction (see below); monitor blood pressure, plasma electrolytes, blood counts, and thyroid function; **interactions:** Appendix 1 (aminoglutethimide)

ADRENAL HYPOFUNCTION. May cause adrenal hypofunction especially under conditions of stress (such as surgery, trauma, or acute illness), therefore corticosteroid replacement therapy is necessary (section 6.3.1). If a synthetic glucocorticoid such as dexamethasone is used instead of hydrocortisone a relatively high dose may be needed (metabolism of synthetic corticosteroids accelerated)

Contra-indications: pregnancy (advise non-hormonal contraceptive methods if appropriate—Appendix 4); breast-feeding; porphyria (section 9.8.2)

Side-effects: see notes above; drowsiness, lethargy, rash (sometimes with fever—usually in first 2 weeks and resolves despite continued administration); occasionally dizziness, nausea; other side-effects reported include ataxia, headache, depression, insomnia, pruritus, urticaria, diarrhoea, vomiting, constipation, anorexia, sweating, hypotension, adrenal insufficiency, hyponatraemia, hypoglycaemia, agranulocytosis, leucopenia, thrombocytopenia, hyperkalaemia, exfoliative dermatitis, Stevens-Johnson syndrome, hypothyroidism, inappropriate ADH-secretion, masculinisation and hirsutism in females, renal impairment, pancytopenia, anaemia, allergy, anaphylactic reactions, allergic alveolitis (withdraw immediately if suspected), cholestatic hepatitis, confusion

Dose: advanced breast or prostate cancer, 250 mg daily, increased once a week to max. 250 mg 4 times daily (in breast cancer 250 mg twice daily has proved sufficient in some patients; in prostate cancer up to 750 mg daily is usually satisfactory); given with a glucocorticoid (and sometimes with a mineralocorticoid as well)

Cushing's syndrome due to malignant disease, 250 mg daily, increased gradually to 1 g daily in divided doses (occasionally 1.5–2 g daily); glucocorticoid given only if necessary

Orimeten® (Novartis) PoM
Tablets, scored, aminoglutethimide 250 mg. Net price 56-tab pack = £24.27. Label: 2

ANASTROZOLE

Indications: adjuvant treatment of oestrogen-receptor-positive early breast cancer in postmenopausal women; advanced breast cancer in postmenopausal women which is oestrogen-receptor positive or responsive to tamoxifen

Cautions: laboratory test for menopause if doubt; susceptibility to osteoporosis (assess bone mineral density before treatment and at regular intervals)

Contra-indications: pregnancy and breast-feeding; moderate or severe hepatic disease; moderate or severe renal impairment; not for premenopausal women

Side-effects: hot flushes, vaginal dryness, vaginal bleeding, hair thinning, anorexia, nausea, vomiting, diarrhoea, headache, arthralgia, bone fractures, rash (including Stevens-Johnson syndrome); asthenia and drowsiness—may initially affect ability to drive or operate machinery; slight increases in total cholesterol levels reported; very rarely allergic reactions including angioedema and anaphylaxis

Dose: 1 mg daily; for early disease, recommended duration 5 years

Arimidex® (AstraZeneca) PoM
Tablets, f/c, anastrozole 1 mg. Net price 28-tab pack = £68.56

EXEMESTANE

Indications: advanced breast cancer in postmenopausal women in whom anti-oestrogen therapy has failed

Cautions: hepatic impairment (Appendix 2); renal impairment (Appendix 3); **interactions:** Appendix 1 (exemestane)

Contra-indications: pregnancy and breast-feeding; not indicated for premenopausal women

Side-effects: nausea, vomiting, abdominal pain, dyspepsia, constipation, anorexia; dizziness, fatigue, headache, depression, insomnia; hot flushes, sweating; alopecia, rash; *less commonly* drowsiness, asthenia, and peripheral oedema; *rarely* thrombocytopenia, leucopenia

Dose: 25 mg daily

Aromasin® (Pharmacia) PoM
Tablets, s/c, exemestane 25 mg, net price 30-tab pack = £88.80, 90-tab pack = £266.40. Label: 21

FULVESTRANT

Indications: treatment of oestrogen-receptor-positive metastatic or locally advanced breast cancer in postmenopausal women in whom disease progresses or relapses while on or after other anti-oestrogen therapy

Cautions: hepatic impairment (avoid if severe; Appendix 2)

Contra-indications: pregnancy (Appendix 4); breast-feeding (Appendix 5)

Side-effects: hot flushes, nausea, vomiting, diarrhoea, anorexia, headache, back pain, rash, asthenia, venous thromboembolism, injection-site reactions, urinary-tract infections; less commonly vaginal haemorrhage, vaginal candidiasis, leucorrhoea, hypersensitivity reactions including angioedema, urticaria

Dose: *by deep intramuscular injection*, 250 mg into gluteal muscle every 4 weeks

Faslodex® (AstraZeneca) ▼ PoM
Injection (oily), fulvestrant 50 mg/mL, net price 5-mL (250-mg) prefilled syringe = £348.27

LETROZOLE

Indications: advanced breast cancer in postmenopausal women (including those in whom other anti-oestrogen therapy has failed); early invasive breast cancer in postmenopausal women after standard adjuvant tamoxifen therapy; pre-operative treatment in postmenopausal women with localised hormone-receptor-positive breast cancer to allow subsequent breast conserving surgery

Cautions: severe renal impairment

Contra-indications: severe hepatic impairment; not indicated for premenopausal women; pregnancy and breast-feeding

Side-effects: hot flushes, nausea, vomiting, fatigue, dizziness, headache, dyspepsia, constipation, diarrhoea, anorexia, appetite increase, alopecia, increased sweating, rash, peripheral oedema, musculoskeletal pain; less frequently hypertension, palpitation, tachycardia, dyspnoea, drowsiness, insomnia, depression, anxiety, memory impairment, dysaesthesia, taste disturbance, pruritus, dry skin, urticaria, thrombophlebitis, abdominal pain, urinary frequency, urinary-tract infection, vaginal bleeding, vaginal discharge, breast pain, pyrexia, mucosal dryness, stomatitis, cataract, eye irritation, blurred vision, tumour pain, leucopenia, hypercholesterolaemia, general oedema; rarely pulmonary embolism, arterial thrombosis, cerebrovascular infarction

Dose: 2.5 mg daily (for 3 years after tamoxifen); discontinue if tumour progression occurs

Femara® (Novartis) PoM
Tablets, f/c, letrozole 2.5 mg. Net price 14-tab pack = £41.58, 28-tab pack = £83.16

TOREMIFENE

Indications: hormone-dependent metastatic breast cancer in postmenopausal women

Cautions: hypercalcaemia may occur (especially if bone metastases and usually at beginning of treatment); **interactions:** Appendix 1 (toremifene)

ENDOMETRIAL CHANGES. There is a risk of increased endometrial changes including hyperplasia, polyps and cancer. Abnormal vaginal bleeding including menstrual irregularities, vaginal discharge and symptoms such as pelvic pain or pressure should be promptly investigated

Contra-indications: endometrial hyperplasia, severe hepatic impairment (Appendix 2), history of severe thromboembolic disease; pregnancy and breast-feeding

Side-effects: hot flushes, vaginal bleeding or discharge (**important:** see also Cautions), dizziness, oedema, sweating, nausea, vomiting, chest or back pain, fatigue, headache, skin discoloration, weight increase, insomnia, constipation, dyspnoea, paresis, tremor, vertigo, pruritus, anorexia, corneal opacity (reversible), asthenia; thromboembolic events reported; rarely dermatitis, alopecia, emotional lability, depression, jaundice, stiffness

Dose: 60 mg daily

Fareston® (Orion) PoM
Tablets, toremifene (as citrate) 60 mg. Net price 30-tab pack = £30.37

8.3.4.2 Prostate cancer and gonadorelin analogues

Metastatic cancer of the prostate usually responds to hormonal treatment aimed at androgen depletion. Standard treatments include bilateral subcapsular orchidectomy or use of a gonadorelin analogue (**buserelin**, **goserelin**, **leuprorelin**, or **triptorelin**). Response in most patients lasts for 12 to 18 months. No entirely satisfactory therapy exists for disease progression despite this treatment (hormone-refractory prostate cancer), but occasional patients respond to other hormone manipulation e.g. with an anti-androgen. Bone disease can often be palliated with irradiation or, if widespread, with strontium, aminoglutethimide (section 8.3.4.1), or prednisolone (section 6.3.2).

Gonadorelin analogues

Gonadorelin analogues are as effective as orchidectomy or **diethylstilbestrol** (section 8.3.1) but are expensive and require parenteral administration, at least initially. They cause initial stimulation then depression of luteinising hormone release by the pituitary. During the initial stage (1–2 weeks) increased production of testosterone may be associated with progression of prostate cancer. In susceptible patients this tumour 'flare' may cause spinal cord compression, ureteric obstruction or increased bone pain. When such problems are anticipated, alternative treatments (e.g. orchidectomy) or concomitant use of an anti-androgen such as cyproterone acetate or flutamide (see below) are recommended; anti-androgen treatment should be started 3 days before the gonadorelin analogue and continued for 3 weeks. Gonadorelin analogues are also used in women for breast cancer (section 8.3.4.1) and other indications (section 6.7.2).

CAUTIONS. Men at risk of tumour 'flare'(see above) should be monitored closely during the first month of therapy. Caution is required in women with metabolic bone disease because decreases in bone mineral density may occur. The injection site should be rotated.

SIDE-EFFECTS. The gonadorelin analogues cause side-effects similar to the menopause in women and orchidectomy in men and include hot flushes and sweating, sexual dysfunction, vaginal dryness or bleeding, and gynaecomastia or changes in breast size. Signs and symptoms of prostate or breast cancer may worsen initially (managed in prostate cancer with anti-androgens, see above). Other side-effects include hypersensitivity reactions (rashes, pruritus, asthma, and rarely anaphylaxis), injection site reactions (see Cautions), headache (rarely migraine), visual disturbances, dizziness, arthralgia and possibly myalgia, hair loss, peripheral oedema, gastro-intestinal disturbances, weight changes, sleep disorders, and mood changes.

Anti-androgens

Cyproterone acetate, **flutamide** and **bicalutamide** are anti-androgens that inhibit the tumour 'flare' which may occur after commencing gonadorelin analogue administration. Cyproterone acetate and flutamide are also licensed for use alone in patients with metastatic prostate cancer refractory to gonadorelin analogue therapy. Bicalutamide is used for prostate cancer either alone or as an adjunct to other therapy, according to the clinical circumstances.

BICALUTAMIDE

Indications: advanced prostate cancer in combination with a gonadorelin analogue or surgical castration; locally advanced prostate cancer either alone or as adjuvant treatment

Cautions: hepatic impairment (Appendix 2), also consider periodic liver function tests; **interactions:** Appendix 1 (bicalutamide)

Side-effects: nausea, vomiting, diarrhoea, asthenia, gynaecomastia, breast tenderness, hot flushes, pruritus, dry skin, alopecia, hirsutism, decreased libido, impotence, weight gain; less commonly hypersensitivity reactions including angioneurotic oedema and urticaria, interstitial lung disease; rarely abdominal pain, cardiovascular disorders (including angina, heart failure and arrhythmias), depression, dyspepsia, haematuria, cholestasis, jaundice, thrombocytopenia

Dose: advanced prostate cancer, with orchidectomy or gonadorelin therapy, 50 mg daily (in gonadorelin therapy, started 3 days beforehand, see also notes above)

Locally advanced prostate cancer, 150 mg once daily

NOTE. The CSM has advised (October 2003) that bicalutamide should no longer be used for the treatment of localised prostate cancer

Casodex® (AstraZeneca) PoM
Tablets, f/c, bicalutamide 50 mg, net price 28-tab pack = £128.00; 150 mg, 28-tab pack = £240.00

BUSERELIN

Indications: advanced prostate cancer; other indications (section 6.7.2)

Cautions: depression, see also notes above

Side-effects: see notes above; worsening hypertension, palpitation, glucose intolerance, altered blood lipids, thrombocytopenia, leucopenia, nervousness, fatigue, memory and concentration disturbances, anxiety, increased thirst, hearing disorders, musculoskeletal pain; nasal irritation, nose bleeds and altered sense of taste and smell (spray formulation only)

Dose: *by subcutaneous injection*, 500 micrograms every 8 hours for 7 days, then *intranasally*, 1 spray into each nostril 6 times daily (see also notes above)

COUNSELLING. Avoid use of nasal decongestants before and for at least 30 minutes after treatment.

Suprefact® (Aventis Pharma) PoM

Injection, buserelin (as acetate) 1 mg/mL. Net price 2 × 5.5-mL vial = £23.69

Nasal spray, buserelin (as acetate) 100 micrograms/metered spray. Net price treatment pack of 4 × 10-g bottle with spray pump = £87.68. Counselling, see above

CYPROTERONE ACETATE

Indications: prostate cancer, see under Dose and also notes above; other indications, see section 6.4.2

Cautions: in prostate cancer, blood counts initially and throughout treatment; hepatic impairment (Appendix 2; see also under side-effects below); monitor hepatic function (liver function tests should be performed before treatment, see also under Side-effects below); monitor adrenocortical function regularly; risk of recurrence of thromboembolic disease; diabetes mellitus, sickle-cell anaemia, severe depression (in other indications some of these are contra-indicated, see section 6.4.2)

DRIVING. Fatigue and lassitude may impair performance of skilled tasks (e.g. driving)

Contra-indications: none in prostate cancer; for contra-indications relating to other indications see section 6.4.2

Side-effects: see section 6.4.2

HEPATOTOXICITY. Direct hepatic toxicity including jaundice, hepatitis and hepatic failure have been reported (usually after several months) in patients treated with cyproterone acetate 200–300 mg daily. Liver function tests should be performed before and regularly during treatment and whenever symptoms suggestive of hepatotoxicity occur—if confirmed cyproterone should normally be withdrawn unless the hepatotoxicity can be explained by another cause such as metastatic disease (in which case cyproterone should be continued only if the perceived benefit exceeds the risk)

Dose: flare with initial gonadorelin therapy, 300 mg daily in 2–3 divided doses, reduced to 200 mg daily in 2–3 divided doses if necesssary

Long-term palliative therapy where gonadorelin analogues or orchidectomy contra-indicated, not tolerated, or where oral therapy preferred, 200–300 mg daily in 2–3 divided doses

Hot flushes with gonadorelin therapy or after orchidectomy, initially 50 mg daily, adjusted according to response to 50–150 mg daily in 1–3 divided doses

Cyproterone Acetate (Non-proprietary) PoM

Tablets, cyproterone acetate 50 mg, net price 56-tab pack = £31.54; 100 mg, 84-tab pack = £91.39. Label: 21, counselling, driving

Cyprostat® (Schering Health) PoM

Tablets, scored, cyproterone acetate 50 mg, net price 168-tab pack = £77.68; 100 mg, 84-tab pack = £77.68. Label: 21, counselling, driving

FLUTAMIDE

Indications: advanced prostate cancer, see also notes above

Cautions: cardiac disease (oedema reported); hepatic impairment, also liver function tests, monthly for first 4 months, periodically thereafter and at the first sign or symptom of liver disorder (e.g. pruritus, dark urine, persistent anorexia, jaundice, abdominal pain, unexplained influenza-like symptoms); avoid excessive alcohol consumption; **interactions:** Appendix 1 (flutamide)

Side-effects: gynaecomastia (sometimes with galactorrhoea); nausea, vomiting, diarrhoea, increased appetite, insomnia, tiredness; other side-effects reported include decreased libido, reduced sperm count, gastric and chest pain, hypertension, headache, dizziness, oedema, blurred vision, thirst, rash, pruritus, haemolytic anaemia, systemic lupus erythematosus-like syndrome, and lymphoedema; hepatic injury (with transaminase abnormalities, cholestatic jaundice, hepatic necrosis, hepatic encephalopathy and occasional fatality) reported

Dose: 250 mg 3 times daily (see also notes above)

Flutamide (Non-proprietary) PoM

Tablets, flutamide 250 mg. Net price 84-tab pack = £68.06

Drogenil® (Schering-Plough) PoM

Tablets, yellow, scored, flutamide 250 mg, net price 84-tab pack = £65.10

GOSERELIN

Indications: prostate cancer; advanced breast cancer; oestrogen-receptor positive early breast cancer (section 8.3.4.1); other indications (section 6.7.2)

Cautions: see notes above; breast-feeding (Appendix 5)

Contra-indications: pregnancy (Appendix 4); undiagnosed vaginal bleeding

Side-effects: see notes above; also transient changes in blood pressure, paraesthesia, rarely hypercalcaemia (in patients with metastatic breast cancer)

Dose: see under preparations below

Zoladex® (AstraZeneca) PoM

Implant, goserelin 3.6 mg (as acetate) in *SafeSystem*® syringe applicator. Net price each = £84.14

Dose: breast cancer and prostate cancer *by subcutaneous injection* into anterior abdominal wall, 3.6 mg every 28 days (see also notes above)

Zoladex® **LA** (AstraZeneca) PoM

Implant, goserelin 10.8 mg (as acetate) in *SafeSystem*® syringe applicator. Net price each = £267.48

Dose: prostate cancer, *by subcutaneous injection* into anterior abdominal wall, 10.8 mg every 12 weeks (see also notes above)

LEUPRORELIN ACETATE

Indications: advanced prostate cancer; other indications (section 6.7.2)

Cautions: see notes above and section 6.7.2

Side-effects: see notes above and section 6.7.2; also fatigue, muscle weakness, paraesthesia, hypertension, palpitation, alteration of glucose tolerance

and of blood lipids; hypotension, jaundice, thrombocytopenia and leucopenia reported
Dose: see under preparations below

Prostap® SR (Wyeth) PoM
Injection (microsphere powder for reconstitution), leuprorelin acetate, net price 3.75-mg vial with 1-mL vehicle-filled syringe = £125.40
Dose: advanced prostate cancer, *by subcutaneous or by intramuscular injection*, 3.75 mg every 4 weeks (see also notes above)

Prostap® 3 (Wyeth) PoM
Injection (microsphere powder for reconstitution), leuprorelin acetate, net price 11.25-mg vial with 2-mL vehicle-filled syringe = £376.20
Dose: advanced prostate cancer, *by subcutaneous injection*, 11.25 mg every three months (see also notes above)

TRIPTORELIN

Indications: advanced prostate cancer; endometriosis, precocious puberty, reduction in size of uterine fibroids (section 6.7.2)
Cautions: see notes above
Side-effects: see notes above; transient hypertension, dry mouth, paraesthesia, increased dysuria, gynaecomastia
Dose: see under preparations below

Decapeptyl® SR (Ipsen) PoM
Injection (powder for suspension), m/r, triptorelin (as acetate), net price 4.2-mg vial (with diluent) = £69.00
Dose: by intramuscular injection, advanced prostate cancer, 3 mg every 4 weeks
Endometriosis and reduction in size of uterine fibroids, 3 mg every 4 weeks starting during first 5 days of menstrual cycle; for uterine fibroids continue treatment for at least 3 months; max. duration of treatment 6 months (do not repeat)
NOTE. Each 4.2-mg vial includes an overage to allow administration of a 3-mg dose
Injection (powder for suspension), m/r, triptorelin (as acetate), net price 15-mg vial (with diluent) = £207.00
Dose: by intramuscular injection, advanced prostate cancer, 11.25 mg every 3 months (see also notes above)
NOTE. Each 15-mg vial includes an overage to allow administration of an 11.25-mg dose

Gonapeptyl Depot® (Ferring) PoM
Injection (powder for suspension), triptorelin (as acetate), net price 3.75-mg prefilled syringe (with prefilled syringe of vehicle) = £85.00
Dose: by subcutaneous or deep intramuscular injection, advanced prostate cancer, 3.75 mg every 4 weeks (see also notes above)
Endometriosis and reduction in size of uterine fibroids, 3.75 mg every 4 weeks starting during first 5 days of menstrual cycle; for uterine fibroids continue treatment for 3 or 4 months; max. duration of treatment 6 months (do not repeat)
Precocious puberty (girls under 9 years, boys under 10 years), initially 3.75 mg every 2 weeks for 3 doses then every 3–4 weeks; dose reduced to 1.875 mg if body-weight under 20 kg or to 2.5 mg if body-weight 20–30 kg; discontinue when bone maturation consistent with age over 12 years in girls or over 13 years in boys

8.3.4.3 Somatostatin analogues

Octreotide and **lanreotide** are analogues of the hypothalamic release-inhibiting hormone somatostatin. They are indicated for the relief of symptoms associated with neuroendocrine (particularly carcinoid) tumours and acromegaly. Additionally, lanreotide is licensed for the treatment of thyroid tumours and octreotide is also licensed for the prevention of complications following pancreatic surgery; octreotide may also be valuable in reducing vomiting in palliative care (see p. 16) and in stopping variceal bleeding [unlicensed indication]—see also vasopressin and terlipressin (section 6.5.2).

CAUTIONS. Growth hormone-secreting pituitary tumours can expand causing serious complications; during treatment with somatostatin analogues patients should be monitored for signs of tumour expansion (e.g. visual field defects). Ultrasound examination of the gallbladder is recommended before treatment and at intervals of 6–12 months during treatment (avoid abrupt withdrawal of short-acting octreotide—see Side-effects below). In insulinoma an increase in the depth and duration of hypoglycaemia may occur (observe patients when initiating treatment and changing doses); in diabetes mellitus, insulin or oral antidiabetic requirements may be reduced.

SIDE-EFFECTS. Gastro-intestinal disturbances including anorexia, nausea, vomiting, abdominal pain and bloating, flatulence, diarrhoea, and steatorrhoea may occur. Postprandial glucose tolerance may be impaired and rarely persistent hyperglycaemia occurs with chronic administration; hypoglycaemia has also been reported. Gallstones have been reported after long-term treatment (abrupt withdrawal of subcutaneous octreotide is associated with biliary colic and pancreatitis). Pain and irritation may occur at the injection site and sites should be rotated. Rarely, pancreatitis has been reported shortly after administration.

OCTREOTIDE

Indications: see under Dose
Cautions: see notes above; hepatic impairment; pregnancy (Appendix 4); breast-feeding (Appendix 5); monitor thyroid function on long-term therapy; **interactions:** Appendix 1 (octreotide)
Side-effects: see notes above; rarely altered liver function tests, hepatitis and transient alopecia
Dose: symptoms associated with carcinoid tumours with features of carcinoid syndrome, VIPomas, glucagonomas, *by subcutaneous injection*, initially 50 micrograms once or twice daily, gradually increased according to response to 200 micrograms 3 times daily (higher doses required exceptionally); maintenance doses variable; in carcinoid tumours discontinue after 1 week if no effect; if rapid response required, initial dose *by intravenous injection* (with ECG monitoring and after dilution to a concentration of 10–50% with sodium chloride 0.9% injection)
Acromegaly, short-term treatment before pituitary surgery *or* long-term treatment in those inadequately controlled by other treatment *or* until radiotherapy becomes fully effective *by subcutaneous injection*, 100–200 micrograms 3 times daily; discontinue if no improvement within 3 months
Prevention of complications following pancreatic surgery, consult product literature

Sandostatin® (Novartis) PoM
Injection, octreotide (as acetate) 50 micrograms/mL, net price 1-mL amp = £3.47; 100 micrograms/mL, 1-mL amp = £6.53; 200 micrograms/mL 5-mL vial = £65.10; 500 micrograms/mL, 1-mL amp = £31.65

■ Depot preparation

Sandostatin Lar® (Novartis) PoM
Injection (microsphere powder for aqueous suspension), octreotide (as acetate) 10-mg vial = £637.50; 20-mg vial = £850.00; 30-mg vial = £1062.50 (all supplied with 2.5-mL diluent-filled syringe)

Dose: acromegaly (test dose *by subcutaneous injection* 50–100 micrograms if subcutaneous octreotide not previously given), neuroendocrine (particularly carcinoid) tumour adequately controlled by subcutaneous octreotide, *by deep intramuscular injection* into gluteal muscle, initially 20 mg every 4 weeks for 3 months then adjusted according to response; max. 30 mg every 4 weeks

For acromegaly, start depot octreotide 1 day after the last dose of subcutaneous octreotide (for pituitary surgery give last dose of depot octreotide at least 3 weeks before surgery); for neuroendocrine tumours, continue subcutaneous octreotide for 2 weeks after first dose of depot octreotide

LANREOTIDE

Indications: see notes above

Cautions: see notes above; pregnancy (Appendix 4); breast-feeding (Appendix 5); **interactions:** Appendix 1 (lanreotide)

Side-effects: see notes above; also reported asthenia, fatigue, raised bilirubin; less commonly skin nodule, hot flushes, leg pain, malaise, headache, tenesmus, decreased libido, drowsiness, pruritus, increased sweating; rarely hypothyroidism (monitor as necessary)

Dose: see under preparations

Somatuline® **LA** (Ipsen) PoM
Injection (copolymer microparticles for aqueous suspension), lanreotide (as acetate) 30-mg vial (with vehicle) = £310.85

Dose: by intramuscular injection, acromegaly and neuroendocrine (particularly carcinoid) tumours, initially 30 mg every 14 days, frequency increased to every 7–10 days according to response

Thyroid tumours, 30 mg every 14 days, frequency increased to every 10 days according to response

Somatuline Autogel® (Ipsen)
Injection, prefilled syringe, lanreotide (as acetate) 60 mg = £525.00; 90 mg = £699.00; 120 mg = £902.00

Dose: by deep subcutaneous injection into the gluteal region, acromegaly (if somatostatin analogue not given previously), initially 60 mg every 28 days, adjusted according to response; for patients treated previously with somatostatin analogue, consult product literature for initial dose

Neuroendocrine (particularly carcinoid) tumours, initially 60–120 mg every 28 days, adjusted according to response

9: Nutrition and blood

9.1 Anaemias and some other blood disorders

Before initiating treatment for anaemia it is essential to determine which type is present. Iron salts may be harmful and result in iron overload if given alone to patients with anaemias other than those due to iron deficiency.

9.1.1 Iron-deficiency anaemias

Treatment with an iron preparation is justified only in the presence of a demonstrable iron-deficiency state. Before starting treatment, it is important to exclude any serious underlying cause of the anaemia (e.g. gastric erosion, gastro-intestinal cancer).

Prophylaxis with an iron preparation is justifiable in individuals who have additional risk factors for iron deficiency (e.g. poor diet). Prophylaxis may also be appropriate in malabsorption, menorrhagia, pregnancy, after subtotal or total gastrectomy, in haemodialysis patients, and in the management of low birth-weight infants such as preterm neonates.

9.1.1.1 Oral iron

Iron salts should be given by mouth unless there are good reasons for using another route.

Ferrous salts show only marginal differences between one another in efficiency of absorption of iron, but ferric salts are much less well absorbed. Haemoglobin regeneration rate is little affected by the type of salt used provided sufficient iron is given, and in most patients the speed of response is not critical. Choice of preparation is thus usually decided by incidence of side-effects and cost.

The oral dose of elemental iron for deficiency should be 100 to 200 mg daily. It is customary to give this as dried **ferrous sulphate**, 200 mg (≡ 65 mg elemental iron) three times daily; a dose of ferrous sulphate 200 mg once or twice daily may be effective for prophylaxis or for mild iron deficiency.

Iron content of different iron salts

Iron salt	Amount	Content of ferrous iron
Ferrous fumarate	200 mg	65 mg
Ferrous gluconate	300 mg	35 mg
Ferrous succinate	100 mg	35 mg
Ferrous sulphate	300 mg	60 mg
Ferrous sulphate, dried	200 mg	65 mg

THERAPEUTIC RESPONSE. The haemoglobin concentration should rise by about 100–200 mg/100 mL (1–2 g/litre) per day *or* 2 g/100 mL (20 g/litre) over 3–4 weeks. When the haemoglobin is in the normal range, treatment should be continued for a further 3 months to replenish the iron stores. Epithelial tissue changes such as atrophic glossitis and koilonychia are usually improved, but the response is often slow.

SIDE-EFFECTS. Gastro-intestinal irritation may occur with iron salts. Nausea and epigastric pain are dose-related but the relationship between dose and altered bowel habit (constipation or diarrhoea) is less clear. Oral iron, particularly modified-release preparations, may exacerbate diarrhoea in patients with inflammatory bowel disease; care is also needed in patients with intestinal strictures and diverticular disease.

Iron preparations taken orally may be constipating, particularly in older patients, occasionally leading to faecal impaction.

If side-effects occur, the dose may be reduced; alternatively, another iron salt may be used but an improvement in tolerance may simply be a result of a lower content of elemental iron. The incidence of side-effects due to ferrous sulphate is no greater than with other iron salts when compared on the basis of equivalent amounts of elemental iron.

Iron preparations are a common cause of accidental overdose in children. For the treatment of **iron overdose**, see Emergency Treatment of Poisoning, p. 32.

COMPOUND PREPARATIONS. Some oral preparations contain ascorbic acid to aid absorption of the iron but the therapeutic advantage of such preparations is minimal and cost may be increased.

There is no justification for the inclusion of other ingredients, such as the B group of vitamins (except folic acid for pregnant women, see Iron and Folic Acid, p. 462 and on p. 464).

MODIFIED-RELEASE PREPARATIONS. Modified-release preparations of iron are licensed for once-daily dosage, but have no therapeutic advantage and should not be used. These preparations are formulated to release iron gradually; the low incidence of side-effects may reflect the small amounts of iron available for absorption as the iron is carried past the first part of the duodenum into an area of the gut where absorption may be poor.

FERROUS SULPHATE

Indications: iron-deficiency anaemia
Cautions: pregnancy (see section 9.1.1); **interactions:** Appendix 1 (iron)
Side-effects: see notes above
Dose: see under preparations below and notes above
COUNSELLING. Although iron preparations are best absorbed on an empty stomach they may be taken after food to reduce gastro-intestinal side-effects; they may discolour stools

Ferrous Sulphate (Non-proprietary)
Tablets, coated, dried ferrous sulphate 200 mg (65 mg iron), net price 28-tab pack = £1.50
Dose: prophylactic, 1 tablet daily; therapeutic, 1 tablet 2–3 times daily

Ironorm® Drops (Wallace Mfg)
Oral drops, ferrous sulphate 625 mg (125 mg iron)/5 mL. Net price 15-mL = £3.35
Dose: ADULT and CHILD over 6 years, 0.6 mL daily; INFANT and CHILD up to 6 years, 0.3 mL daily

■ Modified-release preparations

Feospan® (Intrapharm) NHS
Spansule® (= capsules m/r), clear/red, enclosing green and brown pellets, dried ferrous sulphate 150 mg (47 mg iron). Net price 30-cap pack = £1.43. Label: 25
Dose: 1–2 capsules daily; CHILD over 1 year, 1 capsule daily; can be opened and sprinkled on food

Ferrograd® (Abbott)
Tablets, f/c, m/r, red, dried ferrous sulphate 325 mg (105 mg iron). Net price 30-tab pack = 54p. Label: 25
Dose: ADULT and CHILD over 12 years, 1 tablet daily before food

FERROUS FUMARATE

Indications: iron-deficiency anaemia
Cautions: pregnancy (see section 9.1.1); **interactions:** Appendix 1 (iron)
Side-effects: see notes above
Dose: see under preparations below and notes above

Fersaday® (Goldshield)
Tablets, brown, f/c, ferrous fumarate 322 mg (100 mg iron). Net price 28-tab pack = 66p
Dose: prophylactic, 1 tablet daily; therapeutic, 1 tablet twice daily

Fersamal® (Goldshield)
Tablets, brown, ferrous fumarate 210 mg (68 mg iron). Net price 20 = 29p
Dose: 1–2 tablets 3 times daily
Syrup, brown, ferrous fumarate approx. 140 mg (45 mg iron)/5 mL. Net price 200 mL = £3.00
Dose: 10–20 mL twice daily; PRETERM NEONATE 0.6–2.4 mL/kg daily; CHILD up to 6 years 2.5–5 mL twice daily

Galfer® (Thornton & Ross)
Capsules, red/green, ferrous fumarate 305 mg (100 mg iron). Net price 20 = 36p
Dose: 1 capsule 1–2 times daily before food
Syrup, brown, sugar-free ferrous fumarate 140 mg (45 mg iron)/5 mL. Net price 300 mL = £4.86
Dose: 10 mL 1–2 times daily before food; CHILD (full-term infant and young child) 2.5–5 mL 1–2 times daily

FERROUS GLUCONATE

Indications: iron-deficiency anaemia
Cautions: pregnancy (see section 9.1.1); **interactions:** Appendix 1 (iron)
Side-effects: see notes above
Dose: see under preparation below and notes above

Ferrous Gluconate (Non-proprietary)
Tablets, red, coated, ferrous gluconate 300 mg (35 mg iron). Net price 20 = 73p
Dose: prophylactic, 2 tablets daily before food; therapeutic, 4–6 tablets daily in divided doses before food; CHILD 6–12 years, prophylactic and therapeutic, 1–3 tablets daily

FERROUS GLYCINE SULPHATE

Indications: iron-deficiency anaemia
Cautions: pregnancy (see section 9.1.1); **interactions:** Appendix 1 (iron)
Side-effects: see notes above
Dose: see under preparation below and notes above

Plesmet® (Link)
Syrup, ferrous glycine sulphate equivalent to 25 mg iron/5 mL. Net price 100 mL = 59p
Dose: prophylactic, ADULT and CHILD body-weight over 30 kg, 5 mL 3 times daily; CHILD body-weight 7.5–15 kg, 2.5 mL daily; body-weight 15–30 kg, 2.5 mL 3 times daily
Therapeutic, ADULT and CHILD body-weight over 30 kg, 10 mL 3 times daily; CHILD body-weight 2.5–5 kg, 2.5 mL daily; body-weight 5–7.5 kg, 2.5 mL twice daily; body-weight 7.5–15 kg, 2.5 mL 3 times daily; body-weight 15–30 kg, 5 mL 3 times daily

POLYSACCHARIDE-IRON COMPLEX

Indications: iron-deficiency anaemia
Cautions: pregnancy (see section 9.1.1); **interactions:** Appendix 1 (iron)
Side-effects: see notes above
Dose: see under preparation below and notes above

Niferex® (Tillomed)
Elixir, brown, sugar-free, polysaccharide-iron complex equivalent to 100 mg of iron/5 mL. Net price 240-mL pack = £6.06; NHS[1] 30-mL dropper bottle for paediatric use = £2.16. Counselling, use of dropper
Dose: prophylactic, 2.5 mL daily; therapeutic, 5 mL 1–2 times daily (once daily if required during second and third trimester of pregnancy); PRETERM NEONATE, NEONATE, and INFANT (from dropper bottle) 1 drop (approx. 500 micrograms iron) per 450 g body-weight 3 times daily; CHILD 2–6 years 2.5 mL daily, 6–12 years 5 mL daily

1. except 30 mL paediatric dropper bottle for prophylaxis and treatment of iron deficiency in infants born prematurely; endorse prescription 'SLS'

SODIUM FEREDETATE

(Sodium ironedetate)
Indications: iron-deficiency anaemia
Cautions: pregnancy (see section 9.1.1); **interactions:** Appendix 1 (iron)
Side-effects: see notes above
Dose: see under preparation below and notes above

Sytron® (Link)
Elixir, sugar-free, sodium feredetate 190 mg equivalent to 27.5 mg of iron/5 mL. Net price 100 mL = 89p
Dose: 5 mL increasing gradually to 10 mL 3 times daily; PRETERM NEONATE, NEONATE, and INFANT under 1 year 2.5 mL twice daily (smaller doses should be used initially); CHILD 1–5 years 2.5 mL 3 times daily, 6–12 years 5 mL 3 times daily

Iron and folic acid

These preparations are used during pregnancy in women who are at high risk of developing iron and folic acid deficiency; they should be distinguished from those used for the prevention of neural tube defects in women planning a pregnancy (see p. 464).

It is important to note that the small doses of folic acid contained in these preparations are inadequate for the treatment of megaloblastic anaemias.

Fefol® (Intrapharm) NHS
Spansule® (= capsules m/r), clear/green, enclosing brown, yellow, and white pellets, dried ferrous sulphate 150 mg (47 mg iron), folic acid 500 micrograms. Net price 30-cap pack = £1.69. Label: 25
Dose: 1 capsule daily

Ferrograd Folic® (Abbott)
Tablets, f/c, red/yellow, dried ferrous sulphate 325 mg (105 mg iron) for sustained release, folic acid 350 micrograms. Net price 30-tab pack = 60p. Label: 25
Dose: ADULT and CHILD over 12 years, 1 tablet daily before food

Galfer FA® (Thornton & Ross)
Capsules, red/yellow, ferrous fumarate 305 mg (100 mg iron), folic acid 350 micrograms. Net price 30-cap pack = £1.10
Dose: 1 capsule daily before food

Lexpec with Iron-M® (Rosemont) PoM
Syrup, brown, sugar-free, ferric ammonium citrate equivalent to 80 mg iron, folic acid 500 micrograms/5 mL. Net price 150 mL = £4.09
Dose: 5–10 mL daily before food
NOTE. *Lexpec with Iron-M*® contains five times less folic acid than *Lexpec with Iron*®

Pregaday® (Celltech)
Tablets, brown, f/c, ferrous fumarate equivalent to 100 mg iron, folic acid 350 micrograms. Net price 28-tab pack =£1.25
Dose: 1 tablet daily

■ Higher folic acid content

Appropriate in context of prevention of *recurrence of neural tube defects*, see recommendations on p. 464
Cautions: theoretical possibility of masking anaemia due to vitamin-B_{12} deficiency (which could allow vitamin-B_{12} neuropathy to develop).

Ferfolic SV® (Durbin) PoM NHS
Tablets, pink, ferrous gluconate 250 mg (30 mg iron), folic acid 4 mg, ascorbic acid 10 mg. Net price 100-tab pack = £2.50
Dose: anaemia, 1–3 tablets daily after food
Prophylaxis of neural tube defects in women known to be at risk, 1 tablet daily started before conception and continued for at least first trimester; see also recommendations on p. 464

Lexpec with Iron® (Rosemont) PoM
Syrup, brown, sugar-free, ferric ammonium citrate equivalent to 80 mg iron, folic acid 2.5 mg/5 mL. Net price 150 mL = £4.09
Dose: 5–10 mL daily before food
NOTE. *Lexpec with Iron*® contains five times as much folic acid as *Lexpec with Iron-M*®

Compound iron preparations

There is no justification for prescribing compound iron preparations, except for preparations of iron and folic acid for prophylactic use in pregnancy (see above).

Ferrograd C® (Abbott) NHS
Tablets, f/c, red, dried ferrous sulphate 325 mg (105 mg iron) for sustained release, ascorbic acid 500 mg (as sodium salt). Net price 30-tab pack = £1.71. Label: 25
Dose: ADULT and CHILD over 12 years, 1 tablet daily before food

Givitol® (Galen) NHS
Capsules, red/maroon, ferrous fumarate 305 mg (100 mg iron) with vitamins B group and C. Net price 20 = 88p
Dose: 1 capsule daily before food

9.1.1.2 Parenteral iron

Iron may be administered parenterally as iron dextran, or iron sucrose. Parenteral iron is generally reserved for use when oral therapy is unsuccessful because the patient cannot tolerate oral iron, or does not take it reliably, or if there is continuing blood loss, or in malabsorption.

Also, many patients with chronic renal failure who are receiving haemodialysis (and some who are receiving peritoneal dialysis) require iron by the intravenous route on a regular basis (see also Erythropoietin, section 9.1.3).

With the exception of patients with severe renal failure receiving haemodialysis, parenteral iron does not produce a faster haemoglobin response than oral iron provided that the oral iron preparation is taken reliably and is absorbed adequately.

Iron dextran, a complex of ferric hydroxide with dextrans, and **iron sucrose**, a complex of ferric hydroxide with sucrose, are used for the parenteral administration of iron. Anaphylactoid reactions can occur with parenteral administration of iron complexes and patients should be given a small test dose initially.

IRON DEXTRAN

A complex of ferric hydroxide with dextran containing 5% (50 mg/mL) of iron

Indications: iron-deficiency anaemia, see notes above

Cautions: facilities for cardiopulmonary resuscitation must be at hand; increased risk of allergic reaction in immune or inflammatory conditions; hepatic impairment (Appendix 2); renal impairment; oral iron not to be given until 5 days after last injection; pregnancy (Appendix 4)

Contra-indications: history of allergic disorders including asthma and eczema; infection; active rheumatoid arthritis

Side-effects: nausea, vomiting, abdominal pain; flushing, anaphylactoid reactions, dyspnoea, numbness, fever, urticaria, rash, arthralgia, myalgia; blurred vision; injection-site reactions including phlebitis; rarely diarrhoea, arrhythmias, hypotension, chest pain, seizures, tremor, dizziness, fatigue, sweating

Dose: *by deep intramuscular injection* into the gluteal muscle or *by slow intravenous injection* or *by intravenous infusion*, calculated according to body-weight and iron deficit, consult product literature
CHILD under 14 years, not recommended

CosmoFer® (Vitaline) ▼ PoM
Injection, iron (as iron dextran) 50 mg/mL, net price 2-mL amp = £7.97

IRON SUCROSE

A complex of ferric hydroxide with sucrose containing 2% (20 mg/mL) of iron

Indications: iron-deficiency anaemia, see notes above

Cautions: oral iron therapy should not be given until 5 days after last injection; facilities for cardiopulmonary resuscitation must be at hand; pregnancy (Appendix 4)

Contra-indications: history of allergic disorders including asthma, eczema and anaphylaxis; liver disease; infection

Side-effects: taste disturbance; less commonly nausea, vomiting, abdominal pain, diarrhoea, hypotension, tachycardia, palpitation, chest pain, flushing, bronchospasm, dyspnoea, headache, dizziness, fever, myalgia, pruritus, urticaria, rash, injection-site reactions including phlebitis; rarely peripheral oedema, paraesthesia, fatigue, anaphylactoid reactions

Dose: *by slow intravenous injection* or *by intravenous infusion*, calculated according to body-weight and iron deficit, consult product literature
CHILD not recommended

Venofer® (Syner-Med) PoM
Injection, iron (as iron sucrose) 20 mg/mL, net price 5-mL amp = £8.50

9.1.2 Drugs used in megaloblastic anaemias

Most megaloblastic anaemias result from a lack of either vitamin B_{12} or folate, and it is essential to establish in every case which deficiency is present and the underlying cause. In emergencies, where delay might be dangerous, it is sometimes necessary to administer both substances after the bone marrow test while plasma assay results are awaited. Normally, however, appropriate treatment should be instituted only when the results of tests are available.

One cause of megaloblastic anaemia in the UK is *pernicious anaemia* in which lack of gastric intrinsic factor resulting from an auto-immune gastritis causes malabsorption of vitamin B_{12}.

Vitamin B_{12} is also needed in the treatment of megaloblastosis caused by *prolonged nitrous oxide anaesthesia*, which inactivates the vitamin, and in the rare syndrome of *congenital transcobalamin II deficiency*.

Vitamin B_{12} should be given prophylactically after *total gastrectomy* or *total ileal resection* (or after *partial gastrectomy* if a vitamin B_{12} absorption test shows vitamin B_{12} malabsorption).

Apart from dietary deficiency, all other causes of vitamin-B_{12} deficiency are attributable to malabsorption. There is little place for the use of low-dose vitamin B_{12} orally and none for vitamin B_{12} intrinsic factor complexes given by mouth. Vitamin B_{12} in larger oral doses of 1–2 mg daily [unlicensed] may be effective.

Hydroxocobalamin has completely replaced cyanocobalamin as the form of vitamin B_{12} of choice for therapy; it is retained in the body longer than cyanocobalamin and thus for maintenance therapy can be given at intervals of up to 3 months. Treatment is generally initiated with frequent administration of intramuscular injections to replenish the depleted body stores. Thereafter, maintenance treatment, which is usually for life, can be instituted. There is no evidence that doses larger than those recommended provide any additional benefit in vitamin-B_{12} neuropathy.

Folic acid has few indications for long-term therapy since most causes of folate deficiency are self-limiting or will yield to a short course of treatment. It should not be used in undiagnosed megaloblastic anaemia unless vitamin B_{12} is administered concurrently otherwise neuropathy may be precipitated (see above).

In *folate-deficient megaloblastic anaemia* (e.g. because of poor nutrition, pregnancy, or antiepileptics), standard treatment to bring about a haematological remission and replenish body stores, is oral administration of folic acid 5 mg daily for 4 months; up to 15 mg daily may be necessary in malabsorption states. In pregnancy, folic acid 5 mg is continued to term.

For *prophylaxis in chronic haemolytic states or in renal dialysis*, it is sufficient to give folic acid 5 mg daily or even weekly, depending on the diet and the rate of haemolysis.

For *prophylaxis in pregnancy* the dose of folic acid is 200–500 micrograms daily (see Iron and Folic Acid, section 9.1.1.1). See also Prevention of Neural Tube Defects below.

Folinic acid is also effective in the treatment of folate-deficient megaloblastic anaemia but it is generally used in association with cytotoxic drugs (see section 8.1); it is given as calcium folinate.

PREVENTION OF NEURAL TUBE DEFECTS. Recommendations of an expert advisory group of the Department of Health include the advice that:

> To prevent *recurrence of neural tube defect* (in a child of a man or woman with spina bifida or if there is a history of neural tube defect in a previous child) women who wish to become pregnant (or who are at risk of becoming pregnant) should be advised to take folic acid supplements at a dose of 5 mg daily (reduced to 4 mg daily if a suitable preparation becomes available); supplementation should continue until week 12 of pregnancy. Women receiving antiepileptic therapy need individual counselling by their doctor before starting folic acid.
>
> To prevent *first occurrence of neural tube defect* women who are planning a pregnancy should be advised to take folic acid as a medicinal or food supplement at a dose of 400 micrograms daily before conception and during the first 12 weeks of pregnancy. Women who have not been taking supplements and who suspect they are pregnant should start at once and continue until week 12 of pregnancy.

There is **no** justification for prescribing multiple-ingredient vitamin preparations containing vitamin B_{12} or folic acid.

HYDROXOCOBALAMIN

Indications: see under dose below

Cautions: should not be given before diagnosis fully established but see also notes above

Side-effects: nausea, headache, dizziness; fever, hypersensitivity reactions including rash and pruritus; injection-site pain; hypokalaemia during initial treatment

Dose: *by intramuscular injection*, pernicious anaemia and other macrocytic anaemias without neurological involvement, initially 1 mg 3 times a week for 2 weeks then 1 mg every 3 months

Pernicious anaemia and other macrocytic anaemias with neurological involvement, initially 1 mg on alternate days until no further improvement, then 1 mg every 2 months

Prophylaxis of macrocytic anaemias associated with vitamin-B_{12} deficiency, 1 mg every 2–3 months

Tobacco amblyopia and Leber's optic atrophy, initially 1 mg daily for 2 weeks, then 1 mg twice weekly until no further improvement, thereafter 1 mg every 1–3 months

CHILD, doses as for adult

Hydroxocobalamin (Non-proprietary) PoM

Injection, hydroxocobalamin 1 mg/mL. Net price 1-mL amp = £2.46

NOTE. The BP directs that when vitamin B_{12} injection is prescribed or demanded hydroxocobalamin injection shall be dispensed or supplied

Brands include *Cobalin-H*® NHS, *Neo-Cytamen*® NHS

CYANOCOBALAMIN 

Indications: see notes above

Dose: *by mouth*, vitamin-B_{12} deficiency of dietary origin, 50–150 micrograms or more daily taken between meals; CHILD 50–105 micrograms daily in 1–3 divided doses

By intramuscular injection, initially 1 mg repeated 10 times at intervals of 2–3 days, maintenance 1 mg every month, but see notes above

Cyanocobalamin (Non-proprietary)

[1]*Tablets* NHS, cyanocobalamin 50 micrograms. Net price 50-tab pack = £3.04

Brands include *Cytacon*® NHS

Liquid NHS, cyanocobalamin 35 micrograms/ 5 mL. Net price 200 mL = £2.77

Brands include *Cytacon*® NHS

Injection PoM, cyanocobalamin 1 mg/mL. Net price 1-mL amp = £1.67

Brands include *Cytamen*® NHS

NOTE. The BP directs that when vitamin B_{12} injection is prescribed or demanded hydroxocobalamin injection shall be dispensed or supplied

1. NHS except to treat or prevent vitamin-B_{12} deficiency in a patient who is a vegan or who has a proven vitamin-B_{12} deficiency of dietary origin; endorse prescription 'SLS'

FOLIC ACID

Indications: see notes above

Cautions: should never be given alone for pernicious anaemia and other vitamin-B_{12} deficiency states (may precipitate subacute combined degeneration of the spinal cord); **interactions:** Appendix 1 (folates)

Dose: *by mouth*, initially, 5 mg daily for 4 months (see notes above); maintenance, 5 mg every 1–7 days depending on underlying disease; CHILD up to 1 year, 500 micrograms/kg daily; over 1 year, as adult dose

Prevention of neural tube defects, see notes above

[1]**Folic Acid** (Non-proprietary) PoM

Tablets, folic acid 400 micrograms, net price = 90-tab pack = £2.24; 5 mg, 28-tab pack = 81p

Syrup, folic acid 2.5 mg/5 mL, net price 150 mL = £9.16; 400 micrograms/5 mL, 150 mL = £1.40

Brands include *Folicare*®, *Lexpec*® (sugar-free)

Injection, folic acid 15 mg, net price 1-mL amp = £1.34
'Special order' [unlicensed] product; contact BCM Specials

1. Can be sold to the public provided daily doses do not exceed 500 micrograms; brands include *Preconceive*®

9.1.3 Drugs used in hypoplastic, haemolytic, and renal anaemias

Anabolic steroids (section 6.4.3), pyridoxine, antilymphocyte immunoglobulin, and various corticosteroids are used in hypoplastic and haemolytic anaemias.

Antilymphocyte globulin given intravenously through a central line over 12–18 hours each day for 5 days produces a response in about 50% of cases of acquired *aplastic anaemia*; the response rate may be increased when ciclosporin is given as well. Severe reactions are common in the first 2 days and profound immunosuppression can occur; antilymphocyte globulin should be given under specialist supervision with appropriate resuscitation facilities. Alternatively, oxymetholone tablets (available on a named-patient basis only) may be used in aplastic anaemia at a dose of 1–5 mg/kg daily for 3 to 6 months.

It is unlikely that dietary deprivation of **pyridoxine** (section 9.6.2) produces clinically relevant haematological effects. However, certain forms of *sideroblastic anaemia* respond to pharmacological doses, possibly reflecting its role as a co-enzyme during haemoglobin synthesis. Pyridoxine is indicated in both *idiopathic acquired* and *hereditary sideroblastic anaemias*. Although complete cures have not been reported, some increase in haemoglobin may occur; the dose required is usually high, up to 400 mg daily. *Reversible sideroblastic anaemias* respond to treatment of the underlying cause but in pregnancy, haemolytic anaemias, and alcohol dependence, or during isoniazid treatment, pyridoxine is also indicated.

Hydroxycarbamide (hydroxyurea, section 8.1.5) can reduce the frequency of crises in *sickle-cell disease* and reduce the need for blood transfusions [unlicensed indication].

Corticosteroids (see section 6.3) have an important place in the management of a wide variety of haematological disorders. They include conditions with an immune basis such as *autoimmune haemolytic anaemia*, *immune thrombocytopenias* and *neutropenias*, and *major transfusion reactions*. They are also used in chemotherapy schedules for many types of *lymphoma*, *lymphoid leukaemias*, and *paraproteinaemias*, including *multiple myeloma*.

Erythropoietin

Epoetin (recombinant human erythropoietin) is used for the anaemia associated with erythropoietin deficiency in chronic renal failure, to increase the yield of autologous blood in normal individuals and to shorten the period of anaemia in patients receiving cytotoxic chemotherapy. The clinical efficacy of epoetin alfa and epoetin beta is similar. Epoetin beta is also used for the prevention of anaemia in preterm neonates of low birth-weight.

Darbepoetin, is a hyperglycosylated derivative of epoetin which has a longer half-life and may be administered less frequently than epoetin.

Other factors which contribute to the anaemia of chronic renal failure such as iron or folate deficiency should be corrected before treatment and monitored during therapy. Supplemental iron may improve the response in resistant patients. Aluminium toxicity, concurrent infection or other inflammatory disease may impair the response to erythropoietin.

CSM advice. There have been very rare reports of pure red cell aplasia in patients treated with epoetin alfa. The CSM has advised that in patients developing epoetin alfa failure with a diagnosis of pure red cell aplasia, treatment with epoetin alfa must be discontinued and testing for erythropoietin antibodies considered. Patients who develop pure red cell aplasia should **not** be switched to another erythropoietin.

DARBEPOETIN ALFA

Indications: see under Dose below

Cautions: see Epoetin; hepatic disease (Appendix 2); pregnancy (Appendix 4); **interactions:** Appendix 1 (epoetin)

Contra-indications: see Epoetin; breast-feeding (Appendix 5)

Side-effects: see Epoetin; also, peripheral oedema, injection site pain

Dose: anaemia associated with chronic renal failure in patients on dialysis, ADULT and CHILD over 11 years, *by subcutaneous or intravenous injection*, initially 450 nanograms/kg once weekly, adjusted according to response by approx. 25% of initial dose at intervals of at least 4 weeks; maintenance dose (when haemoglobin concentration of 11 g/100 mL achieved), given once weekly *or* once every 2 weeks

Anaemia associated with chronic renal failure in patients not on dialysis, ADULT and CHILD over 11 years, *by subcutaneous or intravenous injection*, initially 450 nanograms/kg once weekly *or by subcutaneous injection*, initially 750 nanograms/kg once every 2 weeks; adjusted according to response by approx. 25% of initial dose at intervals of at least 4 weeks; maintenance dose (when haemoglobin concentration of at least 11 g/100 mL achieved), given once weekly *or* once every 2 weeks *or* once every month

NOTE. Reduce dose by 25–50% if haemoglobin rise exceeds 2.5 g/100 mL per month; suspend if haemoglobin exceeds 14 g/100 mL until it falls below 13 g/100 mL and then restart with dose at 25% below previous dose. When changing route give same dose then adjust according to weekly or fortnightly haemoglobin measurements. Adjust doses at 2-week intervals during maintenance treatment

Anaemia in adults with non-myeloid malignancies receiving chemotherapy, *by subcutaneous injection*, initially 6.75 micrograms/kg once every 3 weeks (if response inadequate after 9 weeks further treatment may not be effective) *or* 2.25 micrograms/kg once weekly (if appropriate rise in haemoglobin not achieved after 4 weeks, double initial dose; if response remains inadequate after 4 weeks at higher dose further treatment may not be effective); haemoglobin should not exceed 13 g/100 mL; if adequate response obtained or if rise in haemoglobin greater than 2 g/100 mL in 4 weeks, reduce dose by 25–50%; continue for approx. 4 weeks after chemotherapy

Aranesp® (Amgen) ▼ PoM
Injection, prefilled syringe, darbepoetin alfa, 25 micrograms/mL, net price 0.4 mL (10 micrograms) = £15.59; 40 micrograms/mL, 0.375 mL (15 micrograms) = £23.38, 0.5 mL (20 micrograms) = £31.17; 100 micrograms/mL, 0.3 mL (30 micrograms) = £46.76, 0.4 mL (40 micrograms) = £62.34, 0.5 mL (50 micrograms) = £77.93; 200 micrograms/mL, 0.3 mL (60 micrograms) = £93.51, 0.4 mL (80 micrograms) = £124.68, 0.5 mL (100 micrograms) = £155.85; 500 micrograms/mL, 0.3 mL (150 micrograms) = £233.78, 0.6 mL (300 micrograms) = £467.55, 1 mL (500 micrograms) = £779.25

Aranesp® **SureClick** (Amgen) ▼ PoM
Injection, prefilled disposable injection device, darbepoetin alfa, 40 micrograms/mL, net price 0.5 mL (20 micrograms) = £31.17; 100 micrograms/mL, net price 0.4 mL (40 micrograms) = £62.34; 200 micrograms/mL, net price 0.3 mL (60 micrograms) = £93.51, 0.4 mL (80 micrograms) = £124.68, 0.5 mL (100 micrograms) = £155.85; 500 micrograms/mL, net price 0.3 mL (150 micrograms) = £233.78, 0.6 mL (300 microrgrams) = £467.55, 1 mL (500 micrograms) = £779.25

EPOETIN ALFA and BETA

(Recombinant human erythropoietins)

NOTE. Although epoetin alfa and beta are clinically indistinguishable the prescriber must specify which is required

Indications: see under preparations, below

Cautions: inadequately treated or poorly controlled blood pressure (monitor closely blood pressure, reticulocyte counts, haemoglobin, and electrolytes), interrupt treatment if blood pressure uncontrolled; sudden stabbing migraine-like pain is warning of hypertensive crisis; sickle-cell disease (lower target haemoglobin concentration may be appropriate), exclude other causes of anaemia (e.g. folic acid or vitamin B_{12} deficiency) and give iron supplements if necessary (see also notes above); ischaemic vascular disease; thrombocytosis (monitor platelet count for first 8 weeks); epilepsy; malignant disease; chronic liver failure (Appendix 2); increase in heparin dose may be needed; risk of thrombosis may be increased when used for anaemia in adults receiving cancer chemotherapy; risk of thrombosis may be increased when used for anaemia before orthopaedic surgery—avoid in cardiovascular disease including recent myocardial infarction or cerebrovascular accident ; pregnancy (Appendix 4) and breast-feeding (Appendix 5); **interactions:** Appendix 1 (epoetin)

Contra-indications: pure red cell aplasia following erythropoietin (see also CSM advice above); uncontrolled hypertension; patients unable to receive thromboprophylaxis; avoid injections containing benzyl alcohol in neonates (see under preparations, below)

Side-effects: dose-dependent increase in blood pressure or aggravation of hypertension; in isolated patients with normal or low blood pressure, hypertensive crisis with encephalopathy-like symptoms and generalised tonic-clonic seizures requiring immediate medical attention; headache; dose-dependent increase in platelet count (but thrombocytosis rare) regressing during treatment; influenza-like symptoms (may be reduced if intravenous injection given over 5 minutes); thromboembolic events; shunt thrombosis especially if tendency to hypotension or arteriovenous shunt complications; very rarely sudden loss of response because of pure red cell aplasia, particularly following subcutaneous administration in patients with chronic renal failure (discontinue erythropoietin therapy)—see also CSM advice above, hyperkalaemia, and skin reactions

Dose: aimed at increasing haemoglobin concentration at rate not exceeding 2 g/100 mL/month to stable level of 10–12 g/100 mL (9.5–11 g/100 mL in children); see under preparations, below

■ Epoetin alfa

Eprex® (Janssen-Cilag) PoM
Injection, epoetin alfa 40 000 units/mL, net price 1-mL (40 000-unit) vial = £318.44
Injection, prefilled syringe, epoetin alfa, net price 1000 units = £7.96; 2000 units = £15.92; 3000 units = £23.88; 4000 units = £31.84; 5000 units = £39.81; 6000 units = £47.77; 8000 units = £63.69; 10 000 units = £79.61. An auto-injector device is available for use with 10 000-units prefilled syringes

Dose: anaemia associated with chronic renal failure in patients on haemodialysis, *by intravenous injection* over 1–5 minutes, initially 50 units/kg 3 times weekly adjusted according to response in steps of 25 units/kg 3 times weekly at intervals of at least 4 weeks; maintenance dose (when haemoglobin concentration of 10–12 g/100 mL achieved), usually a total of 75–300 units/kg weekly (as a single dose or in divided doses); CHILD initially as for adults; maintenance dose (when haemoglobin concentration of 9.5–11 g/100 mL achieved), body-weight under 10 kg usually 75–150 units/kg 3 times weekly, body-weight 10–30 kg usually 60–150 units/kg 3 times weekly, body-weight over 30 kg usually 30–100 units/kg 3 times weekly

IMPORTANT. Subcutaneous injection **contra-indicated** in patients with chronic renal failure

Anaemia associated with chronic renal failure in adults on peritoneal dialysis, *by intravenous injection* over 1–5 minutes, initially 50 units/kg twice weekly; maintenance dose (when haemoglobin concentration of 10–12 g/100 mL achieved), 25–50 units/kg twice weekly

IMPORTANT. Subcutaneous injection **contra-indicated** in patients with chronic renal failure

Severe symptomatic anaemia of renal origin in adults with renal insufficiency not yet on dialysis, *by intravenous injection* over 1–5 minutes, initially 50 units/kg 3 times weekly increased according to response in steps of 25 units/kg 3 times weekly at intervals of at least 4 weeks; maintenance dose (when haemoglobin concentration of 10–12 g/100 mL achieved), 17–33 units/kg 3 times weekly; max. 200 units/kg 3 times weekly;

IMPORTANT. Subcutaneous injection **contra-indicated** in patients with chronic renal failure

Anaemia in adults receiving cancer chemotherapy, *by subcutaneous injection* (max. 1 mL per injection site), initially 150 units/kg 3 times weekly, increased if appropriate rise in haemoglobin (or reticulocyte count) not achieved after 4 weeks to 300 units/kg 3 times weekly; discontinue if inadequate response after 4 weeks at higher dose; reduce dose by 25–50% if haemoglobin rise exceeds 2 g/100 mL per month; suspend if haemoglobin exceeds 14 g/100 mL until it falls below 12 g/100 mL and

reinstate with dose at 25% below previous dose; continue epoetin for 1 month after end of chemotherapy
To increase yield of autologous blood (to avoid homologous blood) in predonation programme in moderate anaemia *either* when large volume of blood required *or* when sufficient blood cannot be saved for elective major surgery, *by intravenous injection* over 1–5 minutes, 600 units/kg twice weekly for 3 weeks before surgery; consult product literature for details and advice on ensuring high iron stores
Moderate anaemia (haemoglobin concentration 10–13 g/100 mL) before elective orthopaedic surgery in adults with expected moderate blood loss to reduce exposure to allogeneic transfusion or if autologous transfusion unavailable, *by subcutaneous injection* (max. 1 mL per injection site), 600 units/kg every week for 3 weeks before surgery and on day of surgery *or* 300 units/kg daily for 15 days starting 10 days before surgery; consult product literature for details

■ Epoetin beta

NeoRecormon® (Roche) PoM

Injection, prefilled syringe, epoetin beta, net price 500 units = £3.90; 1000 units = £7.79; 2000 units = £15.59; 3000 units = £23.38; 4000 units = £31.17; 5000 units = £38.97; 6000 units = £46.76; 10 000 units = £77.93; 20 000 units = £155.87; 30 000 units = £233.81
Excipients: include phenylalanine up to 300 micrograms/syringe (section 9.4.1)

Multidose injection, powder for reconstitution, epoetin beta, net price 50 000-unit vial = £419.01; 100 000-unit vial = £838.01 (both with solvent)
Excipients: include phenylalanine up to 5 mg/vial (section 9.4.1), benzyl alcohol (avoid in neonates, see Excipients p. 2)
NOTE. Avoid contact of reconstituted injection with glass; use only plastic materials

Reco-Pen, (for subcutaneous use), double-chamber cartridges (containing epoetin beta and solvent), net price 10 000-unit cartridge = £77.93; 20 000-unit cartridge = £155.87; 60 000-unit cartridge = £467.61; for use with *Reco-Pen* injection device and needles (both available free from Roche)
Excipients: include phenylalanine up to 500 micrograms/cartridge (section 9.4.1), benzyl alcohol (avoid in neonates, see Excipients, p. 2)

Dose: anaemia associated with chronic renal failure in dialysis patients, symptomatic anaemia of renal origin in patients not yet on dialysis, ADULT and CHILD
By subcutaneous injection, initially 60 units/kg weekly (in 1–7 divided doses) for 4 weeks, increased according to response at intervals of 4 weeks in steps of 60 units/kg; maintenance dose (when haemoglobin concentration of 10–12 g/100 mL achieved), initially reduce dose by half then adjust according to response at intervals of 1–2 weeks; max. 720 units/kg weekly
By intravenous injection over 2 minutes, initially 40 units/kg 3 times weekly for 4 weeks, increased according to response to 80 units/kg 3 times weekly with further increases if needed at intervals of 4 weeks in steps of 20 units/kg 3 times weekly; maintenance dose (when haemoglobin concentration of 10–12 g/100 mL achieved), initially reduce dose by half then adjust according to response at intervals of 1–2 weeks; max. 720 units/kg weekly
Prevention of anaemia of prematurity in neonates with birth-weight of 0.75–1.5 kg and gestational age of less than 34 weeks, *by subcutaneous injection* (of single-dose, unpreserved injection), 250 units/kg 3 times weekly preferably starting within 3 days of birth and continued for 6 weeks
Anaemia in adults with solid tumours receiving platinum-containing chemotherapy, *by subcutaneous injection*, initially 450 units/kg weekly (in 3–7 divided doses), increased if appropriate rise in haemoglobin not achieved after 4 weeks to 900 units/kg weekly (in 3–7 divided doses); reduce dose by half if haemoglobin rise exceeds 2 g/100 mL per month; suspend if haemoglobin exceeds 14 g/100 mL until concentration falls below 12 g/100 mL and reinstate at 50% of the previous weekly dose; continue for up to 3 weeks after end of chemotherapy
NOTE. If haemoglobin concentration falls by more than 1 g/100 mL in the first cycle of chemotherapy despite treatment with epoetin beta, further treatment may not be effective
To increase yield of autologous blood (to avoid homologous blood) in predonation programme in moderate anaemia when blood-conserving procedures are insufficient or unavailable, consult product literature
Anaemia in adults with multiple myeloma, low-grade non-Hodgkin's lymphoma or chronic lymphocytic leukaemia receiving chemotherapy, *by subcutaneous injection*, initially 450 units/kg weekly (as a single dose or in 3–7 divided doses), increased if rise in haemoglobin of at least 1 g/100 mL not achieved after 4 weeks to 900 units/kg weekly (in 2–7 divided doses); reduce dose by half if haemoglobin rise exceeds 2 g/100 mL per month; suspend if haemoglobin exceeds 14 g/100 mL until concentration falls below 13 g/100 mL and reinstate at 50% of previous dose; max. 900 units/kg weekly; continue for up to 4 weeks after end of chemotherapy
NOTE. Discontinue treatment if haemoglobin concentration does not increase by at least 1 g/100 mL after 8 weeks of therapy

Iron overload

Severe tissue iron overload may occur in aplastic and other refractory anaemias, mainly as the result of repeated blood transfusions. It is a particular problem in refractory anaemias with hyperplastic bone marrow, especially *thalassaemia major*, where excessive iron absorption from the gut and inappropriate iron therapy may add to the tissue siderosis.

Iron overload associated with haemochromatosis may be treated with repeated venesection. Venesection may also be used for patients who have received multiple transfusions and whose bone marrow has recovered. Where venesection is contra-indicated, the long-term administration of the iron chelating compound **desferrioxamine mesilate** is useful. Subcutaneous infusions of desferrioxamine are given over 8–12 hours, 3–7 times a week. The dose should reflect the degree of iron overload. For children starting therapy (and who have low iron overload) the dose should not exceed 30 mg/kg. For established overload the dose is usually between 20 and 50 mg/kg daily. Desferrioxamine (up to 2 g per unit of blood) may also be given at the time of blood transfusion, provided that the desferrioxamine is **not** added to the blood and is **not** given through the same line as the blood (but the two may be given through the same cannula).

Iron excretion induced by desferrioxamine is enhanced by administration of ascorbic acid (vitamin C, section 9.6.3) in a dose of 200 mg daily (100 mg in infants); it should be given separately from food since it also enhances iron absorption. Ascorbic acid should not be given to patients with cardiac dysfunction; in patients with normal cardiac function ascorbic acid should be introduced 1 month after starting desferrioxamine.

Infusion of desferrioxamine may be used to treat *aluminium overload* in dialysis patients; theoretically 100 mg of desferrioxamine binds with 4.1 mg of aluminium.

Deferiprone, an oral iron chelator, is licensed for the treatment of iron overload in patients with thalassaemia major in whom desferrioxamine is contra-indicated or is not tolerated. Blood dyscrasias, particularly agranulocytosis, have been reported with deferiprone.

DEFERIPRONE

Indications: see notes above

Cautions: monitor neutrophil count weekly and discontinue treatment if neutropenia develops; monitor plasma-zinc concentration; hepatic impairment (Appendix 2); renal impairment (Appendix 3); limited experience in children 6–10 years

BLOOD DISORDERS. Patients or their carers should be told how to recognise signs of neutropenia and advised to seek immediate medical attention if symptoms such as fever or sore throat develop

Contra-indications: pregnancy (contraception advised in women of child-bearing potential; *important teratogenic risk*: see Appendix 4) and breast-feeding (Appendix 5)

Side-effects: gastro-intestinal disturbances (reducing dose and increasing gradually may improve tolerance); red-brown urine discoloration; neutropenia, agranulocytosis; zinc deficiency; arthropathy

Dose: ADULT and CHILD over 6 years 25 mg/kg (to the nearest 250 mg) 3 times daily (max. 100 mg/kg daily); CHILD under 6 years not recommended

Ferriprox® (Swedish Orphan) PoM
Tablets, f/c, scored, deferiprone 500 mg, net price 100-tab pack = £152.39. Label: 14, counselling, blood disorders

DESFERRIOXAMINE MESILATE

(Deferoxamine Mesilate)

Indications: see notes above; iron poisoning, see Emergency Treatment of Poisoning

Cautions: renal impairment; eye and ear examinations before treatment and at 3-month intervals during treatment; monitor body-weight and height in children at 3-month intervals—risk of growth retardation with excessive doses; aluminium-related encephalopathy (may exacerbate neurological dysfunction); pregnancy (Appendix 4), breast-feeding (Appendix 5); **interactions:** Appendix 1 (desferrioxamine)

Side-effects: hypotension (especially when given too rapidly by intravenous injection), disturbances of hearing and vision (including lens opacity and retinopathy); injection site reactions, gastro-intestinal disturbances, asthma, fever, headache, arthralgia and myalgia; very rarely anaphylaxis, acute respiratory distress syndrome, neurological disturbances (including dizziness, neuropathy and paraesthesia), Yersinia and mucormycosis infections, rash, renal impairment, and blood dyscrasias

Dose: see notes above; iron poisoning, see Emergency Treatment of Poisoning

NOTE. For full details and warnings relating to administration, consult product literature

Desferrioxamine mesilate (Non-proprietary) PoM
Injection, powder for reconstitution, desferrioxamine mesilate, net price 500-mg vial = £4.26; 2-g vial = £17.05

Desferal® (Novartis) PoM
Injection, powder for reconstitution, desferrioxamine mesilate, net price 500-mg vial = £4.44, 2-g vial = £17.77

9.1.4 Drugs used in platelet disorders

It is usual to treat autoimmune (idiopathic) thrombocytopenic purpura with a **corticosteroid**, e.g. prednisolone 1 mg/kg daily, gradually reducing the dose over several weeks. Splenectomy is considered if a satisfactory platelet count is not achieved or if there is a relapse on reducing the dose of corticosteroid or withdrawing it.

Immunoglobulin preparations (section 14.5), are also used in autoimmune thrombocytopenic purpura or where a temporary rapid rise in platelets is needed, as in pregnancy or pre-operatively; they are also used for children often in preference to a corticosteroid. **Anti-D (Rh_0) immunoglobulin** (section 14.5) is effective in raising the platelet count in about 80% of unsplenectomised rhesus-positive individuals; its effects may last longer than normal immunoglobulin for intravenous use, but further doses are usually required. In autoimmune thrombocytopenic purpura refractory to corticosteroid treatment or in chronic cases where splenectomy is inappropriate, **danazol** (section 6.7.2) may be used [unlicensed indication], particularly in older patients. Danazol may also allow the dose of corticosteroid to be reduced.

Other therapy that has been tried in refractory autoimmune thrombocytopenic purpura includes azathioprine (section 8.2.1), cyclophosphamide (section 8.1.1), vincristine (section 8.1.4), and ciclosporin (section 8.2.2). Rituximab (section 8.2.3) may also be effective and in some cases induces prolonged remission. For patients with chronic severe thrombocytopenia refractory to other therapy, tranexamic acid (section 2.11) may be given to reduce the severity of haemorrhage.

Anagrelide reduces platelets in primary thrombocythaemia and in thrombocythaemia secondary to myeloproliferative disorders.

The *Scottish Medicines Consortium* has advised (March 2005) that anagrelide is **not** recommended for use in accordance with the licensed indications for *Xagrid*®.

ANAGRELIDE

Indications: primary thrombocythaemia in at risk patients who have not responded adequately to other therapy or who are intolerant of it (initiated under specialist supervision)

Cautions: cardiac disease; assess cardiac function before and during treatment; concomitant aspirin in patients with a history of haemorrhage or severely raised platelet count; monitor full blood count (monitor platelet count every 2 days for 1 week, then weekly until maintenance dose established), liver function, serum creatinine and urea; hepatic impairment (Appendix 2); renal impairment (Appendix 3); **interactions:** Appendix 1 (anagrelide)

DRIVING. Dizziness may affect performance of skilled tasks (e.g. driving)

Contra-indications: pregnancy (Appendix 4); breast-feeding (Appendix 5)

Side-effects: gastro-intestinal disturbances; palpitation, tachycardia, fluid retention; headache, dizziness, fatigue; anaemia; rash; *less commonly* pancreatitis, gastro-intestinal haemorrhage, congestive heart failure, hypertension, arrhythmias, syncope, chest pain, dyspnoea, sleep disturbances, paraesthesia, hypoaesthesia, depression, confusion, amnesia, fever, weight changes, impotence, blood disorders, myalgia, arthralgia, epistaxis, dry mouth, alopecia, skin discoloration, and pruritus; *rarely* gastritis, colitis, postural hypotension, myocardial infarction, vasodilatation, pulmonary infiltrates, impaired co-ordination, dysarthria, asthenia, tinnitus, renal failure, nocturia, visual disturbances, and gingival bleeding

Dose: initially 500 micrograms twice daily adjusted according to response in steps of 500 micrograms daily at weekly intervals to max. 10 mg daily (max. single dose 2.5 mg); usual dose range 1–3 mg daily in divided doses

Xagrid® (Shire) ▼ PoM

Capsules, anagrelide (as hydrochloride), 500 micrograms, net price 100-cap pack = £337.14. Counselling, driving, see above

9.1.5 G6PD deficiency

Glucose 6-phosphate dehydrogenase (G6PD) deficiency is highly prevalent in individuals originating from most parts of Africa, from most parts of Asia, from Oceania, and from Southern Europe; it can also occur, rarely, in any other individuals.

Individuals with G6PD deficiency are susceptible to developing acute haemolytic anaemia on taking a number of common drugs. They are also susceptible to developing acute haemolytic anaemia upon ingestion of fava beans (broad beans, *Vicia faba*); this is termed *favism* and can be more severe in children or when the fresh fava beans are eaten raw.

When prescribing drugs for patients with G6PD deficiency, the following three points should be kept in mind:

- G6PD deficiency is genetically heterogeneous; susceptibility to the haemolytic risk from drugs varies; thus, a drug found to be safe in some G6PD-deficient individuals may not be equally safe in others;
- manufacturers do not routinely test drugs for their effects in G6PD-deficient individuals;
- the risk and severity of haemolysis is almost always dose-related.

The lists below should be read with these points in mind. Ideally, information about G6PD deficiency should be available before prescribing a drug listed below. However, in the absence of this information, the possibility of haemolysis should be considered, especially if the patient belongs to a group in which G6PD deficiency is common.

A very few G6PD-deficient individuals with chronic non-spherocytic haemolytic anaemia have haemolysis even in the absence of an exogenous trigger. These patients must be regarded as being at high risk of severe exacerbation of haemolysis following administration of any of the drugs listed below.

Drugs with definite risk of haemolysis in most G6PD-deficient individuals. Dapsone and other sulphones (higher doses for dermatitis herpetiformis more likely to cause problems)
Methylthioninium chloride (methylene blue)
Niridazole [not on UK market]
Nitrofurantoin
Pamaquin [not on UK market]
Primaquine (30 mg weekly for 8 weeks has been found to be without undue harmful effects in African and Asian people, see section 5.4.1)
Quinolones (including ciprofloxacin, moxifloxacin, nalidixic acid, norfloxacin, and ofloxacin)
Sulphonamides (including co-trimoxazole; some sulphonamides, e.g. sulfadiazine, have been tested and found not to be haemolytic in many G6PD-deficient individuals)

Drugs with possible risk of haemolysis in some G6PD-deficient individuals. Aspirin (acceptable up to a dose of at least 1 g daily in most G6PD-deficient individuals)
Chloroquine (acceptable in acute malaria)
Menadione, water-soluble derivatives (e.g. menadiol sodium phosphate)
Probenecid [not on UK market]
Quinidine (acceptable in acute malaria)
Quinine (acceptable in acute malaria)

NOTE. Naphthalene in mothballs also causes haemolysis in individuals with G6PD-deficiency.

9.1.6 Drugs used in neutropenia

Recombinant human granulocyte-colony stimulating factor (rhG-CSF) stimulates the production of neutrophils and may reduce the duration of chemotherapy-induced neutropenia and thereby reduce the incidence of associated sepsis; there is as yet no evidence that it improves overall survival. **Filgrastim** (unglycosylated rhG-CSF) and **lenograstim** (glycosylated rhG-CSF) have similar effects; both have been used in a variety of clinical settings but they do not have any clear-cut routine indications. In congenital neutropenia filgrastim usually elevates the neutrophil count with appropriate clinical response. Prolonged use may be associated with an increased risk of myeloid malignancy. **Pegfilgrastim** is a polyethylene glycol-conjugated ('pegylated') derivative of filgrastim; pegylation increases the duration of filgrastim activity.

Treatment with recombinant human growth factors should only be prescribed by those experienced in their use.

CAUTIONS. Recombinant human growth factors should be used with caution in patients with premalignant or malignant myeloid conditions. Full blood counts including differential white cell and platelet counts should be monitored. Treatment should be withdrawn in patients who develop signs of pulmonary infiltration. Splenic rupture following administration of granulocyte-colony stimulating factors has been reported; monitor spleen size. Recombinant human growth factors are not recommended in pregnancy (Appendix 4) or breast-feeding (Appendix 5).

SIDE-EFFECTS. Side-effects of granulocyte-colony stimulating factors include gastro-intestinal disturbances (including nausea, vomiting, and diarrhoea), anorexia, headache, asthenia, fever, musculoskeletal pain, bone pain, rash, alopecia, injection-site reactions, and leucocytosis. Less frequent side-effects include chest pain, hypersensitivity reactions (including anaphylaxis and bronchospasm) and arthralgia. There have been reports of pulmonary infiltrates leading to acute respiratory distress syndrome.

FILGRASTIM

(Recombinant human granulocyte-colony stimulating factor, G-CSF)

Indications: (specialist use only) reduction in duration of neutropenia and incidence of febrile neutropenia in cytotoxic chemotherapy for malignancy (except chronic myeloid leukaemia and myelodysplastic syndromes); reduction in duration of neutropenia (and associated sequelae) in myeloablative therapy followed by bone-marrow transplantation; mobilisation of peripheral blood progenitor cells for harvesting and subsequent autologous or allogeneic infusion; severe congenital neutropenia, cyclic neutropenia, or idiopathic neutropenia and history of severe or recurrent infections (distinguish carefully from other haematological disorders, consult product literature); persistent neutropenia in advanced HIV infection

Cautions: see notes above; also reduced myeloid precursors; regular morphological and cytogenetic bone-marrow examinations recommended in severe congenital neutropenia (possible risk of myelodysplastic syndromes or leukaemia); secondary acute myeloid leukaemia, sickle-cell disease; monitor spleen size (risk of rupture); osteoporotic bone disease (monitor bone density if given for more than 6 months); **interactions:** Appendix 1 (filgrastim)

Contra-indications: severe congenital neutropenia (Kostman's syndrome) with abnormal cytogenetics

Side-effects: see notes above; also splenic enlargement, hepatomegaly, transient hypotension, epistaxis, urinary abnormalities (including dysuria, proteinuria, and haematuria), osteoporosis, exacerbation of rheumatoid arthritis, cutaneous vasculitis, thrombocytopenia, anaemia, transient decrease in blood glucose, raised uric acid

Dose: cytotoxic-induced neutropenia, preferably *by subcutaneous injection or by intravenous infusion* (over 30 minutes), ADULT and CHILD, 500 000 units/kg daily started not less than 24 hours after cytotoxic chemotherapy, continued until neutrophil count in normal range, usually for up to 14 days (up to 38 days in acute myeloid leukaemia)

Myeloablative therapy followed by bone-marrow transplantation, *by intravenous infusion* over 30 minutes or over 24 hours *or by subcutaneous infusion* over 24 hours, 1 million units/kg daily, started not less than 24 hours following cytotoxic chemotherapy (and within 24 hours of bone-marrow infusion), then adjusted according to absolute neutrophil count (consult product literature)

Mobilisation of peripheral blood progenitor cells for autologous infusion, used alone, *by subcutaneous injection or by subcutaneous infusion* over 24 hours, 1 million units/kg daily for 5-7 days; used following adjunctive myelosuppressive chemotherapy (to improve yield), *by subcutaneous injection*, 500 000 units/kg daily, started the day after completion of chemotherapy and continued until neutrophil count in normal range; for timing of leucopheresis consult product literature

Mobilisation of peripheral blood progenitor cells in normal donors for allogeneic infusion, *by subcutaneous injection*, ADULT under 60 years and ADOLESCENT over 16 years, 1 million units/kg daily for 4–5 days; for timing of leucopheresis consult product literature

Severe chronic neutropenia, *by subcutaneous injection*, ADULT and CHILD, in severe congenital neutropenia, initially 1.2 million units/kg daily in single or divided doses (initially 500 000 units/kg daily in idiopathic or cyclic neutropenia), adjusted according to response (consult product literature)

Persistent neutropenia in HIV infection, *by subcutaneous injection*, initially 100 000 units/kg daily, increased as necessary until absolute neutrophil count in normal range (usual max. 400 000 units/kg daily), then adjusted to maintain absolute neutrophil count in normal range (consult product literature)

Neupogen® (Amgen) PoM

Injection, filgrastim 30 million-units (300 micrograms)/mL, net price 1-mL vial = £68.41

Injection (Singleject®), filgrastim 60 million-units (600 micrograms)/mL, net price 0.5-mL prefilled syringe = £68.41; 96 million-units (960 micrograms)/mL, 0.5-mL prefilled syringe = £109.11

LENOGRASTIM

(Recombinant human granulocyte-colony stimulating factor, rHuG-CSF)

Indications: (specialist use only) reduction in the duration of neutropenia and associated complications following bone-marrow transplantation for non-myeloid malignancy or following treatment with cytotoxic chemotherapy associated with a significant incidence of febrile neutropenia; mobilisation of peripheral blood progenitor cells for harvesting and subsequent infusion

Cautions: see notes above; also pre-malignant myeloid conditions; reduced myeloid precursors; sickle cell disease; monitor spleen size (risk of rupture)

Side-effects: see notes above; also splenic rupture, cutaneous vasculitis, Sweet's syndrome, toxic epidermal necrolysis

Dose: following bone-marrow transplantation, *by intravenous infusion*, ADULT and CHILD over 2 years 19.2 million units/m^2 daily started the day after transplantation, continued until neutrophil count stable in acceptable range (max. 28 days)

Cytotoxic-induced neutropenia, *by subcutaneous injection*, ADULT 19.2 million units/m^2 daily started the day after completion of chemotherapy, continued until neutrophil count stable in acceptable range (max. 28 days)

Mobilisation of peripheral blood progenitor cells, used alone, *by subcutaneous injection*, ADULT 1.28 million units/kg daily for 4–6 days (5–6 days in healthy donors); used following adjunctive myelosuppressive chemotherapy (to improve yield), *by subcutaneous injection*, 19.2 million-units/m^2 daily, started the day after completion of chemotherapy and continued until neutrophil count in acceptable range; for timing of leucopheresis consult product literature

Granocyte® (Chugai) PoM
Injection, powder for reconstitution, lenograstim, net price 13.4 million-unit (105-microgram) vial = £42.00; 33.6 million-unit (263-microgram) vial = £67.95 (both with 1-mL prefilled syringe water for injections)

PEGFILGRASTIM

(Pegylated recombinant methionyl human granulocyte-colony stimulating factor)

Indications: (specialist use only) reduction in duration of neutropenia and incidence of febrile neutropenia in cytotoxic chemotherapy for malignancy (except chronic myeloid leukaemia and myelodysplastic syndromes)

Cautions: see notes above; also acute leukaemia and myelosuppressive chemotherapy; sickle-cell disease; monitor spleen size (risk of rupture); **interactions:** Appendix 1 (filgrastim)

Side-effects: see notes above

Dose: (expressed as filgrastim) *by subcutaneous injection*, ADULT over 18 years, 6 mg (0.6 mL) for each chemotherapy cycle, starting 24 hours after chemotherapy

Neulasta® (Amgen) ▼ PoM
Injection, pegfilgrastim (expressed as filgrastim) 10 mg/mL, net price 0.6-mL (6-mg) prefilled syringe = £714.24

9.2 Fluids and electrolytes

The following tables give a selection of useful electrolyte values :

Electrolyte concentrations —intravenous fluids

Intravenous infusion	Millimoles per litre				
	Na^+	K^+	HCO_3^-	Cl^-	Ca^{2+}
Normal plasma values	142	4.5	26	103	2.5
Sodium Chloride 0.9%	150	—	—	150	—
Compound Sodium Lactate (Hartmann's)	131	5	29	111	2
Sodium Chloride 0.18% and Glucose 4%	30	—	—	30	—
Potassium Chloride 0.3% and Glucose 5%	—	40	—	40	—
Potassium Chloride 0.3% and Sodium Chloride 0.9%	150	40	—	190	—
To correct metabolic acidosis					
Sodium Bicarbonate 1.26%	150	—	150	—	—
Sodium Bicarbonate 8.4% for cardiac arrest	1000	—	1000	—	—
Sodium Lactate (m/6)	167	—	167	—	—

Electrolyte content —gastro-intestinal secretions

Type of fluid	Millimoles per litre				
	H^+	Na^+	K^+	HCO_3^-	Cl^-
Gastric	40–60	20–80	5–20	—	100–150
Biliary	—	120–140	5–15	30–50	80–120
Pancreatic	—	120–140	5–15	70–110	40–80
Small bowel	—	120–140	5–15	20–40	90–130

Faeces, vomit, or aspiration should be saved and analysed where possible if abnormal losses are suspected; where this is impracticable the approximations above may be helpful in planning replacement therapy

9.2.1 Oral preparations for fluid and electrolyte imbalance

Sodium and potassium salts, which may be given by mouth to prevent deficiencies or to treat established deficiencies of mild or moderate degree, are discussed in this section. Oral preparations for removing excess potassium and preparations for oral rehydration therapy are also included here. Oral bicarbonate, for metabolic acidosis, is also described in this section.

For reference to calcium, magnesium, and phosphate, see section 9.5.

9.2.1.1 Oral potassium

Compensation for potassium loss is especially necessary:

- in those taking digoxin or anti-arrhythmic drugs, where potassium depletion may induce arrhythmias;
- in patients in whom secondary hyperaldosteronism occurs, e.g. renal artery stenosis, cirrhosis of the liver, the nephrotic syndrome, and severe heart failure;
- in patients with excessive losses of potassium in the faeces, e.g. chronic diarrhoea associated with intestinal malabsorption or laxative abuse.

Measures to compensate for potassium loss may also be required in the elderly since they frequently take inadequate amounts of potassium in the diet (but see below for **warning** on **renal insufficiency**). Measures may also be required during long-term administration of drugs known to induce potassium loss (e.g. corticosteroids). Potassium supplements are **seldom required** with the small doses of diuretics given to treat hypertension; **potassium-sparing diuretics** (rather than potassium supplements) are recommended for prevention of hypokalaemia due to diuretics such as furosemide (frusemide) or the thiazides when these are given to eliminate oedema.

DOSAGE. If potassium salts are used for the *prevention of hypokalaemia*, then doses of potassium chloride 2 to 4 g (approx. 25 to 50 mmol) daily by mouth are suitable in patients taking a normal diet. *Smaller doses* must be used if there is *renal insufficiency (common in the elderly)* otherwise there is **danger of hyperkalaemia**. Potassium salts cause nausea and vomiting therefore poor compliance is a major limitation to their effectiveness; where appropriate, potassium-sparing diuretics are preferable (see also above). When there is *established potassium depletion* larger doses may be necessary, the quantity depending on the severity of any continuing potassium loss (monitoring of plasma-potassium concentration and specialist advice would be required). Potassium depletion is frequently associated with chloride depletion and with metabolic alkalosis, and these disorders require correction.

ADMINISTRATION. Potassium salts are preferably given as a liquid (or effervescent) preparation, rather than modified-release tablets; they should be given as the chloride (the use of effervescent potassium tablets BPC 1968 should be restricted to *hyperchloraemic states*, section 9.2.1.3).

Salt substitutes. A number of salt substitutes which contain significant amounts of potassium chloride are readily available as health food products (e.g. *LoSalt*® and *Ruthmol*®). These should not be used by patients with renal failure as potassium intoxication may result.

POTASSIUM CHLORIDE

Indications: potassium depletion (see notes above)

Cautions: elderly, mild to moderate renal impairment (close monitoring required), intestinal stricture, history of peptic ulcer, hiatus hernia (for sustained-release preparations); **important:** special hazard if given with drugs liable to raise plasma potassium concentration such as potassium-sparing diuretics, ACE inhibitors, or ciclosporin, for other **interactions:** Appendix 1 (potassium salts)

Contra-indications: severe renal impairment, plasma potassium concentrations above 5 mmol/litre

Side-effects: nausea and vomiting (severe symptoms may indicate obstruction), oesophageal or small bowel ulceration

Dose: see notes above

NOTE. Do not confuse Effervescent Potassium Tablets BPC 1968 (section 9.2.1.3) with effervescent potassium chloride tablets. Effervescent Potassium Tablets BPC 1968 do not contain chloride ions and their use should be restricted to hyperchloraemic states (section 9.2.1.3). Effervescent Potassium Chloride Tablets BP are usually available in two strengths, one containing 6.7 mmol each of K^+ and Cl^- (corresponding to *Kloref*®), the other containing 12 mmol K^+ and 8 mmol Cl^- (corresponding to *Sando-K*®). Generic prescriptions must specify the strength required.

Kay-Cee-L® (Geistlich)
Syrup, red, sugar-free, potassium chloride 7.5% (1 mmol/mL each of K^+ and Cl^-). Net price 500 mL = £3.74. Label: 21

Kloref® (Alpharma)
Tablets, effervescent, betaine hydrochloride, potassium benzoate, bicarbonate, and chloride, equivalent to potassium chloride 500 mg (6.7 mmol each of K^+ and Cl^-). Net price 50 = £2.71. Label: 13, 21
NOTE. May be difficult to obtain

Sando-K® (HK Pharma)
Tablets, effervescent, potassium bicarbonate and chloride equivalent to potassium 470 mg (12 mmol of K^+) and chloride 285 mg (8 mmol of Cl^-). Net price 20 = £1.53. Label: 13, 21

■ Modified-release preparations
Avoid unless effervescent tablets or liquid preparations inappropriate

Slow-K® (Alliance) ▬
Tablets, m/r, orange, s/c, potassium chloride 600 mg (8 mmol each of K^+ and Cl^-). Net price 20 = 54p. Label: 25, 27, counselling, swallow whole with fluid during meals while sitting or standing

Potassium removal

Ion-exchange resins may be used to remove excess potassium in *mild hyperkalaemia* or in *moderate hyperkalaemia* when there are no ECG changes; intravenous therapy is required in emergencies (section 9.2.2).

POLYSTYRENE SULPHONATE RESINS

Indications: hyperkalaemia associated with anuria or severe oliguria, and in dialysis patients

Cautions: children (impaction of resin with excessive dosage or inadequate dilution); monitor for electrolyte disturbances (stop if plasma-potassium concentration below 5 mmol/litre); pregnancy and breast-feeding; sodium-containing resin in congestive heart failure, hypertension, renal impairment, and oedema; **interactions:** Appendix 1 (sodium polystyrene sulphonate)

Contra-indications: obstructive bowel disease; oral administration or reduced gut motility in neonates; avoid calcium-containing resin in hyperparathyroidism, multiple myeloma, sarcoidosis, or metastatic carcinoma

Side-effects: rectal ulceration following rectal administration; colonic necrosis reported following enemas containing sorbitol; sodium retention, hypercalcaemia, gastric irritation, anorexia, nausea and vomiting, constipation (discontinue treatment—avoid magnesium-containing laxatives), diarrhoea; calcium-containing resin may cause hypercalcaemia (in dialysed patients and occasionally in those with renal impairment), hypomagnesaemia

Dose: *by mouth*, 15 g 3–4 times daily in water (not fruit squash which has a high potassium content) or as a paste; CHILD 0.5–1 g/kg daily in divided doses
By rectum, as an enema, 30 g in methylcellulose solution, retained for 9 hours followed by irrigation to remove resin from colon; NEONATE and CHILD, 0.5–1 g/kg daily

Calcium Resonium® (Sanofi-Synthelabo)
Powder, buff, calcium polystyrene sulphonate. Net price 300 g = £47.55. Label: 13

Resonium A® (Sanofi-Synthelabo)
Powder, buff, sodium polystyrene sulphonate. Net price 454 g = £58.53. Label: 13

9.2.1.2 Oral sodium and water

Sodium chloride is indicated in states of sodium depletion and usually needs to be given intravenously (section 9.2.2). In chronic conditions associated with mild or moderate degrees of sodium depletion, e.g. in salt-losing bowel or renal disease, oral supplements of sodium chloride or sodium bicarbonate (section 9.2.1.3), according to the acid-base status of the patient, may be sufficient.

SODIUM CHLORIDE

Indications: sodium depletion; see also section 9.2.2

Slow Sodium® (HK Pharma)
Tablets, m/r, sodium chloride 600 mg (approx. 10 mmol each of Na^+ and Cl^-). Net price 100-tab pack = £6.05. Label: 25
Dose: prophylaxis of sodium chloride deficiency 4–8 tablets daily with water (in severe depletion up to max. 20 tablets daily)
Chronic renal salt wasting, up to 20 tablets daily with appropriate fluid intake
CHILD, according to requirements

Oral rehydration therapy (ORT)

As a worldwide problem *diarrhoea* is by far the most important indication for fluid and electrolyte replacement. Intestinal absorption of sodium and water is enhanced by glucose (and other carbohydrates). Replacement of fluid and electrolytes lost through diarrhoea can therefore be achieved by giving solutions containing sodium, potassium, and glucose or another carbohydrate such as rice starch.

Oral rehydration solutions should:

- enhance the absorption of water and electrolytes;
- replace the electrolyte deficit adequately and safely;
- contain an alkalinising agent to counter acidosis;
- be slightly hypo-osmolar (about 250 mmol/litre) to prevent the possible induction of osmotic diarrhoea;
- be simple to use in hospital and at home;
- be palatable and acceptable, especially to children;
- be readily available.

It is the policy of the World Health Organization (WHO) to promote a single oral rehydration solution but to use it flexibly (e.g. by giving extra water between drinks of oral rehydration solution to moderately dehydrated infants).

Oral rehydration solutions used in the UK are lower in sodium (50–60 mmol/litre) than the WHO formulation since, in general, patients suffer less severe sodium loss.

Rehydration should be rapid over 3 to 4 hours (except in hypernatraemic dehydration in which case rehydration should occur more slowly over 12 hours). The patient should be reassessed after initial rehydration and if still dehydrated rapid fluid replacement should continue.

Once rehydration is complete further dehydration is prevented by encouraging the patient to drink normal volumes of an appropriate fluid and by replacing continuing losses with an oral rehydration solution; in infants, breast-feeding or formula feeds should be offered between oral rehydration drinks.

For intravenous rehydration see section 9.2.2.

ORAL REHYDRATION SALTS (ORS)

Indications: fluid and electrolyte loss in diarrhoea, see notes above

Dose: according to fluid loss, usually 200–400 mL solution after every loose motion; INFANT 1–1½ times usual feed volume; CHILD 200 mL after every loose motion

■ UK formulations

NOTE. After reconstitution any unused solution should be discarded no later than 1 hour after preparation unless stored in a refrigerator when it may be kept for up to 24 hours.
Proprietary brands of oral rehydration salts on sale to the public include *Boots Oral Rehydration Treatment*.

Dioralyte® (Rhône-Poulenc Rorer)
Effervescent tablets, sodium chloride 117 mg, sodium bicarbonate 336 mg, potassium chloride 186 mg, citric acid anhydrous 384 mg, anhydrous glucose 1.62 g. Net price 10-tab pack (blackcurrant- or citrus-flavoured) = £1.42
Dose: reconstitute 2 tablets with 200 mL of water (only for adults and for children over 1 year)
NOTE. Ten tablets when reconstituted with 1 litre of water provide Na^+ 60 mmol, K^+ 25 mmol, Cl^- 45 mmol, citrate 20 mmol, and glucose 90 mmol
Oral powder, sodium chloride 470 mg, potassium chloride 300 mg, disodium hydrogen citrate 530 mg, glucose 3.56 g/sachet, net price 6-sachet pack = £2.02, 20-sachet pack (blackcurrant- or citrus-flavoured or natural) = £6.19
Dose: reconstitute one sachet with 200 mL of water (freshly boiled and cooled for infants)
NOTE. Five sachets reconstituted with 1 litre of water provide Na^+ 60 mmol, K^+ 20 mmol, Cl^- 60 mmol, citrate 10 mmol, and glucose 90 mmol

Dioralyte® **Relief** (Rhône-Poulenc Rorer)
Oral powder, sodium chloride 350 mg, potassium chloride 300 mg, sodium citrate 580 mg, cooked rice powder 6 g/sachet, net price 6-sachet pack (apricot-, blackcurrant- or raspberry-flavoured) = £2.26, 20-sachet pack (apricot-flavoured) = £7.42
Dose: reconstitute one sachet with 200 mL of water (freshly boiled and cooled for infants)
NOTE. 5 sachets when reconstitued with 1 litre of water provide Na^+ 60 mmol, K^+ 20 mmol, Cl^- 50 mmol and citrate 10 mmol; contains aspartame (section 9.4.1)

Electrolade® (Baxter)
Oral powder, sodium chloride 236 mg, potassium chloride 300 mg, sodium bicarbonate 500 mg, anhydrous glucose 4 g/sachet (banana-, blackcurrant-, melon-, or orange-flavoured). Net price 6-sachet (plain or multiflavoured) pack = £1.33, 20-sachet (single- or multiflavoured) pack = £4.99
Dose: reconstitute one sachet with 200 mL of water (freshly boiled and cooled for infants)
NOTE. Five sachets when reconstituted with 1 litre of water provide Na^+ 50 mmol, K^+ 20 mmol, Cl^- 40 mmol, HCO_3^- 30 mmol, and glucose 111 mmol

Rapolyte® (Provalis)
Oral powder, sodium chloride 350 mg, potassium chloride 300 mg, sodium citrate 600 mg, anhydrous glucose 4 g, net price 20-sachet pack (blackcurrant-, natural-, raspberry-, or tutti-frutti-flavoured) = £4.60
Dose: reconstitute one sachet with 200 mL of water (freshly boiled and cooled for infants)
NOTE. Five sachets when reconstituted with 1 litre of water provide Na^+ 60 mmol, K^+ 20 mmol, Cl^- 50 mmol, citrate 10 mmol, and glucose 110 mmol

■ WHO formulation

Oral Rehydration Salts (Non-proprietary)
Oral powder, sodium chloride 2.6 g, potassium chloride 1.5 g, sodium citrate 2.9 g, anhydrous glucose 13.5 g. To be dissolved in sufficient water to produce 1 litre (providing Na^+ 75 mmol, K^+

20 mmol, Cl^- 65 mmol, citrate 10 mmol, glucose 75 mmol/litre)

NOTE. Recommended by the WHO and the United Nations Children's Fund but not commonly used in the UK.

9.2.1.3 Oral bicarbonate

Sodium bicarbonate is given by mouth for *chronic acidotic states* such as uraemic acidosis or renal tubular acidosis. The dose for correction of metabolic acidosis is not predictable and the response must be assessed; sodium bicarbonate 4.8 g daily (57 mmol each of Na^+ and HCO_3^-) or more may be required. For severe metabolic acidosis, sodium bicarbonate can be given intravenously (section 9.2.2).

Sodium bicarbonate may also be used to increase the pH of the urine (see section 7.4.3); for use in dyspepsia see section 1.1.1.

Sodium supplements may increase blood pressure or cause fluid retention and pulmonary oedema in those at risk; hypokalaemia may be exacerbated.

Where *hyperchloraemic acidosis* is associated with potassium deficiency, as in some renal tubular and gastro-intestinal disorders it may be appropriate to give oral **potassium bicarbonate**, although acute or severe deficiency should be managed by intravenous therapy.

SODIUM BICARBONATE

Indications: see notes above

Cautions: see notes above; avoid in respiratory acidosis; **interactions:** Appendix 1 (antacids)

Dose: see notes above

Sodium Bicarbonate (Non-proprietary)

Capsules, sodium bicarbonate 500 mg (approx. 6 mmol each of Na^+ and HCO_3^-). Net price 20 = £6.61

Tablets, sodium bicarbonate 600 mg, net price 100 = £2.48

IMPORTANT. Oral solutions of sodium bicarbonate are required occasionally; these need to be obtained on special order and the strength of sodium bicarbonate should be stated on the prescription

POTASSIUM BICARBONATE

Indications: see notes above

Cautions: cardiac disease, renal impairment (Appendix 3); **interactions:** Appendix 1 (potassium salts)

Contra-indications: hypochloraemia; plasma potassium concentration above 5 mmol/litre

Side-effects: nausea and vomiting

Dose: see notes above

Potassium Tablets, Effervescent (Non-proprietary)

Effervescent tablets, potassium bicarbonate 500 mg, potassium acid tartrate 300 mg, each tablet providing 6.5 mmol of K^+. To be dissolved in water before administration. Net price 56 = £4.20. Label: 13, 21

NOTE. These tablets do not contain chloride; for effervescent tablets containing potassium and chloride, see under Potassium Chloride, section 9.2.1.1

9.2.2 Parenteral preparations for fluid and electrolyte imbalance

9.2.2.1 Electrolytes and water

Solutions of electrolytes are given intravenously, to meet normal fluid and electrolyte requirements or to replenish substantial deficits or continuing losses, when the patient is nauseated or vomiting and is unable to take adequate amounts by mouth. When intravenous administration is not possible large volumes of fluid can also be given subcutaneously by hypodermoclysis.

In an individual patient the nature and severity of the electrolyte imbalance must be assessed from the history and clinical and biochemical examination. Sodium, potassium, chloride, magnesium, phosphate, and water depletion can occur singly and in combination with or without disturbances of acid-base balance; for reference to the use of magnesium and phosphates, see section 9.5.

Isotonic solutions may be infused safely into a peripheral vein. Solutions more concentrated than plasma, e.g. 20% glucose, are best given through an indwelling catheter positioned in a large vein.

Intravenous sodium

Sodium chloride in isotonic solution provides the most important extracellular ions in near physiological concentration and is indicated in *sodium depletion* which may arise from such conditions as gastro-enteritis, diabetic ketoacidosis, ileus, and ascites. In a severe deficit of from 4 to 8 litres, 2 to 3 litres of isotonic sodium chloride may be given over 2 to 3 hours; thereafter infusion can usually be at a slower rate. Excessive administration should be avoided; the jugular venous pressure should be assessed, the bases of the lungs should be examined for crepitations, and in elderly or seriously ill patients it is often helpful to monitor the right atrial (central) venous pressure.

Chronic hyponatraemia should ideally be corrected by fluid restriction. However, if sodium chloride is required, the deficit should be corrected slowly to avoid the risk of osmotic demyelination syndrome; the rise in plasma-sodium concentration should be no more than 10 mmol/litre in 24 hours. In severe hyponatraemia, sodium chloride 1.8% may be used cautiously.

Compound sodium lactate (Hartmann's solution) can be used instead of isotonic sodium chloride solution during surgery or in the initial management of the injured or wounded.

Sodium chloride and glucose solutions are indicated when there is combined *water and sodium depletion*. A 1:1 mixture of isotonic sodium chloride and 5% glucose allows some of the water (free of sodium) to enter body cells which suffer most from dehydration while the sodium salt with a volume of water determined by the normal plasma Na^+ remains extracellular. Maintenance fluid should accurately reflect daily requirements and close monitoring is required to avoid fluid and electrolyte imbalance. Illness or injury increase the secretion of anti-diuretic hormone and therefore the ability to excrete excess water may be impaired. Injudicious use of solutions such as sodium chloride 0.18% and glucose 4% may also cause dilutional hyponatraemia especially in children and the elderly; if necessary, guidance should be sought from a clinician experienced in the management of fluid and electrolytes.

Combined sodium, potassium, chloride, and water depletion may occur, for example, with severe diarrhoea or persistent vomiting; replacement is carried out with sodium chloride intravenous infusion 0.9% and glucose intravenous infusion 5% with potassium as appropriate.

SODIUM CHLORIDE

Indications: electrolyte imbalance, also section 9.2.1.2

Cautions: restrict intake in impaired renal function, cardiac failure, hypertension, peripheral and pulmonary oedema, toxaemia of pregnancy

Side-effects: administration of large doses may give rise to sodium accumulation, oedema, and hyperchloraemic acidosis

Dose: see notes above

Sodium Chloride Intravenous Infusion (Non-proprietary) PoM

Intravenous infusion, usual strength sodium chloride 0.9% (9 g, 150 mmol each of Na^+ and Cl^-/litre), this strength being supplied when normal saline for injection is requested. Net price 2-mL amp = 24p; 5-mL amp = 33p; 10-mL amp = 36p; 20-mL amp = £1.04; 50-mL amp = £2.01

In hospitals, 500- and 1000-mL packs, and sometimes other sizes, are available

NOTE. The term 'normal saline' should **not** be used to describe sodium chloride intravenous infusion 0.9%; the term 'physiological saline' is acceptable but it is preferable to give the composition (i.e. sodium chloride intravenous infusion 0.9%).

■ With other ingredients

Sodium Chloride and Glucose Intravenous Infusion (Non-proprietary) PoM

Intravenous infusion, sodium chloride 0.18% (Na^+ and Cl^- each 30 mmol/litre), glucose 4%

In hospitals, usually 500-mL packs and sometimes other sizes are available

Intravenous infusion, sodium chloride 0.9% (Na^+ and Cl^- each 150 mmol/litre), glucose 5%

In hospitals, usually 500-mL packs and sometimes other sizes are available

Intravenous infusion, sodium chloride 0.45% (Na^+ and Cl^- each 75 mmol/litre), glucose 2.5%

In hospitals, usually 500-mL packs and sometimes other sizes are available

NOTE. See above for warning on hyponatraemia especially in children and elderly

Ringer's Solution for Injection PoM

Calcium chloride (dihydrate) 322 micrograms, potassium chloride 300 micrograms, sodium chloride 8.6 mg/mL, providing the following ions (in mmol/litre), Ca^{2+} 2.2, K^+ 4, Na^+ 147, Cl^- 156

In hospitals, 500- and 1000-mL packs, and sometimes other sizes, are available

Sodium Lactate Intravenous Infusion, Compound (Non-proprietary) PoM

(Hartmann's Solution for Injection; Ringer-Lactate Solution for Injection)

Intravenous infusion, sodium chloride 0.6%, sodium lactate 0.25%, potassium chloride 0.04%, calcium chloride 0.027% (containing Na^+ 131 mmol, K^+ 5 mmol, Ca^{2+} 2 mmol, HCO_3^- (as lactate) 29 mmol, Cl^- 111 mmol/litre)

In hospitals, 500- and 1000-mL packs, and sometimes other sizes, are available

Intravenous glucose

Glucose solutions (5%) are mainly used to replace water deficits and should be given alone when there is no significant loss of electrolytes. Average water requirements in a healthy adult are 1.5 to 2.5 litres daily and this is needed to balance unavoidable losses of water through the skin and lungs and to provide sufficient for urinary excretion. Water depletion (dehydration) tends to occur when these losses are not matched by a comparable intake, as may occur in coma or dysphagia or in the elderly or apathetic who may not drink enough water on their own initiative.

Excessive loss of water without loss of electrolytes is uncommon, occurring in fevers, hyperthyroidism, and in uncommon water-losing renal states such as diabetes insipidus or hypercalcaemia. The volume of glucose solution needed to replace deficits varies with the severity of the disorder, but usually lies within the range of 2 to 6 litres.

Glucose solutions are also given in regimens with calcium, bicarbonate, and insulin for the emergency management of *hyperkalaemia*. They are also given, after correction of hyperglycaemia, during treatment of diabetic ketoacidosis, when they must be accompanied by continuing insulin infusion.

GLUCOSE

(Dextrose Monohydrate)

NOTE. Glucose BP is the monohydrate but Glucose Intravenous Infusion BP is a sterile solution of anhydrous glucose or glucose monohydrate, potency being expressed in terms of anhydrous glucose

Indications: fluid replacement (see notes above), provision of energy (section 9.3)

Side-effects: glucose injections especially if hypertonic may have a low pH and may cause venous irritation and thrombophlebitis

Dose: water replacement, see notes above; energy source, 1–3 litres daily of 20–50% solution

Glucose Intravenous Infusion (Non-proprietary) PoM

Intravenous infusion, glucose or anhydrous glucose (potency expressed in terms of anhydrous glucose), usual strength 5% (50 mg/mL). 25% solution, net price 25-mL amp = £2.21; 50% solution, 25-mL amp = £3.80, 50-mL amp = £1.63

In hospitals, 500- and 1000-mL packs, and sometimes other sizes and strengths, are available; also available as *Min-I-Jet® Glucose*, 50% in 50-mL disposable syringe

Intravenous potassium

Potassium chloride and sodium chloride intravenous infusion is the initial treatment for the correction of *severe hypokalaemia* and when sufficient potassium cannot be taken by mouth. Ready-mixed infusion solutions should be used when possible; alternatively, potassium chloride concentrate, as ampoules containing 1.5 g (K^+ 20 mmol) in 10 mL, is **thoroughly mixed** with 500 mL of sodium chloride 0.9% intravenous infusion and given slowly over 2 to 3 hours, with specialist advice and ECG monitoring in difficult cases. Higher concentrations of potassium chloride may be given in very severe depletion, but require specialist advice.

Repeated measurements of plasma-potassium concentration are necessary to determine whether further infusions are required and to avoid the development of hyperkalaemia, which is especially likely in renal impairment.

Initial potassium replacement therapy should **not** involve glucose infusions, because glucose may cause a further decrease in the plasma-potassium concentration.

POTASSIUM CHLORIDE

Indications: electrolyte imbalance; see also oral potassium supplements, section 9.2.1.1

Cautions: for intravenous infusion the concentration of solution should not usually exceed 3.2 g (43 mmol)/litre; specialist advice and ECG monitoring (see notes above); **interactions:** Appendix 1 (potassium salts)

Side-effects: rapid infusion toxic to heart

Dose: *by slow intravenous infusion*, depending on the deficit or the daily maintenance requirements, see also notes above

Potassium Chloride and Glucose Intravenous Infusion (Non-proprietary) PoM
Intravenous infusion, usual strength potassium chloride 0.3% (3 g, 40 mmol each of K^+ and Cl^-/litre) with 5% of anhydrous glucose
In hospitals, 500- and 1000-mL packs, and sometimes other sizes, are available

Potassium Chloride and Sodium Chloride Intravenous Infusion (Non-proprietary) PoM
Intravenous infusion, usual strength potassium chloride 0.3% (3 g/litre) and sodium chloride 0.9% (9 g/litre), containing K^+ 40 mmol, Na^+ 150 mmol, and Cl^- 190 mmol/litre
In hospitals, 500- and 1000-mL packs, and sometimes other sizes, are available

Potassium Chloride, Sodium Chloride, and Glucose Intravenous Infusion (Non-proprietary) PoM
Intravenous infusion, sodium chloride 0.18% (1.8 g, Na^+ 30 mmol/litre) with 4% of anhydrous glucose and usually sufficient potassium chloride to provide K^+ 10–40 mmol/litre (to be specified by the prescriber)
In hospitals, 500- and 1000-mL packs, and sometimes other sizes, are available

Potassium Chloride Concentrate, Sterile (Non-proprietary) PoM
Sterile concentrate, potassium chloride 15% (150 mg, approximately 2 mmol each of K^+ and Cl^-/mL). Net price 10-mL amp = 48p
IMPORTANT. Must be diluted with **not less** than 50 times its volume of sodium chloride intravenous infusion 0.9% or other suitable diluent and **mixed well**
Solutions containing 10 and 20% of potassium chloride are also available in both 5- and 10-mL ampoules

Bicarbonate and lactate

Sodium bicarbonate is used to control severe *metabolic acidosis* (as in renal failure). Since this condition is usually attended by sodium depletion, it is reasonable to correct this first by the administration of isotonic sodium chloride intravenous infusion, provided the kidneys are not primarily affected and the degree of acidosis is not so severe as to impair renal function. In these circumstances, isotonic sodium chloride alone is usually effective as it restores the ability of the kidneys to generate bicarbonate. In renal acidosis or in severe metabolic acidosis of any origin (for example, blood pH < 7.1) sodium bicarbonate (1.26%) may be infused with isotonic sodium chloride when the acidosis remains unresponsive to correction of anoxia or fluid depletion; a total volume of up to 6 litres (4 litres of sodium chloride and 2 litres of sodium bicarbonate) may be necessary in the adult. In severe shock due for example to cardiac arrest (see section 2.7), metabolic acidosis may develop without sodium depletion; in these circumstances sodium bicarbonate is best given in a small volume of hypertonic solution, such as 50 mL of 8.4% solution intravenously; plasma pH should be monitored.

Sodium bicarbonate infusion is also used in the emergency management of *hyperkalaemia* (see also under Glucose).

Sodium lactate intravenous infusion is obsolete in metabolic acidosis, and carries the risk of producing lactic acidosis, particularly in seriously ill patients with poor tissue perfusion or impaired hepatic function.

SODIUM BICARBONATE

Indications: metabolic acidosis

Dose: *by slow intravenous injection*, a strong solution (up to 8.4%), or *by continuous intravenous infusion*, a weaker solution (usually 1.26%), an amount appropriate to the body base deficit (see notes above)

Sodium Bicarbonate Intravenous Infusion PoM
Usual strength sodium bicarbonate 1.26% (12.6 g, 150 mmol each of Na^+ and HCO_3^-/litre); various other strengths available
In hospitals, 500- and 1000-mL packs, and sometimes other sizes, are available

Min-I-Jet® Sodium Bicarbonate (Celltech) PoM
Intravenous injection, sodium bicarbonate in disposable syringe, net price 4.2%, 10 mL = £5.29; 8.4%, 10 mL = £5.71, 50 mL = £7.75

SODIUM LACTATE 

Indications: see notes above

Sodium Lactate (Non-proprietary) PoM
Intravenous infusion, sodium lactate M/6, contains the following ions (in mmol/litre), Na^+ 167, HCO_3^- (as lactate) 167

Water

Water for Injections PoM
Net price 1-mL amp = 18p; 2-mL amp = 17p; 5-mL amp = 28p; 10-mL amp = 31p; 20-mL amp = 55p; 50-mL amp = £1.91; 100-mL vial = 23p

9.2.2.2 Plasma and plasma substitutes

Albumin solutions, prepared from whole blood, contain soluble proteins and electrolytes but no clotting factors, blood group antibodies, or plasma cholinesterases; they may be given without regard to the recipient's blood group.

Albumin should usually be used after the acute phase of illness, to correct a plasma-volume deficit in patients with salt and water retention and oedema; hypoalbuminaemia itself is not an appropriate indication. The use of albumin solutions in acute plasma or blood loss may be wasteful; plasma substitutes are more appropriate. Concentrated albumin solutions may also be used to obtain a diuresis in hypoalbuminaemic patients (e.g. in hepatic cirrhosis).

Recent evidence does not support the previous view that the use of albumin increases mortality.

> Plasma and plasma substitutes are often used in very ill patients whose condition is unstable. Therefore, close monitoring is required and fluid and electrolyte therapy should be adjusted according to the patient's condition at all times.

ALBUMIN SOLUTION

(Human Albumin Solution)

A solution containing protein derived from plasma, serum, or normal placentas; at least 95% of the protein is albumin. The solution may be isotonic (containing 4–5% protein) or concentrated (containing 15–25% protein).

Indications: see under preparations, and also notes above

Cautions: history of cardiac or circulatory disease (administer slowly to avoid rapid rise in blood pressure and cardiac failure, and monitor cardiovascular and respiratory function); increased capillary permeability; correct dehydration when administering concentrated solution

Contra-indications: cardiac failure; severe anaemia

Side-effects: hypersensitivity reactions (including anaphylaxis) with nausea, vomiting, increased salivation, fever, tachycardia, hypotension and chills reported

■ Isotonic solutions

Indications: acute or sub-acute loss of plasma volume e.g. in burns, pancreatitis, trauma, and complications of surgery; plasma exchange

Available as: *Human Albumin Solution 4.5%* (50-, 100-, 250- and 400-mL bottles—Baxter Bioscience); *Human Albumin Solution 5%* (100-, 250- and 500-mL bottles—Grifols); *ALBA® 4.5%* (100- and 400-mL bottles—SNBTS); *Albutein® 5%* (250- and 500-mL bottles—Grifols); *Octalbin® 5%* (100- and 200-mL bottles—Octapharm); *Zenalb® 4.5%* (50-, 100-, 250-, and 500-mL bottles—BPL)

■ Concentrated solutions (20–25%)

Indications: severe hypoalbuminaemia associated with low plasma volume and generalised oedema where salt and water restriction with plasma volume expansion are required; adjunct in the treatment of hyperbilirubinaemia by exchange transfusion in the newborn; paracentesis of large volume ascites associated with portal hypertension

Available as: *Human Albumin Solution 20%* (50- and 100-mL vials—Baxter Bioscience); *Human Albumin Solution 20%* (50- and 100-mL bottles—Grifols); *ALBA® 20%* (50-mL vials—SNBTS); *Albutein® 20%* (50- and 100-mL bottles—Grifols); *Albutein® 25%* (20-, 50-, and 100-mL vials—Grifols); *Octalbin® 20%* (50- and 100-mL bottles—Octapharm); *Zenalb® 20%* (50- and 100-mL bottles—BPL)

Plasma substitutes

Dextrans, **gelatin**, and the etherified starches, **hexastarch**, **hydroxyethyl starch** and **pentastarch** are macromolecular substances which are metabolised slowly; they may be used at the outset to expand and maintain blood volume in shock arising from conditions such as burns or septicaemia. Plasma substitutes may be used as an immediate short-term measure to treat haemorrhage until blood is available. They are rarely needed when shock is due to sodium and water depletion because, in these circumstances, the shock responds to water and electrolyte repletion. See also section 2.7.1 for the management of shock.

Plasma substitutes should **not** be used to maintain plasma volume in conditions such as burns or peritonitis where there is loss of plasma protein, water and electrolytes over periods of several days or weeks. In these situations, plasma or plasma protein fractions containing large amounts of albumin should be given.

Large volumes of *some* plasma substitutes can increase the risk of bleeding through depletion of coagulation factors; however, the risk is reduced if 1–2 litres of a substitute such as hexastarch is used.

Dextran 70 by intravenous infusion is used predominantly for volume expansion. Dextran 40 intravenous infusion is used in an attempt to improve peripheral blood flow in ischaemic disease of the limbs. Dextrans 40 and 70 have also been used in the prophylaxis of thromboembolism but are now rarely used for this purpose.

Dextrans may interfere with blood group cross-matching or biochemical measurements and these should be carried out before infusion is begun.

> Plasma and plasma substitutes are often used in very ill patients whose condition is unstable. Therefore, close monitoring is required and fluid and electrolyte therapy should be adjusted according to the patient's condition at all times.

CAUTIONS. Plasma substitutes should be used with caution in patients with cardiac disease, liver disease, or renal impairment; urine output should be monitored. Care should be taken to avoid haematocrit concentration from falling below 25–30% and the patient should be monitored for hypersensitivity reactions.

SIDE-EFFECTS. Hypersensitivity reactions may occur including, rarely, severe anaphylactoid reactions. Transient increase in bleeding time may occur.

DEXTRAN 40

Dextrans of weight average molecular weight about '40 000'

Indications: conditions associated with peripheral local slowing of the blood flow; prophylaxis of post-surgical thromboembolic disease (but see notes above)

Cautions: see notes above; can interfere with some laboratory tests (see also above); correct dehydration beforehand, give adequate fluids during therapy and, where possible, monitor central venous pressure; pregnancy (Appendix 4)
Side-effects: see notes above
Dose: *by intravenous infusion*, initially 500–1000 mL; further doses are given according to the patient's condition (see notes above)

Dextran 40® (Baxter) PoM
Intravenous infusion, dextran 40 intravenous infusion in glucose intravenous infusion 5% or in sodium chloride intravenous infusion 0.9%. Net price 500-mL bag (both) = £4.56

DEXTRAN 70

Dextrans of weight average molecular weight about '70 000'
Indications: short-term blood volume expansion; prophylaxis of post-surgical thromboembolic disease (but see notes above)
Cautions: see notes above; can interfere with some laboratory tests (see also above); where possible, monitor central venous pressure; pregnancy (Appendix 4)
Side-effects: see notes above
Dose: *by intravenous infusion*, after moderate to severe haemorrhage or in the shock phase of burn injury (initial 48 hours), 500–1000 mL rapidly initially followed by 500 mL later if necessary (see also notes above); total dosage should not exceed 20 mL/kg during initial 24 hours; CHILD total dosage should not exceed 20 mL/kg

Dextran 70® (Baxter) PoM
Intravenous infusion, dextran 70 intravenous infusion in glucose intravenous infusion 5% or in sodium chloride intravenous infusion 0.9%. Net price 500-mL bag (both) = £4.56

■ Hypertonic solution

RescueFlow® (Vitaline) PoM
Intravenous infusion, dextran 70 intravenous infusion 6% in sodium chloride intravenous infusion 7.5%. Net price 250-mL bag = £28.50
Cautions: see notes above; severe hyperglycaemia and hyperosmolality
Dose: initial treatment of hypovolaemia with hypotension induced by traumatic injury, *by intravenous infusion* over 2–5 minutes, 250 mL, followed immediately by administration of isotonic fluids

GELATIN

NOTE. The gelatin is partially degraded
Indications: low blood volume
Cautions: see notes above
Side-effects: see notes above
Dose: *by intravenous infusion*, initially 500–1000 mL of a 3.5–4% solution (see notes above)

Gelofusine® (Braun) PoM
Intravenous infusion, succinylated gelatin (modified fluid gelatin, average molecular weight 30 000) 40 g (4%), Na^+ 154 mmol, Cl^- 120 mmol/litre, net price 500-mL *Ecobag*® = £4.63, 1-litre *Ecobag*® = £9.45

Volplex® (Cambridge) PoM
Intravenous infusion, succinylated gelatin (modified fluid gelatin, average molecular weight 30 000) 40 g (4%), Na^+ 154 mmol, Cl^- 125 mmol/litre, net price 500-mL bag = £5.05

ETHERIFIED STARCH

A starch composed of more than 90% of amylopectin that has been etherified with hydroxyethyl groups; hetastarch has a higher degree of etherification than pentastarch
Indications: low blood volume
Cautions: see notes above; children
Side-effects: see notes above; also pruritus, raised serum amylase
Dose: see under preparations below

■ Hexastarch

eloHAES® (Fresenius Kabi) PoM
Intravenous infusion, hexastarch (weight average molecular weight 200 000) 6% in sodium chloride intravenous infusion 0.9%. Net price 500-mL *Steriflex*® bag = £12.50
Dose: by intravenous infusion, 500–1000 mL; usual daily max. 1500 mL (see notes above)

■ Pentastarch

HAES-steril® (Fresenius Kabi) PoM
Intravenous infusion, pentastarch (weight average molecular weight 200 000), net price (both in sodium chloride intravenous infusion 0.9%) 6%, 500 mL = £10.50; 10%, 500 mL = £16.50
Dose: by intravenous infusion, pentastarch 6%, up to 2500 mL daily; pentastarch 10%, up to 1500 mL daily (see notes above)

Hemohes® (Braun) PoM
Intravenous infusion, pentastarch (weight average molecular weight 200 000), net price (both in sodium chloride intravenous infusion 0.9%) 6%, 500 mL = £12.50; 10%, 500 mL = £16.50
Cautions: see notes above
Dose: by intravenous infusion, pentastarch 6%, up to 2500 mL daily; pentastarch 10 %, up to 1500 mL daily (see notes above)

Infukoll® (Beacon) PoM
Intravenous infusion, pentastarch (hydroxyethyl starch, weight average molecular weight 200 000) 6% in sodium chloride intravenous infusion 0.9%, net price 500-mL bag = £10.00
Dose: by intravenous infusion, up to 2 500 mL daily (see notes above)

■ Tetrastarch

Voluven® (Fresenius Kabi) PoM
Intravenous infusion, hydroxyethyl starch (weight average molecular weight 130 000) 6% in sodium chloride intravenous infusion 0.9%, net price 500-mL bag = £12.50
Dose: by intravenous infusion, up to 50 mL/kg daily (see notes above)

■ Hypertonic solution

HyperHAES® (Fresenius Kabi) PoM
Intravenous infusion, hydroxyethyl starch (weight average molecular weight 200 000) 6% in sodium chloride intravenous infusion 7.2%, net price 250-mL bag = £28.00
Cautions: see notes above; also diabetes
Dose: by intravenous injection over 2–5 minutes, 4 mL/kg as a single dose, followed immediately by administration of appropriate replacement fluids

9.3 Intravenous nutrition

When adequate feeding through the alimentary tract is not possible, nutrients may be given by intravenous infusion. This may be in addition to ordinary oral or tube feeding—**supplemental parenteral**

nutrition, or may be the sole source of nutrition—**total parenteral nutrition** (TPN). Indications for this method include preparation of undernourished patients for surgery, chemotherapy, or radiation therapy; severe or prolonged disorders of the gastro-intestinal tract; major surgery, trauma, or burns; prolonged coma or refusal to eat; and some patients with renal or hepatic failure. The composition of proprietary preparations available is given in the table below.

Total parenteral nutrition requires the use of a solution containing amino acids, glucose, fat, electrolytes, trace elements, and vitamins. This is now commonly provided by the pharmacy in the form of a 3-litre bag. A single dose of vitamin B_{12}, as hydroxocobalamin, is given by intramuscular injection; regular vitamin B_{12} injections are not usually required unless total parenteral nutrition continues for many months. Folic acid is given in a dose of 15 mg once or twice each week, usually in the nutrition solution. Other vitamins are usually given daily; they are generally introduced in the parenteral nutrition solution. Alternatively, if the patient is able to take small amounts by mouth, vitamins may be given orally.

The nutrition solution is infused through a central venous catheter inserted under full surgical precautions. Alternatively infusion through a peripheral vein may be used for supplementary as well as total parenteral nutrition for periods of up to a month, depending on the availability of peripheral veins; factors prolonging cannula life and preventing thrombophlebitis include the use of soft polyurethane paediatric cannulas and use of feeds of low osmolality and neutral pH. Only nutritional fluids should be given by the dedicated intravenous line.

Before starting, the patient should be well oxygenated with a near normal circulating blood volume and attention should be given to renal function and acid-base status. Appropriate biochemical tests should have been carried out beforehand and serious deficits corrected. Nutritional and electrolyte status must be monitored throughout treatment.

Complications of long-term TPN include gall bladder sludging, gall stones, cholestasis and abnormal liver function tests. For details of the prevention and management of TPN complications, specialist literature should be consulted.

Protein is given as mixtures of essential and non-essential synthetic L-amino acids. Ideally, all essential amino acids should be included with a wide variety of non-essential ones to provide sufficient nitrogen together with electrolytes (see also section 9.2.2). Solutions vary in their composition of amino acids; they often contain an energy source (usually glucose) and electrolytes.

Energy is provided in a ratio of 0.6 to 1.1 megajoules (150–250 kcals) per gram of protein nitrogen. Energy requirements must be met if amino acids are to be utilised for tissue maintenance. A mixture of carbohydrate and fat energy sources (usually 30–50% as fat) gives better utilisation of amino acids than glucose alone.

Glucose is the preferred source of carbohydrate, but if more than 180 g is given per day frequent monitoring of blood glucose is required, and insulin may be necessary. Glucose in various strengths from 10 to 50% must be infused through a central venous catheter to avoid thrombosis.

In total parenteral nutrition regimens, it is necessary to provide adequate phosphate in order to allow phosphorylation of the glucose; between 20 and 30 mmol of phosphate is required daily.

Fructose and sorbitol have been used in an attempt to avoid the problem of hyperosmolar hyperglycaemic non-ketotic acidosis but other metabolic problems may occur, as with xylitol and ethanol which are now rarely used.

Fat emulsions have the advantages of a high energy to fluid volume ratio, neutral pH, and iso-osmolarity with plasma, and provide essential fatty acids. Several days of adaptation may be required to attain maximal utilisation. Reactions include occasional febrile episodes (usually only with 20% emulsions) and rare anaphylactic responses. Interference with biochemical measurements such as those for blood gases and calcium may occur if samples are taken before fat has been cleared. Daily checks are necessary to ensure complete clearance from the plasma in conditions where fat metabolism may be disturbed. **Additives may only be mixed with fat emulsions where compatibility is known**.

Administration. Because of the complex requirements relating to parenteral nutrition full details relating to administration have been omitted. In all cases *product literature and other specialist literature should be consulted*.

Supplementary preparations

Compatibility with the infusion solution must be ascertained before adding supplementary preparations.

Addiphos® (Fresenius Kabi) PoM
Solution, sterile, phosphate 40 mmol, K^+ 30 mmol, Na^+ 30 mmol/20 mL. For addition to *Vamin*® solutions and glucose intravenous infusions. Net price 20-mL vial = £1.44

Additrace® (Fresenius Kabi) PoM
Solution, trace elements for addition to *Vamin*® solutions and glucose intravenous infusions, traces of Fe^{3+}, Zn^{2+}, Mn^{2+}, Cu^{2+}, Cr^{3+}, Se^{4+}, Mo^{6+}, F^-, I^-. For adults and children over 40 kg. Net price 10-mL amp = £2.18

Cernevit® (Baxter) PoM
Solution, *dl*-alpha tocopherol 11.2 units, ascorbic acid 125 mg, biotin 69 micrograms, colecalciferol 220 units, cyanocobalamin 6 micrograms, folic acid 414 micrograms, glycine 250 mg, nicotinamide 46 mg, pantothenic acid (as dexpanthenol) 17.25 mg, pyridoxine hydrochloride 5.5 mg, retinol (as palmitate) 3500 units, riboflavin (as dihydrated sodium phosphate) 4.14 mg, thiamine (as cocarboxylase tetrahydrate) 3.51 mg. Dissolve in 5 mL water for injections. Net price per vial = £2.90

Decan® (Baxter) PoM
Solution, trace elements for addition to infusion solutions, Fe^{2+}, Zn^{2+}, Cu^{2+}, Mn^{2+}, F^-, Co^{2+}, I^-, Se^{4+}, Mo^{6+}, Cr^{3+}. For adults and children over 40 kg. Net price 40-mL vial = £2.00

Proprietary Infusion Fluids for Parenteral Feeding

Preparation	Nitrogen g/litre	[1]Energy kJ/litre	Electrolytes mmol/litre					Other components/litre
			K^+	Mg^{2+}	Na^+	$Acet^-$	Cl^-	
Aminoplasmal 5% E (Braun) Net price 500 mL = £9.02	8		25	2.6	43	59	29	dihydrogen phosphate 9 mmol, malic acid 1.01 g
Aminoplasmal 10% (Braun) Net price 500 mL = £17.06	16						57	
Aminoven 25 (Fresenius Kabi) Net price 500 mL = £22.00	25.7							
Clinimix N9G20E (Baxter) Net price (dual compartment bag of amino acids with electrolytes 1000 mL and glucose 20% with calcium 1000 mL) = £29.00	4.55	1680	30	2.5	35	50	40	Ca^{2+} 2.25 mmol, phosphate 15 mmol, anhydrous glucose 100 g
Clinimix N14G30E (Baxter) Net price (dual compartment bag of amino acids with electrolytes 1000 mL and glucose 30% with calcium 1000 mL) = £33.00	7	2520	30	2.5	35	70	40	Ca^{2+} 2.25 mmol, phosphate 15 mmol, anhydrous glucose 150 g
ClinOleic 20% (Baxter) Net price 100 mL = £6.28; 250 mL = £10.08; 500 mL = £13.88		8360						purified olive and soya oil 200 g, glycerol 22.5 g, egg phosphatides 12 g
Compleven (Fresenius Kabi) Net price (triple compartment bag of amino acids 1000 mL; glucose 1000 mL; lipid emulsion 500 mL) 2500 mL = £67.00	4.8	3275	20	2	32		32.4	Ca^{2+} 2 mmol, Zn^{2+} 0.04 mmol, glycerophosphate 8 mmol, anhydrous glucose 96 g, soya oil 40 g, egg lecithin 2.4 g, glycerol 2.4 g
Glamin (Fresenius Kabi) Net price 250 mL = £14.16; 500 mL = £26.38	22.4					62		
Hyperamine 30 (Braun) Net price 500 mL = £23.67	30				5			
Intrafusin 11 (Fresenius Kabi) Net price 1000 mL = £17.80	11.4		40	5	80		76	Ca^{2+} 3 mmol, phosphate 20 mmol, citrate 6 mmol
Intrafusin 22 (Fresenius Kabi) Net price 500 mL = £17.80	22.8							
Intralipid 10% (Fresenius Kabi) Net price 100 mL = £4.70; 500 mL = £10.30		4600						soya oil 100 g, glycerol 22 g, purified egg phospholipids 12 g, phosphate 15 mmol
Intralipid 20% (Fresenius Kabi) Net price 100 mL = £7.05; 250 mL = £11.60; 500 mL = £15.45		8400						soya oil 200 g, glycerol 22 g, purified egg phospholipids 12 g, phosphate 15 mmol
Intralipid 30% (Fresenius Kabi) Net price 333 mL = £17.30		12600						soya oil 300 g, glycerol 16.7 g, purified egg phospholipids 12 g, phosphate 15 mmol
Ivelip 10% (Baxter) Net price 500 mL = £9.08		4600						soya oil 100 g, glycerol 25 g
Ivelip 20% (Baxter) Net price 100 mL = £6.28; 500 mL = £13.88		8400						soya oil 200 g, glycerol 25 g
Kabiven (Fresenius Kabi) Net price (triple compartment bag of amino acids and electrolytes 300 mL, 450 mL, 600 mL, or 750 mL; glucose 526 mL, 790 mL, 1053 mL, or 1316 mL; lipid emulsion 200 mL, 300 mL, 400 mL, or 500 mL) 1026 mL = £35.00, 1540 mL = £50.00, 2053 mL = £67.00, 2566 mL = £70.00	5.3	3275	23	4	31	38	45	Ca^{2+} 2 mmol, phosphate 9.7 mmol, anhydrous glucose 97 g, soya oil 39 g
Kabiven Peripheral (Fresenius Kabi) Net price (triple compartment bag of amino acids and electrolytes 300 mL, 400 mL, or 500 mL; glucose 885 mL, 1180 mL, or 1475 mL; lipid emulsion 255 mL, 340 mL, or 425 mL) 1440 mL = £35.00, 1920 mL = £50.00, 2400 mL = £64.00	3.75	2625	17	2.8	22	27	33	Ca^{2+} 1.4 mmol, phosphate 7.5 mmol, anhydrous glucose 67.5 g, soya oil 35.4 g
Lipofundin MCT/LCT 10% (Braun) Net price 100 mL = £7.70; 500 mL = £12.90		4430						soya oil 50 g, medium chain triglycerides 50 g

1. Excludes protein- or amino acid-derived energy

Note. 1000 kcal = 4200 kJ; 1000 kJ= 238.8 kcal. All entries are PoM

Proprietary Infusion Fluids for Parenteral Feeding

Preparation	Nitrogen g/litre	Energy[1] kJ/litre	Electrolytes mmol/litre					Other components/litre
			K^+	Mg^{2+}	Na^+	$Acet^-$	Cl^-	
Lipofundin MCT/LCT 20% (Braun) Net price 100 mL = £12.51; 250 mL = £11.30; 500 mL = £19.18		8000						soya oil 100 g, medium chain triglycerides 100 g
Lipofundin N 10% (Braun) Net price 100 mL = £7.10; 250 mL = £9.50; 500 mL = £11.76		4470						soya oil 100 g, glycerol 25 g, egg lethicin 8 g
Lipofundin N 20% (Braun) Net price 100 mL = £8.10; 250 mL = £9.99; 500 mL = £18.38		8520						soya oil 200 g, glycerol 25 g, egg lethicin 12 g
Nutracel 400 (Baxter) Net price 500 mL = £2.43		3400		18		0.16	66	Ca^{2+} 15 mmol, Mn^{2+} 0.01 mmol, Zn^{2+} 0.08 mmol, anhydrous glucose 200 g
Nutracel 800 (Baxter) Net price 1000 mL = £4.19		3400		9		0.08	33	Ca^{2+} 7.5 mmol, Mn^{2+} 0.005 mmol, Zn^{2+} 0.04 mmol, anhydrous glucose 200 g
NuTRIflex Lipid basal (Braun) Net price (triple compartment bag of amino acids 500 mL, 750 mL or 1000 mL; glucose 500 mL, 750 mL or 1000 mL; lipid emulsion 20% 250 mL, 375 mL or 500 mL) 1250 mL = £41.50, 1875 mL = £56.20, 2500 mL = £64.00	3.68	3268	28	3.2	40	36	32	Ca^{2+} 3.2 mmol, anhydrous glucose 100 g, phosphate 12 mmol, soya oil 20 g, medium chain trigylcerides 20 g
NuTRIflex Lipid peri (Braun) Net price (triple compartment bag of amino acids 500 mL or 1000 mL; glucose 500 mL or 1000 mL; lipid emulsion 20% 250 mL or 500 mL) 1250 mL = £43.38, 2500 mL = £65.05	4.56	2664	24	2.4	40	32	38.4	Ca^{2+} 2.4 mmol, Zn^{2+} 0.024 mmol, phosphate 6 mmol, anhydrous glucose 64 g, soya oil 20 g, medium chain triglycerides 20 g
NuTRIflex Lipid plus (Braun) Net price (triple compartment bag of amino acids 500 mL, 750 mL or 1000 mL; glucose 500 mL, 750 mL or 1000 mL; lipid emulsion 20% 250 mL, 375 mL or 500 mL) 1250 mL = £47.17, 1875 mL = £60.23, 2500 mL = £69.27	5.44	3600	28	3.2	40	36	36	Ca^{2+} 3.2 mmol, Zn^{2+} 0.024 mmol, phosphate 12 mmol, anhydrous glucose 120 g, soya oil 20 g, medium chain triglycerides 20 g
NuTRIflex Lipid plus without Electrolytes (Braun) Net price (triple compartment bag of amino acids 500 mL, 750 mL or 1000 mL; glucose 500 mL, 750 mL or 1000 mL; lipid emulsion 20% 250 mL, 375 mL or 500 mL) 1250 mL = £47.17, 1875 mL = £60.23, 2500 mL = £69.27	5.44	3600						anhydrous glucose 120 g, soya oil 20 g, medium chain triglycerides 20 g
NuTRIflex Lipid special (Braun) Net price (triple compartment bag of amino acids 500 mL, 750 mL or 1000 mL; glucose 500 mL, 750 mL or 1000 mL; lipid emulsion 20% 250 mL, 375 mL or 500 mL) 1250 mL = £57.69, 1875 mL = £75.58, 2500 mL = £89.21	8	4004	37.6	4.24	53.6	48	48	Ca^{2+} 4.24 mmol, Zn^{2+} 0.032 mmol, phosphate 16 mmol, anhydrous glucose 144 g, soya oil 20 g, medium chain triglycerides 20 g
NuTRIflex Lipid special without Electrolytes (Braun) Net price (triple compartment bag of amino acids 500 mL, 750 mL or 1000 mL; glucose 500 mL, 750 mL or 1000 mL; lipid emulsion 20% 250 mL, 375 mL or 500 mL) 1250 mL = £57.69, 1875 mL = £75.58, 2500 mL = £89.21	8	4004						anhydrous glucose 144 g, soya oil 20 g, medium chain triglycerides 20 g
Nutriflex Basal (Braun) Net price (dual compartment bag of 800 mL and 1200 mL) = £28.35	4.6	2095	30	5.7	49.9	35	50	Ca^{2+} 3.6 mmol, phosphate 12.8 mmol, anhydrous glucose 125 g
Nutriflex Peri (Braun) Net price (dual compartment bag of 800 mL and 1200 mL) = £33.00	5.7	1340	15	4	27	19.5	31.6	Ca^{2+} 2.5 mmol, phosphate 5.7 mmol, anhydrous glucose 80 g
Nutriflex Plus (Braun) Net price (dual compartment bag of 800 mL and 1200 mL) = £39.18	6.8	2510	25	5.7	37.2	22.9	35.5	Ca^{2+} 3.6 mmol, phosphate 20 mmol, anhydrous glucose 150 g
Nutriflex Special (Braun) Net price (dual compartment bag of 750 mL and 750 mL) = £43.30	10	4020	25.7	5	40.5	22	49.5	Ca^{2+} 4.1 mmol, phosphate 15 mmol, anhydrous glucose 240 g

1. Excludes protein- or amino acid-derived energy

Note. 1000 kcal = 4200 kJ; 1000 kJ= 238.8 kcal. All entries are PoM

Proprietary Infusion Fluids for Parenteral Feeding

Preparation	Nitrogen g/litre	[1]Energy kJ/litre	Electrolytes mmol/litre					Other components/litre
			K^+	Mg^{2+}	Na^+	$Acet^-$	Cl^-	
OliClinomel N4-550E (Baxter) Net price (triple compartment bag of amino acids with electrolytes 1000 mL; glucose 20% 1000 mL; lipid emulsion 10% 500 mL) 2500 mL = £69.30	3.6	2184	16	2.2	21	30	33	Ca^{2+} 2 mmol, phosphate 8.5 mmol, refined olive and soya oil 20 g, anhydrous glucose 80 g
OliClinomel N4-720E (Baxter) Net price (triple compartment bag of amino acids with electrolytes 1000 mL; glucose 20% 1000 mL; lipid emulsion 20% 500 mL) 2500 mL = £69.30	3.64	3024	24	2	28	40	40	Ca^{2+} 1.8 mmol, phosphate 8 mmol, refined olive and soya oil 40 g, anhydrous glucose 80 g
OliClinomel N6-900E (Baxter) Net price (triple compartment bag of amino acids with electrolytes 800 mL or 1000 mL; glucose 30% 800 mL or 1000 mL; lipid emulsion 20% 400 mL or 500 mL) 2000 mL = £70.40, 2500 mL = £75.90	5.6	3696	24	2.2	32	53	46	Ca^{2+} 2 mmol, phosphate 10 mmol, refined olive and soya oil 40 g, anhydrous glucose 120 g
OliClinomel N7-1000 (Baxter) Net price (triple compartment bag of amino acids with electrolytes 400 mL or 600 mL; glucose 40% 400 mL or 600 mL; lipid emulsion 20% 200 mL or 300 mL) 1000 mL = £28.75, 1500 mL = £43.70	6.6	4368				37	16	phosphate 3 mmol, refined olive and soya oil 40 g, anhydrous glucose 160 g
Plasma-Lyte 148 (water) (Baxter) Net price 1000 mL = £1.59			5	1.5	140	27	98	gluconate 23 mmol
Plasma-Lyte 148 (dextrose 5%) (Baxter) Net price 1000 mL = £1.59		840	5	1.5	140	27	98	gluconate 23 mmol, anhydrous glucose 50 g
Plasma-Lyte M (dextrose 5%) (Baxter) Net price 1000 mL = £1.33		840	16	1.5	40	12	40	Ca^{2+} 2.5 mmol, lactate 12 mmol, anhydrous glucose 50 g
[2]Primene 10% (Baxter) Net price 100 mL = £5.78, 250 mL = £7.92	15						19	
StructoKabiven Electrolyte Free (Fresenius Kabi) Net price (triple compartment bag of amino acids 750 mL or 1000 mL; glucose 42% 446 mL or 595 mL; lipid emulsion 281 mL or 375 mL) 1477 mL = £69.00, 1970 mL = £74.00	8	3685				74.5		phosphate 2.8 mmol, anhydrous glucose 127 g, glycerol 4.23 g, egg phospholipids 4.56 g, purified structured triglyceride 38.5 g (contains coconut oil, palm kernel oil and soya oil trigylcerides)
Structolipid 20% (Fresenius Kabi) Net price 500 mL = £16.09		8200						purified structured triglyceride 200 g (contains coconut oil, palm kernel oil, and soya oil triglycerides)
Synthamin 9 (Baxter) Net price 500 mL = £6.66; 1000 mL = £12.34	9.1		60	5	70	100	70	acid phosphate 30 mmol
Synthamin 9 EF (electrolyte-free) (Baxter) Net price 500 mL = £6.66; 1000 mL = £12.34	9.1					44	22	
Synthamin 14 (Baxter) Net price 500 mL = £9.64; 1000 mL = £17.13; 3000 mL = £48.98	14		60	5	70	140	70	acid phosphate 30 mmol
Synthamin 14 EF (electrolyte–free) (Baxter) Net price 500 mL = £9.87; 1000 mL = £17.51	14					68	34	
Synthamin 17 (Baxter) Net price 500 mL = £12.66; 1000 mL = £23.00	16.5		60	5	70	150	70	acid phosphate 30 mmol
Synthamin 17 EF (electrolyte–free) (Baxter) Net price 500 mL = £12.66	16.5					82	40	
Vamin 9 (Fresenius Kabi) Net price 500 mL = £7.30; 1000 mL = £12.55	9.4		20	1.5	50		50	Ca^{2+} 2.5 mmol

1. Excludes protein- or amino acid-derived energy
Note. 1000 kcal = 4200 kJ; 1000 kJ= 238.8 kcal. All entries are PoM

2. For use in neonates and children only
Note. 1000 kcal = 4200 kJ; = 238.8 kcal. All entries are PoM

Proprietary Infusion Fluids for Parenteral Feeding

Preparation	Nitrogen g/litre	[1]Energy kJ/litre	Electrolytes mmol/litre					Other components/litre
			K^+	Mg^{2+}	Na^+	$Acet^-$	Cl^-	
Vamin 9 Glucose (Fresenius Kabi) Net price 100 mL = £3.80; 500 mL = £7.70; 1000 mL = £13.40	9.4	1700	20	1.5	50		50	Ca^{2+} 2.5 mmol, anhydrous glucose 100 g
Vamin 14 (Fresenius Kabi) Net price 500 mL = £10.80; 1000 mL = £14.67	13.5		50	8	100	135	100	Ca^{2+} 5 mmol, SO_4^{2-} 8 mmol
Vamin 14 (Electrolyte-Free) (Fresenius Kabi) Net price 500 mL = £10.80; 1000 mL = £18.30	13.5					90		
Vamin 18 (Electrolyte-Free) (Fresenius Kabi) Net price 500 mL = £13.70; 1000 mL = £26.70	18					110		
Vaminolact (Fresenius Kabi) Net price 100 mL = £4.20; 500 mL = £9.70	9.3							
Vitrimix KV (Fresenius Kabi) Net price (combined pack of Intralipid 20% 250 mL and Vamin 9 glucose 750 mL) = £21.00	7	3340	15	1.1	38		38	Ca^{2+} 1.9 mmol, anhydrous glucose 75 g, soya oil 50 g, purified egg phospholipids 3 g, glycerol 5.5 g, phosphate 3.75 mmol

Dipeptiven® (Fresenius Kabi) PoM

Solution, *N*(2)-L-alanyl-L-glutamine 200 mg/mL (providing L-alanine 82 mg, L-glutamine 134.6 mg). For addition to infusion solutions containing amino acids. Net price 50 mL = £15.90, 100 mL = £29.60

Dose: amino acid supplement for hypercatabolic or hypermetabolic states, 300–400 mg/kg daily; max. 400 mg/kg daily, dose not to exceed 20% of total amino acid intake

Glycophos® **Sterile Concentrate** (Fresenius Kabi) PoM

Solution, sterile, phosphate 20 mmol, Na^+ 40 mmol/20 mL. For addition to *Vamin*® and *Vaminolact*® solutions, and glucose intravenous infusions. Net price 20-mL vial = £4.25

Peditrace® (Fresenius Kabi) PoM

Solution, trace elements for addition to *Vaminolact*®, *Vamin*® *14 Electrolyte-Free* solutions and glucose intravenous infusions, traces of Zn^{2+}, Cu^{2+}, Mn^{2+}, Se^{4+}, F^-, I^-. For use in neonates (when kidney function established, usually second day of life), infants, and children. Net price 10-mL vial = £3.88

Cautions: reduced biliary excretion especially in cholestatic liver disease or in markedly reduced urinary excretion (careful biochemical monitoring required); total parenteral nutrition exceeding 1 month (measure serum manganese concentration and check liver function before commencing treatment and regularly during treatment)—discontinue if manganese concentration raised or if cholestasis develops

Solivito N® (Fresenius Kabi) PoM

Solution, powder for reconstitution, biotin 60 micrograms, cyanocobalamin 5 micrograms, folic acid 400 micrograms, glycine 300 mg, nicotinamide 40 mg, pyridoxine hydrochloride 4.9 mg, riboflavin sodium phosphate 4.9 mg, sodium ascorbate 113 mg, sodium pantothenate 16.5 mg, thiamine mononitrate 3.1 mg. Dissolve in water for injections or glucose intravenous infusion for adding to glucose intravenous infusion or *Intralipid*®; dissolve in *Vitlipid N*® or *Intralipid*® for adding to *Intralipid*® only. Net price per vial = £2.19

Vitlipid N® (Fresenius Kabi) PoM

Emulsion, adult, vitamin A 330 units, ergocalciferol 20 units, *dl*-alpha tocopherol 1 unit, phytomenadione 15 micrograms/mL. For addition to *Intralipid*®. For adults and children over 11 years. Net price 10-mL amp = £2.19

Emulsion, infant, vitamin A 230 units, ergocalciferol 40 units, *dl*-alpha tocopherol 0.7 unit, phytomenadione 20 micrograms/mL. For addition to *Intralipid*®. Net price 10-mL amp = £2.19

9.4 Oral nutrition

9.4.1 Foods for special diets

These are preparations that have been modified to eliminate a particular constituent from a food or are nutrient mixtures formulated as substitutes for the food. They are for patients who either cannot tolerate or cannot metabolise certain common constituents of food.

PHENYLKETONURIA. Phenylketonuria (phenylalaninaemia), which results from the inability to metabolise phenylalanine, is managed by restricting its dietary intake to a small amount sufficient for tissue building and repair. Aspartame (as a sweetener in some foods and medicines) contributes to the phenylalanine intake and may affect control of phenylketonuria. Where the presence of aspartame is specified in the product literature this is indicated in the BNF against the preparation.

1. Excludes protein- or amino acid-derived energy

Note. 1000 kcal = 4200 kJ; 1000 kJ= 238.8 kcal. All entries are PoM

COELIAC DISEASE. Coeliac disease, which results from an intolerance to gluten, is managed by completely eliminating gluten from the diet.

ACBS. In certain clinical conditions some foods may have the characteristics of drugs and the Advisory Committee on Borderline Substances advises as to the circumstances in which such foods may be regarded as drugs and so can be prescribed in the NHS. Prescriptions for these foods issued in accordance with the advice of this committee and endorsed 'ACBS' will normally not be investigated. See Appendix 7 for details of these foods and a listing by clinical condition (consult Drug Tariff for late amendments).

■ Preparations

For preparations on the ACBS list see Appendix 7

Forceval Protein Powder® (Alliance)

Powder, strawberry, vanilla and natural flavours, protein (calcium caseinate, providing all essential amino acids) 55%, carbohydrate 30%, with vitamins, minerals, trace elements, fat and low electrolytes (lactose- and gluten-free), net price 14 × 30-g sachets = £15.57; chocolate flavour (as above but protein content is 45%), 14 × 36-g sachets = £15.57.

For hypoproteinaemia, malabsorption states and as an adjunct to nutritional support. Not to be prescribed for any CHILD under 2 years or for those with renal or hepatic failure; unsuitable as a sole source of nutrition

9.4.2 Enteral nutrition

The body's reserves of protein rapidly become exhausted in severely ill patients, especially during chronic illness or in those with severe burns, extensive trauma, pancreatitis, or intestinal fistula. Much can be achieved by frequent meals and by persuading the patient to take supplementary snacks of ordinary food between the meals.

However, extra calories, protein, other nutrients, and vitamins are often best given by supplementing ordinary meals with sip or tube feeds of one of the nutritionally complete foods.

When patients cannot feed normally at all, for example, patients with severe facial injury, oesophageal obstruction, or coma, a diet composed solely of nutritionally complete foods must be given. This is planned by a dietitian who will take into account the protein and total energy requirement of the patient and decide on the form and relative contribution of carbohydrate and fat to the energy requirements.

There are a number of nutritionally complete foods available and their use reduces an otherwise heavy workload in hospital or in the home. Most contain protein derived from milk or soya. Some contain protein hydrolysates or free amino acids and are only appropriate for patients who have diminished ability to break down protein, as may be the case in inflammatory bowel disease or pancreatic insufficiency.

Even when nutritionally complete feeds are being given it may be important to monitor water and electrolyte balance. Extra minerals (e.g. magnesium and zinc) may be needed in patients where gastro-intestinal secretions are being lost. Additional vitamins may also be needed. Regular haematological and biochemical tests may be needed particularly in the unstable patient.

Some feeds are supplemented with vitamin K; for drug interactions of vitamin K see Appendix 1 (vitamins).

CHILDREN. Infants and young children have special requirements and in most situations liquid feeds prepared for adults are totally unsuitable and should not be given. Expert advice should be sought.

■ Preparations

See Appendix 7

9.5 Minerals

See section 9.1.1 for iron salts.

9.5.1 Calcium and magnesium

9.5.1.1 Calcium supplements

Calcium supplements are usually only required where dietary calcium intake is deficient. This dietary requirement varies with age and is relatively greater in childhood, pregnancy, and lactation, due to an increased demand, and in old age, due to impaired absorption. In osteoporosis, a calcium intake which is double the recommended amount reduces the rate of bone loss. If the actual dietary intake is less than the recommended amount, a supplement of as much as 40 mmol is appropriate.

In hypocalcaemic tetany an initial intravenous injection of 10 mL (2.25 mmol) of calcium gluconate injection 10% should be followed by the continuous infusion of about 40 mL (9 mmol) daily, but plasma calcium should be monitored. This regimen can also be used immediately to temporarily reduce the toxic effects of hyperkalaemia.

CALCIUM SALTS

Indications: see notes above; calcium deficiency

Cautions: renal impairment; sarcoidosis; history of nephrolithiasis; avoid calcium chloride in respiratory acidosis or respiratory failure; **interactions:** Appendix 1 (antacids, calcium salts)

Contra-indications: conditions associated with hypercalcaemia and hypercalciuria (e.g. some forms of malignant disease)

Side-effects: gastro-intestinal disturbances; bradycardia, arrhythmias; *with injection*, peripheral vasodilatation, fall in blood pressure, injection-site reactions

Dose: *by mouth*, daily in divided doses, see notes above

By slow intravenous injection, acute hypocalcaemia, calcium gluconate 1–2 g (Ca^{2+} 2.25–4.5 mmol)

CHILD obtain paediatric advice

■ Oral preparations

Calcium Gluconate (Non-proprietary)

Tablets, calcium gluconate 600 mg (calcium 53.4 mg or Ca^{2+} 1.35 mmol), net price 20 = £1.43. Label: 24

Effervescent tablets, calcium gluconate 1 g (calcium 89 mg or Ca^{2+} 2.25 mmol), net price 28-tab pack = £4.62. Label: 13

NOTE. Each tablet usually contains 4.46 mmol Na^+

Calcium Lactate (Non-proprietary)

Tablets, calcium lactate 300 mg (calcium 39 mg or Ca^{2+} 1 mmol), net price 20 = 98p

Adcal® (Strakan)

Chewable tablets, calcium carbonate 1.5 g (calcium 600 mg or Ca^{2+} 15 mmol), net price 100-tab pack = £7.25. Label: 24

Cacit® (Procter & Gamble Pharm.)

Tablets, effervescent, pink, calcium carbonate 1.25 g, providing calcium citrate when dispersed in water (calcium 500 mg or Ca^{2+} 12.6 mmol), net price 76-tab pack = £15.55. Label: 13

Calcichew® (Shire)

Tablets (chewable), calcium carbonate 1.25 g (calcium 500 mg or Ca^{2+} 12.6 mmol), net price 100-tab pack = £9.33

Forte tablets (chewable), scored, calcium carbonate 2.5 g (calcium 1 g or Ca^{2+} 25 mmol), net price 60-tab pack = £13.16. Label: 24

Excipients: include aspartame

Calcium-500 (Martindale)

Tablets, pink, f/c, calcium carbonate 1.25 g (calcium 500 mg or Ca^{2+} 12.5 mmol). Net price 100-tab pack = £9.46. Label: 25

Calcium-Sandoz® (Alliance)

Syrup, calcium glubionate 1.09 g, calcium lactobionate 727 mg (calcium 108.3 mg or Ca^{2+} 2.7 mmol)/5 mL. Net price 300 mL = £3.39

Sandocal® (Novartis Consumer Health)

Sandocal-400 tablets, effervescent, calcium lactate gluconate 930 mg, calcium carbonate 700 mg, anhydrous citric acid 1.189 g, providing calcium 400 mg (Ca^{2+} 10 mmol). Net price 5 × 20-tab pack = £6.87. Label: 13

Excipients: include aspartame (section 9.4.1)

Sandocal-1000 tablets, effervescent, calcium lactate gluconate 2.327 g, calcium carbonate 1.75 g, anhydrous citric acid 2.973 g providing 1 g calcium (Ca^{2+} 25 mmol). Net price 3 × 10-tab pack = £6.17. Label: 13

Excipients: include aspartame (section 9.4.1)

■ Parenteral preparations

Calcium Gluconate (Non-proprietary) PoM

Injection, calcium gluconate 10% (calcium 8.9 mg or Ca^{2+} 220 micromol/mL). Net price 10-mL amp = 60p

Calcium Chloride (Non-proprietary) PoM

Injection, calcium chloride (as calcium chloride dihydrate 10%) 75 mg/mL (calcium 27.3 mg or Ca^{2+} 680 micromol/mL). Net price 10-mL disposable syringe = £4.42

Brands include *Minijet*® *Calcium Chloride 10%*

Injection, calcium chloride (as calcium chloride dihydrate 13.4%) 100 mg/mL (calcium 36 mg or Ca^{2+} 910 micromol/mL). Net price 10-mL amp = £14.94

■ With vitamin D

Section 9.6.4

9.5.1.2 Hypercalcaemia and hypercalciuria

SEVERE HYPERCALCAEMIA. Severe hypercalcaemia calls for urgent treatment before detailed investigation of the cause. Dehydration should be corrected first with intravenous infusion of **sodium chloride 0.9%**. Drugs (such as thiazides and vitamin D compounds) which promote hypercalcaemia, should be discontinued and dietary calcium should be restricted.

If *severe hypercalcaemia persists* drugs which inhibit mobilisation of calcium from the skeleton may be required. The **bisphosphonates** are useful and disodium pamidronate (section 6.6.2) is probably the most effective.

Corticosteroids (section 6.3) are widely given, but may only be useful where hypercalcaemia is due to sarcoidosis or vitamin D intoxication; they often take several days to achieve the desired effect.

Calcitonin (section 6.6.1) is relatively non-toxic but is expensive and its effect can wear off after a few days despite continued use; it is rarely effective where bisphosphonates have failed to reduce serum calcium adequately.

Intravenous chelating drugs such as **trisodium edetate** are rarely used; they usually cause pain in the limb receiving the infusion and may cause renal damage; trisodium edetate should no longer be used for the management of hypercalcaemia.

After treatment of severe hypercalcaemia the underlying cause must be established. *Further treatment* is governed by the same principles as for initial therapy. Salt and water depletion and drugs promoting hypercalcaemia should be avoided; oral administration of a bisphosphonate may be useful.

HYPERPARATHYROIDISM. **Cinacalcet** is licensed for the treatment of secondary hyperparathyroidism in dialysis patients with end-stage renal disease and for the treatment of hypercalcaemia in parathyroid carcinoma. Cinacalcet reduces parathyroid hormone which leads to a decrease in serum calcium concentrations.

Parathyroidectomy may be indicated for hyperparathyroidism.

HYPERCALCIURIA. Hypercalciuria should be investigated for an underlying cause, which should be treated. Where a cause is not identified (idiopathic hypercalciuria), the condition is managed by increasing fluid intake and giving bendroflumethiazide in a dose of 2.5 mg daily (a higher dose is not usually necessary). Reducing dietary calcium intake may be beneficial but severe restriction of calcium intake has not proved beneficial and may even be harmful.

CINACALCET

Indications: see under Dose

Cautions: measure serum-calcium concentration within 1 week of starting treatment or adjusting dose, then every 1–3 months; monitor parathyroid hormone concentration; dose adjustment may be necessary if smoking started or stopped during treatment; hepatic impairment (Appendix 2); pregnancy (Appendix 4); **interactions:** Appendix 1 (cinacalcet)

Contra-indications: breast-feeding (Appendix 5)

Side-effects: nausea, vomiting; anorexia, dizziness, paraesthesia, asthenia; reduced testosterone concentrations; myalgia; rash; *less commonly* dyspepsia, seizures

Dose: secondary hyperparathyroidism in patients with end-stage renal disease on dialysis, ADULT over 18 years, 30 mg once daily, adjusted every 2–4 weeks to max. 180 mg daily

Hypercalcaemia of parathyroid carcinoma, ADULT over 18 years, initially 30 mg twice daily, adjusted every 2–4 weeks to max. 90 mg 4 times daily

Mimpara® (Amgen) ▼ PoM

Tablets, green, f/c, cinacalcet (as hydrochloride) 30 mg, net price 28-tab pack = £126.28; 60 mg, 28-tab pack = £232.96; 90 mg, 28-tab pack = £349.44. Label: 21

TRISODIUM EDETATE

Indications: hypercalcaemia (but see notes above); lime burns in the eye (see under preparations)

Cautions: repeated plasma-calcium determinations important; caution in tuberculosis; avoid rapid infusion, see under Dose

Contra-indications: impaired renal function (Appendix 3)

Side-effects: nausea, diarrhoea, cramp; in overdosage renal damage

Dose: hypercalcaemia, *by intravenous infusion* over 2–3 hours, up to 70 mg/kg daily; CHILD up to 60 mg/kg daily

IMPORTANT. Ensure rate of infusion and concentration correct (see Appendix 6); too rapid a rate or too high a concentration is extremely hazardous and repeated measurements of plasma calcium concentrations are important for control and maintenance of near normal ionised calcium concentrations. Decrease infusion rate on signs of increased muscle reactivity; discontinue if tetany occurs and restart cautiously only after plasma ionised and total calcium concentrations indicate need for further treatment (and tetany has stopped)

Limclair® (Sinclair) PoM

Concentrate for infusion, trisodium edetate 200 mg/mL. Net price 5-mL amp = £7.93

NOTE. For topical use in the eye, dilute 1 mL to 50 mL with sterile purified water

9.5.1.3 Magnesium

Magnesium is an essential constituent of many enzyme systems, particularly those involved in energy generation; the largest stores are in the skeleton.

Magnesium salts are not well absorbed from the gastro-intestinal tract, which explains the use of magnesium sulphate (section 1.6.4) as an osmotic laxative.

Magnesium is excreted mainly by the kidneys and is therefore retained in renal failure, but significant *hypermagnesaemia* (causing muscle weakness and arrhythmias) is rare.

HYPOMAGNESAEMIA. Since magnesium is secreted in large amounts in the gastro-intestinal fluid, excessive losses in diarrhoea, stoma or fistula are the most common causes of *hypomagnesaemia*; deficiency may also occur in alcoholism or diuretic therapy and it has been reported after prolonged treatment with aminoglycosides. Hypomagnesaemia often causes secondary hypocalcaemia (with which it may be confused) and also hypokalaemia and hyponatraemia.

Symptomatic *hypomagnesaemia* is associated with a deficit of 0.5–1 mmol/kg; up to 160 mmol Mg^{2+} over up to 5 days may be required to replace the deficit (allowing for urinary losses). Magnesium is given initially by intravenous infusion or by intramuscular injection of **magnesium sulphate**; the intramuscular injection is painful. Plasma magnesium concentration should be measured to determine the rate and duration of infusion and the dose should be reduced in renal impairment. To prevent *recurrence of the deficit*, magnesium may be given by mouth in a dose of 24 mmol Mg^{2+} daily in divided doses; a suitable preparation is magnesium glycerophosphate tablets [not licensed, available from IDIS and Special Products]. For maintenance (e.g. in intravenous nutrition), parenteral doses of magnesium are of the order of 10–20 mmol Mg^{2+} daily (often about 12 mmol Mg^{2+} daily).

ARRHYTHMIAS. Magnesium sulphate has also been recommended for the emergency treatment of *serious arrhythmias*, especially in the presence of hypokalaemia (when hypomagnesaemia may also be present) and when salvos of rapid ventricular tachycardia show the characteristic twisting wave front known as *torsades de pointes*. The usual dose of magnesium sulphate is intravenous injection of 8 mmol Mg^{2+} over 10–15 minutes (repeated once if necessary).

MYOCARDIAL INFARCTION. Evidence suggesting a sustained reduction in mortality in patients with *suspected myocardial infarction* given an initial intravenous injection of magnesium sulphate 8 mmol Mg^{2+} over 20 minutes followed by an intravenous infusion of 65–72 mmol Mg^{2+} over the following 24 hours, has not been borne out by a larger study. Some, however, continue to hold the view that magnesium is beneficial if given immediately (and for as long as there is a likelihood of reperfusion taking place).

ECLAMPSIA AND PRE-ECLAMPSIA. Magnesium sulphate is the drug of choice for the prevention of recurrent seizures in *eclampsia*; see also Appendix 4. Regimens may vary between hospitals. Calcium gluconate injection is used for the management of magnesium toxicity.

Magnesium sulphate is also of benefit in women with *pre-eclampsia* in whom there is concern about developing eclampsia. The patient should be monitored carefully (see under Magnesium Sulphate).

MAGNESIUM SULPHATE

Indications: see notes above; constipation (section 1.6.4); severe acute asthma (section 3.1); paste for boils (section 13.10.5)

Cautions: see notes above; hepatic impairment (Appendix 2); renal impairment (Appendix 3); in severe hypomagnesaemia administer initially via controlled infusion device (preferably syringe pump); monitor blood pressure, respiratory rate, urinary output and for signs of overdosage (loss of patellar reflexes, weakness, nausea, sensation of warmth, flushing, drowsiness, double vision, and slurred speech); pregnancy (Appendix 4); **interactions:** Appendix 1 (magnesium, parenteral)

Side-effects: generally associated with hypermagnesaemia, nausea, vomiting, thirst, flushing of skin, hypotension, arrhythmias, coma, respiratory depression, drowsiness, confusion, loss of tendon reflexes, muscle weakness; colic and diarrhoea following oral administration

Dose: hypomagnesaemia, see notes above

Prevention of seizure recurrence in eclampsia, initially *by intravenous injection* over 5–15 minutes, 4 g, followed *by intravenous infusion*, 1 g/hour for at least 24 hours after last seizure; if seizure recurs, additional dose *by intravenous injection*, 2 g (4 g if body-weight over 70 kg)

Prevention of seizures in pre-eclampsia [unlicensed indication], initially *by intravenous infusion* over 5–15 minutes, 4 g followed *by intravenous infusion*, 1 g/hour for 24 hours; if seizure occurs, additional dose *by intravenous injection*, 2 g

INTRAVENOUS ADMINISTRATION. For intravenous injection concentration of magnesium sulphate should not exceed 20% (dilute 1 part of magnesium sulphate injection 50% with at least 1.5 parts of water for injections)

NOTE. Magnesium sulphate 1 g equivalent to Mg^{2+} approx. 4 mmol

Magnesium Sulphate (Non-proprietary) PoM
Injection, magnesium sulphate 50% (Mg^{2+} approx. 2 mmol /mL), net price 2-mL (1-g) amp = £2.59, 5-mL (2.5-g) amp = £2.50, 10-mL (5-g) amp = £3.35; prefilled 10-mL (5-g) syringe = £4.95

9.5.2 Phosphorus

9.5.2.1 Phosphate supplements

Oral phosphate supplements may be required in addition to vitamin D in a small minority of patients with hypophosphataemic vitamin D-resistant rickets. Diarrhoea is a common side-effect and should prompt a reduction in dosage.

Phosphate infusion is occasionally needed in alcohol dependence or in phosphate deficiency arising from use of parenteral nutrition deficient in phosphate supplements; phosphate depletion also occurs in severe diabetic ketoacidosis. For *established hypophosphataemia*, monobasic potassium phosphate may be infused at a maximum rate of 9 mmol every 12 hours. Excessive doses of phosphates may cause hypocalcaemia and metastatic calcification; it is **essential** to monitor closely plasma concentrations of calcium, phosphate, potassium, and other electrolytes.

For phosphate requirements in *total parenteral nutrition* regimens, see section 9.3.

Phosphates (Fresenius Kabi) PoM
Intravenous infusion, phosphates (providing PO_4^{3-} 100 mmol/litre), net price 500 mL (*Polyfusor*®) = £3.75.
For the treatment of moderate to severe hypophosphatemia

Phosphate-Sandoz® (HK Pharma)
Tablets, effervescent, anhydrous sodium acid phosphate 1.936 g, sodium bicarbonate 350 mg, potassium bicarbonate 315 mg, equivalent to phosphorus 500 mg (phosphate 16.1 mmol), sodium 468.8 mg (Na^+ 20.4 mmol), potassium 123 mg (K^+ 3.1 mmol). Net price 20 = £3.29. Label: 13
Dose: hypercalcaemia, up to 6 tablets daily adjusted according to response; CHILD under 5 years up to 3 tablets daily
Vitamin D-resistant hypophosphataemic osteomalacia, 4–6 tablets daily; CHILD under 5 years 2–3 tablets daily

9.5.2.2 Phosphate-binding agents

Aluminium-containing and calcium-containing preparations are used as phosphate-binding agents in the management of hyperphosphataemia complicating renal failure. Calcium-containing phosphate-binding agents are contra-indicated in hypercalcaemia or hypercalciuria. Phosphate-binding agents which contain aluminium may increase plasma aluminium in dialysis patients.

Sevelamer is licensed for the treatment of hyperphosphataemia in patients on haemodialysis.

ALUMINIUM HYDROXIDE

Indications: hyperphosphataemia; dyspepsia (section 1.1)

Cautions: hyperaluminaemia; porphyria (section 9.8.2); see also notes above; **interactions:** Appendix 1 (antacids)

Side-effects: see section 1.1.1

Aluminium Hydroxide (Non-proprietary)
Mixture (gel), about 4% w/w Al_2O_3 in water. Net price 200 mL = 41p
Dose: hyperphosphataemia, 20–100 mL according to requirements of patient
NOTE. The brand name *Aludrox*® NHS (Pfizer Consumer) is used for aluminium hydroxide mixture, net price 200 mL = £1.42

Alu-Cap® (3M)
Capsules, green/red, dried aluminium hydroxide 475 mg (low Na^+). Net price 120-cap pack = £3.75
Dose: phosphate-binding agent in renal failure, 4–20 capsules daily in divided doses with meals

CALCIUM SALTS

Indications: hyperphosphataemia

Cautions: see notes above; **interactions:** Appendix 1 (antacids, calcium salts)

Side-effects: hypercalcaemia

Adcal®, section 9.5.1.1

Calcichew®, section 9.5.1.1

Calcium-500, section 9.5.1.1

Phosex® (Vitaline)
Tablets, yellow, calcium acetate 1 g (calcium 250 mg or Ca^{2+} 6.2 mmol), net price 180-tab pack = £19.79. Label: 25
Dose: phosphate-binding agent (with meals) in renal failure, according to the requirements of the patient

SEVELAMER

Indications: hyperphosphataemia in patients on haemodialysis

Cautions: pregnancy (Appendix 4); breast-feeding (Appendix 5); gastro-intestinal disorders

Contra-indications: bowel obstruction

Side-effects: intestinal obstruction

Dose: ADULT over 18 years, initially 2.4–4.8 g daily in 3 divided doses with meals, then adjusted according to plasma-phosphate concentration

Renagel® (Genzyme) PoM

Tablets, f/c, sevelamer 800 mg, net price 180-tab pack = £122.76. Label: 25, C, with meals

9.5.3 Fluoride

Availability of adequate fluoride confers significant resistance to dental caries. It is now considered that the topical action of fluoride on enamel and plaque is more important than the systemic effect.

Where the fluoride content of the drinking water is less than 700 micrograms per litre (0.7 parts per million), daily administration of fluoride tablets or drops is a suitable means of supplementation. Systemic fluoride supplements should not be prescribed without reference to the fluoride content of the local water supply. Infants need not receive fluoride supplements until the age of 6 months.

Dentifrices which incorporate sodium fluoride or monofluorophosphate are also a convenient source of fluoride.

Individuals who are either particularly caries prone or medically compromised may be given additional protection by use of fluoride rinses or by application of fluoride gels. Rinses may be used daily or weekly; daily use of a less concentrated rinse is more effective than weekly use of a more concentrated one. High-strength gels must be applied on a regular basis under professional supervision; extreme caution is necessary to prevent the child from swallowing any excess. Less concentrated gels are available for home use. Varnishes are also available and are particularly valuable for young or disabled children since they adhere to the teeth and set in the presence of moisture.

> Fluoride tablets and oral drops are prescribable on form FP10D (GP14 in Scotland, WP10D in Wales; for details see below).
> There are also arrangements for health authorities to supply fluoride tablets in the course of pre-school dental schemes, and they may also be supplied in school dental schemes.
> Fluoride gels, mouthwashes and toothpastes are not prescribable on form FP10D (GP14 in Scotland, WP10D in Wales) .

FLUORIDES

NOTE. Sodium fluoride 2.2 mg provides approx. 1 mg fluoride ion

Indications: prophylaxis of dental caries—see notes above

Contra-indications: not for areas where drinking water is fluoridated

Side-effects: occasional white flecks on teeth with recommended doses; rarely yellowish-brown discoloration if recommended doses are exceeded

Dose: expressed as fluoride ion (F^-):

Water content less than F^- 300 micrograms/litre (0.3 parts per million), CHILD up to 6 months none; 6 months–3 years F^- 250 micrograms daily, 3–6 years F^- 500 micrograms daily, over 6 years F^- 1 mg daily

Water content between F^- 300 and 700 micrograms/litre (0.3–0.7 parts per million), CHILD up to 3 years none, 3–6 years F^- 250 micrograms daily, over 6 years F^- 500 micrograms daily

Water content above F^- 700 micrograms/litre (0.7 parts per million), supplements not advised

NOTE. These doses reflect the recommendations of the British Dental Association, the British Society of Paediatric Dentistry and the British Association for the Study of Community Dentistry (*Br Dent J* 1997; **182:** 6–7)

■ Tablets

COUNSELLING. Tablets should be sucked or dissolved in the mouth and taken preferably in the evening

En-De-Kay® (Manx)

Fluotabs 3–6 years, orange-flavoured, scored, sodium fluoride 1.1 mg (F^- 500 micrograms). Net price 200-tab pack = £1.80

Fluotabs 6+ years, orange-flavoured, scored, sodium fluoride 2.2 mg (F^- 1 mg). Net price 200-tab pack = £1.80

DENTAL PRESCRIBING ON NHS. May be prescribed as Sodium Fluoride Tablets

Fluor-a-day® (Dental Health)

Tablets, buff, sodium fluoride 1.1 mg (F^- 500 micrograms), net price 200-tab pack = £1.91; 2.2 mg (F^- 1 mg), 200-tab pack = £1.91

DENTAL PRESCRIBING ON NHS. May be prescribed as Sodium Fluoride Tablets

FluoriGard® (Colgate-Palmolive)

Tablets 0.5, purple, grape-flavoured, scored, sodium fluoride 1.1 mg (F^- 500 micrograms). Net price 200-tab pack = £1.91

Tablets 1.0, orange, orange-flavoured, scored, sodium fluoride 2.2 mg (F^- 1 mg). Net price 200-tab pack = £1.91

DENTAL PRESCRIBING ON NHS. May be prescribed as Sodium Fluoride Tablets

■ Oral drops

Note. Fluoride supplements not considered necessary below 6 months of age (see notes above)

En-De-Kay® (Manx)

Fluodrops® (= paediatric drops), sugar-free, sodium fluoride 550 micrograms (F^- 250 micrograms)/ 0.15 mL. Net price 60 mL = £1.82

DENTAL PRESCRIBING ON NHS. Corresponds to Sodium Fluoride Oral Drops DPF 0.37% equivalent to sodium fluoride 80 micrograms (F^- 36 micrograms)/drop

■ Mouthwashes

Rinse mouth for 1 minute and spit out

COUNSELLING. Avoid eating, drinking, or rinsing mouth for 15 minutes after use

Duraphat® (Colgate-Palmolive)

Weekly dental rinse (= mouthwash), blue, sodium fluoride 0.2%. Net price 150 mL = £2.42. Counselling, see above

Dose: CHILD 6 years and over, for *weekly* use, rinse with 10 mL

En-De-Kay® (Manx)

Daily fluoride mouthrinse (= mouthwash), blue, sodium fluoride 0.05%. Net price 250 mL = £1.51

Dose: CHILD 6 years and over, for *daily* use, rinse with 10 mL

Fluorinse PoM (= mouthwash), red, sodium fluoride 2%. Net price 100 mL = £3.97. Counselling, see above

Dose: CHILD 8 years and over, for *daily* use, dilute 5 drops to 10 mL of water; for *weekly* use, dilute 20 drops to 10 mL

FluoriGard® (Colgate-Palmolive)

Daily dental rinse (= mouthwash), blue, sodium fluoride 0.05%. Net price 500 mL = £3.11. Counselling, see above

Dose: CHILD 6 years and over, for *daily* use, rinse with 10 mL

■ Gels

FluoriGard® (Colgate-Palmolive)

Gel-Kam (= gel), stannous fluoride 0.4% in glycerol basis. Net price 100 mL = £3.05. Counselling, see below

Dose: ADULT and CHILD 3 years and over, for *daily* use, using a toothbrush, apply onto all tooth surfaces

COUNSELLING. Swish between teeth for 1 minute before spitting out. Avoid eating, drinking, or rinsing mouth for at least 30 minutes after use

■ Toothpastes

Duraphat® (Colgate-Palmolive) PoM

Toothpaste, sodium fluoride 0.619%. Net price 75 mL = £2.86. Counselling, see below

Dose: ADULT and ADOLESCENT over 16 years, apply 1 cm twice daily using a toothbrush

COUNSELLING. Brush teeth for 1 minute before spitting out. Avoid drinking or rinsing mouth for 30 minutes after use

9.5.4 Zinc

Zinc supplements should be given only when there is good evidence of deficiency (hypoproteinaemia spuriously lowers plasma-zinc concentration) or in zinc-losing conditions. Zinc deficiency can occur as a result of inadequate diet or malabsorption; excessive loss of zinc can occur in trauma, burns and protein-losing conditions. A zinc supplement is given until clinical improvement occurs but it may need to be continued in severe malabsorption, metabolic disease (section 9.8.1) or in zinc-losing states.

Total parenteral nutrition regimens usually include trace amounts of zinc (section 9.3). If necessary, further zinc can be added to intravenous feeding regimens. A suggested dose for intravenous nutrition is elemental zinc 6.5 mg (Zn^{2+} 100 micromol) daily.

ZINC SULPHATE

Indications: zinc deficiency or supplementation in zinc-losing conditions

Cautions: acute renal failure (may accumulate); **interactions:** Appendix 1 (zinc)

Side-effects: abdominal pain, dyspepsia, nausea, vomiting, diarrhoea, gastric irritation, gastritis; irritability, headache, lethargy

Dose: see preparation below and notes above

Zinc Sulphate (Non-proprietary) PoM

Injection, zinc sulphate 14.6 mg/mL (zinc 50 micromol/mL), net price 10 mL vial = £2.50

Solvazinc® (Provalis)

Effervescent tablets, yellow-white, zinc sulphate monohydrate 125 mg (45 mg zinc). Net price 30 = £4.32. Label: 13, 21

Dose: ADULT and CHILD over 30 kg, 1 tablet in water 1–3 times daily after food; CHILD under 10 kg, ½ tablet daily; 10–30 kg, ½ tablet 1–3 times daily

9.6 Vitamins

Vitamins are used for the prevention and treatment of specific deficiency states or where the diet is known to be inadequate; they may be prescribed in the NHS to prevent or treat deficiency but not as dietary supplements.

Their use as general 'pick-me-ups' is of unproven value and, in the case of preparations containing vitamin A or D, may actually be harmful if patients take more than the prescribed dose. The 'fad' for mega-vitamin therapy with water-soluble vitamins, such as ascorbic acid and pyridoxine, is unscientific and can be harmful.

Dietary reference values for vitamins are available in the Department of Health publication:

Dietary Reference Values for Food Energy and Nutrients for the United Kingdom: Report of the Panel on Dietary Reference Values of the Committee on Medical Aspects of Food Policy. *Report on Health and Social Subjects 41*. London: HMSO, 1991

DENTAL PATIENTS. Most patients who develop a nutritional deficiency despite an adequate intake of vitamins have malabsorption and if this is suspected the patient should be referred to a medical practitioner.

It is unjustifiable to treat stomatitis or glossitis with mixtures of vitamin preparations; this delays diagnosis and correct treatment.

9.6.1 Vitamin A

Deficiency of vitamin A (retinol) is associated with ocular defects (particularly xerophthalmia) and an increased susceptibility to infections, but deficiency is rare in the UK (even in disorders of fat absorption).

Massive overdose can cause rough skin, dry hair, an enlarged liver, and a raised erythrocyte sedimentation rate and raised serum calcium and serum alkaline phosphatase concentrations.

In view of evidence suggesting that high levels of vitamin A may cause birth defects, women who are (or may become) pregnant are advised not to take vitamin A supplements (including tablets and fish-liver oil drops), except on the advice of a doctor or an antenatal clinic; nor should they eat liver or products such as liver paté or liver sausage.

VITAMIN A

(Retinol)

Indications: see notes above

Cautions: see notes above; **interactions:** Appendix 1 (vitamins)

Side-effects: see notes above

Dose: see notes above and under preparations

■ Vitamins A and D

Halibut-liver Oil (Non-proprietary)
Capsules, vitamin A 4000 units [also contains vitamin D]. Net price 20 = 18p

Vitamins A and D (Non-proprietary)
Capsules, vitamin A 4000 units, vitamin D 400 units. Net price 20 = 64p

Halycitrol® (LAB) NHS
Emulsion, vitamin A 4600 units, vitamin D 380 units/5 mL. Net price 114 mL = £1.77
Dose: 5 mL daily but see notes above

9.6.2 Vitamin B group

Deficiency of the B vitamins, other than deficiency of vitamin B_{12} (section 9.1.2), is rare in the UK and is usually treated by preparations containing thiamine (B_1), riboflavin (B_2), and nicotinamide, which is used in preference to nicotinic acid, as it does not cause vasodilatation. Other members (or substances traditionally classified as members) of the vitamin B complex such as aminobenzoic acid, biotin, choline, inositol, and pantothenic acid or panthenol may be included in vitamin B preparations but there is no evidence of their value.

The severe deficiency states Wernicke's encephalopathy and Korsakoff's psychosis, especially as seen in chronic alcoholism, are best treated initially by the parenteral administration of B vitamins (*Pabrinex*®), followed by oral administration of thiamine in the longer term. Anaphylaxis has been reported with parenteral B vitamins (see CSM advice, below).

As with other vitamins of the B group, pyridoxine (B_6) deficiency is rare, but it may occur during isoniazid therapy (section 5.1.9) and is characterised by peripheral neuritis. High doses of pyridoxine are given in some metabolic disorders, such as hyperoxaluria, and it is also used in sideroblastic anaemia (section 9.1.3). There is evidence to suggest that pyridoxine in a dose not exceeding 100 mg daily may provide some benefit in premenstrual syndrome. It has been tried for a wide variety of other disorders, but there is little sound evidence to support the claims of efficacy, and overdosage induces toxic effects.

Nicotinic acid inhibits the synthesis of cholesterol and triglyceride (see section 2.12). Folic acid and vitamin B_{12} are used in the treatment of megaloblastic anaemia (section 9.1.2). Folinic acid (available as calcium folinate) is used in association with cytotoxic therapy (section 8.1).

RIBOFLAVIN

(Riboflavine, vitamin B_2)

Indications: see notes above

■ Preparations

Injections of vitamins B and C, see under Thiamine

■ Oral vitamin B complex preparations

See below

THIAMINE

(Vitamin B_1)

> **CSM advice.** Since potentially serious allergic adverse reactions may occur during, or shortly after, parenteral administration, the CSM has recommended that:
>
> 1. Use be restricted to patients in whom parenteral treatment is essential;
> 2. Intravenous injections should be administered slowly (over 10 minutes);
> 3. Facilities for treating anaphylaxis should be available when administered.

Indications: see notes above

Cautions: anaphylactic shock may occasionally follow injection (see CSM advice above)

Dose: mild chronic deficiency, 10–25 mg daily; severe deficiency, 200–300 mg daily

Thiamine (Non-proprietary)
Tablets, thiamine hydrochloride 50 mg, net price 20 = 80p; 100 mg, 20 = £1.23
Brands include *Benerva*® NHS

Pabrinex® (Link) PoM
I/M High potency injection, for intramuscular use only, ascorbic acid 500 mg, nicotinamide 160 mg, pyridoxine hydrochloride 50 mg, riboflavin 4 mg, thiamine hydrochloride 250 mg/7 mL. Net price 7 mL (in 2 amps) = £1.96
I/V High potency injection, for intravenous use only, ascorbic acid 500 mg, anhydrous glucose 1 g, nicotinamide 160 mg, pyridoxine hydrochloride 50 mg, riboflavin 4 mg, thiamine hydrochloride 250 mg/10 mL. Net price 10 mL (in 2 amps) = £1.96
Parenteral vitamins B and C for rapid correction of severe depletion or malabsorption (e.g. in alcoholism, after acute infections, postoperatively, or in psychiatric states), maintenance of vitamins B and C in chronic intermittent haemodialysis
Dose: see CSM advice above
Coma or delirium from alcohol, from opioids, or from barbiturates, collapse following narcosis, by intravenous injection or infusion of *I/V High potency*, 2–3 pairs every 8 hours
Psychosis following narcosis or electroconvulsive therapy, toxicity from acute infections, by intravenous injection or infusion of *I/V High potency* or by deep intramuscular injection into the gluteal muscle of *I/M High potency*, 1 pair twice daily for up to 7 days
Haemodialysis, by intravenous infusion of *I/V High potency* (in sodium chloride intravenous infusion 0.9%) 1 pair every 2 weeks

■ Oral vitamin B complex preparations

See below

PYRIDOXINE HYDROCHLORIDE

(Vitamin B_6)

Indications: see under Dose

Cautions: interactions: Appendix 1 (vitamins)

Dose: deficiency states, 20–50 mg up to 3 times daily

Isoniazid neuropathy, prophylaxis 10 mg daily [or 20 mg daily if suitable product not available]; therapeutic, 50 mg three times daily

Idiopathic sideroblastic anaemia, 100–400 mg daily in divided doses

Premenstrual syndrome, 50–100 mg daily (see notes above)

> **Important.** Concerns about possible toxicity resulting from prolonged use of pyridoxine (vitamin B_6) at high dosage have not yet been resolved. The Royal Pharmaceutical Society of Great Britain has advised that pharmacists should consider how to advise customers requesting preparations containing higher doses and that they should decide their own policy on the display of products containing more than 10 mg per daily dose of pyridoxine.

Pyridoxine (Non-proprietary)

Tablets, pyridoxine hydrochloride 10 mg, net price 20 = 34p; 20 mg, 20 = 34p; 50 mg, 20 = 38p

■ Injections of vitamins B and C

See under Thiamine

NICOTINAMIDE

Indications: see notes above; acne vulgaris, see section 13.6.1

Nicotinamide (Non-proprietary)

Tablets, nicotinamide 50 mg. Net price 20 = £1.37

■ Injections of vitamins B and C

See under Thiamine

Oral vitamin B complex preparations

NOTE. Other multivitamin preparations are in section 9.6.7.

Vitamin B Tablets, Compound

Tablets, nicotinamide 15 mg, riboflavin 1 mg, thiamine hydrochloride 1 mg. Net price 20 = 7p

Dose: prophylactic, 1–2 tablets daily

Vitamin B Tablets, Compound, Strong

Tablets, brown, f/c or s/c, nicotinamide 20 mg, pyridoxine hydrochloride 2 mg, riboflavin 2 mg, thiamine hydrochloride 5 mg. Net price 28-tab pack = 93p

Dose: treatment of vitamin-B deficiency, 1–2 tablets 3 times daily

DENTAL PRESCRIBING ON NHS. Vitamin B Tablets, Compound Strong may be prescribed

Vigranon B® (Wallace Mfg) NHS

Syrup, thiamine hydrochloride 5 mg, riboflavin 2 mg, nicotinamide 20 mg, pyridoxine hydrochloride 2 mg, panthenol 3 mg/5 mL. Net price 150 mL = £2.41

Other compounds

Potassium aminobenzoate has been used in the treatment of various disorders associated with excessive fibrosis such as scleroderma but its therapeutic value is **doubtful**.

Potaba® (Glenwood)

Capsules, potassium aminobenzoate 500 mg. Net price 20 = £1.59. Label: 21

Tablets, potassium aminobenzoate 500 mg. Net price 20 = £1.12. Label: 21

Envules® (= powder in sachets), potassium aminobenzoate 3 g. Net price 40 sachets = £17.21. Label: 13, 21

Dose: Peyronie's disease, scleroderma, 12 g daily in divided doses after food

9.6.3 Vitamin C

(Ascorbic acid)

Vitamin C therapy is essential in scurvy, but less florid manifestations of vitamin C deficiency are commonly found, especially in the elderly. It is rarely necessary to prescribe more than 100 mg daily except early in the treatment of scurvy.

Severe scurvy causes gingival swelling and bleeding margins as well as petechiae on the skin. This is, however, exceedingly rare and a patient with these signs is more likely to have leukaemia. Investigation should not be delayed by a trial period of vitamin treatment.

Claims that vitamin C ameliorates colds or promotes wound healing have not been proved.

ASCORBIC ACID

Indications: prevention and treatment of scurvy

Dose: prophylactic, 25–75 mg daily; therapeutic, not less than 250 mg daily in divided doses

Ascorbic Acid (Non-proprietary)

Tablets, ascorbic acid 50 mg, net price 20 = 84p; 100 mg, 20 = 18p; 200 mg, 20 = 22p; 500 mg (label: 24), 20 = £1.63

Brands include *Redoxon*® NHS

DENTAL PRESCRIBING ON NHS. Ascorbic Acid Tablets may be prescribed

Injection, ascorbic acid 100 mg/mL. Net price 5-mL amp = £2.51

Available from UCB Pharma

■ For children's welfare vitamin drops containing vitamin C with A and D

See vitamin A

9.6.4 Vitamin D

NOTE. The term Vitamin D is used for a range of compounds which possess the property of preventing or curing rickets. They include ergocalciferol (calciferol, vitamin D_2), colecalciferol (vitamin D_3), dihydrotachysterol, alfacalcidol (1α-hydroxycholecalciferol), and calcitriol (1,25-dihydroxycholecalciferol).

Simple vitamin D deficiency can be prevented by taking an oral supplement of only 10 micrograms (400 units) of ergocalciferol (calciferol, vitamin D_2) daily. Vitamin D deficiency is not uncommon in

Asians consuming unleavened bread and in the elderly living alone and can be prevented by taking an oral supplement of 20 micrograms (800 units) of ergocalciferol daily. Since there is no plain tablet of this strength available **calcium and ergocalciferol tablets** can be given (although the calcium is unnecessary).

Vitamin D deficiency caused by *intestinal malabsorption* or *chronic liver disease* usually requires vitamin D in pharmacological doses, such as **calciferol tablets** up to 1 mg (40 000 units) daily; the hypocalcaemia of *hypoparathyroidism* often requires doses of up to 2.5 mg (100 000 units) daily in order to achieve normocalcaemia.

Vitamin D requires hydroxylation by the kidney to its active form therefore the hydroxylated derivatives **alfacalcidol** or **calcitriol** should be prescribed if patients with *severe renal impairment* require vitamin D therapy. Calcitriol is also licensed for the management of postmenopausal osteoporosis.

Paricalcitol, a synthetic vitamin D analogue, is licensed for the prevention and treatment of secondary hyperparathyroidism associated with chronic renal failure.

Important. All patients receiving pharmacological doses of vitamin D should have the plasma-calcium concentration checked at intervals (initially weekly) and whenever nausea or vomiting are present. Breast milk from women taking pharmacological doses of vitamin D may cause hypercalcaemia if given to an infant.

ERGOCALCIFEROL

(Calciferol, Vitamin D_2)

Indications: see notes above

Cautions: take care to ensure correct dose in infants; monitor plasma calcium in patients receiving high doses and in renal impairment; **interactions**: Appendix 1 (vitamins)

Contra-indications: hypercalcaemia; metastatic calcification

Side-effects: symptoms of overdosage include anorexia, lassitude, nausea and vomiting, diarrhoea, weight loss, polyuria, sweating, headache, thirst, vertigo, and raised concentrations of calcium and phosphate in plasma and urine

Dose: see notes above

■ Daily supplements

NOTE. There is no plain vitamin D tablet available for treating simple deficiency (see notes above). Alternatives include vitamins capsules (see 9.6.7), preparations of vitamins A and D (see 9.6.1), and calcium and ergocalciferol tablets (see below).

Calcium and Ergocalciferol (Non-proprietary) (Calcium and Vitamin D)
Tablets, calcium lactate 300 mg, calcium phosphate 150 mg (calcium 97 mg or Ca^{2+} 2.4 mmol), ergocalciferol 10 micrograms (400 units). Net price 28-tab pack = £1.85. Counselling, crush before administration or may be chewed

Adcal-D$_3$® (Strakan)
Tablets (chewable), calcium carbonate 1.5 g (calcium 600 mg or Ca^{2+} 15.1 mmol), colecalciferol 10 micrograms (400 units), net price 100-tab pack = £7.25. Label: 24

Cacit® D3 (Procter & Gamble Pharm.)
Granules, effervescent, calcium carbonate 1.25 g (calcium 500 mg or Ca^{2+} 12.6 mmol), colecalciferol 11 micrograms (440 units)/sachet. Net price 30-sachet pack = £5.35. Label: 13

Calceos® (Provalis)
Tablets (chewable), calcium carbonate 1.25 g (calcium 500 mg or Ca^{2+} 12.6 mmol), colecalciferol 10 micrograms (400 units). Net price 60-tab pack = £5.10. Label: 24

Calcichew-D$_3$® (Shire)
Tablets (chewable), calcium carbonate 1.25 g (calcium 500 mg or Ca^{2+} 12.6 mmol), colecalciferol 5 micrograms (200 units). Net price 100-tab pack = £15.02. Label: 24
Excipients: include aspartame (section 9.4.1)

Calcichew-D$_3$® Forte (Shire)
Tablets (chewable), calcium carbonate 1.25 g (calcium 500 mg or Ca^{2+} 12.6 mmol), colecalciferol 10 micrograms (400 units). Net price 100-tab pack = £7.50. Label: 24
Excipients: include aspartame (section 9.4.1)

Calfovit D3® (Trinity) PoM
Powder, calcium phosphate 3.1 g (calcium 1.2 g or Ca^{2+} 30 mmol), colecalciferol 20 micrograms (800 units), net price 30-sachet pack = £4.32. Label: 13, 21

■ Pharmacological strengths (see notes above)

NOTE. The BP directs that when vitamin D_2 is prescribed or demanded, ergocalciferol should be dispensed or supplied; when calciferol or vitamin D is prescribed or demanded, ergocalciferol or colecalciferol should be dispensed or supplied

Ergocalciferol (Non-proprietary)
Tablets, ergocalciferol 250 micrograms (10 000 units), net price 20 = £4.27; 1.25 mg (50 000 units) may also be available
IMPORTANT. When the strength of the tablets ordered or prescribed is not clear, the intention of the prescriber with respect to the strength (expressed in micrograms or milligrams per tablet) should be ascertained.
Injection PoM, ergocalciferol, 7.5 mg (300 000 units)/mL in oil, net price 1-mL amp = £5.92, 2-mL amp = £7.07

ALFACALCIDOL

(1α-Hydroxycholecalciferol)

Indications: see notes above

Cautions: see under Ergocalciferol

Contra-indications: see under Ergocalciferol

Side-effects: see under Ergocalciferol

Dose: *by mouth or by intravenous injection* over 30 seconds, ADULT and CHILD over 20 kg, initially 1 microgram daily (elderly 500 nanograms), adjusted to avoid hypercalcaemia; maintenance, usually 0.25–1 microgram daily; NEONATE and PRETERM NEONATE initially 50–100 nanograms/kg daily, CHILD under 20 kg initially 50 nanograms/kg daily

Alfacalcidol (Non-proprietary) PoM
Capsules, alfacalcidol 250 nanograms, net price 30-cap pack = £5.86; 500 nanograms 30-cap pack = £9.61; 1 microgram 30-cap pack = £14.65

One-Alpha® (Leo) PoM
Capsules, alfacalcidol 250 nanograms (white), net price 30-cap pack = £3.37; 500 nanograms (red),

30-cap pack = £6.27; 1 microgram (brown), 30-cap pack = £8.75
Excipients: include sesame oil

Oral drops, sugar-free, alfacalcidol 2 micrograms/mL (1 drop contains approx. 100 nanograms), net price 10 mL = £22.49
Excipients: include alcohol
NOTE. The concentration of alfacalcidol in *One-Alpha*® *drops* is **10 times greater** than that of the former presentation *One-Alpha*® *solution*.

Injection, alfacalcidol 2 micrograms/mL, net price 0.5-mL amp = £2.16, 1-mL amp = £4.11
NOTE. Contains propylene glycol and should be used with caution in small preterm neonates

CALCITRIOL

(1,25-Dihydroxycholecalciferol)

Indications: see notes above

Cautions: see under Ergocalciferol; monitor plasma calcium, phosphate, and creatinine during dosage titration

Contra-indications: see under Ergocalciferol

Side-effects: see under Ergocalciferol

Dose: *by mouth*, renal osteodystrophy, initially 250 nanograms daily, or on alternate days (in patients with normal or only slightly reduced plasma-calcium concentration), increased if necessary in steps of 250 nanograms at intervals of 2–4 weeks; usual dose 0.5–1 microgram daily; CHILD not established

Established postmenopausal osteoporosis, 250 nanograms twice daily (monitor plasma-calcium concentration and creatinine, consult product literature)

by intravenous injection (or injection through catheter after haemodialysis), hypocalcaemia in dialysis patients with chronic renal failure, initially 500 nanograms (approx. 10 nanograms/kg) 3 times a week, increased if necessary in steps of 250–500 nanograms at intervals of 2–4 weeks; usual dose 0.5–3 micrograms 3 times a week; CHILD not established

Moderate to severe secondary hyperparathyroidism in dialysis patients, initially 0.5–4 micrograms 3 times a week, increased if necessary in steps of 250–500 nanograms at intervals of 2–4 weeks; max. 8 micrograms 3 times a week

Calcitriol (Non-proprietary) PoM

Capsules, calcitriol 250 nanograms, net price 30-cap pack = £6.18; 500 nanograms, 30-cap pack = £11.05

Rocaltrol® (Roche) PoM

Capsules, calcitriol 250 nanograms (red/white), net price 20 = £3.83; 500 nanograms (red), 20 = £6.85

Calcijex® (Abbott) PoM

Injection, calcitriol 1 microgram/mL, net price 1-mL amp = £5.14; 2 micrograms/mL, 1-mL amp = £10.28

COLECALCIFEROL

(Cholecalciferol, vitamin D_3)

Indications: see under Ergocalciferol—alternative to ergocalciferol in calciferol tablets and injection

Cautions: see under Ergocalciferol

Contra-indications: see under Ergocalciferol

Side-effects: see under Ergocalciferol

DIHYDROTACHYSTEROL

Indications: see under Ergocalciferol

Cautions: see under Ergocalciferol

Contra-indications: see under Ergocalciferol

Side-effects: see under Ergocalciferol

AT 10® (Intrapharm)

Oral solution, dihydrotachysterol 250 micrograms/mL. Net price 15-mL dropper bottle = £22.87
Excipients: include arachis (peanut) oil
Dose: acute, chronic, and latent forms of hypocalcaemic tetany due to hypoparathyroidism, consult product literature

PARICALCITOL

Indications: see notes above

Cautions: monitor plasma calcium and phosphate during dose titration and at least monthly when stabilised; monitor parathyroid hormone concentration; pregnancy (Appendix 4); breast-feeding (Appendix 5); **interactions:** Appendix 1 (vitamins)

Contra-indications: see under Ergocalciferol

Side-effects: see under Ergocalciferol; also hypercalcaemia, hyperphosphataemia; pruritus; taste disturbance

Dose: *by slow intravenous injection*—consult product literature; max. initial dose 40 micrograms

Zemplar® (Abbott) ▼ PoM

Injection, paricalcitol 5 micrograms/mL, net price 5 × 1-mL amp = £62.00, 5 × 2-mL amp = £124.00
Excipients: include propylene glycol

9.6.5 Vitamin E

(Tocopherols)

The daily requirement of vitamin E has not been well defined but is probably about 3 to 15 mg daily. There is little evidence that oral supplements of vitamin E are essential in adults, even where there is fat malabsorption secondary to cholestasis. In young children with congenital cholestasis, abnormally low vitamin E concentrations may be found in association with neuromuscular abnormalities, which usually respond only to the parenteral administration of vitamin E.

Vitamin E has been tried for various other conditions but there is little scientific evidence of its value.

ALPHA TOCOPHERYL ACETATE

Indications: see notes above

Cautions: predisposition to thrombosis; increased risk of necrotising enterocolitis in neonate weighing less than 1.5 kg

Side-effects: diarrhoea and abdominal pain with doses more than 1 g daily

Vitamin E Suspension (Cambridge)

Suspension, alpha tocopheryl acetate 500 mg/5 mL. Net price 100 mL = £17.23
Dose: malabsorption in cystic fibrosis, 100–200 mg daily; CHILD under 1 year 50 mg daily; 1 year and over, 100 mg daily
Malabsorption in abetalipoproteinaemia, ADULT and CHILD 50–100 mg/kg daily
Malabsorption in chronic cholestasis, INFANT 150–200 mg/kg daily

NOTE. Tablets containing tocopheryl acetate 100 mg are available on a named-patient basis from Bell and Croyden (*Ephynal*®)

9.6.6 Vitamin K

Vitamin K is necessary for the production of blood clotting factors and proteins necessary for the normal calcification of bone.

Because vitamin K is fat soluble, patients with fat malabsorption, especially in biliary obstruction or hepatic disease, may become deficient. For oral administration to prevent vitamin-K deficiency in malabsorption syndromes, a water-soluble preparation, **menadiol sodium phosphate** must be used; the usual dose is about 10 mg daily.

Oral coumarin anticoagulants act by interfering with vitamin K metabolism in the hepatic cells and their effects can be antagonised by giving vitamin K; for British Society for Haematology Guidelines, see section 2.8.2.

VITAMIN K DEFICIENCY BLEEDING. Neonates are relatively deficient in vitamin K and those who do not receive supplements of vitamin K are at risk of serious bleeds including intracranial bleeding. The Chief Medical Officer and the Chief Nursing Officer have recommended that all newborn babies should receive vitamin K to prevent vitamin K deficiency bleeding (haemorrhagic disease of the newborn). An appropriate regimen should be selected after discussion with parents in the antenatal period.

Vitamin K (as **phytomenadione**) 1 mg may be given by a single intramuscular injection at birth; this prevents vitamin K deficiency bleeding in virtually all babies. Fears about the safety of parenteral vitamin K appear to be unfounded.

Alternatively, vitamin K may be given by mouth, and arrangements must be in place to ensure the appropriate regimen is followed. Two doses of a colloidal (mixed micelle) preparation of phytomenadione 2 mg should be given in the first week. For breast-fed babies, a third dose of phytomenadione 2 mg is given at 1 month of age; the third dose is omitted in formula-fed babies because formula feeds contain vitamin K.

MENADIOL SODIUM PHOSPHATE

Indications: see notes above

Cautions: G6PD deficiency (section 9.1.5) and vitamin E deficiency (risk of haemolysis); **interactions:** Appendix 1 (vitamins)

Contra-indications: neonates and infants, late pregnancy

Dose: see notes above

Menadiol Phosphate (Cambridge)
Tablets, menadiol sodium phosphate equivalent to 10 mg of menadiol phosphate. Net price 100-tab pack = £37.34

PHYTOMENADIONE

(Vitamin K_1)

Indications: see notes above

Cautions: intravenous injections should be given very slowly (see also below); pregnancy (Appendix 4); **interactions:** Appendix 1 (vitamins)

Dose: see notes above and section 2.8.2

Konakion® (Roche) PoM
Tablets, s/c, phytomenadione 10 mg, net price 10-tab pack = £1.65. To be chewed or allowed to dissolve slowly in the mouth (Label: 24)

Injection (Konakion® Neonatal), phytomenadione 2 mg/mL, net price 0.5-mL amp = 21p
Excipients: include polyoxyl castor oil (risk of anaphylaxis, see Excipients, p. 2)
NOTE. *Konakion® Neonatal* is for use in healthy neonates of over 36 weeks gestation; for intramuscular injection only

■ Colloidal formulation

Konakion® MM (Roche) PoM
Injection, phytomenadione 10 mg/mL in a mixed micelles vehicle. Net price 1-mL amp = 40p
Excipients: include glycocholic acid 54.6 mg/amp, lecithin
CAUTIONS. reduce dose in elderly; liver impairment (glycocholic acid may displace bilirubin); reports of anaphylactoid reactions
NOTE. *Konakion® MM* may be administered by slow intravenous injection or by intravenous infusion in glucose 5% (see Appendix 6); **not** for intramuscular injection

Konakion® MM Paediatric (Roche) PoM
Injection, phytomenadione 10 mg/mL in a mixed micelles vehicle. Net price 0.2-mL amp = £1.44
Excipients: include glycocholic acid 10.9 mg/amp, lecithin
CAUTIONS. parenteral administration in neonate of less than 2.5 kg (increased risk of kernicterus)
NOTE. *Konakion® MM Paediatric* may be administered *by mouth* or *by intramuscular injection* or *by intravenous injection*

9.6.7 Multivitamin preparations

Vitamins
Capsules, ascorbic acid 15 mg, nicotinamide 7.5 mg, riboflavin 500 micrograms, thiamine hydrochloride 1 mg, vitamin A 2500 units, vitamin D 300 units. Net price 20 = 23p

Abidec® (Chefaro UK)
Drops, vitamins A, B group, C, and D. Net price 25 mL (with dropper) = £1.84
Excipients: include arachis (peanut) oil

Dalivit® (LPC)
Oral drops, vitamins A, B group, C, and D, net price 25 mL = £1.60, 50 mL = £2.85

Vitamin and mineral supplements and adjuncts to synthetic diets

Forceval® (Alliance)
Capsules, brown/red, vitamins (ascorbic acid 60 mg, biotin 100 micrograms, cyanocobalamin 3 micrograms, folic acid 400 micrograms, nicotinamide 18 mg, pantothenic acid 4 mg, pyridoxine 2 mg, riboflavin 1.6 mg, thiamine 1.2 mg, vitamin A 2500 units, vitamin D_2 400 units, vitamin E 10 mg, minerals and trace elements (calcium 100 mg, chromium 200 micrograms, copper 2 mg, iodine 140 micrograms, iron 12 mg, magnesium 30 mg, manganese 3 mg, molybdenum 250 micrograms, phosphorus 77 mg, potassium 4 mg, selenium 50 micrograms, zinc 15 mg). Net price 30-cap pack = £4.94, 45-cap pack = £6.47; 90-cap pack = £11.93
Dose: vitamin and mineral deficiency and as adjunct in synthetic diets, 1 capsule daily

Junior capsules, brown, vitamins (ascorbic acid 25 mg, biotin 50 micrograms, cyanocobalamin 2 micrograms, folic acid 100 micrograms, nicotinamide 7.5 mg, pantothenic acid 2 mg, pyridoxine 1 mg, riboflavin 1 mg, thiamine 1.5 mg, vitamin A 1250 units, vitamin D_2 200 units, vitamin E 5 mg, vitamin K_1 25 micrograms), minerals and trace elements (chromium 50 micrograms, copper 1 mg, iodine 75 micrograms, iron 5 mg, magnesium 1 mg, manganese 1.25 mg, molybdenum 50 micrograms, selenium 25 micrograms, zinc 5 mg). Net price 30-cap pack = £3.52, 60-cap pack = £6.69
Dose: vitamin and mineral deficiency and as adjunct in synthetic diets, CHILD over 5 years, 2 capsules daily

Ketovite® (Paines & Byrne)
Tablets PoM, yellow, ascorbic acid 16.6 mg, riboflavin 1 mg, thiamine hydrochloride 1 mg, pyridoxine hydrochloride 330 micrograms, nicotinamide 3.3 mg, calcium pantothenate 1.16 mg, alpha tocopheryl acetate 5 mg, inositol 50 mg, biotin 170 micrograms, folic acid 250 micrograms, acetomenaphthone 500 micrograms. Net price 100-tab pack = £4.17
Dose: prevention of vitamin deficiency in disorders of carbohydrate or amino-acid metabolism and adjunct in restricted, specialised, or synthetic diets, 1 tablet 3 times daily; use with *Ketovite*® *Liquid* for complete vitamin supplementation
Liquid, pink, sugar-free, vitamin A 2500 units, ergocalciferol 400 units, choline chloride 150 mg, cyanocobalamin 12.5 micrograms/5 mL. Net price 150-mL pack = £2.70
Dose: prevention of vitamin deficiency in disorders of carbohydrate or amino-acid metabolism and adjunct in restricted, specialised, or synthetic diets, 5 mL daily; use with *Ketovite*® *Tablets* for complete vitamin supplementation

Vivioptal® (Pharma-Global)
Capsules, brown, vitamins (biotin 50 micrograms, calcium ascorbate 60 mg, colecalciferol 400 units, cyanocobalamin 3 micrograms, dexpanthenol 10 mg, folic acid 400 micrograms, inositol 30 mg, nicotinamide 25 mg, pyridoxine 6.08 mg, riboflavin 3 mg, rutoside 20 mg, thiamine nitrate 5 mg, vitamin A 5000 units, vitamin E 10 mg), minerals and trace elements (calcium hydrogen phosphate 35 mg, cobalt sulphate 100 micrograms, copper sulphate 500 micrograms, iron 3.25 mg, magnesium glycerophosphate 40 mg, manganese sulphate 500 micrograms, potassium sulphate 8 mg, sodium molybdate 80 micrograms, zinc oxide 500 micrograms); also contains adenosine, choline hydrogen tartrate, ethyl linoleate, lecithin, lysine hydrochloride, and orotic acid, net price 30-cap pack = £5.62
Dose: vitamin and mineral deficiency and as an adjunct in synthetic diets, 1 capsule daily
Excipients: include arachis (peanut) oil

9.7 Bitters and tonics

Mixtures containing simple and aromatic bitters, such as alkaline gentian mixture, are traditional remedies for loss of appetite. All depend on suggestion.

Gentian [illegible]ine, BP
(Alkaline Ge[illegible]lution)
Mixture, co[illegible]mpound gentian infusion 10%, sodium [illegible] 5% in a suitable vehicle. Extemporaneo[illegible]ions should be recently prepared accord[illegible] following formula: concentrated com[illegible]entian infusion 1 mL, sodium bicarbona[illegible], double-strength chloroform water 5[illegible]ter to 10 [illegible]
Dose: 1[illegible]L 3 times da[illegible] water before [illegible]

Effico® (P[illegible]est) NHS
Tonic, orange-red, thiami[illegible]ydrochloride 180 micrograms, nicotinam[illegible]e 2 mg, ca[illegible] 20.2 mg, compound gentian [illegible]on 0.31[illegible] 5 mL. Net price 300-mL pack [illegible]2.46, 500[illegible] pack = £3.[illegible]

Labiton® (LA[illegible]) NHS
Tonic, brow[illegible]hiamine hydrochloride 375 micrograms, caff[illegible].5 mg, kola nut dried extract 3.025 mg, alco[illegible]1.4 mL/5 mL. Net price 200 mL = £2.62

Metatone® (W-L) [illegible]
Tonic, thiamine hyd[illegible]loride 500 micrograms, calcium glycerophos[illegible]te 45.6 mg, manganese glycerophosphate 5.7[illegible], potassium glycerophosphate 45.6 mg, sodium glycerophosphate 22.8 mg/5 mL. Net price [illegible]0 mL = £2.79

9.8 Metabolic disorders

This section covers drugs used in metabolic disorders and not readily classified elsewhere.

9.8.1 Drugs used in metabolic disorders

Wilson's disease

Penicillamine (see also section 10.1.3) is used in Wilson's disease (hepatolenticular degeneration) to aid the elimination of copper ions. See below for other indications.

Trientine is used for the treatment of Wilson's disease only in patients intolerant of penicillamine; it is **not** an alternative to penicillamine for rheumatoid arthritis or cystinuria. Penicillamine-induced systemic lupus erythematosus may not resolve on transfer to trientine.

Zinc prevents the absorption of copper in Wilson's disease. Symptomatic patients should be treated initially with a chelating agent because zinc has a slow onset of action. When transferring from chelating treatment to zinc maintenance therapy, chelating treatment should be co-administered for 2–3 weeks until zinc takes maximum effect.

PENICILLAMINE

Indications: see under Dose below

Cautions: see section 10.1.3

Contra-indications: see section 10.1.3

Side-effects: see section 10.1.3

Dose: Wilson's disease, 1.5–2 g daily in divided doses before food; max. 2 g daily for 1 year; maintenance 0.75–1 g daily; ELDERLY 20 mg/kg daily in divided doses adjusted according to response; CHILD up to 12 years, minimum 500 mg daily in divided doses adjusted according to response

Autoimmune hepatitis (used rarely; after disease controlled with corticosteroids), initially 500 mg daily in divided doses increased slowly over 3 months; usual maintenance dose 1.25 g daily; ELDERLY not recommended

Cystinuria, therapeutic, 1–3 g daily in divided doses before food, adjusted to maintain urinary cystine below 200 mg/litre; prophylactic (maintain urinary cystine below 300 mg/litre) 0.5–1 g at bedtime; maintain adequate fluid intake (at least 3 litres daily); CHILD and ELDERLY minimum dose to maintain urinary cystine below 200 mg/litre

Severe active rheumatoid arthritis, section 10.1.3

Copper and lead poisoning, see Emergency Treatment of Poisoning

■ Preparations

Section 10.1.3

TRIENTINE DIHYDROCHLORIDE

Indications: Wilson's disease in patients intolerant of penicillamine

Cautions: see notes above; pregnancy (Appendix 4); **interactions:** Appendix 1 (trientine)

Side-effects: nausea, rash; rarely anaemia

Dose: 1.2–2.4 g daily in 2–4 divided doses before food; CHILD initially 0.6–1.5 g daily in 2–4 divided doses before food, adjusted according to response

Trientine Dihydrochloride (Univar) PoM
Capsules, trientine dihydrochloride 300 mg. Label: 6, 22

NOTE. The CSM has requested that in addition to the usual CSM reporting request, special records should also be kept by the pharmacist

ZINC ACETATE

Indications: Wilson's disease (initiated under specialist supervision)

Cautions: portal hypertension (risk of hepatic decompensation when switching from chelating agent); monitor full blood count and serum cholesterol; pregnancy (Appendix 4); **interactions:** Appendix 1 (zinc)

Contra-indications: breast-feeding

Side-effects: gastric irritation (usually transient; may be reduced if first dose taken mid-morning or with a little protein); *less commonly* sideroblastic anaemia and leucopenia

Dose: dose expressed as elemental zinc

Wilson's disease, 50 mg 3 times daily (max. 50 mg 5 times daily), adjusted according to response; CHILD 1–6 years, 25 mg twice daily; 6–16 years, body-weight under 57 kg, 25 mg 3 times daily, body-weight over 57 kg, 50 mg 3 times daily; ADOLESCENT 16–18 years, 50 mg 3 times daily

Wilzin® (Orphan Europe) ▼ PoM
Capsules, zinc (as acetate) 25 mg (blue), net price 250-cap pack = £123.00; 50 mg (orange), 250-cap pack = £233.00. Label: 23

Carnitine deficiency

Carnitine is available for the management of primary carnitine deficiency due to inborn errors of metabolism or of secondary deficiency in haemodialysis patients.

CARNITINE

Indications: primary and secondary carnitine deficiency

Cautions: diabetes mellitus; renal impairment; monitoring of free and acyl carnitine in blood and urine recommended; pregnancy (but appropriate to use—Appendix 4) and breast-feeding

Side-effects: nausea, vomiting, abdominal pain, diarrhoea, body odour; side-effects may be dose-related—monitor tolerance during first week and after any dose increase

Dose: primary deficiency, *by mouth*, up to 200 mg/kg daily in 2–4 divided doses; higher doses of up to 400 mg/kg daily occasionally required; *by intravenous injection* over 2–3 minutes, up to 100 mg/kg daily in 3–4 divided doses

Secondary deficiency, *by intravenous injection* over 2–3 minutes, 20 mg/kg after each dialysis session (dosage adjusted according to carnitine concentration); maintenance, *by mouth*, 1 g daily

Carnitor® (Shire) PoM
Oral liquid, L-carnitine 1 g/10-mL (10%) single-dose bottle. Net price 10 × 10-mL single-dose bottle = £35.00
Paediatric solution, L-carnitine 30% (3 g/10-mL). Net price 20 mL = £21.00
Excipients: include sorbitol
Injection, L-carnitine 200 mg/mL. Net price 5-mL amp = £11.90

Fabry's disease

Agalsidase beta, an enzyme produced by recombinant DNA technology, is licensed for long-term enzyme replacement therapy in Fabry's disease (a lysosomal storage disorder caused by deficiency of α-galactosidase).

AGALSIDASE BETA

Indications: (specialist use only) Fabry's disease

Cautions: pregnancy (Appendix 4); breast-feeding (Appendix 5); **interactions:** Appendix 1 (agalsidase beta)

HYPERSENSITIVITY REACTIONS. Hypersensitivity reactions common, calling for use of antihistamine, antipyretic and corticosteroid; consult product literature for details

Side-effects: nausea, vomiting, oedema, hypertension, hypersensitivity reactions, fever, headache, tremor, myalgia, injection-site pain; commonly abdominal pain, bradycardia, tachycardia, palpitation, fatigue, drowsiness, paraesthesia, dizziness, anaemia, proteinuria, visual disturbances, and abnormal tear secretion

Dose: *by intravenous infusion*, ADULT and ADOLESCENT over 16 years 1 mg/kg every 2 weeks

Fabrazyme® (Genzyme) ▼ PoM
Intravenous infusion, powder for reconstitution, agalsidase beta, net price 5-mg vial = £325.50; 35-mg vial = £2269.20

Gaucher's disease

Imiglucerase, an enzyme produced by recombinant DNA technology, is administered as enzyme replacement therapy for non-neurological manifestations of type I or type III Gaucher's disease, a familial disorder affecting principally the liver, spleen, bone marrow, and lymph nodes.

Miglustat, an inhibitor of glucosylceramide synthase, is licensed for the treatment of mild to moderate type I Gaucher's disease in patients for whom imiglucerase is unsuitable; it is given by mouth.

IMIGLUCERASE

Indications: (specialist use only) non-neurological manifestations of type I or type III Gaucher's disease

Cautions: pregnancy (Appendix 4); breast-feeding (Appendix 5); monitor for imiglucerase antibodies; when stabilised monitor all parameters and response to treatment at intervals of 6–12 months

Side-effects: hypersensitivity reactions (including urticaria, angioedema, hypotension, flushing, tachycardia); less commonly nausea, vomiting, diarrhoea, abdominal cramps, headache, dizziness, fatigue, fever, injection-site reactions

Dose: *by intravenous infusion*, initially 60 units/kg once every 2 weeks (2.5 units/kg 3 times a week or 15 units/kg once every 2 weeks may improve haematological parameters and organomegaly, but not bone parameters); maintenance, adjust dose according to response

Cerezyme® (Genzyme) PoM
Intravenous infusion, powder for reconstitution, imiglucerase, net price 200-unit vial = £553.35; 400-unit vial = £1106.70

MIGLUSTAT

Indications: mild to moderate type I Gaucher's disease (specialist supervision only)

Cautions: hepatic impairment (Appendix 2); renal impairment (Appendix 3); monitor cognitive and neurological function

Contra-indications: pregnancy (Appendix 4); men should not father a child during or within 3 months of treatment; breast-feeding (Appendix 5)

Side-effects: diarrhoea, flatulence, abdominal pain, constipation, nausea, vomiting, weight changes; tremor, dizziness, headache; leg cramps; visual disturbances; commonly dyspepsia, decreased appetite, peripheral neuropathy, cognitive dysfunction

Dose: ADULT over 18 years, 100 mg 3 times daily; reduced if not tolerated to 100 mg 1–2 times daily

Zavesca® (Actelion) ▼ PoM
Capsules, miglustat 100 mg, net price 84-cap pack = £4480.00 (hospital only)

Mucopolysaccharidosis I

Laronidase, an enzyme produced by recombinant DNA technology, is licensed for long-term replacement therapy in the treatment of non-neurological manifestations of mucopolysaccharidosis I, a lysosomal storage disorder caused by deficiency of α-L-iduronidase.

LARONIDASE

Indications: (specialist use only) non-neurological manifestations of mucopolysaccharidosis I

Cautions: pregnancy (Appendix 4); breast-feeding (Appendix 5); **interactions:** Appendix 1 (laronidase)

INFUSION-RELATED REACTIONS. Infusion-related reactions very common, calling for use of antihistamine and antipyretic; recurrent reactions may require corticosteroid; consult product literature for details

Side-effects: flushing, musculoskeletal pain, rash, headache, abdominal pain

Dose: *by intravenous infusion*, ADULT and CHILD over 5 years 100 units/kg once weekly

Aldurazyme® (Genzyme) ▼ PoM
Concentrate for intravenous infusion, laronidase 100 units/mL, net price 5-mL vial = £460.35

Nephropathic cystinosis

Mercaptamine (cysteamine) is available for the treatment of nephropathic cystinosis.

MERCAPTAMINE

(Cysteamine)

Indications: (specialist use only) nephropathic cystinosis

Cautions: leucocyte-cystine concentration and haematological monitoring required—consult product literature; dose of phosphate supplement may need to be adjusted

Contra-indications: pregnancy and breast-feeding; hypersensitivity to mercaptamine or penicillamine

Side-effects: breath and body odour, nausea, vomiting, diarrhoea, anorexia, lethargy, fever, rash; also reported dehydration, hypertension, abdominal discomfort, gastroenteritis, drowsiness, encephalopathy, headache, nervousness, depression; anaemia, leucopenia, increases in liver enzymes; rarely gastro-intestinal ulceration and bleeding, seizures, hallucinations, urticaria, interstitial nephritis

Dose: initial doses should be one-sixth to one-quarter of the expected maintenance dose, increased gradually over 4–6 weeks

Maintenance, ADULT and CHILD over 50 kg body-weight, 2 g daily in 4 divided doses

CHILD up to 12 years, 1.3 g/m^2 (approx. 50 mg/kg) daily in 4 divided doses

Cystagon® (Orphan Europe) PoM

Capsules, mercaptamine (as bitartrate) 50 mg, net price 100-cap pack = £44.00; 150 mg, 100-cap pack = £125.00

NOTE. CHILD under 6 years at risk of aspiration, capsules can be opened and contents sprinkled on food (at a temperature suitable for eating); avoid adding to acidic drinks (e.g. orange juice)

Urea cycle disorders

Sodium phenylbutyrate is used in the management of urea cycle disorders. It is indicated as adjunctive therapy in all patients with neonatal-onset disease and in those with late-onset disease who have a history of hyperammonaemic encephalopathy.

Carglumic acid is licensed for the treatment of hyperammonaemia due to *N*-acetylglutamate synthase deficiency.

CARGLUMIC ACID

Indications: hyperammonaemia due to *N*-acetylglutamate synthase deficiency (initiated under specialist supervision)

Cautions: pregnancy (Appendix 4) and breast-feeding (Appendix 5)

Side-effects: occasionally, raised serum transaminases, sweating

Dose: ADULT and CHILD initially 100 mg/kg daily in 2–4 divided doses immediately before food (max. 250 mg/kg daily), adjusted according to plasma-ammonia concentration; maintenance 10–100 mg/kg daily in 2–4 divided doses

Carbaglu® (Orphan Europe) ▼ PoM

Dispersible tablets, carglumic acid 200 mg, net price 15-tab pack = £679.00, 60-tab pack = £2685.00. Label: 13

SODIUM PHENYLBUTYRATE

Indications: adjunct in long-term treatment of urea cycle disorders (under specialist supervision)

Cautions: congestive heart failure, hepatic and renal impairment

Contra-indications: pregnancy (Appendix 4); breast-feeding (Appendix 5)

Side-effects: amenorrhoea and irregular menstrual cycles, decreased appetite, body odour, taste disturbances; less commonly nausea, vomiting, abdominal pain, peptic ulcer, pancreatitis, rectal bleeding, arrhythmia, oedema, syncope, depression, headache, rash, weight gain, renal tubular acidosis, aplastic anaemia, ecchymoses

Dose: ADULT and CHILD over 20 kg, 9.9–13 g/m^2 daily in divided doses with meals (max. 20 g daily); CHILD less than 20 kg, 450–600 mg/kg daily in divided doses with meals

Ammonaps® (Orphan Europe) PoM

Tablets, sodium phenylbutyrate 500 mg. Contains Na^+ 2.7 mmol/tablet. Net price 250-tab pack = £493.00

Granules, sodium phenylbutyrate 940 mg/g. Contains Na^+ 5.4 mmol/g. Net price 266-g pack = £860.00

NOTE. Granules should be mixed with food before taking

9.8.2 Acute porphyrias

The acute porphyrias (acute intermittent porphyria, variegate porphyria, hereditary coproporphyria and 5-aminolaevulinic acid dehydratase deficiency porphyria) are hereditary disorders of haem biosynthesis; they have a prevalence of about 1 in 10 000 of the population.

Great care must be taken when prescribing for patients with acute porphyria since many drugs can induce acute porphyric crises. Since acute porphyrias are hereditary, relatives of affected individuals should be screened and advised about the potential danger of certain drugs.

Treatment of serious or life-threatening conditions should not be withheld from patients with acute porphyria. Where there is no safe alternative, urinary porphobilinogen excretion should be measured regularly; if it increases or symptoms occur, the drug can be withdrawn and the acute attack treated.

Haem arginate is administered by short intravenous infusion as haem replacement in moderate, severe or unremitting acute porphyria crises.

Supplies of haem arginate may be obtained outside office hours from the on-call pharmacist at:

St. James's University Hospital, Leeds	(0113) 243 3144
	or (0113) 283 7010
St Thomas' Hospital, London	(020) 7188 7188

HAEM ARGINATE

(Human hemin)

Indications: acute porphyrias (acute intermittent porphyria, porphyria variegata, hereditary coproporphyria)

Cautions: pregnancy (Appendix 4); breast feeding (Appendix 5)

Side-effects: rarely hypersensitivity reactions and fever; pain and thrombophlebitis at injection site

Dose: *by intravenous infusion*, ADULT and CHILD 3 mg/kg once daily (max. 250 mg daily) for 4 days; if response inadequate, repeat 4-day course with close biochemical monitoring

Normosang® (Orphan Europe) ▼ PoM

Concentrate for intravenous infusion, haem arginate 25 mg/mL, net price 10-mL amp = £281.25

Drugs unsafe for use in acute porphyrias

The following list contains drugs on the UK market that have been classified as 'unsafe' in porphyria because they have been shown to be porphyrinogenic in animals or *in vitro*, or have been associated with acute attacks in patients. Absence of a drug from the following lists does not necessarily imply that the drug is safe. For many drugs no information about porphyria is available.

Further information may be obtained from:
www.porphyria-europe.com
and also from:

Welsh Medicines Information Centre
University Hospital of Wales
Cardiff CF14 4XWTelephone (029) 2074 2979/3877

NOTE. Quite modest changes in chemical structure can lead to changes in porphyrinogenicity but where possible general statements have been made about groups of drugs; these should be checked first

Unsafe Drug groups (check first)

Amphetamines	Antihistamines[2]	Ergot Derivatives[5]	Progestogens[4]
Anabolic Steroids	Barbiturates[3]	Gold Salts	Statins[6]
Antidepressants[1]	Contraceptives, hormonal[4]	Hormone Replacement Therapy[4]	Sulphonamides[7]
			Sulphonylureas[8]

Unsafe Drugs (check groups above first)

Aceclofenac	Diazepam[12]	Mefenamic Acid[11]	Porfimer
Alcohol	Diclofenac	Meprobamate	Probenecid
Aminoglutethimide	Doxycycline	Methyldopa	Pyrazinamide
Amiodarone	Econazole	Metoclopramide[11]	Rifabutin[15]
Baclofen	Erythromycin	Metolazone	Rifampicin[15]
Bromocriptine	Etamsylate	Metronidazole[11]	Ritonavir
Busulfan	Ethionamide	Metyrapone	Simvastatin
Cabergoline	Ethosuximide	Miconazole	Spironolactone
Carbamazepine	Etomidate	Mifepristone	Sulfinpyrazone
Carisoprodol	Fenfluramine	Minoxidil[11]	Sulpiride
Chloral Hydrate[9]	Flupentixol	Nalidixic Acid	Tamoxifen
Chlorambucil	Griseofulvin	Nifedipine	Temoporfin
Chloramphenicol	Halothane	Nitrofurantoin	Theophylline[16]
Chloroform[10]	Hydralazine	Orphenadrine	Thioridazine
Clindamycin	Hyoscine	Oxcarbazepine	Tiagabine
Clonidine	Indapamide	Oxybutynin	Tinidazole
Cocaine	Indinavir	Oxycodone	Topiramate
Colistin	Isometheptene Mucate	Oxytetracycline	Triclofos[9]
Cyclophosphamide[11]	Isoniazid	Pentazocine[14]	Trimethoprim
Cycloserine	Ketamine	Pentoxifylline (oxpentifylline)	Valproate[12]
Danazol	Ketoconazole	Phenoxybenzamine	Verapamil
Dapsone	Ketorolac	Phenylbutazone	Xipamide
Dexfenfluramine	Lidocaine (lignocaine)[13]	Phenytoin	Zuclopenthixol
Dextropropoxyphene	Mebeverine	Pivmecillinam	

1. Includes tricyclic (and related) and MAOIs; fluoxetine thought to be safe.
2. Chlorphenamine, ketotifen, loratadine, and alimemazine (trimeprazine) thought to be safe.
3. Includes primidone and thiopental.
4. Progestogens are more porphyrinogenic than oestrogens; oestrogens may be safe at least in replacement doses. Progestogens should be avoided whenever possible by all women susceptible to acute porphyria; however, where non-hormonal contraception is inappropriate, progestogens may be used with extreme caution if the potential benefit outweighs risk. The risk of an acute attack is greatest in women who have had a previous attack or are aged under 30 years. Long-acting progestogen preparations should never be used in those at risk of acute porphyria.
5. Includes ergometrine (oxytocin probably safe), lisuride and pergolide.
6. Rosuvastatin is thought to be safe.
7. Includes co-trimoxazole and sulfasalazine.
8. Glipizide is thought to be safe.
9. Although evidence of hazard is uncertain, manufacturer advises avoid.
10. Small amounts in medicines probably safe.
11. May be used with caution if safer alternative not available.
12. Status epilepticus has been treated successfully with intravenous diazepam.
13. For local anaesthesia, bupivacaine, lidocaine (lignocaine), and prilocaine are thought to be safe.
14. Buprenorphine, codeine, diamorphine, dihydrocodeine, fentanyl, morphine, and pethidine are thought to be safe.
15. Rifamycins have been used in a few patients without evidence of harm—use with caution if safer alternative not available.
16. Includes aminophylline.

10: Musculoskeletal and joint diseases

For treatment of septic arthritis see section 5.1, table 1.

10.1 Drugs used in rheumatic diseases and gout

Rheumatoid arthritis and other inflammatory disorders

A non-steroidal anti-inflammatory drug (NSAID) is indicated for pain and stiffness resulting from inflammatory rheumatic disease. Drugs are also used to influence the disease process itself (section 10.1.3). For rheumatoid arthritis these disease-modifying antirheumatic drugs (DMARDs) include penicillamine, gold salts, antimalarials (chloroquine and hydroxychloroquine), drugs that affect the immune response, and sulfasalazine; corticosteroids may also be of value (section 10.1.2.1). Drugs which may affect the disease process in psoriatic arthritis include sulfasalazine, gold salts, azathioprine, methotrexate (section 10.1.3), and etanercept. For long-term control of gout uricosuric drugs and allopurinol (section 10.1.4) may be used.

Osteoarthritis and soft-tissue disorders

In osteoarthritis (sometimes called degenerative joint disease or osteoarthrosis) non-drug measures such as weight reduction and exercise should be encouraged. For pain relief in osteoarthritis and soft-tissue disorders, paracetamol (section 4.7.1) is often adequate and should be used first. Alternatively a low-dose of a NSAID (e.g. ibuprofen up to 1.2 g daily) may be used. If pain relief with either drug is inadequate, both paracetamol (in a full dose of 4 g daily) and a low-dose of a NSAID may be required; if necessary the dose of the NSAID may be increased or a low dose of an opioid analgesic given with paracetamol (as co-codamol 8/500 or co-dydramol 10/500).

Topical treatment including application of a NSAID or capsaicin 0.025% (section 10.3.2) may provide some pain relief in osteoarthritis.

Intra-articular corticosteroid injections (section 10.1.2.2) may produce temporary benefit in osteoarthritis, especially if associated with soft-tissue inflammation.

Hyaluronic acid and its derivatives are available for osteoarthritis of the knee. Sodium hyaluronate (*Arthrease*®, *Durolane*®, *Fermathron*®, *Hyalgan*®, *Orthovisc*®, *Ostenil*®, *Suplasyn*®), or hylan G-F 20

(*Synvisc*®) is injected intra-articularly to supplement natural hyaluronic acid in the synovial fluid. These injections may reduce pain over 1–6 months but they are associated with short-term increase in knee inflammation.

10.1.1 Non-steroidal anti-inflammatory drugs

In *single doses* non-steroidal anti-inflammatory drugs (NSAIDs) have analgesic activity comparable to that of paracetamol (section 4.7.1), but paracetamol is preferred, particularly in the elderly (see also Prescribing for the Elderly, p. 19).

In regular *full dosage* NSAIDs have both a lasting analgesic and an anti-inflammatory effect which makes them particularly useful for the treatment of continuous or regular pain associated with inflammation. Therefore, although paracetamol often gives adequate pain control in osteoarthritis, NSAIDs are more appropriate than paracetamol or the opioid analgesics in the *inflammatory arthritides* (e.g. rheumatoid arthritis) and in some cases of *advanced osteoarthritis*. They may also be of benefit in the less well defined conditions of *back pain* and *soft-tissue disorders*.

CHOICE. Differences in anti-inflammatory activity between different NSAIDs are small, but there is considerable variation in individual patient tolerance and response. About 60% of patients will respond to any NSAID; of the others, those who do not respond to one may well respond to another. Pain relief starts soon after taking the first dose and a full analgesic effect should normally be obtained within a week, whereas an anti-inflammatory effect may not be achieved (or may not be clinically assessable) for up to 3 weeks. If appropriate responses are not obtained within these times, another NSAID should be tried.

The main differences between NSAIDs are in the incidence and type of side-effects. Before treatment is started the prescriber should weigh efficacy against possible side-effects.

NSAIDs vary in their selectivity for inhibiting different types of cyclo-oxygenase; selective inhibition of cyclo-oxygenase-2 improves gastro-intestinal tolerance. A number of other factors also determine susceptibility to gastro-intestinal effects and a NSAID should be chosen on the basis of the incidence of gastro-intestinal and other side-effects.

Ibuprofen is a propionic acid derivative with anti-inflammatory, analgesic, and antipyretic properties. It has fewer side-effects than other non-selective NSAIDs but its anti-inflammatory properties are weaker. Doses of 1.6 to 2.4 g daily are needed for rheumatoid arthritis and it is unsuitable for conditions where inflammation is prominent such as acute gout.

Other propionic acid derivatives:

Naproxen is one of the first choices because it combines good efficacy with a low incidence of side-effects (but more than ibuprofen, see CSM comment below).

Fenbufen is claimed to be associated with less gastro-intestinal bleeding, but there is a high risk of rashes (see p. 505).

Fenoprofen is as effective as naproxen, and **flurbiprofen** may be slightly more effective. Both are associated with slightly more gastro-intestinal side-effects than ibuprofen.

Ketoprofen has anti-inflammatory properties similar to ibuprofen and has more side-effects (see also CSM comment below). **Dexketoprofen**, an isomer of ketoprofen, has been introduced for the short-term relief of mild to moderate pain.

Tiaprofenic acid is as effective as naproxen; it has more side-effects than ibuprofen (**important:** reports of severe cystitis, see CSM advice on p. 509).

Drugs with properties similar to those of propionic acid derivatives:

Diclofenac and **aceclofenac** have actions similar to that of naproxen; their side-effects are also similar to naproxen.

Diflunisal is an aspirin derivative but its clinical effect more closely resembles that of the propionic acid derivatives than that of its parent compound. Its long duration of action allows twice-daily administration.

Etodolac is comparable in effect to naproxen; it is licensed for symptomatic relief in osteoarthritis and rheumatoid arthritis.

Indometacin (indomethacin) has an action equal to or superior to that of naproxen, but with a high incidence of side-effects including headaches, dizziness, and gastro-intestinal disturbances (see also CSM comment below).

Mefenamic acid has minor anti-inflammatory properties. Occasionally, it has been associated with diarrhoea and haemolytic anaemia which require discontinuation of treatment.

Meloxicam is licensed for the short-term symptomatic relief of osteoarthritis and long-term symptomatic treatment of rheumatoid arthritis and ankylosing spondylitis.

Nabumetone is comparable in effect to naproxen.

Piroxicam is as effective as naproxen and has a prolonged duration of action which permits once-daily administration. It has more gastro-intestinal side-effects than ibuprofen, especially in the elderly (see also CSM comment below).

Sulindac is similar in tolerance to naproxen.

Tenoxicam is similar in activity and tolerance to naproxen. Its long half-life allows once-daily administration.

Tolfenamic acid is licensed for the treatment of migraine (section 4.7.4.1)

Ketorolac and the selective inhibitor of cyclo-oxygenase-2, **parecoxib** are licensed for the short-term management of postoperative pain (section 15.1.4.2).

The selective inhibitors of cyclo-oxygenase-2, **etoricoxib** and **celecoxib**, are as effective as non-selective NSAIDs such as diclofenac and naproxen. Short-term data indicate that the risk of serious upper gastro-intestinal events is lower with selective inhibitors compared to non-selective NSAIDs; this advantage may be lost in patients who require concomitant low-dose aspirin. There are concerns about the cardiovascular safety of cyclo-oxygenase-2 selective inhibitors (see below).

Celecoxib and **etoricoxib** are licensed for symptomatic relief of osteoarthritis and rheumatoid arthritis; **etoricoxib** is also licensed for the relief of pain from acute gout.

Cyclo-oxygenase-2 inhibitors and cardiovascular events. In the light of emerging concerns about cardiovascular safety, cyclo-oxygenase-2 selective inhibitors should be used in preference to standard NSAIDs **only** when specifically indicated (i.e. for patients who are at a particularly high risk of developing gastroduodenal ulcer, perforation, or bleeding) *and* after an assessment of cardiovascular risk. Furthermore, the CSM has advised (December 2004) that patients receiving a cyclo-oxygenase-2 selective inhibitor who have ischaemic heart disease or cerebrovascular disease should be switched to alternative treatment as soon as possible.

DENTAL AND OROFACIAL PAIN. Most mild to moderate dental pain and inflammation is effectively relieved by NSAIDs. Those used for dental pain include **ibuprofen** and **aspirin**. **Diflunisal** is also licensed for dental pain. Postoperative use of diflunisal has been associated with localised osteitis (dry socket) but this remains to be confirmed. Ibuprofen can be used in children.

Like aspirin and diflunisal, ibuprofen causes gastro-intestinal irritation, but in an appraisal of the relative safety of 7 non-selective NSAIDs the CSM has assessed ibuprofen to have the lowest risk of serious gastro-intestinal side-effects (see below).

For further information on the management of dental and orofacial pain, see p. 218.

CAUTIONS AND CONTRA-INDICATIONS. NSAIDs should be used with caution in the elderly (risk of serious side-effects and fatalities, see also Prescribing for the Elderly p. 19), in allergic disorders (they are **contra-indicated** in patients with a history of hypersensitivity to aspirin or any other NSAID—which includes those in whom attacks of asthma, angioedema, urticaria or rhinitis have been precipitated by aspirin or any other NSAID), during pregnancy and breast-feeding (see Appendix 4 and Appendix 5), and in coagulation defects. Long-term use of some NSAIDs is associated with reduced female fertility which is reversible on stopping treatment.

In patients with renal, cardiac, or hepatic impairment caution is required since NSAIDs may impair renal function (see also under Side-effects, below and Appendix 2 and Appendix 3); the dose should be kept as **low as possible** and renal function should be **monitored**.

The selective inhibitors of cyclo-oxygenase-2, celecoxib and etoricoxib are **contra-indicated** in ischaemic heart disease, cerebrovascular disease, peripheral arterial disease, and moderate or severe congestive heart failure. Celecoxib and etoricoxib should be used with caution in patients with a history of cardiac failure, left ventricular dysfunction, hypertension, in patients with oedema for any other reason, and in patients with risk factors for developing heart disease.

The CSM has advised that non-selective NSAIDs are contra-indicated in patients with previous or active peptic ulceration and that selective inhibitors of cyclo-oxygenase-2 are contra-indicated in active peptic ulceration (see also **CSM advice** below). While it is preferable to avoid NSAIDs in patients with active or previous gastro-intestinal ulceration or bleeding, and to withdraw them if gastro-intestinal lesions develop, nevertheless patients with serious rheumatic diseases (e.g. rheumatoid arthritis) are usually dependent on NSAIDs for effective relief of pain and stiffness. For advice on the prophylaxis and treatment of NSAID-associated peptic ulcers, see section 1.3.

For **interactions** of NSAIDs, see Appendix 1 (NSAIDs)

SIDE-EFFECTS. Gastro-intestinal discomfort, nausea, diarrhoea, and occasionally bleeding and ulceration occur (see also CSM advice below). Systemic as well as local effects of NSAIDs contribute to gastro-intestinal damage; taking oral formulations with milk or food, or using enteric-coated formulations, or changing the route of administration may only partially reduce symptoms such as dyspepsia. Those at risk of duodenal or gastric ulceration (including the elderly) who need to continue NSAID treatment should receive either a selective inhibitor of cyclo-oxygenase-2 alone, or a non-selective NSAID with gastroprotective treatment (section 1.3). Other side-effects include hypersensitivity reactions (particularly rashes, angioedema, and bronchospasm—see CSM advice below), headache, dizziness, nervousness, depression, drowsiness, insomnia, vertigo, hearing disturbances such as tinnitus, photosensitivity, and haematuria. Blood disorders have also occurred. Fluid retention may occur (rarely precipitating congestive heart failure in elderly patients); blood pressure may be raised. Renal failure may be provoked by NSAIDs especially in patients with pre-existing renal impairment (**important**, see also under Cautions above). Rarely, papillary necrosis or interstitial fibrosis associated with NSAIDs may lead to renal failure. Hepatic damage, alveolitis, pulmonary eosinophilia, pancreatitis, eye changes, Stevens-Johnson syndrome and toxic epidermal necrolysis are other rare side-effects. Induction of or exacerbation of colitis has been reported. Aseptic meningitis has been reported rarely with NSAIDs; patients with connective-tissue disorders such as systemic lupus erythematosus may be especially susceptible.

Overdosage: see Emergency Treatment of Poisoning, p. 29.

CSM advice (gastro-intestinal side-effects). All NSAIDs are associated with serious gastro-intestinal toxicity; the risk is higher in the elderly. Evidence on the relative safety of 7 **non-selective** NSAIDs indicates differences in the risks of serious upper gastro-intestinal side-effects. **Azapropazone** [discontinued] is associated with the *highest risk* and **ibuprofen** with the *lowest*; **piroxicam**, **ketoprofen**, **indometacin**, **naproxen** and **diclofenac** are associated with *intermediate risks* (possibly higher in the case of piroxicam). **Selective inhibitors of cyclo-oxygenase-2** are associated with a *lower risk* of serious upper gastro-intestinal side-effects than non-selective NSAIDs.

Recommendations are that NSAIDs associated with low risk e.g. ibuprofen are *generally preferred*, to start at the *lowest recommended dose*, *not to use more than one* oral NSAID at a time, and to remember that all NSAIDs (including selective inhibitors of cyclo-oxygenase-2) are *contra-indicated* in patients with active peptic ulceration. The CSM also contra-indicates non-selective NSAIDs in patients with a history of peptic ulceration.

The combination of a NSAID and low-dose aspirin may increase the risk of gastro-intestinal side-effects; this combination should only be used if absolutely necessary and the patient monitored closely

CSM warning (asthma). Any degree of worsening of asthma may be related to the ingestion of NSAIDs, either prescribed or (in the case of ibuprofen and others) purchased over the counter.

IBUPROFEN

Indications: pain and inflammation in rheumatic disease (including juvenile arthritis) and other musculoskeletal disorders; mild to moderate pain including dysmenorrhoea; postoperative analgesia; migraine; fever and pain in children; post-immunisation pyrexia (section 14.1)

Cautions: see notes above; breast-feeding (Appendix 5); **interactions:** Appendix 1 (NSAIDs)

Contra-indications: see notes above

Side-effects: see notes above; **overdosage:** see Emergency Treatment of Poisoning, p. 29

Dose: initially 1.2–1.8 g daily in 3–4 divided doses preferably after food; increased if necessary to max. 2.4 g daily; maintenance dose of 0.6–1.2 g daily may be adequate

Juvenile rheumatoid arthritis, CHILD over 7 kg body-weight 30–40 mg/kg daily in 3–4 divided doses

Fever and pain in children, CHILD over 7 kg body-weight 20–30 mg/kg daily in divided doses *or* 1–2 years 50 mg 3–4 times daily, 3–7 years 100 mg 3–4 times daily, 8–12 years 200 mg 3–4 times daily

Ibuprofen (Non-proprietary) PoM

Tablets, coated, ibuprofen 200 mg, net price 84-tab pack = £1.90; 400 mg, 84-tab pack = £2.74; 600 mg, 84-tab pack = £4.02. Label: 21

Brands include *Arthrofen®*, *Ebufac®*, *Rimafen®*

Oral suspension, ibuprofen 100 mg/5 mL, net price 100 mL = £2.65, 150 mL = £2.71, 500 mL = £8.88. Label: 21

NOTE. Sugar-free versions are available and can be ordered by specifying 'sugar-free' on the prescription

Brands include *Calprofen®*, *Fenpaed®*, *Galprofen®*, *Nurofen® for Children*, *Orbifen® for Children*

DENTAL PRESCRIBING ON NHS. Ibuprofen Tablets and Ibuprofen Oral Suspension Sugar-free may be prescribed

NOTE. Proprietary brands of ibuprofen preparations are on sale to the public; brand names include, *Advil®*, *Anadin Ibuprofen®*, *Anadin Ultra®*, *Arthrofen®*, *Boots Children's 6 years Plus Fever & Pain Relief®*, *Cuprofen®*, *Galprofen®*, *Hedex® Ibuprofen*, *Ibrufhalal®*, *Ibufem®*, *Inoven®*, *Librofem®*, *Migrafen®*, *Novaprin®*, *Nurofen®*, *Nurofen® for Children Singles*, *Nurofen® Long Lasting*, *Nurofen® Meltlets*, *Nurofen® Migraine Pain*, *Nurofen® Mobile*, *Nurofen® Recovery*, *Obifen®*, *Pacifene®*, *PhorPain®*, *Relcofen®*; compound proprietary preparations containing ibuprofen include *Lemsip® Cold & Flu Sinus 12HR*, *Lemsip® Max 12HR* (ibuprofen, pseudoephedrine), *Nurofen® Plus* (ibuprofen, codeine), *Solpaflex®* (ibuprofen, codeine)

Brufen® (Abbott) PoM

Tablets, all magenta, ibuprofen 200 mg (s/c), net price 20 = 82p; 400 mg (s/c), 20 = £1.63; 600 mg (f/c), 20 = £2.45. Label: 21

Syrup, orange, ibuprofen 100 mg/5 mL. Net price 500 mL = £8.07. Label: 21

Granules, effervescent, ibuprofen 600 mg/sachet. Net price 20-sachet pack = £6.80. Label: 13, 21

NOTE. Contains sodium approx. 9 mmol/sachet

■ Topical preparations

Section 10.3.2

■ Modified release

Brufen Retard® (Abbott) PoM

Tablets, m/r, f/c, ibuprofen 800 mg, net price 56-tab pack = £6.74. Label: 25, 27

Dose: 2 tablets daily as a single dose, preferably in the early evening, increased in severe cases to 3 tablets daily in 2 divided doses; CHILD not recommended

Fenbid® (Goldshield) PoM

Spansule® (= capsule m/r), maroon/pink, enclosing off-white pellets, ibuprofen 300 mg. Net price 120-cap pack = £9.64. Label: 25

Dose: 1–3 capsules every 12 hours; CHILD not recommended

■ With codeine

For comment on compound analgesic preparations, see p. 219. For details of the **side-effects**, **cautions**, and **contra-indications** of opioid analgesics, see p. 224 (**important:** the elderly are particularly susceptible to opioid side-effects).

Codafen Continus® (Napp) PoM

Tablets, white/pink, ibuprofen 300 mg (m/r), codeine phosphate 20 mg. Net price 56-tab pack = £4.80; 112-tab pack = £9.59. Label: 2, 21, 25

Dose: 1–2 tablets every 12 hours; max. 3 tablets every 12 hours; CHILD not recommended

ACECLOFENAC

Indications: pain and inflammation in rheumatoid arthritis, osteoarthritis and ankylosing spondylitis

Cautions: see notes above; avoid in porphyria (section 9.8.2); breast-feeding (Appendix 5); **interactions:** Appendix 1 (NSAIDs)

Contra-indications: see notes above

Side-effects: see notes above

Dose: 100 mg twice daily; CHILD not recommended

Preservex® (UCB Pharma) PoM

Tablets, f/c, aceclofenac 100 mg, net price 60-tab pack = £9.63. Label: 21

ACEMETACIN

(Glycolic acid ester of indometacin)

Indications: pain and inflammation in rheumatic disease and other musculoskeletal disorders; postoperative analgesia

Cautions: see under Indometacin and notes above; breast-feeding (Appendix 5); **interactions:** Appendix 1 (NSAIDs)

DRIVING. Dizziness may affect performance of skilled tasks (e.g. driving)

Contra-indications: see notes above

Side-effects: see under Indometacin and notes above

Dose: 120 mg daily in divided doses with food, increased if necessary to 180 mg daily; CHILD not recommended

Emflex® (Merck) PoM

Capsules, yellow/orange, acemetacin 60 mg, net price 90-cap pack = £23.50. Label: 21, counselling, driving

CELECOXIB

Indications: pain and inflammation in osteoarthritis or rheumatoid arthritis

Cautions: see notes above; breast-feeding (Appendix 5); **interactions**: Appendix 1 (NSAIDs)

Contra-indications: see notes above; sulphonamide sensitivity; inflammatory bowel disease

Side-effects: see notes above; flatulence, insomnia, pharyngitis, sinusitis; less frequently stomatitis, constipation, palpitations, fatigue, paraesthesia, muscle cramps; rarely taste alteration, alopecia; very rarely aggravation of epilepsy

Dose: osteoarthritis, 200 mg daily in 1–2 divided doses, increased if necessary to max. 200 mg twice daily; CHILD not recommended

Rheumatoid arthritis, 200–400 mg daily in 2 divided doses; ELDERLY initially 200 mg daily in 2 divided doses; max. 200 mg twice daily; CHILD not recommended

Celebrex® (Pharmacia) PoM
Capsules, celecoxib 100 mg (white/blue), net price 60-cap pack = £21.55; 200 mg (white/gold), 30-cap pack = £21.55

DEXKETOPROFEN

Indications: short-term treatment of mild to moderate pain including dysmenorrhoea

Cautions: see notes above; breast-feeding (Appendix 5); **interactions**: Appendix 1 (NSAIDs)

Contra-indications: see notes above

Side-effects: see notes above

Dose: 12.5 mg every 4–6 hours *or* 25 mg every 8 hours; max. 75 mg daily; ELDERLY initially max. 50 mg daily; CHILD not recommended

Keral® (Menarini) PoM
Tablets, f/c, scored, dexketoprofen (as trometamol) 25 mg, net price 20-tab pack = £3.67, 50-tab pack = £9.18. Label: 22

DICLOFENAC SODIUM

Indications: pain and inflammation in rheumatic disease (including juvenile arthritis) and other musculoskeletal disorders; acute gout; postoperative pain

Cautions: see notes above; breast-feeding (Appendix 5); **interactions:** Appendix 1 (NSAIDs)

Contra-indications: see notes above; porphyria (section 9.8.2)

INTRAVENOUS USE. Additional contra-indications include concomitant NSAID or anticoagulant use (including low-dose heparin), history of haemorrhagic diathesis, history of confirmed or suspected cerebrovascular bleeding, operations with high risk of haemorrhage, history of asthma, moderate or severe renal impairment, hypovolaemia, dehydration

Side-effects: see notes above; suppositories may cause rectal irritation; injection site reactions

Dose: *by mouth*, 75–150 mg daily in 2–3 divided doses

By deep intramuscular injection into the gluteal muscle, acute exacerbations of pain and postoperative pain, 75 mg once daily (twice daily in severe cases) for max. of 2 days

Ureteric colic, 75 mg then a further 75 mg after 30 minutes if necessary

By intravenous infusion (in hospital setting), 75 mg repeated if necessary after 4–6 hours for max. 2 days

Prevention of postoperative pain, initially after surgery 25–50 mg over 15–60 minutes then 5 mg/hour for max. 2 days

By rectum in suppositories, 75–150 mg daily in divided doses

Max. total daily dose by any route 150 mg

CHILD 1–12 years, juvenile arthritis, *by mouth or by rectum*, 1–3 mg/kg daily in divided doses (25 mg e/c tablets, 12.5 mg and 25 mg suppositories only)

Diclofenac Sodium (Non-proprietary) PoM
Tablets, both e/c, diclofenac sodium 25 mg, net price 84-tab pack = £1.72; 50 mg, 84-tab pack = £1.45. Label: 5, 25
NOTE. Other brands include *Acoflam*®, *Defenac*®, *Diclo-flex*®, *Diclovol*®, *Diclozip*®, *Fenactol*®, *Flamrase*®, *Lofensaid*®, *Volraman*®
Suppositories, diclofenac sodium 100 mg, net price 10 = £3.04
Brands include *Econac*®
Injection, diclofenac sodium 25 mg/mL. Net price 3-mL amp = 74p
NOTE. Licensed for intramuscular use

Voltarol® (Novartis) PoM
Tablets, both e/c, diclofenac sodium 25 mg (yellow), net price 84-tab pack = £3.67; 50 mg (brown), 84-tab pack = £5.71. Label: 5, 25
Dispersible tablets, sugar-free, pink, diclofenac, equivalent to diclofenac sodium 50 mg, net price 21-tab pack = £5.63. Label: 13, 21
NOTE. Voltarol Dispersible tablets are more suitable for **short-term** use in acute conditions for which treatment required for no more than 3 months (no information on use beyond 3 months)
Injection, diclofenac sodium 25 mg/mL. Net price 3-mL amp = 83p
Excipients: include benzyl alcohol (see Excipients, p. 2)
Suppositories, diclofenac sodium 12.5 mg, net price 10 = 71p; 25 mg, 10 = £1.26; 50 mg, 10 = £2.07; 100 mg, 10 = £3.70
Emulgel® gel, section 10.3.2

■ Diclofenac potassium

Voltarol® **Rapid** (Novartis) PoM
Tablets, s/c, diclofenac potassium 25 mg (red), net price 28-tab pack = £3.67; 50 mg (brown), 28-tab pack = £7.03
Dose: rheumatic disease, musculoskeletal disorders, acute gout, post-operative pain, 75–150 mg daily in 2–3 divided doses; CHILD over 14 years, 75–100 mg daily in 2–3 divided doses
Migraine, 50 mg at onset, repeated after 2 hours if necessary then after 4–6 hours; max. 200 mg in 24 hours; CHILD not recommended

■ Modified release

Diclomax SR® (Provalis) PoM
Capsules, m/r, yellow, diclofenac sodium 75 mg. Net price 56-cap pack = £12.10. Label: 21, 25
Dose: 1 capsule 1–2 times daily *or* 2 capsules once daily, preferably with food; CHILD not recommended

Diclomax Retard® (Provalis) PoM
Capsules, m/r, diclofenac sodium 100 mg. Net price 28-tab pack = £8.71. Label: 21, 25
Dose: 1 capsule daily preferably with food; CHILD not recommended

Motifene® **75 mg** (Sankyo) PoM
Capsules, e/c, m/r, diclofenac sodium 75 mg (enclosing e/c pellets containing diclofenac sodium 25 mg and m/r pellets containing diclofenac sodium 50 mg). Net price 56-cap pack = £8.00. Label: 25
Dose: 1 capsule 1-2 times daily; CHILD not recommended

Voltarol® 75 mg SR (Novartis) PoM
Tablets, m/r, pink, diclofenac sodium 75 mg. Net price 28-tab pack = £8.08; 56-tab pack = £16.15. Label: 21, 25
Dose: 75 mg 1–2 times daily preferably with food; CHILD not recommended
NOTE. Other brands of modified-release tablets containing diclofenac sodium 75 mg include *Acoflam® 75 SR, Defenac® SR, Dexomon® 75 SR, Dicloflex® 75 SR, Diclovol® SR, Fenactol® 75 mg SR, Flamatak® 75 MR, Flamrase® SR, Flexotard® MR 75, Rheumatac® Retard 75, Rhumalgan® CR, Slofenac® SR, Volsaid® Retard 75*

Voltarol® Retard (Novartis) PoM
Tablets, m/r, red, diclofenac sodium 100 mg. Net price 28-tab pack = £11.84. Label: 21, 25
Dose: 1 tablet daily preferably with food; CHILD not recommended
NOTE. Other brands of modified-release tablets containing diclofenac sodium 100 mg include *Acoflam® Retard, Defenac® Retard, Dexomon® Retard 100, Dicloflex® Retard, Diclovol® Retard, Fenactol® Retard 100 mg, Flamatak® 100 MR, Flamrase® SR, Rhumalgan® CR, Slofenac® SR, Volsaid® Retard 100*

■ With misoprostol

For **cautions**, **contra-indications**, and **side-effects** of misoprostol, see section 1.3.4

Arthrotec® (Pharmacia) PoM
Arthrotec® 50 tablets, diclofenac sodium (in e/c core) 50 mg, misoprostol 200 micrograms. Net price 60-tab pack = £13.31; Label: 21, 25
Dose: prophylaxis against NSAID-induced gastroduodenal ulceration in patients requiring diclofenac for rheumatoid arthritis or osteoarthritis, 1 tablet 2–3 times daily with food; CHILD not recommended
Arthrotec® 75 tablets, diclofenac sodium (in e/c core) 75 mg, misoprostol 200 micrograms. Net price 60-tab pack = £17.59. Label: 21, 25
Dose: prophylaxis against NSAID-induced gastroduodenal ulceration in patients requiring diclofenac for rheumatoid arthritis or osteoarthritis, 1 tablet twice daily with food; CHILD not recommended

DIFLUNISAL

Indications: pain and inflammation in rheumatic disease and other musculoskeletal disorders; mild to moderate pain including dysmenorrhoea
Cautions: see notes above; breast-feeding (Appendix 5); **interactions:** Appendix 1 (NSAIDs)
Contra-indications: see notes above
Side-effects: see notes above
Dose: mild to moderate pain, initially 1 g, then 500 mg every 12 hours (increased to max. 500 mg every 8 hours if necessary)
Osteoarthritis, rheumatoid arthritis, 0.5–1 g daily as a single daily dose *or* in 2 divided doses
Dysmenorrhoea, initially 1 g, then 500 mg every 12 hours
CHILD not recommended

Dolobid® (MSD) PoM
Tablets, both f/c, diflunisal 250 mg (peach), net price 60-tab pack = £5.41; 500 mg (orange), 60-tab pack = £10.82. Label: 21, 25, counselling, avoid aluminium hydroxide
DENTAL PRESCRIBING ON NHS. May be prescribed as Diflusinal Tablets

ETODOLAC

Indications: pain and inflammation in rheumatoid arthritis and osteoarthritis
Cautions: see notes above; breast-feeding (Appendix 5); **interactions:** Appendix 1 (NSAIDs)
Contra-indications: see notes above
Side-effects: see notes above
Dose: 600 mg daily in 1–2 divided doses; CHILD not recommended

Etodolac (Non-proprietary) PoM
Capsules, etodolac 300 mg, net price 60-cap pack = £8.14
Brands include *Eccoxolac®*

■ Modified release

Lodine SR® (Shire) PoM
Tablets, m/r, light-grey, etodolac 600 mg. Net price 30-tab pack = £15.50. Label: 25
Dose: 1 tablet daily; CHILD not recommended

ETORICOXIB

Indications: pain and inflammation in osteoarthritis and in rheumatoid arthritis; acute gout
Cautions: see notes above; monitor blood pressure; breast-feeding (Appendix 5); **interactions:** Appendix 1 (NSAIDs)
Contra-indications: see notes above; inflammatory bowel disease; uncontrolled hypertension
Side-effects: see notes above; also dry mouth, taste disturbance, mouth ulcers, flatulence, constipation, appetite and weight changes, chest pain, fatigue, paraesthesia, influenza-like syndrome, myalgia
Dose: osteoarthritis, ADULT and ADOLESCENT over 16 years, 60 mg once daily
Rheumatoid arthritis, ADULT and ADOLESCENT over 16 years, 90 mg once daily
Acute gout, ADULT and ADOLESCENT over 16 years, 120 mg once daily

Arcoxia® (MSD) ▼ PoM
Tablets, f/c, etoricoxib 60 mg (green), net price 28-tab pack = £22.96; 90 mg (white), 28-tab pack = £22.96; 120 mg (pale green), 7-tab pack = £5.74

FENBUFEN

Indications: pain and inflammation in rheumatic disease and other musculoskeletal disorders
Cautions: see notes above; breast-feeding (Appendix 5); **interactions:** Appendix 1 (NSAIDs)
Contra-indications: see notes above
Side-effects: see notes above, but also high risk of rashes especially in seronegative rheumatoid arthritis, psoriatic arthritis and in women (discontinue immediately); erythema multiforme and Stevens-Johnson syndrome reported; also allergic interstitial lung disorders (may follow rashes)
Dose: 300 mg in the morning and 600 mg at bedtime *or* 450 mg twice daily; CHILD under 14 years not recommended

Fenbufen (Non-proprietary) PoM
Capsules, fenbufen 300 mg, net price 84-cap pack = £20.71. Label: 21
Tablets, fenbufen 300 mg, net price 84-tab pack = £11.77; 450 mg, 56-tab pack = £9.38. Label: 21

Lederfen® (Goldshield) PoM
Capsules, dark blue, fenbufen 300 mg. Net price 84-cap pack = £20.71. Label: 21
Tablets, both light blue, f/c, fenbufen 300 mg, net price 84-tab pack = £20.71; 450 mg, 56-tab pack = £18.83. Label: 21

FENOPROFEN

Indications: pain and inflammation in rheumatic disease and other musculoskeletal disorders; mild to moderate pain

Cautions: see notes above; breast-feeding (Appendix 5); **interactions:** Appendix 1 (NSAIDs)

Contra-indications: see notes above

Side-effects: see notes above; upper respiratory-tract infection, nasopharyngitis, and cystitis also reported

Dose: 300–600 mg 3–4 times daily with food; max. 3 g daily; CHILD not recommended

Fenopron® (Typharm) PoM

Tablets, both orange, fenoprofen (as calcium salt) 300 mg (*Fenopron*® 300), net price 100-tab pack = £9.45; 600 mg (*Fenopron*® 600, scored), 100-tab pack = £18.29. Label: 21

FLURBIPROFEN

Indications: pain and inflammation in rheumatic disease and other musculoskeletal disorders; mild to moderate pain including dysmenorrhoea; migraine; postoperative analgesia; relief of sore throat (section 12.3.1)

Cautions: see notes above; breast-feeding (Appendix 5); **interactions:** Appendix 1 (NSAIDs)

Contra-indications: see notes above

Side-effects: see notes above; suppositories may cause rectal irritation

Dose: *by mouth or by rectum* in suppositories, 150–200 mg, daily in divided doses, increased in acute conditions to 300 mg daily

Dysmenorrhoea, initially 100 mg, then 50–100 mg every 4–6 hours; max. 300 mg daily

CHILD not recommended

Flurbiprofen (Non-proprietary) PoM

Tablets, flurbiprofen 50 mg, net price 20 = £1.98; 100 mg, 20 = £3.76. Label: 21

Froben® (Abbott) PoM

Tablets, both yellow, s/c, flurbiprofen 50 mg, net price 20 = £2.18; 100 mg, 20 = £4.13. Label: 21

■ Modified release

Froben SR® (Abbott) PoM

Capsules, m/r, yellow, enclosing off-white beads, flurbiprofen 200 mg. Net price 30-cap pack = £7.84. Label: 21, 25

Dose: rheumatic disease, 1 capsule daily, preferably in the evening; CHILD not recommended

INDOMETACIN

(Indomethacin)

Indications: pain and moderate to severe inflammation in rheumatic disease and other acute musculoskeletal disorders; acute gout; dysmenorrhoea; closure of ductus arteriosus (section 7.1.1.1)

Cautions: see notes above; also epilepsy, parkinsonism, psychiatric disturbances; during prolonged therapy ophthalmic and blood examinations particularly advisable; avoid rectal administration in proctitis and haemorrhoids; breast-feeding (Appendix 5); **interactions:** Appendix 1 (NSAIDs)

DRIVING. Dizziness may affect performance of skilled tasks (e.g. driving)

Contra-indications: see notes above

Side-effects: see notes above; frequently gastro-intestinal disturbances (including diarrhoea), headache, dizziness, and light-headedness; also gastro-intestinal ulceration and bleeding; rarely, drowsiness, confusion, insomnia, convulsions, psychiatric disturbances, depression, syncope, blood disorders (particularly thrombocytopenia), hypertension, hyperglycaemia, blurred vision, corneal deposits, peripheral neuropathy, and intestinal strictures; suppositories may cause rectal irritation and occasional bleeding

Dose: *by mouth*, rheumatic disease, 50–200 mg daily in divided doses, with food; CHILD not recommended

Acute gout, 150–200 mg daily in divided doses

Dysmenorrhoea, up to 75 mg daily

By rectum in suppositories, 100 mg at night and in the morning if required; CHILD not recommended

Combined oral and rectal treatment, max. total daily dose 150–200 mg

Indometacin (Non-proprietary) PoM

Capsules, indometacin 25 mg, net price 20 = 51p; 50 mg, 20 = 81p. Label: 21, counselling, driving, see above

Brands include *Rimacid*®

Suppositories, indometacin 100 mg. Net price 10 = £1.20. Counselling, driving, see above

■ Modified release

Indometacin m/r preparations PoM

Capsules, m/r, indometacin 75 mg. Label: 21, 25, counselling, driving, see above

Brands include *Indolar SR*®, *Indomax 75 SR*®, *Indomod*®, *Pardelprin*®, *Rheumacin LA*®, *Slo-Indo*®

Dose: 1 capsule 1–2 times daily; CHILD not recommended

Flexin Continus (Napp) PoM

Tablets, m/r, indometacin 25 mg (green), net price 56-tab pack = £5.45; 50 mg (red), 28-tab pack = £5.45; 75 mg (yellow), 28-tab pack = £7.79. Label: 21, 25, counselling, driving, see above

Dose: initially 75 mg daily, adjusted in steps of 25–50 mg; range 25–200 mg daily in 1–2 divided doses; dysmenorrhoea, up to 75 mg daily; CHILD not recommended

KETOPROFEN

Indications: pain and mild inflammation in rheumatic disease and other musculoskeletal disorders, and after orthopaedic surgery; acute gout; dysmenorrhoea

Cautions: see notes above; breast-feeding (Appendix 5); **interactions:** Appendix 1 (NSAIDs)

Contra-indications: see notes above

Side-effects: see notes above; pain may occur at injection site (occasionally tissue damage); suppositories may cause rectal irritation

Dose: *by mouth*, rheumatic disease, 100–200 mg daily in 2–4 divided doses with food; CHILD not recommended

Pain and dysmenorrhoea, 50 mg up to 3 times daily; CHILD not recommended

By rectum in suppositories, rheumatic disease, 100 mg at bedtime; CHILD not recommended

Combined oral and rectal treatment, max. total daily dose 200 mg

By deep intramuscular injection into the gluteal muscle, 50–100 mg every 4 hours (max. 200 mg in 24 hours) for up to 3 days; CHILD not recommended

Ketoprofen (Non-proprietary) PoM
Capsules, ketoprofen 50 mg, net price 28-cap pack = £7.35; 100 mg, 100-cap pack = £13.55. Label: 21

Orudis® (Hawgreen) PoM
Capsules, ketoprofen 50 mg (green/purple), net price 112-cap pack = £16.07; 100 mg (pink), 56-cap pack = £16.12. Label: 21
Suppositories, ketoprofen 100 mg. Net price 10 = £6.92

Oruvail® (Hawgreen) PoM
Injection, ketoprofen 50 mg /mL. Net price 2-mL amp = £1.11
Gel, section 10.3.2

■ Modified release

Oruvail® (Hawgreen) PoM
Capsules, all m/r, enclosing white pellets, ketoprofen 100 mg (pink/purple), net price 56-cap pack = £24.90; 150 mg (pink), 28-cap pack = £14.21; 200 mg (pink/white), 28-cap pack = £24.82. Label: 21, 25
Dose: 100–200 mg once daily with food; CHILD not recommended
NOTE. Other brands of modified-release capsules containing ketoprofen 100 mg and 200 mg include *Ketocid*® 200 mg, *Ketovail*®, *Ketpron XL*® 100 mg, *Ketpron*® 200 mg, *Larafen CR*® 200 mg, *Tiloket*® *CR*

MEFENAMIC ACID

Indications: mild to moderate pain in rheumatoid arthritis (including juvenile arthritis), osteoarthritis, and related conditions; postoperative analgesia; mild to moderate pain; dysmenorrhoea and menorrhagia
Cautions: see notes above; breast-feeding (Appendix 5); porphyria (section 9.8.2); **interactions:** Appendix 1 (NSAIDs)
Contra-indications: see notes above; inflammatory bowel disease
Side-effects: see notes above; drowsiness; diarrhoea or rashes (withdraw treatment); thrombocytopenia, haemolytic anaemia (positive Coombs' test), and aplastic anaemia reported; convulsions in overdosage
Dose: 500 mg 3 times daily preferably after food; CHILD over 6 months, 25 mg/kg daily in divided doses for not longer than 7 days, except in juvenile arthritis

Mefenamic Acid (Non-proprietary) PoM
Capsules, mefenamic acid 250 mg. Net price 20 = 50p. Label: 21
Tablets, mefenamic acid 500 mg, net price 28-tab pack = £2.88. Label: 21
Paediatric oral suspension, mefenamic acid 50 mg/5 mL. Net price 125 mL = £79.98. Label: 21

Ponstan® (Chemidex) PoM
Capsules, blue/white, mefenamic acid 250 mg, net price 100-cap pack = £8.17. Label: 21
Forte tablets, yellow, mefenamic acid 500 mg, net price 100-tab pack = £15.72. Label: 21

MELOXICAM

Indications: pain and inflammation in rheumatic disease; exacerbation of osteoarthritis (short-term); ankylosing spondylitis
Cautions: see notes above; avoid rectal administration in proctitis or haemorrhoids; breast-feeding (Appendix 5); **interactions:** Appendix 1 (NSAIDs)
Contra-indications: see notes above; renal failure (unless receiving dialysis); severe heart failure
Side-effects: see notes above
Dose: *by mouth*, osteoarthritis, 7.5 mg daily with food, increased if necessary to max. 15 mg once daily
Rheumatoid arthritis, ankylosing spondylitis, 15 mg once daily with food, may be reduced to 7.5 mg daily; ELDERLY 7.5 mg daily
By rectum, in suppositories, osteoarthritis, 7.5 mg daily, increased if necessary to max. 15 mg once daily
Rheumatoid arthritis, ankylosing spondylitis, 15 mg once daily, may be reduced to 7.5 mg daily; ELDERLY 7.5 mg daily
CHILD under 15 years not recommended

Mobic® (Boehringer Ingelheim) PoM
Tablets, both yellow, scored, meloxicam 7.5 mg, net price 30-tab pack = £9.70; 15 mg, 30-tab pack = £13.48. Label: 21
Suppositories, meloxicam 7.5 mg, net price 12 = £3.88; 15 mg, 12 = £5.82

NABUMETONE

Indications: pain and inflammation in osteoarthritis and rheumatoid arthritis
Cautions: see notes above; breast-feeding (Appendix 5); **interactions:** Appendix 1 (NSAIDs)
Contra-indications: see notes above
Side-effects: see notes above
Dose: 1 g at night, in severe conditions 0.5–1 g in morning as well; elderly 0.5–1 g daily; CHILD not recommended

Nabumetone (Non-proprietary) PoM
Tablets, nabumetone 500 mg, net price 56-tab pack = £11.89. Label: 21

Relifex® (Meda) PoM
Tablets, red, f/c, nabumetone 500 mg. Net price 56-tab pack = £6.18. Label: 21
Suspension, sugar-free, nabumetone 500 mg/5 mL. Net price 300-mL pack = £24.08. Label: 21

NAPROXEN

Indications: pain and inflammation in rheumatic disease (including juvenile arthritis) and other musculoskeletal disorders; dysmenorrhoea; acute gout
Cautions: see notes above; breast-feeding (Appendix 5); **interactions:** Appendix 1 (NSAIDs)
Contra-indications: see notes above
Side-effects: see notes above
Dose: 0.5–1 g daily in 1–2 divided doses; CHILD (over 5 years), juvenile arthritis, 10 mg/kg daily in 2 divided doses
Acute musculoskeletal disorders and dysmenorrhoea, 500 mg initially, then 250 mg every 6–8 hours as required; max. dose after first day 1.25 g daily; CHILD under 16 years not recommended
Acute gout, 750 mg initially, then 250 mg every 8 hours until attack has passed; CHILD under 16 years not recommended

Naproxen (Non-proprietary) PoM
Tablets, naproxen 250 mg, net price 28-tab pack = £1.34; 500 mg, 28-tab pack = £2.45. Label: 21
Brands include *Arthroxen*®

Tablets, e/c, naproxen 250 mg, net price 56-tab pack = £5.09; 375 mg, 56-tab pack = £6.96; 500 mg, 56-tab pack = £8.63. Label: 5, 25

Naprosyn® (Roche) PoM
Tablets, all scored, naproxen 250 mg (buff), net price 56-tab pack = £4.55; 500 mg (buff), 56-tab pack = £9.09. Label: 21
Tablets, e/c, (*Naprosyn EC*®), naproxen 250 mg, net price 56-tab pack = £4.55; 375 mg, 56-tab pack = £6.82; 500 mg, 56-tab pack = £9.09. Label: 5, 25

Synflex® (Roche) PoM
Tablets, blue, naproxen sodium 275 mg. Net price 60-tab pack = £7.54. Label: 21
NOTE. 275 mg naproxen sodium ≡ 250 mg naproxen
Dose: musculoskeletal disorders, postoperative analgesia, 550 mg twice daily when necessary, preferably after food; max. 1.1 g daily; CHILD under 16 years not recommended
Dysmenorrhoea and acute gout, initially 550 mg then 275 mg every 6–8 hours as required; max. of 1.375 g on first day and 1.1 g daily thereafter; CHILD under 16 years not recommended
Migraine, 825 mg at onset, then 275–550 mg at least 30 minutes after initial dose; max. 1.375 g in 24 hours; CHILD under 16 years not recommended

■ With misoprostol
For **cautions**, **contra-indications**, and **side-effects** of misoprostol, see section 1.3.4

Napratec® (Pharmacia) PoM
Combination pack, 56 yellow scored tablets, naproxen 500 mg; 56 white scored tablets, misoprostol 200 micrograms. Net price = £23.76. Label: 21
Dose: patients requiring naproxen for rheumatoid arthritis, osteoarthritis, or ankylosing spondylitis, with prophylaxis against NSAID-induced gastroduodenal ulceration, 1 naproxen 500-mg tablet and 1 misoprostol 200-microgram tablet taken together twice daily with food; CHILD not recommended

PIROXICAM

Indications: pain and inflammation in rheumatic disease (including juvenile arthritis) and other musculoskeletal disorders; acute gout
Cautions: see notes above; avoid in porphyria (section 9.8.2); breast-feeding (Appendix 5); **interactions:** Appendix 1 (NSAIDs)
Contra-indications: see notes above
Side-effects: see notes above; pain at injection site (occasionally tissue damage); suppositories may cause rectal irritation and occasional bleeding
Dose: *by mouth*, rheumatic disease, initially 20 mg daily, maintenance 10–30 mg daily, in single or divided doses; CHILD (over 6 years), juvenile arthritis, under 15 kg, 5 mg daily; 16–25 kg, 10 mg; 26–45 kg, 15 mg; over 46 kg, 20 mg
Acute musculoskeletal disorders, 40 mg daily in single or divided doses for 2 days, then 20 mg daily for 7–14 days; CHILD not recommended
Acute gout, 40 mg initially, then 40 mg daily in single or divided doses for 4–6 days; CHILD not recommended
By deep intramuscular injection into gluteal muscle, for initial treatment of acute conditions, as dose by mouth (on short-term basis); CHILD not recommended

Piroxicam (Non-proprietary) PoM
Capsules, piroxicam 10 mg, net price 56-cap pack = £3.54; 20 mg, 28-cap pack = £4.14. Label: 21
Dispersible tablets, piroxicam 10 mg, net price 56-tab pack = £9.33; 20 mg, 28-tab pack = £14.75. Label: 13, 21

Feldene® (Pfizer) PoM
Capsules, piroxicam 10 mg (maroon/blue), net price 56-cap pack = £7.20; 20 mg (maroon), 28-cap pack = £7.20. Label: 21
Tablets, (*Feldene Melt*®), piroxicam 20 mg, net price 28-tab pack = £9.83. Label: 10, patient information leaflet, 21
Excipients: include aspartame equivalent to phenylalanine 140 micrograms/tablet (section 9.4.1)
NOTE. *Feldene Melt*® tablets can be taken by placing on tongue or by swallowing
Dispersible tablets, piroxicam 10 mg (scored), net price 56-tab pack = £11.70; 20 mg, 28-tab pack = £11.70. Label: 13, 21
Injection, piroxicam 20 mg/mL. Net price 1-mL amp = 84p
Gel, section 10.3.2

Brexidol® (Trinity) PoM
Tablets, yellow, scored, piroxicam (as betadex) 20 mg, net price 30-tab pack = £12.22. Label: 21
Dose: osteoarthritis, rheumatic disease and acute musculoskeletal disorders, 1 tablet daily (may be halved in elderly); CHILD not recommended

SULINDAC

Indications: pain and inflammation in rheumatic disease and other musculoskeletal disorders; acute gout
Cautions: see notes above; also history of renal stones and ensure adequate hydration; breast-feeding (Appendix 5); **interactions:** Appendix 1 (NSAIDs)
Contra-indications: see notes above
Side-effects: see notes above; jaundice with fever, cholestasis, hepatitis, hepatic failure; also urine discoloration occasionally reported
Dose: 200 mg twice daily with food (may be reduced according to response); max. 400 mg daily; acute gout should respond within 7 days; limit treatment of peri-articular disorders to 7–10 days; CHILD not recommended

Sulindac (Non-proprietary) PoM
Tablets, sulindac 100 mg, net price 56-tab pack = £11.00; 200 mg, 56-tab pack = £20.07. Label: 21

Clinoril® (MSD) PoM
Tablets, both yellow, scored, sulindac 100 mg, net price 60-tab pack = £6.73; 200 mg, 60-tab pack = £12.96. Label: 21

TENOXICAM

Indications: pain and inflammation in rheumatic disease and other musculoskeletal disorders
Cautions: see notes above; breast-feeding (Appendix 5); **interactions:** Appendix 1 (NSAIDs)
Contra-indications: see notes above
Side-effects: see notes above
Dose: *by mouth*, rheumatic disease, 20 mg daily; CHILD not recommended
Acute musculoskeletal disorders, 20 mg daily for 7 days; max. 14 days; CHILD not recommended
By intravenous or intramuscular injection, for initial treatment for 1–2 days, as dose by mouth; CHILD not recommended

Mobiflex® (Roche) PoM
Tablets, yellow, f/c, tenoxicam 20 mg. Net price 30-tab pack = £13.42. Label: 21
Injection, powder for reconstitution, tenoxicam 20 mg. Net price per amp (with solvent) = 82p

TIAPROFENIC ACID

Indications: pain and inflammation in rheumatic disease and other musculoskeletal disorders
Cautions: see notes above; breast-feeding (Appendix 5); **interactions:** Appendix 1 (NSAIDs)
Contra-indications: see notes above; also active bladder or prostate disease (or symptoms) and history of recurrent urinary-tract disorders—if urinary symptoms develop discontinue immediately and perform urine tests and culture; see also CSM advice below

> **CSM advice.** Following reports of **severe cystitis** CSM has recommended that tiaprofenic acid should not be given to patients with urinary-tract disorders and should be stopped if urinary symptoms develop. Patients should be advised to stop taking tiaprofenic acid and to report to their doctor promptly if they develop urinary-tract symptoms (such as increased frequency, nocturia, urgency, pain on urinating, or blood in urine)

Side-effects: see notes above
Dose: 600 mg daily in 2–3 divided doses; CHILD not recommended

Tiaprofenic Acid (Non-proprietary) PoM
Tablets, tiaprofenic acid 200 mg, net price 84-tab pack = £20.48; 300 mg, 56-tab pack = £20.48. Label: 21

Surgam® (Florizel) PoM
Tablets, tiaprofenic acid 200 mg, net price 84-tab pack = £15.56; 300 mg, 56-tab pack = £15.56. Label: 21

■ Modified release

Surgam SA® (Aventis Pharma) PoM
Capsules, m/r, maroon/pink enclosing white pellets, tiaprofenic acid 300 mg. Net price 56-cap pack = £15.56. Label: 25
Dose: 2 capsules once daily; CHILD not recommended

Aspirin

Aspirin was the traditional first choice anti-inflammatory analgesic but most physicians now prefer to start treatment with another NSAID which may be better tolerated and more convenient for the patient.

In regular high dosage aspirin has about the same anti-inflammatory effect as other NSAIDs. The required dose for active inflammatory joint disease is at least 3.6 g daily. There is little anti-inflammatory effect with less than 3 g daily. Gastro-intestinal side-effects such as nausea, dyspepsia, and gastro-intestinal bleeding may occur with any dosage of aspirin but anti-inflammatory doses are associated with a much higher incidence of side-effects. Anti-inflammatory doses of aspirin may also cause mild chronic salicylate intoxication (salicylism) characterised by dizziness, tinnitus, and deafness; these symptoms may be controlled by reducing the dosage.

ASPIRIN

(Acetylsalicylic Acid)

Indications: pain and inflammation in rheumatic disease and other musculoskeletal disorders (including juvenile arthritis); see also section 4.7.1; antiplatelet (section 2.9)
Cautions: asthma, allergic disease, uncontrolled hypertension, hepatic impairment (Appendix 2), renal impairment—avoid if severe (Appendix 3), dehydration, pregnancy (particularly at term; see also Appendix 4), elderly; preferably avoid during fever or viral infection in adolescents (risk of Reye's syndrome, see below); G6PD-deficiency (section 9.1.5); **interactions:** Appendix 1 (aspirin)
REYE'S SYNDROME. Owing to an association with Reye's syndrome the CSM has advised that aspirin-containing preparations should not be given to children and adolescents under 16 years, unless specifically indicated, e.g. for Kawasaki syndrome
Contra-indications: previous or active peptic ulceration; children and adolescents under 16 years (unless specifically indicated e.g. for Kawasaki syndrome) and breast-feeding—risk of Reye's syndrome (Appendix 5), see above; haemophilia and other bleeding disorders; not for treatment of gout
HYPERSENSITIVITY. Aspirin and other NSAIDs **contra-indicated** in history of hypersensitivity to aspirin or any other NSAID—which includes those in whom attacks of asthma, angioedema, urticaria or rhinitis have been precipitated by aspirin or any other NSAID
Side-effects: common with anti-inflammatory doses; gastro-intestinal discomfort or nausea, ulceration with occult bleeding (but occasionally major haemorrhage); also other haemorrhage (e.g. subconjunctival); hearing disturbances such as tinnitus (leading rarely to deafness), vertigo, confusion, hypersensitivity reactions (angioedema, bronchospasm and rashes); increased bleeding time; rarely oedema, blood disorders, particularly thrombocytopenia; **overdosage:** see Emergency Treatment of Poisoning, p. 29
Dose: 0.3–1 g every 4 hours after food; max. in acute conditions 8 g daily; CHILD, juvenile arthritis, up to 80 mg/kg daily in 5–6 divided doses after food, increased in acute exacerbations to 130 mg/kg
NOTE. High doses of aspirin are very rarely required and are now given under specialist supervision only, and with plasma monitoring (especially in children)

■ Preparations
Section 4.7.1

10.1.2 Corticosteroids

10.1.2.1 Systemic corticosteroids

The general actions and uses of the corticosteroids are described in section 6.3. Treatment with corticosteroids in rheumatic diseases should be reserved for specific indications, e.g. when other anti-inflammatory drugs are unsuccessful. Corticosteroids can induce osteoporosis, and prophylaxis should be considered on long-term treatment (section 6.6).

In severe, possibly life-threatening, situations a high initial dose of corticosteroid is given to induce remission and the dose is then reduced gradually and discontinued altogether. Relapse may occur as the dose of corticosteroid is reduced, particularly if the reduction is too rapid. The tendency is therefore to increase the maintenance dose and consequently the patient becomes dependent on corticosteroids. For this reason pulse doses of corticosteroids (e.g. methylprednisolone up to 1 g intravenously on 3 consecutive days) are used to suppress highly active inflammatory disease while longer-term treatment with a disease-modifying drug is commenced.

Prednisolone 7.5 mg daily may reduce the rate of joint destruction in moderate to severe *rheumatoid arthritis* of less than 2 years' duration. The reduction in joint destruction must be distinguished from mere symptomatic improvement (which lasts only 6 to 12 months at this dose) and care should be taken to avoid increasing the dose above 7.5 mg daily. Evidence supports maintenance of this anti-erosive dose for 2–4 years only after which treatment should be tapered off to reduce long-term adverse effects.

Polymyalgia rheumatica and *giant cell (temporal) arteritis* are always treated with corticosteroids. The usual initial dose of prednisolone in polymyalgia rheumatica is 10–15 mg daily and in giant cell arteritis 40–60 mg daily (the higher dose being used if visual symptoms occur). Treatment should be continued until remission of disease activity and doses are then reduced gradually to about 7.5 –10 mg daily for maintenance. Relapse is common if therapy is stopped prematurely. Many patients require treatment for at least 2 years and in some patients it may be necessary to continue long-term low-dose corticosteroid treatment.

Polyarteritis nodosa and *polymyositis* are usually treated with corticosteroids. An initial dose of 60 mg of prednisolone daily is often used and reduced to a maintenance dose of 10–15 mg daily.

Systemic lupus erythematosus is treated with corticosteroids when necessary using a similar dosage regimen to that for polyarteritis nodosa and polymyositis (above). Patients with pleurisy, pericarditis, or other systemic manifestations will respond to corticosteroids. It may then be possible to reduce the dosage; alternate-day treatment is sometimes adequate, and the drug may be gradually withdrawn. In some mild cases corticosteroid treatment may be stopped after a few months. Many mild cases of systemic lupus erythematosus do not require corticosteroid treatment. Alternative treatment with anti-inflammatory analgesics, and possibly chloroquine or hydroxychloroquine, should be considered.

Ankylosing spondylitis should not be treated with long-term corticosteroids; rarely, pulse doses may be needed and may be useful in extremely active disease that does not respond to conventional treatment.

10.1.2.2 Local corticosteroid injections

Corticosteroids are injected locally for an anti-inflammatory effect. In inflammatory conditions of the joints, particularly in rheumatoid arthritis, they are given by *intra-articular injection* to relieve pain, increase mobility, and reduce deformity in one or a few joints. Full aseptic precautions are essential; infected areas should be avoided. Occasionally an acute inflammatory reaction develops after an intra-articular or soft-tissue injection of a corticosteroid. This may be a reaction to the microcrystalline suspension of the corticosteroid used, but must be distinguished from sepsis introduced into the injection site.

Smaller amounts of corticosteroids may also be injected directly into soft tissues for the relief of inflammation in conditions such as *tennis* or *golfer's elbow* or *compression neuropathies*. In *tendinitis*, injections should be made into the tendon sheath and not directly into the tendon (due to the absence of a true tendon sheath, the Achilles tendon should not be injected). A soluble preparation (e.g. containing betamethasone or dexamethasone sodium phosphate) is preferred for injection into the carpal tunnel.

Hydrocortisone acetate or one of the synthetic analogues is generally used for local injection. Flushing has been reported with intra-articular corticosteroid injections. Charcot-like arthropathies have also been reported (particularly following repeated intra-articular injections). Intra-articular injections may affect the hyaline cartilage and each joint should usually be treated **no more** than 3 times in one year.

Corticosteroid injections are also injected into soft tissues for the treatment of skin lesions (see section 13.4).

LOCAL CORTICOSTEROID INJECTIONS

Indications: local inflammation of joints and soft tissues (for details, consult product literature)

Cautions: see notes above and consult product literature; see also section 6.3.2

Contra-indications: see notes above and consult product literature

Side-effects: see notes above and consult product literature

Dose: see under preparations

■ Dose calculated as dexamethasone

Dexamethasone (Organon) PoM

Injection, dexamethasone 4 mg/mL (as sodium phosphate) (≡ dexamethasone sodium phosphate 5.2 mg/mL ≡ dexamethasone phosphate 4.8 mg/mL). Net price 1-mL amp = 83p; 2-mL vial = £1.27

Dose: by intra-articular or intrasynovial injection (for details consult product literature), 0.6–3 mg (calculated as dexamethasone) according to size; where appropriate may be repeated at intervals of 3–21 days according to response

■ Dose calculated as dexamethasone phosphate

Dexamethasone (Mayne) PoM

Injection, dexamethasone phosphate 4 mg/mL (as sodium phosphate) (≡ dexamethasone 3.3 mg/mL ≡ dexamethasone sodium phosphate 4.4 mg/mL), net price 1-mL amp = £1.00; 2-mL vial = £1.98

Dose: by intra-articular or intrasynovial injection (for details consult product literature), 0.4–4 mg (calculated as dexamethasone phosphate) according to size (*soft-tissue infiltration* 2–6 mg); where appropriate may be repeated at intervals of 3–21 days

■ Hydrocortisone acetate

Hydrocortistab® (Sovereign) PoM

Injection, (aqueous suspension), hydrocortisone acetate 25 mg/mL. Net price 1-mL amp = £4.77

Dose: by intra-articular or intrasynovial injection (for details consult product literature), 5–50 mg according to size; where appropriate may be repeated at intervals of 21 days; not more than 3 joints should be treated on any one day; CHILD 5–30 mg (divided)

■ Methylprednisolone acetate

Depo-Medrone® (Pharmacia) PoM

Injection (aqueous suspension), methylprednisolone acetate 40 mg/mL. Net price 1-mL vial = £2.87; 2-mL vial = £5.15; 3-mL vial = £7.47

Dose: by intra-articular or intrasynovial injection (for details consult product literature), 4–80 mg, according to size; where appropriate may be repeated at intervals of 7–35 days; also for *intralesional injection*

Depo-Medrone® **with Lidocaine** (Pharmacia) PoM

Injection (aqueous suspension), methylprednisolone acetate 40 mg, lidocaine hydrochloride 10 mg/mL. Net price 1-mL vial = £3.28; 2-mL vial = £5.88

Dose: by intra-articular or intrasynovial injection (for details consult product literature), 4–80 mg, according to size; where appropriate may be repeated at intervals of 7–35 days

■ Prednisolone acetate

Deltastab® (Sovereign) PoM

Injection (aqueous suspension), prednisolone acetate 25 mg/mL. Net price 1-mL amp = £4.77

Dose: by intra-articular or intrasynovial injection (for details consult product literature), 5–25 mg according to size; not more than 3 joints should be treated on any one day; where appropriate may be repeated when relapse occurs

For *intramuscular injection*, see section 6.3.2

■ Triamcinolone acetonide

Adcortyl® **Intra-articular/Intradermal** (Squibb) PoM

Injection (aqueous suspension), triamcinolone acetonide 10 mg/mL. Net price 1-mL amp = £1.02; 5-mL vial = £4.14

Dose: by intra-articular injection or intrasynovial injection (for details consult product literature), 2.5–15 mg according to size (for larger doses use *Kenalog*®); where appropriate may be repeated when relapse occurs

By intradermal injection, (for details consult product literature): 2–3 mg; max. 5 mg at any one site (total max. 30 mg); where appropriate may be repeated at intervals of 1–2 weeks

CHILD under 6 years not recommended

Kenalog® **Intra-articular/Intramuscular** (Squibb) PoM

Injection (aqueous suspension), triamcinolone acetonide 40 mg/mL, net price 1-mL vial = £1.70; 1-mL prefilled syringe = £2.11; 2-mL prefilled syringe = £3.66

NOTE. Intramuscular needle with prefilled syringe should be replaced for intra-articular injection

Dose: by intra-articular or intrasynovial injection (for details consult product literature), 5–40 mg according to size; total max. 80 mg (for doses below 5 mg use *Adcortyl*® *Intra-articular/Intradermal*); where appropriate may be repeated when relapse occurs; CHILD under 6 years not recommended

For *intramuscular injection*, see section 6.3.2

10.1.3 Drugs which suppress the rheumatic disease process

Certain drugs such as gold, penicillamine, hydroxychloroquine, chloroquine, drugs affecting the immune response, and sulfasalazine may suppress the disease process in *rheumatoid arthritis*, as may sulfasalazine, methotrexate, and possibly gold and azathioprine in *psoriatic arthritis*. They are known as disease-modifying antirheumatic drugs (DMARDs). Unlike NSAIDs they do not produce an immediate therapeutic effect but require 4 to 6 months of treatment for a full response. If one of these drugs does not lead to objective benefit within 6 months of initiating treatment or 3 months after maximum treatment, it should be discontinued and a different drug tried. Response to a disease-modifying antirheumatic drug may allow the dose of the NSAID to be reduced.

Disease-modifying antirheumatic drugs may improve not only the symptoms and signs of inflammatory joint disease but also extra-articular manifestations such as vasculitis. They reduce the erythrocyte sedimentation rate, C-reactive protein, and sometimes the titre of rheumatoid factor. Some (e.g. methotrexate and ciclosporin) are believed to retard erosive damage as judged radiologically.

CHOICE. Since in the first few months, the course of rheumatoid arthritis is unpredictable and the diagnosis uncertain, it is usual to start treatment with an NSAID alone. Disease-modifying antirheumatic drugs are, however, instituted by specialists as soon as diagnosis, progression, and severity of the disease have been confirmed. The choice of a disease-modifying antirheumatic drug should take into account co-morbidity and patient preference. Sulfasalazine, methotrexate, intramuscular gold and penicillamine are similar in efficacy. However, **sulfasalazine** or **methotrexate** are often used first because they may be better tolerated.

Penicillamine and drugs that affect the immune response ('immunomodulators') are also sometimes used in rheumatoid arthritis where there are troublesome extra-articular features such as vasculitis, and in patients who are taking high doses of corticosteroids. Where the response is satisfactory there is often a striking reduction in requirements of both corticosteroids and other drugs. **Gold** and **penicillamine** are effective in *palindromic rheumatism*. *Systemic* and *discoid lupus erythematosus* are sometimes treated with **chloroquine** or **hydroxychloroquine**.

In some circumstances, and under specialist supervision, combining two or more disease-modifying antirheumatic drugs may be considered.

JUVENILE IDIOPATHIC ARTHRITIS. Many children with *juvenile idiopathic arthritis* (juvenile chronic arthritis) do not require disease-modifying antirheumatic drugs. If drug treatment is required, methotrexate is effective [unlicensed indication]; sulfasalazine is an alternative [unlicensed indication] but it should be avoided in systemic-onset juvenile idiopathic arthritis. Gold and penicillamine are used very rarely. For the role of etanercept in polyarticular-course juvenile idiopathic arthritis, see p. 517

Gold

Gold may be given by intramuscular injection as sodium aurothiomalate or by mouth as auranofin.

Sodium aurothiomalate must be given by deep intramuscular injection and the area gently massaged. A test dose of 10 mg must be given followed by doses of 50 mg at weekly intervals until there is definite evidence of remission. Benefit is not to be expected until about 300–500 mg has been given; it should be discontinued if there is no remission after 1 g has been given. In patients who do respond, the interval between injections is then gradually increased to 4 weeks and treatment is continued for up to 5 years after complete remission. If relapse occurs the dosage frequency may be immediately increased to 50 mg weekly and only once control has been obtained again should the dosage frequency be decreased; if no response is seen within 2 months, alternative treatment should be sought. It is important to avoid complete relapse since second courses of gold are not usually effective. Children may be given 1 mg/kg weekly to a maximum of 50 mg weekly, the intervals being gradually increased to 4 weeks according to response; an initial test dose is given corresponding to one-tenth to one-fifth of the calculated dose.

Auranofin is given by mouth. If there is no response after 6 months treatment should be discontinued. Auranofin is less effective than parenteral gold.

Gold therapy should be discontinued in the presence of blood disorders, gastro-intestinal bleeding (associated with ulcerative enterocolitis), or unexplained proteinuria (associated with immune complex nephritis) which is repeatedly above 300 mg/litre. Urine tests and full blood counts (including total and differential white cell and platelet counts) must therefore be performed before starting treatment with gold and before each intramuscular injection; in the case of oral treatment the urine and blood tests should be carried out monthly. Rashes with pruritus often occur after 2 to 6 months of intramuscular treatment and may necessitate discontinuation of treatment; the most common side-effect of oral therapy, diarrhoea with or without nausea or abdominal pain, may respond to bulking agents (such as bran) or temporary reduction in dosage.

SODIUM AUROTHIOMALATE

Indications: active progressive rheumatoid arthritis, juvenile arthritis

Cautions: see notes above; hepatic impairment (Appendix 2), renal impairment (Appendix 3), pregnancy (Appendix 4), breast-feeding (Appendix 5); elderly, history of urticaria, eczema, colitis, drugs which cause blood disorders; annual chest X-ray

Contra-indications: severe renal and hepatic disease (see notes above); history of blood disorders or bone marrow aplasia, exfoliative dermatitis, systemic lupus erythematosus, necrotising enterocolitis, pulmonary fibrosis; porphyria (section 9.8.2)

Side-effects: severe reactions (occasionally fatal) in up to 5% of patients; mouth ulcers, skin reactions (including, on prolonged parenteral treatment, irreversible pigmentation in sun-exposed areas), proteinuria, blood disorders (sometimes sudden and fatal); rarely colitis, peripheral neuritis, pulmonary fibrosis, hepatotoxicity with cholestatic jaundice, nephrotic syndrome, alopecia

Dose: *by deep intramuscular injection*, administered on expert advice, see notes above

COUNSELLING. Warn patient to tell doctor immediately if sore throat, fever, infection, non-specific illness, unexplained bleeding and bruising, purpura, mouth ulcers, metallic taste, or rashes develop; also ask patients to report immediately any breathlessness or cough

Myocrisin® (JHC) PoM

Injection, sodium aurothiomalate 20 mg/mL, net price 0.5-mL (10-mg) amp = £2.94; 40 mg/mL, 0.5-mL (20-mg) amp = £4.28; 100 mg/mL, 0.5-mL (50-mg) amp = £8.71. Counselling, blood disorder symptoms

---

AURANOFIN

Indications: active progressive rheumatoid arthritis

Cautions: see under Sodium Aurothiomalate; hepatic impairment (Appendix 2); pregnancy (Appendix 4); breast-feeding (Appendix 5); also inflammatory bowel disease

BLOOD COUNTS. Withdraw if platelet count falls below 100 000/mm^3 or if signs and symptoms suggestive of thrombocytopenia occur, see also notes above

Contra-indications: see under Sodium Aurothiomalate

Side-effects: diarrhoea most common (reduced by bulking agents such as bran); see also under Sodium Aurothiomalate

Dose: administered on expert advice, 6 mg daily (initially in 2 divided doses then if tolerated as single dose), if response inadequate after 6 months, increase to 9 mg daily (in 3 divided doses), discontinue if no response after a further 3 months; CHILD not recommended

COUNSELLING. Warn patient to tell doctor immediately if sore throat, fever, infection, non-specific illness, unexplained bleeding and bruising, purpura, mouth ulcers, metallic taste, or rashes develop; also ask patients to report immediately any breathlessness or cough

NOTE. The package insert for *Ridaura*® also advises that patients must also report immediately if conjunctivitis or hair loss develops

Ridaura® (Yamanouchi) PoM

Tablets, yellow, f/c, auranofin 3 mg. Net price 60-tab pack = £25.20. Label: 21, counselling, blood disorder symptoms (see above)

Penicillamine

Penicillamine has a similar action to gold, and more patients are able to continue treatment than with gold but side-effects occur frequently. Penicillamine should be discontinued if there is no improvement within 1 year.

Patients should be warned not to expect improvement for at least 6 to 12 weeks after treatment is initiated. If remission has been sustained for 6 months, reduction of dosage by 125 to 250 mg every 12 weeks may be attempted.

Blood counts, including platelets, and urine examinations should be carried out before starting treatment and then every 1 or 2 weeks for the first 2 months then every 4 weeks to detect blood disorders and proteinuria (they should also be carried out in the week after any dose increase). A reduction in platelet count calls for discontinuation with subsequent re-introduction at a lower dosage and then, if possible, gradual increase. Proteinuria, associated with immune complex nephritis, occurs in up to 30% of patients, but may resolve despite continuation of treatment; treatment may be continued provided that renal function tests remain normal, oedema is absent, and the 24-hour urinary excretion of protein does not exceed 2 g.

Nausea may occur but is not usually a problem provided that penicillamine is taken before food or on retiring and that low initial doses are used and only gradually increased. Loss of taste may occur about 6 weeks after treatment is started but usually returns 6 weeks later irrespective of whether or not treatment is discontinued; mineral supplements are not recommended. Rashes are a common side-effect. Those which occur in the first few months of treatment disappear when the drug is stopped and treatment may then be re-introduced at a lower dose level and gradually increased. Late rashes are more resistant and often necessitate discontinuation of treatment.

Patients who are hypersensitive to penicillin may react rarely to penicillamine.

PENICILLAMINE

Indications: see notes above and under Dose

Cautions: see notes above; renal impairment (Appendix 3); pregnancy (Appendix 4); concomitant nephrotoxic drugs (increased risk of toxicity); gold treatment (avoid concomitant use if adverse reactions to gold); **interactions:** Appendix 1 (penicillamine)

BLOOD COUNTS AND URINE TESTS. See notes above. Longer intervals may be adequate in cystinuria and Wilson's disease. Consider withdrawal if platelet count falls below 120 000/mm^3 or white blood cells below 2500/mm^3 or if 3 successive falls within reference range (can restart at reduced dose when counts return to within reference range but permanent withdrawal necessary if recurrence of leucopenia or thrombocytopenia)

COUNSELLING. Warn patient to tell doctor immediately if sore throat, fever, infection, non-specific illness, unexplained bleeding and bruising, purpura, mouth ulcers, or rashes develop

Contra-indications: lupus erythematosus; moderate to severe renal impairment

Side-effects: (see also notes above) initially nausea, anorexia, fever, and skin reactions; taste loss (mineral supplements not recommended); blood disorders including thrombocytopenia, leucopenia, agranulocytosis and aplastic anaemia; proteinuria, rarely haematuria (withdraw immediately); haemolytic anaemia, nephrotic syndrome, lupus erythematosus-like syndrome, myasthenia gravis-like syndrome, polymyositis (rarely with cardiac involvement), dermatomyositis, mouth ulcers, stomatitis, alopecia, bronchiolitis and pneumonitis, pemphigus, Goodpasture's syndrome, and Stevens-Johnson syndrome also reported; male and female breast enlargement reported; in non-rheumatoid conditions rheumatoid arthritis-like syndrome also reported; late rashes (consider withdrawing treatment)

Dose: severe active rheumatoid arthritis, administered on expert advice, ADULT initially 125–250 mg daily before food for 1 month increased by similar amounts at intervals of not less than 4 weeks to usual maintenance of 500–750 mg daily in divided doses; max. 1.5 g daily; ELDERLY initially up to 125 mg daily before food for 1 month increased by similar amounts at intervals of not less than 4 weeks; max. 1 g daily; CHILD maintenance of 15–20 mg/kg daily (initial dose lower and increased at intervals of 4 weeks over a period of 3-6 months)

Wilson's disease, chronic active hepatitis, and cystinuria, section 9.8.1

Lead poisoning, see Emergency Treatment of Poisoning, p. 34

Penicillamine (Non-proprietary) PoM

Tablets, penicillamine 125 mg, net price 20 = £1.96; 250 mg, 20 = £3.41. Label: 6, 22, counselling, blood disorder symptoms (see above)

Distamine® (Alliance) PoM

Tablets, all f/c, penicillamine 125 mg, net price 20 = £1.96; 250 mg, 20 = £3.41. Label: 6, 22, counselling, blood disorder symptoms (see above)

Antimalarials

The antimalarial **hydroxychloroquine** is used to treat rheumatoid arthritis of moderate inflammatory activity; **chloroquine** is also licensed for treating inflammatory disorders but it is used much less frequently and it is generally reserved for use if other drugs have failed. These drugs are effective for mild systemic lupus erythematosus, particularly involving cutaneous and joint manifestations. Chloroquine and hydroxychloroquine should not be used for psoriatic arthritis.

Chloroquine and hydroxychloroquine are better tolerated than gold or penicillamine. Retinopathy (see below) occurs rarely provided that the recommended doses are not exceeded; in the elderly it is difficult to distinguish drug-induced retinopathy from ageing changes.

Mepacrine (section 5.4.4) is sometimes used in discoid lupus erythematosus [unlicensed].

CAUTIONS. Chloroquine and hydroxychloroquine should be used with caution in hepatic impairment (Appendix 2) and in renal impairment (Appendix 3). Manufacturers recommend regular ophthalmological examination but the evidence of practical value is unsatisfactory (see advice of Royal College of Ophthalmologists, below). It is not necessary to withdraw an antimalarial during pregnancy (Appendix 4) if the rheumatic disease is well controlled. Chloroquine and hydroxychloroquine are present in breast milk and breast-feeding (Appendix 5) should be avoided when they are used to treat rheumatic disease; chloroquine can, however, be used for malaria during pregnancy and breast-feeding (section 5.4.1). Both should be used with caution in neurological disorders (especially in those with a history of epilepsy), in severe gastro-intestinal disorders, in G6PD deficiency (section 9.1.5), in porphyria, and in the elderly (see also above). Chloroquine and hydroxychloroquine may exacerbate psoriasis and aggravate myasthenia gravis. Concurrent use of hepatotoxic drugs should be avoided; other **interactions**: Appendix 1 (chloroquine and hydroxychloroquine).

Screening for ocular toxicity

A review group convened by the Royal College of Ophthalmologists has updated guidelines for screening to prevent ocular toxicity on long-term treatment with chloroquine, hydroxychloroquine, and mepacrine (*Ocular toxicity with hydroxychloroquine: guidelines for screening 2004*). Chloroquine should be considered (for treating chronic inflammatory conditions) **only** if other drugs have failed. All patients taking chloroquine should receive ocular examination according to a protocol arranged locally between the prescriber and the ophthalmologist. Mepacrine has negligible ocular toxicity. The following recommendations relate to hydroxychloroquine, which is only rarely associated with toxicity.

Before treatment:

- Assess renal and liver function (adjust dose if impaired)
- Ask patient about visual impairment (not corrected by glasses). If impairment or eye disease present, assessment by an optometrist is advised and any abnormality should be referred to an ophthalmologist
- Record near visual acuity of each eye (with glasses where appropriate) using a standard reading chart
- Initiate hydroxychloroquine treatment if no abnormality detected (at a dose not exceeding hydroxychloroquine sulphate 6.5 mg/kg daily)

During treatment:

- Ask patient about visual symptoms and monitor visual acuity annually using the standard reading chart
- Refer to ophthalmologist if visual acuity changes or if vision blurred and warn patient to stop treatment and seek prescribing doctor's advice
- A child treated for juvenile arthritis should receive slit-lamp examination routinely to check for uveitis
- If long-term treatment is required (more than 5 years), individual arrangement should be agreed with the local ophthalmologist

NOTE. To avoid excessive dosage in obese patients, the dose of hydroxychloroquine and chloroquine should be calculated on the basis of lean body weight. Ocular toxicity is unlikely with chloroquine phosphate not exceeding 4 mg/kg daily (equivalent to chloroquine base approx. 2.5 mg/kg daily)

SIDE-EFFECTS. The side-effects of chloroquine and hydroxychloroquine include gastro-intestinal disturbances, headache and skin reactions (rashes, pruritus); those occurring less frequently include ECG changes, convulsions, visual changes, retinal damage (see above), keratopathy, ototoxicity, hair depigmentation, hair loss, and discoloration of skin, nails, and mucous membranes. Side-effects that occur rarely include blood disorders (including thrombocytopenia, agranulocytosis, and aplastic anaemia), mental changes (including emotional disturbances and psychosis), myopathy (including cardiomyopathy and neuromyopathy), acute generalised exanthematous pustulosis, exfoliative dermatitis, Stevens-Johnson syndrome, photosensitivity, and hepatic damage. **Important**: very toxic in overdosage—immediate advice from poisons centres essential (see also p. 32).

CHLOROQUINE

Indications: active rheumatoid arthritis (including juvenile arthritis), systemic and discoid lupus erythematosus; malaria (section 5.4.1)
Cautions: see notes above
Side-effects: see notes above
Dose: administered on expert advice, *by mouth*, chloroquine (base) 150 mg daily; max. 2.5 mg/kg daily, see recommendations above; CHILD up to 3 mg/kg daily

NOTE. Chloroquine base 150 mg ≡ chloroquine sulphate 200 mg ≡ chloroquine phosphate 250 mg (approx.).

■ Preparations
Section 5.4.1

HYDROXYCHLOROQUINE SULPHATE

Indications: active rheumatoid arthritis (including juvenile arthritis), systemic and discoid lupus erythematosus; dermatological conditions caused or aggravated by sunlight
Cautions: see notes above
Side-effects: see notes above
Dose: administered on expert advice, initially 400 mg daily in divided doses; maintenance 200–400 mg daily; max. 6.5 mg/kg daily (but not exceeding 400 mg daily), see recommendations above; CHILD, up to 6.5 mg/kg daily (max. 400 mg daily)

Plaquenil® (Sanofi-Synthelabo) PoM
Tablets, f/c, hydroxychloroquine sulphate 200 mg. Net price 60-tab pack = £4.55. Label: 5, 21

Drugs affecting the immune response

Methotrexate is a disease-modifying antirheumatic drug suitable for moderate to severe rheumatoid arthritis. **Azathioprine**, **ciclosporin**, **cyclophosphamide**, **leflunomide**, and the **cytokine inhibitors** (adalimumab, anakinra, etanercept, and infliximab) are considered more toxic and they are used in cases that have not responded to other disease-modifying drugs.

Methotrexate is usually given in an initial dose of 7.5 mg by mouth once a week, adjusted according to response to a maximum of 15 mg once a week (occasionally 20 mg once a week). Regular full blood counts (including differential white cell count and platelet count), renal and liver-function tests are required. In patients who experience mucosal or gastro-intestinal side-effects with methotrexate, folic acid 5 mg every week may help to reduce the frequency of such side-effects.

Azathioprine is usually given in a dose of 1.5 to 2.5 mg/kg daily in divided doses. Blood counts are needed to detect possible neutropenia or thrombocytopenia (usually resolved by reducing the dose). Nausea, vomiting, and diarrhoea may occur, usually starting early during the course of treatment, and may necessitate withdrawal of the drug; herpes zoster infection may also occur.

Leflunomide acts on the immune system as a disease-modifying antirheumatic drug. Its therapeutic effect starts after 4–6 weeks and improvement may continue for a further 4–6 months. Leflunomide, which is similar in efficacy to sulfasalazine and methotrexate, may be chosen when these drugs cannot be used. The active metabolite of leflunomide persists for a long period; active procedures to wash the drug out are required in case of serious adverse effects, or before starting treatment with another disease-modifying antirheumatic drug, or, in men or women, before conception. Side-effects of leflunomide include bone-marrow toxicity; its immunosuppressive effects increase the risk of infection and malignancy.

Ciclosporin (cyclosporin) is licensed for severe active rheumatoid arthritis when conventional second-line therapy is inappropriate or ineffective. There is some evidence that ciclosporin may retard the rate of erosive progression and improve symptom control in those who respond only partially to methotrexate.

Cyclophosphamide (section 8.1.1) may be used at a dose of 1 to 1.5 mg/kg daily by mouth for rheumatoid arthritis with severe systemic manifestations [unlicensed indication]; it is toxic and regular blood counts (including platelet count) should be carried out. Cyclophosphamide may also be given intravenously in a dose of 0.5 to 1 g (with prophylactic mesna) for *severe systemic rheumatoid arthritis* and for other connective tissue diseases (especially with active vasculitis), repeated initially at fortnightly then at monthly intervals (according to clinical response and haematological monitoring).

Drugs that affect the immune response are also used in the management of severe cases of *systemic lupus erythematosus* and other connective tissue disorders. They are often given in conjunction with corticosteroids for patients with severe or progressive renal disease. They may be used in cases of *polymyositis* which are resistant to corticosteroids. They are used for their corticosteroid-sparing effect in patients whose corticosteroid requirements are excessive. **Azathioprine** is usually used.

Azathioprine and methotrexate are used in the treatment of *psoriatic arthropathy* [unlicensed indication] for severe or progressive cases which are not controlled with anti-inflammatory drugs.

AZATHIOPRINE

Indications: see notes above; transplantation rejection, see section 8.2.1

Cautions: see section 8.2.1

Contra-indications: see section 8.2.1

Side-effects: see section 8.2.1

Dose: *by mouth*, initially, rarely more than 3 mg/kg daily, reduced according to response; maintenance 1–3 mg/kg daily; consider withdrawal if no improvement within 3 months

■ Preparations
Section 8.2.1

CICLOSPORIN

(Cyclosporin)

Indications: severe active rheumatoid arthritis when conventional second-line therapy inappropriate or ineffective; graft-versus-host disease (section 8.2.2); atopic dermatitis and psoriasis (section 13.5.3).

Cautions: see section 8.2.2

ADDITIONAL CAUTIONS IN RHEUMATOID ARTHRITIS. ***Contra-indicated*** in abnormal renal function, uncontrolled hypertension (see also below), uncontrolled infections, and malignancy. Measure serum creatinine at least twice before treatment and monitor every 2 weeks for first 3 months, then every 4 weeks (or more frequently if dose increased or concomitant NSAIDs introduced or increased (see also ***interactions:*** Appendix 1 (ciclosporin)), reduce dose if serum creatinine increases more than 30% above baseline in more than 1 measurement; if above 50%, reduce dose by 50% (even if within normal range) and discontinue if reduction not successful within 1 month; monitor blood pressure (discontinue if hypertension develops that cannot be controlled by antihypertensive therapy); monitor hepatic function if concomitant NSAIDs given.

Side-effects: see section 8.2.2

Dose: *by mouth*, administered in accordance with expert advice, initially 2.5 mg/kg daily in 2 divided doses, if necessary increased gradually after 6 weeks; max. 4 mg/kg daily (discontinue if response insufficient after 3 months); dose adjusted according to response for maintenance and treatment reviewed after 6 months (continue only if benefits outweigh risks); CHILD and under 18 years, not recommended

IMPORTANT. For preparations and counselling and for advice on conversion between the preparations, see section 8.2.2

■ Preparations
Section 8.2.2

LEFLUNOMIDE

Indications: moderate to severe active rheumatoid arthritis; active psoriatic arthritis

Cautions: renal impairment (Appendix 3); impaired bone-marrow function including anaemia, leucopenia or thrombocytopenia (avoid if significant and due to causes other than rheumatoid arthritis); recent treatment with other hepatotoxic or myelotoxic disease-modifying antirheumatic drugs (avoid concomitant use); history of tuberculosis; exclude pregnancy before treatment; effective contraception **essential** during treatment and for at least 2 years after treatment in women and at least 3 months after treatment in men (plasma concentration monitoring required; waiting time before conception may be reduced with washout procedures—consult product literature and see Washout Procedure below); monitor full blood count (including differential white cell count and platelet count) before treatment and every 2 weeks for 6 months then every 8 weeks; monitor liver function—(see Hepatotoxicity below); monitor blood pressure; washout procedures recommended for serious adverse effects and before switching to other disease-modifying antirheumatic drugs (consult product literature and see below); **interactions:** Appendix 1 (leflunomide)

HEPATOTOXICITY. Potentially life-threatening hepatotoxicity reported usually in the first 6 months; monitor liver function before treatment and every 2 weeks for first 6 months then every 8 weeks. Discontinue treatment (and institute washout procedure—consult product literature and see Washout Procedure below) or reduce dose according to liver-function abnormality; if liver-function abnormality persists after dose reduction, discontinue treatment and institute washout procedure

WASHOUT PROCEDURE. To aid drug elimination in case of serious adverse effect, or before starting another disease-modifying antirheumatic drug, or before conception (see also Appendix 4), stop treatment and give *either* colestyramine 8 g 3 times daily for 11 days *or* activated charcoal 50 g 4 times daily for 11 days; the concentration of the active metabolite after washout should be less than 20 micrograms/litre (measured on 2 occasions 14 days apart) in men or women before conception—consult product literature

Contra-indications: severe immunodeficiency; serious infection; hepatic impairment (Appendix 2); severe hypoproteinaemia; pregnancy (**important teratogenic risk:** see Cautions and Appendix 4); breast-feeding (Appendix 5)

Side-effects: diarrhoea, nausea, vomiting, anorexia, oral mucosal disorders, abdominal pain, weight loss; increase in blood pressure; headache, dizziness, asthenia, paraesthesia; tenosynovitis; alopecia, eczema, dry skin, rash, pruritus; leucopenia; rarely taste disturbances, anxiety, tendon rupture, urticaria, anaemia, thrombocytopenia, eosinophilia, hyperlipidaemia, hypokalaemia, hypophosphataemia, hepatic dysfunction (see Hepatotoxicity above); also reported, pancreatitis, anaphylaxis, interstitial lung disease, severe infection, pancytopenia, vasculitis, Stevens-Johnson syndrome, toxic epidermal necrolysis (discontinue and initiate washout procedure—consult product literature)

Dose: rheumatoid arthritis, ADULT over 18 years, initially 100 mg once daily for 3 days then maintenance, 10–20 mg once daily

Psoriatic arthritis, ADULT over 18 years, initially 100 mg once daily for 3 days then maintenance, 20 mg once daily

Arava® (Aventis Pharma) ▼ PoM
Tablets, f/c, leflunomide 10 mg, net price 30-tab pack = £51.13; 20 mg (ochre), 30-tab pack = £51.13; 100 mg, 3-tab pack = £25.56. Label: 4

METHOTREXATE

Indications: moderate to severe active rheumatoid arthritis; Crohn's disease (section 1.5); malignant disease (section 8.1.3); psoriasis (section 13.5.3)

Cautions: section 8.1; see CSM advice below (blood count, liver and pulmonary toxicity); extreme caution in blood disorders (avoid if severe); renal impairment (avoid in moderate or severe—Appendix 3); peptic ulceration, ulcerative colitis, diarrhoea and ulcerative stomatitis (withdraw if stomatitis develops—may be first sign of gastro-intestinal toxicity); risk of accumulation in pleural effusion or ascites—drain before treatment; porphyria (section 9.8.2); **interactions:** see below and Appendix 1 (methotrexate)

CSM advice. In view of reports of blood dyscrasias (including fatalities) and liver cirrhosis with low-dose methotrexate, the CSM has advised:

- full blood count and renal and liver function tests before starting treatment and repeated weekly until therapy stabilised, thereafter patients should be monitored every 2–3 months
- that patients should be advised to report all symptoms and signs suggestive of infection, especially sore throat

Treatment with folinic acid (as calcium folinate, section 8.1) may be required in acute toxicity

BLOOD COUNT. Haematopoietic suppression may occur abruptly; factors likely to increase toxicity include advanced age, renal impairment and concomitant administration of another anti-folate drug. Any profound drop in white cell or platelet count calls for immediate withdrawal of methotrexate and introduction of supportive therapy

LIVER TOXICITY. Liver cirrhosis reported. Treatment should not be started or should be discontinued if any abnormality of liver function tests or liver biopsy is present or develops during therapy. Abnormalities may return to normal within 2 weeks after which treatment may be recommenced if judged appropriate

PULMONARY TOXICITY. Pulmonary toxicity may be a special problem in rheumatoid arthritis (patient to seek medical attention if dyspnoea, cough or fever); monitor for symptoms at each visit—discontinue if pneumonitis suspected.

ASPIRIN AND OTHER NSAIDS. If aspirin or other NSAIDs are given concurrently the dose of methotrexate should be carefully monitored. Patients should be advised to avoid self-medication with over-the-counter aspirin or ibuprofen

Contra-indications: see Cautions above, hepatic impairment (Appendix 2), pregnancy (following administration to a woman or a man, avoid conception for **at least 3 months** after stopping—Appendix 4), breast-feeding (Appendix 5), active infection and immunodeficiency syndromes

Side-effects: section 8.1; also anorexia, abdominal discomfort, intestinal ulceration and bleeding, diarrhoea, toxic megacolon, hepatotoxicity (see Cautions above); ecchymosis; pulmonary oedema, pleuritic pain, pulmonary fibrosis, interstitial pneumonitis (see Pulmonary Toxicity above); anaphylactic reactions, urticaria; dizziness, drowsiness, malaise, headache, mood changes, abnormal cranial sensations; precipitation of diabetes, osteoporosis; menstrual disturbances, vaginitis, impotence, loss of libido; haematuria, dysuria, renal failure; arthralgia, myalgia, vasculitis, blurred vision; rash, pruritus, Stevens-Johnson syndrome, toxic epidermal necrolysis, photosensitivity, changes of skin pigmentation, telangiectasia

Dose: *by mouth*, 7.5 mg once weekly (as a single dose *or* divided into 3 doses of 2.5 mg given at intervals of 12 hours), adjusted according to response; max. total weekly dose 20 mg

Important. Note that the above dose is a **weekly** dose. The CSM has received reports of prescription and dispensing errors including fatalities. Attention should be paid to the **strength** of methotrexate tablets prescribed and the **frequency** of dosing.

Methotrexate (Non-proprietary) PoM
Tablets, yellow, methotrexate 2.5 mg, net price 28-tab pack = £3.27. Counselling, dose, NSAIDs
Brands include *Maxtrex*®
Tablets, yellow, methotrexate 10 mg, net price 20 (Mayne) = £11.01; (Pharmacia, *Maxtrex*®) = £9.03. Counselling, dose, NSAIDs

Cytokine inhibitors

Cytokine inhibitors should be used under specialist supervision.

Adalimumab, etanercept, and infliximab inhibit the activity of tumour necrosis factor.

NICE guidance (etanercept and infliximab for rheumatoid arthritis). NICE has recommended (March 2002) the use of either etanercept or infliximab for highly active rheumatoid arthritis in adults who have failed to respond to at least 2 standard disease-modifying antirheumatic drugs, including methotrexate (unless methotrexate cannot be used because of intolerance or contra-indications). Etanercept and infliximab should be prescribed (according to the guidelines of the British Society for Rheumatology) and their use monitored by consultant rheumatologists specialising in their use. Infliximab should be given concomitantly with methotrexate.

Etanercept or infliximab should be withdrawn if severe side-effects develop or if there is no response after 3 months. There is no evidence to support treatment for longer than 4 years; a decision to continue therapy should be based on disease activity and clinical effectiveness in individual cases.

Consecutive use of etanercept and infliximab is not recommended.

Prescribers of etanercept and infliximab should register consenting patients with the Biologics Registry of the British Society for Rheumatology.

NICE guidance (etanercept for juvenile idiopathic arthritis). NICE has recommended (March 2002) the use of etanercept in children aged 4–17 years with active polyarticular-course juvenile idiopathic arthritis who have not responded adequately to methotrexate or who are intolerant of it. Etanercept should be used under specialist supervision according to the guidelines of the British Paediatric Rheumatology Group.

Etanercept should be withdrawn if severe side-effects develop or if there is no response after 6 months or if the initial response is not maintained. There is no evidence to support treatment for longer than 2 years; a decision to continue therapy should be based on disease activity and clinical effectiveness in individual cases.

Prescribers of etanercept and infliximab should register consenting patients with the Biologics Registry of the British Paediatric Rheumatology Group.

Adalimumab is licensed for moderate to severe active rheumatoid arthritis when response to other disease-modifying antirheumatic drugs (including methotrexate) has been inadequate. Adalimumab should be used in combination with methotrexate, but it may be given alone if methotrexate is inappropriate. If there is no response after 3 months, adalimumab should be discontinued.

Etanercept is licensed for the treatment of active *rheumatoid arthritis* either alone or in combination with methotrexate when the response to other disease-modifying antirheumatic drugs is inadequate (see also NICE guidelines). It is also licensed for the treatment of active and progressive *psoriatic arthritis* inadequately responsive to other disease-modifying antirheumatic drugs, and for severe *ankylosing spondylitis* inadequately responsive to conventional therapy. For the role of etanercept in psoriasis see section 13.5.3.

Infliximab is licensed for the treatment of active rheumatoid arthritis in combination with methotrexate when the response to other disease-modifying antirheumatic drugs is inadequate (see also NICE guidelines). It is also licensed for the treatment of *ankylosing spondylitis*, in patients with severe axial symptoms who have not responded adequately to conventional therapy and in combination with methotrexate for the treatment of active and progressive *psoriatic arthritis* which has not responded adequately to disease-modifying antirheumatic drugs. The *Scottish Medicines Consortium* has advised (July 2004) that infliximab is not recommended for ankylosing spondylitis.

Adalimumab, etanercept, and infliximab have been associated with infections, sometimes severe, including tuberculosis and septicaemia. Other side-effects include nausea, abdominal pain, worsening heart failure, hypersensitivity reactions, fever, headache, depression, lupus erythematosus-like syndrome, pruritus, injection-site reactions, and blood disorders (including anaemia, leucopenia, thrombocytopenia, pancytopenia, and aplastic anaemia).

Anakinra inhibits the activity of interleukin-1. Anakinra (in combination with methotrexate) is licensed for the treatment of *rheumatoid arthritis* which has not responded to methotrexate alone; it is not, however, recommended for routine management of *rheumatoid arthritis*, see NICE guidance below.

The *Scottish Medicines Consortium* has advised (October 2003) that anakinra is **not** recommended for rheumatoid arthritis.

NICE guidance (anakinra for rheumatoid arthritis). NICE does not recommend (November 2003) anakinra for the treatment of rheumatoid arthritis except when used in a controlled long-term clinical study. Patients receiving anakinra for rheumatoid arthritis should continue treatment until they and their consultant consider it appropriate to stop.

ADALIMUMAB

Indications: see under Cytokine Inhibitors above

Cautions: hepatic impairment; renal impairment; monitor for infections before, during, and for 5 months after treatment (see also Tuberculosis below); not to be initiated until active (including chronic or local) infections controlled; predisposition to infections; heart failure (discontinue if symptoms develop or worsen; avoid in moderate or severe heart failure); demyelinating CNS disorders (risk of exacerbation); **interactions:** Appendix 1 (adalimumab)

TUBERCULOSIS. Check for active and latent tuberculosis before treatment. Tuberculosis chemoprophylaxis must be started before initiating adalimumab in latent tuberculosis (contra-indicated in active tuberculosis). Patients should be instructed to seek medical advice if they develop symptoms suggestive of tuberculosis (such as persistent cough, weight loss, fever). If active tuberculosis suspected, adalimumab should be discontinued until infection either ruled out or treated

Contra-indications: pregnancy (Appendix 4); breast-feeding (Appendix 5); severe infections (see also Cautions)

Side-effects: see under Cytokine Inhibitors and Cautions above; also diarrhoea, constipation, vomiting, oesophagitis, dyspepsia, gastritis, dysphagia, taste disturbances, mouth ulceration, hypertension, vasodilatation, chest pain, ecchymosis, cough, sore throat, asthma, dyspnoea, asthenia, insomnia, drowsiness, dizziness, agitation, tremor, paraesthesia, hypoaesthesia, neuralgia, menorrhagia, urinary frequency, haematuria, proteinuria, arthralgia, myalgia, eye disorders, rash, alopecia, sweating, hyperlipidaemia, hypokalaemia, hyperuricaemia

Dose: *by subcutaneous injection*, ADULT over 18 years, 40 mg on alternate weeks; if necessary increased to 40 mg weekly in patients receiving adalimumab alone

Humira® (Abbott) ▼ PoM

Injection, adalimumab, net price 40-mg prefilled syringe = £357.50. Counselling, tuberculosis

ANAKINRA

Indications: see under Cytokine Inhibitors above

Cautions: renal impairment (Appendix 3); predisposition to infections; history of asthma (risk of serious infection); **interactions:** Appendix 1 (anakinra)

BLOOD DISORDERS. Neutropenia reported commonly. Monitor neutrophil count before treatment, then every month for 6 months, then every 3 months—discontinue if neutropenia develops. Patients should be instructed to seek medical advice if symptoms suggestive of neutropenia (such as fever, sore throat, infection) develop

Contra-indications: pregnancy (Appendix 4); breast-feeding (Appendix 5); neutropenia

Side-effects: injection-site reactions, headache; infections, neutropenia (see also Cautions)

Dose: *by subcutaneous injection*, ADULT over 18 years, 100 mg once daily

Kineret® (Amgen) ▼ PoM
Injection, anakinra, net price 100-mg prefilled syringe = £19.03. Counselling, blood disorder symptoms

---

ETANERCEPT

Indications: see under Cytokine Inhibitors above; severe, active and progressive rheumatoid arthritis in patients not previously treated with methotrexate; psoriasis (section 13.5.3)

Cautions: predisposition to infection (avoid if predisposition to septicaemia); significant exposure to herpes zoster virus—interrupt treatment and consider varicella–zoster immunoglobulin; heart failure (risk of exacerbation); demyelinating CNS disorders (risk of exacerbation); history of blood disorders; **interactions:** Appendix 1 (etanercept)

COUNSELLING. Patients should be advised to seek medical attention if symptoms suggestive of blood disorders (such as fever, sore throat, bruising, or bleeding) develop.

Contra-indications: pregnancy (Appendix 4); breast-feeding (Appendix 5); active infection

Side-effects: see under Cytokine Inhibitors above; also vomiting, oesophagitis, cholecystitis, pancreatitis, gastro-intestinal haemorrhage, myocardial or cerebral ischaemia, venous thromboembolism, hypotension, hypertension, dyspnoea, demyelinating disorders, seizures, bone fracture, renal impairment, polymyositis, bursitis, lymphadenopathy

Dose: *by subcutaneous injection*, rheumatoid arthritis ADULT over 18 years, 25 mg twice weekly *or* 50 mg once weekly

Psoriatic arthritis, ankylosing spondylitis ADULT over 18 years, 25 mg twice weekly

Polyarticular-course juvenile idiopathic arthritis, CHILD and ADOLESCENT 4–17 years, 400 micrograms/kg twice weekly (max. 25 mg twice weekly)

Psoriasis, ADULT over 18 years, initially 25–50 mg twice weekly for up to 12 weeks then reduce to 25 mg twice weekly; max. treatment duration 24 weeks; discontinue if no response after 12 weeks

Enbrel (Wyeth) ▼ PoM
Injection, powder for reconstitution, etanercept, net price 25-mg vial = £89.38, 50-mg vial = £178.75

INFLIXIMAB

Indications: see under Cytokine Inhibitors above; severe, active and progressive rheumatoid arthritis in patients not previously treated with methotrexate; Crohn's disease (section 1.5)

Cautions: hepatic impairment; renal impairment; monitor for infections before, during, and for 6 months after treatment (see also Tuberculosis below); heart failure (discontinue if symptoms develop or worsen; avoid in moderate or severe heart failure); demyelinating CNS disorders (risk of exacerbation); **interactions:** Appendix 1 (infliximab)

TUBERCULOSIS. Tuberculosis (often in extrapulmonary sites) reported. Patients must be evaluated for active and latent tuberculosis before treatment. Tuberculosis chemoprophylaxis must be started before initiating infliximab in latent tuberculosis (contra-indicated in active tuberculosis). Patients should be instructed to seek medical advice if they develop symptoms suggestive of tuberculosis (such as persistent cough, weight loss, fever). If active tuberculosis suspected, infliximab should be discontinued until infection either ruled out or treated

HYPERSENSITIVITY REACTIONS. Hypersensitivity reactions (including fever, chest pain, hypotension, hypertension, dyspnoea, pruritus, urticaria, serum sickness-like reactions, angioedema, anaphylaxis) reported during or within 1–2 hours after infusion (risk greatest during first or second infusion or in patients who discontinue other immunosuppressants. All patients should be observed carefully for 1–2 hours after infusion and resuscitation equipment should be available for immediate use. Prophylactic antipyretics, antihistamines, or hydrocortisone may be administered. Readministration not recommended after infliximab-free interval of more than 16 weeks—risk of delayed hypersensitivity reactions. Patients should be advised to keep Alert card with them at all times and seek medical advice if symptoms of delayed hypersensitivity develop

Contra-indications: pregnancy (Appendix 4); breast-feeding (Appendix 5); severe infections (see also under Cautions)

Side-effects: see under Cytokine Inhibitors and Cautions above; also dyspepsia, diarrhoea, constipation, hepatitis, cholecystitis, diverticulitis, gastro-intestinal haemorrhage, flushing, bradycardia, arrhythmias, palpitation, syncope, vasospasm, peripheral ischaemia, ecchymosis, haematoma, interstitial pneumonitis or fibrosis, fatigue, anxiety, drowsiness, dizziness, insomnia, confusion, agitation, amnesia, seizures, demyelinating disorders, vaginitis, myalgia, arthralgia, endophthalmitis, rash, sweating, hyperkeratosis, skin pigmentation, alopecia

Dose: *by intravenous infusion*, rheumatoid arthritis (in combination with methotrexate), ADULT and ADOLESCENT over 17 years, 3 mg/kg, repeated 2 weeks and 6 weeks after initial infusion, then repeated every 8 weeks

Ankylosing spondylitis, ADULT and ADOLESCENT over 17 years, 5 mg/kg, repeated 2 weeks and 6 weeks after initial infusion, then repeated every 6–8 weeks; discontinue if no response by 6 weeks of initial infusion

Psoriatic arthritis (in combination with methotrexate), ADULT and ADOLESCENT over 17 years, 5 mg/kg, repeated 2 weeks and 6 weeks after initial infusion, then repeated every 8 weeks

Remicade® (Schering-Plough) ▼ PoM
Intravenous infusion, powder for reconstitution, infliximab, net price 100-mg vial = £419.62. Label: 10, alert card, counselling, tuberculosis and hypersensitivity reactions

Sulfasalazine

Sulfasalazine (sulphasalazine) has a beneficial effect in suppressing the inflammatory activity of rheumatoid arthritis. Side-effects include rashes, gastro-intestinal intolerance and, especially in patients with rheumatoid arthritis, occasional leucopenia, neutropenia, and thrombocytopenia. These haematological abnormalities occur usually in the first 3 to 6 months of treatment and are reversible on cessation of treatment. Close monitoring of full blood counts (including differential white cell count and platelet count) is necessary initially, and at monthly intervals during the first 3 months (liver-function tests also being performed at monthly intervals for the first 3 months). Although the manufacturer recommends renal function tests, evidence of practical value is unsatisfactory.

SULFASALAZINE

(Sulphasalazine)

Indications: active rheumatoid arthritis; ulcerative colitis, see section 1.5 and notes above

Cautions: see section 1.5 and notes above

The CSM has recommended that patients should be advised to report any unexplained bleeding, bruising, purpura, sore throat, fever or malaise. A blood count should be performed and the drug stopped immediately if there is suspicion of a blood dyscrasia.

Contra-indications: see section 1.5 and notes above

Side-effects: see section 1.5 and notes above

Dose: *by mouth*, administered on expert advice, as enteric-coated tablets, initially 500 mg daily, increased by 500 mg at intervals of 1 week to a max. of 2–3 g daily in divided doses

Sulfasalazine (Non-proprietary) PoM

Tablets, e/c, sulfasalazine 500 mg. Net price 112-tab pack = £8.43. Label: 5, 14, 25, counselling, blood disorder symptoms (see CSM recommendation above), contact lenses may be stained

Brands include *Sulazine EC*®

Salazopyrin EN-Tabs® (Pharmacia) PoM

Tablets, e/c, yellow, f/c, sulfasalazine 500 mg. Net price 112-tab pack = £8.43. Label: 5, 14, 25, counselling, blood disorder symptoms (see CSM recommendation above), contact lenses may be stained

10.1.4 Gout and cytotoxic-induced hyperuricaemia

It is important to distinguish drugs used for the treatment of acute attacks of gout from those used in the long-term control of the disease. The latter exacerbate and prolong the acute manifestations if started during an attack.

Acute attacks of gout

Acute attacks of gout are usually treated with high doses of **NSAIDs** such as diclofenac, etoricoxib, indometacin, ketoprofen, naproxen, piroxicam, or sulindac (section 10.1.1). Colchicine is an alternative. Aspirin is *not* indicated in gout. Allopurinol and uricosurics are not effective in treating an acute attack and may prolong it indefinitely if started during the acute episode.

Colchicine is probably as effective as NSAIDs. Its use is limited by the development of toxicity at higher doses, but it is of value in patients with heart failure since, unlike NSAIDs, it does not induce fluid retention; moreover, it can be given to patients receiving anticoagulants.

Intra-articular injection of a **corticosteroid** may be used in acute monoarticular gout [unlicensed indication]. A corticosteroid by intramuscular injection can be effective in podagra.

COLCHICINE

Indications: acute gout, short-term prophylaxis during initial therapy with allopurinol and uricosuric drugs; prophylaxis of familial Mediterranean fever (recurrent polyserositis) [unlicensed]

Cautions: breast–feeding (Appendix 5), elderly, gastro-intestinal disease, cardiac, hepatic impairment, renal impairment (Appendix 3); **interactions:** Appendix 1 (colchicine)

Contra-indications: pregnancy (Appendix 4)

Side-effects: most common are nausea, vomiting, and abdominal pain; excessive doses may also cause profuse diarrhoea, gastro-intestinal haemorrhage, rashes, renal and hepatic damage. Rarely peripheral neuritis, myopathy, alopecia, inhibition of spermatogenesis, and with prolonged treatment blood disorders

Dose: treatment of gout, initially 1 mg, then 500 micrograms no more frequently than every 4 hours until pain relieved or vomiting or diarrhoea occur, max. 6 mg per course; course not to be repeated within 3 days

Prevention of gout attacks during initial treatment with allopurinol or uricosuric drugs, 500 micrograms 2–3 times daily

Prophylaxis of familial Mediterranean fever [unlicensed], 0.5–2 mg daily

Colchicine (Non-proprietary) PoM

Tablets, colchicine 500 micrograms, net price 20 = £3.32

Long-term control of gout

Frequent recurrence of acute attacks of gout, the presence of tophi, or signs of chronic gouty arthritis may call for the initiation of long-term ('interval') treatment. For long-term control of gout the formation of uric acid from purines may be reduced with the xanthine-oxidase inhibitor allopurinol, or the uricosuric drug sulfinpyrazone may be used to increase the excretion of uric acid in the urine. Treatment should be continued indefinitely to prevent further attacks of gout by correcting the hyperuricaemia. These drugs should never be started during an acute attack; they are usually started 2–3 weeks after the attack has settled. The initiation of treatment may precipitate an acute attack therefore colchicine or an anti-inflammatory analgesic should be used as a prophylactic and continued for at least one month after the hyperuricaemia has been corrected (usually about 3 months of prophylaxis). However, if an acute attack develops during treatment, then the treatment should continue at the same dosage and the acute attack treated in its own right.

Allopurinol is a well tolerated drug which is widely used. It is especially useful in patients with renal impairment or urate stones where uricosuric drugs cannot be used; it is *not* indicated for the treatment of asymptomatic hyperuricaemia. It is usually given once daily, since the active metabolite of allopurinol has a long half-life, but doses over 300 mg daily should be divided. It may occasionally cause rashes.

Sulfinpyrazone (sulphinpyrazone) can be used instead of allopurinol, or in conjunction with it in cases that are resistant to treatment.

Probenecid (available on a named-patient basis) is a uricosuric drug used to prevent nephrotoxicity associated with cidofovir (section 5.3.2.2).

Crystallisation of urate in the urine may occur with the uricosuric drugs and it is important to ensure an adequate urine output especially in the first few weeks of treatment. As an additional precaution the urine may be rendered alkaline.

Aspirin and salicylates antagonise the uricosuric drugs; they do not antagonise allopurinol but are nevertheless *not* indicated in gout.

ALLOPURINOL

Indications: prophylaxis of gout and of uric acid and calcium oxalate renal stones; prophylaxis of hyperuricaemia associated with cancer chemotherapy

Cautions: administer prophylactic colchicine or NSAID (*not* aspirin or salicylates) until at least 1 month after hyperuricaemia corrected; ensure adequate fluid intake (2–3 litres/day); for hyperuricaemia associated with cancer therapy, allopurinol treatment should be started before cancer therapy; hepatic impairment (Appendix 2); renal impairment (Appendix 3; also monitor liver function); pregnancy (Appendix 4); breast-feeding (Appendix 5); **interactions:** Appendix 1 (allopurinol)

Contra-indications: not a treatment for acute gout but continue if attack develops when already receiving allopurinol, and treat attack separately (see notes above)

Side-effects: rashes (**withdraw** therapy; if rash mild re-introduce cautiously but **discontinue** immediately if recurrence—hypersensitivity reactions occur rarely and include exfoliation, fever, lymphadenopathy, arthralgia, and eosinophilia resembling Stevens-Johnson or Lyell's syndrome, vasculitis, hepatitis, renal impairment, and very rarely seizures); gastro-intestinal disorders; rarely malaise, headache, vertigo, drowsiness, visual and taste disturbances, hypertension, alopecia, hepatotoxicity, paraesthesia and neuropathy, gynaecomastia, blood disorders (including leucopenia, thrombocytopenia, haemolytic anaemia and aplastic anaemia)

Dose: initially 100 mg daily, preferably after food, then adjusted according to plasma or urinary uric acid concentration; usual maintenance dose in mild conditions 100–200 mg daily, in moderately severe conditions 300–600 mg daily, in severe conditions 700–900 mg daily; doses over 300 mg daily given in divided doses; CHILD under 15 years, (in neoplastic conditions, enzyme disorders) 10–20 mg/kg daily (max. 400 mg daily)

Allopurinol (Non-proprietary) PoM
Tablets, allopurinol 100 mg, net price 28-tab pack = £1.28; 300 mg, 28-tab pack = £1.84. Label: 8, 21, 27
Brands include *Caplenal®*, *Cosuric®*, *Rimapurinol®*

Zyloric® (GSK) PoM
Tablets, allopurinol 100 mg, net price 100-tab pack = £10.19; 300 mg, 28-tab pack = £7.31. Label: 8, 21, 27

PROBENECID

Indications: prevention of nephrotoxicity associated with cidofovir (section 5.3.2.2)

Cautions: ensure adequate fluid intake (about 2–3 litres daily) and render urine alkaline if uric acid overload is high; peptic ulceration, renal impairment (avoid if severe—Appendix 3); transient false-positive Benedict's test; G6PD-deficiency (section 9.1.5); **interactions:** Appendix 1 (probenecid)

Contra-indications: history of blood disorders, nephrolithiasis, porphyria (section 9.8.2), acute gout attack; avoid aspirin and salicylates

Side-effects: gastro-intestinal disturbances, urinary frequency, headache, flushing, dizziness, alopecia, anaemia, haemolytic anaemia, sore gums; hypersensitivity reactions including anaphylaxis, dermatitis, pruritus, urticaria, fever and Stevens-Johnson syndrome; rarely nephrotic syndrome, hepatic necrosis, leucopenia, aplastic anaemia; toxic epidermal necrolysis reported with concurrent colchicine

Dose: used with cidofovir, see section 5.3.2.2

Probenecid (Non-proprietary) PoM
Tablets, probenecid 500 mg. Label: 12, 21, 27
Available on named-patient basis from IDIS (*Benuryl®*, *Probecid®*)

SULFINPYRAZONE

(Sulphinpyrazone)

Indications: gout prophylaxis, hyperuricaemia

Cautions: see under Probenecid; regular blood counts advisable; cardiac disease (may cause salt and water retention); renal impairment (Appendix 3); **interactions:** Appendix 1 (sulfinpyrazone)

Contra-indications: see under Probenecid; avoid in hypersensitivity to NSAIDs

Side-effects: gastro-intestinal disturbances, occasionally allergic skin reactions, salt and water retention; rarely blood disorders, gastro-intestinal ulceration and bleeding, acute renal failure, raised liver enzymes, jaundice and hepatitis

Dose: initially 100–200 mg daily with food (or milk) increasing over 2–3 weeks to 600 mg daily (rarely 800 mg daily), continued until serum uric acid concentration normal then reduced for maintenance (maintenance dose may be as low as 200 mg daily)

Anturan® (Amdipharm) PoM
Tablets, both yellow, s/c, sulfinpyrazone 100 mg, net price 84-tab pack = £4.72; 200 mg, 84-tab pack = £9.38. Label: 12, 21

Hyperuricaemia associated with cytotoxic drugs

Allopurinol is used to prevent hyperuricaemia associated with cytotoxic drugs—see section 8.1 (Hyperuricaemia) and Allopurinol above.

Rasburicase is licensed for the prophylaxis and treatment of acute hyperuricaemia, before and during initiation of chemotherapy, in patients with haematological malignancy and a high tumour burden at risk of rapid lysis.

RASBURICASE

Indications: prophylaxis and treatment of acute hyperuricaemia with initial chemotherapy for haematological malignancy

Cautions: monitor closely for hypersensitivity; atopic allergies; may interfere with test for uric acid—consult product literature

Contra-indications: susceptibility to haemolytic anaemia including G6PD deficiency; pregnancy (Appendix 4); breast-feeding (Appendix 5)
Side-effects: fever; nausea, vomiting; less frequently diarrhoea, headache, hypersensitivity reactions (including rash, bronchospasm and anaphylaxis); haemolytic anaemia, methaemoglobinaemia
Dose: *by intravenous infusion,* 200 micrograms/kg once daily for 5–7 days

Fasturtec (Sanofi-Synthelabo) ▼ PoM
Intravenous infusion, powder for reconstitution, rasburicase, net price 1.5-mg vial (with solvent) = £48.24; 7.5-mg vial (with solvent) = £201.00

10.2 Drugs used in neuromuscular disorders

10.2.1 Drugs which enhance neuromuscular transmission

Anticholinesterases are used as first-line treatment in *ocular myasthenia gravis* and as an adjunct to immunosuppressant therapy for *generalised myasthenia gravis*.

Corticosteroids are used when anticholinesterases do not control symptoms completely. A second-line immunosuppressant such as azathioprine is frequently used to reduce the dose of corticosteroid.

Plasmapheresis or infusion of intravenous immunoglobulin [unlicensed indication] may induce temporary remission in severe relapses, particularly where bulbar or respiratory function is compromised or before thymectomy.

Anticholinesterases

Anticholinesterase drugs enhance neuromuscular transmission in voluntary and involuntary muscle in myasthenia gravis. They prolong the action of acetylcholine by inhibiting the action of the enzyme acetylcholinesterase. Excessive dosage of these drugs may impair neuromuscular transmission and precipitate 'cholinergic crises' by causing a depolarising block. This may be difficult to distinguish from a worsening myasthenic state.

Muscarinic side-effects of anticholinesterases include increased sweating, salivary, and gastric secretion, also increased gastro-intestinal and uterine motility, and bradycardia. These parasympathomimetic effects are antagonised by atropine.

Edrophonium has a very brief action and it is therefore used mainly for the diagnosis of myasthenia gravis. However, such testing should be performed only by those experienced in its use; other means of establishing the diagnosis are available. A single test-dose usually causes substantial improvement in muscle power (lasting about 5 minutes) in patients with the disease (if respiration already impaired, *only* in conjunction with someone skilled at intubation).

Edrophonium can also be used to determine whether a patient with myasthenia is receiving inadequate or excessive treatment with cholinergic drugs. If treatment is excessive an injection of edrophonium will either have no effect or will intensify symptoms (if respiration already impaired, *only* in conjunction with someone skilled at intubation). Conversely, transient improvement may be seen if the patient is being inadequately treated. The test is best performed just before the next dose of anticholinesterase.

Neostigmine produces a therapeutic effect for up to 4 hours. Its pronounced muscarinic action is a disadvantage, and simultaneous administration of an antimuscarinic drug such as atropine or propantheline may be required to prevent colic, excessive salivation, or diarrhoea. In severe disease neostigmine may be given every 2 hours. The maximum that most patients can tolerate is 180 mg daily.

Pyridostigmine is less powerful and slower in action than neostigmine but it has a longer duration of action. It is preferable to neostigmine because of its smoother action and the need for less frequent dosage. It is particularly preferred in patients whose muscles are weak on waking. It has a comparatively mild gastro-intestinal effect but an antimuscarinic drug may still be required. It is inadvisable to exceed a total daily dose of 450 mg in order to avoid acetylcholine receptor downregulation. Immunosuppressant therapy is usually considered if the dose of pyridostigmine exceeds 360 mg daily.

Distigmine has the longest action but the danger of a 'cholinergic crisis' caused by accumulation of the drug is greater than with shorter-acting drugs; it is rarely used in the management of myasthenia gravis.

Neostigmine and edrophonium are also used to reverse the actions of the non-depolarising muscle relaxants (see section 15.1.6).

NEOSTIGMINE

Indications: myasthenia gravis; other indications (section 15.1.6)
Cautions: asthma (*extreme* caution), bradycardia, arrhythmias, recent myocardial infarction, epilepsy, hypotension, parkinsonism, vagotonia, peptic ulceration, hyperthyroidism, renal impairment (Appendix 3), pregnancy (Appendix 4), breast-feeding (Appendix 5); atropine or other antidote to muscarinic effects may be necessary (particularly when neostigmine is given by injection), but not given routinely because it may mask signs of overdosage; **interactions:** Appendix 1 (parasympathomimetics)
Contra-indications: intestinal or urinary obstruction
Side-effects: nausea, vomiting, increased salivation, diarrhoea, abdominal cramps (more marked with higher doses); signs of overdosage include bronchoconstriction, increased bronchial secretions, lacrimation, excessive sweating, involuntary defaecation and micturition, miosis, nystagmus, bradycardia, heart block, arrhythmias, hypotension, agitation, excessive dreaming, and weakness eventually leading to fasciculation and paralysis
Dose: *by mouth*, neostigmine bromide 15–30 mg at suitable intervals throughout day, total daily dose 75–300 mg (but see also notes above); NEONATE 1–5 mg every 4 hours, half an hour before feeds; CHILD up to 6 years initially 7.5 mg, 6–12 years initially 15 mg, usual total daily dose 15–90 mg

By subcutaneous or intramuscular injection, neostigmine metilsulfate 1–2.5 mg at suitable intervals throughout day (usual total daily dose 5–20 mg); NEONATE 50–250 micrograms every 4 hours half an hour before feeds; CHILD 200–500 micrograms as required

Neostigmine (Non-proprietary) PoM
Tablets, scored, neostigmine bromide 15 mg. Net price 20 = £4.24
Injection, neostigmine metilsulfate 2.5 mg/mL. Net price 1-mL amp = 58p

DISTIGMINE BROMIDE

Indications: myasthenia gravis (but rarely used); urinary retention and other indications (section 7.4.1)
Cautions: see under Neostigmine; also oesophagitis
Contra-indications: see under Neostigmine; also severe constipation, severe postoperative shock, serious circulatory insufficiency
Side-effects: see under Neostigmine
Dose: initially 5 mg daily half an hour before breakfast, increased at intervals of 3–4 days if necessary to a max. of 20 mg daily; CHILD up to 10 mg daily according to age

■ Preparations
Section 7.4.1

EDROPHONIUM CHLORIDE

Indications: see under Dose and notes above; reversal of non-depolarising neuromuscular blockade and diagnosis of dual block (section 15.1.6)
Cautions: see under Neostigmine; have resuscitation facilities; *extreme* caution in respiratory distress (see notes above) and in asthma
NOTE. Severe cholinergic reactions can be counteracted by injection of atropine sulphate (which should always be available)
Contra-indications: see under Neostigmine
Side-effects: see under Neostigmine
Dose: diagnosis of myasthenia gravis, *by intravenous injection*, 2 mg followed after 30 seconds (if no adverse reaction has occurred) by 8 mg; in adults without suitable veins, *by intramuscular injection*, 10 mg
Detection of overdosage or underdosage of cholinergic drugs, *by intravenous injection*, 2 mg (best before next dose of anticholinesterase, see notes above)
CHILD *by intravenous injection*, 20 micrograms/kg followed after 30 seconds (if no adverse reaction has occurred) by 80 micrograms/kg

Edrophonium (Cambridge) PoM
Injection, edrophonium chloride 10 mg/mL. Net price 1-mL amp = £4.76

PYRIDOSTIGMINE BROMIDE

Indications: myasthenia gravis
Cautions: see under Neostigmine; weaker muscarinic action
Contra-indications: see under Neostigmine
Side-effects: see under Neostigmine
Dose: *by mouth*, 30–120 mg at suitable intervals throughout day, total daily dose 0.3–1.2 g (but see also notes above); NEONATE 5–10 mg every 4 hours, 30–60 minutes before feeds; CHILD up to 6 years initially 30 mg, 6–12 years initially 60 mg, usual total daily dose 30–360 mg

Mestinon® (Valeant) PoM
Tablets, scored, pyridostigmine bromide 60 mg. Net price 20 = £4.81

Immunosuppressant therapy

Corticosteroids (section 6.3) are established as treatment for myasthenia gravis; although they are commonly given on alternate days there is little evidence of benefit over daily administration. Corticosteroid treatment is usually initiated under in-patient supervision and all patients should receive osteoporosis prophylaxis (section 6.6).

In *generalised myasthenia gravis* small initial doses of prednisolone (10 mg on alternate days) are increased in steps of 10 mg on alternate days to 1–1.5 mg/kg (max. 100 mg) on alternate days. When given daily, prednisolone is started at 5 mg daily and then increased in steps of 5 mg daily to 60 mg daily or occasionally up to 80 mg daily (0.75–1 mg/kg daily). About 10% of patients experience a transient but very serious worsening of symptoms in the first 2–3 weeks, especially if the corticosteroid is started at a high dose. However, ventilated patients may be started on 1.5 mg/kg (max. 100 mg) on alternate days. Smaller doses of corticosteroid are usually required in *ocular myasthenia*. Once clinical remission has occurred (usually after 2–6 months), the dose of prednisolone should be reduced slowly to the minimum effective dose (usually 10–40 mg on alternate days).

In generalised myasthenia gravis **azathioprine** (section 8.2.1) is usually started at the same time as the corticosteroid and it allows a lower maintenance dose of the corticosteroid to be used; azathioprine is initiated at a low dose, which is increased over 3–4 weeks to 2–2.5 mg/kg daily. **Ciclosporin** (section 8.2.2), **methotrexate** (section 8.1.3), or **mycophenolate mofetil** (section 8.2.1) may be used in patients unresponsive or intolerant to other treatments [unlicensed indications].

10.2.2 Skeletal muscle relaxants

Drugs described below are used for the relief of chronic muscle spasm or spasticity associated with multiple sclerosis or other neurological damage; they are not indicated for spasm associated with minor injuries. They act principally on the central nervous system with the exception of dantrolene which has a peripheral site of action. They differ in action from the muscle relaxants used in anaesthesia (section 15.1.5) which block transmission at the neuromuscular junction.

The underlying cause of spasticity should be treated and any aggravating factors (e.g. pressure sores, infection) remedied. Skeletal muscle relaxants are effective in most forms of spasticity except the rare alpha variety. The major disadvantage of treatment with these drugs is that reduction in muscle tone can cause a loss of splinting action of the spastic leg and trunk muscles and sometimes lead to an increase in disability.

Dantrolene acts directly on skeletal muscle and produces fewer central adverse effects making it a drug of choice. The dose should be increased slowly.

Baclofen inhibits transmission at spinal level and also depresses the central nervous system. The dose should be increased slowly to avoid the major side-effects of sedation and muscular hypotonia (other adverse events are uncommon).

Diazepam may also be used. Sedation and, occasionally, extensor hypotonus are disadvantages. Other benzodiazepines also have muscle-relaxant properties. Muscle-relaxant doses of benzodiazepines are similar to anxiolytic doses (section 4.1.2).

Tizanidine is an alpha$_2$-adrenoceptor agonist indicated for spasticity associated with multiple sclerosis or spinal cord injury.

BACLOFEN

Indications: chronic severe spasticity resulting from disorders such as multiple sclerosis or traumatic partial section of spinal cord

Cautions: renal impairment (Appendix 3); psychiatric illness, Parkinson's disease, cerebrovascular disease, elderly; respiratory impairment, epilepsy; history of peptic ulcer; diabetes; hypertonic bladder sphincter; pregnancy (Appendix 4); avoid abrupt withdrawal (risk of hyperactive state, may exacerbate spasticity, and precipitate autonomic dysfunction including hyperthermia, psychiatric reactions and convulsions, see also under Withdrawal below); porphyria (section 9.8.2); **interactions:** Appendix 1 (muscle relaxants)

WITHDRAWAL. CSM has advised that serious side-effects can occur on abrupt withdrawal; to minimise risk, discontinue by gradual dose reduction over at least 1–2 weeks (longer if symptoms occur)

DRIVING. Drowsiness may affect performance of skilled tasks (e.g. driving); effects of alcohol enhanced

Contra-indications: peptic ulceration

Side-effects: frequently sedation, drowsiness, muscular hypotonia, nausea, urinary disturbances; occasionally lassitude, confusion, speech disturbance, dizziness, ataxia, hallucinations, nightmares, headache, euphoria, insomnia, depression, anxiety, agitation, tremor, nystagmus, paraesthesias, seizures, myalgia, fever, respiratory or cardiovascular depression, hypotension, dry mouth, gastro-intestinal disturbances, sexual dysfunction, visual disorders, rash, pruritus, urticaria, hyperhidrosis, angioedema; rarely taste alterations, blood sugar changes, and paradoxical increase in spasticity

Dose: *by mouth*, 5 mg 3 times daily, preferably with or after food, gradually increased; max. 100 mg daily (discontinue if no benefit within 6 weeks); CHILD 0.75–2 mg/kg daily (over 10 years, max. 2.5 mg/kg daily) *or* 2.5 mg 4 times daily increased gradually according to age to maintenance: 1–2 years 10–20 mg daily, 2–6 years 20–30 mg daily, 6–10 years 30–60 mg daily

By intrathecal injection, see preparation below

Baclofen (Non-proprietary) PoM

Tablets, baclofen 10 mg, net price 28-tab pack = 76p, 84-tab pack = £2.60. Label: 2, 8

Brands include *Baclospas*®

Oral solution, baclofen 5 mg/5 mL, net price 300 mL = £7.95. Label: 2, 8

Brands include *Lyflex*® (sugar-free)

Lioresal® (Cephalon) PoM

Tablets, scored, baclofen 10 mg. Net price 84-tab pack = £10.84. Label: 2, 8

Excipients: include gluten

Liquid, sugar-free, raspberry-flavoured, baclofen 5 mg/5 mL. Net price 300 mL = £8.95. Label: 2, 8

■ By intrathecal injection

Lioresal® (Novartis) PoM

Intrathecal injection, baclofen, 50 micrograms/mL, net price 1-mL amp (for test dose) = £2.74; 500 micrograms/mL, 20-mL amp (for use with implantable pump) = £60.77; 2 mg/mL, 5-mL amp (for use with implantable pump) = £60.77

Important: consult product literature for details on dose testing and titration—important to monitor patients closely in appropriately equipped and staffed environment during screening and immediately after pump implantation, and to have resuscitation equipment available for immediate use

Dose: by intrathecal injection, specialist use only, severe chronic spasticity unresponsive to oral antispastic drugs (or where side-effects of oral therapy unacceptable) *or* as alternative to ablative neurosurgical procedures, initial *test dose* 25–50 micrograms over at least 1 minute via catheter or lumbar puncture, increased in 25-microgram steps (not more often than every 24 hours) to max. 100 micrograms to determine appropriate dose *then dose-titration phase*, most often using infusion pump (implanted into chest wall or abdominal wall tissues) to establish *appropriate maintenance dose* (ranging from 12 micrograms to 2 mg daily for spasticity of spinal origin *or* 22 micrograms to 1.4 mg daily for spasticity of cerebral origin) retaining some spasticity to avoid sensation of paralysis; CHILD 4–18 years (spasticity of cerebral origin only), initial *test dose* 25 micrograms then titrated as for ADULT to *appropriate maintenance dose* (ranging from 24 micrograms to 1.2 mg daily in children under 12 years)

DANTROLENE SODIUM

Indications: chronic severe spasticity of voluntary muscle; malignant hyperthermia (section 15.1.8)

Cautions: impaired cardiac and pulmonary function; test liver function before and at intervals during therapy; therapeutic effect may take a few weeks to develop but if treatment is ineffective it should be discontinued after 4–6 weeks; avoid when spasticity is useful, for example, locomotion; **interactions:** Appendix 1 (muscle relaxants).

DRIVING. Drowsiness may affect performance of skilled tasks (e.g. driving); effects of alcohol enhanced

Contra-indications: hepatic impairment (may cause severe liver damage); acute muscle spasm; pregnancy (Appendix 4); breast-feeding (Appendix 5)

Side-effects: transient drowsiness, dizziness, weakness, malaise, fatigue, diarrhoea (withdraw if severe, discontinue treatment if recurs on re-introduction), anorexia, nausea, headache, rash; less frequently constipation, dysphagia, speech and visual disturbances, confusion, nervousness, insomnia, depression, seizures, chills, fever, increased urinary frequency; rarely, tachycardia, erratic blood pressure, dyspnoea, haematuria, possible crystalluria, urinary incontinence or retention, pleural effusion, pericarditis, dose-related hepatotoxicity (occasionally fatal) may be more common in women over 30 especially those taking oestrogens

Dose: initially 25 mg daily, may be increased at weekly intervals to max. of 100 mg 4 times daily;

usual dose 75 mg 3 times daily; CHILD not recommended

Dantrium® (Procter & Gamble Pharm.) PoM
Capsules, both orange/brown, dantrolene sodium 25 mg, net price 20 = £2.29; 100 mg, 20 = £8.01. Label: 2

DIAZEPAM

Indications: muscle spasm of varied aetiology, including tetanus; other indications (section 4.1.2, section 4.8, section 15.1.4.1)
Cautions: see section 4.1.2; special precautions for intravenous injection (section 4.8.2)
Contra-indications: see section 4.1.2
Side-effects: see section 4.1.2; also hypotonia
Dose: *by mouth*, 2–15 mg daily in divided doses, increased if necessary in spastic conditions to 60 mg daily according to response
Cerebral spasticity in selected cases, CHILD 2–40 mg daily in divided doses
By intramuscular or by slow intravenous injection (into a large vein at a rate of not more than 5 mg/minute), in acute muscle spasm, 10 mg repeated if necessary after 4 hours
NOTE. Only use intramuscular route when oral and intravenous routes not possible; special precautions for intravenous injection see section 4.8.2
Tetanus, ADULT and CHILD, *by intravenous injection*, 100–300 micrograms/kg repeated every 1–4 hours; *by intravenous infusion* (*or by nasoduodenal tube*), 3–10 mg/kg over 24 hours, adjusted according to response

■ Preparations
Section 4.1.2

TIZANIDINE

Indications: spasticity associated with multiple sclerosis or spinal cord injury or disease
Cautions: elderly, renal impairment (Appendix 3), pregnancy (Appendix 4), breast-feeding (Appendix 5), monitor liver function monthly for first 4 months and in those who develop unexplained nausea, anorexia or fatigue; concomitant administration of drugs that prolong QT interval; **interactions:** Appendix 1 (muscle relaxants)
DRIVING. Drowsiness may affect performance of skilled tasks (e.g. driving); effects of alcohol enhanced
Contra-indications: severe hepatic impairment
Side-effects: drowsiness, fatigue, dizziness, dry mouth, nausea, gastro-intestinal disturbances, hypotension; also reported, bradycardia, insomnia, hallucinations and altered liver enzymes (discontinue if persistently raised—consult product literature); rarely acute hepatitis
Dose: initially 2 mg daily as a single dose increased according to response at intervals of at least 3–4 days in steps of 2 mg daily (and given in divided doses) usually up to 24 mg daily in 3–4 divided doses; max. 36 mg daily; CHILD not recommended

Tizanidine (Non-proprietary) PoM
Tablets, tizanidine (as hydrochloride) 2 mg net price 120-tab pack = £34.68; 4 mg, 120-tab pack = £53.04. Label: 2

Zanaflex® (Zeneus) PoM
Tablets, scored, tizanidine (as hydrochloride) 2 mg, net price 120-tab pack = £63.00; 4 mg, 120-tab pack = £80.00. Label: 2

Other muscle relaxants

The clinical efficacy of carisoprodol, meprobamate (section 4.1.2), and methocarbamol as muscle relaxants is **not** well established although they have been included in compound analgesic preparations.

CARISOPRODOL ▲

Indications: short-term symptomatic relief of muscle spasm (but see notes above)
Cautions: see under Meprobamate (section 4.1.2); breast-feeding (Appendix 5); **interactions:** Appendix 1 (muscle relaxants)
Contra-indications: see under Meprobamate (section 4.1.2); porphyria (section 9.8.2)
Side-effects: see under Meprobamate (section 4.1.2); drowsiness is common
Dose: 350 mg 3 times daily; ELDERLY half adult dose or less

Carisoma® (Forest) PoM ▲
Tablets, carisoprodol 125 mg, net price 100 = £6.65; 350 mg, 100 = £7.45. Label: 2

METHOCARBAMOL ▲

Indications: short-term symptomatic relief of muscle spasm (but see notes above)
Cautions: hepatic impairment (Appendix 2); renal impairment (Appendix 3); pregnancy (Appendix 4); breast-feeding (Appendix 5); **interactions:** Appendix 1 (muscle relaxants)
DRIVING. Drowsiness may affect performance of skilled tasks (e.g. driving); effects of alcohol enhanced
Contra-indications: coma or pre-coma, brain damage, epilepsy, myasthenia gravis
Side-effects: nausea, vomiting, dyspepsia; hypersensitivity reactions (including urticaria, angioedema, anaphylaxis); fever, headache, drowsiness, dizziness, confusion, amnesia, restlessness, anxiety, tremor, seizures; blurred vision, nasal congestion; rash, pruritus; leucopenia, cholestatic jaundice
Dose: 1.5 g 4 times daily; may be reduced to 750 mg 3 times daily; ELDERLY up to 750 mg 4 times daily may be sufficient; CHILD not recommended

Robaxin® (Shire) PoM ▲
750 Tablets, f/c, scored, methocarbamol 750 mg, net price 20 = £2.53. Label: 2

Nocturnal leg cramps

Quinine salts (section 5.4.1) 200–300 mg at bedtime are effective in reducing the frequency of nocturnal leg cramps by about 25% in ambulatory patients. It may take up to 4 weeks for improvement to become apparent and it is then given on a continuous basis if there is benefit. Patients should be monitored closely during the early stages for adverse effects as well as for benefit. Treatment should be interrupted at intervals of approximately 3 months to assess the need for further quinine treatment. Quinine is very toxic in overdosage and accidental fatalities have occurred in children (see also below).

QUININE

Indications: see notes above; malaria (section 5.4.1)
Cautions: see section 5.4.1

Contra-indications: see section 5.4.1
Side-effects: see section 5.4.1; **important:** very toxic in **overdosage**—immediate advice from poison centres essential (see also p. 32)
Dose: see notes above

■ Preparations
Section 5.4.1

10.3 Drugs for the relief of soft-tissue inflammation

10.3.1 Enzymes
10.3.2 Rubefacients and other topical anti-rheumatics

Extravasation

Local guidelines for the management of extravasation should be followed where they exist or specialist advice sought.

Extravasation injury follows leakage of drugs or intravenous fluids from the veins or inadvertent administration into the subcutaneous or subdermal tissue. It must be dealt with **promptly** to prevent tissue necrosis.

Acidic or alkaline preparations and those with an osmolarity greater than that of plasma can cause extravasation injury and excipients including alcohol and polyethylene glycol have also been implicated. Cytotoxic drugs commonly cause extravasation injury. In addition, certain patients such as the very young and the elderly are at increased risk. Those receiving anticoagulants are more likely to lose blood into surrounding tissues if extravasation occurs whilst those receiving sedatives or analgesics may not notice the early signs or symptoms of extravasation.

PREVENTION OF EXTRAVASATION. Precautions should be taken to avoid extravasation; ideally, drugs liable to cause extravasation injury should be given through a central line and patients receiving repeated doses of hazardous drugs peripherally should have the cannula resited at regular intervals. Attention should be paid to the manufacturers' recommendations for administration. Placing a glyceryl trinitrate patch (section 2.6.1) distal to the cannula may improve the patency of the vessel in patients with small veins or in those whose veins are prone to collapse.

Patients should be asked to report any pain or burning at the site of injection immediately.

MANAGEMENT OF EXTRAVASATION. If extravasation is suspected the infusion should be stopped immediately but the cannula should not be removed until after an attempt has been made to aspirate the area (through the cannula) in order to remove as much of the drug as possible. Aspiration is sometimes possible if the extravasation presents with a raised bleb or blister at the injection site and is surrounded by hardened tissue, but it is often unsuccessful if the tissue is soft or soggy. Corticosteroids are usually given to treat inflammation, although there is little evidence to support their use in extravasation. Hydrocortisone or dexamethasone (section 6.3.2) may be given either locally by subcutaneous injection or intravenously at a site distant from the injury. Antihistamines (section 3.4.1) and analgesics (section 4.7) may be required for symptom relief.

The management of extravasation beyond these measures is not well standardised and calls for specialist advice. Treatment depends on the nature of the offending substance; one approach is to localise and neutralise the substance whereas another is to spread and dilute it. The first method may be appropriate following extravasation of vesicant drugs and involves administration of an antidote (if available) and the application of cold compresses 3–4 times a day (consult specialist literature for details of specific antidotes). Spreading and diluting the offending substance involves infiltrating the area with physiological saline, applying warm compresses, elevating the affected limb, and administering hyaluronidase (section 10.3.1). A saline flush-out technique (involving flushing the subcutaneous tissue with physiological saline) may be effective but requires specialist advice. Hyaluronidase should **not** be administered following extravasation of vesicant drugs (unless it is either specifically indicated or used in the saline flush-out technique).

10.3.1 Enzymes

Hyaluronidase is used to render the tissues more easily permeable to injected fluids, e.g. for introduction of fluids by subcutaneous infusion (termed hypodermoclysis).

HYALURONIDASE

Indications: enhance permeation of subcutaneous or intramuscular injections, local anaesthetics and subcutaneous infusions; promote resorption of excess fluids and blood
Cautions: infants or elderly (control speed and total volume and avoid overhydration especially in renal impairment)
Contra-indications: do not apply direct to cornea; avoid sites where infection or malignancy; not for anaesthesia in unexplained premature labour; not to be used to reduce swelling of bites or stings; not for intravenous administration
Side-effects: occasional severe allergy
Dose: With subcutaneous or intramuscular injection, 1500 units dissolved directly in solution to be injected (ensure compatibility)

With local anaesthetics, 1500 units mixed with local anaesthetic solution (ophthalmology, 15 units/mL)

Hypodermoclysis, 1500 units dissolved in 1 mL water for injections or 0.9% sodium chloride injection, administered before start of 500–1000 mL infusion fluid

Extravasation (see notes above) or haematoma, 1500 units dissolved in 1 mL water for injections or 0.9% sodium chloride injection, infiltrated into affected area (as soon as possible after extravasation)

Hyalase® (CP) PoM
Injection, powder for reconstitution, hyaluronidase (ovine). Net price 1500-unit amp = £7.60

10.3.2 Rubefacients and other topical antirheumatics

Rubefacients act by counter-irritation. Pain, whether superficial or deep-seated, is relieved by any method which itself produces irritation of the skin. Counter-irritation is comforting in painful lesions of the muscles, tendons, and joints, and in non-articular rheumatism. Rubefacients probably all act through the same essential mechanism and differ mainly in intensity and duration of action.

The use of a NSAID by mouth is effective for relieving musculoskeletal pain. **Topical NSAIDs** (e.g. felbinac, ibuprofen, ketoprofen and piroxicam) may provide some slight relief of pain in musculoskeletal conditions.

Topical NSAIDs and counter-irritants

CAUTIONS. Apply with gentle massage only. Avoid contact with eyes, mucous membranes, and inflamed or broken skin; discontinue if rash develops. Hands should be washed immediately after use. Not for use with occlusive dressings. Topical application of large amounts may result in systemic effects including hypersensitivity and asthma (renal disease has also been reported). Not generally suitable for children. Patient packs carry a **warning** to avoid during **pregnancy** or **breast-feeding**.

HYPERSENSITIVITY. For NSAID hypersensitivity and asthma warning, see p. 502 and p. 503

PHOTOSENSITIVITY. Patients should be advised against excessive exposure to sunlight of area treated in order to avoid possibility of photosensitivity

Ketoprofen (Non-proprietary) PoM
Gel, ketoprofen 2.5%, net price 30 g = £2.59, 50 g = £3.06, 100 g = £5.89
Dose: apply 2–4 times daily for up to 7 days (usual max. 15 g daily)

Piroxicam (Non-proprietary) PoM
Gel, piroxicam 0.5%, net price 60 g = £3.52; 112 g = £6.01
Dose: apply 3–4 times daily

■ Proprietary preparations

Feldene® (Pfizer) PoM
Gel, piroxicam 0.5%. Net price 60 g = £6.00; 112 g = £9.41 (also 7.5 g starter pack, hosp. only)
Excipients: include benzyl alcohol, propylene glycol
Dose: apply 3–4 times daily; therapy should be reviewed after 4 weeks

Fenbid® **Forte Gel** (Goldshield) PoM
Gel, ibuprofen 10%, net price 100 g = £6.50
Excipients: include benzyl alcohol
Dose: apply up to 4 times daily; therapy should be reviewed after 14 days

Ibugel® **Forte** (Dermal) PoM
Forte gel, ibuprofen 10%, net price 100 g = £6.05
Excipients: none as listed in section 13.1.3
Dose: apply up to 3 times daily

Oruvail® (Rhône-Poulenc Rorer) PoM
Gel, ketoprofen 2.5%. Net price 100 g = £7.12
Excipients: include fragrance
Dose: apply 2–4 times daily for up to 7 days (usual recommended dose 15 g daily)

Pennsaid® (Dimethaid) PoM
Cutaneous solution, diclofenac sodium 16 mg/mL in dimethyl sulfoxide, net price 60 mL = £16.00
Excipients: include propylene glycol
Dose: pain in osteoarthritis of superficial joints, apply 0.5–1 mL 4 times daily

Powergel® (Menarini) PoM
Gel, ketoprofen 2.5%. Net price 50 g = £3.06; 100 g = £5.89
Excipients: include hydroxybenzoates (parabens), fragrance
Dose: apply 2–3 times daily for up to max. 10 days

Traxam® (Goldshield) PoM
Foam, felbinac 3.17%. Net price 100 g = £7.00. Label: 15
Excipients: include cetostearyl alcohol
Gel, felbinac 3%. Net price 100 g = £7.00
Excipients: none as listed in section 13.1.3
Dose: apply 2–4 times daily; max. 25 g daily; therapy should be reviewed after 14 days
NOTE. Felbinac is an active metabolite of the NSAID fenbufen

Voltarol Emulgel® (Novartis) PoM
Gel, diclofenac diethylammonium salt 1.16% (equivalent to diclofenac sodium 1%). Net price 20 g (hosp. only) = £1.55; 100 g = £7.00
Excipients: include propylene glycol, fragrance
Dose: apply 3–4 times daily; therapy should be reviewed after 14 days (or after 28 days for osteoarthritis)

■ Preparations on sale to the public

Topical NSAIDs and counter-irritants on sale to the public together with their significant ingredients include:

Algesal® (diethylamine salicylate),
Balmosa® (camphor, capsicum oleoresin, menthol, methyl salicylate), **Boots Pain Relief Balm**® (ethyl nicotinate, glycol monosalicylate, nonylic acid vanillylamide), **Boots Pain Relief Embrocation**® (camphor, turpentine oil), **Boots Pain Relief Warming Spray**® (camphor, ethyl nicotinate, methyl salicylate)
Cremalgin® (capsicin, glycol salicylate, methyl nicotinate), **Cuprofen**® **Ibutop**® **Gel** (ibuprofen)
Deep Freeze Cold Gel® (menthol), **Deep Freeze Spray**® (levomenthol), **Deep Heat Maximum**® (menthol, methyl salicylate), **Deep Heat Rub**® (eucalyptus oil, menthol, methyl salicylate, turpentine oil), **Deep Heat Spray**® (glycol salicylate, ethyl salicylate, methyl salicylate, methyl nicotinate), **Deep Relief**® (ibuprofen, menthol), **Difflam**® **Cream** (benzydamine), **Difflam**®**-P Cream** (benzydamine), **Dubam Cream**® (methyl salicylate, menthol, cineole), **Dubam Spray**® (ethyl salicylate, methyl salicylate, glycol salicylate, methyl nicotinate), **Dulbalm Cream**® (ethyl nicotinate, methyl nicotinate, benzyl nicotinate, glycol salicylate, oleoresin capsicum)
Elliman's Universal Embrocation® (acetic acid, turpentine oil)
Feldene P® **Gel** (piroxicam), **Fenbid**® **Gel** (ibuprofen), **Fiery Jack Cream**® (capsicum oleoresin, diethylamine salicylate, glycol salicylate, methyl nicotinate), **Fiery Jack Ointment**® (capsicum oleoresin)
Goddard's White Oil Embrocation® (dilute acetic acid, dilute ammonia solution, turpentine oil)
Ibugel® (ibuprofen), **Ibuleve**®, **Ibuleve**® **Maximum Strength**, **Ibuleve Mousse**®, **Ibuleve Sports Gel**® (ibuprofen), **Ibumousse**® (ibuprofen), **Ibuspray**® (ibuprofen),
Lloyds Cream® (diethyl salicylate)
Mentholatum® **Ibuprofen Gel** (ibuprofen), **Movelat**® **Cream** (mucopolysaccharide polysulphate, salicylic acid, thymol), **Movelat**® **Gel** (mucopolysaccharide polysul-

phate, salicylic acid), **Movelat® Relief Cream** (mucopolysaccharide polysulphate, salicylic acid, thymol), **Movelat® Relief Gel** (mucopolysaccharide polysulphate, salicylic acid)

Nella Red Oil® (arachis oil, clove oil, mustard oil, methyl nicotinate), **Nurofen® Gel Maximum Strength** (ibuprofen), **Nurofen Muscular Pain Relief Gel®** (ibuprofen)

Oruvail® Gel (ketoprofen 30-g tube; 100-g tube prescribable on NHS (PoM))

PR Heat Spray® (ethyl nicotinate, methyl salicylate, camphor); **Proflex® Cream** (ibuprofen), **Proflex Pain Relief Cream®** (ibuprofen)

Radian®-B Ibuprofen Gel (ibuprofen), **Radian®-B Muscle Lotion**, **Radian®-B Heat Spray** (ammonium salicylate, camphor, menthol, salicylic acid), **Radian®-B Muscle Rub** (camphor, capsicin, menthol, methyl salicylate), **Ralgex Cream®** (capsicin, glycol monosalicylate, methyl nicotinate), **Ralgex Freeze Spray®** (dimethyl ether, glycol monosalicylate, isopentane), **Ralgex Spray®** (ethyl salicylate, methyl salicylate, glycol monosalicylate, methyl nicotinate), **Ralgex Stick®** (capsicin, ethyl salicylate, methyl salicylate, glycol salicylate, menthol)

Salonpas Plasters® (glycol salicylate, methyl salicylate), **Solpaflex® Gel** (ketoprofen)

Tiger Balm Red® (camphor, clove oil, cajuput oil, menthol), **Tiger Balm White®** (cajuput oil, camphor, clove oil, menthol), **Transvasin Cream®** (ethyl nicotinate, hexyl nicotinate, thurfyl salicylate), **Transvasin Spray®** (diethylamine salicylate, hydroxyethyl salicylate, methyl nicotinate), **Traxam Pain Relief®** (felbinac), **Voltarol Emulgel® P** (diclofenac diethylammonium)

Capsaicin

CAUTIONS. Avoid contact with eyes, and inflamed or broken skin. Hands should be washed immediately after use. Not for use under tight bandages. Avoid taking a hot shower or bath just before or after applying capsaicin—burning sensation enhanced.

SIDE-EFFECTS. Transient burning sensation may occur during initial treatment, particularly if too much cream is used, or if the frequency of administration is less than 3–4 times daily.

Axsain® (Zeneus) PoM
Cream, capsaicin 0.075%. net price 45 g = £12.15.
Excipients: include benzyl alcohol, cetyl alcohol
Dose: post-herpetic neuralgia (**important: after** lesions have healed), apply a small amount up to 3–4 times daily; for painful diabetic neuropathy, under supervision of hospital consultant, apply 3–4 times daily for 8 weeks then review

Zacin® (Zeneus) PoM
Cream, capsaicin 0.025%. net price 45 g = £15.04.
Excipients: include benzyl alcohol, cetyl alcohol
Dose: symptomatic relief in osteoarthritis, apply a small amount 4 times daily

Poultices

Kaolin Poultice
Poultice, heavy kaolin 52.7%, thymol 0.05%, boric acid 4.5%, peppermint oil 0.05%, methyl salicylate 0.2%, glycerol 42.5%. Net price 200 g = £2.12
Dose: warm and apply directly or between layers of muslin; avoid application of overheated poultice

Kaolin Poultice K/L Pack® (K/L)
Kaolin poultice Net price 4 × 100-g pouches = £6.40

11: Eye

11.1 Administration of drugs to the eye

Drugs are most commonly administered to the eye by topical application as eye drops or eye ointments. Where a higher drug concentration is required within the eye, a local injection may be necessary.

Eye-drop dispenser devices are available to aid the instillation of eye drops from plastic bottles especially amongst the elderly, visually impaired, arthritic, or otherwise physically limited patients. Eye-drop dispensers are for use with plastic eye drop bottles, for repeat use by individual patients.

EYE DROPS AND EYE OINTMENTS. Eye drops are generally instilled into the pocket formed by gently pulling down the lower eyelid and keeping the eye closed for as long as possible after application, preferably 1–2 minutes; one drop is all that is needed. A small amount of eye ointment is applied similarly; the ointment melts rapidly and blinking helps to spread it

When two different eye-drop preparations are used at the same time of day, dilution and overflow may occur when one immediately follows the other. The patient should therefore leave an interval of at least 5 minutes between the two.

Systemic effects may arise from absorption of drugs into the general circulation from conjunctival vessels or from the nasal mucosa after the excess preparation has drained down through the tear ducts. The extent of systemic absorption following ocular administration is highly variable; nasal drainage of drugs is associated with eye drops much more often than with eye ointments.

For warnings relating to eye drops and contact lenses, see section 11.9.

EYE LOTIONS. These are solutions for the irrigation of the conjunctival sac. They act mechanically to flush out irritants or foreign bodies as a first-aid treatment. Sterile sodium chloride 0.9% solution (section 11.8.1) is usually used. Clean water will suffice in an emergency.

OTHER PREPARATIONS. Subconjunctival injection may be used to administer anti-infective drugs, mydriatics, or corticosteroids for conditions not responding to topical therapy. The drug diffuses through the cornea and sclera to the anterior and posterior chambers and vitreous humour. However, because the dose-volume is limited (usually not more than 1 mL), this route is suitable only for drugs which are readily soluble.

Drugs such as antimicrobials and corticosteroids may be administered systemically to treat an eye condition. Implants which gradually release a drug over a prolonged period are also available.

PRESERVATIVES AND SENSITISERS. Information on preservatives and on substances identified as skin sensitisers (see section 13.1.3) is provided under preparation entries.

11.2 Control of microbial contamination

Preparations for the eye should be sterile when issued. Eye drops in multiple-application containers include a preservative but care should nevertheless be taken to avoid contamination of the contents during use.

Eye drops in multiple-application containers for *domiciliary use* should not be used for more than 4 weeks after first opening (unless otherwise stated).

Eye drops for use in *hospital wards* are normally discarded 1 week after first opening. Individual containers should be provided for each patient. A separate bottle should be supplied for each eye only if there are special concerns about contamination. Containers used before an operation should be discarded at the time of the operation and fresh containers supplied. A fresh supply should also be provided upon discharge from hospital; in specialist ophthalmology units, it may be acceptable to issue eye-drop bottles that have been dispensed to the patient on the day of discharge.

In *out-patient departments* single-application packs should preferably be used; if multiple-application packs are used, they should be discarded at the end of each day. In clinics for eye diseases and in accident and emergency departments, where the dangers of infection are high, single-application packs should be used; if a multiple-application pack is used, it should be discarded after single use.

Diagnostic dyes (e.g. fluorescein) should be used only from single-application packs.

In *eye surgery* single-application containers should be used if possible; if a multiple-application pack is used, it should be discarded after single use. Preparations used during intra-ocular procedures and others that may penetrate into the anterior chamber must be isotonic and without preservatives and buffered if necessary to a neutral pH. Specially formulated fluids should be used for intra-ocular surgery; intravenous infusion preparations are not suitable for this purpose. For all surgical procedures, a previously unopened container is used for each patient.

11.3 Anti-infective eye preparations

EYE INFECTIONS. Most acute superficial eye infections can be treated topically. Blepharitis and conjunctivitis are often caused by staphylococci; keratitis and endophthalmitis may be bacterial, viral, or fungal.

Bacterial *blepharitis* is treated by application of an antibacterial eye ointment to the conjunctival sac or to the lid margins. Systemic treatment may occasionally be required and is usually undertaken after culturing organisms from the lid margin and determining their antimicrobial sensitivity; antibiotics such as the tetracyclines given for 3 months or longer may be appropriate.

Most cases of acute bacterial conjunctivitis are self-limiting; where treatment is appropriate, antibacterial eye drops or an eye ointment are used. A poor response might indicate viral or allergic conjunctivitis. *Gonococcal conjunctivitis* is treated with systemic and topical antibacterials.

Corneal ulcer and *keratitis* require specialist treatment and may call for subconjunctival or systemic administration of antimicrobials.

Endophthalmitis is a medical emergency which also calls for specialist management and often requires parenteral, subconjunctival, or intra-ocular administration of antimicrobials.

For reference to the treatment of *crab lice of the eyelashes*, see section 13.10.4

11.3.1 Antibacterials

Bacterial infections are generally treated topically with eye drops and eye ointments. Systemic administration is sometimes appropriate in blepharitis. In intra-ocular infection, a variety of routes (intracorneal, intravitreal and systemic) may be used.

Chloramphenicol has a broad spectrum of activity and is the drug of choice for *superficial eye infections*. Chloramphenicol eye drops are well tolerated and the recommendation that chloramphenicol eye drops should be avoided because of an increased risk of aplastic anaemia is not well founded.

Other antibacterials with a broad spectrum of activity include the quinolones, **ciprofloxacin** and **ofloxacin**; **framycetin**, **gentamicin**, and **neomycin** are also active against a wide variety of bacteria. Gentamicin, ciprofloxacin, and ofloxacin are effective for infections caused by *Pseudomonas aeruginosa*.

Ciprofloxacin eye drops are licensed for *corneal ulcers*; intensive application (especially in the first 2 days) is required throughout the day and night.

Trachoma which results from chronic infection with *Chlamydia trachomatis* can be treated with **azithromycin** by mouth [unlicensed indication]; alternatively a combination of an oral and a topical tetracycline can be used.

Fusidic acid is useful for staphylococcal infections.

Propamidine isetionate is of little value in bacterial infections but is specific for the rare but potentially devastating condition of *acanthamoeba keratitis* (see also section 11.9).

WITH CORTICOSTEROIDS. Many antibacterial preparations also incorporate a corticosteroid but such mixtures should **not** be used unless a patient is under close specialist supervision. In particular they should not be prescribed for undiagnosed 'red eye' which is sometimes caused by the herpes simplex virus and may be difficult to diagnose (section 11.4).

ADMINISTRATION.

Eye drops. Apply 1 drop at least every 2 hours then reduce frequency as infection is controlled and continue for 48 hours after healing.

Eye ointment. Apply *either* at night (if eye drops used during the day) *or* 3–4 times daily (if eye ointment used alone).

CHLORAMPHENICOL

Indications: see notes above
Side-effects: transient stinging; see also notes above
Dose: see notes above

[1]**Chloramphenicol** (Non-proprietary) PoM
Eye drops, chloramphenicol 0.5%. Net price 10 mL = £1.23
Eye ointment, chloramphenicol 1%. Net price 4 g = £2.07

1. Chloramphenicol 0.5% eye drops can be sold to the public (in max. pack size 10 mL) for treatment of acute bacterial conjunctivitis in adults and children over 2 years; max. duration of treatment 5 days; proprietary brands on sale to the public include *Optrex Infected Eyes®*

Chloromycetin® (Goldshield) PoM
Redidrops (= eye drops), chloramphenicol 0.5%. Net price 5 mL = £1.65; 10 mL = £2.01
Excipients: include phenylmercuric acetate
Ophthalmic ointment (= eye ointment), chloramphenicol 1%. Net price 4 g = £2.01

■ Single use

Minims® Chloramphenicol (Chauvin) PoM
Eye drops, chloramphenicol 0.5%. Net price 20 × 0.5 mL = £4.92

CIPROFLOXACIN

Indications: superficial bacterial infections, see notes above; corneal ulcers
Cautions: not recommended for children under 1 year; pregnancy (Appendix 4); breast-feeding (Appendix 5)
Side-effects: local burning and itching; lid margin crusting; hyperaemia; taste disturbances; corneal staining, keratitis, lid oedema, lacrimation, photophobia, corneal infiltrates; nausea and visual disturbances reported
Dose: superficial bacterial infection, see notes above

Corneal ulcer, apply throughout day and night, day 1 apply every 15 minutes for 6 hours then every 30 minutes, day 2 apply every hour, days 3–14 apply every 4 hours (max. duration of treatment 21 days)

Ciloxan® (Alcon) PoM
Ophthalmic solution (= eye drops), ciprofloxacin (as hydrochloride) 0.3%. Net price 5 mL = £4.94
Excipients: include benzalkonium chloride

FRAMYCETIN SULPHATE

Indications: see notes above
Dose: see notes above

Soframycin® (Florizel) PoM
Eye drops, framycetin sulphate 0.5%. Net price 10 mL = £4.30
Excipients: include benzalkonium chloride
Eye ointment, framycetin sulphate 0.5%. Net price 5 g = £2.34

FUSIDIC ACID

Indications: see notes above
Dose: see under preparation below

Fucithalmic® (Leo) PoM
Eye drops, m/r, fusidic acid 1% in gel basis (liquifies on contact with eye). Net price 5 g = £2.09
Excipients: include benzalkonium chloride, disodium edetate
Dose: apply twice daily

GENTAMICIN

Indications: see notes above
Dose: see notes above

Genticin® (Roche) PoM
Drops (for ear or eye), gentamicin 0.3% (as sulphate). Net price 10 mL = £1.78
Excipients: include benzalkonium chloride

■ Single use

Minims® Gentamicin Sulphate (Chauvin) PoM
Eye drops, gentamicin 0.3% (as sulphate). Net price 20 × 0.5 mL = £5.75

NEOMYCIN SULPHATE

Indications: see notes above
Dose: see notes above

Neomycin (Non-proprietary) PoM
Eye drops, neomycin sulphate 0.5% (3500 units/mL). Net price 10 mL = £3.11
Eye ointment, neomycin sulphate 0.5% (3500 units/g). Net price 3 g = £2.44

■ With antibacterials

Neosporin® (PLIVA) PoM
Eye drops, gramicidin 25 units, neomycin sulphate 1700 units, polymyxin B sulphate 5000 units/mL. Net price 5 mL = £4.86
Excipients: include thiomersal
Dose: apply 2–4 times daily or more frequently if required

■ With hydrocortisone

Section 12.1.1

OFLOXACIN

Indications: see notes above
Cautions: pregnancy (Appendix 4); breast-feeding (Appendix 5); not to be used for more than 10 days
Side-effects: local irritation including photophobia; dizziness, numbness, nausea and headache reported
Dose: see notes above

Exocin® (Allergan) PoM
Ophthalmic solution (= eye drops), ofloxacin 0.3%. Net price 5 mL = £2.17
Excipients: include benzalkonium chloride

POLYMYXIN B SULPHATE

Indications: see notes above
Side-effects: local irritation and dermatitis
Dose: see notes above

■ With antibacterials

Polyfax® (PLIVA) PoM
Eye ointment, polymyxin B sulphate 10 000 units, bacitracin zinc 500 units/g. Net price 4 g = £3.26

Polytrim® (PLIVA) PoM
Eye drops, trimethoprim 0.1%, polymyxin B sulphate 10 000 units/mL. Net price 5 mL = £3.05
Excipients: include benzalkonium chloride
Eye ointment, trimethoprim 0.5%, polymyxin B sulphate 10 000 units/g. Net price 4 g = £2.90

PROPAMIDINE ISETIONATE

Indications: local treatment of infections (but see notes above)

Brolene® (Aventis Pharma)
Eye drops, propamidine isetionate 0.1%. Net price 10 mL = £2.73
Excipients: include benzalkonium chloride
Dose: apply 4 times daily
NOTE. Eye drops containing propamidine isetionate 0.1% also available from Typharm (*Golden Eye Drops*)
Eye ointment, dibromopropamidine isetionate 0.15%. Net price 5 g = £2.85
Dose: apply 1–2 times daily
NOTE. Eye ointment containing dibromopropamidine isetionate 0.15% also available from Typharm (*Golden Eye Ointment*)

11.3.2 Antifungals

Fungal infections of the cornea are rare but can occur after agricultural injuries, especially in hot and humid climates. Orbital mycosis is rarer, and when it occurs it is usually because of a direct spread of infection from the paranasal sinuses. Increasing age, debility, or immunosuppression may encourage fungal proliferation. The spread of infection through blood occasionally produces a metastatic endophthalmitis.

Many different fungi are capable of producing ocular infection; they may be identified by appropriate laboratory procedures.

Antifungal preparations for the eye are not generally available. Treatment will normally be carried out at specialist centres, but requests for information about supplies of preparations not available commercially should be addressed to the local Health Authority (or equivalent in Scotland or Northern Ireland), or to the nearest hospital ophthalmology unit, or to Moorfields Eye Hospital, City Road, London EC1V 2PD (tel. (020) 7253 3411).

11.3.3 Antivirals

Herpes simplex infections producing, for example, dendritic corneal ulcer can be treated with **aciclovir**. **Ganciclovir** eye drops are licensed for the treatment of acute herpetic keratitis.

Slow-release ocular implants containing **ganciclovir** may be inserted surgically to treat immediate sight-threatening CMV retinitis. Local treatments do not protect against systemic infection or infection in the other eye. For systemic treatment of CMV retinitis, see section 5.3.2.2.

ACICLOVIR

(Acyclovir)

Indications: local treatment of herpes simplex infections

Side-effects: local irritation and inflammation reported

Dose: apply 5 times daily (continue for at least 3 days after complete healing)

Zovirax® (GSK) PoM
Eye ointment, aciclovir 3%. Net price 4.5 g = £9.92
Tablets and *injection*, see section 5.3.2.1
Cream, see section 13.10.3

GANCICLOVIR

Indications: acute herpetic keratitis

Cautions: pregnancy (Appendix 4); breast-feeding (Appendix 5)

Side-effects: ocular irritation, visual disturbances; superficial punctate keratitis

Dose: apply 5 times daily until complete corneal re-epithelialisation, then 3 times daily for 7 days (usual duration of treatment 21 days)

Virgan® (Chauvin) PoM
Eye drops, ganciclovir 0.15 % in gel basis, net price 5 g = £10.64
Excipients: include benzalkonium chloride

11.4 Corticosteroids and other anti-inflammatory preparations

11.4.1 Corticosteroids

Corticosteroids administered locally (as eye drops, eye ointments or subconjunctival injection) or by mouth have an important place in treating anterior segment inflammation, including that which results from surgery.

Topical corticosteroids should normally only be used under expert supervision; three main dangers are associated with their use:

- a 'red eye', where the diagnosis is unconfirmed, may be due to herpes simplex virus, and a corticosteroid may aggravate the condition, leading to corneal ulceration, with possible damage to vision and even loss of the eye. Bacterial, fungal and amoebic infections pose a similar hazard;
- 'steroid glaucoma' may follow the use of corticosteroid eye preparations in susceptible individuals;
- a 'steroid cataract' may follow prolonged use.

Other side-effects include thinning of the cornea and sclera.

Use of a combination product containing a corticosteroid with an anti-infective is rarely justified.

Systemic corticosteroids (section 6.3.2) may be useful for ocular conditions. The risk of producing a 'steroid cataract' is very high (75%) if the equivalent of more than 15 mg prednisolone is given daily for several years.

BETAMETHASONE

Indications: local treatment of inflammation (short-term)

Cautions: see notes above

Side-effects: see notes above

Dose: apply eye drops every 1–2 hours until controlled then reduce frequency, eye ointment 2–4 times daily or at night when used with eye drops

Betnesol® (Celltech) PoM
Drops (for ear, eye, or nose), betamethasone sodium phosphate 0.1%. Net price 10 mL = £2.32
Excipients: include benzalkonium chloride, disodium edetate
Eye ointment, betamethasone sodium phosphate 0.1%. Net price 3 g = £1.41

Vista-Methasone® (Martindale) PoM
Drops (for ear, eye, or nose), betamethasone sodium phosphate 0.1%. Net price 5 mL = £1.02; 10 mL = £1.16
Excipients: include benzalkonium chloride

■ With neomycin

Betnesol-N® (Celltech) PoM
Drops (for ear, eye, or nose), see section 12.1.1
Eye ointment, betamethasone sodium phosphate 0.1%, neomycin sulphate 0.5%. Net price 3 g = £1.28
NOTE. May be difficult to obtain

Vista-Methasone N® (Martindale) PoM
Drops (for ear, eye, or nose), see section 12.1.1

DEXAMETHASONE

Indications: local treatment of inflammation (short-term)
Cautions: see notes above
Side-effects: see notes above
Dose: apply eye drops 4–6 times daily; severe conditions every 30–60 minutes until controlled then reduce frequency

Maxidex® (Alcon) PoM
Eye drops, dexamethasone 0.1%, hypromellose 0.5%. Net price 5 mL = £1.49; 10 mL = £2.95
Excipients: include benzalkonium chloride, disodium edetate, polysorbate 80

■ Single use

Minims® **Dexamethasone** (Chauvin) PoM
Eye drops, dexamethasone sodium phosphate 0.1%. Net price 20 × 0.5 mL = £6.95
Excipients: include disodium edetate

■ With antibacterials

Maxitrol® (Alcon) PoM
Eye drops, dexamethasone 0.1%, hypromellose 0.5%, neomycin 0.35% (as sulphate), polymyxin B sulphate 6000 units/mL. Net price 5 mL = £1.77
Excipients: include benzalkonium chloride, polysorbate 20
Eye ointment, dexamethasone 0.1%, neomycin 0.35% (as sulphate), polymyxin B sulphate 6000 units/g. Net price 3.5 g = £1.52
Excipients: include hydroxybenzoates (parabens), wool fat

Sofradex® (Florizel) PoM
Drops (for ear or eye), see section 12.1.1

Tobradex® (Alcon) PoM
Eye drops, dexamethasone 0.1%, tobramycin 0.3%. Net price 5 mL = £5.65
Excipients: include benzalkonium chloride, disodium edetate

FLUOROMETHOLONE

Indications: local treatment of inflammation (short-term)
Cautions: see notes above
Side-effects: see notes above
Dose: apply eye drops 2–4 times daily (initially every hour for 24–48 hours then reduce frequency)

FML® (Allergan) PoM
Ophthalmic suspension (= eye drops), fluorometholone 0.1%, polyvinyl alcohol (*Liquifilm*®) 1.4%. Net price 5 mL = £1.71; 10 mL = £2.95
Excipients: include benzalkonium chloride, disodium edetate, polysorbate 80

HYDROCORTISONE ACETATE

Indications: local treatment of inflammation (short-term)
Cautions: see notes above
Side-effects: see notes above

Hydrocortisone (Non-proprietary) PoM
Eye drops, hydrocortisone acetate 1%. Net price 10 mL = £3.21
Eye ointment, hydrocortisone acetate 0.5%, net price 3 g = £2.40; 1%, 3 g = £2.42; 2.5%, 3 g = £2.44

■ With neomycin

Neo-Cortef® (PLIVA) PoM
Ointment (for ear or eye), see section 12.1.1
NOTE. May be difficult to obtain

PREDNISOLONE

Indications: local treatment of inflammation (short-term)
Cautions: see notes above
Side-effects: see notes above
Dose: apply eye drops every 1–2 hours until controlled then reduce frequency

Pred Forte® (Allergan) PoM
Eye drops, prednisolone acetate 1%. Net price 5 mL = £1.52; 10 mL = £3.05
Excipients: include benzalkonium chloride, disodium edetate, polysorbate 80
Dose: apply 2–4 times daily

Predsol® (Celltech) PoM
Drops (for ear or eye), prednisolone sodium phosphate 0.5%. Net price 10 mL = £2.00
Excipients: include benzalkonium chloride, disodium edetate

■ Single use

Minims® **Prednisolone Sodium Phosphate** (Chauvin) PoM
Eye drops, prednisolone sodium phosphate 0.5%. Net price 20 × 0.5 mL = £5.75
Excipients: include disodium edetate

■ With neomycin

Predsol-N® (Celltech) PoM
Drops (for ear or eye), see section 12.1.1

RIMEXOLONE

Indications: local treatment of inflammation (short-term)
Cautions: see notes above
Side-effects: see notes above
Dose: postoperative inflammation, apply 4 times daily for 2 weeks, beginning 24 hours after surgery
Steroid-responsive inflammation, apply at least 4 times daily for up to 4 weeks
Uveitis, apply every hour during daytime in week 1, then every 2 hours in week 2, then 4 times daily in week 3, then twice daily for first 4 days of week 4, then once daily for remaining 3 days of week 4

Vexol® (Alcon) ▼ PoM
Eye drops, rimexolone 1%, net price 5 mL = £5.95
Excipients: include benzalkonium chloride, disodium edetate, polysorbate 80

11.4.2 Other anti-inflammatory preparations

Other preparations used for the topical treatment of inflammation and allergic conjunctivitis include antihistamines, lodoxamide, and sodium cromoglicate.

Topical preparations of **antihistamines** such as eye drops containing **antazoline** (with xylometazoline as *Otrivine-Antistin*®), **azelastine**, **epinastine**, **ketotifen**, **levocabastine** and **olopatadine** may be used for allergic conjunctivitis.

Sodium cromoglicate (sodium cromoglycate) and **nedocromil sodium** eye drops may be useful for vernal keratoconjunctivitis and other allergic forms of conjunctivitis.

Lodoxamide eye drops are used for allergic conjunctival conditions including seasonal allergic conjunctivitis.

Diclofenac eye drops (section 11.8.2) and **emedastine** eye drops are also licensed for seasonal allergic conjunctivitis.

ANTAZOLINE SULPHATE

Indications: allergic conjunctivitis

Otrivine-Antistin® (Novartis Consumer Health)
Eye drops, antazoline sulphate 0.5%, xylometazoline hydrochloride 0.05%. Net price 10 mL = £2.35
Excipients: include benzalkonium chloride, disodium edetate
Dose: ADULT and CHILD over 5 years apply 2–3 times daily
NOTE. Xylometazoline is a sympathomimetic; it should be avoided in angle-closure glaucoma; absorption of antazoline and xylometazoline may result in systemic side-effects and the possibility of interaction with other drugs

AZELASTINE HYDROCHLORIDE

Indications: allergic conjunctivitis
Side-effects: mild transient irritation; bitter taste reported
Dose: seasonal allergic conjunctivitis, ADULT and CHILD over 4 years, apply twice daily, increased if necessary to 4 times daily
Perennial conjunctivitis, ADULT and ADOLESCENT over 12 years, apply twice daily, increased if necessary to 4 times daily; max. duration of treatment 6 weeks

[1]**Optilast**® (Viatris) PoM
Eye drops, azelastine hydrochloride 0.05%. Net price 8 mL = £6.40
Excipients: include benzalkonium chloride, disodium edetate

1. Azelastine 0.05% eye drops can be sold to the public (in max. pack size of 6 mL) for treatment of seasonal and perennial allergic conjunctivitis in adults and children over 12 years; proprietary brands on sale to the public include *Aller-eze*®

EMEDASTINE

Indications: seasonal allergic conjunctivitis
Side-effects: transient burning or stinging; blurred vision, local oedema, keratitis, irritation, dry eye, lacrimation, corneal infiltrates (discontinue) and staining; photophobia; headache, and rhinitis occasionally reported
Dose: ADULT and CHILD over 3 years, apply twice daily

Emadine® (Alcon) PoM
Eye drops, emedastine 0.05% (as difumarate), net price 5 mL = £7.69
Excipients: include benzalkonium chloride

EPINASTINE HYDROCHLORIDE

Indications: seasonal allergic conjunctivitis
Side-effects: burning; less commonly dry mouth, taste disturbance; nasal irritation, rhinitis; headache, blepharoptosis, conjunctival oedema and hyperaemia, dry eye, local irritation, photophobia, visual disturbance; pruritus
Dose: ADULT and ADOLESCENT over 12 years, apply twice daily; max. duration of treatment 8 weeks

Relestat® (Allergan) ▼ PoM
Eye drops, epinastine hydrochloride 500 micrograms/mL, net price 5 mL = £14.50
Excipients: include benzalkonium chloride, disodium edetate

KETOTIFEN

Indications: seasonal allergic conjunctivitis
Side-effects: transient burning or stinging, punctate corneal epithelial erosion; less commonly dry eye, subconjunctival haemmorhage, photophobia; headache, drowsiness, skin reactions, and dry mouth also reported
Dose: ADULT and CHILD over 3 years, apply twice daily

Zaditen® (Novartis) PoM
Eye drops, ketotifen (as fumarate) 250 micrograms/mL, net price 5 mL = £9.75
Excipients: include benzalkonium chloride

LEVOCABASTINE

Indications: seasonal allergic conjunctivitis
Side-effects: local irritation, blurred vision, local oedema, urticaria; dyspnoea, headache
Dose: ADULT and CHILD over 9 years, apply twice daily, increased if necessary to 3–4 times daily, discontinue if no improvement within 3 days

[1]**Livostin**® (McNeil) PoM
Eye drops, levocabastine 0.05% (as hydrochloride). Net price 3 mL = £3.28
Excipients: include benzalkonium chloride, disodium edetate, polysorbate 80, propylene glycol
NOTE. May be difficult to obtain

1. Levocabastine 0.05% eye drops can be sold to the public (in max. pack size of 4 mL) for treatment of seasonal allergic conjunctivitis in adults and children over 12 years; proprietary brands on sale to the public include *Livostin*® *Direct*

LODOXAMIDE

Indications: allergic conjunctivitis
Side-effects: mild transient burning, stinging, itching, and lacrimation; flushing and dizziness reported
Dose: ADULT and CHILD over 4 years, apply eye drops 4 times daily

[1]**Alomide**® (Alcon) PoM
Ophthalmic solution (= eye drops), lodoxamide 0.1% (as trometamol). Net price 10 mL = £5.48
Excipients: include benzalkonium chloride, disodium edetate

1. Lodoxamide 0.1% eye drops can be sold to the public for treatment of allergic conjunctivitis in adults and children over 4 years; proprietary brands on sale to the public include *Alomide Allergy*®

NEDOCROMIL SODIUM

Indications: allergic conjunctivitis; vernal kerato-conjunctivitis

Side-effects: transient burning and stinging; distinctive taste reported

Dose: seasonal and perennial conjunctivitis, ADULT and CHILD over 6 years, apply twice daily increased if necessary to 4 times daily; max. 12 weeks treatment for seasonal allergic conjunctivitis

Vernal keratoconjunctivitis, ADULT and CHILD over 6 years, apply 4 times daily

Rapitil® (Aventis Pharma) PoM

Eye drops, nedocromil sodium 2%. Net price 5 mL = £5.12

Excipients: include benzalkonium chloride, disodium edetate

OLOPATADINE

Indications: seasonal allergic conjunctivitis

Side-effects: local irritation; less commonly keratitis, dry eye, local oedema, photophobia; headache, asthenia, dizziness; dry nose also reported

Dose: ADULT and CHILD over 3 years, apply twice daily; max. duration of treatment 4 months

Opatanol® (Alcon) ▼ PoM

Eye drops, olopatadine (as hydrochloride) 1 mg/mL, net price 5 mL = £4.11

Excipients: include benzalkonium chloride

SODIUM CROMOGLICATE

(Sodium cromoglycate)

Indications: allergic conjunctivitis; vernal kerato-conjunctivitis

Side-effects: transient burning and stinging

Dose: ADULT and CHILD apply eye drops 4 times daily

[1]**Sodium Cromoglicate** (Non-proprietary) PoM

Eye drops, sodium cromoglicate 2%. Net price 13.5 mL = £3.46

Brands include *Hay-Crom*® *Aqueous*, *Opticrom*® *Aqueous*, *Vividrin*®)

1. Sodium cromoglicate 2% eye drops can be sold to the public (in max. pack size of 10 mL) for treatment of acute seasonal and perennial allergic conjunctivitis; proprietary brands on sale to the public include *Boots Hayfever Relief*, *Clariteyes*®, *Opticrom*® *Allergy*, *Optrex*® *Allergy*, and *Vivicrom*®

11.5 Mydriatics and cycloplegics

Antimuscarinics dilate the pupil and paralyse the ciliary muscle; they vary in potency and duration of action.

Short-acting, relatively weak mydriatics, such as **tropicamide** 0.5%, facilitate the examination of the fundus of the eye. **Cyclopentolate** 1% or **atropine** are preferable for producing cycloplegia for refraction in young children. Atropine ointment 1% is sometimes preferred for children aged under 5 years because the ointment formulation reduces systemic absorption. Atropine, which has a longer duration of action, is also used for the treatment of anterior uveitis mainly to prevent posterior synechiae, often with phenylephrine 10% eye drops (2.5% in children, the elderly, and those with cardiac disease). **Homatropine** 1% is also used in the treatment of anterior segment inflammation, and may be preferred for its shorter duration of action.

CAUTIONS. Darkly pigmented iris is more resistant to pupillary dilatation and caution should be exercised to avoid overdosage. Mydriasis may precipitate acute angle-closure glaucoma in a very few patients, usually aged over 60 years and hypermetropic (long-sighted), who are predisposed to the condition because of a shallow anterior chamber. Phenylephrine may interact with systemically administered monoamine-oxidase inhibitors; other **interactions:** Appendix 1 (sympathomimetics).

DRIVING. Patients should be warned not to drive for 1–2 hours after mydriasis.

SIDE-EFFECTS. Ocular side-effects of mydriatics and cycloplegics include transient stinging and raised intra-ocular pressure; on prolonged administration, local irritation, hyperaemia, oedema and conjunctivitis may occur. Contact dermatitis (conjunctivitis) is not uncommon with the antimuscarinic mydriatic drugs, especially atropine.

Toxic systemic reactions to atropine and cyclopentolate may occur in the very young and the very old; see under Atropine Sulphate (section 1.2) for systemic side-effects of antimuscarinic drugs.

Antimuscarinics

ATROPINE SULPHATE

Indications: refraction procedures in young children; anterior uveitis—see also notes above

Cautions: risk of systemic effects with eye drops in infants under 3 months—eye ointment preferred; see also notes above

Side-effects: see notes above

Atropine (Non-proprietary) PoM

Eye drops, atropine sulphate 0.5%, net price 10 mL = £2.32; 1%, 10 mL = 91p

Eye ointment, atropine sulphate 1%. Net price 3 g = £2.95

Isopto Atropine® (Alcon) PoM

Eye drops, atropine sulphate 1%, hypromellose 0.5%. Net price 5 mL = 99p

Excipients: include benzalkonium chloride

■ Single use

Minims® **Atropine Sulphate** (Chauvin) PoM

Eye drops, atropine sulphate 1%. Net price 20 × 0.5 mL = £4.92

CYCLOPENTOLATE HYDROCHLORIDE

Indications: see notes above

Cautions: see notes above

Side-effects: see notes above

Mydrilate® (Intrapharm) PoM

Eye drops, cyclopentolate hydrochloride 0.5%, net price 5 mL = 97p; 1%, 5 mL = £1.19

Excipients: include benzalkonium chloride

■ Single use

Minims® **Cyclopentolate Hydrochloride** (Chauvin) PoM

Eye drops, cyclopentolate hydrochloride 0.5 and 1%. Net price 20 × 0.5 mL (both) = £4.92

HOMATROPINE HYDROBROMIDE

Indications: see notes above
Cautions: see notes above
Side-effects: see notes above

Homatropine (Non-proprietary) PoM
Eye drops, homatropine hydrobromide 1%, net price 10 mL = £2.14; 2%, 10 mL = £2.26

TROPICAMIDE

Indications: see notes above
Cautions: see notes above
Side-effects: see notes above

Mydriacyl® (Alcon) PoM
Eye drops, tropicamide 0.5%, net price 5 mL = £1.36; 1%, 5 mL = £1.68
Excipients: include benzalkonium chloride, disodium edetate

■ Single use
Minims® **Tropicamide** (Chauvin) PoM
Eye drops, tropicamide 0.5 and 1%. Net price 20 × 0.5 mL (both) = £5.75

Sympathomimetics

PHENYLEPHRINE HYDROCHLORIDE

Indications: mydriasis; see also notes above
Cautions: children and elderly (avoid 10% strength); cardiovascular disease (avoid or use 2.5% strength only); tachycardia; hyperthyroidism; diabetes; see also notes above
Contra-indications: angle-closure glaucoma
Side-effects: eye pain and stinging; blurred vision, photophobia; systemic effects include arrhythmias, hypertension, coronary artery spasm

Phenylephrine (Non-proprietary)
Eye drops, phenylephrine hydrochloride 10%. Net price 10 mL = £3.38
See also under Hypromellose (section 11.8.1)

■ Single use
Minims® **Phenylephrine Hydrochloride** (Chauvin)
Eye drops, phenylephrine hydrochloride 2.5%, net price 20 × 0.5 mL = £5.75; 10%, 20 × 0.5 mL = £5.75
Excipients: include disodium edetate, sodium metabisulphite

11.6 Treatment of glaucoma

Glaucoma describes a group of disorders characterised by a loss of visual field associated with cupping of the optic disc and optic nerve damage. While glaucoma is generally associated with raised intra-ocular pressure, it can occur when the intra-ocular pressure is within the normal range.

The commonest form of glaucoma is *primary open-angle glaucoma* (chronic simple glaucoma; wide-angle glaucoma), where the obstruction is in the trabecular meshwork. The condition is often asymptomatic and the patient may present with significant loss of visual-field . *Primary angle closure glaucoma* (acute closed-angle glaucoma, narrow-angle glaucoma) results from blockage of aqueous humour flow into the anterior chamber and is a medical emergency.

Only drugs that reduce intra-ocular pressure are available for managing glaucoma; they act by a variety of mechanisms. A topical beta-blocker or a prostaglandin analogue is commonly the drug of first choice. It may be necessary to combine these drugs or add others such as miotics, sympathomimetics and carbonic anhydrase inhibitors to control intra-ocular pressure.

For urgent reduction of intra-ocular pressure and before surgery, mannitol 20% (up to 500 mL) is given by slow intravenous infusion until the intra-ocular pressure has been satisfactorily reduced. Acetazolamide by intravenous injection may also be used for the emergency management of raised intra-ocular pressure.

Standard antiglaucoma therapy is used if supplementary treatment is required after iridotomy, iridectomy or a drainage operation in either primary open-angle or acute closed-angle glaucoma.

Beta-blockers

Topical application of a beta-blocker to the eye reduces intra-ocular pressure effectively in *primary open-angle glaucoma*, probably by reducing the rate of production of aqueous humour. Administration by mouth also reduces intra-ocular pressure but this route is not used since side-effects may be troublesome.

Beta-blockers used as eye drops include **betaxolol**, **carteolol**, **levobunolol**, **metipranolol**, and **timolol**.

CAUTIONS, CONTRA-INDICATIONS AND SIDE-EFFECTS. Systemic absorption may follow topical application therefore eye drops containing a beta-blocker are contra-indicated in patients with bradycardia, heart block, or uncontrolled heart failure. **Important:** for a warning to avoid in asthma see CSM advice below. Consider also other cautions, contra-indications and side-effects of beta-blockers (p. 83). Local side-effects of eye drops include ocular stinging, burning, pain, itching, erythema, dry eyes and allergic reactions including anaphylaxis and blepharoconjunctivitis; occasionally corneal disorders have been reported.
CSM advice. The CSM has advised that beta-blockers, even those with apparent cardioselectivity, should not be used in patients with asthma or a history of obstructive airways disease, unless no alternative treatment is available. In such cases the risk of inducing bronchospasm should be appreciated and appropriate precautions taken.

INTERACTIONS. Since systemic absorption may follow topical application the possibility of interactions, in particular, with drugs such as verapamil should be borne in mind. See also Appendix 1 (beta-blockers).

BETAXOLOL HYDROCHLORIDE

Indications: see notes above
Cautions: see notes above
Contra-indications: see notes above
Side-effects: see notes above
Dose: apply twice daily

Betoptic® (Alcon) PoM
Ophthalmic solution (= eye drops), betaxolol (as hydrochloride) 0.5%, net price 5 mL = £2.00
Excipients: include benzalkonium chloride, disodium edetate

Ophthalmic suspension (= eye drops), m/r, betaxolol (as hydrochloride) 0.25%, net price 5 mL = £2.80
Excipients: include benzalkonium chloride, disodium edetate
Unit dose eye drop suspension, m/r, betaxolol (as hydrochloride) 0.25%, net price 50 × 0.25 mL = £14.49

CARTEOLOL HYDROCHLORIDE

Indications: see notes above
Cautions: see notes above
Contra-indications: see notes above
Side-effects: see notes above
Dose: apply twice daily

Teoptic® (Novartis) PoM
Eye drops, carteolol hydrochloride 1%, net price 5 mL = £4.60; 2%, 5 mL = £5.40
Excipients: include benzalkonium chloride

LEVOBUNOLOL HYDROCHLORIDE

Indications: see notes above
Cautions: see notes above
Contra-indications: see notes above
Side-effects: see notes above; anterior uveitis occasionally reported
Dose: apply once or twice daily

Levobunolol (Non-proprietary) PoM
Eye drops, levobunolol hydrochloride 0.5%. Net price 5 mL = £3.00

Betagan® (Allergan) PoM
Eye drops, levobunolol hydrochloride 0.5%, polyvinyl alcohol (*Liquifilm®*) 1.4%. Net price 5-mL = £2.85
Excipients: include benzalkonium chloride, disodium edetate, sodium metabisulphite
Unit dose eye drops, levobunolol hydrochloride 0.5%, polyvinyl alcohol (*Liquifilm®*) 1.4%. Net price 30 × 0.4 mL = £9.98
Excipients: include disodium edetate

METIPRANOLOL

Indications: see notes above but in chronic open-angle glaucoma **restricted** to patients allergic to preservatives or to those wearing soft contact lenses (in whom benzalkonium chloride should be avoided)
Cautions: see notes above
Contra-indications: see notes above
Side-effects: see notes above; granulomatous anterior uveitis reported (discontinue treatment)
Dose: apply twice daily

Minims® Metipranolol (Chauvin) PoM
Eye drops, metipranolol 0.1%, net price 20 × 0.5 mL = £10.19; 0.3%, 20 × 0.5 mL = £11.09

TIMOLOL MALEATE

Indications: see notes above
Cautions: see notes above
Contra-indications: see notes above
Side-effects: see notes above
Dose: apply twice daily; long-acting preparations, see under preparations below

Timolol (Non-proprietary) PoM
Eye drops, timolol (as maleate) 0.25%, net price 5 mL = £1.70; 0.5%, 5 mL = £2.31

Timoptol® (MSD) PoM
Eye drops, in Ocumeter® metered-dose unit, timolol (as maleate) 0.25%, net price 5 mL = £3.12; 0.5%, 5 mL = £3.12
Excipients: include benzalkonium chloride
Unit dose eye drops, timolol (as maleate) 0.25%, net price 30 × 0.2 mL = £8.45; 0.5%, 30 × 0.2 mL = £9.65

■ Once-daily preparations

Nyogel® (Novartis) PoM
Eye gel (= eye drops), timolol (as maleate) 0.1%, net price 5 mL = £2.85
Excipients: include benzalkonium chloride
Dose: apply eye drops once daily

Timoptol®-LA (MSD) PoM
Ophthalmic gel-forming solution (= eye drops), timolol (as maleate) 0.25%, net price 2.5 mL = £3.12; 0.5%, 2.5 mL = £3.12
Excipients: include benzododecinium bromide
Dose: apply eye drops once daily

■ With brimonidine
See under Brimonidine

■ With dorzolamide
See under Dorzolamide

■ With latanoprost
See under Latanoprost

Prostaglandin analogues

Latanoprost and **travoprost** are prostaglandin analogues which increase uveoscleral outflow; **bimatoprost** is a related drug. They are used to reduce intra-ocular pressure in ocular hypertension or in open-angle glaucoma. Patients receiving prostaglandin analogues should be monitored for any changes to eye coloration since an increase in the brown pigment in the iris may occur; particular care is required in those with mixed coloured irides and those receiving treatment to one eye only.

BIMATOPROST

Indications: raised intra-ocular pressure in open-angle glaucoma and ocular hypertension
Cautions: see under Latanoprost and notes above
Side-effects: see under Latanoprost; also ocular pruritus, allergic conjunctivitis, cataract, conjunctival oedema, eye discharge, photophobia, superficial punctate keratitis, headache; hypertension
Dose: apply once daily, preferably in the evening; CHILD and ADOLESCENT under 18 years, not recommended

Lumigan® (Allergan) ▼ PoM
Eye drops, bimatoprost 300 micrograms/mL, net price 3 mL = £11.46, triple pack (3 × 3 mL) = £32.66
Excipients: include benzalkonium chloride

LATANOPROST

Indications: raised intra-ocular pressure in open-angle glaucoma and ocular hypertension
Cautions: before initiating treatment, advise patients of possible change in eye colour; monitor for eye colour change; aphakia, or pseudophakia with torn posterior lens capsule or anterior chamber lenses; risk factors for cystoid macular oedema; brittle or severe asthma; not to be used within 5

minutes of use of thiomersal-containing preparations; manufacturer advises avoid in pregnancy and in breast-feeding

Side-effects: brown pigmentation particularly in those with mixed-colour irides; blepharitis, ocular irritation and pain; darkening, thickening and lengthening of eye lashes; conjunctival hyperaemia; transient punctate epithelial erosion; skin rash; *less commonly* eye lid oedema and rash; *rarely* dyspnoea, exacerbation of asthma, iritis, uveitis, local oedema, darkening of palpebral skin

Dose: apply once daily, preferably in the evening

Xalatan® (Pharmacia) PoM

Eye drops, latanoprost 50 micrograms/mL, net price 2.5 mL = £11.95

Excipients: include benzalkonium chloride

■ With timolol

For cautions, contra-indications, and side-effects of timolol, see section 11.6, Beta-blockers

Xalacom® (Pharmacia) ▼ PoM

Eye drops, latanoprost 50 micrograms, timolol (as maleate) 5 mg/mL, net price 2.5 mL = £15.07

Excipients: include benzalkonium chloride

Dose: for raised intra-ocular pressure in patients with open-angle glaucoma and ocular hypertension when beta-blocker alone not adequate; apply once daily, in the morning

TRAVOPROST

Indications: raised intra-ocular pressure in open-angle glaucoma and ocular hypertension

Cautions: see under Latanoprost and notes above

Side-effects: see under Latanoprost; also headache, ocular pruritus, photophobia, and keratitis reported; rarely, hypotension, bradycardia, conjunctivitis, browache

Dose: apply once daily, preferably in the evening; CHILD and ADOLESCENT under 18 years, not recommended

Travatan® (Alcon) ▼ PoM

Eye drops, travoprost 40 micrograms/mL, net price 2.5 mL = £11.06

Excipients: include benzalkonium chloride

Sympathomimetics

Dipivefrine is a pro-drug of adrenaline. It is claimed to pass more rapidly than adrenaline through the cornea and is then converted to the active form.

Adrenaline (epinephrine) probably acts both by reducing the rate of production of aqueous humour and by increasing the outflow through the trabecular meshwork. It is contra-indicated in angle-closure glaucoma because it is a mydriatic, unless an iridectomy has been carried out. Side-effects include severe smarting and redness of the eye; adrenaline should be used with caution in patients with hypertension and heart disease.

Brimonidine, a selective alpha$_2$-adrenoceptor stimulant, is licensed for the reduction of intra-ocular pressure in open-angle glaucoma or ocular hypertension in patients for whom beta-blockers are inappropriate; it may also be used as adjunctive therapy when intra-ocular pressure is inadequately controlled by other antiglaucoma therapy.

Apraclonidine (section 11.8.2) is another alpha$_2$-adrenoceptor stimulant. Eye drops containing apraclonidine 0.5% are used for a short term to delay laser treatment or surgery for glaucoma in patients not adequately controlled by another drug; eye drops containing 1% are used for control of intra-ocular pressure after anterior segment laser surgery.

BRIMONIDINE TARTRATE

Indications: raised intra-ocular pressure, see notes above

Cautions: severe cardiovascular disease; cerebral or coronary insufficiency, Raynaud's syndrome, postural hypotension, depression, hepatic or renal impairment; pregnancy, breast-feeding; **interactions:** Appendix 1 (alpha$_2$-adrenoceptor stimulants)

DRIVING. Drowsiness may affect performance of skilled tasks (e.g. driving)

Side-effects: ocular reactions include hyperaemia, burning, stinging, blurring, pruritus, allergy, and conjunctival follicles; occasionally corneal erosion and staining, photophobia, eyelid inflammation, conjunctivitis; headache, dry mouth, taste alteration, fatigue, dizziness, drowsiness reported; rarely depression, nasal dryness, palpitation, and hypersensitivity reactions

Dose: apply twice daily

Alphagan® (Allergan) PoM

Eye drops, brimonidine tartrate 0.2%, net price 5 mL = £8.25

Excipients: include benzalkonium chloride

■ With timolol

For cautions, contra-indications, and side-effects of timolol, see section 11.6, Beta-blockers

Combigan® (Allergan) ▼ PoM

Eye drops, brimonidine tartrate 0.2%, timolol (as maleate) 0.5%, net price 5-mL = £10.00

Excipients: include benzalkonium chloride

Dose: for raised intra-ocular pressure in open-angle glaucoma or ocular hypertension when beta-blocker alone not adequate, apply twice daily

DIPIVEFRINE HYDROCHLORIDE

Indications: see notes above

Contra-indications: see notes above

Side-effects: see notes above

Dose: apply twice daily

Propine® (Allergan) PoM

Eye drops, dipivefrine hydrochloride 0.1%, net price 5 mL = £3.81, 10 mL = £4.77

Excipients: include benzalkonium chloride, disodium edetate

Carbonic anhydrase inhibitors and systemic drugs

The **carbonic anhydrase inhibitors**, acetazolamide and dorzolamide, reduce intra-ocular pressure by reducing aqueous humour production. Systemic use also produces weak diuresis.

Acetazolamide is given by mouth or by intravenous injection (intramuscular injections are painful because of the alkaline pH of the solution). It is used as an adjunct to other treatment for reducing intra-ocular pressure. Acetazolamide is a sulphonamide; blood disorders, rashes and other sulphonamide-related side-effects occur occasionally. It is not generally recommended for long-term use; electrolyte disturbances and metabolic acidosis that occur may be corrected by administering potassium bicarbonate (as effervescent potassium tablets, section 9.2.1.3).

Dorzolamide and **brinzolamide** are topical carbonic anhydrase inhibitors. They are licensed for use in patients resistant to beta-blockers or those in whom beta-blockers are contra-indicated. They are used alone or as an adjunct to a topical beta-blocker. Systemic absorption may rarely give rise to sulphonamide-like side-effects and may require discontinuation if severe.

The **osmotic diuretics**, intravenous hypertonic **mannitol** (section 2.2.5), or **glycerol** by mouth, are useful short-term ocular hypotensive drugs.

ACETAZOLAMIDE

Indications: reduction of intra-ocular pressure in open-angle glaucoma, secondary glaucoma, and peri-operatively in angle-closure glaucoma; diuresis (section 2.2.7); epilepsy

Cautions: not generally recommended for prolonged use but if given monitor blood count and plasma electrolyte concentration; pulmonary obstruction (risk of acidosis); elderly; pregnancy (Appendix 4); avoid extravasation at injection site (risk of necrosis); **interactions:** Appendix 1 (diuretics)

Contra-indications: hypokalaemia, hyponatraemia, hyperchloraemic acidosis; severe hepatic impairment; renal impairment (Appendix 3); sulphonamide hypersensitivity

Side-effects: nausea, vomiting, diarrhoea, taste disturbance; loss of appetite, paraesthesia, flushing, headache, dizziness, fatigue, irritability, depression; thirst, polyuria; reduced libido; metabolic acidosis and electrolyte disturbances on long-term therapy; occasionally, drowsiness, confusion, hearing disturbances, urticaria, malaena, glycosuria, haematuria, abnormal liver function, renal calculi, blood disorders including agranulocytosis and thrombocytopenia, rashes including Stevens-Johnson syndrome and toxic epidermal necrolysis; rarely, photosensitivity, liver damage, flaccid paralysis, convulsions; transient myopia reported

Dose: *by mouth or by intravenous injection*, glaucoma, 0.25–1 g daily in divided doses

Epilepsy, 0.25–1 g daily in divided doses; CHILD 8–30 mg/kg daily, max. 750 mg daily

By intramuscular injection, as for intravenous injection but preferably avoided because of alkalinity

Diamox® (Goldshield) PoM

Tablets, acetazolamide 250 mg. Net price 112-tab pack = £12.68. Label: 3

Sodium Parenteral (= injection), powder for reconstitution, acetazolamide (as sodium salt). Net price 500-mg vial = £14.76

Diamox® **SR** (Goldshield) PoM

Capsules, m/r, two-tone orange, enclosing orange f/c pellets, acetazolamide 250 mg. Net price 28-cap pack = £11.55. Label: 3, 25

Dose: glaucoma, 1–2 capsules daily

BRINZOLAMIDE

Indications: adjunct to beta-blockers or used alone in raised intra-ocular pressure in ocular hypertension and in open-angle glaucoma if beta-blocker alone inadequate or inappropriate

Cautions: hepatic impairment; pregnancy (Appendix 4); **interactions:** Appendix 1 (brinzolamide)

Contra-indications: renal impairment (creatinine clearance less than 30 mL/minute), hyperchloraemic acidosis; breast-feeding

Side-effects: local irritation, taste disturbance; less commonly nausea, dyspepsia, dry mouth, chest pain, epistaxis, haemoptysis, dyspnoea, rhinitis, pharyngitis, bronchitis, paraesthesia, depression, dizziness, headache, dermatitis, alopecia, corneal erosion

Dose: apply twice daily increased to 3 times daily if necessary

Azopt® (Alcon) PoM

Eye drops, brinzolamide 10 mg/mL, net price 5 mL = £6.90

Excipients: include benzalkonium chloride, disodium edetate

DORZOLAMIDE

Indications: raised intra-ocular pressure in ocular hypertension, open-angle glaucoma, pseudo-exfoliative glaucoma *either* as adjunct to beta-blocker *or* used alone in patients unresponsive to beta-blockers or if beta-blockers contra-indicated

Cautions: hepatic impairment; systemic absorption follows topical application; history of renal calculi; chronic corneal defects, history of intra-ocular surgery; **interactions:** Appendix 1 (dorzolamide)

Contra-indications: severe renal impairment or hyperchloraemic acidosis; pregnancy and breast-feeding

Side-effects: ocular burning, stinging and itching, blurred vision, lacrimation, conjunctivitis, superficial punctate keratitis, eyelid inflammation and crusting, anterior uveitis, transient myopia, corneal oedema, iridocyclitis; headache, dizziness, paraesthesia, asthenia, sinusitis, rhinitis, nausea; hypersensitivity reactions (including urticaria, angioedema, bronchospasm); bitter taste, epistaxis, urolithiasis

Dose: used alone, apply 3 times daily; with topical beta-blocker, apply twice daily

Trusopt® (MSD) PoM

Ophthalmic solution (= eye drops), dorzolamide (as hydrochloride) 2%, net price 5 mL = £6.33

Excipients: include benzalkonium chloride

■ With timolol

For cautions, contra-indications, and side-effects of timolol, see section 11.6, Beta-blockers

Cosopt® (MSD) PoM

Ophthalmic solution (= eye drops), dorzolamide (as hydrochloride) 2%, timolol (as maleate) 0.5%, net price 5 mL = £10.05

Excipients: include benzalkonium chloride

Dose: for raised intra-ocular pressure in open-angle glaucoma, or pseudoexfoliative glaucoma when beta-blockers alone not adequate, apply twice daily

Miotics

The small pupil is an unfortunate side-effect of these drugs (except when pilocarpine is used temporarily before an operation for *angle-closure glaucoma*). They act by opening up the inefficient drainage channels in the trabecular meshwork resulting from contraction or spasm of the ciliary muscle.

Miotics used in the management of raised intra-ocular pressure include pilocarpine.

CAUTIONS. A darkly pigmented iris may require higher concentration of the miotic or more frequent administration and care should be taken to avoid overdosage. Retinal detachment has occurred in susceptible individuals and those with retinal disease; therefore fundus examination is advised before starting treatment with a miotic. Care is also required in conjunctival or corneal damage. Intra-ocular pressure and visual fields should be monitored in those with chronic simple glaucoma and those receiving long-term treatment with a miotic. Miotics should be used with caution in cardiac disease, hypertension, asthma, peptic ulceration, urinary-tract obstruction, and Parkinson's disease.

COUNSELLING. Blurred vision may affect performance of skilled tasks (e.g. driving) particularly at night or in reduced lighting

CONTRA-INDICATIONS. Miotics are contra-indicated in conditions where pupillary constriction is undesirable such as acute iritis, anterior uveitis and some forms of secondary glaucoma. They should be avoided in acute inflammatory disease of the anterior segment.

SIDE-EFFECTS. Ciliary spasm leads to headache and browache which may be more severe in the initial 2–4 weeks of treatment (a particular disadvantage in patients under 40 years of age). Ocular side-effects include burning, itching, smarting, blurred vision, conjunctival vascular congestion, myopia, lens changes with chronic use, vitreous haemorrhage, and pupillary block. Systemic side-effects (see under Parasympathomimetics, section 7.4.1) are rare following application to the eye.

PILOCARPINE

Indications: see notes above; dry mouth (section 12.3.5)
Cautions: see notes above
Contra-indications: see notes above
Side-effects: see notes above
Dose: apply up to 4 times daily; long-acting preparations, see under preparations below

Pilocarpine Hydrochloride (Non-proprietary) PoM
Eye drops, pilocarpine hydrochloride 0.5%, net price 10 mL = £1.40; 1%, 10 mL = £2.30; 2%, 10 mL = £2.16; 3%, 10 mL = £1.44; 4%, 10 mL = £2.76

■ Single use

Minims® Pilocarpine Nitrate (Chauvin) PoM
Eye drops, pilocarpine nitrate 2 and 4%, net price 20 × 0.5 mL (both) = £4.92

■ Long acting

Pilogel® (Alcon) PoM
Ophthalmic gel, pilocarpine hydrochloride 4%, carbomer 940 (polyacrylic acid) 3.5%, net price 5 g = £6.86
Excipients: include benzalkonium chloride, disodium edetate
Dose: apply 1–1.5 cm gel once daily at bedtime

11.7 Local anaesthetics

Oxybuprocaine and tetracaine (amethocaine) are probably the most widely used topical local anaesthetics. Proxymetacaine causes less initial stinging and is useful for children. Oxybuprocaine or a combined preparation of lidocaine (lignocaine) and fluorescein is used for tonometry. Tetracaine produces a more profound anaesthesia and is suitable for use before minor surgical procedures, such as the removal of corneal sutures. It has a temporary disruptive effect on the corneal epithelium. Lidocaine, with or without adrenaline (epinephrine), is injected into the eyelids for minor surgery, while retrobulbar or peribulbar injections are used for surgery of the globe itself. Local anaesthetics should never be used for the management of ocular symptoms.

LIDOCAINE HYDROCHLORIDE

(Lignocaine hydrochloride)
Indications: local anaesthetic

Minims® Lignocaine and Fluorescein (Chauvin) PoM
Eye drops, lidocaine hydrochloride 4%, fluorescein sodium 0.25%. Net price 20 × 0.5 mL = £6.93

OXYBUPROCAINE HYDROCHLORIDE

Indications: local anaesthetic

Minims® Benoxinate (Oxybuprocaine) Hydrochloride (Chauvin) PoM
Eye drops, oxybuprocaine hydrochloride 0.4%. Net price 20 × 0.5 mL = £4.92

PROXYMETACAINE HYDROCHLORIDE

Indications: local anaesthetic

Minims® Proxymetacaine (Chauvin) PoM
Eye drops, proxymetacaine hydrochloride 0.5%. Net price 20 × 0.5 mL = £6.95

■ With fluorescein

Minims® Proxymetacaine and Fluorescein (Chauvin) PoM
Eye drops, proxymetacaine hydrochloride 0.5%, fluorescein sodium 0.25%. Net price 20 × 0.5 mL = £7.95

TETRACAINE HYDROCHLORIDE

(Amethocaine hydrochloride)
Indications: local anaesthetic

Minims® Amethocaine Hydrochloride (Chauvin) PoM
Eye drops, tetracaine hydrochloride 0.5 and 1%. Net price 20 × 0.5 mL (both) = £5.75

11.8 Miscellaneous ophthalmic preparations

Certain eye drops, e.g. amphotericin, ceftazidime, cefuroxime, colistin, desferrioxamine, dexamethasone, gentamicin and vancomycin may be prepared aseptically from material supplied for injection; for details on preparation of trisodium edetate eye drops see under *Limclair*® section 9.5.1.2.

11.8.1 Tear deficiency, ocular lubricants, and astringents

Chronic soreness of the eyes associated with reduced or abnormal tear secretion (e.g. in Sjögren's syndrome) often responds to tear replacement therapy or pilocarpine given by mouth (section 12.3.5). The severity of the condition and patient preference will often guide the choice of preparation.

Hypromellose is the traditional choice of treatment for tear deficiency. It may need to be instilled frequently (e.g. hourly) for adequate relief. Ocular surface mucin is often abnormal in tear deficiency and the combination of hypromellose with a mucolytic such as **acetylcysteine** can be helpful.

The ability of **carbomers** to cling to the eye surface may help reduce frequency of application to 4 times daily.

Polyvinyl alcohol increases the persistence of the tear film and is useful when the ocular surface mucin is reduced.

Povidone eye drops are also used in the management of tear deficiency.

Sodium chloride 0.9% drops are sometimes useful in tear deficiency, and can be used as 'comfort drops' by contact lens wearers, and to facilitate lens removal. Special presentations of sodium chloride 0.9% and other irrigation solutions are used routinely for intra-ocular surgery.

Eye ointments containing a **paraffin** may be used to lubricate the eye surface, especially in cases of recurrent corneal epithelial erosion. They may cause temporary visual disturbance and are best suited for application before sleep. Ointments should not be used during contact lens wear.

Zinc sulphate is a traditional astringent that is now little used.

ACETYLCYSTEINE

Indications: tear deficiency, impaired or abnormal mucus production

Dose: apply eye drops 3–4 times daily

Ilube® (Alcon) PoM

Eye drops, acetylcysteine 5%, hypromellose 0.35%. Net price 10 mL = £4.63

Excipients: include benzalkonium chloride, disodium edetate

CARBOMERS

(Polyacrylic acid)

Synthetic high molecular weight polymers of acrylic acid cross-linked with either allyl ethers of sucrose or allyl ethers of pentaerithrityl

Indications: dry eyes including keratoconjunctivitis sicca, unstable tear film

Dose: apply 3–4 times daily or as required

GelTears® (Chauvin)

Gel (= eye drops), carbomer 980 (polyacrylic acid) 0.2%, net price 10 g = £2.80

Excipients: include benzalkonium chloride

Liposic® (Bausch & Lomb)

Gel (= eye drops), carbomer 980 (polyacrylic acid) 0.2%, net price 10 g = £2.96

Excipients: include cetrimide

Liquivisc® (Allergan)

Gel (= eye drops), carbomer 974P (polyacrylic acid) 0.25%, net price 10 g = £1.99

Excipients: include benzalkonium chloride

Viscotears® (Novartis Ophthalmics)

Liquid gel (= eye drops), carbomer 980 (polyacrylic acid) 0.2%, net price 10 g = £3.12

Excipients: include cetrimide, disodium edetate

Liquid gel (= eye drops), carbomer 980 (polyacrylic acid) 0.2%, net price 30 × 0.6-mL single-dose units = £5.75

CARMELLOSE SODIUM

Indications: dry eye conditions

Dose: apply as required

Celluvisc® (Allergan) ▼

Eye drops, carmellose sodium 1%, net price 30 × 0.4 mL = £5.75, 60 × 0.4 mL = £10.99

HYDROXYETHYLCELLULOSE

Indications: tear deficiency

Minims® **Artificial Tears** (Chauvin)

Eye drops, hydroxyethylcellulose 0.44%, sodium chloride 0.35%. Net price 20 × 0.5 mL = £5.75

HYPROMELLOSE

Indications: tear deficiency

NOTE. The Royal Pharmaceutical Society of Great Britain has stated that where it is not possible to ascertain the strength of hypromellose prescribed, the prescriber should be contacted to clarify the strength intended.

Hypromellose (Non-proprietary)

Eye drops, hypromellose 0.3%, net price 10 mL = £1.57

Isopto Alkaline® (Alcon)

Eye drops, hypromellose 1%, net price 10 mL = 99p

Excipients: include benzalkonium chloride

Isopto Plain® (Alcon)

Eye drops, hypromellose 0.5%, net price 10 mL = 85p

Excipients: include benzalkonium chloride

Tears Naturale® (Alcon)

Eye drops, dextran '70' 0.1%, hypromellose 0.3%, net price 15 mL = £1.68

Excipients: include benzalkonium chloride, disodium edetate

■ Single use

Artelac® **SDU** (Pharma-Global)

Eye drops, hypromellose 0.32%, net price 30 × 0.5 mL = £11.88

■ With phenylephrine

NOTE. Phenylephrine (section 11.5) acts to constrict conjunctival vessels, thus producing a whiter eye; it is not recommended for prolonged use

Isopto Frin® (Alcon)

Eye drops, phenylephrine hydrochloride 0.12%, hypromellose 0.5%, net price 10 mL = £1.14

Excipients: include benzethonium chloride

Dose: temporary relief of redness due to minor irritation, apply up to 4 times daily

LIQUID PARAFFIN

Indications: dry eye conditions

Lacri-Lube® (Allergan)
Eye ointment, white soft paraffin 57.3%, liquid paraffin 42.5%, wool alcohols 0.2%. Net price 3.5 g = £1.90, 5 g = £2.47

Lubri-Tears® (Alcon)
Eye ointment, white soft paraffin 60%, liquid paraffin 30%, wool fat 10%. Net price 5 g = £2.29

PARAFFIN, YELLOW, SOFT

Indications: see notes above

Simple Eye Ointment
Ointment, liquid paraffin 10%, wool fat 10%, in yellow soft paraffin. Net price 4 g = £2.68

POLYVINYL ALCOHOL

Indications: tear deficiency

Liquifilm Tears® (Allergan)
Ophthalmic solution (= eye drops), polyvinyl alcohol 1.4%. Net price 15 mL = £1.61
Excipients: include benzalkonium chloride, disodium edetate
Ophthalmic solution (= eye drops), polyvinyl alcohol 1.4%, povidone 0.6%. Net price 30 × 0.4 mL = £5.35

Sno Tears® (Chauvin)
Eye drops, polyvinyl alcohol 1.4%. Net price 10 mL = £1.06
Excipients: include benzalkonium chloride, disodium edetate

POVIDONE

Indications: dry eye conditions
Dose: apply 4 times daily or as required

Oculotect® (Novartis)
Eye drops, povidone 5%. Net price 20 × 0.4 mL = £3.40

SODIUM CHLORIDE

Indications: irrigation, including first-aid removal of harmful substances

Sodium Chloride 0.9% Solutions
See section 13.11.1

Balanced Salt Solution
Solution (sterile), sodium chloride 0.64%, sodium acetate 0.39%, sodium citrate 0.17%, calcium chloride 0.048%, magnesium chloride 0.03%, potassium chloride 0.075%
For intra-ocular or topical irrigation during surgical procedures
Brands include *Iocare*®

■ Single use

Minims® **Saline** (Chauvin)
Eye drops, sodium chloride 0.9%. Net price 20 × 0.5 mL = £4.92

ZINC SULPHATE

Indications: see notes above
Cautions: see notes above

Zinc Sulphate (Non-proprietary)
Eye drops, zinc sulphate 0.25%. Net price 10 mL = £3.15

11.8.2 Ocular diagnostic and peri-operative preparations and photodynamic treatment

Ocular diagnostic preparations

Fluorescein sodium and **rose bengal** are used in diagnostic procedures and for locating damaged areas of the cornea due to injury or disease. Rose bengal is more efficient for the diagnosis of conjunctival epithelial damage but it often stings excessively unless a local anaesthetic is instilled beforehand.

FLUORESCEIN SODIUM

Indications: detection of lesions and foreign bodies

Minims® **Fluorescein Sodium** (Chauvin)
Eye drops, fluorescein sodium 1 or 2%. Net price 20 × 0.5 mL (both) = £4.92

■ With local anaesthetic
Section 11.7

ROSE BENGAL

Indications: detection of lesions and foreign bodies

Minims® **Rose Bengal** (Chauvin)
Eye drops, rose bengal 1%. Net price 20 × 0.5 mL = £5.75

Ocular peri-operative drugs

Drugs used to prepare the eye for surgery and drugs that are injected into the anterior chamber at the time of surgery are included here.

Sodium hyaluronate (*Ophthalin*®) is used during surgical procedures on the eye.

Apraclonidine, an alpha$_2$-adrenoceptor stimulant, reduces intra-ocular pressure possibly by reducing the production of aqueous humour. It is used for short-term treatment only.

Special presentations of **sodium chloride 0.9%** solution are used routinely in intra-ocular surgery (section 11.8.1).

ACETYLCHOLINE CHLORIDE

Indications: cataract surgery, penetrating keratoplasty, iridectomy, and other anterior segment surgery requiring rapid complete miosis

Miochol-E® (Novartis) PoM
Solution for intra-ocular irrigation, acetylcholine chloride 1%, mannitol 3% when reconstituted. Net price 2 mL-vial = £9.10

APRACLONIDINE

NOTE. Apraclonidine is a derivative of clonidine

Indications: control of intra-ocular pressure
Cautions: history of angina, severe coronary insufficiency, recent myocardial infarction, heart failure, cerebrovascular disease, vasovagal attack, chronic renal failure; depression; pregnancy and breast-feeding; monitor intra-ocular pressure and

visual fields; loss of effect may occur over time; suspend treatment if reduction in vision occurs in end-stage glaucoma; monitor for excessive reduction in intra-ocular pressure following peri-operative use; **interactions:** Appendix 1 (alpha$_2$-adrenoceptor stimulants)

DRIVING. Drowsiness may affect performance of skilled tasks (e.g. driving)

Contra-indications: history of severe or unstable and uncontrolled cardiovascular disease

Side-effects: dry mouth, taste disturbance; hyperaemia, ocular pruritus, discomfort and lacrimation (withdraw if ocular intolerance including oedema of lids and conjunctiva); headache, asthenia, dry nose; lid retraction, conjunctival blanching and mydriasis reported after peri-operative use; since absorption may follow topical application systemic effects (see Clonidine Hydrochloride, section 2.5.2) may occur

Dose: see under preparations below

Iopidine® (Alcon) PoM

Ophthalmic solution (= eye drops), apraclonidine 1% (as hydrochloride). Net price 12 × 2 single use 0.25-mL units = £81.90

Dose: control or prevention of postoperative elevation of intra-ocular pressure after anterior segment laser surgery, apply 1 drop 1 hour before laser procedure then 1 drop immediately after completion of procedure; CHILD not recommended

Iopidine 0.5% ophthalmic solution (= eye drops), apraclonidine 0.5% (as hydrochloride). Net price 5 mL = £11.45

Excipients: include benzalkonium chloride

Dose: short-term adjunctive treatment of chronic glaucoma in patients not adequately controlled by another drug (see note below), apply 1 drop 3 times daily usually for max. 1 month; CHILD not recommended

NOTE. May not provide additional benefit if patient already using two drugs that suppress the production of aqueous humour

DICLOFENAC SODIUM

Indications: inhibition of intra-operative miosis during cataract surgery (but does not possess intrinsic mydriatic properties); postoperative inflammation in cataract surgery, strabismus surgery or argon laser trabeculoplasty; pain in corneal epithelial defects after photorefractive keratectomy, radial keratotomy or accidental trauma; seasonal allergic conjunctivitis (section 11.4.2)

Voltarol® **Ophtha Multidose** (Novartis) PoM

Eye drops, diclofenac sodium 0.1%, net price 5 mL = £6.68

Excipients: include benzalkonium chloride, disodium edetate, propylene glycol

■ Single use

Voltarol® **Ophtha** (Novartis) PoM

Eye drops, diclofenac sodium 0.1%. Net price pack of 5 single-dose units = £4.00, 40 single-dose units = £32.00

FLURBIPROFEN SODIUM

Indications: inhibition of intra-operative miosis (but does not possess intrinsic mydriatic properties); anterior segment inflammation following postoperative and post-laser trabeculoplasty when corticosteroids contra-indicated

Ocufen® (Allergan) PoM

Ophthalmic solution (= eye drops), flurbiprofen sodium 0.03%, polyvinyl alcohol (*Liquifilm*®) 1.4%. Net price 40 × 0.4 mL = £37.15

KETOROLAC TROMETAMOL

Indications: prophylaxis and reduction of inflammation and associated symptoms following ocular surgery

Acular® (Allergan) PoM

Eye drops, ketorolac trometamol 0.5%. Net price 5 mL = £5.00

Excipients: include benzalkonium chloride, disodium edetate

Subfoveal choroidal neovascularisation

Verteporfin is licensed for use in the photodynamic treatment of age-related macular degeneration associated with predominantly classic subfoveal choroidal neovascularisation *or* with pathological myopia (see NICE guidance below). It is also licensed for occult subfoveal choroidal neovascularisation with disease progression. Following intravenous infusion, verteporfin is activated by local irradiation using non-thermal red light to produce cytotoxic derivatives. Only specialists experienced in the management of these conditions should use it.

NICE guidance (photodynamic therapy for wet age-related macular degeneration). NICE has recommended (September 2003) photodynamic therapy for wet age-related macular degeneration with a confirmed diagnosis of classic (no occult) subfoveal choroidal neovascularisation and best-corrected visual acuity of 6/60 or better.

Photodynamic therapy is **not** recommended for wet age-related macular degeneration with predominantly classic but partly occult subfoveal choroidal neovascularisation *except* in clinical studies.

VERTEPORFIN

Indications: see notes above—specialist use only

Cautions: photosensitivity—avoid exposure of unprotected skin and eyes to bright light during infusion and for 48 hours afterwards; hepatic impairment (avoid if severe), biliary obstruction; avoid extravasation; pregnancy (Appendix 4)

Contra-indications: porphyria; breast-feeding (Appendix 5)

Side-effects: visual disturbances (including blurred vision, flashing lights, visual-field defects), nausea, back pain, asthenia, pruritus, hypercholesterolaemia, fever; rarely lacrimation disorder, subretinal or vitreous haemorrhage, hypersensitivity reactions (including chest pain, syncope, sweating, changes in blood pressure and in heart rate); injection-site reactions including pain, oedema, inflammation, haemorrhage, discoloration

Dose: *by intravenous infusion* over 10 minutes, 6 mg/m^2

NOTE. For information on administration and light activation, consult product literature

Visudyne® (Novartis) PoM

Injection, powder for reconstitution, verteporfin, net price 15-mg vial = £850.00

11.9 Contact lenses

NOTE. Some recommendations in this section involve non-licensed indications.

For cosmetic reasons many people prefer to wear contact lenses rather than spectacles; contact lenses are also sometimes required for medical indications. Visual defects are corrected by either rigid ('hard' or gas permeable) lenses or soft (hydrogel) lenses; soft lenses are the most popular type, because they are the most comfortable, though they may not give the best vision. Lenses should usually be worn for a specified number of hours each day. Continuous (extended) wear involves much greater risks to eye health and is not recommended except where medically indicated.

Contact lenses require meticulous care. Poor compliance with directions for use, and with daily cleaning and disinfection, may result in complications which include ulcerative keratitis, conjunctival problems (such as purulent or papillary conjunctivitis). One-day disposable lenses, which are worn only once and therefore require no maintenance or storage, are becoming increasingly popular.

Acanthamoeba keratitis, a sight-threatening condition, is associated with ineffective lens cleaning and disinfection or the use of contaminated lens cases. The condition is especially associated with the use of soft lenses (including frequently replaced lenses). Acanthamoeba keratitis is treated by specialists with intensive use of polihexanide (polyhexamethylene biguanide), propamidine isetionate, chlorhexidine and neomycin drops, sometimes in combination.

CONTACT LENSES AND DRUG TREATMENT. Special care is required in prescribing eye preparations for contact lens users. Some drugs and preservatives in eye preparations can accumulate in hydrogel lenses and may induce toxic reactions. Therefore, unless medically indicated, the lenses should be removed before instillation and not worn during the period of treatment. Alternatively, unpreserved drops can be used. Eye drops may, however, be instilled over rigid corneal contact lenses. Ointment preparations should never be used in conjunction with contact lens wear; oily eye drops should also be avoided.

Many drugs given systemically can also have adverse effects on contact lens wear. These include oral contraceptives (particularly those with a higher oestrogen content), drugs which reduce blink rate (e.g. anxiolytics, hypnotics, antihistamines, and muscle relaxants), drugs which reduce lacrimation (e.g. antihistamines, antimuscarinics, phenothiazines and related drugs, some beta-blockers, diuretics, and tricyclic antidepressants), and drugs which increase lacrimation (including ephedrine and hydralazine). Other drugs that may affect contact lens wear are isotretinoin (may cause conjunctival inflammation), aspirin (salicylic acid appears in tears and may be absorbed by contact lenses—leading to irritation), and rifampicin and sulfasalazine (may discolour lenses).

12: Ear, nose, and oropharynx

12.1 Drugs acting on the ear

12.1.1 Otitis externa

Otitis externa is an inflammatory reaction of the meatal skin. It is important to exclude an underlying chronic otitis media before treatment is commenced. Many cases recover after thorough cleansing of the external ear canal by suction, dry mopping, or gentle syringing. A frequent problem in resistant cases is the difficulty in applying lotions and ointments satisfactorily to the relatively inaccessible affected skin. The most effective method is to introduce a ribbon gauze dressing or sponge wick soaked with **corticosteroid** ear drops or with an astringent such as **aluminium acetate** solution. When this is not practical, the ear should be gently cleansed with a probe covered in cotton wool and the patient encouraged to lie with the affected ear uppermost for ten minutes after the canal has been filled with a liberal quantity of the appropriate solution.

If infection is present, a topical anti-infective which is not used systemically (such as **neomycin** or **clioquinol**) may be used, but for only about a week as excessive use may result in fungal infections; these may be difficult to treat and require expert advice. Sensitivity to the anti-infective or solvent may occur and resistance to antibacterials is a possibility with prolonged use. **Chloramphenicol** may also be used but the ear drops contain propylene glycol and cause sensitivity in about 10% of patients. Solutions containing an anti-infective and a corticosteroid (such as *Locorten-Vioform*®) are used for treating cases where infection is present with inflammation and eczema. In view of reports of ototoxicity in patients with a perforated tympanic membrane (eardrum), the CSM has stated that treatment with a topical aminoglycoside antibiotic is contra-indicated in those with a tympanic perforation. However, many specialists do use these drops cautiously in the presence of a perforation in patients with otitis media (section 12.1.2) and where other measures have failed for otitis externa.

A solution of **acetic acid** 2% acts as an antifungal and antibacterial in the external ear canal. It may be used to treat mild otitis externa but in severe cases an anti-inflammatory preparation with or without an anti-infective drug is required. A proprietary preparation containing acetic acid 2% (*EarCalm*® spray) is on sale to the public.

An acute infection may cause severe pain and a systemic antibacterial is required with a simple analgesic such as paracetamol. When a resistant staphylococcal infection (a boil) is present in the external auditory meatus, **flucloxacillin** is the drug of choice (section 5.1, table 1); **ciprofloxacin** (or an aminoglycoside) may be needed in pseudomonal infections which may occur if the patient has diabetes or is immunocompromised.

The skin of the pinna adjacent to the ear canal is often affected by eczema. Topical corticosteroid creams and ointments (see section 13.4) are then required, but prolonged use should be avoided.

Astringent preparations

ALUMINIUM ACETATE

Indications: inflammation in otitis externa (see notes above)

Dose: insert into meatus or apply on a gauze wick which should be kept saturated with the ear drops

Aluminium Acetate (Non-proprietary)
Ear drops 13%, aluminium sulphate 2.25 g, calcium carbonate 1 g, tartaric acid 450 mg, acetic acid (33%) 2.5 mL, purified water 7.5 mL
Available from manufacturers of 'special order' products
Ear drops 8%, dilute 8 parts aluminium acetate ear drops (13%) with 5 parts purified water. Must be freshly prepared

Anti-inflammatory preparations

BETAMETHASONE SODIUM PHOSPHATE

Indications: eczematous inflammation in otitis externa (see notes above)
Cautions: avoid prolonged use
Contra-indications: untreated infection
Side-effects: local sensitivity reactions

Betnesol® (Celltech) PoM
Drops (for ear, eye, or nose), betamethasone sodium phosphate 0.1%. Net price 10 mL = £2.32
Excipients: include benzalkonium chloride, disodium edetate
Dose: ear, apply 2–3 drops every 2–3 hours; reduce frequency when relief obtained; *eye*, see section 11.4.1; *nose*, see section 12.2.1

Vista-Methasone® (Martindale) PoM
Drops (for ear, eye, or nose), betamethasone sodium phosphate 0.1%. Net price 5 mL = £1.10; 10 mL = £1.25
Excipients: include benzalkonium chloride, disodium edetate
Dose: ear, apply 2–3 drops every 3–4 hours; reduce frequency when relief obtained; *eye*, see section 11.4.1; *nose*, see section 12.2.1

■ With antibacterial

Betnesol-N® (Celltech) PoM
Drops (for ear, eye, or nose), betamethasone sodium phosphate 0.1%, neomycin sulphate 0.5%. Net price 10 mL = £2.39
Excipients: include benzalkonium chloride, disodium edetate
Dose: ear, apply 2–3 drops 3–4 times daily; *eye*, see section 11.4.1; *nose*, section 12.2.3

Vista-Methasone N® (Martindale) PoM
Drops (for ear, eye, or nose), betamethasone sodium phosphate 0.1%, neomycin sulphate 0.5%. Net price 5 mL = £1.09; 10 mL = £1.20
Excipients: include thiomersal
Dose: ear, apply 2–3 drops every 3–4 hours; reduce frequency when relief obtained; *eye*, see section 11.4.1; *nose*, section 12.2.3

DEXAMETHASONE

Indications: eczematous inflammation in otitis externa (see notes above)
Cautions: avoid prolonged use
Contra-indications: untreated infection
Side-effects: local sensitivity reactions

■ With antibacterial

Otomize® (GSK Consumer Healthcare) PoM
Ear spray, dexamethasone 0.1%, neomycin sulphate 3250 units/mL, glacial acetic acid 2%. Net price 5-mL pump-action aerosol unit = £4.24
Excipients: include hydroxybenzoates (parabens)
Dose: apply 1 metered spray into the ear 3 times daily

Sofradex® (Florizel) PoM ▲
Drops (for ear or eye), dexamethasone (as sodium metasulphobenzoate) 0.05%, framycetin sulphate 0.5%, gramicidin 0.005%. Net price 10 mL = £4.85
Excipients: include polysorbate 80
Dose: ear, apply 2–3 drops 3–4 times daily; *eye*, see section 11.4.1

FLUMETASONE PIVALATE

(Flumethasone Pivalate)
Indications: eczematous inflammation in otitis externa (see notes above)
Cautions: avoid prolonged use
Contra-indications: untreated infection
Side-effects: local sensitivity reactions

■ With antibacterial

Locorten-Vioform® (Amdipharm) PoM
Ear drops, flumetasone pivalate 0.02%, clioquinol 1%. Net price 7.5 mL = £1.47
Contra-indications: iodine sensitivity
Dose: apply 2–3 drops into the ear twice daily for up to 7–10 days; not recommended for child under 2 years

HYDROCORTISONE

Indications: eczematous inflammation in otitis externa (see notes above)
Cautions: avoid prolonged use
Contra-indications: untreated infection
Side-effects: local sensitivity reactions

■ With antibacterial

Gentisone HC® (Roche) PoM
Ear drops, hydrocortisone acetate 1%, gentamicin 0.3% (as sulphate). Net price 10 mL = £3.69
Excipients: include benzalkonium chloride, disodium edetate
Dose: apply 2–4 drops into the ear 3–4 times daily and at night

Neo-Cortef® (PLIVA) PoM
Ointment (for ear or eye), hydrocortisone acetate 1.5%, neomycin sulphate 0.5%. Net price 3.9 g = £1.53
Excipients: include wool fat
Dose: ear, apply 1–2 times daily; *eye*, see section 11.4.1
NOTE. May be difficult to obtain

Otosporin® (GSK) PoM ▲
Ear drops, hydrocortisone 1%, neomycin sulphate 3400 units, polymyxin B sulphate 10 000 units/mL. Net price 5 mL = £2.00; 10 mL = £4.00
Excipients: include cetostearyl alcohol, hydroxybenzoates (parabens), polysorbate 20
Dose: ADULT and CHILD over 3 years, apply 3 drops into the ear 3–4 times daily

PREDNISOLONE SODIUM PHOSPHATE

Indications: eczematous inflammation in otitis externa (see notes above)
Cautions: avoid prolonged use
Contra-indications: untreated infection
Side-effects: local sensitivity reactions

Predsol® (Celltech) PoM
Drops (for ear or eye), prednisolone sodium phosphate 0.5%. Net price 10 mL = £2.00
Excipients: include benzalkonium chloride, disodium edetate
Dose: ear, apply 2–3 drops every 2–3 hours; reduce frequency when relief obtained; *eye*, see section 11.4.1

■ With antibacterial

Predsol-N® (Celltech) PoM
Drops (for ear or eye), prednisolone sodium phosphate 0.5%, neomycin sulphate 0.5%. Net price 10 mL = £2.36
Excipients: include benzalkonium chloride, disodium edetate
Dose: ear, apply 2–3 drops 3–4 times daily; *eye*, see section 11.4.1

TRIAMCINOLONE ACETONIDE

Indications: eczematous inflammation in otitis externa (see notes above)
Cautions: avoid prolonged use
Contra-indications: untreated infection
Side-effects: local sensitivity reactions

■ With antibacterial

Tri-Adcortyl Otic® (Squibb) PoM
Ear ointment, triamcinolone acetonide 0.1%, gramicidin 0.025%, neomycin 0.25% (as sulphate), nystatin 100 000 units/g in *Plastibase*®. Net price 10 g = £1.58
Dose: apply into the ear 2–3 times daily; CHILD under 1 year not recommended

Anti-infective preparations

CHLORAMPHENICOL

Indications: bacterial infection in otitis externa (but see notes above)
Cautions: avoid prolonged use (see notes above)
Side-effects: high incidence of sensitivity reactions to vehicle

Chloramphenicol (Non-proprietary) PoM
Ear drops, chloramphenicol in propylene glycol, net price 5%, 10 mL = £1.47; 10%, 10 mL = £1.40
Dose: apply 2–3 drops into the ear 2–3 times daily

CLIOQUINOL

Indications: mild bacterial or fungal infections in otitis externa (see notes above)
Cautions: avoid prolonged use (see notes above)
Contra-indications: perforated tympanic membrane
Side-effects: local sensitivity; stains skin and clothing

■ With corticosteroid

Locorten-Vioform®, see Flumetasone

CLOTRIMAZOLE

Indications: fungal infection in otitis externa (see notes above)
Side-effects: occasional local irritation or sensitivity

Canesten® (Bayer Consumer Care)
Solution, clotrimazole 1% in polyethylene glycol 400 (macrogol 400). Net price 20 mL = £2.43
Dose: ear, apply 2–3 times daily continuing for at least 14 days after disappearance of infection; *skin*, see section 13.10.2

FRAMYCETIN SULPHATE

Indications: see under Gentamicin
Cautions: see under Gentamicin
Contra-indications: perforated tympanic membrane (see notes above)
Side-effects: local sensitivity

■ With corticosteroid

Sofradex®, see Dexamethasone

GENTAMICIN

Indications: bacterial infection in otitis externa (see notes above)
Cautions: avoid prolonged use (see notes above)
Contra-indications: perforated tympanic membrane (but see also notes above and section 12.1.2)
Side-effects: local sensitivity

Genticin® (Roche) PoM
Drops (for ear or eye), gentamicin 0.3% (as sulphate). Net price 10 mL = £1.91
Excipients: include benzalkonium chloride
Dose: ear, apply 2–3 drops 3–4 times daily and at night; *eye*, see section 11.3.1

■ With corticosteroid

Gentisone HC® see Hydrocortisone

NEOMYCIN SULPHATE

Indications: bacterial infection in otitis externa (see notes above)
Cautions: avoid prolonged use (see notes above)
Contra-indications: perforated tympanic membrane (see notes above)
Side-effects: local sensitivity

■ With corticosteroid

Betnesol-N® see Betamethasone

Neo-Cortef® see Hydrocortisone

Otomize® see Dexamethasone

Otosporin® see Hydrocortisone

Predsol-N® see Prednisolone

Tri-Adcortyl Otic® see Triamcinolone

Vista-Methasone N® see Betamethasone

Other aural preparations

Choline salicylate is a mild analgesic but it is of doubtful value when applied topically.

Audax® (SSL) NHS
Ear drops, choline salicylate 21.6%, glycerol 12.6%. Net price 10 mL = £2.62
Excipients: include propylene glycol

12.1.2 Otitis media

ACUTE OTITIS MEDIA. Acute otitis media is the commonest cause of severe pain in small children. Many infections, especially those accompanying coryza, are caused by viruses. Most uncomplicated cases resolve without antibacterial treatment and a **simple analgesic**, such as paracetamol, may be sufficient. In children without systemic features, a **systemic antibacterial** may be started after 72 hours if there is no improvement, or earlier if there is deterioration (Table 1, section 5.1). Topical treatment of acute otitis media is ineffective and there is no place for drops containing a local anaesthetic. If the tympanic membrane has perforated, culture and sensitivity testing of any discharge is helpful in selecting an appropriate systemic antibacterial (Table 1, section 5.1).

In *recurrent acute otitis media* prophylaxis with an antibacterial (e.g. amoxicillin) during the winter months can be tried in young children who live at home and do not attend day centres. A full course of a systemic antibacterial is required if otitis media recurs.

OTITIS MEDIA WITH EFFUSION. Otitis media with effusion ('glue ear') occurs in about 10% of children and in 90% of children with cleft palates. Systemic antibacterials are not usually required for otitis media with effusion. If 'glue ear' persists for more than a month or two, the child should be referred for assessment and follow up because of the risk of long-term hearing impairment which can delay language development. Untreated or resistant glue ear may be responsible for some types of *chronic otitis media*.

CHRONIC OTITIS MEDIA. Opportunistic organisms are often present in the debris, keratin, and necrotic bone of the middle ear and mastoid in patients with chronic otitis media. The mainstay of treatment is thorough cleansing with aural microsuction which may completely resolve long-standing infection. Local cleansing of the meatal and middle ear may be followed by treatment with ribbon gauze dressings soaked with corticosteroid ear drops or with an astringent such as aluminium acetate solution; this is particularly beneficial for discharging ears or infections of the mastoid cavity. An antibacterial ear ointment may also be used. Acute exacerbations of chronic infection may also require systemic treatment with amoxicillin (or erythromycin if penicillin-allergic) and metronidazole; treatment is adjusted according to the results of sensitivity testing. Parenteral antibacterials are required if *Pseudomonas aeruginosa* and *Proteus* spp. are present.

The CSM has stated that topical treatment with ototoxic antibacterials is contra-indicated in the presence of a perforation (section 12.1.1). However, many specialists use ear drops containing **aminoglycosides** (e.g. neomycin) or **polymyxins** if the otitis media has failed to settle with systemic antibacterials; it is considered that the pus in the middle ear associated with otitis media carries a higher risk of ototoxicity than the drops themselves. Ciprofloxacin or ofloxacin ear drops [both unlicensed; available on named-patient basis from IDIS] are an effective alternative to aminoglycoside ear drops for chronic otitis media in patients with perforation of the tympanic membrane.

12.1.3 Removal of ear wax

Wax is a normal bodily secretion which provides a protective film on the meatal skin and need only be removed if it causes deafness or interferes with a proper view of the ear drum. Syringing is generally best avoided in young children, in patients with a history of recurrent otitis externa, a history of ear-drum perforation, or previous ear surgery. A person who has hearing in one ear only should not have that ear syringed because even a very slight risk of damage is unacceptable in this situation.

Wax may be removed by syringing with water (warmed to body temperature). If necessary, wax can be softened before syringing with simple remedies such as **sodium bicarbonate** ear drops, **olive oil** ear drops or **almond oil** ear drops, which are safe, effective and inexpensive. If the wax is hard and impacted the drops may be used twice daily for a few days before syringing; otherwise the wax may be softened on the day of syringing. The patient should lie with the affected ear uppermost for 5 to 10 minutes after a generous amount of the softening remedy has been introduced into the ear. Some proprietary preparations containing organic solvents can irritate the meatal skin, and in most cases the simple remedies indicated above are just as effective and less likely to cause irritation. Docusate sodium or urea–hydrogen peroxide are ingredients in a number of proprietary preparations.

Almond Oil (Non-proprietary)
Ear drops, almond oil in a suitable container
Allow to warm to room temperature before use

Olive Oil (Non-proprietary)
Ear drops, olive oil in a suitable container
Allow to warm to room temperature before use

Sodium Bicarbonate (Non-proprietary)
Ear drops, sodium bicarbonate 5%, net price 10 mL = £1.25

Cerumol® (LAB)
Ear drops, chlorobutanol 5%, paradichlorobenzene 2%, arachis (peanut) oil 57.3%. Net price 11 mL = £1.60

Exterol® (Dermal)
Ear drops, urea–hydrogen peroxide complex 5% in glycerol. Net price 8 mL = £1.83

Molcer® (Wallace Mfg)
Ear drops, docusate sodium 5%. Net price 15 mL = £1.90
Excipients: include propylene glycol

Otex® (DDD)
Ear drops, urea–hydrogen peroxide 5%. Net price 8 mL = £2.64

Waxsol® (Norgine)
Ear drops, docusate sodium 0.5%. Net price 10 mL = £1.26

12.2 Drugs acting on the nose

Rhinitis is often self-limiting but bacterial sinusitis may require treatment with antibacterials (Table 1, section 5.1). There are few indications for nasal sprays and drops except in allergic rhinitis and perennial rhinitis (section 12.2.1). Many nasal preparations contain sympathomimetic drugs which may damage the nasal cilia (section 12.2.2). Some specialists use saline sniffs for a short period after endonasal surgery.

NASAL POLYPS. Short-term use of corticosteroid nasal drops helps to produce significant shrinkage of nasal polyps; to be effective, the drops must be administered with the patient in the 'head down' position. The reduction in swelling can be maintained by continuing treatment with a corticosteroid nasal spray. A short course of a systemic corticosteroid may be required initially to shrink large polyps.

12.2.1 Drugs used in nasal allergy

Mild allergic rhinitis is controlled by **antihistamines** (see also section 3.4.1) or topical **nasal corticosteroids**; systemic nasal decongestants are of doubtful value (section 3.10). Topical nasal decongestants can be used for a short period to relieve congestion and allow penetration of a topical nasal corticosteroid.

More persistent symptoms and nasal congestion can be relieved by topical nasal **corticosteroids** and **cromoglicate** (cromoglycate); topical antihistamines (azelastine and levocabastine) are useful for controlling breakthrough symptoms in allergic rhinitis. In seasonal allergic rhinitis (e.g. hay fever), treatment should begin 2 to 3 weeks before the season commences and may have to be continued for several months; treatment may be required for years in perennial rhinitis.

In allergic rhinitis, topical preparations of corticosteroids and cromoglicate have a well-established role; although it may be less effective, cromoglicate is often the first choice in children. Topical antihistamines are considered less effective than topical corticosteroids but probably more effective than cromoglicate.

Sometimes allergic rhinitis is accompanied by vasomotor rhinitis. In this situation, the addition of topical nasal ipratropium bromide (section 12.2.2) can reduce watery rhinorrhoea.

Very disabling symptoms occasionally justify the use of **systemic corticosteroids** for short periods (section 6.3), for example, in students taking important examinations. They may also be used at the beginning of a course of treatment with a corticosteroid spray to relieve severe mucosal oedema and allow the spray to penetrate the nasal cavity.

PREGNANCY. If a pregnant woman cannot tolerate the symptoms of allergic rhinitis, treatment with nasal beclometasone or sodium cromoglicate may be considered.

Antihistamines

AZELASTINE HYDROCHLORIDE

Indications: allergic rhinitis
Side-effects: irritation of nasal mucosa; bitter taste (if applied incorrectly)

[1]**Rhinolast**® (Viatris) PoM
Aqueous nasal spray, azelastine hydrochloride 140 micrograms (0.14 mL)/metered spray. Net price 22 mL (with metered pump) = £11.09
Excipients: include sodium edetate
Dose: ADULT and CHILD over 5 years, apply 140 micrograms (1 spray) into each nostril twice daily

1. Can be sold to the public for nasal administration in aqueous form (other than by aerosol) if supplied for the treatment of seasonal allergic rhinitis or perennial allergic rhinitis in adults and children over 5 years, subject to max. single dose of 140 micrograms per nostril, max. daily dose of 280 micrograms per nostril, and a pack size limit of 36 doses; a proprietary brand (*Aller-eze*®) is on sale to the public

LEVOCABASTINE

Indications: treatment of allergic rhinitis
Cautions: renal impairment (see Appendix 3)
Side-effects: nasal irritation; hypersensitivity reactions, headache, fatigue, drowsiness reported

[1]**Livostin**® (Novartis) PoM
Aqueous nasal spray, levocabastine (as hydrochloride) 0.05%. Net price 10-mL spray pump = £9.74
Excipients: include disodium edetate, propylene glycol, polysorbate 80 and benzalkonium chloride
Dose: ADULT and CHILD over 9 years, apply 2 sprays into each nostril twice daily, increased if necessary to 3–4 times daily

1. Can be sold to the public for nasal administration if supplied for symptomatic treatment of seasonal allergic rhinitis in adults and children over 12 years subject to max. strength of levocabastine 0.05% and max. pack size 10 mL; proprietary brands on sale to the public include *Livostin*® *Direct Nasal Spray*

Corticosteroids

Nasal preparations containing corticosteroids (beclometasone, betamethasone, budesonide, flunisolide, fluticasone, mometasone, and triamcinolone) have a useful role in the prophylaxis and treatment of allergic rhinitis (see notes above).

CAUTIONS. Corticosteroid nasal preparations should be avoided in the presence of untreated nasal infections, and also after nasal surgery (until healing has occurred); they should also be avoided in pulmonary tuberculosis. Patients transferred from systemic corticosteroids may experience exacerbation of some symptoms. Systemic absorption may follow nasal administration particularly if high doses are used or if treatment is prolonged; for cautions and side-effects of systemic corticosteroids, see section 6.3.2. The risk of systemic effects may be greater with nasal drops than with nasal sprays; drops are administered incorrectly more often than sprays. The CSM recommends that the height of children receiving prolonged treatment with nasal corticosteroids is monitored; if growth is slowed, referral to a paediatrician should be considered.

SIDE-EFFECTS. Local side-effects include dryness, irritation of nose and throat, epistaxis and rarely ulceration; nasal septal perforation (usually following nasal surgery) and raised intra-ocular pressure or glaucoma may also occur rarely. Headache, smell and taste disturbances may also occur. Hypersensitivity reactions, including bronchospasm, have been reported.

BECLOMETASONE DIPROPIONATE

(Beclomethasone Dipropionate)

Indications: prophylaxis and treatment of allergic and vasomotor rhinitis
Cautions: see notes above
Side-effects: see notes above
Dose: ADULT and CHILD over 6 years, apply 100 micrograms (2 sprays) into each nostril twice daily *or* 50 micrograms (1 spray) into each nostril 3–4 times daily; max. total 400 micrograms (8 sprays) daily; when symptoms controlled, dose reduced to 50 micrograms (1 spray) into each nostril twice daily

[1]**Beclometasone** (Non-proprietary) PoM
Nasal spray, beclometasone dipropionate 50 micrograms/metered spray. Net price 200-spray unit = £4.20
Brands include *Nasobec Aqueous*®

1. Can be sold to the public for nasal administration (other than by aerosol) if supplied for the prevention and treatment of allergic rhinitis in adults over 18 years subject to max. single dose of 100 micrograms per nostril, max. daily dose of 200 micrograms per nostril for max. 3 months, and a pack size of 20 mg; proprietary brands on sale to the public include *Beclogen*®, *Beconase*® *Allergy*, *Beconase*® *Hayfever*, *Boots Hayfever Relief*®, *Care Hayfever Relief*®, *Nasobec*® *Hayfever*, *Pollenase*® *Hayfever*, *Tesco Hayfever Relief*®, *Vivabec*®

Beconase® (A&H) PoM
Nasal spray (aqueous suspension), beclometasone dipropionate 50 micrograms/metered spray. Net price 200-spray unit with applicator = £2.19
Excipients: include benzalkonium chloride, polysorbate 80

BETAMETHASONE SODIUM PHOSPHATE

Indications: non-infected inflammatory conditions of nose
Cautions: see notes above
Side-effects: see notes above

Betnesol® (Celltech) PoM
Drops (for ear, eye, or nose), betamethasone sodium phosphate 0.1%, net price 10 mL = £2.32
Excipients: include benzalkonium chloride, disodium edetate
Dose: nose, apply 2–3 drops into each nostril 2–3 times daily; *ear*, section 12.1.1; *eye*, see section 11.4.1

Vista-Methasone® (Martindale) PoM
Drops (for ear, eye, or nose), betamethasone sodium phosphate 0.1%. Net price 5 mL = £1.02, 10 mL = £1.16
Excipients: include benzalkonium chloride, disodium edetate
Dose: nose, apply 2–3 drops into each nostril twice daily; *ear*, section 12.1.1; *eye*, see section 11.4.1

BUDESONIDE

Indications: prophylaxis and treatment of allergic and vasomotor rhinitis; nasal polyps
Cautions: see notes above
Side-effects: see notes above
Dose: see preparations

[1]**Budesonide** (Non-proprietary) PoM
Nasal spray, budesonide 100 micrograms/metered spray, net price 100-spray unit = £5.85
Dose: rhinitis, ADULT and CHILD over 12 years, apply 2 sprays into each nostril once daily in the morning *or* 1 spray into each nostril twice daily; when control achieved reduce to 1 spray into each nostril once daily
Nasal polyps, ADULT and CHILD over 12 years, 1 spray into each nostril twice daily for up to 3 months

1. Can be sold to the public for nasal administration (other than by aerosol) if supplied for the prevention and treatment of seasonal allergic rhinitis in adults over 18 years subject to max. single dose of 200 micrograms per nostril, max. daily dose of 200 micrograms per nostril for max. period of 3 months, and a pack size of 10 mg

Rhinocort Aqua® (AstraZeneca) PoM
Nasal spray, budesonide 64 micrograms/metered spray. Net price 120-spray unit = £4.49
Excipients: include disodium edetate, polysorbate 80, potassium sorbate
Dose: rhinitis, ADULT and CHILD over 12 years, apply 2 sprays into each nostril once daily in the morning or 1 spray into each nostril twice daily; when control achieved reduce to 1 spray into each nostril once daily; max. duration of treatment 3 months
Nasal polyps, ADULT and CHILD over 12 years, 1 spray into each nostril twice daily for up to 3 months

DEXAMETHASONE ISONICOTINATE

Indications: treatment of allergic rhinitis
Cautions: see notes above; avoid contact with eyes
Side-effects: see notes above

■ With sympathomimetic

For cautions and side-effects of sympathomimetics see Ephedrine Hydrochloride, section 12.2.2

Dexa-Rhinaspray Duo® (Boehringer Ingelheim) PoM
Nasal spray, dexamethasone isonicotinate 20 micrograms, tramazoline hydrochloride 120 micrograms/metered spray. Net price 110-dose unit = £2.15
Excipients: include benzalkonium chloride, polysorbate 80
Dose: allergic rhinitis, ADULT and CHILD over 12 years, apply 1 spray into each nostril 2–3 times daily, max. 6 times daily; max. duration 14 days; CHILD 5–12 years 1 spray into each nostril up to twice daily; under 5 years not recommended

FLUNISOLIDE

Indications: prophylaxis and treatment of allergic rhinitis
Cautions: see notes above
Side-effects: see notes above

Syntaris® (IVAX) PoM
Aqueous nasal spray, flunisolide 25 micrograms/metered spray. Net price 240-spray unit with pump and applicator = £5.05
Excipients: include benzalkonium chloride, butylated hydroxytoluene, disodium edetate, polysorbate 20, propylene glycol
Dose: ADULT, apply 50 micrograms (2 sprays) into each nostril twice daily, increased if necessary to max. 3 times daily then reduced for maintenance; CHILD 5–14 years initially 25 micrograms (1 spray) into each nostril up to 3 times daily

FLUTICASONE PROPIONATE

Indications: see under preparations below
Cautions: see notes above
Side-effects: see notes above

[1]**Flixonase**® (A&H) PoM
Aqueous nasal spray, fluticasone propionate 50 micrograms/metered spray. Net price 150-spray unit with applicator = £11.69
Excipients: include benzalkonium chloride, polysorbate 80
Dose: prophylaxis and treatment of allergic rhinitis, ADULT and CHILD over 12 years, apply 100 micrograms (2 sprays) into each nostril once daily, preferably in the morning, increased to max. twice daily if required; when control achieved reduce to 50 micrograms (1 spray) into each nostril once daily; CHILD 4–11 years, 50 micrograms (1 spray) into each nostril once daily, increased to max. twice daily if required

1. Can be sold to the public for nasal administration (other than by pressurised nasal spray) if supplied for the prevention and treatment of allergic rhinitis in adults over 18 years, subject to max. single dose of 100 micrograms per nostril, max. daily dose of 200 micrograms per nostril for max. 3 months, and a pack size of 3 mg; proprietary brands on sale to the public include *Flixonase® Allergy*

Flixonase Nasule® (A&H) PoM
Nasal drops, fluticasone propionate 400 micrograms/unit dose, net price 28 × 0.4-mL units = £13.76
Excipients: include polysorbate 20
Dose: nasal polyps, ADULT and ADOLESCENT over 16 years, apply 200 micrograms (approx. 6 drops) into each nostril once or twice daily; consider alternative treatment if no improvement after 4–6 weeks

MOMETASONE FUROATE

Indications: see preparations
Cautions: see notes above
Side-effects: see notes above

Nasonex® (Schering-Plough) PoM
Nasal spray, mometasone furoate 50 micrograms/metered spray. Net price 140-spray unit = £7.83
Excipients: include benzalkonium chloride, polysorbate 80
Dose: prophylaxis and treatment of allergic rhinitis, ADULT and CHILD over 12 years, apply 100 micrograms (2 sprays) into each nostril once daily, increased if necessary to max. 200 micrograms (4 sprays) into each nostril once daily; when control achieved reduce to 50 micrograms (1 spray) into each nostril once daily; CHILD 6–11 years, 50 micrograms (1 spray) into each nostril once daily
Nasal polyps, ADULT over 18 years, apply 100 micrograms (2 sprays) into each nostril once daily, increased if necessary after 5–6 weeks to 100 micrograms (2 sprays) into each nostril twice daily (consider alternative treatment if no improvement after further 5–6 weeks); reduce dose when control achieved

TRIAMCINOLONE ACETONIDE

Indications: prophylaxis and treatment of allergic rhinitis
Cautions: see notes above
Side-effects: see notes above

[1]**Nasacort**® (Aventis Pharma) PoM
Aqueous nasal spray, triamcinolone acetonide 55 micrograms/metered spray. Net price 120-spray unit = £7.39
Excipients: include benzalkonium chloride, disodium edetate, polysorbate 80
Dose: ADULT and CHILD over 12 years apply 110 micrograms (2 sprays) into each nostril once daily; when control achieved, reduce to 55 micrograms (1 spray) into each nostril once daily; CHILD 6–12 years, 55 micrograms (1 spray) into each nostril once daily

1. Can be sold to the public for nasal administration as a non-pressurised nasal spray if supplied for the symptomatic treatment of seasonal allergic rhinitis in adults over 18 years, subject to max. daily dose of 110 micrograms per nostril for max. 3 months, and a pack size of 3.575 mg

Cromoglicate

SODIUM CROMOGLICATE

(Sodium Cromoglycate)
Indications: prophylaxis of allergic rhinitis
Side-effects: local irritation; rarely transient bronchospasm

Rynacrom® (Sanofi-Aventis)
4% aqueous nasal spray, sodium cromoglicate 4% (5.2 mg/squeeze). Net price 22 mL with pump = £17.76
Excipients: include benzalkonium chloride, disodium edetate
Dose: ADULT and CHILD, apply 1 squeeze into each nostril 2–4 times daily

Vividrin® (Pharma-Global)
Nasal spray, sodium cromoglicate 2%. Net price 15 mL = £8.56
Excipients: include benzalkonium chloride, edetic acid, polysorbate 80
Dose: ADULT and CHILD, apply 1 spray into each nostril 4–6 times daily

12.2.2 Topical nasal decongestants

The nasal mucosa is sensitive to changes in atmospheric temperature and humidity and these alone may cause slight nasal congestion. The nose and nasal sinuses produce a litre of mucus in 24 hours and much of this finds its way silently into the stomach via the nasopharynx. Slight changes in the nasal airway, accompanied by an awareness of mucus passing along the nasopharynx causes some patients to be inaccurately diagnosed as suffering from chronic sinusitis. These symptoms are particularly noticeable in the later stages of the common cold. **Sodium chloride** 0.9% given as nasal drops may relieve nasal congestion by helping to liquefy mucous secretions. Corticosteroid nasal drops produce shrinkage of nasal polyps (section 12.2).

Symptoms of nasal congestion associated with vasomotor rhinitis and the common cold can be relieved by the short-term use (usually not longer than 7 days) of decongestant nasal drops and sprays. These all contain sympathomimetic drugs which exert their effect by vasoconstriction of the mucosal blood vessels which in turn reduces oedema of the nasal mucosa. They are of limited value because they can give rise to a rebound congestion (rhinitis medicamentosa) on withdrawal, due to a secondary vasodilation with a subsequent temporary increase in nasal congestion. This in turn tempts the further use of the decongestant, leading to a vicious cycle of events. **Ephedrine nasal drops** is the safest sympathomimetic preparation and can give relief for several hours. The more potent sympathomimetic drugs oxymetazoline, and xylometazoline are more likely to cause a rebound effect. **All** of these preparations may cause a hypertensive crisis if used during treatment with a monoamine-oxidase inhibitor including moclobemide.

Non-allergic watery rhinorrhoea often responds well to treatment with the antimuscarinic **ipratropium bromide**.

Inhalation of **warm moist air** is useful in the treatment of symptoms of acute infective conditions. The addition of volatile substances such as menthol and eucalyptus may encourage the use of warm moist air (section 3.8).

Systemic nasal decongestants—see section 3.10.

SINUSITIS AND ORAL PAIN. Sinusitis affecting the maxillary antrum can cause pain in the upper jaw. Where this is associated with blockage of the opening from the sinus into the nasal cavity, it may be helpful to relieve the congestion with inhalation of warm moist air (section 3.8) or with **ephedrine nasal drops** (see above). For antibacterial treatment of sinusitis, see Table 1, section 5.1.

Sympathomimetics

EPHEDRINE HYDROCHLORIDE

Indications: nasal congestion

Cautions: avoid excessive or prolonged use; caution in infants under 3 months (no good evidence of value—if irritation occurs might narrow nasal passage); **interactions:** Appendix 1 (sympathomimetics)

Side-effects: local irritation, nausea, headache; after excessive use tolerance with diminished effect, rebound congestion; cardiovascular effects also reported

Dose: see below

Ephedrine (Non-proprietary)

Nasal drops, ephedrine hydrochloride 0.5%, net price 10 mL = £1.35; 1%, 10 mL = £1.41

NOTE. The BP directs that if no strength is specified 0.5% drops should be supplied

Dose: instil 1–2 drops into each nostril up to 3 or 4 times daily when required

DENTAL PRESCRIBING ON NHS. Ephedrine nasal drops may be prescribed

XYLOMETAZOLINE HYDROCHLORIDE

Indications: nasal congestion

Cautions: see under Ephedrine Hydrochloride and notes above

Side-effects: see under Ephedrine Hydrochloride and notes above

Dose: see below

Xylometazoline (Non-proprietary)

Nasal drops, xylometazoline hydrochloride 0.1%, net price 10 mL = £1.91

Dose: instil 2–3 drops into each nostril 2–3 times daily when required; max. duration 7 days; not recommended for children under 12 years

Brands include *Otradrops*®, *Otrivine*® NHS

Paediatric nasal drops, xylometazoline hydrochloride 0.05%, net price 10 mL = £1.59

Dose: CHILD over 3 months instil 1–2 drops into each nostril 1–2 times daily when required (not recommended for infants under 3 months of age, doctor's advice only under 2 years); max. duration 7 days

Brands include *Otradrops*®, *Otrivine*® NHS, *Tixycolds*®

Nasal spray, xylometazoline hydrochloride 0.1%, net price 10 mL = £1.91

Dose: apply 1 spray into each nostril 2–3 times daily when required; max. duration 7 days; not recommended for children under 12 years

Brands include *Otraspray*®, *Otrivine*® NHS

■ Preparations on Sale to the Public

Sympathomimetic nasal preparations on sale to the public (not prescribable on the NHS) include:

Afrazine® (oxymetazoline), **Dristan**® (oxymetazoline), **Fenox**® (phenylephrine), **Non Drowsy Sudafed Decongestant Nasal Spray**® (xylometazoline), **Sudafed**® nasal spray (oxymetazoline), **Vicks Sinex**® (oxymetazoline)

Antimuscarinic

IPRATROPIUM BROMIDE

Indications: rhinorrhoea associated with allergic and non-allergic rhinitis

Cautions: see section 3.1.2; avoid spraying near eyes

Side-effects: epistaxis, nasal dryness, and irritation; less frequently nausea, headache, and pharyngitis; *very rarely* antimuscarinic effects such as gastro-intestinal motility disturbances, palpitations, and urinary retention

Dose: apply 42 micrograms (2 sprays) into each nostril 2–3 times daily; CHILD under 12 years not recommended

Rinatec® (Boehringer Ingelheim) PoM

Nasal spray 0.03%, ipratropium bromide 21 micrograms/metered spray. Net price 180-dose unit = £4.55

Excipients: include benzalkonium chloride, disodium edetate

12.2.3 Nasal preparations for infection and epistaxis

There is **no** evidence that topical anti-infective nasal preparations have any therapeutic value in rhinitis or sinusitis; for elimination of nasal staphylococci, see below.

Systemic treatment of sinusitis—see section 5.1, table 1.

Betnesol-N® (Celltech) PoM

Drops (for ear, eye, or nose), betamethasone sodium phosphate 0.1%, neomycin sulphate 0.5%. Net price 10 mL = £2.39

Excipients: include benzalkonium chloride, disodium edetate

Dose: nose, apply 2–3 drops into nostril 2–3 times daily; *eye*, see section 11.4.1; *ear*, see section 12.1.1

[1]**Locabiotal**® (Servier) PoM NHS

Spray, fusafungine 500 micrograms/metered spray. Net price 50-spray unit with nasal (yellow) and oral (white) adapters = £1.44

Excipients: include alcohol

Dose: infection and inflammation of upper respiratory tract (but not recommended, see notes above), 1 spray into each nostril or into mouth every 4 hours; CHILD over 30 months, 1 spray into each nostril or into mouth every 6 hours; withdraw if no improvement after 7 days

1. NHS Except for treatment of infections and inflammation of the oropharynx and endorsed 'SLS'

Vista-Methasone N® (Martindale) PoM
Drops (for ear, eye, or nose), betamethasone sodium phosphate 0.1%, neomycin sulphate 0.5%. Net price 5 mL = £1.09, 10 mL = £1.20
Excipients: include thiomersal
Dose: nose, apply 2–3 drops into each nostril twice daily; *eye*, see section 11.4.1; *ear*, see section 12.1.1

Nasal staphylococci

Elimination of organisms such as staphylococci from the nasal vestibule can be achieved by the use of a cream containing **chlorhexidine and neomycin** (*Naseptin*®), but re-colonisation frequently occurs. Coagulase-positive staphylococci are present in the noses of 40% of the population.

A nasal ointment containing **mupirocin** is also available; it should probably be held in reserve for resistant cases. In hospital or in care establishments, mupirocin nasal ointment should be reserved for the eradication (in both patients and staff) of nasal carriage of methicillin-resistant *Staphylococcus aureus* (MRSA). The ointment should be applied 3 times daily for 5 days and a sample taken 2 days after treatment to confirm eradication. The course may be repeated if the sample is positive (and the throat is not colonised). To avoid the development of resistance, the treatment course should not exceed 7 days and the course should not be repeated on more than one occasion. If the MRSA strain is mupirocin-resistant or does not respond after 2 courses, consider alternative products such as chlorhexidine and neomycin cream.

Bactroban Nasal® (GSK) PoM
Nasal ointment, mupirocin 2% (as calcium salt) in white soft paraffin basis. Net price 3 g = £5.80
Dose: for eradication of nasal carriage of staphylococci, including methicillin-resistant *Staphylococcus aureus* (MRSA), apply 2–3 times daily to the inner surface of each nostril

Naseptin® (Alliance) PoM
Cream, chlorhexidine hydrochloride 0.1%, neomycin sulphate 0.5%, net price 15 g = £1.58
Excipients: include arachis (peanut) oil, cetostearyl alcohol
Dose: for eradication of nasal carriage of staphylococci, apply to nostrils 4 times daily for 10 days; for preventing nasal carriage of staphylococci apply to nostrils twice daily

Epistaxis

Bismuth iodoform paraffin paste (BIPP) is used for packing cavities after ear, nose and oropharyngeal surgery as a mild disinfectant and astringent; it is also used to pack nasal cavities in acute epistaxis. It is available either as a paste, to be applied to ribbon gauze packing, or as BIPP-impregnated ribbon gauze.

BISMUTH SUBNITRATE AND IODOFORM

Indications: packing cavities after ear, nose or oropharyngeal surgery; epistaxis
Cautions: hyperthyroidism
Side-effects: erythematous rash (discontinue use); encephalopathy reported only with large packs or when placed directly on neural tissue

Bismuth Subnitrate and Iodoform (Non-proprietary)
Paste, 30-g sachet, net price = £9.50; 30-g tube = £10.07
Impregnated gauze, sterile, net price 1.25 cm × 100 cm, 10 = £95.08; 1.25 cm × 200 cm, 5 = £65.78; 1.25 cm × 300 cm, 5 = £86.02; 2.5 cm × 100 cm, 10 = £103.03; 2.5 cm × 200 cm, 5 = £74.57; 2.5 cm × 300 cm, 5 = £98.10

12.3 Drugs acting on the oropharynx

12.3.1 Drugs for oral ulceration and inflammation

Ulceration of the oral mucosa may be caused by trauma (physical or chemical), recurrent aphthae, infections, carcinoma, dermatological disorders, nutritional deficiencies, gastro-intestinal disease, haematopoietic disorders, and drug therapy. It is important to establish the diagnosis in each case as the majority of these lesions require specific management in addition to local treatment. Patients with an unexplained mouth ulcer of more than 3 weeks' duration require urgent referral to hospital to exclude oral cancer. Local treatment aims at protecting the ulcerated area, or at relieving pain, or reducing inflammation, or at controlling secondary infection.

SIMPLE MOUTHWASHES. A **saline** mouthwash (section 12.3.4) may relieve the pain of traumatic ulceration. The mouthwash is made up with warm water and used at frequent intervals until the discomfort and swelling subsides.

ANTISEPTIC MOUTHWASHES. Secondary bacterial infection may be a feature of any mucosal ulceration; it can increase discomfort and delay healing. Use of a **chlorhexidine** or **povidone–iodine** mouthwash (section 12.3.4) is often beneficial and may accelerate healing of recurrent aphthae.

MECHANICAL PROTECTION. **Carmellose gelatin paste** may relieve some discomfort arising from ulceration by protecting the ulcer site. The paste adheres to dry mucosa, but is difficult to apply effectively to some parts of the mouth. *Gelclair*® is available for the management of oral lesions; it forms a film of povidone and sodium hyaluronate on the lesion.

CORTICOSTEROIDS. Topical corticosteroid therapy may be used for some forms of oral ulceration. In the case of aphthous ulcers it is most effective if applied in the 'prodromal' phase.

Thrush or other types of candidiasis are recognised complications of corticosteroid treatment.

Hydrocortisone oromucosal tablets are allowed to dissolve next to an ulcer and are useful in recurrent aphthae and erosive lichenoid lesions.

Triamcinolone dental paste is designed to keep the corticosteroid in contact with the mucosa for long enough to permit penetration of the lesion, but is difficult for patients to apply properly.

Beclometasone dipropionate inhaler 50–100 micrograms sprayed twice daily on the oral mucosa is used to manage oral ulceration [unlicensed indication]. Alternatively, **betamethasone** soluble tablet 500 micrograms dissolved in water, may be used as a mouthwash 4 times daily to treat oral ulceration [unlicensed indication]; the solution should not be swallowed in order to minimise the risk of systemic effects.

Systemic corticosteroid therapy (section 6.3.2) is reserved for severe conditions such as pemphigus vulgaris.

LOCAL ANALGESICS. Local analgesics have a limited role in the management of oral ulceration. When applied topically their action is of a relatively short duration so that analgesia cannot be maintained continuously throughout the day. The main indication for a topical local analgesic is to relieve the pain of otherwise intractable oral ulceration particularly when it is due to major aphthae. For this purpose lidocaine (lignocaine) 5% ointment or lozenges containing a local anaesthetic are applied to the ulcer. Lidocaine 10% solution as spray, section 15.2) can be applied thinly to the ulcer [unlicensed indication] using a cotton bud. When local anaesthetics are used in the mouth care must be taken not to produce anaesthesia of the pharynx before meals as this might lead to choking.

Benzydamine mouthwash or spray may be useful in palliating the discomfort associated with a variety of ulcerative conditions. It has also been found to be effective in reducing the discomfort of post-irradiation mucositis. Some patients find the full-strength mouthwash causes some stinging and, for them, it should be diluted with an equal volume of water. **Flurbiprofen** lozenges are licensed for the relief of sore throat.

Choline salicylate dental gel has some analgesic action and may provide relief for recurrent aphthae, but excessive application or confinement under a denture irritates the mucosa and can itself cause ulceration. Benefit in teething may merely be due to pressure of application (comparable with biting a teething ring); excessive use can lead to salicylate poisoning.

OTHER PREPARATIONS. **Carbenoxolone** gel or mouthwash may be of some value for mild oral and perioral lesions. **Doxycycline** rinsed in the mouth may also be of value for recurrent aphthous ulceration.

PERIODONTITIS. Low-dose doxycycline (*Periostat*®) is licensed as an adjunct to scaling and root planing for the treatment of periodontitis; a low dose of doxycycline reduces collagenase activity without inhibiting bacteria associated with periodontitis. For anti-infectives used in the treatment of destructive (refractory) forms of periodontal disease, see section 12.3.2. For mouthwashes used for oral hygiene and plaque inhibition, see section 12.3.4.

BENZYDAMINE HYDROCHLORIDE

Indications: painful inflammatory conditions of oropharynx
Side-effects: occasional numbness or stinging; rarely hypersensitivity reactions

Difflam® (3M)
Oral rinse, green, benzydamine hydrochloride 0.15%, net price 200 mL (*Difflam*® *Sore Throat Rinse*) = £2.63; 300 mL = £4.01
Dose: rinse or gargle, using 15 mL (diluted with water if stinging occurs) every 1½–3 hours as required, usually for not more than 7 days; not suitable for children aged 12 years or under
DENTAL PRESCRIBING ON NHS. May be prescribed as Benzydamine Mouthwash 0.15%
Spray, benzydamine hydrochloride 0.15%. Net price 30-mL unit = £3.17
Dose: ADULT, 4–8 sprays onto affected area every 1½–3 hours; CHILD under 6 years 1 spray per 4 kg body-weight to max. 4 sprays every 1½–3 hours; 6–12 years 4 sprays every 1½–3 hours
DENTAL PRESCRIBING ON NHS. May be prescribed as Benzydamine Oromucosal Spray 0.15%

CARBENOXOLONE SODIUM

Indications: mild oral and perioral lesions

Bioplex® (TEVA UK) PoM
Mouthwash granules, carbenoxolone sodium 1% (20 mg/sachet). Net price 24 × 2-g sachets = £7.23
Dose: for mouth ulcers, rinse with 1 sachet in 30–50 mL of warm water 3 times daily and at bedtime

CARMELLOSE SODIUM

Indications: mechanical protection of oral and perioral lesions

Orabase® (ConvaTec)
Protective paste (= oral paste), carmellose sodium 16.7%, pectin 16.7%, gelatin 16.7%, in *Plastibase*®. Net price 30 g = £1.94; 100 g = £4.32
Dose: apply a thin layer when necessary after meals
DENTAL PRESCRIBING ON NHS. May be prescribed as Carmellose Gelatin Paste

Orahesive® (ConvaTec)
Powder, carmellose sodium, pectin, gelatin, equal parts. Net price 25 g = £2.24
Dose: sprinkle on the affected area

CORTICOSTEROIDS

Indications: oral and perioral lesions
Contra-indications: untreated oral infection; manufacturer of triamcinolone contra-indicates use on tuberculous and viral lesions
Side-effects: occasional exacerbation of local infection; thrush or other candidal infections

[1]**Adcortyl in Orabase**® (Squibb) PoM
Oral paste, triamcinolone acetonide 0.1% in adhesive basis. Net price 10 g = £1.27
Dose: ADULT and CHILD, apply a thin layer 2–4 times daily; do not rub in; use limited to 5 days for children and short-term use also advised for elderly
DENTAL PRESCRIBING ON NHS. May be prescribed as Triamcinolone Dental Paste

1. A 5-g tube (*Adcortyl in Orabase*® *for Mouth Ulcers*) is on sale to the public for the treatment of common mouth ulcers for max. 5 days

Corlan® (Celltech)
Pellets (= oromucosal tablets), hydrocortisone 2.5 mg (as sodium succinate). Net price 20 = £2.54
Dose: ADULT and CHILD, 1 lozenge 4 times daily, allowed to dissolve slowly in the mouth in contact with the ulcer
DENTAL PRESCRIBING ON NHS. May be prescribed as Hydrocortisone Oromucosal Tablets

DOXYCYCLINE

Indications: see preparations; oral herpes (section 12.3.2); other indications (section 5.1.3)
Cautions: section 5.1.3; monitor for superficial fungal infection, particularly, if predisposition to oral candidiasis
Contra-indications: section 5.1.3
Side-effects: section 5.1.3; fungal superinfection
Dose: see preparations

Periostat (Alliance) PoM
Tablets, f/c, doxycycline (as hyclate) 20 mg, net price 56-tab pack = £16.50. Label: 6, 11, 27, counselling, posture
Dose: periodontitis (as an adjunct to gingival scaling and root planing), 20 mg twice daily for 3 months; CHILD under 12 years not recommended
COUNSELLING. Tablets should be swallowed whole with plenty of fluid, while sitting or standing
DENTAL PRESCRIBING ON NHS. May be prescribed as Doxycycline Tablets 20 mg

■ Local application
For recurrent aphthous ulceration, the contents of a 100 mg doxycycline capsule can be stirred into a small amount of water then rinsed around the mouth for 2–3 minutes 4 times daily usually for 3 days; it should preferably not be swallowed [unlicensed indication].
NOTE. Doxycycline stains teeth; avoid in children under 12 years of age

FLURBIPROFEN

Indications: relief of sore throat
Cautions: see section 10.1.1
Contra-indications: see section 10.1.1
Side-effects: taste disturbance, mouth ulcers (move lozenge around mouth); see also section 10.1.1

Strefen® (Crookes)
Lozenges, flurbiprofen 8.75 mg, net price 16 = £2.08
Dose: allow 1 lozenge to dissolve slowly in the mouth every 3–6 hours, max. 5 lozenges in 24 hours, for max. 3 days; CHILD under 12 years not recommended

LOCAL ANAESTHETICS

Indications: relief of pain in oral lesions
Cautions: avoid prolonged use; hypersensitivity; pregnancy (Appendix 4); avoid anaesthesia of the pharynx before meals—risk of choking

Lidocaine (Non-proprietary)
Ointment, lidocaine 5% in a water-miscible basis, net price 15 g = 80p
Dose: rub sparingly and gently on affected areas
DENTAL PRESCRIBING ON NHS. Lidocaine 5% Ointment may be prescribed

■ Other preparations
Local anaesthetics are included in some mouth ulcer preparations, for details see below
Local anaesthetics are also included in some throat lozenges and sprays, see section 12.3.3

SALICYLATES

Indications: mild oral and perioral lesions
Cautions: not to be applied to dentures—leave at least 30 minutes before re-insertion of dentures; frequent application, especially in children, may give rise to salicylate poisoning
NOTE. CSM warning on aspirin and Reye's syndrome does not apply to non-aspirin salicylates or to topical preparations such as teething gels

■ Choline salicylate

Choline Salicylate Dental Gel, BP
Oral gel, choline salicylate 8.7% in a flavoured gel basis, net price 15 g = £1.79
Brands include *Bonjela*® (sugar-free)
Dose: apply ½-inch of gel with gentle massage not more often than every 3 hours; CHILD over 4 months ¼-inch of gel not more often than every 3 hours; max. 6 applications daily
DENTAL PRESCRIBING ON NHS. Choline Salicylate Dental Gel may be prescribed

■ Salicylic acid

Pyralvex® (Norgine)
Oral paint, brown, rhubarb extract (anthraquinone glycosides 0.5%), salicylic acid 1%. Net price 10 mL with brush = £1.69
Dose: apply 3–4 times daily; CHILD under 12 years not recommended

■ Preparations on Sale to the Public
The following list includes topical treatments for mouth ulcers and for teething on sale to the public, together with their active ingredients:
Anbesol Liquid® and **Anbesol Teething gel**® (cetylpyridinium, chlorocresol, lidocaine), **Bansor**® (cetrimide), **Bonjela gel**® (cetalkonium chloride, choline salicylate), **Bonjela Teething gel**® (cetalkonium chloride, lidocaine), **Calgel**® (cetylpyridinium, lidocaine), **Dentinox Teething gel**® (cetylpyridinium, lidocaine), **Frador**® (chlorobutanol, menthol), **Medijel**® (aminoacridine, lidocaine), **Pyralvex**® (anthraquinone glycoside, salicylic acid), **Rinstead Adult gel**® (benzocaine, chloroxylenol), **Rinstead Contact pastilles**® (lidocaine), **Rinstead pastilles**® (cetylpyridinium, menthol), **Woodward's Teething gel**® (cetylpyridinium, lidocaine)

12.3.2 Oropharyngeal anti-infective drugs

The most common cause of a sore throat is a viral infection which does not benefit from anti-infective treatment. Streptococcal sore throats require systemic **penicillin** therapy (Table 1, section 5.1). Acute ulcerative gingivitis (Vincent's infection) responds to systemic **metronidazole** (section 5.1.11).

Preparations administered in the dental surgery for the local treatment of periodontal disease include gels of metronidazole (*Elyzol*®, Colgate-Palmolive) and of minocycline (*Dentomycin*®, Blackwell).

Oropharyngeal fungal infections

Fungal infections of the mouth are usually caused by *Candida* spp. (candidiasis or candidosis). There are different types of oropharyngeal candidiasis.

THRUSH. Acute pseudomembranous candidiasis (thrush), is classically an acute infection but one which may persist for months in patients receiving inhaled corticosteroids, cytotoxics or broad-specrum antibacterials. Thrush is also associated with serious systemic disease associated with reduced immunity such as leukaemia, other malignancies, and HIV infection. The predisposing cause should be dealt with. When associated with corticosteroid inhalers, rinsing the mouth with water (or cleaning a child's teeth) immediately after using the inhaler may avoid the problem. Treatment with **nystatin**, **amphotericin**, or **miconazole** may be needed. **Fluconazole** (section 5.2) is effective for unresponsive infections or if a topical antifungal drug cannot be used or if the patient has dry mouth.

ACUTE ERYTHEMATOUS CANDIDIASIS. Acute erythematous (atrophic) candidiasis is a relatively uncommon condition associated with corticosteroid and broad-spectrum antibacterial use and with HIV disease. It is usually treated with **fluconazole** (section 5.2).

DENTURE STOMATITIS. Patients with denture stomatitis (chronic atrophic candidiasis), should cleanse their dentures thoroughly and leave them out as often as possible during the treatment period. To prevent recurrence of the problem, dentures should not normally be worn at night. New dentures may be required if these measures fail despite good compliance.

Miconazole oral gel can be applied to the fitting surface of the denture before insertion (for short periods only). Alternatively, **nystatin** pastilles or **amphotericin** lozenges can be allowed to dissolve slowly in the mouth but they are less effective at resolving the stomatitis. Denture stomatitis is not always associated with candidiasis and other factors such as mechanical or chemical irritation, bacterial infection, or rarely allergy to the dental base material, may be the cause.

CHRONIC HYPERPLASTIC CANDIDIASIS. Chronic hyperplastic candidiasis (candidal leucoplakia) carries an increased risk of malignancy; biopsy is essential—this type of candidiasis may be associated with varying degrees of dysplasia, with oral cancer present in a high proportion of cases. Chronic hyperplastic candidiasis is treated with a systemic antifungal such as **fluconazole** (section 5.2) to eliminate candidal overlay. Patients should avoid the use of tobacco.

ANGULAR CHEILITIS. Angular cheilitis (angular stomatitis) is characterised by soreness, erythema and fissuring at the angles of the mouth. It is commonly associated with denture stomatitis but may represent a nutritional deficiency or it may be related to orofacial granulomatosis or HIV infection. Both yeasts (*Candida* spp.) and bacteria (*Staphylococcus aureus* and beta-haemolytic streptococci) are commonly involved as interacting, infective factors. A reduction in facial height related to ageing and tooth loss with maceration in the deep occlusive folds that may subsequently arise, predisposes to such infection. While the underlying cause is being identified and treated, it is often helpful to apply **miconazole** and **hydrocortisone** cream or ointment (see p. 567), **nystatin** ointment (see p. 592), or **sodium fusidate** ointment (see p. 591).

IMMUNOCOMPROMISED PATIENTS. For advice on prevention of fungal infections in immunocompromised patients see p. 307.

DRUGS USED IN OROPHARYNGEAL CANDIDIASIS. **Amphotericin** and **nystatin** are not absorbed from the gastro-intestinal tract and are applied locally (as lozenges or suspension) to the mouth for treating local fungal infections. Nystatin ointment is available for perioral lesions (see p. 592). **Miconazole** is used by local application (as an oral gel) in the mouth but it is also absorbed to the extent that potential interactions need to be considered. Miconazole may be more effective than amphotericin or nystatin for some types of candidiasis, particularly chronic hyperplastic candidiasis or chronic mucocutaneous candidiasis (chronic thrush). Miconazole also has some activity against Gram-positive bacteria including streptococci and staphylococci. **Fluconazole** and **itraconazole** (section 5.2) are absorbed when taken by mouth; they are used for oropharyngeal candidiasis that does not respond to topical therapy.

If candidal infection fails to respond to 1 to 2 weeks of treatment with antifungal drugs the patient should be sent for investigation to eliminate the possibility of underlying disease. Persistent infection may also be caused by reinfection from the genito-urinary or gastro-intestinal tract. The infection can be eliminated from these sources by appropriate anticandidal therapy but calls for referral to the patient's medical practitioner; the patient's partner may also require treatment to prevent reinfection.

For the role of antiseptic mouthwashes in the prevention of oral candidiasis in immunocompromised patients and treatment of denture stomatitis, see section 12.3.4.

AMPHOTERICIN

Indications: oral and perioral fungal infections
Side-effects: mild gastro-intestinal disturbances reported

Fungilin® (Squibb) PoM

Lozenges, yellow, amphotericin 10 mg. Net price 60-lozenge pack = £3.67. Label: 9, 24, counselling, after food

Dose: allow 1 lozenge to dissolve slowly in the mouth 4 times daily for 10–15 days (continued for 48 hours after lesions have resolved); increase to 8 daily if infection severe

DENTAL PRESCRIBING ON NHS. May be prescribed as Amphotericin Lozenges

Oral suspension, yellow, sugar-free, amphotericin 100 mg/mL. Net price 12 mL with pipette = £2.15. Label: 9, counselling, use of pipette, hold in mouth, after food

Dose: place 1 mL in the mouth after food and retain near lesions 4 times daily for 14 days (continued for 48 hours after lesions have resolved)

DENTAL PRESCRIBING ON NHS. May be prescribed as Amphotericin Oral Suspension

---

MICONAZOLE

Indications: see under Preparations; intestinal fungal infections (section 5.2)
Cautions: pregnancy (Appendix 4) and breast-feeding; avoid in porphyria (section 9.8.2); **interactions:** Appendix 1 (antifungals, imidazole)
Contra-indications: hepatic impairment
Side-effects: nausea and vomiting, diarrhoea (with long-term treatment); rarely allergic reactions; isolated reports of hepatitis

[1]**Daktarin**® (Janssen-Cilag) PoM
Oral gel, sugar-free, orange-flavoured, miconazole 24 mg/mL (20 mg/g). Net price 15-g tube = £2.45, 80-g tube = £4.75. Label: 9, counselling, hold in mouth, after food
Dose: prevention and treatment of oral fungal infections, place 5–10 mL in the mouth after food and retain near lesions 4 times daily; CHILD under 2 years 2.5 mL twice daily, 2–6 years 5 mL twice daily, over 6 years 5 mL 4 times daily; treatment continued for 48 hours after lesions have resolved
Localised lesions, smear small amount on affected area with clean finger 4 times daily (dental prostheses should be removed at night and brushed with gel)
NOTE. Not licensed for use in NEONATES
DENTAL PRESCRIBING ON NHS. May be prescribed as Miconazole Oromucosal Gel

1. 15-g tube can be sold to the public

NYSTATIN

Indications: oral and perioral fungal infections
Side-effects: oral irritation and sensitisation, nausea reported; see also section 5.2
Dose: (as pastilles or as suspension) ADULT and CHILD, 100 000 units 4 times daily after food, usually for 7 days (continued for 48 hours after lesions have resolved)
NOTE. Unlicensed for treating candidiasis in NEONATE under 1 month. Immunosuppressed ADULT and CHILD over 1 month may require higher doses (e.g. 500 000 units 4 times daily)
Prophylaxis, NEONATE 100 000 units once daily

Nystatin (Non-proprietary) PoM
Oral suspension, nystatin 100 000 units/mL. Net price 30 mL = £1.95. Label: 9, counselling, hold in mouth, after food
Brands include *Nystamont*®, (sugar-free)
NOTE. Sugar-free versions are available and can be ordered by specifying 'sugar-free' on the prescription
DENTAL PRESCRIBING ON NHS. Nystatin Oral Suspension may be prescribed

Nystan® (Squibb) PoM
Pastilles, yellow/brown, nystatin 100 000 units. Net price 28-pastille pack = £3.24. Label: 9, 24, counselling, after food
DENTAL PRESCRIBING ON NHS. May be prescribed as Nystatin Pastilles
Oral suspension, yellow, nystatin 100 000 units/mL. Net price 30 mL with pipette = £2.05. Label: 9, counselling, use of pipette, hold in mouth, after food

Oropharyngeal viral infections

The management of primary herpetic gingivostomatitis is a soft diet, adequate fluid intake, and analgesics as required, including local use of **benzydamine** (section 12.3.1). The use of chlorhexidine mouthwash (section 12.3.4) will control plaque accumulation if toothbrushing is painful and will also help to control secondary infection in general.

In the case of severe herpetic stomatitis, a systemic antiviral such as aciclovir is required (section 5.3.2.1). Valaciclovir and famciclovir are suitable alternatives for oral lesions associated with herpes zoster. Aciclovir and valaciclovir are also used for the prevention of frequently recurring herpes simplex lesions of the mouth, particularly when implicated in the initiation of erythema multiforme. See section 13.10.3 for the treatment of labial herpes simplex infections.

Herpes infections of the mouth may also respond to rinsing the mouth with **doxycycline** (section 12.3.1).

12.3.3 Lozenges and sprays

There is no convincing evidence that antiseptic lozenges and sprays have a beneficial action and they sometimes irritate and cause sore tongue and sore lips. Some of these preparations also contain local anaesthetics which relieve pain but may cause sensitisation.

■ Preparations on Sale to the Public

The following list includes throat lozenges and sprays on sale to the public, together with their significant ingredients.

AAA® (benzocaine), **Beechams Throat Plus**® (benzalkonium, hexylresorcinol), **Bradosol**® (benzalkonium), **Bradosol Plus**® (domiphen, lidocaine), **Dequacaine**® (benzocaine, dequalinium), **Dequadin**® (dequalinium), **Dequaspray**® (lidocaine), **Eludril**® spray (tetracaine, chlorhexidine), **Labosept**® (dequalinium), **Meggezones**® (menthol), **Mentholatum**® lozenges (amylmetacresol, menthol), **Merocaine**® (benzocaine, cetylpyridinium), **Merocets**® lozenges (cetylpyridinium), **Merocets Plus**® lozenges (cetylpyridinium, menthol), **Strepsils**® lozenges (amylmetacresol, dichlorobenzyl alcohol), **Strepsils Extra**® lozenges (hexylresorcinol), **TCP**® **sore throat** lozenges (hexylresorcinol), **Tyrozets**® (benzocaine, tyrothricin), **Vicks Ultra Chloraseptic**® (benzocaine)

12.3.4 Mouthwashes, gargles, and dentifrices

Superficial infections of the mouth are often helped by warm mouthwashes which have a mechanical cleansing effect and cause some local hyperaemia. However, to be effective, they must be used frequently and vigorously. A warm saline mouthwash is ideal and can be prepared either by dissolving half a teaspoonful of salt in a glassful of warm water or by diluting **compound sodium chloride mouthwash** with an equal volume of warm water. **Mouthwash solution-tablets** are used to remove unpleasant tastes.

Mouthwashes containing an oxidising agent, such as **hydrogen peroxide**, may be useful in the treatment of acute ulcerative gingivitis (Vincent's infection) since the organisms involved are anaerobes. It also has a mechanical cleansing effect arising from frothing when in contact with oral debris.

Chlorhexidine is an effective antiseptic which has the advantage of inhibiting plaque formation on the teeth. It does not, however, completely control plaque deposition and is not a substitute for effective toothbrushing. Moreover, chlorhexidine preparations do not penetrate significantly into stagnation areas and are therefore of little value in the control of dental caries or of periodontal disease once pocketing has developed. Chlorhexidine mouthwash is used in the treatment of denture stomatitis. It is also used in the prevention of oral candidiasis in immunocompromised patients.

Chlorhexidine can be used as a mouthwash, spray or gel for secondary infection in mucosal ulceration and for controlling gingivitis, as an adjunct to other oral hygiene measures. These preparations may also be used instead of toothbrushing where there is a painful periodontal condition (e.g. primary herpetic stomatitis) or if the patient has a haemorrhagic disorder, or is disabled. Chlorhexidine preparations are of little value in the control of acute necrotising ulcerative gingivitis.

Povidone–iodine mouthwash is licensed for oral mucosal infections but does not inhibit plaque accumulation. It should not be used for longer than 14 days because a significant amount of iodine is absorbed. As with chlorhexidine, povidone–iodine mouthwash is of little value in the control of acute necrotising ulcerative gingivitis.

There is no convincing evidence that gargles are effective.

CHLORHEXIDINE GLUCONATE

Indications: see under preparations below

Side-effects: mucosal irritation (if desquamation occurs, discontinue treatment or dilute mouthwash with an equal volume of water); taste disturbance; reversible brown staining of teeth, and of silicate or composite restorations; tongue discoloration; parotid gland swelling reported

NOTE. Chlorhexidine gluconate may be incompatible with some ingredients in toothpaste; leave an interval of at least 30 minutes between using mouthwash and toothpaste

Chlorhexidine (Non-proprietary)

Mouthwash, chlorhexidine gluconate 0.2%, net price 300 mL = £1.77

Dose: oral hygiene and plaque inhibition, rinse mouth with 10 mL for about 1 minute twice daily

Denture stomatitis, cleanse and soak dentures in mouthwash solution for 15 minutes twice daily

Prophylaxis of endocarditis for dental procedures (as adjunct to antibacterial prophylaxis), Table 2, section 5.1

DENTAL PRESCRIBING ON NHS. Chlorhexidine Mouthwash may be prescribed

Chlorohex® (Colgate-Palmolive)

Chlorohex 1200® *mouthwash*, chlorhexidine gluconate 0.12% (mint-flavoured). Net price 300 mL = £2.20

Dose: oral hygiene and plaque inhibition, rinse mouth with 15 mL for about 30 seconds twice daily

Corsodyl® (GSK Consumer Healthcare)

Dental gel, chlorhexidine gluconate 1%. Net price 50 g = £1.21

Dose: oral hygiene and plaque inhibition and gingivitis, brush on the teeth once or twice daily

Oral candidiasis and management of aphthous ulcers, apply to affected areas once or twice daily

Prophylaxis of endocarditis for dental procedures (as adjunct to antibacterial prophylaxis), Table 2, section 5.1

DENTAL PRESCRIBING ON NHS. May be prescribed as Chlorhexidine Gluconate Gel 1%

Mouthwash, chlorhexidine gluconate 0.2%. Net price 300 mL (original or mint) = £1.81, 600 mL (mint) = £3.62

Dose: oral hygiene and plaque inhibition, oral candidiasis, gingivitis, and management of aphthous ulcers, rinse mouth with 10 mL for about 1 minute twice daily

Denture stomatitis, cleanse and soak dentures in mouthwash solution for 15 minutes twice daily

Prophylaxis of endocarditis for dental procedures (as adjunct to antibacterial prophylaxis), Table 2, section 5.1

Oral spray, chlorhexidine gluconate 0.2% (mint-flavoured). Net price 60 mL = £4.10

Dose: oral hygiene and plaque inhibition, oral candidiasis, gingivitis, and management of aphthous ulcers, apply as required to tooth, gingival, or ulcer surfaces using up to 12 actuations (approx. 0.14 mL/actuation) twice daily

DENTAL PRESCRIBING ON NHS. May be prescribed as Chlorhexidine Oral Spray

■ With chlorobutanol

Eludril® (Ceuta)

Mouthwash or *gargle*, chlorhexidine gluconate 0.1%, chlorobutanol 0.5% (mint-flavoured), net price 90 mL = £1.22, 250 mL = £2.56, 500 mL = £4.64

Dose: oral hygiene, plaque inhibition, minor throat infections, use 10–15 mL (diluted with warm water in measuring cup provided) 2–3 times daily

Denture disinfection, soak previously cleansed dentures in mouthwash (diluted with 2 volumes of water) for 60 minutes

HEXETIDINE

Indications: oral hygiene

Side-effects: local irritation; *very rarely* taste disturbance and transient anaesthesia

Oraldene® (Warner Lambert)

Mouthwash or *gargle*, red, hexetidine 0.1%. Net price 100 mL = £1.31; 200 mL = £2.02

Dose: ADULT and CHILD over 6 years, use 15 mL undiluted 2–3 times daily

OXIDISING AGENTS

Indications: oral hygiene, see notes above

Hydrogen Peroxide Mouthwash, BP

Mouthwash, consists of Hydrogen Peroxide Solution 6% (= approx. 20 volume) BP

Dose: rinse the mouth for 2–3 minutes with 15 mL diluted in half a tumblerful of warm water 2–3 times daily

DENTAL PRESCRIBING ON NHS. Hydrogen Peroxide Mouthwash may be prescribed

Peroxyl® (Colgate-Palmolive)

Mouthwash, hydrogen peroxide 1.5%, net price 300 mL = £2.81

Dose: rinse the mouth with 10 mL for about 1 minute up to 4 times daily (after meals and at bedtime)

POVIDONE–IODINE

Indications: oral hygiene

Cautions: pregnancy (Appendix 4); breast-feeding (Appendix 5); see also notes above

Contra-indications: avoid regular use in patients with thyroid disorders or those receiving lithium therapy

Side-effects: idiosyncratic mucosal irritation and hypersensitivity reactions; may interfere with thyroid-function tests and with tests for occult blood

Betadine® (Medlock)

Mouthwash or *gargle*, amber, povidone-iodine 1%. Net price 250 mL = £1.12

Dose: adults and children over 6 years, up to 10 mL undiluted or diluted with an equal quantity of warm water for up to 30 seconds up to 4 times daily for up to 14 days

SODIUM CHLORIDE

Indications: oral hygiene, see notes above

Sodium Chloride Mouthwash, Compound, BP
Mouthwash, sodium bicarbonate 1%, sodium chloride 1.5% in a suitable vehicle with a peppermint flavour.
Dose: extemporaneous preparations should be prepared according to the following formula: sodium chloride 1.5 g, sodium bicarbonate 1 g, concentrated peppermint emulsion 2.5 mL, double-strength chloroform water 50 mL, water to 100 mL
To be diluted with an equal volume of warm water
DENTAL PRESCRIBING ON NHS. Compound Sodium Chloride Mouthwash may be prescribed

THYMOL

Indications: oral hygiene, see notes above

Mouthwash Solution-tablets
Consist of tablets which may contain antimicrobial, colouring, and flavouring agents in a suitable soluble effervescent basis to make a mouthwash suitable for dental purposes.
Dose: dissolve 1 tablet in a tumblerful of warm water
NOTE. Mouthwash solution tablets may contain ingredients such as thymol
DENTAL PRESCRIBING ON NHS. Mouthwash Solution-tablets may be prescribed

12.3.5 Treatment of dry mouth

Dry mouth (xerostomia) may be caused by drugs with antimuscarinic (anticholinergic) side-effects (e.g. antispasmodics, tricyclic antidepressants, and some antipsychotics), by irradiation of the head and neck region or by damage to or disease of the salivary glands. Patients with a persistently dry mouth may develop a burning or scalded sensation and have poor oral hygiene; they may develop increased dental caries, periodontal disease, intolerance of dentures, and oral infections (particularly candidiasis). Dry mouth may be relieved in many patients by simple measures such as frequent sips of cool drinks or sucking pieces of ice or sugar-free fruit pastilles. Sugar-free chewing gum stimulates salivation in patients with residual salivary function.

Artificial saliva can provide useful relief of dry mouth. A properly balanced artificial saliva should be of a neutral pH and contain electrolytes (including fluoride) to correspond approximately to the composition of saliva. The pH of some artificial saliva products may be inappropriate. Of the proprietary preparations, *Luborant*® is licensed for any condition giving rise to a dry mouth; *Biotène Oralbalance*® *BioXtra*®, *Glandosane*®, *Saliva Orthana*®, and *Saliveze*®, have ACBS approval for dry mouth associated only with radiotherapy or sicca syndrome. *Salivix*® pastilles, which act locally as salivary stimulants, are also available and have similar ACBS approval. *SST* tablets may be prescribed for dry mouth in patients with salivary gland impairment (and patent salivary ducts).

Pilocarpine tablets are licensed for the treatment of xerostomia following irradiation for head and neck cancer and for dry mouth and dry eyes (xerophthalmia) in Sjögren's syndrome. They are effective only in patients who have some residual salivary gland function, and therefore should be withdrawn if there is no response.

Local treatment

AS Saliva Orthana® (AS Pharma)
Oral spray, gastric mucin 3.5%, xylitol 2%, sodium fluoride 4.2 mg/litre, with preservatives and flavouring agents. Net price 50-mL bottle = £4.25; 450-mL refill = £29.69
Lozenges, mucin 65 mg, xylitol 59 mg, in a sorbitol basis. Net price 45-lozenge pack = £3.02
Dose: ACBS: patients suffering from dry mouth as a result of having (or having undergone) radiotherapy, or sicca syndrome, spray 2–3 times onto oral and pharyngeal mucosa, when required
NOTE. *AS Saliva Orthana*® lozenges do not contain fluoride
DENTAL PRESCRIBING ON NHS. *AS Saliva Orthana*® Oral Spray and Lozenges may be prescribed

Glandosane® (Fresenius Kabi)
Aerosol spray, carmellose sodium 500 mg, sorbitol 1.5 g, potassium chloride 60 mg, sodium chloride 42.2 mg, magnesium chloride 2.6 mg, calcium chloride 7.3 mg, and dipotassium hydrogen phosphate 17.1 mg/50 g. Net price 50-mL unit (neutral, lemon or peppermint flavoured) = £4.48
Dose: ACBS: patients suffering from dry mouth as a result of having (or having undergone) radiotherapy, or sicca syndrome, spray onto oral and pharyngeal mucosa as required
DENTAL PRESCRIBING ON NHS. *Glandosane*® Aerosol Spray may be prescribed

Luborant® (Goldshield)
Oral spray, pink, sorbitol 1.8 g, carmellose sodium (sodium carboxymethylcellulose) 390 mg, dibasic potassium phosphate 48.23 mg, potassium chloride 37.5 mg, monobasic potassium phosphate 21.97 mg, calcium chloride 9.972 mg, magnesium chloride 3.528 mg, sodium fluoride 258 micrograms/60 mL, with preservatives and colouring agents. Net price 60-mL unit = £3.96
Dose: saliva deficiency, 2–3 sprays onto oral mucosa up to 4 times daily, or as directed
NOTE. May be difficult to obtain
DENTAL PRESCRIBING ON NHS. *Luborant*® Oral Spray may be prescribed as Artificial Saliva

Biotène Oralbalance® (Anglian)
Saliva replacement gel, lactoperoxidase, lactoferrin, lysozyme, glucose oxidase, xylitol in a gel basis, net price 50-g tube = £4.10; 24 × 9-mL tube = £35.76
Dose: ACBS: patients suffering from dry mouth as a result of having (or having undergone) radiotherapy, or sicca syndrome, apply to gums and tongue as required
NOTE. Avoid use with toothpastes containing detergents (including foaming agents)
DENTAL PRESCRIBING ON NHS. *Biotene Oralbalance*® Saliva Replacement Gel may be prescribed

BioXtra® (Molar)
Gel, lactoperoxidase, lactoferrin, lysozyme, whey colostrum, xylitol and other ingredients, net price 40-mL tube = £2.25
Dose: ACBS: patients suffering from dry mouth as a result of having (or having undergone) radiotherapy, or sicca syndrome, apply to oral mucosa as required
DENTAL PRESCRIBING ON NHS. *BioXtra*® Gel may be prescribed

Saliveze® (Wyvern)

Oral spray, carmellose sodium (sodium carboxymethylcellulose), calcium chloride, magnesium chloride, potassium chloride, sodium chloride, and dibasic sodium phosphate. Net price 50-mL bottle (mint-flavoured) = £3.50

Dose: ACBS: patients suffering from dry mouth as a result of having (or having undergone) radiotherapy, or sicca syndrome, 1 spray onto oral mucosa as required

DENTAL PRESCRIBING ON NHS. *Saliveze*® Oral Spray may be prescribed

Salivix® (Provalis)

Pastilles, sugar-free, reddish-amber, acacia, malic acid and other ingredients. Net price 50-pastille pack = £2.86

Dose: ACBS: patients suffering from dry mouth as a result of having (or having undergone) radiotherapy, or sicca syndrome, suck 1 pastille when required

DENTAL PRESCRIBING ON NHS. *Salivix*® Pastilles may be prescribed

SST (Medac)

Tablets, sugar-free, citric acid, malic acid and other ingredients in a sorbitol base, net price 100-tab pack = £4.86

Dose: symptomatic treatment of dry mouth in patients with impaired salivary gland function and patent salivary ducts, allow 1 tablet to dissolve slowly in the mouth when required

Systemic treatment

PILOCARPINE HYDROCHLORIDE

Indications: xerostomia following irradiation for head and neck cancer (see also notes above); dry mouth and dry eyes in Sjögren's syndrome

Cautions: asthma and chronic obstructive pulmonary disease (avoid if uncontrolled, see Contra-indications), cardiovascular disease (avoid if uncontrolled); cholelithiasis or biliary-tract disease, peptic ulcer, hepatic impairment (Appendix 2), renal impairment; risk of increased urethral smooth muscle tone and renal colic; maintain adequate fluid intake to avoid dehydration associated with excessive sweating; cognitive or psychiatric disturbances; angle-closure glaucoma; **interactions:** Appendix 1 (parasympathomimetics)

COUNSELLING. Blurred vision or dizziness may affect performance of skilled tasks (e.g. driving) particularly at night or in reduced lighting

Contra-indications: uncontrolled asthma and chronic obstructive pulmonary disease (increased bronchial secretions and increased airways resistance); uncontrolled cardiorenal disease; acute iritis; pregnancy (Appendix 4); breast-feeding

Side-effects: headache, influenza-like syndrome, increased urinary frequency, sweating; less frequently, nausea, vomiting, abdominal pain, dyspepsia, diarrhoea, constipation, flushing, hypertension, palpitations, rhinitis, dizziness, asthenia, lacrimation, conjunctivitis, visual disturbances, ocular pain, rash, pruritus; rarely, flatulence, urinary urgency

Dose: xerostomia following irradiation for head and neck cancer, 5 mg 3 times daily with or immediately after meals (last dose always with evening meal); if tolerated but response insufficient after 4 weeks, may be increased to max. 30 mg daily in divided doses; max. therapeutic effect normally within 4–8 weeks; discontinue if no improvement after 2–3 months; CHILD not recommended

Dry mouth and dry eyes in Sjögren's syndrome, 5 mg 4 times daily (with meals and at bedtime); if tolerated but response insufficient, may be increased to max. 30 mg daily in divided doses; discontinue if no improvement after 2–3 months; CHILD not recommended

Salagen® (Novartis) PoM

Tablets, f/c, pilocarpine hydrochloride 5 mg. Net price 84-tab pack = £51.43. Label: 21, 27, counselling, driving

13: Skin

13.1 Management of skin conditions

13.1.1 Vehicles

Both vehicle and active ingredients are important in the treatment of skin conditions; the vehicle alone may have more than a mere placebo effect. The vehicle affects the degree of hydration of the skin, has a mild anti-inflammatory effect, and aids the penetration of active drug.

Applications are usually viscous solutions, emulsions, or suspensions for application to the skin (including the scalp) or nails.

Collodions are painted on the skin and allowed to dry to leave a flexible film over the site of application.

Creams are emulsions of oil and water and are generally well absorbed into the skin. They may contain an antimicrobial preservative unless the active ingredient or basis is intrinsically bactericidal and fungicidal. Generally, creams are cosmetically more acceptable than ointments because they are less greasy and easier to apply.

Gels consist of active ingredients in suitable hydrophilic or hydrophobic bases; they generally have a high water content. Gels are particularly suitable for application to the face and scalp.

Lotions have a cooling effect and may be preferred to ointments or creams for application over a hairy area. Lotions in alcoholic basis can sting if used on broken skin. *Shake lotions* (such as calamine lotion) contain insoluble powders which leave a deposit on the skin surface.

Ointments are greasy preparations which are normally anhydrous and insoluble in water, and are more occlusive than creams. They are particularly suitable for chronic, dry lesions. The most commonly used ointment bases consist of soft paraffin or a combination of soft, liquid and hard paraffin. Some ointment bases have both *hydrophilic and lipophilic* properties; they may have occlusive properties on the skin surface, encourage hydration, and also be miscible with water; they often have a mild anti-inflammatory effect. *Water-soluble ointments* contain macrogols which are freely soluble in water and are therefore readily washed off; they have a limited but useful role where ready removal is desirable.

Pastes are stiff preparations containing a high proportion of finely powdered solids such as zinc oxide and starch suspended in an ointment. They are used for circumscribed lesions such as those which occur in lichen simplex, chronic eczema, or psoriasis. They are less occlusive than ointments and can be used to protect inflamed, lichenified, or excoriated skin.

Dusting powders are used only rarely. They reduce friction between opposing skin surfaces. Dusting powders should not be applied to moist areas because they can cake and abrade the skin. Talc is a lubricant but it does not absorb moisture whereas starch is less lubricant but absorbs water.

DILUTION. The BP directs that creams and ointments should **not** normally be diluted but that should dilution be necessary care should be taken, in particular, to prevent microbial contamination. The appropriate diluent should be used and heating should be avoided during mixing; excessive dilution may affect the stability of some creams. Diluted creams should normally be used within 2 weeks of their preparation.

13.1.2 Suitable quantities for prescribing

Suitable quantities of dermatological preparations to be prescribed for specific areas of the body:

	Creams and Ointments	Lotions
Face	15–30 g	100 mL
Both hands	25–50 g	200 mL
Scalp	50–100 g	200 mL
Both arms or both legs	100–200 g	200 mL
Trunk	400 g	500 mL
Groins and genitalia	15–25 g	100 mL

These amounts are usually suitable for an adult for twice daily application for 1 week. The recommendations do not apply to corticosteroid preparations—for suitable quantities of corticosteroid preparations see section 13.4.

13.1.3 Excipients and sensitisation

Excipients in topical products rarely cause problems. If a patch test indicates allergy to an excipient, then products containing the substance should be avoided. The following excipients in topical preparations may rarely be associated with sensitisation; the presence of these excipients is indicated in the entries for topical products.

Beeswax	Imidurea
Benzyl alcohol	Isopropyl palmitate
Butylated hydroxyanisole	N-(3-Chloroallyl) hexaminium chloride (quaternium 15)
Butylated hydroxytoluene	Polysorbates
Cetostearyl alcohol (including cetyl and stearyl alcohol)	Propylene glycol
Chlorocresol	Sodium metabisulphite
Edetic acid (EDTA)	Sorbic acid
Ethylenediamine	Wool fat and related substances including lanolin[1]
Fragrances	
Hydroxybenzoates (parabens)	

1. Purified versions of wool fat have reduced the problem

13.2 Emollient and barrier preparations

BORDERLINE SUBSTANCES. The preparations marked 'ACBS' are regarded as drugs when prescribed in accordance with the advice of the Advisory Committee on Borderline Substances for the clinical conditions listed. Prescriptions issued in accordance with this advice and endorsed 'ACBS' will normally not be investigated. See Appendix 7 for listing by clinical condition.

13.2.1 Emollients

Emollients soothe, smooth and hydrate the skin and are indicated for all dry or scaling disorders. Their effects are short-lived and they should be applied frequently even after improvement occurs. They are useful in dry and eczematous disorders, and to a lesser extent in psoriasis (section 13.5.2). Light emollients such as **aqueous cream** are suitable for many patients with dry skin but a wide range of more greasy preparations including **white soft paraffin**, **emulsifying ointment**, and **liquid and white soft paraffin ointment** are available; the severity of the condition, patient preference and site of application will often guide the choice of emollient; emollients should be applied in the direction of hair growth. Some ingredients may rarely cause sensitisation (section 13.1.3) and this should be suspected if an eczematous reaction occurs.

Preparations such as **aqueous cream** and **emulsifying ointment** can be used as soap substitutes for hand washing and in the bath; the preparation is rubbed on the skin before rinsing off completely. The addition of a bath oil (section 13.2.1.1) may also be helpful.

Preparations containing an antibacterial should be avoided unless infection is present (section 13.10) or is a frequent complication.

Urea is employed as a hydrating agent. It is used in scaling conditions and may be useful in elderly patients. It is occasionally used with other topical agents such as corticosteroids to enhance penetration.

■ Non-proprietary emollient preparations

Aqueous Cream, BP
Cream, emulsifying ointment 30%, [1]phenoxyethanol 1% in freshly boiled and cooled purified water, net price 100 g = 50p
Excipients: include cetostearyl alcohol

1. The BP permits use of alternative antimicrobials provided their identity and concentration are stated on the label

Emulsifying Ointment, BP
Ointment, emulsifying wax 30%, white soft paraffin 50%, liquid paraffin 20%, net price 100 g = 65p
Excipients: include cetostearyl alcohol

Hydrous Ointment, BP
Ointment, (oily cream), dried magnesium sulphate 0.5%, phenoxyethanol 1%, wool alcohols ointment 50%, in freshly boiled and cooled purified water, net price 100 g = 40p

Liquid and White Soft Paraffin Ointment, NPF
Ointment, liquid paraffin 50%, white soft paraffin 50%, net price 250 g = £3.24

Paraffin, White Soft, BP
White petroleum jelly, net price 100 g = 52p

Paraffin, Yellow Soft, BP
Yellow petroleum jelly, net price 100 g = 33p

■ Proprietary emollient preparations

Aveeno® (J&J)
Cream, colloidal oatmeal in emollient basis, net price 100 mL = £3.78
Excipients: include benzyl alcohol, cetyl alcohol, isopropyl palmitate
ACBS: For endogenous and exogenous eczema, xeroderma, ichthyosis, and senile pruritus (pruritus of the elderly) associated with dry skin
Lotion, colloidal oatmeal in emollient basis, net price 400-mL pump pack = £6.42
Excipients: include benzyl alcohol, cetyl alcohol, isopropyl palmitate
ACBS: as for *Aveeno*® *Cream*

Cetraben® (Sankyo)
Emollient cream, white soft paraffin 13.2%, light liquid paraffin 10.5%, net price 50 g = £1.17, 125 g = £2.38, 500-g pump pack = £5.61
Excipients: include cetostearyl alcohol, hydroxybenzoates (parabens)
For inflamed, damaged, dry or chapped skin including eczema

Decubal® **Clinic** (Alpharma)
Cream, isopropyl myristate 17%, glycerol 8.5%, wool fat 6%, dimeticone 5%, net price 50 g = £1.02, 100 g = £1.98
Excipients: include cetyl alcohol, polysorbates, sorbic acid, wool fat
For dry skin conditions including ichthyosis, psoriasis, dermatitis and hyperkeratosis

Dermamist® (Yamanouchi)
Spray application, white soft paraffin 10% in a basis containing liquid paraffin, fractionated coconut oil, net price 250-mL pressurised aerosol unit = £9.22
Excipients: none as listed in section 13.1.3
For dry skin conditions including eczema, ichthyosis, pruritus of the elderly
NOTE. Flammable

Diprobase® (Schering-Plough)
Cream, cetomacrogol 2.25%, cetostearyl alcohol 7.2%, liquid paraffin 6%, white soft paraffin 15%, water-miscible basis used for *Diprosone*® cream, net price 50 g = £1.43; 500-g dispenser = £6.15
Excipients: include cetostearyl alcohol, chlorocresol
For dry skin conditions
Ointment, liquid paraffin 5%, white soft paraffin 95%, basis used for *Diprosone*® ointment, net price 50 g = £1.54
Excipients: none as listed in section 13.1.3
For dry skin conditions

Doublebase® (Dermal)
Gel, isopropyl myristate 15%, liquid paraffin 15%, net price 100 g = £2.77, 500 g = £6.09
Excipients: none as listed in section 13.1.3
For dry chapped or itchy skin conditions

Drapolene®
Section 13.2.2

E45® (Crookes)
Cream, light liquid paraffin 12.6%, white soft paraffin 14.5%, hypoallergenic hydrous wool fat (hypoallergenic lanolin) 1% in self-emulsifying monostearin, net price 50 g = £1.18, 125 g = £2.39, 350 g = £4.14, 500-g pump pack = £6.20
Excipients: include cetyl alcohol, hydroxybenzoates (parabens)
For dry skin conditions
Emollient Wash Cream, soap substitute, zinc oxide 5% in an emollient basis, net price 250-mL pump pack = £2.95
Excipients: none as listed in section 13.1.3
ACBS: for endogenous and exogenous eczema, xeroderma, ichthyosis and senile pruritus (pruritus of the elderly) associated with dry skin
Lotion, light liquid paraffin 4%, cetomacrogol, white soft paraffin 10%, hypoallergenic anhydrous wool fat (hypoallergenic lanolin) 1% in glyceryl monostearate, net price 200 mL = £2.40, 500-mL pump pack = £4.50
Excipients: include isopropyl palmitate, hydroxybenzoates (parabens), benzyl alcohol
ACBS: for symptomatic relief of dry skin conditions, such as those associated with atopic eczema and contact dermatitis

Epaderm® (Medlock)
Ointment, emulsifying wax 30%, yellow soft paraffin 30%, liquid paraffin 40%, net price 125 g = £3.48, 500 g = £5.90
Excipients: include cetostearyl alcohol
For use as an emollient or soap substitute

Gammaderm® (Linderma)
Cream, evening primrose oil 20%, net price 50 g = £2.83, 250 g = £8.20
Excipients: include beeswax, hydroxybenzoates (parabens), propylene glycol
Cautions: epilepsy (but hazard unlikely with topical preparations)
For dry skin conditions

Hewletts® (Kestrel)
Cream, hydrous wool fat 4%, zinc oxide 8%, arachis (peanut) oil, oleic acid, white soft paraffin, net price 35 g = £1.43, 400 g = £6.69
Excipients: include fragrance
For nursing hygiene and care of skin, and chapped hands

Hydromol® (Ferndale)
Cream, sodium pidolate 2.5%, net price 50 g = £2.04, 100 g = £3.80, 500 g = £12.60
Excipients: include cetostearyl alcohol, hydroxybenzoates (parabens)
For dry skin conditions
Ointment, yellow soft paraffin 30%, emulsifying wax 30%, net price 125 g = £2.79, 500 g = £4.74
Excipients: include cetostearyl alcohol
For use as an emollient or as a bath additive

Kamillosan® (Goldshield)
Ointment, chamomile extracts 10.5% in a basis containing wool fat, net price 50 g = £2.50, 100 g = £5.00
Excipients: include beeswax, cetostearyl alcohol, hydroxybenzoates (parabens)
For nappy rash, sore nipples and chapped hands

Keri® (Bristol-Myers Squibb)
Lotion, mineral oil 16%, with lanolin oil, net price 190-mL pump pack = £3.56, 380-mL pump pack = £5.81
Excipients: include fragrance, hydroxybenzoates (parabens), *N*-(3-chloroallyl)hexaminium chloride (quaternium 15), propylene glycol
For dry skin conditions and nappy rash

LactiCare® (Stiefel)
Lotion, lactic acid 5%, sodium pidolate 2.5%, net price 150 mL = £3.19
Excipients: include cetostearyl alcohol, imidurea, isopropyl palmitate, fragrance
For dry skin conditions

Lipobase® (Yamanouchi)
Cream, fatty cream basis used for *Locoid Lipocream*®, net price 50 g = £2.08
Excipients: include cetostearyl alcohol, hydroxybenzoates (parabens)
For dry skin conditions, also for use during treatment with topical corticosteroid and as diluent for *Locoid Lipocream*®

Neutrogena® **Dermatological Cream** (J&J)
Cream, glycerol 40% in an emollient basis, net price 100 g = £3.77
Excipients: include cetostearyl alcohol, hydroxybenzoates (parabens)
For dry skin conditions

Oilatum® (Stiefel)
Cream, light liquid paraffin 6%, white soft paraffin 15%, net price 40 g = £1.79, 150 g = £3.38
Excipients: include benzyl alcohol, cetostearyl alcohol
For dry skin conditions
Shower emollient (gel), light liquid paraffin 70%, net price 150 g = £5.15
Excipients: include fragrance
For dry skin conditions including dermatitis

Ultrabase® (Schering Health)
Cream, water-miscible, containing liquid paraffin and white soft paraffin, net price 50 g = 89p, 500-g dispenser = £6.44
Excipients: include fragrance, hydroxybenzoates (parabens), disodium edetate, stearyl alcohol
For dry skin conditions

Unguentum M® (Crookes)
Cream, containing saturated neutral oil, liquid paraffin, white soft paraffin, net price 50 g = £1.59, 100 g = £3.13, 200-mL dispenser = £6.19, 500 g = £9.55
Excipients: include cetostearyl alcohol, polysorbate 40, propylene glycol, sorbic acid
For dry skin conditions and nappy rash

Vaseline Dermacare® (Elida Fabergé)
Cream, dimeticone 1%, white soft paraffin 15%, net price 150 mL = £2.11
Excipients: include hydroxybenzoates (parabens)
ACBS: for endogenous and exogenous eczema, xeroderma, ichthyosis and senile pruritus (pruritus of the elderly) associated with dry skin
Lotion, dimeticone 1%, liquid paraffin 4%, white soft paraffin 5% in an emollient basis, net price 75 mL = 78p, 200 mL = £1.49
Excipients: include disodium edetate, hydroxybenzoates (parabens), wool fat
ACBS: as for *Vaseline Dermacare*® *Cream*

Zerobase® (Zeroderma)
Cream, liquid paraffin 11%, net price 500-g dispenser = £5.99
Excipients: include cetostearyl alcohol, chlorocresol
For dry skin conditions

■ Preparations containing urea

Aquadrate® (Alliance)
Cream, urea 10%, net price 30 g = £1.37, 100 g = £3.64
Excipients: none as listed in section 13.1.3
Dose: for dry, scaling and itching skin, apply thinly and rub into area when required

Balneum® **Plus** (Crookes)
Cream, urea 5%, lauromacrogols 3%, net price 100 g = £5.58, 175-g pump pack = £7.81, 500-g pump pack = £19.50
Excipients: include benzyl alcohol, polysorbates
Dose: for dry, scaling and itching skin, apply twice daily

Calmurid® (Galderma)
Cream, urea 10%, lactic acid 5%. Diluent aqueous cream, life of diluted cream 14 days, net price 100 g = £6.84, 500-g dispenser = £25.78
Excipients: none as listed in section 13.1.3
Dose: for dry, scaling and itching skin, apply a thick layer for 3–5 minutes, massage into area, and remove excess, usually twice daily. Use half-strength cream for 1 week if stinging occurs

E45® **Itch Relief Cream** (Crookes)
Cream, urea 5%, macrogol lauryl ether 3%, net price 50 g = £2.16, 100 g = £3.47
Excipients: include benzyl alcohol, polysorbates
Dose: for dry, scaling, and itching skin, apply twice a day

Eucerin® (Beiersdorf)
Cream, urea 10%, net price 50 mL = £5.85, 150 mL = £9.23
Excipients: include benzyl alcohol, isopropyl palmitate, wool fat
Dose: for dry skin conditions including eczema, ichthyosis, xeroderma, hyperkeratosis, apply thinly and rub into area twice daily
Lotion, urea 10%, net price 250 mL = £7.69
Excipients: include benzyl alcohol, isopropyl palmitate
Dose: for dry skin conditions including eczema, ichthyosis, xeroderma, hyperkeratosis, apply sparingly and rub into area twice daily

Nutraplus® (Galderma)
Cream, urea 10%, net price 100 g = £4.37
Excipients: include hydroxybenzoates (parabens), propylene glycol
Dose: for dry, scaling and itching skin, apply 2–3 times daily

■ With antimicrobials

Dermol® (Dermal)
Cream, benzalkonium chloride 0.1%, chlorhexidine hydrochloride 0.1%, isopropyl myristate 10%, liquid paraffin 10%, net price 100-g tube = £3.22, 500-g bottle = £7.45
Excipients: include cetostearyl alcohol
Dose: for dry and pruritic skin conditions including eczema and dermatitis, apply to skin or use as soap substitute
Dermol® *500 Lotion*, benzalkonium chloride 0.1%, chlorhexidine hydrochloride 0.1%, liquid paraffin 2.5%, isopropyl myristate 2.5%, net price 500-mL dispenser = £6.31
Excipients: include cetostearyl alcohol
Dose: for dry and pruritic skin conditions including eczema and dermatitis, apply to skin or use as soap substitute
Dermol® *200 Shower Emollient*, benzalkonium chloride 0.1%, chlorhexidine hydrochloride 0.1%, liquid paraffin 2.5%, isopropyl myristate 2.5%, net price 200 mL = £3.71
Excipients: include cetostearyl alcohol
Dose: for dry and pruritic skin conditions including eczema and dermatitis, apply to skin or use as soap substitute

13.2.1.1 Emollient bath additives

Alpha Keri Bath® (Bristol-Myers Squibb)
Bath oil, liquid paraffin 91.7%, oil-soluble fraction of wool fat 3%, net price 240 mL = £3.45, 480 mL = £6.43
Excipients: include fragrance
Dose: for dry skin conditions including ichthyosis and pruritus of the elderly, add 10–20 mL/bath (INFANT 5 mL)

Aveeno® (J&J)

Aveeno® Bath oil, colloidal oatmeal, white oat fraction in emollient basis, net price 250 mL = £4.28

Excipients: include beeswax, fragrance

Dose: ACBS: for endogenous and exogenous eczema, xeroderma, ichthyosis, and senile pruritus (pruritus of the elderly) associated with dry skin, add 30 mL/bath

Aveeno Colloidal® Bath additive, oatmeal, white oat fraction in emollient basis, net price 10 × 50-g sachets = £7.33

Excipients: none as listed in section 13.1.3

Dose: ACBS: as for Aveeno® Bath oil; add 1 sachet/bath (INFANT half sachet)

Balneum® (Crookes)

Balneum® bath oil, soya oil 84.75%, net price 200 mL = £2.79, 500 mL = £6.06, 1 litre = £11.70

Excipients: include butylated hydroxytoluene, propylene glycol, fragrance

Dose: for dry skin conditions including those associated with dermatitis and eczema; add 20 mL/bath (INFANT 5 mL)

Balneum Plus® bath oil, soya oil 82.95%, mixed lauromacrogols 15%, net price 500 mL = £7.50

Excipients: include butylated hydroxytoluene, propylene glycol, fragrance

Dose: for dry skin conditions including those associated with dermatitis and eczema where pruritus also experienced; add 20 mL/bath (INFANT 5 mL)

Cetraben® (Sankyo)

Emollient bath additive, light liquid paraffin 82.8%, net price 500 mL = £5.25

Dose: for dry skin conditions, including eczema, add 1–2 capfuls/bath (CHILD ½–1 capful)

Dermalo® (Dermal)

Bath emollient, acetylated wool alcohols 5%, liquid paraffin 65%, net price 500 mL = £3.60

Excipients: none as listed in section 13.1.3

Dose: for dermatitis, dry skin conditions including ichthyosis and pruritus of the elderly; add 15–20 mL/bath (INFANT and CHILD 5–10 mL)

Diprobath® (Schering-Plough)

Bath additive, isopropyl myristate 39%, light liquid paraffin 46%, net price 500 mL = £6.97

Excipients: none as listed in section 13.1.3

Dose: for dry skin conditions including dermatitis and eczema; add 25 mL/bath (INFANT 10 mL)

E45® (Crookes)

Emollient bath oil, cetyl dimeticone 5%, liquid paraffin 91%, net price 250 mL = £2.95, 500 mL = £4.70

Excipients: none as listed in section 13.1.3

Dose: ACBS: for endogenous and exogenous eczema, xeroderma, ichthyosis, and senile pruritus (pruritus of the elderly) associated with dry skin; add 15 mL/bath (CHILD 5–10 mL)

Emollient Medicinal Bath Oil (Ashbourne)

Emollient bath oil, liquid paraffin 65%, acetylated wool alcohols 5%, net price 250 mL = £2.75, 500 mL = £5.46

Dose: for dry skin conditions including dermatitis, pruritus of the elderly, and ichthyosis, add 15–20 mL/bath (INFANT and CHILD 5–10 mL added to a small bath or washbasin)

Hydromol Emollient® (Ferndale)

Bath additive, isopropyl myristate 13%, light liquid paraffin 37.8%, net price 150 mL = £1.87, 350 mL = £3.80, 1 litre = £9.00

Excipients: none as listed in section 13.1.3

Dose: for dry skin conditions including eczema, ichthyosis and pruritus of the elderly; add 1–3 capfuls/bath (INFANT ½–2 capfuls)

Imuderm® (Goldshield)

Bath oil, almond oil 30%, light liquid paraffin 69.6%, net price 250 mL = £3.75

Excipients: include butylated hydroxyanisole

Dose: for dry skin conditions including dermatitis, eczema, pruritus of the elderly, and ichthyosis, add 15–30 mL/bath (INFANT and CHILD 7.5–15 mL)

Oilatum® (Stiefel)

Oilatum® Emollient bath additive (emulsion), acetylated wool alcohols 5%, liquid paraffin 63.4%, net price 250 mL = £2.75, 500 mL = £4.57

Excipients: include isopropyl palmitate, fragrance

Dose: for dry skin conditions including dermatitis, pruritus of the elderly and ichthyosis; add 1–3 capfuls/bath (INFANT 0.5–2 capfuls)

Oilatum® Fragrance Free Junior bath additive, light liquid paraffin 63.4%, net price 250 mL = £3.25, 500 mL = £5.75, 1 litre = £11.50

Excipients: include wool fat, isopropyl palmitate

Dose: for dry skin conditions including dermatitis, pruritus of the elderly and ichthyosis; add 1–3 capfuls/bath (INFANT 0.5–2 capfuls)

■ With antimicrobials

Dermol® (Dermal)

Dermol® 600 Bath Emollient, benzalkonium chloride 0.5%, liquid paraffin 25%, isopropyl myristate 25%, net price 600 mL = £7.90

Excipients: include polysorbate 60

Dose: for dry and pruritic skin conditions including eczema and dermatitis, add up to 30 mL/bath (INFANT up to 15 mL)

Emulsiderm® (Dermal)

Liquid emulsion, liquid paraffin 25%, isopropyl myristate 25%, benzalkonium chloride 0.5%, net price 300 mL (with 15-mL measure) = £4.03, 1 litre (with 30-mL measure) = £12.55

Excipients: include polysorbate 60

Dose: for dry skin conditions including eczema and ichthyosis; add 7–30 mL/bath

Oilatum® (Stiefel)

Oilatum® Plus bath additive, benzalkonium chloride 6%, triclosan 2%, light liquid paraffin 52.5%, net price 500 mL = £6.98, 1 litre = £13.59

Excipients: include wool fat, isopropyl palmitate

Dose: for topical treatment of eczema including eczema at risk from infection; add 1–2 capfuls/bath (INFANT over 6 months 1 mL)

13.2.2 Barrier preparations

Barrier preparations often contain water-repellent substances such as **dimeticone** (dimethicone) or other silicones. They are used on the skin around stomas, bedsores, and pressure areas in the elderly where the skin is intact. Where the skin has broken down, barrier preparations have a limited role in protecting adjacent skin. They are no substitute for adequate nursing care and it is doubtful if they are any more effective than the traditional compound **zinc ointments**.

NAPPY RASH. Barrier creams and ointments are used for protection against nappy rash which is usually a local dermatitis. The first line of treatment is to ensure that nappies are changed frequently and that tightly fitting water-proof pants are avoided. The rash may clear when left exposed to the air and a barrier preparation may be helpful. If the rash is associated with a fungal infection, an antifungal cream such as clotrimazole cream (section 13.10.2) is useful. A mild corticosteroid such as hydrocortisone 1% may be useful but treatment should be limited to a week or less; the occlusive effect of nappies and water-proof pants may increase absorption (for cautions, see p. 567).

■ Non-proprietary barrier preparations

Zinc Cream, BP
Cream, zinc oxide 32%, arachis (peanut) oil 32%, calcium hydroxide 0.045%, oleic acid 0.5%, wool fat 8%, in freshly boiled and cooled purified water, net price 50 g = 50p
For nappy and urinary rash and eczematous conditions

Zinc Ointment, BP
Ointment, zinc oxide 15%, in Simple Ointment BP 1988 (which contains wool fat 5%, hard paraffin 5%, cetostearyl alcohol 5%, white soft paraffin 85%), net price 25 g = 16p
For nappy and urinary rash and eczematous conditions

Zinc and Castor Oil Ointment, BP
Ointment, zinc oxide 7.5%, castor oil 50%, arachis (peanut) oil 30.5%, white beeswax 10%, cetostearyl alcohol 2%, net price 25 g = 14p
For nappy and urinary rash

■ Proprietary barrier preparations

Conotrane® (Yamanouchi)
Cream, benzalkonium chloride 0.1%, dimeticone '350' 22%, net price 100 g = 74p, 500 g = £3.51
Excipients: include cetostearyl alcohol, fragrance
For nappy and urinary rash and pressure sores

Drapolene® (Warner Lambert)
Cream, benzalkonium chloride 0.01%, cetrimide 0.2% in a basis containing white soft paraffin, cetyl alcohol and wool fat, net price 100 g = £1.43, 200 g = £2.38, 350 g = £3.66
Excipients: include cetyl alcohol, chlorocresol, wool fat
For nappy and urinary rash; minor wounds

Medicaid® (LPC)
Cream, cetrimide 0.5% in a basis containing light liquid paraffin, white soft paraffin, cetostearyl alcohol, glyceryl monostearate, net price 50 g = £1.69
Excipients: include cetostearyl alcohol, fragrance, hydroxybenzoates (parabens), wool fat
For nappy rash, minor burns and abrasions

Metanium® (Ransom)
Ointment, titanium dioxide 20%, titanium peroxide 5%, titanium salicylate 3% in a basis containing dimeticone, light liquid paraffin, white soft paraffin, and benzoin tincture, net price 30 g = £2.01
Excipients: none as listed in section 13.1.3
For nappy rash and related disorders

Morhulin® (Thornton & Ross)
Ointment, cod-liver oil 11.4%, zinc oxide 38%, in a basis containing liquid paraffin and yellow soft paraffin, net price 50 g = £1.62
Excipients: include wool fat derivative
For minor wounds, varicose ulcers, pressure sores, eczema and nappy rash

Siopel® (Centrapharm)
Barrier cream, dimeticone '1000' 10%, cetrimide 0.3%, arachis (peanut) oil, net price 50 g = £1.66
Excipients: include butylated hydroxytoluene, cetostearyl alcohol, hydroxybenzoates (parabens)
For protection against water-soluble irritants

Sprilon® (Ayrton Saunders)
Spray application, dimeticone 1.04%, zinc oxide 12.5%, in a basis containing wool alcohols, cetostearyl alcohol, dextran, white soft paraffin, liquid paraffin, propellants, net price 115-g pressurised aerosol unit = £3.54
Excipients: include cetostearyl alcohol, hydroxybenzoates (parabens), wool fat
For urinary rash, pressure sores, leg ulcers, moist eczema, fissures, fistulae and ileostomy care
NOTE. Flammable

Sudocrem® (Forest)
Cream, benzyl alcohol 0.39%, benzyl benzoate 1.01%, benzyl cinnamate 0.15%, hydrous wool fat (hypoallergenic lanolin) 4%, zinc oxide 15.25%, net price 30 g = £1.01, 60 g = £1.07, 125 g = £1.62, 250 g = £2.75, 400 g = £3.88
Excipients: include beeswax (synthetic), propylene glycol, fragrance
For nappy rash and pressure sores

Vasogen® (Forest)
Barrier cream, dimeticone 20%, calamine 1.5%, zinc oxide 7.5%, net price 50 g = 80p, 100 g = £1.36
Excipients: include hydroxybenzoates (parabens), wool fat
For nappy rash, pressure sores, ileostomy and colostomy care

13.3 Topical local anaesthetics and antipruritics

Pruritus may be caused by systemic disease (such as drug hypersensitivity, obstructive jaundice, endocrine disease, and certain malignant diseases) as well as by skin disease (e.g. psoriasis, eczema, urticaria, and scabies). Where possible the underlying causes should be treated. An **emollient** (section 13.2.1) may be of value where the pruritus is associated with dry skin. Pruritus that occurs in otherwise healthy elderly people can also be treated with an emollient. For advice on the treatment of pruritus in palliative care, see p. 16.

Preparations containing **crotamiton** are sometimes used but are of uncertain value. Preparations containing **calamine** are often ineffective.

A topical preparation containing **doxepin** 5% is licensed for the relief of pruritus in eczema; it can cause drowsiness and there may be a risk of sensitisation.

Pruritus is common in biliary obstruction, especially in primary biliary cirrhosis and drug-induced cholestasis. Oral administration of **colestyramine** (cholestyramine) is the treatment of choice (section 1.9.2).

Topical antihistamines and local anaesthetics are only marginally effective and may occasionally cause sensitisation. A short course of a topical corticosteroid is appropriate in treating *insect stings*. Insect stings should not be treated with calamine preparations.

A short treatment with a **sedating antihistamine** (section 3.4.1) may help in insect stings and in intractable pruritus where sedation is desirable.

For preparations used in *pruritus ani*, see section 1.7.1.

CALAMINE

Indications: pruritus

Calamine (Non-proprietary)
Aqueous cream, calamine 4%, zinc oxide 3%, liquid paraffin 20%, self-emulsifying glyceryl monostearate 5%, cetomacrogol emulsifying wax 5%,

phenoxyethanol 0.5%, freshly boiled and cooled purified water 62.5%, net price 100 mL = 59p

Lotion (= cutaneous suspension), calamine 15%, zinc oxide 5%, glycerol 5%, bentonite 3%, sodium citrate 0.5%, liquefied phenol 0.5%, in freshly boiled and cooled purified water, net price 200 mL = 63p

Oily lotion (BP 1980), calamine 5%, arachis (peanut) oil 50%, oleic acid 0.5%, wool fat 1%, in calcium hydroxide solution, net price 200 mL = £1.58

CROTAMITON

Indications: pruritus (including pruritus after scabies—section 13.10.4); see notes above

Cautions: avoid use near eyes and broken skin; use on doctor's advice for children under 3 years

Contra-indications: acute exudative dermatoses

Dose: pruritus, apply 2–3 times daily; CHILD below 3 years, apply once daily

Eurax® (Novartis Consumer Health)

Cream, crotamiton 10%, net price 30 g = £2.27, 100 g = £3.95

Excipients: include beeswax, fragrance, hydroxybenzoates (parabens), stearyl alcohol

Lotion, crotamiton 10%, net price 100 mL = £2.99

Excipients: include cetyl alcohol, fragrance, propylene glycol, sorbic acid, stearyl alcohol

DOXEPIN HYDROCHLORIDE

Indications: pruritus in eczema; depressive illness (section 4.3.1)

Cautions: glaucoma, urinary retention, severe liver impairment, mania; avoid application to large areas; pregnancy and breast-feeding; **interactions:** Appendix 1 (antidepressants, tricyclic)

DRIVING. Drowsiness may affect performance of skilled tasks (e.g. driving); effects of alcohol enhanced

Side-effects: drowsiness; local burning, stinging, irritation, tingling and rash; dry mouth and other systemic side-effects reported (section 4.3.1)

Dose: apply thinly 3–4 times daily; usual max. 3 g per application; usual total max. 12 g daily; coverage should be less than 10% of body surface area; CHILD under 12 years not recommended

Xepin® (CHS) PoM

Cream, doxepin hydrochloride 5%, net price 30 g = £11.70. Label: 2, 10, patient information leaflet

Excipients: include benzyl alcohol

TOPICAL LOCAL ANAESTHETICS

Indications: relief of local pain, see notes above. See section 15.2 for use in surface anaesthesia

Cautions: occasionally cause hypersensitivity

NOTE. Topical local anaesthetic preparations may be absorbed, especially through mucosal surfaces, therefore excessive application should be avoided and they should preferably not be used for more than about 3 days; not generally suitable for young children

■ Preparations on sale to the public

The following is a list of topical local anaesthetic preparations on sale to the public, together with their significant ingredients:

Anethaine® (tetracaine), **Anthisan**® **Plus** (benzocaine, mepyramine), **BurnEze**® (benzocaine), **Dermidex**® (lidocaine, alcloxa, cetrimide, chlorobutanol), **Lanacane**® **cream** (benzocaine, chlorothymol), **Vagisil**® **cream** (lidocaine), **Wasp-Eze**® **spray** (benzocaine, mepyramine)

TOPICAL ANTIHISTAMINES

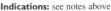

Indications: see notes above

Cautions: may cause hypersensitivity; avoid in eczema; photosensitivity (diphenhydramine); not recommended for longer than 3 days

■ Preparations on sale to the public

The following is a list of topical antihistamine preparations on sale to the public, together with their significant ingredients:

Anthisan® (mepyramine), **Anthisan**® **Bite and Sting** (mepyramine), **Anthisan**® **Plus** (mepyramine, benzocaine), **Benadryl**® **Skin Allergy Relief cream** (diphenhydramine, camphor), **Benadryl**® **Skin Allergy Relief lotion** (diphenhydramine, camphor), **Boots Bite & Sting Relief Antihistamine cream** (mepyramine), **R.B.C.**® (antazoline, calamine, camphor, cetrimide, menthol), **Wasp-Eze**® **ointment** (antazoline), **Wasp-Eze**® **spray** (mepyramine, benzocaine)

13.4 Topical corticosteroids

Topical corticosteroids are used for the treatment of inflammatory conditions of the skin (other than those arising from an infection) in particular eczema (section 13.5.1), contact dermatitis, insect stings (p. 36), and eczema of scabies (section 13.10.4). Corticosteroids suppress the inflammatory reaction during use; they are not curative and on discontinuation a rebound exacerbation of the condition may occur. They are generally used to relieve symptoms and suppress signs of the disorder when other measures such as emollients are ineffective.

Topical corticosteroids are of no value in the treatment of urticaria and they are **contra-indicated** in rosacea; they may worsen ulcerated or secondarily infected lesions. They should not be used indiscriminately in pruritus (where they will only benefit if inflammation is causing the itch) and are **not** recommended for acne vulgaris.

Systemic or potent topical corticosteroids should be avoided or given only under specialist supervision in *psoriasis* because, although they may suppress the psoriasis in the short term, relapse or vigorous rebound occurs on withdrawal (sometimes precipitating severe pustular psoriasis). Topical use of potent corticosteroids on widespread psoriasis can lead to systemic as well as to local side-effects. It is reasonable, however, to prescribe a mild to moderate topical corticosteroid for a short period (2–4 weeks) for *flexural* and *facial psoriasis*. In the case of scalp psoriasis it is reasonable to use a more potent corticosteroid such as betamethasone or fluocinonide (see below for cautions in psoriasis).

In general, the most potent topical corticosteroids should be reserved for recalcitrant dermatoses such as *chronic discoid lupus erythematosus*, *lichen simplex chronicus*, *hypertrophic lichen planus*, and *palmoplantar pustulosis*. Potent corticosteroids should generally be avoided on the face and skin flexures, but specialists occasionally prescribe them for these areas in certain circumstances.

When topical treatment has failed, intralesional corticosteroid injections (section 10.1.2.2) may be used. These are more effective than the very potent topical corticosteroid preparations and should be reserved for severe cases where there are localised lesions such as *keloid scars*, *hypertrophic lichen planus*, or *localised alopecia areata*.

PERIORAL LESIONS. **Hydrocortisone** cream 1% can be used for a limited time to treat uninfected inflammatory lesions on the lips and on the skin surrounding the mouth. **Hydrocortisone and miconazole** cream or ointment is useful where infection by susceptible organisms and inflammation co-exist, particularly for initial treatment (up to about 7 days) e.g. in angular cheilitis (see also p. 555). Organisms susceptible to miconazole include *Candida* spp. and many Gram-positive bacteria including streptococci and staphylococci.

CHILDREN. Children, especially infants, are particularly susceptible to side-effects. However, concern about the safety of topical corticosteroids in children should not result in the child being undertreated. The aim is to control the condition as well as possible; inadequate treatment will perpetuate the condition. A mild corticosteroid such as hydrocortisone 1% ointment or cream is useful for treating nappy rash (section 13.2.2) and for atopic eczema in childhood (section 13.5.1). A moderately potent or potent corticosteroid may be appropriate for severe atopic eczema on the limbs, for 1–2 weeks only, switching to a less potent preparation as the condition improves. In an acute flare-up of atopic eczema, it may be appropriate to use more potent formulations of topical corticosteroids for a short period to regain control of the condition. Continuous daily application of a mild corticosteroid such as hydrocortisone 1% is equivalent to a potent corticosteroid such as betamethasone 0.1% applied intermittently. Carers of young children should be advised that treatment should **not** necessarily be reserved to 'treat only the worst areas' and they may need to be advised that patient information leaflets may contain inappropriate advice for the patient's condition.

CHOICE OF FORMULATION. Water-miscible corticosteroid *creams* are suitable for moist or weeping lesions whereas *ointments* are generally chosen for dry, lichenified or scaly lesions or where a more occlusive effect is required. *Lotions* may be useful when minimal application to a large or hair-bearing area is required or for the treatment of exudative lesions. *Occlusive polythene or hydrocolloid dressings* increase absorption, but also increase the risk of side-effects; they are therefore used only under supervision on a short-term basis for areas of very thick skin (such as the palms and soles). The inclusion of urea or salicylic acid also increases the penetration of the corticosteroid.

In the BNF topical corticosteroids for the skin are categorised as 'mild', 'moderately potent', 'potent' or 'very potent' (see p. 568); the **least potent** preparation which is effective should be chosen but dilution should be avoided whenever possible.

CAUTIONS. Avoid prolonged use of a topical corticosteroid on the face (and keep away from eyes). In children avoid prolonged use and use potent or very potent corticosteroids under specialist supervision; extreme caution is required in dermatoses of infancy including nappy rash—treatment should be limited to 5–7 days.

PSORIASIS. The use of potent or very potent corticosteroids in psoriasis can result in rebound relapse, development of generalised pustular psoriasis, and local and systemic toxicity.

CONTRA-INDICATIONS. Topical corticosteroids are contra-indicated in untreated bacterial, fungal, or viral skin lesions, in acne rosacea, and in perioral dermatitis; potent corticosteroids are contra-indicated in widespread plaque psoriasis (see notes above).

SIDE-EFFECTS. *Mild* and *moderately potent* topical corticosteroids are associated with few side-effects but care is required in the use of *potent* and *very potent* corticosteroids. Absorption through the skin can rarely cause adrenal suppression and even Cushing's syndrome (section 6.3.2), depending on the area of the body being treated and the duration of treatment. Absorption is greatest where the skin is thin or raw, and from intertriginous areas; it is increased by occlusion. Local side-effects include:

- spread and worsening of untreated infection;
- thinning of the skin which may be restored over a period after stopping treatment but the original structure may never return;
- irreversible striae atrophicae and telangiectasia;
- contact dermatitis;
- perioral dermatitis;
- acne, or worsening of acne or acne rosacea;
- mild depigmentation which may be reversible;
- hypertrichosis also reported

In order to minimise the side-effects of a topical corticosteroid, it is important to apply it **thinly** to affected areas **only**, no more frequently than **twice daily**, and to use the least potent formulation which is fully effective.

APPLICATION. Topical corticosteroid preparations should be applied no more frequently than twice daily; once daily is often sufficient.

Topical corticosteroids are spread thinly on the skin; the length of cream or ointment expelled from a tube may be used to specify the quantity to be applied to a given area of skin. This length can be measured in terms of a *fingertip unit* (the distance from the tip of the adult index finger to the first crease). One fingertip unit (approximately 500 mg) is sufficient to cover an area that is twice that of the flat adult palm.

Suitable quantities of corticosteroid preparations to be prescribed for specific areas of the body are:

	Creams and Ointments
Face and neck	15 to 30 g
Both hands	15 to 30 g
Scalp	15 to 30 g
Both arms	30 to 60 g
Both legs	100 g
Trunk	100 g
Groins and genitalia	15 to 30 g

These amounts are usually suitable for an adult for a single daily application for 2 weeks

Mixing topical preparations on the skin should be avoided where possible; at least 30 minutes should elapse between application of different preparations. The practice of using an emollient immediately before a topical corticosteroid is inappropriate.

COMPOUND PREPARATIONS. The advantages of including other substances (such as antibacterials or antifungals) with corticosteroids in topical preparations are uncertain, but such combinations may have a place where inflammatory skin conditions are associated with bacterial or fungal infection, such as infected eczema. In these cases the antimicrobial drug should be chosen according to the sensitivity of the infecting organism and used regularly for a short period (typically twice daily for 1 week). Longer use increases the likelihood of resistance and of sensitisation.

Topical corticosteroid preparation potencies

Potency of a topical corticosteroid preparation is a result of the formulation as well as the corticosteroid. Therefore, proprietary names are shown below.

Mild

Hydrocortisone 0.1–2.5%, *Dioderm*, *Efcortelan*, *Mildison*

- Mild with antimicrobials: *Canesten HC*, *Daktacort*, *Econacort*, *Fucidin H*, *Nystaform-HC*, *Synalar 1 in 10 Dilution*, *Timodine*, *Vioform-Hydrocortisone*
- Mild with crotamiton: *Eurax-Hydrocortisone*

Moderate

Betnovate-RD, *Eumovate*, *Haelan*, *Modrasone*, *Synalar 1 in 4 Dilution*, *Ultralanum Plain*

- Moderate with antimicrobials: *Trimovate*
- Moderate with urea: *Alphaderm*, *Calmurid HC*

Potent

Betamethasone valerate 0.1%, *Betacap*, *Betta-mousse*, *Betnovate*, *Cutivate*, *Diprosone*, *Elocon*, *Locoid*, *Locoid Crelo*, *Metosyn*, *Nerisone*, *Propaderm*, *Synalar*

- Potent with antimicrobials: *Acorvio Plus*, *Aureocort*, *Betnovate-C*, *Betnovate-N*, *FuciBET*, *Locoid C*, *Lotriderm*, *Synalar C*, *Synalar N*, *Tri-Adcortyl*
- Potent with salicylic acid: *Diprosalic*

Very potent

Dermovate, *Halciderm Topical*, *Nerisone Forte*

- Very potent with antimicrobials: *Dermovate-NN*

HYDROCORTISONE

Indications: mild inflammatory skin disorders such as eczemas (but for over-the-counter preparations, see below); nappy rash, see notes above and section 13.2.2
Cautions: see notes above
Contra-indications: see notes above
Side-effects: see notes above
Dose: apply thinly 1–2 times daily

Hydrocortisone (Non-proprietary) PoM
Cream, hydrocortisone 0.5%, net price, 15 g = 80p, 30 g = 61p; 1%, 15 g = £1.24 Label: 28. Potency: mild
DENTAL PRESCRIBING ON NHS. Hydrocortisone Cream 1% 15 g may be prescribed
Ointment, hydrocortisone 0.5%, net price 15 g = £1.03 , 30 g = 61p; 1%, 15 g = 84p. Label: 28. Potency: mild
When hydrocortisone cream or ointment is prescribed and no strength is stated, the 1% strength should be supplied

■ Over-the-counter hydrocortisone products
The following skin creams and ointments contain hydrocortisone (alone or with other ingredients) and can be sold to the public for the treatment of allergic contact dermatitis, irritant dermatitis, insect bite reactions and mild to moderate eczema
Cautions: not for children under 10 years or in pregnancy, without medical advice
Contra-indications: eyes/face, anogenital region, broken or infected skin (including cold sores, acne, and athlete's foot)
Dose: apply sparingly over small area 1–2 times daily for max. 1 week
Dermacort® (hydrocortisone 0.1%, cream), **Eurax Hc**® (hydrocortisone 0.25%; crotamiton 10%, cream), **Hc45**® (hydrocortisone acetate 1%, cream), **Lanacort**® (hydrocortisone acetate 1%, cream and ointment), **Zenoxone**® (hydrocortisone 1%, cream)

■ Proprietary hydrocortisone preparations
NOTE. The following preparations are PoM; those on sale to the public (with restrictions) are listed above

Dioderm® (Dermal) PoM
Cream, hydrocortisone 0.1%, net price 30 g = £2.50. Label: 28. Potency: mild
Excipients: include cetostearyl alcohol, propylene glycol
NOTE. Although this contains only 0.1% hydrocortisone, the formulation is designed to provide a clinical activity comparable to that of Hydrocortisone Cream 1% BP

Efcortelan® (GSK) PoM
Cream, hydrocortisone 0.5%, net price, 30 g = 61p; 1%, 30 g = 75p; 2.5%, 30 g = £1.70. Label: 28. Potency: mild
Excipients: include cetostearyl alcohol, chlorocresol
Ointment, hydrocortisone 0.5%, net price, 30 g = 61p; 1%, 30 g = 75p; 2.5%, 30 g = £1.70. Label: 28. Potency: mild
Excipients: none as listed in section 13.1.3

Mildison® (Yamanouchi) PoM
Lipocream, hydrocortisone 1%, net price 30 g = £2.45. Label: 28. Potency: mild
Excipients: include cetostearyl alcohol, hydroxybenzoates (parabens)

■ Compound preparations
Compound preparations with coal tar see section 13.5.2

Alphaderm® (Alliance) PoM
Cream, hydrocortisone 1%, urea 10%, net price 30 g = £1.98; 100 g = £5.86. Label: 28. Potency: moderate
Excipients: none as listed in section 13.1.3

Calmurid HC® (Galderma) PoM
Cream, hydrocortisone 1%, urea 10%, lactic acid 5%, net price 30 g = £2.80, 50 g = £4.67. Label: 28. Potency: moderate
Excipients: none as listed in section 13.1.3
NOTE. Manufacturer advises dilute to half-strength with aqueous cream for 1 week if stinging occurs then transfer to undiluted preparation (but see section 13.1.1 for advice to avoid dilution where possible)

[1]**Eurax-Hydrocortisone**® (Novartis Consumer Health) PoM
Cream, hydrocortisone 0.25%, crotamiton 10%, net price 30 g = 87p. Label: 28. Potency: mild
Excipients: include fragrance, hydroxybenzoates (parabens), propylene glycol, stearyl alcohol

1. A 15-g tube is on sale to the public for treatment of contact dermatitis and insect bites (*Eurax Hc*®)

■ With antimicrobials

See notes above for comment on compound preparations

[1]**Canesten HC**® (Bayer Consumer Care) PoM
Cream, hydrocortisone 1%, clotrimazole 1%, net price 30 g = £2.15. Label: 28. Potency: mild
Excipients: include benzyl alcohol, cetostearyl alcohol

1. A 15-g tube is on sale to the public for the treatment of athlete's foot and fungal infection of skin folds with associated inflammation (*Canesten*® *Hydrocortisone*)

[1]**Daktacort**® (Janssen-Cilag) PoM
Cream, hydrocortisone 1%, miconazole nitrate 2%, net price 30 g = £2.13. Label: 28. Potency: mild
Excipients: include butylated hydroxyanisole, disodium edetate
Ointment, hydrocortisone 1%, miconazole nitrate 2%, net price 30 g = £2.14. Label: 28. Potency: mild
Excipients: none as listed in section 13.1.3

DENTAL PRESCRIBING ON NHS. May be prescribed as Hydrocortisone and Miconazole Cream or Ointment for max. 7 days

1. A 15-g tube is on sale to the public for the treatment of athlete's foot and candidal intertrigo (*Daktacort*® *HC*)

Econacort® (Squibb) PoM
Cream, hydrocortisone 1%, econazole nitrate 1%, net price 30 g = £2.25. Label: 28. Potency: mild
Excipients: include butylated hydroxyanisole

Fucidin H® (Leo) PoM
Cream, hydrocortisone acetate 1%, fusidic acid 2%, net price 30 g = £5.30, 60 g = £10.60. Label: 28. Potency: mild
Excipients: include butylated hydroxyanisole, cetyl alcohol, potassium sorbate
Ointment, hydrocortisone acetate 1%, sodium fusidate 2%, net price 30 g = £3.26, 60 g = £6.53. Label: 28. Potency: mild
Excipients: include cetyl alcohol, wool fat

Nystaform-HC® (Typharm) PoM
Cream, hydrocortisone 0.5%, nystatin 100 000 units/g, chlorhexidine hydrochloride 1%, net price 30 g = £2.66. Label: 28. Potency: mild
Excipients: include benzyl alcohol, cetostearyl alcohol, polysorbate '60'
Ointment, hydrocortisone 1%, nystatin 100 000 units/g, chlorhexidine acetate 1%, net price 30 g = £2.66. Label: 28. Potency: mild
Excipients: none as listed in section 13.1.3

Timodine® (R&C) PoM
Cream, hydrocortisone 0.5%, nystatin 100 000 units/g, benzalkonium chloride solution 0.2%, dimeticone '350' 10%, net price 30 g = £2.38. Label: 28. Potency: mild
Excipients: include butylated hydroxyanisole, cetostearyl alcohol, hydroxybenzoates (parabens), sodium metabisulphite, sorbic acid

Vioform-Hydrocortisone® (Novartis Consumer Health) PoM
Cream, hydrocortisone 1%, clioquinol 3%, net price 30 g = £1.46. Label: 28. Potency: mild
Excipients: include cetostearyl alcohol
Ointment, hydrocortisone 1%, clioquinol 3%, net price 30 g = £1.46. Label: 28. Potency: mild
Excipients: none as listed in section 13.1.3
NOTE. Stains clothing

HYDROCORTISONE BUTYRATE

Indications: severe inflammatory skin disorders such as eczemas unresponsive to less potent corticosteroids; psoriasis, see notes above
Cautions: see notes above
Contra-indications: see notes above
Side-effects: see notes above
Dose: apply thinly 1–2 times daily

Locoid® (Yamanouchi) PoM
Cream, hydrocortisone butyrate 0.1%, net price 30 g = £2.29, 100 g = £7.05. Label: 28. Potency: potent
Excipients: include cetostearyl alcohol, hydroxybenzoates (parabens)
Lipocream, hydrocortisone butyrate 0.1%, net price 30 g = £2.41, 100 g = £7.38. Label: 28. Potency: potent
Excipients: include cetostearyl alcohol, hydroxybenzoates (parabens)
NOTE. For bland cream basis see *Lipobase*®, section 13.2.1
Ointment, hydrocortisone butyrate 0.1%, net price 30 g = £2.29, 100 g = £7.05. Label: 28. Potency: potent
Excipients: none as listed in section 13.1.3
Scalp lotion, hydrocortisone butyrate 0.1%, in an aqueous isopropyl alcohol basis, net price 100 mL = £9.76. Label: 15, 28. Potency: potent
Excipients: none as listed in section 13.1.3

Locoid Crelo® (Yamanouchi) PoM
Lotion (topical emulsion), hydrocortisone butyrate 0.1% in a water-miscible basis, net price 100 g (with applicator nozzle) = £8.44. Label: 28. Potency: potent
Excipients: include butylated hydroxytoluene, cetostearyl alcohol, hydroxybenzoates (parabens), propylene glycol

■ With antimicrobials

See notes above for comment on compound preparations

Locoid C® (Yamanouchi) PoM
Cream, hydrocortisone butyrate 0.1%, chlorquinaldol 3%, net price 30 g = £3.00. Label: 28. Potency: potent
Excipients: include cetostearyl alcohol
NOTE. Stains clothing and can darken skin and hair
Ointment, ingredients as for cream, in a greasy basis, net price 30 g = £3.00. Label: 28. Potency: potent
Excipients: none as listed in section 13.1.3
NOTE. Stains clothing and can darken skin and hair

ALCLOMETASONE DIPROPIONATE

Indications: inflammatory skin disorders such as eczemas
Cautions: see notes above
Contra-indications: see notes above
Side-effects: see notes above
Dose: apply thinly 1–2 times daily

Modrasone® (PLIVA) PoM
Cream, alclometasone dipropionate 0.05%, net price 50 g = £2.68. Label: 28. Potency: moderate
Excipients: include cetostearyl alcohol, chlorocresol, propylene glycol
Ointment, alclometasone dipropionate 0.05%, net price 50 g = £2.68. Label: 28. Potency: moderate
Excipients: include beeswax, propylene glycol

BECLOMETASONE DIPROPIONATE

(Beclomethasone dipropionate)

Indications: severe inflammatory skin disorders such as eczemas unresponsive to less potent corticosteroids; psoriasis, see notes above

Cautions: see notes above

Contra-indications: see notes above

Side-effects: see notes above

Dose: apply thinly 1–2 times daily

Propaderm® (GSK) PoM

Cream, beclometasone dipropionate 0.025%, net price 30 g = £1.77. Label: 28. Potency: potent

Excipients: include cetostearyl alcohol, chlorocresol

Ointment, beclometasone dipropionate 0.025%, net price 30 g = £1.77. Label: 28. Potency: potent

Excipients: include propylene glycol

BETAMETHASONE ESTERS

Indications: severe inflammatory skin disorders such as eczemas unresponsive to less potent corticosteroids; psoriasis, see notes above

Cautions: see notes above; use of more than 100 g per week of 0.1% preparation likely to cause adrenal suppression

Contra-indications: see notes above

Side-effects: see notes above

Dose: apply thinly 1–2 times daily

Betamethasone Valerate (Non-proprietary) PoM

Cream, betamethasone (as valerate) 0.1%, net price 30 g = £1.43. Label: 28. Potency: potent

Ointment, betamethasone (as valerate) 0.1%, net price 30 g = £1.68. Label: 28. Potency: potent

Betacap® (Dermal) PoM

Scalp application, betamethasone (as valerate) 0.1% in a water-miscible basis containing coconut oil derivative, net price 100 mL = £3.92. Label: 15, 28. Potency: potent

Excipients: none as listed in section 13.1.3

Betnovate® (GSK) PoM

Cream, betamethasone (as valerate) 0.1% in a water-miscible basis, net price 30 g = £1.43, 100 g = £4.05. Label: 28. Potency: potent

Excipients: include cetostearyl alcohol, chlorocresol

Ointment, betamethasone (as valerate) 0.1% in an anhydrous paraffin basis, net price 30 g = £1.43, 100 g = £4.05. Label: 28. Potency: potent

Excipients: none as listed in section 13.1.3

Lotion, betamethasone (as valerate) 0.1%, net price 100 mL = £4.86. Label: 28. Potency: potent

Excipients: include cetostearyl alcohol, hydroxybenzoates (parabens)

Scalp application, betamethasone (as valerate) 0.1% in a water-miscible basis, net price 100 mL = £5.30. Label: 15, 28. Potency: potent

Excipients: none as listed in section 13.1.3

Betnovate-RD® (GSK) PoM

Cream, betamethasone (as valerate) 0.025% in a water-miscible basis (1 in 4 dilution of *Betnovate*® cream), net price 100 g = £3.34. Label: 28. Potency: moderate

Excipients: include cetostearyl alcohol, chlorocresol

Ointment, betamethasone (as valerate) 0.025% in an anhydrous paraffin basis (1 in 4 dilution of *Betnovate*® ointment), net price 100 g = £3.34. Label: 28. Potency: moderate

Excipients: none as listed in section 13.1.3

Bettamousse® (Celltech) PoM

Foam (= scalp application), betamethasone valerate 0.12% (≡ betamethasone 0.1%), net price 100 g = £9.75. Label: 28. Potency: potent

Excipients: include cetyl alcohol, polysorbate 60, propylene glycol, stearyl alcohol

NOTE. Flammable

Diprosone® (Schering-Plough) PoM

Cream, betamethasone (as dipropionate) 0.05%, net price 30 g = £2.24, 100 g = £6.36. Label: 28. Potency: potent

Excipients: include cetostearyl alcohol, chlorocresol

Ointment, betamethasone (as dipropionate) 0.05%, net price 30 g = £2.24, 100 g = £6.36. Label: 28. Potency: potent

Excipients: none as listed in section 13.1.3

Lotion, betamethasone (as dipropionate) 0.05%, net price 30 mL = £2.83, 100 mL = £8.10. Label: 28. Potency: potent

Excipients: none as listed in section 13.1.3

■ With salicylic acid

See notes above for comment on compound preparations

Diprosalic® (Schering-Plough) PoM

Ointment, betamethasone (as dipropionate) 0.05%, salicylic acid 3%, net price 30 g = £3.30, 100 g = £9.50. Label: 28. Potency: potent

Excipients: none as listed in section 13.1.3

Dose: apply thinly 1–2 times daily; max. 60 g per week

Scalp application, betamethasone (as dipropionate) 0.05%, salicylic acid 2%, in an alcoholic basis, net price 100 mL = £10.50. Label: 28. Potency: potent

Excipients: include disodium edetate

Dose: apply a few drops 1–2 times daily

■ With antimicrobials

See notes above for comment on compound preparations

Betnovate-C® (GSK) PoM

Cream, betamethasone (as valerate) 0.1%, clioquinol 3%, net price 30 g = £1.76. Label: 28. Potency: potent

Excipients: include cetostearyl alcohol, chlorocresol

NOTE. Stains clothing

Ointment, betamethasone (as valerate) 0.1%, clioquinol 3%, net price 30 g = £1.76. Label: 28. Potency: potent

Excipients: none as listed in section 13.1.3

NOTE. Stains clothing

Betnovate-N® (GSK) PoM

Cream, betamethasone (as valerate) 0.1%, neomycin sulphate 0.5%, net price 30 g = £1.76, 100 g = £4.88. Label: 28. Potency: potent

Excipients: include cetostearyl alcohol, chlorocresol

Ointment, betamethasone (as valerate) 0.1%, neomycin sulphate 0.5%, net price 30 g = £1.76, 100 g = £4.88. Label: 28. Potency: potent

Excipients: none as listed in section 13.1.3

FuciBET® (Leo) PoM

Cream, betamethasone (as valerate) 0.1%, fusidic acid 2%, net price 30 g = £5.62, 60 g = £11.23. Label: 28. Potency: potent

Excipients: include cetostearyl alcohol, chlorocresol

Lotriderm® (PLIVA) PoM

Cream, betamethasone dipropionate 0.064% (≡ betamethasone 0.05%), clotrimazole 1%, net price 30 g = £6.34. Label: 28. Potency: potent

Excipients: include benzyl alcohol, cetostearyl alcohol, propylene glycol

CLOBETASOL PROPIONATE

Indications: short-term treatment only of severe resistant inflammatory skin disorders such as

recalcitrant eczemas unresponsive to less potent corticosteroids; psoriasis, see notes above
Cautions: see notes above
Contra-indications: see notes above
Side-effects: see notes above
Dose: apply thinly 1–2 times daily for up to 4 weeks; max. 50 g of 0.05% preparation per week

Dermovate® (GSK) PoM
Cream, clobetasol propionate 0.05%, net price 30 g = £2.86, 100 g = £8.39. Label: 28. Potency: very potent
Excipients: include beeswax (or beeswax substitute), cetostearyl alcohol, chlorocresol, propylene glycol
Ointment, clobetasol propionate 0.05%, net price 30 g = £2.86, 100 g = £8.39. Label: 28. Potency: very potent
Excipients: include propylene glycol
Scalp application, clobetasol propionate 0.05%, in a thickened alcoholic basis, net price 30 mL = £3.26, 100 mL = £11.06. Label: 15, 28. Potency: very potent
Excipients: none as listed in section 13.1.3

■ With antimicrobials
See notes above for comment on compound preparations

Dermovate-NN® (GSK) PoM
Cream, clobetasol propionate 0.05%, neomycin sulphate 0.5%, nystatin 100 000 units/g, net price 30 g = £3.91. Label: 28. Potency: very potent
Excipients: include arachis (peanut) oil, beeswax substitute
Ointment, ingredients as for cream, in a paraffin basis, net price 30 g = £3.91. Label: 28. Potency: very potent
Excipients: none as listed in section 13.1.3

CLOBETASONE BUTYRATE

Indications: eczemas and dermatitis of all types; maintenance between courses of more potent corticosteroids
Cautions: see notes above
Contra-indications: see notes above
Side-effects: see notes above
Dose: apply thinly 1–2 times daily

[1]**Eumovate**® (GSK) PoM
Cream, clobetasone butyrate 0.05%, net price 30 g = £1.97, 100 g = £5.77. Label: 28. Potency: moderate
Excipients: include beeswax substitute, cetostearyl alcohol, chlorocresol
Ointment, clobetasone butyrate 0.05%, net price 30 g = £1.97, 100 g = £5.77. Label: 28. Potency: moderate
Excipients: none as listed in section 13.1.3

1. Cream can be sold to the public for short-term symptomatic treatment and control of patches of eczema and dermatitis (but not seborrhoeic dermatitis) in adults and children over 12 years provided pack does not contain more than 15 g

■ With antimicrobials
See notes above for comment on compound preparations

Trimovate® (GSK) PoM
Cream, clobetasone butyrate 0.05%, oxytetracycline 3% (as calcium salt), nystatin 100 000 units/g, net price 30 g = £3.49. Label: 28. Potency: moderate
Excipients: include cetostearyl alcohol, chlorocresol, sodium metabisulphite
NOTE. Stains clothing

DIFLUCORTOLONE VALERATE

Indications: severe inflammatory skin disorders such as eczemas unresponsive to less potent corticosteroids; high strength (0.3%), short-term treatment of severe exacerbations; psoriasis, see notes above
Cautions: see notes above
Contra-indications: see notes above
Side-effects: see notes above
Dose: apply thinly 1–2 times daily for up to 4 weeks (0.1% preparations) or 2 weeks (0.3% preparations), reducing strength as condition responds; max. 60 g of 0.3% per week

Nerisone® (Meadow) PoM
Cream, diflucortolone valerate 0.1%, net price 30 g = £1.59. Label: 28. Potency: potent
Excipients: include disodium edetate, hydroxybenzoates (parabens), stearyl alcohol
Oily cream, diflucortolone valerate 0.1%, net price 30 g = £2.56. Label: 28. Potency: potent
Excipients: include beeswax
Ointment, diflucortolone valerate 0.1%, net price 30 g = £1.59. Label: 28. Potency: potent
Excipients: none as listed in section 13.1.3

Nerisone Forte® (Meadow) PoM
Oily cream, diflucortolone valerate 0.3%, net price 15 g = £2.09. Label: 28. Potency: very potent
Excipients: include beeswax
Ointment, diflucortolone valerate 0.3%, net price 15 g = £2.09. Label: 28. Potency: very potent
Excipients: none as listed in section 13.1.3

FLUDROXYCORTIDE

(Flurandrenolone)
Indications: inflammatory skin disorders such as eczemas
Cautions: see notes above
Contra-indications: see notes above
Side-effects: see notes above
Dose: apply thinly 1–2 times daily

Haelan® (Typharm) PoM
Cream, fludroxycortide 0.0125%, net price 60 g = £3.26. Label: 28. Potency: moderate
Excipients: include cetyl alcohol, propylene glycol
Ointment, fludroxycortide 0.0125%, net price 60 g = £3.26. Label: 28. Potency: moderate
Excipients: include beeswax, cetyl alcohol, polysorbate
Tape, polythene adhesive film impregnated with fludroxycortide 4 micrograms/cm^2, net price 7.5 cm × 50 cm = £9.27, 7.5 cm × 200 cm = £24.95
Dose: for chronic localised recalcitrant dermatoses (but not acute or weeping), cut tape to fit lesion, apply to clean, dry skin shorn of hair, usually for 12 of each 24 hours

FLUOCINOLONE ACETONIDE

Indications: inflammatory skin disorders such as eczemas; psoriasis, see notes above
Cautions: see notes above
Contra-indications: see notes above
Side-effects: see notes above
Dose: apply thinly 1–2 times daily, reducing strength as condition responds

Synalar® (GP Pharma) PoM
Cream, fluocinolone acetonide 0.025%, net price 30 g = £2.26, 100 g = £6.42. Label: 28. Potency: potent
Excipients: include benzyl alcohol, cetostearyl alcohol, polysorbates, propylene glycol
Gel, fluocinolone acetonide 0.025%, net price 30 g = £3.34. For use on scalp and other hairy areas. Label: 28. Potency: potent
Excipients: include hydroxybenzoates (parabens), propylene glycol

Ointment, fluocinolone acetonide 0.025%, net price 30 g = £2.26, 100 g = £6.42. Label: 28. Potency: potent
Excipients: include propylene glycol, wool fat

Synalar 1 in 4 Dilution® (GP Pharma) PoM
Cream, fluocinolone acetonide 0.00625%, net price 50 g = £2.64. Label: 28. Potency: moderate
Excipients: include benzyl alcohol, cetostearyl alcohol, polysorbates, propylene glycol
Ointment, fluocinolone acetonide 0.00625%, net price 50 g = £2.64. Label: 28. Potency: moderate
Excipients: include propylene glycol, wool fat

Synalar 1 in 10 Dilution® (GP Pharma) PoM
Cream, fluocinolone acetonide 0.0025%, net price 50 g = £2.50. Label: 28. Potency: mild
Excipients: include benzyl alcohol, cetostearyl alcohol, polysorbates, propylene glycol

■ With antibacterials

See notes above for comment on compound preparations

Synalar C® (GP Pharma) PoM
Cream, fluocinolone acetonide 0.025%, clioquinol 3%, net price 15 g = £1.46. Label: 28. Potency: potent
Excipients: include cetostearyl alcohol, disodium edetate, hydroxybenzoates (parabens), polysorbates, propylene glycol
Ointment, ingredients as for cream, net price 15 g = £1.46. Label: 28. Potency: potent.
NOTE. stains clothing
Excipients: include propylene glycol, wool fat

Synalar N® (GP Pharma) PoM
Cream, fluocinolone acetonide 0.025%, neomycin sulphate 0.5%, net price 30 g = £2.38. Label: 28. Potency: potent
Excipients: include cetostearyl alcohol, hydroxybenzoates (parabens), polysorbates, propylene glycol
Ointment, ingredients as for cream, in a greasy basis, net price 30 g = £2.38. Label: 28. Potency: potent
Excipients: include propylene glycol, wool fat

FLUOCINONIDE

Indications: severe inflammatory skin disorders such as eczemas unresponsive to less potent corticosteroids; psoriasis, see notes above
Cautions: see notes above
Contra-indications: see notes above
Side-effects: see notes above
Dose: apply thinly 1–2 times daily

Metosyn® (GP Pharma) PoM
FAPG cream, fluocinonide 0.05%, net price 25 g = £1.98, 100 g = £6.68. Label: 28. Potency: potent
Excipients: include propylene glycol
Ointment, fluocinonide 0.05%, net price 25 g = £1.76, 100 g = £6.59. Label: 28. Potency: potent
Excipients: include propylene glycol, wool fat

FLUOCORTOLONE

Indications: severe inflammatory skin disorders such as eczemas unresponsive to less potent corticosteroids; psoriasis, see notes above
Cautions: see notes above
Contra-indications: see notes above
Side-effects: see notes above
Dose: apply thinly 1–2 times daily, reducing strength as condition responds

Ultralanum Plain® (Meadow) PoM
Cream, fluocortolone caproate 0.25%, fluocortolone pivalate 0.25%, net price 50 g = £2.95. Label: 28. Potency: moderate
Excipients: include disodium edetate, fragrance, hydroxybenzoates (parabens), stearyl alcohol
Ointment, fluocortolone 0.25%, fluocortolone caproate 0.25%, net price 50 g = £2.95. Label: 28. Potency: moderate
Excipients: include wool fat, fragrance

FLUPREDNIDENE ACETATE

Indications: see notes above
Cautions: see notes above
Contra-indications: see notes above
Side-effects: see notes above
Dose: see preparation below

■ With antimicrobials

Acorvio® **Plus** (Ferndale) PoM
Cream, fluprednidene acetate 0.1%, miconazole nitrate 2%, net price 20 g = £5.25, 45 g = £ 8.10. Label: 28. Potency: potent
Excipients: include propylene glycol, stearyl alcohol
Dose: inflammatory dermatophyte, candidal and fungal skin conditions, apply thinly twice daily for up to 1 week (max. 2 weeks)

FLUTICASONE PROPIONATE

Indications: inflammatory skin disorders such as dermatitis and eczemas unresponsive to less potent corticosteroids
Cautions: see notes above
Contra-indications: see notes above
Side-effects: see notes above
Dose: apply thinly 1–2 times daily

Cutivate® (GSK) PoM
Cream, fluticasone propionate 0.05%, net price 15 g = £2.41, 50 g = £7.11. Label: 28. Potency: potent
Excipients: include cetostearyl alcohol, imidurea, propylene glycol
Ointment, fluticasone propionate 0.005%, net price 15 g = £2.41, 50 g = £7.11. Label: 28. Potency: potent
Excipients: include propylene glycol

HALCINONIDE

Indications: short-term treatment only of severe resistant inflammatory skin disorders such as recalcitrant eczemas unresponsive to less potent corticosteroids; psoriasis, see notes above
Cautions: see notes above
Contra-indications: see notes above
Side-effects: see notes above
Dose: apply thinly 1–2 times daily

Halciderm Topical® (Squibb) PoM
Cream, halcinonide 0.1%, net price 30 g = £3.16. Label: 28. Potency: very potent
Excipients: include propylene glycol

MOMETASONE FUROATE

Indications: severe inflammatory skin disorders such as eczemas unresponsive to less potent corticosteroids; psoriasis, see notes above
Cautions: see notes above
Contra-indications: see notes above
Side-effects: see notes above
Dose: apply thinly once daily (to scalp in case of lotion)

Elocon® (Schering-Plough) PoM
Cream, mometasone furoate 0.1%, net price 30 g = £4.54, 100 g = £13.07. Label: 28. Potency: potent
Excipients: include stearyl alcohol
Ointment, mometasone furoate 0.1%, net price 30 g = £4.54, 100 g = £13.07. Label: 28. Potency: potent
Excipients: none as listed in section 13.1.3

Scalp lotion, mometasone furoate 0.1% in an aqueous isopropyl alcohol basis, net price 30 mL = £4.54. Label: 28. Potency: potent
Excipients: include propylene glycol

TRIAMCINOLONE ACETONIDE

Indications: severe inflammatory skin disorders such as eczemas unresponsive to less potent corticosteroids; psoriasis, see notes above
Cautions: see notes above
Contra-indications: see notes above
Side-effects: see notes above
Dose: apply thinly 1–2 times daily

■ With antimicrobials
See notes above for comment on compound preparations

Aureocort® (Lederle) PoM
Ointment, triamcinolone acetonide 0.1%, chlortetracycline hydrochloride 3%, in an anhydrous greasy basis containing wool fat and white soft paraffin, net price 15 g = £2.70. Label: 28. Potency: potent
Excipients: include wool fat
NOTE. Stains clothing

Tri-Adcortyl® (Squibb) PoM
Cream, triamcinolone acetonide 0.1%, gramicidin 0.025%, neomycin (as sulphate) 0.25%, nystatin 100 000 units/g, net price 30 g = £3.15. Label: 28. Potency: potent
Excipients: include benzyl alcohol, ethylenediamine, propylene glycol, fragrance
Ointment, triamcinolone acetonide 0.1%, gramicidin 0.025%, neomycin (as sulphate) 0.25%, nystatin 100 000 units/g, net price 30 g = £3.15. Label: 28. Potency: potent
Excipients: none as listed in section 13.1.3
NOTE. Not recommended owing to presence of ethylenediamine in the cream and also because combination of antibacterial with antifungal not considered useful in either the cream or ointment

13.5 Preparations for eczema and psoriasis

13.5.1 Preparations for eczema

Eczema (dermatitis) has several causes, which may influence treatment. The main types of eczema are irritant, allergic contact, atopic, venous and discoid; different types may co-exist. Lichenification, due to scratching and rubbing, may complicate any chronic eczema. *Atopic eczema* is the most common type and it usually involves dry skin as well as infection and lichenification.

Management of eczema involves the removal or treatment of contributory factors including occupational and domestic irritants. Known or suspected contact allergens should be avoided. Rarely, ingredients in topical medicinal products may sensitise the skin; the BNF lists active ingredients together with excipients that have been associated with skin sensitisation.

Skin dryness and the consequent irritant eczema requires **emollients** (section 13.2.1) applied regularly and liberally to the affected area; this may be supplemented with bath or shower emollients. The use of emollients should continue even if the eczema improves or if other treatment is being used.

Topical corticosteroids (section 13.4) are also required in the management of eczema; the potency of the corticosteroid should be appropriate to the severity and site of the condition. Mild corticosteroids are generally used on the face and on flexures; potent corticosteroids are generally required for use on adults with discoid or lichenified eczema or with eczema on the scalp, limbs, and trunk. Treatment should be reviewed regularly, especially if a potent corticosteroid is required. Bandages (including those containing **zinc** and **ichthammol**) are sometimes applied over topical corticosteroids to treat eczema of the limbs.

INFECTION. Bacterial infection (commonly with *Staphylococcus aureus* and occasionally with *Streptococcus pyogenes*) can exacerbate eczema and requires treatment with topical or systemic **antibacterial drugs** (section 13.10.1 and section 5.1). Antibacterial drugs, particularly fusidic acid, should be used in short courses (typically 1 week) to reduce the risk of drug resistance or skin sensitisation. Associated eczema is treated simultaneously with a topical corticosteroid usually of moderate or high potency.

Eczema involving widespread or recurrent infection requires the use of a systemic antibacterial that is active against the infecting organism. Products that combine an antiseptic with an emollient application (section 13.2.1) and with a bath emollient (section 13.2.1.1) may also be used; antiseptic shampoos (section 13.9) may be used on the scalp.

Intertriginous eczema commonly involves candida and bacteria; it is best treated with a mild or moderately potent topical corticosteroid and a suitable antimicrobial drug.

Widespread herpes simplex infection may complicate atopic eczema and treatment with a systemic antiviral drug (section 5.3.2.1) is indicated.

The management of *seborrhoeic dermatitis* is described below.

MANAGEMENT OF OTHER FEATURES OF ECZEMA. *Lichenification*, which results from repeated scratching is treated initially with a potent corticosteroid. Bandages containing **ichthammol paste** (to reduce pruritus) and other substances such as **zinc oxide** may be applied over the corticosteroid. **Coal tar** (section 13.5.2) and **ichthammol** can be useful in some cases of *chronic eczema*.

Antihistamines (section 3.4.1) may be of some value in relieving the itch of eczema, usually because of their sedating effect.

Exudative ('*weeping*') *eczema* requires a potent corticosteroid initially; infection may also be present and require specific treatment (see above). **Potassium permanganate** solution (1 in 10 000) can be used in exudating eczema for its antiseptic and astringent effect; treatment should be stopped when exudation stops.

Severe refractory eczema is best managed under specialist supervision; it may require phototherapy, systemic corticosteroids (section 6.3.2), or other drugs acting on the immune system (section 13.5.3).

SEBORRHOEIC DERMATITIS. *Seborrhoeic dermatitis (seborrhoeic eczema)* is associated with species of the yeast *Malassezia* and affects the scalp, paranasal areas, and eyebrows. Shampoos active against the yeast (including those containing ketoconazole and coal tar, section 13.9) and combinations of mild corticosteroids with suitable antimicrobials (section 13.4) are used.

ICHTHAMMOL

Indications: chronic lichenified eczema
Side-effects: skin irritation
Dose: apply 1–3 times daily

Ichthammol Ointment, BP 1980
Ointment, ichthammol 10%, yellow soft paraffin 45%, wool fat 45%, net price 25 g = 53p

Zinc and Ichthammol Cream, BP
Cream, ichthammol 5%, cetostearyl alcohol 3%, wool fat 10%, in zinc cream, net price 100 g = 79p

Zinc Paste and Ichthammol Bandage, BP 1993
See Appendix 8 (section A8.2.9)

13.5.2 Preparations for psoriasis

Psoriasis is characterised by epidermal thickening and scaling. It commonly affects extensor surfaces and the scalp. For mild psoriasis, reassurance and treatment with an emollient may be all that is necessary.

Occasionally psoriasis is provoked or exacerbated by drugs such as lithium, chloroquine and hydroxychloroquine, beta-blockers, non-steroidal anti-inflammatory drugs, and ACE inhibitors. Psoriasis may not be seen until the drug has been taken for weeks or months.

Emollients (section 13.2.1), in addition to their effects on dryness, scaling and cracking, may have an antiproliferative effect in psoriasis. They are particularly useful in *inflammatory psoriasis* and in *plaque psoriasis of palms and soles*, in which irritant factors can perpetuate the condition. Emollients are useful adjuncts to other more specific treatment.

More specific treatment for *chronic stable plaque psoriasis* on extensor surfaces of trunk and limbs involves the use of **vitamin D analogues, coal tar, dithranol**, and the retinoid **tazarotene**. However, they can irritate the skin and they are not suitable for the more inflammatory forms of psoriasis; their use should be suspended during an inflammatory phase of psoriasis. The efficacy and the irritancy of each substance varies between patients. If a substance irritates significantly, it should be stopped or the concentration reduced; if it is tolerated, its effects should be assessed after 4 to 6 weeks and treatment continued if it is effective.

Widespread *unstable psoriasis* of erythrodermic or generalised pustular type requires urgent specialist assessment. Initial topical treatment should be limited to using emollients frequently and generously; emollients should be prescribed in quantities of 1 kg or more. More localised acute or subacute *inflammatory psoriasis* with hot, spreading or itchy lesions, should be treated topically with emollients or with a corticosteroid of medium potency.

Calcipotriol and **tacalcitol** are analogues of vitamin D that affect cell division and differentiation. **Calcitriol** is an active form of vitamin D. Vitamin D and its analogues do not smell or stain and they may be more acceptable than tar or dithranol products. Of the vitamin D analogues, tacalcitol and calcitriol are less likely to irritate.

Coal tar has anti-inflammatory properties that are useful in chronic plaque psoriasis; it also has antiscaling properties. Crude coal tar (coal tar, BP) is the most effective form, typically in a concentration of 1 to 10% in a soft paraffin base, but few outpatients tolerate the smell and mess. Cleaner extracts of coal tar included in proprietary preparations, are more practicable for home use but they are less effective and improvement takes longer. Contact of coal tar products with normal skin is not normally harmful and they can be used for widespread small lesions; however, irritation, contact allergy, and sterile folliculitis can occur. The milder tar extracts can be used on the face and flexures. Tar baths and tar shampoos are also helpful.

Dithranol is effective for chronic plaque psoriasis. Its major disadvantages are irritation (for which individual susceptibility varies) and staining of skin and of clothing. It should be applied to chronic extensor plaques only, carefully avoiding normal skin. Dithranol is not generally suitable for widespread small lesions nor should it be used in the flexures or on the face. Treatment should be started with a low concentration such as dithranol 0.1%, and the strength increased gradually every few days up to 3%, according to tolerance. Proprietary preparations are more suitable for home use; they are usually washed off after 5 to 60 minutes ('short contact'). Specialist nurses may apply intensive treatment with dithranol paste which is covered by stockinette dressings and usually retained overnight. Dithranol should be discontinued if even a low concentration causes acute inflammation; continued use can result in the psoriasis becoming unstable. When applying dithranol, hands should be protected by gloves or they should be washed thoroughly afterwards.

Tazarotene, a retinoid, is effective in psoriasis. It is clean and odourless. Irritation is common but it is minimised by applying tazarotene sparingly to the plaques and avoiding normal skin.

A topical **corticosteroid** (section 13.4) is not generally suitable as the sole treatment of extensive chronic plaque psoriasis; any early improvement is not usually maintained and there is a risk of the condition deteriorating or of precipitating an unstable form of psoriasis (e.g. erythrodermic psoriasis or generalised pustular psoriasis). However, it may be appropriate to treat psoriasis in specific sites such as the face and flexures usually with a mild corticosteroid, and psoriasis of the scalp, hands and feet with a potent corticosteroid.

Combining the use of a corticosteroid with another specific topical treatment may be beneficial in chronic plaque psoriasis; the drugs may be used separately at different times of the day or used together in a single formulation. *Eczema* co-existing with psoriasis may be treated with a corticosteroid, or coal tar, or both.

Scalp psoriasis is usually scaly, and the scale may be thick and adherent. This requires softening with an emollient ointment, cream, or oil and usually combined with **salicylic acid** as a keratolytic.

Some preparations prescribed for psoriasis affecting the scalp combine salicylic acid with coal tar or **sulphur**. Preparations containing salicylic acid, sulphur, and coal tar are available as proprietary products. The product should be applied generously and an adequate quantity should be prescribed. It should be left on for at least an hour, often more conveniently overnight, before washing it off. If a corticosteroid lotion or gel is required (e.g. for itch), it can be used in the morning.

PHOTOTHERAPY. **Ultraviolet B** (UVB) radiation is usually effective for *chronic stable psoriasis* and for *guttate psoriasis*. It may be considered for patients with moderately severe psoriasis in whom topical treatment has failed, but it may irritate inflammatory psoriasis. Narrow-band UVB is more effective and it is less likely to burn than conventional broad-band therapy.

Photochemotherapy combining long-wave ultraviolet A radiation with a psoralen (PUVA) is available in dermatology centres. The psoralen, which enhances the effect of the irradiation, is administered either by mouth or topically. PUVA is effective in most forms of psoriasis, including the *unstable forms of psoriasis* and *localised palmoplantar pustular psoriasis*. Early adverse effects include phototoxicity and pruritus. Higher cumulative doses exaggerate signs of skin ageing, increase the risk of dysplastic and neoplastic skin lesions especially squamous cancer, and pose a theoretical risk of cataracts.

SYSTEMIC TREATMENT. **Systemic treatment** is required for severe, resistant, unstable or complicated forms of psoriasis, and it should be initiated only under specialist supervision. Systemic drugs for psoriasis include acitretin and drugs that act on the immune system (such as ciclosporin, hydroxycarbamide, and methotrexate, section 13.5.3).

Systemic corticosteroids should be used only rarely in psoriasis because rebound deterioration may occur on reducing the dose.

The main indication for **acitretin** is *psoriasis*, but it is also used in disorders of keratinisation such as severe *Darier's disease* (keratosis follicularis), and some forms of *ichthyosis*. Acitretin, a metabolite of etretinate, is a retinoid (vitamin A derivative). Although a minority of cases of psoriasis respond well to acitretin alone, it is only moderately effective in many cases and it is combined with other treatments. A therapeutic effect occurs after 2 to 4 weeks and the maximum benefit after 4 to 6 weeks or longer. Acitretin is prescribed by specialists and its availability is limited to hospital pharmacies or to a small number of specified retail pharmacies.

Apart from teratogenicity, which remains a risk for 2 years after stopping, acitretin is the least toxic systemic treatment for psoriasis; in women with a potential for child-bearing, the possibility of pregnancy must be excluded before treatment and pregnancy must be avoided during treatment and for a period of 2 years afterwards. Common side effects derive from its widespread but reversible effects on epithelia, such as dry and cracking lips, dry skin and mucosal surfaces, hair thinning, paronychia, and soft and sticky palms and soles. Liver function and blood lipid concentration should be monitored.

Topical preparations for psoriasis

Vitamin D and analogues

Calcipotriol, **calcitriol**, and **tacalcitol** are used for the management of *plaque psoriasis*. They should be avoided by those with calcium metabolism disorders, and used with caution in *generalised pustular* or *erythrodermic exfoliative psoriasis* (enhanced risk of hypercalcaemia). Local skin reactions (itching, erythema, burning, paraesthesia, dermatitis) are common. Hands should be washed thoroughly after application to avoid inadvertent transfer to other body areas. Aggravation of psoriasis has also been reported.

CALCIPOTRIOL

Indications: plaque psoriasis
Cautions: see notes above; pregnancy (Appendix 4); avoid use on face; if used with UV treatment apply at least 2 hours before UV exposure
Contra-indications: see notes above
Side-effects: see notes above; also photosensitivity; rarely facial or perioral dermatitis, skin atrophy
Dose: *cream* or *ointment* apply once or twice daily; max. 100 g weekly (less with *scalp solution*, see below); CHILD over 6 years, apply twice daily; 6–12 years max. 50 g weekly; over 12 years max. 75 g weekly
NOTE. Patient information leaflets for *Dovonex*® cream and ointment advise liberal application (but note max. recommended weekly dose, above)

Dovonex® (Leo) PoM
Cream, calcipotriol 50 micrograms/g, net price 60 g = £13.04, 120 g = £26.07
Excipients: include cetostearyl alcohol, disodium edetate
Ointment, calcipotriol 50 micrograms/g, net price 60 g = £12.02, 120 g = £26.07
Excipients: include disodium edetate, propylene glycol
Scalp solution, calcipotriol 50 micrograms/mL, net price 60 mL = £13.04, 120 mL = £26.07
Excipients: include propylene glycol
Dose: scalp psoriasis, apply to scalp twice daily; max. 60 mL weekly (less with cream or ointment, see below); CHILD not recommended
NOTE. When preparations used together max. total calcipotriol 5 mg in any one week (e.g. scalp solution 60 mL with cream or ointment 30 g *or* cream or ointment 60 g with scalp solution 30 mL)

■ With betamethasone
For cautions, contra-indications, side-effects, and for comment on the limited role of corticosteroids in psoriasis, see section 13.4.

Dovobet® (LEO) PoM
Ointment, betamethasone 0.05% (as dipropionate), calcipotriol 50 micrograms/g, net price 60 g = £35.00. Label: 28
Excipients: none as listed in section 13.1.3
Dose: initial treatment of stable plaque psoriasis, apply once daily to max. 30% of body surface for up to 4 weeks; max. 15 g daily, max. 100 g weekly; CHILD and ADOLESCENT under 18 years not recommended

CALCITRIOL

(1,25-Dihydroxycholecalciferol)
Indications: mild to moderate plaque psoriasis
Cautions: see notes above; liver impairment (Appendix 2), renal impairment (Appendix 3); pregnancy (Appendix 4)

Contra-indications: see notes above; do not apply under occlusion
Side-effects: see notes above
Dose: apply twice daily; not more than 35% of body surface to be treated daily, max. 30 g daily; CHILD not recommended

Silkis® (Galderma) ▼ PoM
Ointment, calcitriol 3 micrograms/g, net price 30 g = £5.76, 100 g = £16.34
Excipients: none as listed in section 13.1.3

TACALCITOL

Indications: plaque psoriasis
Cautions: see notes above; pregnancy (Appendix 4), breast-feeding (Appendix 5); avoid eyes; monitor plasma calcium if risk of hypercalcaemia or in renal impairment; if used in conjunction with UV treatment, UV radiation should be given in the morning and tacalcitol applied at bedtime
Contra-indications: see notes above
Side-effects: see notes above
Dose: apply daily preferably at bedtime; max. 10 g daily; CHILD not recommended

Curatoderm® (Crookes) PoM
Ointment, tacalcitol (as monohydrate) 4 micrograms/g, net price 30 g = £15.09, 60 g = £26.06, 100 g = £34.75
Excipients: none as listed in section 13.1.3

Tazarotene

TAZAROTENE

Indications: mild to moderate plaque psoriasis affecting up to 10% of skin area
Cautions: wash hands immediately after use, avoid contact with eyes, face, intertriginous areas, hair-covered scalp, eczematous or inflamed skin; avoid excessive exposure to UV light (including sunlight, solariums, PUVA or UVB treatment); do not apply emollients or cosmetics within 1 hour of application
Contra-indications: pregnancy—advise women of child-bearing age to ensure adequate contraceptive protection; breast-feeding (Appendix 5)
Side-effects: local irritation (more common with higher concentration and may require discontinuation), pruritus, burning, erythema, desquamation, non-specific rash, contact dermatitis, and worsening of psoriasis; rarely stinging and inflamed, dry or painful skin
Dose: apply once daily in the evening usually for up to 12 weeks; CHILD under 18 years not recommended

Zorac® (Allergan) PoM
Gel, tazarotene 0.05%, net price 30 g = £14.09; 0.1%, 30 g = £14.80
Excipients: include benzyl alcohol, butylated hydroxyanisole, butylated hydroxytoluene, disodium edetate, polysorbate 40

Coal tar

COAL TAR

Indications: psoriasis and occasionally chronic atopic eczema
Cautions: avoid eyes, mucosa, genital or rectal areas, and broken or inflamed skin; use suitable chemical protection gloves for extemporaneous preparation
Contra-indications: not for use in sore, acute, or pustular psoriasis or in presence of infection
Side-effects: skin irritation and acne-like eruptions, photosensitivity; stains skin, hair, and fabric
Dose: apply 1–3 times daily starting with low-strength preparations

NOTE. For shampoo preparations see section 13.9; impregnated dressings see Appendix 8 (section A8.2.9)

■ Non-proprietary preparations

May be difficult to obtain—some patients may find newer proprietary preparations more acceptable

Calamine and Coal Tar Ointment, BP
Ointment, calamine 12.5 g, strong coal tar solution 2.5 g, zinc oxide 12.5 g, hydrous wool fat 25 g, white soft paraffin 47.5 g
Excipients: include wool fat
Dose: apply 1–2 times daily

Coal Tar and Salicylic Acid Ointment, BP
Ointment, coal tar 2 g, salicylic acid 2 g, emulsifying wax 11.4 g, white soft paraffin 19 g, coconut oil 54 g, polysorbate '80' 4 g, liquid paraffin 7.6 g
Excipients: include cetostearyl alcohol
Dose: apply 1–2 times daily

Coal Tar Paste, BP
Paste, strong coal tar solution 7.5%, in compound zinc paste
Dose: apply 1–2 times daily

Zinc and Coal Tar Paste, BP
Paste, zinc oxide 6%, coal tar 6%, emulsifying wax 5%, starch 38%, yellow soft paraffin 45%
Excipients: include cetostearyl alcohol
Dose: apply 1–2 times daily

■ Proprietary preparations

Carbo-Dome® (Sandoz)
Cream, coal tar solution 10%, in a water-miscible basis, net price 30 g = £4.77, 100 g = £16.38
Excipients: include beeswax, hydroxybenzoates (parabens)
Dose: psoriasis, apply to skin 2–3 times daily

Clinitar® (CHS)
Cream, coal tar extract 1%, net price 100 g = £10.99
Excipients: include cetostearyl alcohol, isopropyl palmitate, propylene glycol
Dose: psoriasis and eczema, apply to skin 1–2 times daily

Cocois® (Celltech)
Scalp ointment, coal tar solution 12%, salicylic acid 2%, precipitated sulphur 4%, in a coconut oil emollient basis, net price 40 g (with applicator nozzle) = £6.65, 100 g = £12.30
Excipients: include cetostearyl alcohol
Dose: scaly scalp disorders including psoriasis, eczema, seborrhoeic dermatitis and dandruff, apply to scalp once weekly as necessary (if severe use daily for first 3–7 days), shampoo off after 1 hour; CHILD 6–12 years, medical supervision required (not recommended under 6 years)
NOTE. Brands of ointment containing coal tar solution 12%, salicylic acid 2%, precipitated sulphur 4% include *Sebco*®

Exorex® (Forest)
Lotion, prepared coal tar 1% in an emollient basis, net price 100 mL = £8.11, 250 mL = £16.24
Excipients: include hydroxybenzoates (parabens), polysorbate 80
Dose: psoriasis, apply to skin or scalp 2–3 times daily; CHILD and ELDERLY, dilute with a few drops of water before applying

Pragmatar® (Alliance)
Cream, cetyl alcohol-coal tar distillate 4%, salicylic acid 3%, sulphur (precipitated) 3%, net price 25 g = £3.04, 100 g = £9.82
Excipients: include cetyl alcohol, fragrance
Dose: scaly skin disorders, apply thinly once daily; dandruff and other seborrhoeic conditions, apply to scalp once weekly or in severe cases daily; INFANT dilute with a few drops of water before application

Psoriderm® (Dermal)
Cream, coal tar 6%, lecithin 0.4%, net price 225 mL = £3.30
Excipients: include isopropyl palmitate, propylene glycol
Dose: psoriasis, apply to skin or scalp 1–2 times daily
Scalp lotion—section 13.9

■ Bath preparations

Coal Tar Solution, BP
Solution, coal tar 20%, polysorbate '80' 5%, in alcohol (96%), net price 100 mL = 91p
Excipients: include polysorbates
Dose: use 100 mL in a bath
NOTE. Strong Coal Tar Solution BP contains coal tar 40%

Polytar Emollient® (Stiefel)
Bath additive, coal tar solution 2.5%, arachis (peanut) oil extract of coal tar 7.5%, tar 7.5%, cade oil 7.5%, liquid paraffin 35%, net price 500 mL = £5.78
Excipients: include isopropyl palmitate
Dose: psoriasis, eczema, atopic and pruritic dermatoses, use 2–4 capfuls (15–30 mL) in bath and soak for 20 minutes

Psoriderm® (Dermal)
Bath emulsion, coal tar 40%, net price 200 mL = £2.87
Excipients: include polysorbate 20
Dose: psoriasis, use 30 mL in a bath and soak for 5 minutes

■ With corticosteroids

Alphosyl HC® (GSK Consumer Healthcare) PoM
Cream, coal tar extract 5%, hydrocortisone 0.5%, allantoin 2%, net price 100 g = £3.54. Label: 28. Potency: mild
Excipients: include beeswax, cetyl alcohol, hydroxybenzoates (parabens), isopropyl palmitate, wool fat
Dose: psoriasis, apply thinly 1–2 times daily; CHILD under 5 years not recommended

Dithranol

DITHRANOL

(Anthralin)

Indications: subacute and chronic psoriasis, see notes above

Cautions: avoid use near eyes and sensitive areas of skin; see also notes above

Contra-indications: hypersensitivity; acute and pustular psoriasis

Side-effects: local burning sensation and irritation; stains skin, hair, and fabrics

Dose: see notes above and under preparations
NOTE. Some of these dithranol preparations also contain coal tar or salicylic acid—for cautions and side-effects see under Coal Tar (above) or under Salicylic Acid

■ Non-proprietary preparations

[1]**Dithranol Ointment, BP** PoM
Ointment, dithranol, in yellow soft paraffin; usual strengths 0.1–2%. Part of basis may be replaced by hard paraffin if a stiffer preparation is required. Label: 28

1. PoM if dithranol content more than 1%, otherwise may be sold to the public

Dithranol Paste, BP
Paste, dithranol in zinc and salicylic acid (Lassar's) paste. Usual strengths 0.1–1% of dithranol. Label: 28

■ Proprietary preparations

Dithrocream® (Dermal)
Cream, dithranol 0.1%, net price 50 g = £3.94; 0.25%, 50 g = £4.23; 0.5%, 50 g = £4.87; 1%, 50 g = £5.67; PoM 2%, 50 g = £7.10. Label: 28
Excipients: include cetostearyl alcohol, chlorocresol
Dose: for application to skin or scalp; 0.1–0.5% suitable for overnight treatment, 1–2% for max. 1 hour

Micanol® (GP Pharma)
Cream, dithranol 1% in a lipid-stabilised basis, net price 50 g = £10.37; PoM 3%, 50 g = £12.92. Label: 28
Excipients: none as listed in section 13.1.3
Dose: for application to skin, for up to 30 minutes, if necessary 3% cream may be used under medical supervision; apply to scalp for up to 30 minutes
NOTE. At the end of contact time use plenty of lukewarm (not hot) water to rinse off cream; soap should not be used

Psorin® (LPC)
Ointment, dithranol 0.11%, coal tar 1%, salicylic acid 1.6%, net price 50 g = £8.20, 100 g = £16.35. Label: 28
Excipients: include beeswax, wool fat
Dose: for application to skin up to twice daily

Scalp gel, dithranol 0.25%, salicylic acid 1.6% in gel basis containing methyl salicylate, net price 50 g = £6.25. Label: 28
Excipients: none as listed in section 13.1.3
Dose: for application to scalp, initially apply on alternate days for 10–20 minutes; may be increased to daily application for max. 1 hour and then wash off

Salicylic acid

SALICYLIC ACID

For coal tar preparations containing salicylic acid, see under Coal Tar p. 576; for dithranol preparations containing salicylic acid see under Dithranol, above

Indications: hyperkeratotic skin disorders; acne (section 13.6.1); warts and calluses (section 13.7); scalp conditions (section 13.9); fungal nail infections (section 13.10.2)

Cautions: see notes above; avoid broken or inflamed skin
SALICYLATE TOXICITY. If large areas of skin are treated, salicylate toxicity may be a hazard

Side-effects: sensitivity, excessive drying, irritation, systemic effects after widespread use (see under Cautions)

Zinc and Salicylic Acid Paste, BP
Paste, (Lassar's Paste), zinc oxide 24%, salicylic acid 2%, starch 24%, white soft paraffin 50%, net price 25 g = 17p
Dose: apply twice daily

Oral retinoids for psoriasis

ACITRETIN

NOTE. Acitretin is a metabolite of etretinate

Indications: severe extensive psoriasis resistant to other forms of therapy; palmoplantar pustular psoriasis; severe congenital ichthyosis; severe Darier's disease (keratosis follicularis)

Cautions: exclude pregnancy before starting (test for pregnancy within 2 weeks before treatment and monthly thereafter; start treatment on day 2 or 3 of menstrual cycle)—women (including those with history of infertility) should avoid pregnancy for at least 1 month before, during, and for at least 2 years after treatment; patients should avoid concomitant tetracycline or methotrexate, high doses of vitamin A (more than 4000–5000 units daily) and use of keratolytics, and should not donate blood during or for at least 1 year after stopping therapy (teratogenic risk); check liver function at start, then every 1–2 weeks for 2 months, then every 3 months; monitor plasma lipids; diabetes (can alter glucose tolerance—initial frequent blood glucose checks); radiographic assessment on long-term treatment; investigate atypical musculoskeletal symptoms; in children use only in exceptional circumstances (premature epiphyseal closure reported); avoid excessive exposure to sunlight and unsupervised use of sunlamps; **interactions:** Appendix 1 (retinoids)

Contra-indications: hepatic impairment (Appendix 2); renal impairment (Appendix 3); hyperlipidaemia, pregnancy (**important teratogenic risk:** see Cautions above); breast-feeding

Side-effects: dryness of mucous membranes (sometimes erosion), of skin (sometimes scaling, thinning, erythema especially of face, and pruritus), and of conjunctiva (sometimes conjunctivitis and decreased tolerance of contact lenses); sticky skin, dermatitis; other side-effects reported include palmoplantar exfoliation, epistaxis, epidermal and nail fragility, oedema, paronychia, granulomatous lesions, bullous eruptions, reversible hair thinning and alopecia, myalgia and arthralgia, occasional nausea, headache, malaise, drowsiness, rhinitis, sweating, taste disturbance, and gingivitis; benign intracranial hypertension (discontinue if severe headache, vomiting, diarrhoea, abdominal pain, and visual disturbance occur; **avoid** concomitant tetracyclines); photosensitivity, corneal ulceration, raised liver enzymes, rarely jaundice and hepatitis (**avoid** concomitant methotrexate); raised triglycerides; decreased night vision reported; skeletal hyperostosis and extra-osseous calcification reported following long-term administration of etretinate (and premature epiphyseal closure in children, see Cautions)

Dose: under expert supervision, initially 25–30 mg daily (Darier's disease 10 mg daily) for 2–4 weeks, then adjusted according to response, usual range 25–50 mg daily (max. 75 mg daily) for further 6–8 weeks (in Darier's disease and ichthyosis not more than 50 mg daily for up to 6 months); CHILD (**important:** exceptional circumstances only, see Cautions), 500 micrograms/kg daily (occasionally up to 1 mg/kg daily to max. 35 mg daily for limited periods) with careful monitoring of musculoskeletal development

Neotigason® (Roche) PoM
Capsules, acitretin 10 mg (brown/white), net price 60-cap pack = £25.25; 25 mg (brown/yellow), 60-cap pack = £58.59 (hosp. or specified retail pharmacy only—consult product literature for details, specialist dermatological supervision). Label: 10, patient information leaflet, 21

13.5.3 Drugs affecting the immune response

Drugs affecting the immune response are used for eczema or psoriasis. Systemic drugs acting on the immune system are generally used by **specialists** in a hospital setting.

Ciclosporin (cyclosporin) by mouth can be used for *severe psoriasis* and for *severe eczema*. **Azathioprine** (section 8.2.1) or **mycophenolate mofetil** (section 8.2.1) are used for severe refractory eczema [unlicensed indication]. **Hydroxycarbamide** (hydroxyurea) (section 8.1.5) is used by mouth for severe psoriasis [unlicensed indication].

Methotrexate may be used for *severe psoriasis*, the dose being adjusted according to severity of the condition and haematological and biochemical measurements; the usual dose is methotrexate 10 to 25 mg **once weekly**, by mouth. Folic acid may be given to reduce the possibility of methotrexate toxicity. For *severe psoriasis* refractory to other systemic treatment and photochemotherapy or if other treatments are not tolerated, **efalizumab**, which inhibits T-cell activation and is licensed for moderate and severe *chronic plaque psoriasis*, or the cytokine inhibitor **etanercept** (section 10.1.3) may be used; etanercept and infliximab (section 10.1.3) are licensed for *psoriatic arthritis*.

Pimecrolimus by topical application is licensed for *mild to moderate atopic eczema* for short-term use to treat signs and symptoms and for intermittent use to prevent flares. **Tacrolimus** is licensed for topical use in *moderate to severe atopic eczema*. Both are drugs whose long-term safety and place in therapy is still being evaluated and they should not usually be considered first-line treatments unless there is a specific reason to avoid or reduce the use of topical corticosteroids.

For the role of corticosteroids in eczema see section 13.5.1 and for comment on their limited role in psoriasis see section 13.4.

NICE guidance (tacrolimus and pimecrolimus for atopic eczema). NICE has recommended (August 2004) that topical pimecrolimus and tacrolimus are options for atopic eczema not controlled by maximal topical corticosteroid treatment or if there is a risk of important corticosteroid side-effects (particularly skin atrophy).
Topical pimecrolimus is recommended for moderate atopic eczema on the face and neck of children aged 2–16 years and topical tacrolimus is recommended for moderate to severe atopic eczema in adults and children over 2 years. Pimecrolimus and tacrolimus should be used within their licensed indications.

CICLOSPORIN

(Cyclosporin)

Indications: see under Dose; transplantation and graft-versus-host disease (section 8.2.2)

Cautions: see section 8.2.2

ADDITIONAL CAUTIONS IN ATOPIC DERMATITIS AND PSORIASIS. ***Contra-indicated*** in abnormal renal function, hypertension not under control (see also below), infections not under control, and malignancy (see also below). Dermatological and physical examination, including blood pressure and renal function measurements required at least twice before starting; discontinue if hypertension develops that cannot be controlled by dose reduction or antihypertensive therapy; avoid excessive exposure to sunlight and use of UVB or PUVA; *in atopic dermatitis*, also allow herpes simplex infections to clear before starting (if they occur during treatment withdraw if severe); *Staphylococcus aureus* skin infections not absolute contra-indication providing controlled (but avoid erythromycin unless no other alternative—see also **interactions**: Appendix 1 (ciclosporin)); monitor serum creatinine every 2 weeks during treatment; *in psoriasis*, also exclude malignancies (including those of skin and cervix) before starting (biopsy any lesions not typical of psoriasis) and treat patients with malignant or pre-malignant conditions of skin only after appropriate treatment (and if no other option); monitor serum creatinine every 2 weeks for first 3 months then every 2 months (monthly if dose more than 2.5 mg/kg daily), reducing dose by 25–50% if increases more than 30% above baseline (even if within normal range) and discontinuing if reduction not successful within 1 month; also discontinue if lymphoproliferative disorder develops

Side-effects: see section 8.2.2

Dose: ADULT over 16 years *by mouth*, administered in accordance with expert advice

Short-term treatment (max. 8 weeks) of severe atopic dermatitis where conventional therapy ineffective or inappropriate, initially 2.5 mg/kg daily in 2 divided doses, if good initial response not achieved within 2 weeks, increase rapidly to max. 5 mg/kg daily; initial dose of 5 mg/kg daily in 2 divided doses if very severe; CHILD under 16 years not recommended

Severe psoriasis where conventional therapy ineffective or inappropriate, initially 2.5 mg/kg daily in 2 divided doses, increased gradually to max. 5 mg/kg daily if no improvement within 1 month (discontinue if response still insufficient after 6 weeks); initial dose of 5 mg/kg daily justified if condition requires rapid improvement; CHILD under 16 years not recommended

IMPORTANT. For preparations and counselling and for advice on conversion between the preparations, see section 8.2.2

■ Preparations

Section 8.2.2

EFALIZUMAB

Indications: moderate to severe chronic plaque psoriasis for those whose disease is unresponsive to, or who are intolerant of other systemic therapy or photochemotherapy

Cautions: low platelet count (monitor platelet count before treatment, monthly during initial therapy then every 3 months), hepatic impairment, renal impairment; **interactions:** Appendix 1 (efalizumab)

Contra-indications: immunodeficiency, severe infection, active tuberculosis; history of malignancy; pregnancy and breast-feeding (Appendix 5)

Side-effects: influenza-like symptoms, leucocytosis, arthralgia, exacerbation of psoriasis or development of variant forms including psoriatic arthritis (discontinue treatment), *less commonly* thrombocytopenia and injection-site reactions

Dose: *by subcutaneous injection*, initially 700 micrograms/kg then 1 mg/kg *weekly*; discontinue if inadequate response after 12 weeks; CHILD and ADOLESCENT not recommended

Raptiva® (Serono) ▼ PoM

Injection, powder for reconstitution, efalizumab, net price 125-mg vial = £169.20 (with 1.3 mL water for injections in prefilled syringe)

METHOTREXATE

Indications: severe psoriasis unresponsive to conventional therapy (specialist use only); Crohn's disease (section 1.5); malignant disease (section 8.1.3); rheumatoid arthritis (section 10.1.3)

Cautions: section 10.1.3; also photosensitivity—psoriasis lesions aggravated by UV radiation (skin ulceration reported)

Contra-indications: section 10.1.3

Side-effects: section 10.1.3

Dose: *by mouth*, 10–25 mg once weekly, adjusted according to response; ELDERLY consider dose reduction (extreme caution); CHILD not recommended

> **Important.** Note that the above dose is a **weekly** dose. The CSM has received reports of prescription and dispensing errors including fatalities. Attention should be paid to the **strength** of methotrexate tablets prescribed and the **frequency** of dosing.

■ Preparations

Section 10.1.3

PIMECROLIMUS

Indications: acute treatment of mild to moderate atopic eczema (including flares)

Cautions: UV light (avoid excessive exposure to sunlight and sunlamps), avoid other topical treatments except emollients at treatment site

Contra-indications: contact with eyes and mucous membranes, application under occlusion, infection at treatment site; congenital epidermal barrier defects; generalised erythroderma

Side-effects: burning sensation, pruritus, erythema, skin infections (including folliculitis and rarely impetigo, herpes simplex and zoster, molluscum contagiosum); rarely papilloma; local reactions including pain, paraesthesia, peeling, dryness, oedema, and worsening of eczema

Dose: apply twice daily until symptoms resolve; CHILD under 2 years not recommended

Elidel® (Novartis) ▼ PoM

Cream, pimecrolimus 1%, net price 30 g = £19.69, 60 g = £37.41, 100 g = £59.07. Label: 28

Excipients: include benzyl alcohol, cetyl alcohol, propylene glycol, stearyl alcohol

TACROLIMUS

Indications: moderate to severe atopic eczema unresponsive to conventional therapy (prescribed by physicians experienced in treating atopic eczema); other indications section 8.2.2

Cautions: infection at treatment site, UV light (avoid excessive exposure to sunlight and sunlamps)

Contra-indications: avoid contact with eyes and mucous membranes, application under occlusion; congenital epidermal barrier defects; generalised erythroderma; pregnancy and breast-feeding

Side-effects: burning or tingling sensation, pruritus, erythema, folliculitis, acne, herpes simplex infection, increased sensitivity to hot and cold, alcohol intolerance; lymphadenopathy also reported

Dose: ADULT and ADOLESCENT over 16 years initially apply 0.1% ointment thinly twice daily until lesion clears (consider other treatment options if no improvement after 2 weeks); reduce to once daily or switch to 0.03% ointment if clinical condition allows; CHILD 2–15 years, initially apply 0.03% ointment twice daily for up to 3 weeks then reduce to once daily until lesion clears

Protopic® (Fujisawa) ▼ PoM

Ointment, tacrolimus (as monohydrate) 0.03%, net price 30 g = £19.44, 60 g = £36.94; 0.1%, 30 g = £21.60, 60 g = £41.04. Label: 4, 11, 28

Excipients: include beeswax

13.6 Acne and rosacea

ACNE. Treatment of acne should be commenced early to prevent scarring. Patients should be counselled that an improvement may not be seen for at least a couple of months. The choice of treatment depends on whether the acne is predominantly inflammatory or comedonal and its severity.

Mild to moderate acne is generally treated with topical preparations (section 13.6.1). Systemic treatment (section 13.6.2) with oral antibiotics is generally used for *moderate to severe acne* or where topical preparations are not tolerated or are ineffective or where application to the site is difficult. Another oral preparation used for acne is the hormone treatment co-cyprindiol (cyproterone acetate with ethinylestradiol); it is for women only.

Severe acne, acne unresponsive to prolonged courses of oral antibiotics, scarring, or acne associated with psychological problems calls for early referral to a consultant dermatologist who may prescribe isotretinoin for administration by mouth.

ROSACEA. Rosacea is not comedonal (but may exist with acne which may be comedonal). The pustules and papules of rosacea respond to topical metronidazole (section 13.10.1.2) or to oral administration of oxytetracycline or tetracycline 500 mg twice daily (section 5.1.3) or of erythromycin 500 mg twice daily (section 5.1.5); courses usually last 6–12 weeks and are repeated intermittently. Alternatively, doxycycline (section 5.1.3) in a dose of 100 mg once daily may be used [unlicensed indication] if oxytetracycline or tetracycline is inappropriate (e.g. in renal impairment). Isotretinoin is occasionally given in refractory cases [unlicensed indication]. Camouflagers (section 13.8.2) may be required for the redness.

13.6.1 Topical preparations for acne

Significant comedonal acne responds well to topical retinoids (see p. 581), whereas both comedones and inflamed lesions respond well to benzoyl peroxide or azelaic acid (see below). Alternatively, topical application of an antibiotic such as erythromycin or clindamycin may be effective for inflammatory acne. If topical preparations prove inadequate oral preparations may be needed (section 13.6.2).

Benzoyl peroxide and azelaic acid

Benzoyl peroxide is effective in mild to moderate acne. Both comedones and inflamed lesions respond well to benzoyl peroxide. The lower concentrations seem to be as effective as higher concentrations in reducing inflammation. It is usual to start with a lower strength and to increase the concentration of benzoyl peroxide gradually. Adverse effects include local skin irritation, particularly when therapy is initiated, but the scaling and redness often subside with treatment continued at a reduced frequency of application. If the acne does not respond after 2 months then use of a topical antibacterial should be considered.

Azelaic acid has antimicrobial and anticomedonal properties. It may be an alternative to benzoyl peroxide or to a topical retinoid for treating mild to moderate comedonal acne, particularly of the face. Some patients prefer it because it is less likely to cause local irritation than benzoyl peroxide.

BENZOYL PEROXIDE

Indications: acne vulgaris

Cautions: avoid contact with eyes, mouth, and mucous membranes; may bleach fabrics and hair; avoid excessive exposure to sunlight

Side-effects: skin irritation (reduce frequency or suspend use until irritation subsides and re-introduce at reduced frequency)

Dose: apply 1–2 times daily preferably after washing with soap and water, start treatment with lower-strength preparations

NOTE. May bleach clothing

Brevoxyl® (Stiefel)

Cream, benzoyl peroxide 4% in an aqueous basis, net price 40 g = £3.30

Excipients: include cetyl alcohol, fragrance, stearyl alcohol

PanOxyl® (Stiefel)

Aquagel (= aqueous gel), benzoyl peroxide 2.5%, net price 40 g = £1.76; 5%, 40 g = £1.92; 10%, 40 g = £2.07

Excipients: include propylene glycol

Cream, benzoyl peroxide 5% in a non-greasy basis, net price 40 g = £1.51

Excipients: include isopropyl palmitate, propylene glycol

Gel, benzoyl peroxide 5% in an aqueous alcoholic basis, net price 40 g = £1.51; 10%, 40 g = £1.69

Excipients: include fragrance

Wash, benzoyl peroxide 10% in a detergent basis, net price 150 mL = £4.00

Excipients: include imidurea

■ With antimicrobials

Benzamycin® (Schwarz) PoM
Gel, pack for reconstitution, providing erythromycin 3% and benzoyl peroxide 5% in an alcoholic basis, net price per pack to provide 46.6 g = £15.62
Excipients: none as listed in section 13.1.3
Dose: apply twice daily (very fair skin, initially once daily at night)

Duac® **Once Daily** (Stiefel) PoM
Gel, benzoyl peroxide 5%, clindamycin 1% (as phosphate) in an aqueous basis, net price 25 g = £9.95, 50 g = £19.90
Excipients: include disodium edetate
Dose: apply once daily in the evening

Quinoderm® (Ferndale)
Cream, benzoyl peroxide 5%, potassium hydroxyquinoline sulphate 0.5%, in an astringent vanishing-cream basis, net price 50 g = £2.21
Excipients: include cetostearyl alcohol, edetic acid (EDTA)
Cream, benzoyl peroxide 10%, potassium hydroxyquinoline sulphate 0.5%, in an astringent vanishing-cream basis, net price 25 g = £1.30, 50 g = £2.49
Excipients: include cetostearyl alcohol, edetic acid (EDTA)

AZELAIC ACID

Indications: acne vulgaris
Cautions: pregnancy, breast-feeding; avoid contact with eyes
Side-effects: local irritation (reduce frequency or discontinue use temporarily); rarely photosensitisation

Skinoren® (Schering Health) PoM
Cream, azelaic acid 20%, net price 30 g = £3.74
Excipients: include propylene glycol
Dose: apply twice daily (sensitive skin, once daily for first week). Extended treatment may be required but manufacturer advises period of treatment should not exceed 6 months

Topical antibacterials for acne

For many patients with mild to moderate inflammatory acne, topical antibacterials may be no more effective than topical benzoyl peroxide or tretinoin. Topical antibacterials are probably best reserved for patients who wish to avoid oral antibacterials or who cannot tolerate them. Topical preparations of **erythromycin** and **clindamycin** are effective for inflammatory acne; topical preparations of tetracycline may also be effective. Topical antibacterials can produce mild irritation of the skin, and on rare occasions cause sensitisation.

Antibacterial resistance of *Propionibacterium acnes* is increasing; there is cross-resistance between erythromycin and clindamycin. To avoid development of resistance:

- when possible use non-antibiotic antimicrobials (such as benzoyl peroxide or azelaic acid);
- avoid concomitant treatment with different oral and topical antibiotics;
- if a particular antibiotic is effective, use it for repeat courses if needed (short intervening courses of a topical antibacterial, such as benzoyl peroxide or azelaic acid, may eliminate any resistant propionibacteria);
- do not continue treatment for longer than necessary (however, treatment with a topical preparation should be continued for at least 6 months)

ANTIBIOTICS

Indications: acne vulgaris
Cautions: some manufacturers advise preparations containing alcohol are not suitable for use with benzoyl peroxide

Benzamycin® PoM
See under Benzoyl Peroxide above

Dalacin T® (Pharmacia) PoM
Topical solution, clindamycin 1% (as phosphate), in an aqueous alcoholic basis, net price (both with applicator) 30 mL = £4.34, 50 mL = £7.23
Excipients: include propylene glycol
Dose: apply twice daily
Lotion, clindamycin 1% (as phosphate) in an aqueous basis, net price 30 mL = £5.08, 50 mL = £8.47
Excipients: include cetostearyl alcohol, hydroxybenzoates (parabens)
Dose: apply twice daily

Stiemycin® (Stiefel) PoM
Solution, erythromycin 2% in an alcoholic basis, net price 50 mL = £8.00
Excipients: include propylene glycol
Dose: apply twice daily

Topicycline® (Shire) PoM
Solution, powder for reconstitution, tetracycline hydrochloride, 4-epitetracycline hydrochloride, providing tetracycline hydrochloride 2.2 mg/mL when reconstituted with solvent containing *n*-decyl methyl sulphoxide and citric acid in 40% alcohol. Net price per pack of powder and solvent to provide 70 mL = £6.15
Excipients: none as listed in section 13.1.3
Dose: apply twice daily

Zindaclin® (Strakan) PoM
Gel, clindamycin 1% (as phosphate), net price 30 g = £8.66
Excipients: include propylene glycol
Dose: apply once daily

Zineryt® (Yamanouchi) PoM
Topical solution, powder for reconstitution, erythromycin 40 mg, zinc acetate 12 mg/mL when reconstituted with solvent containing ethanol, net price per pack of powder and solvent to provide 30 mL = £7.71, 90 mL = £22.24
Excipients: none as listed in section 13.1.3
Dose: apply twice daily

Topical retinoids and related preparations for acne

Tretinoin and its isomer **isotretinoin** are useful in treating comedonal acne but patients should be warned that some redness and skin peeling might occur initially but settles with time. Several months of treatment may be needed to achieve an optimal response and the treatment should be continued until no new lesions develop.

Topical **isotretinoin** is licensed to treat non-inflammatory and inflammatory lesions in patients with mild to moderate acne. Isotretinoin is also given by mouth; see section 13.6.2 for **warnings** relating to use by mouth.

Adapalene, a retinoid-like drug, is licensed for mild to moderate acne. It is less irritant than topical retinoids.

CAUTIONS. Topical retinoids should be avoided in severe acne involving large areas. Contact with eyes, nostrils, mouth and mucous membranes, eczematous, broken or sunburned skin should be avoided. These drugs should be used with caution in sensitive areas such as the neck, and accumulation in angles of the nose should be avoided. Exposure to UV light (including sunlight, solariums) should be avoided; if sun exposure is unavoidable, an appropriate sunscreen or protective clothing should be used. Use of retinoids with abrasive cleaners, comedogenic or astringent cosmetics should be avoided. Allow peeling (e.g. resulting from use of benzoyl peroxide) to subside before using a topical retinoid; alternating a preparation that causes peeling with a topical retinoid may give rise to contact dermatitis (reduce frequency of retinoid application).

CONTRA-INDICATIONS. Topical retinoids are contra-indicated in pregnancy (Appendix 4); women of child-bearing age should take adequate contraceptive precautions. Tretinoin is contra-indicated in personal or familial history of cutaneous epithelioma.

SIDE-EFFECTS. Local reactions include burning, erythema, stinging, pruritus, dry or peeling skin (discontinue if severe). Increased sensitivity to UVB light or sunlight occurs. Temporary changes of skin pigmentation have been reported. Eye irritation and oedema, and blistering or crusting of skin have been reported rarely.

ADAPALENE

Indications: mild to moderate acne
Cautions: see notes above
Contra-indications: see notes above
Side-effects: see notes above
Dose: apply thinly once daily before retiring

Differin® (Galderma) PoM
Cream, adapalene 0.1%, net price 30 g = £6.86, 45 g = £11.40
Excipients: include disodium edetate, hydroxybenzoates (parabens)
Gel, adapalene 0.1%, net price 30 g = £6.86, 45 g = £11.40
Excipients: include disodium edetate, hydroxybenzoates (parabens), propylene glycol

TRETINOIN

NOTE. Tretinoin is the acid form of vitamin A
Indications: see under preparations below; photodamage (section 13.8.1); malignant disease (section 8.1.5)
Cautions: see notes above
Contra-indications: see notes above
Side-effects: see notes above
Dose: see under preparations below

Retin-A® (Janssen-Cilag) PoM
Cream, tretinoin 0.025%, net price 60 g = £5.73
Excipients: include butylated hydroxytoluene, sorbic acid, stearyl alcohol
Dose: acne vulgaris, for dry or fair skin, apply thinly 1–2 times daily
Gel, tretinoin 0.01%, net price 60 g = £5.73; 0.025%, 60 g = £5.73
Excipients: include butylated hydroxytoluene
Dose: acne vulgaris and other keratotic conditions, apply thinly 1–2 times daily
Lotion, tretinoin 0.025%, net price 100 mL = £6.59
Excipients: include butylated hydroxytoluene
Dose: acne vulgaris, apply thinly 1–2 times daily

■ With antibacterial

Aknemycin® **Plus** (Crookes) PoM
Solution, tretinoin 0.025%, erythromycin 4% in an alcoholic basis, net price 25 mL = £7.94
Dose: acne, apply thinly 1–2 times daily
Excipients: none as listed in section 13.1.3

ISOTRETINOIN

NOTE. Isotretinoin is an isomer of tretinoin
IMPORTANT. For **indications, cautions, contra-indications** and **side-effects** of isotretinoin **when given by mouth**, see p. 584
Indications: see notes above; oral treatment (see section 13.6.2)
Cautions: (*topical application* **only**) see notes above
Contra-indications: (*topical application* **only**) see notes above
Dose: apply thinly 1–2 times daily

Isotrex® (Stiefel) PoM
Gel, isotretinoin 0.05%, net price 30 g = £6.18
Excipients: include butylated hydroxytoluene

■ With antibacterial

Isotrexin® (Stiefel) PoM
Gel, isotretinoin 0.05%, erythromycin 2% in ethanolic basis, net price 30 g = £7.78
Excipients: include butylated hydroxytoluene

Other topical preparations for acne

Salicylic acid is available in various preparations for sale direct to the public for the treatment of mild acne. Other products are more suitable for acne; salicylic acid is used mainly for its keratolytic effect.

Preparations containing **sulphur** and **abrasive agents** are not considered beneficial in acne.

Topical **corticosteroids** should **not** be used in acne.

A topical preparation of **nicotinamide** is available for inflammatory acne.

ABRASIVE AGENTS

Indications: acne vulgaris (but see notes above)
Cautions: avoid contact with eyes; discontinue use temporarily if skin becomes irritated
Contra-indications: superficial venules, telangiectasia

Brasivol® (Stiefel)
Paste No. 1, aluminium oxide 38.09% in fine particles, in a soap-detergent basis, net price 75 g = £2.21
Excipients: include fragrance, *N*-(3-Chloroallyl)hexaminium chloride (quaternium 15)
Dose: use instead of soap 1–3 times daily

CORTICOSTEROIDS

Indications: use in acne not recommended (see notes above)
Cautions: see section 13.4 and notes above
Contra-indications: see section 13.4 and notes above
Side-effects: see section 13.4 and notes above

Actinac® (Peckforton) PoM
Lotion (powder for reconstitution with solvent), chloramphenicol 40 mg, hydrocortisone acetate 40 mg, allantoin 24 mg, butoxyethyl nicotinate 24 mg, precipitated sulphur 320 mg/g. Discard 21 days after reconstitution, net price 2 × 6.25-g

bottles powder with 2 × 20-mL bottles solvent = £16.28. Label: 28. Potency: mild
Excipients: none as listed in section 13.1.3

NICOTINAMIDE

Indications: see under preparation
Cautions: avoid contact with eyes and mucous membranes (including nose and mouth); reduce frequency of application if excessive dryness, irritation or peeling
Side-effects: dryness of skin; also pruritus, erythema, burning and irritation

Nicam® (Dermal)
Gel, nicotinamide 4%, net price 60 g = £7.42
Excipients: none as listed in section 13.1.3
Dose: inflammatory acne vulgaris, apply twice daily; reduce to once daily or on alternate days if irritation occurs
NOTE. Formerly marketed as *Papulex*®

SALICYLIC ACID

Indications: acne; psoriasis (section 13.5.2); warts and calluses (section 13.7); fungal nail infections (section 13.10.2)
Cautions: avoid contact with mouth, eyes, mucous membranes; systemic effects after excessive use (see Aspirin and the salicylates, section 10.1.1)
Side-effects: local irritation

Acnisal® (Alliance)
Topical solution, salicylic acid 2% in a detergent and emollient basis, net price 177 mL = £4.03.
Excipients: include benzyl alcohol
Dose: use up to 3 times daily

SULPHUR

Cautions: avoid contact with eyes, mouth, and mucous membranes; causes skin irritation

■ With resorcinol

Prolonged application of resorcinol may interfere with thyroid function, therefore not recommended

Eskamel® (Goldshield) NHS
Cream, resorcinol 2%, sulphur 8%, in a non-greasy flesh-coloured basis, net price 25 g = £3.03
Excipients: include propylene glycol, fragrance

13.6.2 Oral preparations for acne

Oral antibacterials for acne

Systemic antibacterial treatment is useful for inflammatory acne if topical treatment is not adequately effective or if it is inappropriate. Anticomedonal treatment (e.g. with topical benzoyl peroxide) may also be required.

Either **oxytetracycline** or **tetracycline** (section 5.1.3) is usually given for acne in a dose of 500 mg twice daily. If there is no improvement after the first 3 months another oral antibacterial should be used. Maximum improvement usually occurs after 4 to 6 months but in more severe cases treatment may need to be continued for 2 years or longer.

Doxycycline and **minocycline** (section 5.1.3) are alternatives to tetracycline. Doxycycline may be used in a dose of 100 mg daily. Minocycline offers less likelihood of bacterial resistance but may sometimes cause irreversible pigmentation; it is given in a dose of 100 mg daily (in one or two divided doses).

Erythromycin (section 5.1.5) in a dose of 500 mg twice daily is an alternative for the management of acne but propionibacteria strains resistant to erythromycin are becoming widespread and this may explain poor response.

Trimethoprim (section 5.1.8) in a dose of 300 mg twice daily may be used for acne resistant to other antibacterials [unlicensed indication]. Prolonged treatment with trimethoprim may depress haematopoiesis; it should generally be initiated by specialists.

Concomitant use of different topical and systemic antibacterials is undesirable owing to the increased likelihood of the development of bacterial resistance.

Hormone treatment for acne

Co-cyprindiol (cyproterone acetate with ethinylestradiol) contains an anti-androgen. It is no more effective than an oral broad-spectrum antibacterial but is useful in women who also wish to receive oral contraception.

Improvement of acne with co-cyprindiol probably occurs because of decreased sebum secretion which is under androgen control. Some women with moderately severe hirsutism may also benefit because hair growth is also androgen-dependent. Contra-indications of co-cyprindiol include pregnancy and a predisposition to thrombosis.

CSM advice. Venous thromboembolism occurs more frequently in women taking co-cyprindiol than those taking a low-dose combined oral contraceptive. The CSM has reminded prescribers that co-cyprindiol is licensed for use in women with severe acne which has not responded to oral antibacterials and for moderately severe hirsutism; it should not be used solely for contraception. It is contra-indicated in those with a personal or close family history of venous thromboembolism. Women with severe acne or hirsutism may have an inherently increased risk of cardiovascular disease.

CO-CYPRINDIOL

A mixture of cyproterone acetate and ethinylestradiol in the mass proportions 2000 parts to 35 parts, respectively

Indications: severe acne in women refractory to prolonged oral antibacterial therapy (but see notes above); moderately severe hirsutism
Cautions: see under Combined Hormonal Contraceptives, section 7.3.1
Contra-indications: see under Combined Hormonal Contraceptives, section 7.3.1
Side-effects: see under Combined Hormonal Contraceptives, section 7.3.1
Dose: 1 tablet daily for 21 days starting on day 1 of menstrual cycle and repeated after a 7-day interval, usually for several months; withdraw when acne or hirsutism completely resolved (repeat courses may be given if recurrence)

Co-cyprindiol (Non-proprietary) PoM
Tablets, co-cyprindiol 2000/35 (cyproterone acetate 2 mg, ethinylestradiol 35 micrograms), net price 21-tab pack = £3.70
Brands include *Acnocin*®

Dianette® (Schering Health) PoM
Tablets, beige, s/c, co-cyprindiol 2000/35 (cyproterone acetate 2 mg, ethinylestradiol 35 micrograms), net price 21-tab pack = £3.11

Oral retinoid for acne

The retinoid **isotretinoin** (*Roaccutane*®) reduces sebum secretion. It is used for the systemic treatment of nodulo-cystic and conglobate acne, severe acne, scarring, acne which has not responded to an adequate course of a systemic antibacterial, or acne which is associated with psychological problems. It is also useful in women who develop acne in the third or fourth decades of life, since late onset acne is frequently unresponsive to antibacterials.

Isotretinoin is a toxic drug that should be prescribed **only** by, or under the supervision of, a consultant dermatologist. It is given for at least 16 weeks; repeat courses are not normally required.

Side-effects of isotretinoin include severe dryness of the skin and mucous membranes, nose bleeds, and joint pains. The drug is **teratogenic** and must **not** be given to women of child-bearing age unless they practise effective contraception and then only after detailed assessment and explanation by the physician and they are registered with a pregnancy prevention programme (see under Cautions below).

ISOTRETINOIN

NOTE. Isotretinoin is an isomer of tretinoin

Indications: see notes above

Cautions: exclude pregnancy before starting (perform pregnancy test 2–3 days before expected menstruation, start treatment on day 2 or 3 of menstrual cycle)—effective contraception must be practised at least 1 month before, during, and for at least 1 month after treatment; avoid blood donation during treatment and for at least 1 month after treatment; history of depression; measure hepatic function before treatment, 1 month after starting and then every 3 months (reduce dose or discontinue if transaminase raised above normal); measure serum lipids before treatment, 1 month after starting, then at end of treatment (reduce dose or discontinue if raised), discontinue if uncontrolled hypertriglyceridaemia or pancreatitis; diabetes; dry eye syndrome (associated with risk of keratitis); avoid keratolytics; renal impairment (Appendix 3) **interactions:** Appendix 1 (retinoids)

COUNSELLING. Warn patient to avoid wax epilation (risk of epidermal stripping), dermabrasion, and laser skin treatments (risk of scarring) during treatment and for at least 6 months after stopping; patient should avoid exposure to UV light (including sunlight) and use sunscreen and emollient (including lip balm) preparations from the start of treatment.

Contra-indications: pregnancy (**important teratogenic risk:** see Cautions above); breast-feeding; hepatic impairment (Appendix 2); hypervitaminosis A, hyperlipidaemia

Side-effects: dryness of skin (with dermatitis, scaling, thinning, erythema, pruritus), epidermal fragility (trauma may cause blistering), dryness of lips (sometimes cheilitis), dryness of eyes (with blepharitis and conjunctivitis), dryness of pharyngeal mucosa (with hoarseness), dryness of nasal mucosa (with epistaxis), headache, myalgia and arthralgia, raised plasma concentration of triglycerides, of glucose, of serum transaminases, and of cholesterol (risk of pancreatitis if triglycerides above 8 g/litre), haematuria and proteinuria, thrombocytopenia, thrombocytosis, neutropenia and anaemia; *rarely* irreversible mood changes (depression, suicidal ideation, aggressive behaviour, anxiety)—expert referral required, exacerbation of acne, acne fulminans, allergic skin reactions, and hypersensitivity, alopecia; *very rarely* nausea, inflammatory bowel disease, diarrhoea (discontinue if severe), benign intracranial hypertension (avoid concomitant tetracyclines), convulsions, malaise, drowsiness, lymphadenopathy, increased sweating, hyperuricaemia, raised serum creatinine concentration and glomerulonephritis, hepatitis, tendonitis, bone changes (including reduced bone density, early epiphyseal closure, and skeletal hyperostosis following long-term administration), visual disturbances (papilloedema, corneal opacities, cataracts, decreased night vision, photophobia, blurred vision, colour blindness)—expert referral required and consider withdrawal, decreased tolerance to contact lenses and keratitis, impaired hearing, Gram-positive infections of skin and mucous membranes, allergic vasculitis and granulomatous lesions, paronychia, hirsutism, nail dystrophy, skin hyperpigmentation, photosensitivity

Dose: 500 micrograms/kg daily increased if necessary to 1 mg/kg (in 1–2 divided doses) for 16–24 weeks (8 weeks if failure or relapse after first course); max. cumulative dose 150 mg/kg per course; CHILD not recommended

Isotretinoin (Non-proprietary) PoM
Capsules, isotretinoin 5 mg, net price 56-cap pack = £18.00; 20 mg, 56-cap pack = £50.00 (hosp. only). Label: 10, patient information leaflet, 11, 21

Roaccutane® (Roche) PoM
Capsules, isotretinoin 5 mg (red-violet/white), net price 30-cap pack = £9.08; 20 mg (red-violet/white), 30-cap pack = £25.02 (hosp. or specified retail pharmacy only). Label: 10, patient information card, 11, 21
Excipients: include arachis (peanut) oil

13.7 Preparations for warts and calluses

Warts (verrucas) are caused by a human papillomavirus, which most frequently affects the hands, feet (plantar warts), and the anogenital region (see below); treatment usually relies on local tissue destruction. Warts may regress on their own and treatment is required only if the warts are painful, unsightly, persistent, or cause distress.

Preparations of **salicylic acid, formaldehyde, gluteraldehyde** or **silver nitrate** are available for purchase by the public; they are suitable for the removal of warts on hands and feet. **Salicylic acid** is a useful keratolytic which may be considered first; it is also suitable for the removal of *corns and calluses*. Colloidal preparations of salicylic acid are available but some patients may develop an allergy to colophony in the formulation. An ointment combining **salicylic acid** with **podophyllum resin** (*Posalfilin*®) is available for treating plantar warts.

SALICYLIC ACID

Indications: see under preparations; psoriasis (section 13.5.2); acne (section 13.6.1); fungal nail infections (section 13.10.2)

Cautions: significant peripheral neuropathy, patients with diabetes at risk of neuropathic ulcers; protect surrounding skin and avoid broken skin; not suitable for application to face, anogenital region, or large areas

Side-effects: skin irritation, see notes above

Dose: see under preparations; advise patient to apply carefully to wart and to protect surrounding skin (e.g. with soft paraffin or specially designed plaster); rub wart surface gently with file or pumice stone once weekly; treatment may need to be continued for up to 3 months

Cuplex® (Crawford)
Gel, salicylic acid 11%, lactic acid 4%, in a collodion basis, net price 5 g = £2.23. Label: 15
Dose: for plantar and mosaic warts, corns, and calluses, apply twice daily

Duofilm® (Stiefel)
Paint, salicylic acid 16.7%, lactic acid 16.7%, in flexible collodion, net price 15 mL (with applicator) = £1.74. Label: 15
Dose: for plantar and mosaic warts, apply daily

Occlusal® (Alliance)
Application, salicylic acid 26% in polyacrylic solution, net price 10 mL (with applicator) = £3.39. Label: 15
Dose: for common and plantar warts, apply daily

Salactol® (Dermal)
Paint, salicylic acid 16.7%, lactic acid 16.7%, in flexible collodion, net price 10 mL (with applicator) = £1.79. Label: 15
Dose: for warts, particularly plantar warts, verrucas, corns, and calluses, apply daily

Salatac® (Dermal)
Gel, salicylic acid 12%, lactic acid 4% in a collodion basis, net price 8 g (with applicator) = £3.12. Label: 15
Dose: for warts, verrucas, corns, and calluses, apply daily

Verrugon® (Pickles)
Ointment, salicylic acid 50% in a paraffin basis, net price 6 g = £2.83
Dose: for plantar warts, apply daily

■ With podophyllum

Posalfilin® (Norgine)
Ointment, podophyllum resin 20%, salicylic acid 25%, net price 10 g = £3.51
Dose: for plantar warts apply daily
NOTE. Owing to the salicylic acid content, not suitable for anogenital warts; owing to the podophyllum content also contra-indicated in pregnancy and breast-feeding

FORMALDEHYDE

Indications: see under preparations

Cautions: see under Salicylic Acid

Side-effects: see under Salicylic Acid

Veracur® (Typharm)
Gel, formaldehyde 0.75% in a water-miscible gel basis, net price 15 g = £2.41.
Dose: for warts, particularly plantar warts, apply twice daily

GLUTARALDEHYDE

Indications: warts, particularly plantar warts

Cautions: protect surrounding skin; not for application to face, mucosa, or anogenital areas

Side-effects: rashes, skin irritation (discontinue if severe); stains skin brown

Dose: apply twice daily (see also under Salicylic acid)

Glutarol® (Dermal)
Solution (= application), glutaraldehyde 10%, net price 10 mL (with applicator) = £2.17

SILVER NITRATE

Indications: see under preparation

Cautions: protect surrounding skin and avoid broken skin; not suitable for application to face, ano-genital region, or large areas

Side-effects: stains skin and fabric

Dose: see under preparation; instructions in proprietary packs generally incorporate advice to remove dead skin before use by gentle filing and to cover with adhesive dressing after application

AVOCA® (Bray)
Caustic pencil, tip containing silver nitrate 95%, potassium nitrate 5%, net price, treatment pack (including emery file, 6 adhesive dressings and protector pads) = £1.89.
Dose: for common warts and verrucas, apply moistened caustic pencil tip for 1–2 minutes; repeat after 24 hours up to max. 3 applications for warts *or* max. 6 applications for verrucas

Anogenital warts

The treatment of anogenital warts (condylomata acuminata) should be accompanied by screening for other sexually transmitted diseases. **Podophyllum** and **podophyllotoxin** (the major active ingredient of podophyllum) may be used for *soft, non-keratinised* external anogenital warts; these preparations can cause considerable irritation of the treated area. They can also cause severe systemic toxicity on excessive application including gastro-intestinal, renal, haematological, and CNS effects. Patients with a limited number of external warts or *keratinised* lesions may be better treated with cryotherapy or other forms of physical ablation.

Imiquimod cream is licensed for the treatment of external anogenital warts; it may be used for both keratinised and non-keratinised lesions. It is also licensed for the treatment of superficial basal cell carcinoma.

Inosine pranobex (section 5.3.2.1) is licensed for adjunctive treatment of genital warts but it has been superseded by more effective drugs.

IMIQUIMOD

Indications: external genital and perianal warts; superficial basal cell carcinoma

Cautions: avoid normal skin, inflamed skin and open wounds; not suitable for internal genital warts; uncircumcised males (risk of phimosis or stricture of foreskin); pregnancy

Side-effects: local reactions including itching, pain, erythema, erosion, oedema, and excoriation; less commonly local ulceration and scabbing; permanent hypopigmentation or hyperpigmentation and dysuria in women reported

Dose: warts, apply thinly 3 times a week at night until lesions resolve (max. 16 weeks)

Superficial basal cell carcinoma, apply to lesion (and 1 cm beyond it) on 5 days each week for 6 weeks; assess response after a further 12 weeks

CHILD not recommended

IMPORTANT. Should be rubbed in and allowed to stay on the treated area for 6–10 hours for warts or for 8 hours for basal cell carcinoma then washed off with mild soap and water (uncircumcised males treating warts under foreskin should wash the area daily). The cream should be washed off before sexual contact

Aldara® (3M) PoM

Cream, imiquimod 5%, net price 12-sachet pack = £51.32. Label: 10, patient information leaflet

Excipients: include benzyl alcohol, cetyl alcohol, hydroxybenzoates (parabens), polysorbate 60, stearyl alcohol

Condoms: may damage latex condoms and diaphragms

PODOPHYLLUM

Indications: see under preparations

Cautions: avoid normal skin and open wounds; keep away from face; very irritant to eyes; **important:** see also warnings below

Contra-indications: pregnancy and breast-feeding; children

Side-effects: see notes above

Podophyllin Paint, Compound, BP PoM

(podophyllum resin 15% in compound benzoin tincture), podophyllum resin 1.5 g, compound benzoin tincture to 10 mL; 5 mL to be dispensed unless otherwise directed. Label: 15

Dose: external genital warts, applied weekly in genitourinary clinic (or at a general practitioner's surgery by trained nurses after screening for other sexually transmitted diseases)

IMPORTANT. Should be allowed to stay on the treated area for not longer than 6 hours and then washed off. Care should be taken to avoid splashing the surrounding skin during application (which must be covered with soft paraffin as a protection). Where there are a large number of warts only a few should be treated at any one time as **severe toxicity** caused by absorption of podophyllin has been reported

■ Podophyllotoxin

Condyline® (Ardern) PoM

Solution, podophyllotoxin 0.5% in alcoholic basis, net price 3.5 mL (with applicators) = £14.49. Label: 15

Dose: condylomata acuminata affecting the penis or the female external genitalia, apply twice daily for 3 consecutive days; treatment may be repeated at weekly intervals if necessary for a total of five 3-day treatment courses; direct medical supervision for lesions in the female and for lesions greater than 4 cm^2 in the male; max. 50 single applications ('loops') per session (consult product literature)

Warticon® (Stiefel) PoM

Cream, podophyllotoxin 0.15%, net price 5 g (with mirror) = £15.46

Excipients: include butylated hydroxyanisole, cetyl alcohol, hydroxybenzoates (parabens), sorbic acid, stearyl alcohol

Dose: condylomata acuminata affecting the penis or the female external genitalia, apply twice daily for 3 consecutive days; treatment may be repeated at weekly intervals if necessary for a total of four 3-day treatment courses; direct medical supervision for lesions greater than 4 cm^2

Solution, blue, podophyllotoxin 0.5% in alcoholic basis, net price 3 mL (with applicators—*Warticon*® [for men]; with applicators and mirror—*Warticon Fem*® [for women]) = £12.88. Label: 15

Dose: condylomata acuminata affecting the penis or the female external genitalia, apply twice daily for 3 consecutive days; treatment may be repeated at weekly intervals if necessary for a total of four 3-day treatment courses; direct medical supervision for lesions greater than 4 cm^2; max. 50 single applications ('loops') per session (consult product literature)

13.8 Sunscreens and camouflagers

13.8.1 Sunscreen preparations

Solar ultraviolet irradiation can be harmful to the skin. It is responsible for disorders such as *polymorphic light eruption, solar urticaria*, and it provokes the various *cutaneous porphyrias*. It also provokes (or at least aggravates) skin lesions of *lupus erythematosus* and may aggravate *rosacea* and some other *dermatoses*. Sunlight may also cause photosensitivity in patients taking some drugs such as demeclocycline, phenothiazines, or amiodarone. All these conditions (as well as *sunburn*) may occur after relatively short periods of exposure to the sun. Solar ultraviolet irradiation may provoke attacks of recurrent herpes labialis (but it is not known whether the effect of sunlight exposure is local or systemic).

The effects of exposure over longer periods include *ageing changes* and more importantly the initiation of *skin cancer*.

Solar ultraviolet radiation is approximately 200–400 nm in wavelength. The medium wavelengths (290–320 nm, known as UVB) cause sunburn and contribute to the long-term changes responsible for skin cancer and ageing. The long wavelengths (320–400 nm, known as UVA) do not cause sunburn but are responsible for many *photosensitivity reactions* and *photodermatoses*. Both UVA and UVB contribute to long-term *photodamage* and to the pathogenesis of *skin cancer*.

Sunscreen preparations contain substances that protect the skin against UVB and hence against sunburn, but they are no substitute for covering the skin and avoiding sunlight. The sun protection factor (SPF, usually indicated in the preparation title) provides guidance on the degree of protection offered against UVB; it indicates the multiples of protection provided against burning, compared with unprotected skin; for example, an SPF of 8 should enable a person to remain 8 times longer in the sun without burning. However, in practice users do not apply sufficient sunscreen product and the protection is lower than that found in experimental studies. Sunscreen preparations, do not prevent long-term damage associated with UVA, which might not become apparent for 10 to 20 years. Preparations that also contain reflective substances, such as titanium dioxide, provide the most effective protection against UVA. Some products use a star rating system to indicate the protection against UVA relative to protection against UVB for the same product. Four stars indicate that the product offers balanced UVA and UVB protection; products with 3, 2, or 1 star rating indicate that greater protection is offered against UVB than against UVA. However, the usefulness of the star rating system remains controversial.

Some sunscreen preparations, particularly aminobenzoates, may rarely cause photosensitivity reactions.

> For optimum photoprotection, sunscreen preparations should be applied **thickly** and **frequently** (approximately 2 hourly). In photodermatoses, they should be used from spring to autumn. As maximum protection from sunlight is desirable, preparations with the highest SPF should be prescribed.

BORDERLINE SUBSTANCES. The preparations marked 'ACBS' are regarded as drugs when prescribed for skin protection against ultraviolet radiation in abnormal cutaneous photosensitivity resulting from genetic disorders or photodermatoses, including vitiligo and those resulting from radiotherapy; chronic or recurrent herpes simplex labialis. Preparations with SPF less than 15 are not prescribable. See also Appendix 7.

Ambre Solaire® (Garnier)

Total Screen Sun Intolerant Skin Lotion (UVA and UVB protection; UVB-SPF 60), octocrylene 10%, titanium dioxide 5.3%, drometrizole trisiloxane 2.5%, avobenzone 2.5%, terephthalydene dicamphor sulfonic acid 0.5%, net price 200 mL = £7.98. ACBS

Excipients: include disodium edetate, hydroxybenzoates (parabens), propylene glycol

Delph® (Fenton)

Lotion, (UVA and UVB protection; UVB-SPF 15), ethylhexyl *p*-methoxycinnamate 7.5%, oxybenzone 3%, titanium dioxide 0.6%, net price 200 mL = £1.99. ACBS

Excipients: include cetostearyl alcohol, fragrance, hydroxybenzoates (parabens), imidurea

Lotion, (UVA and UVB protection; UVB-SPF 20), ethylhexyl *p*-methoxycinnamate 7.5%, oxybenzone 3%, titanium dioxide 1.6%, net price 200 mL = £1.99. ACBS

Excipients: include cetostearyl alcohol, fragrance, hydroxybenzoates (parabens), imidurea

Lotion, (UVA and UVB protection; UVB-SPF 25), avobenzone 4%, ethylhexyl *p*-methoxycinnamate 3.5%, titanium dioxide 2.1%, oxybenzone 1.3%, net price 200 mL = £2.85. ACBS

Excipients: include cetostearyl alcohol, fragrance, hydroxybenzoates (parabens), imidurea

Lotion, (UVA and UVB protection; UVB-SPF 30), ethylhexyl *p*-methoxycinnamate 4.8%, avobenzone 4%, titanium dioxide 2.5%, oxybenzone 1.5%, net price 200 mL = £2.85. ACBS

Excipients: include cetostearyl alcohol, fragrance, hydroxybenzoates (parabens), imidurea

E45 Sun® (Crookes)

Reflective Sunscreen (UVA and UVB protection; UVB-SPF 25), waterproof, titanium dioxide 3.6%, zinc oxide 13.9%, net price 150 mL = £6.56. ACBS

Excipients: include hydroxybenzoates (parabens), isopropyl palmitate

Reflective Sunscreen (UVA and UVB protection; UVB-SPF 50), waterproof, titanium dioxide 6.4%, zinc oxide 16%, net price 150 mL = £7.09. ACBS

Excipients: include hydroxybenzoates (parabens), isopropyl palmitate

RoC Sante Soleil® (J&J)

Cream (UVA and UVB protection; UVB-SPF 25), containing avobenzone 2%, ethylhexyl *p*-methoxycinnamate 7.5%, titanium dioxide 5.5%, net price 50 mL = £4.06. ACBS

Excipients: include beeswax, cetostearyl alcohol, disodium edetate, hydroxybenzoates (parabens)

SpectraBan® (Stiefel)

Lotion (UVB protection; UVB-SPF 25), aminobenzoic acid 5%, padimate-O 3.2%, in an alcoholic basis, net price 150 mL = £3.45. ACBS

Excipients: include fragrance

NOTE. Flammable; stains clothing

Ultra lotion (UVA and UVB protection; UVB-SPF 28), water resistant, avobenzone 2%, oxybenzone 3%, padimate-O 8%, titanium dioxide 2%, net price 150 mL = £5.45. ACBS

Excipients: include benzyl alcohol, disodium edetate, sorbic acid, fragrance

Sunsense® **Ultra** (Typharm)

Lotion (UVA and UVB protection; UVB-SPF 60), ethylhexyl *p*-methoxycinnamate 7.5% oxybenzone 3%, titanium dioxide 3.5%, net price 50-mL bottle with roll-on applicator = £3.11, 125 mL = £5.10. ACBS

Excipients: include butylated hydroxytoluene, cetyl alcohol, fragrance, hydroxybenzoates (parabens), propylene glycol

Uvistat® (LPC)

Cream (UVA and UVB protection; UVB-SPF 22 but marketed as 'factor 20'), water-resistant, ethylhexyl *p*-methoxycinnamate 7%, avobenzone 4%, titanium dioxide 4.5%, net price 125 g = £5.10. ACBS

Excipients: include disodium edetate, fragrance, hydroxybenzoates (parabens)

Ultrablock cream (UVA and UVB protection; UVB-SPF 30), water-resistant, ethylhexyl *p*-methoxycinnamate 7.5%, avobenzone 4%, titanium dioxide 6.5%, net price 125 g = £5.10. ACBS

Excipients: include disodium edetate, fragrance, hydroxybenzoates (parabens)

Photodamage

Diclofenac gel is licensed for *actinic keratosis*. Treatment should continue for 60 to 90 days (optimal therapeutic effect may not be seen until 30 days after stopping). **Fluorouracil** cream (section 8.1.3) is also licensed for actinic keratosis. **Methyl-5-aminolevulinate** cream (*Metvix*®, available from Galderma), followed by irradiation with red light, is licensed for treating thin non-hyperkeratotic actinic keratoses of the face and scalp when other treatments are less appropriate, or for treating superficial or nodular basal cell carcinoma that is considered unsuitable for other therapies; it is used in specialist centres.

Application of **tretinoin** 0.05% cream is reported to be associated with gradual improvement in *photodamaged skin* (usually within 3–4 months of starting).

DICLOFENAC SODIUM

Indications: actinic keratosis

Cautions: as for topical NSAIDs, see section 10.3.2

Contra-indications: as for topical NSAIDs, see section 10.3.2

Side-effects: as for topical NSAIDs, see section 10.3.2; also paraesthesia; application of large amounts may result in systemic effects, see section 10.1

Dose: apply thinly twice daily for 60–90 days; max. 8 g daily

Solaraze® (Shire) PoM

Gel, diclofenac sodium 3%, net price 25 g = £16.65

Excipients: include benzyl alcohol

TRETINOIN

NOTE. Tretinoin is the acid form of vitamin A

Indications: mottled hyperpigmentation, roughness and fine wrinkling of photodamaged skin due to chronic sun exposure; acne vulgaris (section 13.6); malignant disease (section 8.1.5)

Cautions: see section 13.6.1

Contra-indications: see section 13.6.1

Side-effects: see section 13.6.1

Dose: apply thinly at night, then reduce to 1–3 nights weekly

Retinova® (Janssen-Cilag) PoM NHS
Cream, tretinoin 0.05%, net price 20 g = £13.75.
Excipients: include fragrance

13.8.2 Camouflagers

Disfigurement of the skin can be very distressing to patients and may have a marked psychological effect. In skilled hands, or with experience, camouflage cosmetics can be very effective in concealing scars and birthmarks. The depigmented patches in vitiligo are also very disfiguring and camouflage creams are of great cosmetic value.

BORDERLINE SUBSTANCES. The preparations marked 'ACBS' are regarded as drugs when prescribed for postoperative scars and other deformities and as an adjunctive therapy in the relief of emotional disturbances due to disfiguring skin disease, such as vitiligo. See also Appendix 7.

Covermark® (Epiderm)
Classic foundation (masking cream), net price 15 mL (10 shades) = £10.75. ACBS
Excipients: include beeswax, hydroxybenzoates (parabens), fragrance
Finishing powder, net price 60 g = £10.55. ACBS
Excipients: include beeswax, hydroxybenzoates (parabens), fragrance

Dermablend® (Brodie & Stone)
Cover creme, net price 10.7 g (15 shades) = £8.76; 28.4 g (11 shades) = £13.47. ACBS
Excipients: include beeswax, hydroxybenzoates (parabens)
Leg and body cover, (9 shades), net price 64 g = £12.25. ACBS
Excipients: include beeswax, hydroxybenzoates (parabens)
Setting powder, net price 28 g = £11.13. ACBS
Excipients: include hydroxybenzoates (parabens)

Dermacolor® (Fox)
Camouflage creme, (100 shades), net price 25 g = £8.10. ACBS
Excipients: include beeswax, butylated hydroxytoluene, fragrance, propylene glycol, stearyl alcohol, wool fat
Fixing powder, (7 shades), net price 60 g = £6.55. ACBS
Excipients: include fragrance

Keromask® (Network)
Masking cream, (2 shades), net price 15 mL = £5.67. ACBS
Excipients: include butylated hydroxyanisole, hydroxybenzoates (parabens), wool fat, propylene glycol
Finishing powder, net price 20 g = £5.67. ACBS
Excipients: include butylated hydroxytoluene, hydroxybenzoates (parabens)

Veil® (Blake)
Cover cream, (20 shades), net price 19 g = £8.23, 44 g = £13.90, 70 g = £18.44. ACBS
Excipients: include hydroxybenzoates (parabens), wool fat derivative
Finishing powder, translucent, net price 35 g = £8.79. ACBS
Excipients: include butylated hydroxyanisole, hydroxybenzoates (parabens)

13.9 Shampoos and other preparations for scalp and hair conditions

Dandruff is considered to be a mild form of seborrhoeic dermatitis (see also section 13.5.1). Shampoos containing antimicrobial agents such as **pyrithione zinc** (which are widely available) and **selenium sulphide** may have beneficial effects. Shampoos containing **tar** extracts may be useful and they are also used in *psoriasis*. **Ketoconazole** shampoo should be considered for more persistent or severe dandruff or for seborrhoeic dermatitis of the scalp.

Corticosteroid gels and lotions (section 13.4) can also be used.

Shampoos containing **coal tar** and **salicylic acid** may also be useful. A cream or an ointment containing coal tar and salicylic acid is very helpful in *psoriasis* that affects the scalp (section 13.5.2). Patients who do not respond to these treatments may need to be referred to exclude the possibility of other skin conditions.

Cradle cap in infants may be treated with **olive oil** or **arachis oil** (ground-nut oil, peanut oil) applications followed by shampooing.

See below for male-pattern baldness and also section 13.5 (psoriasis and eczema), section 13.10.4 (lice), and section 13.10.2 (ringworm).

■ Shampoos

[1]**Ketoconazole** (Non-proprietary) PoM
Cream—section 13.10.2
Shampoo, ketoconazole 2%, net price 120 mL = £5.11
Excipients: include imidurea
Brands include *Dandrazol*® *2% Shampoo*, *Nizoral*®
Dose: treatment of seborrhoeic dermatitis and dandruff apply twice weekly for 2–4 weeks (prophylaxis apply once every 1–2 weeks); treatment of pityriasis versicolor apply once daily for max. 5 days (prophylaxis apply once daily for up to 3 days before sun exposure); leave preparation on for 3–5 minutes before rinsing

1. Can be sold to the public for the prevention and treatment of dandruff and seborrhoeic dermatitis of the scalp as a shampoo formulation containing ketoconazole max. 2%, in a pack containing max. 120 mL and labelled to show a max. frequency of application of once every 3 days; brands on sale to the public include *Dandrazol*® *Antidandruff 2% Shampoo*, *Nizoral*® *Dandruff Shampoo*, and *Nizoral*® *Anti-Dandruff Shampoo*

Alphosyl 2 in 1® (GSK Consumer Healthcare)
Shampoo, alcoholic coal tar extract 5%, net price 125 mL = £1.81, 250 mL = £3.43
Excipients: include hydroxybenzoates (parabens), fragrance
Dose: dandruff, use once or twice weekly as necessary; psoriasis, seborrhoeic dermatitis, scaling and itching, use every 2–3 days

Betadine® (Medlock)
Skin disinfectants—section 13.11.4
Shampoo, povidone–iodine 4%, in a surfactant solution, net price 250 mL = £2.32
Excipients: include fragrance
Dose: seborrhoeic scalp conditions associated with excessive dandruff, pruritus, scaling, exudation and erythema, infected scalp lesions (recurrent furunculosis, infective folliculitis, impetigo), apply 1–2 times weekly; CHILD under 2 years not recommended
Cautions; Contra-indications; Side-effects: section 13.11.4, Povidone-Iodine

Capasal® (Dermal)
Shampoo, coal tar 1%, coconut oil 1%, salicylic acid 0.5%, net price 250 mL = £4.91
Excipients: none as listed in section 13.1.3
Dose: scaly scalp disorders including psoriasis, seborrhoeic dermatitis, dandruff, and cradle cap, apply daily as necessary

Ceanel Concentrate® (Ferndale)
Shampoo, cetrimide 10%, undecenoic acid 1%, phenylethyl alcohol 7.5%, net price 150 mL = £3.40, 500 mL = £9.80
Excipients: none as listed in section 13.1.3
Dose: scalp psoriasis, seborrhoeic dermatitis, dandruff, apply 3 times in first week then twice weekly

Clinitar® (CHS)
Shampoo, coal tar extract 2%, net price 100 g = £2.50
Excipients: include polysorbates, fragrance
Dose: scalp psoriasis, seborrhoeic dermatitis, and dandruff, apply up to 3 times weekly

Meted® (Alliance)
Shampoo, salicylic acid 3%, sulphur 5%, net price 120 mL = £3.80
Excipients: include fragrance
Dose: scaly scalp disorders including psoriasis, seborrhoeic dermatitis, and dandruff, apply at least twice weekly

Pentrax® (Alliance)
Shampoo, coal tar 4.3%, net price 120 mL = £3.80
Excipients: none as listed in section 13.1.3
Dose: scaly scalp disorders including psoriasis, seborrhoeic dermatitis, and dandruff, apply at least twice weekly

Polytar AF® (Stiefel)
Shampoo, arachis (peanut) oil extract of coal tar 0.3%, cade oil 0.3%, coal tar solution 0.1%, pine tar 0.3%, pyrithione zinc 1%, net price 150 mL = £3.91
Excipients: include fragrance, imidurea
Dose: scaly scalp disorders including psoriasis, seborrhoeic dermatitis, and dandruff, apply 2–3 times weekly for at least 3 weeks

Psoriderm® (Dermal)
Scalp lotion (= shampoo), coal tar 2.5%, lecithin 0.3%, net price 250 mL = £4.96
Excipients: include disodium edetate
Dose: scalp psoriasis, use as necessary

Selsun® (Abbott)
Shampoo, selenium sulphide 2.5%, net price 50 mL = £1.44, 100 mL = £1.96, 150 mL = £2.75
Excipients: include fragrance
Dose: seborrhoeic dermatitis and dandruff, apply twice weekly for 2 weeks then once weekly for 2 weeks and then as necessary; CHILD under 5 years not recommended; pityriasis versicolor, section 13.10.2 [unlicensed indication]
Cautions: avoid using 48 hours before or after applying hair colouring, straightening or waving preparations

T/Gel® (Neutrogena)
Shampoo, coal tar extract 2%, net price 125 mL = £3.18, 250 mL = £4.78
Excipients: include fragrance, hydroxybenzoates (parabens), imidurea, tetrasodium edetate
Dose: scalp psoriasis, seborrhoeic dermatitis, dandruff, apply as necessary

■ Other scalp preparations

Cocois®
Section 13.5.2

Polytar® (Stiefel)
Liquid, arachis (peanut) oil extract of coal tar 0.3%, cade oil 0.3%, coal tar solution 0.1%, oleyl alcohol 1%, tar 0.3%, net price 250 mL = £2.23
Excipients: include fragrance, imidurea, polysorbate 80
Dose: scalp disorders including psoriasis, seborrhoea, eczema, pruritus, and dandruff, apply 1–2 times weekly

Polytar Plus® (Stiefel)
Liquid, ingredients as *Polytar*® liquid with hydrolysed animal protein 3%, net price 500 mL = £3.91
Excipients: include fragrance, imidurea, polysorbate 80
Dose: scalp disorders including psoriasis, seborrhoea, eczema, pruritus, and dandruff, apply 1–2 times weekly

Pragmatar®
Section 13.5.2

Hirsutism

Hirsutism may result from hormonal disorders or as a side-effect of drugs such as minoxidil, corticosteroids, anabolic steroids, androgens, danazol, and progestogens.

When hirsutism co-exists with acne (e.g. in polycystic ovary syndrome) co-cyprindiol (section 13.6.2) may be effective.

Eflornithine, an antiprotozoal drug, inhibits the enzyme ornithine decarboxylase in hair follicles and topical application can reduce the growth of unwanted facial hair. It must be used indefinitely to prevent regrowth. Continuous use for 8 weeks is required before benefit is seen. Eflornithine should be discontinued in the absence of improvement after treatment for 4 months.

EFLORNITHINE

Indications: facial hirsutism in women
Contra-indications: pregnancy (Appendix 4); breast-feeding (Appendix 5)
Side-effects: acne, application site reactions including burning and stinging sensation, rash
Dose: apply thinly twice daily; CHILD under 12 years not recommended
NOTE. Preparation must be rubbed in thoroughly; cosmetics may be applied over treated area 5 minutes after eflornithine; do not wash treated area for 4 hours after application

Vaniqa® (Shire) ▼ PoM
Cream, eflornithine (as hydrochloride) 11.5%, net price 30 g = £26.04
Excipients: include cetostearyl alcohol, hydroxybenzoates, stearyl alcohol
NOTE. The *Scottish Medicines Consortium* has advised (May 2005) that *Vaniqa*® is not recommended for the treatment of facial hirsutism in women

Male-pattern baldness

Finasteride is licensed for the treatment of male-pattern baldness in men. Continuous use for 3–6 months is required before benefit is seen, and effects are reversed 6–12 months after treatment is discontinued.

Topical application of **minoxidil** may stimulate limited hair growth in a small proportion of adults but only for as long as it is used.

FINASTERIDE

Indications: male-pattern baldness in men
Cautions: see section 6.4.2

Side-effects: see section 6.4.2
Dose: 1 mg daily

Propecia® (MSD) ▼ PoM NHS
Tablets, f/c, beige, finasteride 1 mg, net price 28-tab pack = £26.99

MINOXIDIL

Indications: male-pattern baldness (men and women)
Cautions: section 2.5.1 (only about 1.4–1.7% absorbed); avoid contact with eyes, mouth and mucous membranes, broken, infected, shaved, or inflamed skin; avoid inhalation of spray mist; avoid occlusive dressings and topical drugs which enhance absorption
Contra-indications: section 2.5.1
Side-effects: section 2.5.1; irritant dermatitis, allergic contact dermatitis, discontinue if hair loss persists for more than 2 weeks
Dose: apply 1 mL twice daily to dry hair and scalp (discontinue if no improvement after 1 year); 5% strength for use in men only

Regaine® (Pharmacia) NHS
Regaine® Regular Strength topical solution, minoxidil 2% in an aqueous alcoholic basis, net price 60-mL bottle with applicators = £14.16
Excipients: include propylene glycol
Regaine® Extra Strength topical solution, minoxidil 5% in an aqueous alcoholic basis, net price 60-mL bottle with applicators = £17.00, 3 × 60-mL bottles = £34.03
Excipients: include propylene glycol
Cautions: flammable; wash hands after application

13.10 Anti-infective skin preparations

13.10.1 Antibacterial preparations

For many skin infections such as *erysipelas* and *cellulitis* systemic antibacterial treatment is more appropriate because the infection is too deeply seated for adequate penetration of topical preparations. For details of suitable treatment see section 5.1, table 1.

In the community acute *impetigo* on small areas of the skin may be treated by short-term topical application of **fusidic acid**; **mupirocin** should be used only to treat methicillin-resistant *Staphylococcus aureus*. If the impetigo is extensive or long-standing, an oral antibacterial such as **flucloxacillin** (or **erythromycin** in penicillin-allergy) (section 5.1, Table 1) should be used. Mild antiseptics such as **povidone–iodine** (section 13.11.4) are used to soften crusts and exudate.

Although there are a great many antibacterial drugs presented in topical preparations some are potentially hazardous and frequently their use is not necessary if adequate hygienic measures can be taken. Moreover, not all skin conditions that are oozing, crusted, or characterised by pustules are actually infected. Topical antibacterials should be **avoided** on *leg ulcers* unless used in short courses for defined infections; treatment of bacterial colonisation is generally inappropriate.

To minimise the development of resistant organisms it is advisable to limit the choice of antibacterials applied topically to those not used systemically. Unfortunately some of these, for example neomycin, may cause sensitisation, and there is cross-sensitivity with other aminoglycoside antibiotics, such as gentamicin. If *large areas of skin* are being treated, ototoxicity may also be a hazard with aminoglycoside antibiotics (and also with polymyxins), particularly in children, in the elderly, and in those with renal impairment. *Resistant organisms* are more common in hospitals, and whenever possible swabs should be taken for bacteriological examination before beginning treatment.

Mupirocin is not related to any other antibacterial in use; it is effective for skin infections, particularly those due to Gram-positive organisms but it is not indicated for pseudomonal infection. Although *Staphylococcus aureus* strains with low-level resistance to mupirocin are emerging, it is generally useful in infections resistant to other antibacterials. To avoid the development of resistance, mupirocin or fusidic acid should not be used for longer than 10 days and local microbiology advice should be sought before using it in hospital. In the presence of mupirocin-resistant MRSA infection, a polymyxin or an antiseptic like povidone-iodine, chlorhexidine, and alcohol can be used; their use should be discussed with the local microbiologist.

Silver sulfadiazine (silver sulphadiazine) is used in the treatment of infected burns.

13.10.1.1 Antibacterial preparations only used topically

MUPIROCIN

Indications: bacterial skin infections (see also notes above)
Side-effects: local reactions including urticaria, pruritus, burning sensation, rash
Dose: apply up to 3 times daily for up to 10 days; INFANT under 1 year not recommended

Bactroban® (GSK) PoM
Cream, mupirocin (as mupirocin calcium) 2%, net price 15 g = £4.38
Excipients: include benzyl alcohol, cetyl alcohol, stearyl alcohol
Ointment, mupirocin 2%, net price 15 g = £4.38
Excipients: none as listed in section 13.1.3
NOTE. Contains macrogol and manufacturer advises caution in renal impairment; may sting
Nasal ointment—section 12.2.3

NEOMYCIN SULPHATE

Indications: bacterial skin infections
Cautions: large areas, see below
LARGE AREAS. If large areas of skin are being treated ototoxicity may be a hazard, particularly in children, in the elderly, and in those with renal impairment
Contra-indications: neonates
Side-effects: sensitisation (see also notes above)

Neomycin Cream BPC PoM
Cream, neomycin sulphate 0.5%, cetomacrogol emulsifying ointment 30%, chlorocresol 0.1%, disodium edetate 0.01%, in freshly boiled and cooled purified water, net price 15 g = £2.27
Excipients: include cetostearyl alcohol, edetic acid (EDTA)
Dose: apply up to 3 times daily (short-term use)

Cicatrin® (GSK) PoM
Cream, neomycin sulphate 3300 units, bacitracin zinc 250 units, cysteine 2 mg, glycine 10 mg, threonine 1 mg/g, net price 15 g = 92p, 30 g = £1.84
Excipients: include wool fat derivative, polysorbates
Dose: superficial bacterial infection of skin, ADULT and CHILD over 2 years, apply up to 3 times daily (short-term use)
Dusting powder, neomycin sulphate 3300 units, bacitracin zinc 250 units, cysteine 2 mg, glycine 10 mg, threonine 1 mg/g, net price 15 g = 92p, 50 g = £3.07
Excipients: none as listed in section 13.1.3
Dose: superficial bacterial infection of skin, ADULT and CHILD over 2 years, apply up to 3 times daily (short-term use)

Graneodin® (Squibb) PoM
Ointment, neomycin sulphate 0.25%, gramicidin 0.025%, net price 25 g = £1.37
Excipients: none as listed in section 13.1.3
Dose: superficial bacterial infection of skin, apply 2–4 times daily (for max. 7 days—possibly longer for sycosis barbae)

POLYMYXINS

(Includes colistin sulphate and polymyxin B sulphate)
Indications: bacterial skin infections
Cautions: large areas, see below
LARGE AREAS. If large areas of skin are being treated nephrotoxicity and neurotoxicity may be a hazard, particularly in children, in the elderly, and in those with renal impairment
Side-effects: sensitisation (see also notes above)

Polyfax® (PLIVA) PoM
Ointment, polymyxin B sulphate 10 000 units, bacitracin zinc 500 units/g, net price 20 g = £4.62
Excipients: none as listed in section 13.1.3
Dose: apply twice daily or more frequently if required

Colomycin® (Forest) PoM
Powder, sterile, for making topical preparations (usually 1%), colistin sulphate, net price 1-g vial = £17.22
Excipients: none as listed in section 13.1.3

SILVER SULFADIAZINE

(Silver sulphadiazine)
Indications: prophylaxis and treatment of infection in burn wounds; as an adjunct to short-term treatment of infection in leg ulcers and pressure sores; as an adjunct to prophylaxis of infection in skin graft donor sites and extensive abrasions; for conservative management of finger-tip injuries
Cautions: hepatic and renal impairment; G6PD deficiency; pregnancy and breast-feeding (avoid in late pregnancy and in neonate—see also Appendix 4); may inactivate enzymatic debriding agents—concomitant use may be inappropriate; for large amounts see also **interactions:** Appendix 1 (sulphonamides)
LARGE AREAS. Plasma-sulfadiazine concentrations may approach therapeutic levels with *side-effects* and *interactions* as for sulphonamides (see section 5.1.8) if large areas of skin are treated. Owing to the association of sulphonamides with severe blood and skin disorders treatment should be stopped immediately if blood disorders or rashes develop—but leucopenia developing 2–3 days after starting treatment of burns patients is reported usually to be self-limiting and silver sulfadiazine need not usually be discontinued provided blood counts are monitored carefully to ensure return to normality within a few days. Argyria may also occur if large areas of skin are treated (or if application is prolonged).
Contra-indications: pregnancy (Appendix 4) and breast-feeding (Appendix 5); sensitivity to sulphonamides; not recommended for neonates (see also Appendix 4)
Side-effects: allergic reactions including burning, itching and rashes; argyria reported following prolonged use; leucopenia reported (monitor blood levels)

Flamazine® (S&N Hlth.) PoM
Cream, silver sulfadiazine 1%, net price 20 g = £2.91, 50 g = £3.85, 250 g = £10.32, 500 g = £18.27
Excipients: include cetyl alcohol, polysorbates, propylene glycol
Dose: apply with sterile applicator; burns, apply daily or more frequently if very exudative; leg ulcers or pressure sores, apply daily or on alternate days (not recommended if ulcer very exudative); finger-tip injuries, apply every 2–3 days; consult product literature for details

13.10.1.2 Antibacterial preparations also used systemically

Sodium fusidate is a narrow-spectrum antibacterial used for staphylococcal infections. For the role of sodium fusidate in the treatment of impetigo see p. 590.

Metronidazole is used topically for acne rosacea and to reduce the odour associated with anerobic infections; oral metronidazole (section 5.1.11) is used to treat wounds infected with anaerobic bacteria.

ANGULAR CHEILITIS. An ointment containing sodium fusidate is used in the fissures of angular cheilitis when associated with staphylococcal infection. For further information on angular cheilitis, see section 12.3.2.

FUSIDIC ACID

Indications: staphylococcal skin infections; penicillin-resistant staphylococcal infections (section 5.1.7); staphylococcal eye infections (section 11.3.1)
Cautions: see notes above; avoid contact with eyes
Side-effects: rarely hypersensitivity reactions
Dose: apply 3–4 times daily

Fucidin® (Leo) PoM
Cream, fusidic acid 2%, net price 15 g = £2.00, 30 g = £3.79
Excipients: include butylated hydroxyanisole, cetyl alcohol
Ointment, sodium fusidate 2%, net price 15 g = £2.23, 30 g = £3.79
Excipients: include cetyl alcohol, wool fat
DENTAL PRESCRIBING ON NHS. May be prescribed as Sodium Fusidate ointment

METRONIDAZOLE

Indications: see preparations; *Helicobacter pylori* eradication (section 1.3); anaerobic infections (section 5.1.11 and section 7.2.2); protozoal infections (section 5.4.2)

Cautions: avoid exposure to strong sunlight or UV light

Side-effects: skin irritation

Dose: see preparations

■ Rosacea (see also section 13.6)

Metrogel® (Novartis) PoM

Gel, metronidazole 0.75%, net price 40 g = £19.90. Label: 10, patient information leaflet

Excipients: include hydroxybenzoates (parabens), propylene glycol

Dose: acute inflammatory exacerbations of acne rosacea, apply thinly twice daily for 8–9 weeks

Metrosa® (Linderma) PoM

Gel, metronidazole 0.75%, net price 40 g = £19.90. Label: 10, patient information leaflet

Excipients: include propylene glycol

Dose: acute exacerbation of acne rosacea, apply thinly twice daily for up to 8 weeks

Noritate® (Aventis Pharma) PoM

Cream, metronidazole 1%, net price 30 g = £19.08. Label: 10, patient information leaflet

Excipients: include hydroxybenzoates (parabens)

Dose: acne rosacea, apply once daily for 8 weeks

Rozex® (Galderma) PoM

Cream, metronidazole 0.75%, net price 30 g = £10.00, 40 g = £15.28. Label: 10, patient information leaflet

Excipients: include benzyl alcohol, isopropyl palmitate

Gel, metronidazole 0.75%, net price 30 g = £10.00, 40 g = £15.28. Label: 10, patient information leaflet

Excipients: include disodium edetate, hydroxybenzoates (parabens), propylene glycol

Dose: inflammatory papules, pustules and erythema of acne rosacea, apply twice daily for 3–4 months

Zyomet® (Goldshield) PoM

Gel, metronidazole 0.75%, net price 30 g = £12.00. Label: 10, patient information leaflet

Excipients: include benzyl alcohol, disodium edetate, propylene glycol

Dose: acute inflammatory exacerbations of acne rosacea, apply thinly twice daily for 8–9 weeks

■ Malodorous tumours and skin ulcers

Anabact® (CHS) PoM

Gel, metronidazole 0.75%, net price 15 g = £4.47, 30 g = £7.89

Excipients: include hydroxybenzoates (parabens), propylene glycol

Dose: malodorous fungating tumours and malodorous gravitational and decubitus ulcers, apply to clean wound 1–2 times daily and cover with non-adherent dressing

Metrotop® (Medlock) PoM

Gel, metronidazole 0.8%, net price 15 g = £4.73, 30 g = £8.36

Excipients: none as listed in section 13.1.3

Dose: malodorous fungating tumours and malodorous gravitational and decubitus ulcers, apply to clean wound 1–2 times daily and cover (flat wounds, apply liberally; cavities, smear on paraffin gauze and pack loosely)

13.10.2 Antifungal preparations

Most localised fungal infections are treated with topical preparations. Systemic therapy (section 5.2) is necessary for nail or scalp infection or if the skin infection is widespread, disseminated or intractable. Skin scrapings should be examined if systemic therapy is being considered or where there is doubt about the diagnosis.

DERMATOPHYTOSES. Ringworm infection can affect the scalp (tinea capitis), body (tinea corporis), groin (tinea cruris), hand (tinea manuum), foot (tinea pedis, athlete's foot), or nail (tinea unguium). Scalp infection requires systemic treatment (section 5.2); additional topical application of an antifungal may reduce the risk of transmission. Most other local ringworm infections can be treated adequately with topical antifungal preparations (including shampoos, section 13.9). The imidazole antifungals **clotrimazole, econazole, ketoconazole, miconazole**, and **sulconazole** are all effective. **Terbinafine** cream is also effective but it is more expensive. Other topical antifungals include **amorolfine**, **griseofulvin**, and the **undecenoates**. **Compound benzoic acid ointment** (Whitfield's ointment) has been used for ringworm infections but it is cosmetically less acceptable than proprietary preparations. Topical preparations for athlete's foot containing **tolnaftate** are on sale to the public.

Antifungal dusting powders are of little therapeutic value in the treatment of fungal skin infections and may cause skin irritation; they may have some role in preventing re-infection.

Tinea infection of the nail is almost always treated systemically (section 5.2); topical application of **amorolfine** or **tioconazole** may be effective for treating early onychomycosis when involvement is limited to mild distal disease in up to 2 nails.

PITYRIASIS VERSICOLOR. Pityriasis (tinea) versicolor may be treated with **ketoconazole** shampoo (section 13.9). Alternatively, **selenium sulphide** shampoo [unlicensed indication] (section 13.9) may be used as a lotion (diluted with water to reduce irritation) and left on for at least 30 minutes or overnight; it is applied 2–7 times over a fortnight and the course repeated if necessary.

Topical imidazole antifungals **clotrimazole**, **econazole**, **ketoconazole**, **miconazole**, and **sulconazole** and topical **terbinafine** are alternatives but large quantities may be required.

If topical therapy fails, or if the infection is widespread, pityriasis versicolor is treated systemically with an azole antifungal (section 5.2). Relapse is common, especially in the immunocompromised.

CANDIDIASIS. Candidal skin infections may be treated with topical imidazole antifungals **clotrimazole**, **econazole**, **ketoconazole**, **miconazole**, and **sulconazole**; topical terbinafine is an alternative. Topical application of **nystatin** is also effective for candidiasis but it is ineffective against dermatophytosis. Refractory candidiasis requires systemic treatment (section 5.2) generally with a triazole such as fluconazole; systemic treatment with terbinafine is **not appropriate** for refractory candidiasis.

ANGULAR CHEILITIS. Nystatin ointment is used in the fissures of angular cheilitis when associated with *Candida*. For further information on angular cheilitis, see p. 555.

COMPOUND TOPICAL PREPARATIONS. Combination of an imidazole and a mild corticosteroid (such as hydrocortisone 1%) (section 13.4) may be of value in the treatment of eczematous intertrigo and, in the first few days only, of a severely inflamed patch of ringworm. Combination of a mild corticosteroid with either an imidazole or nystatin may be of use in the treatment of intertrigo associated with candida.

CAUTIONS. Contact with eyes and mucous membranes should be avoided.

SIDE-EFFECTS. Occasional local irritation and hypersensitivity reactions include mild burning sensation, erythema, and itching. Treatment should be discontinued if these are severe.

AMOROLFINE

Indications: see under preparations
Cautions: see notes above; also avoid contact with ears; pregnancy and breast-feeding
Side-effects: see notes above

Loceryl® (Galderma) PoM
Cream, amorolfine (as hydrochloride) 0.25%, net price 20 g = £4.83. Label: 10, patient information leaflet
Excipients: include cetostearyl alcohol, disodium edetate
Dose: fungal skin infections, apply once daily after cleansing in the evening for at least 2–3 weeks (up to 6 weeks for foot infection) continuing for 3–5 days after lesions have healed
Nail lacquer, amorolfine (as hydrochloride) 5%, net price 5-mL pack (with nail files, spatulas and cleansing swabs) = £21.43. Label: 10, patient information leaflet
Excipients: none as listed in section 13.1.3
Dose: fungal nail infections, apply to infected nails 1–2 times weekly after filing and cleansing; allow to dry (approx. 3 minutes); treat finger nails for 6 months, toe nails for 9–12 months (review at intervals of 3 months); avoid nail varnish or artificial nails during treatment

BENZOIC ACID

Indications: ringworm (tinea), but see notes above

Benzoic Acid Ointment, Compound, BP (Whitfield's ointment)
Ointment, benzoic acid 6%, salicylic acid 3%, in emulsifying ointment
Dose: apply twice daily
Excipients: include cetostearyl alcohol

CLOTRIMAZOLE

Indications: fungal skin infections; vaginal candidiasis (section 7.2.2); otitis externa (section 12.1.1)
Cautions: see notes above
Side-effects: see notes above
Dose: apply 2–3 times daily

Clotrimazole (Non-proprietary)
Cream, clotrimazole 1%, net price 20 g = £2.12
Brands include *Candiden*®

[1]**Canesten**® (Bayer Consumer Care)
Cream, clotrimazole 1%, net price 20 g = £2.14, 50 g = £3.80. On sale to the public as *Canesten*® *AF* cream
Excipients: include benzyl alcohol, cetostearyl alcohol, polysorbate 60
Powder, clotrimazole 1%, net price 30 g = £1.52. On sale to the public as *Canesten*® *AF* powder
Excipients: none as listed in section 13.1.3
Solution, clotrimazole 1% in macrogol 400 (polyethylene glycol 400), net price 20 mL = £2.43. For hairy areas
Excipients: none as listed in section 13.1.3
Spray, clotrimazole 1%, in 30% isopropyl alcohol, net price 40-mL atomiser = £4.99. Label: 15. For large or hairy areas. On sale to the public as *Canesten*® *AF* spray
Excipients: include propylene glycol

1. The brand name *Canesten*® *AF Once Daily* is used for bifonazole

ECONAZOLE NITRATE

Indications: fungal skin infections; vaginal candidiasis (section 7.2.2)
Cautions: see notes above
Side-effects: see notes above
Dose: skin infections apply twice daily; nail infections, apply once daily under occlusive dressing

Ecostatin® (Squibb)
Cream, econazole nitrate 1%, net price 15 g = £1.49; 30 g = £2.75
Excipients: include butylated hydroxyanisole, fragrance

Pevaryl® (Janssen-Cilag)
Cream, econazole nitrate 1%, net price 30 g = £2.65
Excipients: include butylated hydroxyanisole, fragrance

GRISEOFULVIN

Indications: tinea pedis; resistant fungal infections (section 5.2)
Cautions: see notes above
Side-effects: see notes above
Dose: apply 400 micrograms (1 spray) to an area approx. 13 cm^2 once daily, increased to 1.2 mg (3 sprays, allowing each spray to dry between applications) once daily if necessary; max. treatment duration 4 weeks

Grisol® (Transdermal)
Spray, griseofulvin 400 micrograms/metered spray, net price 20-mL (400-dose) spray = £4.80. Label: 15
Excipients: include benzyl alcohol

KETOCONAZOLE

Indications: fungal skin infections; systemic or resistant fungal infections (section 5.2); vulval candidiasis (section 7.2.2)
Cautions: see notes above; do **not** use within 2 weeks of a topical corticosteroid for seborrhoeic dermatitis—risk of skin sensitisation
Side-effects: see notes above
Dose: tinea pedis, apply twice daily; other fungal infections, apply 1–2 times daily

[1]**Nizoral**® (Janssen-Cilag) PoM
[2]*Cream*, ketoconazole 2%, net price 30 g = £3.62
Excipients: include cetyl alcohol, polysorbates, propylene glycol, stearyl alcohol
Shampoo—section 13.9

1. A 15-g tube is available for sale to the public for the treatment of tinea pedis, tinea cruris, and candidal intertrigo (*Daktarin*® *Gold*)
2. NHS except for seborrhoeic dermatitis and pityriasis versicolor and endorsed 'SLS'

MICONAZOLE NITRATE

Indications: fungal skin infections; intestinal fungal infections (section 5.2); oral fungal infections (section 12.3.2); vaginal candidiasis (section 7.2.2)
Cautions: see notes above
Side-effects: see notes above

Dose: apply twice daily continuing for 10 days after lesions have healed; nail infections, apply 1–2 times daily

Miconazole (Non-proprietary)
Cream, miconazole nitrate 2%, net price 20 g = £2.05, 45 g = £1.97
Brands include *Acorvio*® (*excipients: include* cetostearyl alcohol, polysorbate 40, propylene glycol)

Daktarin® (Janssen-Cilag)
Cream, miconazole nitrate 2%, net price 30 g = £1.97. Also on sale to the public as *Daktarin*® *Dual Action cream* for athlete's foot
Excipients: include butylated hydroxyanisole
NOTE. A 15-g tube [NHS] is on sale to the public.
Powder [NHS], miconazole nitrate 2%, net price 20 g = £1.81. Also on sale to the public as *Daktarin*® *Dual Action powder* for athlete's foot
Excipients: include none as listed in section 13.1.3
Dual Action Spray powder, miconazole nitrate 0.16%, in an aerosol basis, net price 100 g = £2.27
Excipients: none as listed in section 13.1.3

NYSTATIN

Indications: skin infections due to *Candida* spp.; intestinal candidiasis (section 5.2); vaginal candidiasis (section 7.2.2); oral fungal infections (section 12.3.2)
Cautions: see notes above
Side-effects: see notes above

Nystaform® (Typharm) [PoM]
Cream, nystatin 100 000 units/g, chlorhexidine hydrochloride 1%, net price 30 g = £2.62
Excipients: include benzyl alcohol, cetostearyl alcohol, polysorbate 60
Dose: apply 2–3 times daily continuing for 7 days after lesions have healed.

Nystan® (Squibb) [PoM]
Cream, nystatin 100 000 units/g, net price 30 g = £2.18
Excipients: include benzyl alcohol, propylene glycol, fragrance
Dose: apply 2–4 times daily
Ointment, nystatin 100 000 units/g, in *Plastibase*®, net price 30 g = £1.75
Excipients: none as listed in section 13.1.3
Dose: apply 2–4 times daily
DENTAL PRESCRIBING ON NHS. May be prescribed as Nystatin Ointment

Tinaderm-M® (Schering-Plough) [PoM]
Cream, nystatin 100 000 units/g, tolnaftate 1%, net price 20 g = £1.83
Excipients: include butylated hydroxytoluene, cetostearyl alcohol, hydroxybenzoates (parabens), fragrance
Dose: apply 2–3 times daily

SALICYLIC ACID

Indications: fungal nail infections, particularly tinea; hyperkeratotic skin disorders (section 13.5.2); acne vulgaris (section 13.6.1); warts and calluses (section 13.7)
Contra-indications: pregnancy
Side-effects: see notes above
Dose: apply twice daily; CHILD under 5 years not recommended

Phytex® (Wynlit) [black triangle]
Paint, salicylic acid 1.46% (total combined), tannic acid 4.89% and boric acid 3.12% (as borotannic complex), in a vehicle containing alcohol and ethyl acetate, net price 25 mL (with brush) = £1.56
Excipients: none as listed in section 13.1.3
NOTE. Flammable

SULCONAZOLE NITRATE

Indications: fungal skin infections
Cautions: see notes above
Side-effects: see notes above; also blistering
Dose: apply 1–2 times daily continuing for 2–3 weeks after lesions have healed

Exelderm® (Centrapharm)
Cream, sulconazole nitrate 1%, net price 30 g = £3.00
Excipients: include cetyl alcohol, polysorbates, propylene glycol, stearyl alcohol

TERBINAFINE

Indications: fungal skin infections
Cautions: pregnancy, breast-feeding; avoid contact with eyes
Side-effects: redness, itching, or stinging; rarely allergic reactions (discontinue)

[1]**Lamisil**® (Novartis) [PoM]
Cream, terbinafine hydrochloride 1%, net price 15 g = £4.86, 30 g = £8.76
Dose: apply thinly 1–2 times daily for up to 1 week in tinea pedis, 1–2 weeks in tinea corporis and tinea cruris, 2 weeks in cutaneous candidiasis and pityriasis versicolor; review after 2 weeks; CHILD not recommended
Excipients: include benzyl alcohol, cetyl alcohol, polysorbate 60, stearyl alcohol
Tablets—section 5.2

1. Can be sold to the public for external use for the treatment of tinea pedis and tinea cruris as a cream containing terbinafine hydrochloride max. 1% in a pack containing max. 15 g (*Lamisil*® *AT* cream); also for the treatment of tinea pedis, tinea cruris, and tinea corporis as a spray containing terbinafine hydrochloride max. 1% in a pack containing max. 30 mL (*Lamisil*® *AT* spray) or max. 30 g (*Lamisil*® *AT* gel)

TIOCONAZOLE

Indications: fungal nail infections
Cautions: see notes above
Contra-indications: pregnancy
Side-effects: see notes above; also local oedema, dry skin, nail discoloration, periungual inflammation, nail pain, rash, exfoliation
Dose: apply to nails and surrounding skin twice daily for up to 6 months (may be extended to 12 months)

Trosyl® (Pfizer) [PoM]
Cutaneous solution, tioconazole 28%, net price 12 mL (with applicator brush) = £27.38
Excipients: none as listed in section 13.1.3

UNDECENOATES

Indications: see under preparations below
Side-effects: see notes above
Dose: see under preparations below

Monphytol® (LAB) [black triangle]
Paint, methyl undecenoate 5%, propyl undecenoate 0.7%, salicylic acid 3%, methyl salicylate 25%, propyl salicylate 5%, chlorobutanol 3%, net price 18 mL (with brush) = £1.77
Excipients: none as listed in section 13.1.3
Dose: fungal skin and nail infections, apply twice daily

Mycota® (Thornton & Ross)
Cream, zinc undecenoate 20%, undecenoic acid 5%, net price 25 g = £1.31
Excipients: include fragrance
Dose: treatment of athlete's foot, apply twice daily continuing for 7 days after lesions have healed
Prevention of athlete's foot, apply once daily

Powder, zinc undecenoate 20%, undecenoic acid 2%, net price 70 g = £1.87
Excipients: include fragrance
Dose: treatment of athlete's foot, apply twice daily continuing for 7 days after lesions have healed
Prevention of athlete's foot, apply once daily

Spray application, undecenoic acid 2.5%, dichlorophen 0.25% (pressurised aerosol pack), net price 100 mL = £2.13
Excipients: include fragrance
Dose: treatment of athlete's foot, apply twice daily continuing for 7 days after lesions have healed
Prevention of athlete's foot, apply once daily

13.10.3 Antiviral preparations

Aciclovir cream is licensed for the treatment of initial and recurrent labial and genital *herpes simplex infections*; treatment should begin as early as possible. Systemic treatment is necessary for buccal or vaginal infections and for *herpes zoster (shingles)* (for details of systemic use see section 5.3.2.1).

Idoxuridine solution (5% in dimethyl sulfoxide) is of little value.

HERPES LABIALIS. **Aciclovir** cream can be used for the treatment of initial and recurrent labial herpes simplex infections (cold sores). It is best applied at the earliest possible stage, usually when prodromal changes of sensation are felt in the lip and before vesicles appear.

Penciclovir cream is also licensed for the treatment of herpes labialis; it needs to be applied more frequently than aciclovir cream. These creams should not be used in the mouth.

Systemic treatment is necessary if cold sores recur frequently or for infections in the mouth (see p. 321).

ACICLOVIR

(Acyclovir)

Indications: see notes above; herpes simplex and varicella–zoster infections (section 5.3.2.1); eye infections (section 11.3.3)

Cautions: avoid contact with eyes and mucous membranes

Side-effects: transient stinging or burning; occasionally erythema, itching or drying of the skin

Dose: apply to lesions every 4 hours (5 times daily) for 5–10 days, starting at first sign of attack

[1]**Aciclovir** (Non-proprietary) PoM
Cream, aciclovir 5%, net price 2 g = £1.85, 10 g = £5.98
Excipients: include propylene glycol
Brands include *Zuvogen*® (*excipients* also include cetyl alcohol, propylene glycol)
DENTAL PRESCRIBING ON NHS. Aciclovir Cream may be prescribed

1. A 2-g tube and a pump pack are on sale to the public for the treatment of cold sores (*Zovirax*® *Cold Sore Cream*); other brands on sale to the public include *Action*® *Cold Sore*, *Aviral*®, *Boots Cold Sore*®, *Clearsore*®, *Herpetad*®, *Soothelip*®, *Viralief*®, and *Virasorb*®

Zovirax® (GSK) PoM
Cream, aciclovir 5%, net price 2 g = £4.92, 10 g = £14.82
Excipients: include cetostearyl alcohol, propylene glycol
Eye ointment—section 11.3.3
Tablets—section 5.3.2.1

PENCICLOVIR

Indications: see notes above

Cautions: avoid contact with eyes and mucous membranes

Side-effects: transient stinging, burning, numbness

Vectavir® (Novartis Consumer Health) PoM
Cream, penciclovir 1%, net price 2 g = £4.20
Excipients: include cetostearyl alcohol, propylene glycol
Dose: herpes labialis, apply to lesions every 2 hours during waking hours for 4 days, starting at first sign of attack; CHILD under 12 years, not recommended
DENTAL PRESCRIBING ON NHS. May be prescribed as Penciclovir Cream

IDOXURIDINE IN DIMETHYL SULFOXIDE

Indications: herpes simplex and herpes zoster infection but of little value

Cautions: avoid contact with the eyes, mucous membranes, and textiles; breast-feeding (Appendix 5)

Contra-indications: pregnancy (Appendix 4); **not** to be used in mouth

Side-effects: stinging on application, changes in taste; overuse may cause maceration

Herpid® (Yamanouchi) PoM
Application, idoxuridine 5% in dimethyl sulfoxide, net price 5 mL (with applicator) = £6.33
Dose: apply to lesions 4 times daily for 4 days, starting at first sign of attack; CHILD under 12 years, not recommended

13.10.4 Parasiticidal preparations

Suitable quantities of parasiticidal preparations

	Skin creams	Lotions	Cream rinses
Scalp (headlice)	—	50–100 mL	50–100 mL
Body (scabies)	30–60 g	100 mL	—
Body (crab lice)	30–60 g	100 mL	—

These amounts are usually suitable for an adult for single application.

Scabies

Permethrin is effective for the treatment of *scabies* (*Sarcoptes scabiei*); **malathion** can be used if permethrin is inappropriate.

Aqueous preparations are preferable to alcoholic lotions, which are not recommended owing to irritation of excoriated skin and the genitalia.

Older preparations include **benzyl benzoate**, which is an irritant and should be avoided in children; it is less effective than malathion and permethrin.

Ivermectin (available on a named patient basis from IDIS) in a single dose of 200 micrograms/kg by mouth has been used, in combination with topical drugs, for the treatment of hyperkeratotic (crusted or 'Norwegian') scabies that does not respond to topical treatment alone.

APPLICATION. Although acaricides have traditionally been applied after a hot bath, this is **not** necessary and there is even evidence that a hot bath may increase absorption into the blood, removing them from their site of action on the skin.

All members of the affected household should be treated simultaneously. Treatment should be applied to the whole body including the scalp, neck, face, and ears. Particular attention should be paid to the webs of the fingers and toes and lotion brushed under the ends of nails. It is now recommended that malathion and permethrin should be applied twice, one week apart; in the case of benzyl benzoate up to 3 applications on consecutive days may be needed. It is important to warn users to reapply treatment to the hands if they are washed. Patients with hyperkeratotic scabies may require 2 or 3 applications of acaricide on consecutive days to ensure that enough penetrates the skin crusts to kill all the mites.

ITCHING. The *itch* and *eczema* of scabies persists for some weeks after the infestation has been eliminated and treatment for pruritus and eczema (section 13.5.1) may be required. Application of **crotamiton** can be used to control itching after treatment with more effective acaricides. A topical corticosteroid may help to reduce itch and inflammation after scabies has been treated successfully; however, persistent symptoms suggest that scabies eradication was not successful. Oral administration of a **sedating antihistamine** (section 3.4.1) at night may also be useful.

Head lice

Carbaryl, **malathion**, and the **pyrethroids** (permethrin and phenothrin) are effective against head lice (*Pediculus humanus capitis*) but lice in some districts have developed resistance; resistance to two or more parasiticidal preparations has also been reported. Benzyl benzoate is licensed for the treatment of head lice but it is less effective than other drugs.

Head lice infestation (pediculosis) should be treated using lotion or liquid formulations. Shampoos are diluted too much in use to be effective. Alcoholic formulations are effective but aqueous formulations are preferred in severe eczema, for patients with asthma, and small children. A contact time of 12 hours or overnight treatment is recommended for lotions and liquids; a 2-hour treatment is not sufficient to kill eggs.

In general, a course of treatment for head lice should be 2 applications of product 7 days apart to prevent lice emerging from any eggs that survive the first application.

The policy of rotating insecticides on a district-wide basis is now considered outmoded. To overcome the development of resistance, a mosaic strategy is required whereby, if a course of treatment fails to cure, a different insecticide is used for the next course. If a course of treatment with either permethrin or phenothrin fails, then a non-pyrethroid parasiticidal product should be used for the next course.

WET COMBING METHODS. Several products are available which require the use of a plastic detection comb and hair conditioner; a head lice device (*Bug Buster® Kit*) is prescribable on the NHS. The methods typically involve meticulous combing with the detection comb (probably for at least 30 minutes each time) over the whole scalp at 4-day intervals for a minimum of 2 weeks.

Crab lice

Carbaryl [unlicensed for crab lice], **permethrin, phenothrin**, and **malathion** are effective for *crab lice* (*Pthirus pubis*). An aqueous preparation should be applied, allowed to dry naturally and washed off after 12 hours; a second treatment is needed after 7 days to kill lice emerging from surviving eggs. All surfaces of the body should be treated, including the scalp, neck, ears, and face (paying particular attention to the eyebrows and any beard). A different insecticide should be used if a course of treatment fails. Alcoholic lotions are not recommended (owing to irritation of excoriated skin and the genitalia).

Aqueous **malathion** lotion is effective for *crab lice of the eye lashes* [unlicensed use].

Benzyl benzoate

Benzyl benzoate is effective for *scabies* but is not a first-choice for *scabies* (see notes above).

BENZYL BENZOATE

Indications: scabies (but see notes above)

Cautions: children (not recommended, see also under Dose, below), avoid contact with eyes and mucous membranes; do not use on broken or secondarily infected skin; breast-feeding (suspend feeding until product has been washed off)

Side-effects: skin irritation, burning sensation especially on genitalia and excoriations, occasionally rashes

Dose: apply over the whole body; repeat without bathing on the following day and wash off 24 hours later; a third application may be required in some cases

NOTE. Not recommended for children—dilution to reduce irritant effect also reduces efficacy. Some manufacturers recommend application to the body but to exclude the head and neck. However, application should be extended to the scalp, neck, face, and ears

Benzyl Benzoate Application, BP (Non-proprietary)

Application, benzyl benzoate 25% in an emulsion basis, net price 500 mL = £2.47

Brands include *Ascabiol®* (*excipients: include* triethanolamine)

Carbaryl

Carbaryl is recommended for *head lice*; an aqueous preparation is recommended for *crab lice* (see notes above) but a suitable product is not currently licensed for this indication. In the light of experimental data in *animals* it would be prudent to consider carbaryl as a potential human carcinogen and it has been restricted to prescription only use. The Department of Health has emphasised that the risk is a theoretical one and that any risk from the intermittent use of head lice preparations is likely to be exceedingly small.

CARBARYL

(Carbaril)

Indications: see notes above and under preparations

Cautions: avoid contact with eyes; do not use on broken or secondarily infected skin; do not use more than once a week for 3 consecutive weeks; children under 6 months, medical supervision required; alcoholic lotion **not** recommended for pediculosis in asthma, in severe eczema or in small children

Side-effects: skin irritation

Dose: head lice, rub into dry hair and scalp, allow to dry naturally, shampoo after 12 hours, and comb wet hair (see also notes above); repeat application after 7 days [unlicensed use]

Crab lice [unlicensed indication], apply aqueous solution over whole body (see notes above), allow to dry naturally and wash off after 12 hours or overnight; repeat application after 7 days

Carylderm® (SSL) PoM

Liquid, carbaryl 1% in an aqueous basis, net price 50 mL = £2.28

Excipients: include cetostearyl alcohol, hydroxybenzoates (parabens)

Lotion, carbaryl 0.5%, in an alcoholic basis, net price 50 mL = £2.28. Label: 15

Excipients: include fragrance

Malathion

Malathion is recommended for *scabies*, *head lice* and *crab lice* (for details see notes above).

The risk of systemic effects associated with 1–2 applications of malathion is considered to be very low; however, applications of lotion repeated at intervals of less than 1 week *or* application for more than 3 consecutive weeks should be **avoided** since the likelihood of eradication of lice is not increased.

MALATHION

Indications: see notes above and under preparations

Cautions: avoid contact with eyes; do not use on broken or secondarily infected skin; do not use lotion more than once a week for 3 consecutive weeks; children under 6 months, medical supervision required; alcoholic lotions **not** recommended for head lice in severe eczema, asthma or in small children, or for scabies or crab lice

Side-effects: skin irritation

Dose: head lice, rub 0.5% preparation into dry hair and scalp, allow to dry naturally, remove by washing after 12 hours (see also notes above); repeat application after 7 days [unlicensed use]

Crab lice, apply 0.5% aqueous preparation over whole body, allow to dry naturally, wash off after 12 hours or overnight; repeat application after 7 days [unlicensed use]

Scabies, apply 0.5% preparation over whole body, and wash off after 24 hours; if hands are washed with soap within 24 hours, they should be retreated; see also notes above; repeat application after 7 days [unlicensed use]

NOTE. For scabies, manufacturer recommends application to the body but not necessarily to the head and neck. However, application should be extended to the scalp, neck, face, and ears

Derbac-M® (SSL)

Liquid, malathion 0.5% in an aqueous basis, net price 50 mL = £2.22, 200 mL = £5.70

Excipients: include cetostearyl alcohol, fragrance, hydroxybenzoates (parabens)

For crab lice, head lice, and scabies

Prioderm® (SSL)

Lotion, malathion 0.5%, in an alcoholic basis, net price 50 mL = £2.22, 200 mL = £5.70. Label: 15

Excipients: include fragrance

For head lice (alcoholic formulation, see notes above)

Cream shampoo NHS, malathion 1%, net price 40 g = £2.77

Excipients: include cetostearyl alcohol, fragrance, hydroxybenzoates (parabens), sodium edetate, wool fat

Dose: head and crab lice, not recommended, therefore no dose stated (product too diluted in use and insufficient contact time)

Quellada M® (GSK Consumer Healthcare)

Liquid, malathion 0.5% in an aqueous basis, net price 50 mL = £1.85, 200 mL = £4.62

Excipients: include cetostearyl alcohol, fragrance, hydroxybenzoates (parabens)

For crab lice, head lice, and scabies

Cream shampoo, malathion 1%, net price 40 g = £2.18

Excipients: include cetostearyl alcohol, fragrance, hydroxybenzoates (parabens), sodium edetate, wool fat

Dose: head and crab lice, not recommended, therefore no dose stated (product too diluted in use and insufficient contact time)

Suleo-M® (SSL)

Lotion, malathion 0.5%, in an alcoholic basis, net price 50 mL = £2.22, 200 mL = £5.70. Label: 15

Excipients: include fragrance

For head lice (alcoholic formulation, see notes above)

Permethrin

Permethrin is effective for *scabies* and *crab lice* (for details see notes above). Permethrin is active against *head lice* but the formulation and licensed methods of application of the current products make them unsuitable for the treatment of head lice.

PERMETHRIN

Indications: see notes above and under Dose

Cautions: avoid contact with eyes; do not use on broken or secondarily infected skin; children under 6 months, medical supervision required for cream rinse (head lice); children aged 2 months–2 years, medical supervision required for dermal cream (scabies)

Side-effects: pruritus, erythema, and stinging; rarely rashes and oedema

Dose: scabies, apply 5% preparation over whole body and wash off after 8–12 hours; CHILD (see also Cautions, above) apply over whole body including face, neck, scalp and ears; if hands washed with soap within 8 hours of application, they should be treated again with cream (see notes above); repeat application after 7 days

NOTE. Manufacturer recommends application to the body but to exclude head and neck. However, application should be extended to the scalp, neck, face, and ears

Larger patients may require up to two 30-g packs for adequate treatment

Crab lice, ADULT over 18 years, apply 5% cream over whole body, allow to dry naturally and wash off after 12 hours or after leaving on overnight; repeat application after 7 days

Permethrin (Non-proprietary)
Cream, permethrin 5%, net price 30 g = £5.52

Lyclear® Creme Rinse (Chefaro UK)
Cream rinse, permethrin 1% in basis containing isopropyl alcohol 20%, net price 59 mL = £2.38, 2 × 59-mL pack = £4.32
Excipients: include cetyl alcohol
Dose: head lice, not recommended, therefore no dose stated (insufficient contact time)

Lyclear® Dermal Cream (Chefaro UK)
Dermal cream, permethrin 5%, net price 30 g = £5.52. Label: 10, patient information leaflet
Excipients: include butylated hydroxytoluene, wool fat derivative

Phenothrin

Phenothrin is recommended for *head lice* and *crab lice* (for details see notes above).

PHENOTHRIN

Indications: see notes above and under preparations
Cautions: avoid contact with eyes; do not use on broken or secondarily infected skin; do not use more than once a week for 3 weeks at a time; children under 6 months, medical supervision required; alcoholic preparations **not** recommended for head lice in severe eczema, in asthma, in small children, or for crab lice (see notes above)
Side-effects: skin irritation
Dose: see under preparations

Full Marks® (SSL)
Liquid, phenothrin 0.5% in an aqueous basis, net price 50 mL = £2.22, 200 mL = £5.70
Excipients: include cetostearyl alcohol, fragrance, hydroxybenzoates (parabens)
Dose: head lice, apply to dry hair, allow to dry naturally; shampoo after 12 hours or next day, comb wet hair; repeat application after 7 days [unlicensed use]
Lotion, phenothrin 0.2% in basis containing isopropyl alcohol 69.3%, net price 50 mL = £2.22, 200 mL = £5.70. Label: 15
Excipients: include fragrance
Dose: crab lice and head lice (alcoholic formulation, see notes above), apply to dry hair, allow to dry naturally; shampoo after 12 hours [unlicensed contact duration], comb wet hair; repeat application after 7 days [unlicensed use]
Mousse (= foam application), phenothrin 0.5% in an alcoholic basis, net price 50 g = £2.44, 150 g = £6.11. Label: 15
Excipients: include cetostearyl alcohol
Dose: head lice (alcoholic formulation, see notes above), apply to dry hair, shampoo after 30 minutes, comb wet hair—but product not recommended because it is too diluted in use and insufficient contact time (longer contact time not recommended because of risk of irritation)

13.10.5 Preparations for minor cuts and abrasions

Some of the preparations listed are used in minor burns, and abrasions. They are applied as necessary. Preparations containing camphor and sulphonamides should be **avoided**. Preparations such as magnesium sulphate paste are also listed but are now rarely used to treat carbuncles and boils as these are best treated with antibiotics (section 5.1.1.2).

Cetrimide Cream, BP
Cream, cetrimide 0.5% in a suitable water-miscible basis such as cetostearyl alcohol 5%, liquid paraffin 50% in freshly boiled and cooled purified water, net price 50 g = 76p

Proflavine Cream, BPC
Cream, proflavine hemisulphate 0.1%, yellow beeswax 2.5%, chlorocresol 0.1%, liquid paraffin 67.3%, freshly boiled and cooled purified water 25%, wool fat 5%, net price 100 mL = 85p
Excipients: include beeswax, wool fat
NOTE. Stains clothing

■ Preparations for boils

Magnesium Sulphate Paste, BP
Paste, dried magnesium sulphate 45 g, glycerol 55 g, phenol 500 mg, net price 25 g = 59p, 50 g = 72p
NOTE. Should be stirred before use
Dose: apply under dressing

Collodion

Flexible collodion may be used to seal minor cuts and wounds that have partially healed.

Collodion, Flexible, BP
Collodion, castor oil 2.5%, colophony 2.5% in a collodion basis, prepared by dissolving pyroxylin (10%) in a mixture of 3 volumes of ether and 1 volume of alcohol (90%), net price 10 mL = 27p. Label: 15

Skin tissue adhesive

Tissue adhesives are used for closure of minor skin wounds and for additional suture support. They should be applied by an appropriately trained healthcare professional.

Dermabond® (Ethicon)
Topical skin adhesive, sterile, ocrilate, net price 0.5 mL = £10.18

Epiglu® (Valeant)
Tissue adhesive, sterile, ethyl-2-cyanoacrylate 954.5 mg/g, polymethylmethacrylate, net price 4 × 3-g vials = £95.00 (with dispensing pipettes and pallete)

Indermil® (Tyco)
Tissue adhesive, sterile, enbucrilate, net price 5 × 500-mg units = £32.50, 20 × 500-mg units = £130.00

Histoacryl® (Braun)
Tissue adhesive, sterile, enbucrilate, net price 5 × 200-mg unit (blue) = £32.00, 10 × 200-mg unit (blue) = £67.20, 5 × 500-mg unit (clear or blue) = £34.65, 10 × 500-mg unit (blue) = £69.30

LiquiBand® (MedLogic)
Tissue adhesive, sterile, enbucrilate, net price 0.5-g amp = £5.50

13.11 Skin cleansers and antiseptics

Soap or detergent is used with water to cleanse intact skin; emollient preparations such as aqueous cream or emulsifying ointment (section 13.2.1) that do not irritate the skin are best used for cleansing dry skin.

An antiseptic is used for skin that is infected or that is susceptible to recurrent infection. Detergent preparations containing **chlorhexidine**, **triclosan**, or **povidone–iodine**, which should be thoroughly rinsed off, are used. Emollients may also contain antiseptics (section 13.2.1).

Antiseptics such as **chlorhexidine** or **povidone–iodine** are used on intact skin before surgical procedures; their antiseptic effect is enhanced by an alcoholic solvent. **Cetrimide** solution may be used if a detergent effect is also required.

For irrigating ulcers or wounds, lukewarm sterile sodium chloride 0.9% solution is used but tap water is often appropriate.

Potassium permanganate solution 1 in 10 000, a mild antiseptic with astringent properties, can be used for exudative eczematous areas; it should be stopped when the skin becomes dry. It can stain skin and nails especially with prolonged use.

13.11.1 Alcohols and saline

ALCOHOL

Indications: skin preparation before injection

Cautions: flammable; avoid broken skin; patients have suffered severe burns when diathermy has been preceded by application of alcoholic skin disinfectants

Industrial Methylated Spirit, BP
Solution, 19 volumes of ethanol and 1 volume approved wood naphtha, net price '66 OP' (containing 95% by volume alcohol) 100 mL = 32p; '74 OP' (containing 99% by volume alcohol) 100 mL = 32p. Label: 15

Surgical Spirit, BP
Spirit, methyl salicylate 0.5 mL, diethyl phthalate 2%, castor oil 2.5%, in industrial methylated spirit, net price 100 mL = 20p. Label: 15

SODIUM CHLORIDE

Indications: see notes above; nebuliser diluent (section 3.1.5); eye (section 11.8.1)

Sodium Chloride (Non-proprietary)
Solution (sterile), sodium chloride 0.9%, net price 10 × 10-mL unit = £3.60; 10 × 20-mL unit = £10.36; 10 × 30-mL unit = £3.00

Flowfusor® (Fresenius Kabi)
Solution (sterile), sodium chloride 0.9%, net price 120-mL Bellows Pack = £1.55

Irriclens® (ConvaTec)
Solution in aerosol can (sterile), sodium chloride 0.9%, net price 240-mL can = £3.00

Irripod® (C D Medical)
Solution (sterile), sodium chloride 0.9%, net price 25 × 20-mL sachet = £5.50

Miniversol® (Aguettant)
Solution (sterile), sodium chloride 0.9%, net price 30 × 45-mL unit = £15.00; 30 × 100-mL unit = £21.30

Normasol® (Medlock)
Solution (sterile), sodium chloride 0.9%, net price 25 × 25-mL sachet = £5.95; 10 × 100-mL sachet = £7.28

Stericlens® (C D Medical)
Solution in aerosol can (sterile), sodium chloride 0.9%, net price 100-mL can = £1.94, 240-mL can = £2.95

Steripod® Sodium Chloride (Medlock)
Solution (sterile), sodium chloride 0.9%, net price 25 × 20-mL sachet = £6.95

Versol® (Aguettant)
Solution, (sterile), sodium chloride 0.9%, net price 500 mL = 90p, 1 litre = 95p

13.11.2 Chlorhexidine salts

CHLORHEXIDINE

Indications: see under preparations; bladder irrigation and catheter patency solutions (see section 7.4.4)

Cautions: avoid contact with eyes, brain, meninges and middle ear; not for use in body cavities; alcoholic solutions not suitable before diathermy

Side-effects: occasional sensitivity

Chlorhexidine 0.05% (Baxter)
2000 Solution (sterile), pink, chlorhexidine acetate 0.05%, net price 500 mL = 72p, 1000 mL = 77p
For cleansing and disinfecting wounds and burns

Cepton® (LPC)
Skin wash (= solution), red, chlorhexidine gluconate 1%, net price 150 mL = £1.99
For use as skin wash in acne
Lotion, blue, chlorhexidine gluconate 0.1%, net price 150 mL = £1.99
For skin disinfection in acne

CX Antiseptic Dusting Powder® (Adams Hlth.)
Dusting powder, sterile, chlorhexidine acetate 1%, net price 15 g = £2.52
For skin disinfection

Hibiscrub® (SSL)
Cleansing solution, red, chlorhexidine gluconate solution 20% (≡ 4% chlorhexidine gluconate), perfumed, in a surfactant solution, net price 250 mL = £1.10, 500 mL = £1.60, 5 litres = £12.70
Excipients: include fragrance
Use instead of soap for pre-operative hand and skin preparation and for general hand and skin disinfection

Hibisol® (SSL)
Solution, chlorhexidine gluconate solution 2.5% (≡ 0.5% chlorhexidine gluconate), in isopropyl

alcohol 70% with emollients, net price 500 mL = £1.70
To be used undiluted for hand and skin disinfection

Hibitane Obstetric® (Centrapharm)
Cream, chlorhexidine gluconate solution 5% (≡ 1% chlorhexidine gluconate), in a pourable water-miscible basis, net price 250 mL = £2.89
For use in obstetrics and gynaecology as an antiseptic and lubricant (for application to skin around vulva and perineum and to hands of midwife or doctor)

Hydrex® (Adams Hlth.)
Solution, chlorhexidine gluconate solution 2.5% (≡ chlorhexidine gluconate 0.5%), in an alcoholic solution, net price 600 mL (clear) = £1.94; 600 mL (pink) = £1.94, 200-mL spray = £1.77, 500-mL spray = £3.01; 600 mL (blue) = £2.12
For pre-operative skin disinfection
NOTE. Flammable
Surgical scrub, chlorhexidine gluconate 4% in a surfactant solution, net price 250 mL = £1.82, 500 mL = £1.92
For pre-operative hand and skin preparation and for general hand disinfection

Unisept® (Medlock)
Solution (sterile), pink, chlorhexidine gluconate 0.05%, net price 25 × 25-mL sachet = £5.59; 10 × 100-mL sachet = £6.84
For cleansing and disinfecting wounds and burns and swabbing in obstetrics

■ With cetrimide

Tisept® (Medlock)
Solution (sterile), yellow, chlorhexidine gluconate 0.015%, cetrimide 0.15%, net price 25 × 25-mL sachet = £5.59; 10 × 100-mL sachet = £6.84
To be used undiluted for general skin disinfection and wound cleansing

Travasept 100® (Baxter)
Solution (sterile), yellow, chlorhexidine acetate 0.015%, cetrimide 0.15%, net price 500 mL = 72p, 1 litre = 77p
To be used undiluted in skin disinfection such as wound cleansing and obstetrics

Concentrates

Hibitane 5% Concentrate® (SSL)
Solution, red, chlorhexidine gluconate solution 25% (≡ 5% chlorhexidine gluconate), in a perfumed aqueous solution, net price 5 litres = £11.50
Dose: to be used diluted 1 in 10 (0.5%) with alcohol 70% for pre-operative skin preparation, or 1 in 100 (0.05%) with water for general skin disinfection
NOTE. Alcoholic solutions not suitable before diathermy (see Alcohol, p. 599)

■ With cetrimide

Hibicet Hospital Concentrate® (SSL)
Solution, orange, chlorhexidine gluconate solution 7.5% (≡ chlorhexidine gluconate 1.5%), cetrimide 15%, net price 5 litres = £8.55
Dose: to be used diluted 1 in 100 (1%) to 1 in 30 with water for skin disinfection and wound cleansing, and diluted 1 in 30 in alcohol 70% for pre-operative skin preparation
NOTE. Alcoholic solutions not suitable before diathermy (see Alcohol, p. 599)

13.11.3 Cationic surfactants and soaps

CETRIMIDE

Indications: skin disinfection
Cautions: avoid contact with eyes; avoid use in body cavities
Side-effects: skin irritation and occasionally sensitisation

■ Preparations

Ingredient of *Hibicet Hospital Concentrate*®, *Steripod*®, *Tisept*®, and *Travasept*® *100*, see above

13.11.4 Iodine

POVIDONE–IODINE

Indications: skin disinfection; vaginal infections (section 7.2.2); oral hygiene (section 12.3.4)
Cautions: pregnancy (Appendix 4), breast-feeding (Appendix 5); broken skin (see below); renal impairment (Appendix 3)
LARGE OPEN WOUNDS. The application of povidone–iodine to large wounds or severe burns may produce systemic adverse effects such as metabolic acidosis, hypernatraemia and impairment of renal function.
Contra-indications: avoid regular use in patients with thyroid disorders or those receiving lithium therapy
Side-effects: rarely sensitivity; may interfere with thyroid function tests

Betadine® (Medlock)
Antiseptic paint, povidone–iodine 10% in an alcoholic solution, net price 8 mL (with applicator brush) = £1.01
Dose: apply undiluted to minor wounds and infections, twice daily
Alcoholic solution, povidone–iodine 10%, net price 500 mL = £1.91
Dose: apply undiluted in pre- and post-operative skin disinfection; NEONATE not recommended for regular use (contra-indicated if birthweight below 1.5 kg)
NOTE. Flammable—caution in procedures involving hot wire cautery and diathermy
Antiseptic solution, povidone–iodine 10% in aqueous solution, net price 500 mL = £1.75
Dose: apply undiluted in pre- and post-operative skin disinfection; NEONATE not recommended for regular use (and contra-indicated if birthweight below 1.5 kg)
NOTE. Not for body cavity irrigation
Dry powder spray, povidone–iodine 2.5% in a pressurised aerosol unit, net price 150-g unit = £2.79
For skin disinfection, particularly minor wounds and infections; INFANT under 2 years not recommended
NOTE. Not for use in serous cavities
Ointment, povidone–iodine 10%, in a water-miscible basis, net price 20 g = £1.39, 80 g = £2.79
Excipients: none as listed in section 13.1.3
For skin disinfection, particularly minor wounds and infections; INFANT under 2 years not recommended
Skin cleanser solution, povidone–iodine 4%, in a surfactant basis, net price 250 mL = £2.14
Dose: for infective conditions of the skin. Retain on skin for 3–5 minutes before rinsing; repeat twice daily; INFANT under 2 years max. treatment duration 3 days

Surgical scrub, povidone–iodine 7.5%, in a non-ionic surfactant basis, net price 500 mL = £1.58
To be used as a pre-operative scrub for hands and skin; NEONATE not recommended for regular use (contra-indicated if birthweight below 1.5 kg)

Savlon® Dry Antiseptic (Novartis Consumer Health)
Powder spray, povidone–iodine 1.14% in a pressurised aerosol unit, net price 50-mL unit = £2.39
For minor wounds

Videne® (Adams Hlth.)
Alcoholic tincture, povidone–iodine 10%, net price 500 mL = £2.35
To be applied undiluted in pre-operative skin disinfection
Antiseptic solution, povidone–iodine 10% in aqueous solution, net price 500 mL = £2.35
To be applied undiluted in pre-operative skin disinfection and general antisepsis
Surgical scrub, povidone–iodine 7.5% in aqueous solution, net price 500 mL = £2.35
To be used as a pre-operative scrub for hand and skin disinfection

13.11.5 Phenolics

TRICLOSAN

Indications: skin disinfection
Cautions: avoid contact with eyes

Aquasept® (Medlock)
Skin cleanser, blue, triclosan 2%, net price 250 mL = £1.10, 500 mL = £1.68
Excipients: include chlorocresol, propylene glycol, fragrance, tetrasodium edetate
For disinfection and pre-operative hand preparation

Manusept® (Medlock)
Antibacterial hand rub, triclosan 0.5%, isopropyl alcohol 70%, net price 250 mL = £1.07, 500 mL = £1.56
Excipients: none as listed in section 13.1.3
For disinfection and pre-operative hand preparation
NOTE. Flammable

Ster-Zac Bath Concentrate® (Medlock)
Solution, triclosan 2%, net price 28.5 mL = 40p, 500 mL = £2.24
Dose: for prevention of cross-infection use 28.5 mL/bath
Excipients: include trisodium edetate

13.11.6 Astringents, oxidisers, and dyes

HYDROGEN PEROXIDE

Indications: see under preparations below
Cautions: large or deep wounds; avoid on healthy skin and eyes; bleaches fabric; incompatible with products containing iodine or potassium permanganate

Hydrogen Peroxide Solution, BP
Solution 6% (20 vols), net price 100 mL = 17p
Solution 3% (10 vols), net price 100 mL = 18p
For skin disinfection, particularly cleansing and deodorising wounds and ulcers
NOTE. The BP directs that when hydrogen peroxide is prescribed, hydrogen peroxide solution 6% (20 vols) should be dispensed.
IMPORTANT. Strong solutions of hydrogen peroxide which contain 27% (90 vols) and 30% (100 vols) are only for the preparation of weaker solutions

Crystacide® (GP Pharma)
Cream, hydrogen peroxide 1%, net price 10 g = £3.71, 25 g = £6.21
Dose: superficial bacterial skin infection, apply 2-3 times daily for up to 3 weeks
Excipients: include edetic acid (EDTA), propylene glycol

Hioxyl®
Section 13.11.7

POTASSIUM PERMANGANATE

Indications: cleansing and deodorising suppurating eczematous reactions and wounds
Cautions: irritant to mucous membranes
Dose: wet dressings or baths, approx. 0.01% solution
NOTE. Stains skin and clothing

Potassium Permanganate Solution
Solution, potassium permanganate 0.1% (1 in 1000) in water
Dose: to be diluted 1 in 10 to provide a 0.01% (1 in 10 000) solution

Permitabs® (Centrapharm)
Solution tablets, for preparation of topical solution, potassium permanganate 400 mg, net price 30-tab pack = £6.22
NOTE. 1 tablet dissolved in 4 litres of water provides a 0.01% (1 in 10 000) solution

13.11.7 Preparations for promotion of wound healing

Desloughing agents

Desloughing agents for ulcers are second-line treatment and the underlying causes should be treated. The main beneficial effect is removal of slough and clot and the ablation of local infection. Preparations which absorb or help promote the removal of exudate may also help (Appendix 8). It should be noted that substances applied to an open area are easily absorbed and perilesional skin is easily sensitised. Gravitational dermatitis may be complicated by superimposed contact sensitivity to substances such as neomycin or lanolin. Enzyme preparations such as streptokinase-streptodornase or, alternatively, dextranomer (Appendix 8) are designed for applying to sloughing ulcers. Sterile larvae (maggots) (*LarvE®*, Biosurgical Research Unit) are also used for managing sloughing wounds and are prescribable on the NHS.

Aserbine® (Goldshield)
Solution, benzoic acid 0.15%, malic acid 2.25%, propylene glycol 40%, salicylic acid 0.0375%, net price 500 mL = £3.61
Excipients: include fragrance
Dose: use as wash before each application of cream (or use as wet dressing)

Hioxyl® (Ferndale)
Cream, hydrogen peroxide (stabilised) 1.5%, net price 25 g = £2.16, 100 g = £6.76
Excipients: include cetostearyl alcohol
For leg ulcers and pressure sores
Dose: apply when necessary and if necessary cover with a dressing

Varidase Topical® (Wyeth) PoM
Powder, streptokinase 100 000 units, streptodornase 25 000 units. For preparing solutions for topical use, net price with sterile physiological saline 20 mL (combi-pack) = £10.06
Excipients: none as listed in section 13.1.3
Dose: reconstitute with 20 mL sterile physiological saline (or water for injections) and apply as wet dressing 1–2 times daily; cover with semi-occlusive dressing; irrigate lesion thoroughly with physiological saline and remove loosened material before next application; also used to dissolve clots in the bladder or urinary catheters
Contra-indications: active haemorrhage, severe hypertension
Side-effects: infrequent allergic reactions (reduced by careful and frequent removal of exudate and thorough irrigation with physiological saline); fever, transient burning, haemorrhage, and hypersensitivity reactions including shock reported

Growth factor

A topical preparation of **becaplermin** (recombinant human platelet-derived growth factor) is licensed as an adjunct treatment of full-thickness, neuropathic, diabetic ulcers.

Regranex® (Janssen-Cilag) PoM
Gel, becaplermin (recombinant human platelet-derived growth factor) 0.01%, net price 15 g = £275
Excipients: include hydroxybenzoates
Dose: full-thickness, neuropathic, diabetic ulcers (no larger than 5 cm^2), apply thin layer daily and cover with gauze dressing moistened with physiological saline; max. duration of treatment 20 weeks (reassess if no healing after first 10 weeks)
Cautions: malignant disease; avoid on sites with infection, malignancy, peripheral arteriopathy, or osteomyelitis
Side-effects: irritation, rarely bullous eruption, oedema

13.12 Antiperspirants

Aluminium chloride is a potent antiperspirant used in the treatment of hyperhidrosis. Aluminium salts are also incorporated in preparations used for minor fungal skin infections associated with hyperhidrosis.

In more severe cases specialists use **glycopyrronium bromide** as a 0.05% solution in the iontophoretic treatment of hyperhidrosis of plantar and palmar areas. **Botulinum A toxin-haemagglutinin complex** (section 4.9.3) is licensed for use intradermally for severe hyperhidrosis of the axillae unresponsive to topical antiperspirant or other antihidrotic treatment.

ALUMINIUM SALTS

Indications: see under Dose below
Cautions: avoid contact with eyes or mucous membranes; avoid use on broken or irritated skin; do not shave axillae or use depilatories within 12 hours of application; avoid contact with clothing
Side-effects: skin irritation
Dose: hyperhidrosis affecting axillae, hands or feet, apply liquid formulation at night to dry skin, wash off the following morning, initially daily then reduce frequency as condition improves—do not bathe immediately before use
Hyperhidrosis, bromidrosis, intertrigo, and prevention of tinea pedis and related conditions, apply powder to dry skin

Anhydrol Forte® (Dermal)
Solution (= application), aluminium chloride hexahydrate 20% in an alcoholic basis, net price 60-mL bottle with roll-on applicator = £2.62. Label: 15
Excipients: none as listed in section 13.1.3

[1]**Driclor®** (Stiefel)
Application, aluminium chloride hexahydrate 20% in an alcoholic basis, net price 60-mL bottle with roll-on applicator = £2.82. Label: 15
Excipients: none as listed in section 13.1.3

1. A 30-mL pack is on sale to the public (*Driclor® Solution*)

ZeaSORB® (Stiefel)
Dusting powder, aldioxa 0.22%, chloroxylenol 0.5%, net price 50 g = £2.15
Excipients: include fragrance

GLYCOPYRRONIUM BROMIDE

Indications: iontophoretic treatment of hyperhidrosis; other indications section 15.1.3
Cautions: see section 15.1.3 (but poorly absorbed and systemic effects unlikely)
Contra-indications: see section 15.1.3 (but poorly absorbed and systemic effects unlikely), infections affecting the treatment site
Side-effects: see section 15.1.3 (but poorly absorbed and systemic effects unlikely), tingling at administration site
Dose: consult product literature; only 1 site to be treated at a time, max. 2 sites treated in any 24 hours, treatment not to be repeated within 7 days

Robinul® (Antigen) PoM
Powder, glycopyrronium bromide, net price 3 g = £110.00

13.13 Wound management products and Elastic Hosiery

■ Preparations
See Appendix 8

13.14 Topical circulatory preparations

These preparations are used to improve circulation in conditions such as bruising, superficial thrombophlebitis, chilblains and varicose veins but are of little value. Chilblains are best managed by avoidance of exposure to cold; neither systemic nor topical vasodilator therapy is established as being effective. Sclerotherapy of varicose veins is described in section 2.13.

Rubefacients are described in section 10.3.2.

Hirudoid® (Sankyo)

Cream, heparinoid 0.3% in a vanishing-cream basis, net price 50 g = £1.39

Excipients: include cetostearyl alcohol, hydroxybenzoates (parabens)

Gel, heparinoid 0.3%, net price 50 g = £1.39

Excipients: include propylene glycol, fragrance

Dose: apply up to 4 times daily in superficial soft-tissue injuries and superficial thrombophlebitis

Lasonil® (Bayer Consumer Care)

Ointment, heparinoid 0.8% in white soft paraffin, net price 40 g = £1.08

Excipients: include wool fat derivative

Dose: apply 2–3 times daily in superficial soft-tissue injuries

14: Immunological products and vaccines

Post-immunisation pyrexia in infants. The parent should be advised that if pyrexia develops after childhood immunisation, the infant can be given a dose of paracetamol and, if necessary, a second dose given 6 hours later; ibuprofen may be used if paracetamol is unsuitable. The parent should be warned to seek medical advice if the pyrexia persists.
For post-immunisation pyrexia in an infant aged 2–3 months, the dose of paracetamol is 60 mg; the dose of ibuprofen is 50 mg (on doctor's advice). An oral syringe can be obtained from any pharmacy to give the small volume required.

14.1 Active immunity

Vaccines may consist of:

1. a *live attenuated* form of a virus (e.g. rubella or measles vaccine) or bacteria (e.g. BCG vaccine)
2. *inactivated* preparations of the virus (e.g. influenza vaccine) or bacteria, or
3. *extracts of* or *detoxified exotoxins* produced by a micro-organism (e.g. tetanus vaccine).

They stimulate production of antibodies and other components of the immune mechanism.

Live attenuated vaccines usually produce a durable immunity but not always as long-lasting as that of the natural infection. When two live virus vaccines are required (and are not available as a combined preparation) they should be given either simultaneously at different sites or separated by an interval of at least 3 weeks.

Inactivated vaccines may require a primary series of injections of vaccine to produce adequate antibody response and in most cases booster (reinforcing) injections are required; the duration of immunity varies from months to many years. Some inactivated vaccines are adsorbed onto an adjuvant (such as aluminium hydroxide) to enhance the antibody response.

Advice in this chapter reflects that in the handbook *Immunisation against Infectious Disease* (1996), which in turn reflects the guidance of the Joint Committee on Vaccination and Immunisation (JCVI). Chapters from the handbook are available at www.dh.gov.uk
The advice incorporates changes announced by the Chief Medical Officer and Health Department Updates.

SIDE-EFFECTS. Some vaccines (e.g. poliomyelitis) produce very few reactions, while others (e.g. measles and rubella) may produce a very mild form of the disease. Some vaccines may produce discomfort at the site of injection and mild fever and malaise. Occasionally there are more serious untoward reactions and these should always be reported to the CSM. Anaphylactic reactions are very rare but can be fatal (see section 3.4.3 for management). The product literature should be consulted for full details of side-effects.

CONTRA-INDICATIONS. Most vaccines have some basic contra-indication to their use, and the product literature and *Immunisation against Infectious Disease* should be consulted for details. In general, vaccination should be postponed if the individual is suffering from an *acute illness*. Minor illnesses without fever or systemic upset are not contra-indications. Anaphylaxis with a preceding dose of a vaccine (or vaccine component) is a contra-indication to further doses.

Hypersensitivity to egg contra-indicates influenza vaccine and tick-borne encephalitis vaccine (residual egg protein present) and, if evidence of previous anaphylactic reaction, also yellow fever vaccine. Some viral vaccines contain small quantities of antibacterials; such vaccines may need to be withheld from individuals who are *extremely sensitive to the antibacterial*. Other excipients in vaccines may also rarely cause allergic reactions. The presence of the following excipients in vaccines and immunological products has been noted under the relevant entries:

Gelatin	Polymyxin B
Gentamicin	Streptomycin
Neomycin	Thiomersal
Penicillins	

Live vaccines should not be administered routinely to *pregnant women* because of possible harm to the fetus but where there is a significant risk of exposure (e.g. to yellow fever), the need for vaccination outweighs any possible risk to the fetus. Live vaccines should not be given to individuals with *impaired immune response*, whether caused by disease (for special reference to *HIV infection*, see below) or treatment with high doses of corticosteroids or other immunosuppressive drugs. They should not be given to those being treated for *malignant conditions* with chemotherapy or generalised radiotherapy[1,2]. The response to vaccines may be reduced

1. Live vaccines should be postponed until at least 3 months after stopping corticosteroids or other immunosuppressive drugs and 6 months after stopping chemotherapy or generalised radiotherapy.

2. Use of normal immunoglobulin should be considered after exposure to measles (see p. 621) and varicella–zoster immunoglobulin considered after exposure to chickenpox or herpes zoster (see p. 621).

and there is risk of generalised infection with live vaccines.

The Royal College of Paediatrics and Child Health has produced a statement, *Immunisation of the Immunocompromised Child (2002)* (available at www.rcpch.ac.uk).

The intramuscular route should not be used in patients with bleeding disorders such as haemophilia or thrombocytopenia. Vaccines that are usually given by the intramuscular route may be given by subcutaneous injection in those with bleeding disorders.

NOTE. The Department of Health has advised *against the use of jet guns* for vaccination owing to the risk of transmitting blood-borne infections, such as HIV.

VACCINES AND HIV INFECTION. HIV-positive individuals with or without symptoms can receive the following live vaccines:

MMR (but not whilst severely immunosuppressed), varicella-zoster (but avoid if immunity significantly impaired—consult product literature);[1,2]

and the following inactivated vaccines:

cholera (oral), diphtheria, haemophilus influenzae type b, hepatitis A, hepatitis B, influenza, meningococcal, pertussis, pneumococcal, poliomyelitis[3], rabies, tetanus, typhoid (injection).

HIV-positive individuals should **not** receive:

BCG, yellow fever[4]

NOTE. The above advice differs from that for other immunocompromised patients.

VACCINES AND ASPLENIA. The following vaccines are recommended for asplenic patients or those with splenic dysfunction:

haemophilus influenzae type b, meningococcal group C, pneumococcal, influenza.

For antibiotic prophylaxis in asplenia see p. 272.

Immunisation schedule

Vaccines for the childhood immunisation schedule should be obtained from **local health authorities** or **direct from Farillon**—not to be prescribed on FP10 (HS21 in Northern Ireland; GP10 in Scotland; WP10 in Wales).

During first year of life

Diphtheria, Tetanus, Pertussis (Acellular, Component), Poliomyelitis (Inactivated) and Haemophilus Type b Conjugate Vaccine (Adsorbed)

3 doses at intervals of 4 weeks; first dose at 2 months of age

plus

Meningococcal Group C Conjugate Vaccine

3 doses at intervals of 4 weeks; first dose at 2 months of age

BCG Vaccine (for neonates at risk only)

See section 14.4, BCG Vaccines

1. Use of normal immunoglobulin should be considered after exposure to measles (see p. 621) and varicella–zoster immunoglobulin considered after exposure to chickenpox or herpes zoster (see p. 621).

2. The Royal College of Paediatrics and Child Health recommends that MMR is not given to a child with HIV infection whilst severely immunosuppressed.

3. Inactivated poliomyelitis vaccine is now used instead of oral poliomyelitis vaccine for routine immunisation of children.

4. Because insufficient evidence of safety.

During second year of life

Measles, Mumps and Rubella Vaccine, Live (MMR)

Single dose at 12–15 months of age

Before school or nursery school entry

Adsorbed Diphtheria [low dose], **Tetanus, Pertussis (Acellular, Component) and Inactivated Poliomyelitis Vaccine**

or

Adsorbed Diphtheria, Tetanus, Pertussis (Acellular, Component) and Inactivated Poliomyelitis Vaccine

Single booster dose

Preferably allow interval of at least 3 years after completing basic course; can be given at same session as MMR Vaccine but use separate syringe and needle, and give in different limb

plus

Measles, Mumps and Rubella Vaccine, Live (MMR)

Single booster dose

Can be given at same session as Adsorbed Diphtheria [low dose], Tetanus, Pertussis (Acellular, Component) and Inactivated Poliomyelitis Vaccine but use separate syringe and needle, and use different limb

Before leaving school or before employment or further education

Adsorbed Diphtheria [low dose], **Tetanus and Inactivated Poliomyelitis Vaccine**

Single booster dose

During adult life

Measles, Mumps and Rubella Vaccine, Live (MMR) (for women of child-bearing age susceptible to rubella)

Single dose

Women of child-bearing age should be tested for rubella antibodies and sero-negative women offered rubella immunisation (using the MMR vaccine)—exclude pregnancy before immunisation, but see also section 14.4, Measles, Mumps and Rubella Vaccine

Adsorbed Diphtheria [low dose], **Tetanus and Inactivated Poliomyelitis Vaccine** (if not previously immunised)

3 doses at intervals of 4 weeks

Booster dose at least 1 year after primary course and again 5–10 years later

High-risk groups

For information on high-risk groups, see section 14.4 under individual vaccines

BCG Vaccines
Hepatitis A Vaccine
Hepatitis B Vaccine
Influenza Vaccine
Pneumococcal Vaccines
Tetanus Vaccines

14.2 Passive immunity

Immunity with immediate protection against certain infective organisms can be obtained by injecting preparations made from the plasma of immune individuals with adequate levels of antibody to the disease for which protection is sought (see under Immunoglobulin section 14.5). This passive immunity lasts only a few weeks; where necessary passive immunisation can be repeated.

Antibodies of human origin are usually termed *immunoglobulins*. The term *antiserum* is applied to material prepared in animals. Because of serum sickness and other allergic-type reactions that may follow injections of antisera, this therapy has been replaced wherever possible by the use of immunoglobulins. Reactions are theoretically possible after injection of human immunoglobulins but reports of such reactions are very rare.

14.3 Storage and use

Care must be taken to store all vaccines and other immunological products under the conditions recommended in the product literature, otherwise the preparation may become ineffective. **Refrigerated storage** is usually necessary; many vaccines need to be stored at 2–8°C and not allowed to freeze. Vaccines should be protected from light. Unused vaccine in multidose vials without preservative (most live virus vaccines) should be discarded within 1 hour of first use; those containing a preservative (including oral poliomyelitis vaccine) should be discarded within 3 hours or at the end of a session. Unused vaccines should be disposed of by incineration at a registered disposal contractor.

Particular attention must be paid to instructions on the use of diluents. Vaccines which are liquid suspensions or are reconstituted before use should be adequately mixed to ensure uniformity of the material to be injected.

14.4 Vaccines and antisera

AVAILABILITY. Anthrax and yellow fever vaccines, botulism antitoxin, diphtheria antitoxin, and snake and spider venom antitoxins are available from local designated holding centres.

For antivenom, see Emergency Treatment of Poisoning, p. 36.

Enquiries for vaccines not available commercially can also be made to:

Immunisation and Communicable Diseases Branch
Department of Health
Skipton House
80 London Road
London SE1 6LH
Tel: (020) 7972 1522

In Scotland information about availability of vaccines can be obtained from a Specialist in Pharmaceutical Public Health. In Wales enquiries should be directed to:

Welsh Medicines Information Centre
University Hospital of Wales
Cardiff CF14 4XW
Tel: (029) 2074 2979

and in Northern Ireland:

Regional Pharmacist (procurement co-ordination)
United Hospitals Trust Pharmacy Dept
Whiteabbey Hospital
Doagh Road
Newtownabbey BT37 9RH
Tel: (028) 9086 5181 ext 2386

For further details of availability, see under individual vaccines.

Anthrax vaccine

Anthrax immunisation is indicated for individuals who handle infected animals, for those exposed to imported infected animal products, and for laboratory staff who work with *Bacillus anthracis*.

In the event of possible contact with *B. anthracis*, post-exposure immunisation may be indicated, in addition to antimicrobial prophylaxis (section 5.1.12). Advice on the use of anthrax vaccine must be obtained from the Communicable Disease Surveillance Centre, Health Protection Agency (CDSC) (tel. 020 8200 6868)

The vaccine is the alum precipitate of an antigen from *B. anthracis* and, following the primary course of injections, booster doses should be given at about yearly intervals.

Anthrax Vaccine PoM

Dose: initial course 3 doses of 0.5 mL *by intramuscular injection* at intervals of 3 weeks followed by a fourth dose after an interval of 6 months; for post-exposure prophylaxis [unlicensed use], fifth dose recommended 1 year after exposure

Booster doses: 0.5 mL annually

NOTE. Advice on post-exposure prophylaxis must be obtained from CDSC

Available from CDSC (*excipients include* thiomersal)

BCG vaccines

BCG (Bacillus Calmette-Guérin) is a live attenuated strain derived from *Mycobacterium bovis* which stimulates the development of hypersensitivity to *M. tuberculosis*. BCG vaccine should be given intradermally by operators skilled in the technique (see below).

Within 2–6 weeks a small swelling appears at the injection site which progresses to a papule or to a benign ulcer about 10 mm in diameter and heals in 6–12 weeks. A dry dressing may be used if the ulcer discharges, but air should **not** be excluded.

Serious reactions with BCG are uncommon and most often consist of prolonged ulceration or subcutaneous abscess formation due to faulty injection technique.

BCG is recommended for the following groups if BCG immunisation, as evidenced by a characteristic scar, has not previously been carried out and they are negative for tuberculoprotein hypersensitivity:

- all infants living in areas where the incidence of tuberculosis is greater than 40 per 100 000;
- infants with a parent or grandparent born in a country with an incidence of tuberculosis greater than 40 per 100 000;
- previously unvaccinated new immigrants from countries with a high incidence of tuberculosis;
- contacts of those with active respiratory tuberculosis;
- health service staff (including medical students, hospital medical staff, nurses, physiotherapists, radiographers, technical staff in pathology departments and any others considered to be at special risk because of the likelihood of contact with infective patients or their sputum; particularly important to test staff in contact with the immunocompromised, e.g. in trans-

plant, oncology and HIV units, and staff in maternity and paediatric departments);

- veterinary and other staff who handle animal species known to be susceptible to tuberculosis;
- staff working in prisons, in residential homes and in hostels for refugees and the homeless;
- those intending to stay for more than 1 month in countries with a high incidence of tuberculosis (section 14.6);
- neonates, infants, children or adults where immunisation is requested.

Apart from neonates and infants of up to 12 months, any person being considered for BCG immunisation must first be given a skin test for hypersensitivity to tuberculoprotein (see under Diagnostic agents, below).

BCG vaccine may be given simultaneously with another live vaccine (see also section 14.1), but if they are not given at the same time, an interval of 4 weeks should normally be allowed between them. When BCG is given to infants, there is no need to delay routine primary immunisations.

See section 14.1 for general contra-indications. BCG is also contra-indicated in individuals with generalised septic skin conditions (in the case of eczema, a vaccination site free from lesions should be chosen).

Bladder instillations of BCG are licensed for the management of bladder carcinoma (section 8.2.4).

For advice on chemoprophylaxis against tuberculosis, see section 5.1.9.

■ Intradermal

Bacillus Calmette-Guérin Vaccine ▼ PoM

BCG Vaccine, Dried Tub/Vac/BCG

A freeze-dried preparation of live bacteria of a strain derived from the bacillus of Calmette and Guérin.

Dose: by intradermal injection, 0.1 mL (NEONATE and INFANT under 12 months 0.05 mL)

Available from health authorities or direct from Farillon (SSI brand, multidose vial with diluent)

INTRADERMAL INJECTION TECHNIQUE. After swabbing with spirit and allowing to dry, skin is stretched between thumb and forefinger and needle (size 25G or 26G) inserted (bevel upwards) for about 2 mm into superficial layers of dermis (almost parallel with surface). Needle should be short with short bevel (can usually be seen through epidermis during insertion). Raised blanched bleb showing tips of hair follicles is sign of correct injection; 7 mm bleb ≡ 0.1 mL injection; if considerable resistance not felt, needle is removed and reinserted before giving more vaccine.

To be injected at insertion of deltoid muscle onto humerus (keloid formation more likely with sites higher on arm); tip of shoulder should be **avoided**; for cosmetic reasons, upper and lateral surface of thigh may be preferred (but in neonates, upper arm **must** be used).

Diagnostic agents

The *Mantoux test* is recommended for tuberculin skin testing, but no licensed preparation is currently available. Guidance for healthcare professionals is available at www.immunisation.nhs.uk.

In the Mantoux test, the diagnostic dose is by intradermal injection of Tuberculin Purified Protein Derivative (PPD).

The *Heaf test* (involving the use of multiple-puncture apparatus) is no longer available.

NOTE. Tuberculin testing should not be carried out within 3 weeks of receiving a live viral vaccine since response to tuberculin may be inhibited.

Botulism antitoxin

A trivalent botulism antitoxin is available for the post-exposure prophylaxis of botulism and for the treatment of persons thought to be suffering from botulism. It specifically neutralises the toxins produced by *Clostridium botulinum* types A, B, and E. It is not effective against infantile botulism as the toxin (type A) is seldom, if ever, found in the blood in this type of infection.

Hypersensitivity reactions are a problem. It is essential to read the contra-indications, warnings, and details of sensitivity tests on the package insert. Prior to treatment checks should be made regarding previous administration of any antitoxin and history of any allergic condition, e.g. asthma, hay fever, etc. All patients should be tested for sensitivity (diluting the antitoxin if history of allergy).

Botulism Antitoxin PoM

A preparation containing the specific antitoxic globulins that have the power of neutralising the toxins formed by types A, B, and E of *Clostridium botulinum*.

NOTE. The BP title Botulinum Antitoxin is not used because the preparation currently in use may have a different specification.

Dose: prophylaxis, consult product literature

Available from local designated centres, for details see TOXBASE (requires registration) www.spib.axl.co.uk. For supplies outside working hours apply to other designated centres and, as a last resort, to Department of Health Duty Officer (Tel (020) 7210 3000).

Cholera vaccine

Cholera vaccine (oral) contains inactivated Inaba (including El-Tor biotype) and Ogawa strains of *Vibrio cholerae*, serotype O1 together with recombinant B-subunit of the cholera toxin produced in Inaba strains of *V.cholerae*, serotype O1.

Oral cholera vaccine is licensed for travellers to endemic or epidemic areas on the basis of current recommendations (see also section 14.6). Immunisation should be completed at least 1 week before potential exposure. However, there is no requirement for cholera vaccination for international travel.

Immunisation with cholera vaccine does not provide complete protection and all travellers to a country where cholera exists should be warned that scrupulous attention to food, water, and personal hygiene is **essential**.

CAUTIONS and SIDE-EFFECTS. Food, drink, and other oral medicines should be avoided 1 hour before and after vaccination. Side-effects of oral cholera vaccine include diarrhoea, abdominal pain, headache; rarely nausea, vomiting, loss of appetite, dizziness, fever, and respiratory symptoms can also occur.

See section 14.1 for general contra-indications.

Injectable cholera vaccine provides unreliable protection and is no longer available in the UK

Dukoral® (Chiron) ▼ PoM

Oral suspension, for dilution with solution of effervescent sodium bicarbonate granules, heat- and formaldehyde-inactivated Inaba (including El-Tor biotype) and Ogawa strains of *Vibrio cholerae* bacteria and recombinant cholera toxin B-subunit produced in *V. cholerae*, net price 2-dose pack = £16.00

Dose: ADULT and CHILD over 6 years 2 doses separated by an interval of 1 week; CHILD 2–6 years 3 doses each separated by an interval of 1 week (consult product literature for dilution and administration)

Booster dose can be given after 2 years for adults and children over 6 years, and after 6 months for children 2–6 years

Diphtheria vaccines

Diphtheria vaccines are prepared from the toxin of *Corynebacterium diphtheriae* and adsorption on aluminium hydroxide or aluminium phosphate improves antigenicity. The vaccine stimulates the production of the protective antitoxin. Single-antigen diphtheria vaccine is not available and adsorbed diphtheria vaccine is given as a combination product containing other vaccines.

For primary immunisation *of children aged between 2 months and 10 years* vaccination is recommended usually in the form of 3 doses (separated by 1-month intervals) of **diphtheria, tetanus, pertussis (acellular, component), poliomyelitis (inactivated) and haemophilus type b conjugate vaccine (adsorbed)** (see schedule, section 14.1). In unimmunised individuals aged *over 10 years* the primary course comprises of 3 doses of **adsorbed diphtheria** [low dose], **tetanus and inactivated poliomyelitis vaccine**.

A booster dose should be given 3 years after the primary course. Children *under 10 years* should receive *either* **adsorbed diphtheria, tetanus, pertussis (acellular, component) and inactivated poliomyelitis vaccine** *or* **adsorbed diphtheria** [low dose], **tetanus, pertussis (acellular, component) and inactivated poliomyelitis vaccine**. Individuals aged *over 10 years* should receive **adsorbed diphtheria** [low dose], **tetanus, and inactivated poliomyelitis vaccine**.

A second booster dose of adsorbed diphtheria [low dose], tetanus and inactivated poliomyelitis vaccine should be given 10 years after the previous booster dose.

Those intending to travel to areas with a risk of diphtheria infection should be fully immunised according to the UK schedule. If more than 10 years have lapsed since completion of the UK schedule, a dose of **adsorbed diphtheria** [low dose], **tetanus and inactivated poliomyelitis vaccine** should be administered.

Staff in contact with diphtheria patients or with potentially pathogenic clinical specimens or working directly with *C. diphtheriae* or *C. ulcerans* should receive a booster dose if fully immunised (with 5 doses of diphtheria-containing vaccine given at appropriate intervals); further doses should be given at 10-year intervals if risk persists. Individuals at risk who are not fully immunised should complete the primary course; a booster dose should be given after 5 years and then at 10-year intervals. **Adsorbed diphtheria** [low dose], **tetanus and inactivated poliomyelitis vaccine** is used for this purpose; immunity should be checked by antibody testing at least 3 months after completion of immunisation.

Advice on the management of cases, carriers, contacts and outbreaks must be sought from health protection units. The immunisation history of infected individuals and their contacts should be determined; those who have been incompletely immunised should complete their immunisation and fully immunised individuals should receive a reinforcing dose. For advice on antibacterial treatment to prevent a secondary case of diphtheria in a non-immune individual, see Table 2, section 5.1.

See section 14.1 for general contra-indications.

Diphtheria vaccines for children under 10 years

IMPORTANT. **Not** recommended for persons *aged 10 years or over* (see Diphtheria Vaccines for Children over 10 years and Adults, below)

Diphtheria, Tetanus, Pertussis (Acellular, Component), Poliomyelitis (Inactivated) and Haemophilus Type b Conjugate Vaccine (Adsorbed) PoM

Injection, suspension of diphtheria toxoid, tetanus toxoid, acellular pertussis, inactivated poliomyelitis and *Haemophilus influenzae* type b (conjugated to tetanus protein), net price 0.5-mL prefilled syringe = £19.94

Excipients: include neomycin, polymyxin B and streptomycin

Dose: CHILD up to 10 years, *by intramuscular injection* 0.5 mL; primary immunisation, 3 doses at intervals of 1 month (see schedule, section 14.1)

Available as part of childhood immunisation schedule, from health authorities or Farillon; brands include ▼*Pediacel*®

Adsorbed Diphtheria, Tetanus, Pertussis (Acellular, Component) and Inactivated Poliomyelitis Vaccine PoM

Injection, suspension of diphtheria toxoid, tetanus toxoid, acellular pertussis and inactivated poliomyelitis vaccine components adsorbed on a mineral carrier, net price 0.5-mL prefilled syringe = £17.56

Excipients: include neomycin and polymyxin B

Dose: CHILD 3–10 years, *by intramuscular injection*, 0.5 mL (see schedule, section 14.1)

Available as part of childhood immunisation schedule, from health authorities or Farillon; brands include ▼ *Infanrix-IPV*®

Adsorbed Diphtheria [low dose], Tetanus, Pertussis (Acellular, Component) and Inactivated Poliomyelitis Vaccine PoM

Injection, suspension of diphtheria toxoid [low dose], tetanus toxoid, acellular pertussis and inactivated poliomyelitis vaccine components adsorbed on a mineral carrier, net price 0.5-mL prefilled syringe = £11.98

Excipients: include neomycin, polymyxin B and streptomycin

Dose: CHILD 3–10 years, *by intramuscular injection*, 0.5 mL (see schedule, section 14.1)

Available as part of childhood immunisation schedule, from health authorities or Farillon; brands include ▼*Repevax*®

Diphtheria vaccines for children over 10 years and adults

A low dose of diphtheria toxoid is sufficient to recall immunity in individuals previously immunised against diphtheria but whose immunity may have diminished with time; it is insufficient to cause serious reactions that may occur when a higher-dose vaccine is used in an individual who is already immune. Preparations containing low dose diphtheria should be used for adults and children *over 10 years*, whether for primary immunisation or for booster doses.

Adsorbed Diphtheria [low dose], Tetanus and Inactivated Poliomyelitis Vaccine PoM

Injection, suspension of diphtheria toxoid [low dose], tetanus toxoid and inactivated poliomyelitis vaccine components adsorbed on a mineral carrier, net price 0.5-mL prefilled syringe = £6.74

Excipients: include neomycin, polymyxin B and streptomycin

Dose: primary immunisation in ADULT and CHILD over 10 years, *by intramuscular injection*, 3 doses each of 0.5 mL separated by intervals of 4 weeks; booster, 0.5 mL after 5 years, repeated 10 years later (see schedule, section 14.1)

Available as part of childhood schedule, from health authorities or Farillon; brands include ▼*Revaxis*®

Adsorbed Diphtheria [low dose] and Tetanus Vaccine for Adults and Adolescents PoM

DT/Vac/Ads(Adult)

Injection, suspension of diphtheria formol toxoid and tetanus formol toxoid adsorbed on a mineral carrier, net price 0.5-mL prefilled syringe = £2.48

NOTE. Not recommended for routine use (vaccines which also protect against poliomyelitis should be used for primary immunisation and for boosters)

Brands include *Diftavax*®

Diphtheria antitoxin

Diphtheria antitoxin is used for passive immunisation. It is derived from horse serum and reactions are common after administration; resuscitation facilities should be available immediately.

It is now only used in suspected cases of diphtheria (without waiting for bacteriological confirmation); tests for hypersensitivity should be first carried out.

It is no longer used for prophylaxis because of the risk of hypersensitivity; unimmunised contacts should be promptly investigated and given antibacterial prophylaxis (section 5.1, table 2) and vaccine (see notes above).

Diphtheria Antitoxin PoM

Dip/Ser

Dose: prophylaxis, not recommended therefore no dose stated (see notes above)

Treatment, *by intravenous infusion*, nasal diphtheria, 10 000–20 000 units; tonsillar diphtheria, 15 000–25 000 units; pharyngeal or laryngeal diphtheria, 20 000–40 000 units; combined types or delayed diagnosis, 40 000–60 000 units; severe diphtheria, 40 000–100 000 units; CHILD under 10 years half adult dose

Available from Communicable Disease Surveillance Centre (Tel (020) 8200 6868) or in Northern Ireland from Public Health Laboratory, Belfast City Hospital (Tel (028) 9032 9241)

Haemophilus influenzae type B vaccine

Haemophilus influenzae type b (Hib) vaccine is made from capsular polysaccharide; it is conjugated with a protein such as diphtheria toxin or tetanus toxoid to increase immunogenicity, especially in young children. Haemophilus influenzae type b vaccine is a component of the primary course of childhood immunisation (see schedule, section 14.1); it is combined with diphtheria, tetanus, pertussis (acellular component) and inactivated poliomyelitis vaccine (see under Diphtheria Vaccines). For infants under 1 year, the course consists of 3 doses of a vaccine containing haemophilus influenzae type b component with an interval of 1 month between doses. Unimmunised children over 12 months need receive only 1 dose of the vaccine, but for full protection against other diseases, 3 doses should be given of diphtheria, tetanus, pertussis (acellular, component), poliomyelitis (inactivated) and haemophilus type b conjugate vaccine (adsorbed). The risk of infection falls sharply in older children and the vaccine is not normally required for children over 10 years.

Haemophilus influenzae type b vaccine may be given to those over 10 years who are considered to be at increased risk of invasive *H. influenzae* type b disease (such as those with sickle-cell disease and those receiving treatment for malignancy). Also, children and adults with asplenia or splenic dysfunction, irrespective of age or the time laspsed since splenectomy, should receive a single dose of haemophilus influenzae type b vaccine; those under 1 year should be given 3 doses. Individuals vaccinated in infancy who have had a splenectomy or develop splenic dysfunction should receive a single booster dose of haemophilus influenzae type b vaccine after the age of 1 year. For elective splenectomy, the vaccine should ideally be given at least 2 weeks before surgery.

Side-effects of haemophilus influenzae type b vaccine include fever, restlessness, prolonged crying, loss of appetite, vomiting, and diarrhoea; hypersensitivity reactions (including anaphylaxis) and collapse have been reported.

See section 14.1 for general contra-indications

■ Single component

Hiberix® (GSK) PoM

Injection, powder for reconstitution, capsular polysaccharide of *Haemophilus influenzae* type b (conjugated to tetanus protein), net price single-dose vial = £8.97

Dose: children and adults at risk because of asplenia (and where combination vaccination not required), *by intramuscular injection*, 0.5 mL

■ Combined vaccines

See Diphtheria vaccines

Hepatitis A vaccine

Hepatitis A vaccine is prepared from formaldehyde-inactivated hepatitis A virus grown in human diploid cells.

Immunisation is recommended for:

- laboratory staff who work directly with the virus;
- patients with haemophilia treated with Factor VIII or Factor IX concentrates or who have liver disease or who have been infected with hepatitis B or hepatitis C;
- travellers to high-risk areas (see p. 624);
- individuals who are at risk due to their sexual behaviour.

Immunisation should be considered for :

- patients with chronic liver disease;
- staff and residents of homes for those with severe learning difficulties;
- workers at risk of exposure to untreated sewage;
- prevention of secondary cases in close contacts of confirmed cases of hepatitis A, within 7 days of onset of disease in the primary case;
- parenteral drug abusers.

Side-effects of hepatitis A vaccine, usually mild, include transient soreness, erythema, and induration at the injection site. Less common effects include fever, malaise, fatigue, headache, nausea, diarrhoea, and loss of appetite; arthralgia, myalgia, and, generalised rashes are occasionally reported.

See section 14.1 for general contra-indications.

■ Single component

Avaxim® (Aventis Pasteur) PoM

Injection, suspension of formaldehyde-inactivated hepatitis A virus (GBM grown in human diploid cells) 320 antigen units/mL adsorbed onto aluminium hydroxide, net price 0.5-mL prefilled syringe = £19.19

Excipients: include neomycin

Dose: by intramuscular injection (see note below), 0.5 mL as a single dose; booster dose 0.5 mL 6–12 months after initial dose; further booster doses, 0.5 mL every 10 years; CHILD under 16 years, not recommended

NOTE. Booster dose may be delayed by up to 3 years if not given after recommended interval following primary dose with *Avaxim*®. The deltoid region is the preferred site of injection. The subcutaneous route may be used for patients with bleeding disorders

Epaxal® (MASTA) PoM

Injection, suspension of formaldehyde-inactivated hepatitis A virus (RG-SB grown in human diploid cells) at least 48 units/mL, net price 0.5-mL prefilled syringe = £23.81

Dose: by intramuscular injection (see note below), ADULT and CHILD over 1 year, 0.5 mL as a single dose; booster dose 0.5 mL 6–12 months after initial dose (1–6 months if splenectomised)

NOTE. Booster dose may be delayed by up to 4 years in adults if not given after recommended interval following primary dose. The deltoid region is the preferred site of injection. The subcutaneous route may be used for patients with bleeding disorders

IMPORTANT. *Epaxal*® contains influenza virus haemagglutinin grown in the allantoic cavity of chick embryos, therefore contra-indicated in those hypersensitive to eggs or chicken protein.

Havrix Monodose® (GSK) PoM

Injection, suspension of formaldehyde-inactivated hepatitis A virus (HM 175 grown in human diploid cells) 1440 ELISA units/mL adsorbed onto aluminium hydroxide, net price 1-mL prefilled syringe = £22.14, 0.5-mL (720 ELISA units) prefilled syringe (*Havrix Junior Monodose*®) = £16.77

Excipients: include neomycin

Dose: by intramuscular injection (see note below), 1 mL as a single dose; booster dose, 1 mL 6–12 months after initial dose; CHILD 1–15 years 0.5 mL; booster dose, 0.5 mL 6–12 months after initial dose

NOTE. Booster dose may be delayed by up to 3 years if not given after recommended interval following primary dose with *Havrix Monodose*®. The deltoid region is the preferred site of injection. The subcutaneous route may be used for patients with bleeding disorders

Vaqta® **Paediatric** (Aventis Pasteur) PoM

Injection, suspension of formaldehyde-inactivated hepatitis A virus (grown in human diploid cells) 50 antigen units/mL adsorbed onto aluminium hydroxide, net price 0.5-mL vial = £14.55

Dose: by intramuscular injection (see note below) CHILD and ADOLESCENT 2–17 years, 0.5 mL as a single dose; booster dose 0.5 mL 6–18 months after initial dose; under 2 years, not recommended

NOTE. The deltoid region is the preferred site of injection

■ With hepatitis B vaccine

Twinrix® (GSK) PoM

Injection, inactivated hepatitis A virus 720 ELISA units and recombinant (DNA) hepatitis B surface antigen 20 micrograms/mL adsorbed onto aluminium hydroxide and aluminium phosphate, net price 1-mL prefilled syringe (*Twinrix*® *Adult*) = £27.76, 0.5-mL prefilled syringe (*Twinrix*® *Paediatric*) = £20.79

Excipients: include neomycin and thiomersal

Dose: by intramuscular injection (see note below); primary course of 3 doses of 1 mL, the second 1 month and the third 6 months after the first dose; CHILD 1–15 years *by intramuscular injection*, 3 doses of 0.5 mL Accelerated schedule (e.g. for travellers departing within 1 month), ADULT, second dose 7 days after first dose, third dose after further 14 days and a fourth dose after 12 months

NOTE. Primary course should be completed with *Twinrix*® (single component vaccines given at appropriate intervals may be used for booster dose); the deltoid region is the preferred site of injection in adults and older children; anterolateral thigh is preferred site in infants; not to be injected into the buttock (vaccine efficacy reduced); subcutaneous route used for patients with bleeding disorders (but immune response may be reduced).

IMPORTANT. *Twinrix*® **not** recommended for post-exposure prophylaxis following percutaneous (needle-stick), ocular or mucous membrane exposure to hepatitis B virus.

■ With typhoid vaccine

Hepatyrix® (GSK) PoM

Injection, suspension of inactivated hepatitis A virus (grown in human diploid cells) 1440 ELISA units/mL adsorbed onto aluminium hydroxide, combined with typhoid vaccine containing 25 micrograms/mL virulence polysaccharide antigen of *Salmonella typhi*, net price 1-mL prefilled syringe = £32.08

Excipients: include neomycin

Dose: by intramuscular injection (see note below), ADULT and ADOLESCENT over 15 years, 1 mL as a single dose; booster doses, see under single component hepatitis A vaccine and under polysaccharide typhoid vaccine

NOTE. The deltoid region is the preferred site of injection. The subcutaneous route may be used for patients with bleeding disorders

ViATIM® (Aventis Pasteur) PoM

Injection, suspension of inactivated hepatitis A virus (grown in human diploid cells) 160 antigen units/mL adsorbed onto aluminium hydroxide, combined with typhoid vaccine containing 25 micrograms/mL virulence polysaccharide antigen of *Salmonella typhi*, net price 1-mL prefilled syringe = £30.22

Dose: by intramuscular injection (see note below), ADULT and ADOLESCENT over 16 years, 1 mL as a single dose; booster doses, see under single component hepatitis A vaccine and under polysaccharide typhoid vaccine

NOTE. The deltoid region is the preferred site of injection. The subcutaneous route may be used for patients with bleeding disorders

Hepatitis B vaccine

Hepatitis B vaccine contains inactivated hepatitis B virus surface antigen (HBsAg) adsorbed on aluminium hydroxide adjuvant. It is made biosynthetically using recombinant DNA technology. The vaccine is used in individuals at high risk of contracting hepatitis B.

In the UK, high-risk groups include:

- parenteral drug abusers;
- individuals who change sexual partners frequently;
- close family contacts of a case or carrier;
- infants born to mothers who *either* have had hepat-

itis B during pregnancy, *or* are positive for both hepatitis B surface antigen and hepatitis B e-antigen *or* are surface antigen positive without e markers (or where they have not been determined); active immunisation of the infant is started immediately after delivery and *hepatitis B immunoglobulin* (see p. 621) is given at the same time as the vaccine (but preferably at a different site). Infants born to mothers who are positive for hepatitis B surface antigen and for e-antigen antibody should receive the vaccine but not the immunoglobulin;

- individuals with haemophilia, those receiving regular blood transfusions or blood products, and carers responsible for the administration of such products;
- patients with chronic renal failure including those on haemodialysis. Haemodialysis patients should be monitored for antibodies annually and re-immunised if necessary. Home carers (of dialysis patients) who are negative for hepatitis B surface antigen should be vaccinated;
- healthcare personnel (including trainees) who have direct contact with blood or blood-stained body fluids or with patients' tissues;
- other occupational risk groups such as morticians and embalmers;
- staff and patients of day-care or residential accommodation for those with severe learning difficulties;
- inmates of custodial institutions;
- those travelling to areas of high prevalence who are at increased risk or who plan to remain there for lengthy periods (see p. 624);
- families adopting children from countries with a high prevalence of hepatitis B.

Immunisation takes up to 6 months to confer adequate protection; the duration of immunity is not known precisely, but a single booster 5 years after the primary course may be sufficient to maintain immunity for those who continue to be at risk.

More detailed guidance is given in the memorandum *Immunisation against Infectious Disease*. Immunisation does not eliminate the need for commonsense precautions for avoiding the risk of infection from known carriers by the routes of infection which have been clearly established, consult *Guidance for Clinical Health Care Workers: Protection against Infection with Blood-borne Viruses* (available at www.dh.gov.uk). Accidental inoculation of hepatitis B virus-infected blood into a wound, incision, needle-prick, or abrasion may lead to infection, whereas it is unlikely that indirect exposure to a carrier will do so.

Specific **hepatitis B immunoglobulin** ('HBIG') is available for use with the vaccine in those accidentally infected and in neonates at special risk of infection (section 14.5).

A combined hepatitis A and hepatitis B vaccine is also available.

See section 14.1 for general contra-indications.

■ Single component

Engerix B® (GSK) PoM

Injection, suspension of hepatitis B surface antigen (rby, prepared from yeast cells by recombinant DNA technique) 20 micrograms/mL adsorbed onto aluminium hydroxide, net price 0.5-mL (paediatric) vial = £9.16, 0.5-mL (paediatric) prefilled syringe = £9.67, 1-mL vial = £12.34, 1-mL prefilled syringe = £12.99

Excipients: include thiomersal

Dose: by intramuscular injection (see note below), 3 doses of 1 mL (20 micrograms), the second 1month and the third 6 months after the first dose; CHILD birth to 15 years 3 doses of 0.5 mL (10 micrograms); if compliance likely to be low in CHILD 10–15 years increase dose to 1 mL (20 micrograms)

Accelerated schedule, third dose 2 months after first dose and a fourth dose at 12 months; exceptionally (e.g. for travellers departing within 1 month), ADULT, second dose 7 days after first dose, third dose after a further 14 days and a fourth dose after 12 months

NEONATE born to hepatitis B surface antigen-positive mothers (see also notes above), 4 doses of 0.5 mL (10 micrograms), first dose at birth with hepatitis B immunoglobulin injection (separate site) the second 1 month, the third 2 months and the fourth 12 months after the first dose

Chronic haemodialysis patients, *by intramuscular injection* (see note below) 4 doses of 2 mL (40 micrograms), the second 1 month, the third 2 months and the fourth 6 months after the first dose; adjustment of immunisation schedule and booster doses may be required in those with low antibody concentration

NOTE. Deltoid muscle is preferred site of injection in adults and older children; anterolateral thigh is preferred site in neonates, infants and young children; not to be injected into the buttock (vaccine efficacy reduced); subcutaneous route used for patients with bleeding disorders

HBvaxPRO® (Aventis Pasteur) PoM

Injection, suspension of hepatitis B surface antigen (prepared from yeast cells by recombinant DNA technique) 10 micrograms/mL adsorbed onto aluminium hydroxyphosphate sulphate, net price 0.5-mL (5-microgram) vial = £9.02, 1-mL (10-microgram) vial = £12.00; 40 micrograms/mL, 1-mL (40-microgram) vial = £29.30

Dose: by intramuscular injection (see note below), ADULT and ADOLESCENT over 16 years, 3 doses of 10 micrograms, the second 1 month and the third 6 months after the first dose; CHILD under 16 years, 3 doses of 5 micrograms

Accelerated schedule, third dose 2 months after first dose with fourth dose at 12 months

Booster doses may be required in immunocompromised patients with low antibody concentration

NEONATE born to hepatitis B surface antigen-positive mothers (see also notes above), 0.5 mL (5 micrograms), first dose at birth with hepatitis B immunoglobulin injection (separate site), subsequent doses according to local policy

Chronic haemodialysis patients, *by intramuscular injection* (see note below) 3 doses of 40 micrograms, the second 1 month and the third 6 months after the first dose; booster doses may be required in those with low antibody concentration

NOTE. Deltoid muscle is preferred site of injection in adults and older children; anterolateral thigh is preferred site in neonates and infants; not to be injected into the buttock (vaccine efficacy reduced); subcutaneous route used for patients with bleeding disorders

■ With hepatitis A vaccine

See Hepatitis A Vaccine

Influenza vaccine

While most viruses are antigenically stable, the influenza viruses A and B (especially A) are constantly altering their antigenic structure as indicated by changes in the haemagglutinins (H) and neuraminidases (N) on the surface of the viruses. It is essential that influenza vaccines in use contain the H and N components of the prevalent strain or strains. Every year the World Health Organization recommends which strains should be included.

The recommended strains are grown in the allantoic cavity of chick embryos (therefore **contra-indicated** in those hypersensitive to eggs).

Since **influenza vaccines** will not control epidemics they are recommended *only for persons at high risk*. Annual immunisation is strongly recommended for individuals aged over 6 months with the following conditions:

- chronic respiratory disease, including asthma;
- chronic heart disease;
- chronic liver disease;
- chronic renal disease;
- diabetes mellitus;
- immunosuppression because of disease (including asplenia or splenic dysfunction) or treatment (including prolonged corticosteroid treatment);
- HIV infection (regardless of immune status).

Influenza immunisation is also recommended for all persons aged over 65 years, for residents of nursing or residential homes for the elderly and other long-stay facilities, and for carers of persons whose welfare may be at risk if the carer falls ill.

As part of the winter planning, NHS employers should offer vaccination to healthcare workers directly involved in patient care. Employers of social care workers should consider similar action.

Interactions: Appendix 1 (vaccines).

See section 14.1 for general contra-indications.

Inactivated Influenza Vaccine (Split Virion) (Non-proprietary) PoM

Injection, suspension of formaldehyde-inactivated influenza virus (split virion) Flu/Vac/Split, net price 0.5-mL prefilled syringe = £6.29

Excipients: may include neomycin and polymyxin

Dose: by intramuscular injection, ADULT and CHILD over 13 years 0.5 mL as a single dose; CHILD 6–35 months 0.25–0.5 mL, 3–12 years 0.5 mL, in children dose repeated after 4–6 weeks if not previously vaccinated

NOTE. Subcutaneous route used for patients with bleeding disorders

Inactivated Influenza Vaccine (Surface Antigen) (Non-proprietary) PoM

Injection, suspension of propiolactone-inactivated influenza virus (surface antigen) Flu/Vac/SA, net price 0.5-mL prefilled syringe = £3.98

Excipients: include neomycin, polymyxin B and thiomersal

Dose: by intramuscular injection, ADULT and CHILD over 13 years 0.5 mL as a single dose; CHILD 6–35 months 0.25–0.5 mL, 3–12 years 0.5 mL, in children dose repeated after 4–6 weeks if not previously vaccinated

NOTE. Subcutaneous route used for patients with bleeding disorders

Agrippal® (Wyeth) PoM

Injection, suspension of formaldehyde-inactivated influenza virus (surface antigen) Flu/Vac/SA, net price 0.5-mL prefilled syringe = £5.03

Excipients: include neomycin

Dose: by intramuscular injection, ADULT and CHILD over 13 years 0.5 mL as a single dose; CHILD 6–35 months 0.25–0.5 mL, 3–12 years 0.5 mL, in children dose repeated after 4–6 weeks if not previously vaccinated

NOTE. Subcutaneous route used for patients with bleeding disorders

Begrivac® (Wyeth) PoM

Injection, suspension of formaldehyde-inactivated influenza virus (split virion) Flu/Vac/Split, net price 0.5-mL prefilled syringe = £5.03

Excipients: include polymyxin B

Dose: by intramuscular injection, ADULT and CHILD over 13 years 0.5 mL as a single dose; CHILD 6–35 months 0.25–0.5 mL, 3–12 years 0.5 mL, in children dose repeated after 4–6 weeks if not previously vaccinated

NOTE. Subcutaneous route used for patients with bleeding disorders

Enzira® (Chiron Vaccines) ▼ PoM

Injection, suspension of inactivated influenza virus (split virion) Flu/Vac/Split, net price 0.5-mL prefilled syringe = £6.59

Excipients: include neomycin and polymyxin B

Dose: by intramuscular injection, ADULT and CHILD over 13 years 0.5 mL as a single dose; CHILD 6–35 months 0.25–0.5 mL, 3–12 years 0.5 mL, in children dose repeated after 4–6 weeks if not previously vaccinated

NOTE. Subcutaneous route used for patients with bleeding disorders

Fluarix® (GSK) PoM

Injection, suspension of formaldehyde-inactivated influenza virus (split virion) Flu/Vac/Split, net price 0.5-mL prefilled syringe = £4.49

Excipients: include gentamicin

Dose: by intramuscular injection, ADULT and CHILD over 13 years 0.5 mL as a single dose; CHILD 6–35 months 0.25–0.5 mL, 3–12 years 0.5 mL, in children dose repeated after 4–6 weeks if not previously vaccinated

NOTE. Subcutaneous route used for patients with bleeding disorders

Inflexal® V (Aventis Pasteur) PoM

Injection, suspension of inactivated influenza virus (surface antigen) Flu/Vac/SA, net price 0.5-mL prefilled syringe = £6.13

Excipients: include neomycin and polymyxin B

Dose: by intramuscular injection, ADULT and CHILD over 13 years 0.5 mL as a single dose; CHILD 6–35 months 0.25–0.5 mL, 3–12 years 0.5 mL, in children dose repeated after 4–6 weeks if not previously vaccinated

NOTE. Subcutaneous route used for patients with bleeding disorders

Influvac Sub-unit® (Solvay) PoM

Injection, suspension of formaldehyde-inactivated influenza virus (surface antigen) Flu/Vac/SA, net price 0.5-mL prefilled syringe = £5.22

Excipients: include gentamicin

Dose: by intramuscular injection, ADULT and CHILD over 13 years 0.5 mL as a single dose; CHILD 6–35 months 0.25–0.5 mL, 3–12 years 0.5 mL, in children dose repeated after 4–6 weeks if not previously vaccinated

NOTE. Subcutaneous route used for patients with bleeding disorders

Invivac® (Solvay) PoM

Injection, suspension of inactivated influenza virus (surface antigen) Flu/Vac/SA, net price 0.5-mL prefilled syringe = £6.59

Excipients: include gentamicin

Dose: by intramuscular (or deep subcutaneous) injection, ADULT 0.5 mL as a single dose

NOTE. Subcutaneous route used for patients with bleeding disorders

Mastaflu® (MASTA) PoM

Injection, suspension of formaldehyde-inactivated influenza virus (surface antigen) Flu/Vac/SA, net price 0.5-mL prefilled syringe = £6.50

Excipients: include gentamicin

Dose: by intramuscular injection, ADULT and CHILD over 13 years 0.5 mL as a single dose; CHILD 6–35 months 0.25–0.5 mL, 3–12 years 0.5 mL, in children dose repeated after 4–6 weeks if not previously vaccinated

NOTE. Subcutaneous route used for patients with bleeding disorders

Measles vaccine

Measles vaccine has been replaced by a combined live measles, mumps and rubella vaccine (MMR vaccine) for all eligible children.

Administration of a measles-containing vaccine to children may be associated with a mild measles-like syndrome with a measles-like rash and pyrexia about a week after injection. Much less commonly, convulsions and, very rarely, encephalitis have been reported. Convulsions in infants are much less frequently associated with measles vaccines than with other conditions leading to febrile episodes.

MMR vaccine may be used in the control of outbreaks of measles (see under MMR Vaccine).

■ Single antigen vaccine
No longer available in the UK

■ Combined vaccines
See MMR vaccine

Measles, Mumps and Rubella (MMR) vaccine

A combined live **measles, mumps, and rubella vaccine** (MMR vaccine) aims to eliminate rubella (and congenital rubella syndrome), measles, and mumps. Every child should receive two doses of MMR vaccine by entry to primary school, unless there is a valid contra-indication (see below) or parental refusal. MMR vaccine should be given irrespective of previous measles, mumps or rubella infection.

The first dose of MMR vaccine is given to children aged 12–15 months. A second (booster) dose is given before starting school at 3–5 years of age (see schedule, section 14.1). Children presenting for pre-school booster who have not received the first dose of MMR vaccine should be given a dose of MMR vaccine followed 3 months later by a second dose. At school-leaving age or at entry into further education, MMR immunisation should be offered to individuals of both sexes who have not received it. In a young adult who has received only a single dose of MMR in childhood, a second dose is recommended to acheive full protection.

MMR vaccine should be used to protect against rubella in *seronegative women of child-bearing age* (see schedule, section 14.1); unimmunised health-care workers who might put pregnant women at risk of rubella should be vaccinated. MMR vaccine may also be offered to previously *unimmunised and seronegative post-partum women*. Vaccination a few days after delivery is important because about 60% of congenital abnormalities from rubella infection occur in babies of women who have borne more than one child. Immigrants arriving after the age of school immunisation are particularly likely to require immunisation.

MMR vaccine may also be used in the control of outbreaks of measles and should be offered to susceptible children aged over 6 months who are contacts of a case, within 3 days of exposure to infection; these children should still receive routine MMR vaccinations at the recommended ages. Household contacts of a case, aged between 6 and 9 months may receive normal immunoglobulin (section 14.5). MMR vaccine is **not suitable** for prophylaxis following exposure to mumps or rubella since the antibody response to the mumps and rubella components is too slow for effective prophylaxis.

Children with impaired immune response should not receive live vaccines (for advice on HIV see section 14.1). If they have been exposed to measles infection they should be given normal immunoglobulin (section 14.5).

Fever or a rash may occur after the first dose of MMR vaccine, most commonly about a week after vaccination and lasting about 2 to 3 days (section 14.1). Leaflets are available for parents on advice for reducing fever (including the use of paracetamol). Parotid swelling occurs occasionally, usually in the third week. Adverse reactions are considerably less common after the second dose of MMR vaccine than after the first dose.

Idiopathic thrombocytopenic purpura has occurred rarely following MMR vaccination, usually within 6 weeks of the first dose. The risk of developing idiopathic thrombocytopenic purpura after MMR vaccine is much less than the risk of developing it after infection with wild measles, mumps or rubella virus. The CSM has recommended that children who develop idiopathic thrombocytopenic purpura within 6 weeks of the first dose of MMR should undergo serological testing before the second dose is due; if the results suggest incomplete immunity against measles, mumps or rubella then a second dose of MMR is recommended. The Specialist and Reference Microbiology Division, Health Protection Agency offers free serological testing for children who develop idiopathic thrombocytopenic purpura *within 6 weeks* of the first dose of MMR.

Post-vaccination meningoencephalitis was reported (rarely and with complete recovery) following vaccination with MMR vaccine containing Urabe mumps vaccine, which has now been discontinued; no cases have been confirmed in association with the currently used Jeryl Lynn mumps vaccine. Children with post-vaccination symptoms are not infectious.

> Reviews undertaken on behalf of the CSM and the Medical Research Council have not found any evidence of a link between MMR vaccination and bowel disease or autism. The Chief Medical Officers have advised that the MMR vaccine is the safest and best way to protect children against measles, mumps, and rubella. Information (including fact sheets and a list of references) may be obtained from:
> www.immunisation.nhs.uk and
> www.mmrthefacts.nhs.uk

Contra-indications to MMR include:

- children with untreated malignant disease or altered immunity (for advice on vaccines and HIV see section 14.1), and those receiving immunosuppressive drugs or radiotherapy, or high-dose corticosteroids;
- children who have received another live vaccine by injection within 3 weeks;
- children with allergies to excipients such as gelatin and neomycin;
- children with acute febrile illness (vaccination should be deferred);
- if given to women, pregnancy should be avoided for 1 month;
- should not be given within 3 months of an immunoglobulin injection.

The Department of Health recommends avoiding rubella vaccination during pregnancy. However, if given inadvertently during pregnancy, then termination is not recommended because extensive studies have failed to link rubella vaccination in early pregnancy with fetal damage.

NOTE. Children with a personal or close family history of convulsions should be given MMR vaccine, provided the parents understand that there may be a febrile response; doctors should seek specialist paediatric advice rather than withhold vaccination; there is increasing evidence that MMR vaccine can be given safely even when the child has had an anaphylactic reaction to food containing egg (dislike of egg or refusal to eat egg is not a contra-indication).

MMR Vaccine PoM

Live measles, mumps, and rubella vaccine

Dose: by deep subcutaneous or by intramuscular injection, 0.5 mL (see schedule, section 14.1)

Available from health authorities or direct from Farillon as *MMR II*® (*excipients include* gelatin and neomycin) or *Priorix*® (*excipients include* neomycin)

Meningococcal vaccines

Almost all childhood meningococcal disease in the UK is caused by *Neisseria meningitidis* serogroups B and C. **Meningococcal Group C conjugate vaccine** protects only against infection by serogroup C; it can be given from 2 months of age. After early adulthood the risk of meningococcal disease declines, and immunisation is not generally recommended after the age of 25 years.

CHILDHOOD IMMUNISATION. **Meningococcal Group C conjugate vaccine** provides long-term protection against infection by serogroup C of *Neisseria meningitidis* in children from 2 months of age; it is now a component of the primary course of childhood immunisation. The recommended schedule consists of 3 doses starting at 2 months of age with an interval of 1 month between each dose (see schedule, section 14.1). Infants aged 5–12 months not previously vaccinated should receive 2 doses, with an interval of 1 month between doses. It is recommended that meningococcal group C conjugate vaccine be given to anyone aged under 25 years who has not been vaccinated previously with this vaccine; those over 1 year receive a single dose.

Meningococcal group C conjugate vaccine is also recommended for individuals with a dysfunctional or absent spleen.

IMMUNISATION FOR TRAVELLERS. Individuals travelling to countries of risk (see below) should be immunised with a meningococcal polysaccharide vaccine that covers serotypes **A, C, W135 and Y**. Vaccination is particularly important for those living or working with local people or visiting an area of risk during outbreaks.

Outbreaks of infection with the W135 strain of meningococcus have occurred in Burkina Faso, West Africa and there have been cases in a number of other African countries. Countries with risk in Africa are listed below but outbreaks may also occur in countries not listed:

Angola, Benin, Burkina Faso, Burundi, Cameroon, Central African Republic, Chad, Democratic Republic of Congo, Eritrea, Ethiopia, Gambia, Ghana, Guinea, Guinea Bissau, Ivory Coast, Kenya, Mali, Mozambique, Namibia, Niger, Nigeria, Rwanda, Senegal, Sierra Leone, Somalia, Sudan, Tanzania, Togo, Uganda, and Zambia

Proof of vaccination with the tetravalent (A, C, W135 and Y) meningococcal vaccine is required for those travelling to Saudi Arabia during the Hajj and Umrah pilgrimages (where outbreaks of the W135 strain have occurred).

Travellers should be immunised with the meningococcal polysaccharide vaccine that covers serogroups A, C, W135 and Y, even if they have already received meningococcal group C conjugate vaccine. The response to serotype C in unconjugated meningococcal polysaccharide vaccines given to children aged under 18 months is not as good as in adults.

CONTACTS OF INFECTED INDIVIDUALS AND LABORATORY WORKERS. For advice on the immunisation of *close contacts* of cases of meningococcal disease in the UK and on the role of the vaccine in the control of *local outbreaks*, consult Guidelines for Public Health Management of Meningococcal Disease in the UK in *Commun Dis Public Health* 2002; **5**: 187–204. See section 5.1 Table 2 for antibacterial prophylaxis to prevent a secondary case of meningococcal meningitis

The need for immunisation of laboratory staff who work directly with *Neisseria meningitidis* should be considered.

SIDE-EFFECTS. Side-effects of meningococcal Group C conjugate vaccine include redness, swelling, and pain at the site of the injection, mild fever, irritability, drowsiness, dizziness, nausea, vomiting, diarrhoea, headache, myalgia, rash, urticaria, pruritus, malaise, lymphadenopathy, hypotonia, paraesthesia, hypoaesthesia, and syncope. Hypersensitivity reactions (including anaphylaxis, bronchospasm, and angioedema) and seizures have been reported rarely. Symptoms of meningism have also been reported rarely, but there is no evidence that the vaccine causes meningococcal C meningitis. There have been very rare reports of Stevens-Johnson syndrome. The CSM has advised that vaccination provides benefit in terms of lives saved and disabilities prevented.

Meningococcal polysaccharide A, C, W135 and Y vaccine is associated with injection-site reactions and very rarely headache, fatigue, fever, and drowsiness. Hypersensitivity reactions including anaphylaxis have been reported.

See section 14.1 for general contra-indications.

■ Meningococcal Group C conjugate vaccine

Meningitec® (Wyeth) PoM

Injection, suspension of capsular polysaccharide antigen of *Neisseria meningitidis* group C (conjugated to *Corynebacterium diphtheriae* protein), adsorbed onto aluminium phosphate, net price 0.5-mL vial = £17.95

Dose: by intramuscular (or deep subcutaneous) injection, ADULT and CHILD over 1 year 0.5 mL as a single dose; for routine immunisation in INFANT under 1 year, 3 doses (each of 0.5 mL) at intervals of 1 month (but see notes above and schedule, section 14.1)

Available as part of childhood immunisation schedule from Farillon

NOTE. Subcutaneous route used for patients with bleeding disorders

Menjugate® (Chiron) PoM
Injection, powder for reconstitution, capsular polysaccharide antigen of *Neisseria meningitidis* group C (conjugated to *Corynebacterium diphtheriae* protein), adsorbed onto aluminium hydroxide, single-dose and 10-dose vials
Dose: by intramuscular (or deep subcutaneous) injection, ADULT and CHILD over 1 year 0.5 mL as a single dose; for routine immunisation in INFANT under 1 year, 3 doses (each of 0.5 mL) at intervals of 1 month (but see notes above and schedule, section 14.1)
NOTE. Subcutaneous route used for patients with bleeding disorders

NeisVac-C® (Baxter) PoM
Injection, suspension of polysaccharide antigen of *Neisseria meningitidis* group C (conjugated to tetanus toxoid protein), adsorbed onto aluminium hydroxide, 0.5-mL prefilled syringe
Dose: by intramuscular (or deep subcutaneous) injection, ADULT and CHILD over 1 year 0.5 mL as a single dose; for routine immunisation in INFANT under 1 year, 3 doses (each of 0.5 mL) at intervals of 1 month (but see notes above and schedule, section 14.1)
Available from Farillon
NOTE. Subcutaneous route used for patients with bleeding disorders
The dose in the BNF may differ from that in product literature

■ Meningococcal polysaccharide A, C, W135 and Y vaccine

ACWY Vax® (GSK) PoM
Injection, powder for reconstitution, capsular polysaccharide antigens of *Neisseria meningitidis* groups A, C, W135 and Y, net price single-dose vial (with syringe containing diluent) = £16.73
Dose: by deep subcutaneous injection, ADULT and CHILD over 2 years 0.5 mL
NOTE. May be given to INFANT 2 months–2 years [unlicensed] but antibody response may be suboptimal

Mumps vaccine

■ Single antigen vaccine
No longer available in the UK

■ Combined vaccine
See MMR Vaccine

Pertussis vaccine

Pertussis vaccine is usually given as a combination preparation containing other vaccines (see under Diphtheria Vaccines). Acellular vaccines are derived from highly purified components of *Bordetella pertussis*.

For the routine immunisation of infants, primary immunisation with pertussis (whooping cough) vaccine is recommended usually in the form of 3 doses (separated by 1-month intervals) of **diphtheria, tetanus, pertussis (acellular, component), poliomyelitis (inactivated) and haemophilus type b conjugate vaccine (adsorbed)** (see schedule, section 14.1).

A booster dose should be given 3 years after the primary course; children *under 10 years* should receive *either* **adsorbed diphtheria, tetanus, pertussis (acellular, component) and inactivated poliomyelitis vaccine** *or* **adsorbed diphtheria** [low dose], **tetanus, pertussis (acellular, component) and inactivated poliomyelitis vaccine**.

Acellular pertussis vaccine components in the combination products offer adequate protection for primary immunisation and the incidence of local and systemic effects is lower than with the whole-cell pertussis vaccine used previously.

The vaccine should not be withheld from children with a history to a preceding dose of:

- fever, irrespective of severity;
- persistent crying or screaming for more than 3 hours;
- severe local reaction, irrespective of extent.

These side-effects were associated with whole-cell pertussis vaccine. Such reactions occur less frequently with the acellular pertussis vaccines.

PREDISPOSITION TO NEUROLOGICAL PROBLEMS. When there is a personal or family history of *febrile* convulsions, there is an increased risk of these occurring during fever from any cause including immunisation. In such children, immunisation is *recommended* but advice on the *prevention of fever* (see Post-immunisation pyrexia, p. 604) should be given before immunisation.

When a child has had a convulsion not associated with fever and the neurological condition is not deteriorating, immunisation is *recommended*.

Where there is a *still evolving neurological problem* including poorly controlled epilepsy, immunisation should be *deferred* and the child referred to a specialist. Immunisation is recommended if a cause for the neurological disorder is found. If a cause is not found, immunisation should be deferred until the condition is stable.

Children with stable neurological disorders (e.g. spina bifida, congenital brain abnormality, and perinatal hypoxic ischaemic encephalopathy) should be immunised according to the recommended schedule.

OLDER CHILDREN. All children up to the age of 10 years should receive primary immunisation with diphtheria, tetanus, pertussis (acellular, component), poliomyelitis (inactivated) and haemophilus type b conjugate vaccine (adsorbed). Primary immunisation against pertussis is not currently recommended in individuals over 10 years of age.

■ Combined vaccines
Combined vaccines, see under Diphtheria vaccines

Pneumococcal vaccines

Pneumococcal vaccines protect against infection with *Streptococcus pneumoniae* (pneumococcus); the vaccines contain polysaccharide from capsular pneumococci. Pneumococcal polysaccharide vaccine contains purified polysaccharide from 23 capsular types of pneumococci whereas pneumococcal polysaccharide conjugated vaccine contains polysaccharide from 7 capsular types, the polysaccharide being conjugated to protein.

Pneumococcal vaccination is recommended for individuals at special risk as follows:

- age over 65 years;
- asplenia or splenic dysfunction (including homozygous sickle cell disease and coeliac

disease which could lead to splenic dysfunction);
- chronic respiratory disease (includes asthma treated with continuous or frequent use of a systemic corticosteroid);
- chronic heart disease;
- chronic renal disease;
- chronic liver disease;
- diabetes mellitus;
- immune deficiency because of disease (e.g. HIV infection) or treatment (including prolonged systemic corticosteroid treatment);
- presence of cochlear implant;
- presence of CSF shunt or other condition where leakage of cerebrospinal fluid may occur;
- child under 5 years with a history of invasive pneumococcal disease.

Where possible, the vaccine should be given at least 2 weeks before splenectomy, surgery to insert a CSF shunt, cochlear implant surgery, and chemotherapy; patients should be given advice about increased risk of pneumococcal infection. A patient card and information leaflet for patients with asplenia are available from the Department of Health or in Scotland from the Scottish Executive, Public Health Division 1 (Tel (0131) 244 2501). Prophylactic antibacterial therapy against pneumococcal infection should not be stopped after immunisation.

CHOICE OF VACCINE. A single dose of the 23-valent unconjugated **pneumococcal polysaccharide vaccine** is used to immunise individuals over 5 years who are at special risk of pneumococcal disease. Children under 5 years who are at special risk should receive the 7-valent **pneumococcal polysaccharide conjugated vaccine** as follows:

- infants from 2 months to under 6 months should receive 3 doses (separated by 1-month intervals) of pneumococcal polysaccharide conjugated vaccine, starting at 2 months of age; a further dose is given after the first birthday;
- unimmunised infants 6–11 months should receive 2 doses (separated by 1 month) of pneumococcal polysaccharide conjugated vaccine; a further dose is given after the first birthday and at least 1 month after the previous dose;
- children 1–5 years should receive 2 doses (separated by 2 months) of pneumococcal polysaccharide conjugated vaccine.

All children who have received the pneumococcal polysaccharide conjugated vaccine should receive a single dose of the 23-valent pneumococcal polysaccharide vaccine after their second birthday and at least 2 months after the final dose of the 7-valent pneumococcal polysaccharide conjugated vaccine.

REVACCINATION. In individuals with higher concentrations of antibodies to pneumococcal polysaccharides, revaccination with the 23-valent pneumococcal polysaccharide vaccine more commonly produces adverse reactions. Revaccination is therefore not recommended, except every 5 years in individuals in whom the antibody concentration is likely to decline rapidly (e.g. asplenia, splenic dysfunction and nephrotic syndrome). If there is doubt, the need for revaccination should be discussed with a haematologist, immunologist, or microbiologist.

See section 14.1 for general contra-indications.

■ Pneumococcal polysaccharide vaccines

Pneumovax® II (Aventis Pasteur) PoM

Polysaccharide from each of 23 capsular types of pneumococcus, net price 0.5-mL vial = £8.83

Dose: by intramuscular injection, 0.5 mL; revaccination, see notes above; INFANT under 2 years, not recommended (suboptimal response and also safety and efficacy not established)

■ Pneumococcal polysaccharide conjugated vaccine

Prevenar® (Wyeth) ▼ PoM

Polysaccharide from each of 7 capsular types of pneumococcus (conjugated to diphtheria toxoid) adsorbed onto aluminium phosphate, net price 0.5-mL vial = £34.50

Dose: by intramuscular injection, INFANT 2–6 months 3 doses each of 0.5 mL separated by intervals of 1 month and a further dose in second year of life; 6–11 months 2 doses each of 0.5 mL separated by an interval of 1 month and a further dose in second year of life; CHILD 1–5 years 2 doses each of 0.5 mL separated by an interval of 2 months

NOTE. Deltoid muscle is preferred site of injection in young children; anterolateral thigh is preferred site in infants

The dose in the BNF may differ from that in product literature

Poliomyelitis vaccines

There are two types of poliomyelitis vaccine, inactivated poliomyelitis vaccine and live (oral) poliomyelitis vaccine. **Inactivated poliomyelitis vaccine** is now recommended for routine immunisation; it is given by injection and contains inactivated strains of human poliovirus types 1, 2 and 3.

A course of primary immunisation consists of 3 doses of a combined preparation containing inactivated poliomyelitis vaccine (see under Diphtheria Vaccines), starting at 2 months of age with intervals of 1 month between doses (see schedule, section 14.1). A course of 3 doses should also be given to all unimmunised adults; no adult should remain unimmunised against poliomyelitis.

Two booster doses of a preparation containing inactivated poliomyelitis vaccine are recommended, the first before school entry and the second before leaving school (see schedule, section 14.1). Booster doses for adults are not necessary except for those at special risk such as travellers to endemic areas, or laboratory staff likely to be exposed to the viruses, or healthcare workers in possible contact with cases; booster doses should be given to such individuals every 10 years.

Preparations containing inactivated poliomyelitis vaccine may be used to complete an immunisation course initiated with the live (oral) poliomyelitis vaccine. Live (oral) poliomyelitis vaccine is available only for use during outbreaks. The live (oral) vaccine poses a very rare risk of vaccine-associated paralytic polio because the attenuated strain of the virus can revert to a virulent form. For this reason the live (oral) vaccine must **not** be used for immunosuppressed individuals or their household contacts. The use of inactivated poliomyelitis vaccine removes the risk of vaccine-associated paralytic polio altogether.

TRAVELLERS. Unimmunised travellers to areas with a high incidence of poliomyelitis should receive a full course of a preparation containing inactivated poliomyelitis vaccine. Those who have not been vaccinated in the last 10 years should receive a booster dose of adsorbed diphtheria [low dose], tetanus and inactivated poliomyelitis vaccine. A list of countries with a high incidence of poliomyelitis can be obtained from www.travax.scot.nhs.uk or by contacting the National Travel Health Network and Centre.

■ Inactivated (Salk)

Combined vaccines, see under Diphtheria Vaccines

Poliomyelitis Vaccine, Inactivated (Non-proprietary) ▼ PoM

Pol/Vac (Inact)

Injection, inactivated suspension of suitable strains of poliomyelitis virus, types 1, 2, and 3, net price 0.5-mL prefilled syringe = £10.35

Excipients: may include neomycin, polymyxin B and streptomycin

NOTE. Not recommended for routine use—combination vaccines are recommended for primary immunisation and for boosters (see schedule, section 14.1)

■ Live (oral) (Sabin)

Poliomyelitis Vaccine, Live (Oral) (GSK) PoM

[1]Pol/Vac (Oral)

A suspension of suitable live attenuated strains of poliomyelitis virus, types 1, 2, and 3. Available in single-dose and 10-dose containers

Excipients: include neomycin and polymyxin B

Dose: control of outbreaks, 3 drops; may be given on a lump of sugar; not to be given with foods which contain preservatives

NOTE. Live poliomyelitis vaccine loses potency once the container has been opened—any vaccine remaining at the end of an immunisation session should be discarded; whenever possible sessions should be arranged to avoid undue wastage.

1. BP permits code OPV for vaccine in single doses provided it also appears on pack.

Rabies vaccine

The licensed rabies vaccines, the human diploid cell vaccine and the purified chick embryo cell vaccine are both cell-derived.

PRE-EXPOSURE PROPHYLAXIS. Immunisation should be offered to those at high risk of exposure to rabies—laboratory staff who handle the rabies virus, those working in quarantine stations, animal handlers, veterinary surgeons and field workers who are likely to be bitten by infected wild animals, certain port officials, and bat handlers. Transmission of rabies by humans has not been recorded but it is advised that those caring for patients with the disease should be vaccinated.

Immunisation against rabies is also recommended where there is limited access to prompt medical care for those living in areas where rabies is enzootic, for those travelling to such areas for longer than 1 month, and for those on shorter visits who may be exposed to unusual risk.

Immunisation against rabies is indicated during pregnancy if there is substantial risk of exposure to rabies and rapid access to post-exposure prophylaxis is likely to be limited.

Up-to-date country-by-country information on the incidence of rabies can be obtained from the National Travel Health Network and Centre (www.nathnac.org) and, in Scotland, from Health Protection Scotland (www.hps.scot.nhs.uk).

Immunisation against rabies requires 3 doses of rabies vaccine, with further booster doses for those who remain at continued risk (see under preparations below for details of regimens). To ensure protection in persons at high risk (e.g. laboratory workers), the concentration of antirabies antibodies in plasma is used to determine the intervals between doses.

POST-EXPOSURE PROPHYLAXIS. Following potential exposure to rabies, the wound or site of exposure (e.g. mucous membrane) should be cleansed under running water and washed for several minutes with soapy water as soon as possible after exposure. Disinfectant and a simple dressing may be applied, but suturing should be delayed because it may increase the risk of introducing rabies virus into the nerves.

Post-exposure prophylaxis against rabies depends on the level of risk in the country, the nature of exposure, and the individual's immunity. In each case, expert risk assessment and advice on appropriate management should be obtained from the Health Protection Agency Virus Reference Department, Colindale, London (tel. (020) 8200 4400) or the Communicable Disease Surveillance Centre (tel. (020) 8200 6868), in Scotland from the Scottish Centre for Infection and Environmental Health (tel. (0141) 300 1100), in Northern Ireland from the Public Health Laboratory, Belfast City Hospital (tel. (028) 9032 9241).

There are no specific contra-indications to the use of rabies vaccine for post-exposure prophylaxis and its use should be considered whenever a patient has been attacked by an animal in a country where rabies is enzootic, even if there is no direct evidence of rabies in the attacking animal. Because of the potential consequences of untreated rabies exposure and because rabies vaccination has not been associated with fetal abnormalities, pregnancy is not considered a contra-indication to post-exposure prophylaxis.

For post-exposure prophylaxis of *fully immunised* individuals (who have previously received pre-exposure or post-exposure prophylaxis with cell-derived rabies vaccine), 2 doses of cell-derived vaccine, separated by 3 days, are likely to be sufficient. Rabies immunoglobulin is not necessary in such cases.

Post-exposure treatment for *unimmunised individuals* (or those whose prophylaxis is possibly incomplete) comprises 5 doses of rabies vaccine given over 1 month (on days 0, 3, 7, 14, and 30); also, depending on the level of risk (determined by factors such as the nature of the bite and the country where it was sustained), rabies immunoglobulin is given on day 0 (section 14.5). The course may be discontinued if it is proved that the individual was not at risk.

Rabies Vaccine (Aventis Pasteur) PoM

Freeze-dried inactivated Wistar rabies virus strain PM/WI 38 1503-3M cultivated in human diploid cells, net price single-dose vial with syringe containing diluent = £22.15

Excipients: include neomycin

Dose: prophylactic, *by deep subcutaneous or intramuscular injection* in the deltoid region, 1 mL on days 0, 7, and 28; also booster doses every 2–3 years to those at continued risk

Post-exposure, *by deep subcutaneous or intramuscular injection* in the deltoid region, 1 mL, see notes above

Also available from local designated centres (special workers and post-exposure treatment)

Rabipur® (Chiron Vaccines) PoM

Freeze-dried inactivated Flury LEP rabies virus strain cultivated in chick embryo cells, net price single-dose vial = £22.15

Excipients: include neomycin

Dose: prophylactic, *by intramuscular injection* in the deltoid muscle or anterolateral thigh in small children, 1 mL on days 0, 7 and 21 or 28; also booster doses every 2–5 years for those at continued risk

Post-exposure, *by intramuscular injection* in the deltoid muscle or anterolateral thigh in small children, 1 mL, see notes above

Rubella vaccine

A combined measles, mumps and rubella vaccine (MMR vaccine) aims to eliminate rubella (German measles) and congenital rubella syndrome. MMR vaccine is used for childhood vaccination as well as for vaccinating adults (including women of child-bearing age) who do not have immunity against rubella.

■ Single antigen vaccine

No longer available in the UK; the combined live measles, mumps and rubella vaccine is a suitable alternative (see MMR vaccine, p. 613)

■ Combined vaccines

see MMR vaccine

Smallpox vaccine

Limited supplies of **smallpox vaccine** are held at the Specialist and Reference Microbiology Division, Health Protection Agency (Tel. (020) 8200 4400) for the exclusive use of workers in laboratories where pox viruses (such as vaccinia) are handled.

If a wider use of the vaccine is being considered, *Guidelines for smallpox response and management in the post-eradication era* should be consulted at www.dh.gov.uk

Tetanus vaccines

Tetanus vaccines stimulate production of a protective antitoxin. In general, adsorption on aluminium hydroxide or aluminium phosphate improves antigenicity.

Primary immunisation for children under 10 years usually consists of 3 doses of a combined preparation containing adsorbed tetanus vaccine, with an interval of 1 month between doses (see schedule, section 14.1).

The recommended schedule of tetanus vaccination not only gives protection against tetanus in childhood but also gives the basic immunity for subsequent booster doses (see schedule, section 14.1).

For primary immunisation of adults and children over 10 years previously unimmunised against tetanus, 3 doses of adsorbed diphtheria [low dose], tetanus and inactivated poliomyelitis vaccine are given with an interval of 1 month between doses (see under Diphtheria Vaccines).

Following routine childhood vaccination, 2 booster doses of a preparation containing adsorbed tetanus vaccine are recommended, the first before school entry and the second before leaving school.

If an individual presents for a booster dose but has been vaccinated following a tetanus-prone wound, the vaccine preparation administered at the time of injury should be determined. If this is not possible, the booster should still be given to ensure adequate protection against all antigens in the booster vaccine. An adult who has received 5 doses of tetanus vaccine is likely to have life-long immunity. Active immunisation is important for individuals who may not have completed a course of immunisation. Adults and children over 10 years may be given a course of adsorbed diphtheria [low dose], tetanus and inactivated poliomyelitis vaccine.

Very rarely, tetanus has developed after abdominal surgery; patients awaiting elective surgery should be asked about tetanus immunisation and immunised if necessary. Parenteral drug abuse is also associated with tetanus; those abusing drugs by injection should be vaccinated if unimmunised. Booster doses should be given if there is any doubt about the immunisation status. All laboratory staff should be offered a primary course if unimmunised.

For travel recommendations see section 14.6.

WOUNDS. Wounds are considered to be tetanus-prone if they are sustained more than 6 hours before surgical treatment *or* at any interval after injury and are puncture-type (particularly if contaminated with soil or manure) *or* show much devitalised tissue *or* are septic *or* are compound fractures *or* contain foreign bodies. All wounds should receive thorough cleansing.

- For *clean wounds*, fully immunised individuals (those who have received a total of 5 doses of a tetanus-containing vaccine at appropriate intervals) and those whose primary immunisation is complete (with boosters up to date), do not require tetanus vaccine; individuals whose primary immunisation is incomplete or whose boosters are not up to date require a reinforcing dose of a tetanus-containing vaccine (followed by further doses as required to complete the schedule); non-immunised individuals (or whose immunisation status is not known or who have been fully immunised but are now immunocompromised) should be given a dose of the appropriate tetanus-containing vaccine immediately (followed by completion of the full course of the vaccine if records confirm the need).
- For *tetanus-prone wounds*, management is as for clean wounds with the addition of a dose of tetanus immunoglobulin (section 14.5) given at a different site; in fully immunised individuals and those whose primary immunisation is complete (see above) the immunoglobulin is needed only if the risk of infection is especially high (e.g. contamination with manure). Antibacterial prophylaxis (with benzylpenicillin, co-amoxiclav, or metronidazole) may also be required for tetanus-prone wounds.

See section 14.1 for general contra-indications.

■ Combined vaccines

See Diphtheria Vaccines

Tick-borne encephalitis vaccine

Tick-borne encephalitis vaccine is licensed for immunisation of those in high-risk areas based on official recommendations (see section 14.6). Those working, walking or camping in warm forested areas of Central and Eastern Europe and Scandinavia, particularly from April to October when ticks are most prevalent, are at greatest risk of tick-borne encephalitis. Ideally, immunisation should be completed at least one month before travel.

Fever exceeding 40°C may occur, particularly after the first dose of tick-borne encephalitis vaccine. Other side effects include arrhythmias; the vaccine should be used with caution in those with cardiovascular disease. Tick-borne encephalitis vaccine is **contra-indicated** in those with acute febrile infection and severe hypersensitivity to egg protein. See section 14.1 for general contra-indications and side-effects.

FSME-IMMUN® (MASTA) PoM
Injection, suspension, inactivated Neudörfl tick-borne encephalitis virus strain, cultivated in chick embryo cells, net price 0.5-mL prefilled syringe = £32.00
Excipients: include gentamicin and neomycin
Dose: ADULT and ADOLESCENT over 16 years *by intramuscular injection* in deltoid muscle, 3 doses each of 0.5 mL , second dose after 1–3 months and third dose after further 5–12 months; ELDERLY over 60 years and immunocompromised (including those receiving immunosuppressants), antibody concentration may be measured 4 weeks after second dose and dose repeated if protective levels not achieved
NOTE. To achieve more rapid protection, second dose may be given 14 days after first dose
First booster dose given within 3 years after third dose, subsequent boosters after 3–5 years

Typhoid vaccines

Typhoid immunisation is advised for travellers to countries where sanitation standards may be poor, although it is not a substitute for scrupulous personal hygiene (see p. 624). Immunisation is also advised for laboratory workers handling specimens from suspected cases.

Capsular **polysaccharide typhoid vaccine** is given by *intramuscular or deep subcutaneous injection*; further doses are needed every 3 years on continued exposure. Local reactions, including pain, swelling or erythema, may appear 48–72 hours after administration.

For general contra-indications to vaccines, see section 14.1.

■ Polysaccharide vaccine for injection

Typherix® (GSK) PoM
Injection, Vi capsular polysaccharide typhoid vaccine, 50 micrograms/mL virulence polysaccharide antigen of *Salmonella typhi*, net price 0.5-mL prefilled syringe = £9.93
Dose: by intramuscular injection, 0.5 mL; CHILD under 2 years may show suboptimal response

Typhim Vi® (Aventis Pasteur) PoM
Injection, Vi capsular polysaccharide typhoid vaccine, 50 micrograms/mL virulence polysaccharide antigen of *Salmonella typhi*, net price 0.5-mL prefilled syringe = £9.49
Dose: by deep subcutaneous or by intramuscular injection, 0.5 mL; CHILD under 18 months may show suboptimal response

■ Polysaccharide vaccine with hepatitis A vaccine
See Hepatitis A Vaccine

Varicella–zoster vaccine

Varicella–zoster vaccine (live) is licensed for immunisation against varicella in seronegative individuals. It is not recommended for routine use in children but may be given to seronegative healthy children over 1 year who come into close contact with individuals at high risk of severe varicella infections. The Department of Health recommends varicella–zoster vaccine for seronegative healthcare workers who come into direct contact with patients. Those with a history of chickenpox or shingles can be considered immune, but healthcare workers with a negative or uncertain history should be tested.

Varicella–zoster vaccine is contra-indicated in pregnancy (avoid pregnancy for 3 months after vaccination) and during breast-feeding. It must not be given to individuals with primary or acquired immunodeficiency or to individuals receiving immunosuppressive therapy. For further contra-indications, see section 14.1.

Rarely, the varicella–zoster vaccine virus has been transmitted from the vaccinated individual to close contacts. Therefore, contact with the following should be avoided if a vaccine-related cutaneous rash develops within 4–6 weeks of the first or second dose:

- varicella-susceptible pregnant women;
- individuals at high risk of severe varicella, including those with immunodeficiency or those receiving immunosuppressive therapy.

Healthcare workers who develop a generalised papular or vesicular rash on vaccination should avoid contact with patients until the lesions have crusted. Those who develop a localised rash after vaccination should cover the lesions and be allowed to continue working unless in contact with patients at high risk of severe varicella.

For reference to specific **varicella–zoster immunoglobulin** see section 14.5.

Varilrix® (GSK) ▼ PoM
Injection, powder for reconstitution, live attenuated varicella–zoster virus (Oka strain) propagated in human diploid cells, net price 0.5-mL vial (with diluent) = £27.31
Excipients: include neomycin
Dose: by subcutaneous injection preferably into deltoid region, ADULT and ADOLESCENT over 13 years (see notes above), 2 doses of 0.5 mL separated by an interval of 8 weeks (minimum 6 weeks); CHILD 1–12 years (but see notes above), 0.5 mL as a single dose

Varivax® (Aventis Pasteur) ▼ PoM
Injection powder for reconstitution, live attenuated varicella-zoster virus (Oka/Merck strain) propagated in human diploid cells, net price 0.5-mL vial (with diluent) = £32.14
Excipients: include gelatin and neomycin
Dose: by subcutaneous injection into deltoid region or higher anterolateral thigh, ADULT and ADOLESCENT over 13 years (see notes above), 2 doses of 0.5 mL separated by 4–8 weeks; CHILD 1–12 years (but see notes above), 0.5 mL as a single dose (2 doses separated by 12 weeks in children with asymptomatic HIV infection)

Yellow fever vaccine

Live yellow fever vaccine is indicated for those travelling or living in areas where infection is endemic (see p. 624) and for laboratory staff who handle the virus or who handle clinical material from suspected cases. Infants under 9 months of age should be vaccinated only if the risk of yellow fever is unavoidable because there is a small risk of encephalitis. The vaccine should not be given to those with impaired immune responsiveness, or who have had an anaphylactic reaction to egg; it should not be given during pregnancy (but where there is a significant risk of exposure the need for immunisation outweighs any risk to the fetus). See section 14.1 for further contra-indications. Headache, fever, tiredness, and stiffness may occur 4–7 days after vaccination. Other side-effects include myalgia, asthenia, lymphadenopathy, rash, urticaria, and injection-site reactions.The immunity which probably lasts for life is officially accepted for 10 years starting from 10 days after primary immunisation and for a further 10 years immediately after revaccination.

Yellow Fever Vaccine, Live PoM
Yel/Vac

Injection, powder for reconstitution, preparation of 17D strain of yellow fever virus grown in fertilized hens eggs

Dose: by subcutaneous injection, 0.5 mL

Available (only to designated Yellow Fever Vaccination centres) as *Arilvax*® (*excipients: include* gelatin) and *Stamaril*®

14.5 Immunoglobulins

Human immunoglobulins have replaced immunoglobulins of animal origin (antisera) which were frequently associated with hypersensitivity. Injection of immunoglobulins produces immediate protection lasting for several weeks.

Immunoglobulins are produced from pooled human plasma or serum, and are tested and found non-reactive for hepatitis B surface antigen and for antibodies against hepatitis C virus and human immunodeficiency virus (types 1 and 2)

The two types of human immunoglobulin preparation are **normal immunoglobulin** and **specific immunoglobulins**.

Further information about immunoglobulins is included in *Immunisation against Infectious Disease* (see section 14.1) and in the Health Protection Agency's *Immunoglobulin Handbook*: www.hpa.org.uk.

AVAILABILITY. **Normal immunoglobulin** is available from Health Protection and microbiology laboratories only for contacts and the control of outbreaks. It is available commercially for other purposes.

Specific immunoglobulins are available from Health Protection and microbiology laboratories with the exception of **tetanus immunoglobulin** which is distributed through BPL to hospital pharmacies or blood transfusion departments and is also available to general medical practitioners. **Rabies immunoglobulin** is available from the Specialist and Reference Microbiology Division, Health Protection Agency. The large amounts of **hepatitis B immunoglobulin** required by transplant centres should be obtained commercially.

In Scotland all immunoglobulins are available from the *Blood Transfusion Service*. **Tetanus immunoglobulin** is distributed by the *Blood Transfusion Service* to hospitals and general medical practitioners on demand.

Normal immunoglobulin

Human **normal immunoglobulin** ('HNIG') is prepared from pools of at least 1000 donations of human plasma; it contains antibody to measles, mumps, varicella, hepatitis A, and other viruses that are currently prevalent in the general population.

CAUTIONS and SIDE-EFFECTS. Side-effects of immunoglobulins include malaise, chills, fever, and rarely anaphylaxis. Normal immunoglobulin is **contra-indicated** in patients with known class specific antibody to immunoglobulin A (IgA).

Normal immunoglobulin may **interfere with the immune response to live virus vaccines** which should therefore only be given **at least 3 weeks before or 3 months after** an injection of normal immunoglobulin (this does not apply to yellow fever vaccine since normal immunoglobulin does not contain antibody to this virus). For travellers, if there is insufficient time, the recommended interval may have to be ignored.

USES. Normal immunoglobulin is administered by intramuscular injection for the protection of susceptible contacts against **hepatitis A** virus (infectious hepatitis), **measles** and, to a lesser extent, **rubella**.

Special formulations of immunoglobulins for intravenous administration are available for *replacement therapy* for patients with congenital agammaglobulinaemia and hypogammaglobulinaemia, for the treatment of idiopathic thrombocytopenic purpura and Kawasaki syndrome, and for the prophylaxis of infection following bone-marrow transplantation and in children with symptomatic HIV infection who have recurrent bacterial infections. Normal immunoglobulin may also be given intramuscularly or subcutaneously for replacement therapy, but intravenous formulations are normally preferred.

Intravenous immunoglobulin is also used in the treatment of Guillain-Barré syndrome in preference to plasma exchange.

HEPATITIS A. **Hepatitis A vaccine** is preferred for individuals at risk of infection (see p. 609) including those visiting areas where the disease is highly endemic (all countries excluding Northern and Western Europe, North America, Japan, Australia, and New Zealand). In unimmunised individuals, transmission of hepatitis A is reduced by good hygiene. Intramuscular normal immunoglobulin is no longer recommended for routine prophylaxis in travellers but it may be indicated for immunocompromised patients if their antibody response to vaccine is unlikely to be adequate.

Intramuscular normal immunoglobulin is of value in the prevention of infection in close contact of confirmed cases of hepatitis A where there has been a delay in identifying cases or for individuals at high risk of severe disease.

MEASLES. Intramuscular normal immunoglobulin may be given to prevent or attenuate an attack of measles in individuals who do not have adequate immunity. Children and adults with compromised immunity who have come into contact with measles should receive intramuscular normal immunoglobulin as soon as possible after exposure. It is most effective if given within 72 hours but can be effective if given within 6 days. For individuals receiving intravenous immunoglobulin, 100 mg/kg given within 3 weeks before measles exposure should prevent measles. Intramuscular normal immunoglobulin should also be considered for the following individuals if they have been in contact with a confirmed case of measles or with a person associated with a local outbreak:

- non-immune pregnant women
- infants under 9 months

Further advice should be sought from the Communicable Disease Surveillance Centre, Health Protection Agency (tel. (020) 8200 6868).

Individuals with normal immunity who are not in the above categories and who have not been fully immunised against measles, can be given MMR vaccine (section 14.4) for prophylaxis following exposure to measles.

RUBELLA. Intramuscular immunoglobulin after exposure to rubella does **not** prevent infection in non-immune contacts and is **not** recommended for protection of pregnant women exposed to rubella. It may, however, reduce the likelihood of a clinical attack which may possibly reduce the risk to the fetus. It should be used only if termination of pregnancy would be unacceptable to the pregnant woman, when it should be given as soon as possible after exposure. Serological follow-up of recipients is essential. For routine prophylaxis, see MMR vaccine (p. 613).

■ For intramuscular use

Normal Immunoglobulin PoM

Normal immunoglobulin injection. 250-mg vial; 750-mg vial

Dose: by deep intramuscular injection, to control outbreaks of hepatitis A (see notes above), 500 mg; CHILD under 10 years 250 mg

Measles prophylaxis, CHILD under 1 year 250 mg, 1–2 years 500 mg, 3 years and over 750 mg; to allow attenuated attack, CHILD under 1 year 100 mg, 1 year and over 250 mg

Rubella in pregnancy, prevention of clinical attack, 750 mg

Available from the Communicable Disease Surveillance Centre and other regional Health Protection Agency offices (for contacts and control of outbreaks only, see above) and from SNBTS (as *Liberim*® *IM*, 250-mg strength only)

■ For subcutaneous use

Subcuvia® (Baxter BioScience) PoM

Normal immunoglobulin injection, net price 5-mL vial = £29.60, 10-mL vial = £59.20

Dose: by subcutaneous injection, antibody deficiency syndromes, consult product literature

NOTE. May be administered by intramuscular injection (if subcutaneous route not possible) but **not** for patients with thrombocytopenia or other bleeding disorders

Subgam® (BPL) PoM

Normal immunoglobulin injection, net price 2-mL vial = £11.20, 5-mL vial = £28.00, 10-mL vial = £56.00

Dose: by subcutaneous injection, antibody deficiency syndromes, consult product literature

NOTE. May be administered by intramuscular injection (if subcutaneous route not possible) but **not** for patients with thrombocytopenia or other bleeding disorders

Vivaglobin® (ZLB Behring) PoM

Normal immunoglobulin injection, net price 10-mL vial = £59.20

Dose: by subcutaneous injection, antibody deficiency syndromes, consult product literature

■ For intravenous use

Normal Immunoglobulin for Intravenous Use PoM

Brands include *Flebogamma*® *5%* (0.5 g, 2.5 g, 5 g, 10 g); *Gammagard*® *S/D* (0.5 g, 2.5 g, 5 g, 10 g); Human Immunoglobulin (3 g, 5 g, 10 g); *Octagam*® (2.5 g, 5 g, 10 g); *Sandoglobulin*® (1 g, 3 g, 6 g, 12 g); *Sandoglobulin*® NF Liquid (6 g, 12 g); *Vigam*®*S* (2.5 g, 5 g); *Vigam*®*Liquid* (2.5 g, 5 g, 10 g)

Dose: consult product literature

Specific immunoglobulins

Specific immunoglobulins are prepared by pooling the plasma of selected donors with high levels of the specific antibody required.

Although a hepatitis B vaccine is now available for those at high risk of infection, specific **hepatitis B immunoglobulin** ('HBIG') is available for use in association with hepatitis B vaccine for the prevention of infection in laboratory and other personnel who have been accidentally inoculated with hepatitis B virus, and in infants born to mothers who have become infected with this virus in pregnancy or who are high-risk carriers (see Hepatitis B Vaccine, p. 610).

Following exposure of an unimmunised individual to an animal in or from a high-risk country, the site of the bite should be washed with soapy water and specific **rabies immunoglobulin** of human origin administered; as much of the dose as possible should be injected in and around the cleansed wound. Rabies vaccine should also be given (for details see Rabies Vaccine, p. 617).

For the management of tetanus-prone wounds, **tetanus immunoglobulin** of human origin ('HTIG') should be used in addition to wound cleansing and, where appropriate, antibacterial prophylaxis and a tetanus-containing vaccine (section 14.4). Tetanus immunoglobulin, together with metronidazole (section 5.1.11) and wound cleansing, should also be used for the treatment of established cases of tetanus.

Varicella–zoster immunoglobulin (VZIG) is recommended for individuals who are at increased risk of severe varicella *and* who have no antibodies to varicella–zoster virus *and* who have significant exposure to chickenpox or herpes zoster. Those at increased risk include neonates of women who develop chickenpox in the period 7 days before to 7 days after delivery, women exposed at any stage of pregnancy (but when supplies of VZIG are short, only issued to those exposed in the first 20 weeks' gestation or to those near term), and the immunosuppressed including those who have received corticosteroids in the previous 3 months at the following dose equivalents of prednisolone: *children* 2 mg/kg daily for at least 1 week or 1 mg/kg daily for 1 month; *adults* about 40 mg daily for more than 1 week. (**Important:** for full details consult *Immunisation against Infectious Disease*). **Varicella–zoster vaccine** is available—see section 14.4

Cytomegalovirus (CMV) immunoglobulin (available on a named-patient basis from SNBTS) is indicated for prophylaxis in patients receiving immunosuppressive treatment.

■ Hepatitis B

Hepatitis B Immunoglobulin PoM

See notes above

Dose: by intramuscular injection (as soon as possible after exposure), ADULT and CHILD over 10 years 500 units; CHILD under 5 years 200 units, 5–9 years 300 units; NEONATE 200 units as soon as possible after birth; for full details consult *Immunisation against Infectious Disease*

Available from selected Health Protection Agency and NHS laboratories (except for Transplant Centres, see p. 620), also available from BPL and SNBTS (as *Liberim® HB*)

NOTE. Hepatitis B immunoglobulin for intravenous use is available from BPL and SNBTS on a named-patient basis.

■ Rabies

Rabies Immunoglobulin PoM

(Antirabies Immunoglobulin Injection)

See notes above

Dose: 20 units/kg *by infiltration* in and around the cleansed wound; if wound not visible or healed or if infiltration of whole volume not possible, give remainder *by intramuscular injection* into anterolateral thigh (remote from vaccination site)

Available from Specialist and Reference Microbiology Division, Health Protection Agency (also from BPL and SNBTS)

■ Tetanus

Tetanus Immunoglobulin PoM

(Antitetanus Immunoglobulin Injection)

See notes above

Dose: by intramuscular injection, prophylactic 250 units, increased to 500 units if more than 24 hours have elapsed or there is risk of heavy contamination or following burns

Therapeutic, 150 units/kg (multiple sites)

Available from BPL and from SNBTS (as *Liberim® T*, licensed only for tetanus prophylaxis)

Tetabulin® (Baxter BioScience) PoM

Tetanus immunoglobulin, net price 250-unit prefilled syringe = £14.80

Dose: by intramuscular injection, prophylactic, 250 units, increased to 500 units if wound older than 12 hours or if risk of heavy contamination or if patient weighs more than 90 kg; second dose of 250 units given after 3–4 weeks if patient immunosuppressed or if active immunisation with tetanus vaccine contra-indicated

Therapeutic, 150 units/kg (multiple sites)

Tetanus Immunoglobulin for Intravenous Use PoM

Used for proven or suspected clinical tetanus

Dose: by intravenous infusion, 5000–10 000 units

Available from BPL and SNBTS on a named-patient basis and from the Northern Ireland Blood Transfusion Service

■ Varicella–zoster

Varicella–Zoster Immunoglobulin PoM

(Antivaricella–zoster Immunoglobulin)

See notes above

Dose: by deep intramuscular injection, prophylaxis (as soon as possible—not later than 10 days after exposure), NEONATE, INFANT and CHILD up to 5 years 250 mg, 6–10 years 500 mg, 11–14 years 750 mg, over 15 years 1 g; give second dose if further exposure occurs more than 3 weeks after first dose

NOTE. No evidence that effective in treatment of severe disease. Normal immunoglobulin for intravenous use may be used to provide an immediate source of antibody.

Available from selected Health Protection Agency and NHS laboratories (also from BPL, and SNBTS as *Liberim® Z*)

Anti-D (Rh_0) immunoglobulin

Anti-D (Rh_0) immunoglobulin is available to prevent a rhesus-negative mother from forming antibodies to fetal rhesus-positive cells which may pass into the maternal circulation. The objective is to protect any subsequent child from the hazard of haemolytic disease of the newborn.

Anti-D immunoglobulin should be administered following any sensitising episode (e.g. abortion, miscarriage and birth); it should be injected within 72 hours of the episode but even if a longer period has elapsed it may still give protection and should be administered. The dose of anti-D immunoglobulin is determined according to the level of exposure to rhesus-positive blood.

For routine antenatal prophylaxis (see also NICE guidance below), two doses of at least 500 units of anti-D immunoglobulin should be given, the first at 28 weeks' gestation and the second at 34 weeks.

NICE Guidance (routine antenatal anti-D prophylaxis for rhesus-negative women). NICE has recommended (May 2002) that routine antenatal anti-D prophylaxis be offered to all non-sensitised pregnant women who are rhesus negative.

Use of routine *antenatal* anti-D prophylaxis should not be affected by previous anti-D prophylaxis for a sensitising event early in the same pregnancy. Similarly, *postpartum* anti-D prophylaxis should not be affected by previous routine antenatal anti-D prophylaxis or by antenatal anti-D prophylaxis for a sensitising event.

Note. MMR vaccine may be given in the postpartum period with anti-D (Rh_0) immunoglobulin injection provided that separate syringes are used and the products are administered into different limbs. If blood is transfused, the antibody response to the vaccine may be inhibited—measure rubella antibodies after 8 weeks and revaccinate if necessary.

Anti-D (Rh_0) Immunoglobulin (Non-proprietary) PoM

Injection, anti-D (Rh_0) immunoglobulin, net price 250-unit vial = £14.95, 500-unit vial = £19.50, 2500-unit vial = £94.40

Dose: by deep intramuscular injection, to rhesus-negative woman for prevention of Rh_0(D) sensitisation:

Following birth of rhesus-positive infant, 500 units immediately or within 72 hours; for transplacental bleed of over 4 mL fetal red cells, extra 100–125 units per mL fetal red cells

Following any potentially sensitising episode (e.g. stillbirth, abortion, amniocentesis) up to 20 weeks' gestation 250 units per episode (after 20 weeks, 500 units) immediately or within 72 hours

Antenatal prophylaxis, 500 units given at weeks 28 and 34 of pregnancy; a further dose is still needed immediately or within 72 hours of delivery

NOTE. Some UK authorities recommend different doses for antenatal prophylaxis (see notes above)

Following Rh_0(D) incompatible blood transfusion, 100–125 units per mL transfused rhesus-positive red cells

Available from Blood Centres and from BPL (*D-Gam®*) and SNBTS (as *Liberim® D250*, *Liberim® D500*)

Partobulin SDF® (Baxter BioScience) PoM
Injection, anti-D (Rh_0) immunoglobulin 1250 units/mL (250 micrograms/mL), net price 1-mL prefilled syringe = £35.00
Dose: by intramuscular injection, to rhesus-negative woman for prevention of Rh_0 (D) sensitisation:
Following birth of rhesus-positive infant, 1000–1650 units immediately or within 72 hours; for large transplacental blood loss, 50–125 units per mL of fetal red cells
Antenatal prophylaxis, 1000–1650 units given at weeks 28 and 34 of pregnancy; if infant rhesus-positive, further dose is needed immediately or within 72 hours of delivery
Following abortion, ectopic pregnancy or hydatidiform mole up to 12 weeks' gestation, 600–750 units (after 12 weeks, 1250–1650 units) immediately or within 72 hours
Following amniocentesis or chorionic villous sampling, 1250–1650 units immediately or within 72 hours
NOTE. Some UK authorities recommend different doses for antenatal prophylaxis (see notes above)
Following Rh_0 (D) incompatible blood or red cell transfusion, 1250 units per 10 mL of transfused rhesus-positive red cells immediately or within 72 hours

Rhophylac® (ZLB) PoM
Injection, anti-D (Rh_0) immunoglobulin 750 units/mL (150 micrograms/mL), net price 2-mL (1500-unit) prefilled syringe = £50.00.
Dose: by intramuscular or intravenous injection, to rhesus-negative woman for prevention of Rh_0(D) sensitisation:
Following birth of rhesus-positive infant, 1000–1500 units immediately or within 72 hours; for large transplacental bleed, extra 100 units per mL fetal red cells (preferably by intravenous injection)
Following any potentially sensitising episode (e.g. abortion, amniocentesis, chorionic villous sampling) up to 12 weeks' gestation 1000 units per episode (after 12 weeks, higher doses may be required) immediately or within 72 hours
Antenatal prophylaxis, 1500 units given between weeks 28–30 of pregnancy; a further dose is still needed immediately or within 72 hours of delivery
NOTE. Some UK authorities recommend different doses for antenatal prophylaxis (see notes above)
Following Rh_0(D) incompatible blood transfusion, *by intravenous injection*, 50 units per mL transfused rhesus-positive blood (or 100 units per mL of erythrocyte concentrate)

WinRho SDF® (Baxter BioScience) PoM
Injection, anti-D (Rh_0) immunoglobulin, powder for reconstitution, net price 1500-unit (300-microgram) vial (with diluent) = £313.50, 5000-unit (1-mg) vial (with diluent) = £1045.00
Dose: to rhesus-negative woman for prevention of Rh_0(D) sensitisation:
Following birth of rhesus-positive infant, *by intramuscular injection*, 1500 units *or by intravenous injection*, 600 units immediately or within 72 hours; for transplacental bleed of over 25 mL fetal blood, *by intramuscular injection*, extra 50 units per mL fetal blood
Following any potentially sensitising episode (e.g. abortion, amniocentesis, chorionic villous sampling) up to 12 weeks' gestation, *by intramuscular injection*, 600 units per episode (after 12 weeks, 1500 units) immediately or within 72 hours
Antenatal prophylaxis, *by intramuscular or intravenous injection*, 1500 units given at week 28 of pregnancy; a further dose is still needed immediately or within 72 hours of delivery
Following Rh_0(D) incompatible thrombocyte transfusion in rhesus-negative woman of child-bearing age, *by intravenous injection*, 1500 units
NOTE. Some UK authorities recommend different doses for antenatal prophylaxis (see notes above)
Following Rh_0(D) incompatible blood transfusion, *by intramuscular injection*, at least 600 units per 10 mL transfused rhesus-positive blood, given in divided doses over several days
Autoimmune (idiopathic) thrombocytopenic purpura, consult product literature

Interferons

Interferon gamma-1b is licensed to reduce the frequency of serious infection in chronic granulomatous disease and in severe malignant osteopetrosis.

INTERFERON GAMMA-1b

(Immune interferon)

Indications: see notes above

Cautions: severe hepatic impairment (Appendix 2) or severe renal impairment (Appendix 3); seizure disorders (including seizures associated with fever); cardiac disease (including ischaemia, congestive heart failure, and arrhythmias); monitor before and during treatment: haematological tests (including full blood count, differential white cell count, and platelet count), blood chemistry tests (including renal and liver function tests) and urinalysis; avoid simultaneous administration of foreign proteins including immunological products (risk of exaggerated immune response); pregnancy (Appendix 4); breast-feeding (Appendix 5); **interactions:** Appendix 1 (interferons)
DRIVING. May impair ability to drive or operate machinery; effects may be enhanced by alcohol

Side-effects: fever, headache, chills, myalgia, fatigue; nausea, vomiting, arthralgia, rashes and injection-site reactions reported

Dose: see under Preparations

Immukin® (Boehringer Ingelheim) PoM
Injection, recombinant human interferon gamma-1b 200 micrograms/mL, net price 0.5-mL vial = £88.00
Dose: by subcutaneous injection, 50 micrograms/m^2 3 times a week; patients with body surface area of 0.5 m^2 or less, 1.5 micrograms/kg 3 times a week; not yet recommended for children under 6 months with chronic granulomatous disease

14.6 International travel

NOTE. For advice on **malaria chemoprophylaxis**, see section 5.4.1.

No special immunisation is required for travellers to the United States, Europe, Australia, or New Zealand although all travellers should have immunity to tetanus and poliomyelitis (and childhood immunisations should be up to date). Certain special precautions are required in non-European areas surrounding the Mediterranean, in Africa, the Middle East, Asia, and South America.

Long-term travellers to areas that have a high incidence of **poliomyelitis** or **tuberculosis** should be immunised with the appropriate vaccine; in the case of poliomyelitis previously immunised adults may be given a booster dose of a preparation containing inactivated poliomyelitis vaccine. BCG immunisation is recommended for travellers proposing to stay for longer than one month (or in close contact with the local population) in Asia, Africa, or Central and South America; it should preferably be given three months or more before departure.

Yellow fever immunisation is recommended for travel to the endemic zones of Africa and South America. Many countries require an International Certificate of Vaccination from individuals arriving from, or who have been travelling through, endemic areas, whilst other countries require a certificate from all entering travellers (consult the Department of Health handbook, *Health Information for Overseas Travel*, www.dh.gov.uk).

Immunisation against **meningococcal meningitis** is recommended for a number of areas of the world (for details, see p. 614).

Protection against **hepatitis A** is recommended for travellers to high-risk areas outside Northern and Western Europe, North America, Japan, Australia and New Zealand. Hepatitis A vaccine (see p. 609) is preferred and it is likely to be effective even if given shortly before departure; normal immunoglobulin is no longer given routinely but may be indicated in the immunocompromised (see p. 620). Special care must also be taken with food hygiene (see below).

Hepatitis B vaccine (see p. 610) is recommended for those travelling to areas of high prevalence who intend to seek employment as healthcare workers or who plan to remain there for lengthy periods and who may therefore be at increased risk of acquiring infection as the result of medical or dental procedures carried out in those countries. Short-term tourists or business travellers are not generally at increased risk of infection but may place themselves at risk by their sexual behaviour when abroad.

Prophylactic immunisation against **rabies** (see p. 617) is recommended for travellers to enzootic areas on long journeys or to areas out of reach of immediate medical attention.

Travellers who have not had a **tetanus** booster in the last 10 years and are visiting areas where medical attention may not be accessible should receive a booster dose of adsorbed diphtheria [low dose], tetanus and inactivated poliomyelitis vaccine (see p. 608), even if they have received 5 doses of a tetanus-containing vaccine previously.

Typhoid vaccine is indicated for travellers to those countries where typhoid is endemic but the vaccine is no substitute for personal precautions (see below).

There is no requirement for cholera vaccination as a condition for entry into any country, but **oral cholera vaccine** (see p. 607) may be considered for backpackers and those travelling to situations where the risk is greatest (e.g. refugee camps). Regardless of vaccination, travellers to areas where cholera is endemic should take special care with food hygiene (see below).

Advice on **diphtheria**, on **Japanese encephalitis** (NHS vaccine available on named-patient basis from Sanofi Pasteur and MASTA) and on **tick-borne encephalitis** is included in *Health Information for Overseas Travel*, see below.

FOOD HYGIENE. In areas where sanitation is poor, good food hygiene is important to help prevent hepatitis A, typhoid, cholera, and other diarrhoeal diseases (including travellers' diarrhoea). Food should be freshly prepared and hot, and uncooked vegetables (including green salads) should be avoided; only fruits which can be peeled should be eaten. Only suitable bottled water, or tap water that has been boiled, or treated with sterilising tablets should be used for drinking.

Information on health advice for travellers. The Department of Health booklet, *Health Advice For Travellers* (code: T6) includes information on immunisation requirements (or recommendations) around the world. The booklet can be obtained from travel agents, post-offices or by telephoning 0800 555 777 (24-hour service); also available on the Internet at: www.dh.gov.uk

The Department of Health handbook, *Health Information for Overseas Travel* (2001), which draws together essential information *for healthcare professionals* regarding health advice for travellers, can be obtained from
The Stationery Office
PO Box 29, Norwich NR3 1GN
Telephone orders, 0870 600 5522
Fax: 0870 600 5533
www.tso.co.uk

Immunisation requirements change from time to time, and information on the current requirements for any particular country may be obtained from:

National Travel Health Network and Centre
Hospital for Tropical Diseases
Mortimer Market Centre
Capper Street, off Tottenham Court Road
London WC1E 6AU
Tel: (020) 7380 9234
(9 a.m.–noon, 2–4.30 p.m. weekdays for healthcare professionals **only**)
www.nathnac.org

Scottish Centre for Infection and Environmental Health
Clifton House
Clifton Place
Glasgow G3 7LN
Tel: (0141) 300 1130
(14.00–16.00 hours weekdays)
www.travax.scot.nhs.uk (registration required. Annual fee may be payable for users outside NHS Scotland)

Welsh Medicines Information Centre
University Hospital of Wales
Cardiff CF14 4XW
Tel: (029) 2074 2979 (for health professionals **only**)

Department of Health and Social Services
Castle Buildings
Stormont
Belfast BT4 3PP
Tel: (028) 9052 0000

or from the embassy or legation of the appropriate country.

15: Anaesthesia

15.1 General anaesthesia

> NOTE. The drugs in section 15.1 should be used only by experienced personnel and where adequate resuscitation equipment is available.

It is common practice to administer several drugs with different actions to produce surgical anaesthesia. An intravenous anaesthetic is usually used for induction, followed by maintenance with an inhalational anaesthetic, perhaps supplemented by other drugs administered intravenously. Specific drugs are often used to produce muscle relaxation; these drugs interfere with spontaneous respiration and intermittent positive-pressure ventilation is commonly employed.

SURGERY AND LONG-TERM MEDICATION. The risk of stopping long-term medication before surgery is often greater than the risk of continuing it during surgery; however, surgery itself may alter the need for continued drug therapy of certain conditions. It is vital that the anaesthetist knows about **all** drugs that a patient is (or has been) taking.

Patients with adrenal atrophy resulting from long-term corticosteroid use (section 6.3.2) may suffer a precipitous fall in blood pressure unless corticosteroid cover is provided during anaesthesia and in the immediate postoperative period. Anaesthetists must therefore know whether a patient is, or has been, receiving corticosteroids (including high-dose inhaled corticosteroids).

Other drugs that should normally not be stopped before surgery include antiepileptics, antiparkinsonian drugs, antipsychotics, anxiolytics, bronchodilators, cardiovascular drugs, glaucoma drugs, immunosuppressants, drugs of dependence, and thyroid or antithyroid drugs. Expert advice is required for patients receiving antivirals for HIV infection. For general advice on surgery in diabetic patients see section 6.1.1.

Patients on oral anticoagulant therapy present with increased risk for anaesthesia and surgery. In these circumstances, the anaesthetist and surgeon should assess the relative risks and decide jointly whether the anticoagulant should be stopped or replaced with heparin therapy.

Drugs that are stopped before surgery include combined oral contraceptives (see Surgery, section 7.3.1 for details); for advice on hormone replacement therapy, see section 6.4.1.1. If antidepressants need to be stopped, they should be withdrawn gradually to avoid withdrawal symptoms. In view of their hazardous interactions MAOIs should normally be stopped 2 weeks before surgery. Tricyclic antidepressants need not be stopped, but there may be an increased risk of arrhythmias and hypotension (and dangerous interaction with vasopressor drugs); therefore, the anaesthetist should be informed if they are not stopped. Lithium should be stopped 24 hours before major surgery but the normal dose can be continued for minor surgery (with careful monitoring of fluids and electrolytes). Potassium-sparing diuretics may need to be withheld on the morning of surgery because hyperkalaemia may develop if renal perfusion is impaired or if there is tissue damage.

ANAESTHESIA AND DRIVING. Patients given sedatives and analgesics during minor outpatient procedures should be very carefully warned about the risk of driving afterwards. For intravenous benzodiazepines and for a short general anaesthetic the risk extends to **at least 24 hours** after administration. Responsible persons should be available to take patients home. The dangers of taking **alcohol** should also be emphasised.

PROPHYLAXIS OF ACID ASPIRATION. Regurgitation and aspiration of gastric contents (Mendelson's syndrome) is an important complication of general anaesthesia, particularly in obstetrics and emergency surgery.

An **H_2-receptor antagonist** (section 1.3.1) or a **proton pump inhibitor** (section 1.3.5) such as omeprazole may be used before surgery to increase the pH and reduce the volume of gastric fluid. They do not affect the pH of fluid already in the stomach and this limits their value in emergency procedures; oral H_2-receptor antagonists can be given 1–2 hours before the procedure but omeprazole must be given at least 12 hours earlier. Antacids are frequently used to neutralise the acidity of the fluid already in the stomach; 'clear' (non-particulate) antacids such as sodium citrate are preferred.

Anaesthesia, sedation and resuscitation in dental practice

> **Anaesthesia, sedation and resuscitation in dental practice.**
> For details see *A Conscious Decision: A review of the use of general anaesthesia and conscious sedation in primary dental care*. Report by a group chaired by the Chief Medical Officer and Chief Dental Officer, July 2000 (www.dh.gov.uk), and associated documents.
> Guidance is also included in *Maintaining Standards: Guidance to Dentists on Professional and Personal Conduct*, London, General Dental Council, May 1999 (and as amended subsequently).

Gas cylinders

Each gas cylinder bears a label with the name of the gas contained in the cylinder. The name or chemical symbol of the gas appears on the shoulder of the cylinder and is also clearly and indelibly stamped on the cylinder valve.

The colours on the valve end of the cylinder extend down to the shoulder; in the case of mixed gases the colours for the individual gases are applied in four segments, two for each colour.

Gas cylinders should be stored in a cool well-ventilated room, free from flammable materials.

No lubricant of any description should be used on the cylinder valves.

15.1.1 Intravenous anaesthetics

Intravenous anaesthetics may be used either to induce anaesthesia or for maintenance of anaesthesia throughout surgery. Intravenous anaesthetics nearly all produce their effect in one arm-brain circulation time and can cause apnoea and hypotension, and so adequate resuscitative facilities **must** be available. They are **contra-indicated** if the anaesthetist is not confident of being able to maintain the airway (e.g. in the presence of a tumour in the pharynx or larynx). Extreme care is required in surgery of the mouth, pharynx, or larynx and in patients with acute circulatory failure (shock) or fixed cardiac output.

Individual requirements vary considerably and the recommended dosage is only a guide. Smaller dosage is indicated in ill, shocked, or debilitated patients and in significant hepatic impairment, while robust individuals may require more. To facilitate tracheal intubation, induction is followed by a neuromuscular blocking drug (section 15.1.5).

TOTAL INTRAVENOUS ANAESTHESIA. This is a technique in which major surgery is carried out with all anaesthetic drugs given intravenously. Respiration is controlled, the lungs being inflated with oxygen-enriched air. Muscle relaxants are used to provide relaxation and prevent reflex muscle movements. The main problem to be overcome is the assessment of depth of anaesthesia.

ANAESTHESIA AND DRIVING. See section 15.1.

Barbiturates

Thiopental sodium (thiopentone sodium) is used widely, but it has no analgesic properties. Induction is generally smooth and rapid, but owing to its potency, overdosage with cardiorespiratory depression may occur.

Awakening from a moderate dose of thiopental is rapid due to redistribution of the drug into other tissues. However, metabolism is slow and some sedative effects may persist for 24 hours. Repeated doses have a cumulative effect.

THIOPENTAL SODIUM

(Thiopentone sodium)

Indications: induction of general anaesthesia; anaesthesia of short duration; reduction of raised intracranial pressure if ventilation controlled

Cautions: see notes above; cardiovascular disease; hepatic impairment (Appendix 2); reconstituted solution is highly alkaline—extravasation causes tissue necrosis and severe pain; avoid intra-arterial injection; pregnancy (Appendix 4); **interactions:** Appendix 1 (anaesthetics, general)

Contra-indications: see notes above; porphyria (section 9.8.2); myotonic dystrophy; breast-feeding (Appendix 5)

Side-effects: arrhythmias, myocardial depression, laryngeal spasm, cough, sneezing, hypersensitivity reactions, rash, injection-site reactions

Dose: induction of general anaesthesia, *by intravenous injection* usually as a 2.5% (25 mg/mL) solution, in fit premedicated adults, initially 100–150 mg (reduced in elderly or debilitated) over 10–15 seconds (longer in elderly or debilitated), followed by further quantity if necessary according to response after 30–60 seconds; *or* up to 4 mg/kg (max. 500mg); CHILD induction 2–7 mg/kg

Raised intracranial pressure, *by intravenous injection*, 1.5–3 mg/kg, repeated as required

Thiopental (Link) PoM

Injection, powder for reconstitution, thiopental sodium, net price 500-mg vial = £3.06

Other intravenous anaesthetics

Etomidate is an induction agent associated with rapid recovery without a hangover effect. It causes less hypotension than other drugs used for induction. There is a high incidence of extraneous muscle movement which can be minimised by an opioid analgesic or a short-acting benzodiazepine given just before induction. Pain on injection can be reduced by the use of a larger vein or by an opioid analgesic given just before induction. Etomidate may suppress adrenocortical function, particularly on continuous administration, and it should not be used for maintenance of anaesthesia.

Propofol is associated with rapid recovery without a hangover effect and it is very widely used. There is sometimes pain on intravenous injection and significant extraneous muscle movements may occur. Convulsions, anaphylaxis, and delayed recovery from anaesthesia have occurred after propofol administration; since the onset of convulsions can be delayed the CSM has advised special caution after day surgery. Propofol has been associated with bradycardia, occasionally profound; intravenous administration of an antimuscarinic drug may be necessary to prevent this.

Ketamine is rarely used now; it can be given by the intravenous or the intramuscular route and it has good analgesic properties at sub-anaesthetic dosage. The maximum effect occurs after more than one arm-brain circulation time. There is a high incidence of extraneous muscle movements; also cardiovascular stimulation and arterial pressure may rise with tachycardia. The main disadvantage of ketamine is the high incidence of hallucinations and other transient psychotic sequelae. The incidence of psychotic effects can be reduced when drugs such as diazepam are also used. Ketamine is **contra-indicated** in patients with hypertension and is best avoided in those prone to hallucinations. It is used mainly for paediatric anaesthesia, particularly when repeated administration is required. Recovery is relatively slow.

ETOMIDATE

Indications: induction of anaesthesia

Cautions: see notes above; avoid in porphyria (section 9.8.2); pregnancy (Appendix 4); breast-feeding (Appendix 5); **interactions:** Appendix 1 (anaesthetics, general)

Contra-indications: see notes above

Side-effects: see notes above

Dose: see under preparations

Etomidate-Lipuro® (Braun) PoM

Injection (emulsion), etomidate 2 mg/mL, net price 10-mL amp = £1.53

Dose: ADULT and CHILD, *by slow intravenous injection*, 150–300 micrograms/kg; CHILD under 10 years may need up to 400 micrograms/kg; ELDERLY 150–200 micrograms/kg

Hypnomidate® (Janssen-Cilag) PoM

Injection, etomidate 2 mg/mL, net price 10-mL amp = £1.50

Excipients: include propylene glycol (see Excipients, p. 2)

Dose: ADULT and CHILD, *by slow intravenous injection*, 300 micrograms/kg; ELDERLY 150–200 micrograms/kg; max. total dose 60 mg

KETAMINE

Indications: induction and maintenance of anaesthesia

Cautions: see notes above; pregnancy (Appendix 4); **interactions:** Appendix 1 (anaesthetics, general)

Contra-indications: see notes above; also porphyria (section 9.8.2)

Side-effects: see notes above

Dose: *by intramuscular injection*, short procedures, initially 6.5–13 mg/kg (10 mg/kg usually produces 12–25 minutes of surgical anaesthesia)

Diagnostic manoeuvres and procedures not involving intense pain, initially 4 mg/kg

By intravenous injection over at least 60 seconds, short procedures, initially 1–4.5 mg/kg (2 mg/kg usually produces 5–10 minutes of surgical anaesthesia)

By intravenous infusion of a solution containing 1 mg/mL, longer procedures, induction, total dose of 0.5–2 mg/kg; maintenance (using microdrip infusion), 10–45 micrograms/kg/minute, rate adjusted according to response

Ketalar® (Pfizer) PoM

Injection, ketamine (as hydrochloride) 10 mg/mL, net price 20-mL vial = £4.22; 50 mg/mL, 10-mL vial = £8.77; 100 mg/mL, 10-mL vial = £16.10

PROPOFOL

Indications: see under dose

Cautions: see notes above; monitor blood-lipid concentration if risk of fat overload or if sedation longer than 3 days; pregnancy (Appendix 4); **interactions:** Appendix 1 (anaesthetics, general)

Contra-indications: see notes above; not to be used for sedation of ventilated children and adolescents under 17 years (risk of potentially fatal effects including metabolic acidosis, cardiac failure, rhabdomyolysis, hyperlipidaemia and hepatomegaly)

Side-effects: see notes above; also flushing; transient apnoea during induction; *less commonly* thrombosis, phlebitis; *very rarely* pancreatitis, pulmonary oedema, sexual disinhibition, and discoloration of urine; serious and sometimes fatal side-effects reported with prolonged infusion of doses exceeding 5 mg/kg/hour, including metabolic acidosis, rhabdomyolysis, hyperkalaemia, and cardiac failure

Dose: *1% injection*

Induction of anaesthesia, *by intravenous injection or infusion*, 1.5–2.5 mg/kg (less in those over

55 years) at a rate of 20–40 mg every 10 seconds; CHILD over 1 month, administer slowly until response (usual dose in child over 8 years 2.5 mg/kg, may need more in younger child e.g. 2.5–4 mg/kg)
Maintenance of anaesthesia, *by intravenous injection*, 25–50 mg repeated according to response *or by intravenous infusion*, 4–12 mg/kg/hour; CHILD over 3 years, *by intravenous infusion*, 9–15 mg/kg/hour

NOTE. *Propofol-Lipuro*® may be used for maintenance of anaesthesia in CHILD over 1 month, *by intravenous infusion*, 9–15 mg/kg/hour

Sedation in intensive care, *by intravenous infusion*, ADULT over 17 years, 0.3–4 mg/kg/hour
Sedation for surgical and diagnostic procedures, initially *by intravenous injection* over 1–5 minutes, 0.5–1 mg/kg; maintenance, *by intravenous infusion*, 1.5–4.5 mg/kg/hour (additionally, if rapid increase in sedation required, *by intravenous injection*, 10–20 mg); those over 55 years may require lower dose; CHILD and ADOLESCENT under 17 years not recommended

2% injection
Induction of anaesthesia, *by intravenous infusion*, 1.5–2.5 mg/kg (less in those over 55 years) at a rate of 20–40 mg every 10 seconds; CHILD over 3 years, administer slowly until response (usual dose in child over 8 years 2.5 mg/kg, may need more in younger child e.g. 2.5–4 mg/kg)
Maintenance of anaesthesia, *by intravenous infusion*, 4–12 mg/kg/hour; CHILD over 3 years, *by intravenous infusion*, 9–15 mg/kg/hour
Sedation in intensive care, *by intravenous infusion*, ADULT over 17 years, 0.3–4 mg/kg/hour

Propofol (Non-proprietary) PoM
1% injection (emulsion), propofol 10 mg/mL, net price 20-mL amp = £2.33, 50-mL bottle = £5.82, 100-mL bottle = £11.64
2% injection (emulsion), propofol 20 mg/mL, net price 50-mL vial = £11.64
Brands include *Propofol-Lipuro*®

Diprivan® (AstraZeneca) PoM
1% injection (emulsion), propofol 10 mg/mL, net price 20-mL amp = £3.88, 50-mL vial = £9.70, 50-mL prefilled syringe (for use with *Diprifusor*® *TCI* system) = £10.67, 100-mL vial = £19.40
2% injection (emulsion), propofol 20 mg/mL, net price 50-mL vial = £19.40, 50-mL prefilled syringe (for use with *Diprifusor*® *TCI* system) = £20.37
NOTE. *Diprifusor*® *TCI* ('target controlled infusion') system is for use **only** for induction and maintenance of general anaesthesia in adults

15.1.2 Inhalational anaesthetics

Inhalational anaesthetics may be gases or volatile liquids. They can be used both for induction and maintenance of anaesthesia and may also be used following induction with an intravenous anaesthetic (section 15.1.1).

Gaseous anaesthetics require suitable equipment for storage and administration. They may be supplied via hospital pipelines or from metal cylinders. *Volatile liquid anaesthetics* are administered using calibrated vaporisers, using air, oxygen, or nitrous oxide–oxygen mixtures as the carrier gas. It should be noted that they can all trigger malignant hyperthermia (section 15.1.8).

To prevent hypoxia inhalational anaesthetics must be given with concentrations of oxygen greater than in air.

ANAESTHESIA AND DRIVING. See section 15.1.

Volatile liquid anaesthetics

Halothane is a volatile liquid anaesthetic. Its advantages are that it is potent, induction is smooth, the vapour is non-irritant, pleasant to inhale, and seldom induces coughing or breath-holding. Despite these advantages, however, halothane is much less widely used than previously owing to its association with *severe hepatotoxicity* (**important:** see CSM advice, below).

Halothane causes cardiorespiratory depression. Respiratory depression results in elevation of arterial carbon dioxide tension and perhaps ventricular arrhythmias. Halothane also depresses the cardiac muscle fibres and may cause bradycardia. The result is diminished cardiac output and fall of arterial pressure. Adrenaline (epinephrine) infiltrations should be avoided in patients anaesthetised with halothane as ventricular arrhythmias may result.

Halothane produces moderate muscle relaxation, but this may be inadequate for major abdominal surgery and specific muscle relaxants are then used.

CSM advice (halothane hepatotoxicity). In a publication on findings confirming that *severe hepatotoxicity* can follow halothane anaesthesia the CSM has reported that this occurs more frequently after repeated exposures to halothane and has a high mortality. The risk of severe hepatotoxicity appears to be increased by repeated exposures within a short time interval, but even after a long interval (sometimes of several years) susceptible patients have been reported to develop jaundice. Since there is no reliable way of identifying susceptible patients the CSM recommends the following precautions prior to use of halothane:

1. a careful anaesthetic history should be taken to determine previous exposure and previous reactions to halothane;
2. repeated exposure to halothane within a period of **at least** 3 months should be **avoided** unless there are **overriding** clinical circumstances;
3. a history of unexplained jaundice or pyrexia in a patient following exposure to halothane is an absolute **contra-indication** to its future use in that patient.

Isoflurane is a less potent anaesthetic than halothane. Heart rhythm is generally stable during isoflurane anaesthesia, but heart-rate may rise, particularly in younger patients. Systemic arterial pressure may fall, owing to a decrease in systemic vascular resistance and with less decrease in cardiac output than occurs with halothane. Respiration is depressed. Muscle relaxation is produced and muscle relaxant drugs potentiated. Isoflurane may also cause hepatotoxicity in those sensitised to halogenated anaesthetics but the risk is appreciably smaller than with halothane.

Desflurane is reported to have about one-fifth the potency of isoflurane. Owing to limited experience it is not recommended in neurosurgical patients. It is not recommended for induction in children because cough, breath-holding, apnoea, laryngospasm and increased secretions can occur. The risk of hepatotoxicity with desflurane in those sensitised to halogenated anaesthetics appears to be remote.

Sevoflurane is a rapid acting volatile liquid anaesthetic. Patients may require early postoperative pain relief as emergence and recovery are particularly rapid. Sevoflurane can interact with carbon dioxide absorbents to form compound A, a potentially nephrotoxic vinyl ether. However, in spite of extensive use, no cases of sevoflurane-induced permanent renal injury have been reported and the carbon dioxide absorbents used in the UK produce very low concentrations of compound A, even in low-flow anaesthetic systems.

DESFLURANE

Indications: see notes above

Cautions: see notes above; hepatic impairment (Appendix 2); renal impairment (Appendix 3); pregnancy (Appendix 4); **interactions:** Appendix 1 (anaesthetics, general)

Contra-indications: see notes above; susceptibility to malignant hyperthermia

Side-effects: see notes above

Dose: using a specifically calibrated vaporiser, *induction*, 4–11%; CHILD not recommended for induction

Maintenance, 2–6% in nitrous oxide; 2.5–8.5% in oxygen or oxygen-enriched air; max. 17%

Suprane® (Baxter) PoM
Desflurane, net price 240 mL = £44.41

HALOTHANE

Indications: see notes above

Cautions: see notes above (**important:** CSM advice, see notes above); avoid for dental procedures in those under 18 years unless treated in hospital (high risk of arrhythmia); avoid in porphyria (section 9.8.2); pregnancy (Appendix 4); breast-feeding (Appendix 5); **interactions:** Appendix 1 (anaesthetics, general)

Contra-indications: see notes above; susceptibility to malignant hyperthermia

Side-effects: see notes above

Dose: using a specifically calibrated vaporiser, *induction*, increased gradually to 2–4% in oxygen or nitrous oxide–oxygen; CHILD (see cautions) 1.5–2%

Maintenance, 0.5–2%

Halothane (Concord)
Halothane, net price 250 mL = £20.57

ISOFLURANE

Indications: see notes above

Cautions: see notes above; pregnancy (Appendix 4); **interactions:** Appendix 1 (anaesthetics, general)

Contra-indications: susceptibility to malignant hyperthermia

Side-effects: see notes above

Dose: using a specifically calibrated vaporiser, *induction*, increased gradually from 0.5% to 3%, in oxygen or nitrous oxide–oxygen

Maintenance, 1–2.5% in nitrous oxide–oxygen; an additional 0.5–1% may be required when given with oxygen alone; caesarean section, 0.5–0.75% in nitrous oxide–oxygen

Isoflurane (Abbott)
Isoflurane, net price 250 mL = £47.50

Aerrane® (Baxter)
Isoflurane, net price 100 mL = £7.98, 250 mL = £30.00

SEVOFLURANE

Indications: see notes above

Cautions: see notes above; renal impairment (Appendix 3); pregnancy (Appendix 4); **interactions:** Appendix 1 (anaesthetics, general)

Contra-indications: see notes above; susceptibility to malignant hyperthermia

Side-effects: see notes above; also agitation occurs frequently in children

Dose: using a specifically calibrated vaporiser, *induction*, up to 5% in oxygen or nitrous oxide–oxygen; CHILD up to 7%

Maintenance, 0.5–3%

Sevoflurane (Abbott) PoM
Sevoflurane, net price 250 mL = £123.00

Nitrous oxide

Nitrous oxide is used for maintenance of anaesthesia and, in sub-anaesthetic concentrations, for analgesia. For anaesthesia it is commonly used in a concentration of 50 to 70% in oxygen as part of a balanced technique in association with other inhalational or intravenous agents. Nitrous oxide is unsatisfactory as a sole anaesthetic owing to lack of potency, but is useful as part of a combination of drugs since it allows a significant reduction in dosage.

A mixture of nitrous oxide and oxygen containing 50% of each gas (*Entonox*®, *Equanox*®) is used to produce analgesia without loss of consciousness. Self-administration using a demand valve is popular in obstetric practice, for changing painful dressings, as an aid to postoperative physiotherapy, and in emergency ambulances.

Nitrous oxide may have a deleterious effect if used in patients with an air-containing closed space since nitrous oxide diffuses into such a space with a resulting increase in pressure. This effect may be dangerous in the presence of a pneumothorax which may enlarge to compromise respiration.

Special care is needed to avoid hypoxia if an anaesthetic machine is being used; machines should incorporate an anti-hypoxia device. Exposure of patients to nitrous oxide for prolonged periods, either by continuous or by intermittent administration, may result in megaloblastic anaemia owing to interference with the action of vitamin B_{12}. For the same reason, exposure of theatre staff to nitrous oxide should be minimised. Depression of white cell formation may also occur.

NITROUS OXIDE

Indications: see notes above

Cautions: see notes above; pregnancy (Appendix 4); **interactions:** Appendix 1 (anaesthetics, general)

Side-effects: see notes above

Dose: using suitable anaesthetic apparatus, *maintenance* of light anaesthesia, as a mixture with 25–30% oxygen

Analgesic, as a mixture with 50% oxygen, according to the patient's needs

15.1.3 Antimuscarinic drugs

Antimuscarinic drugs are used (less commonly nowadays) as premedicants to dry bronchial and salivary secretions which are increased by intubation, by surgery to the upper airways, and by some inhalational anaesthetics. They are also used before or with neostigmine (section 15.1.6) to prevent bradycardia, excessive salivation, and other muscarinic actions of neostigmine. They also prevent bradycardia and hypotension associated with drugs such as halothane, propofol, and suxamethonium.

Atropine is now rarely used for premedication but still has an emergency role in the treatment of vagotonic side-effects. For its role in acute arrhythmias after myocardial infarction, see section 2.3.1; see also cardiopulmonary resuscitation, section 2.7.3.

Hyoscine reduces secretions and also provides a degree of amnesia, sedation and anti-emesis. Unlike atropine it may produce bradycardia rather than tachycardia. In some patients, especially the elderly, hyoscine may cause the central anticholinergic syndrome (excitement, ataxia, hallucinations, behavioural abnormalities, and drowsiness).

Glycopyrronium reduces salivary secretions. When given intravenously it produces less tachycardia than atropine. It is widely used with neostigmine for reversal of non-depolarising muscle relaxants (section 15.1.5).

Phenothiazines do not effectively reduce secretions when used alone.

ATROPINE SULPHATE

Indications: drying secretions; reversal of excessive bradycardia; with neostigmine for reversal of non-depolarising neuromuscular block; antidote to organophosphorous poisoning (see Emergency Treatment of Poisoning p. 36), antispasmodic (section 1.2); bradycardia (section 2.3.1); cardiopulmonary resuscitation (section 2.7.3); eye (section 11.5)

Cautions: cardiovascular disease; see also section 1.2; **interactions:** Appendix 1 (antimuscarinics)

DURATION OF ACTION. Since atropine has a shorter duration of action than neostigmine, late unopposed bradycardia may result; close monitoring of the patient is necessary

Contra-indications: see section 1.2

Side-effects: see section 1.2

Dose: premedication, *by intravenous injection*, 300–600 micrograms immediately before induction of anaesthesia; CHILD 20 micrograms/kg (max. 600 micrograms)

By subcutaneous or *intramuscular injection*, 300–600 micrograms 30–60 minutes before induction; CHILD 20 micrograms/kg (max. 600 micrograms)

Intra-operative bradycardia, *by intravenous injection*, 300–600 micrograms (larger doses in emergencies); CHILD [unlicensed indication] 1–12 years 10–20 micrograms/kg

Control of muscarinic side-effects of neostigmine in reversal of competitive neuromuscular block, *by intravenous injection*, 0.6–1.2 mg; CHILD under 12 years (but rarely used) 20 micrograms/kg (max. 600 micrograms) with neostigmine 50 micrograms/kg

Arrhythmias after myocardial infarction, see section 2.3.1; see also cardiopulmonary resuscitation algorithm, inside back cover

[1]**Atropine** (Non-proprietary) PoM

Injection, atropine sulphate 600 micrograms/mL, net price 1-mL amp = 50p

NOTE. Other strengths also available

Injection, prefilled disposable syringe, atropine sulphate 100 micrograms/mL, net price 5 mL = £4.16, 10 mL = £4.66, 30 mL = £8.52

Brands include *Minijet® Atropine Sulphate*

Injection, prefilled disposable syringe, atropine sulphate 200 micrograms/mL, net price 5 mL = £4.67; 300 micrograms/mL, 10 mL = £4.67; 600 micrograms/mL, 1 mL = £4.67

1. PoM restriction does not apply where administration is for saving life in emergency

GLYCOPYRRONIUM BROMIDE

(Glycopyrrolate)

Indications: drying secretions; reversal of excessive bradycardia; with neostigmine for reversal of non-depolarising neuromuscular block; hyperhidrosis (section 13.12)

Cautions: cardiovascular disease; see also Atropine sulphate (section 1.2); **interactions:** Appendix 1 (antimuscarinics)

Side-effects: see under Atropine Sulphate

Dose: premedication, *by intramuscular or intravenous injection*, 200–400 micrograms, *or* 4–5 micrograms/kg to a max. of 400 micrograms; CHILD *by intramuscular or* preferably *by intravenous injection*, 4–8 micrograms/kg to a max. of 200 micrograms

Intra-operative use, *by intravenous injection*, as for premedication, repeated if necessary

Control of muscarinic side-effects of neostigmine in reversal of non-depolarising neuromuscular block, *by intravenous injection*, 200 micrograms per 1 mg of neostigmine, *or* 10–15 micrograms/kg with neostigmine 50 micrograms/kg; CHILD 10 micrograms/kg with neostigmine 50 micrograms/kg

Robinul® (Anpharm) PoM

Injection, glycopyrronium bromide 200 micrograms/mL, net price 1-mL amp = 60p; 3-mL amp = £1.01

Available as a generic from Antigen

■ With neostigmine metilsulphate

Section 15.1.6

HYOSCINE HYDROBROMIDE

(Scopolamine hydrobromide)

Indications: drying secretions, amnesia; other indications (section 4.6)

Cautions: see under Hyoscine Hydrobromide (section 4.6); also paralytic ileus, myasthenia gravis, epilepsy, prostatic enlargement; avoid in the elderly (see notes above)

Contra-indications: porphyria (section 9.8.2); angle-closure glaucoma

Side-effects: see under Atropine Sulphate; bradycardia

Dose: premedication, *by subcutaneous or intramuscular injection*, 200–600 micrograms 30–60 minutes before induction of anaesthesia; CHILD 15 micrograms/kg

Hyoscine (Non-proprietary) PoM
Injection, hyoscine hydrobromide 400 micrograms/mL, net price 1-mL amp = £2.71; 600 micrograms/mL, 1-mL amp = £2.81

■ With papaveretum
See under papaveretum (section 4.7.2)

15.1.4 Sedative and analgesic peri-operative drugs

These drugs are given to allay the apprehension of the patient in the pre-operative period (including the night before operation), to relieve pain and discomfort when present, and to augment the action of subsequent anaesthetic agents. A number of the drugs used also provide some degree of pre-operative amnesia. The choice will vary with the individual patient, the nature of the operative procedure, the anaesthetic to be used and other prevailing circumstances such as outpatients, obstetrics, recovery facilities etc. The choice would also vary in elective and emergency operations.

PREMEDICATION IN CHILDREN. Oral administration is preferred to injections where possible but is not altogether satisfactory; the rectal route should only be used in exceptional circumstances. Oral alimemazine (trimeprazine, section 3.4.1) is still used but when given alone it may cause postoperative restlessness when pain is present.

Atropine or hyoscine is often given orally to children, but may be given intravenously immediately before induction.

The use of a suitable local anaesthetic cream (section 15.2) should be considered to avoid pain at injection site.

ANAESTHESIA AND DRIVING. See section 15.1.

15.1.4.1 Anxiolytics and neuroleptics

Anxiolytic benzodiazepines are widely used whereas neuroleptics such as **chlorpromazine** (section 4.2.1) are rarely used in the UK for premedication although chlorpromazine was used to prevent shivering in induction of hypothermia. **Alimemazine (trimeprazine)** (section 3.4.1) is still occasionally used as a premedicant for children (but see section 15.1.4).

Benzodiazepines

Benzodiazepines possess useful properties for premedication including relief of anxiety, sedation, and amnesia; short-acting benzodiazepines taken by mouth are the most common premedicants. They have no analgesic effect so an opioid analgesic may sometimes be required for pain.

Benzodiazepines can alleviate anxiety at doses that do not necessarily cause excessive sedation and they are of particular value during short procedures or during operations under local anaesthesia (including dentistry). Amnesia reduces the likelihood of any unpleasant memories of the procedure (although benzodiazepines, particularly when used for more profound sedation, can sometimes induce sexual fantasies). Benzodiazepines are also used in intensive care units for sedation, particularly in those receiving assisted ventilation.

Benzodiazepines may occasionally cause marked respiratory depression and facilities for its treatment are essential; flumazenil (section 15.1.7) is used to antagonise the effects of benzodiazepines. They are best avoided in myasthenia gravis, especially peri-operatively.

Diazepam is used to produce mild sedation with amnesia. It is a long-acting drug with active metabolites and a second period of drowsiness can occur several hours after its administration. Peri-operative use of diazepam in children is not generally recommended; its effect and timing of response are unreliable and paradoxical effects may occur.

Diazepam is relatively insoluble in water and preparations formulated in organic solvents are painful on intravenous injection and give rise to a high incidence of venous thrombosis (which may not be noticed for several days after the injection). Intramuscular injection of diazepam is painful and absorption is erratic. An emulsion preparation for intravenous injection is less irritant and is followed by a negligible incidence of venous thrombosis; it is not suitable for intramuscular injection. Diazepam is also available as a rectal solution.

Temazepam is given by mouth and has a shorter duration of action and a more rapid onset than diazepam given by mouth. It has been used as a premedicant in inpatient and day-case surgery; anxiolytic and sedative effects last about 90 minutes although there may be residual drowsiness.

Lorazepam produces more prolonged sedation than temazepam and it has marked amnesic effects. It is used as a premedicant the night before major surgery; a further, smaller dose may be required the following morning if any delay in starting surgery is anticipated. Alternatively the first dose may be given early in the morning on the day of operation.

Midazolam is a water-soluble benzodiazepine which is often used in preference to intravenous diazepam; recovery is faster than from diazepam. Midazolam is associated with profound sedation when high doses are given intravenously or when used with certain other drugs.

DENTAL PROCEDURES. Anxiolytics diminish feelings of tension, anxiety and panic, and may benefit anxious patients. However, their use is no substitute for sympathy and reassurance.

Diazepam and temazepam are effective anxiolytics for dental treatment in adults, but they are less suitable for children. Diazepam has a longer duration of action than temazepam. When given at night diazepam is associated with more residual effects the following day; patients should be very carefully warned **not** to drive (**important**: for general advice on anaesthesia and driving see p. 626). For further information on hypnotics and anxiolytics, see section 4.1. For further information on hypnotics used for dental procedures, see section 4.1.1.

DIAZEPAM

Indications: premedication; sedation with amnesia, and in conjunction with local anaesthesia; other indications (section 4.1.2, section 4.8.2, and section 10.2.2)

Cautions: see notes above and section 4.1.2 and section 4.8.2

Contra-indications: see notes above and section 4.1.2

Side-effects: see notes above and section 4.1.2

Dose: *by mouth*, 5 mg on night before minor or dental surgery then 5 mg 2 hours before procedure; ELDERLY (or debilitated), half adult dose

By intravenous injection, into a large vein 10–20 mg over 2–4 minutes as sedative cover for minor surgical and medical procedures; premedication 100–200 micrograms/kg

By rectum in solution, 10 mg; ELDERLY 5 mg; CHILD not recommended (see notes above)

NOTE. Diazepam rectal solution doses in the BNF may differ from those in the product literature

■ Preparations
Section 4.1.2

LORAZEPAM

Indications: sedation with amnesia; premedication; other indications (section 4.1.2 and section 4.8.2)

Cautions: see notes above and section 4.1.2; **interactions:** Appendix 1 (anxiolytics and hypnotics)

Contra-indications: see notes above and under Diazepam (section 4.1.2)

Side-effects: see notes above and under Diazepam (section 4.1.2)

Dose: *by mouth*, 2–3 mg the night before operation; 2–4 mg 1–2 hours before operation

By slow intravenous injection, preferably diluted with an equal volume of sodium chloride intravenous infusion 0.9% or water for injections, 50 micrograms/kg 30–45 minutes before operation

By intramuscular injection, diluted as above, 50 micrograms/kg 60–90 minutes before operation

■ Preparations
Section 4.1.2

MIDAZOLAM

Indications: sedation with amnesia; sedation in intensive care; premedication, induction of anaesthesia; status epilepticus [unlicensed use], section 4.8.2

Cautions: hepatic impairment (Appendix 2); renal impairment (Appendix 3); pregnancy (Appendix 4) and breastfeeding (Appendix 5); cardiac disease; respiratory disease; children (particularly if cardiovascular impairment); history of drug or alcohol abuse; reduce dose in elderly and debilitated; avoid prolonged use (and abrupt withdrawal thereafter); concentration of midazolam in children under 15 kg not to exceed 1 mg/mL; **interactions:** Appendix 1 (anxiolytics and hypnotics)

Contra-indications: myasthenia gravis; severe respiratory depression; acute pulmonary insufficiency

Side-effects: gastro-intestinal disturbances, increased appetite, jaundice; hypotension, cardiac arrest, heart rate changes, anaphylaxis, thrombosis; laryngospasm, bronchospasm, respiratory depression and respiratory arrest (particularly with high doses or on rapid injection); drowsiness, confusion, ataxia, amnesia, headache, euphoria, hallucinations, fatigue, dizziness, vertigo, involuntary movements, paradoxical excitement and aggression (especially in children and elderly), dysarthria; urinary retention, incontinence, changes in libido; blood disorders; muscle weakness; visual disturbances; salivation changes; skin reactions; on intravenous injection, pain, thrombophlebitis

Dose: conscious sedation, *by slow intravenous injection* (approx. 2 mg/minute), initially 2–2.5 mg (ELDERLY 0.5–1 mg), increased if necessary in steps of 1 mg (ELDERLY 0.5–1 mg); usual range 3.5–7.5 mg, ELDERLY max. 3.5 mg; CHILD *by intravenous injection* over 2–3 minutes, 6 months–5 years initially 50–100 micrograms/kg, dose increased if necessary in small steps (max. total dose 6 mg), 6–12 years initially 25–50 micrograms/kg, dose increased if necessary in small steps (max. total dose 10 mg)

By intramuscular injection, CHILD 1–15 years 50–150 micrograms/kg; max. 10 mg

By rectum (see note below), CHILD over 6 months 300–500 micrograms/kg

Sedative in combined anaesthesia, *by intravenous injection*, 30–100 micrograms/kg repeated as required or *by intravenous infusion*, 30–100 micrograms/kg/hour (ELDERLY lower doses needed); CHILD not recommended

Premedication, *by deep intramuscular injection*, 70–100 micrograms/kg (ELDERLY 25–50 micrograms/kg) 20–60 minutes before induction, usual dose 2–3 mg; CHILD 1–15 years 80–200 micrograms/kg

By rectum, CHILD over 6 months 300–500 micrograms/kg 15–30 minutes before induction

Induction, *by slow intravenous injection*, with premedication, 150–200 micrograms/kg (ELDERLY 100–200 micrograms/kg); without premedication, 300–350 micrograms/kg (ELDERLY 150–300 micrograms/kg); doses increased in steps not greater than 5 mg every 2 minutes; max. 600 micrograms/kg; CHILD over 7 years 150 micrograms/kg

Sedation of patients receiving intensive care, *by slow intravenous injection*, initially 30–300 micrograms/kg given in steps of 1–2.5 mg every 2 minutes, then *by slow intravenous injection or by intravenous infusion*, 30–200 micrograms/kg/hour; reduce dose (or omit initial dose) in hypovolaemia, vasoconstriction, or hypothermia; lower doses may be adequate if opioid analgesic also used; NEONATE under 32 weeks gestational age *by intravenous infusion*, 30 micrograms/kg/hour, NEONATE over 32 weeks gestational age and CHILD under 6 months 60 micrograms/kg/hour, over 6 months *by slow intravenous injection*, initially 50–200 micrograms/kg, then *by intravenous infusion*, 60–120 micrograms/kg/hour

NOTE. For rectal administration of the injection solution, attach a plastic applicator onto the end of a syringe; if the volume to be given rectally is too small, water for injection may be added to give a total volume of 10 mL

Midazolam (Non-proprietary) PoM

Injection, midazolam (as hydrochloride) 1 mg/mL, net price 50-mL vial = £6.30; 5 mg/mL, 2-mL amp = 79p, 5-mL amp = 91p, 10-mL amp = £4.70, 18-mL amp = £6.80

Hypnovel® (Roche) PoM
Injection, midazolam (as hydrochloride) 2 mg/mL, net price 5-mL amp = 75p; 5 mg/mL, 2-mL amp = 90p

TEMAZEPAM

Indications: premedication before surgery; anxiety before investigatory procedures; hypnotic (section 4.1.1)
Cautions: see notes above and under Diazepam (section 4.1.2 and section 4.8.2); **interactions:** Appendix 1 (anxiolytics and hypnotics)
Contra-indications: see notes above and under Diazepam (section 4.1.2)
Side-effects: see notes above and under Diazepam (section 4.1.2)
Dose: *by mouth*, premedication, 20–40 mg (elderly, 10–20 mg) 1 hour before operation; CHILD 1 mg/kg (max. 30 mg)

■ Preparations
Section 4.1.1

15.1.4.2 Non-opioid analgesics

Since non-steroidal anti-inflammatory drugs (NSAIDs) do not depress respiration, do not impair gastro-intestinal motility, and do not cause dependence, they may be useful alternatives (or adjuncts) to the use of opioids for the relief of postoperative pain. NSAIDs may be inadequate for the relief of severe pain.

Acemetacin, **diclofenac**, **flurbiprofen**, **ibuprofen**, **ketoprofen**, (section 10.1.1), **parecoxib**, and **ketorolac** are licensed for postoperative use. Diclofenac, ketoprofen, and ketorolac can be given by injection as well as by mouth. Intramuscular injections of diclofenac and ketoprofen are given deep into the gluteal muscle to minimise pain and tissue damage; diclofenac can also be given by intravenous infusion for the treatment or prevention of postoperative pain. Ketorolac is less irritant on intramuscular injection but pain has been reported; it can also be given by intravenous injection. Parecoxib (a selective inhibitor of cyclo-oxygenase-2) can be given by intramuscular or intravenous injection (but see also Cyclo-oxygenase-2 inhibitors and Cardiovascular Events, section 10.1.1).

The *Scottish Medicines Consortium* has advised (January 2003) that parecoxib should **not** be used because there is no evidence of a reduction in postoperative haemorrhagic or gastro-intestinal complications compared with non-selective NSAIDs.

Suppositories of diclofenac and ketoprofen may be effective alternatives to the parenteral use of these drugs. Flurbiprofen is also available as suppositories.

KETOROLAC TROMETAMOL

Indications: short-term management of moderate to severe acute postoperative pain **only**
Cautions: see section 10.1.1; avoid in porphyria (section 9.8.2); **interactions:** Appendix 1 (NSAIDs)
Contra-indications: see section 10.1.1; also history of asthma, complete or partial syndrome of nasal polyps, angioedema or bronchospasm; history of peptic ulceration or gastro-intestinal bleeding; haemorrhagic diatheses (including coagulation disorders) and following operations with high risk of haemorrhage or incomplete haemostasis; confirmed or suspected cerebrovascular bleeding; moderate or severe renal impairment; hypovolaemia or dehydration; pregnancy (including labour and delivery); breast-feeding
Side-effects: see section 10.1.1; also anaphylaxis, dry mouth, excessive thirst, psychotic reactions, convulsions, myalgia, hyponatraemia, hyperkalaemia, flushing or pallor, bradycardia, hypertension, palpitations, chest pain, purpura, postoperative wound haemorrhage, haematoma, epistaxis; pain at injection site
Dose: *by mouth*, 10 mg every 4–6 hours (ELDERLY every 6–8 hours); max. 40 mg daily; max. duration of treatment 7 days; CHILD under 16 years, not recommended

By intramuscular injection or by intravenous injection over not less than 15 seconds, initially 10 mg, then 10–30 mg every 4–6 hours when required (every 2 hours in initial postoperative period); max. 90 mg daily (ELDERLY and patients weighing less than 50 kg max. 60 mg daily); max. duration of treatment 2 days by either route; CHILD under 16 years, not recommended

NOTE. Pain relief may not occur for over 30 minutes after intravenous or intramuscular injection. When converting from parenteral to oral administration, total combined dose on the day of converting should not exceed 90 mg (60 mg in the elderly and patients weighing less than 50 kg) of which the oral component should not exceed 40 mg; patients should be converted to oral route as soon as possible

Toradol® (Roche) PoM
Tablets, ivory, f/c, ketorolac trometamol 10 mg, net price 20-tab pack = £5.79. Label: 17, 21
Injection, ketorolac trometamol 10 mg/mL, net price 1-mL amp = 94p; 30 mg/mL, 1-mL amp = £1.14

PARECOXIB

NOTE. Parecoxib is a pro-drug of valdecoxib

Indications: short-term management of acute postoperative pain
Cautions: see section 10.1.1; dehydration; following coronary artery bypass graft surgery; **interactions:** Appendix 1 (NSAIDs)
Contra-indications: see section 10.1.1; sulphonamide hypersensitivity, inflammatory bowel disease; severe congestive heart failure
Side-effects: see section 10.1.1; also flatulence; hypertension, hypotension, peripheral oedema; pharyngitis, respiratory insufficiency; hypoaesthesia; alveolar osteitis; oliguria; postoperative anaemia, hypokalaemia; back pain; pruritus; *less commonly* bradycardia, cerebrovascular disorders, increased blood urea nitrogen, ecchymosis, thrombocytopenia, rash (discontinue—risk of serious reactions including Stevens-Johnson syndrome and toxic epidermal necrolysis)
Dose: *by deep intramuscular injection or by intravenous injection*, initially 40 mg, then 20–40 mg every 6–12 hours when required; max. 80 mg daily; ELDERLY weighing less than 50 kg, initially 20 mg, then max. 40 mg daily; CHILD and ADOLESCENT under 18 years, not recommended

Dynastat® (Pharmacia) ▼ PoM
Injection, powder for reconstitution, parecoxib (as sodium salt), net price 40-mg vial = £4.96, 40-mg vial (with solvent) = £5.67

15.1.4.3 Opioid analgesics

Opioid analgesics are now rarely used as premedicants; they are more likely to be administered at induction. Pre-operative use of opioid analgesics is generally limited to those patients who require control of existing pain. The main side-effects of opioid analgesics are respiratory depression, cardiovascular depression, nausea, and vomiting; for general notes on opioid analgesics and their use in postoperative pain, see section 4.7.2.

For the management of opioid-induced respiratory depression, see section 15.1.7.

INTRA-OPERATIVE ANALGESIA. Opioid analgesics given in small doses before or with induction reduce the dose requirement of some drugs used during anaesthesia. Pethidine, morphine and papaveretum have been used for this purpose, but shorter-acting and more potent drugs such as alfentanil, fentanyl, and remifentanil are now preferred.

Alfentanil, **fentanyl** and **remifentanil** are particularly useful because they act within 1–2 minutes. The initial doses of alfentanil or fentanyl are followed either by successive intravenous injections or by an intravenous infusion; prolonged infusions increase the duration of effect. Repeated intra-operative doses of alfentanil or fentanyl should be given with care since the respiratory depression can persist into the postoperative period and occasionally it may become apparent for the first time postoperatively when monitoring of the patient might be less intensive.

In contrast to other opioids which are metabolised in the liver, remifentanil undergoes rapid metabolism by non-specific blood and tissue esterases; its short duration of action allows prolonged administration at high dosage, without accumulation, and with little risk of residual postoperative respiratory depression. Remifentanil should not be given as a bolus injection intra-operatively, but it is well suited to continuous infusion; a supplemental analgesic will often be required after stopping the infusion.

ALFENTANIL

Indications: analgesia especially during short operative procedure and outpatient surgery; enhancement of anaesthesia; analgesia and suppression of respiratory activity in patients receiving intensive care, with assisted ventilation, for up to 4 days

Cautions: see under Morphine Salts (section 4.7.2) and notes above

Contra-indications: see section 4.7.2 and notes above

Side-effects: see section 4.7.2 and notes above; also hypertension, myoclonic movements; *less commonly* arrhythmias, cough, hiccup, laryngospasm, visual disturbances

Dose:

> To avoid excessive dosage in obese patients, dose may need to be calculated on the basis of ideal body-weight

By intravenous injection, spontaneous respiration, ADULT, initially up to 500 micrograms over 30 seconds; supplemental, 250 micrograms

With assisted ventilation, ADULT and CHILD, initially 30–50 micrograms/kg; supplemental, 15 micrograms/kg

By intravenous infusion, with assisted ventilation, ADULT and CHILD, initially 50–100 micrograms/kg over 10 minutes *or* as a bolus, followed by maintenance of 0.5–1 micrograms/kg/minute

Analgesia and suppression of respiratory activity during intensive care, with assisted ventilation, *by intravenous infusion*, initially 2 mg/hour subsequently adjusted according to response (usual range 0.5–10 mg/hour); more rapid initial control may be obtained with an intravenous dose of 5 mg given in divided portions over 10 minutes (slowing if hypotension or bradycardia occur); additional doses of 0.5–1 mg may be given by intravenous injection during short painful procedures

Rapifen® (Janssen-Cilag) CD

Injection, alfentanil (as hydrochloride) 500 micrograms/mL. Net price 2-mL amp = 69p; 10-mL amp = £3.14

Intensive care injection, alfentanil (as hydrochloride) 5 mg/mL. To be diluted before use. Net price 1-mL amp = £2.52

FENTANYL

Indications: analgesia during operation, enhancement of anaesthesia; respiratory depressant in assisted respiration; analgesia in other situations (section 4.7.2)

Cautions: see under Morphine Salts (section 4.7.2) and notes above

Contra-indications: see section 4.7.2 and notes above

Side-effects: see section 4.7.2 and notes above

Dose: *By intravenous injection*, with spontaneous respiration, 50–200 micrograms, then 50 micrograms as required; CHILD 3–5 micrograms/kg, then 1 microgram/kg as required

With assisted ventilation, 0.3–3.5 mg, then 100–200 micrograms as required; CHILD 15 micrograms/kg, then 1–3 micrograms/kg as required

By intravenous infusion, with spontaneous respiration, ADULT and CHILD, 50–80 nanograms/kg/minute adjusted according to response

With assisted ventilation, ADULT and CHILD, initially 10 micrograms/kg over 10 minutes then 100 nanograms/kg/minute; up to 3 micrograms/kg/minute may be required in cardiac surgery

Fentanyl (Non-proprietary) CD

Injection, fentanyl (as citrate) 50 micrograms/mL, net price 2-mL amp = 54p, 10-mL amp = £1.65

Sublimaze® (Janssen-Cilag) CD

Injection, fentanyl (as citrate) 50 micrograms/mL, net price 2-mL amp = 23p, 10-mL amp = £1.11

REMIFENTANIL

Indications: supplementation of general anaesthesia during induction and analgesia during maintenance of anaesthesia (consult product literature for use in patients undergoing cardiac surgery); analgesia and sedation in ventilated, intensive care patients

Cautions: see under Morphine Salts (section 4.7.2) and notes above

Contra-indications: see section 4.7.2 and notes above

Side-effects: see section 4.7.2 and notes above

Dose:

> To avoid excessive dosage in obese patients, dose should be calculated on the basis of ideal body-weight

Induction, *by intravenous infusion*, 0.5–1 micrograms/kg/minute, *with or without* an initial bolus *by intravenous injection* (of a solution containing 20–250 micrograms/mL) over not less than 30 seconds, 1 microgram/kg
NOTE. If patient is to be intubated more than 8 minutes after start of intravenous infusion, initial intravenous injection dose is unnecessary
Maintenance in ventilated patients, *by intravenous infusion*, 0.05–2 micrograms/kg/minute according to anaesthetic technique and adjusted according to response; supplemental doses in light anaesthesia, *by intravenous injection* every 2–5 minutes
Maintenance in spontaneous respiration anaesthesia, *by intravenous infusion*, initially 40 nanograms/kg/minute adjusted according to response, usual range 25–100 nanograms/kg/minute
CHILD 1–12 years, maintenance, *by intravenous infusion*, 0.05–1.3 micrograms/kg/minute (*with or without* an initial bolus *by intravenous injection* over not less than 30 seconds, 1 microgram/kg/minute) according to anaesthetic technique and adjusted according to response
Analgesia and sedation in ventilated, intensive care patients, *by intravenous infusion*, ADULT over 18 years initially 100–150 nanograms/kg/minute adjusted according to response, usual range 6–740 nanograms/kg/minute; if an infusion rate of 200 nanograms/kg/minute does not produce adequate sedation add another sedative (consult product literature for details); additional analgesia during stimulating or painful procedures, *by intravenous infusion*, ADULT over 18 years maintain infusion of at least 100 nanograms/kg/minute for at least 5 minutes before procedure and adjust every 2–5 minutes according to requirements, usual range 250–750 nanograms/kg/minute

Ultiva® (GSK) CD
Injection, powder for reconstitution, remifentanil (as hydrochloride), net price 1-mg vial = £5.50; 2-mg vial = £11.00; 5-mg vial = £27.50

15.1.5 Muscle relaxants

Muscle relaxants used in anaesthesia are also known as **neuromuscular blocking drugs**. By specific blockade of the neuromuscular junction they enable light levels of anaesthesia to be employed with adequate relaxation of the muscles of the abdomen and diaphragm. They also relax the vocal cords and allow the passage of a tracheal tube. Their action differs from the muscle relaxants acting on the spinal cord or brain which are used in musculoskeletal disorders (section 10.2.2).

Patients who have received a muscle relaxant should **always** have their respiration assisted or controlled until the drug has been inactivated or antagonised (section 15.1.6).

Non-depolarising muscle relaxants

Non-depolarising muscle relaxants (also known as competitive muscle relaxants) compete with acetylcholine for receptor sites at the neuromuscular junction and their action may be reversed with anticholinesterases such as neostigmine (section 15.1.6). Non-depolarising muscle relaxants may be divided into the **aminosteroid** group which includes pancuronium, rocuronium and vecuronium, and the **benzylisoquinolinium** group which includes atracurium, cisatracurium, gallamine and mivacurium.

Non-depolarising muscle relaxants have a slower onset of action than suxamethonium. These drugs can be classified by their duration of action as short-acting (15–30 minutes), intermediate-acting (30–40 minutes) and long-acting (60–120 minutes), although duration of action is dose-dependent. Drugs with a shorter or intermediate duration of action, such as atracurium and vecuronium, are more widely employed than those with a longer duration of action such as pancuronium.

Non-depolarising muscle relaxants have no sedative or analgesic effects and are not considered to be a triggering factor for malignant hyperthermia.

For patients receiving intensive care and who require tracheal intubation and mechanical ventilation, a non-depolarising muscle relaxant is chosen according to its onset of effect, duration of action and side-effects. Rocuronium, with a rapid onset of effect, may facilitate intubation. Atracurium or cisatracurium may be suitable for long-term muscle relaxation since their duration of action is not dependent on elimination by the liver or the kidneys.

CAUTIONS. Allergic cross-reactivity between neuromuscular blocking agents has been reported; caution is advised in cases of hypersensitivity to these drugs. Their activity is prolonged in patients with myasthenia gravis and in hypothermia, therefore lower doses are required. Resistance may develop in patients with burns who may require increased doses; low plasma cholinesterase activity in these patients requires dose titration for mivacurium. **Interactions:** Appendix 1 (muscle relaxants).

SIDE-EFFECTS. Benzylisoquinolinium non-depolarising muscle relaxants (except cisatracurium) are associated with histamine release which can cause skin flushing, hypotension, tachycardia, bronchospasm and rarely, anaphylactoid reactions. Most aminosteroid muscle relaxants produce minimal histamine release. Drugs possessing vagolytic activity can counteract any bradycardia that occurs during surgery.

Atracurium is a mixture of 10 isomers and is a benzylisoquinolinium muscle relaxant with an intermediate duration of action. It undergoes non-enzymatic metabolism which is independent of liver and kidney function, thus allowing its use in patients with hepatic or renal impairment. Cardiovascular effects are associated with significant histamine release.

Cisatracurium is a single isomer of atracurium. It is more potent and has a slightly longer duration of action than atracurium and provides greater cardiovascular stability because cisatracurium lacks histamine-releasing effects.

Mivacurium, a benzylisoquinolinium muscle relaxant, has a short duration of action. It is metabolised by plasma cholinesterase and muscle paralysis is prolonged in individuals deficient in this enzyme. It is not associated with vagolytic activity or ganglionic blockade although histamine release may occur, particularly with rapid injection.

Pancuronium, an aminosteroid muscle relaxant, has a long duration of action and is often used in patients receiving long-term mechanical ventilation in intensive care units. It lacks a histamine-releasing effect, but vagolytic and sympathomimetic effects can cause tachycardia and hypertension.

Rocuronium exerts an effect within 2 minutes and has the most rapid onset of any of the competitive muscle relaxants. It is an aminosteroid muscle relaxant with an intermediate duration of action. It is reported to have minimal cardiovascular effects; high doses produce mild vagolytic activity.

Vecuronium, an aminosteroid muscle relaxant, has an intermediate duration of action. It does not generally produce histamine release and lacks cardiovascular effects.

Gallamine has vagolytic and sympathomimetic properties and frequently increases pulse rate and blood pressure. It is rarely used since the other neuromuscular blocking drugs have a more predictable response and it should be avoided in patients with renal impairment.

ATRACURIUM BESILATE

(Atracurium besylate)

Indications: muscle relaxation (short to intermediate duration) for surgery or during intensive care

Cautions: see notes above; pregnancy (Appendix 4); breast-feeding (Appendix 5)

Side-effects: see notes above

Dose: surgery or intubation, ADULT and CHILD over 1 month, *by intravenous injection*, initially 300–600 micrograms/kg; maintenance, *by intravenous injection*, 100–200 micrograms/kg as required *or by intravenous infusion*, 5–10 micrograms/kg/minute (300–600 micrograms/kg/hour)

Intensive care, ADULT and CHILD over 1 month, *by intravenous injection*, initially 300–600 micrograms/kg (optional) then *by intravenous infusion* 4.5–29.5 micrograms/kg/minute (usual dose 11–13 micrograms/kg/minute)

Atracurium (Non-proprietary) PoM

Injection, atracurium besilate 10 mg/mL, net price 2.5-mL amp = £1.85; 5-mL amp = £3.37; 25-mL amp = £14.45

Tracrium® (GSK) PoM

Injection, atracurium besilate 10 mg/mL, net price 2.5-mL amp = £1.66; 5-mL amp = £3.00; 25-mL amp = £12.91

CISATRACURIUM

Indications: muscle relaxation (intermediate duration) for surgery or during intensive care

Cautions: see notes above; pregnancy (Appendix 4)

Side-effects: see notes above

Dose: intubation, *by intravenous injection*, ADULT and CHILD over 1 month, initially 150 micrograms/kg; maintenance, *by intravenous injection*, 30 micrograms/kg approx. every 20 minutes; CHILD 2–12 years, 20 micrograms/kg approx. every 9 minutes; or maintenance, *by intravenous infusion*, ADULT and CHILD over 2 years, initially, 3 micrograms/kg/minute, *then after stabilisation*, 1–2 micrograms/kg/minute; dose reduced by up to 40% if used with isoflurane

Intensive care, *by intravenous infusion*, ADULT 0.5–10.2 micrograms/kg/minute (usual dose 3 micrograms/kg/minute)

NOTE. Lower doses can be used for children over 2 years when *not* for intubation

Nimbex® (GSK) PoM

Injection, cisatracurium (as besilate) 2 mg/mL, net price 2.5-mL amp = £2.04, 5-mL amp = £3.91, 10-mL amp = £7.55

Forte injection, cisatracurium (as besilate) 5 mg/mL, net price 30-mL vial = £31.09

GALLAMINE TRIETHIODIDE

Indications: muscle relaxation (intermediate duration) for surgery

Cautions: see notes above

Contra-indications: renal impairment (Appendix 3)

Side-effects: see notes above

Dose: *by intravenous injection*, 80–120 mg, then 20–40 mg as required; NEONATE 600 micrograms/kg; CHILD 1.5 mg/kg

Gallamine (Concord) PoM

Injection, gallamine triethiodide 40 mg/mL, net price 2-mL amp = £4.97

MIVACURIUM

Indications: muscle relaxation (short duration) for surgery

Cautions: see notes above; low plasma cholinesterase activity; elderly; hepatic impairment (Appendix 2); renal impairment (Appendix 3); pregnancy (Appendix 4)

Side-effects: see notes above

Dose:

> To avoid excessive dosage in obese patients, dose should be calculated on the basis of ideal body-weight

By intravenous injection, 70–250 micrograms/kg; maintenance 100 micrograms/kg every 15 minutes; CHILD 2–6 months initially 150 micrograms/kg, 7 months–12 years initially 200 micrograms/kg; maintenance (CHILD 2 months–12 years) 100 micrograms/kg every 6–9 minutes

NOTE. Doses up to 150 micrograms/kg may be given over 5–15 seconds, higher doses should be given over 30 seconds. In patients with asthma, cardiovascular disease or those who are sensitive to falls in arterial blood pressure give over 60 seconds

By intravenous infusion, maintenance of block, 8–10 micrograms/kg/minute, adjusted if necessary every 3 minutes by 1 microgram/kg/minute to usual dose of 6–7 micrograms/kg/minute; CHILD 2 months–12 years, usual dose 11–14 micrograms/kg/minute

Mivacron® (GSK) PoM

Injection, mivacurium (as chloride) 2 mg/mL, net price 5-mL amp = £2.79; 10-mL amp = £4.51

PANCURONIUM BROMIDE

Indications: muscle relaxation (long duration) for surgery or during intensive care

Cautions: see notes above; hepatic impairment (Appendix 2); renal impairment (Appendix 3); pregnancy (Appendix 4) and breast-feeding (Appendix 5)

Side-effects: see notes above

Dose:

> To avoid excessive dosage in obese patients, dose should be calculated on the basis of ideal body-weight

By intravenous injection, initially for intubation 50–100 micrograms/kg then 10–20 micrograms/kg as required; CHILD initially 60–100 micrograms/kg, then 10–20 micrograms/kg, NEONATE 30–40 micrograms/kg initially then 10–20 micrograms/kg

Intensive care, *by intravenous injection*, 60 micrograms/kg every 60–90 minutes

Pancuronium (Non-proprietary) PoM
Injection, pancuronium bromide 2 mg/mL, net price 2-mL amp = 65p

ROCURONIUM BROMIDE

Indications: muscle relaxation (intermediate duration) for surgery or during intensive care
Cautions: see notes above; hepatic impairment (Appendix 2); renal impairment (Appendix 3); pregnancy (Appendix 4) and breast-feeding (Appendix 5)
Side-effects: see notes above
Dose:

> To avoid excessive dosage in obese patients, dose should be calculated on the basis of ideal body-weight

Intubation, ADULT and CHILD over 1 month, *by intravenous injection*, initially 600 micrograms/kg; maintenance *by intravenous injection*, 150 micrograms/kg (ELDERLY 75–100 micrograms/kg) *or* maintenance *by intravenous infusion*, 300–600 micrograms/kg/hour (ELDERLY up to 400 micrograms/kg/hour)
Intensive care, *by intravenous injection*, ADULT initially 600 micrograms/kg; maintenance *by intravenous infusion*, 300–600 micrograms/kg/hour for first hour, then adjusted according to response

Esmeron® (Organon) PoM
Injection, rocuronium bromide 10 mg/mL, net price 5-mL vial = £3.01, 10-mL vial = £6.01

VECURONIUM BROMIDE

Indications: muscle relaxation (intermediate duration) for surgery
Cautions: see notes above; pregnancy (Appendix 4)
Side-effects: see notes above
Dose:

> To avoid excessive dosage in obese patients, dose should be calculated on the basis of ideal body-weight

By intravenous injection, intubation, 80–100 micrograms/kg; maintenance 20–30 micrograms/kg according to response; NEONATE and INFANT up to 4 months, initially 10–20 micrograms/kg then incremental doses to achieve response; CHILD over 5 months, as adult dose (up to 1 year onset more rapid and high intubation dose may not be required)
By intravenous infusion, 0.8–1.4 micrograms/kg/minute (after initial intravenous injection of 40–100 micrograms/kg)

Norcuron® (Organon) PoM
Injection, powder for reconstitution, vecuronium bromide, net price 10-mg vial = £3.95 (with water for injections)

Depolarising muscle relaxants

Suxamethonium has the most rapid onset of action of any of the muscle relaxants and is ideal if fast onset and brief duration of action are required e.g. with tracheal intubation. Its duration of action is about 2 to 6 minutes following intravenous doses of about 1 mg/kg; repeated doses can be used for longer procedures.

Suxamethonium acts by mimicking acetylcholine at the neuromuscular junction but hydrolysis is much slower than for acetylcholine; depolarisation is therefore prolonged, resulting in neuromuscular blockade. Unlike the non-depolarising muscle relaxants, its action cannot be reversed and recovery is spontaneous; anticholinesterases such as neostigmine potentiate the neuromuscular block.

Suxamethonium should be given after anaesthetic induction because paralysis is usually preceded by painful muscle fasciculations. While tachycardia occurs with single use, bradycardia may occur with repeated doses in adults and with the first dose in children. Premedication with atropine reduces bradycardia as well as the excessive salivation associated with suxamethonium use.

Prolonged paralysis may occur in **dual block**, which occurs with high or repeated doses of suxamethonium and is caused by the development of a non-depolarising block following the initial depolarising block; edrophonium (section 15.1.6) may be used to confirm the diagnosis of dual block. Individuals with myasthenia gravis are resistant to suxamethonium but can develop dual block resulting in delayed recovery. Prolonged paralysis may also occur in those with low or atypical plasma cholinesterase. Assisted ventilation should be continued until muscle function is restored.

SUXAMETHONIUM CHLORIDE

Indications: muscle relaxation (rapid onset, short duration)

Cautions: see notes above; pregnancy (Appendix 4); patients with cardiac, respiratory or neuromuscular disease; raised intra-ocular pressure (avoid in penetrating eye injury); severe sepsis (risk of hyperkalaemia); **interactions:** Appendix 1 (muscle relaxants)

Contra-indications: family history of malignant hyperthermia, low plasma cholinesterase activity (including severe liver disease) (Appendix 2), hyperkalaemia; major trauma, severe burns, neurological disease involving acute wasting of major muscle, prolonged immobilisation—risk of hyperkalaemia, personal or family history of congenital myotonic disease, Duchenne muscular dystrophy

Side-effects: see notes above; also postoperative muscle pain, myoglobinuria, myoglobinaemia; tachycardia, arrhythmias, cardiac arrest, hypertension, hypotension; bronchospasm, apnoea, prolonged respiratory depression, anaphylactic reactions; hyperkalaemia; hyperthermia; increased gastric pressure; rash, flushing

Dose: *by intravenous injection*, initially 1 mg/kg; maintenance, usually 0.5–1 mg/kg at 5–10 minute intervals; max. 500 mg/hour; NEONATE and INFANT under 1 year, 2 mg/kg; CHILD over 1 year, 1 mg/kg

By intravenous infusion of a solution containing 1–2 mg/mL (0.1–0.2%), 2.5–4 mg/minute; max. 500 mg/hour; CHILD reduce infusion rate according to body-weight

By intramuscular injection, INFANT under 1 year, up to 4–5 mg/kg; CHILD over 1 year, up to 4 mg/kg; max. 150 mg

Suxamethonium Chloride (Non-proprietary) PoM
Injection, suxamethonium chloride 50 mg/mL, net price 2-mL amp = 70p, 2-mL prefilled syringe = £7.35

Anectine® (GSK) PoM
Injection, suxamethonium chloride 50 mg/mL, net price 2-mL amp = 71p

15.1.6 Anticholinesterases used in anaesthesia

Anticholinesterases reverse the effects of the non-depolarising (competitive) muscle relaxant drugs such as pancuronium but they prolong the action of the depolarising muscle relaxant drug suxamethonium.

Edrophonium has a transient action and may be used in the diagnosis of suspected dual block due to suxamethonium.

Neostigmine has a longer duration of action than edrophonium. It is the specific drug for reversal of non-depolarising (competitive) blockade. It acts within one minute of intravenous injection and lasts for 20 to 30 minutes; a second dose may then be necessary. Atropine or preferably glycopyrronium (section 15.1.3) should be given before or with neostigmine in order to prevent bradycardia, excessive salivation, and other muscarinic actions of neostigmine.

EDROPHONIUM CHLORIDE

Indications: see under Dose; myasthenia gravis (section 10.2.1)
Cautions: see section 10.2.1 and notes above; atropine should also be given
Contra-indications: see section 10.2.1 and notes above
Side-effects: see section 10.2.1 and notes above
Dose: brief reversal of non-depolarising neuromuscular blockade, *by intravenous injection* over several minutes, 500–700 micrograms/kg (after or with atropine sulphate 600 micrograms)
Diagnosis of dual block, *by intravenous injection*, 10 mg

Edrophonium (Cambridge) PoM
Injection, edrophonium chloride 10 mg/mL, net price 1-mL amp = £4.76

NEOSTIGMINE METILSULFATE

(Neostigmine methylsulphate)
Indications: see under Dose
Cautions: see section 10.2.1 and notes above; atropine should also be given
Contra-indications: see section 10.2.1 and notes above
Side-effects: see section 10.2.1 and notes above
Dose: reversal of non-depolarising neuromuscular blockade, *by intravenous injection* over 1 minute, 50–70 micrograms/kg (max. 5 mg) after or with atropine sulphate 0.6–1.2 mg
Myasthenia gravis, see section 10.2.1

Neostigmine (Non-proprietary) PoM
Injection, neostigmine metilsulfate 2.5 mg/mL, net price 1-mL amp = 58p

■ With glycopyrronium
Robinul-Neostigmine® (Anpharm) PoM
Injection, neostigmine metilsulfate 2.5 mg, glycopyrronium bromide 500 micrograms/mL, net price 1-mL amp = £1.01
Dose: reversal of non-depolarising neuromuscular blockade *by intravenous injection* over 10–30 seconds, 1–2 mL *or* 0.02 mL/kg, dose may be repeated if required (total max. 2 mL); CHILD 0.02 mL/kg (*or* 0.2 mL/kg of a 1 in 10 dilution using water for injections or sodium chloride injection 0.9%), dose may be repeated if required (total max. 2 mL)

15.1.7 Antagonists for central and respiratory depression

Respiratory depression is a major concern with opioid analgesics and it may be treated by artificial ventilation or be reversed by **naloxone**. Naloxone will immediately reverse opioid-induced respiratory depression but the dose may have to be repeated because of the short duration of action of naloxone; however, naloxone will also antagonise the analgesic effect.

Flumazenil is a benzodiazepine antagonist for the reversal of the central sedative effects of benzodiazepines after anaesthetic and similar procedures. Flumazenil has a shorter half-life than that of diazepam and midazolam (and there is a risk that patients may become resedated).

Doxapram (section 3.5.1) is a central and respiratory stimulant but is of limited value.

FLUMAZENIL

Indications: reversal of sedative effects of benzodiazepines in anaesthetic, intensive care, and diagnostic procedures
Cautions: short-acting (repeat doses may be necessary—benzodiazepine effects may persist for at least 24 hours); benzodiazepine dependence (may precipitate withdrawal symptoms); prolonged benzodiazepine therapy for epilepsy (risk of convulsions); history of panic disorders (risk of recurrence); ensure neuromuscular blockade cleared before giving; avoid rapid injection in high-risk or anxious patients and following major surgery; hepatic impairment; head injury (rapid reversal of benzodiazepine sedation may cause convulsions); elderly, children, pregnancy (Appendix 4), breast-feeding
Contra-indications: life-threatening condition (e.g. raised intracranial pressure, status epilepticus) controlled by benzodiazepines
Side-effects: nausea, vomiting, and flushing; if wakening too rapid, agitation, anxiety, and fear; transient increase in blood pressure and heart-rate in intensive care patients; very rarely convulsions (particularly in epileptics)
Dose: *by intravenous injection*, 200 micrograms over 15 seconds, then 100 micrograms at 60-second intervals if required; usual dose range, 300–600 micrograms; max. total dose 1 mg (2 mg in intensive care); question aetiology if no response to repeated doses
By intravenous infusion, if drowsiness recurs after injection, 100–400 micrograms/hour, adjusted according to level of arousal

Flumazenil (Non-proprietary) PoM
Injection, flumazenil 100 micrograms/mL, net price 5-mL amp = £14.49

Anexate® (Roche) PoM
Injection, flumazenil 100 micrograms/mL, net price 5-mL amp = £14.49

NALOXONE HYDROCHLORIDE

Indications: reversal of opioid-induced respiratory depression; reversal of neonatal respiratory depression resulting from opioid administration to mother during labour; overdosage with opioids (see Emergency Treatment of Poisoning)
Cautions: cardiovascular disease or those receiving cardiotoxic drugs (serious adverse cardiovascular effects reported); physical dependence on opioids (precipitates withdrawal); pain (see also under Titration of Dose, below); has short duration of action (repeated doses or infusion may be necessary to reverse effects of opioids with longer duration of action); pregnancy (Appendix 4)
TITRATION OF DOSE. In postoperative use, the dose should be titrated for each patient in order to obtain sufficient respiratory response; however, naloxone antagonises analgesia
Side-effects: nausea and vomiting reported; tachycardia and fibrillation also reported
Dose: *by intravenous injection*, 100–200 micrograms (1.5–3 micrograms/kg); if response inadequate, increments of 100 micrograms every 2 minutes; further doses *by intramuscular injection* after 1–2 hours if required
CHILD *by intravenous injection*, 10 micrograms/kg; subsequent dose of 100 micrograms/kg if no response; if intravenous route not possible, may be given in divided doses by *intramuscular or subcutaneous injection*
NEONATE, reversal of respiratory depression resulting from opioid administration to mother, *by subcutaneous, intramuscular, or intravenous injection*, 10 micrograms/kg, repeated every 2–3 minutes *or by intramuscular injection*, 200 micrograms (60 micrograms/kg) as a single dose at birth (onset of action slower)

Naloxone PoM
See under Emergency Treatment of Poisoning p. 31

Narcan® PoM
See under Emergency Treatment of Poisoning p. 31

Narcan Neonatal® (Bristol-Myers Squibb) PoM
Injection, naloxone hydrochloride 20 micrograms/mL, net price 2-mL amp = £3.32

15.1.8 Drugs for malignant hyperthermia

Malignant hyperthermia is a rare but potentially lethal complication of anaesthesia. It is characterised by a rapid rise in temperature, increased muscle rigidity, tachycardia, and acidosis. The most common triggers of malignant hyperthermia are the volatile anaesthetics. Suxamethonium has also been implicated, but malignant hyperthermia is more likely if it is given following a volatile anaesthetic. Known trigger agents should be avoided during anaesthesia.

Dantrolene is used in the treatment of malignant hyperthermia. It acts on skeletal muscle cells by interfering with calcium efflux, thereby stopping the contractile process.

DANTROLENE SODIUM

Indications: malignant hyperthermia; chronic severe spasticity of voluntary muscle (section 10.2.2)
Cautions: avoid extravasation; pregnancy (Appendix 4); **interactions:** Appendix 1 (muscle relaxants)
Contra-indications: breast-feeding (Appendix 5)
Dose: *by rapid intravenous injection*, 1 mg/kg, repeated as required to a cumulative max. of 10 mg/kg

Dantrium Intravenous® (Procter & Gamble Pharm.) PoM
Injection, powder for reconstitution, dantrolene sodium, net price 20-mg vial = £15.08 (hosp. only)

15.2 Local anaesthesia

The use of local anaesthetics by injection or by application to mucous membranes to produce local analgesia is discussed in this section.

See also section 1.7 (anus), section 11.7 (eye), section 12.3 (oropharynx), and section 13.3 (skin).

USE OF LOCAL ANAESTHETICS. Local anaesthetic drugs act by causing a reversible block to conduction along nerve fibres. The drugs used vary widely in their potency, toxicity, duration of action, stability, solubility in water, and ability to penetrate mucous membranes. These variations determine their suitability for use by various routes, e.g. topical (surface), infiltration, plexus, epidural (extradural) or spinal block. Local anaesthetics may also be used for postoperative pain relief, thereby reducing the need for analgesics such as opioids.

ADMINISTRATION. In estimating the safe dosage of these drugs it is important to take account of the rate at which they are absorbed and excreted as well as their potency. The patient's age, weight, physique, and clinical condition, the degree of vascularity of the area to which the drug is to be applied, and the duration of administration are other factors which must be taken into account.

Local anaesthetics do not rely on the circulation to transport them to their sites of action, but uptake into the systemic circulation is important in terminating their action and producing toxicity. Following most regional anaesthetic procedures, maximum arterial plasma concentrations of anaesthetic develop within about 10 to 25 minutes, so **careful surveillance** for toxic effects is necessary during the first 30 minutes after injection. Great care must be taken to avoid accidental intravascular injection. Local anaesthesia around the oral cavity may impair swallowing and therefore increase the risk of aspiration.

Epidural anaesthesia is commonly used during surgery, often combined with general anaesthesia, because of its protective effect against the stress response of surgery. It is often used when good postoperative pain relief is essential (e.g. aortic aneurysm surgery or major gut surgery).

TOXICITY. Toxic effects associated with local anaesthetics usually result from excessively high plasma concentrations; single application of topical lidocaine preparations does not generally cause systemic side-effects. Effects initially include a feeling of inebriation and lightheadedness followed by sedation, circumoral paraesthesia and twitching; convulsions can occur in severe reactions. On intravenous injection convulsions and cardiovascular collapse may occur very rapidly. Hypersensitivity reactions occur mainly with the ester-type local anaesthetics such as benzocaine, cocaine, procaine, and tetracaine (amethocaine); reactions are less frequent with the amide types such as lidocaine (lignocaine), bupivacaine, prilocaine, and ropivacaine.

When prolonged analgesia is required, a long-acting local anaesthetic is preferred to minimise the likelihood of cumulative systemic toxicity. Local anaesthetic injections should be given slowly in order to detect inadvertent intravascular administration. Local anaesthetics should **not** be injected into inflamed or infected tissues nor should they be applied to the traumatised urethra. In such cases absorption into the blood may increase the possibility of systemic side-effects. The local anaesthetic effect may also be reduced by the altered local pH.

USE OF VASOCONSTRICTORS. Most local anaesthetics, with the exception of cocaine, cause dilation of blood vessels. The addition of a vasoconstrictor such as **adrenaline** (**epinephrine**) diminishes local blood flow, slows the rate of absorption of the local anaesthetic, and prolongs its local effect. Adrenaline must be used in a low concentration (e.g. 1 in 200 000) for this purpose and it should **not** be given with a local anaesthetic injection in digits and appendages; it may produce ischaemic necrosis.

When adrenaline is included the final concentration should be 1 in 200 000 (5 micrograms/mL). In dental surgery, up to 1 in 80 000 (12.5 micrograms/mL) of adrenaline is used with local anaesthetics. There is no justification for using higher concentrations.

The total dose of adrenaline should **not** exceed 500 micrograms and it is essential not to exceed a concentration of 1 in 200 000 (5 micrograms/mL) if more than 50 mL of the mixture is to be injected. For general cautions associated with the use of adrenaline, see section 2.7.3. For drug interactions, see Appendix 1 (sympathomimetics).

DENTAL ANAESTHESIA. **Lidocaine** (lignocaine) is widely used in dental procedures; it is most often used in combination with **adrenaline** (epinephrine). Lidocaine 2% with adrenaline 1 in 80 000 is a safe and effective preparation that has been used for many years.

The local anaesthetics **articaine** (carticaine) and **mepivacaine** are also used in dentistry; they are available in cartridges suitable for dental use. Mepivacaine is available with or without adrenaline (as *Scandonest*®) and articaine is available with adrenaline (as *Septanest*®).

In patients with severe hypertension or unstable cardiac rhythm, the use of adrenaline in a local anaesthetic may be hazardous. For these patients **prilocaine** with or without felypressin can be used but there is no evidence that it is any safer.

Great care should be taken to avoid inadvertent intravenous administration of a preparation containing adrenaline.

There is no clinical evidence of dangerous interactions between adrenaline-containing local anaesthetics and monoamine-oxidase inhibitors (MAOIs) or tricyclic antidepressants.

Lidocaine

Lidocaine (lignocaine) is effectively absorbed from mucous membranes and is a useful surface anaesthetic in concentrations of 2 to 4%. Except for surface anaesthesia, solutions should not usually exceed 1% in strength. The duration of the block (with adrenaline) is about 90 minutes.

LIDOCAINE HYDROCHLORIDE

(Lignocaine hydrochloride)

Indications: see under Dose; also dental anaesthesia (see p. 641); ventricular arrhythmias (section 2.3.2)

Cautions: epilepsy, respiratory impairment, impaired cardiac conduction, bradycardia, severe shock; porphyria (section 9.8.2); myasthenia gravis; reduce dose in elderly or debilitated; resuscitative equipment should be available; see section 2.3.2 for effects on heart; hepatic impairment (Appendix 2); renal impairment (Appendix 3); pregnancy (Appendix 4); **interactions:** Appendix 1 (lidocaine)

Contra-indications: hypovolaemia, complete heart block; do not use solutions containing adrenaline for anaesthesia in appendages

Side-effects: CNS effects include confusion, respiratory depression and convulsions; hypotension and bradycardia (may lead to cardiac arrest); hypersensitivity reported; see also notes above and section 2.3.2

Dose: infiltration anaesthesia, *by injection*, according to patient's weight and nature of procedure, max. 200 mg (or 500 mg if given in solutions containing adrenaline)—see also Administration on p. 639 and see also **important** warning below

Intravenous regional anaesthesia and nerve blocks, seek expert advice

Surface anaesthesia, usual strengths 2–4%, see preparations below

> **Important.** The licensed doses stated above may not be appropriate in some settings and expert advice should be sought

■ Lidocaine hydrochloride injections

Lidocaine (Non-proprietary) PoM

Injection 0.5%, lidocaine hydrochloride 5 mg/mL, net price 10-mL amp = 35p

Injection 1%, lidocaine hydrochloride 10 mg/mL, net price 2-mL amp = 21p; 5-mL amp = 23p; 10-mL amp = 35p; 10-mL prefilled syringe = £4.53; 20-mL amp =58p

Injection 2%, lidocaine hydrochloride 20 mg/mL, net price 2-mL amp = 28p; 5-mL amp = 25p

Xylocaine® (AstraZeneca) PoM

Injection 1% with adrenaline 1 in 200 000, anhydrous lidocaine hydrochloride 10 mg/mL, adrenaline 1 in 200 000 (5 micrograms/mL), net price 20-mL vial = 76p

Injection 2% with adrenaline 1 in 200 000, anhydrous lidocaine hydrochloride 20 mg/mL, adrenaline 1 in 200 000 (5 micrograms/mL), net price 20-mL vial = 81p

■ Lidocaine injections for dental use

NOTE. Consult expert dental sources for specific advice in relation to dose of lidocaine for dental anaesthesia

A variety of lidocaine injections with adrenaline is available in dental cartridges; brands include *Lignospan Special®*, *Lignostab® A*, *Rexocaine®* and *Xylocaine®*

■ Lidocaine for surface anaesthesia

Important. Rapid and extensive absorption may result in systemic side-effects

Lidocaine (Non-proprietary)

Gel, lidocaine hydrochloride 1%, net price 15 mL = £1.30; 2%, 15 mL = £1.30

Dose: urethral catheterisation, into urethra at least 5 minutes before catheter insertion, MEN 10 mL followed by further 3–5 mL; WOMEN 3–5 mL; CHILD 1–5 mL
Mucocutaneous anaesthesia, 2–3 mL applied when necessary; CHILD 1–2 mL
Major aphthae in immunocompromised patients, 2–3 mL applied when necessary, max. 15 mL in 24 hours; CHILD 1–2 mL, max. 8 mL in 24 hours

Ointment, lidocaine hydrochloride 5%, net price 15 g = 88p

Dose: dental practice, rub gently into dry gum
Sore nipples from breast-feeding, apply using gauze and wash off immediately before feed
Pain relief (in anal fissures, haemorrhoids, pruritus ani, pruritus vulvae, herpes zoster, or herpes labialis), 1–2 mL applied when necessary; avoid long-term use

Solution, lidocaine hydrochloride 4%, net price 25 mL = £1.35

Dose: biopsy in mouth, 3–4 mL with suitable spray *or* swab (with adrenaline if necessary); max. 5 mL, ELDERLY lower max. dose, CHILD max. 3 mg/kg
Puncture of maxillary sinus or polypectomy, apply with swab for 2–3 minutes (with adrenaline); max. 5 mL, ELDERLY lower max. dose, CHILD max. 3 mg/kg
Bronchoscopy and bronchography, 2–3 mL with suitable spray; max. 5 mL, ELDERLY lower max. dose, CHILD max. 3 mg/kg

Lidocaine and chlorhexidine (Non-proprietary)

Gel, lidocaine hydrochloride 1%, chlorhexidine gluconate solution 0.25%, net price 15 mL = 70p; lidocaine hydrochloride 2%, chlorhexidine gluconate solution 0.25%, 15 mL = 70p

Dose: urethral catheterisation, into urethra at least 5 minutes before catheter insertion, MEN 10 mL followed by further 3–5 mL; WOMEN 3–5 mL; CHILD 1–5 mL
Mucocutaneous anaesthesia, 2–3 mL applied when necessary; CHILD 1–2 mL
Major aphthae in immunocompromised patients, 2–3 mL applied when necessary, max. 15 mL in 24 hours; CHILD 1–2 mL, max. 8 mL in 24 hours

Emla® (AstraZeneca)

Drug Tariff cream, lidocaine 2.5%, prilocaine 2.5%, net price 5-g tube = £1.73

Surgical pack cream, lidocaine 2.5%, prilocaine 2.5%, net price 30-g tube = £10.25

Premedication pack cream, lidocaine 2.5%, prilocaine 2.5%, net price 5 × 5-g tube with 12 occlusive dressings = £9.75

Cautions: not for wounds, mucous membranes (except genital warts in adults), or atopic dermatitis; avoid use near eyes or middle ear; although systemic absorption low, caution in anaemia, in congenital or acquired methaemoglobinaemia or in G6PD deficiency (see also Prilocaine, p. 642)

Side-effects: include transient paleness, redness, and oedema

Dose: anaesthesia before minor skin procedures including venepuncture, apply thick layer under occlusive dressing 1–5 hours before procedure (2–5 hours before procedures on large areas e.g. split skin grafting); INFANT 1–12 months [unlicensed use] single application on intact skin under specialist supervision, under 1 month not recommended (risk of methaemoglobinaemia, see Cautions above)
Removal of warts from genital mucosa in adults, apply up to 10 g 5–10 minutes before removal

Instillagel® (CliniMed)

Gel, lidocaine hydrochloride 2%, chlorhexidine gluconate solution 0.25%, in a sterile lubricant basis in disposable syringe, net price 6-mL syringe = £1.41, 11-mL syringe = £1.58

Excipients: include hydroxybenzoates (parabens)

Dose: 6–11 mL into urethra

Laryngojet® (Celltech) PoM

Jet spray 4% (disposable kit for laryngotracheal anaesthesia), lidocaine hydrochloride 40 mg/mL, net price per unit (4-mL vial and disposable sterile cannula with cover and vial injector) = £5.10

Cautions: may be rapidly and almost completely absorbed from respiratory tract and systemic side-effects may occur; extreme caution if mucosa has been traumatised or if sepsis present

Dose: usually 160 mg (4 mL) as a single dose instilled as jet spray into lumen of larynx and trachea or applied with a swab (reduce dose according to size, age and condition of patient), max. 200 mg (5 mL); CHILD up to 3 mg/kg

Xylocaine® (AstraZeneca)

Spray (= pump spray), lidocaine 10% (100 mg/g) supplying 10 mg lidocaine/dose; 500 spray doses per container. Net price 50-mL bottle = £3.13

Dose: dental practice, 1–5 doses
Maxillary sinus puncture, 3 doses
During delivery in obstetrics, up to 20 doses
Procedures in pharynx, larynx, and trachea, up to 20 doses
Lidocaine can damage plastic cuffs of endotracheal tubes

Topical 4%, anhydrous lidocaine hydrochloride 40 mg/mL, net price 30-mL bottle = £1.21

Excipients: include hydroxybenzoates (parabens)

Dose: bronchoscopy, laryngoscopy, oesophagoscopy, endotracheal intubation, 1–7.5 mL with suitable spray; max. 5 mL when applied to larynx, trachea, or bronchi (max. 7.5 mL when applied to oesophagus); max. 10 mL when nebulised or when used for prolonged procedures (over 5 minutes); CHILD under 12 years, max. 0.075 mL/kg (3 mg/kg)
Biopsy in mouth, 3–4 mL with suitable spray *or* swab (with adrenaline if necessary)

■ Lidocaine for ear, nose, and oropharyngeal use

Lidocaine with Phenylephrine (Non-proprietary)

Topical solution, lidocaine hydrochloride 5%, phenylephrine hydrochloride 0.5%, net price 2.5 mL (with nasal applicator) = £8.73. For cautions, contra-indications and side-effects of phenylephrine, see section 2.7.2

Bupivacaine

The advantage of bupivacaine over other local anaesthetics is its longer duration of action. It has a slow onset of action, taking up to 30 minutes for full effect. It is often used in lumbar epidural blockade and is particularly suitable for continuous epidural analgesia in labour. It is the principal drug used for spinal anaesthesia.

BUPIVACAINE HYDROCHLORIDE

Indications: see under Dose

Cautions: see under Lidocaine Hydrochloride and notes above; myocardial depression may be more severe and more resistant to treatment; **interactions:** Appendix 1 (bupivacaine)

Contra-indications: see under Lidocaine Hydrochloride and notes above; intravenous regional anaesthesia (Bier's block)

Side-effects: see under Lidocaine Hydrochloride and notes above

Dose: adjusted according to patient's physical status and nature of procedure—**important**: see also under Administration, above

Local infiltration, 0.25% (up to 60 mL)

Peripheral nerve block, 0.25% (max. 60 mL), 0.5% (max. 30 mL)

Epidural block,

Surgery, *lumbar*, 0.5% (max. 20 mL)

Surgery, *caudal*, 0.5% (max. 30 mL); CHILD (up to 10 years) using 0.25% solution, up to lower-thoracic (T10) 0.3–0.4 mL/kg, up to mid-thoracic (T6) 0.4–0.8 mL/kg

Labour, *lumbar*, 0.25–0.5% (max. 12 mL); *caudal*, but rarely used, 0.25–0.5% (max. 20 mL)

Sympathetic block, 0.25% (max. 50 mL)

Intrathecal anaesthesia, see under preparations

> **Important.** The licensed doses stated above may not be appropriate in some settings and expert advice should be sought

Bupivacaine (Non-proprietary) PoM

Injection, anhydrous bupivacaine hydrochloride 2.5 mg/mL (0.25%), net price 10 mL = 82p; 5 mg/mL (0.5%), 10 mL = 94p

NOTE. Bupivacaine hydrochloride injection 0.25% and 0.5% are available in glass or plastic ampoules, and sterile-wrapped glass ampoules

Infusion, anhydrous bupivacaine hydrochloride 1 mg/mL (0.1%), net price 100 mL = £8.41, 250 mL = £10.59; 1.25 mg/mL (0.125%), 250 mL = £10.80

Dose: Continuous lumbar epidural infusion during labour (once epidural block established), 10–15 mg/hour of 0.1% or 0.125% solution; max. 2 mg/kg over 4 hours and total of 400 mg in 24 hours

Continuous thoracic, upper abdominal, or lower abdominal epidural infusion for post-operative pain (once epidural block established), 4–15 mg/hour of 0.1% or 0.125% solution; max. 2 mg/kg over 4 hours and total of 400 mg in 24 hours; not recommended for use in children

Marcain® (AstraZeneca) PoM

Injection, anhydrous bupivacaine hydrochloride 2.5 mg/mL (*Marcain*® *0.25%*), net price 10-mL *Polyamp*® = £1.06; 5 mg/mL (*Marcain*® *0.5%*), 10-mL *Polyamp*® = £1.21

Marcain Heavy® (AstraZeneca) PoM

Injection, anhydrous bupivacaine hydrochloride 5 mg, glucose 80 mg/mL, net price 4-mL amp = 93p

Dose: intrathecal anaesthesia for surgery, 2–4 mL (dose may need to be reduced in elderly and in late pregnancy)

■ With adrenaline

Bupivacaine and Adrenaline (Non-proprietary) PoM

Injection, anhydrous bupivacaine hydrochloride 2.5 mg/mL (0.25%), adrenaline 1 in 200 000 (5 micrograms/mL), net price 10-mL amp = £1.23

Injection, anhydrous bupivacaine hydrochloride 5 mg/mL (0.5%), adrenaline 1 in 200 000 (5 micrograms/mL), net price 10-mL amp = £1.40

Levobupivacaine

Levobupivacaine, an isomer of bupivacaine, has anaesthetic and analgesic properties similar to bupivacaine.

LEVOBUPIVACAINE HYDROCHLORIDE

NOTE. Levobupivacaine is an isomer of bupivacaine

Indications: see under Dose

Cautions: see under Lidocaine Hydrochloride and notes above; **interactions:** Appendix 1 (levobupivacaine)

Contra-indications: see under Lidocaine Hydrochloride and notes above; intravenous regional anaesthesia (Bier's block); paracervical block in obstetrics

Side-effects: see under Lidocaine Hydrochloride and notes above

Dose: adjusted according to patient's physical status and nature of procedure—**important:** see also under Administration, above

Surgical anaesthesia,

lumbar epidural, 10–20 mL (50–150 mg) of 5 or 7.5 mg/mL solution over 5 minutes; caesarean section, 15–30 mL (75–150 mg) of 5 mg/mL solution over 15–20 minutes

intrathecal, 3 mL (15 mg) of 5 mg/mL solution

peripheral nerve block, 1–40 mL of 2.5 or 5 mg/mL solution (max. 150 mg)

ilioinguinal/iliohypogastric block, CHILD 0.25–0.5 mL/kg (1.25–2.5 mg/kg) of a 2.5 mg/mL or 5 mg/mL solution

peribulbar block, 5–15 mL (37.5–112.5 mg) of 7.5 mg/mL solution

local infiltration, 1–60 mL (max. 150 mg) of 2.5 mg/mL solution

Acute pain,

lumbar epidural, 6–10 mL (15–25 mg) of 2.5 mg/mL solution at intervals of at least 15 minutes *or* 4–10 mL/hour (5–12.5 mg/hour) of 1.25 mg/mL solution as a continuous epidural infusion for labour pain, *or* 10–15 mL/hour (12.5–18.75 mg/hour) of 1.25 mg/mL solution or 5–7.5 mL/hour (12.5–18.75 mg/hour) of 2.5 mg/mL solution as a continuous epidural infusion for postoperative pain

NOTE. 7.5 mg/mL **contra-indicated** for use in obstetrics; for 1.25 mg/mL concentration dilute standard solutions with sodium chloride 0.9%.

> **Important.** The licensed doses stated above may not be appropriate in some settings and expert advice should be sought

Chirocaine® (Abbott) ▼ PoM

Injection, levobupivacaine hydrochloride 2.5 mg/mL, net price 10-mL amp = £1.66; 5 mg/mL, 10-mL amp = £1.90; 7.5 mg/mL, 10-mL amp = £2.85

Infusion, levobupivacaine hydrochloride 625 micrograms/mL, net price 100 mL = £7.80, 200 mL = £10.40; 1.25 mg/mL, net price 100 mL = £8.54, 200 mL = £12.20

Prilocaine

Prilocaine is a local anaesthetic of low toxicity which is similar to lidocaine (lignocaine). If used in high doses, methaemoglobinaemia may occur which can be treated with intravenous injection of methylthioninium chloride (methylene blue) 1% using a dose of 1 mg/kg. Infants under 6 months are particularly susceptible to methaemoglobinaemia.

PRILOCAINE HYDROCHLORIDE

Indications: infiltration anaesthesia (higher strengths for dental use only), nerve block

Cautions: see under Lidocaine Hydrochloride and notes above; severe or untreated hypertension, severe heart disease; concomitant drugs which cause methaemoglobinaemia; reduce dose in elderly or debilitated; hepatic impairment; renal impairment; pregnancy (Appendix 4); **interactions:** Appendix 1 (prilocaine)

Contra-indications: see under Lidocaine Hydrochloride and notes above; anaemia or congenital or acquired methaemoglobinaemia

Side-effects: see under Lidocaine Hydrochloride and notes above; ocular toxicity (including blindness) reported with excessive strengths used for ophthalmic procedures

Dose: see under preparations

Citanest® (AstraZeneca) PoM
Injection 1%, prilocaine hydrochloride 10 mg/mL, net price 50-mL multidose vial = £2.01
Dose: adjusted according to site of administration and response, 100–200 mg/minute, or in incremental doses, to max. total dose 400 mg; CHILD over 6 months up to 5 mg/kg

■ For dental use

Citanest® (Dentsply) PoM
Injection 4%, prilocaine hydrochloride 40 mg/mL, net price 2-mL cartridge = 16p
Dose: dental infiltration and dental nerve block, adjusted according to response, ADULT, 1–2 mL (max. 10 mL); CHILD under 10 years, 1 mL

Citanest with Octapressin® (Dentsply) PoM
Injection 3%, prilocaine hydrochloride 30 mg/mL, felypressin 0.03 unit/mL, net price 2-mL cartridge and self-aspirating cartridge (both) = 16p
Dose: dental infiltration and dental nerve block, adjusted according to response 1–5 mL (max. 10 mL); CHILD under 10 years, 1–2 mL

Procaine

Procaine is now seldom used. It is as potent as lidocaine (lignocaine) but has a shorter duration of action. It provides less intense analgesia because of reduced spread through the tissues. It is of no value as a surface anaesthetic.

PROCAINE HYDROCHLORIDE 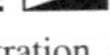

Indications: local anaesthesia by infiltration and regional routes (but see notes above)

Cautions: see notes above; pregnancy (Appendix 4)

Side-effects: see notes above

Dose: adjusted according to site of operation and patient's response

By injection, up to 1 g (200 mL of 0.5% solution or 100 mL of 1%) with adrenaline 1 in 200 000

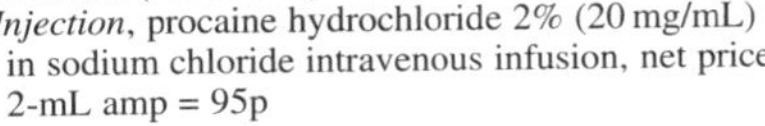

Procaine (Martindale) PoM
Injection, procaine hydrochloride 2% (20 mg/mL) in sodium chloride intravenous infusion, net price 2-mL amp = 95p

Ropivacaine

Ropivacaine is an amide-type local anaesthetic agent.

ROPIVACAINE HYDROCHLORIDE

Indications: see under Dose

Cautions: see Lidocaine Hydrochloride and notes above; **interactions:** Appendix 1 (ropivacaine)

Contra-indications: see Lidocaine Hydrochloride and notes above; intravenous regional anaesthesia (Bier's block); paracervical block in obstetrics

Side-effects: see Lidocaine Hydrochloride and notes above

Dose: adjust according to patient's physical status and nature of procedure—see also under Administration on p. 639

Surgical anaesthesia,
lumbar epidural, 15–20 mL of 10 mg/mL solution *or* 15–25 mL of 7.5 mg/mL solution; caesarean section, 15–20 mL of 7.5 mg/mL solution in incremental doses (max. total dose 150 mg)
thoracic epidural (to establish block for postoperative pain), 5–15 mL of 7.5 mg/mL solution
major nerve block (brachial plexus block), 30–40 mL of 7.5 mg/mL solution
field block, up to 30 mL of 7.5 mg/mL solution

Acute pain,
lumbar epidural, 10–20 mL of 2 mg/mL solution followed by 10–15 mL of 2 mg/mL solution at intervals of at least 30 minutes *or* 6–10 mL/hour of 2 mg/mL solution as a continuous epidural infusion for labour pain *or* 6–14 mL/hour of 2 mg/mL solution as a continuous epidural infusion for postoperative pain
thoracic epidural, 6–14 mL/hour of 2 mg/mL solution as a continuous infusion
field block, up to 100 mL of 2 mg/mL solution
peripheral nerve block, 5–10 mL/hour of 2 mg/mL solution as a continuous infusion *or* by intermittent injection
CHILD over 1 year (body-weight up to 25 kg), *caudal epidural* (for pre- and post-operative pain only), 2 mg/kg of 2 mg/mL solution

Naropin® (AstraZeneca) PoM
Injection, ropivacaine hydrochloride 2 mg/mL, net price 10-mL *Polyamp*® = £1.37; 7.5 mg/mL, 10-mL *Polyamp*® = £2.65; 10 mg/mL, 10-mL *Polyamp*® = £3.20
Epidural infusion, ropivacaine hydrochloride 2 mg/mL, net price 200-mL *Polybag*® = £14.45

Tetracaine

Tetracaine (amethocaine) is an effective local anaesthetic for topical application; a 4% gel is indicated for anaesthesia prior to venepuncture or venous cannulation. It is rapidly absorbed from mucous membranes and should **never** be applied to inflamed, traumatised, or highly vascular surfaces. It should **never** be used to provide anaesthesia for bronchoscopy or cystoscopy, as lidocaine (lignocaine) is a safer alternative. It is used in ophthalmology (section 11.7) and in skin preparations (section 13.3). Hypersensitivity to tetracaine has been reported.

TETRACAINE

(Amethocaine)

Indications: see under preparation below

Cautions: see notes above

Contra-indications: see notes above

Side-effects: see notes above; also erythema, oedema and pruritus; very rarely blistering

Important. Rapid and extensive absorption may result in systemic side-effects (see also notes above)

Ametop® (S&N Hlth.)

Gel, tetracaine 4%, net price 1.5-g tube = £1.08

Dose: apply contents of tube to site of venepuncture or venous cannulation and cover with occlusive dressing; remove gel and dressing after 30 minutes for venepuncture and after 45 minutes for venous cannulation; PRETERM NEONATE and INFANT under 1 month not recommended

Other local anaesthetics

Benzocaine is a local anaesthetic of low potency and toxicity. It is used in concentrations of up to 20% for topical anaesthesia of the oral mucosa before injection. It is an ingredient of some proprietary topical preparations for musculoskeletal conditions (section 10.3.2), mouth-ulcer preparations (section 12.3.1), and throat lozenges (section 12.3.3).

Cocaine readily penetrates mucous membranes and is an effective surface anaesthetic with an intense vasoconstrictor action. However, apart from its use in otolaryngology (see below), it has now been replaced by less toxic alternatives. It has marked sympathomimetic activity and should **never** be given by injection because of its toxicity. As a result of its intense stimulant effect it is a drug of addiction. In otolaryngology cocaine is applied to the nasal mucosa in concentrations of 4 to 10% (40–100 mg/mL); an oromucosal solution and nasal spray both containing cocaine hydrochloride 10% are available (Aurum). In order to avoid systemic effects, the maximum dose recommended for application to the nasal mucosa in fit adults is a total of 1.5 mg/kg, which is equivalent to a total topical dose of approximately 100 mg for an adult male; this dose relates to direct application of cocaine (application on gauze may reduce systemic absorption). It should be used only by those skilled in the precautions needed to *minimise absorption* and the *consequent risk of arrhythmias*. Although cocaine interacts with other drugs liable to induce arrhythmias, including adrenaline, some otolaryngologists consider that combined use of topical cocaine with topical adrenaline (in the form of a paste or a solution) improves the operative field and may possibly reduce absorption. Cocaine is a mydriatic as well as a local anaesthetic but owing to corneal toxicity it is now little used in ophthalmology. Cocaine should be avoided in porphyria (section 9.8.2).

Appendix 1: Interactions

Two or more drugs given at the same time may exert their effects independently or may interact. The interaction may be potentiation or antagonism of one drug by another, or occasionally some other effect. Adverse drug interactions should be reported to the CSM as for other adverse drug reactions.

Drug interactions may be **pharmacodynamic** or **pharmacokinetic**.

Pharmacodynamic interactions

These are interactions between drugs which have similar or antagonistic pharmacological effects or side-effects. They may be due to competition at receptor sites, or occur between drugs acting on the same physiological system. They are usually predictable from a knowledge of the pharmacology of the interacting drugs; in general, those demonstrated with one drug are likely to occur with related drugs. They occur to a greater or lesser extent in most patients who receive the interacting drugs.

Pharmacokinetic interactions

These occur when one drug alters the absorption, distribution, metabolism, or excretion of another, thus increasing or reducing the amount of drug available to produce its pharmacological effects. They are not easily predicted and many of them affect only a small proportion of patients taking the combination of drugs. Pharmacokinetic interactions occurring with one drug cannot be assumed to occur with related drugs unless their pharmacokinetic properties are known to be similar.

Pharmacokinetic interactions are of several types:

AFFECTING ABSORPTION. The rate of absorption or the total amount absorbed can both be altered by drug interactions. Delayed absorption is rarely of clinical importance unless high peak plasma concentrations are required (e.g. when giving an analgesic). Reduction in the total amount absorbed, however, may result in ineffective therapy.

DUE TO CHANGES IN PROTEIN BINDING. To a variable extent most drugs are loosely bound to plasma proteins. Protein-binding sites are non-specific and one drug can displace another thereby increasing its proportion free to diffuse from plasma to its site of action. This only produces a detectable increase in effect if it is an extensively bound drug (more than 90%) that is not widely distributed throughout the body. Even so displacement rarely produces more than transient potentiation because this increased concentration of free drug results in an increased rate of elimination.

Displacement from protein binding plays a part in the potentiation of warfarin by sulphonamides, and tolbutamide but the importance of these interactions is due mainly to the fact that warfarin metabolism is also inhibited.

AFFECTING METABOLISM. Many drugs are metabolised in the liver. Induction of the hepatic microsomal enzyme system by one drug can gradually increase the rate of metabolism of another, resulting in lower plasma concentrations and a reduced effect. On withdrawal of the inducer plasma concentrations increase and toxicity may occur. Barbiturates, griseofulvin, many antiepileptics, and rifampicin are the most important enzyme inducers. Drugs affected include warfarin and the oral contraceptives.

Conversely when one drug inhibits the metabolism of another higher plasma concentrations are produced, rapidly resulting in an increased effect with risk of toxicity. Some drugs which potentiate warfarin and phenytoin do so by this mechanism.

AFFECTING RENAL EXCRETION. Drugs are eliminated through the kidney both by glomerular filtration and by active tubular secretion. Competition occurs between those which share active transport mechanisms in the proximal tubule. For example, salicylates and some other NSAIDs delay the excretion of methotrexate; serious methotrexate toxicity is possible.

Relative importance of interactions

Many drug interactions are harmless and many of those which are potentially harmful only occur in a small proportion of patients; moreover, the severity of an interaction varies from one patient to another. Drugs with a small therapeutic ratio (e.g. phenytoin) and those which require careful control of dosage (e.g. anticoagulants, antihypertensives, and antidiabetics) are most often involved.

Patients at increased risk from drug interactions include the elderly and those with impaired renal or liver function.

HAZARDOUS INTERACTIONS. The symbol • has been placed against interactions that are **potentially hazardous** and where combined administration of the drugs involved should be **avoided** (or only undertaken with caution and appropriate monitoring).

Interactions that have no symbol do not usually have serious consequences.

List of drug interactions

The following is an alphabetical list of drugs and their interactions; to avoid excessive cross-referencing each drug or group is listed twice: in the alphabetical list and also against the drug or group with which it interacts; changes in the interactions lists since BNF No. 49 (March 2005) are underlined.

For explanation of symbol • see above

Abacavir
- Analgesics: abacavir possibly reduces plasma concentration of methadone
- Antibacterials: plasma concentration of abacavir possibly reduced by rifampicin
- Antiepileptics: plasma concentration of abacavir possibly reduced by phenytoin
- Barbiturates: plasma concentration of abacavir possibly reduced by phenobarbital

Acarbose *see* Antidiabetics

ACE Inhibitors

Alcohol: enhanced hypotensive effect when ACE inhibitors given with alcohol

Aldesleukin: enhanced hypotensive effect when ACE inhibitors given with aldesleukin

Allopurinol: increased risk of toxicity when captopril given with allopurinol especially in renal impairment

Alpha-blockers: enhanced hypotensive effect when ACE inhibitors given with alpha-blockers

Analgesics: increased risk of renal impairment when ACE inhibitors given with NSAIDs, also hypotensive effect antagonised; increased risk of hyperkalaemia when ACE inhibitors given with ketorolac; risk of renal impairment when ACE inhibitors given with aspirin (in doses over 300 mg daily), also hypotensive effect antagonised

Angiotensin-II Receptor Antagonists: enhanced hypotensive effect when ACE inhibitors given with angiotensin-II receptor antagonists

Antacids: absorption of ACE inhibitors possibly reduced by antacids; absorption of captopril, enalapril and fosinopril reduced by antacids

Anti-arrhythmics: increased risk of toxicity when captopril given with procainamide especially in renal impairment

Antibacterials: plasma concentration of active metabolite of imidapril reduced by rifampicin (reduced antihypertensive effect); quinapril tablets reduce absorption of tetracyclines (quinapril tablets contain magnesium carbonate)

Anticoagulants: increased risk of hyperkalaemia when ACE inhibitors given with heparins

Antidepressants: hypotensive effect of ACE inhibitors possibly enhanced by MAOIs

Antidiabetics: ACE inhibitors possibly enhance hypoglycaemic effect of insulin, metformin and sulphonylureas

Antipsychotics: enhanced hypotensive effect when ACE inhibitors given with antipsychotics

Anxiolytics and Hypnotics: enhanced hypotensive effect when ACE inhibitors given with anxiolytics and hypnotics

Beta-blockers: enhanced hypotensive effect when ACE inhibitors given with beta-blockers

Calcium-channel Blockers: enhanced hypotensive effect when ACE inhibitors given with calcium-channel blockers

Cardiac Glycosides: captopril possibly increases plasma concentration of digoxin

• Ciclosporin: increased risk of hyperkalaemia when ACE inhibitors given with •ciclosporin

Clonidine: enhanced hypotensive effect when ACE inhibitors given with clonidine; antihypertensive effect of captopril possibly delayed by previous treatment with clonidine

Corticosteroids: hypotensive effect of ACE inhibitors antagonised by corticosteroids

Cytotoxics: increased risk of leucopenia when captopril given with azathioprine

Diazoxide: enhanced hypotensive effect when ACE inhibitors given with diazoxide

• Diuretics: enhanced hypotensive effect when ACE inhibitors given with •diuretics; increased risk of severe hyperkalaemia when ACE inhibitors given with •potassium-sparing diuretics and aldosterone antagonists (monitor potassium concentration with low-dose spironolactone in heart failure)

Dopaminergics: enhanced hypotensive effect when ACE inhibitors given with levodopa

Epoetin: antagonism of hypotensive effect and increased risk of hyperkalaemia when ACE inhibitors given with epoetin

ACE Inhibitors *(continued)*

• Lithium: ACE inhibitors reduce excretion of •lithium (increased plasma concentration)

Methyldopa: enhanced hypotensive effect when ACE inhibitors given with methyldopa

Moxisylyte (thymoxamine): enhanced hypotensive effect when ACE inhibitors given with moxisylyte

Moxonidine: enhanced hypotensive effect when ACE inhibitors given with moxonidine

Muscle Relaxants: enhanced hypotensive effect when ACE inhibitors given with baclofen or tizanidine

Nitrates: enhanced hypotensive effect when ACE inhibitors given with nitrates

Oestrogens: hypotensive effect of ACE inhibitors antagonised by oestrogens

• Potassium Salts: increased risk of severe hyperkalaemia when ACE inhibitors given with •potassium salts

Probenecid: excretion of captopril reduced by probenecid

Progestogens: risk of hyperkalaemia when ACE inhibitors given with drospirenone (monitor serum potassium during first cycle)

Prostaglandins: enhanced hypotensive effect when ACE inhibitors given with alprostadil

Vasodilator Antihypertensives: enhanced hypotensive effect when ACE inhibitors given with hydralazine, minoxidil or nitroprusside

Acebutolol *see* Beta-blockers

Aceclofenac *see* NSAIDs

Acemetacin *see* NSAIDs

Acenocoumarol (nicoumalone) *see* Coumarins

Acetazolamide *see* Diuretics

Aciclovir

Note. Interactions do not apply to topical aciclovir preparations

Note. Valaciclovir interactions as for aciclovir

Cytotoxics: plasma concentration of aciclovir increased by mycophenolate mofetil, also plasma concentration of inactive metabolite of mycophenolate mofetil increased

Probenecid: excretion of aciclovir reduced by probenecid (increased plasma concentration)

Acitretin *see* Retinoids

Acrivastine *see* Antihistamines

Adalimumab

• Anakinra: avoid concomitant use of adalimumab with •anakinra

• Vaccines: avoid concomitant use of adalimumab with live •vaccines (see p. 604)

Adenosine

Note. Possibility of interaction with drugs tending to impair myocardial conduction

Anaesthetics, Local: increased myocardial depression when anti-arrhythmics given with bupivacaine, levobupivacaine or prilocaine

• Anti-arrhythmics: increased myocardial depression when anti-arrhythmics given with other •anti-arrhythmics

• Antihistamines: increased risk of ventricular arrhythmias when anti-arrhythmics given with •terfenadine

• Antipsychotics: increased risk of ventricular arrhythmias when anti-arrhythmics that prolong the QT interval given with •antipsychotics that prolong the QT interval

• Beta-blockers: increased myocardial depression when anti-arrhythmics given with •beta-blockers

• Dipyridamole: effect of adenosine enhanced and extended by •dipyridamole (important risk of toxicity)

Adenosine *(continued)*

5HT$_3$ Antagonists: caution with anti-arrhythmics advised by manufacturer of tropisetron (risk of ventricular arrhythmias)

Theophylline: anti-arrhythmic effect of adenosine antagonised by theophylline

Adrenaline (epinephrine) *see* Sympathomimetics

Adrenergic Neurone Blockers

Alcohol: enhanced hypotensive effect when adrenergic neurone blockers given with alcohol

Alpha-blockers: enhanced hypotensive effect when adrenergic neurone blockers given with alpha-blockers

• Anaesthetics, General: enhanced hypotensive effect when adrenergic neurone blockers given with •general anaesthetics

Analgesics: hypotensive effect of adrenergic neurone blockers antagonised by NSAIDs

Angiotensin-II Receptor Antagonists: enhanced hypotensive effect when adrenergic neurone blockers given with angiotensin-II receptor antagonists

Antidepressants: enhanced hypotensive effect when adrenergic neurone blockers given with MAOIs; hypotensive effect of adrenergic neurone blockers antagonised by tricyclics

Antipsychotics: hypotensive effect of adrenergic neurone blockers antagonised by haloperidol; hypotensive effect of adrenergic neurone blockers antagonised by higher doses of chlorpromazine; enhanced hypotensive effect when adrenergic neurone blockers given with phenothiazines

Anxiolytics and Hypnotics: enhanced hypotensive effect when adrenergic neurone blockers given with anxiolytics and hypnotics

Beta-blockers: enhanced hypotensive effect when adrenergic neurone blockers given with beta-blockers

Calcium-channel Blockers: enhanced hypotensive effect when adrenergic neurone blockers given with calcium-channel blockers

Clonidine: enhanced hypotensive effect when adrenergic neurone blockers given with clonidine

Corticosteroids: hypotensive effect of adrenergic neurone blockers antagonised by corticosteroids

Diazoxide: enhanced hypotensive effect when adrenergic neurone blockers given with diazoxide

Diuretics: enhanced hypotensive effect when adrenergic neurone blockers given with diuretics

Dopaminergics: enhanced hypotensive effect when adrenergic neurone blockers given with levodopa

Methyldopa: enhanced hypotensive effect when adrenergic neurone blockers given with methyldopa

Moxisylyte (thymoxamine): enhanced hypotensive effect when adrenergic neurone blockers given with moxisylyte

Moxonidine: enhanced hypotensive effect when adrenergic neurone blockers given with moxonidine

Muscle Relaxants: enhanced hypotensive effect when adrenergic neurone blockers given with baclofen or tizanidine

Nitrates: enhanced hypotensive effect when adrenergic neurone blockers given with nitrates

Oestrogens: hypotensive effect of adrenergic neurone blockers antagonised by oestrogens

Pizotifen: hypotensive effect of adrenergic neurone blockers antagonised by pizotifen

Prostaglandins: enhanced hypotensive effect when adrenergic neurone blockers given with alprostadil

• Sympathomimetics: hypotensive effect of adrenergic neurone blockers antagonised by •ephedrine, •isometheptene, •metaraminol, •methylphenidate, •noradrenaline (norepinephrine), •oxymetazoline, •phenylephrine, •phenylpropanolamine, •pseudoephedrine and •xylometazoline

Vasodilator Antihypertensives: enhanced hypotensive effect when adrenergic neurone blockers given with hydralazine, minoxidil or nitroprusside

Adsorbents *see* Kaolin

Agalsidase Beta

Anti-arrhythmics: effects of agalsidase beta possibly inhibited by amiodarone (manufacturer of agalsidase beta advises avoid concomitant use)

Antibacterials: effects of agalsidase beta possibly inhibited by gentamicin (manufacturer of agalsidase beta advises avoid concomitant use)

Antimalarials: effects of agalsidase beta possibly inhibited by chloroquine and hydroxychloroquine (manufacturer of agalsidase beta advises avoid concomitant use)

Alcohol

ACE Inhibitors: enhanced hypotensive effect when alcohol given with ACE inhibitors

Adrenergic Neurone Blockers: enhanced hypotensive effect when alcohol given with adrenergic neurone blockers

Alpha-blockers: increased sedative effect when alcohol given with indoramin; enhanced hypotensive effect when alcohol given with alpha-blockers

Analgesics: enhanced hypotensive and sedative effects when alcohol given with opioid analgesics

Angiotensin-II Receptor Antagonists: enhanced hypotensive effect when alcohol given with angiotensin-II receptor antagonists

• Antibacterials: disulfiram-like reaction when alcohol given with metronidazole; possibility of disulfiram-like reaction when alcohol given with tinidazole; increased risk of convulsions when alcohol given with •cycloserine

• Anticoagulants: major changes in consumption of alcohol may affect anticoagulant control with •coumarins or •phenindione

• Antidepressants: some beverages containing alcohol and some dealcoholised beverages contain tyramine which interacts with •MAOIs (hypertensive crisis)—if no tyramine, enhanced hypotensive effect; sedative effects possibly increased when alcohol given with SSRIs; increased sedative effect when alcohol given with •mirtazapine, •tricyclic-related antidepressants or •tricyclics

Antidiabetics: alcohol enhances hypoglycaemic effect of antidiabetics; increased risk of lactic acidosis when alcohol given with metformin; flushing, in susceptible subjects, when alcohol given with chlorpropamide

Antiepileptics: alcohol possibly increases CNS side-effects of carbamazepine; increased sedative effect when alcohol given with primidone

Antifungals: effects of alcohol possibly enhanced by griseofulvin

Antihistamines: increased sedative effect when alcohol given with antihistamines (possibly less effect with non-sedating antihistamines)

Antimuscarinics: increased sedative effect when alcohol given with hyoscine

Antipsychotics: increased sedative effect when alcohol given with antipsychotics

Anxiolytics and Hypnotics: increased sedative effect when alcohol given with anxiolytics and hypnotics

Barbiturates: increased sedative effect when alcohol given with barbiturates

Beta-blockers: enhanced hypotensive effect when alcohol given with beta-blockers

Alcohol *(continued)*

Calcium-channel Blockers: enhanced hypotensive effect when alcohol given with calcium-channel blockers; plasma concentration of alcohol possibly increased by verapamil

Clonidine: enhanced hypotensive effect when alcohol given with clonidine

Cytotoxics: disulfiram-like reaction when alcohol given with procarbazine

Diazoxide: enhanced hypotensive effect when alcohol given with diazoxide

Disulfiram: disulfiram reaction when alcohol given with disulfiram (see p. 260)

Diuretics: enhanced hypotensive effect when alcohol given with diuretics

Dopaminergics: alcohol reduces tolerance to bromocriptine

Levamisole: possibility of disulfiram-like reaction when alcohol given with levamisole

Lofexidine: increased sedative effect when alcohol given with lofexidine

Methyldopa: enhanced hypotensive effect when alcohol given with methyldopa

Moxonidine: enhanced hypotensive effect when alcohol given with moxonidine

Muscle Relaxants: increased sedative effect when alcohol given with baclofen, methocarbamol or tizanidine

Nabilone: increased sedative effect when alcohol given with nabilone

Nicorandil: alcohol possibly enhances hypotensive effect of nicorandil

Nitrates: enhanced hypotensive effect when alcohol given with nitrates

• Paraldehyde: increased sedative effect when alcohol given with •paraldehyde

Retinoids: presence of alcohol causes etretinate to be formed from acitretin

Vasodilator Antihypertensives: enhanced hypotensive effect when alcohol given with hydralazine, minoxidil or nitroprusside

Aldesleukin

ACE Inhibitors: enhanced hypotensive effect when aldesleukin given with ACE inhibitors

Alpha-blockers: enhanced hypotensive effect when aldesleukin given with alpha-blockers

Angiotensin-II Receptor Antagonists: enhanced hypotensive effect when aldesleukin given with angiotensin-II receptor antagonists

Beta-blockers: enhanced hypotensive effect when aldesleukin given with beta-blockers

Calcium-channel Blockers: enhanced hypotensive effect when aldesleukin given with calcium-channel blockers

Clonidine: enhanced hypotensive effect when aldesleukin given with clonidine

Diazoxide: enhanced hypotensive effect when aldesleukin given with diazoxide

Diuretics: enhanced hypotensive effect when aldesleukin given with diuretics

Methyldopa: enhanced hypotensive effect when aldesleukin given with methyldopa

Moxonidine: enhanced hypotensive effect when aldesleukin given with moxonidine

Nitrates: enhanced hypotensive effect when aldesleukin given with nitrates

Vasodilator Antihypertensives: enhanced hypotensive effect when aldesleukin given with hydralazine, minoxidil or nitroprusside

Alendronic Acid *see* Bisphosphonates

Alfentanil *see* Opioid Analgesics

Alfuzosin *see* Alpha-blockers

Alimemazine (trimeprazine) *see* Antihistamines

Alkylating Drugs *see* Busulfan, Cyclophosphamide, Ifosfamide, Melphalan, and Thiotepa

Allopurinol

ACE Inhibitors: increased risk of toxicity when allopurinol given with captopril especially in renal impairment

Antibacterials: increased risk of rash when allopurinol given with amoxicillin or ampicillin

Anticoagulants: allopurinol possibly enhances anticoagulant effect of coumarins

Antivirals: allopurinol possibly increases plasma concentration of didanosine

Ciclosporin: allopurinol possibly increases plasma concentration of ciclosporin (risk of nephrotoxicity)

• Cytotoxics: allopurinol enhances effects and increases toxicity of •azathioprine and •mercaptopurine (reduce dose of azathioprine and mercaptopurine); avoidance of allopurinol advised by manufacturer of •capecitabine

Theophylline: allopurinol possibly increases plasma concentration of theophylline

Almotriptan *see* $5HT_1$ Agonists

Alpha$_2$-adrenoceptor Stimulants

Antidepressants: manufacturer of apraclonidine and brimonidine advises avoid concomitant use with MAOIs; manufacturer of apraclonidine and brimonidine advises avoid concomitant use with tricyclic-related antidepressants; manufacturer of apraclonidine and brimonidine advises avoid concomitant use with tricyclics

Alpha-blockers

ACE Inhibitors: enhanced hypotensive effect when alpha-blockers given with ACE inhibitors

Adrenergic Neurone Blockers: enhanced hypotensive effect when alpha-blockers given with adrenergic neurone blockers

Alcohol: enhanced hypotensive effect when alpha-blockers given with alcohol; increased sedative effect when indoramin given with alcohol

Aldesleukin: enhanced hypotensive effect when alpha-blockers given with aldesleukin

• Anaesthetics, General: enhanced hypotensive effect when alpha-blockers given with •general anaesthetics

Analgesics: hypotensive effect of alpha-blockers antagonised by NSAIDs

Angiotensin-II Receptor Antagonists: enhanced hypotensive effect when alpha-blockers given with angiotensin-II receptor antagonists

• Antidepressants: enhanced hypotensive effect when alpha-blockers given with MAOIs; manufacturer of indoramin advises avoid concomitant use with •MAOIs

Antipsychotics: enhanced hypotensive effect when alpha-blockers given with antipsychotics

Anxiolytics and Hypnotics: enhanced hypotensive and sedative effects when alpha-blockers given with anxiolytics and hypnotics

• Beta-blockers: enhanced hypotensive effect when alpha-blockers given with •beta-blockers, also increased risk of first-dose hypotension with post-synaptic alpha-blockers such as prazosin

• Calcium-channel Blockers: enhanced hypotensive effect when alpha-blockers given with •calcium-channel blockers, also increased risk of first-dose hypotension with post-synaptic alpha-blockers such as prazosin

Cardiac Glycosides: prazosin increases plasma concentration of digoxin

Clonidine: enhanced hypotensive effect when alpha-blockers given with clonidine

Alpha-blockers *(continued)*

Corticosteroids: hypotensive effect of alpha-blockers antagonised by corticosteroids
Diazoxide: enhanced hypotensive effect when alpha-blockers given with diazoxide
• Diuretics: enhanced hypotensive effect when alpha-blockers given with •diuretics, also increased risk of first-dose hypotension with post-synaptic alpha-blockers such as prazosin
Dopaminergics: enhanced hypotensive effect when alpha-blockers given with levodopa
Methyldopa: enhanced hypotensive effect when alpha-blockers given with methyldopa
• Moxisylyte (thymoxamine): possible severe postural hypotension when alpha-blockers given with •moxisylyte
Moxonidine: enhanced hypotensive effect when alpha-blockers given with moxonidine
Muscle Relaxants: enhanced hypotensive effect when alpha-blockers given with baclofen or tizanidine
Nitrates: enhanced hypotensive effect when alpha-blockers given with nitrates
Oestrogens: hypotensive effect of alpha-blockers antagonised by oestrogens
Prostaglandins: enhanced hypotensive effect when alpha-blockers given with alprostadil
Sildenafil: enhanced hypotensive effect when alpha-blockers given with sildenafil (avoid alpha-blockers for 4 hours after sildenafil)
• Sympathomimetics: avoid concomitant use of tolazoline with •adrenaline (epinephrine) or •dopamine
• Tadalafil: enhanced hypotensive effect when alpha-blockers given with •tadalafil—avoid concomitant use
• Ulcer-healing Drugs: effects of tolazoline antagonised by •cimetidine and •ranitidine
• Vardenafil: possible increased hypotensive effect when alpha-blockers given with •vardenafil—avoid concomitant use
Vasodilator Antihypertensives: enhanced hypotensive effect when alpha-blockers given with hydralazine, minoxidil or nitroprusside

Alpha-blockers (post-synaptic) *see* Alpha-blockers

Alprazolam *see* Anxiolytics and Hypnotics

Alprostadil *see* Prostaglandins

Aluminium Hydroxide *see* Antacids

Amantadine

Antimuscarinics: increased risk of antimuscarinic side-effects when amantadine given with antimuscarinics
Antipsychotics: increased risk of extrapyramidal side-effects when amantadine given with antipsychotics
Bupropion: increased risk of side-effects when amantadine given with bupropion
Domperidone: increased risk of extrapyramidal side-effects when amantadine given with domperidone
• Memantine: increased risk of CNS toxicity when amantadine given with •memantine (manufacturer of memantine advises avoid concomitant use); effects of dopaminergics possibly enhanced by memantine
Methyldopa: increased risk of extrapyramidal side-effects when amantadine given with methyldopa; antiparkinsonian effect of dopaminergics antagonised by methyldopa
Metoclopramide: increased risk of extrapyramidal side-effects when amantadine given with metoclopramide
Tetrabenazine: increased risk of extrapyramidal side-effects when amantadine given with tetrabenazine

Amikacin *see* Aminoglycosides

Amiloride *see* Diuretics

Aminoglutethimide

• Anticoagulants: aminoglutethimide accelerates metabolism of •coumarins and •phenindione (reduced anticoagulant effect)
Antidiabetics: manufacturer of aminoglutethimide advises that metabolism of biguanides and sulphonylureas possibly accelerated
Cardiac Glycosides: aminoglutethimide accelerates metabolism of digitoxin (reduced effect)
Corticosteroids: aminoglutethimide accelerates metabolism of corticosteroids (reduced effect)
Diuretics: increased risk of hyponatraemia when aminoglutethimide given with diuretics
Hormone Antagonists: aminoglutethimide reduces plasma concentration of tamoxifen
Progestogens: aminoglutethimide reduces plasma concentration of medroxyprogesterone
Theophylline: aminoglutethimide accelerates metabolism of theophylline (reduced effect)

Aminoglycosides

Agalsidase Beta: gentamicin possibly inhibits effects of agalsidase beta (manufacturer of agalsidase beta advises avoid concomitant use)
Analgesics: plasma concentration of amikacin and gentamicin in neonates possibly increased by indometacin
Antibacterials: neomycin reduces absorption of phenoxymethylpenicillin; increased risk of nephrotoxicity when aminoglycosides given with colistin or polymyxins; increased risk of nephrotoxicity and ototoxicity when aminoglycosides given with capreomycin, teicoplanin or vancomycin
• Anticoagulants: experience in anticoagulant clinics suggests that INR possibly altered when neomycin (given for local action on gut) is given with •coumarins or •phenindione
Antidiabetics: neomycin possibly enhances hypoglycaemic effect of acarbose, also severity of gastro-intestinal effects increased
Antifungals: increased risk of nephrotoxicity when aminoglycosides given with amphotericin
Bisphosphonates: increased risk of hypocalcaemia when aminoglycosides given with bisphosphonates
Cardiac Glycosides: gentamicin possibly increases plasma concentration of digoxin; neomycin reduces absorption of digoxin
• Ciclosporin: increased risk of nephrotoxicity when aminoglycosides given with •ciclosporin
• Cytotoxics: neomycin possibly reduces absorption of methotrexate; increased risk of nephrotoxicity and possibly of ototoxicity when aminoglycosides given with •platinum compounds
• Diuretics: increased risk of otoxicity when aminoglycosides given with •loop diuretics
• Muscle Relaxants: aminoglycosides enhance effects of •non-depolarising muscle relaxants and •suxamethonium
Oestrogens: broad-spectrum antibacterials possibly reduce contraceptive effect of oestrogens (risk probably small, see p. 407)
• Parasympathomimetics: aminoglycosides antagonise effects of •neostigmine and •pyridostigmine
• Tacrolimus: increased risk of nephrotoxicity when aminoglycosides given with •tacrolimus
Vitamins: neomycin possibly reduces absorption of vitamin A

Aminophylline *see* Theophylline

Aminosalicylates

Cardiac Glycosides: sulfasalazine possibly reduces absorption of digoxin

Cytotoxics: possible increased risk of leucopenia when aminosalicylates given with azathioprine or mercaptopurine

Folates: sulfasalazine possibly reduces absorption of folic acid

Amiodarone

Note. Amiodarone has a long half-life; there is a potential for drug interactions to occur for several weeks (or even months) after treatment with it has been stopped

Agalsidase Beta: amiodarone possibly inhibits effects of agalsidase beta (manufacturer of agalsidase beta advises avoid concomitant use)

Anaesthetics, Local: increased myocardial depression when anti-arrhythmics given with bupivacaine, levobupivacaine or prilocaine

• Anti-arrhythmics: increased myocardial depression when anti-arrhythmics given with other •anti-arrhythmics; increased risk of ventricular arrhythmias when amiodarone given with •disopyramide—avoid concomitant use; amiodarone increases plasma concentration of •flecainide (halve dose of flecainide); amiodarone increases plasma concentration of •procainamide and •quinidine (increased risk of ventricular arrhythmias—avoid concomitant use)

• Antibacterials: increased risk of ventricular arrhythmias when amiodarone given with parenteral •erythromycin—avoid concomitant use; increased risk of ventricular arrhythmias when amiodarone given with •moxifloxacin—avoid concomitant use; increased risk of ventricular arrhythmias when amiodarone given with •sulfamethoxazole and •trimethoprim (as co-trimoxazole)—avoid concomitant use of co-trimoxazole

• Anticoagulants: amiodarone inhibits metabolism of •coumarins and •phenindione (enhanced anticoagulant effect)

• Antidepressants: increased risk of ventricular arrhythmias when amiodarone given with •tricyclics—avoid concomitant use

• Antiepileptics: amiodarone inhibits metabolism of •phenytoin (increased plasma concentration)

• Antihistamines: increased risk of ventricular arrhythmias when amiodarone given with •mizolastine or •terfenadine—avoid concomitant use; increased risk of ventricular arrhythmias when anti-arrhythmics given with •terfenadine

• Antimalarials: avoidance of amiodarone advised by manufacturer of •artemether/lumefantrine (risk of ventricular arrhythmias); increased risk of ventricular arrhythmias when amiodarone given with •chloroquine and hydroxychloroquine, •mefloquine or •quinine—avoid concomitant use

• Antipsychotics: increased risk of ventricular arrhythmias when anti-arrhythmics that prolong the QT interval given with •antipsychotics that prolong the QT interval; increased risk of ventricular arrhythmias when amiodarone given with •amisulpride, •haloperidol, •phenothiazines, •pimozide or •sertindole—avoid concomitant use

• Antivirals: plasma concentration of amiodarone possibly increased by •amprenavir (increased risk of ventricular arrhythmias—avoid concomitant use); plasma concentration of amiodarone possibly increased by •atazanavir; increased risk of ventricular arrhythmias when amiodarone given with •nelfinavir—avoid concomitant use; plasma concentration of amiodarone increased by •ritonavir (increased risk of ventricular arrhythmias—avoid concomitant use)

Amiodarone *(continued)*

• Beta-blockers: increased risk of bradycardia, AV block and myocardial depression when amiodarone given with •beta-blockers; increased myocardial depression when anti-arrhythmics given with •beta-blockers; increased risk of ventricular arrhythmias when amiodarone given with •sotalol—avoid concomitant use

• Calcium-channel Blockers: increased risk of bradycardia, AV block and myocardial depression when amiodarone given with •diltiazem or •verapamil

• Cardiac Glycosides: amiodarone increases plasma concentration of •digoxin (halve dose of digoxin)

Ciclosporin: amiodarone possibly increases plasma concentration of ciclosporin

Diuretics: increased cardiac toxicity with amiodarone if hypokalaemia occurs with acetazolamide, loop diuretics or thiazides and related diuretics; amiodarone increases plasma concentration of eplerenone (reduce dose of eplerenone)

• Dolasetron: increased risk of ventricular arrhythmias when amiodarone given with •dolasetron—avoid concomitant use

$5HT_3$ Antagonists: caution with anti-arrhythmics advised by manufacturer of tropisetron (risk of ventricular arrhythmias)

• Lipid-regulating Drugs: increased risk of myopathy when amiodarone given with •simvastatin

• Lithium: manufacturer of amiodarone advises avoid concomitant use with •lithium (risk of ventricular arrhythmias)

Orlistat: plasma concentration of amiodarone possibly reduced by orlistat

• Pentamidine Isetionate: increased risk of ventricular arrhythmias when amiodarone given with •pentamidine isetionate—avoid concomitant use

Thyroid Hormones: for concomitant use of amiodarone and thyroid hormones see p. 79

Ulcer-healing Drugs: plasma concentration of amiodarone increased by cimetidine

Amisulpride *see* Antipsychotics

Amitriptyline *see* Antidepressants, Tricyclic

Amlodipine *see* Calcium-channel Blockers

Amobarbital *see* Barbiturates

Amoxapine *see* Antidepressants, Tricyclic

Amoxicillin *see* Penicillins

Amphotericin

Note. Close monitoring required with concomitant administration of nephrotoxic drugs or cytotoxics

Antibacterials: increased risk of nephrotoxicity when amphotericin given with aminoglycosides or polymyxins; possible increased risk of nephrotoxicity when amphotericin given with vancomycin

Antifungals: amphotericin reduces renal excretion and increases cellular uptake of flucytosine (toxicity possibly increased); effects of amphotericin possibly antagonised by imidazoles and triazoles

• Cardiac Glycosides: hypokalaemia caused by amphotericin increases cardiac toxicity with •cardiac glycosides

• Ciclosporin: increased risk of nephrotoxicity when amphotericin given with •ciclosporin

• Corticosteroids: increased risk of hypokalaemia when amphotericin given with •corticosteroids—avoid concomitant use unless corticosteroids needed to control reactions

Diuretics: increased risk of hypokalaemia when amphotericin given with loop diuretics or thiazides and related diuretics

Pentamidine Isetionate: possible increased risk of nephrotoxicity when amphotericin given with pentamidine isetionate

Amphotericin *(continued)*
- Tacrolimus: increased risk of nephrotoxicity when amphotericin given with •tacrolimus

Ampicillin *see* Penicillins

Amprenavir
Note. Fosamprenavir is a prodrug of amprenavir—see also Amprenavir
Analgesics: amprenavir reduces plasma concentration of methadone
Antacids: absorption of amprenavir possibly reduced by antacids
- Anti-arrhythmics: amprenavir possibly increases plasma concentration of •amiodarone, •flecainide, •propafenone and •quinidine (increased risk of ventricular arrhythmias—avoid concomitant use); amprenavir possibly increases plasma concentration of •lidocaine (lignocaine)—avoid concomitant use
- Antibacterials: plasma concentration of both drugs increased when amprenavir given with erythromycin; amprenavir increases plasma concentration of •rifabutin (reduce dose of rifabutin); plasma concentration of amprenavir significantly reduced by •rifampicin—avoid concomitant use; amprenavir possibly increases plasma concentration of dapsone

Anticoagulants: amprenavir may enhance or reduce anticoagulant effect of coumarins
- Antidepressants: plasma concentration of amprenavir reduced by •St John's wort—avoid concomitant use; amprenavir possibly increases side-effects of tricyclics

Antiepileptics: amprenavir possibly increases plasma concentration of carbamazepine; plasma concentration of amprenavir possibly reduced by phenytoin
Antifungals: amprenavir increases plasma concentration of ketoconazole; amprenavir possibly increases plasma concentration of itraconazole
- Antihistamines: amprenavir possibly increases plasma concentration of loratadine; increased risk of ventricular arrhythmias when amprenavir given with •terfenadine—avoid concomitant use

Antimuscarinics: avoidance of amprenavir advised by manufacturer of tolterodine
- Antipsychotics: amprenavir possibly inhibits metabolism of •aripiprazole (reduce dose of aripiprazole); amprenavir possibly increases plasma concentration of clozapine; amprenavir increases plasma concentration of •pimozide and •sertindole (increased risk of ventricular arrhythmias—avoid concomitant use)

Antivirals: plasma concentration of amprenavir reduced by efavirenz; plasma concentration of amprenavir reduced by lopinavir, effect on lopinavir plasma concentration not predictable; plasma concentration of amprenavir possibly reduced by nevirapine; plasma concentration of amprenavir increased by ritonavir
- Anxiolytics and Hypnotics: increased risk of prolonged sedation and respiratory depression when amprenavir given with •alprazolam, clonazepam, •clorazepate, •diazepam, •flurazepam or •midazolam

Barbiturates: plasma concentration of amprenavir possibly reduced by phenobarbital
Calcium-channel Blockers: amprenavir possibly increases plasma concentration of diltiazem, nicardipine, nifedipine and nimodipine
- Cilostazol: amprenavir possibly increases plasma concentration of •cilostazol—avoid concomitant use

Amprenavir *(continued)*
- Ergot Alkaloids: increased risk of ergotism when amprenavir given with •ergotamine and methysergide—avoid concomitant use
- Lipid-regulating Drugs: possible increased risk of myopathy when amprenavir given with atorvastatin; amprenavir possibly increases plasma concentration of •simvastatin—avoid concomitant use

Oestrogens: amprenavir possibly reduces contraceptive effect of oestrogens
Progestogens: amprenavir possibly reduces contraceptive effect of progestogens
Sildenafil: amprenavir possibly increases plasma concentration of sildenafil— reduce initial dose of sildenafil
Ulcer-healing Drugs: amprenavir possibly increases plasma concentration of cimetidine
Vardenafil: amprenavir possibly increases plasma concentration of vardenafil

Anabolic Steroids
- Anticoagulants: anabolic steroids enhance anticoagulant effect of •coumarins and •phenindione

Antidiabetics: anabolic steroids possibly enhance hypoglycaemic effect of antidiabetics

Anaesthetics, General
Note. See also Surgery and Long-term Medication, p. 625
- Adrenergic Neurone Blockers: enhanced hypotensive effect when general anaesthetics given with •adrenergic neurone blockers
- Alpha-blockers: enhanced hypotensive effect when general anaesthetics given with •alpha-blockers

Angiotensin-II Receptor Antagonists: enhanced hypotensive effect when general anaesthetics given with angiotensin-II receptor antagonists
Antibacterials: general anaesthetics possibly potentiate hepatotoxicity of isoniazid; effects of thiopental enhanced by sulphonamides; hypersensitivity-like reactions can occur when general anaesthetics given with intravenous vancomycin
- Antidepressants: Because of hazardous interactions between general anaesthetics and •MAOIs, MAOIs should normally be stopped 2 weeks before surgery; increased risk of arrhythmias and hypotension when general anaesthetics given with tricyclics
- Antipsychotics: enhanced hypotensive effect when general anaesthetics given with •antipsychotics

Anxiolytics and Hypnotics: increased sedative effect when general anaesthetics given with anxiolytics and hypnotics
Beta-blockers: enhanced hypotensive effect when general anaesthetics given with beta-blockers
- Calcium-channel Blockers: enhanced hypotensive effect when general anaesthetics or isoflurane given with calcium-channel blockers; general anaesthetics enhance hypotensive effect of •verapamil (also AV delay)

Clonidine: enhanced hypotensive effect when general anaesthetics given with clonidine
- Cytotoxics: nitrous oxide increases antifolate effect of •methotrexate—avoid concomitant use

Diazoxide: enhanced hypotensive effect when general anaesthetics given with diazoxide
Diuretics: enhanced hypotensive effect when general anaesthetics given with diuretics
- Dopaminergics: increased risk of arrhythmias when volatile liquid general anaesthetics given with •levodopa

Ergot Alkaloids: halothane reduces effects of ergometrine on the parturient uterus

Anaesthetics, General *(continued)*
- • Memantine: increased risk of CNS toxicity when ketamine given with •memantine (manufacturer of memantine advises avoid concomitant use)
- Methyldopa: enhanced hypotensive effect when general anaesthetics given with methyldopa
- Moxonidine: enhanced hypotensive effect when general anaesthetics given with moxonidine
- Muscle Relaxants: volatile liquid general anaesthetics enhance effects of non-depolarising muscle relaxants and suxamethonium
- Nitrates: enhanced hypotensive effect when general anaesthetics given with nitrates
- Oxytocin: oxytocic effect possibly reduced, also enhanced hypotensive effect and risk of arrhythmias when volatile liquid general anaesthetics given with oxytocin
- • Sympathomimetics: increased risk of arrhythmias when volatile liquid general anaesthetics given with •adrenaline (epinephrine); increased risk of hypertension when volatile liquid general anaesthetics given with •methylphenidate
- Theophylline: increased risk of convulsions when ketamine given with theophylline; increased risk of arrhythmias when halothane given with theophylline
- Vasodilator Antihypertensives: enhanced hypotensive effect when general anaesthetics given with hydralazine, minoxidil or nitroprusside

Anaesthetics, General (intravenous) *see* Anaesthetics, General

Anaesthetics, General (volatile liquids) *see* Anaesthetics, General

Anaesthetics, Local *see* Bupivacaine, Levobupivacaine, Lidocaine (lignocaine), Prilocaine, and Ropivacaine

Anagrelide
- • Cilostazol: manufacturer of anagrelide advises avoid concomitant use with •cilostazol
- • Phosphodiesterase Inhibitors: manufacturer of anagrelide advises avoid concomitant use with •enoximone and •milrinone

Anakinra
- • Adalimumab: avoid concomitant use of anakinra with •adalimumab
- • Etanercept: increased risk of side-effects when anakinra given with •etanercept—avoid concomitant use
- • Infliximab: avoid concomitant use of anakinra with •infliximab
- • Vaccines: avoid concomitant use of anakinra with live •vaccines (see p. 604)

Analgesics *see* Aspirin, Nefopam, NSAIDs, Opioid Analgesics, and Paracetamol

Angiotensin-II Receptor Antagonists
- ACE Inhibitors: enhanced hypotensive effect when angiotensin-II receptor antagonists given with ACE inhibitors
- Adrenergic Neurone Blockers: enhanced hypotensive effect when angiotensin-II receptor antagonists given with adrenergic neurone blockers
- Alcohol: enhanced hypotensive effect when angiotensin-II receptor antagonists given with alcohol
- Aldesleukin: enhanced hypotensive effect when angiotensin-II receptor antagonists given with aldesleukin
- Alpha-blockers: enhanced hypotensive effect when angiotensin-II receptor antagonists given with alpha-blockers
- Anaesthetics, General: enhanced hypotensive effect when angiotensin-II receptor antagonists given with general anaesthetics
- Analgesics: increased risk of renal impairment when angiotensin-II receptor antagonists given with NSAIDs, also hypotensive effect antagonised; increased risk of hyperkalaemia when angiotensin-II receptor antagonists given with ketorolac; risk of renal impairment when angiotensin-II receptor antagonists given with aspirin (in doses over 300 mg daily), also hypotensive effect antagonised
- Anticoagulants: increased risk of hyperkalaemia when angiotensin-II receptor antagonists given with heparin
- Antidepressants: hypotensive effect of angiotensin-II receptor antagonists possibly enhanced by MAOIs
- Antipsychotics: enhanced hypotensive effect when angiotensin-II receptor antagonists given with antipsychotics
- Anxiolytics and Hypnotics: enhanced hypotensive effect when angiotensin-II receptor antagonists given with anxiolytics and hypnotics
- Beta-blockers: enhanced hypotensive effect when angiotensin-II receptor antagonists given with beta-blockers
- Calcium-channel Blockers: enhanced hypotensive effect when angiotensin-II receptor antagonists given with calcium-channel blockers
- • Cardiac Glycosides: telmisartan increases plasma concentration of •digoxin
- • Ciclosporin: increased risk of hyperkalaemia when angiotensin-II receptor antagonists given with •ciclosporin
- Clonidine: enhanced hypotensive effect when angiotensin-II receptor antagonists given with clonidine
- Corticosteroids: hypotensive effect of angiotensin-II receptor antagonists antagonised by corticosteroids
- Diazoxide: enhanced hypotensive effect when angiotensin-II receptor antagonists given with diazoxide
- • Diuretics: enhanced hypotensive effect when angiotensin-II receptor antagonists given with •diuretics; increased risk of hyperkalaemia when angiotensin-II receptor antagonists given with •potassium-sparing diuretics and aldosterone antagonists
- Dopaminergics: enhanced hypotensive effect when angiotensin-II receptor antagonists given with levodopa
- Epoetin: antagonism of hypotensive effect and increased risk of hyperkalaemia when angiotensin-II receptor antagonists given with epoetin
- • Lithium: angiotensin-II receptor antagonists reduce excretion of •lithium (increased plasma concentration)
- Methyldopa: enhanced hypotensive effect when angiotensin-II receptor antagonists given with methyldopa
- Moxisylyte (thymoxamine): enhanced hypotensive effect when angiotensin-II receptor antagonists given with moxisylyte
- Moxonidine: enhanced hypotensive effect when angiotensin-II receptor antagonists given with moxonidine
- Muscle Relaxants: enhanced hypotensive effect when angiotensin-II receptor antagonists given with baclofen or tizanidine
- Nitrates: enhanced hypotensive effect when angiotensin-II receptor antagonists given with nitrates
- Oestrogens: hypotensive effect of angiotensin-II receptor antagonists antagonised by oestrogens

Angiotensin-II Receptor Antagonists *(continued)*

- Potassium Salts: increased risk of hyperkalaemia when angiotensin-II receptor antagonists given with •potassium salts

Progestogens: risk of hyperkalaemia when angiotensin-II receptor antagonists given with drospirenone (monitor serum potassium during first cycle)

Prostaglandins: enhanced hypotensive effect when angiotensin-II receptor antagonists given with alprostadil

Vasodilator Antihypertensives: enhanced hypotensive effect when angiotensin-II receptor antagonists given with hydralazine, minoxidil or nitroprusside

Anion-exchange Resins *see* Colestipol and Colestyramine

Antacids

Note. Antacids should preferably not be taken at the same time as other drugs since they may impair absorption

ACE Inhibitors: antacids possibly reduce absorption of ACE inhibitors; antacids reduce absorption of captopril, enalapril and fosinopril

Analgesics: antacids reduce absorption of diflunisal; alkaline urine due to some antacids increases excretion of aspirin

Anti-arrhythmics: alkaline urine due to some antacids reduces excretion of quinidine (plasma concentration of quinidine occasionally increased)

Antibacterials: antacids reduce absorption of azithromycin, cefaclor, cefpodoxime, ciprofloxacin, isoniazid, levofloxacin, moxifloxacin, norfloxacin, ofloxacin, rifampicin and tetracyclines; oral magnesium salts (as magnesium trisilicate) reduce absorption of nitrofurantoin

Antiepileptics: antacids reduce absorption of gabapentin and phenytoin

Antifungals: antacids reduce absorption of itraconazole and ketoconazole

Antihistamines: antacids reduce absorption of fexofenadine

Antimalarials: antacids reduce absorption of chloroquine and hydroxychloroquine; oral magnesium salts (as magnesium trisilicate) reduce absorption of proguanil

Antipsychotics: antacids reduce absorption of phenothiazines and sulpiride

Antivirals: antacids possibly reduce absorption of amprenavir; antacids possibly reduce plasma concentration of atazanavir; antacids reduce absorption of zalcitabine

Bile Acids: antacids possibly reduce absorption of bile acids

Bisphosphonates: antacids reduce absorption of bisphosphonates

Cardiac Glycosides: antacids possibly reduce absorption of digoxin

Corticosteroids: antacids reduce absorption of deflazacort

Cytotoxics: antacids reduce absorption of mycophenolate mofetil

Dipyridamole: antacids possibly reduce absorption of dipyridamole

Iron: oral magnesium salts (as magnesium trisilicate) reduce absorption of *oral* iron

Lipid-regulating Drugs: antacids reduce absorption of rosuvastatin

Lithium: sodium bicarbonate increases excretion of lithium (reduced plasma concentration)

Penicillamine: antacids reduce absorption of penicillamine

Ulcer-healing Drugs: antacids possibly reduce absorption of lansoprazole

Antazoline *see* Antihistamines

Anti-arrhythmics *see* Adenosine, Amiodarone, Bretylium, Disopyramide, Flecainide, Lidocaine (lignocaine), Mexiletine, Procainamide, Propafenone, and Quinidine

Antibacterials *see* individual drugs

Antibiotics (cytotoxic) *see* Bleomycin, Doxorubicin, Epirubicin

Anticoagulants *see* Coumarins, Heparins, and Phenindione

Antidepressants *see* Antidepressants, SSRI; Antidepressants, Tricyclic; Antidepressants, Tricyclic (related); MAOIs; Mirtazapine; Moclobemide; Reboxetine; St John's Wort; Tryptophan; Venlafaxine

Antidepressants, Noradrenaline Re-uptake Inhibitors *see* Reboxetine

Antidepressants, SSRI

Alcohol: sedative effects possibly increased when SSRIs given with alcohol

Anaesthetics, Local: fluvoxamine inhibits metabolism of ropivacaine—avoid prolonged administration of ropivacaine

- Analgesics: increased risk of bleeding when SSRIs given with •NSAIDs or •aspirin; fluvoxamine possibly increases plasma concentration of methadone; increased risk of CNS toxicity when SSRIs given with •tramadol
- Anti-arrhythmics: fluoxetine increases plasma concentration of flecainide; fluvoxamine inhibits metabolism of •mexiletine (increased risk of toxicity); paroxetine possibly inhibits metabolism of propafenone (increased risk of toxicity)
- Anticoagulants: SSRIs possibly enhance anticoagulant effect of •coumarins
- Antidepressants: avoidance of fluvoxamine advised by manufacturer of •reboxetine; possible increased serotonergic effects when SSRIs given with duloxetine; fluvoxamine inhibits metabolism of •duloxetine—avoid concomitant use; citalopram, escitalopram, fluvoxamine or paroxetine should not be started until 2 weeks after stopping •MAOIs, also MAOIs should not be started until at least 1 week after stopping citalopram, escitalopram, fluvoxamine or paroxetine; fluoxetine should not be started until 2 weeks after stopping •MAOIs, also MAOIs should not be started until at least 5 weeks after stopping fluoxetine; CNS effects of SSRIs increased by •MAOIs (risk of serious toxicity); sertraline should not be started until 2 weeks after stopping •MAOIs, also MAOIs should not be started until at least 2 weeks after stopping sertraline; increased risk of CNS toxicity when escitalopram given with •moclobemide, preferably avoid concomitant use; after stopping citalopram, fluvoxamine or paroxetine do not start •moclobemide for at least 1 week; after stopping fluoxetine do not start •moclobemide for 5 weeks; after stopping sertraline do not start •moclobemide for 2 weeks; increased serotonergic effects when SSRIs given with •St John's wort—avoid concomitant use; SSRIs increase plasma concentration of some •tricyclics; agitation and nausea may occur when SSRIs given with •tryptophan
- Antiepileptics: SSRIs antagonise anticonvulsant effect of •antiepileptics (convulsive threshold lowered); fluoxetine and fluvoxamine increase plasma concentration of •carbamazepine; plasma concentration of paroxetine reduced by carbamazepine, phenytoin and primidone; fluoxetine and fluvoxamine increase plasma concentration of •phenytoin

Antidepressants, SSRI *(continued)*

- Antihistamines: increased risk of ventricular arrhythmias when citalopram, fluoxetine or fluvoxamine given with •terfenadine—avoid concomitant use; antidepressant effect of SSRIs possibly antagonised by cyproheptadine
- Antimalarials: avoidance of antidepressants advised by manufacturer of •artemether/lumefantrine

Antimuscarinics: paroxetine increases plasma concentration of procyclidine

- Antipsychotics: fluoxetine increases plasma concentration of •clozapine, •haloperidol, risperidone, •sertindole and •zotepine; paroxetine inhibits metabolism of perphenazine (reduce dose of perphenazine); fluoxetine and paroxetine possibly inhibit metabolism of •aripiprazole (reduce dose of aripiprazole); fluvoxamine, paroxetine and sertraline increase plasma concentration of •clozapine; fluvoxamine increases plasma concentration of olanzapine; sertraline increases plasma concentration of •pimozide (increased risk of ventricular arrhythmias—avoid concomitant use); paroxetine increases plasma concentration of •sertindole
- Antivirals: plasma concentration of sertraline reduced by efavirenz; plasma concentration of SSRIs possibly increased by •ritonavir

Anxiolytics and Hypnotics: fluvoxamine increases plasma concentration of some benzodiazepines; sedative effects possibly increased when sertraline given with zolpidem

Barbiturates: SSRIs antagonise anticonvulsant effect of barbiturates (convulsive threshold lowered); plasma concentration of paroxetine reduced by phenobarbital

Beta-blockers: fluvoxamine increases plasma concentration of propranolol

- Dopaminergics: caution with paroxetine advised by manufacturer of entacapone; increased risk of hypertension and CNS excitation when paroxetine or sertraline given with •selegiline (selegiline should not be started until 2 weeks after stopping paroxetine or sertraline, avoid paroxetine or sertraline for 2 weeks after stopping selegiline); increased risk of hypertension and CNS excitation when fluvoxamine given with •selegiline (selegiline should not be started until 1 week after stopping fluvoxamine, avoid fluvoxamine for 2 weeks after stopping selegiline); increased risk of hypertension and CNS excitation when fluoxetine given with •selegiline (selegiline should not be started until 5 weeks after stopping fluoxetine, avoid fluoxetine for 2 weeks after stopping selegiline); theoretical risk of serotonin syndrome if citalopram given with selegiline (especially if dose of selegiline exceeds 10 mg daily); manufacturer of escitalopram advises caution with selegiline
- $5HT_1$ Agonists: possible increased serotonergic effects when SSRIs given with frovatriptan; fluvoxamine possibly inhibits metabolism of frovatriptan; increased risk of CNS toxicity when citalopram, escitalopram, fluoxetine, fluvoxamine or paroxetine given with •sumatriptan; increased risk of CNS toxicity when sertraline given with •sumatriptan (manufacturer of sertraline advises avoid concomitant use); fluvoxamine possibly inhibits metabolism of zolmitriptan (reduce dose of zolmitriptan)
- Lithium: Increased risk of CNS effects when SSRIs given with •lithium (lithium toxicity reported)

Parasympathomimetics: paroxetine increases plasma concentration of galantamine

Antidepressants, SSRI *(continued)*

- Sibutramine: increased risk of CNS toxicity when SSRIs given with •sibutramine (manufacturer of sibutramine advises avoid concomitant use)

Sympathomimetics: metabolism of SSRIs possibly inhibited by methylphenidate

- Theophylline: fluvoxamine increases plasma concentration of •theophylline (concomitant use should usually be avoided, but where not possible halve theophylline dose and monitor plasma-theophylline concentration)

Ulcer-healing Drugs: plasma concentration of sertraline increased by cimetidine

Antidepressants, SSRI (related) *see* Duloxetine and Venlafaxine

Antidepressants, Tricyclic

Adrenergic Neurone Blockers: tricyclics antagonise hypotensive effect of adrenergic neurone blockers

- Alcohol: increased sedative effect when tricyclics given with •alcohol

Alpha$_2$-adrenoceptor Stimulants: avoidance of tricyclics advised by manufacturer of apraclonidine and brimonidine

Anaesthetics, General: increased risk of arrhythmias and hypotension when tricyclics given with general anaesthetics

- Analgesics: increased risk of CNS toxicity when tricyclics given with •tramadol; side-effects possibly increased when tricyclics given with nefopam; sedative effects possibly increased when tricyclics given with opioid analgesics
- Anti-arrhythmics: increased risk of ventricular arrhythmias when tricyclics given with •amiodarone—avoid concomitant use; increased risk of ventricular arrhythmias when tricyclics given with •disopyramide, •flecainide, •procainamide or •quinidine; increased risk of arrhythmias when tricyclics given with •propafenone
- Antibacterials: increased risk of ventricular arrhythmias when tricyclics given with •moxifloxacin—avoid concomitant use; plasma concentration of tricyclics possibly reduced by rifampicin
- Anticoagulants: tricyclics may enhance or reduce anticoagulant effect of •coumarins
- Antidepressants: possible increased serotonergic effects when amitriptyline or clomipramine given with duloxetine; increased risk of hypertension and CNS excitation when tricyclics given with •MAOIs, tricyclics should not be started until 2 weeks after stopping MAOIs (3 weeks if starting clomipramine or imipramine), also MAOIs should not be started for at least 1–2 weeks after stopping tricyclics (3 weeks in the case of clomipramine or imipramine); after stopping tricyclics do not start •moclobemide for at least 1 week; plasma concentration of some tricyclics increased by •SSRIs; plasma concentration of amitriptyline reduced by St John's wort
- Antiepileptics: tricyclics antagonise anticonvulsant effect of •antiepileptics (convulsive threshold lowered); metabolism of tricyclics accelerated by •carbamazepine (reduced plasma concentration and reduced effect); plasma concentration of tricyclics possibly reduced by •phenytoin; tricyclics antagonises anticonvulsant effect of •primidone (convulsive threshold lowered), also metabolism of tricyclics possibly accelerated (reduced plasma concentration)

Antifungals: plasma concentration of imipramine and nortriptyline possibly increased by terbinafine

- Antihistamines: increased risk of ventricular arrhythmias when tricyclics given with •terfenadine—avoid concomitant use; increased antimuscarinic

Antidepressants, Tricyclic

- Antihistamines *(continued)* and sedative effects when tricyclics given with antihistamines
- Antimalarials: avoidance of antidepressants advised by manufacturer of •artemether/lumefantrine

Antimuscarinics: increased risk of antimuscarinic side-effects when tricyclics given with antimuscarinics

- Antipsychotics: plasma concentration of tricyclics increased by •antipsychotics—possibly increased risk of ventricular arrhythmias; possibly increased antimuscarinic side-effects when tricyclics given with clozapine; increased risk of antimuscarinic side-effects when tricyclics given with phenothiazines; increased risk of ventricular arrhythmias when tricyclics given with •pimozide—avoid concomitant use
- Antivirals: side-effects of tricyclics possibly increased by amprenavir; plasma concentration of tricyclics possibly increased by •ritonavir

Anxiolytics and Hypnotics: increased sedative effect when tricyclics given with anxiolytics and hypnotics

- Barbiturates: tricyclics antagonises anticonvulsant effect of •barbiturates (convulsive threshold lowered), also metabolism of tricyclics possibly accelerated (reduced plasma concentration)
- Beta-blockers: increased risk of ventricular arrhythmias when tricyclics given with •sotalol

Calcium-channel Blockers: plasma concentration of imipramine increased by diltiazem and verapamil; plasma concentration of tricyclics possibly increased by diltiazem and verapamil

- Clonidine: tricyclics antagonise hypotensive effect of •clonidine, also increased risk of hypertension on clonidine withdrawal

Disulfiram: metabolism of tricyclics inhibited by disulfiram (increased plasma concentration); concomitant amitriptyline reported to increase disulfiram reaction with alcohol

Diuretics: increased risk of postural hypotension when tricyclics given with diuretics

- Dopaminergics: caution with tricyclics advised by manufacturer of entacapone; CNS toxicity reported when tricyclics given with •selegiline

Lithium: risk of toxicity when tricyclics given with lithium

Muscle Relaxants: tricyclics enhance muscle relaxant effect of baclofen

Nicorandil: tricyclics possibly enhance hypotensive effect of nicorandil

Nitrates: tricyclics reduce effects of sublingual tablets of nitrates (failure to dissolve under tongue owing to dry mouth)

Oestrogens: antidepressant effect of tricyclics antagonised by oestrogens (but side-effects of tricyclics possibly increased due to increased plasma concentration)

- Sibutramine: increased risk of CNS toxicity when tricyclics given with •sibutramine (manufacturer of sibutramine advises avoid concomitant use)
- Sympathomimetics: increased risk of hypertension and arrhythmias when tricyclics given with •adrenaline (epinephrine) (but local anaesthetics with adrenaline appear to be safe); metabolism of tricyclics possibly inhibited by methylphenidate; increased risk of hypertension and arrhythmias when tricyclics given with •noradrenaline (norepinephrine)

Thyroid Hormones: effects of tricyclics possibly enhanced by thyroid hormones; effects of amitriptyline and imipramine enhanced by thyroid hormones

Ulcer-healing Drugs: plasma concentration of tricyclics possibly increased by cimetidine; metabolism of amitriptyline, doxepin, imipramine and nortriptyline inhibited by cimetidine (increased plasma concentration)

Antidepressants, Tricyclic (related)

- Alcohol: increased sedative effect when tricyclic-related antidepressants given with •alcohol

Alpha$_2$-adrenoceptor Stimulants: avoidance of tricyclic-related antidepressants advised by manufacturer of apraclonidine and brimonidine

- Antidepressants: tricyclic-related antidepressants should not be started until 2 weeks after stopping •MAOIs, also MAOIs should not be started until at least 1–2 weeks after stopping tricyclic-related antidepressants; after stopping tricyclic-related antidepressants do not start •moclobemide for at least 1 week
- Antiepileptics: tricyclic-related antidepressants possibly antagonise anticonvulsant effect of •antiepileptics (convulsive threshold lowered); plasma concentration of mianserin reduced by •carbamazepine and •phenytoin; metabolism of mianserin accelerated by •primidone (reduced plasma concentration)

Antihistamines: possible increased antimuscarinic and sedative effects when tricyclic-related antidepressants given with antihistamines

- Antimalarials: avoidance of antidepressants advised by manufacturer of •artemether/lumefantrine

Antimuscarinics: possibly increased antimuscarinic side-effects when tricyclic-related antidepressants given with antimuscarinics

- Antipsychotics: increased risk of ventricular arrhythmias when maprotiline given with •pimozide—avoid concomitant use

Anxiolytics and Hypnotics: increased sedative effect when tricyclic-related antidepressants given with anxiolytics and hypnotics

- Barbiturates: tricyclic-related antidepressants possibly antagonise anticonvulsant effect of •barbiturates (convulsive threshold lowered); metabolism of mianserin accelerated by •phenobarbital (reduced plasma concentration)

Diazoxide: enhanced hypotensive effect when tricyclic-related antidepressants given with diazoxide

Dopaminergics: caution with maprotiline advised by manufacturer of entacapone

Nitrates: tricyclic-related antidepressants possibly reduce effects of sublingual tablets of nitrates (failure to dissolve under tongue owing to dry mouth)

- Sibutramine: increased risk of CNS toxicity when tricyclic-related antidepressants given with •sibutramine (manufacturer of sibutramine advises avoid concomitant use)

Vasodilator Antihypertensives: enhanced hypotensive effect when tricyclic-related antidepressants given with hydralazine or nitroprusside

Antidiabetics

ACE Inhibitors: hypoglycaemic effect of insulin, metformin and sulphonylureas possibly enhanced by ACE inhibitors

Alcohol: hypoglycaemic effect of antidiabetics enhanced by alcohol; increased risk of lactic acidosis when metformin given with alcohol; flushing, in susceptible subjects, when chlorpropamide given with alcohol

Antidiabetics *(continued)*

Anabolic Steroids: hypoglycaemic effect of antidiabetics possibly enhanced by anabolic steroids

- Analgesics: effects of sulphonylureas possibly enhanced by •NSAIDs
- Antibacterials: hypoglycaemic effect of acarbose possibly enhanced by neomycin, also severity of gastro-intestinal effects increased; effects of repaglinide enhanced by clarithromycin; effects of glibenclamide possibly enhanced by ciprofloxacin and norfloxacin; plasma concentration of nateglinide and repaglinide reduced by rifampicin; plasma concentration of rosiglitazone reduced by •rifampicin—consider increasing dose of rosiglitazone; effects of sulphonylureas enhanced by •chloramphenicol; metabolism of chlorpropamide and tolbutamide accelerated by •rifamycins (reduced effect); metabolism of sulphonylureas possibly accelerated by •rifamycins (reduced effect); effects of sulphonylureas rarely enhanced by sulphonamides and trimethoprim
- Anticoagulants: hypoglycaemic effect of sulphonylureas possibly enhanced by •coumarins, also possible changes to anticoagulant effect

Antidepressants: hypoglycaemic effect of insulin, metformin and sulphonylureas enhanced by MAOIs; hypoglycaemic effect of antidiabetics possibly enhanced by MAOIs

Antiepileptics: tolbutamide transiently increases plasma concentration of phenytoin (possibility of toxicity)

- Antifungals: plasma concentration of sulphonylureas increased by •fluconazole and •miconazole; hypoglycaemic effect of gliclazide and glipizide enhanced by •miconazole— avoid concomitant use; hypoglycaemic effect of nateglinide possibly enhanced by fluconazole; plasma concentration of sulphonylureas possibly increased by voriconazole

Antihistamines: thrombocyte count depressed when metformin given with ketotifen

Antipsychotics: hypoglycaemic effect of sulphonylureas possibly antagonised by phenothiazines

Antivirals: plasma concentration of tolbutamide possibly increased by ritonavir

Aprepitant: plasma concentration of tolbutamide reduced by aprepitant

Beta-blockers: warning signs of hypoglycaemia (such as tremor) with antidiabetics may be masked when given with beta-blockers; hypoglycaemic effect of insulin enhanced by beta-blockers

- Bosentan: plasma concentration of both drugs reduced when glibenclamide given with •bosentan (avoid concomitant use)

Calcium-channel Blockers: glucose tolerance occasionally impaired when insulin given with nifedipine

Cardiac Glycosides: acarbose possibly reduces plasma concentration of digoxin

Corticosteroids: hypoglycaemic effect of antidiabetics antagonised by corticosteroids

Cytotoxics: metabolism of rosiglitazone possibly inhibited by paclitaxel

Diazoxide: hypoglycaemic effect of antidiabetics antagonised by diazoxide

Diuretics: hypoglycaemic effect of antidiabetics antagonised by loop diuretics and thiazides and related diuretics; increased risk of hyponatraemia when chlorpropamide given with potassium-sparing diuretics and aldosterone antagonists plus *thiazide*; increased risk of hyponatraemia when chlorpropamide given with thiazides and related diuretics plus potassium-sparing diuretic

Antidiabetics *(continued)*

Hormone Antagonists: possible acceleration of the metabolism of biguanides and sulphonylureas advised by manufacturer of aminoglutethimide; requirements for insulin, metformin, repaglinide and sulphonylureas possibly reduced by lanreotide; requirements for insulin, metformin, repaglinide and sulphonylureas possibly reduced by octreotide

Leflunomide: hypoglycaemic effect of tolbutamide possibly enhanced by leflunomide

- Lipid-regulating Drugs: hypoglycaemic effect of acarbose possibly enhanced by colestyramine; hypoglycaemic effect of nateglinide possibly enhanced by gemfibrozil; increased risk of severe hypoglycaemia when repaglinide given with •gemfibrozil—avoid concomitant use; plasma concentration of rosiglitazone increased by •gemfibrozil (consider reducing dose of rosiglitazone); may be improved glucose tolerance and an additive effect when insulin or sulphonylureas given with fibrates

Oestrogens: hypoglycaemic effect of antidiabetics antagonised by oestrogens

Orlistat: avoidance of acarbose advised by manufacturer of orlistat

Pancreatin: hypoglycaemic effect of acarbose antagonised by pancreatin

Probenecid: hypoglycaemic effect of chlorpropamide possibly enhanced by probenecid

Progestogens: hypoglycaemic effect of antidiabetics antagonised by progestogens

- Sulfinpyrazone: effects of sulphonylureas enhanced by •sulfinpyrazone

Testosterone: hypoglycaemic effect of antidiabetics possibly enhanced by testosterone

Ulcer-healing Drugs: excretion of metformin reduced by cimetidine (increased plasma concentration); hypoglycaemic effect of sulphonylureas enhanced by cimetidine

Antiepileptics *see* Carbamazepine, Ethosuximide, Gabapentin, Lamotrigine, Levetiracetam, Oxcarbazepine, Phenytoin, Primidone, Tiagabine, Topiramate, Valproate, Vigabatrin, and Zonisamide

Antifungals *see* Amphotericin; Antifungals, Imidazole; Antifungals, Triazole; Caspofungin; Flucytosine; Griseofulvin; Terbinafine

Antifungals, Imidazole

- Analgesics: ketoconazole inhibits metabolism of alfentanil (risk of prolonged or delayed respiratory depression); ketoconazole inhibits metabolism of •buprenorphine (reduce dose of buprenorphine)

Antacids: absorption of ketoconazole reduced by antacids

- Anti-arrhythmics: miconazole increases plasma concentration of •quinidine (increased risk of ventricular arrhythmias—avoid concomitant use)
- Antibacterials: metabolism of ketoconazole accelerated by •rifampicin (reduced plasma concentration), also plasma concentration of rifampicin may be reduced by ketoconazole; plasma concentration of ketoconazole possibly reduced by isoniazid
- Anticoagulants: ketoconazole enhances anticoagulant effect of •coumarins; miconazole enhances anticoagulant effect of •coumarins (miconazole oral gel and possibly vaginal formulations absorbed)
- Antidepressants: avoidance of imidazoles advised by manufacturer of •reboxetine; ketoconazole increases plasma concentration of mirtazapine
- Antidiabetics: miconazole enhances hypoglycaemic effect of •gliclazide and •glipizide— avoid concomitant use; miconazole increases plasma concentration of •sulphonylureas

Antifungals, Imidazole *(continued)*

- Antiepileptics: miconazole possibly increases plasma concentration of carbamazepine; plasma concentration of ketoconazole reduced by •phenytoin; miconazole enhances anticonvulsant effect of •phenytoin (plasma concentration of phenytoin increased)

Antifungals: imidazoles possibly antagonise effects of amphotericin

- Antihistamines: manufacturer of loratadine advises ketoconazole possibly increases plasma concentration of loratadine; imidazoles possibly inhibit metabolism of •mizolastine (avoid concomitant use); ketoconazole inhibits metabolism of •mizolastine—avoid concomitant use; imidazoles inhibit metabolism of •terfenadine—risk of ventricular arrhythmias, avoid concomitant use of systemic or topical preparations
- Antimalarials: avoidance of imidazoles advised by manufacturer of •artemether/lumefantrine

Antimuscarinics: absorption of ketoconazole reduced by antimuscarinics; ketoconazole increases plasma concentration of solifenacin; avoidance of ketoconazole advised by manufacturer of tolterodine

- Antipsychotics: ketoconazole inhibits metabolism of •aripiprazole (reduce dose of aripiprazole); increased risk of ventricular arrhythmias when imidazoles given with •pimozide—avoid concomitant use; imidazoles possibly increase plasma concentration of quetiapine (reduce dose of quetiapine); increased risk of ventricular arrhythmias when ketoconazole given with •sertindole—avoid concomitant use; possible increased risk of ventricular arrhythmias when imidazoles given with •sertindole—avoid concomitant use
- Antivirals: plasma concentration of ketoconazole increased by amprenavir; ketoconazole inhibits the metabolism of indinavir; plasma concentration of ketoconazole reduced by •nevirapine—avoid concomitant use; combination of ketoconazole with •ritonavir may increase plasma concentration of either drug (or both); ketoconazole increases plasma concentration of saquinavir; imidazoles possibly increase plasma concentration of saquinavir
- Anxiolytics and Hypnotics: ketoconazole increases plasma concentration of •midazolam (risk of prolonged sedation)

Aprepitant: ketoconazole increases plasma concentration of aprepitant

Bosentan: ketoconazole possibly increases plasma concentration of bosentan

- Calcium-channel Blockers: ketoconazole inhibits metabolism of •felodipine (increased plasma concentration); avoidance of ketoconazole advised by manufacturer of lercanidipine; ketoconazole possibly inhibits metabolism of dihydropyridines (increased plasma concentration)
- Ciclosporin: ketoconazole inhibits metabolism of •ciclosporin (increased plasma concentration); miconazole possibly inhibits metabolism of •ciclosporin (increased plasma concentration)
- Cilostazol: ketoconazole possibly increases plasma concentration of •cilostazol—avoid concomitant use

Cinacalcet: ketoconazole inhibits metabolism of cinacalcet (increased plasma concentration)

Corticosteroids: ketoconazole possibly inhibits metabolism of corticosteroids; ketoconazole inhibits the metabolism of methylprednisolone; ketoconazole increases plasma concentration of inhaled mometasone

Antifungals, Imidazole *(continued)*

Cytotoxics: *in vitro* studies suggest a possible interaction between ketoconazole and docetaxel (consult docetaxel product literature); ketoconazole increases plasma concentration of imatinib

- Diuretics: ketoconazole increases plasma concentration of •eplerenone—avoid concomitant use
- Ergot Alkaloids: increased risk of ergotism when imidazoles given with •ergotamine and methysergide—avoid concomitant use
- $5HT_1$ Agonists: ketoconazole increases plasma concentration of •eletriptan (risk of toxicity)—avoid concomitant use
- Lipid-regulating Drugs: possible increased risk of myopathy when imidazoles given with atorvastatin or simvastatin; increased risk of myopathy when ketoconazole given with •simvastatin (avoid concomitant use); possible increased risk of myopathy when miconazole given with •simvastatin—avoid concomitant use

Oestrogens: anecdotal reports of contraceptive failure when imidazoles or ketoconazole given with oestrogens

Parasympathomimetics: ketoconazole increases plasma concentration of galantamine

Sildenafil: ketoconazole increases plasma concentration of sildenafil—reduce initial dose of sildenafil

- Sirolimus: ketoconazole increases plasma concentration of •sirolimus—avoid concomitant use; miconazole increases plasma concentration of •sirolimus
- Tacrolimus: imidazoles possibly increase plasma concentration of •tacrolimus; ketoconazole increases plasma concentration of •tacrolimus

Tadalafil: ketoconazole increases plasma concentration of tadalafil

- Theophylline: ketoconazole possibly increases plasma concentration of •theophylline

Ulcer-healing Drugs: absorption of ketoconazole reduced by histamine H_2-antagonists, proton pump inhibitors and sucralfate

- Vardenafil: ketoconazole increases plasma concentration of •vardenafil—avoid concomitant use

Antifungals, Polyene *see* Amphotericin

Antifungals, Triazole

Note. In general, fluconazole interactions relate to multiple-dose treatment

- Analgesics: fluconazole increases plasma concentration of celecoxib (halve dose of celecoxib); fluconazole increases plasma concentration of parecoxib (reduce dose of parecoxib); fluconazole inhibits metabolism of alfentanil (risk of prolonged or delayed respiratory depression); itraconazole possibly inhibits metabolism of alfentanil; voriconazole increases plasma concentration of •methadone (consider reducing dose of methadone)

Antacids: absorption of itraconazole reduced by antacids

- Anti-arrhythmics: itraconazole and voriconazole increase plasma concentration of •quinidine (increased risk of ventricular arrhythmias—avoid concomitant use)
- Antibacterials: plasma concentration of itraconazole increased by clarithromycin; triazoles possibly increase plasma concentration of •rifabutin (increased risk of uveitis—reduce rifabutin dose); voriconazole increases plasma concentration of •rifabutin, also rifabutin reduces plasma concentration of voriconazole (increase dose of voriconazole and also monitor for rifabutin toxicity); fluconazole increases plasma concentration of •rifabutin (increased risk of uveitis—reduce

Antifungals, Triazole

- Antibacterials *(continued)* rifabutin dose); plasma concentration of itraconazole reduced by •rifabutin—avoid concomitant use; plasma concentration of voriconazole reduced by •rifampicin—avoid concomitant use; metabolism of fluconazole and itraconazole accelerated by •rifampicin (reduced plasma concentration)
- Anticoagulants: fluconazole, itraconazole and voriconazole enhance anticoagulant effect of •coumarins
- Antidepressants: avoidance of triazoles advised by manufacturer of •reboxetine
- Antidiabetics: fluconazole possibly enhances hypoglycaemic effect of nateglinide; fluconazole increases plasma concentration of •sulphonylureas; voriconazole possibly increases plasma concentration of sulphonylureas
- Antiepileptics: plasma concentration of voriconazole possibly reduced by •carbamazepine and •primidone—avoid concomitant use; plasma concentration of itraconazole possibly reduced by carbamazepine; fluconazole increases plasma concentration of •phenytoin (consider reducing dose of phenytoin); voriconazole increases plasma concentration of •phenytoin, also phenytoin reduces plasma concentration of voriconazole (increase dose of voriconazole and also monitor for phenytoin toxicity); plasma concentration of itraconazole reduced by •phenytoin—avoid concomitant use

Antifungals: triazoles possibly antagonise effects of amphotericin

- Antihistamines: itraconazole inhibits metabolism of •mizolastine—avoid concomitant use; triazoles inhibit metabolism of •terfenadine—risk of ventricular arrhythmias, avoid concomitant use of systemic or topical preparations
- Antimalarials: avoidance of triazoles advised by manufacturer of •artemether/lumefantrine

Antimuscarinics: itraconazole increases plasma concentration of solifenacin; avoidance of itraconazole advised by manufacturer of tolterodine

- Antipsychotics: itraconazole possibly inhibits metabolism of •aripiprazole (reduce dose of aripiprazole); increased risk of ventricular arrhythmias when triazoles given with •pimozide—avoid concomitant use; triazoles possibly increase plasma concentration of quetiapine (reduce dose of quetiapine); possible increased risk of ventricular arrhythmias when triazoles given with •sertindole—avoid concomitant use; increased risk of ventricular arrhythmias when itraconazole given with •sertindole—avoid concomitant use
- Antivirals: plasma concentration of itraconazole possibly increased by amprenavir; plasma concentration of voriconazole reduced by •efavirenz, also plasma concentration of efavirenz increased (avoid concomitant use); itraconazole increases plasma concentration of •indinavir (consider reducing dose of indinavir); fluconazole increases plasma concentration of •nevirapine and ritonavir; plasma concentration of voriconazole reduced by •ritonavir—avoid concomitant use; combination of itraconazole with •ritonavir may increase plasma concentration of either drug (or both); triazoles possibly increase plasma concentration of saquinavir; fluconazole increases plasma concentration of •zidovudine (increased risk of toxicity)
- Anxiolytics and Hypnotics: itraconazole increases plasma concentration of alprazolam; fluconazole and itraconazole increase plasma concentration of •midazolam (risk of prolonged sedation); itraconazole increases plasma concentration of buspirone (reduce dose of buspirone)
- Barbiturates: plasma concentration of itraconazole possibly reduced by phenobarbital; plasma concentration of voriconazole possibly reduced by •phenobarbital—avoid concomitant use
- Bosentan: fluconazole increases plasma concentration of •bosentan—avoid concomitant use; itraconazole possibly increases plasma concentration of bosentan
- Calcium-channel Blockers: negative inotropic effect possibly increased when itraconazole given with calcium-channel blockers; itraconazole inhibits metabolism of •felodipine (increased plasma concentration); avoidance of itraconazole advised by manufacturer of lercanidipine; itraconazole possibly inhibits metabolism of dihydropyridines (increased plasma concentration)
- Cardiac Glycosides: itraconazole increases plasma concentration of •digoxin
- Ciclosporin: fluconazole, itraconazole and voriconazole inhibit metabolism of •ciclosporin (increased plasma concentration)

Corticosteroids: itraconazole possibly inhibits metabolism of methylprednisolone

- Cytotoxics: itraconazole inhibits metabolism of busulfan (increased risk of toxicity); itraconazole possibly inhibits metabolism of •vincristine (increased risk of neurotoxicity)
- Diuretics: fluconazole increases plasma concentration of eplerenone (reduce dose of eplerenone); itraconazole increases plasma concentration of •eplerenone—avoid concomitant use; plasma concentration of fluconazole increased by hydrochlorothiazide
- Ergot Alkaloids: increased risk of ergotism when triazoles given with •ergotamine and methysergide—avoid concomitant use
- $5HT_1$ Agonists: itraconazole increases plasma concentration of •eletriptan (risk of toxicity)—avoid concomitant use
- Lipid-regulating Drugs: possible increased risk of myopathy when triazoles given with atorvastatin or simvastatin; increased risk of myopathy when itraconazole given with •atorvastatin or •simvastatin (avoid concomitant use)

Oestrogens: anecdotal reports of contraceptive failure when fluconazole or itraconazole given with oestrogens

Sildenafil: itraconazole increases plasma concentration of sildenafil—reduce initial dose of sildenafil

- Sirolimus: itraconazole and voriconazole increase plasma concentration of •sirolimus—avoid concomitant use
- Tacrolimus: triazoles possibly increase plasma concentration of •tacrolimus; fluconazole and voriconazole increase plasma concentration of •tacrolimus

Tadalafil: itraconazole possibly increases plasma concentration of tadalafil

- Theophylline: fluconazole possibly increases plasma concentration of •theophylline

Ulcer-healing Drugs: voriconazole increases plasma concentration of omeprazole (reduce dose of omeprazole); absorption of itraconazole reduced by histamine H_2-antagonists and proton pump inhibitors

- Vardenafil: itraconazole possibly increases plasma concentration of •vardenafil—avoid concomitant use

Antihistamines

Note. Sedative interactions apply to a lesser extent to the non-sedating antihistamines. Interactions do not generally apply to antihistamines used for topical action (including inhalation)

Alcohol: increased sedative effect when antihistamines given with alcohol (possibly less effect with non-sedating antihistamines)

Antacids: absorption of fexofenadine reduced by antacids

• Anti-arrhythmics: increased risk of ventricular arrhythmias when terfenadine given with •anti-arrhythmics; increased risk of ventricular arrhythmias when mizolastine or terfenadine given with •amiodarone—avoid concomitant use; increased risk of ventricular arrhythmias when mizolastine or terfenadine given with •disopyramide—avoid concomitant use; increased risk of ventricular arrhythmias when mizolastine or terfenadine given with •flecainide—avoid concomitant use; increased risk of ventricular arrhythmias when mizolastine or terfenadine given with •mexiletine—avoid concomitant use; increased risk of ventricular arrhythmias when mizolastine or terfenadine given with •procainamide—avoid concomitant use; increased risk of ventricular arrhythmias when mizolastine or terfenadine given with •propafenone—avoid concomitant use; increased risk of ventricular arrhythmias when mizolastine or terfenadine given with •quinidine—avoid concomitant use

• Antibacterials: metabolism of terfenadine inhibited by •clarithromycin (avoid concomitant use—increased risk of ventricular arrhythmias); manufacturer of loratadine advises plasma concentration possibly increased by erythromycin; metabolism of mizolastine inhibited by •erythromycin—avoid concomitant use; metabolism of terfenadine inhibited by •erythromycin—risk of ventricular arrhythmias, avoid concomitant use of systemic or topical preparations; increased risk of ventricular arrhythmias when mizolastine or terfenadine given with •moxifloxacin—avoid concomitant use; metabolism of mizolastine possibly inhibited by •macrolides (avoid concomitant use); increased risk of ventricular arrhythmias when terfenadine given with •quinupristin/dalfopristin or •telithromycin—avoid concomitant use

• Antidepressants: increased risk of ventricular arrhythmias when terfenadine given with •citalopram, •fluoxetine, •fluvoxamine or •tricyclics—avoid concomitant use; increased antimuscarinic and sedative effects when antihistamines given with MAOIs or tricyclics; cyproheptadine possibly antagonises antidepressant effect of SSRIs; possible increased antimuscarinic and sedative effects when antihistamines given with tricyclic-related antidepressants

Antidiabetics: thrombocyte count depressed when ketotifen given with metformin

• Antifungals: manufacturer of loratadine advises plasma concentration possibly increased by ketoconazole; metabolism of mizolastine inhibited by •itraconazole or •ketoconazole—avoid concomitant use; metabolism of terfenadine inhibited by •imidazoles and •triazoles—risk of ventricular arrhythmias, avoid concomitant use of systemic or topical preparations; metabolism of mizolastine possibly inhibited by •imidazoles (avoid concomitant use)

• Antimalarials: avoidance of terfenadine advised by manufacturer of •artemether/lumefantrine (risk of ventricular arrhythmias); increased risk of ventricular arrhythmias when terfenadine given with •quinine—avoid concomitant use

Antimuscarinics: increased risk of antimuscarinic side-effects when antihistamines given with antimuscarinics

• Antipsychotics: increased risk of ventricular arrhythmias when terfenadine given with •antipsychotics; increased risk of ventricular arrhythmias when terfenadine given with •pimozide or •sertindole—avoid concomitant use

• Antivirals: increased risk of ventricular arrhythmias when terfenadine given with •amprenavir, •efavirenz, •indinavir, •nelfinavir, •ritonavir or •saquinavir—avoid concomitant use; plasma concentration of loratadine possibly increased by amprenavir; plasma concentration of terfenadine possibly increased by •atazanavir—avoid concomitant use; plasma concentration of chlorphenamine (chlorpheniramine) possibly increased by lopinavir; plasma concentration of non-sedating antihistamines possibly increased by ritonavir

Anxiolytics and Hypnotics: increased sedative effect when antihistamines given with anxiolytics and hypnotics

• Aprepitant: avoidance of terfenadine advised by manufacturer of •aprepitant

• Beta-blockers: increased risk of ventricular arrhythmias when mizolastine or terfenadine given with •sotalol—avoid concomitant use

Betahistine: antihistamines theoretically antagonise effect of betahistine

Cytotoxics: *in vitro* studies suggest a possible interaction between terfenadine and docetaxel (consult docetaxel product literature)

• Diuretics: risk of ventricular arrhythmias with terfenadine increased by hypokalaemia or other electrolyte imbalance caused by •diuretics

• Grapefruit Juice: plasma concentration of terfenadine increased by •grapefruit juice—avoid concomitant use

• Hormone Antagonists: avoidance of terfenadine advised by manufacturer of •bicalutamide

Leukotriene Antagonists: terfenadine reduces plasma concentration of zafirlukast

• Pentamidine Isetionate: increased risk of ventricular arrhythmias when terfenadine given with •pentamidine isetionate—avoid concomitant use

Ulcer-healing Drugs: manufacturer of loratadine advises plasma concentration possibly increased by cimetidine

Antihistamines, Non-sedating *see* Antihistamines

Antihistamines, Sedating *see* Antihistamines

Antimalarials *see* Artemether with Lumefantrine, Chloroquine and Hydroxychloroquine, Mefloquine, Primaquine, Proguanil, and Quinine

Antimetabolites *see* Cytarabine, Fludarabine, Fluorouracil, Mercaptopurine, Methotrexate, and Tioguanine

Antimuscarinics

Note. Many drugs have antimuscarinic effects; concomitant use of two or more such drugs can increase side-effects such as dry mouth, urine retention, and constipation; concomitant use can also lead to confusion in the elderly. Interactions do not generally apply to antimuscarinics used by inhalation

Alcohol: increased sedative effect when hyoscine given with alcohol

Analgesics: increased risk of antimuscarinic side-effects when antimuscarinics given with nefopam

Anti-arrhythmics: increased risk of antimuscarinic side-effects when antimuscarinics given with

Antimuscarinics

Anti-arrhythmics *(continued)*
disopyramide; atropine delays absorption of mexiletine

Antibacterials: manufacturer of tolterodine advises avoid concomitant use with clarithromycin and erythromycin

Antidepressants: plasma concentration of procyclidine increased by paroxetine; increased risk of antimuscarinic side-effects when antimuscarinics given with MAOIs or tricyclics; possibly increased antimuscarinic side-effects when antimuscarinics given with tricyclic-related antidepressants

Antifungals: antimuscarinics reduce absorption of ketoconazole; plasma concentration of solifenacin increased by itraconazole and ketoconazole; manufacturer of tolterodine advises avoid concomitant use with itraconazole and ketoconazole

Antihistamines: increased risk of antimuscarinic side-effects when antimuscarinics given with antihistamines

Antipsychotics: antimuscarinics possibly reduce effects of haloperidol; increased risk of antimuscarinic side-effects when antimuscarinics given with clozapine; antimuscarinics reduce plasma concentration of phenothiazines, but risk of antimuscarinic side-effects increased

Antivirals: manufacturer of tolterodine advises avoid concomitant use with amprenavir, indinavir, lopinavir, nelfinavir, ritonavir and saquinavir; plasma concentration of solifenacin increased by nelfinavir and ritonavir

Domperidone: antimuscarinics antagonise effects of domperidone on gastro-intestinal activity

Dopaminergics: increased risk of antimuscarinic side-effects when antimuscarinics given with amantadine; antimuscarinics possibly reduce absorption of levodopa

Memantine: effects of antimuscarinics possibly enhanced by memantine

Metoclopramide: antimuscarinics antagonise effects of metoclopramide on gastro-intestinal activity

Nitrates: antimuscarinics possibly reduce effects of sublingual tablets of nitrates (failure to dissolve under tongue owing to dry mouth)

Parasympathomimetics: antimuscarinics antagonise effects of parasympathomimetics

Antipsychotics

Note. Increased risk of toxicity with myelosuppressive drugs

Note. Avoid concomitant use of clozapine with drugs that have a substantial potential for causing agranulocytosis

ACE Inhibitors: enhanced hypotensive effect when antipsychotics given with ACE inhibitors

Adrenergic Neurone Blockers: enhanced hypotensive effect when phenothiazines given with adrenergic neurone blockers; higher doses of chlorpromazine antagonise hypotensive effect of adrenergic neurone blockers; haloperidol antagonises hypotensive effect of adrenergic neurone blockers

Adsorbents: absorption of phenothiazines possibly reduced by kaolin

Alcohol: increased sedative effect when antipsychotics given with alcohol

Alpha-blockers: enhanced hypotensive effect when antipsychotics given with alpha-blockers

• Anaesthetics, General: enhanced hypotensive effect when antipsychotics given with •general anaesthetics

Analgesics: possible severe drowsiness when haloperidol given with indometacin; increased risk of convulsions when antipsychotics given with tramadol; enhanced hypotensive and sedative effects when antipsychotics given with opioid analgesics

Angiotensin-II Receptor Antagonists: enhanced hypotensive effect when antipsychotics given with angiotensin-II receptor antagonists

Antacids: absorption of phenothiazines and sulpiride reduced by antacids

• Anti-arrhythmics: increased risk of ventricular arrhythmias when antipsychotics that prolong the QT interval given with •anti-arrhythmics that prolong the QT interval; increased risk of ventricular arrhythmias when amisulpride, haloperidol, phenothiazines, pimozide or sertindole given with •amiodarone—avoid concomitant use; increased risk of ventricular arrhythmias when amisulpride, pimozide or sertindole given with •disopyramide—avoid concomitant use; increased risk of ventricular arrhythmias when phenothiazines given with •disopyramide, •procainamide or •quinidine; increased risk of arrhythmias when clozapine given with •flecainide; increased risk of ventricular arrhythmias when amisulpride, pimozide or sertindole given with •procainamide—avoid concomitant use; increased risk of ventricular arrhythmias when amisulpride, pimozide or sertindole given with •quinidine—avoid concomitant use; metabolism of aripiprazole inhibited by •quinidine (reduce dose of aripiprazole)

• Antibacterials: increased risk of ventricular arrhythmias when pimozide given with •clarithromycin, •moxifloxacin or •telithromycin—avoid concomitant use; increased risk of ventricular arrhythmias when sertindole given with •erythromycin or •moxifloxacin—avoid concomitant use; increased risk of ventricular arrhythmias when amisulpride given with parenteral •erythromycin—avoid concomitant use; plasma concentration of clozapine possibly increased by •erythromycin (possible increased risk of convulsions); possible increased risk of ventricular arrhythmias when pimozide given with •erythromycin—avoid concomitant use; increased risk of ventricular arrhythmias when haloperidol or phenothiazines given with •moxifloxacin—avoid concomitant use; plasma concentration of aripiprazole possibly reduced by •rifabutin and •rifampicin—increase dose of aripiprazole; plasma concentration of clozapine possibly reduced by rifampicin; metabolism of haloperidol accelerated by •rifampicin (reduced plasma concentration); avoid concomitant use of clozapine with •chloramphenicol or •sulphonamides (increased risk of agranulocytosis); plasma concentration of quetiapine possibly increased by macrolides (reduce dose of quetiapine); possible increased risk of ventricular arrhythmias when sertindole given with •macrolides—avoid concomitant use

• Antidepressants: metabolism of aripiprazole possibly inhibited by •fluoxetine and •paroxetine (reduce dose of aripiprazole); plasma concentration of clozapine, haloperidol, risperidone, sertindole and zotepine increased by •fluoxetine; plasma concentration of clozapine and olanzapine increased by •fluvoxamine; plasma concentration of clozapine and sertindole increased by •paroxetine; metabolism of perphenazine inhibited by paroxetine (reduce dose of perphenazine); plasma concentration of clozapine increased by •sertraline and •venlafaxine; plasma concentra-

Antipsychotics

- Antidepressants *(continued)*
  tion of pimozide increased by •sertraline (increased risk of ventricular arrhythmias—avoid concomitant use); plasma concentration of haloperidol increased by venlafaxine; increased risk of ventricular arrhythmias when pimozide given with •maprotiline or •tricyclics—avoid concomitant use; clozapine possibly increases CNS effects of •MAOIs; plasma concentration of aripiprazole possibly reduced by •St John's wort—increase dose of aripiprazole; possibly increased antimuscarinic side-effects when clozapine given with tricyclics; antipsychotics increase plasma concentration of •tricyclics—possibly increased risk of ventricular arrhythmias; increased risk of antimuscarinic side-effects when phenothiazines given with tricyclics

  Antidiabetics: phenothiazines possibly antagonise hypoglycaemic effect of sulphonylureas

- Antiepileptics: metabolism of clozapine accelerated by •carbamazepine (reduced plasma concentration), also avoid concomitant use of drugs with substantial potential for causing agranulocytosis; metabolism of haloperidol, olanzapine, quetiapine, risperidone and sertindole accelerated by carbamazepine (reduced plasma concentration); plasma concentration of aripiprazole reduced by •carbamazepine—increase dose of aripiprazole; antipsychotics antagonise anticonvulsant effect of •carbamazepine, •ethosuximide, •oxcarbazepine, •phenytoin, •primidone and •valproate (convulsive threshold lowered); metabolism of clozapine, quetiapine and sertindole accelerated by phenytoin (reduced plasma concentration); plasma concentration of aripiprazole possibly reduced by •phenytoin and •primidone—increase dose of aripiprazole; metabolism of haloperidol accelerated by primidone (reduced plasma concentration); increased risk of neutropenia when olanzapine given with •valproate
- Antifungals: metabolism of aripiprazole inhibited by •ketoconazole (reduce dose of aripiprazole); increased risk of ventricular arrhythmias when sertindole given with •itraconazole or •ketoconazole—avoid concomitant use; metabolism of aripiprazole possibly inhibited by •itraconazole (reduce dose of aripiprazole); possible increased risk of ventricular arrhythmias when sertindole given with •imidazoles or •triazoles—avoid concomitant use; plasma concentration of quetiapine possibly increased by imidazoles and triazoles (reduce dose of quetiapine); increased risk of ventricular arrhythmias when pimozide given with •imidazoles or •triazoles—avoid concomitant use
- Antihistamines: increased risk of ventricular arrhythmias when antipsychotics given with •terfenadine; increased risk of ventricular arrhythmias when pimozide or sertindole given with •terfenadine—avoid concomitant use
- Antimalarials: avoidance of antipsychotics advised by manufacturer of •artemether/lumefantrine; increased risk of ventricular arrhythmias when pimozide given with •mefloquine or •quinine—avoid concomitant use

  Antimuscarinics: increased risk of antimuscarinic side-effects when clozapine given with antimuscarinics; plasma concentration of phenothiazines reduced by antimuscarinics, but risk of antimuscarinic side-effects increased; effects of haloperidol possibly reduced by antimuscarinics

- Antipsychotics: avoid concomitant use of clozapine with depot formulation of •flupentixol, •fluphenazine, •haloperidol, •pipotiazine or •zuclopenthixol as cannot be withdrawn quickly if neutropenia occurs; increased risk of ventricular arrhythmias when sertindole given with •amisulpride—avoid concomitant use; increased risk of ventricular arrhythmias when pimozide given with •phenothiazines—avoid concomitant use

Antipsychotics

- Antipsychotics *(continued)*
- Antivirals: plasma concentration of pimozide and sertindole increased by •amprenavir (increased risk of ventricular arrhythmias—avoid concomitant use); plasma concentration of clozapine possibly increased by amprenavir; metabolism of aripiprazole possibly inhibited by •amprenavir, •atazanavir, •indinavir, •lopinavir, •nelfinavir, •ritonavir and •saquinavir (reduce dose of aripiprazole); plasma concentration of pimozide possibly increased by •atazanavir—avoid concomitant use; plasma concentration of aripiprazole possibly reduced by •efavirenz and •nevirapine—increase dose of aripiprazole; plasma concentration of pimozide possibly increased by •efavirenz, •indinavir, •nelfinavir and •saquinavir (increased risk of ventricular arrhythmias—avoid concomitant use); plasma concentration of sertindole increased by •indinavir, •lopinavir, •nelfinavir, •ritonavir and •saquinavir (increased risk of ventricular arrhythmias—avoid concomitant use); plasma concentration of clozapine increased by •ritonavir (increased risk of toxicity)—avoid concomitant use; plasma concentration of antipsychotics possibly increased by •ritonavir; plasma concentration of pimozide increased by •ritonavir (increased risk of ventricular arrhythmias—avoid concomitant use)
- Anxiolytics and Hypnotics: increased sedative effect when antipsychotics given with anxiolytics and hypnotics; plasma concentration of zotepine increased by diazepam; increased risk of hypotension, bradycardia and respiratory depression when intramuscular olanzapine given with parenteral •benzodiazepines; plasma concentration of haloperidol increased by buspirone
- Aprepitant: avoidance of pimozide advised by manufacturer of •aprepitant
- Barbiturates: antipsychotics antagonise anticonvulsant effect of •barbiturates (convulsive threshold lowered); metabolism of haloperidol accelerated by phenobarbital (reduced plasma concentration); plasma concentration of aripiprazole possibly reduced by •phenobarbital—increase dose of aripiprazole
- Beta-blockers: enhanced hypotensive effect when phenothiazines given with beta-blockers; plasma concentration of both drugs may increase when chlorpromazine given with •propranolol; increased risk of ventricular arrhythmias when amisulpride, phenothiazines, pimozide or sertindole given with •sotalol

  Calcium-channel Blockers: enhanced hypotensive effect when antipsychotics given with calcium-channel blockers

  Clonidine: enhanced hypotensive effect when phenothiazines given with clonidine

- Cytotoxics: avoid concomitant use of clozapine with •cytotoxics (increased risk of agranulocytosis)

  Desferrioxamine: manufacturer of levomepromazine (methotrimeprazine) advises avoid concomitant use with desferrioxamine; avoidance of prochlorperazine advised by manufacturer of desferrioxamine

Antipsychotics *(continued)*

Diazoxide: enhanced hypotensive effect when phenothiazines given with diazoxide

• Diuretics: risk of ventricular arrhythmias with amisulpride or sertindole increased by hypokalaemia caused by •diuretics; risk of ventricular arrhythmias with pimozide increased by hypokalaemia caused by •diuretics (avoid concomitant use); enhanced hypotensive effect when phenothiazines given with diuretics

Dopaminergics: increased risk of extrapyramidal side-effects when antipsychotics given with amantadine; antipsychotics antagonise effects of apomorphine, levodopa, lisuride and pergolide; antipsychotics antagonise hypoprolactinaemic and antiparkinsonian effects of bromocriptine and cabergoline; manufacturer of amisulpride advises avoid concomitant use of levodopa (antagonism of effect); avoidance of antipsychotics advised by manufacturer of pramipexole and ropinirole (antagonism of effect)

• Lithium: increased risk of ventricular arrhythmias when sertindole given with •lithium—avoid concomitant use; increased risk of extrapyramidal side-effects and possibly neurotoxicity when clozapine, haloperidol or phenothiazines given with lithium; increased risk of extrapyramidal side-effects when sulpiride given with lithium

Memantine: effects of antipsychotics possibly reduced by memantine

Methyldopa: enhanced hypotensive effect when antipsychotics given with methyldopa (also increased risk of extrapyramidal effects)

Metoclopramide: increased risk of extrapyramidal side-effects when antipsychotics given with metoclopramide

Moxonidine: enhanced hypotensive effect when phenothiazines given with moxonidine

Muscle Relaxants: promazine possibly enhances effects of suxamethonium

Nitrates: enhanced hypotensive effect when phenothiazines given with nitrates

• Penicillamine: avoid concomitant use of clozapine with •penicillamine (increased risk of agranulocytosis)

• Pentamidine Isetionate: increased risk of ventricular arrhythmias when amisulpride given with •pentamidine isetionate—avoid concomitant use

• Sibutramine: increased risk of CNS toxicity when antipsychotics given with •sibutramine (manufacturer of sibutramine advises avoid concomitant use)

Sodium Benzoate: haloperidol possibly reduces effects of sodium benzoate

Sodium Phenylbutyrate: haloperidol possibly reduces effects of sodium phenylbutyrate

Sympathomimetics: antipsychotics antagonise hypertensive effect of sympathomimetics

Tetrabenazine: increased risk of extrapyramidal side-effects when antipsychotics given with tetrabenazine

• Ulcer-healing Drugs: effects of antipsychotics, chlorpromazine and clozapine possibly enhanced by cimetidine; increased risk of ventricular arrhythmias when sertindole given with •cimetidine—avoid concomitant use; absorption of sulpiride reduced by sucralfate

Vasodilator Antihypertensives: enhanced hypotensive effect when phenothiazines given with hydralazine, minoxidil or nitroprusside

Antivirals *see* Abacavir, Aciclovir, Amprenavir, Atazanavir, Cidofovir, Didanosine, Efavirenz, Emtricitabine, Famciclovir, Foscarnet, Ganciclovir, Indinavir, Lamivudine, Lopinavir, Nelfinavir, Nevirapine, Ribavirin, Ritonavir, Saquinavir, Stavudine, Tenofovir, Valaciclovir, Zalcitabine, and Zidovudine

Anxiolytics and Hypnotics

ACE Inhibitors: enhanced hypotensive effect when anxiolytics and hypnotics given with ACE inhibitors

Adrenergic Neurone Blockers: enhanced hypotensive effect when anxiolytics and hypnotics given with adrenergic neurone blockers

Alcohol: increased sedative effect when anxiolytics and hypnotics given with alcohol

Alpha-blockers: enhanced hypotensive and sedative effects when anxiolytics and hypnotics given with alpha-blockers

Anaesthetics, General: increased sedative effect when anxiolytics and hypnotics given with general anaesthetics

Analgesics: increased sedative effect when anxiolytics and hypnotics given with opioid analgesics

Angiotensin-II Receptor Antagonists: enhanced hypotensive effect when anxiolytics and hypnotics given with angiotensin-II receptor antagonists

• Antibacterials: metabolism of midazolam inhibited by •clarithromycin, •erythromycin, •quinupristin/dalfopristin and •telithromycin (increased plasma concentration with increased sedation); plasma concentration of buspirone increased by erythromycin (reduce dose of buspirone); metabolism of zopiclone inhibited by erythromycin and quinupristin/dalfopristin; metabolism of benzodiazepines possibly accelerated by rifampicin (reduced plasma concentration); metabolism of diazepam accelerated by rifampicin (reduced plasma concentration); metabolism of buspirone and zaleplon possibly accelerated by rifampicin; metabolism of zolpidem accelerated by rifampicin (reduced plasma concentration and reduced effect); metabolism of diazepam inhibited by isoniazid

Anticoagulants: chloral and triclofos may transiently enhance anticoagulant effect of coumarins

Antidepressants: plasma concentration of some benzodiazepines increased by fluvoxamine; sedative effects possibly increased when zolpidem given with sertraline; manufacturer of buspirone advises avoid concomitant use with MAOIs; increased sedative effect when anxiolytics and hypnotics given with mirtazapine, tricyclic-related antidepressants or tricyclics

Antiepileptics: plasma concentration of clonazepam often reduced by carbamazepine, phenytoin and primidone; diazepam increases or decreases plasma concentration of phenytoin; benzodiazepines possibly increase or decrease plasma concentration of phenytoin

• Antifungals: plasma concentration of midazolam increased by •fluconazole, •itraconazole and •ketoconazole (risk of prolonged sedation); plasma concentration of alprazolam increased by itraconazole; plasma concentration of buspirone increased by itraconazole (reduce dose of buspirone)

Antihistamines: increased sedative effect when anxiolytics and hypnotics given with antihistamines

• Antipsychotics: increased sedative effect when anxiolytics and hypnotics given with antipsychotics; buspirone increases plasma concentration of haloperidol; increased risk of hypotension, bradycardia and respiratory depression when parenteral benzodiazepines given with intramuscular •olanzapine; diazepam increases plasma concentration of zotepine

Anxiolytics and Hypnotics *(continued)*

- Antivirals: increased risk of prolonged sedation and respiratory depression when alprazolam, clonazepam, clorazepate, diazepam, flurazepam or midazolam given with •amprenavir; increased risk of prolonged sedation when midazolam given with •efavirenz, •indinavir or •nelfinavir—avoid concomitant use; increased risk of prolonged sedation when alprazolam given with •indinavir—avoid concomitant use; plasma concentration of buspirone increased by ritonavir (increased risk of toxicity); plasma concentration of alprazolam, clorazepate, diazepam, flurazepam, midazolam and zolpidem possibly increased by •ritonavir (risk of extreme sedation and respiratory depression — avoid concomitant use); plasma concentration of anxiolytics and hypnotics possibly increased by •ritonavir; plasma concentration of midazolam increased by •saquinavir (risk of prolonged sedation)

Barbiturates: plasma concentration of clonazepam often reduced by phenobarbital

Beta-blockers: enhanced hypotensive effect when anxiolytics and hypnotics given with beta-blockers

Calcium-channel Blockers: enhanced hypotensive effect when anxiolytics and hypnotics given with calcium-channel blockers; midazolam increases absorption of lercanidipine; plasma concentration of buspirone increased by diltiazem and verapamil (reduce dose of buspirone); metabolism of midazolam inhibited by diltiazem and verapamil (increased plasma concentration with increased sedation)

Cardiac Glycosides: alprazolam increases plasma concentration of digoxin (increased risk of toxicity)

Clonidine: enhanced hypotensive effect when anxiolytics and hypnotics given with clonidine

Diazoxide: enhanced hypotensive effect when anxiolytics and hypnotics given with diazoxide

Disulfiram: metabolism of benzodiazepines inhibited by disulfiram (increased sedative effects); increased risk of temazepam toxicity when given with disulfiram

Diuretics: enhanced hypotensive effect when anxiolytics and hypnotics given with diuretics; administration of chloral or triclofos with parenteral furosemide (frusemide) may displace thyroid hormone from binding sites

Dopaminergics: benzodiazepines possibly antagonise effects of levodopa

Grapefruit Juice: plasma concentration of buspirone increased by grapefruit juice

Lofexidine: increased sedative effect when anxiolytics and hypnotics given with lofexidine

Methyldopa: enhanced hypotensive effect when anxiolytics and hypnotics given with methyldopa

Moxonidine: enhanced hypotensive effect when anxiolytics and hypnotics given with moxonidine; sedative effects possibly increased when benzodiazepines given with moxonidine

Muscle Relaxants: increased sedative effect when anxiolytics and hypnotics given with baclofen or tizanidine

Nabilone: increased sedative effect when anxiolytics and hypnotics given with nabilone

Nitrates: enhanced hypotensive effect when anxiolytics and hypnotics given with nitrates

Theophylline: effects of benzodiazepines possibly reduced by theophylline

Ulcer-healing Drugs: metabolism of benzodiazepines, clomethiazole and zaleplon inhibited by cimetidine (increased plasma concentration); metabolism of diazepam possibly inhibited by esomeprazole and omeprazole (increased plasma concentration)

Vasodilator Antihypertensives: enhanced hypotensive effect when anxiolytics and hypnotics given with hydralazine, minoxidil or nitroprusside

Apomorphine

Antipsychotics: effects of apomorphine antagonised by antipsychotics

Dopaminergics: effects of apomorphine possibly enhanced by entacapone

Memantine: effects of dopaminergics possibly enhanced by memantine

Methyldopa: antiparkinsonian effect of dopaminergics antagonised by methyldopa

Nitrates: sublingual apomorphine enhances hypotensive effect of nitrates

Apraclonidine *see* Alpha$_2$-adrenoceptor Stimulants

Aprepitant

Antibacterials: plasma concentration of aprepitant possibly increased by clarithromycin and telithromycin; plasma concentration of aprepitant reduced by rifampicin

Anticoagulants: aprepitant possibly reduces anticoagulant effect of warfarin

- Antidepressants: manufacturer of aprepitant advises avoid concomitant use with •St John's wort

Antidiabetics: aprepitant reduces plasma concentration of tolbutamide

Antiepileptics: plasma concentration of aprepitant possibly reduced by carbamazepine and phenytoin

Antifungals: plasma concentration of aprepitant increased by ketoconazole

- Antihistamines: manufacturer of aprepitant advises avoid concomitant use with •terfenadine
- Antipsychotics: manufacturer of aprepitant advises avoid concomitant use with •pimozide

Antivirals: plasma concentration of aprepitant possibly increased by ritonavir

Barbiturates: plasma concentration of aprepitant possibly reduced by phenobarbital

Corticosteroids: aprepitant inhibits metabolism of dexamethasone and methylprednisolone (reduce dose of dexamethasone and methylprednisolone)

- Oestrogens: aprepitant possibly causes contraceptive failure of hormonal contraceptives containing •oestrogens (alternative contraception recommended)
- Progestogens: aprepitant possibly causes contraceptive failure of hormonal contraceptives containing •progestogens (alternative contraception recommended)

Aripiprazole *see* Antipsychotics

Artemether with Lumefantrine

- Anti-arrhythmics: manufacturer of artemether/lumefantrine advises avoid concomitant use with •amiodarone, •disopyramide, •flecainide, •procainamide or •quinidine (risk of ventricular arrhythmias)
- Antibacterials: manufacturer of artemether/lumefantrine advises avoid concomitant use with •macrolides and •quinolones
- Antidepressants: manufacturer of artemether/lumefantrine advises avoid concomitant use with •antidepressants
- Antifungals: manufacturer of artemether/lumefantrine advises avoid concomitant use with •imidazoles and •triazoles
- Antihistamines: manufacturer of artemether/lumefantrine advises avoid concomitant use with •terfenadine (risk of ventricular arrhythmias)

Artemether with Lumefantrine *(continued)*
- • Antimalarials: manufacturer of artemether/lumefantrine advises avoid concomitant use with •antimalarials
- • Antipsychotics: manufacturer of artemether/lumefantrine advises avoid concomitant use with •antipsychotics
- • Beta-blockers: manufacturer of artemether/lumefantrine advises avoid concomitant use with •metoprolol and •sotalol
- • Grapefruit Juice: metabolism of artemether/lumefantrine possibly inhibited by •grapefruit juice (avoid concomitant use)

Aspirin
- ACE Inhibitors: risk of renal impairment when aspirin (in doses over 300 mg daily) given with ACE inhibitors, also hypotensive effect antagonised
- Adsorbents: absorption of aspirin possibly reduced by kaolin
- • Analgesics: avoid concomitant use of aspirin with •NSAIDs (increased side-effects); antiplatelet effect of aspirin possibly reduced by ibuprofen
- Angiotensin-II Receptor Antagonists: risk of renal impairment when aspirin (in doses over 300 mg daily) given with angiotensin-II receptor antagonists, also hypotensive effect antagonised
- Antacids: excretion of aspirin increased by alkaline urine due to some antacids
- • Anticoagulants: increased risk of bleeding when aspirin given with •coumarins or •phenindione (due to antiplatelet effect); aspirin enhances anticoagulant effect of •heparins
- • Antidepressants: increased risk of bleeding when aspirin given with •SSRIs or •venlafaxine
- Antiepileptics: aspirin enhances effects of phenytoin and valproate
- Cilostazol: manufacturer of cilostazol recommends dose of aspirin should not exceed 80 mg daily when given with cilostazol
- Clopidogrel: increased risk of bleeding when aspirin given with clopidogrel
- Corticosteroids: increased risk of gastro-intestinal bleeding and ulceration when aspirin given with corticosteroids, also corticosteroids reduce plasma concentration of salicylate
- • Cytotoxics: aspirin reduces excretion of •methotrexate (increased risk of toxicity)
- Diuretics: aspirin antagonises diuretic effect of spironolactone; increased risk of toxicity when high-dose aspirin given with carbonic anhydrase inhibitors
- Iloprost: increased risk of bleeding when aspirin given with iloprost
- Leukotriene Antagonists: aspirin increases plasma concentration of zafirlukast
- Metoclopramide: rate of absorption of aspirin increased by metoclopramide (enhanced effect)
- Mifepristone: avoidance of aspirin advised by manufacturer of mifepristone
- Probenecid: aspirin antagonises effects of probenecid
- Sibutramine: increased risk of bleeding when aspirin given with sibutramine
- Sulfinpyrazone: aspirin antagonises effects of sulfinpyrazone

Atazanavir
- Antacids: plasma concentration of atazanavir possibly reduced by antacids
- • Anti-arrhythmics: atazanavir possibly increases plasma concentration of •amiodarone and •lidocaine (lignocaine); atazanavir possibly increases plasma concentration of •quinidine—avoid concomitant use

Atazanavir *(continued)*
- • Antibacterials: plasma concentration of both drugs increased when atazanavir given with clarithromycin; atazanavir increases plasma concentration of •rifabutin (reduce dose of rifabutin); plasma concentration of atazanavir reduced by •rifampicin—avoid concomitant use
- Anticoagulants: atazanavir may enhance or reduce anticoagulant effect of warfarin
- • Antidepressants: plasma concentration of atazanavir reduced by •St John's wort—avoid concomitant use
- • Antihistamines: atazanavir possibly increases plasma concentration of •terfenadine—avoid concomitant use
- • Antipsychotics: atazanavir possibly inhibits metabolism of •aripiprazole (reduce dose of aripiprazole); atazanavir possibly increases plasma concentration of •pimozide—avoid concomitant use
- • Antivirals: plasma concentration of atazanavir reduced by efavirenz—increase dose of atazanavir; avoid concomitant use of atazanavir with •indinavir; plasma concentration of atazanavir possibly reduced by •nevirapine—avoid concomitant use; plasma concentration of atazanavir reduced by tenofovir
- • Calcium-channel Blockers: atazanavir increases plasma concentration of •diltiazem (reduce dose of diltiazem); atazanavir possibly increases plasma concentration of verapamil
- • Ciclosporin: atazanavir possibly increases plasma concentration of •ciclosporin
- • Cytotoxics: atazanavir possibly inhibits metabolism of •irinotecan (increased risk of toxicity)
- • Ergot Alkaloids: atazanavir possibly increases plasma concentration of •ergot alkaloids—avoid concomitant use
- • Lipid-regulating Drugs: possible increased risk of myopathy when atazanavir given with atorvastatin; increased risk of myopathy when atazanavir given with •simvastatin (avoid concomitant use)
- • Oestrogens: atazanavir increases plasma concentration of •ethinylestradiol—avoid concomitant use
- • Sildenafil: atazanavir possibly increases side-effects of •sildenafil
- • Sirolimus: atazanavir possibly increases plasma concentration of •sirolimus
- • Tacrolimus: atazanavir possibly increases plasma concentration of •tacrolimus
- • Ulcer-healing Drugs: plasma concentration of atazanavir significantly reduced by •omeprazole—avoid concomitant use; plasma concentration of atazanavir possibly reduced by •proton pump inhibitors—avoid concomitant use

Atenolol *see* Beta-blockers

Atomoxetine
- • Antidepressants: atomoxetine should not be started until 2 weeks after stopping •MAOIs, also MAOIs should not be started until at least 2 weeks after stopping atomoxetine

Atorvastatin *see* Statins

Atovaquone
- • Antibacterials: plasma concentration of atovaquone reduced by •rifabutin and •rifampicin (possible therapeutic failure of atovaquone); plasma concentration of atovaquone reduced by tetracycline
- Antivirals: atovaquone possibly reduces plasma concentration of indinavir; atovaquone possibly inhibits metabolism of zidovudine (increased plasma concentration)
- Metoclopramide: plasma concentration of atovaquone reduced by metoclopramide

Atracurium *see* Muscle Relaxants

Atropine *see* Antimuscarinics

Azathioprine

ACE Inhibitors: increased risk of leucopenia when azathioprine given with captopril

• Allopurinol: enhanced effects and increased toxicity of azathioprine when given with •allopurinol (reduce dose of azathioprine)

Aminosalicylates: possible increased risk of leucopenia when azathioprine given with aminosalicylates

• Antibacterials: increased risk of haematological toxicity when azathioprine given with •sulfamethoxazole (as co-trimoxazole); increased risk of haematological toxicity when azathioprine given with •trimethoprim (also with co-trimoxazole)

• Anticoagulants: azathioprine possibly reduces anticoagulant effect of •warfarin

Antiepileptics: cytotoxics possibly reduce absorption of phenytoin

• Antipsychotics: avoid concomitant use of cytotoxics with •clozapine (increased risk of agranulocytosis)

Azelastine *see* Antihistamines

Azithromycin *see* Macrolides

Aztreonam

• Anticoagulants: aztreonam possibly enhances anticoagulant effect of •coumarins

Oestrogens: broad-spectrum antibacterials possibly reduce contraceptive effect of oestrogens (risk probably small, see p. 407)

Baclofen *see* Muscle Relaxants

Balsalazide *see* Aminosalicylates

Bambuterol *see* Sympathomimetics, $Beta_2$

Barbiturates

Alcohol: increased sedative effect when barbiturates given with alcohol

Anti-arrhythmics: barbiturates accelerate metabolism of disopyramide and quinidine (reduced plasma concentration)

• Antibacterials: barbiturates accelerate metabolism of •chloramphenicol, doxycycline and metronidazole (reduced plasma concentration); phenobarbital reduces plasma concentration of •telithromycin (avoid during and for 2 weeks after phenobarbital)

• Anticoagulants: barbiturates accelerate metabolism of •coumarins (reduced anticoagulant effect)

• Antidepressants: phenobarbital reduces plasma concentration of paroxetine; phenobarbital accelerates metabolism of •mianserin (reduced plasma concentration); anticonvulsant effect of barbiturates possibly antagonised by MAOIs and •tricyclic-related antidepressants (convulsive threshold lowered); anticonvulsant effect of barbiturates antagonised by SSRIs (convulsive threshold lowered); plasma concentration of phenobarbital reduced by •St John's wort—avoid concomitant use; anticonvulsant effect of barbiturates antagonised by •tricyclics (convulsive threshold lowered), also metabolism of tricyclics possibly accelerated (reduced plasma concentration)

Antiepileptics: phenobarbital reduces plasma concentration of carbamazepine, lamotrigine, tiagabine and zonisamide; phenobarbital possibly reduces plasma concentration of ethosuximide; plasma concentration of phenobarbital increased by oxcarbazepine, also plasma concentration of an active metabolite of oxcarbazepine reduced; plasma concentration of phenobarbital often increased by phenytoin, plasma concentration of phenytoin often reduced but may be increased; increased sedative effect when barbiturates given with primidone; plasma concentration of phenobarbital increased by valproate (also plasma concentration of valproate reduced); plasma concentration of phenobarbital possibly reduced by vigabatrin

Barbiturates

Antiepileptics *(continued)*

• Antifungals: phenobarbital possibly reduces plasma concentration of itraconazole; phenobarbital possibly reduces plasma concentration of •voriconazole—avoid concomitant use; phenobarbital reduces absorption of griseofulvin (reduced effect)

• Antipsychotics: anticonvulsant effect of barbiturates antagonised by •antipsychotics (convulsive threshold lowered); phenobarbital accelerates metabolism of haloperidol (reduced plasma concentration); phenobarbital possibly reduces plasma concentration of •aripiprazole—increase dose of aripiprazole

• Antivirals: phenobarbital possibly reduces plasma concentration of abacavir, amprenavir and •lopinavir; barbiturates possibly reduce plasma concentration of •indinavir, •nelfinavir and •saquinavir

Anxiolytics and Hypnotics: phenobarbital often reduces plasma concentration of clonazepam

Aprepitant: phenobarbital possibly reduces plasma concentration of aprepitant

• Calcium-channel Blockers: barbiturates reduce effects of •felodipine and •isradipine; barbiturates probably reduce effects of •dihydropyridines, •diltiazem and •verapamil

Cardiac Glycosides: barbiturates accelerate metabolism of digitoxin (reduced effect)

• Ciclosporin: barbiturates accelerate metabolism of •ciclosporin (reduced effect)

• Corticosteroids: barbiturates accelerate metabolism of •corticosteroids (reduced effect)

Cytotoxics: phenobarbital possibly reduces plasma concentration of etoposide

• Diuretics: phenobarbital reduces plasma concentration of •eplerenone—avoid concomitant use; increased risk of osteomalacia when phenobarbital given with carbonic anhydrase inhibitors

Folates: plasma concentration of phenobarbital possibly reduced by folates

Hormone Antagonists: barbiturates accelerate metabolism of gestrinone (reduced plasma concentration); barbiturates possibly accelerate metabolism of toremifene (reduced plasma concentration)

$5HT_3$ Antagonists: phenobarbital reduces plasma concentration of tropisetron

Leukotriene Antagonists: phenobarbital reduces plasma concentration of montelukast

Memantine: effects of barbiturates possibly reduced by memantine

• Oestrogens: barbiturates accelerate metabolism of •oestrogens (reduced contraceptive effect—see p. 407)

• Progestogens: barbiturates accelerate metabolism of •progestogens (reduced contraceptive effect—see p. 407)

Sympathomimetics: plasma concentration of phenobarbital possibly increased by methylphenidate

Theophylline: barbiturates accelerate metabolism of theophylline (reduced effect)

Thyroid Hormones: barbiturates accelerate metabolism of thyroid hormones (may increase requirements for thyroid hormones in hypothyroidism)

Tibolone: barbiturates accelerate metabolism of tibolone (reduced plasma concentration)

Vitamins: barbiturates possibly increase requirements for vitamin D

Beclometasone *see* Corticosteroids
Belladonna Alkaloids *see* Antimuscarinics
Bendroflumethiazide (bendrofluazide) *see* Diuretics
Benperidol *see* Antipsychotics
Benzatropine (benztropine) *see* Antimuscarinics
Benzodiazepines *see* Anxiolytics and Hypnotics
Benzthiazide *see* Diuretics
Benzylpenicillin *see* Penicillins
Beta-blockers

Note. Since systemic absorption may follow topical application of beta-blockers to the eye the possibility of interactions, in particular, with drugs such as verapamil should be borne in mind

ACE Inhibitors: enhanced hypotensive effect when beta-blockers given with ACE inhibitors

Adrenergic Neurone Blockers: enhanced hypotensive effect when beta-blockers given with adrenergic neurone blockers

Alcohol: enhanced hypotensive effect when beta-blockers given with alcohol

Aldesleukin: enhanced hypotensive effect when beta-blockers given with aldesleukin

• Alpha-blockers: enhanced hypotensive effect when beta-blockers given with •alpha-blockers, also increased risk of first-dose hypotension with post-synaptic alpha-blockers such as prazosin

Anaesthetics, General: enhanced hypotensive effect when beta-blockers given with general anaesthetics

• Anaesthetics, Local: propranolol increases risk of •bupivacaine toxicity

Analgesics: hypotensive effect of beta-blockers antagonised by NSAIDs; plasma concentration of esmolol possibly increased by morphine

Angiotensin-II Receptor Antagonists: enhanced hypotensive effect when beta-blockers given with angiotensin-II receptor antagonists

• Anti-arrhythmics: increased myocardial depression when beta-blockers given with •anti-arrhythmics; increased risk of bradycardia, AV block and myocardial depression when beta-blockers given with •amiodarone; increased risk of ventricular arrhythmias when sotalol given with •amiodarone, •disopyramide, •procainamide or •quinidine—avoid concomitant use; increased risk of myocardial depression and bradycardia when beta-blockers given with •flecainide; propranolol increases risk of •lidocaine (lignocaine) toxicity; plasma concentration of metoprolol and propranolol increased by propafenone

• Antibacterials: increased risk of ventricular arrhythmias when sotalol given with •moxifloxacin—avoid concomitant use; metabolism of bisoprolol and propranolol accelerated by rifampicin (plasma concentration significantly reduced)

• Antidepressants: plasma concentration of propranolol increased by fluvoxamine; enhanced hypotensive effect when beta-blockers given with MAOIs; increased risk of ventricular arrhythmias when sotalol given with •tricyclics

Antidiabetics: beta-blockers may mask warning signs of hypoglycaemia (such as tremor) with antidiabetics; beta-blockers enhance hypoglycaemic effect of insulin

• Antihistamines: increased risk of ventricular arrhythmias when sotalol given with •mizolastine or •terfenadine—avoid concomitant use

• Antimalarials: avoidance of metoprolol and sotalol advised by manufacturer of •artemether/lumefantrine; increased risk of bradycardia when beta-blockers given with mefloquine

Beta-blockers *(continued)*

• Antipsychotics: plasma concentration of both drugs may increase when propranolol given with •chlorpromazine; increased risk of ventricular arrhythmias when sotalol given with •amisulpride, •phenothiazines, •pimozide or •sertindole; enhanced hypotensive effect when beta-blockers given with phenothiazines

Anxiolytics and Hypnotics: enhanced hypotensive effect when beta-blockers given with anxiolytics and hypnotics

• Calcium-channel Blockers: enhanced hypotensive effect when beta-blockers given with calcium-channel blockers; possible severe hypotension and heart failure when beta-blockers given with •nifedipine or •nisoldipine; increased risk of AV block and bradycardia when beta-blockers given with •diltiazem; asystole, severe hypotension and heart failure when beta-blockers given with •verapamil (see p. 113)

Cardiac Glycosides: increased risk of AV block and bradycardia when beta-blockers given with cardiac glycosides

• Ciclosporin: carvedilol increases plasma concentration of •ciclosporin

• Clonidine: increased risk of withdrawal hypertension when beta-blockers given with •clonidine (withdraw beta-blockers several days before slowly withdrawing clonidine)

Corticosteroids: hypotensive effect of beta-blockers antagonised by corticosteroids

Diazoxide: enhanced hypotensive effect when beta-blockers given with diazoxide

• Diuretics: enhanced hypotensive effect when beta-blockers given with diuretics; risk of ventricular arrhythmias with sotalol increased by hypokalaemia caused by •loop diuretics or •thiazides and related diuretics

• Dolasetron: increased risk of ventricular arrhythmias when sotalol given with •dolasetron—avoid concomitant use

Dopaminergics: enhanced hypotensive effect when beta-blockers given with levodopa

Ergot Alkaloids: increased peripheral vasoconstriction when beta-blockers given with ergotamine and methysergide

$5HT_1$ Agonists: propranolol possibly increases plasma concentration of rizatriptan (reduce dose of rizatriptan)

$5HT_3$ Antagonists: caution with beta-blockers advised by manufacturer of tropisetron (risk of ventricular arrhythmias)

Methyldopa: enhanced hypotensive effect when beta-blockers given with methyldopa

• Moxisylyte (thymoxamine): possible severe postural hypotension when beta-blockers given with •moxisylyte

Moxonidine: enhanced hypotensive effect when beta-blockers given with moxonidine

Muscle Relaxants: propranolol enhances effects of muscle relaxants; enhanced hypotensive effect when beta-blockers given with baclofen; possible enhanced hypotensive effect and bradycardia when beta-blockers given with tizanidine

Nitrates: enhanced hypotensive effect when beta-blockers given with nitrates

Oestrogens: hypotensive effect of beta-blockers antagonised by oestrogens

Parasympathomimetics: propranolol antagonises effects of neostigmine and pyridostigmine; increased risk of arrhythmias when beta-blockers given with pilocarpine

Prostaglandins: enhanced hypotensive effect when beta-blockers given with alprostadil

Beta-blockers *(continued)*

- Sympathomimetics: severe hypertension when beta-blockers given with •adrenaline (epinephrine) or •noradrenaline (norepinephrine) especially with non-selective beta-blockers; possible severe hypertension when beta-blockers given with •dobutamine especially with non-selective beta-blockers

Ulcer-healing Drugs: plasma concentration of labetalol, metoprolol and propranolol increased by cimetidine

Vasodilator Antihypertensives: enhanced hypotensive effect when beta-blockers given with hydralazine, minoxidil or nitroprusside

Betahistine

Antihistamines: effect of betahistine theoretically antagonised by antihistamines

Betamethasone *see* Corticosteroids

Betaxolol *see* Beta-blockers

Bethanechol *see* Parasympathomimetics

Bexarotene

Antiepileptics: cytotoxics possibly reduce absorption of phenytoin

- Antipsychotics: avoid concomitant use of cytotoxics with •clozapine (increased risk of agranulocytosis)
- Lipid-regulating Drugs: plasma concentration of bexarotene increased by •gemfibrozil—avoid concomitant use

Bezafibrate *see* Fibrates

Bicalutamide

Anticoagulants: bicalutamide possibly enhances anticoagulant effect of coumarins

- Antihistamines: manufacturer of bicalutamide advises avoid concomitant use with •terfenadine

Biguanides *see* Antidiabetics

Bile Acids *see* Ursodeoxycholic Acid

Bisoprolol *see* Beta-blockers

Bisphosphonates

Analgesics: bioavailability of tiludronic acid increased by indometacin

Antacids: absorption of bisphosphonates reduced by antacids

Antibacterials: increased risk of hypocalcaemia when bisphosphonates given with aminoglycosides

Calcium Salts: absorption of bisphosphonates reduced by calcium salts

Iron: absorption of bisphosphonates reduced by *oral* iron

Bleomycin

Antiepileptics: cytotoxics possibly reduce absorption of phenytoin

- Antipsychotics: avoid concomitant use of cytotoxics with •clozapine (increased risk of agranulocytosis)
- Cytotoxics: increased pulmonary toxicity when bleomycin given with •cisplatin

Bosentan

Anticoagulants: manufacturer of bosentan recommends monitoring anticoagulant effect of coumarins

- Antidiabetics: plasma concentration of both drugs reduced when bosentan given with •glibenclamide (avoid concomitant use)
- Antifungals: plasma concentration of bosentan possibly increased by itraconazole and ketoconazole; plasma concentration of bosentan increased by •fluconazole—avoid concomitant use

Antivirals: plasma concentration of bosentan possibly increased by ritonavir

- Ciclosporin: plasma concentration of bosentan increased by •ciclosporin (also plasma concentration of ciclosporin reduced—avoid concomitant use)

Bosentan *(continued)*

Lipid-regulating Drugs: bosentan reduces plasma concentration of simvastatin

- Oestrogens: bosentan possibly causes contraceptive failure of hormonal contraceptives containing •oestrogens (alternative contraception recommended)
- Progestogens: bosentan possibly causes contraceptive failure of hormonal contraceptives containing •progestogens (alternative contraception recommended)

Brimonidine *see* Alpha$_2$-adrenoceptor Stimulants

Brinzolamide *see* Diuretics

Bromocriptine

Alcohol: tolerance of bromocriptine reduced by alcohol

Antibacterials: plasma concentration of bromocriptine increased by erythromycin (increased risk of toxicity); plasma concentration of bromocriptine possibly increased by macrolides (increased risk of toxicity)

Antipsychotics: hypoprolactinaemic and antiparkinsonian effects of bromocriptine antagonised by antipsychotics

Domperidone: hypoprolactinaemic effect of bromocriptine possibly antagonised by domperidone

Hormone Antagonists: plasma concentration of bromocriptine increased by octreotide

Memantine: effects of dopaminergics possibly enhanced by memantine

Methyldopa: antiparkinsonian effect of dopaminergics antagonised by methyldopa

Metoclopramide: hypoprolactinaemic effect of bromocriptine antagonised by metoclopramide

- Sympathomimetics: risk of toxicity when bromocriptine given with •isometheptene or •phenylpropanolamine

Buclizine *see* Antihistamines

Budesonide *see* Corticosteroids

Bumetanide *see* Diuretics

Bupivacaine

Anti-arrhythmics: increased myocardial depression when bupivacaine given with anti-arrhythmics

- Beta-blockers: increased risk of bupivacaine toxicity when given with •propranolol

Buprenorphine *see* Opioid Analgesics

Bupropion

Note. Bupropion should be administered with extreme caution to patients receiving other medication known to lower the seizure threshold—see CSM advice p. 261 and Cautions, Contra-indications and Side-effects of individual drugs

- Antidepressants: manufacturer of bupropion advises avoid for 2 weeks after stopping •MAOIs; manufacturer of bupropion advises avoid concomitant use with •moclobemide

Antiepileptics: plasma concentration of bupropion reduced by carbamazepine and phenytoin; metabolism of bupropion inhibited by valproate

- Antivirals: plasma concentration of bupropion increased by •ritonavir (risk of toxicity)—avoid concomitant use

Dopaminergics: increased risk of side-effects when bupropion given with amantadine or levodopa

Buspirone *see* Anxiolytics and Hypnotics

Busulfan

Analgesics: metabolism of *intravenous* busulfan possibly inhibited by paracetamol (manufacturer of *intravenous* busulfan advises caution within 72 hours of paracetamol)

Antiepileptics: cytotoxics possibly reduce absorption of phenytoin

Antifungals: metabolism of busulfan inhibited by itraconazole (increased risk of toxicity)

Busulfan *(continued)*

- • Antipsychotics: avoid concomitant use of cytotoxics with •clozapine (increased risk of agranulocytosis)
- Cytotoxics: increased risk of hepatotoxicity when busulfan given with tioguanine

Butobarbital *see* Barbiturates

Butyrophenones *see* Antipsychotics

Cabergoline

- Antibacterials: plasma concentration of cabergoline increased by erythromycin (increased risk of toxicity); plasma concentration of cabergoline possibly increased by macrolides (increased risk of toxicity)
- Antipsychotics: hypoprolactinaemic and antiparkinsonian effects of cabergoline antagonised by antipsychotics
- Domperidone: hypoprolactinaemic effect of cabergoline possibly antagonised by domperidone
- Memantine: effects of dopaminergics possibly enhanced by memantine
- Methyldopa: antiparkinsonian effect of dopaminergics antagonised by methyldopa
- Metoclopramide: hypoprolactinaemic effect of cabergoline antagonised by metoclopramide

Calcium Salts

Note. see also Antacids

- Antibacterials: calcium salts reduce absorption of ciprofloxacin and tetracycline
- Bisphosphonates: calcium salts reduce absorption of bisphosphonates
- Cardiac Glycosides: large intravenous doses of calcium salts can precipitate arrhythmias when given with cardiac glycosides
- Corticosteroids: absorption of calcium salts reduced by corticosteroids
- Diuretics: increased risk of hypercalcaemia when calcium salts given with thiazides and related diuretics
- Fluorides: calcium salts reduce absorption of fluorides
- Iron: calcium salts reduce absorption of *oral* iron
- Thyroid Hormones: calcium salts reduce absorption of levothyroxine (thyroxine)
- Zinc: calcium salts reduce absorption of zinc

Calcium-channel Blockers

Note. Dihydropyridine calcium-channel blockers include amlodipine, felodipine, isradipine, lacidipine, lercanidipine, nicardipine, nifedipine, nimodipine, and nisoldipine

- ACE Inhibitors: enhanced hypotensive effect when calcium-channel blockers given with ACE inhibitors
- Adrenergic Neurone Blockers: enhanced hypotensive effect when calcium-channel blockers given with adrenergic neurone blockers
- Alcohol: enhanced hypotensive effect when calcium-channel blockers given with alcohol; verapamil possibly increases plasma concentration of alcohol
- Aldesleukin: enhanced hypotensive effect when calcium-channel blockers given with aldesleukin
- • Alpha-blockers: enhanced hypotensive effect when calcium-channel blockers given with •alpha-blockers, also increased risk of first-dose hypotension with post-synaptic alpha-blockers such as prazosin
- • Anaesthetics, General: enhanced hypotensive effect when calcium-channel blockers given with general anaesthetics or isoflurane; hypotensive effect of verapamil enhanced by •general anaesthetics (also AV delay)
- Analgesics: hypotensive effect of calcium-channel blockers antagonised by NSAIDs; diltiazem inhibits metabolism of alfentanil (risk of prolonged or delayed respiratory depression)

Calcium-channel Blockers *(continued)*

- Angiotensin-II Receptor Antagonists: enhanced hypotensive effect when calcium-channel blockers given with angiotensin-II receptor antagonists
- • Anti-arrhythmics: increased risk of bradycardia, AV block and myocardial depression when diltiazem or verapamil given with •amiodarone; increased risk of myocardial depression and asystole when verapamil given with •disopyramide or •flecainide; verapamil increases plasma concentration of •quinidine (extreme hypotension may occur); nifedipine reduces plasma concentration of quinidine
- • Antibacterials: metabolism of felodipine possibly inhibited by erythromycin (increased plasma concentration); manufacturer of lercanidipine advises avoid concomitant use with erythromycin; metabolism of diltiazem, nifedipine, nimodipine and verapamil accelerated by •rifampicin (plasma concentration significantly reduced); metabolism of isradipine, nicardipine and nisoldipine possibly accelerated by •rifampicin (possible significantly reduced plasma concentration); plasma concentration of nifedipine increased by •quinupristin/dalfopristin
- Antidepressants: diltiazem and verapamil increase plasma concentration of imipramine; enhanced hypotensive effect when calcium-channel blockers given with MAOIs; diltiazem and verapamil possibly increase plasma concentration of tricyclics
- Antidiabetics: glucose tolerance occasionally impaired when nifedipine given with insulin
- • Antiepileptics: effects of dihydropyridines, nicardipine and nifedipine probably reduced by carbamazepine; diltiazem and verapamil enhance effects of •carbamazepine; effects of felodipine and isradipine reduced by carbamazepine; plasma concentration of nisoldipine reduced by phenytoin; effects of dihydropyridines, nicardipine and nifedipine probably reduced by •phenytoin; effects of felodipine, isradipine and verapamil reduced by phenytoin; diltiazem increases plasma concentration of •phenytoin but also effect of diltiazem reduced; effects of felodipine and isradipine reduced by •primidone; effects of dihydropyridines, diltiazem and verapamil probably reduced by •primidone
- • Antifungals: metabolism of dihydropyridines possibly inhibited by itraconazole and ketoconazole (increased plasma concentration); metabolism of felodipine inhibited by •itraconazole and •ketoconazole (increased plasma concentration); manufacturer of lercanidipine advises avoid concomitant use with itraconazole and ketoconazole; negative inotropic effect possibly increased when calcium-channel blockers given with itraconazole
- Antimalarials: possible increased risk of bradycardia when calcium-channel blockers given with mefloquine
- Antipsychotics: enhanced hypotensive effect when calcium-channel blockers given with antipsychotics
- • Antivirals: plasma concentration of diltiazem, nicardipine, nifedipine and nimodipine possibly increased by amprenavir; plasma concentration of diltiazem increased by •atazanavir (reduce dose of diltiazem); plasma concentration of verapamil possibly increased by atazanavir; manufacturer of lercanidipine advises avoid concomitant use with ritonavir; plasma concentration of calcium-channel blockers possibly increased by •ritonavir

Calcium-channel Blockers *(continued)*

Anxiolytics and Hypnotics: enhanced hypotensive effect when calcium-channel blockers given with anxiolytics and hypnotics; diltiazem and verapamil inhibit metabolism of midazolam (increased plasma concentration with increased sedation); absorption of lercanidipine increased by midazolam; diltiazem and verapamil increase plasma concentration of buspirone (reduce dose of buspirone)

• Barbiturates: effects of dihydropyridines, diltiazem and verapamil probably reduced by •barbiturates; effects of felodipine and isradipine reduced by •barbiturates

• Beta-blockers: enhanced hypotensive effect when calcium-channel blockers given with beta-blockers; increased risk of AV block and bradycardia when diltiazem given with •beta-blockers; asystole, severe hypotension and heart failure when verapamil given with •beta-blockers (see p. 113); possible severe hypotension and heart failure when nifedipine or nisoldipine given with •beta-blockers

Calcium-channel Blockers: plasma concentration of both drugs may increase when diltiazem given with nifedipine

• Cardiac Glycosides: diltiazem, lercanidipine and nicardipine increase plasma concentration of •digoxin; verapamil increases plasma concentration of •digoxin, also increased risk of AV block and bradycardia; nifedipine possibly increases plasma concentration of •digoxin

• Ciclosporin: diltiazem, nicardipine and verapamil increase plasma concentration of •ciclosporin; combination of lercanidipine with •ciclosporin may increase plasma concentration of either drug (or both)—avoid concomitant use; plasma concentration of nifedipine possibly increased by ciclosporin (increased risk of toxicity including gingival hyperplasia)

• Cilostazol: diltiazem increases plasma concentration of •cilostazol—avoid concomitant use

Clonidine: enhanced hypotensive effect when calcium-channel blockers given with clonidine

Corticosteroids: hypotensive effect of calcium-channel blockers antagonised by corticosteroids

Cytotoxics: nifedipine possibly inhibits metabolism of vincristine

Diazoxide: enhanced hypotensive effect when calcium-channel blockers given with diazoxide

Diuretics: enhanced hypotensive effect when calcium-channel blockers given with diuretics; diltiazem and verapamil increase plasma concentration of eplerenone (reduce dose of eplerenone)

Dopaminergics: enhanced hypotensive effect when calcium-channel blockers given with levodopa

Grapefruit Juice: plasma concentration of felodipine, isradipine, lacidipine, lercanidipine, nicardipine, nifedipine, nimodipine, nisoldipine and verapamil increased by grapefruit juice

Hormone Antagonists: diltiazem and verapamil increase plasma concentration of dutasteride

• Lipid-regulating Drugs: possible increased risk of myopathy when diltiazem given with simvastatin; increased risk of myopathy when verapamil given with •simvastatin

Lithium: neurotoxicity may occur when diltiazem or verapamil given with lithium without increased plasma concentration of lithium

• Magnesium (parenteral): profound hypotension reported with concomitant use of nifedipine and •parenteral magnesium in pre-eclampsia

Methyldopa: enhanced hypotensive effect when calcium-channel blockers given with methyldopa

Calcium-channel Blockers *(continued)*

Moxisylyte (thymoxamine): enhanced hypotensive effect when calcium-channel blockers given with moxisylyte

Moxonidine: enhanced hypotensive effect when calcium-channel blockers given with moxonidine

Muscle Relaxants: verapamil enhances effects of non-depolarising muscle relaxants and suxamethonium; enhanced hypotensive effect when calcium-channel blockers given with baclofen or tizanidine; risk of arrhythmias when diltiazem given with intravenous dantrolene; hypotension, myocardial depression, and hyperkalaemia when verapamil given with intravenous dantrolene; nifedipine enhances effects of non-depolarising muscle relaxants

Nitrates: enhanced hypotensive effect when calcium-channel blockers given with nitrates

Oestrogens: hypotensive effect of calcium-channel blockers antagonised by oestrogens

Prostaglandins: enhanced hypotensive effect when calcium-channel blockers given with alprostadil

Sildenafil: enhanced hypotensive effect when amlodipine given with sildenafil

• Sirolimus: diltiazem increases plasma concentration of •sirolimus; plasma concentration of both drugs increased when verapamil given with •sirolimus

• Tacrolimus: diltiazem and nifedipine increase plasma concentration of •tacrolimus; felodipine possibly increases plasma concentration of tacrolimus

• Theophylline: calcium-channel blockers possibly increase plasma concentration of •theophylline (enhanced effect); diltiazem increases plasma concentration of theophylline; verapamil increases plasma concentration of •theophylline (enhanced effect)

Ulcer-healing Drugs: metabolism of calcium-channel blockers possibly inhibited by cimetidine (increased plasma concentration)

Vardenafil: enhanced hypotensive effect when nifedipine given with vardenafil

Vasodilator Antihypertensives: enhanced hypotensive effect when calcium-channel blockers given with hydralazine, minoxidil or nitroprusside

Calcium-channel Blockers (dihydropyridines) *see* Calcium-channel Blockers

Candesartan *see* Angiotensin-II Receptor Antagonists

Capecitabine *see* Fluorouracil

Capreomycin

Antibacterials: increased risk of nephrotoxicity when capreomycin given with colistin or polymyxins; increased risk of nephrotoxicity and ototoxicity when capreomycin given with aminoglycosides or vancomycin

Cytotoxics: increased risk of nephrotoxicity and ototoxicity when capreomycin given with platinum compounds

Oestrogens: broad-spectrum antibacterials possibly reduce contraceptive effect of oestrogens (risk probably small, see p. 407)

Captopril *see* ACE Inhibitors

Carbamazepine

Alcohol: CNS side-effects of carbamazepine possibly increased by alcohol

• Analgesics: effects of carbamazepine enhanced by •dextropropoxyphene; carbamazepine reduces plasma concentration of methadone; carbamazepine reduces effects of tramadol

• Antibacterials: plasma concentration of carbamazepine increased by •clarithromycin and •erythromycin; plasma concentration of carbamazepine reduced by •rifabutin; carbamazepine accelerates

Carbamazepine

- Antibacterials *(continued)* metabolism of doxycycline (reduced effect); plasma concentration of carbamazepine increased by •isoniazid (also possibly increased isoniazid hepatotoxicity); carbamazepine reduces plasma concentration of •telithromycin (avoid during and for 2 weeks after carbamazepine)
- Anticoagulants: carbamazepine accelerates metabolism of •coumarins (reduced anticoagulant effect)
- Antidepressants: plasma concentration of carbamazepine increased by •fluoxetine and •fluvoxamine; carbamazepine reduces plasma concentration of •mianserin, mirtazapine and paroxetine; manufacturer of carbamazepine advises avoid for 2 weeks after stopping •MAOIs, also antagonism of anticonvulsant effect; anticonvulsant effect of antiepileptics possibly antagonised by MAOIs and •tricyclic-related antidepressants (convulsive threshold lowered); anticonvulsant effect of antiepileptics antagonised by •SSRIs and •tricyclics (convulsive threshold lowered); plasma concentration of carbamazepine reduced by •St John's wort—avoid concomitant use; carbamazepine accelerates metabolism of •tricyclics (reduced plasma concentration and reduced effect)

Antiepileptics: carbamazepine possibly reduces plasma concentration of ethosuximide; carbamazepine often reduces plasma concentration of lamotrigine, also plasma concentration of an active metabolite of carbamazepine sometimes raised (but evidence is conflicting); plasma concentration of carbamazepine sometimes reduced by oxcarbazepine (but concentration of an active metabolite of carbamazepine may be increased), also plasma concentration of an active metabolite of oxcarbazepine often reduced; plasma concentration of both drugs often reduced when carbamazepine given with phenytoin, also plasma concentration of phenytoin may be increased; plasma concentration of carbamazepine often reduced by primidone, also plasma concentration of primidone sometimes reduced (but concentration of an active metabolite of primidone often increased); carbamazepine reduces plasma concentration of tiagabine; carbamazepine often reduces plasma concentration of topiramate; carbamazepine reduces plasma concentration of valproate, also plasma concentration of active metabolite of carbamazepine increased; carbamazepine reduces plasma concentration of zonisamide, effect on carbamazepine plasma concentration not predictable

- Antifungals: plasma concentration of carbamazepine possibly increased by miconazole; carbamazepine possibly reduces plasma concentration of itraconazole; carbamazepine possibly reduces plasma concentration of •voriconazole—avoid concomitant use; carbamazepine possibly reduces plasma concentration of caspofungin—consider increasing dose of caspofungin
- Antimalarials: possible increased risk of convulsions when antiepileptics given with chloroquine and hydroxychloroquine; anticonvulsant effect of antiepileptics and carbamazepine antagonised by •mefloquine
- Antipsychotics: anticonvulsant effect of carbamazepine antagonised by •antipsychotics (convulsive threshold lowered); carbamazepine accelerates metabolism of haloperidol, olanzapine, quetiapine, risperidone and sertindole (reduced plasma concentration); carbamazepine reduces plasma concentration of •aripiprazole—increase dose of aripiprazole; carbamazepine accelerates metabolism of •clozapine (reduced plasma concentration), also avoid concomitant use of drugs with substantial potential for causing agranulocytosis
- Antivirals: plasma concentration of carbamazepine possibly increased by amprenavir and •ritonavir; carbamazepine possibly reduces plasma concentration of indinavir, lopinavir, nelfinavir and saquinavir

Anxiolytics and Hypnotics: carbamazepine often reduces plasma concentration of clonazepam

Aprepitant: carbamazepine possibly reduces plasma concentration of aprepitant

Barbiturates: plasma concentration of carbamazepine reduced by phenobarbital

Bupropion: carbamazepine reduces plasma concentration of bupropion

- Calcium-channel Blockers: carbamazepine reduces effects of felodipine and isradipine; carbamazepine probably reduces effects of dihydropyridines, nicardipine and nifedipine; effects of carbamazepine enhanced by •diltiazem and •verapamil

Cardiac Glycosides: carbamazepine accelerates metabolism of digitoxin (reduced effect)

- Ciclosporin: carbamazepine accelerates metabolism of •ciclosporin (reduced plasma concentration)
- Corticosteroids: carbamazepine accelerates metabolism of •corticosteroids (reduced effect)
- Diuretics: increased risk of hyponatraemia when carbamazepine given with diuretics; plasma concentration of carbamazepine increased by •acetazolamide; carbamazepine reduces plasma concentration of •eplerenone—avoid concomitant use
- Hormone Antagonists: metabolism of carbamazepine inhibited by •danazol (increased risk of toxicity); carbamazepine accelerates metabolism of gestrinone (reduced plasma concentration); carbamazepine possibly accelerates metabolism of toremifene (reduced plasma concentration)

5HT$_3$ Antagonists: carbamazepine accelerates metabolism of ondansetron (reduced effect)

Lithium: neurotoxicity may occur when carbamazepine given with lithium without increased plasma concentration of lithium

Muscle Relaxants: carbamazepine antagonises muscle relaxant effect of non-depolarising muscle relaxants (accelerated recovery from neuromuscular blockade)

- Oestrogens: carbamazepine accelerates metabolism of •oestrogens (reduced contraceptive effect—see p. 407)
- Progestogens: carbamazepine accelerates metabolism of •progestogens (reduced contraceptive effect—see p. 407)

Retinoids: plasma concentration of carbamazepine possibly reduced by isotretinoin

Theophylline: carbamazepine accelerates metabolism of theophylline (reduced effect)

Thyroid Hormones: carbamazepine accelerates metabolism of thyroid hormones (may increase requirements for thyroid hormones in hypothyroidism)

Tibolone: carbamazepine accelerates metabolism of tibolone (reduced plasma concentration)

- Ulcer-healing Drugs: metabolism of carbamazepine inhibited by •cimetidine (increased plasma concentration)

Vitamins: carbamazepine possibly increases requirements for vitamin D

Carbapenems *see* Ertapenem, Imipenem with Cilastatin, and Meropenem

Carbonic Anhydrase Inhibitors *see* Diuretics

Carboplatin *see* Platinum Compounds

Carboprost *see* Prostaglandins

Cardiac Glycosides

ACE Inhibitors: plasma concentration of digoxin possibly increased by captopril

Alpha-blockers: plasma concentration of digoxin increased by prazosin

Aminosalicylates: absorption of digoxin possibly reduced by sulfasalazine

Analgesics: plasma concentration of cardiac glycosides possibly increased by NSAIDs, also possible exacerbation of heart failure and reduction of renal function

• Angiotensin-II Receptor Antagonists: plasma concentration of digoxin increased by •telmisartan

Antacids: absorption of digoxin possibly reduced by antacids

• Anti-arrhythmics: plasma concentration of digoxin increased by •amiodarone, •propafenone and •quinidine (halve dose of digoxin)

Antibacterials: plasma concentration of digoxin possibly increased by gentamicin, telithromycin and trimethoprim; absorption of digoxin reduced by neomycin; plasma concentration of digoxin possibly reduced by rifampicin; plasma concentration of digoxin increased by macrolides (increased risk of toxicity); metabolism of digitoxin accelerated by rifamycins (reduced effect)

• Antidepressants: plasma concentration of digoxin reduced by •St John's wort—avoid concomitant use

Antidiabetics: plasma concentration of digoxin possibly reduced by acarbose

Antiepileptics: metabolism of digitoxin accelerated by carbamazepine, phenytoin and primidone (reduced effect); plasma concentration of digoxin possibly reduced by phenytoin

• Antifungals: increased cardiac toxicity with cardiac glycosides if hypokalaemia occurs with •amphotericin; plasma concentration of digoxin increased by •itraconazole

• Antimalarials: plasma concentration of digoxin possibly increased by •chloroquine and hydroxychloroquine; possible increased risk of bradycardia when digoxin given with mefloquine; plasma concentration of digoxin increased by •quinine

Anxiolytics and Hypnotics: plasma concentration of digoxin increased by alprazolam (increased risk of toxicity)

Barbiturates: metabolism of digitoxin accelerated by barbiturates (reduced effect)

Beta-blockers: increased risk of AV block and bradycardia when cardiac glycosides given with beta-blockers

Calcium Salts: arrhythmias can be precipitated when cardiac glycosides given with large intravenous doses of calcium salts

• Calcium-channel Blockers: plasma concentration of digoxin increased by •diltiazem, •lercanidipine and •nicardipine; plasma concentration of digoxin possibly increased by •nifedipine; plasma concentration of digoxin increased by •verapamil, also increased risk of AV block and bradycardia

• Ciclosporin: plasma concentration of digoxin increased by •ciclosporin (increased risk of toxicity)

Corticosteroids: increased risk of hypokalaemia when cardiac glycosides given with corticosteroids

Cardiac Glycosides *(continued)*

• Diuretics: increased cardiac toxicity with cardiac glycosides if hypokalaemia occurs with •acetazolamide, •loop diuretics or •thiazides and related diuretics; plasma concentration of digitoxin possibly affected by spironolactone; plasma concentration of digoxin increased by •spironolactone

Hormone Antagonists: metabolism of digitoxin accelerated by aminoglutethimide (reduced effect)

Lipid-regulating Drugs: absorption of cardiac glycosides possibly reduced by colestipol and colestyramine; plasma concentration of digoxin possibly increased by atorvastatin

Muscle Relaxants: risk of ventricular arrhythmias when cardiac glycosides given with suxamethonium; possible increased risk of bradycardia when cardiac glycosides given with tizanidine

Penicillamine: plasma concentration of digoxin possibly reduced by penicillamine

Sympathomimetics, $Beta_2$: plasma concentration of digoxin possibly reduced by salbutamol

Ulcer-healing Drugs: plasma concentration of digoxin possibly slightly increased by proton pump inhibitors; absorption of cardiac glycosides possibly reduced by sucralfate

Carisoprodol *see* Muscle Relaxants

Carteolol *see* Beta-blockers

Carvedilol *see* Beta-blockers

Caspofungin

Antibacterials: plasma concentration of caspofungin initially increased and then reduced by rifampicin (consider increasing dose of caspofungin)

Antiepileptics: plasma concentration of caspofungin possibly reduced by carbamazepine and phenytoin—consider increasing dose of caspofungin

Antivirals: plasma concentration of caspofungin possibly reduced by efavirenz and nevirapine—consider increasing dose of caspofungin

• Ciclosporin: plasma concentration of caspofungin increased by •ciclosporin (manufacturer of caspofungin recommends monitoring liver enzymes)

Corticosteroids: plasma concentration of caspofungin possibly reduced by dexamethasone—consider increasing dose of caspofungin

• Tacrolimus: caspofungin reduces plasma concentration of •tacrolimus

Cefaclor *see* Cephalosporins

Cefadroxil *see* Cephalosporins

Cefalexin *see* Cephalosporins

Cefixime *see* Cephalosporins

Cefotaxime *see* Cephalosporins

Cefpirome *see* Cephalosporins

Cefpodoxime *see* Cephalosporins

Cefprozil *see* Cephalosporins

Cefradine *see* Cephalosporins

Ceftazidime *see* Cephalosporins

Ceftriaxone *see* Cephalosporins

Cefuroxime *see* Cephalosporins

Celecoxib *see* NSAIDs

Celiprolol *see* Beta-blockers

Cephalosporins

Antacids: absorption of cefaclor and cefpodoxime reduced by antacids

• Anticoagulants: cephalosporins possibly enhance anticoagulant effect of •coumarins

Oestrogens: broad-spectrum antibacterials possibly reduce contraceptive effect of oestrogens (risk probably small, see p. 407)

Probenecid: excretion of cephalosporins reduced by probenecid (increased plasma concentration)

Ulcer-healing Drugs: absorption of cefpodoxime reduced by histamine H_2-antagonists

Cetirizine *see* Antihistamines

Chloral *see* Anxiolytics and Hypnotics

Chloramphenicol

Antibacterials: metabolism of chloramphenicol accelerated by rifampicin (reduced plasma concentration)
- Anticoagulants: chloramphenicol enhances anticoagulant effect of •coumarins
- Antidiabetics: chloramphenicol enhances effects of •sulphonylureas
- Antiepileptics: chloramphenicol increases plasma concentration of •phenytoin (increased risk of toxicity); metabolism of chloramphenicol accelerated by •primidone (reduced plasma concentration)
- Antipsychotics: avoid concomitant use of chloramphenicol with •clozapine (increased risk of agranulocytosis)
- Barbiturates: metabolism of chloramphenicol accelerated by •barbiturates (reduced plasma concentration)
- Ciclosporin: chloramphenicol possibly increases plasma concentration of •ciclosporin

Hydroxocobalamin: chloramphenicol reduces response to hydroxocobalamin

Oestrogens: broad-spectrum antibacterials possibly reduce contraceptive effect of oestrogens (risk probably small, see p. 407)
- Tacrolimus: chloramphenicol possibly increases plasma concentration of •tacrolimus

Chlordiazepoxide *see* Anxiolytics and Hypnotics

Chloroquine and Hydroxychloroquine

Adsorbents: absorption of chloroquine and hydroxychloroquine reduced by kaolin

Agalsidase Beta: chloroquine and hydroxychloroquine possibly inhibit effects of agalsidase beta (manufacturer of agalsidase beta advises avoid concomitant use)

Antacids: absorption of chloroquine and hydroxychloroquine reduced by antacids
- Anti-arrhythmics: increased risk of ventricular arrhythmias when chloroquine and hydroxychloroquine given with •amiodarone—avoid concomitant use
- Antibacterials: increased risk of ventricular arrhythmias when chloroquine and hydroxychloroquine given with •moxifloxacin—avoid concomitant use

Antiepileptics: possible increased risk of convulsions when chloroquine and hydroxychloroquine given with antiepileptics
- Antimalarials: avoidance of antimalarials advised by manufacturer of •artemether/lumefantrine; increased risk of convulsions when chloroquine and hydroxychloroquine given with •mefloquine
- Cardiac Glycosides: chloroquine and hydroxychloroquine possibly increase plasma concentration of •digoxin
- Ciclosporin: chloroquine and hydroxychloroquine increase plasma concentration of •ciclosporin (increased risk of toxicity)

Laronidase: chloroquine and hydroxychloroquine possibly inhibit effects of laronidase (manufacturer of laronidase advises avoid concomitant use)

Parasympathomimetics: chloroquine and hydroxychloroquine have potential to increase symptoms of myasthenia gravis and thus diminish effect of neostigmine and pyridostigmine

Ulcer-healing Drugs: metabolism of chloroquine and hydroxychloroquine inhibited by cimetidine (increased plasma concentration)

Chlorothiazide *see* Diuretics

Chlorphenamine (chlorpheniramine) *see* Antihistamines

Chlorpromazine *see* Antipsychotics

Chlorpropamide *see* Antidiabetics

Chlortalidone *see* Diuretics

Chlortetracycline *see* Tetracyclines

Ciclesonide *see* Corticosteroids

Ciclosporin
- ACE Inhibitors: increased risk of hyperkalaemia when ciclosporin given with •ACE inhibitors

Allopurinol: plasma concentration of ciclosporin possibly increased by allopurinol (risk of nephrotoxicity)
- Analgesics: increased risk of nephrotoxicity when ciclosporin given with •NSAIDs; ciclosporin increases plasma concentration of •diclofenac (halve dose of diclofenac)
- Angiotensin-II Receptor Antagonists: increased risk of hyperkalaemia when ciclosporin given with •angiotensin-II receptor antagonists

Anti-arrhythmics: plasma concentration of ciclosporin possibly increased by amiodarone and propafenone
- Antibacterials: metabolism of ciclosporin inhibited by •clarithromycin and •erythromycin (increased plasma concentration); metabolism of ciclosporin accelerated by •rifampicin (reduced plasma concentration); plasma concentration of ciclosporin possibly reduced by •sulfadiazine; plasma concentration of ciclosporin possibly increased by •chloramphenicol, •doxycycline and •telithromycin; increased risk of nephrotoxicity when ciclosporin given with •aminoglycosides, •polymyxins, •quinolones, •sulphonamides or •vancomycin; metabolism of ciclosporin possibly inhibited by •macrolides (increased plasma concentration); plasma concentration of ciclosporin increased by •quinupristin/dalfopristin; increased risk of nephrotoxicity when ciclosporin given with •trimethoprim, also plasma concentration of ciclosporin reduced by intravenous trimethoprim
- Antidepressants: plasma concentration of ciclosporin reduced by •St John's wort—avoid concomitant use
- Antiepileptics: metabolism of ciclosporin accelerated by •carbamazepine and •phenytoin (reduced plasma concentration); metabolism of ciclosporin accelerated by •primidone (reduced effect)
- Antifungals: metabolism of ciclosporin inhibited by •fluconazole, •itraconazole, •ketoconazole and •voriconazole (increased plasma concentration); metabolism of ciclosporin possibly inhibited by •miconazole (increased plasma concentration); increased risk of nephrotoxicity when ciclosporin given with •amphotericin; ciclosporin increases plasma concentration of •caspofungin (manufacturer of caspofungin recommends monitoring liver enzymes); plasma concentration of ciclosporin possibly reduced by griseofulvin
- Antimalarials: plasma concentration of ciclosporin increased by •chloroquine and hydroxychloroquine (increased risk of toxicity)
- Antivirals: plasma concentration of ciclosporin possibly increased by •atazanavir, •nelfinavir and •ritonavir; plasma concentration of both drugs increased when ciclosporin given with •saquinavir
- Barbiturates: metabolism of ciclosporin accelerated by •barbiturates (reduced effect)
- Beta-blockers: plasma concentration of ciclosporin increased by •carvedilol
- Bile Acids: absorption of ciclosporin increased by •ursodeoxycholic acid
- Bosentan: ciclosporin increases plasma concentration of •bosentan (also plasma concentration of ciclosporin reduced—avoid concomitant use)

Ciclosporin *(continued)*
- Calcium-channel Blockers: combination of ciclosporin with •lercanidipine may increase plasma concentration of either drug (or both)—avoid concomitant use; plasma concentration of ciclosporin increased by •diltiazem, •nicardipine and •verapamil; ciclosporin possibly increases plasma concentration of nifedipine (increased risk of toxicity including gingival hyperplasia)
- Cardiac Glycosides: ciclosporin increases plasma concentration of •digoxin (increased risk of toxicity)
- Colchicine: possible increased risk of nephrotoxicity and myotoxicity when ciclosporin given with •colchicine (increased plasma concentration of ciclosporin)
- Corticosteroids: plasma concentration of ciclosporin increased by high-dose •methylprednisolone (risk of convulsions); ciclosporin increases plasma concentration of prednisolone
- Cytotoxics: increased risk of nephrotoxicity when ciclosporin given with •melphalan; increased risk of neurotoxicity when ciclosporin given with •doxorubicin; risk of toxicity when ciclosporin given with •methotrexate; *in vitro* studies suggest a possible interaction between ciclosporin and docetaxel (consult docetaxel product literature); ciclosporin possibly increases plasma concentration of etoposide (increased risk of toxicity)
- Diuretics: increased risk of hyperkalaemia when ciclosporin given with •potassium-sparing diuretics and aldosterone antagonists
- Grapefruit Juice: plasma concentration of ciclosporin increased by •grapefruit juice (increased risk of toxicity)
- Hormone Antagonists: metabolism of ciclosporin inhibited by •danazol (increased plasma concentration); plasma concentration of ciclosporin reduced by lanreotide and •octreotide
- Lipid-regulating Drugs: increased risk of renal impairment when ciclosporin given with fenofibrate; increased risk of myopathy when ciclosporin given with •rosuvastatin (avoid concomitant use); increased risk of myopathy when ciclosporin given with •statins; ciclosporin increases plasma concentration of ezetimibe
- Metoclopramide: plasma concentration of ciclosporin increased by •metoclopramide
- Modafinil: plasma concentration of ciclosporin reduced by •modafinil

  Oestrogens: plasma concentration of ciclosporin possibly increased by oestrogens
- Orlistat: absorption of ciclosporin possibly reduced by •orlistat
- Potassium Salts: increased risk of hyperkalaemia when ciclosporin given with •potassium salts
- Progestogens: metabolism of ciclosporin inhibited by •progestogens (increased plasma concentration)

  Sirolimus: ciclosporin increases plasma concentration of sirolimus
- Tacrolimus: plasma concentration of ciclosporin increased by •tacrolimus (increased risk of toxicity)—avoid concomitant use
- Ulcer-healing Drugs: plasma concentration of ciclosporin possibly increased by •cimetidine; plasma concentration of ciclosporin possibly affected by omeprazole

Cidofovir
  Antivirals: combination of cidofovir with tenofovir may increase plasma concentration of either drug (or both)

Cilazapril *see* ACE Inhibitors

Cilostazol
- Anagrelide: avoidance of cilostazol advised by manufacturer of •anagrelide

  Analgesics: manufacturer of cilostazol recommends dose of concomitant aspirin should not exceed 80 mg daily
- Antibacterials: plasma concentration of cilostazol increased by •erythromycin (also plasma concentration of erythromycin reduced)—avoid concomitant use
- Antifungals: plasma concentration of cilostazol possibly increased by •ketoconazole—avoid concomitant use
- Antivirals: plasma concentration of cilostazol possibly increased by •amprenavir, •indinavir, •lopinavir, •nelfinavir, •ritonavir and •saquinavir—avoid concomitant use
- Calcium-channel Blockers: plasma concentration of cilostazol increased by •diltiazem—avoid concomitant use
- Ulcer-healing Drugs: plasma concentration of cilostazol possibly increased by •cimetidine and •lansoprazole—avoid concomitant use; plasma concentration of cilostazol increased by •omeprazole (risk of toxicity)—avoid concomitant use

Cimetidine *see* Histamine H_2-antagonists

Cinacalcet
  Antifungals: metabolism of cinacalcet inhibited by ketoconazole (increased plasma concentration)
  Tobacco: metabolism of cinacalcet increased by tobacco smoking (reduced plasma concentration)

Cinnarizine *see* Antihistamines
Ciprofibrate *see* Fibrates
Ciprofloxacin *see* Quinolones
Cisatracurium *see* Muscle Relaxants
Cisplatin *see* Platinum Compounds
Citalopram *see* Antidepressants, SSRI
Clarithromycin *see* Macrolides
Clemastine *see* Antihistamines

Clindamycin
- Muscle Relaxants: clindamycin enhances effects of •non-depolarising muscle relaxants and •suxamethonium

  Oestrogens: broad-spectrum antibacterials possibly reduce contraceptive effect of oestrogens (risk probably small, see p. 407)
  Parasympathomimetics: clindamycin antagonises effects of neostigmine and pyridostigmine

Clobazam *see* Anxiolytics and Hypnotics
Clomethiazole *see* Anxiolytics and Hypnotics
Clomipramine *see* Antidepressants, Tricyclic
Clonazepam *see* Anxiolytics and Hypnotics

Clonidine
  ACE Inhibitors: enhanced hypotensive effect when clonidine given with ACE inhibitors; previous treatment with clonidine possibly delays antihypertensive effect of captopril
  Adrenergic Neurone Blockers: enhanced hypotensive effect when clonidine given with adrenergic neurone blockers
  Alcohol: enhanced hypotensive effect when clonidine given with alcohol
  Aldesleukin: enhanced hypotensive effect when clonidine given with aldesleukin
  Alpha-blockers: enhanced hypotensive effect when clonidine given with alpha-blockers
  Anaesthetics, General: enhanced hypotensive effect when clonidine given with general anaesthetics
  Analgesics: hypotensive effect of clonidine antagonised by NSAIDs
  Angiotensin-II Receptor Antagonists: enhanced hypotensive effect when clonidine given with angiotensin-II receptor antagonists

Clonidine *(continued)*

- • Antidepressants: enhanced hypotensive effect when clonidine given with MAOIs; hypotensive effect of clonidine antagonised by •tricyclics, also increased risk of hypertension on clonidine withdrawal
- Antipsychotics: enhanced hypotensive effect when clonidine given with phenothiazines
- Anxiolytics and Hypnotics: enhanced hypotensive effect when clonidine given with anxiolytics and hypnotics
- • Beta-blockers: increased risk of withdrawal hypertension when clonidine given with •beta-blockers (withdraw beta-blockers several days before slowly withdrawing clonidine)
- Calcium-channel Blockers: enhanced hypotensive effect when clonidine given with calcium-channel blockers
- Corticosteroids: hypotensive effect of clonidine antagonised by corticosteroids
- Diazoxide: enhanced hypotensive effect when clonidine given with diazoxide
- Diuretics: enhanced hypotensive effect when clonidine given with diuretics
- Dopaminergics: enhanced hypotensive effect when clonidine given with levodopa
- Methyldopa: enhanced hypotensive effect when clonidine given with methyldopa
- Moxisylyte (thymoxamine): enhanced hypotensive effect when clonidine given with moxisylyte
- Moxonidine: enhanced hypotensive effect when clonidine given with moxonidine
- Muscle Relaxants: enhanced hypotensive effect when clonidine given with baclofen or tizanidine
- Nitrates: enhanced hypotensive effect when clonidine given with nitrates
- Oestrogens: hypotensive effect of clonidine antagonised by oestrogens
- Prostaglandins: enhanced hypotensive effect when clonidine given with alprostadil
- • Sympathomimetics: possible risk of hypertension when clonidine given with adrenaline (epinephrine) or noradrenaline (norepinephrine); serious adverse events reported with concomitant use of clonidine and •methylphenidate (causality not established)
- Vasodilator Antihypertensives: enhanced hypotensive effect when clonidine given with hydralazine, minoxidil or nitroprusside

Clopamide *see* Diuretics

Clopidogrel

- Analgesics: increased risk of bleeding when clopidogrel given with NSAIDs or aspirin
- • Anticoagulants: manufacturer of clopidogrel advises avoid concomitant use with •warfarin; antiplatelet action of clopidogrel enhances anticoagulant effect of •coumarins and •phenindione; increased risk of bleeding when clopidogrel given with heparins
- Dipyridamole: increased risk of bleeding when clopidogrel given with dipyridamole
- Iloprost: increased risk of bleeding when clopidogrel given with iloprost

Clorazepate *see* Anxiolytics and Hypnotics

Clotrimazole *see* Antifungals, Imidazole

Clozapine *see* Antipsychotics

Co-amoxiclav *see* Penicillins

Co-beneldopa *see* Levodopa

Co-careldopa *see* Levodopa

Codeine *see* Opioid Analgesics

Co-fluampicil *see* Penicillins

Colchicine

- • Ciclosporin: possible increased risk of nephrotoxicity and myotoxicity when colchicine given with •ciclosporin (increased plasma concentration of ciclosporin)

Colestipol

Note. Other drugs should be taken at least 1 hour before or 4-6 hours after colestipol to reduce possible interference with absorption

- Bile Acids: colestipol possibly reduces absorption of bile acids
- Cardiac Glycosides: colestipol possibly reduces absorption of cardiac glycosides
- Diuretics: colestipol reduces absorption of thiazides and related diuretics (give at least 2 hours apart)
- Thyroid Hormones: colestipol reduces absorption of thyroid hormones

Colestyramine

Note. Other drugs should be taken at least 1 hour before or 4-6 hours after colestyramine to reduce possible interference with absorption

- Analgesics: colestyramine increases the excretion of meloxicam; colestyramine reduces absorption of paracetamol
- Antibacterials: colestyramine antagonises effects of oral vancomycin
- • Anticoagulants: colestyramine may enhance or reduce anticoagulant effect of •coumarins and •phenindione
- Antidiabetics: colestyramine possibly enhances hypoglycaemic effect of acarbose
- Antiepileptics: colestyramine possibly reduces absorption of valproate
- Bile Acids: colestyramine possibly reduces absorption of bile acids
- Cardiac Glycosides: colestyramine possibly reduces absorption of cardiac glycosides
- Cytotoxics: colestyramine reduces absorption of mycophenolate mofetil
- Diuretics: colestyramine reduces absorption of thiazides and related diuretics (give at least 2 hours apart)
- Leflunomide: colestyramine significantly decreases effect of leflunomide (enhanced elimination)—avoid unless drug elimination desired
- Raloxifene: colestyramine reduces absorption of raloxifene (manufacturer of raloxifene advises avoid concomitant administration)
- Thyroid Hormones: colestyramine reduces absorption of thyroid hormones

Colistin *see* Polymyxins

Contraceptives, oral *see* Oestrogens and Progestogens

Corticosteroids

Note. Interactions do not generally apply to corticosteroids used for topical action (including inhalation) unless specified

- ACE Inhibitors: corticosteroids antagonise hypotensive effect of ACE inhibitors
- Adrenergic Neurone Blockers: corticosteroids antagonise hypotensive effect of adrenergic neurone blockers
- Alpha-blockers: corticosteroids antagonise hypotensive effect of alpha-blockers
- Analgesics: increased risk of gastro-intestinal bleeding and ulceration when corticosteroids given with NSAIDs; increased risk of gastro-intestinal bleeding and ulceration when corticosteroids given with aspirin, also corticosteroids reduce plasma concentration of salicylate
- Angiotensin-II Receptor Antagonists: corticosteroids antagonise hypotensive effect of angiotensin-II receptor antagonists
- Antacids: absorption of deflazacort reduced by antacids

Corticosteroids *(continued)*

• Antibacterials: plasma concentration of methylprednisolone possibly increased by clarithromycin; metabolism of corticosteroids possibly inhibited by erythromycin; metabolism of methylprednisolone inhibited by erythromycin; metabolism of corticosteroids accelerated by •rifamycins (reduced effect)

• Anticoagulants: corticosteroids may enhance or reduce anticoagulant effect of •coumarins (high-dose corticosteroids enhance anticoagulant effect)

Antidiabetics: corticosteroids antagonise hypoglycaemic effect of antidiabetics

• Antiepileptics: metabolism of corticosteroids accelerated by •carbamazepine, •phenytoin and •primidone (reduced effect)

• Antifungals: metabolism of corticosteroids possibly inhibited by ketoconazole; plasma concentration of inhaled mometasone increased by ketoconazole; metabolism of methylprednisolone inhibited by ketoconazole; increased risk of hypokalaemia when corticosteroids given with •amphotericin—avoid concomitant use unless amphotericin needed to control reactions; metabolism of methylprednisolone possibly inhibited by itraconazole; dexamethasone possibly reduces plasma concentration of caspofungin—consider increasing dose of caspofungin

• Antivirals: dexamethasone possibly reduces plasma concentration of indinavir, lopinavir and saquinavir; plasma concentration of corticosteroids, dexamethasone and prednisolone possibly increased by ritonavir; plasma concentration of inhaled and intranasal budesonide and fluticasone increased by •ritonavir

Aprepitant: metabolism of dexamethasone and methylprednisolone inhibited by aprepitant (reduce dose of dexamethasone and methylprednisolone)

• Barbiturates: metabolism of corticosteroids accelerated by •barbiturates (reduced effect)

Beta-blockers: corticosteroids antagonise hypotensive effect of beta-blockers

Calcium Salts: corticosteroids reduce absorption of calcium salts

Calcium-channel Blockers: corticosteroids antagonise hypotensive effect of calcium-channel blockers

Cardiac Glycosides: increased risk of hypokalaemia when corticosteroids given with cardiac glycosides

• Ciclosporin: high-dose methylprednisolone increases plasma concentration of •ciclosporin (risk of convulsions); plasma concentration of prednisolone increased by ciclosporin

Clonidine: corticosteroids antagonise hypotensive effect of clonidine

• Cytotoxics: increased risk of haematological toxicity when corticosteroids given with •methotrexate

Diazoxide: corticosteroids antagonise hypotensive effect of diazoxide

Diuretics: corticosteroids antagonise diuretic effect of diuretics; increased risk of hypokalaemia when corticosteroids given with acetazolamide, loop diuretics or thiazides and related diuretics

Hormone Antagonists: metabolism of corticosteroids accelerated by aminoglutethimide (reduced effect)

Methyldopa: corticosteroids antagonise hypotensive effect of methyldopa

Mifepristone: effect of corticosteroids (including inhaled corticosteroids) may be reduced for 3–4 days after mifepristone

Moxonidine: corticosteroids antagonise hypotensive effect of moxonidine

Corticosteroids *(continued)*

Nitrates: corticosteroids antagonise hypotensive effect of nitrates

Oestrogens: plasma concentration of corticosteroids increased by oral contraceptives containing oestrogens

Sodium Benzoate: corticosteroids possibly reduce effects of sodium benzoate

Sodium Phenylbutyrate: corticosteroids possibly reduce effects of sodium phenylbutyrate

Somatropin: corticosteroids may inhibit growth-promoting effect of somatropin

Sympathomimetics: metabolism of dexamethasone accelerated by ephedrine

Sympathomimetics, Beta_2: increased risk of hypokalaemia when corticosteroids given with high doses of beta_2 sympathomimetics—for CSM advice (hypokalaemia) see p. 143

Theophylline: increased risk of hypokalaemia when corticosteroids given with theophylline

• Vaccines: high doses of corticosteroids impair immune response to •vaccines, avoid concomitant use with live vaccines (see p. 604)

Vasodilator Antihypertensives: corticosteroids antagonise hypotensive effect of hydralazine, minoxidil and nitroprusside

Cortisone *see* Corticosteroids

Co-trimoxazole *see* Trimethoprim and Sulfamethoxazole

Coumarins

Note. Change in patient's clinical condition, particularly associated with liver disease, intercurrent illness, or drug administration, necessitates more frequent testing. Major changes in diet (especially involving salads and vegetables) and in alcohol consumption may also affect anticoagulant control

• Alcohol: anticoagulant control with coumarins may be affected by major changes in consumption of •alcohol

Allopurinol: anticoagulant effect of coumarins possibly enhanced by allopurinol

• Anabolic Steroids: anticoagulant effect of coumarins enhanced by •anabolic steroids

• Analgesics: anticoagulant effect of coumarins possibly enhanced by •NSAIDs, •celecoxib, •dextropropoxyphene, •diflunisal, •etodolac, •etoricoxib, •flurbiprofen, •ibuprofen, •mefenamic acid, •meloxicam, •parecoxib, •piroxicam and •sulindac; anticoagulant effect of coumarins possibly enhanced by •diclofenac, also increased risk of haemorrhage with intravenous diclofenac (avoid concomitant use); increased risk of bleeding when coumarins given with •ketorolac (avoid concomitant use); anticoagulant effect of coumarins enhanced by •tramadol; increased risk of bleeding when coumarins given with •aspirin (due to antiplatelet effect); anticoagulant effect of coumarins possibly enhanced by prolonged regular use of paracetamol

• Anti-arrhythmics: metabolism of coumarins inhibited by •amiodarone (enhanced anticoagulant effect); anticoagulant effect of coumarins enhanced by •propafenone; anticoagulant effect of coumarins possibly enhanced by •quinidine

• Antibacterials: experience in anticoagulant clinics suggests that INR possibly altered when coumarins are given with •neomycin (given for local action on gut); anticoagulant effect of coumarins enhanced by •chloramphenicol, •ciprofloxacin, •clarithromycin, •erythromycin, •metronidazole, •nalidixic acid, •norfloxacin, •ofloxacin and •sulphonamides; anticoagulant effect of coumarins possibly enhanced by •aztreonam, •cephalosporins, levofloxacin, •macrolides,

Coumarins

- Antibacterials *(continued)* •tetracyclines and trimethoprim; studies have failed to demonstrate an interaction with coumarins, but common experience in anticoagulant clinics is that INR can be altered by a course of broad-spectrum penicillins such as ampicillin; metabolism of coumarins accelerated by •rifamycins (reduced anticoagulant effect)
- Antidepressants: anticoagulant effect of warfarin possibly enhanced by •venlafaxine; anticoagulant effect of coumarins possibly enhanced by •SSRIs; anticoagulant effect of warfarin reduced by •St John's wort (avoid concomitant use); anticoagulant effect of warfarin enhanced by mirtazapine; anticoagulant effect of coumarins may be enhanced or reduced by •tricyclics
- Antidiabetics: coumarins possibly enhance hypoglycaemic effect of •sulphonylureas, also possible changes to anticoagulant effect
- Antiepileptics: metabolism of coumarins accelerated by •carbamazepine and •primidone (reduced anticoagulant effect); metabolism of coumarins accelerated by •phenytoin (possibility of reduced anticoagulant effect, but enhancement also reported); anticoagulant effect of coumarins possibly enhanced by valproate
- Antifungals: anticoagulant effect of coumarins enhanced by •fluconazole, •itraconazole, •ketoconazole and •voriconazole; anticoagulant effect of coumarins enhanced by •miconazole (miconazole oral gel and possibly vaginal formulations absorbed); anticoagulant effect of coumarins reduced by •griseofulvin

Antimalarials: isolated reports that anticoagulant effect of warfarin may be enhanced by proguanil

- Antivirals: anticoagulant effect of coumarins may be enhanced or reduced by amprenavir; anticoagulant effect of warfarin may be enhanced or reduced by atazanavir, •nevirapine and •ritonavir; anticoagulant effect of coumarins possibly enhanced by •ritonavir

Anxiolytics and Hypnotics: anticoagulant effect of coumarins may transiently be enhanced by chloral and triclofos

Aprepitant: anticoagulant effect of warfarin possibly reduced by aprepitant

- Barbiturates: metabolism of coumarins accelerated by •barbiturates (reduced anticoagulant effect)

Bosentan: monitoring anticoagulant effect of coumarins recommended by manufacturer of bosentan

- Clopidogrel: anticoagulant effect of coumarins enhanced due to antiplatelet action of •clopidogrel; avoidance of warfarin advised by manufacturer of •clopidogrel
- Corticosteroids: anticoagulant effect of coumarins may be enhanced or reduced by •corticosteroids (high-dose corticosteroids enhance anticoagulant effect)
- Cranberry Juice: anticoagulant effect of warfarin possibly enhanced by •cranberry juice—avoid concomitant use
- Cytotoxics: anticoagulant effect of coumarins possibly enhanced by •etoposide, •fluorouracil and •ifosfamide; anticoagulant effect of warfarin possibly reduced by •azathioprine and •mercaptopurine; replacement of warfarin with a heparin advised by manufacturer of imatinib (possibility of enhanced warfarin effect)
- Dipyridamole: anticoagulant effect of coumarins enhanced due to antiplatelet action of •dipyridamole

Coumarins *(continued)*

- Disulfiram: anticoagulant effect of coumarins enhanced by •disulfiram
- Dopaminergics: anticoagulant effect of warfarin enhanced by •entacapone
- Enteral Foods: anticoagulant effect of coumarins antagonised by vitamin K (present in some •enteral feeds)
- Hormone Antagonists: metabolism of coumarins accelerated by •aminoglutethimide (reduced anticoagulant effect); anticoagulant effect of coumarins possibly enhanced by bicalutamide and •toremifene; metabolism of coumarins inhibited by •danazol (enhanced anticoagulant effect); anticoagulant effect of coumarins enhanced by •flutamide and •tamoxifen

Iloprost: anticoagulant effect of coumarins possibly enhanced by iloprost

Leflunomide: anticoagulant effect of warfarin possibly enhanced by leflunomide

Leukotriene Antagonists: anticoagulant effect of warfarin enhanced by zafirlukast

- Levamisole: anticoagulant effect of warfarin possibly enhanced by •levamisole
- Lipid-regulating Drugs: anticoagulant effect of coumarins may be enhanced or reduced by •colestyramine; anticoagulant effect of warfarin may be transiently reduced by atorvastatin; anticoagulant effect of coumarins enhanced by •fibrates, •fluvastatin and simvastatin; anticoagulant effect of coumarins possibly enhanced by •rosuvastatin
- Oestrogens: anticoagulant effect of coumarins antagonised by •oestrogens

Orlistat: monitoring anticoagulant effect of coumarins recommended by manufacturer of orlistat

- Progestogens: anticoagulant effect of coumarins antagonised by •progestogens

Raloxifene: anticoagulant effect of coumarins antagonised by raloxifene

- Retinoids: anticoagulant effect of coumarins possibly reduced by •acitretin

Sibutramine: increased risk of bleeding when anticoagulants given with sibutramine

- Sulfinpyrazone: anticoagulant effect of coumarins enhanced by •sulfinpyrazone
- Sympathomimetics: anticoagulant effect of coumarins possibly enhanced by •methylphenidate

Terpene Mixture: anticoagulant effect of coumarins possibly reduced by Rowachol®

- Testolactone: anticoagulant effect of coumarins enhanced by •testolactone
- Testosterone: anticoagulant effect of coumarins enhanced by •testosterone
- Thyroid Hormones: anticoagulant effect of coumarins enhanced by •thyroid hormones
- Ulcer-healing Drugs: metabolism of coumarins inhibited by •cimetidine (enhanced anticoagulant effect); anticoagulant effect of coumarins possibly enhanced by •esomeprazole and •omeprazole; absorption of coumarins possibly reduced by •sucralfate (reduced anticoagulant effect)

Vaccines: anticoagulant effect of warfarin possibly enhanced by influenza vaccine

- Vitamins: anticoagulant effect of coumarins antagonised by •vitamin K

Cranberry Juice

- Anticoagulants: cranberry juice possibly enhances anticoagulant effect of •warfarin—avoid concomitant use

Cyclizine *see* Antihistamines

Cyclopenthiazide *see* Diuretics

Cyclopentolate *see* Antimuscarinics

Cyclophosphamide
Antiepileptics: cytotoxics possibly reduce absorption of phenytoin
• Antipsychotics: avoid concomitant use of cytotoxics with •clozapine (increased risk of agranulocytosis)
• Cytotoxics: increased toxicity when high-dose cyclophosphamide given with •pentostatin—avoid concomitant use
Muscle Relaxants: cyclophosphamide enhances effects of suxamethonium

Cycloserine
• Alcohol: increased risk of convulsions when cycloserine given with •alcohol
Antibacterials: increased risk of CNS toxicity when cycloserine given with isoniazid
Oestrogens: broad-spectrum antibacterials possibly reduce contraceptive effect of oestrogens (risk probably small, see p. 407)

Cyproheptadine *see* Antihistamines

Cytarabine
Antiepileptics: cytotoxics possibly reduce absorption of phenytoin
Antifungals: cytarabine possibly reduces plasma concentration of flucytosine
• Antipsychotics: avoid concomitant use of cytotoxics with •clozapine (increased risk of agranulocytosis)
Cytotoxics: intracellular concentration of cytarabine increased by fludarabine

Cytotoxics *see* individual drugs

Dairy Products
Antibacterials: dairy products reduces absorption of ciprofloxacin and norfloxacin; dairy products reduces absorption of tetracyclines (except doxycycline and minocycline)

Dalteparin *see* Heparins

Danazol
• Anticoagulants: danazol inhibits metabolism of •coumarins (enhanced anticoagulant effect)
• Antiepileptics: danazol inhibits metabolism of •carbamazepine (increased risk of toxicity)
• Ciclosporin: danazol inhibits metabolism of •ciclosporin (increased plasma concentration)
Tacrolimus: danazol possibly increases plasma concentration of tacrolimus

Dantrolene *see* Muscle Relaxants

Dapsone
Antibacterials: plasma concentration of dapsone reduced by rifamycins; plasma concentration of both drugs may increase when dapsone given with trimethoprim
Antivirals: plasma concentration of dapsone possibly increased by amprenavir
Oestrogens: broad-spectrum antibacterials possibly reduce contraceptive effect of oestrogens (risk probably small, see p. 407)
Probenecid: excretion of dapsone reduced by probenecid (increased risk of side-effects)

Darbepoetin *see* Epoetin

Deflazacort *see* Corticosteroids

Demeclocycline *see* Tetracyclines

Desferrioxamine
Antipsychotics: avoidance of desferrioxamine advised by manufacturer of levomepromazine (methotrimeprazine); manufacturer of desferrioxamine advises avoid concomitant use with prochlorperazine

Desflurane *see* Anaesthetics, General

Desloratadine *see* Antihistamines

Desmopressin
Analgesics: effects of desmopressin enhanced by indometacin
Loperamide: plasma concentration of *oral* desmopressin increased by loperamide

Desogestrel *see* Progestogens

Dexamethasone *see* Corticosteroids

Dexamfetamine *see* Sympathomimetics

Dexketoprofen *see* NSAIDs

Dextromethorphan *see* Opioid Analgesics

Dextropropoxyphene *see* Opioid Analgesics

Diamorphine *see* Opioid Analgesics

Diazepam *see* Anxiolytics and Hypnotics

Diazoxide
ACE Inhibitors: enhanced hypotensive effect when diazoxide given with ACE inhibitors
Adrenergic Neurone Blockers: enhanced hypotensive effect when diazoxide given with adrenergic neurone blockers
Alcohol: enhanced hypotensive effect when diazoxide given with alcohol
Aldesleukin: enhanced hypotensive effect when diazoxide given with aldesleukin
Alpha-blockers: enhanced hypotensive effect when diazoxide given with alpha-blockers
Anaesthetics, General: enhanced hypotensive effect when diazoxide given with general anaesthetics
Analgesics: hypotensive effect of diazoxide antagonised by NSAIDs
Angiotensin-II Receptor Antagonists: enhanced hypotensive effect when diazoxide given with angiotensin-II receptor antagonists
Antidepressants: enhanced hypotensive effect when diazoxide given with MAOIs or tricyclic-related antidepressants
Antidiabetics: diazoxide antagonises hypoglycaemic effect of antidiabetics
Antiepileptics: diazoxide reduces plasma concentration of phenytoin, also effect of diazoxide may be reduced
Antipsychotics: enhanced hypotensive effect when diazoxide given with phenothiazines
Anxiolytics and Hypnotics: enhanced hypotensive effect when diazoxide given with anxiolytics and hypnotics
Beta-blockers: enhanced hypotensive effect when diazoxide given with beta-blockers
Calcium-channel Blockers: enhanced hypotensive effect when diazoxide given with calcium-channel blockers
Clonidine: enhanced hypotensive effect when diazoxide given with clonidine
Corticosteroids: hypotensive effect of diazoxide antagonised by corticosteroids
Diuretics: enhanced hypotensive effect when diazoxide given with diuretics
Dopaminergics: enhanced hypotensive effect when diazoxide given with levodopa
Methyldopa: enhanced hypotensive effect when diazoxide given with methyldopa
Moxisylyte (thymoxamine): enhanced hypotensive effect when diazoxide given with moxisylyte
Moxonidine: enhanced hypotensive effect when diazoxide given with moxonidine
Muscle Relaxants: enhanced hypotensive effect when diazoxide given with baclofen or tizanidine
Nitrates: enhanced hypotensive effect when diazoxide given with nitrates
Oestrogens: hypotensive effect of diazoxide antagonised by oestrogens
Prostaglandins: enhanced hypotensive effect when diazoxide given with alprostadil
Vasodilator Antihypertensives: enhanced hypotensive effect when diazoxide given with hydralazine, minoxidil or nitroprusside

Diclofenac *see* NSAIDs

Dicycloverine (dicyclomine) *see* Antimuscarinics

Didanosine

Note. Antacids in tablet formulation may affect absorption of other drugs

Allopurinol: plasma concentration of didanosine possibly increased by allopurinol

• Antivirals: plasma concentration of didanosine possibly increased by ganciclovir; plasma concentration of didanosine increased by •tenofovir (increased risk of toxicity)—avoid concomitant use

Diflunisal *see* NSAIDs

Digitoxin *see* Cardiac Glycosides

Digoxin *see* Cardiac Glycosides

Dihydrocodeine *see* Opioid Analgesics

Diltiazem *see* Calcium-channel Blockers

Dimercaprol

• Iron: avoid concomitant use of dimercaprol with •iron

Dinoprostone *see* Prostaglandins

Diphenhydramine *see* Antihistamines

Diphenoxylate *see* Opioid Analgesics

Diphenylpyraline *see* Antihistamines

Dipipanone *see* Opioid Analgesics

Dipivefrine *see* Sympathomimetics

Dipyridamole

Antacids: absorption of dipyridamole possibly reduced by antacids

• Anti-arrhythmics: dipyridamole enhances and extends the effects of •adenosine (important risk of toxicity)

• Anticoagulants: antiplatelet action of dipyridamole enhances anticoagulant effect of •coumarins and •phenindione; dipyridamole enhances anticoagulant effect of heparins

Clopidogrel: increased risk of bleeding when dipyridamole given with clopidogrel

Cytotoxics: dipyridamole possibly reduces effects of fludarabine

Disodium Etidronate *see* Bisphosphonates

Disodium Pamidronate *see* Bisphosphonates

Disopyramide

Anaesthetics, Local: increased myocardial depression when anti-arrhythmics given with bupivacaine, levobupivacaine or prilocaine

• Anti-arrhythmics: increased myocardial depression when anti-arrhythmics given with other •anti-arrhythmics; increased risk of ventricular arrhythmias when disopyramide given with •amiodarone—avoid concomitant use

• Antibacterials: plasma concentration of disopyramide possibly increased by •clarithromycin (increased risk of toxicity); plasma concentration of disopyramide increased by •erythromycin (increased risk of toxicity); increased risk of ventricular arrhythmias when disopyramide given with •moxifloxacin or •quinupristin/dalfopristin—avoid concomitant use; metabolism of disopyramide accelerated by •rifamycins (reduced plasma concentration)

• Antidepressants: increased risk of ventricular arrhythmias when disopyramide given with •tricyclics

Antiepileptics: plasma concentration of disopyramide reduced by phenytoin; metabolism of disopyramide accelerated by primidone (reduced plasma concentration)

• Antihistamines: increased risk of ventricular arrhythmias when disopyramide given with •mizolastine or •terfenadine—avoid concomitant use; increased risk of ventricular arrhythmias when anti-arrhythmics given with •terfenadine

• Antimalarials: avoidance of disopyramide advised by manufacturer of •artemether/lumefantrine (risk of ventricular arrhythmias)

Disopyramide *(continued)*

Antimuscarinics: increased risk of antimuscarinic side-effects when disopyramide given with antimuscarinics

• Antipsychotics: increased risk of ventricular arrhythmias when anti-arrhythmics that prolong the QT interval given with •antipsychotics that prolong the QT interval; increased risk of ventricular arrhythmias when disopyramide given with •amisulpride, •pimozide or •sertindole—avoid concomitant use; increased risk of ventricular arrhythmias when disopyramide given with •phenothiazines

• Antivirals: plasma concentration of disopyramide possibly increased by •ritonavir (increased risk of toxicity)

Barbiturates: metabolism of disopyramide accelerated by barbiturates (reduced plasma concentration)

• Beta-blockers: increased myocardial depression when anti-arrhythmics given with •beta-blockers; increased risk of ventricular arrhythmias when disopyramide given with •sotalol—avoid concomitant use

• Calcium-channel Blockers: increased risk of myocardial depression and asystole when disopyramide given with •verapamil

• Diuretics: increased cardiac toxicity with disopyramide if hypokalaemia occurs with •acetazolamide, •loop diuretics or •thiazides and related diuretics

• Dolasetron: increased risk of ventricular arrhythmias when disopyramide given with •dolasetron—avoid concomitant use

$5HT_3$ Antagonists: caution with anti-arrhythmics advised by manufacturer of tropisetron (risk of ventricular arrhythmias)

Nitrates: disopyramide reduces effects of sublingual tablets of nitrates (failure to dissolve under tongue owing to dry mouth)

Distigmine *see* Parasympathomimetics

Disulfiram

Alcohol: disulfiram reaction when disulfiram given with alcohol (see p. 260)

Antibacterials: psychotic reaction reported when disulfiram given with metronidazole

• Anticoagulants: disulfiram enhances anticoagulant effect of •coumarins

Antidepressants: increased disulfiram reaction with alcohol reported with concomitant amitriptyline; disulfiram inhibits metabolism of tricyclics (increased plasma concentration)

• Antiepileptics: disulfiram inhibits metabolism of •phenytoin (increased risk of toxicity)

Anxiolytics and Hypnotics: disulfiram increases risk of temazepam toxicity; disulfiram inhibits metabolism of benzodiazepines (increased sedative effects)

• Paraldehyde: risk of toxicity when disulfiram given with •paraldehyde

Theophylline: disulfiram inhibits metabolism of theophylline (increased risk of toxicity)

Diuretics

Note. Since systemic absorption may follow topical application of brinzolamide to the eye, the possibility of interactions should be borne in mind

Note. Since systemic absorption may follow topical application of dorzolamide to the eye, the possibility of interactions should be borne in mind

• ACE Inhibitors: enhanced hypotensive effect when diuretics given with •ACE inhibitors; increased risk of severe hyperkalaemia when potassium-sparing diuretics and aldosterone antagonists given with •ACE inhibitors (monitor potassium con-

Diuretics

- ACE Inhibitors *(continued)*
  centration with low-dose spironolactone in heart failure)

  Adrenergic Neurone Blockers: enhanced hypotensive effect when diuretics given with adrenergic neurone blockers

  Alcohol: enhanced hypotensive effect when diuretics given with alcohol

  Aldesleukin: enhanced hypotensive effect when diuretics given with aldesleukin
- Alpha-blockers: enhanced hypotensive effect when diuretics given with •alpha-blockers, also increased risk of first-dose hypotension with post-synaptic alpha-blockers such as prazosin

  Anaesthetics, General: enhanced hypotensive effect when diuretics given with general anaesthetics
- Analgesics: diuretics increase risk of nephrotoxicity of NSAIDs, also antagonism of diuretic effect; possibly increased risk of hyperkalaemia when potassium-sparing diuretics and aldosterone antagonists given with NSAIDs; effects of diuretics antagonised by indometacin and ketorolac; increased risk of hyperkalaemia when potassium-sparing diuretics and aldosterone antagonists given with indometacin; occasional reports of reduced renal function when triamterene given with •indometacin—avoid concomitant use; increased risk of toxicity when carbonic anhydrase inhibitors given with high-dose aspirin; diuretic effect of spironolactone antagonised by aspirin
- Angiotensin-II Receptor Antagonists: enhanced hypotensive effect when diuretics given with •angiotensin-II receptor antagonists; increased risk of hyperkalaemia when potassium-sparing diuretics and aldosterone antagonists given with •angiotensin-II receptor antagonists
- Anti-arrhythmics: plasma concentration of eplerenone increased by amiodarone (reduce dose of eplerenone); hypokalaemia caused by acetazolamide, loop diuretics or thiazides and related diuretics increases cardiac toxicity with amiodarone; hypokalaemia caused by acetazolamide, loop diuretics or thiazides and related diuretics increases cardiac toxicity with •disopyramide; hypokalaemia caused by acetazolamide, loop diuretics or thiazides and related diuretics increases cardiac toxicity with •flecainide; hypokalaemia caused by acetazolamide, loop diuretics or thiazides and related diuretics antagonises action of •lidocaine (lignocaine); hypokalaemia caused by acetazolamide, loop diuretics or thiazides and related diuretics antagonises action of •mexiletine; hypokalaemia caused by loop diuretics or thiazides and related diuretics increases cardiac toxicity with •quinidine; acetazolamide possibly reduces excretion of •quinidine (increased plasma concentration), also cardiotoxicity of quinidine increased in hypokalaemia
- Antibacterials: plasma concentration of eplerenone increased by •clarithromycin and •telithromycin—avoid concomitant use; plasma concentration of eplerenone increased by erythromycin (reduce dose of eplerenone); plasma concentration of eplerenone reduced by •rifampicin—avoid concomitant use; avoidance of diuretics advised by manufacturer of lymecycline; increased risk of otoxicity when loop diuretics given with •aminoglycosides, •polymyxins or •vancomycin; acetazolamide antagonises effects of •methenamine; increased risk of hyperkalaemia when eplerenone given with trimethoprim

Diuretics *(continued)*

- Antidepressants: possible increased risk of hypokalaemia when loop diuretics or thiazides and related diuretics given with reboxetine; enhanced hypotensive effect when diuretics given with MAOIs; plasma concentration of eplerenone reduced by •St John's wort—avoid concomitant use; increased risk of postural hypotension when diuretics given with tricyclics

  Antidiabetics: loop diuretics and thiazides and related diuretics antagonise hypoglycaemic effect of antidiabetics; increased risk of hyponatraemia when thiazides and related diuretics plus potassium-sparing diuretic given with chlorpropamide; increased risk of hyponatraemia when potassium-sparing diuretics and aldosterone antagonists plus *thiazide* given with chlorpropamide
- Antiepileptics: acetazolamide increases plasma concentration of •carbamazepine; plasma concentration of eplerenone reduced by •carbamazepine and •phenytoin—avoid concomitant use; increased risk of hyponatraemia when diuretics given with carbamazepine; increased risk of osteomalacia when carbonic anhydrase inhibitors given with phenytoin or primidone; acetazolamide possibly reduces plasma concentration of primidone
- Antifungals: plasma concentration of eplerenone increased by •itraconazole and •ketoconazole—avoid concomitant use; increased risk of hypokalaemia when loop diuretics or thiazides and related diuretics given with amphotericin; hydrochlorothiazide increases plasma concentration of fluconazole; plasma concentration of eplerenone increased by fluconazole (reduce dose of eplerenone)
- Antihistamines: hypokalaemia or other electrolyte imbalance with diuretics increases risk of ventricular arrhythmias with •terfenadine
- Antipsychotics: hypokalaemia caused by diuretics increases risk of ventricular arrhythmias with •amisulpride or •sertindole; enhanced hypotensive effect when diuretics given with phenothiazines; hypokalaemia caused by diuretics increases risk of ventricular arrhythmias with •pimozide (avoid concomitant use)
- Antivirals: plasma concentration of eplerenone increased by •nelfinavir and •ritonavir—avoid concomitant use; plasma concentration of eplerenone increased by saquinavir (reduce dose of eplerenone)

  Anxiolytics and Hypnotics: enhanced hypotensive effect when diuretics given with anxiolytics and hypnotics; administration of parenteral furosemide (frusemide) with chloral or triclofos may displace thyroid hormone from binding sites
- Barbiturates: increased risk of osteomalacia when carbonic anhydrase inhibitors given with phenobarbital; plasma concentration of eplerenone reduced by •phenobarbital—avoid concomitant use
- Beta-blockers: enhanced hypotensive effect when diuretics given with beta-blockers; hypokalaemia caused by loop diuretics or thiazides and related diuretics increases risk of ventricular arrhythmias with •sotalol

  Calcium Salts: increased risk of hypercalcaemia when thiazides and related diuretics given with calcium salts

  Calcium-channel Blockers: enhanced hypotensive effect when diuretics given with calcium-channel blockers; plasma concentration of eplerenone increased by diltiazem and verapamil (reduce dose of eplerenone)

Diuretics *(continued)*

- Cardiac Glycosides: hypokalaemia caused by acetazolamide, loop diuretics or thiazides and related diuretics increases cardiac toxicity with •cardiac glycosides; spironolactone possibly affects plasma concentration of digitoxin; spironolactone increases plasma concentration of •digoxin
- Ciclosporin: increased risk of hyperkalaemia when potassium-sparing diuretics and aldosterone antagonists given with •ciclosporin

Clonidine: enhanced hypotensive effect when diuretics given with clonidine

Corticosteroids: diuretic effect of diuretics antagonised by corticosteroids; increased risk of hypokalaemia when acetazolamide, loop diuretics or thiazides and related diuretics given with corticosteroids

Cytotoxics: increased risk of nephrotoxicity and ototoxicity when diuretics given with platinum compounds

Diazoxide: enhanced hypotensive effect when diuretics given with diazoxide

Diuretics: increased risk of hypokalaemia when loop diuretics or thiazides and related diuretics given with acetazolamide; profound diuresis possible when metolazone given with furosemide (frusemide); increased risk of hypokalaemia when thiazides and related diuretics given with loop diuretics

Dopaminergics: enhanced hypotensive effect when diuretics given with levodopa

Hormone Antagonists: increased risk of hyponatraemia when diuretics given with aminoglutethimide; increased risk of hypercalcaemia when thiazides and related diuretics given with toremifene; increased risk of hyperkalaemia when potassium-sparing diuretics and aldosterone antagonists given with trilostane

Lipid-regulating Drugs: absorption of thiazides and related diuretics reduced by colestipol and colestyramine (give at least 2 hours apart)

- Lithium: loop diuretics and thiazides and related diuretics reduce excretion of •lithium (increased plasma concentration and risk of toxicity)—loop diuretics safer than thiazides; potassium-sparing diuretics and aldosterone antagonists reduce excretion of •lithium (increased plasma concentration and risk of toxicity); acetazolamide increases the excretion of •lithium

Methyldopa: enhanced hypotensive effect when diuretics given with methyldopa

Moxisylyte (thymoxamine): enhanced hypotensive effect when diuretics given with moxisylyte

Moxonidine: enhanced hypotensive effect when diuretics given with moxonidine

Muscle Relaxants: enhanced hypotensive effect when diuretics given with baclofen or tizanidine

Nitrates: enhanced hypotensive effect when diuretics given with nitrates

Oestrogens: diuretic effect of diuretics antagonised by oestrogens

- Potassium Salts: increased risk of hyperkalaemia when potassium-sparing diuretics and aldosterone antagonists given with •potassium salts

Progestogens: risk of hyperkalaemia when potassium-sparing diuretics and aldosterone antagonists given with drospirenone (monitor serum potassium during first cycle)

Prostaglandins: enhanced hypotensive effect when diuretics given with alprostadil

Sympathomimetics, $Beta_2$: increased risk of hypokalaemia when acetazolamide, loop diuretics or thiazides and related diuretics given with high doses of $beta_2$ sympathomimetics—for CSM advice (hypokalaemia) see p. 143

- Tacrolimus: increased risk of hyperkalaemia when potassium-sparing diuretics and aldosterone antagonists given with •tacrolimus

Theophylline: increased risk of hypokalaemia when acetazolamide, loop diuretics or thiazides and related diuretics given with theophylline

Vasodilator Antihypertensives: enhanced hypotensive effect when diuretics given with hydralazine, minoxidil or nitroprusside

Vitamins: increased risk of hypercalcaemia when thiazides and related diuretics given with vitamin D

Diuretics, Loop *see* Diuretics

Diuretics, Potassium-sparing and Aldosterone Antagonists *see* Diuretics

Diuretics, Thiazide and related *see* Diuretics

Dobutamine *see* Sympathomimetics

Docetaxel

Antibacterials: *in vitro* studies suggest a possible interaction between docetaxel and erythromycin (consult docetaxel product literature)

Antiepileptics: cytotoxics possibly reduce absorption of phenytoin

Antifungals: *in vitro* studies suggest a possible interaction between docetaxel and ketoconazole (consult docetaxel product literature)

Antihistamines: *in vitro* studies suggest a possible interaction between docetaxel and terfenadine (consult docetaxel product literature)

- Antipsychotics: avoid concomitant use of cytotoxics with •clozapine (increased risk of agranulocytosis)

Ciclosporin: *in vitro* studies suggest a possible interaction between docetaxel and ciclosporin (consult docetaxel product literature)

Dolasetron

- Anti-arrhythmics: increased risk of ventricular arrhythmias when dolasetron given with •amiodarone, •disopyramide, •flecainide, •lidocaine (lignocaine), •mexiletine, •procainamide or •propafenone—avoid concomitant use
- Beta-blockers: increased risk of ventricular arrhythmias when dolasetron given with •sotalol—avoid concomitant use

Domperidone

Analgesics: effects of domperidone on gastro-intestinal activity antagonised by opioid analgesics

Antimuscarinics: effects of domperidone on gastro-intestinal activity antagonised by antimuscarinics

Dopaminergics: increased risk of extrapyramidal side-effects when domperidone given with amantadine; domperidone possibly antagonises hypoprolactinaemic effects of bromocriptine and cabergoline

Donepezil *see* Parasympathomimetics

Dopamine *see* Sympathomimetics

Dopaminergics *see* Amantadine, Apomorphine, Bromocriptine, Cabergoline, Entacapone, Levodopa, Lisuride, Pergolide, Pramipexole, Quinagolide, Ropinirole, Selegiline, and Tolcapone

Dopexamine *see* Sympathomimetics

Dorzolamide *see* Diuretics

Dosulepin (dothiepin) *see* Antidepressants, Tricyclic

Doxapram

Antidepressants: effects of doxapram enhanced by MAOIs

Sympathomimetics: increased risk of hypertension when doxapram given with sympathomimetics

Doxapram *(continued)*
Theophylline: increased CNS stimulation when doxapram given with theophylline
Doxazosin *see* Alpha-blockers
Doxepin *see* Antidepressants, Tricyclic
Doxorubicin
Antiepileptics: cytotoxics possibly reduce absorption of phenytoin
• Antipsychotics: avoid concomitant use of cytotoxics with •clozapine (increased risk of agranulocytosis)
Antivirals: doxorubicin possibly inhibits effects of stavudine
• Ciclosporin: increased risk of neurotoxicity when doxorubicin given with •ciclosporin
Doxycycline *see* Tetracyclines
Doxylamine *see* Antihistamines
Drospirenone *see* Progestogens
Drotrecogin Alfa
• Anticoagulants: manufacturer of drotrecogin alfa advises avoid concomitant use with high doses of •heparin—consult product literature
Duloxetine
Analgesics: possible increased serotonergic effects when duloxetine given with pethidine or tramadol
• Antibacterials: metabolism of duloxetine inhibited by •ciprofloxacin—avoid concomitant use
• Antidepressants: metabolism of duloxetine inhibited by •fluvoxamine—avoid concomitant use; possible increased serotonergic effects when duloxetine given with SSRIs, St John's wort, amitriptyline, clomipramine, •moclobemide, tryptophan or venlafaxine; duloxetine should not be started until 2 weeks after stopping •MAOIs, also MAOIs should not be started until at least 5 days after stopping duloxetine; after stopping SSRI-related antidepressants do not start •moclobemide for at least 1 week
• Antimalarials: avoidance of antidepressants advised by manufacturer of •artemether/lumefantrine
$5HT_1$ Agonists: possible increased serotonergic effects when duloxetine given with $5HT_1$ agonists
• Sibutramine: increased risk of CNS toxicity when SSRI-related antidepressants given with •sibutramine (manufacturer of sibutramine advises avoid concomitant use)
Dutasteride
Calcium-channel Blockers: plasma concentration of dutasteride increased by diltiazem and verapamil
Dydrogesterone *see* Progestogens
Edrophonium *see* Parasympathomimetics
Efalizumab
• Vaccines: discontinue efalizumab 8 weeks before and until 2 weeks after vaccination with live or live-attenuated •vaccines
Efavirenz
Analgesics: efavirenz reduces plasma concentration of methadone
Antibacterials: increased risk of rash when efavirenz given with clarithromycin; efavirenz reduces plasma concentration of rifabutin—increase dose of rifabutin; plasma concentration of efavirenz reduced by rifampicin—increase dose of efavirenz
• Antidepressants: efavirenz reduces plasma concentration of sertraline; plasma concentration of efavirenz reduced by •St John's wort—avoid concomitant use
• Antifungals: efavirenz reduces plasma concentration of •voriconazole, also plasma concentration of efavirenz increased (avoid concomitant use); efavirenz possibly reduces plasma concentration of caspofungin—consider increasing dose of caspofungin

Efavirenz *(continued)*
• Antihistamines: increased risk of ventricular arrhythmias when efavirenz given with •terfenadine—avoid concomitant use
• Antipsychotics: efavirenz possibly reduces plasma concentration of •aripiprazole—increase dose of aripiprazole; efavirenz possibly increases plasma concentration of •pimozide (increased risk of ventricular arrhythmias—avoid concomitant use)
Antivirals: efavirenz reduces plasma concentration of amprenavir, indinavir and lopinavir; efavirenz reduces plasma concentration of atazanavir—increase dose of atazanavir; plasma concentration of efavirenz reduced by nevirapine; toxicity of efavirenz increased by ritonavir, monitor liver function tests; efavirenz significantly reduces plasma concentration of saquinavir
• Anxiolytics and Hypnotics: increased risk of prolonged sedation when efavirenz given with •midazolam—avoid concomitant use
• Ergot Alkaloids: increased risk of ergotism when efavirenz given with •ergot alkaloids—avoid concomitant use
Grapefruit Juice: plasma concentration of efavirenz possibly increased by grapefruit juice
Oestrogens: efavirenz possibly reduces contraceptive effect of oestrogens
Eletriptan *see* $5HT_1$ Agonists
Emtricitabine
Antivirals: manufacturer of emtricitabine advises avoid concomitant use with lamivudine and zalcitabine
Enalapril *see* ACE Inhibitors
Enoxaparin *see* Heparins
Enoximone *see* Phosphodiesterase Inhibitors
Entacapone
• Anticoagulants: entacapone enhances anticoagulant effect of •warfarin
• Antidepressants: manufacturer of entacapone advises caution with maprotiline, moclobemide, paroxetine, tricyclics and venlafaxine; avoid concomitant use of entacapone with non-selective •MAOIs
Dopaminergics: entacapone possibly enhances effects of apomorphine; manufacturer of entacapone advises max. dose of 10 mg selegiline if used concomitantly
Iron: absorption of entacapone reduced by *oral* iron
Memantine: effects of dopaminergics possibly enhanced by memantine
Methyldopa: entacapone possibly enhances effects of methyldopa; antiparkinsonian effect of dopaminergics antagonised by methyldopa
Sympathomimetics: entacapone possibly enhances effects of adrenaline (epinephrine), dobutamine, dopamine and noradrenaline (norepinephrine)
Enteral Foods
• Anticoagulants: the presence of vitamin K in some enteral feeds can antagonise the anticoagulant effect of •coumarins and •phenindione
Antiepileptics: enteral feeds possibly reduce absorption of phenytoin
Ephedrine *see* Sympathomimetics
Epinephrine (adrenaline) *see* Sympathomimetics
Epirubicin
Antiepileptics: cytotoxics possibly reduce absorption of phenytoin
• Antipsychotics: avoid concomitant use of cytotoxics with •clozapine (increased risk of agranulocytosis)
• Ulcer-healing Drugs: plasma concentration of epirubicin increased by •cimetidine
Eplerenone *see* Diuretics

Epoetin

ACE Inhibitors: antagonism of hypotensive effect and increased risk of hyperkalaemia when epoetin given with ACE inhibitors

Angiotensin-II Receptor Antagonists: antagonism of hypotensive effect and increased risk of hyperkalaemia when epoetin given with angiotensin-II receptor antagonists

Eprosartan *see* Angiotensin-II Receptor Antagonists

Eptifibatide

Iloprost: increased risk of bleeding when eptifibatide given with iloprost

Ergometrine *see* Ergot Alkaloids

Ergot Alkaloids

Anaesthetics, General: effects of ergometrine on the parturient uterus reduced by halothane

● Antibacterials: increased risk of ergotism when ergotamine and methysergide given with ●macrolides or ●telithromycin—avoid concomitant use; avoidance of ergotamine and methysergide advised by manufacturer of ●quinupristin/dalfopristin; increased risk of ergotism when ergotamine and methysergide given with tetracyclines

Antidepressants: possible risk of hypertension when ergotamine and methysergide given with reboxetine

● Antifungals: increased risk of ergotism when ergotamine and methysergide given with ●imidazoles or ●triazoles—avoid concomitant use

● Antivirals: increased risk of ergotism when ergotamine and methysergide given with ●amprenavir, ●indinavir, ●nelfinavir, ●ritonavir or ●saquinavir—avoid concomitant use; plasma concentration of ergot alkaloids possibly increased by ●atazanavir—avoid concomitant use; increased risk of ergotism when ergot alkaloids given with ●efavirenz—avoid concomitant use

Beta-blockers: increased peripheral vasoconstriction when ergotamine and methysergide given with beta-blockers

● $5HT_1$ Agonists: increased risk of vasospasm when ergotamine and methysergide given with ●almotriptan, ●rizatriptan, ●sumatriptan or ●zolmitriptan (avoid ergotamine and methysergide for 6 hours after almotriptan, rizatriptan, sumatriptan or zolmitriptan, avoid almotriptan, rizatriptan, sumatriptan or zolmitriptan for 24 hours after ergotamine and methysergide); increased risk of vasospasm when ergotamine and methysergide given with ●eletriptan or ●frovatriptan (avoid ergotamine and methysergide for 24 hours after eletriptan or frovatriptan, avoid eletriptan or frovatriptan for 24 hours after ergotamine and methysergide)

Sympathomimetics: increased risk of ergotism when ergotamine and methysergide given with sympathomimetics

● Ulcer-healing Drugs: increased risk of ergotism when ergotamine and methysergide given with ●cimetidine—avoid concomitant use

Ergotamine and Methysergide *see* Ergot Alkaloids

Ertapenem

Antiepileptics: ertapenem possibly reduces plasma concentration of valproate

Oestrogens: broad-spectrum antibacterials possibly reduce contraceptive effect of oestrogens (risk probably small, see p. 407)

Erythromycin *see* Macrolides

Erythropoetin *see* Epoetin

Escitalopram *see* Antidepressants, SSRI

Esmolol *see* Beta-blockers

Esomeprazole *see* Proton Pump Inhibitors

Estradiol *see* Oestrogens

Estriol *see* Oestrogens

Estrone *see* Oestrogens

Estropipate *see* Oestrogens

Etanercept

● Anakinra: increased risk of side-effects when etanercept given with ●anakinra—avoid concomitant use

● Vaccines: avoid concomitant use of etanercept with live ●vaccines (see p. 604)

Ethinylestradiol *see* Oestrogens

Ethosuximide

● Antibacterials: metabolism of ethosuximide inhibited by ●isoniazid (increased plasma concentration and risk of toxicity)

● Antidepressants: anticonvulsant effect of antiepileptics possibly antagonised by MAOIs and ●tricyclic-related antidepressants (convulsive threshold lowered); anticonvulsant effect of antiepileptics antagonised by ●SSRIs and ●tricyclics (convulsive threshold lowered)

● Antiepileptics: plasma concentration of ethosuximide possibly reduced by carbamazepine and primidone; plasma concentration of ethosuximide possibly reduced by ●phenytoin, also plasma concentration of phenytoin possibly increased; plasma concentration of ethosuximide possibly increased by valproate

● Antimalarials: possible increased risk of convulsions when antiepileptics given with chloroquine and hydroxychloroquine; anticonvulsant effect of antiepileptics antagonised by ●mefloquine

● Antipsychotics: anticonvulsant effect of ethosuximide antagonised by ●antipsychotics (convulsive threshold lowered)

Barbiturates: plasma concentration of ethosuximide possibly reduced by phenobarbital

Etodolac *see* NSAIDs

Etomidate *see* Anaesthetics, General

Etonogestrel *see* Progestogens

Etoposide

● Anticoagulants: etoposide possibly enhances anticoagulant effect of ●coumarins

Antiepileptics: cytotoxics possibly reduce absorption of phenytoin; plasma concentration of etoposide possibly reduced by phenytoin

● Antipsychotics: avoid concomitant use of cytotoxics with ●clozapine (increased risk of agranulocytosis)

Barbiturates: plasma concentration of etoposide possibly reduced by phenobarbital

Ciclosporin: plasma concentration of etoposide possibly increased by ciclosporin (increased risk of toxicity)

Etoricoxib *see* NSAIDs

Etynodiol *see* Progestogens

Exemestane

Antibacterials: plasma concentration of exemestane possibly reduced by rifampicin

Ezetimibe

Ciclosporin: plasma concentration of ezetimibe increased by ciclosporin

● Lipid-regulating Drugs: manufacturer of ezetimibe advises avoid concomitant use with ●fibrates

Famciclovir

Probenecid: excretion of famciclovir possibly reduced by probenecid (increased plasma concentration)

Famotidine *see* Histamine H_2-antagonists

Felodipine *see* Calcium-channel Blockers

Fenbufen *see* NSAIDs

Fenofibrate *see* Fibrates

Fenoprofen *see* NSAIDs

Fenoterol *see* Sympathomimetics, $Beta_2$

Fentanyl *see* Opioid Analgesics
Ferrous Salts *see* Iron
Fexofenadine *see* Antihistamines
Fibrates
- Anticoagulants: fibrates enhance anticoagulant effect of •coumarins and •phenindione
- Antidiabetics: gemfibrozil increases plasma concentration of •rosiglitazone (consider reducing dose of rosiglitazone); fibrates may improve glucose tolerance and have an additive effect with insulin or sulphonylureas; gemfibrozil possibly enhances hypoglycaemic effect of nateglinide; increased risk of severe hypoglycaemia when gemfibrozil given with •repaglinide—avoid concomitant use

Ciclosporin: increased risk of renal impairment when fenofibrate given with ciclosporin
- Cytotoxics: gemfibrozil increases plasma concentration of •bexarotene—avoid concomitant use
- Lipid-regulating Drugs: increased risk of myopathy when fibrates given with •rosuvastatin or •statins; avoidance of fibrates advised by manufacturer of •ezetimibe; increased risk of myopathy when gemfibrozil given with •statins (preferably avoid concomitant use)

Filgrastim
Note. Pegfilgrastim interactions as for filgrastim
Cytotoxics: neutropenia possibly exacerbated when filgrastim given with fluorouracil
Flavoxate *see* Antimuscarinics
Flecainide
Anaesthetics, Local: increased myocardial depression when anti-arrhythmics given with bupivacaine, levobupivacaine or prilocaine
- Anti-arrhythmics: increased myocardial depression when anti-arrhythmics given with other •anti-arrhythmics; plasma concentration of flecainide increased by •amiodarone (halve dose of flecainide)
- Antidepressants: plasma concentration of flecainide increased by fluoxetine; increased risk of ventricular arrhythmias when flecainide given with •tricyclics
- Antihistamines: increased risk of ventricular arrhythmias when flecainide given with •mizolastine or •terfenadine—avoid concomitant use; increased risk of ventricular arrhythmias when anti-arrhythmics given with •terfenadine
- Antimalarials: avoidance of flecainide advised by manufacturer of •artemether/lumefantrine (risk of ventricular arrhythmias); plasma concentration of flecainide increased by •quinine
- Antipsychotics: increased risk of ventricular arrhythmias when anti-arrhythmics that prolong the QT interval given with •antipsychotics that prolong the QT interval; increased risk of arrhythmias when flecainide given with •clozapine
- Antivirals: plasma concentration of flecainide possibly increased by •amprenavir (increased risk of ventricular arrhythmias—avoid concomitant use); plasma concentration of flecainide increased by •ritonavir (increased risk of ventricular arrhythmias—avoid concomitant use)
- Beta-blockers: increased risk of myocardial depression and bradycardia when flecainide given with •beta-blockers; increased myocardial depression when anti-arrhythmics given with •beta-blockers
- Calcium-channel Blockers: increased risk of myocardial depression and asystole when flecainide given with •verapamil
- Diuretics: increased cardiac toxicity with flecainide if hypokalaemia occurs with •acetazolamide, •loop diuretics or •thiazides and related diuretics

Flecainide *(continued)*
- Dolasetron: increased risk of ventricular arrhythmias when flecainide given with •dolasetron—avoid concomitant use

$5HT_3$ Antagonists: caution with anti-arrhythmics advised by manufacturer of tropisetron (risk of ventricular arrhythmias)
Ulcer-healing Drugs: metabolism of flecainide inhibited by cimetidine (increased plasma concentration)
Flucloxacillin *see* Penicillins
Fluconazole *see* Antifungals, Triazole
Flucytosine
Antifungals: renal excretion of flucytosine decreased and cellular uptake increased by amphotericin (toxicity possibly increased)
Cytotoxics: plasma concentration of flucytosine possibly reduced by cytarabine
Fludarabine
Antiepileptics: cytotoxics possibly reduce absorption of phenytoin
- Antipsychotics: avoid concomitant use of cytotoxics with •clozapine (increased risk of agranulocytosis)
- Cytotoxics: fludarabine increases intracellular concentration of cytarabine; increased pulmonary toxicity when fludarabine given with •pentostatin (unacceptably high incidence of fatalities)

Dipyridamole: effects of fludarabine possibly reduced by dipyridamole
Fludrocortisone *see* Corticosteroids
Flunisolide *see* Corticosteroids
Fluorides
Calcium Salts: absorption of fluorides reduced by calcium salts
Fluorouracil
Note. Capecitabine is a prodrug of fluorouracil
Note. Tegafur is a prodrug of fluorouracil
- Allopurinol: manufacturer of capecitabine advises avoid concomitant use with •allopurinol

Antibacterials: metabolism of fluorouracil inhibited by metronidazole (increased toxicity)
- Anticoagulants: fluorouracil possibly enhances anticoagulant effect of •coumarins

Antiepileptics: fluorouracil possibly inhibits metabolism of phenytoin (increased risk of toxicity); cytotoxics possibly reduce absorption of phenytoin
- Antipsychotics: avoid concomitant use of cytotoxics with •clozapine (increased risk of agranulocytosis)

Filgrastim: neutropenia possibly exacerbated when fluorouracil given with filgrastim
- Temoporfin: increased skin photosensitivity when topical fluorouracil used with •temoporfin

Ulcer-healing Drugs: metabolism of fluorouracil inhibited by cimetidine (increased plasma concentration)
Fluoxetine *see* Antidepressants, SSRI
Flupentixol *see* Antipsychotics
Fluphenazine *see* Antipsychotics
Flurazepam *see* Anxiolytics and Hypnotics
Flurbiprofen *see* NSAIDs
Flutamide
- Anticoagulants: flutamide enhances anticoagulant effect of •coumarins

Fluticasone *see* Corticosteroids
Fluvastatin *see* Statins
Fluvoxamine *see* Antidepressants, SSRI
Folates
Aminosalicylates: absorption of folic acid possibly reduced by sulfasalazine
Antiepileptics: folates possibly reduce plasma concentration of phenytoin and primidone
Barbiturates: folates possibly reduce plasma concentration of phenobarbital

Folic Acid *see* Folates
Folinic Acid *see* Folates
Formoterol (eformoterol) *see* Sympathomimetics, Beta$_2$
Fosamprenavir *see* Amprenavir
Foscarnet
Antivirals: avoidance of foscarnet advised by manufacturer of lamivudine
Fosinopril *see* ACE Inhibitors
Fosphenytoin *see* Phenytoin
Framycetin *see* Aminoglycosides
Frovatriptan *see* 5HT$_1$ Agonists
Furosemide (frusemide) *see* Diuretics
Fusidic Acid
Antivirals: plasma concentration of both drugs may increase when fusidic acid given with ritonavir
Lipid-regulating Drugs: possible increased risk of myopathy when fusidic acid given with atorvastatin or simvastatin
Oestrogens: broad-spectrum antibacterials possibly reduce contraceptive effect of oestrogens (risk probably small, see p. 407)
Gabapentin
Antacids: absorption of gabapentin reduced by antacids
• Antidepressants: anticonvulsant effect of antiepileptics possibly antagonised by MAOIs and •tricyclic-related antidepressants (convulsive threshold lowered); anticonvulsant effect of antiepileptics antagonised by •SSRIs and •tricyclics (convulsive threshold lowered)
• Antimalarials: possible increased risk of convulsions when antiepileptics given with chloroquine and hydroxychloroquine; anticonvulsant effect of antiepileptics antagonised by •mefloquine
Galantamine *see* Parasympathomimetics
Ganciclovir
Note. Increased risk of myelosuppression with other myelosuppressive drugs—consult product literature
Note. Valganciclovir interactions as for ganciclovir
• Antibacterials: increased risk of convulsions when ganciclovir given with •imipenem with cilastatin
• Antivirals: ganciclovir possibly increases plasma concentration of didanosine; avoidance of intravenous ganciclovir advised by manufacturer of lamivudine; profound myelosuppression when ganciclovir given with •zidovudine (if possible avoid concomitant administration, particularly during initial ganciclovir therapy)
Cytotoxics: plasma concentration of ganciclovir possibly increased by mycophenolate mofetil, also plasma concentration of inactive metabolite of mycophenolate mofetil possibly increased
Probenecid: excretion of ganciclovir reduced by probenecid (increased plasma concentration and risk of toxicity)
Gemeprost *see* Prostaglandins
Gemfibrozil *see* Fibrates
Gentamicin *see* Aminoglycosides
Gestodene *see* Progestogens
Gestrinone
Antibacterials: metabolism of gestrinone accelerated by rifampicin (reduced plasma concentration)
Antiepileptics: metabolism of gestrinone accelerated by carbamazepine, phenytoin and primidone (reduced plasma concentration)
Barbiturates: metabolism of gestrinone accelerated by barbiturates (reduced plasma concentration)
Glibenclamide *see* Antidiabetics
Gliclazide *see* Antidiabetics
Glimepiride *see* Antidiabetics
Glipizide *see* Antidiabetics
Gliquidone *see* Antidiabetics
Glyceryl Trinitrate *see* Nitrates
Glycopyrronium *see* Antimuscarinics
Grapefruit Juice
• Antihistamines: grapefruit juice increases plasma concentration of •terfenadine—avoid concomitant use
• Antimalarials: grapefruit juice possibly inhibits metabolism of •artemether/lumefantrine (avoid concomitant use)
Antivirals: grapefruit juice possibly increases plasma concentration of efavirenz
Anxiolytics and Hypnotics: grapefruit juice increases plasma concentration of buspirone
Calcium-channel Blockers: grapefruit juice increases plasma concentration of felodipine, isradipine, lacidipine, lercanidipine, nicardipine, nifedipine, nimodipine, nisoldipine and verapamil
• Ciclosporin: grapefruit juice increases plasma concentration of •ciclosporin (increased risk of toxicity)
• Lipid-regulating Drugs: grapefruit juice increases plasma concentration of •simvastatin—avoid concomitant use
Sildenafil: grapefruit juice possibly increases plasma concentration of sildenafil
• Sirolimus: grapefruit juice increases plasma concentration of •sirolimus—avoid concomitant use
• Tacrolimus: grapefruit juice increases plasma concentration of •tacrolimus
Tadalafil: grapefruit juice possibly increases plasma concentration of tadalafil
• Vardenafil: grapefruit juice possibly increases plasma concentration of •vardenafil—avoid concomitant use
Griseofulvin
Alcohol: griseofulvin possibly enhances effects of alcohol
• Anticoagulants: griseofulvin reduces anticoagulant effect of •coumarins
Antiepileptics: absorption of griseofulvin reduced by primidone (reduced effect)
Barbiturates: absorption of griseofulvin reduced by phenobarbital (reduced effect)
Ciclosporin: griseofulvin possibly reduces plasma concentration of ciclosporin
• Oestrogens: griseofulvin accelerates metabolism of •oestrogens (reduced contraceptive effect—see p. 407)
• Progestogens: griseofulvin accelerates metabolism of •progestogens (reduced contraceptive effect—see p. 407)
Guanethidine *see* Adrenergic Neurone Blockers
Haloperidol *see* Antipsychotics
Halothane *see* Anaesthetics, General
Heparin *see* Heparins
Heparins
ACE Inhibitors: increased risk of hyperkalaemia when heparins given with ACE inhibitors
• Analgesics: possible increased risk of bleeding when heparins given with NSAIDs; increased risk of haemorrhage when heparins given with intravenous •diclofenac (avoid concomitant use, including low-dose heparin); increased risk of haemorrhage when heparins given with •ketorolac (avoid concomitant use, including low-dose heparin); anticoagulant effect of heparins enhanced by •aspirin
Angiotensin-II Receptor Antagonists: increased risk of hyperkalaemia when heparin given with angiotensin-II receptor antagonists
Clopidogrel: increased risk of bleeding when heparins given with clopidogrel
Dipyridamole: anticoagulant effect of heparins enhanced by dipyridamole

Heparins *(continued)*
- Drotrecogin Alfa: avoidance of concomitant use of high doses of heparin with drotrecogin alfa advised by manufacturer of •drotrecogin alfa—consult product literature

Iloprost: anticoagulant effect of heparins possibly enhanced by iloprost
- Nitrates: anticoagulant effect of heparins reduced by infusion of •glyceryl trinitrate

Sibutramine: increased risk of bleeding when anticoagulants given with sibutramine

Histamine H_2-antagonists
- Alpha-blockers: cimetidine and ranitidine antagonise effects of •tolazoline

Analgesics: cimetidine inhibits metabolism of opioid analgesics (increased plasma concentration)
- Anti-arrhythmics: cimetidine increases plasma concentration of amiodarone, •procainamide, •propafenone and •quinidine; cimetidine inhibits metabolism of flecainide (increased plasma concentration); cimetidine increases plasma concentration of •lidocaine (lignocaine) (increased risk of toxicity)

Antibacterials: histamine H_2-antagonists reduce absorption of cefpodoxime; cimetidine increases plasma concentration of erythromycin (increased risk of toxicity, including deafness); cimetidine inhibits metabolism of metronidazole (increased plasma concentration); metabolism of cimetidine accelerated by rifampicin (reduced plasma concentration); ranitidine bismuth citrate reduces absorption of tetracyclines
- Anticoagulants: cimetidine inhibits metabolism of •coumarins (enhanced anticoagulant effect)

Antidepressants: cimetidine increases plasma concentration of mirtazapine and sertraline; cimetidine inhibits metabolism of amitriptyline, doxepin, imipramine and nortriptyline (increased plasma concentration); cimetidine increases plasma concentration of moclobemide (halve dose of moclobemide); cimetidine possibly increases plasma concentration of tricyclics

Antidiabetics: cimetidine reduces excretion of metformin (increased plasma concentration); cimetidine enhances hypoglycaemic effect of sulphonylureas
- Antiepileptics: cimetidine inhibits metabolism of •carbamazepine, •phenytoin and •valproate (increased plasma concentration)

Antifungals: histamine H_2-antagonists reduce absorption of itraconazole and ketoconazole; cimetidine increases plasma concentration of terbinafine

Antihistamines: manufacturer of loratadine advises cimetidine possibly increases plasma concentration of loratadine

Antimalarials: cimetidine inhibits metabolism of chloroquine and hydroxychloroquine and quinine (increased plasma concentration)
- Antipsychotics: cimetidine possibly enhances effects of antipsychotics, chlorpromazine and clozapine; increased risk of ventricular arrhythmias when cimetidine given with •sertindole—avoid concomitant use

Antivirals: plasma concentration of cimetidine possibly increased by amprenavir; cimetidine possibly increases plasma concentration of zalcitabine

Anxiolytics and Hypnotics: cimetidine inhibits metabolism of benzodiazepines, clomethiazole and zaleplon (increased plasma concentration)

Beta-blockers: cimetidine increases plasma concentration of labetalol, metoprolol and propranolol

Histamine H_2-antagonists *(continued)*

Calcium-channel Blockers: cimetidine possibly inhibits metabolism of calcium-channel blockers (increased plasma concentration)
- Ciclosporin: cimetidine possibly increases plasma concentration of •ciclosporin
- Cilostazol: cimetidine possibly increases plasma concentration of •cilostazol—avoid concomitant use
- Cytotoxics: cimetidine increases plasma concentration of •epirubicin; cimetidine inhibits metabolism of fluorouracil (increased plasma concentration)

Dopaminergics: cimetidine reduces excretion of pramipexole (increased plasma concentration)
- Ergot Alkaloids: increased risk of ergotism when cimetidine given with •ergotamine and methysergide—avoid concomitant use

Hormone Antagonists: absorption of cimetidine possibly delayed by octreotide

$5HT_1$ Agonists: cimetidine inhibits metabolism of zolmitriptan (reduce dose of zolmitriptan)

Mebendazole: cimetidine possibly inhibits metabolism of mebendazole (increased plasma concentration)

Sildenafil: cimetidine increases plasma concentration of sildenafil (reduce initial dose of sildenafil)
- Theophylline: cimetidine inhibits metabolism of •theophylline (increased plasma concentration)

Thyroid Hormones: cimetidine reduces absorption of levothyroxine (thyroxine)

Homatropine *see* Antimuscarinics

Hormone Antagonists *see* Aminoglutethimide, Bicalutamide, Danazol, Dutasteride, Exemestane, Flutamide, Gestrinone, Lanreotide, Octreotide, Tamoxifen, Toremifene, and Trilostane

$5HT_1$ Agonists
- Antibacterials: plasma concentration of eletriptan increased by •clarithromycin and •erythromycin (risk of toxicity)—avoid concomitant use; metabolism of zolmitriptan possibly inhibited by quinolones (reduce dose of zolmitriptan)
- Antidepressants: increased risk of CNS toxicity when sumatriptan given with •citalopram, •escitalopram, •fluoxetine, •fluvoxamine or •paroxetine; metabolism of frovatriptan possibly inhibited by fluvoxamine; metabolism of zolmitriptan possibly inhibited by fluvoxamine (reduce dose of zolmitriptan); increased risk of CNS toxicity when sumatriptan given with •sertraline (manufacturer of sertraline advises avoid concomitant use); possible increased serotonergic effects when $5HT_1$ agonists given with duloxetine; increased risk of CNS toxicity when zolmitriptan given with •MAOIs; risk of CNS toxicity when rizatriptan or sumatriptan given with •MAOIs (avoid rizatriptan or sumatriptan for 2 weeks after MAOIs); risk of CNS toxicity when rizatriptan or sumatriptan given with •moclobemide (avoid rizatriptan or sumatriptan for 2 weeks after moclobemide); risk of CNS toxicity when zolmitriptan given with •moclobemide (reduce dose of zolmitriptan); possible increased serotonergic effects when frovatriptan given with SSRIs; increased serotonergic effects when $5HT_1$ agonists given with •St John's wort—avoid concomitant use
- Antifungals: plasma concentration of eletriptan increased by •itraconazole and •ketoconazole (risk of toxicity)—avoid concomitant use
- Antivirals: plasma concentration of eletriptan increased by •indinavir, •nelfinavir and •ritonavir (risk of toxicity)—avoid concomitant use

5HT$_1$ Agonists *(continued)*

Beta-blockers: plasma concentration of rizatriptan possibly increased by propranolol (reduce dose of rizatriptan)

• Ergot Alkaloids: increased risk of vasospasm when eletriptan or frovatriptan given with •ergotamine and methysergide (avoid ergotamine and methysergide for 24 hours after eletriptan or frovatriptan, avoid eletriptan or frovatriptan for 24 hours after ergotamine and methysergide); increased risk of vasospasm when almotriptan, rizatriptan, sumatriptan or zolmitriptan given with •ergotamine and methysergide (avoid ergotamine and methysergide for 6 hours after almotriptan, rizatriptan, sumatriptan or zolmitriptan, avoid almotriptan, rizatriptan, sumatriptan or zolmitriptan for 24 hours after ergotamine and methysergide)

Ulcer-healing Drugs: metabolism of zolmitriptan inhibited by cimetidine (reduce dose of zolmitriptan)

5HT$_3$ Antagonists *see* Ondansetron and Tropisetron

Hydralazine *see* Vasodilator Antihypertensives

Hydrochlorothiazide *see* Diuretics

Hydrocortisone *see* Corticosteroids

Hydroflumethiazide *see* Diuretics

Hydromorphone *see* Opioid Analgesics

Hydrotalcite *see* Antacids

Hydroxocobalamin

Antibacterials: response to hydroxocobalamin reduced by chloramphenicol

Hydroxychloroquine *see* Chloroquine and Hydroxychloroquine

Hydroxyzine *see* Antihistamines

Hyoscine *see* Antimuscarinics

Ibandronic Acid *see* Bisphosphonates

Ibuprofen *see* NSAIDs

Ifosfamide

• Anticoagulants: ifosfamide possibly enhances anticoagulant effect of •coumarins

Antiepileptics: cytotoxics possibly reduce absorption of phenytoin

• Antipsychotics: avoid concomitant use of cytotoxics with •clozapine (increased risk of agranulocytosis)

Iloprost

Analgesics: increased risk of bleeding when iloprost given with NSAIDs or aspirin

Anticoagulants: iloprost possibly enhances anticoagulant effect of coumarins and heparins; increased risk of bleeding when iloprost given with phenindione

Clopidogrel: increased risk of bleeding when iloprost given with clopidogrel

Eptifibatide: increased risk of bleeding when iloprost given with eptifibatide

Tirofiban: increased risk of bleeding when iloprost given with tirofiban

Imatinib

• Antibacterials: plasma concentration of imatinib reduced by •rifampicin—avoid concomitant use

Anticoagulants: manufacturer of imatinib advises replacement of warfarin with a heparin (possibility of enhanced warfarin effect)

• Antiepileptics: plasma concentration of imatinib reduced by •phenytoin—avoid concomitant use; cytotoxics possibly reduce absorption of phenytoin

Antifungals: plasma concentration of imatinib increased by ketoconazole

• Antipsychotics: avoid concomitant use of cytotoxics with •clozapine (increased risk of agranulocytosis)

Lipid-regulating Drugs: imatinib increases plasma concentration of simvastatin

Imidapril *see* ACE Inhibitors

Imipenem with Cilastatin

• Antivirals: increased risk of convulsions when imipenem with cilastatin given with •ganciclovir

Oestrogens: broad-spectrum antibacterials possibly reduce contraceptive effect of oestrogens (risk probably small, see p. 407)

Imipramine *see* Antidepressants, Tricyclic

Immunoglobulins

Note. For advice on immunoglobulins and live virus vaccines, see under Normal Immunoglobulin, p. 620

Immunosuppressants (antiproliferative) *see* Azathioprine and Mycophenolate Mofetil

Indapamide *see* Diuretics

Indinavir

• Antibacterials: indinavir increases plasma concentration of •rifabutin, also plasma concentration of indinavir decreased (reduce dose of rifabutin and increase dose of indinavir); metabolism of indinavir accelerated by •rifampicin (reduced plasma concentration—avoid concomitant use)

• Antidepressants: plasma concentration of indinavir reduced by •St John's wort—avoid concomitant use

• Antiepileptics: plasma concentration of indinavir possibly reduced by carbamazepine, phenytoin and •primidone

• Antifungals: metabolism of indinavir inhibited by ketoconazole; plasma concentration of indinavir increased by •itraconazole (consider reducing dose of indinavir)

• Antihistamines: increased risk of ventricular arrhythmias when indinavir given with •terfenadine—avoid concomitant use

Antimuscarinics: avoidance of indinavir advised by manufacturer of tolterodine

• Antipsychotics: indinavir possibly inhibits metabolism of •aripiprazole (reduce dose of aripiprazole); indinavir possibly increases plasma concentration of •pimozide (increased risk of ventricular arrhythmias—avoid concomitant use); indinavir increases plasma concentration of •sertindole (increased risk of ventricular arrhythmias—avoid concomitant use)

• Antivirals: avoid concomitant use of indinavir with •atazanavir; plasma concentration of indinavir reduced by efavirenz and nevirapine; combination of indinavir with nelfinavir may increase plasma concentration of either drug (or both); plasma concentration of indinavir increased by ritonavir; indinavir increases plasma concentration of saquinavir

• Anxiolytics and Hypnotics: increased risk of prolonged sedation when indinavir given with •alprazolam or •midazolam—avoid concomitant use

Atovaquone: plasma concentration of indinavir possibly reduced by atovaquone

• Barbiturates: plasma concentration of indinavir possibly reduced by •barbiturates

• Cilostazol: indinavir possibly increases plasma concentration of •cilostazol—avoid concomitant use

Corticosteroids: plasma concentration of indinavir possibly reduced by dexamethasone

• Ergot Alkaloids: increased risk of ergotism when indinavir given with •ergotamine and methysergide—avoid concomitant use

• 5HT$_1$ Agonists: indinavir increases plasma concentration of •eletriptan (risk of toxicity)—avoid concomitant use

• Lipid-regulating Drugs: possible increased risk of myopathy when indinavir given with atorvastatin; increased risk of myopathy when indinavir given with •simvastatin (avoid concomitant use)

Indinavir *(continued)*
Sildenafil: indinavir increases plasma concentration of sildenafil—reduce initial dose of sildenafil
• Vardenafil: indinavir increases plasma concentration of •vardenafil—avoid concomitant use

Indometacin *see* NSAIDs
Indoramin *see* Alpha-blockers
Infliximab
• Anakinra: avoid concomitant use of infliximab with •anakinra
• Vaccines: avoid concomitant use of infliximab with live •vaccines (see p. 604)

Influenza Vaccine *see* Vaccines
Insulin *see* Antidiabetics
Interferon Alfa *see* Interferons
Interferon Gamma *see* Interferons
Interferons
Note. Peginterferon alfa interactions as for interferon alfa
Theophylline: interferon alfa inhibits metabolism of theophylline (increased plasma concentration)
Vaccines: manufacturer of interferon gamma advises avoid concomitant use with vaccines

Ipratropium *see* Antimuscarinics
Irbesartan *see* Angiotensin-II Receptor Antagonists
Irinotecan
Antiepileptics: cytotoxics possibly reduce absorption of phenytoin
• Antipsychotics: avoid concomitant use of cytotoxics with •clozapine (increased risk of agranulocytosis)
• Antivirals: metabolism of irinotecan possibly inhibited by •atazanavir (increased risk of toxicity)

Iron
Antacids: absorption of *oral* iron reduced by oral magnesium salts (as magnesium trisilicate)
Antibacterials: *oral* iron reduces absorption of ciprofloxacin, levofloxacin, moxifloxacin, norfloxacin and ofloxacin; *oral* iron reduces absorption of tetracyclines, also absorption of *oral* iron reduced by tetracyclines
Bisphosphonates: *oral* iron reduces absorption of bisphosphonates
Calcium Salts: absorption of *oral* iron reduced by calcium salts
• Dimercaprol: avoid concomitant use of iron with •dimercaprol
Dopaminergics: *oral* iron reduces absorption of entacapone; *oral* iron possibly reduces absorption of levodopa
Methyldopa: *oral* iron antagonises hypotensive effect of methyldopa
Penicillamine: *oral* iron reduces absorption of penicillamine
Thyroid Hormones: *oral* iron reduces absorption of levothyroxine (thyroxine) (give at least 2 hours apart)
Trientine: absorption of *oral* iron reduced by trientine
Zinc: *oral* iron reduces absorption of zinc, also absorption of *oral* iron reduced by zinc

Isocarboxazid *see* MAOIs
Isoflurane *see* Anaesthetics, General
Isometheptene *see* Sympathomimetics
Isoniazid
Anaesthetics, General: hepatotoxicity of isoniazid possibly potentiated by general anaesthetics
Antacids: absorption of isoniazid reduced by antacids
Antibacterials: increased risk of CNS toxicity when isoniazid given with cycloserine
• Antiepileptics: isoniazid increases plasma concentration of •carbamazepine (also possibly increased isoniazid hepatotoxicity); isoniazid inhibits metabolism of •ethosuximide (increased plasma concentration and risk of toxicity); isoniazid

Isoniazid
• Antiepileptics *(continued)*
inhibits metabolism of •phenytoin (increased plasma concentration)
Antifungals: isoniazid possibly reduces plasma concentration of ketoconazole
Anxiolytics and Hypnotics: isoniazid inhibits the metabolism of diazepam
Oestrogens: broad-spectrum antibacterials possibly reduce contraceptive effect of oestrogens (risk probably small, see p. 407)
Theophylline: isoniazid possibly increases plasma concentration of theophylline

Isosorbide Dinitrate *see* Nitrates
Isosorbide Mononitrate *see* Nitrates
Isotretinoin *see* Retinoids
Isradipine *see* Calcium-channel Blockers
Itraconazole *see* Antifungals, Triazole
Kaolin
Analgesics: kaolin possibly reduces absorption of aspirin
Anti-arrhythmics: kaolin possibly reduces absorption of quinidine
Antibacterials: kaolin possibly reduces absorption of tetracyclines
Antimalarials: kaolin reduces absorption of chloroquine and hydroxychloroquine
Antipsychotics: kaolin possibly reduces absorption of phenothiazines

Ketamine *see* Anaesthetics, General
Ketoconazole *see* Antifungals, Imidazole
Ketoprofen *see* NSAIDs
Ketorolac *see* NSAIDs
Ketotifen *see* Antihistamines
Labetalol *see* Beta-blockers
Lacidipine *see* Calcium-channel Blockers
Lamivudine
Antibacterials: plasma concentration of lamivudine increased by trimethoprim (as co-trimoxazole)—avoid concomitant use of high-dose co-trimoxazole
Antivirals: avoidance of lamivudine advised by manufacturer of emtricitabine; manufacturer of lamivudine advises avoid concomitant use with foscarnet; manufacturer of lamivudine advises avoid concomitant use of intravenous ganciclovir; lamivudine possibly inhibits effects of zalcitabine (manufacturers advise avoid concomitant use)

Lamotrigine
• Antidepressants: anticonvulsant effect of antiepileptics possibly antagonised by MAOIs and •tricyclic-related antidepressants (convulsive threshold lowered); anticonvulsant effect of antiepileptics antagonised by •SSRIs and •tricyclics (convulsive threshold lowered)
Antiepileptics: plasma concentration of lamotrigine often reduced by carbamazepine, also plasma concentration of an active metabolite of carbamazepine sometimes raised (but evidence is conflicting); plasma concentration of lamotrigine reduced by phenytoin and primidone; plasma concentration of lamotrigine increased by valproate
• Antimalarials: possible increased risk of convulsions when antiepileptics given with chloroquine and hydroxychloroquine; anticonvulsant effect of antiepileptics antagonised by •mefloquine
Barbiturates: plasma concentration of lamotrigine reduced by phenobarbital

Lanreotide
Antidiabetics: lanreotide possibly reduces requirements for insulin, metformin, repaglinide and sulphonylureas

Lanreotide *(continued)*
Ciclosporin: lanreotide reduces plasma concentration of ciclosporin

Lansoprazole *see* Proton Pump Inhibitors

Laronidase
Anaesthetics, Local: effects of laronidase possibly inhibited by procaine (manufacturer of laronidase advises avoid concomitant use)
Antimalarials: effects of laronidase possibly inhibited by chloroquine and hydroxychloroquine (manufacturer of laronidase advises avoid concomitant use)

Leflunomide
Note. Increased risk of toxicity with other haematotoxic and hepatotoxic drugs
Anticoagulants: leflunomide possibly enhances anticoagulant effect of warfarin
Antidiabetics: leflunomide possibly enhances hypoglycaemic effect of tolbutamide
Antiepileptics: leflunomide possibly increases plasma concentration of phenytoin
Lipid-regulating Drugs: the effect of leflunomide is significantly decreased by colestyramine (enhanced elimination)—avoid unless drug elimination desired
• Vaccines: avoid concomitant use of leflunomide with live •vaccines (see p. 604)

Lercanidipine *see* Calcium-channel Blockers

Leukotriene Antagonists
Analgesics: plasma concentration of zafirlukast increased by aspirin
Antibacterials: plasma concentration of zafirlukast reduced by erythromycin
Anticoagulants: zafirlukast enhances anticoagulant effect of warfarin
Antiepileptics: plasma concentration of montelukast reduced by primidone
Antihistamines: plasma concentration of zafirlukast reduced by terfenadine
Barbiturates: plasma concentration of montelukast reduced by phenobarbital
Theophylline: zafirlukast possibly increases plasma concentration of theophylline, also plasma concentration of zafirlukast reduced

Levamisole
Alcohol: possibility of disulfiram-like reaction when levamisole given with alcohol
• Anticoagulants: levamisole possibly enhances anticoagulant effect of •warfarin
Antiepileptics: levamisole possibly increases plasma concentration of phenytoin

Levetiracetam
• Antidepressants: anticonvulsant effect of antiepileptics possibly antagonised by MAOIs and •tricyclic-related antidepressants (convulsive threshold lowered); anticonvulsant effect of antiepileptics antagonised by •SSRIs and •tricyclics (convulsive threshold lowered)
• Antimalarials: possible increased risk of convulsions when antiepileptics given with chloroquine and hydroxychloroquine; anticonvulsant effect of antiepileptics antagonised by •mefloquine

Levobunolol *see* Beta-blockers

Levobupivacaine
Anti-arrhythmics: increased myocardial depression when levobupivacaine given with anti-arrhythmics

Levocabastine *see* Antihistamines

Levocetirizine *see* Antihistamines

Levodopa
ACE Inhibitors: enhanced hypotensive effect when levodopa given with ACE inhibitors
Adrenergic Neurone Blockers: enhanced hypotensive effect when levodopa given with adrenergic neurone blockers

Levodopa *(continued)*
Alpha-blockers: enhanced hypotensive effect when levodopa given with alpha-blockers
• Anaesthetics, General: increased risk of arrhythmias when levodopa given with •volatile liquid general anaesthetics
Angiotensin-II Receptor Antagonists: enhanced hypotensive effect when levodopa given with angiotensin-II receptor antagonists
• Antidepressants: risk of hypertensive crisis when levodopa given with •MAOIs, avoid levodopa for at least two weeks after stopping MAOIs; increased risk of side-effects when levodopa given with moclobemide
Antiepileptics: effects of levodopa possibly reduced by phenytoin
Antimuscarinics: absorption of levodopa possibly reduced by antimuscarinics
Antipsychotics: effects of levodopa antagonised by antipsychotics; avoidance of levodopa advised by manufacturer of amisulpride (antagonism of effect)
Anxiolytics and Hypnotics: effects of levodopa possibly antagonised by benzodiazepines
Beta-blockers: enhanced hypotensive effect when levodopa given with beta-blockers
Bupropion: increased risk of side-effects when levodopa given with bupropion
Calcium-channel Blockers: enhanced hypotensive effect when levodopa given with calcium-channel blockers
Clonidine: enhanced hypotensive effect when levodopa given with clonidine
Diazoxide: enhanced hypotensive effect when levodopa given with diazoxide
Diuretics: enhanced hypotensive effect when levodopa given with diuretics
Dopaminergics: enhanced effects and increased toxicity of levodopa when given with selegiline (reduce dose of levodopa)
Iron: absorption of levodopa possibly reduced by *oral* iron
Memantine: effects of dopaminergics possibly enhanced by memantine
Methyldopa: enhanced hypotensive effect when levodopa given with methyldopa; antiparkinsonian effect of dopaminergics antagonised by methyldopa
Moxonidine: enhanced hypotensive effect when levodopa given with moxonidine
Muscle Relaxants: possible agitation, confusion and hallucinations when levodopa given with baclofen
Nitrates: enhanced hypotensive effect when levodopa given with nitrates
Vasodilator Antihypertensives: enhanced hypotensive effect when levodopa given with hydralazine, minoxidil or nitroprusside
Vitamins: effects of levodopa reduced by pyridoxine when given without dopa-decarboxylase inhibitor

Levofloxacin *see* Quinolones

Levomepromazine (methotrimeprazine) *see* Antipsychotics

Levonorgestrel *see* Progestogens

Levothyroxine (thyroxine) *see* Thyroid Hormones

Lidocaine (lignocaine)
Note. Interactions less likely when lidocaine used topically
Anaesthetics, Local: increased myocardial depression when anti-arrhythmics given with bupivacaine, levobupivacaine or prilocaine
• Anti-arrhythmics: increased myocardial depression when anti-arrhythmics given with other •anti-arrhythmics

Lidocaine (lignocaine) *(continued)*

- Antibacterials: increased risk of ventricular arrhythmias when lidocaine (lignocaine) given with •quinupristin/dalfopristin—avoid concomitant use
- Antihistamines: increased risk of ventricular arrhythmias when anti-arrhythmics given with •terfenadine
- Antipsychotics: increased risk of ventricular arrhythmias when anti-arrhythmics that prolong the QT interval given with •antipsychotics that prolong the QT interval
- Antivirals: plasma concentration of lidocaine (lignocaine) possibly increased by •amprenavir—avoid concomitant use; plasma concentration of lidocaine (lignocaine) possibly increased by •atazanavir and lopinavir
- Beta-blockers: increased myocardial depression when anti-arrhythmics given with •beta-blockers; increased risk of lidocaine (lignocaine) toxicity when given with •propranolol
- Diuretics: action of lidocaine (lignocaine) antagonised by hypokalaemia caused by •acetazolamide, •loop diuretics or •thiazides and related diuretics
- Dolasetron: increased risk of ventricular arrhythmias when lidocaine (lignocaine) given with •dolasetron—avoid concomitant use

$5HT_3$ Antagonists: caution with anti-arrhythmics advised by manufacturer of tropisetron (risk of ventricular arrhythmias)

Muscle Relaxants: neuromuscular blockade enhanced and prolonged when lidocaine (lignocaine) given with suxamethonium

- Ulcer-healing Drugs: plasma concentration of lidocaine (lignocaine) increased by •cimetidine (increased risk of toxicity)

Linezolid

Note. Linezolid is a reversible, non-selective MAO inhibitor—see interactions of MAOIs

Oestrogens: broad-spectrum antibacterials possibly reduce contraceptive effect of oestrogens (risk probably small, see p. 407)

Liothyronine *see* Thyroid Hormones

Lipid-regulating Drugs *see* Colestipol, Colestyramine, Ezetimibe, Fibrates, Nicotinic Acid, and Statins

Lisinopril *see* ACE Inhibitors

Lisuride

Antipsychotics: effects of lisuride antagonised by antipsychotics

Memantine: effects of dopaminergics possibly enhanced by memantine

Methyldopa: antiparkinsonian effect of dopaminergics antagonised by methyldopa

Lithium

- ACE Inhibitors: excretion of lithium reduced by •ACE inhibitors (increased plasma concentration)
- Analgesics: excretion of lithium probably reduced by •NSAIDs (increased risk of toxicity); excretion of lithium reduced by •diclofenac, •ibuprofen, •indometacin, •mefenamic acid, •naproxen, •parecoxib and •piroxicam (increased risk of toxicity); excretion of lithium reduced by •ketorolac (increased risk of toxicity)—avoid concomitant use
- Angiotensin-II Receptor Antagonists: excretion of lithium reduced by •angiotensin-II receptor antagonists (increased plasma concentration)

Antacids: excretion of lithium increased by sodium bicarbonate (reduced plasma concentration)

- Anti-arrhythmics: avoidance of lithium advised by manufacturer of •amiodarone (risk of ventricular arrhythmias)

Lithium *(continued)*

Antibacterials: increased risk of lithium toxicity when given with metronidazole

- Antidepressants: increased risk of CNS effects when lithium given with •SSRIs (lithium toxicity reported); risk of toxicity when lithium given with tricyclics

Antiepileptics: neurotoxicity may occur when lithium given with carbamazepine or phenytoin without increased plasma concentration of lithium

- Antipsychotics: increased risk of extrapyramidal side-effects and possibly neurotoxicity when lithium given with clozapine, haloperidol or phenothiazines; increased risk of ventricular arrhythmias when lithium given with •sertindole—avoid concomitant use; increased risk of extrapyramidal side-effects when lithium given with sulpiride

Calcium-channel Blockers: neurotoxicity may occur when lithium given with diltiazem or verapamil without increased plasma concentration of lithium

- Diuretics: excretion of lithium increased by •acetazolamide; excretion of lithium reduced by •loop diuretics and •thiazides and related diuretics (increased plasma concentration and risk of toxicity)—loop diuretics safer than thiazides; excretion of lithium reduced by •potassium-sparing diuretics and aldosterone antagonists (increased plasma concentration and risk of toxicity)
- Methyldopa: neurotoxicity may occur when lithium given with •methyldopa without increased plasma concentration of lithium

Muscle Relaxants: lithium enhances effects of muscle relaxants; hyperkinesis caused by lithium possibly aggravated by baclofen

Parasympathomimetics: lithium antagonises effects of neostigmine and pyridostigmine

Theophylline: excretion of lithium increased by theophylline (reduced plasma concentration)

Lofepramine *see* Antidepressants, Tricyclic

Lofexidine

Alcohol: increased sedative effect when lofexidine given with alcohol

Anxiolytics and Hypnotics: increased sedative effect when lofexidine given with anxiolytics and hypnotics

Loperamide

Desmopressin: loperamide increases plasma concentration of *oral* desmopressin

Lopinavir

Note. In combination with ritonavir as Kaletra® (ritonavir is present to inhibit lopinavir metabolism and increase plasma-lopinavir concentration)—see also Ritonavir

Anti-arrhythmics: lopinavir possibly increases plasma concentration of lidocaine (lignocaine)

- Antibacterials: plasma concentration of lopinavir reduced by •rifampicin—avoid concomitant use
- Antidepressants: plasma concentration of lopinavir reduced by •St John's wort—avoid concomitant use
- Antiepileptics: plasma concentration of lopinavir possibly reduced by carbamazepine, phenytoin and •primidone

Antihistamines: lopinavir possibly increases plasma concentration of chlorphenamine (chlorpheniramine)

Antimuscarinics: avoidance of lopinavir advised by manufacturer of tolterodine

- Antipsychotics: lopinavir possibly inhibits metabolism of •aripiprazole (reduce dose of aripiprazole); lopinavir increases plasma concentration of •sertindole (increased risk of ventricular arrhythmias—avoid concomitant use)

Lopinavir *(continued)*

Antivirals: lopinavir reduces plasma concentration of amprenavir, effect on lopinavir plasma concentration not predictable; plasma concentration of lopinavir reduced by efavirenz; plasma concentration of lopinavir reduced by nelfinavir, also plasma concentration of active metabolite of nelfinavir increased; plasma concentration of lopinavir possibly reduced by nevirapine; lopinavir increases plasma concentration of saquinavir and tenofovir

• Barbiturates: plasma concentration of lopinavir possibly reduced by •phenobarbital

• Cilostazol: lopinavir possibly increases plasma concentration of •cilostazol—avoid concomitant use

Corticosteroids: plasma concentration of lopinavir possibly reduced by dexamethasone

Lipid-regulating Drugs: possible increased risk of myopathy when lopinavir given with atorvastatin

Sirolimus: lopinavir possibly increases plasma concentration of sirolimus

Loprazolam *see* Anxiolytics and Hypnotics

Loratadine *see* Antihistamines

Lorazepam *see* Anxiolytics and Hypnotics

Lormetazepam *see* Anxiolytics and Hypnotics

Losartan *see* Angiotensin-II Receptor Antagonists

Lumefantrine *see* Artemether with Lumefantrine

Lymecycline *see* Tetracyclines

Macrolides

Note. See also Telithromycin

Note. Interactions do not apply to small amounts of erythromycin used topically

Analgesics: erythromycin increases plasma concentration of alfentanil

Antacids: absorption of azithromycin reduced by antacids

• Anti-arrhythmics: increased risk of ventricular arrhythmias when parenteral erythromycin given with •amiodarone—avoid concomitant use; clarithromycin possibly increases plasma concentration of •disopyramide (increased risk of toxicity); erythromycin increases plasma concentration of •disopyramide (increased risk of toxicity); increased risk of ventricular arrhythmias when parenteral erythromycin given with •quinidine; increased risk of ventricular arrhythmias when clarithromycin given with •quinidine

• Antibacterials: increased risk of ventricular arrhythmias when parenteral erythromycin given with •moxifloxacin—avoid concomitant use; macrolides possibly increase plasma concentration of •rifabutin (increased risk of uveitis—reduce rifabutin dose); clarithromycin increases plasma concentration of •rifabutin (increased risk of uveitis—reduce rifabutin dose)

• Anticoagulants: clarithromycin and erythromycin enhance anticoagulant effect of •coumarins; macrolides possibly enhance anticoagulant effect of •coumarins

• Antidepressants: avoidance of macrolides advised by manufacturer of •reboxetine

Antidiabetics: clarithromycin enhances effects of repaglinide

• Antiepileptics: clarithromycin and erythromycin increase plasma concentration of •carbamazepine; clarithromycin inhibits metabolism of phenytoin (increased plasma concentration); erythromycin possibly inhibits metabolism of valproate (increased plasma concentration)

Antifungals: clarithromycin increases plasma concentration of itraconazole

• Antihistamines: manufacturer of loratadine advises erythromycin possibly increases plasma concentration of loratadine; macrolides possibly inhibit metabolism of •mizolastine (avoid concomitant use); erythromycin inhibits metabolism of •mizolastine—avoid concomitant use; clarithromycin inhibits metabolism of •terfenadine (avoid concomitant use—increased risk of ventricular arrhythmias); erythromycin inhibits metabolism of •terfenadine—risk of ventricular arrhythmias, avoid concomitant use of systemic or topical preparations

• Antimalarials: avoidance of macrolides advised by manufacturer of •artemether/lumefantrine

Antimuscarinics: avoidance of clarithromycin and erythromycin advised by manufacturer of tolterodine

• Antipsychotics: increased risk of ventricular arrhythmias when parenteral erythromycin given with •amisulpride—avoid concomitant use; erythromycin possibly increases plasma concentration of •clozapine (possible increased risk of convulsions); increased risk of ventricular arrhythmias when clarithromycin given with •pimozide—avoid concomitant use; possible increased risk of ventricular arrhythmias when erythromycin given with •pimozide—avoid concomitant use; macrolides possibly increase plasma concentration of quetiapine (reduce dose of quetiapine); increased risk of ventricular arrhythmias when erythromycin given with •sertindole—avoid concomitant use; possible increased risk of ventricular arrhythmias when macrolides given with •sertindole—avoid concomitant use

• Antivirals: plasma concentration of both drugs increased when erythromycin given with amprenavir; plasma concentration of both drugs increased when clarithromycin given with atazanavir; increased risk of rash when clarithromycin given with efavirenz; plasma concentration of azithromycin and erythromycin possibly increased by ritonavir; plasma concentration of clarithromycin increased by •ritonavir (reduce dose of clarithromycin in renal impairment); clarithromycin tablets reduce absorption of zidovudine

• Anxiolytics and Hypnotics: clarithromycin and erythromycin inhibit metabolism of •midazolam (increased plasma concentration with increased sedation); erythromycin increases plasma concentration of buspirone (reduce dose of buspirone); erythromycin inhibits the metabolism of zopiclone

Aprepitant: clarithromycin possibly increases plasma concentration of aprepitant

Calcium-channel Blockers: erythromycin possibly inhibits metabolism of felodipine (increased plasma concentration); avoidance of erythromycin advised by manufacturer of lercanidipine

Cardiac Glycosides: macrolides increase plasma concentration of digoxin (increased risk of toxicity)

• Ciclosporin: macrolides possibly inhibit metabolism of •ciclosporin (increased plasma concentration); clarithromycin and erythromycin inhibit metabolism of •ciclosporin (increased plasma concentration)

• Cilostazol: erythromycin increases plasma concentration of •cilostazol (also plasma concentration of erythromycin reduced)—avoid concomitant use

Corticosteroids: erythromycin possibly inhibits metabolism of corticosteroids; erythromycin inhibits the metabolism of methylprednisolone; clarithromycin possibly increases plasma concentration of methylprednisolone

Macrolides *(continued)*
- Cytotoxics: *in vitro* studies suggest a possible interaction between erythromycin and docetaxel (consult docetaxel product literature); erythromycin increases toxicity of •vinblastine—avoid concomitant use
- Diuretics: clarithromycin increases plasma concentration of •eplerenone—avoid concomitant use; erythromycin increases plasma concentration of eplerenone (reduce dose of eplerenone)

Dopaminergics: macrolides possibly increase plasma concentration of bromocriptine and cabergoline (increased risk of toxicity); erythromycin increases plasma concentration of bromocriptine and cabergoline (increased risk of toxicity)
- Ergot Alkaloids: increased risk of ergotism when macrolides given with •ergotamine and methysergide—avoid concomitant use
- $5HT_1$ Agonists: clarithromycin and erythromycin increase plasma concentration of •eletriptan (risk of toxicity)—avoid concomitant use

Leukotriene Antagonists: erythromycin reduces plasma concentration of zafirlukast
- Lipid-regulating Drugs: clarithromycin increases plasma concentration of atorvastatin; possible increased risk of myopathy when erythromycin given with atorvastatin; erythromycin reduces plasma concentration of rosuvastatin; increased risk of myopathy when clarithromycin or erythromycin given with •simvastatin (avoid concomitant use)

Oestrogens: broad-spectrum antibacterials possibly reduce contraceptive effect of oestrogens (risk probably small, see p. 407)

Parasympathomimetics: erythromycin increases plasma concentration of galantamine

Sildenafil: erythromycin increases plasma concentration of sildenafil—reduce initial dose of sildenafil
- Sirolimus: clarithromycin increases plasma concentration of •sirolimus—avoid concomitant use; plasma concentration of both drugs increased when erythromycin given with •sirolimus
- Tacrolimus: clarithromycin and erythromycin increase plasma concentration of •tacrolimus

Tadalafil: clarithromycin and erythromycin possibly increase plasma concentration of tadalafil
- Theophylline: azithromycin possibly increases plasma concentration of theophylline; clarithromycin inhibits metabolism of •theophylline (increased plasma concentration); erythromycin inhibits metabolism of •theophylline (increased plasma concentration), if erythromycin given by mouth, also decreased plasma-erythromycin concentration

Ulcer-healing Drugs: plasma concentration of erythromycin increased by cimetidine (increased risk of toxicity, including deafness); plasma concentration of both drugs increased when clarithromycin given with omeprazole

Vardenafil: erythromycin increases plasma concentration of vardenafil (reduce dose of vardenafil)

Magnesium (parenteral)
- Calcium-channel Blockers: profound hypotension reported with concomitant use of parenteral magnesium and •nifedipine in pre-eclampsia

Muscle Relaxants: parenteral magnesium enhances effects of non-depolarising muscle relaxants and suxamethonium

Magnesium Salts (oral) *see* Antacids

MAOIs

Note. For interactions of reversible MAO-A inhibitors (RIMAs) see Moclobemide, and for interactions of MAO-B inhibitors see Selegiline; the antibacterial linezolid is a reversible, non-selective MAO inhibitor

ACE Inhibitors: MAOIs possibly enhance hypotensive effect of ACE inhibitors

Adrenergic Neurone Blockers: enhanced hypotensive effect when MAOIs given with adrenergic neurone blockers
- Alcohol: MAOIs interact with tyramine found in some beverages containing •alcohol and some dealcoholised beverages (hypertensive crisis)—if no tyramine, enhanced hypotensive effect

$Alpha_2$-adrenoceptor Stimulants: avoidance of MAOIs advised by manufacturer of apraclonidine and brimonidine
- Alpha-blockers: avoidance of MAOIs advised by manufacturer of •indoramin; enhanced hypotensive effect when MAOIs given with alpha-blockers
- Anaesthetics, General: Because of hazardous interactions between MAOIs and •general anaesthetics, MAOIs should normally be stopped 2 weeks before surgery
- Analgesics: CNS excitation or depression (hypertension or hypotension) when MAOIs given with •pethidine—avoid concomitant use and for 2 weeks after stopping MAOIs; avoidance of MAOIs advised by manufacturer of •nefopam; possible CNS excitation or depression (hypertension or hypotension) when MAOIs given with •opioid analgesics—avoid concomitant use and for 2 weeks after stopping MAOIs

Angiotensin-II Receptor Antagonists: MAOIs possibly enhance hypotensive effect of angiotensin-II receptor antagonists
- Antidepressants: increased risk of hypertension and CNS excitation when MAOIs given with •reboxetine (MAOIs should not be started until 1 week after stopping reboxetine, avoid reboxetine for 2 weeks after stopping MAOIs); after stopping MAOIs do not start •citalopram, •escitalopram, •fluvoxamine or •paroxetine for 2 weeks, also MAOIs should not be started until at least 1 week after stopping citalopram, escitalopram, fluvoxamine or paroxetine; after stopping MAOIs do not start •fluoxetine for 2 weeks, also MAOIs should not be started until at least 5 weeks after stopping fluoxetine; after stopping MAOIs do not start •mirtazapine or •sertraline for 2 weeks, also MAOIs should not be started until at least 2 weeks after stopping mirtazapine or sertraline; after stopping MAOIs do not start •duloxetine for 2 weeks, also MAOIs should not be started until at least 5 days after stopping duloxetine; enhanced CNS effects and toxicity when MAOIs given with •venlafaxine (venlafaxine should not be started until 2 weeks after stopping MAOIs, avoid MAOIs for 1 week after stopping venlafaxine); MAOIs can cause increased risk of hypertension and CNS excitation when given with other •MAOIs (avoid for at least 2 weeks after stopping previous MAOIs and then start at a reduced dose); after stopping MAOIs do not start •moclobemide for at least 1 week; MAOIs increase CNS effects of •SSRIs (risk of serious toxicity); after stopping MAOIs do not start •tricyclic-related antidepressants for 2 weeks, also MAOIs should not be started until at least 1–2 weeks after stopping tricyclic-related antidepressants; increased risk of hypertension and CNS excitation when MAOIs given with •tricyclics, tricyclics should not be started until 2 weeks after stopping MAOIs (3 weeks if starting clomipramine or imipramine), also MAOIs should not be started for at least 1–2 weeks after stopping tricyclics (3 weeks in the case of clomipramine or

MAOIs

- Antidepressants *(continued)* imipramine); CNS excitation and confusion when MAOIs given with •tryptophan (reduce dose of tryptophan)
  Antidiabetics: MAOIs possibly enhance hypoglycaemic effect of antidiabetics; MAOIs enhance hypoglycaemic effect of insulin, metformin and sulphonylureas
- Antiepileptics: MAOIs possibly antagonise anticonvulsant effect of antiepileptics (convulsive threshold lowered); avoidance for 2 weeks after stopping MAOIs advised by manufacturer of •carbamazepine, also antagonism of anticonvulsant effect; avoidance of MAOIs advised by manufacturer of •oxcarbazepine
  Antihistamines: increased antimuscarinic and sedative effects when MAOIs given with antihistamines
- Antimalarials: avoidance of antidepressants advised by manufacturer of •artemether/lumefantrine
  Antimuscarinics: increased risk of antimuscarinic side-effects when MAOIs given with antimuscarinics
- Antipsychotics: CNS effects of MAOIs possibly increased by •clozapine
  Anxiolytics and Hypnotics: avoidance of MAOIs advised by manufacturer of buspirone
- Atomoxetine: after stopping MAOIs do not start •atomoxetine for 2 weeks, also MAOIs should not be started until at least 2 weeks after stopping atomoxetine
  Barbiturates: MAOIs possibly antagonise anticonvulsant effect of barbiturates (convulsive threshold lowered)
  Beta-blockers: enhanced hypotensive effect when MAOIs given with beta-blockers
- Bupropion: avoidance of bupropion for 2 weeks after stopping MAOIs advised by manufacturer of •bupropion
  Calcium-channel Blockers: enhanced hypotensive effect when MAOIs given with calcium-channel blockers
  Clonidine: enhanced hypotensive effect when MAOIs given with clonidine
  Diazoxide: enhanced hypotensive effect when MAOIs given with diazoxide
  Diuretics: enhanced hypotensive effect when MAOIs given with diuretics
- Dopaminergics: avoid concomitant use of non-selective MAOIs with •entacapone; risk of hypertensive crisis when MAOIs given with •levodopa, avoid levodopa for at least two weeks after stopping MAOIs; enhanced hypotensive effect when MAOIs given with selegiline; avoid concomitant use of MAOIs with tolcapone
  Doxapram: MAOIs enhance effects of doxapram
- $5HT_1$ Agonists: risk of CNS toxicity when MAOIs given with •rizatriptan or •sumatriptan (avoid rizatriptan or sumatriptan for 2 weeks after MAOIs); increased risk of CNS toxicity when MAOIs given with •zolmitriptan
- Methyldopa: avoidance of MAOIs advised by manufacturer of •methyldopa
  Moxonidine: enhanced hypotensive effect when MAOIs given with moxonidine
  Muscle Relaxants: phenelzine enhances effects of suxamethonium
  Nicorandil: enhanced hypotensive effect when MAOIs given with nicorandil
  Nitrates: enhanced hypotensive effect when MAOIs given with nitrates

MAOIs *(continued)*

- Sibutramine: increased CNS toxicity when MAOIs given with •sibutramine (manufacturer of sibutramine advises avoid concomitant use), also avoid sibutramine for 2 weeks after stopping MAOIs
- Sympathomimetics: risk of hypertensive crisis when MAOIs given with •dexamfetamine, •dopamine, •dopexamine, •ephedrine, •isometheptene, •methylphenidate, •phenylephrine, •phenylpropanolamine, •pseudoephedrine or •sympathomimetics
- Tetrabenazine: risk of CNS excitation and hypertension when MAOIs given with •tetrabenazine
  Vasodilator Antihypertensives: enhanced hypotensive effect when MAOIs given with hydralazine, minoxidil or nitroprusside

MAOIs, reversible *see* Moclobemide

Maprotiline *see* Antidepressants, Tricyclic (related)

Mebendazole

  Ulcer-healing Drugs: metabolism of mebendazole possibly inhibited by cimetidine (increased plasma concentration)

Meclozine *see* Antihistamines

Medroxyprogesterone *see* Progestogens

Mefenamic Acid *see* NSAIDs

Mefloquine

- Anti-arrhythmics: increased risk of ventricular arrhythmias when mefloquine given with •amiodarone—avoid concomitant use; increased risk of ventricular arrhythmias when mefloquine given with •quinidine
- Antibacterials: increased risk of ventricular arrhythmias when mefloquine given with •moxifloxacin—avoid concomitant use
- Antiepileptics: mefloquine antagonises anticonvulsant effect of •antiepileptics, •carbamazepine and •valproate
- Antimalarials: avoidance of antimalarials advised by manufacturer of •artemether/lumefantrine; increased risk of convulsions when mefloquine given with •chloroquine and hydroxychloroquine; increased risk of convulsions when mefloquine given with •quinine (but should not prevent the use of intravenous quinine in severe cases)
- Antipsychotics: increased risk of ventricular arrhythmias when mefloquine given with •pimozide—avoid concomitant use
  Beta-blockers: increased risk of bradycardia when mefloquine given with beta-blockers
  Calcium-channel Blockers: possible increased risk of bradycardia when mefloquine given with calcium-channel blockers
  Cardiac Glycosides: possible increased risk of bradycardia when mefloquine given with digoxin

Megestrol *see* Progestogens

Meloxicam *see* NSAIDs

Melphalan

  Antibacterials: increased risk of melphalan toxicity when given with nalidixic acid
  Antiepileptics: cytotoxics possibly reduce absorption of phenytoin
- Antipsychotics: avoid concomitant use of cytotoxics with •clozapine (increased risk of agranulocytosis)
- Ciclosporin: increased risk of nephrotoxicity when melphalan given with •ciclosporin

Memantine

- Anaesthetics, General: increased risk of CNS toxicity when memantine given with •ketamine (manufacturer of memantine advises avoid concomitant use)
- Analgesics: increased risk of CNS toxicity when memantine given with •dextromethorphan (manufacturer of memantine advises avoid concomitant use)

Memantine *(continued)*
Antiepileptics: memantine possibly reduces effects of primidone
Antimuscarinics: memantine possibly enhances effects of antimuscarinics
Antipsychotics: memantine possibly reduces effects of antipsychotics
Barbiturates: memantine possibly reduces effects of barbiturates
• Dopaminergics: memantine possibly enhances effects of dopaminergics and selegiline; increased risk of CNS toxicity when memantine given with •amantadine (manufacturer of memantine advises avoid concomitant use)
Muscle Relaxants: memantine possibly modifies effects of baclofen and dantrolene

Mepacrine
Antimalarials: mepacrine increases plasma concentration of primaquine (increased risk of toxicity)

Meprobamate *see* Anxiolytics and Hypnotics
Meptazinol *see* Opioid Analgesics

Mercaptopurine
• Allopurinol: enhanced effects and increased toxicity of mercaptopurine when given with •allopurinol (reduce dose of mercaptopurine)
Aminosalicylates: possible increased risk of leucopenia when mercaptopurine given with aminosalicylates
• Antibacterials: increased risk of haematological toxicity when mercaptopurine given with •sulfamethoxazole (as co-trimoxazole); increased risk of haematological toxicity when mercaptopurine given with •trimethoprim (also with co-trimoxazole)
• Anticoagulants: mercaptopurine possibly reduces anticoagulant effect of •warfarin
Antiepileptics: cytotoxics possibly reduce absorption of phenytoin
• Antipsychotics: avoid concomitant use of cytotoxics with •clozapine (increased risk of agranulocytosis)

Meropenem
Antiepileptics: meropenem reduces plasma concentration of valproate
Oestrogens: broad-spectrum antibacterials possibly reduce contraceptive effect of oestrogens (risk probably small, see p. 407)
Probenecid: excretion of meropenem reduced by probenecid (manufacturers of meropenem advise avoid concomitant use)

Mesalazine *see* Aminosalicylates
Mestranol *see* Oestrogens
Metaraminol *see* Sympathomimetics
Metformin *see* Antidiabetics
Methadone *see* Opioid Analgesics

Methenamine
• Antibacterials: increased risk of crystalluria when methenamine given with •sulphonamides
• Diuretics: effects of methenamine antagonised by •acetazolamide
Oestrogens: broad-spectrum antibacterials possibly reduce contraceptive effect of oestrogens (risk probably small, see p. 407)
Potassium Salts: avoid concomitant use of methenamine with potassium citrate

Methocarbamol *see* Muscle Relaxants

Methotrexate
• Anaesthetics, General: antifolate effect of methotrexate increased by •nitrous oxide—avoid concomitant use
• Analgesics: excretion of methotrexate probably reduced by •NSAIDs (increased risk of toxicity); excretion of methotrexate reduced by •aspirin, •diclofenac, •ibuprofen, •indometacin, •ketoprofen, •meloxicam and •naproxen (increased risk of toxicity)
• Antibacterials: absorption of methotrexate possibly reduced by neomycin; excretion of methotrexate possibly reduced by ciprofloxacin (increased risk of toxicity); increased risk of haematological toxicity when methotrexate given with •sulfamethoxazole (as co-trimoxazole); increased risk of methotrexate toxicity when given with doxycycline, sulphonamides or tetracycline; excretion of methotrexate reduced by penicillins (increased risk of toxicity); increased risk of haematological toxicity when methotrexate given with •trimethoprim (also with co-trimoxazole)
Antiepileptics: antifolate effect of methotrexate increased by phenytoin; cytotoxics possibly reduce absorption of phenytoin
• Antimalarials: antifolate effect of methotrexate increased by •pyrimethamine
• Antipsychotics: avoid concomitant use of cytotoxics with •clozapine (increased risk of agranulocytosis)
• Ciclosporin: risk of toxicity when methotrexate given with •ciclosporin
• Corticosteroids: increased risk of haematological toxicity when methotrexate given with •corticosteroids
• Cytotoxics: increased pulmonary toxicity when methotrexate given with •cisplatin
• Probenecid: excretion of methotrexate reduced by •probenecid (increased risk of toxicity)
• Retinoids: plasma concentration of methotrexate increased by •acitretin (also increased risk of hepatotoxicity)—avoid concomitant use
Theophylline: methotrexate possibly increases plasma concentration of theophylline
Ulcer-healing Drugs: excretion of methotrexate possibly reduced by omeprazole (increased risk of toxicity)

Methoxamine *see* Sympathomimetics

Methyldopa
ACE Inhibitors: enhanced hypotensive effect when methyldopa given with ACE inhibitors
Adrenergic Neurone Blockers: enhanced hypotensive effect when methyldopa given with adrenergic neurone blockers
Alcohol: enhanced hypotensive effect when methyldopa given with alcohol
Aldesleukin: enhanced hypotensive effect when methyldopa given with aldesleukin
Alpha-blockers: enhanced hypotensive effect when methyldopa given with alpha-blockers
Anaesthetics, General: enhanced hypotensive effect when methyldopa given with general anaesthetics
Analgesics: hypotensive effect of methyldopa antagonised by NSAIDs
Angiotensin-II Receptor Antagonists: enhanced hypotensive effect when methyldopa given with angiotensin-II receptor antagonists
• Antidepressants: manufacturer of methyldopa advises avoid concomitant use with •MAOIs
Antipsychotics: enhanced hypotensive effect when methyldopa given with antipsychotics (also increased risk of extrapyramidal effects)
Anxiolytics and Hypnotics: enhanced hypotensive effect when methyldopa given with anxiolytics and hypnotics
Beta-blockers: enhanced hypotensive effect when methyldopa given with beta-blockers
Calcium-channel Blockers: enhanced hypotensive effect when methyldopa given with calcium-channel blockers

Methyldopa *(continued)*

Clonidine: enhanced hypotensive effect when methyldopa given with clonidine

Corticosteroids: hypotensive effect of methyldopa antagonised by corticosteroids

Diazoxide: enhanced hypotensive effect when methyldopa given with diazoxide

Diuretics: enhanced hypotensive effect when methyldopa given with diuretics

Dopaminergics: methyldopa antagonises antiparkinsonian effect of dopaminergics; increased risk of extrapyramidal side-effects when methyldopa given with amantadine; effects of methyldopa possibly enhanced by entacapone; enhanced hypotensive effect when methyldopa given with levodopa

Iron: hypotensive effect of methyldopa antagonised by *oral* iron

• Lithium: neurotoxicity may occur when methyldopa given with •lithium without increased plasma concentration of lithium

Moxisylyte (thymoxamine): enhanced hypotensive effect when methyldopa given with moxisylyte

Moxonidine: enhanced hypotensive effect when methyldopa given with moxonidine

Muscle Relaxants: enhanced hypotensive effect when methyldopa given with baclofen or tizanidine

Nitrates: enhanced hypotensive effect when methyldopa given with nitrates

Oestrogens: hypotensive effect of methyldopa antagonised by oestrogens

Prostaglandins: enhanced hypotensive effect when methyldopa given with alprostadil

• Sympathomimetics, $Beta_2$: acute hypotension reported when methyldopa given with infusion of •salbutamol

Vasodilator Antihypertensives: enhanced hypotensive effect when methyldopa given with hydralazine, minoxidil or nitroprusside

Methylphenidate *see* Sympathomimetics

Methylprednisolone *see* Corticosteroids

Methysergide *see* Ergot Alkaloids

Metipranolol *see* Beta-blockers

Metoclopramide

Analgesics: metoclopramide increases rate of absorption of aspirin (enhanced effect); effects of metoclopramide on gastro-intestinal activity antagonised by opioid analgesics; metoclopramide increases rate of absorption of paracetamol

Antimuscarinics: effects of metoclopramide on gastro-intestinal activity antagonised by antimuscarinics

Antipsychotics: increased risk of extrapyramidal side-effects when metoclopramide given with antipsychotics

Atovaquone: metoclopramide reduces plasma concentration of atovaquone

• Ciclosporin: metoclopramide increases plasma concentration of •ciclosporin

Dopaminergics: increased risk of extrapyramidal side-effects when metoclopramide given with amantadine; metoclopramide antagonises hypoprolactinaemic effects of bromocriptine and cabergoline; metoclopramide antagonises antiparkinsonian effect of pergolide; metoclopramide antagonises antiparkinsonian effect of ropinirole (manufacturers of ropinirole advise avoid concomitant use)

Muscle Relaxants: metoclopramide enhances effects of suxamethonium

Tetrabenazine: increased risk of extrapyramidal side-effects when metoclopramide given with tetrabenazine

Metolazone *see* Diuretics

Metoprolol *see* Beta-blockers

Metronidazole

Alcohol: disulfiram-like reaction when metronidazole given with alcohol

• Anticoagulants: metronidazole enhances anticoagulant effect of •coumarins

• Antiepileptics: metronidazole inhibits metabolism of •phenytoin (increased plasma concentration); metabolism of metronidazole accelerated by primidone (reduced plasma concentration)

Barbiturates: metabolism of metronidazole accelerated by barbiturates (reduced plasma concentration)

Cytotoxics: metronidazole inhibits metabolism of fluorouracil (increased toxicity)

Disulfiram: psychotic reaction reported when metronidazole given with disulfiram

Lithium: metronidazole increases risk of lithium toxicity

Oestrogens: broad-spectrum antibacterials possibly reduce contraceptive effect of oestrogens (risk probably small, see p. 407)

Ulcer-healing Drugs: metabolism of metronidazole inhibited by cimetidine (increased plasma concentration)

Mexiletine

Anaesthetics, Local: increased myocardial depression when anti-arrhythmics given with bupivacaine, levobupivacaine or prilocaine

Analgesics: absorption of mexiletine delayed by opioid analgesics

• Anti-arrhythmics: increased myocardial depression when anti-arrhythmics given with other •anti-arrhythmics

Antibacterials: metabolism of mexiletine accelerated by rifampicin (reduced plasma concentration)

• Antidepressants: metabolism of mexiletine inhibited by •fluvoxamine (increased risk of toxicity)

Antiepileptics: metabolism of mexiletine accelerated by phenytoin (reduced plasma concentration)

• Antihistamines: increased risk of ventricular arrhythmias when mexiletine given with •mizolastine or •terfenadine—avoid concomitant use; increased risk of ventricular arrhythmias when anti-arrhythmics given with •terfenadine

Antimuscarinics: absorption of mexiletine delayed by atropine

• Antipsychotics: increased risk of ventricular arrhythmias when anti-arrhythmics that prolong the QT interval given with •antipsychotics that prolong the QT interval

• Antivirals: plasma concentration of mexiletine possibly increased by •ritonavir (increased risk of toxicity)

• Beta-blockers: increased myocardial depression when anti-arrhythmics given with •beta-blockers

• Diuretics: action of mexiletine antagonised by hypokalaemia caused by •acetazolamide, •loop diuretics or •thiazides and related diuretics

• Dolasetron: increased risk of ventricular arrhythmias when mexiletine given with •dolasetron—avoid concomitant use

$5HT_3$ Antagonists: caution with anti-arrhythmics advised by manufacturer of tropisetron (risk of ventricular arrhythmias)

Theophylline: mexiletine increases plasma concentration of theophylline

Mianserin *see* Antidepressants, Tricyclic (related)

Miconazole *see* Antifungals, Imidazole

Midazolam *see* Anxiolytics and Hypnotics

Mifepristone
Analgesics: manufacturer of mifepristone advises avoid concomitant use with NSAIDs and aspirin
Corticosteroids: mifepristone may reduce effect of corticosteroids (including inhaled corticosteroids) for 3–4 days

Milrinone *see* Phosphodiesterase Inhibitors

Minocycline *see* Tetracyclines

Minoxidil *see* Vasodilator Antihypertensives

Mirtazapine
• Alcohol: increased sedative effect when mirtazapine given with •alcohol
Anticoagulants: mirtazapine enhances anticoagulant effect of warfarin
• Antidepressants: mirtazapine should not be started until 2 weeks after stopping •MAOIs, also MAOIs should not be started until at least 2 weeks after stopping mirtazapine; after stopping mirtazapine do not start •moclobemide for at least 1 week
Antiepileptics: plasma concentration of mirtazapine reduced by carbamazepine and phenytoin
Antifungals: plasma concentration of mirtazapine increased by ketoconazole
• Antimalarials: avoidance of antidepressants advised by manufacturer of •artemether/lumefantrine
Anxiolytics and Hypnotics: increased sedative effect when mirtazapine given with anxiolytics and hypnotics
• Sibutramine: increased risk of CNS toxicity when mirtazapine given with •sibutramine (manufacturer of sibutramine advises avoid concomitant use)
Ulcer-healing Drugs: plasma concentration of mirtazapine increased by cimetidine

Mivacurium *see* Muscle Relaxants

Mizolastine *see* Antihistamines

Moclobemide
• Analgesics: possible CNS excitation or depression (hypertension or hypotension) when moclobemide given with •dextromethorphan or •pethidine—avoid concomitant use; possible CNS excitation or depression (hypertension or hypotension) when moclobemide given with •opioid analgesics
• Antidepressants: moclobemide should not be started for at least 1 week after stopping •MAOIs, •SSRI-related antidepressants, •citalopram, •fluvoxamine, •mirtazapine, •paroxetine, •tricyclic-related antidepressants or •tricyclics; increased risk of CNS toxicity when moclobemide given with •escitalopram, preferably avoid concomitant use; moclobemide should not be started until 5 weeks after stopping •fluoxetine; moclobemide should not be started until 2 weeks after stopping •sertraline; possible increased serotonergic effects when moclobemide given with •duloxetine
• Antimalarials: avoidance of antidepressants advised by manufacturer of •artemether/lumefantrine
• Bupropion: avoidance of moclobemide advised by manufacturer of •bupropion
• Dopaminergics: caution with moclobemide advised by manufacturer of entacapone; increased risk of side-effects when moclobemide given with levodopa; avoid concomitant use of moclobemide with •selegiline
• $5HT_1$ Agonists: risk of CNS toxicity when moclobemide given with •rizatriptan or •sumatriptan (avoid rizatriptan or sumatriptan for 2 weeks after moclobemide); risk of CNS toxicity when moclobemide given with •zolmitriptan (reduce dose of zolmitriptan)
• Sibutramine: increased CNS toxicity when moclobemide given with •sibutramine (manufacturer of sibutramine advises avoid concomitant use), also

Moclobemide
• Sibutramine *(continued)*
avoid sibutramine for 2 weeks after stopping moclobemide
• Sympathomimetics: risk of hypertensive crisis when moclobemide given with •dexamfetamine, •dopamine, •dopexamine, •ephedrine, •isometheptene, •methylphenidate, •phenylephrine, •phenylpropanolamine, •pseudoephedrine or •sympathomimetics
Ulcer-healing Drugs: plasma concentration of moclobemide increased by cimetidine (halve dose of moclobemide)

Modafinil
Antiepileptics: modafinil possibly increases plasma concentration of phenytoin
• Ciclosporin: modafinil reduces plasma concentration of •ciclosporin
• Oestrogens: modafinil accelerates metabolism of •oestrogens (reduced contraceptive effect—see p. 407)

Moexipril *see* ACE Inhibitors

Mometasone *see* Corticosteroids

Monobactams *see* Aztreonam

Montelukast *see* Leukotriene Antagonists

Morphine *see* Opioid Analgesics

Moxifloxacin *see* Quinolones

Moxisylyte (thymoxamine)
ACE Inhibitors: enhanced hypotensive effect when moxisylyte given with ACE inhibitors
Adrenergic Neurone Blockers: enhanced hypotensive effect when moxisylyte given with adrenergic neurone blockers
• Alpha-blockers: possible severe postural hypotension when moxisylyte given with •alpha-blockers
Angiotensin-II Receptor Antagonists: enhanced hypotensive effect when moxisylyte given with angiotensin-II receptor antagonists
• Beta-blockers: possible severe postural hypotension when moxisylyte given with •beta-blockers
Calcium-channel Blockers: enhanced hypotensive effect when moxisylyte given with calcium-channel blockers
Clonidine: enhanced hypotensive effect when moxisylyte given with clonidine
Diazoxide: enhanced hypotensive effect when moxisylyte given with diazoxide
Diuretics: enhanced hypotensive effect when moxisylyte given with diuretics
Methyldopa: enhanced hypotensive effect when moxisylyte given with methyldopa
Moxonidine: enhanced hypotensive effect when moxisylyte given with moxonidine
Nitrates: enhanced hypotensive effect when moxisylyte given with nitrates
Vasodilator Antihypertensives: enhanced hypotensive effect when moxisylyte given with hydralazine, minoxidil or nitroprusside

Moxonidine
ACE Inhibitors: enhanced hypotensive effect when moxonidine given with ACE inhibitors
Adrenergic Neurone Blockers: enhanced hypotensive effect when moxonidine given with adrenergic neurone blockers
Alcohol: enhanced hypotensive effect when moxonidine given with alcohol
Aldesleukin: enhanced hypotensive effect when moxonidine given with aldesleukin
Alpha-blockers: enhanced hypotensive effect when moxonidine given with alpha-blockers
Anaesthetics, General: enhanced hypotensive effect when moxonidine given with general anaesthetics

Moxonidine *(continued)*

Analgesics: hypotensive effect of moxonidine antagonised by NSAIDs

Angiotensin-II Receptor Antagonists: enhanced hypotensive effect when moxonidine given with angiotensin-II receptor antagonists

Antidepressants: enhanced hypotensive effect when moxonidine given with MAOIs

Antipsychotics: enhanced hypotensive effect when moxonidine given with phenothiazines

Anxiolytics and Hypnotics: enhanced hypotensive effect when moxonidine given with anxiolytics and hypnotics; sedative effects possibly increased when moxonidine given with benzodiazepines

Beta-blockers: enhanced hypotensive effect when moxonidine given with beta-blockers

Calcium-channel Blockers: enhanced hypotensive effect when moxonidine given with calcium-channel blockers

Clonidine: enhanced hypotensive effect when moxonidine given with clonidine

Corticosteroids: hypotensive effect of moxonidine antagonised by corticosteroids

Diazoxide: enhanced hypotensive effect when moxonidine given with diazoxide

Diuretics: enhanced hypotensive effect when moxonidine given with diuretics

Dopaminergics: enhanced hypotensive effect when moxonidine given with levodopa

Methyldopa: enhanced hypotensive effect when moxonidine given with methyldopa

Moxisylyte (thymoxamine): enhanced hypotensive effect when moxonidine given with moxisylyte

Muscle Relaxants: enhanced hypotensive effect when moxonidine given with baclofen or tizanidine

Nitrates: enhanced hypotensive effect when moxonidine given with nitrates

Oestrogens: hypotensive effect of moxonidine antagonised by oestrogens

Prostaglandins: enhanced hypotensive effect when moxonidine given with alprostadil

Vasodilator Antihypertensives: enhanced hypotensive effect when moxonidine given with hydralazine, minoxidil or nitroprusside

Muscle Relaxants

ACE Inhibitors: enhanced hypotensive effect when baclofen or tizanidine given with ACE inhibitors

Adrenergic Neurone Blockers: enhanced hypotensive effect when baclofen or tizanidine given with adrenergic neurone blockers

Alcohol: increased sedative effect when baclofen, methocarbamol or tizanidine given with alcohol

Alpha-blockers: enhanced hypotensive effect when baclofen or tizanidine given with alpha-blockers

Anaesthetics, General: effects of non-depolarising muscle relaxants and suxamethonium enhanced by volatile liquid general anaesthetics

Analgesics: excretion of baclofen possibly reduced by NSAIDs (increased risk of toxicity); excretion of baclofen reduced by ibuprofen (increased risk of toxicity)

Angiotensin-II Receptor Antagonists: enhanced hypotensive effect when baclofen or tizanidine given with angiotensin-II receptor antagonists

• Anti-arrhythmics: neuromuscular blockade enhanced and prolonged when suxamethonium given with lidocaine (lignocaine); effects of muscle relaxants enhanced by •procainamide and •quinidine

• Antibacterials: effects of non-depolarising muscle relaxants and suxamethonium enhanced by piperacillin; effects of non-depolarising muscle relaxants and suxamethonium enhanced by

Muscle Relaxants

• Antibacterials *(continued)*

•aminoglycosides; effects of non-depolarising muscle relaxants and suxamethonium enhanced by •clindamycin; effects of non-depolarising muscle relaxants and suxamethonium enhanced by •polymyxins; effects of suxamethonium enhanced by •vancomycin

Antidepressants: effects of suxamethonium enhanced by phenelzine; muscle relaxant effect of baclofen enhanced by tricyclics

Antiepileptics: muscle relaxant effect of non-depolarising muscle relaxants antagonised by carbamazepine and phenytoin (accelerated recovery from neuromuscular blockade)

Antimalarials: effects of suxamethonium possibly enhanced by quinine

Antipsychotics: effects of suxamethonium possibly enhanced by promazine

Anxiolytics and Hypnotics: increased sedative effect when baclofen or tizanidine given with anxiolytics and hypnotics

Beta-blockers: enhanced hypotensive effect when baclofen given with beta-blockers; possible enhanced hypotensive effect and bradycardia when tizanidine given with beta-blockers; effects of muscle relaxants enhanced by propranolol

Calcium-channel Blockers: enhanced hypotensive effect when baclofen or tizanidine given with calcium-channel blockers; effects of non-depolarising muscle relaxants enhanced by nifedipine and verapamil; risk of arrhythmias when intravenous dantrolene given with diltiazem; hypotension, myocardial depression, and hyperkalaemia when intravenous dantrolene given with verapamil; effects of suxamethonium enhanced by verapamil

Cardiac Glycosides: possible increased risk of bradycardia when tizanidine given with cardiac glycosides; risk of ventricular arrhythmias when suxamethonium given with cardiac glycosides

Clonidine: enhanced hypotensive effect when baclofen or tizanidine given with clonidine

Cytotoxics: effects of suxamethonium enhanced by cyclophosphamide and thiotepa

Diazoxide: enhanced hypotensive effect when baclofen or tizanidine given with diazoxide

Diuretics: enhanced hypotensive effect when baclofen or tizanidine given with diuretics

Dopaminergics: possible agitation, confusion and hallucinations when baclofen given with levodopa

Lithium: effects of muscle relaxants enhanced by lithium; baclofen possibly aggravates hyperkinesis caused by lithium

Magnesium (parenteral): effects of non-depolarising muscle relaxants and suxamethonium enhanced by parenteral magnesium

Memantine: effects of baclofen and dantrolene possibly modified by memantine

Methyldopa: enhanced hypotensive effect when baclofen or tizanidine given with methyldopa

Metoclopramide: effects of suxamethonium enhanced by metoclopramide

Moxonidine: enhanced hypotensive effect when baclofen or tizanidine given with moxonidine

Nitrates: enhanced hypotensive effect when baclofen or tizanidine given with nitrates

Parasympathomimetics: effects of suxamethonium possibly enhanced by donepezil; effects of non-depolarising muscle relaxants possibly antagonised by donepezil; effects of suxamethonium enhanced by edrophonium, galantamine, neostigmine, pyridostigmine and rivastigmine; effects of non-depolarising muscle relaxants antagonised

Muscle Relaxants

Parasympathomimetics *(continued)*
by edrophonium, neostigmine, pyridostigmine and rivastigmine

Sympathomimetics, $Beta_2$: effects of suxamethonium enhanced by bambuterol

Vasodilator Antihypertensives: enhanced hypotensive effect when baclofen or tizanidine given with hydralazine; enhanced hypotensive effect when baclofen or tizanidine given with minoxidil; enhanced hypotensive effect when baclofen or tizanidine given with nitroprusside

Muscle Relaxants, depolarising *see* Muscle Relaxants

Muscle Relaxants, non-depolarising *see* Muscle Relaxants

Mycophenolate Mofetil

Antacids: absorption of mycophenolate mofetil reduced by antacids

Antiepileptics: cytotoxics possibly reduce absorption of phenytoin

• Antipsychotics: avoid concomitant use of cytotoxics with •clozapine (increased risk of agranulocytosis)

Antivirals: mycophenolate mofetil increases plasma concentration of aciclovir, also plasma concentration of inactive metabolite of mycophenolate mofetil increased; mycophenolate mofetil possibly increases plasma concentration of ganciclovir, also plasma concentration of inactive metabolite of mycophenolate mofetil possibly increased

Lipid-regulating Drugs: absorption of mycophenolate mofetil reduced by colestyramine

Nabilone

Alcohol: increased sedative effect when nabilone given with alcohol

Anxiolytics and Hypnotics: increased sedative effect when nabilone given with anxiolytics and hypnotics

Nabumetone *see* NSAIDs

Nadolol *see* Beta-blockers

Nalidixic Acid *see* Quinolones

Nandrolone *see* Anabolic Steroids

Naproxen *see* NSAIDs

Naratriptan *see* $5HT_1$ Agonists

Nateglinide *see* Antidiabetics

Nebivolol *see* Beta-blockers

Nefopam

• Antidepressants: manufacturer of nefopam advises avoid concomitant use with •MAOIs; side-effects possibly increased when nefopam given with tricyclics

Antimuscarinics: increased risk of antimuscarinic side-effects when nefopam given with antimuscarinics

Nelfinavir

Analgesics: nelfinavir reduces plasma concentration of methadone

• Anti-arrhythmics: increased risk of ventricular arrhythmias when nelfinavir given with •amiodarone or •quinidine—avoid concomitant use

• Antibacterials: nelfinavir increases plasma concentration of •rifabutin (halve dose of rifabutin); plasma concentration of nelfinavir significantly reduced by •rifampicin—avoid concomitant use

• Antidepressants: plasma concentration of nelfinavir reduced by •St John's wort—avoid concomitant use

• Antiepileptics: plasma concentration of nelfinavir possibly reduced by carbamazepine and •primidone; nelfinavir reduces plasma concentration of phenytoin

Nelfinavir *(continued)*

• Antihistamines: increased risk of ventricular arrhythmias when nelfinavir given with •terfenadine—avoid concomitant use

Antimuscarinics: nelfinavir increases plasma concentration of solifenacin; avoidance of nelfinavir advised by manufacturer of tolterodine

• Antipsychotics: nelfinavir possibly inhibits metabolism of •aripiprazole (reduce dose of aripiprazole); nelfinavir possibly increases plasma concentration of •pimozide (increased risk of ventricular arrhythmias—avoid concomitant use); nelfinavir increases plasma concentration of •sertindole (increased risk of ventricular arrhythmias—avoid concomitant use)

Antivirals: combination of nelfinavir with indinavir, ritonavir or saquinavir may increase plasma concentration of either drug (or both); nelfinavir reduces plasma concentration of lopinavir, also plasma concentration of active metabolite of nelfinavir increased

• Anxiolytics and Hypnotics: increased risk of prolonged sedation when nelfinavir given with •midazolam—avoid concomitant use

• Barbiturates: plasma concentration of nelfinavir possibly reduced by •barbiturates

• Ciclosporin: nelfinavir possibly increases plasma concentration of •ciclosporin

• Cilostazol: nelfinavir possibly increases plasma concentration of •cilostazol—avoid concomitant use

Cytotoxics: nelfinavir increases plasma concentration of paclitaxel

• Diuretics: nelfinavir increases plasma concentration of •eplerenone—avoid concomitant use

• Ergot Alkaloids: increased risk of ergotism when nelfinavir given with •ergotamine and methysergide—avoid concomitant use

• $5HT_1$ Agonists: nelfinavir increases plasma concentration of •eletriptan (risk of toxicity)—avoid concomitant use

• Lipid-regulating Drugs: possible increased risk of myopathy when nelfinavir given with atorvastatin; increased risk of myopathy when nelfinavir given with •simvastatin (avoid concomitant use)

• Oestrogens: nelfinavir accelerates metabolism of •oestrogens (reduced contraceptive effect—see p. 407)

Progestogens: nelfinavir possibly reduces contraceptive effect of progestogens

Sildenafil: nelfinavir possibly increases plasma concentration of sildenafil— reduce initial dose of sildenafil

• Tacrolimus: nelfinavir possibly increases plasma concentration of •tacrolimus

Neomycin *see* Aminoglycosides

Neostigmine *see* Parasympathomimetics

Netilmicin *see* Aminoglycosides

Nevirapine

Analgesics: nevirapine possibly reduces plasma concentration of methadone

• Antibacterials: plasma concentration of nevirapine reduced by •rifampicin—avoid concomitant use

• Anticoagulants: nevirapine may enhance or reduce anticoagulant effect of •warfarin

• Antidepressants: plasma concentration of nevirapine reduced by •St John's wort—avoid concomitant use

• Antifungals: nevirapine reduces plasma concentration of •ketoconazole—avoid concomitant use; plasma concentration of nevirapine increased by •fluconazole; nevirapine possibly reduces plasma concentration of caspofungin—consider increasing dose of caspofungin

Nevirapine *(continued)*

- Antipsychotics: nevirapine possibly reduces plasma concentration of •aripiprazole—increase dose of aripiprazole
- Antivirals: nevirapine possibly reduces plasma concentration of amprenavir and lopinavir; nevirapine possibly reduces plasma concentration of •atazanavir—avoid concomitant use; nevirapine reduces plasma concentration of efavirenz and indinavir
- Oestrogens: nevirapine accelerates metabolism of •oestrogens (reduced contraceptive effect—see p. 407)
- Progestogens: nevirapine accelerates metabolism of •progestogens (reduced contraceptive effect—see p. 407)

Nicardipine *see* Calcium-channel Blockers

Nicorandil

Alcohol: hypotensive effect of nicorandil possibly enhanced by alcohol

Antidepressants: enhanced hypotensive effect when nicorandil given with MAOIs; hypotensive effect of nicorandil possibly enhanced by tricyclics

- Sildenafil: hypotensive effect of nicorandil significantly enhanced by •sildenafil (avoid concomitant use)
- Tadalafil: hypotensive effect of nicorandil significantly enhanced by •tadalafil (avoid concomitant use)
- Vardenafil: possible increased hypotensive effect when nicorandil given with •vardenafil—avoid concomitant use

Vasodilator Antihypertensives: possible enhanced hypotensive effect when nicorandil given with hydralazine, minoxidil or nitroprusside

Nicotinic Acid

Note. Interactions apply to lipid-regulating doses of nicotinic acid

- Lipid-regulating Drugs: increased risk of myopathy when nicotinic acid given with •statins (applies to lipid regulating doses of nicotinic acid)

Nifedipine *see* Calcium-channel Blockers

Nimodipine *see* Calcium-channel Blockers

Nisoldipine *see* Calcium-channel Blockers

Nitrates

ACE Inhibitors: enhanced hypotensive effect when nitrates given with ACE inhibitors

Adrenergic Neurone Blockers: enhanced hypotensive effect when nitrates given with adrenergic neurone blockers

Alcohol: enhanced hypotensive effect when nitrates given with alcohol

Aldesleukin: enhanced hypotensive effect when nitrates given with aldesleukin

Alpha-blockers: enhanced hypotensive effect when nitrates given with alpha-blockers

Anaesthetics, General: enhanced hypotensive effect when nitrates given with general anaesthetics

Analgesics: hypotensive effect of nitrates antagonised by NSAIDs

Angiotensin-II Receptor Antagonists: enhanced hypotensive effect when nitrates given with angiotensin-II receptor antagonists

Anti-arrhythmics: effects of sublingual tablets of nitrates reduced by disopyramide (failure to dissolve under tongue owing to dry mouth)

- Anticoagulants: infusion of glyceryl trinitrate reduces anticoagulant effect of •heparins

Antidepressants: enhanced hypotensive effect when nitrates given with MAOIs; effects of sublingual tablets of nitrates possibly reduced by tricyclic-related antidepressants (failure to dissolve under tongue owing to dry mouth); effects of sublingual

Nitrates

Antidepressants *(continued)*
tablets of nitrates reduced by tricyclics (failure to dissolve under tongue owing to dry mouth)

Antimuscarinics: effects of sublingual tablets of nitrates possibly reduced by antimuscarinics (failure to dissolve under tongue owing to dry mouth)

Antipsychotics: enhanced hypotensive effect when nitrates given with phenothiazines

Anxiolytics and Hypnotics: enhanced hypotensive effect when nitrates given with anxiolytics and hypnotics

Beta-blockers: enhanced hypotensive effect when nitrates given with beta-blockers

Calcium-channel Blockers: enhanced hypotensive effect when nitrates given with calcium-channel blockers

Clonidine: enhanced hypotensive effect when nitrates given with clonidine

Corticosteroids: hypotensive effect of nitrates antagonised by corticosteroids

Diazoxide: enhanced hypotensive effect when nitrates given with diazoxide

Diuretics: enhanced hypotensive effect when nitrates given with diuretics

Dopaminergics: hypotensive effect of nitrates enhanced by sublingual apomorphine; enhanced hypotensive effect when nitrates given with levodopa

Methyldopa: enhanced hypotensive effect when nitrates given with methyldopa

Moxisylyte (thymoxamine): enhanced hypotensive effect when nitrates given with moxisylyte

Moxonidine: enhanced hypotensive effect when nitrates given with moxonidine

Muscle Relaxants: enhanced hypotensive effect when nitrates given with baclofen or tizanidine

Oestrogens: hypotensive effect of nitrates antagonised by oestrogens

Prostaglandins: enhanced hypotensive effect when nitrates given with alprostadil

- Sildenafil: hypotensive effect of nitrates significantly enhanced by •sildenafil (avoid concomitant use)
- Tadalafil: hypotensive effect of nitrates significantly enhanced by •tadalafil (avoid concomitant use)
- Vardenafil: possible increased hypotensive effect when nitrates given with •vardenafil—avoid concomitant use

Vasodilator Antihypertensives: enhanced hypotensive effect when nitrates given with hydralazine, minoxidil or nitroprusside

Nitrazepam *see* Anxiolytics and Hypnotics

Nitrofurantoin

Antacids: absorption of nitrofurantoin reduced by oral magnesium salts (as magnesium trisilicate)

Oestrogens: broad-spectrum antibacterials possibly reduce contraceptive effect of oestrogens (risk probably small, see p. 407)

Probenecid: excretion of nitrofurantoin reduced by probenecid (increased risk of side-effects)

Sulfinpyrazone: excretion of nitrofurantoin reduced by sulfinpyrazone (increased risk of toxicity)

Nitroimidazoles *see* Metronidazole and Tinidazole

Nitroprusside *see* Vasodilator Antihypertensives

Nitrous Oxide *see* Anaesthetics, General

Nizatidine *see* Histamine H_2-antagonists

Noradrenaline (norepinephrine) *see* Sympathomimetics

Norelgestromin *see* Progestogens

Norepinephrine (noradrenaline) *see* Sympathomimetics

Norethisterone *see* Progestogens

Norfloxacin *see* Quinolones
Norgestimate *see* Progestogens
Norgestrel *see* Progestogens
Nortriptyline *see* Antidepressants, Tricyclic

NSAIDs

Note. See also Aspirin. Interactions do not generally apply to topical NSAIDs

ACE Inhibitors: increased risk of renal impairment when NSAIDs given with ACE inhibitors, also hypotensive effect antagonised; increased risk of hyperkalaemia when ketorolac given with ACE inhibitors

Adrenergic Neurone Blockers: NSAIDs antagonise hypotensive effect of adrenergic neurone blockers

Alpha-blockers: NSAIDs antagonise hypotensive effect of alpha-blockers

• Analgesics: avoid concomitant use of NSAIDs with •NSAIDs or •aspirin (increased side-effects); avoid concomitant use of NSAIDs with •ketorolac (increased side-effects and haemorrhage); ibuprofen possibly reduces antiplatelet effect of aspirin

Angiotensin-II Receptor Antagonists: increased risk of renal impairment when NSAIDs given with angiotensin-II receptor antagonists, also hypotensive effect antagonised; increased risk of hyperkalaemia when ketorolac given with angiotensin-II receptor antagonists

Antacids: absorption of diflunisal reduced by antacids

• Antibacterials: indometacin possibly increases plasma concentration of amikacin and gentamicin in neonates; plasma concentration of etoricoxib reduced by rifampicin; possible increased risk of convulsions when NSAIDs given with •quinolones

• Anticoagulants: celecoxib, diflunisal, etodolac, etoricoxib, flurbiprofen, ibuprofen, mefenamic acid, meloxicam, parecoxib, piroxicam and sulindac possibly enhance anticoagulant effect of •coumarins; NSAIDs possibly enhance anticoagulant effect of •coumarins and •phenindione; increased risk of bleeding when ketorolac given with •coumarins (avoid concomitant use); diclofenac possibly enhances anticoagulant effect of •coumarins, also increased risk of haemorrhage with intravenous diclofenac (avoid concomitant use); possible increased risk of bleeding when NSAIDs given with heparins; increased risk of haemorrhage when ketorolac given with •heparins (avoid concomitant use, including low-dose heparin); increased risk of haemorrhage when intravenous diclofenac given with •heparins (avoid concomitant use, including low-dose heparin); ketorolac enhances anticoagulant effect of •phenindione (increased risk of haemorrhage—avoid concomitant use); diclofenac enhances anticoagulant effect of •phenindione, also increased risk of haemorrhage with intravenous diclofenac (avoid concomitant use)

• Antidepressants: increased risk of bleeding when NSAIDs given with •SSRIs or •venlafaxine

• Antidiabetics: NSAIDs possibly enhance effects of •sulphonylureas

• Antiepileptics: NSAIDs possibly enhance effects of •phenytoin

Antifungals: plasma concentration of parecoxib increased by fluconazole (reduce dose of parecoxib); plasma concentration of celecoxib increased by fluconazole (halve dose of celecoxib)

Antipsychotics: possible severe drowsiness when indometacin given with haloperidol

• Antivirals: plasma concentration of piroxicam increased by •ritonavir (risk of toxicity)—avoid concomitant use; plasma concentration of NSAIDs possibly increased by ritonavir; increased risk of haematological toxicity when NSAIDs given with zidovudine

Beta-blockers: NSAIDs antagonise hypotensive effect of beta-blockers

Bisphosphonates: indometacin increases bioavailability of tiludronic acid

Calcium-channel Blockers: NSAIDs antagonise hypotensive effect of calcium-channel blockers

Cardiac Glycosides: NSAIDs possibly increase plasma concentration of cardiac glycosides, also possible exacerbation of heart failure and reduction of renal function

• Ciclosporin: increased risk of nephrotoxicity when NSAIDs given with •ciclosporin; plasma concentration of diclofenac increased by •ciclosporin (halve dose of diclofenac)

Clonidine: NSAIDs antagonise hypotensive effect of clonidine

Clopidogrel: increased risk of bleeding when NSAIDs given with clopidogrel

Corticosteroids: increased risk of gastro-intestinal bleeding and ulceration when NSAIDs given with corticosteroids

• Cytotoxics: NSAIDs probably reduce excretion of •methotrexate (increased risk of toxicity); diclofenac, ibuprofen, indometacin, ketoprofen, meloxicam and naproxen reduce excretion of •methotrexate (increased risk of toxicity)

Desmopressin: indometacin enhances effects of desmopressin

Diazoxide: NSAIDs antagonise hypotensive effect of diazoxide

• Diuretics: risk of nephrotoxicity of NSAIDs increased by diuretics, also antagonism of diuretic effect; indometacin and ketorolac antagonise effects of diuretics; occasional reports of reduced renal function when indometacin given with •triamterene—avoid concomitant use; possibly increased risk of hyperkalaemia when NSAIDs given with potassium-sparing diuretics and aldosterone antagonists; increased risk of hyperkalaemia when indometacin given with potassium-sparing diuretics and aldosterone antagonists

Iloprost: increased risk of bleeding when NSAIDs given with iloprost

Lipid-regulating Drugs: excretion of meloxicam increased by colestyramine

• Lithium: NSAIDs probably reduce excretion of •lithium (increased risk of toxicity); diclofenac, ibuprofen, indometacin, mefenamic acid, naproxen, parecoxib and piroxicam reduce excretion of •lithium (increased risk of toxicity); ketorolac reduces excretion of •lithium (increased risk of toxicity)—avoid concomitant use

Methyldopa: NSAIDs antagonise hypotensive effect of methyldopa

Mifepristone: avoidance of NSAIDs advised by manufacturer of mifepristone

Moxonidine: NSAIDs antagonise hypotensive effect of moxonidine

Muscle Relaxants: NSAIDs possibly reduce excretion of baclofen (increased risk of toxicity); ibuprofen reduces excretion of baclofen (increased risk of toxicity)

Nitrates: NSAIDs antagonise hypotensive effect of nitrates

Oestrogens: etoricoxib increases plasma concentration of ethinylestradiol

Penicillamine: possible increased risk of nephrotoxicity when NSAIDs given with penicillamine

NSAIDs *(continued)*

- Pentoxifylline (oxpentifylline): possible increased risk of bleeding when NSAIDs given with pentoxifylline (oxpentifylline); increased risk of bleeding when ketorolac given with •pentoxifylline (oxpentifylline) (avoid concomitant use)
- Probenecid: excretion of indometacin, ketoprofen and naproxen reduced by •probenecid (increased plasma concentration); excretion of ketorolac reduced by •probenecid (increased plasma concentration)—avoid concomitant use

Progestogens: risk of hyperkalaemia when NSAIDs given with drospirenone (monitor serum potassium during first cycle)

Sibutramine: increased risk of bleeding when NSAIDs given with sibutramine

- Tacrolimus: possible increased risk of nephrotoxicity when NSAIDs given with tacrolimus; increased risk of nephrotoxicity when ibuprofen given with •tacrolimus

Vasodilator Antihypertensives: NSAIDs antagonise hypotensive effect of hydralazine, minoxidil and nitroprusside

Octreotide

Antidiabetics: octreotide possibly reduces requirements for insulin, metformin, repaglinide and sulphonylureas

- Ciclosporin: octreotide reduces plasma concentration of •ciclosporin

Dopaminergics: octreotide increases plasma concentration of bromocriptine

Ulcer-healing Drugs: octreotide possibly delays absorption of cimetidine

Oestrogens

Note. Interactions of combined oral contraceptives may also apply to combined contraceptive patches; in case of hormone replacement therapy low dose unlikely to induce interactions

ACE Inhibitors: oestrogens antagonise hypotensive effect of ACE inhibitors

Adrenergic Neurone Blockers: oestrogens antagonise hypotensive effect of adrenergic neurone blockers

Alpha-blockers: oestrogens antagonise hypotensive effect of alpha-blockers

Analgesics: plasma concentration of ethinylestradiol increased by etoricoxib

Angiotensin-II Receptor Antagonists: oestrogens antagonise hypotensive effect of angiotensin-II receptor antagonists

- Antibacterials: contraceptive effect of oestrogens possibly reduced by broad-spectrum antibacterials (risk probably small, see p. 407); metabolism of oestrogens accelerated by •rifamycins (reduced contraceptive effect—see p. 407)
- Anticoagulants: oestrogens antagonise anticoagulant effect of •coumarins and •phenindione
- Antidepressants: contraceptive effect of oestrogens reduced by •St John's wort (avoid concomitant use); oestrogens antagonise antidepressant effect of tricyclics (but side-effects of tricyclics possibly increased due to increased plasma concentration)

Antidiabetics: oestrogens antagonise hypoglycaemic effect of antidiabetics

- Antiepileptics: metabolism of oestrogens accelerated by •carbamazepine, •oxcarbazepine, •phenytoin, •primidone and •topiramate (reduced contraceptive effect—see p. 407)
- Antifungals: anecdotal reports of contraceptive failure when oestrogens given with fluconazole, imidazoles, itraconazole or ketoconazole; metabolism of oestrogens accelerated by •griseofulvin (reduced contraceptive effect—see p. 407); occasional reports of breakthrough bleeding when oestrogens (used for contraception) given with terbinafine

Oestrogens

- Antivirals: contraceptive effect of oestrogens possibly reduced by amprenavir and efavirenz; plasma concentration of ethinylestradiol increased by •atazanavir—avoid concomitant use; metabolism of oestrogens accelerated by •nelfinavir, •nevirapine and •ritonavir (reduced contraceptive effect—see p. 407)
- Aprepitant: possible contraceptive failure of hormonal contraceptives containing oestrogens when given with •aprepitant (alternative contraception recommended)
- Barbiturates: metabolism of oestrogens accelerated by •barbiturates (reduced contraceptive effect—see p. 407)

Beta-blockers: oestrogens antagonise hypotensive effect of beta-blockers

Bile Acids: elimination of cholesterol in bile increased when oestrogens given with bile acids

- Bosentan: possible contraceptive failure of hormonal contraceptives containing oestrogens when given with •bosentan (alternative contraception recommended)

Calcium-channel Blockers: oestrogens antagonise hypotensive effect of calcium-channel blockers

Ciclosporin: oestrogens possibly increase plasma concentration of ciclosporin

Clonidine: oestrogens antagonise hypotensive effect of clonidine

Corticosteroids: oral contraceptives containing oestrogens increase plasma concentration of corticosteroids

Diazoxide: oestrogens antagonise hypotensive effect of diazoxide

Diuretics: oestrogens antagonise diuretic effect of diuretics

Dopaminergics: oestrogens increase plasma concentration of ropinirole

Lipid-regulating Drugs: plasma concentration of ethinylestradiol increased by rosuvastatin

Methyldopa: oestrogens antagonise hypotensive effect of methyldopa

- Modafinil: metabolism of oestrogens accelerated by •modafinil (reduced contraceptive effect—see p. 407)

Moxonidine: oestrogens antagonise hypotensive effect of moxonidine

Nitrates: oestrogens antagonise hypotensive effect of nitrates

Somatropin: oestrogens (when used as oral replacement therapy) may increase dose requirements of somatropin

Tacrolimus: contraceptive effect of oestrogens possibly reduced by tacrolimus

Theophylline: oestrogens reduce excretion of theophylline (increased plasma concentration)

Vasodilator Antihypertensives: oestrogens antagonise hypotensive effect of hydralazine, minoxidil and nitroprusside

Oestrogens, conjugated *see* Oestrogens

Ofloxacin *see* Quinolones

Olanzapine *see* Antipsychotics

Olmesartan *see* Angiotensin-II Receptor Antagonists

Olsalazine *see* Aminosalicylates

Omeprazole *see* Proton Pump Inhibitors

Ondansetron

Analgesics: ondansetron possibly antagonises effects of tramadol

Ondansetron *(continued)*

Antibacterials: metabolism of ondansetron accelerated by rifampicin (reduced effect)

Antiepileptics: metabolism of ondansetron accelerated by carbamazepine and phenytoin (reduced effect)

Opioid Analgesics

Alcohol: enhanced hypotensive and sedative effects when opioid analgesics given with alcohol

Anti-arrhythmics: opioid analgesics delay absorption of mexiletine

Antibacterials: plasma concentration of alfentanil increased by erythromycin; avoidance of premedication with opioid analgesics advised by manufacturer of ciprofloxacin (reduced plasma concentration of ciprofloxacin) when ciprofloxacin used for surgical prophylaxis; metabolism of methadone accelerated by rifampicin (reduced effect)

• Anticoagulants: tramadol enhances anticoagulant effect of •coumarins; dextropropoxyphene possibly enhances anticoagulant effect of •coumarins

• Antidepressants: plasma concentration of methadone possibly increased by fluvoxamine; possible increased serotonergic effects when pethidine or tramadol given with duloxetine; CNS excitation or depression (hypertension or hypotension) when pethidine given with •MAOIs—avoid concomitant use and for 2 weeks after stopping MAOIs; possible CNS excitation or depression (hypertension or hypotension) when opioid analgesics given with •MAOIs—avoid concomitant use and for 2 weeks after stopping MAOIs; possible CNS excitation or depression (hypertension or hypotension) when opioid analgesics given with •moclobemide; possible CNS excitation or depression (hypertension or hypotension) when dextromethorphan or pethidine given with •moclobemide—avoid concomitant use; increased risk of CNS toxicity when tramadol given with •SSRIs or •tricyclics; sedative effects possibly increased when opioid analgesics given with tricyclics

• Antiepileptics: effects of tramadol reduced by carbamazepine; plasma concentration of methadone reduced by carbamazepine; dextropropoxyphene enhances effects of •carbamazepine; metabolism of methadone accelerated by phenytoin (reduced effect and risk of withdrawal effects)

• Antifungals: metabolism of alfentanil inhibited by fluconazole and ketoconazole (risk of prolonged or delayed respiratory depression); metabolism of buprenorphine inhibited by •ketoconazole (reduce dose of buprenorphine); metabolism of alfentanil possibly inhibited by itraconazole; plasma concentration of methadone increased by •voriconazole (consider reducing dose of methadone)

Antipsychotics: enhanced hypotensive and sedative effects when opioid analgesics given with antipsychotics; increased risk of convulsions when tramadol given with antipsychotics

• Antivirals: plasma concentration of methadone possibly reduced by abacavir and nevirapine; plasma concentration of methadone reduced by amprenavir, efavirenz, nelfinavir and ritonavir; plasma concentration of pethidine reduced by •ritonavir, but plasma concentration of toxic pethidine metabolite increased (avoid concomitant use); plasma concentration of fentanyl increased by •ritonavir; plasma concentration of dextropropoxyphene increased by •ritonavir (risk of toxicity)—avoid concomitant use; plasma concentration of opioid analgesics (except methadone) possibly increased by •ritonavir; methadone

Opioid Analgesics

• Antivirals *(continued)*

possibly increases plasma concentration of zidovudine

Anxiolytics and Hypnotics: increased sedative effect when opioid analgesics given with anxiolytics and hypnotics

Beta-blockers: morphine possibly increases plasma concentration of esmolol

Calcium-channel Blockers: metabolism of alfentanil inhibited by diltiazem (risk of prolonged or delayed respiratory depression)

Domperidone: opioid analgesics antagonise effects of domperidone on gastro-intestinal activity

• Dopaminergics: hyperpyrexia and CNS toxicity reported when pethidine given with •selegiline (avoid concomitant use); caution with tramadol advised by manufacturer of selegiline

$5HT_3$ Antagonists: effects of tramadol possibly antagonised by ondansetron

• Memantine: increased risk of CNS toxicity when dextromethorphan given with •memantine (manufacturer of memantine advises avoid concomitant use)

Metoclopramide: opioid analgesics antagonise effects of metoclopramide on gastro-intestinal activity

Ulcer-healing Drugs: metabolism of opioid analgesics inhibited by cimetidine (increased plasma concentration)

Orciprenaline *see* Sympathomimetics

Orlistat

Anti-arrhythmics: orlistat possibly reduces plasma concentration of amiodarone

Anticoagulants: manufacturer of orlistat recommends monitoring anticoagulant effect of coumarins

Antidiabetics: manufacturer of orlistat advises avoid concomitant use with acarbose

• Ciclosporin: orlistat possibly reduces absorption of •ciclosporin

Orphenadrine *see* Antimuscarinics

Oxaliplatin *see* Platinum Compounds

Oxandrolone *see* Anabolic Steroids

Oxazepam *see* Anxiolytics and Hypnotics

Oxcarbazepine

• Antidepressants: manufacturer of oxcarbazepine advises avoid concomitant use with •MAOIs; anticonvulsant effect of antiepileptics possibly antagonised by MAOIs and •tricyclic-related antidepressants (convulsive threshold lowered); anticonvulsant effect of antiepileptics antagonised by •SSRIs and •tricyclics (convulsive threshold lowered)

Antiepileptics: oxcarbazepine sometimes reduces plasma concentration of carbamazepine (but concentration of an active metabolite of carbamazepine may be increased), also plasma concentration of an active metabolite of oxcarbazepine often reduced; oxcarbazepine increases plasma concentration of phenytoin, also plasma concentration of an active metabolite of oxcarbazepine reduced; oxcarbazepine increases plasma concentration of an active metabolite of primidone, also plasma concentration of an active metabolite of oxcarbazepine reduced; plasma concentration of an active metabolite of oxcarbazepine sometimes reduced by valproate

• Antimalarials: possible increased risk of convulsions when antiepileptics given with chloroquine and hydroxychloroquine; anticonvulsant effect of antiepileptics antagonised by •mefloquine

Oxcarbazepine *(continued)*
- • Antipsychotics: anticonvulsant effect of oxcarbazepine antagonised by •antipsychotics (convulsive threshold lowered)
- Barbiturates: oxcarbazepine increases plasma concentration of phenobarbital, also plasma concentration of an active metabolite of oxcarbazepine reduced
- • Oestrogens: oxcarbazepine accelerates metabolism of •oestrogens (reduced contraceptive effect—see p. 407)
- • Progestogens: oxcarbazepine accelerates metabolism of •progestogens (reduced contraceptive effect—see p. 407)

Oxprenolol *see* Beta-blockers
Oxybutynin *see* Antimuscarinics
Oxycodone *see* Opioid Analgesics
Oxymetazoline *see* Sympathomimetics
Oxytetracycline *see* Tetracyclines

Oxytocin
- Anaesthetics, General: oxytocic effect possibly reduced, also enhanced hypotensive effect and risk of arrhythmias when oxytocin given with volatile liquid general anaesthetics
- Prostaglandins: uterotonic effect of oxytocin potentiated by prostaglandins
- Sympathomimetics: risk of hypertension when oxytocin given with vasoconstrictor sympathomimetics (due to enhanced vasopressor effect)

Paclitaxel
- Antidiabetics: paclitaxel possibly inhibits metabolism of rosiglitazone
- Antiepileptics: cytotoxics possibly reduce absorption of phenytoin
- • Antipsychotics: avoid concomitant use of cytotoxics with •clozapine (increased risk of agranulocytosis)
- Antivirals: plasma concentration of paclitaxel increased by nelfinavir and ritonavir

Pancreatin
- Antidiabetics: pancreatin antagonises hypoglycaemic effect of acarbose

Pancuronium *see* Muscle Relaxants
Pantoprazole *see* Proton Pump Inhibitors
Papaveretum *see* Opioid Analgesics

Paracetamol
- Anticoagulants: prolonged regular use of paracetamol possibly enhances anticoagulant effect of coumarins
- Cytotoxics: paracetamol possibly inhibits metabolism of *intravenous* busulfan (manufacturer of *intravenous* busulfan advises caution within 72 hours of paracetamol)
- Lipid-regulating Drugs: absorption of paracetamol reduced by colestyramine
- Metoclopramide: rate of absorption of paracetamol increased by metoclopramide

Paraldehyde
- • Alcohol: increased sedative effect when paraldehyde given with •alcohol
- • Disulfiram: risk of toxicity when paraldehyde given with •disulfiram

Parasympathomimetics
- Anti-arrhythmics: effects of neostigmine and pyridostigmine antagonised by procainamide; effects of neostigmine and pyridostigmine possibly antagonised by propafenone; effects of neostigmine and pyridostigmine antagonised by quinidine
- • Antibacterials: plasma concentration of galantamine increased by erythromycin; effects of neostigmine and pyridostigmine antagonised by •aminoglycosides; effects of neostigmine and pyridostigmine antagonised by clindamycin; effects of neostigmine and pyridostigmine antagonised by •polymyxins
- Antidepressants: plasma concentration of galantamine increased by paroxetine
- Antifungals: plasma concentration of galantamine increased by ketoconazole
- Antimalarials: effects of neostigmine and pyridostigmine may be diminished because of potential for chloroquine and hydroxychloroquine to increase symptoms of myasthenia gravis
- Antimuscarinics: effects of parasympathomimetics antagonised by antimuscarinics
- Beta-blockers: increased risk of arrhythmias when pilocarpine given with beta-blockers; effects of neostigmine and pyridostigmine antagonised by propranolol
- Lithium: effects of neostigmine and pyridostigmine antagonised by lithium
- Muscle Relaxants: donepezil possibly enhances effects of suxamethonium; edrophonium, galantamine, neostigmine, pyridostigmine and rivastigmine enhance effects of suxamethonium; donepezil possibly antagonises effects of non-depolarising muscle relaxants ; edrophonium, neostigmine, pyridostigmine and rivastigmine antagonise effects of non-depolarising muscle relaxants

Parecoxib *see* NSAIDs
Paroxetine *see* Antidepressants, SSRI
Pegfilgrastim *see* Filgrastim
Peginterferon Alfa *see* Interferons

Penicillamine
- Analgesics: possible increased risk of nephrotoxicity when penicillamine given with NSAIDs
- Antacids: absorption of penicillamine reduced by antacids
- • Antipsychotics: avoid concomitant use of penicillamine with •clozapine (increased risk of agranulocytosis)
- Cardiac Glycosides: penicillamine possibly reduces plasma concentration of digoxin
- Iron: absorption of penicillamine reduced by *oral* iron
- Zinc: penicillamine reduces absorption of zinc, also absorption of penicillamine reduced by zinc

Penicillins
- Allopurinol: increased risk of rash when amoxicillin or ampicillin given with allopurinol
- Antibacterials: absorption of phenoxymethylpenicillin reduced by neomycin
- Anticoagulants: common experience in anticoagulant clinics is that INR can be altered by a course of broad-spectrum penicillins such as ampicillin, although studies have failed to demonstrate an interaction with coumarins or phenindione
- Cytotoxics: penicillins reduce excretion of methotrexate (increased risk of toxicity)
- Muscle Relaxants: piperacillin enhances effects of non-depolarising muscle relaxants and suxamethonium
- Oestrogens: broad-spectrum antibacterials possibly reduce contraceptive effect of oestrogens (risk probably small, see p. 407)
- Probenecid: excretion of penicillins reduced by probenecid (increased plasma concentration)

Pentamidine Isetionate
- • Anti-arrhythmics: increased risk of ventricular arrhythmias when pentamidine isetionate given with •amiodarone—avoid concomitant use

Pentamidine Isetionate *(continued)*
- Antibacterials: increased risk of ventricular arrhythmias when pentamidine isetionate given with •moxifloxacin—avoid concomitant use

Antifungals: possible increased risk of nephrotoxicity when pentamidine isetionate given with amphotericin
- Antihistamines: increased risk of ventricular arrhythmias when pentamidine isetionate given with •terfenadine—avoid concomitant use
- Antipsychotics: increased risk of ventricular arrhythmias when pentamidine isetionate given with •amisulpride—avoid concomitant use

Pentazocine *see* Opioid Analgesics

Pentostatin

Antiepileptics: cytotoxics possibly reduce absorption of phenytoin
- Antipsychotics: avoid concomitant use of cytotoxics with •clozapine (increased risk of agranulocytosis)
- Cytotoxics: increased toxicity when pentostatin given with high-dose •cyclophosphamide—avoid concomitant use; increased pulmonary toxicity when pentostatin given with •fludarabine (unacceptably high incidence of fatalities)

Pentoxifylline (oxpentifylline)
- Analgesics: possible increased risk of bleeding when pentoxifylline (oxpentifylline) given with NSAIDs; increased risk of bleeding when pentoxifylline (oxpentifylline) given with •ketorolac (avoid concomitant use)

Theophylline: pentoxifylline (oxpentifylline) increases plasma concentration of theophylline

Pergolide

Antipsychotics: effects of pergolide antagonised by antipsychotics

Memantine: effects of dopaminergics possibly enhanced by memantine

Methyldopa: antiparkinsonian effect of dopaminergics antagonised by methyldopa

Metoclopramide: antiparkinsonian effect of pergolide antagonised by metoclopramide

Pericyazine *see* Antipsychotics

Perindopril *see* ACE Inhibitors

Perphenazine *see* Antipsychotics

Pethidine *see* Opioid Analgesics

Phenazocine *see* Opioid Analgesics

Phenelzine *see* MAOIs

Phenindione

Note. Change in patient's clinical condition particularly associated with liver disease, intercurrent illness, or drug administration, necessitates more frequent testing. Major changes in diet (especially involving salads and vegetables) and in alcohol consumption may also affect anticoagulant control
- Alcohol: anticoagulant control with phenindione may be affected by major changes in consumption of •alcohol
- Anabolic Steroids: anticoagulant effect of phenindione enhanced by •anabolic steroids
- Analgesics: anticoagulant effect of phenindione possibly enhanced by •NSAIDs; anticoagulant effect of phenindione enhanced by •diclofenac, also increased risk of haemorrhage with intravenous diclofenac (avoid concomitant use); anticoagulant effect of phenindione enhanced by •ketorolac (increased risk of haemorrhage—avoid concomitant use); increased risk of bleeding when phenindione given with •aspirin (due to antiplatelet effect)
- Anti-arrhythmics: metabolism of phenindione inhibited by •amiodarone (enhanced anticoagulant effect)
- Antibacterials: experience in anticoagulant clinics suggests that INR possibly altered when phenindione is given with •neomycin (given for local action on gut); anticoagulant effect of phenindione possibly enhanced by levofloxacin and •tetracyclines; studies have failed to demonstrate an interaction with phenindione, but common experience in anticoagulant clinics is that INR can be altered by a course of broad-spectrum penicillins such as ampicillin
- Antivirals: anticoagulant effect of phenindione possibly enhanced by •ritonavir
- Clopidogrel: anticoagulant effect of phenindione enhanced due to antiplatelet action of •clopidogrel
- Dipyridamole: anticoagulant effect of phenindione enhanced due to antiplatelet action of •dipyridamole
- Enteral Foods: anticoagulant effect of phenindione antagonised by vitamin K (present in some •enteral feeds)
- Hormone Antagonists: metabolism of phenindione accelerated by •aminoglutethimide (reduced anticoagulant effect)

Iloprost: increased risk of bleeding when phenindione given with iloprost
- Lipid-regulating Drugs: anticoagulant effect of phenindione may be enhanced or reduced by •colestyramine; anticoagulant effect of phenindione possibly enhanced by •rosuvastatin; anticoagulant effect of phenindione enhanced by •fibrates
- Oestrogens: anticoagulant effect of phenindione antagonised by •oestrogens
- Progestogens: anticoagulant effect of phenindione antagonised by •progestogens

Sibutramine: increased risk of bleeding when anticoagulants given with sibutramine
- Testolactone: anticoagulant effect of phenindione enhanced by •testolactone
- Testosterone: anticoagulant effect of phenindione enhanced by •testosterone
- Thyroid Hormones: anticoagulant effect of phenindione enhanced by •thyroid hormones
- Vitamins: anticoagulant effect of phenindione antagonised by •vitamin K

Phenobarbital *see* Barbiturates

Phenoperidine *see* Opioid Analgesics

Phenothiazines *see* Antipsychotics

Phenoxybenzamine *see* Alpha-blockers

Phenoxymethylpenicillin *see* Penicillins

Phentolamine *see* Alpha-blockers

Phenylephrine *see* Sympathomimetics

Phenylpropanolamine *see* Sympathomimetics

Phenytoin
- Analgesics: effects of phenytoin possibly enhanced by •NSAIDs; phenytoin accelerates metabolism of methadone (reduced effect and risk of withdrawal effects); effects of phenytoin enhanced by aspirin

Antacids: absorption of phenytoin reduced by antacids
- Anti-arrhythmics: metabolism of phenytoin inhibited by •amiodarone (increased plasma concentration); phenytoin reduces plasma concentration of disopyramide; phenytoin accelerates metabolism of mexiletine and •quinidine (reduced plasma concentration)
- Antibacterials: metabolism of phenytoin inhibited by clarithromycin, •isoniazid and •metronidazole (increased plasma concentration); plasma concentration of phenytoin increased or decreased by ciprofloxacin; phenytoin accelerates metabolism of doxycycline (reduced plasma concentration); plasma concentration of phenytoin increased by

Phenytoin

- Antibacterials *(continued)*
  •chloramphenicol (increased risk of toxicity); metabolism of phenytoin accelerated by •rifamycins (reduced plasma concentration); plasma concentration of phenytoin possibly increased by sulphonamides; phenytoin reduces plasma concentration of •telithromycin (avoid during and for 2 weeks after phenytoin); plasma concentration of phenytoin increased by •trimethoprim (also increased antifolate effect)
- Anticoagulants: phenytoin accelerates metabolism of •coumarins (possibility of reduced anticoagulant effect, but enhancement also reported)
- Antidepressants: plasma concentration of phenytoin increased by •fluoxetine and •fluvoxamine; phenytoin reduces plasma concentration of •mianserin, mirtazapine and paroxetine; anticonvulsant effect of antiepileptics possibly antagonised by MAOIs and •tricyclic-related antidepressants (convulsive threshold lowered); anticonvulsant effect of antiepileptics antagonised by •SSRIs and •tricyclics (convulsive threshold lowered); plasma concentration of phenytoin reduced by •St John's wort—avoid concomitant use; phenytoin possibly reduces plasma concentration of •tricyclics

Antidiabetics: plasma concentration of phenytoin transiently increased by tolbutamide (possibility of toxicity)

- Antiepileptics: plasma concentration of both drugs often reduced when phenytoin given with carbamazepine, also plasma concentration of phenytoin may be increased; plasma concentration of phenytoin possibly increased by •ethosuximide, also plasma concentration of ethosuximide possibly reduced; phenytoin reduces plasma concentration of lamotrigine, tiagabine and zonisamide; plasma concentration of phenytoin increased by oxcarbazepine, also plasma concentration of an active metabolite of oxcarbazepine reduced; phenytoin possibly reduces plasma concentration of primidone (but concentration of an active metabolite increased), plasma concentration of phenytoin often reduced but may be increased; plasma concentration of phenytoin increased by •topiramate (also plasma concentration of topiramate reduced); plasma concentration of phenytoin increased or possibly reduced when given with valproate, also plasma concentration of valproate reduced; plasma concentration of phenytoin reduced by vigabatrin
- Antifungals: phenytoin reduces plasma concentration of •ketoconazole; anticonvulsant effect of phenytoin enhanced by •miconazole (plasma concentration of phenytoin increased); plasma concentration of phenytoin increased by •fluconazole (consider reducing dose of phenytoin); phenytoin reduces plasma concentration of •itraconazole—avoid concomitant use; plasma concentration of phenytoin increased by •voriconazole, also phenytoin reduces plasma concentration of voriconazole (increase dose of voriconazole and also monitor for phenytoin toxicity); phenytoin possibly reduces plasma concentration of caspofungin—consider increasing dose of caspofungin
- Antimalarials: possible increased risk of convulsions when antiepileptics given with chloroquine and hydroxychloroquine; anticonvulsant effect of antiepileptics antagonised by •mefloquine; anticonvulsant effect of phenytoin antagonised by •pyrimethamine, also increased antifolate effect

Phenytoin *(continued)*

- Antipsychotics: anticonvulsant effect of phenytoin antagonised by •antipsychotics (convulsive threshold lowered); phenytoin possibly reduces plasma concentration of •aripiprazole—increase dose of aripiprazole; phenytoin accelerates metabolism of clozapine, quetiapine and sertindole (reduced plasma concentration)

Antivirals: phenytoin possibly reduces plasma concentration of abacavir, amprenavir, indinavir, lopinavir and saquinavir; plasma concentration of phenytoin reduced by nelfinavir; plasma concentration of phenytoin increased or decreased by zidovudine

Anxiolytics and Hypnotics: phenytoin often reduces plasma concentration of clonazepam; plasma concentration of phenytoin increased or decreased by diazepam; plasma concentration of phenytoin possibly increased or decreased by benzodiazepines

Aprepitant: phenytoin possibly reduces plasma concentration of aprepitant

Barbiturates: phenytoin often increases plasma concentration of phenobarbital, plasma concentration of phenytoin often reduced but may be increased

Bupropion: phenytoin reduces plasma concentration of bupropion

- Calcium-channel Blockers: phenytoin reduces effects of felodipine, isradipine and verapamil; phenytoin probably reduces effects of dihydropyridines, nicardipine and •nifedipine; phenytoin reduces plasma concentration of nisoldipine; plasma concentration of phenytoin increased by •diltiazem but also effect of diltiazem reduced

Cardiac Glycosides: phenytoin accelerates metabolism of digitoxin (reduced effect); phenytoin possibly reduces plasma concentration of digoxin

- Ciclosporin: phenytoin accelerates metabolism of •ciclosporin (reduced plasma concentration)
- Corticosteroids: phenytoin accelerates metabolism of •corticosteroids (reduced effect)
- Cytotoxics: metabolism of phenytoin possibly inhibited by fluorouracil (increased risk of toxicity); phenytoin increases antifolate effect of methotrexate; absorption of phenytoin possibly reduced by cytotoxics; phenytoin possibly reduces plasma concentration of etoposide; phenytoin reduces plasma concentration of •imatinib—avoid concomitant use

Diazoxide: plasma concentration of phenytoin reduced by diazoxide, also effect of diazoxide may be reduced

- Disulfiram: metabolism of phenytoin inhibited by •disulfiram (increased risk of toxicity)
- Diuretics: phenytoin reduces plasma concentration of •eplerenone—avoid concomitant use; increased risk of osteomalacia when phenytoin given with carbonic anhydrase inhibitors

Dopaminergics: phenytoin possibly reduces effects of levodopa

Enteral Foods: absorption of phenytoin possibly reduced by enteral feeds

Folates: plasma concentration of phenytoin possibly reduced by folates

Hormone Antagonists: phenytoin accelerates metabolism of gestrinone (reduced plasma concentration); phenytoin possibly accelerates metabolism of toremifene

$5HT_3$ Antagonists: phenytoin accelerates metabolism of ondansetron (reduced effect)

Leflunomide: plasma concentration of phenytoin possibly increased by leflunomide

Phenytoin *(continued)*
Levamisole: plasma concentration of phenytoin possibly increased by levamisole
Lipid-regulating Drugs: combination of phenytoin with fluvastatin may increase plasma concentration of either drug (or both)
Lithium: neurotoxicity may occur when phenytoin given with lithium without increased plasma concentration of lithium
Modafinil: plasma concentration of phenytoin possibly increased by modafinil
Muscle Relaxants: phenytoin antagonises muscle relaxant effect of non-depolarising muscle relaxants (accelerated recovery from neuromuscular blockade)
• Oestrogens: phenytoin accelerates metabolism of •oestrogens (reduced contraceptive effect—see p. 407)
• Progestogens: phenytoin accelerates metabolism of •progestogens (reduced contraceptive effect—see p. 407)
• Sulfinpyrazone: plasma concentration of phenytoin increased by •sulfinpyrazone
Sympathomimetics: plasma concentration of phenytoin increased by methylphenidate
• Theophylline: plasma concentration of both drugs reduced when phenytoin given with •theophylline
Thyroid Hormones: phenytoin accelerates metabolism of thyroid hormones (may increase requirements in hypothyroidism), also plasma concentration of phenytoin possibly increased
Tibolone: phenytoin accelerates metabolism of tibolone
• Ulcer-healing Drugs: metabolism of phenytoin inhibited by •cimetidine (increased plasma concentration); effects of phenytoin enhanced by •esomeprazole; effects of phenytoin possibly enhanced by omeprazole; absorption of phenytoin reduced by •sucralfate
Vaccines: effects of phenytoin enhanced by influenza vaccine
Vitamins: phenytoin possibly increases requirements for vitamin D

Phosphodiesterase Inhibitors
• Anagrelide: avoidance of enoximone and milrinone advised by manufacturer of •anagrelide

Physostigmine *see* Parasympathomimetics
Pilocarpine *see* Parasympathomimetics
Pimozide *see* Antipsychotics
Pindolol *see* Beta-blockers
Pioglitazone *see* Antidiabetics
Piperacillin *see* Penicillins
Pipotiazine *see* Antipsychotics
Piroxicam *see* NSAIDs
Pivmecillinam *see* Penicillins

Pizotifen
Adrenergic Neurone Blockers: pizotifen antagonises hypotensive effect of adrenergic neurone blockers

Platinum Compounds
• Antibacterials: increased risk of nephrotoxicity and possibly of ototoxicity when platinum compounds given with •aminoglycosides or •polymyxins; increased risk of nephrotoxicity and ototoxicity when platinum compounds given with capreomycin; increased risk of nephrotoxicity and possibly of ototoxicity when cisplatin given with vancomycin
Antiepileptics: cytotoxics possibly reduce absorption of phenytoin
• Antipsychotics: avoid concomitant use of cytotoxics with •clozapine (increased risk of agranulocytosis)
• Cytotoxics: increased pulmonary toxicity when cisplatin given with •bleomycin and •methotrexate

Platinum Compounds *(continued)*
Diuretics: increased risk of nephrotoxicity and ototoxicity when platinum compounds given with diuretics

Polymyxin B *see* Polymyxins

Polymyxins
Antibacterials: increased risk of nephrotoxicity when colistin or polymyxins given with aminoglycosides; increased risk of nephrotoxicity when colistin or polymyxins given with capreomycin; increased risk of nephrotoxicity and ototoxicity when colistin given with teicoplanin or vancomycin; increased risk of nephrotoxicity when polymyxins given with vancomycin
Antifungals: increased risk of nephrotoxicity when polymyxins given with amphotericin
• Ciclosporin: increased risk of nephrotoxicity when polymyxins given with •ciclosporin
• Cytotoxics: increased risk of nephrotoxicity and possibly of ototoxicity when polymyxins given with •platinum compounds
• Diuretics: increased risk of otoxicity when polymyxins given with •loop diuretics
• Muscle Relaxants: polymyxins enhance effects of •non-depolarising muscle relaxants and •suxamethonium
Oestrogens: broad-spectrum antibacterials possibly reduce contraceptive effect of oestrogens (risk probably small, see p. 407)
• Parasympathomimetics: polymyxins antagonise effects of •neostigmine and •pyridostigmine

Potassium Aminobenzoate
Antibacterials: potassium aminobenzoate inhibits effects of sulphonamides

Potassium Bicarbonate *see* Potassium Salts
Potassium Chloride *see* Potassium Salts
Potassium Citrate *see* Potassium Salts

Potassium Salts
Note. Includes salt substitutes
• ACE Inhibitors: increased risk of severe hyperkalaemia when potassium salts given with •ACE inhibitors
• Angiotensin-II Receptor Antagonists: increased risk of hyperkalaemia when potassium salts given with •angiotensin-II receptor antagonists
Antibacterials: avoid concomitant use of potassium citrate with methenamine
• Ciclosporin: increased risk of hyperkalaemia when potassium salts given with •ciclosporin
• Diuretics: increased risk of hyperkalaemia when potassium salts given with •potassium-sparing diuretics and aldosterone antagonists
• Tacrolimus: increased risk of hyperkalaemia when potassium salts given with •tacrolimus

Pramipexole
Antipsychotics: manufacturer of pramipexole advises avoid concomitant use of antipsychotics (antagonism of effect)
Memantine: effects of dopaminergics possibly enhanced by memantine
Methyldopa: antiparkinsonian effect of dopaminergics antagonised by methyldopa
Ulcer-healing Drugs: excretion of pramipexole reduced by cimetidine (increased plasma concentration)

Pravastatin *see* Statins
Prazosin *see* Alpha-blockers
Prednisolone *see* Corticosteroids

Prilocaine
Anti-arrhythmics: increased myocardial depression when prilocaine given with anti-arrhythmics
Antibacterials: increased risk of methaemoglobinaemia when prilocaine given with sulphonamides

Primaquine

- • Antimalarials: avoidance of antimalarials advised by manufacturer of •artemether/lumefantrine
- Mepacrine: plasma concentration of primaquine increased by mepacrine (increased risk of toxicity)

Primidone

- Alcohol: increased sedative effect when primidone given with alcohol
- Anti-arrhythmics: primidone accelerates metabolism of disopyramide and quinidine (reduced plasma concentration)
- • Antibacterials: primidone accelerates metabolism of •chloramphenicol, doxycycline and metronidazole (reduced plasma concentration); primidone reduces plasma concentration of •telithromycin (avoid during and for 2 weeks after primidone)
- • Anticoagulants: primidone accelerates metabolism of •coumarins (reduced anticoagulant effect)
- • Antidepressants: primidone reduces plasma concentration of paroxetine; primidone accelerates metabolism of •mianserin (reduced plasma concentration); anticonvulsant effect of antiepileptics possibly antagonised by MAOIs and •tricyclic-related antidepressants (convulsive threshold lowered); anticonvulsant effect of antiepileptics antagonised by •SSRIs and •tricyclics (convulsive threshold lowered); plasma concentration of active metabolite of primidone reduced by •St John's wort—avoid concomitant use; anticonvulsant effect of primidone antagonised by •tricyclics (convulsive threshold lowered), also metabolism of tricyclics possibly accelerated (reduced plasma concentration)
- • Antiepileptics: primidone often reduces plasma concentration of carbamazepine, also plasma concentration of primidone sometimes reduced (but concentration of an active metabolite of primidone often increased); primidone possibly reduces plasma concentration of ethosuximide; primidone reduces plasma concentration of lamotrigine and tiagabine; plasma concentration of an active metabolite of primidone increased by oxcarbazepine, also plasma concentration of an active metabolite of oxcarbazepine reduced; plasma concentration of primidone possibly reduced by phenytoin (but concentration of an active metabolite increased), plasma concentration of phenytoin often reduced but may be increased; plasma concentration of primidone possibly increased by •valproate (plasma concentration of active metabolite of primidone increased), also plasma concentration of valproate reduced; plasma concentration of primidone possibly reduced by vigabatrin
- • Antifungals: primidone possibly reduces plasma concentration of •voriconazole—avoid concomitant use; primidone reduces absorption of griseofulvin (reduced effect)
- • Antimalarials: possible increased risk of convulsions when antiepileptics given with chloroquine and hydroxychloroquine; anticonvulsant effect of antiepileptics antagonised by •mefloquine
- • Antipsychotics: anticonvulsant effect of primidone antagonised by •antipsychotics (convulsive threshold lowered); primidone accelerates metabolism of haloperidol (reduced plasma concentration); primidone possibly reduces plasma concentration of •aripiprazole—increase dose of aripiprazole
- • Antivirals: primidone possibly reduces plasma concentration of •indinavir, •lopinavir, •nelfinavir and •saquinavir

Primidone *(continued)*

- Anxiolytics and Hypnotics: primidone often reduces plasma concentration of clonazepam
- Barbiturates: increased sedative effect when primidone given with barbiturates
- • Calcium-channel Blockers: primidone reduces effects of •felodipine and •isradipine; primidone probably reduces effects of •dihydropyridines, •diltiazem and •verapamil
- Cardiac Glycosides: primidone accelerates metabolism of digitoxin (reduced effect)
- • Ciclosporin: primidone accelerates metabolism of •ciclosporin (reduced effect)
- • Corticosteroids: primidone accelerates metabolism of •corticosteroids (reduced effect)
- Diuretics: plasma concentration of primidone possibly reduced by acetazolamide; increased risk of osteomalacia when primidone given with carbonic anhydrase inhibitors
- Folates: plasma concentration of primidone possibly reduced by folates
- Hormone Antagonists: primidone accelerates metabolism of gestrinone and toremifene (reduced plasma concentration)
- $5HT_3$ Antagonists: primidone reduces plasma concentration of tropisetron
- Leukotriene Antagonists: primidone reduces plasma concentration of montelukast
- Memantine: effects of primidone possibly reduced by memantine
- • Oestrogens: primidone accelerates metabolism of •oestrogens (reduced contraceptive effect—see p. 407)
- • Progestogens: primidone accelerates metabolism of •progestogens (reduced contraceptive effect—see p. 407)
- Sympathomimetics: plasma concentration of primidone possibly increased by methylphenidate
- Theophylline: primidone accelerates metabolism of theophylline (reduced effect)
- Thyroid Hormones: primidone accelerates metabolism of thyroid hormones (may increase requirements for thyroid hormones in hypothyroidism)
- Tibolone: primidone accelerates metabolism of tibolone (reduced plasma concentration)
- Vitamins: primidone possibly increases requirements for vitamin D

Probenecid

- ACE Inhibitors: probenecid reduces excretion of captopril
- • Analgesics: probenecid reduces excretion of •indometacin, •ketoprofen and •naproxen (increased plasma concentration); probenecid reduces excretion of •ketorolac (increased plasma concentration)—avoid concomitant use; effects of probenecid antagonised by aspirin
- Antibacterials: probenecid reduces excretion of meropenem (manufacturers of meropenem advise avoid concomitant use); probenecid reduces excretion of cephalosporins, ciprofloxacin, nalidixic acid, norfloxacin and penicillins (increased plasma concentration); probenecid reduces excretion of dapsone and nitrofurantoin (increased risk of side-effects); effects of probenecid antagonised by pyrazinamide
- Antidiabetics: probenecid possibly enhances hypoglycaemic effect of chlorpropamide
- Antivirals: probenecid reduces excretion of aciclovir (increased plasma concentration); probenecid possibly reduces excretion of famciclovir and zalcitabine (increased plasma concentration); probenecid reduces excretion of ganciclovir and zidovudine (increased plasma concentration and risk of toxicity)

Probenecid *(continued)*
- Cytotoxics: probenecid reduces excretion of •methotrexate (increased risk of toxicity)
  Sodium Benzoate: probenecid possibly reduces excretion of conjugate formed by sodium benzoate
  Sodium Phenylbutyrate: probenecid possibly reduces excretion of conjugate formed by sodium phenylbutyrate

Procainamide
  ACE Inhibitors: increased risk of toxicity when procainamide given with captopril especially in renal impairment
  Anaesthetics, Local: increased myocardial depression when anti-arrhythmics given with bupivacaine, levobupivacaine or prilocaine
- Anti-arrhythmics: increased myocardial depression when anti-arrhythmics given with other •anti-arrhythmics; plasma concentration of procainamide increased by •amiodarone (increased risk of ventricular arrhythmias—avoid concomitant use)
- Antibacterials: increased risk of ventricular arrhythmias when procainamide given with •moxifloxacin—avoid concomitant use; plasma concentration of procainamide increased by trimethoprim
- Antidepressants: increased risk of ventricular arrhythmias when procainamide given with •tricyclics
- Antihistamines: increased risk of ventricular arrhythmias when procainamide given with •mizolastine or •terfenadine—avoid concomitant use; increased risk of ventricular arrhythmias when anti-arrhythmics given with •terfenadine
- Antimalarials: avoidance of procainamide advised by manufacturer of •artemether/lumefantrine (risk of ventricular arrhythmias)
- Antipsychotics: increased risk of ventricular arrhythmias when anti-arrhythmics that prolong the QT interval given with •antipsychotics that prolong the QT interval; increased risk of ventricular arrhythmias when procainamide given with •amisulpride, •pimozide or •sertindole—avoid concomitant use; increased risk of ventricular arrhythmias when procainamide given with •phenothiazines
- Beta-blockers: increased myocardial depression when anti-arrhythmics given with •beta-blockers; increased risk of ventricular arrhythmias when procainamide given with •sotalol—avoid concomitant use
- Dolasetron: increased risk of ventricular arrhythmias when procainamide given with •dolasetron—avoid concomitant use
  $5HT_3$ Antagonists: caution with anti-arrhythmics advised by manufacturer of tropisetron (risk of ventricular arrhythmias)
- Muscle Relaxants: procainamide enhances effects of •muscle relaxants
  Parasympathomimetics: procainamide antagonises effects of neostigmine and pyridostigmine
- Ulcer-healing Drugs: plasma concentration of procainamide increased by •cimetidine

Procaine
  Laronidase: procaine possibly inhibits effects of laronidase (manufacturer of laronidase advises avoid concomitant use)

Procarbazine
  Alcohol: disulfiram-like reaction when procarbazine given with alcohol
  Antiepileptics: cytotoxics possibly reduce absorption of phenytoin
- Antipsychotics: avoid concomitant use of cytotoxics with •clozapine (increased risk of agranulocytosis)

Prochlorperazine *see* Antipsychotics
Procyclidine *see* Antimuscarinics

Progesterone *see* Progestogens
Progestogens
  Note. Interactions of combined oral contraceptives may also apply to combined contraceptive patches
  ACE Inhibitors: risk of hyperkalaemia when drospirenone given with ACE inhibitors (monitor serum potassium during first cycle)
  Analgesics: risk of hyperkalaemia when drospirenone given with NSAIDs (monitor serum potassium during first cycle)
  Angiotensin-II Receptor Antagonists: risk of hyperkalaemia when drospirenone given with angiotensin-II receptor antagonists (monitor serum potassium during first cycle)
- Antibacterials: metabolism of progestogens accelerated by •rifamycins (reduced contraceptive effect—see p. 407)
- Anticoagulants: progestogens antagonise anticoagulant effect of •coumarins and •phenindione
- Antidepressants: contraceptive effect of progestogens reduced by •St John's wort (avoid concomitant use)
  Antidiabetics: progestogens antagonise hypoglycaemic effect of antidiabetics
- Antiepileptics: metabolism of progestogens accelerated by •carbamazepine, •oxcarbazepine, •phenytoin, •primidone and •topiramate (reduced contraceptive effect—see p. 407)
- Antifungals: metabolism of progestogens accelerated by •griseofulvin (reduced contraceptive effect—see p. 407); occasional reports of breakthrough bleeding when progestogens (used for contraception) given with terbinafine
- Antivirals: contraceptive effect of progestogens possibly reduced by amprenavir and nelfinavir; metabolism of progestogens accelerated by •nevirapine (reduced contraceptive effect—see p. 407)
- Aprepitant: possible contraceptive failure of hormonal contraceptives containing progestogens when given with •aprepitant (alternative contraception recommended)
- Barbiturates: metabolism of progestogens accelerated by •barbiturates (reduced contraceptive effect—see p. 407)
- Bosentan: possible contraceptive failure of hormonal contraceptives containing progestogens when given with •bosentan (alternative contraception recommended)
- Ciclosporin: progestogens inhibit metabolism of •ciclosporin (increased plasma concentration)
  Diuretics: risk of hyperkalaemia when drospirenone given with potassium-sparing diuretics and aldosterone antagonists (monitor serum potassium during first cycle)
  Hormone Antagonists: plasma concentration of medroxyprogesterone reduced by aminoglutethimide
  Lipid-regulating Drugs: plasma concentration of norgestrel increased by rosuvastatin
- Retinoids: efficacy of low dose progestogens may be reduced by •tretinoin but need not affect prescribing of combined oral contraceptives, there is no compelling evidence of interaction between isotretinoin and combined oral contraceptives
  Tacrolimus: contraceptive effect of progestogens possibly reduced by tacrolimus

Proguanil
  Antacids: absorption of proguanil reduced by oral magnesium salts (as magnesium trisilicate)
  Anticoagulants: isolated reports that proguanil may enhance anticoagulant effect of warfarin
- Antimalarials: avoidance of antimalarials advised by manufacturer of •artemether/lumefantrine;

Proguanil
- Antimalarials *(continued)*
  increased antifolate effect when proguanil given with pyrimethamine

Promazine *see* Antipsychotics
Promethazine *see* Antihistamines
Propafenone
  Anaesthetics, Local: increased myocardial depression when anti-arrhythmics given with bupivacaine, levobupivacaine or prilocaine
- Anti-arrhythmics: increased myocardial depression when anti-arrhythmics given with other •anti-arrhythmics; plasma concentration of propafenone increased by quinidine
- Antibacterials: metabolism of propafenone accelerated by •rifampicin (reduced effect)
- Anticoagulants: propafenone enhances anticoagulant effect of •coumarins
- Antidepressants: metabolism of propafenone possibly inhibited by paroxetine (increased risk of toxicity); increased risk of arrhythmias when propafenone given with •tricyclics
- Antihistamines: increased risk of ventricular arrhythmias when propafenone given with •mizolastine or •terfenadine—avoid concomitant use; increased risk of ventricular arrhythmias when anti-arrhythmics given with •terfenadine
- Antipsychotics: increased risk of ventricular arrhythmias when anti-arrhythmics that prolong the QT interval given with •antipsychotics that prolong the QT interval
- Antivirals: plasma concentration of propafenone possibly increased by •amprenavir (increased risk of ventricular arrhythmias—avoid concomitant use); plasma concentration of propafenone increased by •ritonavir (increased risk of ventricular arrhythmias—avoid concomitant use)
- Beta-blockers: increased myocardial depression when anti-arrhythmics given with •beta-blockers; propafenone increases plasma concentration of metoprolol and propranolol
- Cardiac Glycosides: propafenone increases plasma concentration of •digoxin (halve dose of digoxin)

  Ciclosporin: propafenone possibly increases plasma concentration of ciclosporin
- Dolasetron: increased risk of ventricular arrhythmias when propafenone given with •dolasetron—avoid concomitant use

  $5HT_3$ Antagonists: caution with anti-arrhythmics advised by manufacturer of tropisetron (risk of ventricular arrhythmias)

  Parasympathomimetics: propafenone possibly antagonises effects of neostigmine and pyridostigmine

  Theophylline: propafenone increases plasma concentration of theophylline
- Ulcer-healing Drugs: plasma concentration of propafenone increased by •cimetidine

Propantheline *see* Antimuscarinics
Propiverine *see* Antimuscarinics
Propofol *see* Anaesthetics, General
Propranolol *see* Beta-blockers
Prostaglandins
  ACE Inhibitors: enhanced hypotensive effect when alprostadil given with ACE inhibitors
  Adrenergic Neurone Blockers: enhanced hypotensive effect when alprostadil given with adrenergic neurone blockers
  Alpha-blockers: enhanced hypotensive effect when alprostadil given with alpha-blockers
  Angiotensin-II Receptor Antagonists: enhanced hypotensive effect when alprostadil given with angiotensin-II receptor antagonists

Prostaglandins *(continued)*
  Beta-blockers: enhanced hypotensive effect when alprostadil given with beta-blockers
  Calcium-channel Blockers: enhanced hypotensive effect when alprostadil given with calcium-channel blockers
  Clonidine: enhanced hypotensive effect when alprostadil given with clonidine
  Diazoxide: enhanced hypotensive effect when alprostadil given with diazoxide
  Diuretics: enhanced hypotensive effect when alprostadil given with diuretics
  Methyldopa: enhanced hypotensive effect when alprostadil given with methyldopa
  Moxonidine: enhanced hypotensive effect when alprostadil given with moxonidine
  Nitrates: enhanced hypotensive effect when alprostadil given with nitrates
  Oxytocin: prostaglandins potentiate uterotonic effect of oxytocin
  Vasodilator Antihypertensives: enhanced hypotensive effect when alprostadil given with hydralazine, minoxidil or nitroprusside

Proton Pump Inhibitors
  Antacids: absorption of lansoprazole possibly reduced by antacids
  Antibacterials: plasma concentration of both drugs increased when omeprazole given with clarithromycin
- Anticoagulants: esomeprazole and omeprazole possibly enhance anticoagulant effect of •coumarins
- Antiepileptics: esomeprazole enhances effects of •phenytoin; omeprazole possibly enhances effects of phenytoin

  Antifungals: proton pump inhibitors reduce absorption of itraconazole and ketoconazole; plasma concentration of omeprazole increased by voriconazole (reduce dose of omeprazole)
- Antivirals: omeprazole significantly reduces plasma concentration of •atazanavir—avoid concomitant use; proton pump inhibitors possibly reduce plasma concentration of •atazanavir—avoid concomitant use

  Anxiolytics and Hypnotics: esomeprazole and omeprazole possibly inhibit metabolism of diazepam (increased plasma concentration)
  Cardiac Glycosides: proton pump inhibitors possibly slightly increase plasma concentration of digoxin
  Ciclosporin: omeprazole possibly affects plasma concentration of ciclosporin
- Cilostazol: omeprazole increases plasma concentration of •cilostazol (risk of toxicity)—avoid concomitant use; lansoprazole possibly increases plasma concentration of •cilostazol—avoid concomitant use

  Cytotoxics: omeprazole possibly reduces excretion of methotrexate (increased risk of toxicity)
  Tacrolimus: omeprazole possibly increases plasma concentration of tacrolimus
  Ulcer-healing Drugs: absorption of lansoprazole possibly reduced by sucralfate

Pseudoephedrine *see* Sympathomimetics
Pyrazinamide
  Oestrogens: broad-spectrum antibacterials possibly reduce contraceptive effect of oestrogens (risk probably small, see p. 407)
  Probenecid: pyrazinamide antagonises effects of probenecid
  Sulfinpyrazone: pyrazinamide antagonises effects of sulfinpyrazone

Pyridostigmine *see* Parasympathomimetics
Pyridoxine *see* Vitamins

Pyrimethamine
- Antibacterials: increased antifolate effect when pyrimethamine (includes Fansidar®) given with •sulphonamides; increased antifolate effect when pyrimethamine given with •trimethoprim
- Antiepileptics: pyrimethamine antagonises anticonvulsant effect of •phenytoin, also increased antifolate effect
- Antimalarials: avoidance of antimalarials advised by manufacturer of •artemether/lumefantrine; increased antifolate effect when pyrimethamine given with proguanil

Antivirals: increased antifolate effect when pyrimethamine given with zidovudine
- Cytotoxics: pyrimethamine increases antifolate effect of •methotrexate

Quetiapine *see* Antipsychotics
Quinagolide

Memantine: effects of dopaminergics possibly enhanced by memantine

Methyldopa: antiparkinsonian effect of dopaminergics antagonised by methyldopa

Quinapril *see* ACE Inhibitors
Quinidine

Adsorbents: absorption of quinidine possibly reduced by kaolin

Anaesthetics, Local: increased myocardial depression when anti-arrhythmics given with bupivacaine, levobupivacaine or prilocaine

Antacids: excretion of quinidine reduced by alkaline urine due to some antacids (plasma concentration of quinidine occasionally increased)
- Anti-arrhythmics: increased myocardial depression when anti-arrhythmics given with other •anti-arrhythmics; plasma concentration of quinidine increased by •amiodarone (increased risk of ventricular arrhythmias—avoid concomitant use); quinidine increases plasma concentration of propafenone
- Antibacterials: increased risk of ventricular arrhythmias when quinidine given with •clarithromycin; increased risk of ventricular arrhythmias when quinidine given with parenteral •erythromycin; increased risk of ventricular arrhythmias when quinidine given with •moxifloxacin or •quinupristin/dalfopristin—avoid concomitant use; metabolism of quinidine accelerated by •rifamycins (reduced plasma concentration)
- Anticoagulants: quinidine possibly enhances anticoagulant effect of •coumarins
- Antidepressants: increased risk of ventricular arrhythmias when quinidine given with •tricyclics
- Antiepileptics: metabolism of quinidine accelerated by •phenytoin and primidone (reduced plasma concentration)
- Antifungals: plasma concentration of quinidine increased by •itraconazole, •miconazole and •voriconazole (increased risk of ventricular arrhythmias—avoid concomitant use)
- Antihistamines: increased risk of ventricular arrhythmias when quinidine given with •mizolastine or •terfenadine—avoid concomitant use; increased risk of ventricular arrhythmias when anti-arrhythmics given with •terfenadine
- Antimalarials: avoidance of quinidine advised by manufacturer of •artemether/lumefantrine (risk of ventricular arrhythmias); increased risk of ventricular arrhythmias when quinidine given with •mefloquine
- Antipsychotics: increased risk of ventricular arrhythmias when anti-arrhythmics that prolong the QT interval given with •antipsychotics that prolong the QT interval; increased risk of ventricular

Quinidine
- Antipsychotics *(continued)* arrhythmias when quinidine given with •amisulpride, •pimozide or •sertindole—avoid concomitant use; quinidine inhibits metabolism of •aripiprazole (reduce dose of aripiprazole); increased risk of ventricular arrhythmias when quinidine given with •phenothiazines
- Antivirals: plasma concentration of quinidine possibly increased by •amprenavir (increased risk of ventricular arrhythmias—avoid concomitant use); plasma concentration of quinidine possibly increased by •atazanavir—avoid concomitant use; increased risk of ventricular arrhythmias when quinidine given with •nelfinavir—avoid concomitant use; plasma concentration of quinidine increased by •ritonavir (increased risk of ventricular arrhythmias—avoid concomitant use)

Barbiturates: metabolism of quinidine accelerated by barbiturates (reduced plasma concentration)
- Beta-blockers: increased myocardial depression when anti-arrhythmics given with •beta-blockers; increased risk of ventricular arrhythmias when quinidine given with •sotalol—avoid concomitant use
- Calcium-channel Blockers: plasma concentration of quinidine reduced by nifedipine; plasma concentration of quinidine increased by •verapamil (extreme hypotension may occur)
- Cardiac Glycosides: quinidine increases plasma concentration of •digoxin (halve dose of digoxin)
- Diuretics: excretion of quinidine possibly reduced by •acetazolamide (increased plasma concentration), also cardiotoxicity of quinidine increased in hypokalaemia; increased cardiac toxicity with quinidine if hypokalaemia occurs with •loop diuretics or •thiazides and related diuretics

$5HT_3$ Antagonists: caution with anti-arrhythmics advised by manufacturer of tropisetron (risk of ventricular arrhythmias)
- Muscle Relaxants: quinidine enhances effects of •muscle relaxants

Parasympathomimetics: quinidine antagonises effects of neostigmine and pyridostigmine
- Ulcer-healing Drugs: plasma concentration of quinidine increased by •cimetidine

Quinine
- Anti-arrhythmics: increased risk of ventricular arrhythmias when quinine given with •amiodarone—avoid concomitant use; quinine increases plasma concentration of •flecainide
- Antibacterials: increased risk of ventricular arrhythmias when quinine given with •moxifloxacin—avoid concomitant use
- Antihistamines: increased risk of ventricular arrhythmias when quinine given with •terfenadine—avoid concomitant use
- Antimalarials: avoidance of antimalarials advised by manufacturer of •artemether/lumefantrine; increased risk of convulsions when quinine given with •mefloquine (but should not prevent the use of intravenous quinine in severe cases)
- Antipsychotics: increased risk of ventricular arrhythmias when quinine given with •pimozide—avoid concomitant use
- Cardiac Glycosides: quinine increases plasma concentration of •digoxin

Muscle Relaxants: quinine possibly enhances effects of suxamethonium

Ulcer-healing Drugs: metabolism of quinine inhibited by cimetidine (increased plasma concentration)

Quinolones

- Analgesics: possible increased risk of convulsions when quinolones given with •NSAIDs; manufacturer of ciprofloxacin advises avoid premedication with opioid analgesics (reduced plasma concentration of ciprofloxacin) when ciprofloxacin used for surgical prophylaxis

Antacids: absorption of ciprofloxacin, levofloxacin, moxifloxacin, norfloxacin and ofloxacin reduced by antacids

- Anti-arrhythmics: increased risk of ventricular arrhythmias when moxifloxacin given with •amiodarone, •disopyramide, •procainamide or •quinidine—avoid concomitant use
- Antibacterials: increased risk of ventricular arrhythmias when moxifloxacin given with parenteral •erythromycin—avoid concomitant use
- Anticoagulants: ciprofloxacin, nalidixic acid, norfloxacin and ofloxacin enhance anticoagulant effect of •coumarins; levofloxacin possibly enhances anticoagulant effect of coumarins and phenindione
- Antidepressants: ciprofloxacin inhibits metabolism of •duloxetine—avoid concomitant use; increased risk of ventricular arrhythmias when moxifloxacin given with •tricyclics—avoid concomitant use

Antidiabetics: ciprofloxacin and norfloxacin possibly enhance effects of glibenclamide

Antiepileptics: ciprofloxacin increases or decreases plasma concentration of phenytoin

- Antihistamines: increased risk of ventricular arrhythmias when moxifloxacin given with •mizolastine or •terfenadine—avoid concomitant use
- Antimalarials: avoidance of quinolones advised by manufacturer of •artemether/lumefantrine; increased risk of ventricular arrhythmias when moxifloxacin given with •chloroquine and hydroxychloroquine, •mefloquine or •quinine—avoid concomitant use
- Antipsychotics: increased risk of ventricular arrhythmias when moxifloxacin given with •haloperidol, •phenothiazines, •pimozide or •sertindole—avoid concomitant use
- Beta-blockers: increased risk of ventricular arrhythmias when moxifloxacin given with •sotalol—avoid concomitant use

Calcium Salts: absorption of ciprofloxacin reduced by calcium salts

- Ciclosporin: increased risk of nephrotoxicity when quinolones given with •ciclosporin

Cytotoxics: nalidixic acid increases risk of melphalan toxicity; ciprofloxacin possibly reduces excretion of methotrexate (increased risk of toxicity)

Dairy Products: absorption of ciprofloxacin and norfloxacin reduced by dairy products

$5HT_1$ Agonists: quinolones possibly inhibit metabolism of zolmitriptan (reduce dose of zolmitriptan)

Iron: absorption of ciprofloxacin, levofloxacin, moxifloxacin, norfloxacin and ofloxacin reduced by *oral* iron

Oestrogens: broad-spectrum antibacterials possibly reduce contraceptive effect of oestrogens (risk probably small, see p. 407)

- Pentamidine Isetionate: increased risk of ventricular arrhythmias when moxifloxacin given with •pentamidine isetionate—avoid concomitant use

Probenecid: excretion of ciprofloxacin, nalidixic acid and norfloxacin reduced by probenecid (increased plasma concentration)

Quinolones *(continued)*

Strontium Ranelate: absorption of quinolones reduced by strontium ranelate (manufacturer of strontium ranelate advises avoid concomitant use)

- Theophylline: possible increased risk of convulsions when quinolones given with •theophylline; ciprofloxacin and norfloxacin increase plasma concentration of •theophylline

Ulcer-healing Drugs: absorption of ciprofloxacin, levofloxacin, moxifloxacin, norfloxacin and ofloxacin reduced by sucralfate

Zinc: absorption of ciprofloxacin, levofloxacin, moxifloxacin, norfloxacin and ofloxacin reduced by zinc

Quinupristin with Dalfopristin

- Anti-arrhythmics: increased risk of ventricular arrhythmias when quinupristin/dalfopristin given with •disopyramide, •lidocaine (lignocaine) or •quinidine—avoid concomitant use

Antibacterials: manufacturer of quinupristin/dalfopristin recommends monitoring liver function when given with rifampicin

- Antihistamines: increased risk of ventricular arrhythmias when quinupristin/dalfopristin given with •terfenadine—avoid concomitant use

Antivirals: quinupristin/dalfopristin possibly increases plasma concentration of saquinavir

- Anxiolytics and Hypnotics: quinupristin/dalfopristin inhibits metabolism of •midazolam (increased plasma concentration with increased sedation); quinupristin/dalfopristin inhibits the metabolism of zopiclone
- Calcium-channel Blockers: quinupristin/dalfopristin increases plasma concentration of •nifedipine
- Ciclosporin: quinupristin/dalfopristin increases plasma concentration of •ciclosporin
- Ergot Alkaloids: manufacturer of quinupristin/dalfopristin advises avoid concomitant use with •ergotamine and methysergide

Oestrogens: broad-spectrum antibacterials possibly reduce contraceptive effect of oestrogens (risk probably small, see p. 407)

- Tacrolimus: quinupristin/dalfopristin increases plasma concentration of •tacrolimus

Rabeprazole *see* Proton Pump Inhibitors

Raloxifene

Anticoagulants: raloxifene antagonises anticoagulant effect of coumarins

Lipid-regulating Drugs: absorption of raloxifene reduced by colestyramine (manufacturer of raloxifene advises avoid concomitant administration)

Ramipril *see* ACE Inhibitors

Ranitidine *see* Histamine H_2-antagonists

Ranitidine Bismuth Citrate *see* Histamine H_2-antagonists

Reboxetine

- Antibacterials: manufacturer of reboxetine advises avoid concomitant use with •macrolides
- Antidepressants: manufacturer of reboxetine advises avoid concomitant use with •fluvoxamine; increased risk of hypertension and CNS excitation when reboxetine given with •MAOIs (MAOIs should not be started until 1 week after stopping reboxetine, avoid reboxetine for 2 weeks after stopping MAOIs)
- Antifungals: manufacturer of reboxetine advises avoid concomitant use with •imidazoles and •triazoles
- Antimalarials: avoidance of antidepressants advised by manufacturer of •artemether/lumefantrine

Diuretics: possible increased risk of hypokalaemia when reboxetine given with loop diuretics or thiazides and related diuretics

Reboxetine *(continued)*
Ergot Alkaloids: possible risk of hypertension when reboxetine given with ergotamine and methysergide
• Sibutramine: increased risk of CNS toxicity when noradrenaline re-uptake inhibitors given with •sibutramine (manufacturer of sibutramine advises avoid concomitant use)

Remifentanil *see* Opioid Analgesics
Repaglinide *see* Antidiabetics
Retinoids
Alcohol: etretinate formed from acitretin in presence of alcohol
• Antibacterials: possible increased risk of benign intracranial hypertension when retinoids given with •tetracyclines (avoid concomitant use)
• Anticoagulants: acitretin possibly reduces anticoagulant effect of •coumarins
Antiepileptics: isotretinoin possibly reduces plasma concentration of carbamazepine
• Cytotoxics: acitretin increases plasma concentration of •methotrexate (also increased risk of hepatotoxicity)—avoid concomitant use
• Progestogens: oral tretinoin may reduce contraceptive efficacy of low dose •progestogens but need not affect prescribing of combined oral contraceptives, there is no compelling evidence of interaction between isotretinoin and combined oral contraceptives
Vitamins: risk of hypervitaminosis A when retinoids given with vitamin A

Reviparin *see* Heparins
Ribavirin
• Antivirals: ribavirin possibly inhibits effects of •stavudine; ribavirin possibly inhibits effects of •zidovudine (manufacturer of zidovudine advises avoid concomitant use)

Rifabutin *see* Rifamycins
Rifampicin *see* Rifamycins
Rifamycins
ACE Inhibitors: rifampicin reduces plasma concentration of active metabolite of imidapril (reduced antihypertensive effect)
Analgesics: rifampicin reduces plasma concentration of etoricoxib; rifampicin accelerates metabolism of methadone (reduced effect)
Antacids: absorption of rifampicin reduced by antacids
• Anti-arrhythmics: rifamycins accelerate metabolism of •disopyramide and •quinidine (reduced plasma concentration); rifampicin accelerates metabolism of mexiletine (reduced plasma concentration); rifampicin accelerates metabolism of •propafenone (reduced effect)
• Antibacterials: plasma concentration of rifabutin increased by •clarithromycin (increased risk of uveitis—reduce rifabutin dose); rifampicin accelerates metabolism of chloramphenicol (reduced plasma concentration); rifamycins reduce plasma concentration of dapsone; plasma concentration of rifabutin possibly increased by •macrolides (increased risk of uveitis—reduce rifabutin dose); monitoring of liver function with rifampicin recommended by manufacturer of quinupristin/dalfopristin; rifampicin reduces plasma concentration of •telithromycin (avoid during and for 2 weeks after rifampicin)
• Anticoagulants: rifamycins accelerate metabolism of •coumarins (reduced anticoagulant effect)
Antidepressants: rifampicin possibly reduces plasma concentration of tricyclics
• Antidiabetics: rifamycins accelerate metabolism of •chlorpropamide and •tolbutamide (reduced effect); rifampicin reduces plasma concentration of •rosiglitazone—consider increasing dose of rosiglitazone; rifampicin reduces plasma concentration of nateglinide and repaglinide; rifamycins possibly accelerate metabolism of •sulphonylureas (reduced effect)

Rifamycins
• Antidiabetics *(continued)*

• Antiepileptics: rifabutin reduces plasma concentration of •carbamazepine; rifamycins accelerate metabolism of •phenytoin (reduced plasma concentration)
• Antifungals: rifampicin accelerates metabolism of •ketoconazole (reduced plasma concentration), also plasma concentration of rifampicin may be reduced by ketoconazole; plasma concentration of rifabutin increased by •fluconazole (increased risk of uveitis—reduce rifabutin dose); rifampicin accelerates metabolism of •fluconazole and •itraconazole (reduced plasma concentration); rifabutin reduces plasma concentration of •itraconazole—avoid concomitant use; plasma concentration of rifabutin increased by •voriconazole, also rifabutin reduces plasma concentration of voriconazole (increase dose of voriconazole and also monitor for rifabutin toxicity); rifampicin reduces plasma concentration of •voriconazole—avoid concomitant use; rifampicin initially increases and then reduces plasma concentration of caspofungin (consider increasing dose of caspofungin); rifampicin reduces plasma concentration of terbinafine; plasma concentration of rifabutin possibly increased by •triazoles (increased risk of uveitis—reduce rifabutin dose)
• Antipsychotics: rifampicin accelerates metabolism of •haloperidol (reduced plasma concentration); rifabutin and rifampicin possibly reduce plasma concentration of •aripiprazole—increase dose of aripiprazole; rifampicin possibly reduces plasma concentration of clozapine
• Antivirals: rifampicin possibly reduces plasma concentration of abacavir; plasma concentration of rifabutin increased by •amprenavir and •atazanavir (reduce dose of rifabutin); rifampicin significantly reduces plasma concentration of •amprenavir, •nelfinavir and •saquinavir—avoid concomitant use; rifampicin reduces plasma concentration of •atazanavir, •lopinavir and •nevirapine—avoid concomitant use; rifampicin reduces plasma concentration of efavirenz—increase dose of efavirenz; plasma concentration of rifabutin reduced by efavirenz—increase dose of rifabutin; rifampicin accelerates metabolism of •indinavir (reduced plasma concentration—avoid concomitant use); plasma concentration of rifabutin increased by •indinavir, also plasma concentration of indinavir decreased (reduce dose of rifabutin and increase dose of indinavir); plasma concentration of rifabutin increased by •nelfinavir (halve dose of rifabutin); plasma concentration of rifabutin increased by •ritonavir (risk of uveitis—avoid concomitant use); rifabutin significantly reduces plasma concentration of •saquinavir—avoid concomitant use unless another protease inhibitor also given e.g. ritonavir; avoidance of rifampicin advised by manufacturer of zidovudine
Anxiolytics and Hypnotics: rifampicin accelerates metabolism of diazepam (reduced plasma concentration); rifampicin possibly accelerates metabolism of benzodiazepines (reduced plasma concentration); rifampicin possibly accelerates metabolism of buspirone and zaleplon; rifampicin

Rifamycins

Anxiolytics and Hypnotics *(continued)* accelerates metabolism of zolpidem (reduced plasma concentration and reduced effect)

Aprepitant: rifampicin reduces plasma concentration of aprepitant

• Atovaquone: rifabutin and rifampicin reduce plasma concentration of •atovaquone (possible therapeutic failure of atovaquone)

Beta-blockers: rifampicin accelerates metabolism of bisoprolol and propranolol (plasma concentration significantly reduced)

• Calcium-channel Blockers: rifampicin possibly accelerates metabolism of •isradipine, •nicardipine and •nisoldipine (possible significantly reduced plasma concentration); rifampicin accelerates metabolism of •diltiazem, •nifedipine, •nimodipine and •verapamil (plasma concentration significantly reduced)

Cardiac Glycosides: rifamycins accelerate metabolism of digitoxin (reduced effect); rifampicin possibly reduces plasma concentration of digoxin

• Ciclosporin: rifampicin accelerates metabolism of •ciclosporin (reduced plasma concentration)

• Corticosteroids: rifamycins accelerate metabolism of •corticosteroids (reduced effect)

• Cytotoxics: rifampicin reduces plasma concentration of •imatinib—avoid concomitant use

• Diuretics: rifampicin reduces plasma concentration of •eplerenone—avoid concomitant use

Hormone Antagonists: rifampicin possibly reduces plasma concentration of exemestane; rifampicin accelerates metabolism of gestrinone (reduced plasma concentration)

$5HT_3$ Antagonists: rifampicin reduces plasma concentration of tropisetron; rifampicin accelerates metabolism of ondansetron (reduced effect)

Lipid-regulating Drugs: rifampicin accelerates metabolism of fluvastatin (reduced effect)

• Oestrogens: rifamycins accelerate metabolism of •oestrogens (reduced contraceptive effect—see p. 407); broad-spectrum antibacterials possibly reduce contraceptive effect of oestrogens (risk probably small, see p. 407)

• Progestogens: rifamycins accelerate metabolism of •progestogens (reduced contraceptive effect—see p. 407)

• Sirolimus: rifabutin and rifampicin reduce plasma concentration of •sirolimus—avoid concomitant use

• Tacrolimus: rifampicin reduces plasma concentration of •tacrolimus

Tadalafil: rifampicin reduces plasma concentration of tadalafil

Theophylline: rifampicin accelerates metabolism of theophylline (reduced plasma concentration)

Thyroid Hormones: rifampicin accelerates metabolism of levothyroxine (thyroxine) (may increase requirements for levothyroxine (thyroxine) in hypothyroidism)

Tibolone: rifampicin accelerates metabolism of tibolone (reduced plasma concentration)

Ulcer-healing Drugs: rifampicin accelerates metabolism of cimetidine (reduced plasma concentration)

Risedronate Sodium *see* Bisphosphonates

Risperidone *see* Antipsychotics

Ritodrine *see* Sympathomimetics, $Beta_2$

Ritonavir

• Analgesics: ritonavir possibly increases plasma concentration of NSAIDs; ritonavir increases plasma concentration of •dextropropoxyphene and •piroxicam (risk of toxicity)—avoid concomitant use; ritonavir increases plasma concentration of •fentanyl; ritonavir reduces plasma concentration of methadone; ritonavir reduces plasma concentration of •pethidine, but increases plasma concentration of toxic metabolite of pethidine (avoid concomitant use); ritonavir possibly increases plasma concentration of •opioid analgesics (except methadone)

• Anti-arrhythmics: ritonavir increases plasma concentration of •amiodarone, •flecainide, •propafenone and •quinidine (increased risk of ventricular arrhythmias—avoid concomitant use); ritonavir possibly increases plasma concentration of •disopyramide and •mexiletine (increased risk of toxicity)

• Antibacterials: ritonavir possibly increases plasma concentration of azithromycin and erythromycin; ritonavir increases plasma concentration of •clarithromycin (reduce dose of clarithromycin in renal impairment); ritonavir increases plasma concentration of •rifabutin (risk of uveitis—avoid concomitant use); plasma concentration of both drugs may increase when ritonavir given with fusidic acid

• Anticoagulants: ritonavir may enhance or reduce anticoagulant effect of •warfarin; ritonavir possibly enhances anticoagulant effect of •coumarins and •phenindione

• Antidepressants: ritonavir possibly increases plasma concentration of •SSRIs and •tricyclics; plasma concentration of ritonavir reduced by •St John's wort—avoid concomitant use

Antidiabetics: ritonavir possibly increases plasma concentration of tolbutamide

• Antiepileptics: ritonavir possibly increases plasma concentration of •carbamazepine

• Antifungals: combination of ritonavir with •itraconazole or •ketoconazole may increase plasma concentration of either drug (or both); plasma concentration of ritonavir increased by fluconazole; ritonavir reduces plasma concentration of •voriconazole—avoid concomitant use

• Antihistamines: increased risk of ventricular arrhythmias when ritonavir given with •terfenadine—avoid concomitant use; ritonavir possibly increases plasma concentration of non-sedating antihistamines

Antimuscarinics: ritonavir increases plasma concentration of solifenacin; avoidance of ritonavir advised by manufacturer of tolterodine

• Antipsychotics: ritonavir possibly increases plasma concentration of •antipsychotics; ritonavir possibly inhibits metabolism of •aripiprazole (reduce dose of aripiprazole); ritonavir increases plasma concentration of •clozapine (increased risk of toxicity)—avoid concomitant use; ritonavir increases plasma concentration of •pimozide and •sertindole (increased risk of ventricular arrhythmias—avoid concomitant use)

• Antivirals: ritonavir increases plasma concentration of amprenavir, indinavir and •saquinavir; ritonavir increases toxicity of efavirenz, monitor liver function tests; combination of ritonavir with nelfinavir may increase plasma concentration of either drug (or both)

• Anxiolytics and Hypnotics: ritonavir possibly increases plasma concentration of •anxiolytics and hypnotics; ritonavir possibly increases plasma concentration of •alprazolam, •clorazepate, •diazepam, •flurazepam, •midazolam and •zolpidem (risk of extreme sedation and respiratory

Ritonavir

- Anxiolytics and Hypnotics *(continued)* depression —avoid concomitant use); ritonavir increases plasma concentration of buspirone (increased risk of toxicity)

  Aprepitant: ritonavir possibly increases plasma concentration of aprepitant

  Bosentan: ritonavir possibly increases plasma concentration of bosentan
- Bupropion: ritonavir increases plasma concentration of •bupropion (risk of toxicity)—avoid concomitant use
- Calcium-channel Blockers: ritonavir possibly increases plasma concentration of •calcium-channel blockers; avoidance of ritonavir advised by manufacturer of lercanidipine
- Ciclosporin: ritonavir possibly increases plasma concentration of •ciclosporin
- Cilostazol: ritonavir possibly increases plasma concentration of •cilostazol—avoid concomitant use
- Corticosteroids: ritonavir possibly increases plasma concentration of corticosteroids, dexamethasone and prednisolone; ritonavir increases plasma concentration of inhaled and intranasal budesonide and •fluticasone

  Cytotoxics: ritonavir increases plasma concentration of paclitaxel
- Diuretics: ritonavir increases plasma concentration of •eplerenone—avoid concomitant use
- Ergot Alkaloids: increased risk of ergotism when ritonavir given with •ergotamine and methysergide—avoid concomitant use
- $5HT_1$ Agonists: ritonavir increases plasma concentration of •eletriptan (risk of toxicity)—avoid concomitant use
- Lipid-regulating Drugs: possible increased risk of myopathy when ritonavir given with atorvastatin; increased risk of myopathy when ritonavir given with •simvastatin (avoid concomitant use)
- Oestrogens: ritonavir accelerates metabolism of •oestrogens (reduced contraceptive effect—see p. 407)
- Sildenafil: ritonavir significantly increases plasma concentration of •sildenafil—avoid concomitant use

  Sympathomimetics: ritonavir possibly increases plasma concentration of dexamfetamine
- Tacrolimus: ritonavir possibly increases plasma concentration of •tacrolimus

  Tadalafil: ritonavir increases plasma concentration of tadalafil
- Theophylline: ritonavir accelerates metabolism of •theophylline (reduced plasma concentration)
- Vardenafil: ritonavir possibly increases plasma concentration of •vardenafil—avoid concomitant use

Rivastigmine *see* Parasympathomimetics

Rizatriptan *see* $5HT_1$ Agonists

Rocuronium *see* Muscle Relaxants

Ropinirole

Antipsychotics: manufacturer of ropinirole advises avoid concomitant use of antipsychotics (antagonism of effect)

Memantine: effects of dopaminergics possibly enhanced by memantine

Methyldopa: antiparkinsonian effect of dopaminergics antagonised by methyldopa

Metoclopramide: antiparkinsonian effect of ropinirole antagonised by metoclopramide (manufacturers of ropinirole advise avoid concomitant use)

Oestrogens: plasma concentration of ropinirole increased by oestrogens

Ropivacaine

Antidepressants: metabolism of ropivacaine inhibited by fluvoxamine—avoid prolonged administration of ropivacaine

Rosiglitazone *see* Antidiabetics

Rosuvastatin *see* Statins

Rowachol®

Anticoagulants: Rowachol® possibly reduces anticoagulant effect of coumarins

St John's Wort

- Antibacterials: St John's wort reduces plasma concentration of •telithromycin (avoid during and for 2 weeks after St John's wort)
- Anticoagulants: St John's wort reduces anticoagulant effect of •warfarin (avoid concomitant use)
- Antidepressants: possible increased serotonergic effects when St John's wort given with duloxetine; St John's wort reduces plasma concentration of amitriptyline; increased serotonergic effects when St John's wort given with •SSRIs—avoid concomitant use
- Antiepileptics: St John's wort reduces plasma concentration of •carbamazepine and •phenytoin—avoid concomitant use; St John's wort reduces plasma concentration of active metabolite of •primidone—avoid concomitant use
- Antimalarials: avoidance of antidepressants advised by manufacturer of •artemether/lumefantrine
- Antipsychotics: St John's wort possibly reduces plasma concentration of •aripiprazole—increase dose of aripiprazole
- Antivirals: St John's wort reduces plasma concentration of •amprenavir, •atazanavir, •efavirenz, •indinavir, •lopinavir, •nelfinavir, •nevirapine, •ritonavir and •saquinavir—avoid concomitant use
- Aprepitant: avoidance of St John's wort advised by manufacturer of •aprepitant
- Barbiturates: St John's wort reduces plasma concentration of •phenobarbital—avoid concomitant use
- Cardiac Glycosides: St John's wort reduces plasma concentration of •digoxin—avoid concomitant use
- Ciclosporin: St John's wort reduces plasma concentration of •ciclosporin—avoid concomitant use
- Diuretics: St John's wort reduces plasma concentration of •eplerenone—avoid concomitant use
- $5HT_1$ Agonists: increased serotonergic effects when St John's wort given with •$5HT_1$ agonists—avoid concomitant use

  Lipid-regulating Drugs: St John's wort reduces plasma concentration of simvastatin
- Oestrogens: St John's wort reduces contraceptive effect of •oestrogens (avoid concomitant use)
- Progestogens: St John's wort reduces contraceptive effect of •progestogens (avoid concomitant use)
- Tacrolimus: St John's wort reduces plasma concentration of •tacrolimus—avoid concomitant use
- Theophylline: St John's wort reduces plasma concentration of •theophylline—avoid concomitant use

Salbutamol *see* Sympathomimetics, $Beta_2$

Salmeterol *see* Sympathomimetics, $Beta_2$

Saquinavir

- Antibacterials: plasma concentration of saquinavir significantly reduced by •rifabutin—avoid concomitant use unless another protease inhibitor also given e.g. ritonavir; plasma concentration of saquinavir significantly reduced by •rifampicin—avoid concomitant use; plasma concentration of saquinavir possibly increased by quinupristin/dalfopristin

Saquinavir *(continued)*

- Antidepressants: plasma concentration of saquinavir reduced by •St John's wort—avoid concomitant use
- Antiepileptics: plasma concentration of saquinavir possibly reduced by carbamazepine, phenytoin and •primidone

  Antifungals: plasma concentration of saquinavir increased by ketoconazole; plasma concentration of saquinavir possibly increased by imidazoles and triazoles
- Antihistamines: increased risk of ventricular arrhythmias when saquinavir given with •terfenadine—avoid concomitant use

  Antimuscarinics: avoidance of saquinavir advised by manufacturer of tolterodine
- Antipsychotics: saquinavir possibly inhibits metabolism of •aripiprazole (reduce dose of aripiprazole); saquinavir possibly increases plasma concentration of •pimozide (increased risk of ventricular arrhythmias—avoid concomitant use); saquinavir increases plasma concentration of •sertindole (increased risk of ventricular arrhythmias—avoid concomitant use)
- Antivirals: plasma concentration of saquinavir significantly reduced by efavirenz; plasma concentration of saquinavir increased by indinavir, lopinavir and •ritonavir; combination of saquinavir with nelfinavir may increase plasma concentration of either drug (or both)
- Anxiolytics and Hypnotics: saquinavir increases plasma concentration of •midazolam (risk of prolonged sedation)
- Barbiturates: plasma concentration of saquinavir possibly reduced by •barbiturates
- Ciclosporin: plasma concentration of both drugs increased when saquinavir given with •ciclosporin
- Cilostazol: saquinavir possibly increases plasma concentration of •cilostazol—avoid concomitant use

  Corticosteroids: plasma concentration of saquinavir possibly reduced by dexamethasone

  Diuretics: saquinavir increases plasma concentration of eplerenone (reduce dose of eplerenone)
- Ergot Alkaloids: increased risk of ergotism when saquinavir given with •ergotamine and methysergide—avoid concomitant use
- Lipid-regulating Drugs: possible increased risk of myopathy when saquinavir given with atorvastatin; increased risk of myopathy when saquinavir given with •simvastatin (avoid concomitant use)

  Sildenafil: saquinavir possibly increases plasma concentration of sildenafil— reduce initial dose of sildenafil

  Tadalafil: saquinavir possibly increases plasma concentration of tadalafil— reduce initial dose of tadalafil

  Vardenafil: saquinavir possibly increases plasma concentration of vardenafil— reduce initial dose of vardenafil

Secobarbital *see* Barbiturates

Selegiline

Note. Selegiline is a MAO-B inhibitor

- Analgesics: hyperpyrexia and CNS toxicity reported when selegiline given with •pethidine (avoid concomitant use); manufacturer of selegiline advises caution with tramadol
- Antidepressants: theoretical risk of serotonin syndrome if selegiline given with citalopram (especially if dose of selegiline exceeds 10 mg daily); caution with selegiline advised by manufacturer of escitalopram; increased risk of hypertension and CNS excitation when selegiline given with •fluoxetine (selegiline should not be started

Selegiline

- Antidepressants *(continued)* until 5 weeks after stopping fluoxetine, avoid fluoxetine for 2 weeks after stopping selegiline); increased risk of hypertension and CNS excitation when selegiline given with •fluvoxamine or •venlafaxine (selegiline should not be started until 1 week after stopping fluvoxamine or venlafaxine, avoid fluvoxamine or venlafaxine for 2 weeks after stopping selegiline); increased risk of hypertension and CNS excitation when selegiline given with •paroxetine or •sertraline (selegiline should not be started until 2 weeks after stopping paroxetine or sertraline, avoid paroxetine or sertraline for 2 weeks after stopping selegiline); enhanced hypotensive effect when selegiline given with MAOIs; avoid concomitant use of selegiline with •moclobemide; CNS toxicity reported when selegiline given with •tricyclics

  Dopaminergics: max. dose of 10 mg selegiline advised by manufacturer of entacapone if used concomitantly; selegiline enhances effects and increases toxicity of levodopa (reduce dose of levodopa)

  Memantine: effects of dopaminergics and selegiline possibly enhanced by memantine

  Methyldopa: antiparkinsonian effect of dopaminergics antagonised by methyldopa

Sertindole *see* Antipsychotics

Sertraline *see* Antidepressants, SSRI

Sevoflurane *see* Anaesthetics, General

Sibutramine

  Analgesics: increased risk of bleeding when sibutramine given with NSAIDs or aspirin

  Anticoagulants: increased risk of bleeding when sibutramine given with anticoagulants
- Antidepressants: increased CNS toxicity when sibutramine given with •MAOIs or •moclobemide (manufacturer of sibutramine advises avoid concomitant use), also avoid sibutramine for 2 weeks after stopping MAOIs or moclobemide; increased risk of CNS toxicity when sibutramine given with •SSRI-related antidepressants, •SSRIs, •mirtazapine, •noradrenaline re-uptake inhibitors, •tricyclic-related antidepressants, •tricyclics or •tryptophan (manufacturer of sibutramine advises avoid concomitant use)
- Antipsychotics: increased risk of CNS toxicity when sibutramine given with •antipsychotics (manufacturer of sibutramine advises avoid concomitant use)

Sildenafil

  Alpha-blockers: enhanced hypotensive effect when sildenafil given with alpha-blockers (avoid alpha-blockers for 4 hours after sildenafil)

  Antibacterials: plasma concentration of sildenafil increased by erythromycin—reduce initial dose of sildenafil

  Antifungals: plasma concentration of sildenafil increased by itraconazole and ketoconazole—reduce initial dose of sildenafil
- Antivirals: plasma concentration of sildenafil possibly increased by amprenavir, nelfinavir and saquinavir— reduce initial dose of sildenafil; side-effects of sildenafil possibly increased by •atazanavir; plasma concentration of sildenafil increased by indinavir—reduce initial dose of sildenafil; plasma concentration of sildenafil significantly increased by •ritonavir—avoid concomitant use

  Calcium-channel Blockers: enhanced hypotensive effect when sildenafil given with amlodipine

  Grapefruit Juice: plasma concentration of sildenafil possibly increased by grapefruit juice

Sildenafil *(continued)*
- Nicorandil: sildenafil significantly enhances hypotensive effect of •nicorandil (avoid concomitant use)
- Nitrates: sildenafil significantly enhances hypotensive effect of •nitrates (avoid concomitant use)

Ulcer-healing Drugs: plasma concentration of sildenafil increased by cimetidine (reduce initial dose of sildenafil)

Simvastatin *see* Statins

Sirolimus
- Antibacterials: plasma concentration of sirolimus increased by •clarithromycin and •telithromycin—avoid concomitant use; plasma concentration of both drugs increased when sirolimus given with •erythromycin; plasma concentration of sirolimus reduced by •rifabutin and •rifampicin—avoid concomitant use
- Antifungals: plasma concentration of sirolimus increased by •itraconazole, •ketoconazole and •voriconazole—avoid concomitant use; plasma concentration of sirolimus increased by •miconazole
- Antivirals: plasma concentration of sirolimus possibly increased by •atazanavir and lopinavir
- Calcium-channel Blockers: plasma concentration of sirolimus increased by •diltiazem; plasma concentration of both drugs increased when sirolimus given with •verapamil

Ciclosporin: plasma concentration of sirolimus increased by ciclosporin
- Grapefruit Juice: plasma concentration of sirolimus increased by •grapefruit juice—avoid concomitant use

Sodium Benzoate

Antiepileptics: effects of sodium benzoate possibly reduced by valproate

Antipsychotics: effects of sodium benzoate possibly reduced by haloperidol

Corticosteroids: effects of sodium benzoate possibly reduced by corticosteroids

Probenecid: excretion of conjugate formed by sodium benzoate possibly reduced by probenecid

Sodium Bicarbonate *see* Antacids

Sodium Clodronate *see* Bisphosphonates

Sodium Phenylbutyrate

Antiepileptics: effects of sodium phenylbutyrate possibly reduced by valproate

Antipsychotics: effects of sodium phenylbutyrate possibly reduced by haloperidol

Corticosteroids: effects of sodium phenylbutyrate possibly reduced by corticosteroids

Probenecid: excretion of conjugate formed by sodium phenylbutyrate possibly reduced by probenecid

Sodium Polystyrene Sulphonate

Thyroid Hormones: sodium polystyrene sulphonate reduces absorption of levothyroxine (thyroxine)

Sodium Valproate *see* Valproate

Solifenacin *see* Antimuscarinics

Somatropin

Corticosteroids: growth-promoting effect of somatropin may be inhibited by corticosteroids

Oestrogens: increased doses of somatropin may be needed when given with oestrogens (when used as oral replacement therapy)

Sotalol *see* Beta-blockers

Spironolactone *see* Diuretics

Statins

Antacids: absorption of rosuvastatin reduced by antacids
- Anti-arrhythmics: increased risk of myopathy when simvastatin given with •amiodarone

Statins *(continued)*
- Antibacterials: plasma concentration of atorvastatin increased by clarithromycin; increased risk of myopathy when simvastatin given with •clarithromycin, •erythromycin or •telithromycin (avoid concomitant use); plasma concentration of rosuvastatin reduced by erythromycin; possible increased risk of myopathy when atorvastatin given with erythromycin or fusidic acid; metabolism of fluvastatin accelerated by rifampicin (reduced effect); possible increased risk of myopathy when simvastatin given with fusidic acid; increased risk of myopathy when atorvastatin given with •telithromycin (avoid concomitant use)
- Anticoagulants: atorvastatin may transiently reduce anticoagulant effect of warfarin; fluvastatin and simvastatin enhance anticoagulant effect of •coumarins; rosuvastatin possibly enhances anticoagulant effect of •coumarins and •phenindione

Antidepressants: plasma concentration of simvastatin reduced by St John's wort
- Antiepileptics: combination of fluvastatin with phenytoin may increase plasma concentration of either drug (or both)
- Antifungals: increased risk of myopathy when simvastatin given with •itraconazole or •ketoconazole (avoid concomitant use); possible increased risk of myopathy when simvastatin given with •miconazole—avoid concomitant use; increased risk of myopathy when atorvastatin given with •itraconazole (avoid concomitant use); possible increased risk of myopathy when atorvastatin or simvastatin given with imidazoles; possible increased risk of myopathy when atorvastatin or simvastatin given with triazoles
- Antivirals: plasma concentration of simvastatin possibly increased by •amprenavir—avoid concomitant use; possible increased risk of myopathy when atorvastatin given with amprenavir, atazanavir, indinavir, lopinavir, nelfinavir, ritonavir or saquinavir; increased risk of myopathy when simvastatin given with •atazanavir, •indinavir, •nelfinavir, •ritonavir or •saquinavir (avoid concomitant use)

Bosentan: plasma concentration of simvastatin reduced by bosentan
- Calcium-channel Blockers: possible increased risk of myopathy when simvastatin given with diltiazem; increased risk of myopathy when simvastatin given with •verapamil

Cardiac Glycosides: atorvastatin possibly increases plasma concentration of digoxin
- Ciclosporin: increased risk of myopathy when statins given with •ciclosporin; increased risk of myopathy when rosuvastatin given with •ciclosporin (avoid concomitant use)

Cytotoxics: plasma concentration of simvastatin increased by imatinib
- Grapefruit Juice: plasma concentration of simvastatin increased by •grapefruit juice—avoid concomitant use
- Lipid-regulating Drugs: increased risk of myopathy when statins given with •gemfibrozil (preferably avoid concomitant use); increased risk of myopathy when rosuvastatin or statins given with •fibrates; increased risk of myopathy when statins given with •nicotinic acid (applies to lipid regulating doses of nicotinic acid)

Oestrogens: rosuvastatin increases plasma concentration of ethinylestradiol

Progestogens: rosuvastatin increases plasma concentration of norgestrel

Stavudine
- Antivirals: effects of stavudine possibly inhibited by •ribavirin; effects of stavudine possibly inhibited by •zidovudine (manufacturers advise avoid concomitant use)

  Cytotoxics: effects of stavudine possibly inhibited by doxorubicin

Streptomycin *see* Aminoglycosides

Strontium Ranelate

  Antibacterials: strontium ranelate reduces absorption of quinolones and tetracyclines (manufacturer of strontium ranelate advises avoid concomitant use)

Sucralfate

  Antibacterials: sucralfate reduces absorption of ciprofloxacin, levofloxacin, moxifloxacin, norfloxacin, ofloxacin and tetracyclines
- Anticoagulants: sucralfate possibly reduces absorption of •coumarins (reduced anticoagulant effect)
- Antiepileptics: sucralfate reduces absorption of •phenytoin

  Antifungals: sucralfate reduces absorption of ketoconazole

  Antipsychotics: sucralfate reduces absorption of sulpiride

  Cardiac Glycosides: sucralfate possibly reduces absorption of cardiac glycosides

  Thyroid Hormones: sucralfate reduces absorption of levothyroxine (thyroxine)

  Ulcer-healing Drugs: sucralfate possibly reduces absorption of lansoprazole

Sulfadiazine *see* Sulphonamides

Sulfadoxine *see* Sulphonamides

Sulfamethoxazole *see* Sulphonamides

Sulfasalazine *see* Aminosalicylates

Sulfinpyrazone

  Analgesics: effects of sulfinpyrazone antagonised by aspirin

  Antibacterials: sulfinpyrazone reduces excretion of nitrofurantoin (increased risk of toxicity); effects of sulfinpyrazone antagonised by pyrazinamide
- Anticoagulants: sulfinpyrazone enhances anticoagulant effect of •coumarins
- Antidiabetics: sulfinpyrazone enhances effects of •sulphonylureas
- Antiepileptics: sulfinpyrazone increases plasma concentration of •phenytoin

  Theophylline: sulfinpyrazone reduces plasma concentration of theophylline

Sulindac *see* NSAIDs

Sulphonamides

  Anaesthetics, General: sulphonamides enhance effects of thiopental

  Anaesthetics, Local: increased risk of methaemoglobinaemia when sulphonamides given with prilocaine
- Anti-arrhythmics: increased risk of ventricular arrhythmias when sulfamethoxazole (as co-trimoxazole) given with •amiodarone—avoid concomitant use of co-trimoxazole
- Antibacterials: increased risk of crystalluria when sulphonamides given with •methenamine
- Anticoagulants: sulphonamides enhance anticoagulant effect of •coumarins

  Antidiabetics: sulphonamides rarely enhance the effects of sulphonylureas

  Antiepileptics: sulphonamides possibly increase plasma concentration of phenytoin
- Antimalarials: increased antifolate effect when sulphonamides given with •pyrimethamine (includes Fansidar®)
- Antipsychotics: avoid concomitant use of sulphonamides with •clozapine (increased risk of agranulocytosis)

Sulphonamides *(continued)*
- Ciclosporin: increased risk of nephrotoxicity when sulphonamides given with •ciclosporin; sulfadiazine possibly reduces plasma concentration of •ciclosporin
- Cytotoxics: increased risk of haematological toxicity when sulfamethoxazole (as co-trimoxazole) given with •azathioprine, •mercaptopurine or •methotrexate; sulphonamides increase risk of methotrexate toxicity

  Oestrogens: broad-spectrum antibacterials possibly reduce contraceptive effect of oestrogens (risk probably small, see p. 407)

  Potassium Aminobenzoate: effects of sulphonamides inhibited by potassium aminobenzoate

Sulphonylureas *see* Antidiabetics

Sulpiride *see* Antipsychotics

Sumatriptan *see* $5HT_1$ Agonists

Suxamethonium *see* Muscle Relaxants

Sympathomimetics
- Adrenergic Neurone Blockers: ephedrine, isometheptene, metaraminol, methylphenidate, noradrenaline (norepinephrine), oxymetazoline, phenylephrine, phenylpropanolamine, pseudoephedrine and xylometazoline antagonise hypotensive effect of •adrenergic neurone blockers
- Alpha-blockers: avoid concomitant use of adrenaline (epinephrine) or dopamine with •tolazoline
- Anaesthetics, General: increased risk of hypertension when methylphenidate given with •volatile liquid general anaesthetics; increased risk of arrhythmias when adrenaline (epinephrine) given with •volatile liquid general anaesthetics
- Anticoagulants: methylphenidate possibly enhances anticoagulant effect of •coumarins
- Antidepressants: risk of hypertensive crisis when dexamfetamine, dopamine, dopexamine, ephedrine, isometheptene, methylphenidate, phenylephrine, phenylpropanolamine, pseudoephedrine or sympathomimetics given with •MAOIs; risk of hypertensive crisis when dexamfetamine, dopamine, dopexamine, ephedrine, isometheptene, methylphenidate, phenylephrine, phenylpropanolamine, pseudoephedrine or sympathomimetics given with •moclobemide; methylphenidate possibly inhibits metabolism of SSRIs and tricyclics; increased risk of hypertension and arrhythmias when noradrenaline (norepinephrine) given with •tricyclics; increased risk of hypertension and arrhythmias when adrenaline (epinephrine) given with •tricyclics (but local anaesthetics with adrenaline appear to be safe)

  Antiepileptics: methylphenidate increases plasma concentration of phenytoin; methylphenidate possibly increases plasma concentration of primidone

  Antipsychotics: hypertensive effect of sympathomimetics antagonised by antipsychotics

  Antivirals: plasma concentration of dexamfetamine possibly increased by ritonavir

  Barbiturates: methylphenidate possibly increases plasma concentration of phenobarbital
- Beta-blockers: severe hypertension when adrenaline (epinephrine) or noradrenaline (norepinephrine) given with •beta-blockers especially with non-selective beta-blockers; possible severe hypertension when dobutamine given with •beta-blockers especially with non-selective beta-blockers
- Clonidine: possible risk of hypertension when adrenaline (epinephrine) or noradrenaline (norepinephrine) given with clonidine; serious adverse events reported with concomitant use of methyl-

Sympathomimetics
- Clonidine *(continued)* phenidate and •clonidine (causality not established)
  Corticosteroids: ephedrine accelerates metabolism of dexamethasone
- Dopaminergics: risk of toxicity when isometheptene or phenylpropanolamine given with •bromocriptine; effects of adrenaline (epinephrine), dobutamine, dopamine and noradrenaline (norepinephrine) possibly enhanced by entacapone
  Doxapram: increased risk of hypertension when sympathomimetics given with doxapram
  Ergot Alkaloids: increased risk of ergotism when sympathomimetics given with ergotamine and methysergide
  Oxytocin: risk of hypertension when vasoconstrictor sympathomimetics given with oxytocin (due to enhanced vasopressor effect)
- Sympathomimetics: effects of adrenaline (epinephrine) possibly enhanced by •dopexamine; dopexamine possibly enhances effects of •noradrenaline (norepinephrine)

Sympathomimetics, Beta$_2$
  Cardiac Glycosides: salbutamol possibly reduces plasma concentration of digoxin
  Corticosteroids: increased risk of hypokalaemia when high doses of beta$_2$ sympathomimetics given with corticosteroids—for CSM advice (hypokalaemia) see p. 143
  Diuretics: increased risk of hypokalaemia when high doses of beta$_2$ sympathomimetics given with acetazolamide, loop diuretics or thiazides and related diuretics—for CSM advice (hypokalaemia) see p. 143
- Methyldopa: acute hypotension reported when infusion of salbutamol given with •methyldopa
  Muscle Relaxants: bambuterol enhances effects of suxamethonium
  Theophylline: increased risk of hypokalaemia when high doses of beta$_2$ sympathomimetics given with theophylline—for CSM advice (hypokalaemia) see p. 143

Tacrolimus
- Analgesics: possible increased risk of nephrotoxicity when tacrolimus given with NSAIDs; increased risk of nephrotoxicity when tacrolimus given with •ibuprofen
- Antibacterials: plasma concentration of tacrolimus increased by •clarithromycin, •erythromycin and •quinupristin/dalfopristin; plasma concentration of tacrolimus reduced by •rifampicin; increased risk of nephrotoxicity when tacrolimus given with •aminoglycosides; plasma concentration of tacrolimus possibly increased by •chloramphenicol and •telithromycin
- Antidepressants: plasma concentration of tacrolimus reduced by •St John's wort—avoid concomitant use
- Antifungals: plasma concentration of tacrolimus increased by •fluconazole, •ketoconazole and •voriconazole; increased risk of nephrotoxicity when tacrolimus given with •amphotericin; plasma concentration of tacrolimus reduced by •caspofungin; plasma concentration of tacrolimus possibly increased by •imidazoles and •triazoles
- Antivirals: plasma concentration of tacrolimus possibly increased by •atazanavir, •nelfinavir and •ritonavir
- Calcium-channel Blockers: plasma concentration of tacrolimus possibly increased by felodipine;

Tacrolimus
- Calcium-channel Blockers *(continued)* plasma concentration of tacrolimus increased by •diltiazem and •nifedipine
- Ciclosporin: tacrolimus increases plasma concentration of •ciclosporin (increased risk of toxicity)—avoid concomitant use
- Diuretics: increased risk of hyperkalaemia when tacrolimus given with •potassium-sparing diuretics and aldosterone antagonists
- Grapefruit Juice: plasma concentration of tacrolimus increased by •grapefruit juice
  Hormone Antagonists: plasma concentration of tacrolimus possibly increased by danazol
  Oestrogens: tacrolimus possibly reduces contraceptive effect of oestrogens
- Potassium Salts: increased risk of hyperkalaemia when tacrolimus given with •potassium salts
  Progestogens: tacrolimus possibly reduces contraceptive effect of progestogens
  Ulcer-healing Drugs: plasma concentration of tacrolimus possibly increased by omeprazole

Tadalafil
- Alpha-blockers: enhanced hypotensive effect when tadalafil given with •alpha-blockers—avoid concomitant use
  Antibacterials: plasma concentration of tadalafil possibly increased by clarithromycin and erythromycin; plasma concentration of tadalafil reduced by rifampicin
  Antifungals: plasma concentration of tadalafil increased by ketoconazole; plasma concentration of tadalafil possibly increased by itraconazole
  Antivirals: plasma concentration of tadalafil increased by ritonavir; plasma concentration of tadalafil possibly increased by saquinavir—reduce initial dose of tadalafil
  Grapefruit Juice: plasma concentration of tadalafil possibly increased by grapefruit juice
- Nicorandil: tadalafil significantly enhances hypotensive effect of •nicorandil (avoid concomitant use)
- Nitrates: tadalafil significantly enhances hypotensive effect of •nitrates (avoid concomitant use)

Tamoxifen
- Anticoagulants: tamoxifen enhances anticoagulant effect of •coumarins
  Hormone Antagonists: plasma concentration of tamoxifen reduced by aminoglutethimide

Tamsulosin *see* Alpha-blockers

Taxanes *see* Docetaxel and Paclitaxel

Tegafur with uracil *see* Fluorouracil

Teicoplanin
  Antibacterials: increased risk of nephrotoxicity and ototoxicity when teicoplanin given with aminoglycosides or colistin
  Oestrogens: broad-spectrum antibacterials possibly reduce contraceptive effect of oestrogens (risk probably small, see p. 407)

Telithromycin
- Antibacterials: plasma concentration of telithromycin reduced by •rifampicin (avoid during and for 2 weeks after rifampicin)
- Antidepressants: plasma concentration of telithromycin reduced by •St John's wort (avoid during and for 2 weeks after St John's wort)
- Antiepileptics: plasma concentration of telithromycin reduced by •carbamazepine, •phenytoin and •primidone (avoid during and for 2 weeks after carbamazepine, phenytoin and primidone)
- Antihistamines: increased risk of ventricular arrhythmias when telithromycin given with •terfenadine—avoid concomitant use

Telithromycin *(continued)*
- Antipsychotics: increased risk of ventricular arrhythmias when telithromycin given with •pimozide—avoid concomitant use
- Anxiolytics and Hypnotics: telithromycin inhibits metabolism of •midazolam (increased plasma concentration with increased sedation)

Aprepitant: telithromycin possibly increases plasma concentration of aprepitant
- Barbiturates: plasma concentration of telithromycin reduced by •phenobarbital (avoid during and for 2 weeks after phenobarbital)

Cardiac Glycosides: telithromycin possibly increases plasma concentration of digoxin
- Ciclosporin: telithromycin possibly increases plasma concentration of •ciclosporin
- Diuretics: telithromycin increases plasma concentration of •eplerenone—avoid concomitant use
- Ergot Alkaloids: increased risk of ergotism when telithromycin given with •ergotamine and methysergide—avoid concomitant use
- Lipid-regulating Drugs: increased risk of myopathy when telithromycin given with •atorvastatin or •simvastatin (avoid concomitant use)

Oestrogens: broad-spectrum antibacterials possibly reduce contraceptive effect of oestrogens (risk probably small, see p. 407)
- Sirolimus: telithromycin increases plasma concentration of •sirolimus—avoid concomitant use
- Tacrolimus: telithromycin possibly increases plasma concentration of •tacrolimus

Telmisartan *see* Angiotensin-II Receptor Antagonists

Temazepam *see* Anxiolytics and Hypnotics

Temoporfin
- Cytotoxics: increased skin photosensitivity when temoporfin given with topical •fluorouracil

Temozolomide

Antiepileptics: cytotoxics possibly reduce absorption of phenytoin; plasma concentration of temozolomide increased by valproate
- Antipsychotics: avoid concomitant use of cytotoxics with •clozapine (increased risk of agranulocytosis)

Tenofovir
- Antivirals: tenofovir reduces plasma concentration of atazanavir; combination of tenofovir with cidofovir may increase plasma concentration of either drug (or both); tenofovir increases plasma concentration of •didanosine (increased risk of toxicity)—avoid concomitant use; plasma concentration of tenofovir increased by lopinavir

Tenoxicam *see* NSAIDs

Terazosin *see* Alpha-blockers

Terbinafine

Antibacterials: plasma concentration of terbinafine reduced by rifampicin

Antidepressants: terbinafine possibly increases plasma concentration of imipramine and nortriptyline

Oestrogens: occasional reports of breakthrough bleeding when terbinafine given with oestrogens (when used for contraception)

Progestogens: occasional reports of breakthrough bleeding when terbinafine given with progestogens (when used for contraception)

Ulcer-healing Drugs: plasma concentration of terbinafine increased by cimetidine

Terbutaline *see* Sympathomimetics, $Beta_2$

Terfenadine *see* Antihistamines

Terpene Mixture *see* Rowachol®

Testolactone
- Anticoagulants: testolactone enhances anticoagulant effect of •coumarins and •phenindione

Testosterone
- Anticoagulants: testosterone enhances anticoagulant effect of •coumarins and •phenindione

Antidiabetics: testosterone possibly enhances hypoglycaemic effect of antidiabetics

Tetrabenazine
- Antidepressants: risk of CNS excitation and hypertension when tetrabenazine given with •MAOIs

Antipsychotics: increased risk of extrapyramidal side-effects when tetrabenazine given with antipsychotics

Dopaminergics: increased risk of extrapyramidal side-effects when tetrabenazine given with amantadine

Metoclopramide: increased risk of extrapyramidal side-effects when tetrabenazine given with metoclopramide

Tetracosactide *see* Corticosteroids

Tetracycline *see* Tetracyclines

Tetracyclines

ACE Inhibitors: absorption of tetracyclines reduced by quinapril tablets (quinapril tablets contain magnesium carbonate)

Adsorbents: absorption of tetracyclines possibly reduced by kaolin

Antacids: absorption of tetracyclines reduced by antacids
- Anticoagulants: tetracyclines possibly enhance anticoagulant effect of •coumarins and •phenindione

Antiepileptics: metabolism of doxycycline accelerated by carbamazepine (reduced effect); metabolism of doxycycline accelerated by phenytoin and primidone (reduced plasma concentration)

Atovaquone: tetracycline reduces plasma concentration of atovaquone

Barbiturates: metabolism of doxycycline accelerated by barbiturates (reduced plasma concentration)

Calcium Salts: absorption of tetracycline reduced by calcium salts
- Ciclosporin: doxycycline possibly increases plasma concentration of •ciclosporin

Cytotoxics: doxycycline or tetracycline increase risk of methotrexate toxicity

Dairy Products: absorption of tetracyclines (except doxycycline and minocycline) reduced by dairy products

Diuretics: manufacturer of lymecycline advises avoid concomitant use with diuretics

Ergot Alkaloids: increased risk of ergotism when tetracyclines given with ergotamine and methysergide

Iron: absorption of tetracyclines reduced by *oral* iron, also absorption of *oral* iron reduced by tetracyclines

Oestrogens: broad-spectrum antibacterials possibly reduce contraceptive effect of oestrogens (risk probably small, see p. 407)
- Retinoids: possible increased risk of benign intracranial hypertension when tetracyclines given with •retinoids (avoid concomitant use)

Strontium Ranelate: absorption of tetracyclines reduced by strontium ranelate (manufacturer of strontium ranelate advises avoid concomitant use)

Ulcer-healing Drugs: absorption of tetracyclines reduced by ranitidine bismuth citrate, sucralfate and tripotassium dicitratobismuthate

Zinc: absorption of tetracyclines reduced by zinc, also absorption of zinc reduced by tetracyclines

Theophylline

Allopurinol: plasma concentration of theophylline possibly increased by allopurinol

Theophylline *(continued)*

Anaesthetics, General: increased risk of convulsions when theophylline given with ketamine; increased risk of arrhythmias when theophylline given with halothane

Anti-arrhythmics: theophylline antagonises anti-arrhythmic effect of adenosine; plasma concentration of theophylline increased by mexiletine and propafenone

• Antibacterials: plasma concentration of theophylline possibly increased by azithromycin and isoniazid; metabolism of theophylline inhibited by •clarithromycin (increased plasma concentration); metabolism of theophylline inhibited by •erythromycin (increased plasma concentration), if erythromycin given by mouth, also decreased plasma-erythromycin concentration; plasma concentration of theophylline increased by •ciprofloxacin and •norfloxacin; metabolism of theophylline accelerated by rifampicin (reduced plasma concentration); possible increased risk of convulsions when theophylline given with •quinolones

• Antidepressants: plasma concentration of theophylline increased by •fluvoxamine (concomitant use should usually be avoided, but where not possible halve theophylline dose and monitor plasma-theophylline concentration); plasma concentration of theophylline reduced by •St John's wort—avoid concomitant use

• Antiepileptics: metabolism of theophylline accelerated by carbamazepine and primidone (reduced effect); plasma concentration of both drugs reduced when theophylline given with •phenytoin

• Antifungals: plasma concentration of theophylline possibly increased by •fluconazole and •ketoconazole

• Antivirals: metabolism of theophylline accelerated by •ritonavir (reduced plasma concentration)

Anxiolytics and Hypnotics: theophylline possibly reduces effects of benzodiazepines

Barbiturates: metabolism of theophylline accelerated by barbiturates (reduced effect)

• Calcium-channel Blockers: plasma concentration of theophylline possibly increased by •calcium-channel blockers (enhanced effect); plasma concentration of theophylline increased by diltiazem; plasma concentration of theophylline increased by •verapamil (enhanced effect)

Corticosteroids: increased risk of hypokalaemia when theophylline given with corticosteroids

Cytotoxics: plasma concentration of theophylline possibly increased by methotrexate

Disulfiram: metabolism of theophylline inhibited by disulfiram (increased risk of toxicity)

Diuretics: increased risk of hypokalaemia when theophylline given with acetazolamide, loop diuretics or thiazides and related diuretics

Doxapram: increased CNS stimulation when theophylline given with doxapram

Hormone Antagonists: metabolism of theophylline accelerated by aminoglutethimide (reduced effect)

Interferons: metabolism of theophylline inhibited by interferon alfa (increased plasma concentration)

Leukotriene Antagonists: plasma concentration of theophylline possibly increased by zafirlukast, also plasma concentration of zafirlukast reduced

Lithium: theophylline increases excretion of lithium (reduced plasma concentration)

Oestrogens: excretion of theophylline reduced by oestrogens (increased plasma concentration)

Pentoxifylline (oxpentifylline): plasma concentration of theophylline increased by pentoxifylline (oxpentifylline)

Theophylline *(continued)*

Sulfinpyrazone: plasma concentration of theophylline reduced by sulfinpyrazone

Sympathomimetics, $Beta_2$: increased risk of hypokalaemia when theophylline given with high doses of $beta_2$ sympathomimetics—for CSM advice (hypokalaemia) see p. 143

Tobacco: metabolism of theophylline increased by tobacco smoking (reduced plasma concentration)

• Ulcer-healing Drugs: metabolism of theophylline inhibited by •cimetidine (increased plasma concentration)

Vaccines: plasma concentration of theophylline possibly increased by influenza vaccine

Thiazolidinediones *see* Antidiabetics

Thiopental *see* Anaesthetics, General

Thiotepa

Antiepileptics: cytotoxics possibly reduce absorption of phenytoin

• Antipsychotics: avoid concomitant use of cytotoxics with •clozapine (increased risk of agranulocytosis)

Muscle Relaxants: thiotepa enhances effects of suxamethonium

Thioxanthenes *see* Antipsychotics

Thyroid Hormones

Anti-arrhythmics: for concomitant use of thyroid hormones and amiodarone see p. 79

Antibacterials: metabolism of levothyroxine (thyroxine) accelerated by rifampicin (may increase requirements for levothyroxine (thyroxine) in hypothyroidism)

• Anticoagulants: thyroid hormones enhance anticoagulant effect of •coumarins and •phenindione

Antidepressants: thyroid hormones enhance effects of amitriptyline and imipramine; thyroid hormones possibly enhance effects of tricyclics

Antiepileptics: metabolism of thyroid hormones accelerated by carbamazepine and primidone (may increase requirements for thyroid hormones in hypothyroidism); metabolism of thyroid hormones accelerated by phenytoin (may increase requirements in hypothyroidism), also plasma concentration of phenytoin possibly increased

Barbiturates: metabolism of thyroid hormones accelerated by barbiturates (may increase requirements for thyroid hormones in hypothyroidism)

Calcium Salts: absorption of levothyroxine (thyroxine) reduced by calcium salts

Iron: absorption of levothyroxine (thyroxine) reduced by *oral* iron (give at least 2 hours apart)

Lipid-regulating Drugs: absorption of thyroid hormones reduced by colestipol and colestyramine

Sodium Polystyrene Sulphonate: absorption of levothyroxine (thyroxine) reduced by sodium polystyrene sulphonate

Ulcer-healing Drugs: absorption of levothyroxine (thyroxine) reduced by cimetidine and sucralfate

Tiagabine

• Antidepressants: anticonvulsant effect of antiepileptics possibly antagonised by MAOIs and •tricyclic-related antidepressants (convulsive threshold lowered); anticonvulsant effect of antiepileptics antagonised by •SSRIs and •tricyclics (convulsive threshold lowered)

Antiepileptics: plasma concentration of tiagabine reduced by carbamazepine, phenytoin and primidone

• Antimalarials: possible increased risk of convulsions when antiepileptics given with chloroquine and hydroxychloroquine; anticonvulsant effect of antiepileptics antagonised by •mefloquine

Barbiturates: plasma concentration of tiagabine reduced by phenobarbital

Tiaprofenic Acid *see* NSAIDs

Tibolone
Antibacterials: metabolism of tibolone accelerated by rifampicin (reduced plasma concentration)
Antiepileptics: metabolism of tibolone accelerated by carbamazepine and primidone (reduced plasma concentration); metabolism of tibolone accelerated by phenytoin
Barbiturates: metabolism of tibolone accelerated by barbiturates (reduced plasma concentration)

Ticarcillin *see* Penicillins
Tiludronic Acid *see* Bisphosphonates
Timolol *see* Beta-blockers

Tinidazole
Alcohol: possibility of disulfiram-like reaction when tinidazole given with alcohol
Oestrogens: broad-spectrum antibacterials possibly reduce contraceptive effect of oestrogens (risk probably small, see p. 407)

Tinzaparin *see* Heparins

Tioguanine
Antiepileptics: cytotoxics possibly reduce absorption of phenytoin
• Antipsychotics: avoid concomitant use of cytotoxics with •clozapine (increased risk of agranulocytosis)
Cytotoxics: increased risk of hepatotoxicity when tioguanine given with busulfan

Tiotropium *see* Antimuscarinics

Tirofiban
Iloprost: increased risk of bleeding when tirofiban given with iloprost

Tizanidine *see* Muscle Relaxants

Tobacco
Cinacalcet: tobacco smoking increases cinacalcet metabolism (reduced plasma concentration)
Theophylline: tobacco smoking increases theophylline metabolism (reduced plasma concentration)

Tobramycin *see* Aminoglycosides
Tolazoline *see* Alpha-blockers
Tolbutamide *see* Antidiabetics

Tolcapone
Antidepressants: avoid concomitant use of tolcapone with MAOIs
Memantine: effects of dopaminergics possibly enhanced by memantine
Methyldopa: antiparkinsonian effect of dopaminergics antagonised by methyldopa

Tolfenamic Acid *see* NSAIDs
Tolterodine *see* Antimuscarinics

Topiramate
• Antidepressants: anticonvulsant effect of antiepileptics possibly antagonised by MAOIs and •tricyclic-related antidepressants (convulsive threshold lowered); anticonvulsant effect of antiepileptics antagonised by •SSRIs and •tricyclics (convulsive threshold lowered)
• Antiepileptics: plasma concentration of topiramate often reduced by carbamazepine; topiramate increases plasma concentration of •phenytoin (also plasma concentration of topiramate reduced)
• Antimalarials: possible increased risk of convulsions when antiepileptics given with chloroquine and hydroxychloroquine; anticonvulsant effect of antiepileptics antagonised by •mefloquine
• Oestrogens: topiramate accelerates metabolism of •oestrogens (reduced contraceptive effect—see p. 407)
• Progestogens: topiramate accelerates metabolism of •progestogens (reduced contraceptive effect—see p. 407)

Torasemide *see* Diuretics

Toremifene
• Anticoagulants: toremifene possibly enhances anticoagulant effect of •coumarins
Antiepileptics: metabolism of toremifene possibly accelerated by carbamazepine (reduced plasma concentration); metabolism of toremifene possibly accelerated by phenytoin; metabolism of toremifene accelerated by primidone (reduced plasma concentration)
Barbiturates: metabolism of toremifene possibly accelerated by barbiturates (reduced plasma concentration)
Diuretics: increased risk of hypercalcaemia when toremifene given with thiazides and related diuretics

Tramadol *see* Opioid Analgesics
Trandolapril *see* ACE Inhibitors
Tranylcypromine *see* MAOIs
Trazodone *see* Antidepressants, Tricyclic (related)
Tretinoin *see* Retinoids
Triamcinolone *see* Corticosteroids
Triamterene *see* Diuretics
Triclofos *see* Anxiolytics and Hypnotics

Trientine
Iron: trientine reduces absorption of *oral* iron
Zinc: trientine reduces absorption of zinc, also absorption of trientine reduced by zinc

Trifluoperazine *see* Antipsychotics
Trihexyphenidyl (benzhexol) *see* Antimuscarinics

Trilostane
Diuretics: increased risk of hyperkalaemia when trilostane given with potassium-sparing diuretics and aldosterone antagonists

Trimethoprim
• Anti-arrhythmics: increased risk of ventricular arrhythmias when trimethoprim (as co-trimoxazole) given with •amiodarone—avoid concomitant use of co-trimoxazole; trimethoprim increases plasma concentration of procainamide
Antibacterials: plasma concentration of both drugs may increase when trimethoprim given with dapsone
Anticoagulants: trimethoprim possibly enhances anticoagulant effect of coumarins
Antidiabetics: trimethoprim rarely enhances the effects of sulphonylureas
• Antiepileptics: trimethoprim increases plasma concentration of •phenytoin (also increased antifolate effect)
• Antimalarials: increased antifolate effect when trimethoprim given with •pyrimethamine
Antivirals: trimethoprim (as co-trimoxazole) increases plasma concentration of lamivudine—avoid concomitant use of high-dose co-trimoxazole; trimethoprim possibly increases plasma concentration of zalcitabine
Cardiac Glycosides: trimethoprim possibly increases plasma concentration of digoxin
• Ciclosporin: increased risk of nephrotoxicity when trimethoprim given with •ciclosporin, also plasma concentration of ciclosporin reduced by intravenous trimethoprim
• Cytotoxics: increased risk of haematological toxicity when trimethoprim (also with co-trimoxazole) given with •azathioprine, •mercaptopurine or •methotrexate
Diuretics: increased risk of hyperkalaemia when trimethoprim given with eplerenone
Oestrogens: broad-spectrum antibacterials possibly reduce contraceptive effect of oestrogens (risk probably small, see p. 407)

Trimipramine *see* Antidepressants, Tricyclic

Tripotassium Dicitratobismuthate
Antibacterials: tripotassium dicitratobismuthate reduces absorption of tetracyclines
Triprolidine *see* Antihistamines
Tropicamide *see* Antimuscarinics
Tropisetron
Anti-arrhythmics: manufacturer of tropisetron advises caution with anti-arrhythmics (risk of ventricular arrhythmias)
Antibacterials: plasma concentration of tropisetron reduced by rifampicin
Antiepileptics: plasma concentration of tropisetron reduced by primidone
Barbiturates: plasma concentration of tropisetron reduced by phenobarbital
Beta-blockers: manufacturer of tropisetron advises caution with beta-blockers (risk of ventricular arrhythmias)
Trospium *see* Antimuscarinics
Tryptophan
• Antidepressants: possible increased serotonergic effects when tryptophan given with duloxetine; CNS excitation and confusion when tryptophan given with •MAOIs (reduce dose of tryptophan); agitation and nausea may occur when tryptophan given with •SSRIs
• Antimalarials: avoidance of antidepressants advised by manufacturer of •artemether/lumefantrine
• Sibutramine: increased risk of CNS toxicity when tryptophan given with •sibutramine (manufacturer of sibutramine advises avoid concomitant use)
Ulcer-healing Drugs *see* Histamine H_2-antagonists, Proton Pump Inhibitors, Sucralfate, and Tripotassium Dicitratobismuthate
Ursodeoxycholic Acid
Antacids: absorption of bile acids possibly reduced by antacids
• Ciclosporin: ursodeoxycholic acid increases absorption of •ciclosporin
Lipid-regulating Drugs: absorption of bile acids possibly reduced by colestipol and colestyramine
Oestrogens: elimination of cholesterol in bile increased when bile acids given with oestrogens
Vaccines
Note. For a general warning on live vaccines and high doses of corticosteroids or other immunosuppressive drugs, see p. 604 ; for advice on live vaccines and immunoglobulins, see under Normal Immunoglobulin, p. 620
• Adalimumab: avoid concomitant use of live vaccines with •adalimumab (see p. 604)
• Anakinra: avoid concomitant use of live vaccines with •anakinra (see p. 604)
Anticoagulants: influenza vaccine possibly enhances anticoagulant effect of warfarin
Antiepileptics: influenza vaccine enhances effects of phenytoin
• Corticosteroids: immune response to vaccines impaired by high doses of •corticosteroids, avoid concomitant use with live vaccines (see p. 604)
• Efalizumab: live or live-attenuated vaccines should be given 2 weeks before •efalizumab or withheld until 8 weeks after discontinuation
• Etanercept: avoid concomitant use of live vaccines with •etanercept (see p. 604)
• Infliximab: avoid concomitant use of live vaccines with •infliximab (see p. 604)
Interferons: avoidance of vaccines advised by manufacturer of interferon gamma
• Leflunomide: avoid concomitant use of live vaccines with •leflunomide (see p. 604)
Theophylline: influenza vaccine possibly increases plasma concentration of theophylline
Valaciclovir *see* Aciclovir
Valganciclovir *see* Ganciclovir
Valproate
Analgesics: effects of valproate enhanced by aspirin
Antibacterials: plasma concentration of valproate possibly reduced by ertapenem; plasma concentration of valproate reduced by meropenem; metabolism of valproate possibly inhibited by erythromycin (increased plasma concentration)
Anticoagulants: valproate possibly enhances anticoagulant effect of coumarins
• Antidepressants: anticonvulsant effect of antiepileptics possibly antagonised by MAOIs and •tricyclic-related antidepressants (convulsive threshold lowered); anticonvulsant effect of antiepileptics antagonised by •SSRIs and •tricyclics (convulsive threshold lowered)
• Antiepileptics: plasma concentration of valproate reduced by carbamazepine, also plasma concentration of active metabolite of carbamazepine increased; valproate possibly increases plasma concentration of ethosuximide; valproate increases plasma concentration of lamotrigine; valproate sometimes reduces plasma concentration of an active metabolite of oxcarbazepine; valproate increases or possibly decreases plasma concentration of phenytoin, also plasma concentration of valproate reduced; valproate possibly increases plasma concentration of •primidone (plasma concentration of active metabolite of primidone increased), also plasma concentration of valproate reduced
• Antimalarials: possible increased risk of convulsions when antiepileptics given with chloroquine and hydroxychloroquine; anticonvulsant effect of antiepileptics and valproate antagonised by •mefloquine
• Antipsychotics: anticonvulsant effect of valproate antagonised by •antipsychotics (convulsive threshold lowered); increased risk of neutropenia when valproate given with •olanzapine
Antivirals: valproate possibly increases plasma concentration of zidovudine (increased risk of toxicity)
Barbiturates: valproate increases plasma concentration of phenobarbital (also plasma concentration of valproate reduced)
Bupropion: valproate inhibits the metabolism of bupropion
Cytotoxics: valproate increases plasma concentration of temozolomide
Lipid-regulating Drugs: absorption of valproate possibly reduced by colestyramine
Sodium Benzoate: valproate possibly reduces effects of sodium benzoate
Sodium Phenylbutyrate: valproate possibly reduces effects of sodium phenylbutyrate
• Ulcer-healing Drugs: metabolism of valproate inhibited by •cimetidine (increased plasma concentration)
Valsartan *see* Angiotensin-II Receptor Antagonists
Vancomycin
Anaesthetics, General: hypersensitivity-like reactions can occur when intravenous vancomycin given with general anaesthetics
Antibacterials: increased risk of nephrotoxicity and ototoxicity when vancomycin given with aminoglycosides, capreomycin or colistin; increased risk of nephrotoxicity when vancomycin given with polymyxins
Antifungals: possible increased risk of nephrotoxicity when vancomycin given with amphotericin
• Ciclosporin: increased risk of nephrotoxicity when vancomycin given with •ciclosporin

Vancomycin *(continued)*
Cytotoxics: increased risk of nephrotoxicity and possibly of ototoxicity when vancomycin given with cisplatin
- Diuretics: increased risk of otoxicity when vancomycin given with •loop diuretics
Lipid-regulating Drugs: effects of oral vancomycin antagonised by colestyramine
- Muscle Relaxants: vancomycin enhances effects of •suxamethonium
Oestrogens: broad-spectrum antibacterials possibly reduce contraceptive effect of oestrogens (risk probably small, see p. 407)

Vardenafil
- Alpha-blockers: possible increased hypotensive effect when vardenafil given with •alpha-blockers—avoid concomitant use
Antibacterials: plasma concentration of vardenafil increased by erythromycin (reduce dose of vardenafil)
- Antifungals: plasma concentration of vardenafil increased by •ketoconazole—avoid concomitant use; plasma concentration of vardenafil possibly increased by •itraconazole—avoid concomitant use
- Antivirals: plasma concentration of vardenafil possibly increased by amprenavir; plasma concentration of vardenafil increased by •indinavir—avoid concomitant use; plasma concentration of vardenafil possibly increased by •ritonavir—avoid concomitant use; plasma concentration of vardenafil possibly increased by saquinavir— reduce initial dose of vardenafil
Calcium-channel Blockers: enhanced hypotensive effect when vardenafil given with nifedipine
- Grapefruit Juice: plasma concentration of vardenafil possibly increased by •grapefruit juice—avoid concomitant use
- Nicorandil: possible increased hypotensive effect when vardenafil given with •nicorandil—avoid concomitant use
- Nitrates: possible increased hypotensive effect when vardenafil given with •nitrates—avoid concomitant use

Vasodilator Antihypertensives
ACE Inhibitors: enhanced hypotensive effect when hydralazine, minoxidil or nitroprusside given with ACE inhibitors
Adrenergic Neurone Blockers: enhanced hypotensive effect when hydralazine, minoxidil or nitroprusside given with adrenergic neurone blockers
Alcohol: enhanced hypotensive effect when hydralazine, minoxidil or nitroprusside given with alcohol
Aldesleukin: enhanced hypotensive effect when hydralazine, minoxidil or nitroprusside given with aldesleukin
Alpha-blockers: enhanced hypotensive effect when hydralazine, minoxidil or nitroprusside given with alpha-blockers
Anaesthetics, General: enhanced hypotensive effect when hydralazine, minoxidil or nitroprusside given with general anaesthetics
Analgesics: hypotensive effect of hydralazine, minoxidil and nitroprusside antagonised by NSAIDs
Angiotensin-II Receptor Antagonists: enhanced hypotensive effect when hydralazine, minoxidil or nitroprusside given with angiotensin-II receptor antagonists
Antidepressants: enhanced hypotensive effect when hydralazine, minoxidil or nitroprusside given with MAOIs; enhanced hypotensive effect when hydralazine or nitroprusside given with tricyclic-related antidepressants
Antipsychotics: enhanced hypotensive effect when hydralazine, minoxidil or nitroprusside given with phenothiazines
Anxiolytics and Hypnotics: enhanced hypotensive effect when hydralazine, minoxidil or nitroprusside given with anxiolytics and hypnotics
Beta-blockers: enhanced hypotensive effect when hydralazine, minoxidil or nitroprusside given with beta-blockers
Calcium-channel Blockers: enhanced hypotensive effect when hydralazine, minoxidil or nitroprusside given with calcium-channel blockers
Clonidine: enhanced hypotensive effect when hydralazine, minoxidil or nitroprusside given with clonidine
Corticosteroids: hypotensive effect of hydralazine, minoxidil and nitroprusside antagonised by corticosteroids
Diazoxide: enhanced hypotensive effect when hydralazine, minoxidil or nitroprusside given with diazoxide
Diuretics: enhanced hypotensive effect when hydralazine, minoxidil or nitroprusside given with diuretics
Dopaminergics: enhanced hypotensive effect when hydralazine, minoxidil or nitroprusside given with levodopa
Methyldopa: enhanced hypotensive effect when hydralazine, minoxidil or nitroprusside given with methyldopa
Moxisylyte (thymoxamine): enhanced hypotensive effect when hydralazine, minoxidil or nitroprusside given with moxisylyte
Moxonidine: enhanced hypotensive effect when hydralazine, minoxidil or nitroprusside given with moxonidine
Muscle Relaxants: enhanced hypotensive effect when hydralazine, minoxidil or nitroprusside given with baclofen; enhanced hypotensive effect when hydralazine, minoxidil or nitroprusside given with tizanidine
Nicorandil: possible enhanced hypotensive effect when hydralazine, minoxidil or nitroprusside given with nicorandil
Nitrates: enhanced hypotensive effect when hydralazine, minoxidil or nitroprusside given with nitrates
Oestrogens: hypotensive effect of hydralazine, minoxidil and nitroprusside antagonised by oestrogens
Prostaglandins: enhanced hypotensive effect when hydralazine, minoxidil or nitroprusside given with alprostadil
Vasodilator Antihypertensives: enhanced hypotensive effect when hydralazine given with minoxidil or nitroprusside; enhanced hypotensive effect when minoxidil given with nitroprusside

Vecuronium *see* Muscle Relaxants

Venlafaxine
- Analgesics: increased risk of bleeding when venlafaxine given with •NSAIDs or •aspirin
- Anticoagulants: venlafaxine possibly enhances anticoagulant effect of •warfarin
- Antidepressants: possible increased serotonergic effects when venlafaxine given with duloxetine; enhanced CNS effects and toxicity when venlafaxine given with •MAOIs (venlafaxine should not be started until 2 weeks after stopping MAOIs, avoid MAOIs for 1 week after stopping venlafax-

Venlafaxine
- Antidepressants *(continued)* ine); after stopping SSRI-related antidepressants do not start •moclobemide for at least 1 week
- Antimalarials: avoidance of antidepressants advised by manufacturer of •artemether/lumefantrine
- Antipsychotics: venlafaxine increases plasma concentration of •clozapine and haloperidol
- Dopaminergics: caution with venlafaxine advised by manufacturer of entacapone; increased risk of hypertension and CNS excitation when venlafaxine given with •selegiline (selegiline should not be started until 1 week after stopping venlafaxine, avoid venlafaxine for 2 weeks after stopping selegiline)
- Sibutramine: increased risk of CNS toxicity when SSRI-related antidepressants given with •sibutramine (manufacturer of sibutramine advises avoid concomitant use)

Verapamil *see* Calcium-channel Blockers

Vigabatrin
- Antidepressants: anticonvulsant effect of antiepileptics possibly antagonised by MAOIs and •tricyclic-related antidepressants (convulsive threshold lowered); anticonvulsant effect of antiepileptics antagonised by •SSRIs and •tricyclics (convulsive threshold lowered)

  Antiepileptics: vigabatrin reduces plasma concentration of phenytoin; vigabatrin possibly reduces plasma concentration of primidone
- Antimalarials: possible increased risk of convulsions when antiepileptics given with chloroquine and hydroxychloroquine; anticonvulsant effect of antiepileptics antagonised by •mefloquine

  Barbiturates: vigabatrin possibly reduces plasma concentration of phenobarbital

Vinblastine
- Antibacterials: toxicity of vinblastine increased by •erythromycin—avoid concomitant use

  Antiepileptics: cytotoxics possibly reduce absorption of phenytoin
- Antipsychotics: avoid concomitant use of cytotoxics with •clozapine (increased risk of agranulocytosis)

Vincristine

Antiepileptics: cytotoxics possibly reduce absorption of phenytoin
- Antifungals: metabolism of vincristine possibly inhibited by •itraconazole (increased risk of neurotoxicity)
- Antipsychotics: avoid concomitant use of cytotoxics with •clozapine (increased risk of agranulocytosis)

  Calcium-channel Blockers: metabolism of vincristine possibly inhibited by nifedipine

Vitamin A *see* Vitamins

Vitamin D *see* Vitamins

Vitamin K (Phytomenadione) *see* Vitamins

Vitamins

Antibacterials: absorption of vitamin A possibly reduced by neomycin
- Anticoagulants: vitamin K antagonises anticoagulant effect of •coumarins and •phenindione

  Antiepileptics: vitamin D requirements possibly increased when given with carbamazepine, phenytoin or primidone

  Barbiturates: vitamin D requirements possibly increased when given with barbiturates

  Diuretics: increased risk of hypercalcaemia when vitamin D given with thiazides and related diuretics

  Dopaminergics: pyridoxine reduces effects of levodopa when given without dopa-decarboxylase inhibitor

Vitamins *(continued)*

Retinoids: risk of hypervitaminosis A when vitamin A given with retinoids

Voriconazole *see* Antifungals, Triazole

Warfarin *see* Coumarins

Xipamide *see* Diuretics

Xylometazoline *see* Sympathomimetics

Zafirlukast *see* Leukotriene Antagonists

Zalcitabine

Note. Clinical data limited. Avoid use with other drugs which have a potential to cause peripheral neuropathy or pancreatitis—for further details consult product literature

Antacids: absorption of zalcitabine reduced by antacids

Antibacterials: plasma concentration of zalcitabine possibly increased by trimethoprim

Antivirals: avoidance of zalcitabine advised by manufacturer of emtricitabine; effects of zalcitabine possibly inhibited by lamivudine (manufacturers advise avoid concomitant use)

Probenecid: excretion of zalcitabine possibly reduced by probenecid (increased plasma concentration)

Ulcer-healing Drugs: plasma concentration of zalcitabine possibly increased by cimetidine

Zaleplon *see* Anxiolytics and Hypnotics

Zidovudine

Note. Increased risk of toxicity with nephrotoxic and myelosuppressive drugs - for further details consult product literature

Analgesics: increased risk of haematological toxicity when zidovudine given with NSAIDs; plasma concentration of zidovudine possibly increased by methadone

Antibacterials: absorption of zidovudine reduced by clarithromycin tablets; manufacturer of zidovudine advises avoid concomitant use with rifampicin

Antiepileptics: zidovudine increases or decreases plasma concentration of phenytoin; plasma concentration of zidovudine possibly increased by valproate (increased risk of toxicity)
- Antifungals: plasma concentration of zidovudine increased by •fluconazole (increased risk of toxicity)

  Antimalarials: increased antifolate effect when zidovudine given with pyrimethamine
- Antivirals: profound myelosuppression when zidovudine given with •ganciclovir (if possible avoid concomitant administration, particularly during initial ganciclovir therapy); effects of zidovudine possibly inhibited by •ribavirin (manufacturer of zidovudine advises avoid concomitant use); zidovudine possibly inhibits effects of •stavudine (manufacturers advise avoid concomitant use)

  Atovaquone: metabolism of zidovudine possibly inhibited by atovaquone (increased plasma concentration)

  Probenecid: excretion of zidovudine reduced by probenecid (increased plasma concentration and risk of toxicity)

Zinc

Antibacterials: zinc reduces absorption of ciprofloxacin, levofloxacin, moxifloxacin, norfloxacin and ofloxacin; zinc reduces absorption of tetracyclines, also absorption of zinc reduced by tetracyclines

Calcium Salts: absorption of zinc reduced by calcium salts

Iron: absorption of zinc reduced by *oral* iron, also absorption of *oral* iron reduced by zinc

Penicillamine: absorption of zinc reduced by penicillamine, also absorption of penicillamine reduced by zinc

Zinc *(continued)*
Trientine: absorption of zinc reduced by trientine, also absorption of trientine reduced by zinc
Zoledronic Acid *see* Bisphosphonates
Zolmitriptan *see* $5HT_1$ Agonists
Zolpidem *see* Anxiolytics and Hypnotics
Zonisamide
• Antidepressants: anticonvulsant effect of antiepileptics possibly antagonised by MAOIs and •tricyclic-related antidepressants (convulsive threshold lowered); anticonvulsant effect of antiepileptics antagonised by •SSRIs and •tricyclics (convulsive threshold lowered)
Antiepileptics: plasma concentration of zonisamide reduced by carbamazepine, effect on carbamazepine plasma concentration not predictable; plasma concentration of zonisamide reduced by phenytoin
• Antimalarials: possible increased risk of convulsions when antiepileptics given with chloroquine and hydroxychloroquine; anticonvulsant effect of antiepileptics antagonised by •mefloquine
Barbiturates: plasma concentration of zonisamide reduced by phenobarbital
Zopiclone *see* Anxiolytics and Hypnotics
Zotepine *see* Antipsychotics
Zuclopenthixol *see* Antipsychotics

Appendix 2: Liver disease

Liver disease may alter the response to drugs in several ways as indicated below, and drug prescribing should be kept to a minimum in all patients with severe liver disease. The main problems occur in patients with jaundice, ascites, or evidence of encephalopathy.

IMPAIRED DRUG METABOLISM. Metabolism by the liver is the main route of elimination for many drugs, but the hepatic reserve appears to be large and liver disease has to be severe before important changes in drug metabolism occur. Routine liver-function tests are a poor guide to the capacity of the liver to metabolise drugs, and in the individual patient it is not possible to predict the extent to which the metabolism of a particular drug may be impaired.

A few drugs, e.g. rifampicin and fusidic acid, are excreted in the bile unchanged and may accumulate in patients with intrahepatic or extrahepatic obstructive jaundice.

HYPOPROTEINAEMIA. The hypoalbuminaemia in severe liver disease is associated with reduced protein binding and increased toxicity of some highly protein-bound drugs such as phenytoin and prednisolone.

REDUCED CLOTTING. Reduced hepatic synthesis of blood-clotting factors, indicated by a prolonged prothrombin time, increases the sensitivity to oral anticoagulants such as warfarin and phenindione.

HEPATIC ENCEPHALOPATHY. In severe liver disease many drugs can further impair cerebral function and may precipitate hepatic encephalopathy. These include all sedative drugs, opioid analgesics, those diuretics that produce hypokalaemia, and drugs that cause constipation.

FLUID OVERLOAD. Oedema and ascites in chronic liver disease may be exacerbated by drugs that give rise to fluid retention, e.g. NSAIDs, corticosteroids, and carbenoxolone.

HEPATOTOXIC DRUGS. Hepatotoxicity is either dose-related or unpredictable (idiosyncratic). Drugs causing dose-related toxicity may do so at lower doses than in patients with normal liver function, and some drugs producing reactions of the idiosyncratic kind do so more frequently in patients with liver disease. These drugs should be avoided or used very carefully.

Table of drugs to be avoided or used with caution in liver disease

The list of drugs given below is not comprehensive and is based on current information concerning the use of these drugs in therapeutic dosage. Products introduced or amended since publication of BNF No. 49 (March 2005) are underlined.

Drug	Comment
Abacavir	Avoid in moderate hepatic impairment unless essential; avoid in severe hepatic impairment
Abciximab	Avoid in severe liver disease—increased risk of bleeding
Acamprosate	Avoid in severe liver disease
Acarbose	Avoid
ACE inhibitors	Use of prodrugs such as cilazapril, enalapril, fosinopril, imidapril, moexipril, perindopril, quinapril, ramipril, and trandolapril requires close monitoring in patients with impaired liver function
Aceclofenac	*see* NSAIDs
Acemetacin	*see* NSAIDs
Acenocoumarol (nicoumalone)	*see* Anticoagulants, Oral
Acitretin	Avoid—further impairment of liver function may occur
Alfentanil	*see* Opioid Analgesics
Alfuzosin	Reduce dose in mild to moderate liver disease; avoid if severe
Alimemazine (trimeprazine)	Avoid—may precipitate coma in severe liver disease; hepatotoxic
Allopurinol	Reduce dose
Almotriptan	Manufacturer advises caution in mild to moderate liver disease; avoid in severe liver disease
Alprazolam	*see* Anxiolytics and Hypnotics
Alteplase	Avoid in severe hepatic impairment
Amfebutamone	*see* Bupropion
Aminophylline	*see* Theophylline
Amitriptyline	*see* Antidepressants, Tricyclic (and related)
Amlodipine	Half-life prolonged—may need dose reduction
Amoxapine	*see* Antidepressants, Tricyclic (and related)
Amprenavir	Avoid oral solution due to high propylene glycol content; reduce dose of capsules to 450 mg every 12 hours in moderate hepatic impairment and reduce dose to 300 mg every 12 hours in severe impairment
Amsacrine	Reduce dose
Anabolic steroids	Preferably avoid—dose-related toxicity
<u>Anagrelide</u>	Manufacturer advises caution in mild to moderate hepatic impairment; avoid in severe impairment

Drug	Comment
Analgesics	*see* Aspirin, NSAIDs, Opioid Analgesics and Paracetamol
Anastrozole	Avoid in moderate to severe liver disease
Androgens	Preferably avoid—dose-related toxicity with some, and produce fluid retention
Antacids	In patients with fluid retention, avoid those containing large amounts of sodium, e.g. magnesium trisilicate mixture, *Gaviscon*®
	Avoid those causing constipation—can precipitate coma
Anticoagulants, oral	Avoid in severe liver disease, especially if prothrombin time already prolonged
Antidepressants, MAOI	May cause idiosyncratic hepatotoxicity; see also Moclobemide
Antidepressants, SSRI	Reduce dose or avoid
Antidepressants, tricyclic (and related)	Tricyclics preferable to MAOIs but sedative effects increased (avoid in severe liver disease)
Antihistamines	*see* individual entries
Antipsychotics	All can precipitate coma; phenothiazines are hepatotoxic; *see also* Aripiprazole, Clozapine, Olanzapine, Quetiapine, Risperidone and Sertindole
Anxiolytics and hypnotics	All can precipitate coma; small dose of oxazepam or temazepam probably safest; reduce oral dose of clomethiazole; reduce dose of zaleplon to 5 mg (avoid if severe); reduce dose of zolpidem to 5 mg (avoid if severe); reduce dose of zopiclone (avoid if severe); *see also* Chloral Hydrate
Apomorphine	Low sublingual doses may be used with caution for erectile dysfunction
Aprepitant	Manufacturer advises caution in moderate to severe hepatic impairment
Aripiprazole	Manufacturer advises use with caution in severe impairment
Artemether [ingredient]	*see Riamet*®
Aspirin	Avoid in severe hepatic impairment—increased risk of gastro-intestinal bleeding
Atazanavir	Manufacturer advises caution in mild hepatic impairment; avoid in moderate to severe hepatic impairment
Atomoxetine	Halve dose in moderate liver disease; quarter dose in severe liver disease
Atorvastatin	*see* Statins
Atosiban	No information available
Atovaquone	Manufacturer advises caution—monitor more closely
Auranofin	Caution in mild to moderate liver disease; avoid in severe liver disease
Azathioprine	May need dose reduction
Azithromycin	Avoid; jaundice reported
Bambuterol	Avoid in severe liver disease
Bemiparin	Manufacturer advises avoid in severe liver disease
Bendrofluazide	*see* Thiazides and Related Diuretics
Bendroflumethiazide (bendrofluazide)	*see* Thiazides and Related Diuretics
Benperidol	*see* Antipsychotics
Benzthiazide	*see* Thiazides and Related Diuretics
Bexarotene	Avoid
Bezafibrate	Avoid in severe liver disease
Bicalutamide	Increased accumulation possible in moderate to severe hepatic impairment
Bisoprolol	Max. 10 mg daily in severe liver impairment
Bortezomib	Manufacturer advises caution in mild to moderate hepatic impairment—consider dose reduction; avoid in severe hepatic impairment
Bosentan	Avoid in moderate and severe hepatic impairment
Bromocriptine	Dose reduction may be necessary
Buclizine	Sedation inappropriate in severe liver disease—avoid
Budesonide	Plasma-budesonide concentration may increase on oral administration
Bumetanide	*see* Loop Diuretics
Bupivacaine	*see* Lidocaine
Buprenorphine	*see* Opioid Analgesics
Bupropion	Manufacturer recommends 150 mg daily; avoid in severe hepatic cirrhosis
Buspirone	Reduce dose in mild to moderate liver disease; avoid in severe liver disease
Cabergoline	Reduce dose in severe hepatic impairment
Calcitriol	Manufacturer of topical calcitriol advises avoid in severe liver disease
Candesartan	For hypertension, initially 2 mg once daily in mild or moderate hepatic impairment (no initial dose adjustment necessary in heart failure); avoid in severe hepatic impairment
Capecitabine	Manufacturer advises avoid in severe hepatic impairment
Carbamazepine	Metabolism impaired in advanced liver disease
Carvedilol	Avoid
Caspofungin	70 mg on first day then 35 mg once daily in moderate hepatic impairment; no information available for severe hepatic impairment
Ceftriaxone	Reduce dose and monitor plasma concentration if both hepatic and severe renal impairment
Celecoxib	*see* NSAIDs
Cetrorelix	Manufacturer advises avoid in moderate or severe liver impairment

Drug	Comment
Chloral hydrate	Reduce dose in mild to moderate hepatic impairment; avoid in severe impairment; *see also* Anxiolytics and Hypnotics
Chlorambucil	Manufacturer advises consider dose reduction in severe hepatic impairment—limited information available
Chloramphenicol	Avoid if possible—increased risk of bone-marrow depression; reduce dose and monitor plasma-chloramphenicol concentration
Chlordiazepoxide	*see* Anxiolytics and Hypnotics
Chlorphenamine (chlorpheniramine)	Sedation inappropriate in severe liver disease—avoid
Chlorpheniramine	*see* Chorphenamine
Chlorpromazine	*see* Antipsychotics
Chlorpropamide	*see* Sulphonylureas
Chlortalidone	*see* Thiazides and Related Diuretics
Chlortetracycline	*see* Tetracyclines
Ciclosporin	May need dose adjustment
Cilazapril	*see* ACE Inhibitors
Cilostazol	Avoid in moderate or severe liver disease
Cimetidine	Increased risk of confusion; reduce dose
Cinacalcet	Manufacturer advises caution in moderate to severe hepatic impairment—monitor closely especially when increasing dose
Cinnarizine	Sedation inappropriate in severe liver disease—avoid
Ciprofibrate	Avoid in severe liver disease
Citalopram	Use doses at lower end of range
Cladribine	Regular monitoring recommended
Clarithromycin	Hepatic dysfunction including jaundice reported
Clavulanic acid [ingredient]	*see* Co-amoxiclav, below and *Timentin®*, p. 733
Clemastine	Sedation inappropriate in severe liver disease—avoid
Clindamycin	Reduce dose
Clobazam	*see* Anxiolytics and Hypnotics
Clomethiazole	*see* Anxiolytics and Hypnotics
Clomifene	Avoid in severe liver disease
Clomipramine	*see* Antidepressants, Tricyclic (and related)
Clonazepam	Reduce dose in mild to moderate impairment; avoid in severe liver impairment; *see also* Anxiolytics and Hypnotics
Clopamide	*see* Thiazides and Related Diuretics
Clopidogrel	Manufacturer advises caution (risk of bleeding); avoid in severe hepatic impairment
Clorazepate	*see* Anxiolytics and Hypnotics
Clozapine	Initial dose 12.5 mg daily increased slowly with regular monitoring of liver function; avoid in symptomatic or progressive liver disease or hepatic failure
Co-amoxiclav	Monitor liver function in liver disease. Cholestatic jaundice, *see* p. 277
Codeine	*see* Opioid Analgesics
Colestyramine	Interferes with absorption of fat-soluble vitamins and may aggravate malabsorption in primary biliary cirrhosis; likely to be ineffective in complete biliary obstruction
Contraceptives, oral	Avoid in active liver disease and if history of pruritus or cholestasis during pregnancy
Co-trimoxazole	Manufacturer advises avoid in severe liver disease
Cyclizine	Sedation inappropriate in severe liver disease—avoid
Cyclopenthiazide	*see* Thiazides and Related Diuretics
Cyclophosphamide	Reduce dose
Cyclosporin	*see* Ciclosporin
Cyproheptadine	Sedation inappropriate in severe liver disease—avoid
Cyproterone acetate	Dose-related toxicity; *see also* side-effects of cyproterone, section 8.3.4.2
Cytarabine	Reduce dose
Dacarbazine	Dose reduction may be required in mild to moderate liver disease; avoid if severe
Dalfopristin [ingredient]	*see Synercid®*
Dalteparin	*see* Heparin
Danaparoid	Use with caution in moderate hepatic impairment (increased risk of bleeding); avoid in severe hepatic impairment unless patient has heparin-induced thrombocytopenia and no alternative
Dantrolene	Avoid oral use—may cause severe liver damage; injection may be used in emergency for malignant hyperthermia
Darbepoetin	Manufacturer advises caution
Daunorubicin	Reduce dose
Deferiprone	Manufacturer advises monitor liver function—interrupt treatment if persistent elevation in serum alanine aminotransferase
Demeclocycline	*see* Tetracyclines
Desflurane	Reduce dose
Desogestrel	Avoid; *see also* Contraceptives, Oral
Deteclo®	*see* Tetracyclines
Dexketoprofen	*see* NSAIDs
Dextromethorphan	*see* Opioid Analgesics
Dextropropoxyphene	*see* Opioid Analgesics
Diamorphine	*see* Opioid Analgesics
Diazepam	*see* Anxiolytics and Hypnotics
Diclofenac	*see* NSAIDs
Didanosine	Insufficient information but monitor for toxicity
Diethylstilbestrol	Avoid; *see also* Contraceptives, Oral
Diflunisal	*see* NSAIDs
Dihydrocodeine	*see* Opioid Analgesics
Diltiazem	Reduce dose
Diphenhydramine	Caution in mild to moderate liver disease; avoid in severe disease if sedation is inappropriate
Diphenoxylate	*see* Opioid Analgesics

Drug	Comment
Dipipanone	*see* Opioid Analgesics
Disodium pamidronate	Manufacturer advises caution in severe hepatic impairment—no information available
Disopyramide	Half-life prolonged—may need dose reduction
Docetaxel	Monitor liver function—reduce dose according to liver enzymes; avoid in severe hepatic impairment
Domperidone	Avoid
Dosulepin (dothiepin)	*see* Antidepressants, Tricyclic (and related)
Dothiepin	*see* Antidepressants, Tricyclic (and related)
Doxazosin	No information—manufacturer advises caution
Doxepin	*see* Antidepressants, Tricyclic (and related)
Doxorubicin	Reduce dose according to bilirubin concentration
Doxycycline	*see* Tetracyclines
Doxylamine	Caution in mild to moderate liver disease; avoid in severe disease if sedation is inappropriate
Drotrecogin alfa (activated)	Avoid in chronic severe liver disease
Dutasteride	Manufacturer advises avoid in severe liver impairment—no information available
Dydrogesterone	Avoid; *see also* Contraceptives, Oral
Efavirenz	In mild to moderate liver disease, monitor for dose related side-effects (e.g. CNS effects) and monitor liver function; avoid in severe hepatic impairment
Eformoterol	*see* Formoterol
Eletriptan	Manufacturer advises avoid in severe hepatic impairment
Enalapril	*see* ACE Inhibitors
Enfuvirtide	Manufacturer advises caution—no information available
Enoxaparin	*see* Heparin
Entacapone	Avoid
Epirubicin	Reduce dose according to bilirubin concentration
Eplerenone	Avoid in severe liver disease
Epoetin	Manufacturers advise caution in chronic hepatic failure
Eprosartan	Halve initial dose in mild or moderate liver disease; avoid if severe
Eptifibatide	Avoid in severe liver disease—increased risk of bleeding
Ergometrine	Avoid in severe liver disease
Ergotamine	Avoid in severe liver disease—risk of toxicity increased
Erythromycin	May cause idiosyncratic hepatotoxicity
Escitalopram	Initial dose 5 mg daily (for 2 weeks), increased to 10 mg daily according to response
Esomeprazole	In severe liver disease dose should not exceed 20 mg daily
Estradiol	Avoid; *see also* Contraceptives, Oral
Estramustine	Manufacturer advises caution and regular liver function tests; avoid in severe liver disease
Estriol	Avoid; *see also* Contraceptives, Oral
Estrone	Avoid; *see also* Contraceptives, Oral
Estropipate	Avoid; *see also* Contraceptives, Oral
Ethinylestradiol	Avoid; *see also* Contraceptives, Oral
Etodolac	*see* NSAIDs
Etoposide	Avoid in severe hepatic impairment
Etynodiol diacetate	Avoid; *see also* Contraceptives, Oral
Exemestane	Manufacturer advises caution
Ezetimibe	Avoid in moderate and severe hepatic impairment—may accumulate
Famciclovir	Usual dose in well compensated liver disease (information not available on decompensated)
Felodipine	Reduce dose
Fenbufen	*see* NSAIDs
Fenofibrate	Avoid in severe liver disease
Fenoprofen	*see* NSAIDs
Fentanyl	*see* Opioid Analgesics
Flecainide	Avoid (or reduce dose) in severe liver disease
Flucloxacillin	Caution in hepatic impairment (risk of cholestatic jaundice and hepatitis, *see* p. 274)
Fluconazole	Toxicity with related drugs
Fluorouracil	Manufacturer advises caution
Fluoxetine	*see* Antidepressants, SSRI
Flupentixol	*see* Antipsychotics
Fluphenazine	*see* Antipsychotics
Flurazepam	*see* Anxiolytics and Hypnotics
Flurbiprofen	*see* NSAIDs
Flutamide	Use with caution (hepatotoxic)
Fluvastatin	*see* Statins
Fluvoxamine	*see* Antidepressants, SSRI
Fondaparinux sodium	Caution in severe hepatic impairment (increased risk of bleeding)
Formoterol (eformoterol)	Metabolism possibly reduced in severe cirrhosis
Fosamprenavir	Manufacturer advises caution in mild to moderate hepatic impairment; avoid in severe hepatic impairment
Fosinopril	*see* ACE Inhibitors
Fosphenytoin	Consider 10–25% reduction in dose or infusion rate (except initial dose for status epilepticus)
Frovatriptan	Avoid in severe hepatic impairment
Frusemide	*see* Loop Diuretics
Fulvestrant	Manufacturer advises caution in mild to moderate hepatic impairment; avoid in severe hepatic impairment
Furosemide (frusemide)	*see* Loop Diuretics
Fusidic acid	*see* Sodium Fusidate
Galantamine	Reduce dose in moderate hepatic impairment; avoid in severe impairment

Drug	Comment
Ganirelix	Manufacturer advises avoid in moderate or severe hepatic impairment
Gemcitabine	Manufacturer advises caution
Gemfibrozil	Avoid in liver disease
Gestodene	Avoid; *see also* Contraceptives, Oral
Gestrinone	Avoid in severe liver disease
Glibenclamide	*see* Sulphonylureas
Gliclazide	*see* Sulphonylureas
Glimepiride	Manufacturer advises avoid in severe hepatic impairment
Glipizide	*see* Sulphonylureas
Gliquidone	*see* Sulphonylureas
Griseofulvin	Avoid in severe liver disease
Haloperidol	*see* Antipsychotics
Halothane	Avoid if history of unexplained pyrexia or jaundice following previous exposure to halothane
Heparin	Reduce dose in severe liver disease
Hydralazine	Reduce dose
Hydrochlorothiazide	*see* Thiazides and Related Diuretics
Hydroflumethiazide	*see* Thiazides and Related Diuretics
Hydromorphone	*see* Opioid Analgesics
Hydroxyzine	Sedation inappropriate in severe liver disease—avoid
Hyoscine hydrobromide	Manufacturer advises caution
Hypnotics	*see* Anxiolytics and Hypnotics
Ibandronic acid	Manufacturer advises caution in severe hepatic impairment—limited information available
Ibuprofen	*see* NSAIDs
Idarubicin	Reduce dose according to bilirubin concentration
Ifosfamide	Avoid
Iloprost	Elimination reduced in hepatic impairment—initially 2.5 micrograms no more frequently than every 3 hours (max. 6 times daily), adjusted according to response (consult product literature)
Imidapril	*see* ACE Inhibitors
Imipramine	*see* Antidepressants, Tricyclic (and related)
Indapamide	*see* Thiazides and Related Diuretics
Indinavir	Increased risk of nephrolithiasis; reduce dose to 600 mg every 8 hours in mild to moderate hepatic impairment; not studied in severe impairment
Indometacin	*see* NSAIDs
Indoramin	Manufacturer advises caution
Interferon alfa	Close monitoring in mild to moderate hepatic impairment; avoid if severe
Interferon beta	Avoid in decompensated liver disease
Interferon gamma-1b	Manufacturer advises caution in severe liver disease
Irinotecan	Monitor closely for neutropenia if plasma-bilirubin concentration up to 1.5 times upper limit of normal range; avoid if plasma-bilirubin concentration greater than 1.5 times upper limit of normal range
Iron dextran	Avoid in severe hepatic impairment
Iron sorbital	Avoid
Iron sucrose	Avoid
Isocarboxazid	*see* Antidepressants, MAOI
Isometheptene [ingredient]	*see Midrid*®
Isoniazid	Use with caution; monitor liver function regularly and particularly frequently in the first 2 months; *see also* p. 299
Isotretinoin	Avoid—further impairment of liver function may occur
Isradipine	Reduce dose
Itraconazole	Use only if potential benefit outweighs risk of hepatotoxicity (*see* p. 311); dose reduction may be necessary
Kaletra®	Avoid oral solution because of propylene glycol content; manufacturer advises avoid capsules in severe hepatic impairment
Ketoconazole	Avoid
Ketoprofen	*see* NSAIDs
Ketorolac	*see* NSAIDs
Ketotifen	Sedation inappropriate in severe liver disease—avoid
Labetalol	Avoid—severe hepatocellular injury reported
Lacidipine	Antihypertensive effect possibly increased
Lamotrigine	Halve dose in moderate liver disease; quarter dose in severe liver disease
Lansoprazole	In severe liver disease dose should not exceed 30 mg daily
Leflunomide	Avoid—active metabolite may accumulate
Lepirudin	No information—manufacturer advises that cirrhosis may affect renal excretion
Lercanidipine	Avoid in severe liver disease
Levetiracetam	Halve dose in severe hepatic impairment (due to concomitant renal impairment)
Levobupivacaine	Manufacturer advises caution in liver disease
Levomepromazine (methotrimeprazine)	*see* Antipsychotics
Levonorgestrel	Avoid; *see also* Contraceptives, Oral
Lidocaine (lignocaine)	Avoid (or reduce dose) in severe liver disease
Lignocaine	*see* Lidocaine
Linezolid	In severe hepatic impairment manufacturer advises use only if potential benefit outweighs risk
Lofepramine	*see* Antidepressants, Tricyclic (and related)

Drug	Comment
Loop diuretics	Hypokalaemia may precipitate coma (use potassium-sparing diuretic to prevent this); increased risk of hypomagnesaemia in alcoholic cirrhosis
Lopinavir [ingredient]	*see Kaletra®*
Loprazolam	*see* Anxiolytics and Hypnotics
Lorazepam	*see* Anxiolytics and Hypnotics
Lormetazepam	*see* Anxiolytics and Hypnotics
Losartan	Consider lower dose
Lumefantrine [ingredient]	*see Riamet®*
Lymecycline	*see* Tetracyclines
Magnesium salts	Avoid in hepatic coma if risk of renal failure
Maprotiline	*see* Antidepressants, Tricyclic (and related)
Meclozine	Sedation inappropriate in severe liver disease—avoid
Medroxyprogesterone	Avoid; *see also* Contraceptives, Oral
Mefenamic acid	*see* NSAIDs
Mefloquine	Avoid for prophylaxis in severe liver disease
Megestrol	Avoid; *see also* Contraceptives, Oral
Meloxicam	*see* NSAIDs
Meprobamate	*see* Anxiolytics and Hypnotics
Meptazinol	*see* Opioid Analgesics
Mercaptopurine	May need dose reduction
Meropenem	Monitor transaminase and bilirubin concentrations
Mesterolone	*see* Androgens
Mestranol	Avoid; *see also* Contraceptives, Oral
Metformin	Withdraw if tissue hypoxia likely—manufacturers advise avoid
Methadone	*see* Opioid Analgesics
Methenamine	Avoid
Methionine	May precipitate coma
Methocarbamol	Manufacturer advises caution; half-life may be prolonged
Methotrexate	Dose-related toxicity—avoid in non-malignant conditions (e.g. psoriasis); avoid for all indications in severe hepatic impairment
Methotrimeprazine	*see* Antipsychotics
Methoxsalen	Avoid or reduce dose
Methyldopa	Manufacturer advises caution in history of liver disease; avoid in active liver disease
Methysergide	Avoid
Metoclopramide	Reduce dose
Metolazone	*see* Thiazides and Related Diuretics
Metoprolol	Reduce oral dose
Metronidazole	In severe liver disease reduce total daily dose to one-third, and give once daily
Mexiletine	Avoid (or reduce dose) in severe liver disease
Mianserin	*see* Antidepressants, Tricyclic (and related)
Miconazole	Avoid
Midazolam	*see* Anxiolytics and Hypnotics
Midrid®	Avoid in severe liver disease; *see also* Paracetamol
Miglustat	No information available—manufacturer advises caution
Minocycline	*see* Tetracyclines
Mirtazapine	Manufacturer advises caution
Mitoxantrone	Manufacturer advises caution in severe hepatic impairment
Mivacurium	Reduce dose in severe liver impairment
Mizolastine	Manufacturer recommends avoid in significant hepatic impairment
Moclobemide	Reduce dose in severe liver disease
Modafinil	Halve dose in severe liver disease
Moexipril	*see* ACE Inhibitors
Morphine	*see* Opioid Analgesics
Moxifloxacin	Manufacturer advises avoid in severe hepatic impairment
Moxonidine	Avoid in severe liver disease
Nabilone	Avoid in severe liver disease
Nabumetone	*see* NSAIDs
Nalidixic acid	Manufacturer advises caution in liver disease
Nandrolone	*see* Anabolic Steroids
Naproxen	*see* NSAIDs
Naratriptan	Max. 2.5 mg in 24 hours in moderate hepatic impairment; avoid if severe
Nateglinide	Manufacturer advises caution in moderate hepatic impairment; avoid in severe impairment—no information available
Nebivolol	No information available—manufacturer advises avoid
Nelfinavir	No information available—manufacturer advises caution
Neomycin	Absorbed from gastro-intestinal tract in liver disease—increased risk of ototoxicity
Nevirapine	Manufacturer advises caution in moderate hepatic impairment; avoid in severe hepatic impairment; *see also* p. 320
Nicardipine	Half-life prolonged in severe hepatic impairment—may need dose reduction
Nicotinic acid	Manufacturer advises monitor liver function in mild to moderate hepatic impairment and avoid in severe impairment; discontinue if severe abnormalities in liver function tests
Nicoumalone	*see* Anticoagulants, Oral
Nifedipine	Reduce dose in severe liver disease
Nimodipine	Elimination reduced in cirrhosis—monitor blood pressure
Nisoldipine	Formulation not suitable in hepatic impairment
Nitrazepam	*see* Anxiolytics and Hypnotics
Nitrofurantoin	Cholestatic jaundice and chronic active hepatitis reported
Nitroprusside	*see* Sodium Nitroprusside
Nizatidine	Manufacturer advises caution
Norethisterone	Avoid; *see also* Contraceptives, Oral

Drug	Comment
Norgestimate	Avoid; *see also* Contraceptives, Oral
Norgestrel	Avoid; *see also* Contraceptives, Oral
Nortriptyline	*see* Antidepressants, Tricyclic (and related)
NSAIDs	Increased risk of gastro-intestinal bleeding and can cause fluid retention; avoid in severe liver disease; aceclofenac, initially 100 mg daily; celecoxib, halve initial dose in moderate liver disease; etoricoxib, max. 60 mg daily in mild hepatic impairment (max. 60 mg on alternate days in moderate hepatic impairment); parecoxib, halve dose in moderate hepatic impairment (max. 40 mg daily)
Oestrogens	Avoid; *see also* Contraceptives, Oral
Ofloxacin	Elimination may be reduced in severe hepatic impairment
Olanzapine	Consider initial dose of 5 mg daily
Olmesartan	No information available—manufacturer advises avoid
Omega-3-acid ethyl esters	Monitor liver function
Omeprazole	In liver disease not more than 20 mg daily should be needed
Ondansetron	Reduce dose; not more than 8 mg daily in severe liver disease
Opioid analgesics	Avoid or reduce dose—may precipitate coma
Oral contraceptives	*see* Contraceptives, Oral
Oxazepam	*see* Anxiolytics and Hypnotics
Oxcarbazepine	No dosage adjustment required in mild to moderate hepatic impairment; no information in severe impairment
Oxprenolol	Reduce dose
Oxybutynin	Manufacturer advises caution
Oxycodone	*see* Opioid Analgesics
Oxytetracycline	*see* Tetracyclines
Paclitaxel	Avoid in severe liver disease
Pancuronium	Possibly slower onset, higher dose requirement and prolonged recovery time
Pantoprazole	Max. 20 mg daily in severe hepatic impairment and cirrhosis—monitor liver function (discontinue if deterioration)
Papaveretum	*see* Opioid Analgesics
Paracetamol	Dose-related toxicity—avoid large doses
Parecoxib	*see* NSAIDs
Paroxetine	*see* Antidepressants, SSRI
Peginterferon alfa	Avoid in severe hepatic impairment
Pentazocine	*see* Opioid Analgesics
Pericyazine	*see* Antipsychotics
Perindopril	*see* ACE Inhibitors
Perphenazine	*see* Antipsychotics
Pethidine	*see* Opioid Analgesics
Phenazocine	*see* Opioid Analgesics
Phenelzine	*see* Antidepressants, MAOI
Phenindione	*see* Anticoagulants, Oral
Phenobarbital	May precipitate coma
Phenothiazines	*see* Antipsychotics
Phenytoin	Reduce dose to avoid toxicity
Pholcodine	*see* Opioid Analgesics
Pilocarpine	Reduce initial oral dose in moderate or severe cirrhosis
Pimozide	*see* Antipsychotics
Pioglitazone	Avoid
Piperazine	Manufacturer advises avoid
Pipotiazine	*see* Antipsychotics
Piracetam	Avoid
Piroxicam	*see* NSAIDs
Pravastatin	*see* Statins
Prazosin	Initially 500 micrograms daily; increased with caution
Prednisolone	Side-effects more common
Primidone	Reduce dose; may precipitate coma
Procainamide	Avoid or reduce dose
Procarbazine	Avoid in severe hepatic impairment
Prochlorperazine	*see* Antipsychotics
Progesterone	Avoid; *see also* Contraceptives, Oral
Progestogens	Avoid; *see also* Contraceptives, Oral
Promazine	*see* Antipsychotics
Promethazine	Avoid—may precipitate coma in severe liver disease; hepatotoxic
Propafenone	Reduce dose
Propantheline	Manufacturer advises caution
Propiverine	Avoid
Propranolol	Reduce oral dose
Propylthiouracil	Reduce dose
Pyrazinamide	Monitor hepatic function—idiosyncratic hepatotoxicity more common; avoid in severe hepatic impairment; *see also* p. 300
Pyrimethamine	Manufacturer advises caution
Quetiapine	Manufacturer advises initial dose of 25 mg daily, increased daily in steps of 25–50 mg
Quinagolide	Manufacturer advises avoid—no information available
Quinapril	*see* ACE Inhibitors
Quinupristin [ingredient]	*see Synercid®*
Rabeprazole	Manufacturer advises caution in severe hepatic dysfunction
Raloxifene	Manufacturer advises avoid
Raltitrexed	Caution in mild or moderate disease; avoid if severe
Ramipril	*see* ACE Inhibitors
Reboxetine	Initial dose 2 mg twice daily, increased according to tolerance
Remifentanil	*see* Opioid Analgesics
Repaglinide	Manufacturer advises avoid in severe liver disease
Reteplase	Avoid in severe hepatic impairment
Reviparin	Manufacturer advises avoid in severe hepatic impairment
Riamet®	Manufacturer advises caution in severe hepatic impairment—monitor ECG and plasma potassium concentration

Drug	Comment
Ribavirin	No dosage adjustment required; avoid oral administration in severe hepatic dysfunction or decompensated cirrhosis
Rifabutin	Reduce dose in severe hepatic impairment
Rifampicin	Impaired elimination; monitor liver function; avoid or do not exceed 8 mg/kg daily; *see also* p. 300
Riluzole	Avoid
Risperidone	Manufacturer advises initial oral dose of 500 micrograms twice daily increased in steps of 500 micrograms twice daily to 1–2 mg twice daily; if an oral dose of at least 2 mg daily tolerated, 25 mg as a depot injection can be given every 2 weeks
Ritonavir	Avoid in severe hepatic impairment
Rivastigmine	No information available—manufacturer advises avoid in severe liver disease
Rizatriptan	Reduce dose to 5 mg in mild to moderate liver disease; avoid in severe liver disease
Rocuronium	Reduce dose
Ropinirole	Avoid in severe hepatic impairment
Ropivacaine	Manufacturer advises caution in severe liver disease
Rosiglitazone	Avoid
Rosuvastatin	*see* Statins
Saquinavir	Manufacturer advises caution in moderate hepatic impairment; avoid in severe impairment
Sertindole	Slower titration and lower maintenance dose in mild to moderate hepatic impairment; avoid in severe hepatic impairment; *see also* Antipsychotics
Sertraline	*see* Antidepressants, SSRI
Sibutramine	Increased plasma-sibutramine concentration; manufacturer advises caution in mild to moderate hepatic impairment; avoid if severe impairment
Sildenafil	Initial dose 25 mg; manufacturer advises avoid in severe hepatic impairment
Simvastatin	*see* Statins
Sirolimus	Monitor blood-sirolimus trough concentration
Sodium aurothiomalate	Caution in mild to moderate liver disease; avoid in severe liver disease
Sodium bicarbonate	*see* Antacids
Sodium fusidate	Impaired biliary excretion; possibly increased risk of hepatotoxicity; avoid or reduce dose
Sodium nitroprusside	Avoid in severe liver disease
Sodium phenylbutyrate	Manufacturer advises caution
Sodium valproate	*see* Valproate
Solifenacin	Max. 5 mg daily in moderate liver disease; avoid if severe
Statins	Avoid in active liver disease or unexplained persistent elevations in serum transaminases
Stilboestrol (diethylstilbestrol)	Avoid; *see also* Contraceptives, Oral
Streptokinase	Avoid in severe hepatic impairment
Sulindac	*see* NSAIDs
Sulphonylureas	Increased risk of hypoglycaemia in severe liver disease; avoid or use small dose; can produce jaundice; *see also* Glimepiride
Sulpiride	*see* Antipsychotics
Sumatriptan	Manufacturer advises 50 mg oral dose in hepatic impairment; avoid in severe hepatic impairment
Suxamethonium	Prolonged apnoea may occur in severe liver disease due to reduced hepatic synthesis of pseudocholinesterase
Synercid®	Consider reducing dose to 5 mg/kg every 8 hours in moderate hepatic impairment, adjusted according to clinical response; avoid in severe hepatic impairment or if plasma-bilirubin concentration greater than 3 times upper limit of reference range
Tacrolimus	Reduce dose
Tadalafil	Max. dose 10 mg; manufacturer advises monitor patient in severe hepatic impairment
Tamsulosin	Avoid in severe hepatic impairment
Tegafur with uracil	*see Uftoral*®
Telmisartan	20–40 mg once daily in mild or moderate impairment; avoid in severe hepatic impairment or biliary obstruction
Temazepam	*see* Anxiolytics and Hypnotics
Tenecteplase	Avoid in severe hepatic impairment
Tenoxicam	*see* NSAIDs
Terbinafine	Manufacturer advises avoid—elimination reduced
Terfenadine	Avoid—risk of arrhythmias
Testosterone and esters	*see* Androgens
Tetracyclines	Avoid (or use with caution); tetracycline, demeclocycline, and *Deteclo*® max. 1 g daily in divided doses
Theophylline	Reduce dose
Thiazides and related diuretics	Avoid in severe liver disease; hypokalaemia may precipitate coma (potassium-sparing diuretic can prevent); increased risk of hypomagnesaemia in alcoholic cirrhosis
Thiopental	Reduce dose for induction in severe liver disease
Tiagabine	Maintenance dose 5–10 mg 1–2 times daily initially in mild to moderate hepatic impairment; avoid in severe impairment
Tiaprofenic acid	*see* NSAIDs
Tibolone	Avoid in severe liver disease
Ticarcillin [ingredient]	*see* Timentin®

Drug	Comment
Timentin®	Cholestatic jaundice, *see* under Co-amoxiclav p. 277
Timolol	Dose reduction may be necessary
Tinzaparin	*see* Heparin
Tirofiban	Caution in mild to moderate liver disease; avoid in severe liver disease—increased risk of bleeding
Tizanidine	Avoid in severe liver disease
Tolbutamide	*see* Sulphonylureas
Tolcapone	Avoid
Tolfenamic acid	*see* NSAIDs
Tolterodine	Reduce dose to 1 mg twice daily
Topiramate	Use with caution in hepatic impairment—clearance may be decreased
Topotecan	Avoid in severe hepatic impairment
Torasemide	*see* Loop Diuretics
Toremifene	Elimination decreased in hepatic impairment—avoid if severe
Tramadol	*see* Opioid Analgesics
Trandolapril	*see* ACE Inhibitors
Tranylcypromine	*see* Antidepressants, MAOI
Trazodone	*see* Antidepressants, Tricyclic (and related)
Tretinoin (oral)	Reduce dose
Tribavirin	*see* Ribavirin
Triclofos	*see* Anxiolytics and Hypnotics
Trifluoperazine	*see* Antipsychotics
Trimeprazine	*see* Alimemazine
Trimetrexate	Manufacturer advises caution; interrupt treatment if severe abnormalities in liver function tests (consult product literature)
Trimipramine	*see* Antidepressants, Tricyclic (and related)
Triprolidine	Sedation inappropriate in severe liver disease—avoid
Trospium	Manufacturer advises avoid—no information available
Uftoral®	Manufacturer advises monitor liver function in mild to moderate hepatic impairment and avoid in severe impairment
Ursodeoxycholic acid	Avoid in chronic liver disease (but used in primary biliary cirrhosis)
Valaciclovir	Manufacturer advises caution with high doses used for preventing cytomegalovirus disease—no information available
Valproate	Avoid if possible—hepatotoxicity and hepatic failure may occasionally occur (usually in first 6 months); *see also* p. 245
Valproic acid	*see* Valproate
Valsartan	Halve dose in mild to moderate hepatic impairment; avoid if severe
Vardenafil	Initial dose 5 mg in mild to moderate hepatic impairment, increased subsequently according to response (max. 10 mg in moderate hepatic impairment); manufacturer advises avoid in severe hepatic impairment
Venlafaxine	Halve dose in moderate hepatic impairment; avoid if severe
Verapamil	Reduce oral dose
Verteporfin	Avoid in severe hepatic impairment
Vinblastine	Dose reduction may be necessary
Vincristine	Dose reduction may be necessary
Vindesine	Dose reduction may be necessary
Vinorelbine	Dose reduction may be required in significant hepatic impairment
Voriconazole	In mild to moderate hepatic cirrhosis use normal loading dose then halve normal maintenance dose; no information available for severe hepatic cirrhosis—manufacturer advises use only if potential benefit outweighs risk
Warfarin	*see* Anticoagulants, Oral
Xipamide	*see* Thiazides and Related Diuretics
Zafirlukast	Manufacturer advises avoid
Zalcitabine	Further impairment of liver function may occur
Zaleplon	*see* Anxiolytics and Hypnotics
Zidovudine	Accumulation may occur
Zoledronic acid	Manufacturer advises caution in severe hepatic impairment—limited information available
Zolmitriptan	Max. 5 mg in 24 hours in moderate or severe hepatic impairment
Zolpidem	*see* Anxiolytics and Hypnotics
Zonisamide	Initially, increase dose at 2-week intervals if mild or moderate hepatic impairment; avoid in severe impairment
Zopiclone	*see* Anxiolytics and Hypnotics
Zotepine	Initial dose 25 mg twice daily, increased gradually according to response (max. 75 mg twice daily); monitor liver function at weekly intervals for first 3 months
Zuclopenthixol	*see* Antipsychotics

Appendix 3: Renal impairment

The use of drugs in patients with reduced renal function can give rise to problems for several reasons:

- failure to excrete a drug or its metabolites may produce toxicity;
- sensitivity to some drugs is increased even if elimination is unimpaired;
- many side-effects are tolerated poorly by patients in renal failure;
- some drugs cease to be effective when renal function is reduced.

Many of these problems can be avoided by reducing the dose or by using alternative drugs.

Principles of dose adjustment in renal impairment

The level of renal function below which the dose of a drug must be reduced depends on whether the drug is eliminated entirely by renal excretion or is partly metabolised, and on how toxic it is.

For many drugs with only minor or no dose-related side-effects very precise modification of the dose regimen is unnecessary and a simple scheme for dose reduction is sufficient.

For more toxic drugs with a small safety margin dose regimens based on glomerular filtration rate should be used. For those where both efficacy and toxicity are closely related to plasma concentrations recommended regimens should be seen only as a guide to initial treatment; subsequent treatment must be adjusted according to clinical response and plasma concentration.

The total daily maintenance dose of a drug can be reduced either by reducing the size of the individual doses or by increasing the interval between doses. For some drugs, if the size of the maintenance dose is reduced it will be important to give a loading dose if an immediate effect is required. This is because when a patient is given a regular dose of any drug it takes more than five times the half-life to achieve steady-state plasma concentrations. As the plasma half-life of drugs excreted by the kidney is prolonged in renal failure it may take many days for the reduced dosage to achieve a therapeutic plasma concentration. The loading dose should usually be the same size as the initial dose for a patient with normal renal function.

Nephrotoxic drugs should, if possible, be avoided in patients with renal disease because the consequences of nephrotoxicity are likely to be more serious when the renal reserve is already reduced.

Use of dosage table

Dose recommendations are based on the severity of renal impairment. This is expressed in terms of glomerular filtration rate (GFR), usually measured by the **creatinine clearance** (best calculated from a 24-hour urine collection). The serum-creatinine concentration is sometimes used instead as a measure of renal function but is only a **rough guide** even when corrected for age, weight, and sex. Nomograms are available for making the correction and should be used where accuracy is important.

For *prescribing purposes* renal impairment is arbitrarily divided into 3 grades (definitions vary for grades of renal impairment; therefore, where the product literature does not correspond with this grading, values for creatinine clearance or another measure of renal function are included):

Grade	*GFR*	*Serum creatinine (approx.)* (but see above)
Mild	20–50 mL/minute	150–300 micromol/litre
Moderate	10–20 mL/minute	300–700 micromol/litre
Severe	$<$ 10 mL/minute	$>$ 700 micromol/litre

NOTE. Conversion factors are:
Litres/24 hours = mL/minute × 1.44
mL/minute = Litres/24 hours × 0.69

Dialysis. For prescribing in patients on continuous ambulatory peritoneal dialysis (CAPD) or haemodialysis, consult specialist literature.

Renal function declines with age; many elderly patients have a glomerular filtration rate below 50 mL/minute which, because of reduced muscle mass, may not be indicated by a raised serum creatinine. It is wise to assume at least mild impairment of renal function when prescribing for the elderly.

The following table may be used as a guide to drugs which are known to require a reduction in dose in renal impairment, and to those which are potentially harmful or are ineffective. Drug prescribing should be kept to the minimum in all patients with severe renal disease.

If even mild renal impairment is considered likely on clinical grounds, renal function should be checked before prescribing **any** drug which requires dose modification.

Table of drugs to be avoided or used with caution in renal impairment

Products introduced or amended since publication of BNF No. 49 (March 2005) are underlined.

Drug and degree of impairment	Comment
Abacavir	
Severe	Manufacturer advises avoid
Abciximab	
Severe	Avoid—increased risk of bleeding
Acamprosate	
Mild	Avoid; excreted in urine
Acarbose	
Moderate to severe	Manufacturer advises avoid—no information available

Drug and degree of impairment	Comment
ACE inhibitors	
Mild to moderate	Use with caution and monitor response (see also p. 97). Hyperkalaemia and other side-effects more common. *Initial doses*: captopril 12.5 mg twice daily, cilazapril 500 micrograms once daily, enalapril 2.5 mg once daily if creatinine clearance less than 30 mL/minute, imidapril 2.5 mg once daily (avoid if creatinine clearance less than 30 mL/minute), lisinopril 2.5–5 mg, moexipril 3.75 mg once daily, perindopril 2 mg once daily (2 mg once daily on alternate days in moderate impairment), quinapril 2.5 mg once daily, ramipril 1.25 mg once daily, trandolapril 500 micrograms once daily (max. 2 mg daily if creatinine clearance less than 10 mL/minute)
Acebutolol	*see* Beta-blockers
Aceclofenac	*see* NSAIDs
Acemetacin	*see* NSAIDs
Acenocoumarol (nicoumalone)	*see* Anticoagulants, Oral
Acetazolamide	
Mild	Avoid; metabolic acidosis
Aciclovir	
Mild	Reduce intravenous dose
Moderate to severe	Reduce dose
Acipimox	Reduce dose if creatinine clearance 30–60 mL/minute; avoid if creatinine clearance less than 30 mL/minute
Acitretin	
Mild	Avoid; increased risk of toxicity
Acrivastine	
Moderate	Avoid; excreted by kidney
Adefovir dipivoxil	
Mild	10 mg every 48 hours
Moderate	10 mg every 72 hours
Severe	No information available
Adrenergic neurone blockers	
Moderate to severe	Avoid; increased postural hypotension; decrease in renal blood flow
Alendronic acid	
Mild	Manufacturer advises avoid if creatinine clearance less than 35 mL/minute
Alfentanil	*see* Opioid Analgesics
Alfuzosin	Start at 2.5 mg twice daily and adjust according to response
Alimemazine (trimeprazine)	
Severe	Avoid
Allopurinol	
Moderate	100–200 mg daily; increased toxicity; rashes
Severe	100 mg on alternate days (max. 100 mg daily)
Almotriptan	
Severe	Max. 12.5 mg in 24 hours
Alprazolam	*see* Anxiolytics and Hypnotics
Alteplase	
Moderate	Risk of hyperkalaemia
Aluminium salts	
Severe	Aluminium is absorbed and may accumulate

NOTE. Absorption of aluminium from aluminium salts is increased by citrates, which are contained in many effervescent preparations (such as effervescent analgesics)

Drug and degree of impairment	Comment
Amantadine	Reduce dose; avoid if creatinine clearance less than 15 mL/minute (60 mL/minute in elderly)
Amfebutamone	*see* Bupropion
Amikacin	*see* Aminoglycosides
Amiloride	*see* Potassium-sparing Diuretics
Aminoglycosides	
Mild	Reduce dose; monitor serum concentrations; *see also* section 5.1.4
Amisulpride	
Mild	Manufacturer advises use half normal dose
Moderate	Manufacturer advises use one-third of normal dose
Severe	Manufacturer advises dose reduction and intermittent treatment
Amoxicillin	
Mild to moderate	Risk of crystalluria with high doses (particularly during parenteral therapy)
Severe	Reduce dose; rashes more common and risk of crystalluria
Amphotericin	
Mild	Use only if no alternative; nephrotoxicity may be reduced with use of lipid formulations
Ampicillin	
Severe	Reduce dose; rashes more common
Amprenavir	
Mild to moderate	Use oral solution with caution due to high propylene glycol content
Severe	Avoid oral solution
Amsacrine	Reduce dose
Anagrelide	Manufacturer advises avoid if creatinine clearance less than 30 mL/minute
Anakinra	Manufacturer advises caution if creatinine clearance 30–50 mL/minute; avoid if creatinine clearance less than 30 mL/minute
Analgesics	*see* Opioid Analgesics and NSAIDs
Anastrozole	
Moderate to severe	Avoid—no information available
Angeliq®	
Severe	Manufacturer advises avoid
Anticoagulants, oral	
Severe	Avoid
Antipsychotics	
Severe	Start with small doses; increased cerebral sensitivity; *see also* Amisulpride, Clozapine, Olanzapine, Quetiapine, Risperidone and Sulpiride

Drug and degree of impairment	Comment
Anxiolytics and hypnotics	
Severe	Start with small doses; increased cerebral sensitivity; *see also* chloral hydrate
Apomorphine	
Severe	Use with caution; max. sublingual dose 2 mg
Arsenic trioxide	Manufacturer advises caution—risk of accumulation
Artemether [ingredient]	*see Riamet®*
Aspirin	
Severe	Avoid; sodium and water retention; deterioration in renal function; increased risk of gastro-intestinal bleeding
Atenolol	*see* Beta-blockers
Atosiban	No information available
Atovaquone	Manufacturer advises caution—monitor more closely
Auranofin	*see* Sodium Aurothiomalate
Azathioprine	
Severe	Reduce dose
Aztreonam	If creatinine clearance 10–30 mL/minute, usual initial dose, then half normal dose; if creatinine clearance less than 10 mL/minute usual initial dose, then one-quarter normal dose
Baclofen	
Mild	Use smaller doses (e.g. 5 mg daily); excreted by kidney
Balsalazide	
Moderate to severe	Manufacturer advises avoid
Bambuterol	
Mild	Reduce dose
Barbiturates	
Severe	Reduce dose; *see also* Phenobarbital
Bemiparin	*see* Heparin
Bendrofluazide	*see* Thiazides and Related Diuretics
Bendroflumethiazide (bendrofluazide)	*see* Thiazides and Related Diuretics
Benperidol	*see* Antipsychotics
Benzodiazepines	*see* Anxiolytics and Hypnotics
Benzylpenicillin	
Severe	Max. 6 g daily; neurotoxicity—high doses may cause convulsions
Beta-blockers	
Mild	Atenolol 50 mg daily (10 mg on alternate days *intravenously*) if creatinine clearance 15–35 mL/minute; start with 2.5 mg of nebivolol; reduce dose of celiprolol if creatinine clearance less than 40 mL/minute; halve dose of sotalol if creatinine clearance 30–60 mL/minute
Moderate	Start with small dose of acebutolol (active metabolite accumulates); reduce dose of atenolol (see above), bisoprolol, nadolol, pindolol (all excreted unchanged); avoid celiprolol if creatinine clearance less than 15 mL/minute; use one-quarter normal dose of sotalol if creatinine clearance 10–30 mL/minute
Severe	Start with small dose; may reduce renal blood flow and adversely affect renal function in severe impairment; manufacturer advises avoid celiprolol and sotalol; atenolol 25 mg daily (10 mg every 4 days *intravenously*) if creatinine clearance less than 15 mL/minute
Bezafibrate	Reduce dose to 400 mg daily if creatinine clearance 40–60 mL/minute; reduce dose to 200 mg every 1–2 days if creatinine clearance 15–40 mL/minute; avoid if creatinine clearance less than 15 mL/minute
Bisoprolol	*see* Beta-blockers
Bivalirudin	Reduce dose of infusion to 1.4 mg/kg/hour if creatinine clearance 30–60 mL/minute; avoid if creatinine clearance less than 30 mL/minute
Bleomycin	
Moderate	Reduce dose
Bortezomib	Manufacturer advises caution—consider dose reduction
Bumetanide	
Moderate	May need high doses
Buprenorphine	*see* Opioid Analgesics
Bupropion	Manufacturer recommends 150 mg daily
Buspirone	
Mild	Reduce dose
Moderate to severe	Avoid
Calcitriol	
Severe	Manufacturer of topical calcitriol advises avoid—no information available
Candesartan	Initially 4 mg daily
Capecitabine	
Mild	Use three-quarters of starting dose if creatinine clearance 30–50 mL/minute; avoid if creatinine clearance less than 30 mL/minute
Capreomycin	
Mild	Reduce dose; nephrotoxic; ototoxic
Captopril	*see* ACE Inhibitors

Drug and degree of impairment	Comment
Carbamazepine	Manufacturer advises caution
Carboplatin	
Mild	Reduce dose and monitor haematological parameters and renal function
Moderate to severe	Avoid
Cefaclor	No dose adjustment required—manufacturer advises caution
Cefadroxil	
Moderate	Reduce dose
Cefalexin	Max. 3 g daily if creatinine clearance 40–50 mL/minute; max. 1.5 g daily if creatinine clearance 10–40 mL/minute; max. 750 mg daily if creatinine clearance less than 10 mL/minute
Cefixime	
Moderate	Reduce dose
Cefotaxime	If creatinine clearance less than 5 mL/minute, initial dose of 1 g then use half normal dose
Cefpirome	
Mild	Usual initial dose, then use half normal dose
Moderate to severe	Usual initial dose, then use one-quarter normal dose
Cefpodoxime	
Mild	Reduce dose
Cefprozil	Usual initial dose, then use half normal dose
Cefradine	
Moderate to severe	Reduce dose
Ceftazidime	
Mild	Reduce dose
Ceftriaxone	
Severe	Max. 2 g daily; also monitor plasma concentration if both hepatic and severe renal impairment
Cefuroxime	
Moderate to severe	Reduce parenteral dose
Celecoxib	*see* NSAIDs
Celiprolol	*see* Beta-blockers
Cetirizine	
Moderate	Use half normal dose
Cetrorelix	
Moderate to severe	Manufacturer advises avoid
Chloral hydrate	Avoid in severe renal impairment
Chloramphenicol	
Severe	Avoid unless no alternative; dose-related depression of haematopoiesis
Chlordiazepoxide	*see* Anxiolytics and Hypnotics
Chloroquine	
Mild to moderate	Reduce dose (but for malaria prophylaxis see section 5.4.1)
Severe	Avoid (but for malaria prophylaxis see section 5.4.1)
Chlorpromazine	*see* Antipsychotics
Chlorpropamide	Avoid
Chlortalidone	*see* Thiazides and Related Diuretics
Chlortetracycline	*see* Tetracyclines
Ciclosporin	*see* p. 446 (*see also* p. 579 if used in atopic dermatitis or psoriasis and p. 515 if used in rheumatoid arthritis)

Drug and degree of impairment	Comment
Cidofovir	
Mild	Avoid; nephrotoxic
Cilastatin [ingredient]	*see Primaxin*®
Cilazapril	*see* ACE Inhibitors
Cilostazol	Avoid if creatinine clearance less than 25 mL/minute
Cimetidine	
Mild to moderate	600–800 mg daily; occasional risk of confusion
Severe	400 mg daily
Ciprofibrate	
Moderate	100 mg on alternate days
Severe	Avoid
Ciprofloxacin	
Moderate	Use half normal dose
Cisplatin	
Mild	Avoid if possible; nephrotoxic and neurotoxic
Citalopram	
Moderate to severe	No information available
Citramag®	
Severe	Avoid—risk of hypermagnesaemia
Citrates	Absorption of aluminium from aluminium salts is increased by citrates, which are contained in many effervescent preparations (such as effervescent analgesics)
Cladribine	Regular monitoring recommended
Clarithromycin	Use half normal dose if creatinine clearance less than 30 mL/minute; avoid *Klaricid XL*® if creatinine clearance less than 30 mL/minute
Clavulanic acid [ingredient]	*see* Co-amoxiclav and *Timentin*®
Clobazam	*see* Anxiolytics and Hypnotics
Clodronate sodium	*see* Sodium Clodronate
Clomethiazole	*see* Anxiolytics and Hypnotics
Clopamide	*see* Thiazides and Related Diuretics
Clopidogrel	Manufacturer advises caution
Clorazepate	*see* Anxiolytics and Hypnotics
Clozapine	
Mild to moderate	Initial dose 12.5 mg daily increased slowly
Severe	Avoid
Co-amoxiclav	Risk of crystalluria with high doses (particularly during parenteral therapy); reduce dose if creatinine clearance less than 30 mL/minute
Codeine	*see* Opioid Analgesics
Colchicine	
Moderate	Reduce dose
Severe	Avoid or reduce dose if no alternative
Colistin	
Mild	Reduce dose; nephrotoxic; neurotoxic
Co-trimoxazole	Use half normal dose if creatinine clearance 15–30 mL/minute; avoid if creatinine clearance less than 15 mL/minute and if plasma-sulfamethoxazole concentration cannot be monitored

Drug and degree of impairment	Comment
Cyclopenthiazide	*see* Thiazides and Related Diuretics
Cyclophosphamide	Reduce dose
Cycloserine	
Mild to moderate	Reduce dose
Severe	Avoid
Cyclosporin	*see* Ciclosporin
Dacarbazine	
Mild to moderate	Dose reduction may be required
Severe	Avoid
Dalteparin	*see* Heparin
Danaparoid	
Moderate	Increased risk of bleeding (monitor anti-Factor Xa activity)
Severe	Avoid unless patient has heparin-induced thrombocytopenia and no alternative
Daunorubicin	
Mild to moderate	Reduce dose
Deferiprone	Manufacturer advises caution—no information available
Demeclocycline	*see* Tetracyclines
Desflurane	
Moderate	Reduce dose
Desloratadine	
Severe	Manufacturer advises caution
Desmopressin	Antidiuretic effect may be reduced
Dexketoprofen	*see* NSAIDs
Dextromethorphan	*see* Opioid Analgesics
Dextropropoxyphene	*see* Opioid Analgesics
Diamorphine	*see* Opioid Analgesics
Diazepam	*see* Anxiolytics and Hypnotics
Diazoxide	
Severe	75–150 mg i/v; increased sensitivity to hypotensive effect
Diclofenac	*see* NSAIDs
Didanosine	
Mild	Reduce dose; consult product literature
Diflunisal	see NSAIDs (excreted by kidney)
Digitoxin	
Severe	Max. 100 micrograms daily
Digoxin	
Mild	Reduce dose; toxicity increased by electrolyte disturbances
Dihydrocodeine	*see* Opioid Analgesics
Diltiazem	Start with smaller dose
Diphenoxylate	*see* Opioid Analgesics
Dipipanone	*see* Opioid Analgesics
Disodium etidronate	
Mild	Reduce dose
Moderate to severe	Avoid
Disodium pamidronate	Max. infusion rate 20 mg/hour; except in life-threatening hypercalcaemia, manufacturer advises avoid if creatinine clearance less than 30 mL/minute; if renal function deteriorates in patients with bone metastases, withhold dose until serum creatinine returns to within 10% of baseline value
Disopyramide	
Mild	100 mg every 8 hours *or* 150 mg every 12 hours
Moderate	100 mg every 12 hours
Severe	150 mg every 24 hours
NOTE. Sustained-release preparations may be unsuitable; monitor plasma-disopyramide concentrations	
Diuretics, potassium-sparing	*see* Potassium-sparing Diuretics
Domperidone	Manufacturer advises reduce dose
Doxycycline	*see* Tetracyclines
Drospirenone [ingredient]	*see Yasmin*® and *Angeliq*®
Duloxetine	Avoid if creatinine clearance less than 30 mL/minute
Efavirenz	
Severe	Manufacturer advises caution—no information available
Eletriptan	Reduce initial dose to 20 mg; max. 40 mg in 24 hours; avoid if creatinine clearance less than 30 mL/minute
Emtricitabine	
Mild	Reduce dose
Enalapril	*see* ACE Inhibitors
Enfuvirtide	Manufacturer advises caution if creatinine clearance less than 35 mL/minute—no information available
Enoxaparin	Consider switching to heparin if creatinine clearance less than 30 mL/minute; alternatively adjust dose according to plasma concentration of anti-factor Xa
Enoximone	Consider dose reduction
Ephedrine	
Severe	Avoid; increased CNS toxicity
Eplerenone	Increased risk of hyperkalaemia—close monitoring required; avoid if creatinine clearance less than 50 mL/minute
Eprosartan	
Mild	Halve initial dose
Eptifibatide	Avoid if creatinine clearance less than 30 mL/minute
Ergometrine	
Severe	Manufacturer advises avoid
Ergotamine	
Moderate	Avoid; nausea and vomiting; risk of renal vasoconstriction
Ertapenem	Manufacturer advises avoid if creatinine clearance less than 30 mL/minute
Erythromycin	
Severe	Max. 1.5 g daily (ototoxicity)
Escitalopram	
Mild	Manufacturer advises caution
Esmolol	*see* Beta-blockers
Esomeprazole	
Severe	Manufacturer advises caution
Estramustine	Manufacturer advises caution

Drug and degree of impairment	Comment
Ethambutol	
Mild	Reduce dose; if creatinine clearance less than 30 mL/minute monitor plasma-ethambutol concentration; optic nerve damage
Etidronate disodium	*see* Disodium Etidronate
Etodolac	*see* NSAIDs
Etoposide	Consider dose reduction
Etoricoxib	*see* NSAIDs
Exemestane	Manufacturer advises caution
Famciclovir	Reduce dose; consult product literature
Famotidine	
Severe	Max. 20 mg at night
Fenbufen	*see* NSAIDs
Fenofibrate	
Mild	134 mg daily
Moderate	67 mg daily
Severe	Avoid
Fenoprofen	*see* NSAIDs
Fentanyl	*see* Opioid Analgesics
Flecainide	
Mild	Max. initial dose 100 mg daily
Fleet Phospho-soda®	
Severe	Avoid
Flucloxacillin	
Severe	Reduce dose
Fluconazole	
Mild to moderate	Usual initial dose then halve subsequent doses
Flucytosine	Reduce dose and monitor plasma-flucytosine concentration—consult product literature
Fludarabine	
Mild	Reduce dose; avoid if creatinine clearance less than 30 mL/ minute
Fluoxetine	
Mild to moderate	Reduce dose (give on alternate days)
Severe	Avoid
Flupentixol	*see* Antipsychotics
Fluphenazine	*see* Antipsychotics
Flurazepam	*see* Anxiolytics and Hypnotics
Flurbiprofen	*see* NSAIDs
Fluvoxamine	
Moderate	Start with smaller dose
Fondaparinux	Increased risk of bleeding; use with caution if creatinine clearance 30–50 mL/minute; for treatment avoid if creatinine clearance less than 30 mL/ minute; for prophylaxis reduce dose to 1.5 mg daily if creatinine clearance 20–30 mL/minute, avoid if less than 20 mL/minute
Foscarnet	
Mild	Reduce dose; consult product literature
Fosinopril	*see* ACE Inhibitors
Fosphenytoin	Consider 10–25% reduction in dose or infusion rate (except initial dose for status epilepticus)
Frusemide	*see* Furosemide
Furosemide (frusemide)	
Moderate	May need high doses; deafness may follow rapid i/v injection

Drug and degree of impairment	Comment
Fybogel Mebeverine®	
Severe	Avoid; contains 7 mmol potassium per sachet
Gabapentin	
Mild	Reduce dose; consult product literature
Galantamine	
Severe	Avoid
Gallamine	
Moderate	Avoid; prolonged paralysis
Ganciclovir	
Mild	Reduce dose; consult product literature
Ganirelix	
Moderate to severe	Manufacturer advises avoid
Gaviscon®	
Severe	Avoid; high sodium content
Gemcitabine	Manufacturer advises caution
Gemeprost	Manufacturer advises avoid
Gemfibrozil	Start with 900 mg daily if creatinine clearance 30–80 mL/ minute; avoid if creatinine clearance less than 30 mL/ minute
Gentamicin	*see* Aminoglycosides
Gestrinone	
Severe	Avoid
Glatiramer	No information available—manufacturer advises caution
Glibenclamide	
Severe	Avoid
Gliclazide	
Mild to moderate	Reduce dose
Severe	Avoid if possible; if no alternative reduce dose and monitor closely
Glimepiride	
Severe	Avoid
Glipizide	
Mild to moderate	Increased risk of hypoglycaemia; avoid if hepatic impairment also present
Severe	Avoid
Gliquidone	Avoid in renal failure
Guanethidine	*see* Adrenergic Neurone Blockers
Haloperidol	*see* Antipsychotics
Heparin	
Severe	Risk of bleeding increased
Hetastarch	
Severe	Avoid; excreted by kidney
Hydralazine	Reduce dose if creatinine clearance less than 30 mL/minute
Hydrochlorothiazide	*see* Thiazides and Related Diuretics
Hydroflumethiazide	*see* Thiazides and Related Diuretics
Hydromorphone	*see* Opioid Analgesics
Hydroxychloroquine	
Mild to moderate	Reduce dose; only on prolonged use
Severe	Avoid
Hydroxyzine	Use half normal dose
Hyoscine hydrobromide	Manufacturer advises caution
Hypnotics	*see* Anxiolytics and Hypnotics

Drug and degree of impairment	Comment
Ibandronic acid	For repeated doses, if creatinine clearance less than 30 mL/minute, reduce intravenous dose to 2 mg every 3–4 weeks and reduce oral dose to 50 mg once weekly
Ibuprofen	*see* NSAIDs
Idarubicin	
Mild	Reduce dose
Ifosfamide	
Mild	Avoid if serum creatinine concentration greater than 120 micromol/litre
Imidapril	*see* ACE Inhibitors
Imipenem [ingredient]	*see Primaxin®*
Indapamide	*see* Thiazides and Related Diuretics
Indometacin	*see* NSAIDs
Indoramin	Manufacturer advises caution
Inosine pranobex	
Mild	Avoid; metabolised to uric acid
Insulin	
Severe	May need dose reduction; insulin requirements fall; compensatory response to hypoglycaemia is impaired
Interferon alfa	
Mild to moderate	Close monitoring required
Severe	Avoid
Interferon beta	No information available—monitoring advised
Interferon gamma-1b	
Severe	Manufacturer advises caution
Irinotecan	No information available
Isometheptene [ingredient]	see Midrid®
Isoniazid	
Severe	Max. 200 mg daily; peripheral neuropathy
Isotretinoin	
Severe	Start with 10 mg daily and increased if necessary to max. 1 mg/kg daily
Itraconazole	Risk of congestive heart failure; bioavailability of oral formulations possibly reduced; use intravenous infusion with caution if creatinine clearance 30–50 mL/minute (monitor renal function); avoid intravenous infusion if creatinine clearance less than 30 mL/minute
Kaletra®	Avoid oral solution due to propylene glycol content; use capsules with caution in severe impairment
Ketoprofen	*see* NSAIDs
Ketorolac	*see* NSAIDs
Lamivudine	
Mild	Reduce dose; consult product literature
Lamotrigine	
Moderate to severe	Metabolite may accumulate
Leflunomide	
Moderate to severe	Manufacturer advises avoid—no information available
Lepirudin	
Mild to moderate	Manufacturer advises reducing initial dose by 50% and subsequent doses by 50–85%
Severe	Avoid or stop infusion (unless APTT is below therapeutic levels when alternate day administration may be considered)
Lercanidipine	
Severe	Avoid
Levetiracetam	Max. 2 g daily if creatinine clearance 50–80 mL/minute; max. 1.5 g daily if creatinine clearance 30–50 mL/minute; max. 1 g daily if creatinine clearance less than 30 mL/minute
Levocabastine	
Severe	Manufacturer advises avoid
Levocetirizine	5 mg on alternate days if creatinine clearance 30–50 mL/minute; 5 mg every 3 days if creatinine clearance 10–30 mL/minute; avoid if creatinine clearance less than 10 mL/minute
Levofloxacin	
Mild	Usual initial dose, then use half normal dose
Moderate to severe	Reduce dose; consult product literature
Levomepromazine (methotrimeprazine)	*see* Antipsychotics
Lidocaine	
Severe	Caution
Linezolid	Manufacturer advises metabolites may accumulate if creatinine clearance less than 30 mL/minute
Lisinopril	*see* ACE Inhibitors
Lithium salts	
Mild	Avoid if possible or reduce dose and monitor plasma concentration carefully
Moderate	Avoid
Lofepramine	
Severe	Avoid
Lopinavir [ingredient]	*see Kaletra®*
Loprazolam	*see* Anxiolytics and Hypnotics
Lorazepam	*see* Anxiolytics and Hypnotics
Lormetazepam	*see* Anxiolytics and Hypnotics
Losartan	
Moderate to severe	Start with 25 mg once daily
Lumefantrine [ingredient]	*see Riamet®*
Lymecycline	*see* Tetracyclines
Magnesium salts	
Moderate	Avoid or reduce dose; increased risk of toxicity; magnesium carbonate mixture and magnesium trisilicate mixture also have high sodium content
Malarone®	Avoid for malaria prophylaxis (and if possible for malaria treatment) if creatinine clearance less than 30 mL/minute
Mefenamic acid	*see* NSAIDs

Drug and degree of impairment	Comment
Meloxicam	*see* NSAIDs
Melphalan	Reduce dose initially; avoid high doses in moderate to severe impairment
Memantine	
Mild	Reduce dose to 10 mg daily if creatinine clearance 40–60 mL/minute
Moderate to severe	Manufacturer advises avoid—no information available
Meprobamate	*see* Anxiolytics and Hypnotics
Meptazinol	*see* Opioid Analgesics
Mercaptopurine	
Moderate	Reduce dose
Meropenem	
Mild	Increase dose interval to every 12 hours
Moderate	Use half normal dose every 12 hours
Severe	Use half normal dose every 24 hours
Mesalazine	
Moderate	Use with caution
Severe	Manufacturers advise avoid
Metformin	
Mild	Avoid; increased risk of lactic acidosis
Methadone	*see* Opioid Analgesics
Methenamine	
Severe	Avoid—risk of hippurate crystalluria
Methocarbamol	Manufacturer advises caution
Methotrexate	
Mild	Reduce dose; accumulates; nephrotoxic
Moderate	Avoid
Methotrimeprazine	*see* Antipsychotics
Methyldopa	
Moderate	Start with small dose; increased sensitivity to hypotensive and sedative effect
Methysergide	Avoid
Metoclopramide	
Severe	Avoid or use small dose; increased risk of extrapyramidal reactions
Metolazone	*see* Thiazides and Related Diuretics
Metoprolol	*see* Beta-blockers
Midazolam	*see* Anxiolytics and Hypnotics
Midrid®	
Severe	Avoid
Miglustat	Initially 100 mg twice daily if creatinine clearance 50–70 mL/minute; initially 100 mg once daily if creatinine clearance 30–50 mL/minute; avoid if creatinine clearance less than 30 mL/minute
Milrinone	
Mild	Reduce dose and monitor response
Minocycline	*see* Tetracyclines
Mirtazapine	Manufacturer advises caution
Mivacurium	
Severe	Reduce dose; prolonged paralysis

Drug and degree of impairment	Comment
Modafinil	
Severe	Use half normal dose
Moexipril	*see* ACE Inhibitors
Morphine	*see* Opioid Analgesics
Moxonidine	
Mild	Max. single dose 200 micrograms and max. daily dose 400 micrograms
Moderate to severe	Avoid
Nabumetone	*see* NSAIDs
Nadolol	*see* Beta-blockers
Nalidixic acid	
Moderate to severe	Use half normal dose; ineffective in renal failure because concentration in urine is inadequate
Naproxen	*see* NSAIDs
Naratriptan	
Moderate	Max. 2.5 mg in 24 hours
Severe	Avoid
Narcotic analgesics	*see* Opioid Analgesics
Nebivolol	*see* Beta-blockers
Nelfinavir	No information available—manufacturer advises caution
Neomycin	
Mild	Avoid; ototoxic; nephrotoxic
Neostigmine	
Moderate	May need dose reduction
Netilmicin	*see* Aminoglycosides
Nicardipine	
Moderate	Start with small dose
Nicotine	
Severe	May affect clearance of nicotine or its metabolites
Nicoumalone	*see* Anticoagulants, Oral
Nimodipine	Manufacturer advises caution with intravenous administration
Nitrazepam	*see* Anxiolytics and Hypnotics
Nitrofurantoin	
Mild	Avoid; peripheral neuropathy; ineffective because of inadequate urine concentrations
Nitroprusside	*see* Sodium Nitroprusside
Nizatidine	
Mild	Use half normal dose
Moderate	Use one-quarter normal dose
Norfloxacin	Use half normal dose if creatinine clearance less than 30 mL/minute
NSAIDs	
Mild	Use lowest effective dose and monitor renal function; sodium and water retention; deterioration in renal function possibly leading to renal failure; deterioration also reported after topical use
Moderate to severe	Avoid if possible
Ofloxacin	
Mild	Usual initial dose, then use half normal dose
Moderate	Usual initial dose, then 100 mg every 24 hours
Olanzapine	Consider initial dose of 5 mg daily
Olmesartan	Max. 20 mg daily if creatinine clearance 20–60 mL/minute; avoid if creatinine clearance less than 20 mL/minute

Drug and degree of impairment	Comment
Olsalazine	
Moderate	Use with caution
Severe	Manufacturer advises avoid
Opioid analgesics	
Moderate to severe	Reduce doses or avoid; increased and prolonged effect; increased cerebral sensitivity
Oseltamivir	Reduce dose if creatinine clearance 10–30 mL/minute; avoid if creatinine clearance less than 10 mL/minute
Oxaliplatin	
Mild	Manufacturer advises avoid if creatinine clearance less than 30 mL/minute
Oxazepam	*see* Anxiolytics and Hypnotics
Oxcarbazepine	Use half initial dose if creatinine clearance less than 30 mL/minute; increase according to response at intervals of at least 1 week
Oxpentifylline	*see* Pentoxifylline
Oxprenolol	*see* Beta-blockers
Oxybutynin	Manufacturer advises caution
Oxycodone	*see* Opioid Analgesics
Oxytetracycline	*see* Tetracyclines
Pamidronate disodium	*see* Disodium Pamidronate
Pancuronium	
Severe	Prolonged duration of block
Pantoprazole	Max. 40 mg daily
Papaveretum	*see* Opioid Analgesics
Paracetamol	Increase *infusion* dose interval to every 6 hours if creatinine clearance less than 30 mL/minute
Parecoxib	*see* NSAIDs
Paroxetine	Reduce dose if creatinine clearance less than 30 mL/minute
Peginterferon alfa	Close monitoring required—reduce dose if necessary
Penicillamine	
Mild	Reduce dose and monitor renal function (consult product literature)
Moderate to severe	Avoid
Pentamidine	
Mild	Reduce dose; consult product literature
Pentazocine	*see* Opioid Analgesics
Pentoxifylline (oxpentifylline)	Reduce dose by 30–50% if creatinine clearance less than 30 mL/minute
Pericyazine	*see* Antipsychotics
Perindopril	*see* ACE Inhibitors
Perphenazine	*see* Antipsychotics
Pethidine	*see* Opioid Analgesics
Phenazocine	*see* Opioid Analgesics
Phenindione	*see* Anticoagulants, Oral
Phenobarbital	
Severe	Avoid large doses
Phenothiazines	*see* Antipsychotics
Pholcodine	*see* Opioid Analgesics
Picolax®	
Severe	Avoid—risk of hypermagnesaemia
Pilocarpine	Manufacturer advises caution with tablets
Pimozide	*see* Antipsychotics
Pindolol	*see* Beta-blockers
Piperacillin [ingredient]	*see Tazocin*®
Piperazine	
Severe	Avoid—neurotoxic
Pipotiazine	*see* Antipsychotics
Piracetam	
Mild	Use half normal dose
Moderate	Use one-quarter normal dose
Severe	Avoid
Piroxicam	*see* NSAIDs
Potassium salts	
Moderate	Avoid routine use; high risk of hyperkalaemia
Potassium-sparing diuretics	
Mild	Monitor plasma K^+; high risk of hyperkalaemia in renal impairment; amiloride excreted by kidney unchanged
Moderate	Avoid
Povidone–iodine	
Severe	Avoid regular application to inflamed or broken mucosa
Pramipexole	
Mild	Initially 88 micrograms twice daily; if renal function declines, reduce dose further
Moderate to severe	Initially 88 micrograms daily; if renal function declines, reduce dose further
Pravastatin	
Moderate to severe	Start at lower end of dosage range
Prazosin	
Moderate to severe	Initially 500 micrograms daily; increased with caution
Pregabalin	
Mild	Reduce dose; consult product literature
Primaxin®	
Mild	Reduce dose
Primidone	*see* Phenobarbital
Probenecid	
Moderate	Avoid; ineffective and toxicity increased
Procainamide	
Mild	Avoid or reduce dose
Procarbazine	
Severe	Avoid
Prochlorperazine	*see* Antipsychotics
Proguanil	
Mild	100 mg once daily
Moderate	50 mg on alternate days
Severe	50 mg once weekly; increased risk of haematological toxicity
Promazine	*see* Antipsychotics
Propantheline	Manufacturer advises caution
Propiverine	
Severe	Avoid
Propranolol	*see* Beta-blockers
Propylthiouracil	
Mild to moderate	Use three-quarters normal dose
Severe	Use half normal dose
Pseudoephedrine	
Severe	Avoid; increased CNS toxicity
Pyridostigmine	
Moderate	Reduce dose; excreted by kidney

Drug and degree of impairment	Comment
Pyrimethamine	Manufacturer advises caution
Quetiapine	Manufacturer advises initial dose of 25 mg daily, increased daily in steps of 25–50 mg
Quinagolide	Manufacturer advises avoid—no information available
Quinapril	*see* ACE Inhibitors
Quinine	Reduce parenteral maintenance dose for malaria treatment, *see* section 5.4.1
Raloxifene	
Severe	Avoid
Raltitrexed	
Mild	Reduce dose and increase dosing interval
Moderate to severe	Avoid
Ramipril	*see* ACE Inhibitors
Ranitidine	
Severe	Use half normal dose; occasional risk of confusion
Ranitidine bismuth citrate	Avoid if creatinine clearance less than 25 mL/minute
Reboxetine	Initial dose 2 mg twice daily, increased according to tolerance
Regulan®	
Severe	Avoid; contains 6.4 mmol potassium per sachet
Reviparin	
Severe	Manufacturer advises avoid
Riamet®	Manufacturer advises caution in severe renal impairment—monitor ECG and plasma potassium concentration
Ribavirin	
Mild	Plasma-ribavirin concentration increased; manufacturer advises avoid oral ribavirin unless essential—monitor haemoglobin concentration closely
Rifabutin	Use half normal dose if creatinine clearance less than 30 mL/minute
Riluzole	No information available—manufacturer advises avoid
Risedronate sodium	Manufacturer advises avoid if creatinine clearance less than 30 mL/minute
Risperidone	Manufacturer advises initial oral dose of 500 micrograms twice daily increased in steps of 500 micrograms twice daily to 1–2 mg twice daily; if an oral dose of at least 2 mg daily tolerated, 25 mg as a depot injection can be given every 2 weeks
Ritonavir [ingredient]	*see Kaletra®*
Rivastigmine	Manufacturer advises caution
Rizatriptan	
Mild to moderate	Reduce dose to 5 mg
Severe	Avoid
Rocuronium	
Moderate	Reduce dose; prolonged paralysis
Ropinirole	
Severe	Avoid
Rosiglitazone	Manufacturer advises caution, if creatinine clearance less than 30 mL/minute
Rosuvastatin	Avoid if creatinine clearance less than 30 mL/minute; avoid dose of 40 mg daily if creatinine clearance less than 60 mL/minute
Saquinavir	
Severe	Dose adjustment possibly required
Sertraline	Manufacturer advises caution
Sevoflurane	Manufacturer advises caution
Sibutramine	
Mild to moderate	Manufacturer advises caution
Severe	Avoid
Sildenafil	Initial dose 25 mg if creatinine clearance less than 30 mL/minute
Simvastatin	Doses above 10 mg daily should be used with caution if creatinine clearance less than 30 mL/minute
Sirolimus	Adjust immunosuppressant regimen in patients with raised serum creatinine
Sodium aurothiomalate	Caution; nephrotoxic
Sodium bicarbonate	
Severe	Avoid; specialised role in some forms of renal disease
Sodium clodronate	
Mild to moderate	Use half normal dose and monitor serum creatinine
Severe	Avoid
Sodium nitroprusside	
Moderate	Avoid prolonged use
Sodium valproate	*see* Valproate
Solifenacin	Max. 5 mg daily if creatinine clearance less than 30 mL/minute
Solpadeine®	
Severe	Avoid effervescent tablet preparations; contains 18.5 mmol sodium per tablet
Solpadol®	
Severe	Avoid effervescent tablets; contains 16.9 mmol sodium per tablet
Sotalol	*see* Beta-blockers
Spironolactone	*see* Potassium-sparing Diuretics
Stavudine	
Mild	20 mg twice daily (15 mg if $<$ 60 kg)
Moderate to severe	20 mg once daily (15 mg if $<$ 60 kg)
Streptomycin	*see* Aminoglycosides
Strontium ranelate	Manufacturer advises no dose adjustment required if creatinine clearance 30–70 mL/minute; avoid if creatinine clearance less than 30 mL/minute
Sucralfate	
Severe	Avoid; aluminium is absorbed and may accumulate
Sulfadiazine	
Severe	Avoid; high risk of crystalluria
Sulfasalazine	
Moderate	Risk of toxicity including crystalluria—ensure high fluid intake
Severe	Avoid

Drug and degree of impairment	Comment
Sulfinpyrazone	
Moderate	Avoid; ineffective as uricosuric
Sulindac	*see* NSAIDs
Sulphonamides	
Moderate	Ensure high fluid intake; rashes and blood disorders; crystalluria a risk
Sulphonylureas	*see under* individual drugs
Sulpiride	
Moderate	Avoid if possible, or reduce dose
Tacalcitol	Monitor serum calcium concentration
Tadalafil	Max. dose 10 mg if creatinine clearance less than 30 mL/minute
Tamsulosin	
Severe	Manufacturer advises caution
Tazobactam [ingredient]	*see Tazocin®*
Tazocin®	Max. 4.5 g every 8 hours if creatinine clearance 20–80 mL/minute; max. 4.5 g every 12 hours if creatinine clearance less than 20 mL/minute; child under 12 years: Consult product literature
Teicoplanin	On day 4 use half normal dose if creatinine clearance is 40–60 mL/minute and use one-third normal dose if creatinine clearance is less than 40 mL/minute
Telithromycin	Use half normal dose if creatinine clearance less than 30 mL/minute
Telmisartan	
Severe	Initially 20 mg once daily
Temazepam	*see* Anxiolytics and Hypnotics
Tenofovir	Monitor renal function —interrupt treatment if further deterioration; 245 mg every 2 days if creatinine clearance 30–50 mL/minute; 245 mg every 3–4 days if creatinine clearance 10–30 mL/minute
Tenoxicam	*see* NSAIDs
Terbinafine	
Mild	Use half normal dose
Terfenadine	Use half normal dose if creatinine clearance less than 40 mL/minute
Tetracyclines	
Mild	Avoid tetracyclines except doxycycline or minocycline which may be used cautiously (avoid excessive doses)
Thiazides and related diuretics	
Moderate	Avoid; ineffective (metolazone remains effective but risk of excessive diuresis)
Tiaprofenic acid	*see* NSAIDs
Ticarcillin [ingredient]	*see Timentin®*
Tiludronic acid	
Moderate to severe	Avoid
Timentin®	
Mild	Reduce dose
Timolol	*see* Beta-blockers
Tinzaparin	
Severe	May need dose reduction
Tioguanine	
Moderate	Reduce dose
Tiotropium	Plasma-tiotropium concentration raised; manufacturer advises caution
Tirofiban	Use half normal dose if creatinine clearance less than 30 mL/minute
Tizanidine	Initially 2 mg once daily if creatinine clearance less than 25 mL/minute; increase once-daily dose gradually according to response before increasing frequency
Tobramycin	*see* Aminoglycosides
Tolbutamide	
Mild to moderate	Reduce dose
Severe	Avoid if possible; if no alternative reduce dose and monitor closely
Tolfenamic acid	*see* NSAIDs
Tolterodine	Reduce dose to 1 mg twice daily if creatinine clearance less than 30 mL/minute
Topiramate	
Moderate to severe	Longer time to steady-state plasma concentrations
Topotecan	
Moderate	Reduce dose
Severe	Avoid
Torasemide	
Moderate	May need high doses
Tramadol	*see* Opioid Analgesics
Trandolapril	*see* ACE Inhibitors
Tranexamic acid	
Mild to moderate	Reduce dose
Severe	Avoid
Tretinoin (oral)	
Mild	Reduce dose
Triamterene	*see* Potassium-sparing Diuretics
Tribavirin	*see* Ribavirin
Triclofos	*see* Anxiolytics and Hypnotics
Trifluoperazine	*see* Antipsychotics
Trimeprazine	*see* Alimemazine
Trimethoprim	Use half normal dose after 3 days if creatinine clearance 15–30 mL/minute; use half normal dose if creatinine clearance less than 15 mL/minute; avoid if creatinine clearance less than 10 mL/minute (unless plasma-trimethoprim concentration monitored)
Tripotassium dicitratobismuthate	
Severe	Avoid
Trisodium edetate	
Mild	Avoid
Trospium	
Mild to moderate	Reduce dose to 20 mg once daily or 20 mg on alternate days if creatinine clearance 10–30 mL/minute
Severe	Avoid

Drug and degree of impairment	Comment
Truvada®	Monitor renal function; use normal dose every 48 hours if creatinine clearance 30–50 mL/minute; avoid if creatinine clearance less than 30 mL/minute
Tylex®	
Moderate to severe	Avoid effervescent tablets; contain 13.6 mmol sodium per tablet
Ultramol®	Avoid; contains 15.7 mmol sodium per tablet
Valaciclovir	
Mild	Reduce treatment dose for herpes zoster; reduce dose according to creatinine clearance for cytomegalovirus prophylaxis following renal transplantation
Moderate to severe	Reduce dose for all indications
Valganciclovir	Reduce dose; consult product literature
Valproate	
Mild to moderate	Reduce dose
Severe	Alter dosage according to free serum valproic acid concentration
Valproic acid	*see* Valproate
Valsartan	Initially 40 mg once daily if creatinine clearance less than 20 mL/minute
Vancomycin	
Mild	Reduce dose—monitor plasma-vancomycin concentration and renal function regularly
Vardenafil	Initial dose 5 mg if creatinine clearance less than 30 mL/minute; avoid in endstage renal disease requiring dialysis
Venlafaxine	Use half normal dose if creatinine clearance 10–30 mL/minute; avoid if creatinine clearance less than 10 mL/minute
Vigabatrin	
Mild	Excreted by kidney—lower maintenance dose may be required
Voriconazole	Intravenous vehicle may accumulate if creatinine clearance less than 50 mL/minute—manufacturer advises use intravenous infusion only if potential benefit outweighs risk, and monitor renal function; alternatively, use tablets or oral suspension (no dose adjustment required)
Warfarin	*see* Anticoagulants, Oral
Xipamide	*see* Thiazides and Related Diuretics
Yasmin®	
Severe	Manufacturer advises avoid
Zafirlukast	
Moderate to severe	Manufacturer advises caution
Zalcitabine	
Mild to moderate	750 micrograms every 12 hours
Severe	750 micrograms daily
Zidovudine	
Severe	Reduce dose; manufacturer advises oral dose of 300–400 mg daily in divided doses or intravenous dose of 1 mg/kg 3–4 times daily
Zoledronic acid	Avoid if serum creatinine above 400 micromol/litre in tumor-induced hypercalcaemia; in cancer and bone metastases, if creatinine clearance 50–60 mL/minute reduce dose to 3.5 mg every 3–4 weeks, if creatinine clearance 40–50 mL/minute reduce dose to 3.3 mg every 3–4 weeks, if creatinine clearance 30–40 mL/minute reduce dose to 3 mg every 3–4 weeks, and avoid if creatinine clearance below 30 mL/minute (or if serum creatinine above 265 micromol/litre); if renal function deteriorates in patients with bone metastases, withhold dose until serum creatinine returns to within 10% of baseline value
Zonisamide	Initially increase dose at 2-week intervals; discontinue if renal function deteriorates
Zopiclone	*see* Anxiolytics and Hypnotics
Zotepine	Initial dose 25 mg twice daily, increased gradually according to response (max. 75 mg twice daily)
Zuclopenthixol	*see* Antipsychotics

Appendix 4: Pregnancy

Drugs can have harmful effects on the fetus at any time during pregnancy. It is important to bear this in mind when prescribing for a woman of *childbearing age* or for men *trying* to *father* a child.

During the *first trimester* drugs may produce congenital malformations (teratogenesis), and the period of greatest risk is from the third to the eleventh week of pregnancy.

During the *second* and *third trimesters* drugs may affect the growth and functional development of the fetus or have toxic effects on fetal tissues; and drugs given shortly before term or during labour may have adverse effects on labour or on the neonate after delivery.

The following list includes drugs which:

- may have harmful effects in pregnancy and indicates the trimester of risk
- are not known to be harmful in pregnancy

The list is based on human data but information on *animal* studies has been included for some drugs when its omission might be misleading.

> Drugs should be prescribed in pregnancy only if the expected benefit to the mother is thought to be greater than the risk to the fetus, and all drugs should be avoided if possible during the first trimester. Drugs which have been extensively used in pregnancy and appear to be usually safe should be prescribed in preference to new or untried drugs; and the smallest effective dose should be used.
>
> Few drugs have been shown conclusively to be teratogenic in man but no drug is safe beyond all doubt in early pregnancy. Screening procedures are available where there is a known risk of certain defects.
>
> Absence of a drug from the list does not imply safety. It should be noted that the BNF provides independent advice and may not always agree with the product literature.
>
> Information on drugs and pregnancy is also available from the National Teratology Information Service
> Telephone: (0191) 232 1525
> (0191) 223 1307 (out of hours emergency only)
> www.nyrdtc.nhs.uk/Services/teratology/teratology.html

Table of drugs to be avoided or used with caution in pregnancy

Products introduced or amended since publication of BNF No. 49 (March 2005) are underlined.

Drug (trimester of risk)	Comment
Abacavir	Manufacturer advises avoid (toxicity in *animal* studies)
Abciximab	Manufacturer advises use only if potential benefit outweighs risk—no information available
Acamprosate	Manufacturer advises avoid
Acarbose	Manufacturer advises avoid; insulin is normally substituted in all diabetics
ACE inhibitors	
(1, 2, 3)	Avoid; may adversely affect fetal and neonatal blood pressure control and renal function; also possible skull defects and oligohydramnios; toxicity in *animal* studies
Acebutolol	*see* Beta-blockers
Aceclofenac	*see* NSAIDs
Acemetacin	*see* NSAIDs
Acenocoumarol (nicoumalone)	*see* Anticoagulants, Oral
Acetazolamide	*see* Diuretics
Aciclovir	Not known to be harmful—manufacturers advise use only when potential benefit outweighs risk; limited absorption from topical aciclovir preparations
Acipimox	Manufacturer advises avoid
Acitretin	
(1, 2, 3)	Teratogenic; effective contraception must be used for at least 1 month before treatment, during treatment, and for at least 2 years after stopping
Acrivastine	*see* Antihistamines
Adalimumab	Avoid; manufacturer advises adequate contraception during and for at least 5 months after last dose
Adapalene	Manufacturer advises teratogenicity in *animal* studies and recommends effective contraception during treatment
Adefovir dipivoxil	Toxicity in *animal* studies—manufacturer advises use only if potential benefit outweighs risk; effective contraception required during treatment
Agalsidase beta	Manufacturer advises avoid unless essential—no information available
Alclometasone	*see* Corticosteroids
Alcohol	
(1, 2)	Regular daily drinking is teratogenic (fetal alcohol syndrome) and may cause growth restriction; occasional single drinks are probably safe
(3)	Withdrawal syndrome may occur in babies of alcoholic mothers
Alemtuzumab	Avoid; manufacturer advises effective contraception during and for 6 months after administration to men or women
Alendronic acid	*see* Bisphosphonates
Alfentanil	*see* Opioid Analgesics

Drug (trimester of risk)	Comment
Alimemazine (trimeprazine)	*see* Antihistamines
Allopurinol	Toxicity not reported; manufacturer advises avoid; use only if no safer alternative and disease carries risk for mother or child
Almotriptan	*see* $5HT_1$ Agonists
Alpha-blockers, post-synaptic	No evidence of teratogenicity; manufacturers advise use only when potential benefit outweighs risk
Alprazolam	*see* Benzodiazepines
Alprostadil (urethral application only)	Manufacturer advises barrier contraception if partner pregnant
Alteplase	*see* Streptokinase
Amantadine	Avoid; toxicity in *animal* studies
Amfebutamone	*see* Bupropion
Amikacin	*see* Aminoglycosides
Amiloride	*see* Diuretics
Aminoglutethimide	Avoid; toxicity in *animal* studies and may affect fetal sexual development
Aminoglycosides (2, 3)	Auditory or vestibular nerve damage; risk greatest with streptomycin; probably very small with gentamicin and tobramycin, but avoid unless essential (if given, serum-aminoglycoside concentration monitoring essential)
Aminophylline	*see* Theophylline
Amiodarone (2, 3)	Possible risk of neonatal goitre; use only if no alternative
Amisulpride	Manufacturer advises avoid
Amitriptyline	*see* Antidepressants, Tricyclic (and related)
Amlodipine	No information available—manufacturer advises avoid, but risk to fetus should be balanced against risk of uncontrolled maternal hypertension
Amobarbital	*see* Barbiturates
Amorolfine	Systemic absorption very low, but manufacturer advises avoid—no information available
Amoxapine	*see* Antidepressants, Tricyclic (and related)
Amoxicillin	*see* Penicillins
Amphotericin	Not known to be harmful but manufacturers advise avoid unless potential benefit outweighs risk
Ampicillin	*see* Penicillins
Amprenavir	Avoid oral solution due to high propylene glycol content; manufacturer advises use capsules only if potential benefit outweighs risk
Amsacrine	Avoid (teratogenic and toxic in *animal* studies); may reduce fertility; *see also* section 8.1
Anabolic steroids (1, 2, 3)	Masculinisation of female fetus
Anaesthetics, general (3)	Depress neonatal respiration; dose of thiopental should not exceed 250 mg
Anaesthetics, local (3)	With large doses, neonatal respiratory depression, hypotonia, and bradycardia after paracervical or epidural block; neonatal methaemoglobinaemia with prilocaine and procaine; lower doses of bupivacaine for intrathecal use during late pregnancy
Anagrelide	Manufacturer advises avoid (toxicity in *animal* studies)
Anakinra	Manufacturer advises avoid; effective contraception must be used during treatment
Analgesics	*see* Opioid Analgesics, Nefopam, NSAIDs, and Paracetamol
Androgens (1, 2, 3)	Masculinisation of female fetus
Anticoagulants, oral (1, 2, 3)	Congenital malformations; fetal and neonatal haemorrhage; *see also* section 2.8.2
Antidepressants, MAOI (1, 2, 3)	No evidence of harm but manufacturers advise avoid unless compelling reasons
Antidepressants, SSRI	Manufacturers advise use only if potential benefit outweighs risk (no evidence of teratogenicity); risk of neonatal withdrawl, particularly with fluoxetine and paroxetine; toxicity in *animal* studies with escitalopram and paroxetine
Antidepressants, tricyclic (and related) (3)	Tachycardia, irritability, and muscle spasms in neonate reported with imipramine
Antiepileptics	Benefit of treatment outweighs risk to fetus; risk of teratogenicity greater if more than one drug used; **important:** *see also* Carbamazepine, Ethosuximide, Phenobarbital, Phenytoin, Valproate, Vigabatrin, and p. 238
Antihistamines	No evidence of teratogenicity; embryotoxicity in *animal* studies with high doses of hydroxyzine and loratadine; manufacturers of cetirizine, desloratadine, hydroxyzine, loratadine, mizolastine and terfenadine advise avoid
Antimalarials (1, 3)	Benefit of prophylaxis and treatment in malaria outweighs risk; **important:** *see also* individual drugs and p. 330 and p. 331
Antipsychotics	*See also* Amisulpride, Clozapine, Olanzapine, Quetiapine, Risperidone, Sertindole, Zotepine
(3)	Extrapyramidal effects in neonate occasionally reported

Drug (trimester of risk)	Comment
Apomorphine	Avoid
Aprepitant (1, 2, 3)	Manufacturer advises avoid unless potential benefit outweighs risk—no information available
Aprotonin	Manufacturer advises use only if potential benefit outweighs risk; possibly reduced fibrinolytic activity in newborn
Aripiprazole (1, 2, 3)	Manufacturer advises use only if potential benefit outweighs risk—no information available
Arsenic trioxide	Avoid (teratogenic and embryotoxic in *animal* studies); manufacturer advises effective contraception during administration to men or women; *see also* section 8.1
Artemether [ingredient]	*see Riamet®*
Aspirin (3)	Impaired platelet function and risk of haemorrhage; delayed onset and increased duration of labour with increased blood loss; avoid analgesic doses if possible in last few weeks (low doses probably not harmful); with high doses, closure of fetal ductus arteriosus *in utero* and possibly persistent pulmonary hypertension of newborn; kernicterus in jaundiced neonates
Atazanavir	Manufacturer advises use only if potential benefit outweighs risk; theoretical risk of hyperbilirubinaemia in neonate if used at term
Atenolol	*see* Beta-blockers
Atomoxetine	Manufacturer advises avoid unless potential benefit outweighs risk—no information available
Atorvastatin	*see* Statins
Atosiban	For use in premature labour *see* section 7.1.3
Atovaquone	Manufacturer advises avoid unless potential benefit outweighs risk—no information available
Atracurium	Does not cross placenta in significant amounts but manufacturer advises use only if potential benefit outweighs risk
Atropine	Not known to be harmful; manufacturer advises caution
Auranofin	Manufacturer advises avoid (effective contraception should be used during and for at least 6 months after treatment) but limited data suggests usually not necessary to withdraw if condition well controlled—consider reducing dose and frequency
Azathioprine	*see* p. 444
Azelastine	*see* Antihistamines
Azithromycin	Manufacturer advises use only if adequate alternatives not available
Aztreonam	Manufacturer advises avoid—no information available
Baclofen	Manufacturer advises use only if potential benefit outweighs risk (toxicity in *animal* studies)
Balsalazide	Manufacturer advises avoid
Bambuterol	*see* section 3.1
Barbiturates (3)	Withdrawal effects in neonate; *see also* Phenobarbital
Basiliximab	Avoid; adequate contraception must be used during treatment and for 8 weeks after last dose
Beclometasone	*see* Corticosteroids
Bemiparin	Manufacturer advises avoid unless essential—no information available
Bendrofluazide	*see* Diuretics
Bendroflumethiazide (bendrofluazide)	*see* Diuretics
Benperidol	*see* Antipsychotics
Benzodiazepines	Avoid regular use (risk of neonatal withdrawal symptoms); use only if clear indication such as seizure control (high doses during late pregnancy or labour may cause neonatal hypothermia, hypotonia and respiratory depression)
Benzylpenicillin	*see* Penicillins
Beta-blockers	May cause intra-uterine growth restriction, neonatal hypoglycaemia, and bradycardia; risk greater in severe hypertension; *see also* section 2.5
Betamethasone	*see* Corticosteroids
Bethanechol	Manufacturer advises avoid—no information available
Bevacizumab	Manufacturer advises avoid—toxicity in *animal* studies; effective contraception required during and for at least 6 months after treatment in women (*see also* section 8.1)
Bexarotene	Avoid; manufacturer advises effective contraception during and for at least 1 month after administration to men or women; *see also* section 8.1
Bezafibrate	*see* Fibrates
Bimatoprost	Manufacturer advises use only if potential benefit outweighs risk
Bisoprolol	*see* Beta-blockers
Bisphosphonates	Manufacturers advise avoid
Bivalirudin	Manufacturer advises avoid unless potential benefit outweighs risk—no information available
Bleomycin	Avoid (teratogenic and carcinogenic in *animal* studies); *see also* section 8.1
Bosentan	Avoid (teratogenic in *animal* studies); effective contraception required during and for at least 3 months after administration

Drug (trimester of risk)	Comment
Botulinum toxin	Manufacturers advise avoid; toxicity in *animal* studies
Brinzolamide	Manufacturer advises avoid unless essential
Buclizine	*see* Anthistamines
Budesonide	*see* Corticosteroids
Bumetanide	*see* Diuretics
Bupivacaine	*see* Anaesthetics, Local
Buprenorphine	*see* Opioid Analgesics
Bupropion	Manufacturer advises avoid—no information available
Buserelin	Avoid
Buspirone	Manufacturer advises avoid
Busulfan	Avoid (teratogenic in *animals*); manufacturer advises effective contraception during administration to men or women; *see also* section 8.1
Cabergoline	No evidence of harm; manufacturer advises discontinuation one month before intended conception and avoidance during pregnancy; *see also* section 6.7.1
Calcipotriol	Manufacturer advises avoid if possible
Calcitonin (salmon) (salcatonin)	Manufacturer advises avoid unless potential benefit outweighs risk (toxicity in *animal* studies)
Calcitriol	*see* Vitamin D
Calcium folinate	Manufacturer advises use only if potential benefit outweighs risk
Calcium levofolinate	*see* Calcium Folinate
Candesartan	*As for* ACE Inhibitors
Capecitabine	Avoid (teratogenic in animal studies); *see also* section 8.1
Capreomycin	Manufacturer advises use only if potential benefit outweighs risk—teratogenic in *animal* studies
Captopril	*see* ACE Inhibitors
Carbamazepine	
(1)	Risk of teratogenesis including increased risk of neural tube defects (counselling and screening and adequate folate supplements advised, e.g. 5 mg daily); *see also* Antiepileptics and p. 238
(3)	May possibly cause vitamin K deficiency and risk of neonatal bleeding; if vitamin K not given at birth, neonate should be monitored closely for signs of bleeding
Carbimazole	
(2, 3)	Neonatal goitre and hypothyroidism; has been associated with aplasia cutis of the neonate
Carbocisteine	
(1)	Manufacturer advises avoid
Carboplatin	Avoid (teratogenic and embryotoxic in *animal* studies); *see also* section 8.1
Carglumic acid	Manufacturer advises avoid unless essential—no information available
Carmustine	Avoid (teratogenic and embryotoxic in *animals*); manufacturer advises effective contraception during administration to men or women; *see also* section 8.1
Carnitine	No evidence of teratogenicity in *animal* studies; consider serious consequence of discontinuing treatment
Carvedilol	*see* Beta-blockers
Caspofungin	Manufacturer advises avoid unless essential—toxicity in *animal* studies
Cefaclor	Not known to be harmful
Cefadroxil	Not known to be harmful
Cefalexin	Not known to be harmful
Cefixime	Not known to be harmful
Cefotaxime	Not known to be harmful
Cefpirome	Manufacturer advises avoid
Cefpodoxime	Not known to be harmful
Cefprozil	Not known to be harmful
Cefradine	Not known to be harmful
Ceftazidime	Not known to be harmful
Ceftriaxone	Not known to be harmful
Cefuroxime	Not known to be harmful
Celecoxib	Manufacturer advises avoid (teratogenic in *animal* studies); *see also* NSAIDs
Celiprolol	*see* Beta-blockers
Cetirizine	*see* Antihistamines
Cetrorelix	Manufacturer advises avoid in confirmed pregnancy
Cetuximab	Manufacturer advises use only if potential benefit outweighs risk—no information available
Chloral hydrate	Avoid
Chlorambucil	Avoid; manufacturer advises effective contraception during administration to men or women; *see also* section 8.1
Chloramphenicol	
(3)	Neonatal 'grey' syndrome
Chlordiazepoxide	*see* Benzodiazepines
Chloroquine	*see* Antimalarials
Chlorphenamine (chlorpheniramine)	*see* Anthistamines
Chlorpheniramine	*see* Antihistamines
Chlorpromazine	*see* Antipsychotics
Chlorpropamide	*see* Sulphonylureas
Chlortalidone	*see* Diuretics
Chlortetracycline	*see* Tetracyclines
Ciclosporin	*see* p. 444
Cidofovir	Avoid (toxicity in *animal* studies); effective contraception required during and for 1 month after treatment; also men should avoid fathering a child during and for 3 months after treatment
Cilastatin [ingredient]	*see Primaxin*®
Cilazapril	*see* ACE Inhibitors
Cilostazol	Avoid—toxicity in *animal* studies
Cimetidine	Manufacturer advises avoid unless essential

Drug (trimester of risk)	Comment
Cinacalcet	Manufacturer advises use only if potential benefit outweighs risk—no information available
Cinnarizine	*see* Anthistamines
Ciprofibrate	*see* Fibrates
Ciprofloxacin	*see* Quinolones
Cisatracurium	Manufacturer advises avoid—no information available
Cisplatin	Avoid (teratogenic and toxic in *animal* studies); *see also* section 8.1
Citalopram	*see* Antidepressants, SSRI
Cladribine	Avoid (teratogenic in *animal* studies); *see also* section 8.1
Clarithromycin	Manufacturer advises avoid unless potential benefit outweighs risk
Clavulanic acid [ingredient]	*see* Co-amoxiclav, *Timentin*®
Clemastine	*see* Anthistamines
Clindamycin	Not known to be harmful
Clobazam	*see* Benzodiazepines
Clobetasol	*see* Corticosteroids
Clobetasone	*see* Corticosteroids
Clodronate sodium	*see* Bisphosphonates
Clomethiazole	Avoid if possible—especially during first and third trimesters
Clomifene	Possible effects on fetal development
Clomipramine	*see* Antidepressants, Tricyclic (and related)
Clonazepam	*see* Benzodiazepines
Clonidine	May lower fetal heart rate, but risk should be balanced against risk of uncontrolled maternal hypertension; avoid intravenous injection
Clopidogrel	Manufacturer advises avoid—no information available
Clorazepate	*see* Benzodiazepines
Clozapine	Manufacturer advises avoid
Co-amoxiclav	*see* Penicillins
Co-beneldopa	*see* Levodopa
Co-careldopa	*see* Levodopa
Co-cyprindiol (1, 2, 3)	Feminisation of male fetus (due to cyproterone)
Codeine	*see* Opioid Analgesics
Co-fluampicil	*see* Penicillins
Colchicine	Avoid—teratogenicity in animal studies
Colistin (2, 3)	Avoid—possible risk of fetal toxicity
Contraceptives, oral	Epidemiological evidence suggests no harmful effects on fetus
Corticosteroids	Benefit of treatment, e.g. in asthma, outweighs risk (*see also* CSM advice, section 6.3.2); risk of intra-uterine growth restriction on prolonged or repeated systemic treatment; corticosteroid cover required by mother during labour; monitor closely if fluid retention

Drug (trimester of risk)	Comment
Co-trimoxazole	
(1)	Teratogenic risk (trimethoprim a folate antagonist)
(3)	Neonatal haemolysis and methaemoglobinaemia; fear of increased risk of kernicterus in neonates appears to be unfounded
Crisantaspase	Avoid; *see also* section 8.1
Cromoglicate	*see* Sodium Cromoglicate
Cyclizine	*see* Antihistamines
Cyclopenthiazide	*see* Diuretics
Cyclophosphamide	Avoid (manufacturer advises effective contraception during and for at least 3 months after administration to men or women); *see also* section 8.1
Cycloserine	Manufacturer advises use only if potential benefit outweighs risk—crosses the placenta
Cyclosporin	*see* p. 444
Cyproheptadine	*see* Antihistamines
Cyproterone [ingredient]	*see* Co-cyprindiol
Cytarabine	Avoid (teratogenic in *animal* studies); *see also* section 8.1
Dacarbazine	Avoid (carcinogenic and teratogenic in *animal* studies); ensure effective contraception during and for at least 6 months after administration to men or women; *see also* section 8.1
Daclizumab	Avoid
Dactinomycin	Avoid (teratogenic in *animal* studies); *see also* section 8.1
Dalfopristin [ingredient]	*see Synercid*®
Dalteparin	Not known to be harmful
Danaparoid	Limited information available but not known to be harmful—manufacturer advises avoid
Danazol (1, 2, 3)	Avoid; has weak androgenic effects and virilisation of female fetus reported
Dantrolene	Use only for malignant hyperthermia if potential benefit outweighs risk; avoid use in chronic spasticity—embryotoxic in *animal* studies
Dantron (danthron)	Manufacturer advises avoid—no information available
Dapsone (3)	Neonatal haemolysis and methaemoglobinaemia; folic acid 5 mg daily should be given to mother
Darbepoetin	No evidence of harm in *animal* studies—manufacturer advises caution
Daunorubicin	Avoid (teratogenic and carcinogenic in *animal* studies); *see also* section 8.1

Drug (trimester of risk)	Comment
Deferiprone	Manufacturer advises avoid before intended conception and during pregnancy—teratogenic and embryotoxic in *animal* studies; contraception advised in women of child-bearing potential
Deflazacort	*see* Corticosteroids
Demeclocycline	*see* Tetracyclines
Desferrioxamine	Teratogenic in *animal* studies; manufacturer advises use only if potential benefit outweighs risk
Desflurane	*see* Anaesthetics, General
Desloratadine	*see* Antihistamines
Desmopressin	
(3)	Small oxytocic effect in third trimester; increased risk of pre-eclampsia
Desogestrel	*see* Contraceptives, Oral
Dexamethasone	*see* Corticosteroids
Dexamfetamine	Manufacturer advises avoid (retrospective evidence of uncertain significance suggesting possible embryotoxicity)
Dexketoprofen	*see* NSAIDs
Dextran	Avoid—reports of anaphylaxis in mother causing fetal anoxia, neurological damage and death
Dextromethorphan	*see* Opioid Analgesics
Dextropropoxyphene	*see* Opioid Analgesics
Diamorphine	*see* Opioid Analgesics
Diazepam	*see* Benzodiazepines
Diazoxide	
(2, 3)	Prolonged use may produce alopecia and impaired glucose tolerance in neonate; inhibits uterine activity during labour
Diclofenac	*see* NSAIDs
Didanosine	Manufacturer advises use only if potential benefit outweighs risk—no information available
Diethylstilbestrol	
(1)	High doses associated with vaginal carcinoma, urogenital abnormalities, and reduced fertility in female offspring; increased risk of hypospadias in male offspring
Diflucortolone	*see* Corticosteroids
Diflunisal	*see* NSAIDs
Digoxin	May need dosage adjustment
Dihydrocodeine	*see* Opioid Analgesics
Diloxanide	Manufacturer advises avoid—no information available
Diltiazem	Avoid
Diphenhydramine	*see* Antihistamines
Diphenoxylate	*see* Opioid Analgesics
Dipipanone	*see* Opioid Analgesics
Dipyridamole	Not known to be harmful
Disodium etidronate	*see* Bisphosphonates
Disodium pamidronate	*see* Bisphosphonates
Disopyramide	
(3)	May induce labour
Distigmine	Manufacturer advises avoid (may stimulate uterine contractions)
Disulfiram	
(1)	High concentrations of acetaldehyde which occur in presence of alcohol may be teratogenic
Diuretics	Not used to treat hypertension in pregnancy
(1)	Manufacturers advise avoid acetazolamide and torasemide (toxicity in *animal* studies)
(3)	Thiazides may cause neonatal thrombocytopenia
Docetaxel	Avoid (toxicity and reduced fertility in *animal* studies); manufacturer advises effective contraception during and for at least 3 months after administration; *see also* section 8.1
Docusate sodium	Not known to be harmful—manufacturer advises caution
Dolasetron	Manufacturer advises avoid unless potential benefit outweighs risk—no information available
Domperidone	Manufacturer advises avoid
Dornase alfa	No evidence of teratogenicity; manufacturer advises use only if potential benefit outweighs risk
Dosulepin (dothiepin)	*see* Antidepressants, Tricyclic (and related)
Dothiepin	*see* Antidepressants, Tricyclic (and related)
Doxazosin	*see* Alpha-blockers, Post-synaptic
Doxepin	*see* Antidepressants, Tricyclic (and related)
Doxorubicin	Avoid (teratogenic and toxic in *animal* studies); manufacturer of liposomal product advises effective contraception during and for at least 6 months after administration to men or women; *see also* section 8.1
Doxycycline	*see* Tetracyclines
Doxylamine	*see* Antihistamines
Drotrecogin alfa (activated)	Manufacturer advises avoid unless benefit outweighs risk—no information available
Duloxetine	Toxicity in *animal* studies—manufacturer advises avoid in patients with stress urinary incontinence and use only if potential benefit outweighs risk in depression; risk of neonatal withdrawal symptoms if used near term
Dutasteride	
(1, 2, 3)	Avoid unprotected intercourse (*see* section 6.4.2). May cause feminisation of male fetus
Dydrogesterone	Not known to be harmful
Econazole	Not known to be harmful
Edrophonium	Manufacturer advises use only if potential benefit outweighs risk
Efalizumab	Manufacturer advises avoid

Drug (trimester of risk)	Comment
Efavirenz	Toxicity in *animal* studies; manufacturer advises use only if potential benefit outweighs risk and no alternative options available
Eflornithine	Toxicity in *animal* studies—manufacturer advises avoid
Eformoterol	*see* Formoterol
Eletriptan	*see* $5HT_1$ Agonists
Emtricitabine	No information available—manufacturer advises use only if essential
Enalapril	*see* ACE Inhibitors
Enfuvirtide	Manufacturer advises use only if potential benefit outweighs risk
Enoxaparin	Manufacturer advises avoid unless no safer alternative
Enoximone	Manufacturer advises use only if potential benefit outweighs risk
Entacapone	Manufacturer advises avoid—no information available
Ephedrine	Increased fetal heart rate reported with parenteral ephedrine
Epinastine	*see* Antihistamines
Epirubicin	Avoid (carcinogenic in *animal* studies); *see also* section 8.1
Eplerenone	Manufacturer advises caution—no information available
Epoetin	No evidence of harm; benefits probably outweigh risk of anaemia and of transfusion in pregnancy
Epoprostenol	Manufacturer advises use with caution—no information available
Eprosartan	*As for* ACE Inhibitors
Eptifibatide	Manufacturer advises use only if potential benefit outweighs risk—no information available
Ergotamine	
(1, 2, 3)	Oxytocic effects on the pregnant uterus
Ertapenem	Manufacturer advises avoid unless potential benefit outweighs risk
Erythromycin	Not known to be harmful
Escitalopram	*see* Antidepressants, SSRI
Esmolol	*see* Beta-blockers
Esomeprazole	Manufacturer advises caution—no information available
Etanercept	Manufacturer advises avoid—no information available
Ethambutol	Not known to be harmful; *see also* p. 297
Ethinylestradiol	*see* Contraceptives, Oral
Ethionamide	
(1)	May be teratogenic
Ethosuximide	
(1)	May possibly be teratogenic; *see* Antiepileptics
Etidronate disodium	*see* Bisphosphonates
Etodolac	*see* NSAIDs
Etomidate	*see* Anaesthetics, General
Etoposide	Avoid (teratogenic in *animal* studies); *see also* section 8.1
Etoricoxib	*see* NSAIDs
Etynodiol	*see* Contraceptives, Oral
Ezetimibe	Manufacturer advises use only if potential benefit outweighs risk—no information available
Famciclovir	*see* Aciclovir
Famotidine	Manufacturer advises avoid unless potential benefit outweighs risk
Fansidar®	
(1)	Possible teratogenic risk (pyrimethamine a folate antagonist)
(3)	Neonatal haemolysis and methaemoglobinaemia; fear of increased risk of kernicterus in neonates appears to be unfounded
	see also Antimalarials
Felodipine	Avoid; toxicity in *animal* studies; may inhibit labour
Fenbufen	*see* NSAIDs
Fenofibrate	*see* Fibrates
Fenoprofen	*see* NSAIDs
Fenoterol	*see* section 3.1
Fentanyl	*see* Opioid Analgesics
Fenticonazole	Manufacturer advises avoid unless essential
Fexofenadine	*see* Antihistamines
Fibrates	Embryotoxicity in *animal* studies—manufacturers advise avoid
Filgrastim	Toxicity in *animal* studies; manufacturer advises use only if potential benefit outweighs risk
Finasteride	
(1, 2, 3)	Avoid unprotected intercourse (*see* section 6.4.2). May cause feminisation of male fetus
Flavoxate	Manufacturer advises avoid unless no safer alternative
Flecainide	Manufacturer advises toxicity in *animal* studies
Flucloxacillin	*see* Penicillins
Fluconazole	Manufacturer advises avoid—multiple congenital abnormalities reported with long-term high doses
Flucytosine	Teratogenic in *animal* studies; manufacturer advises use only if potential benefit outweighs risk
Fludarabine	Avoid (embryotoxic and teratogenic in *animal* studies); manufacturer advises effective contraception during and for at least 6 months after administration to men or women; *see also* section 8.1
Fludrocortisone	*see* Corticosteroids
Fludroxycortide (flurandrenolone)	*see* Corticosteroids
Flumazenil	May cross placenta in small amounts—manufacturer advises avoid unless potential benefit outweighs risk
Flunisolide	*see* Corticosteroids
Fluocinolone	*see* Corticosteroids
Fluocinonide	*see* Corticosteroids
Fluocortolone	*see* Corticosteroids

Drug (trimester of risk)	Comment
Fluorometholone	*see* Corticosteroids
Fluorouracil	Avoid (teratogenic); *see also* section 8.1
Fluoxetine	*see* Antidepressants, SSRI
Flupentixol	*see* Antipsychotics
Fluphenazine	*see* Antipsychotics
Flurandrenolone	*see* Corticosteroids
Flurazepam	*see* Benzodiazepines
Flurbiprofen	*see* NSAIDs
Fluticasone	*see* Corticosteroids
Fluvastatin	*see* Statins
Fluvoxamine	*see* Antidepressants, SSRI
Follitropin alfa and beta	Avoid
Fondaparinux	Manufacturer advises avoid unless potential benefit outweighs possible risk—no information available
Formoterol (eformoterol)	Manufacturers advise use only if potential benefit outweighs risk; *see also* section 3.1
Fosamprenavir	Toxicity in *animal* studies; manufacturer advises use only if potential benefit outweighs risk
Foscarnet	Manufacturer advises avoid
Fosinopril	*see* ACE Inhibitors
Fosphenytoin	*see* Phenytoin
Framycetin	*see* Aminoglycosides
Frovatriptan	*see* $5HT_1$ Agonists
Frusemide	*see* Diuretics
Fulvestrant	Manufacturer advises avoid—increased incidence of fetal abnormalities and death in *animal* studies
Furosemide (frusemide)	*see* Diuretics
Fusidic acid	*see* Sodium Fusidate
Gabapentin	*see* Antiepileptics
Galantamine	Developmental delay in *animal* studies
Ganciclovir	Avoid—teratogenic risk; *see also* p. 324
Ganirelix	Manufacturer advises avoid in confirmed pregnancy—toxicity in *animal* studies
Gemcitabine	Avoid (teratogenic in *animal* studies); *see also* section 8.1
Gemfibrozil	*see* Fibrates
Gentamicin	*see* Aminoglycosides
Gestodene	*see* Contraceptives, Oral
Gestrinone (1, 2, 3)	Avoid
Glatiramer	Manufacturer advises avoid—no information available
Glibenclamide	*see* Sulphonylureas
Gliclazide	*see* Sulphonylureas
Glimepiride	*see* Sulphonylureas
Glipizide	*see* Sulphonylureas
Gliquidone	*see* Sulphonylureas
Goserelin	Manufacturer advises avoid in pregnancy—exclude pregnancy before treatment and use non-hormonal contraceptives during treatment
Granisetron	Manufacturer advises use only when compelling reasons—no information available
Griseofulvin	Avoid (fetotoxicity and teratogenicity in *animals*); effective contraception required during and for at least 1 month after administration (**important:** effectiveness of oral contraceptives reduced, see p. 407); also men should avoid fathering a child during and for at least 6 months after administration
Guanethidine (3)	Postural hypotension and reduced uteroplacental perfusion; should not be used to treat hypertension in pregnancy
Haem arginate	Manufacturer advises avoid unless essential
Halcinonide	*see* Corticosteroids
Haloperidol	*see* Antipsychotics
Halothane	*see* Anaesthetics, General
Heparin (1, 2, 3)	Maternal osteoporosis reported after prolonged use; multidose vials may contain benzyl alcohol—some manufacturers advise avoid; *see also* Bemiparin, Dalteparin, Enoxaparin, Reviparin, and Tinzaparin
$5HT_1$ agonists	Limited experience—manufacturers advise avoid unless potential benefit outweighs risk
Human menopausal gonadotrophins	Avoid
Hydralazine (1, 2)	Manufacturer advises avoid before third trimester; no reports of serious harm following use in third trimester
Hydrochlorothiazide	*see* Diuretics
Hydrocortisone	*see* Corticosteroids
Hydroflumethiazide	*see* Diuretics
Hydromorphone	*see* Opioid Analgesics
Hydroxycarbamide (hydroxyurea)	Avoid (teratogenic in *animal* studies); manufacturer advises effective contraception before and during administration; *see also* section 8.1
Hydroxychloroquine	Manufacturer advises avoid but see p. 513
Hydroxyurea	*see* Hydroxycarbamide
Hydroxyzine	*see* Antihistamines
Hyoscine butylbromide	Manufacturer advises use only if potential benefit outweighs risk
Hyoscine hydrobromide	Manufacturer advises use only if potential benefit outweighs risk; injection may depress neonatal respiration
Ibandronic acid	*see* Bisphosphonates
Ibuprofen	*see* NSAIDs
Idarubicin	Avoid (teratogenic and toxic in *animal* studies); *see also* section 8.1
Idoxuridine	Teratogenic in *animal* studies—manufacturer advises avoid

Drug (trimester of risk)	Comment
Ifosfamide	Avoid (teratogenic and carcinogenic in *animals*); manufacturer advises adequate contraception during and for at least 6 months after administration to men or women; *see also* section 8.1
Iloprost	Manufacturer advises avoid (toxicity in *animal* studies); effective contraception must be used during treatment
Imatinib	Manufacturer advises avoid unless potential benefit outweighs risk; *see also* section 8.1
Imidapril	*see* ACE Inhibitors
Imiglucerase	Manufacturer advises use only if potential benefit outweighs risk—no information available
Imipenem [ingredient]	*see Primaxin*®
Imipramine	*see* Antidepressants, Tricyclic (and related)
Imiquimod	No evidence of teratogenicity or toxicity in *animal* studies; manufacturer advises caution
Indapamide	*see* Diuretics
Indinavir	Toxicity in *animal* studies; manufacturer advises use only if potential benefit outweighs risk; theoretical risk of hyperbilirubinaemia and renal stones in neonate if used at term
Indometacin	*see* NSAIDs
Infliximab	Avoid; manufacturer advises adequate contraception during and for at least 6 months after last dose
Influenza vaccine	Not known to be harmful
Inosine	Manufacturer advises avoid
Inositol nicotinate	No information available—manufacturer advises avoid unless potential benefit outweighs risk
Insulin (1, 2, 3)	Insulin requirements should be assessed frequently by an experienced diabetes physician; limited evidence of safety of newer insulin analogues
Interferons	Manufacturers recommend avoid unless compelling reasons; effective contraception to be used by men and women receiving treatment
Iodine and iodides (2, 3)	Neonatal goitre and hypothyroidism
Iodine, radioactive (1, 2, 3)	Permanent hypothyroidism—avoid
Iodoform	*see* Povidone–iodine
Ipratropium	Not known to be harmful; *see* section 3.1
Irbesartan	*As for* ACE Inhibitors
Irinotecan	Avoid (teratogenic and toxic in *animal* studies); manufacturer advises effective contraception during and for at least 3 months after administration; *see also* section 8.1
Iron (parenteral)	Avoid in early pregnancy
Isocarboxazid	*see* Antidepressants, MAOI
Isoflurane	*see* Anaesthetics, General
Isometheptene [ingredient]	*see* Midrid®
Isoniazid	Not known to be harmful; *see also* p. 297
Isotretinoin (1, 2, 3)	Teratogenic; effective contraception must be used for at least 1 month before oral treatment, during treatment and for at least 1 month after stopping; also avoid topical treatment
Isradipine	May inhibit labour; risk to fetus should be balanced against risk of uncontrolled maternal hypertension
Itraconazole	Manufacturer advises use only in life-threatening situations (toxicity at high doses in *animal* studies); ensure effective contraception during treatment and until the next menstrual period following end of treatment
Kaletra®	Avoid oral solution due to high propylene glycol content; manufacturer advises use capsules only if potential benefit outweighs risk (toxicity in *animal* studies)
Ketamine	*see* Anaesthetics, General
Ketoconazole	Manufacturer advises teratogenicity in *animal* studies; packs carry a warning to avoid in pregnancy
Ketoprofen	*see* NSAIDs
Ketorolac	*see* NSAIDs
Ketotifen	*see* Antihistamines
Labetalol	*see* Beta-blockers
Lacidipine	Manufacturer advises avoid; may inhibit labour
Lactulose	Not known to be harmful
Lamivudine (1)	Manufacturer advises avoid during first trimester—no information available
Lamotrigine	*see* Antiepileptics
Lanreotide	Manufacturer advises use only if potential benefit outweighs risk
Lansoprazole	Manufacturer advises avoid
Laronidase	Manufacturer advises avoid unless essential—no information available
Latanoprost	Manufacturer advises avoid

Drug (trimester of risk)	Comment
Leflunomide	Avoid—active metabolite teratogenic in *animal* studies; effective contraception essential during treatment and for at least 2 years after treatment in women and at least 3 months after treatment in men (*see also* Leflunomide section 10.1.3)
Lenograstim	Toxicity in *animal* studies; manufacturer advises use only if potential benefit outweighs risk
Lepirudin	Avoid
Lercanidipine	Manufacturer advises avoid—no information available
Leuprorelin	Avoid—teratogenic in *animal* studies
Levetiracetam	Toxicity in *animal* studies—manufacturer advises use only if potential benefit outweighs risk; *see also* Antiepileptics
Levobupivacaine	
(1)	Manufacturer advises avoid if possible—toxicity in *animal* studies; *see also* Anaesthetics, Local
Levocabastine	*see* Antihistamines
Levocetirizine	*see* Antihistamines
Levodopa	Manufacturers advise toxicity in *animal* studies
Levofloxacin	*see* Quinolones
Levomepromazine (methotrimeprazine)	*see* Antipsychotics
Levonorgestrel	*see* Contraceptives, Oral
Levothyroxine (thyroxine)	Monitor maternal serum-thyrotrophin concentration—levothyroxine may cross the placenta and excessive maternal concentration can be detrimental to fetus
Lidocaine (lignocaine)	*see* Anaesthetics, Local
Lignocaine	*see* Anaesthetics, Local
Linezolid	Manufacturer advises use only if potential benefit outweighs risk—no information available
Liothyronine	Does not cross the placenta in significant amounts; monitor maternal thyroid function tests—dosage adjustment may be necessary
Lisinopril	*see* ACE Inhibitors
Lithium salts	
(1)	Avoid if possible (risk of teratogenicity, including cardiac abnormalities)
(2, 3)	Dose requirements increased (but on delivery return to normal abruptly); close monitoring of serum-lithium concentration advised (risk of toxicity in neonate)
Lofepramine	*see* Antidepressants, Tricyclic (and related)
Loperamide	Manufacturers advise avoid—no information available
Lopinavir [ingredient]	*see Kaletra®*
Loprazolam	*see* Benzodiazepines
Loratadine	Embryotoxic in *animal* studies; *see also* Antihistamines
Lorazepam	*see* Benzodiazepines
Lormetazepam	*see* Benzodiazepines
Losartan	*As for* ACE Inhibitors
Lumefantrine [ingredient]	*see Riamet®*
Lymecycline	*see* Tetracyclines
Magnesium sulphate	
(3)	Not known to be harmful for short-term intravenous administration in eclampsia but excessive doses cause neonatal respiratory depression
Malarone®	Manufacturer advises avoid unless essential
Maprotiline	*see* Antidepressants, Tricyclic (and related)
Mebendazole	Manufacturer advises toxicity in *animal* studies
Mebeverine	Not known to be harmful; manufacturers advise caution
Medroxyprogesterone	Avoid—genital malformations and cardiac defects reported in male and female fetuses
Mefenamic acid	*see* NSAIDs
Mefloquine	
(1)	Manufacturer advises teratogenicity in *animal* studies, but *see* p. 330, and p. 331
Meloxicam	*see* NSAIDs
Melphalan	Avoid (manufacturer advises adequate contraception during administration to men or women); *see also* section 8.1
Memantine	Manufacturer advises avoid unless essential—intra-uterine growth restriction in *animal* studies
Menadiol	
(3)	Neonatal haemolytic anaemia, hyperbilirubinaemia and increased risk of kernicterus in jaundiced infants
Menotrophin	Avoid
Meprobamate	Manufacturer advises avoid if possible
Meptazinol	*see* Opioid Analgesics
Mercaptamine	Manufacturer advises avoid
Mercaptopurine	Avoid (teratogenic); *see also* section 8.1
Meropenem	Manufacturer advises use only if potential benefit outweighs risk—no information available
Mesalazine	Negligible quantities cross placenta
Mesna	Not known to be harmful; *see also* section 8.1
Mesterolone	*see* Androgens
Mestranol	*see* Contraceptives, Oral
Metaraminol	May reduce placental perfusion—manufacturer advises use only if potential benefit outweighs risk
Metformin	
(1, 2, 3)	Avoid; insulin is normally substituted in all diabetics

Drug (trimester of risk)	Comment
Methadone	*see* Opioid Analgesics
Methocarbamol	Manufacturer advises avoid unless potential benefit outweighs risk
Methotrexate	Avoid (teratogenic; fertility may be reduced during therapy but this may be reversible); manufacturer advises effective contraception during and for at least 3 months after administration to men or women; *see also* section 8.1
Methotrimeprazine	*see* Antipsychotics
Methyldopa	Not known to be harmful
Methylphenidate	Limited experience—manufacturer advises avoid unless potential benefit outweighs risk; toxicity in *animals*
Methylprednisolone	*see* Corticosteroids
Methysergide	Manufacturer advises avoid
Metoclopramide	Not known to be harmful but manufacturer advises use only when compelling reasons
Metolazone	*see* Diuretics
Metoprolol	*see* Beta-blockers
Metronidazole	Manufacturer advises avoidance of high-dose regimens
Metyrapone	Avoid (may impair biosynthesis of fetal-placental steroids)
Mexiletine	Manufacturer advises avoid unless potential benefit outweighs risk
Mianserin	*see* Antidepressants, Tricyclic (and related)
Miconazole	Manufacturer advises avoid unless essential
Midazolam	*see* Benzodiazepines
Midrid®	Manufacturer advises avoid
Mifepristone	Manufacturer advises that if treatment fails, essential that pregnancy be terminated by another method
Miglustat	Manufacturer advises avoid (toxicity in *animal* studies)—effective contraception must be used during treatment; also men should avoid fathering a child during and for 3 months after treatment
Milrinone	Manufacturer advises use only if potential benefit outweighs risk
Minocycline	*see* Tetracyclines
Minoxidil	
(3)	Neonatal hirsutism reported
Misoprostol	
(1, 2, 3)	Avoid—potent uterine stimulant (has been used to induce abortion) and may be teratogenic
Mitomycin	Avoid (teratogenic in *animal* studies); *see also* section 8.1
Mitoxantrone (mitozantrone)	Avoid; manufacturer advises effective contraception during and for at least 6 months after administration to men or women; *see also* section 8.1
Mitozantrone	*see* Mitoxantrone
Mivacurium	Manufacturer advises avoid—no information available
Mizolastine	Manufacturer advises avoid; *see also* Antihistamines
Moclobemide	*see* Antidepressants, MAOI
Modafinil	Manufacturer advises avoid
Moexipril	*see* ACE Inhibitors
Montelukast	Manufacturer advises avoid unless essential
Morphine	*see* Opioid Analgesics
Movicol®	Manufacturer advises use only if essential—no information available
Moxifloxacin	*see* Quinolones
Moxisylyte (thymoxamine)	Manufacturer advises avoid
Moxonidine	Manufacturer advises avoid—no information available
Mupirocin	Manufacturer advises avoid unless potential benefit outweighs risk—no information available
Mycophenolate mofetil	Manufacturer advises avoid—toxicity in *animal* studies; effective contraception required during and for 6 weeks after discontinuation of treatment
Nabilone	Manufacturer advises avoid unless essential
Nabumetone	*see* NSAIDs
Nadolol	*see* Beta-blockers
Nafarelin	Avoid
Nalidixic acid	*see* Quinolones
Naloxone	Manufacturer advises use only if potential benefit outweighs risk
Nandrolone	*see* Anabolic Steroids
Naproxen	*see* NSAIDs
Naratriptan	*see* $5HT_1$ Agonists
Narcotic analgesics	*see* Opioid Analgesics
Nateglinide	Manufacturer advises avoid—toxicity in *animal* studies; insulin is normally substituted in all diabetics
Nebivolol	*see* Beta-blockers
Nedocromil	*see* section 3.1
Nefopam	No information available—manufacturer advises avoid unless no safer treatment
Nelfinavir	No information available—manufacturer advises use only if potential benefit outweighs risk
Neomycin	*see* Aminoglycosides
Neostigmine	Manufacturer advises use only if potential benefit outweighs risk
Netilmicin	*see* Aminoglycosides
Nevirapine	Although manufacturers advise avoid, may be appropriate to use if clearly indicated; *see also* p. 314
Nicardipine	May inhibit labour; manufacturer advises avoid, but risk to fetus should be balanced against risk of uncontrolled maternal hypertension
Nicorandil	Manufacturer advises use only if potential benefit outweighs risk—no information available

Drug (trimester of risk)	Comment
Nicotine	Use only if smoking cessation without nicotine replacement fails; avoid liquorice-flavoured nicotine products; patient information for some products contra-indicates use
Nicotinic acid	No information available—manufacturer advises avoid unless potential benefit outweighs risk
Nicoumalone	*see* Anticoagulants, Oral
Nifedipine	May inhibit labour; manufacturer advises avoid, but risk to fetus should be balanced against risk of uncontrolled maternal hypertension
Nimodipine	Manufacturer advises use only if potential benefit outweighs risk
Nisoldipine	Avoid (toxicity in *animal* studies)
Nitrazepam	*see* Benzodiazepines
Nitrofurantoin	
(3)	May produce neonatal haemolysis if used at term
Nitroprusside	*see* Sodium Nitroprusside
Nitrous oxide	*see* Anaesthetics, General
Nizatidine	Manufacturer advises avoid unless essential
Noradrenaline (norepinephrine) (1, 2, 3)	Avoid—may reduce placental perfusion
Norethisterone	Masculinisation of female fetuses and other defects reported; *see also* Contraceptives, Oral
Norfloxacin	*see* Quinolones
Norgestimate	*see* Contraceptives, Oral
Norgestrel	*see* Contraceptives, Oral
Nortriptyline	*see* Antidepressants, Tricyclic (and related)
NSAIDs	Most manufacturers advise avoid (or avoid unless potential benefit outweighs risk); ketorolac contra-indicated during pregnancy, labour and delivery
(3)	With regular use closure of fetal ductus arteriosus *in utero* and possibly persistent pulmonary hypertension of the newborn. Delayed onset and increased duration of labour
Nystatin	No information available, but absorption from gastro-intestinal tract negligible
Octreotide	
(1, 2, 3)	Possible effect on fetal growth; manufacturer advises use only if potential benefit outweighs risk
Oestrogens	*see* Contraceptives, Oral
Ofloxacin	*see* Quinolones
Olanzapine	
(3)	Manufacturer advises use only if potential benefit outweighs risk; neonatal lethargy, tremor, and hypertonia reported
Olmesartan	*As for* ACE inhibitors
Olsalazine	Manufacturer advises avoid unless potential benefit outweighs risk
Omega-3-acid ethyl esters	Manufacturer advises use only if potential benefit outweighs risk—no information available
Omeprazole	Not known to be harmful
Ondansetron	No information available; manufacturer advises avoid unless potential benefit outweighs risk
Opioid analgesics	
(3)	Depress neonatal respiration; withdrawal effects in neonates of dependent mothers; gastric stasis and risk of inhalation pneumonia in mother during labour; *see also* Tramadol
Oral contraceptives	*see* Contraceptives, Oral
Orlistat	Manufacturer advises avoid—no information available
Orphenadrine	Manufacturer advises caution
Oseltamivir	Manufacturer advises avoid unless potential benefit outweighs risk
Oxaliplatin	Manufacturer advises avoid—no information available; *see also* section 8.1
Oxazepam	*see* Benzodiazepines
Oxcarbazepine	
(1)	Risk of teratogenesis including increased risk of neural tube defects (counselling and screening and adequate folate supplements advised, e.g. 5 mg daily); *see also* Antiepileptics and p. 238
(3)	Because of neonatal bleeding tendency associated with some antiepileptics, manufacturer advises prophylactic vitamin K_1 for mother before delivery (as well as for neonate)
Oxprenolol	*see* Beta-blockers
Oxybutynin	Manufacturer advises avoid unless potential benefit outweighs risk—toxicity in *animal* studies
Oxycodone	*see* Opioid Analgesics
Oxytetracycline	*see* Tetracyclines
Paclitaxel	Avoid (toxicity in *animal* studies); ensure effective contraception during and for at least 6 months after administration to men or women; *see also* section 8.1
Palonosetron	Manufacturer advises avoid—no information available
Pamidronate disodium	*see* Bisphosphonates
Pancreatin	Not known to be harmful
Pancuronium	Manufacturer advises avoid unless potential benefit outweighs risk—no information available
Pantoprazole	Manufacturer advises avoid unless potential benefit outweighs risk—fetotoxic in *animals*

Drug (trimester of risk)	Comment
Papaveretum	*see* Opioid Analgesics
Paracetamol	Not known to be harmful
Paraldehyde	Manufacturer advises avoid unless essential—crosses the placenta
Parecoxib	*see* NSAIDS
Paricalcitol	Toxicity in *animal* studies—manufacturer advises avoid unless potential benefit outweighs risk; *see also* Vitamin D
Paroxetine	*see* Antidepressants, SSRI
Pegfilgrastim	Toxicity in *animal* studies; manufacturer advises use only if potential benefit ouweighs risk
Pemetrexed	Avoid (toxicity in *animal* studies); manufacturer advises effective contraception during treatment; men must avoid fathering a child during and for at least 6 months after treatment; *see also* section 8.1
Penicillamine (1, 2, 3)	Fetal abnormalities reported rarely; avoid if possible
Penicillins	Not known to be harmful
Pentamidine isetionate	Manufacturer advises avoid unless essential
Pentazocine	*see* Opioid Analgesics
Pentostatin	Avoid (teratogenic in *animal* studies); manufacturer advises that men should not father children during and for 6 months after administration; *see also* section 8.1
Pergolide	Manufacturer advises use only if potential benefit outweighs risk
Pericyazine	*see* Antipsychotics
Perindopril	*see* ACE Inhibitors
Perphenazine	*see* Antipsychotics
Pethidine	*see* Opioid Analgesics
Phenelzine	*see* Antidepressants, MAOI
Phenindione	*see* Anticoagulants, Oral
Phenobarbital (1, 3)	Congenital malformations. May possibly cause vitamin K deficiency and risk of neonatal bleeding; if vitamin K not given at birth, neonate should be monitored closely for signs of bleeding; *see also* Antiepileptics
Phenothiazines	*see* Antipsychotics
Phenoxybenzamine	Hypotension may occur in newborn
Phenoxymethylpenicillin	*see* Penicillins
Phentolamine	Use with caution—may cause marked decrease in maternal blood pressure with resulting fetal anoxia
Phenylephrine (1)	Malformations reported
(3)	Avoid if possible—fetal hypoxia and bradycardia reported in late pregnancy and labour
Phenytoin (1, 3)	Congenital malformations (screening advised); adequate folate supplements should be given to mother (e.g. folic acid 5 mg daily). May possibly cause vitamin K deficiency and risk of neonatal bleeding; if vitamin K not given at birth, neonate should be monitored closely for signs of bleeding. Caution in interpreting plasma concentrations—bound may be reduced but free (i.e. effective) unchanged; *see also* Antiepileptics
Pholcodine	*see* Opioid Analgesics
Phytomenadione	Manufacturer advises use only if potential benefit outweighs risk—no specific information available
Pilocarpine	Avoid—smooth muscle stimulant; toxicity in *animal* studies
Pimozide	*see* Antipsychotics
Pindolol	*see* Beta-blockers
Pioglitazone	Manufacturer advises avoid—toxicity in *animal* studies; insulin is normally substituted in all diabetics
Piperacillin [ingredient]	*see Tazocin*®
Piperazine	Not known to be harmful but manufacturer advises avoid in first trimester
Pipotiazine	*see* Antipsychotics
Piracetam	Manufacturer advises avoid
Piroxicam	*see* NSAIDs
Pivmecillinam	*see* Penicillins
Podophyllum	Avoid—neonatal death and teratogenesis have been reported
Polystyrene sulphonate resins	Manufacturers advise use only if potential benefit outweighs risk—no information available
Porfimer	Manufacturer advises avoid unless essential
Povidone–iodine (2, 3)	Sufficient iodine may be absorbed to affect the fetal thyroid
Pramipexole	Manufacturer advises use only if potential benefit outweighs risk—no information available
Pravastatin	*see* Statins
Prazosin	*see* Alpha-blockers, Post-synaptic
Prednisolone	*see* Corticosteroids
Pregabalin	Toxicity in *animal* studies—manufacturer advises use only if potential benefit outweighs risk
Prilocaine (3)	Neonatal methaemoglobinaemia reported after paracervical block or pudendal block; *see also* Anaesthetics, Local
Primaquine (3)	Neonatal haemolysis and methaemoglobinaemia; *see also* Antimalarials

Drug (trimester of risk)	Comment
Primaxin®	Manufacturer advises avoid unless potential benefit outweighs risk (toxicity in *animal* studies)
Primidone	*see* Phenobarbital
Procainamide	Manufacturer advises avoid unless potential benefit outweighs risk
Procaine	
(3)	Neonatal methaemoglobinaemia; *see also* Anaesthetics, Local
Procarbazine	Avoid (teratogenic in *animal* studies and isolated reports in humans); *see also* section 8.1
Prochlorperazine	*see* Antipsychotics
Progesterone	Not known to be harmful
Proguanil	Adequate folate supplements should be given to mother; *see also* Antimalarials
Promazine	*see* Antipsychotics
Promethazine	*see* Antihistamines
Propafenone	Manufacturer advises avoid—no information available
Propantheline	Manufacturer advises avoid—no information available
Propiverine	Manufacturer advises avoid (restriction of skeletal development in *animals*)
Propofol	*see* Anaesthetics, General
Propranolol	*see* Beta-blockers
Propylthiouracil	
(2, 3)	Neonatal goitre and hypothyroidism
Protionamide	
(1)	May be teratogenic
Pseudoephedrine	Not known to be harmful
Pyrazinamide	Manufacturer advises use only if potential benefit outweighs risk; see also p. 297
Pyridostigmine	Manufacturer advises use only if potential benefit outweighs risk
Pyrimethamine	
(1)	Theoretical teratogenic risk (folate antagonist); adequate folate supplements should be given to mother; *see also* Antimalarials
Quetiapine	Manufacturer advises use only if potential benefit outweighs risk
Quinagolide	Manufacturer advises discontinue when pregnancy confirmed unless medical reason for continuing
Quinapril	*see* ACE Inhibitors
Quinidine	Not known to be harmful at therapeutic doses but manufacturer advises avoid
Quinine	
(1)	High doses are teratogenic; but in malaria benefit of treatment outweighs risk
Quinolones	
(1, 2, 3)	Avoid—arthropathy in *animal* studies; safer alternatives available
Quinupristin [ingredient]	*see Synercid®*

Drug (trimester of risk)	Comment
Rabeprazole	Manufacturer advises avoid—no information available
Raltitrexed	Pregnancy must be excluded before treatment; ensure effective contraception during and for at least 6 months after administration to men or women; *see also* section 8.1
Ramipril	*see* ACE Inhibitors
Ranitidine	Manufacturer advises avoid unless essential, but not known to be harmful
Ranitidine bismuth citrate	Safety not established
Rasburicase	Manufacturer advises avoid—no information available
Reboxetine	Manufacturer advises avoid (and discontinue if pregnancy occurs)—no information available
Remifentanil	No information available; *see also* Opioid Analgesics
Repaglinide	Manufacturer advises avoid; insulin is normally substituted in all diabetics
Reteplase	*see* Streptokinase
Reviparin	Manufacturer advises avoid—no information available
Riamet®	Toxicity in *animal* studies with artemether; manufacturer advises use only if potential benefit outweighs risk
Ribavirin	Avoid; teratogenicity in *animal* studies; ensure effective contraception during oral administration and for 6 months after treatment in women and in men; *see also* Ribavirin section 5.3.5
Rifabutin	Manufacturer advises avoid—no information available
Rifampicin	
(1)	Manufacturers advise very high doses teratogenic in *animal* studies; *see also* p. 297
(3)	Risk of neonatal bleeding may be increased
Riluzole	No information available; manufacturer advises avoid
Risedronate sodium	*see* Bisphosphonates
Risperidone	Manufacturer advises use only if potential benefit outweighs risk
Ritodrine	For use in premature labour *see* section 7.1.3
Ritonavir	Manufacturer advises use only if potential benefit outweighs risk—no information available
Rituximab	Avoid unless potential benefit to mother outweighs risk of B-lymphocyte depletion in fetus—effective contraception required during and for 12 months after treatment
Rivastigmine	Manufacturer advises use only if potential benefit outweighs risk
Rizatriptan	*see* $5HT_1$ Agonists
Rocuronium	Manufacturer advises avoid unless potential benefit outweighs risk

Drug (trimester of risk)	Comment
Ropivacaine	Safety not established but not known to be harmful
Rosiglitazone	Manufacturer advises avoid—toxicity in *animal* studies; insulin is normally substituted in all diabetics
Rosuvastatin	*see* Statins
Salbutamol	For use in asthma *see* section 3.1
(3)	For use in premature labour *see* section 7.1.3
Salcatonin	*see* Calcitonin (salmon)
Salmeterol	*see* section 3.1
Saquinavir	Manufacturer advises use only if potential benefit outweighs risk
Selegiline	Manufacturer advises avoid—no information available
Sertindole	Manufacturer advises avoid
Sertraline	*see* Antidepressants, SSRI
Sevelamer	Manufacturer advises use only if potential benefit outweighs risk
Sevoflurane	*see* Anaesthetics, General
Sibutramine	Manufacturer advises avoid—toxicity in *animal* studies
Silver sulfadiazine	*see* Sulphonamides
Simvastatin	*see* Statins
Sirolimus	Manufacturer advises avoid (toxicity in *animal* studies); effective contraception must be used during treatment and for 12 weeks after stopping
Sodium aurothiomalate	Manufacturer advises avoid but limited data suggests usually not necessary to withdraw if condition well controlled—consider reducing dose and frequency
Sodium clodronate	*see* Bisphosphonates
Sodium cromoglicate	Not known to be harmful; *see also* section 3.1
Sodium fusidate	Not known to be harmful; manufacturer advises use only if potential benefit outweighs risk
Sodium nitroprusside	Potential for accumulation of cyanide in fetus—avoid prolonged use
Sodium phenylbutyrate	Avoid (toxicity in *animal* studies); manufacturer advises adequate contraception during administration
Sodium valproate	*see* Valproate
Solifenacin	Manufacturer advises caution—no information available
Somatropin	Discontinue if pregnancy occurs—no information available but theoretical risk
Sotalol	*see* Beta-blockers
Spironolactone	Manufacturers advise toxicity in *animal* studies
Statins	Avoid—congenital anomalies reported; decreased synthesis of cholesterol possibly affects fetal development
Stavudine	Manufacturer advises use only if potential benefit outweighs risk
Streptokinase (1, 2, 3)	Possibility of premature separation of placenta in first 18 weeks; theoretical possibility of fetal haemorrhage throughout pregnancy; risk of maternal haemorrhage on post-partum use
Streptomycin	*see* Aminoglycosides
Strontium ranelate	Avoid—toxicity in *animal* studies
Sulfadiazine	*see* Sulphonamides
Sulfadoxine	*see* Sulphonamides
Sulfasalazine (3)	Theoretical risk of neonatal haemolysis; adequate folate supplements should be given to mother
Sulindac	*see* NSAIDs
Sulphonamides (3)	Neonatal haemolysis and methaemoglobinaemia; fear of increased risk of kernicterus in neonates appears to be unfounded
Sulphonylureas (3)	Neonatal hypoglycaemia; insulin is normally substituted in all diabetics; if oral drugs are used therapy should be stopped at least 2 days before delivery
Sulpiride	*see* Antipsychotics
Sumatriptan	*see* $5HT_1$ Agonists
Suxamethonium	Mildly prolonged maternal paralysis may occur
Synercid®	Manufacturer advises avoid unless potential benefit outweighs risk—no information available
Tacalcitol	Manufacturer advises avoid unless no safer alternative—no information available
Tacrolimus	Avoid; manufacturer advises toxicity in *animal* studies following systemic administration
Tamoxifen	Avoid—possible effects on fetal development; effective contraception must be used during treatment and for 2 months after stopping
Tazarotene	Avoid; effective contraception required
Tazobactam [ingredient]	*see Tazocin*®
Tazocin®	Manufacturer advises use only if potential benefit outweighs risk
Tegafur with uracil	*see Uftoral*®
Teicoplanin	Manufacturer advises use only if potential benefit outweighs risk
Telithromycin	Toxicity in animal studies—manufacturer advises use only if potential benefit outweighs risk
Telmisartan	*As for* ACE Inhibitors
Temazepam	*see* Benzodiazepines

Drug (trimester of risk)	Comment
Temozolomide	Avoid (teratogenic and embryotoxic in *animal* studies); manufacturer advises adequate contraception during administration; *see also* section 8.1; also men should avoid fathering a child during and for at least 6 months after treatment
Tenecteplase	*see* Streptokinase
Tenofovir	No information available—manufacturer advises use only if potential benefit outweighs risk
Tenoxicam	*see* NSAIDs
Terazosin	*see* Alpha-blockers, Post-synaptic
Terbinafine	Manufacturer advises use only if potential benefit outweighs risk—no information available
Terbutaline	For use in asthma *see* section 3.1
(3)	For use in premature labour *see* section 7.1.3
Terfenadine	*see* Antihistamines
Testosterone	*see* Androgens
Tetrabenazine	Inadequate information but no evidence of harm
Tetracyclines	
(1)	Effects on skeletal development in *animal* studies
(2, 3)	Dental discoloration; maternal hepatotoxicity with large parenteral doses
Theophylline	
(3)	Neonatal irritability and apnoea have been reported
Thiazides and related diuretics	*see* Diuretics
Thiopental	*see* Anaesthetics, General
Thiotepa	Avoid (teratogenic and embryotoxic in *animals*); *see also* section 8.1
Thymoxamine	*see* Moxisylyte
Thyroxine	*see* Levothyroxine
Tiagabine	Manufacturer advises avoid unless potential benefit outweighs risk
Tiaprofenic acid	*see* NSAIDs
Ticarcillin [ingredient]	*see* Penicillins
Tiludronic acid	*see* Bisphosphonates
Timentin®	*see* Penicillins
Timolol	*see* Beta-blockers
Tinidazole	Manufacturer advises avoid in first trimester
Tinzaparin	Manufacturer advises avoid unless no safer alternative
Tioconazole	Manufacturer advises avoid
Tioguanine	Avoid (teratogenicity reported when men receiving tioguanine have fathered children); ensure effective contraception during administration to men or women; *see also* section 8.1
Tiotropium	Toxicity in *animal* studies—manufacturer advises use only if potential benefit outweighs risk
Tirofiban	Manufacturer advises use only if potential benefit outweighs risk—no information available
Tizanidine	Manufacturer advises use only if potential benefit outweighs risk—no information available
Tobramycin	*see* Aminoglycosides
Tocopheryl acetate	
(1, 2, 3)	No evidence of safety of high doses
Tolbutamide	*see* Sulphonylureas
Tolcapone	Toxicity in *animal* studies—manufacturer advises use only if potential benefit outweighs risk
Tolfenamic acid	*see* NSAIDs
Tolterodine	Manufacturer advises avoid—toxicity in *animal* studies
Topiramate	Manufacturer advises avoid unless potential benefit outweighs potential risk; *see also* Antiepileptics
Topotecan	Avoid (teratogenicity and fetal loss in *animal* studies); *see also* section 8.1
Torasemide	*see* Diuretics
Tramadol	Embryotoxic in animal studies—manufacturers advise avoid; *see also* Opioid Analgesics
Trandolapril	*see* ACE Inhibitors
Tranexamic acid	No evidence of teratogenicity in *animal* studies; manufacturer advises use only if potential benefit outweighs risk—crosses the placenta
Tranylcypromine	*see* Antidepressants, MAOI
Trastuzumab	Avoid unless potential benefit outweighs risk
Travoprost	Manufacturer advises use only if potential benefit outweighs risk
Trazodone	*see* Antidepressants, Tricyclic (and related)
Treosulfan	Avoid; *see also* section 8.1
Tretinoin	
(1, 2, 3)	Teratogenic; effective contraception must be used for at least 1 month before oral treatment, during treatment and for at least 1 month after stopping; also avoid topical treatment
Triamcinolone	*see* Corticosteroids
Triamterene	*see* Diuretics
Tribavirin	*see* Ribavirin
Triclofos	Avoid
Trientine	Manufacturer advises use only if potential benefit outweighs risk; monitor maternal and neonatal serum-copper concentration; teratogenic in *animal* studies
Trifluoperazine	*see* Antipsychotics
Trilostane	
(1, 2, 3)	Interferes with placental sex hormone production
Trimeprazine	*see* Antihistamines
Trimethoprim	
(1)	Teratogenic risk (folate antagonist); manufacturers advise avoid

Drug (trimester of risk)	Comment
Trimipramine	*see* Antidepressants, Tricyclic (and related)
Tripotassium dicitratobismuthate	Manufacturer advises avoid on theoretical grounds
Triprolidine	*see* Antihistamines
Triptorelin	Manufacturers advise avoid
Tropisetron	Manufacturer advises toxicity in *animal* studies
Trospium	Manufacturer advises caution—no information available
Uftoral®	Avoid; manufacturer advises effective contraception during and for 3 months after administration to men or women
Ursodeoxycholic acid	No evidence of harm but manufacturer advises avoid
Vaccines (live) (1)	Theoretical risk of congenital malformations, but need for vaccination may outweigh possible risk to fetus (*see also* p. 604); avoid MMR vaccine but *see* p. 618
Valaciclovir	*see* Aciclovir
Valganciclovir	*see* Ganciclovir
Valproate (1, 3)	Increased risk of congenital malformations and developmental delay (counselling and screening advised—**important:** *see also* p. 238); neonatal bleeding (related to hypofibrinaemia) and neonatal hepatotoxicity also reported
Valproic acid	*see* Valproate
Valsartan	*As for* ACE Inhibitors
Vancomycin	Manufacturer advises use only if potential benefit outweighs risk—plasma-vancomycin concentration monitoring essential to reduce risk of fetal toxicity
Vasopressin	Oxytocic effect in third trimester
Vecuronium	Manufacturer advises avoid unless potential benefit outweighs risk—no information available
Venlafaxine	Manufacturer advises avoid—no information available
Verapamil	May reduce uterine blood flow with fetal hypoxia; manufacturer advises avoid in first trimester unless absolutely necessary; may inhibit labour
Verteporfin	Manufacturer advises use only if potential benefit outweighs risk (teratogenic in *animal* studies)
Vigabatrin	Congenital anomalies reported—manufacturer advises avoid unless potential benefit outweighs risk; *see also* Antiepileptics
Vinblastine	Avoid (limited experience suggests fetal harm; teratogenic in *animal* studies); *see also* section 8.1
Vincristine	Avoid (teratogenicity and fetal loss in *animal* studies); *see also* section 8.1
Vindesine	Avoid (teratogenic in *animal* studies); *see also* section 8.1
Vinorelbine	Avoid (teratogenicity and fetal loss in *animal* studies); *see also* section 8.1
Vitamin A (1)	Excessive doses may be teratogenic; *see also* p. 489
Vitamin D	High systemic doses teratogenic in *animals* but therapeutic doses unlikely to be harmful; manufacturer of *topical* calcitriol advises avoid; *see also* Calcipotriol and Tacalcitol
Voriconazole	Toxicity in *animal* studies—manufacturer advises avoid unless potential benefit outweighs risk; effective contraception required during treatment
Warfarin	*see* Anticoagulants, Oral
Xipamide	*see* Diuretics
Zafirlukast	Manufacturer advises use only if potential benefit outweighs risk
Zalcitabine	Manufacturer advises use only if potential benefit outweighs risk—toxicity in *animal* studies; women of childbearing age should use effective contraception during treatment
Zaleplon	Manufacturer advises avoid in early pregnancy—no information available; risk of neonatal withdrawal symptoms if used in late pregnancy
Zanamivir	Manufacturer advises use only if potential benefit outweighs risk—no information available
Zidovudine	Limited information available; manufacturer advises use only if clearly indicated; *see also* p. 314
Zinc acetate	Usual dose 25 mg 3 times daily adjusted according to plasma-copper concentration and urinary copper excretion
Zinc sulphate	Safety not established—crosses placenta
Zoledronic acid	Manufacturer advises avoid—toxicity in *animal* studies
Zolmitriptan	*see* $5HT_1$ Agonists
Zolpidem	*see* Benzodiazepines
Zonisamide	Toxicity in *animal* studies—manufacturer advises use only if potential benefit outweighs risk
Zopiclone	*see* Benzodiazepines
Zotepine	Manufacturer advises avoid unless potential benefit outweighs risk
Zuclopenthixol	*see* Antipsychotics

Appendix 5: Breast-feeding

Administration of some drugs (e.g. ergotamine) to nursing mothers may harm the infant, whereas administration of others (e.g. digoxin) has little effect. Some drugs inhibit lactation (e.g. bromocriptine).

Toxicity to the infant can occur if the drug enters the milk in pharmacologically significant quantities. The concentration in milk of some drugs (e.g. iodides) may exceed the concentration in maternal plasma so that therapeutic doses in the mother may cause toxicity to the infant. Some drugs inhibit the infant's sucking reflex (e.g. phenobarbital). Drugs in breast milk may, at least theoretically, cause hypersensitivity in the infant even when concentration is too low for a pharmacological effect. The following table lists drugs:

- which should be used with caution or which are contra-indicated in breast-feeding for the reasons given above;
- which, on present evidence, may be given to the mother during breast-feeding, because they appear in milk in amounts which are too small to be harmful to the infant;
- which are not known to be harmful to the infant although they are present in milk in significant amounts.

> For many drugs insufficient evidence is available to provide guidance and it is advisable to administer only essential drugs to a mother during breast-feeding. Because of the inadequacy of information on drugs in breast milk the following table should be used only as a guide; absence from the table does not imply safety.

Table of drugs present in breast milk

Products introduced or amended since publication of BNF No. 49 (March 2005) are underlined.

Drug	Comment
Abacavir	Breast-feeding not advised in HIV infection
Abciximab	Manufacturer advises avoid—no information available
Acamprosate	Manufacturer advises avoid
Acarbose	Manufacturer advises avoid
Acebutolol	*see* Beta-blockers
Aceclofenac	Manufacturer advises avoid—no information available
Acemetacin	Manufacturer advises avoid
Acenocoumarol (nicoumalone)	*see* Anticoagulants, Oral
Acetazolamide	Amount too small to be harmful
Aciclovir	Significant amount in milk after systemic administration—not known to be harmful but manufacturer advises caution
Acipimox	Manufacturer advises avoid
Acitretin	Avoid
Acrivastine	*see* Antihistamines
Adalimumab	Avoid; manufacturer advises avoid for at least 5 months after last dose
Adapalene	Manufacturer advises avoid (if used, avoid application to chest)—no information available
Adefovir dipivoxil	Manufacturer advises avoid—no information available
Agalsidase beta	Manufacturer advises avoid—no information available
Alcohol	Large amounts may affect infant and reduce milk consumption
Alemtuzumab	Avoid; manufacturer advises avoid breast-feeding for at least 4 weeks after administration
Alendronic acid	No information available
Alfacalcidol	*see* Vitamin D
Alfentanil	Present in milk—manufacturer advises withhold breast-feeding for 24 hours
Alimemazine (trimeprazine)	*see* Antihistamines
Allopurinol	Present in milk—not known to be harmful
Almotriptan	Present in milk in *animal* studies—withhold breast-feeding for 24 hours
Alprazolam	*see* Benzodiazepines
Alverine	Manufacturer advises avoid—little information available
Amantadine	Avoid; present in milk; toxicity in infant reported
Amethocaine	*see* Tetracaine
Amfebutamone	*see* Bupropion
Amiloride	Manufacturer advises avoid—no information available
Aminoglutethimide	Avoid
Aminophylline	*see* Theophylline
Amiodarone	Avoid; present in milk in significant amounts; theoretical risk from release of iodine; *see also* Iodine
Amisulpride	Manufacturer advises avoid—no information available
Amitriptyline	*see* Antidepressants, Tricyclic (and related)
Amlodipine	Manufacturer advises avoid—no information available
Amobarbital	*see* Barbiturates
Amorolfine	Manufacturer advises avoid—no information available
Amoxapine	*see* Antidepressants, Tricyclic (and related)
Amoxicillin	*see* Penicillins
Amphetamines	Significant amount in milk. Avoid
Amphotericin	No information available
Ampicillin	*see* Penicillins
Amprenavir	Breast-feeding not advised in HIV infection
Amsacrine	*see* Cytotoxic Drugs
<u>Anagrelide</u>	Manufacturer advises avoid—no information available

Drug	Comment
Anakinra	Manufacturer advises avoid—no information available
Analgesics	*see* Aspirin, NSAIDs, Opioid Analgesics and Paracetamol
Androgens	Avoid; may cause masculinisation in the female infant or precocious development in the male infant; high doses suppress lactation
Anthraquinones	Avoid; large doses may cause increased gastric motility and diarrhoea (particularly cascara and dantron)
Anticoagulants, oral	Risk of haemorrhage; increased by vitamin-K deficiency; warfarin appears safe but phenindione should be avoided; manufacturer of acenocoumarol (nicoumalone) recommends prophylactic vitamin K for the infant (consult product literature)
Antidepressants, SSRI	*see* individual entries
Antidepressants, tricyclic (and related)	Amount of tricyclic antidepressants (including related drugs such as mianserin and trazodone) too small to be harmful but most manufacturers advise avoid; accumulation of doxepin metabolite may cause sedation and respiratory depression
Antihistamines	Significant amount of some antihistamines present in milk; although not known to be harmful manufacturers of alimemazine, cetirizine, cyproheptadine, desloratadine, fexofenadine, hydroxyzine, loratadine, mizolastine and terfenadine advise avoid; adverse effects in infant reported with clemastine
Antipsychotics	Although amount present in milk probably too small to be harmful, *animal* studies indicate possible adverse effects of these drugs on developing nervous system therefore avoid unless absolutely necessary; *see also* Amisulpride, Chlorpromazine, Clozapine, Olanzapine, Quetiapine, Risperidone, Sertindole, Sulpiride, Zotepine
Apomorphine	Manufacturer advises avoid—no information available
Aprepitant	Manufacturer advises avoid—present in milk in *animal* studies
Aripiprazole	Manufacturer advises avoid—present in milk in *animal* studies
Arsenic trioxide	*see* Cytotoxic Drugs
Artemether [ingredient]	*see Riamet*®
Aspirin	Avoid—possible risk of Reye's syndrome; regular use of high doses could impair platelet function and produce hypoprothrombinaemia in infant if neonatal vitamin K stores low
Atazanavir	Breast-feeding not advised in HIV infection
Atenolol	*see* Beta-blockers
Atomoxetine	Manufacturer advises avoid—present in milk in *animal* studies
Atorvastatin	*see* Statins
Atosiban	Small amounts present in milk
Atovaquone	Manufacturer advises avoid—no information available
Atracurium	Breast-feeding unlikely to be harmful following recovery from neuromuscular block; some manufacturers advise avoiding breast-feeding for 24 hours after administration
Atropine	Small amount present in milk—manufacturer advises caution
Auranofin	Present in milk; manufacturer advises avoid
Azathioprine	*see* Cytotoxic Drugs
Azithromycin	Present in milk; manufacturer advises use only if no suitable alternative
Aztreonam	Amount probably too small to be harmful—manufacturer advises avoid
Baclofen	Amount too small to be harmful
Balsalazide	Manufacturer advises avoid
Barbiturates	Avoid if possible (*see also* Phenobarbital); large doses may produce drowsiness
Basiliximab	Avoid
Beclometasone	*see* Corticosteroids
Bemiparin	Manufacturer advises avoid—no information available
Bendrofluazide	*see* Thiazides and Related Diuretics
Bendroflumethiazide (bendrofluazide)	*see* Thiazides and Related Diuretics
Benperidol	*see* Antipsychotics
Benzodiazepines	Present in milk—avoid if possible
Benzylpenicillin	*see* Penicillins
Beta-blockers	Monitor infant; possible toxicity due to beta-blockade but amount of most beta-blockers present in milk too small to affect infant; acebutolol, atenolol, nadolol, and sotalol are present in greater amounts than other beta-blockers; manufacturers advise avoid celiprolol and nebivolol
Betamethasone	*see* Corticosteroids
Bethanechol	Manufacturer advises avoid
Bevacizumab	Manufacturer advises avoid breast-feeding during and for at least 6 months after treatment
Bexarotene	*see* Cytotoxic Drugs
Bezafibrate	Manufacturer advises avoid—no information available
Bimatoprost	Manufacturer advises avoid
Bisoprolol	*see* Beta-blockers
Bivalirudin	Manufacturer advises caution—no information available
Bleomycin	*see* Cytotoxic Drugs
Bosentan	Manufacturer advises avoid—no information available
Botulinum toxin	Manufacturers advise avoid—no information available
Bromocriptine	Suppresses lactation
Buclizine	*see* Antihistamines
Budesonide	*see* Corticosteroids

Drug	Comment
Bumetanide	Manufacturer advises avoid if possible—no information available
Bupivacaine	Amount too small to be harmful
Buprenorphine	Amount too small to be harmful; manufacturer advises contra-indicated in the treatment of opioid dependence
Bupropion	Present in milk—manufacturer advises avoid
Buserelin	Small amount present in milk—manufacturer advises avoid
Buspirone	Manufacturer advises avoid
Busulfan	*see* Cytotoxic Drugs
Butobarbital	*see* Barbiturates
Cabergoline	Suppresses lactation
Caffeine	Regular intake of large amounts can affect infant
Calciferol	*see* Vitamin D
Calcipotriol	No information available
Calcitonin (salmon) (salcatonin)	Avoid; inhibits lactation in *animals*
Calcitriol	*see* Vitamin D
Calcium folinate	Manufacturer advises caution—no information available
Calcium levofolinate	*see* Calcium Folinate
Candesartan	Manufacturer advises avoid—no information available
Capecitabine	Discontinue breast-feeding
Capreomycin	Manufacturer advises caution—no information available
Captopril	Present in milk— manufacturers advise avoid
Carbamazepine	Amount probably too small to be harmful but severe skin reaction reported in 1 infant
Carbimazole	Amounts in milk may be sufficient to affect neonatal thyroid function therefore lowest effective dose should be used (*see also* section 6.2.2)
Carbocisteine	No information available
Carboplatin	*see* Cytotoxic Drugs
Carglumic acid	Manufacturer advises avoid unless essential—no information available
Carisoprodol	Concentrated in milk; no adverse effects reported but best avoided
Carmustine	*see* Cytotoxic Drugs
Carvedilol	*see* Beta-blockers
Cascara	*see* Anthraquinones
Caspofungin	Present in milk in *animal* studies—manufacturer advises avoid
Cefaclor	Present in milk in low concentration
Cefadroxil	Present in milk in low concentration
Cefalexin	Present in milk in low concentration
Cefixime	Manufacturer advises avoid—no information available
Cefotaxime	Present in milk in low concentration
Cefpirome	Present in milk—manufacturer advises avoid
Cefpodoxime	Present in milk in low concentration
Cefprozil	Present in milk in low concentration
Cefradine	Present in milk in low concentration
Ceftazidime	Present in milk in low concentration
Ceftriaxone	Present in milk in low concentration
Cefuroxime	Present in milk in low concentration
Celecoxib	Manufacturer advises avoid—no information available
Celiprolol	*see* Beta-blockers
Cetirizine	*see* Antihistamines
Cetrorelix	Manufacturer advises avoid
Cetuximab	Manufacturer advises avoid breast-feeding during and for one month after treatment—no information available
Chloral hydrate	Sedation in infant—manufacturer advises avoid
Chlorambucil	*see* Cytotoxic Drugs
Chloramphenicol	Use another antibiotic; may cause bone-marrow toxicity in infant; concentration in milk usually insufficient to cause 'grey syndrome'
Chlordiazepoxide	*see* Benzodiazepines
Chloroquine	Amount probably too small to be harmful when used for malaria prophylaxis; inadequate for reliable protection against malaria, *see* section 5.4.1; avoid breast-feeding when used for rheumatic diseases
Chlorphenamine (chlorpheniramine)	*see* Antihistamines
Chlorpheniramine	*see* Antihistamines
Chlorpromazine	Drowsiness in infant reported; *see* Antipsychotics
Chlorpropamide	*see* Sulphonylureas
Chlortalidone	*see* Thiazides and Related Diuretics
Chlortetracycline	*see* Tetracyclines
Ciclosporin	Present in milk—manufacturer advises avoid
Cidofovir	Manufacturer advises avoid
Cilastatin [ingredient]	*see Primaxin*®
Cilazapril	No information available—manufacturer advises avoid
Cilostazol	Present in milk in *animal* studies—manufacturer advises avoid
Cimetidine	Significant amount—not known to be harmful but manufacturer advises avoid
Cinacalcet	Manufacturer advises avoid—present in milk in *animal* studies
Ciprofibrate	Manufacturer advises avoid—present in milk in *animal* studies
Ciprofloxacin	Avoid—high concentrations in breast milk
Cisatracurium	No information available
Cisplatin	*see* Cytotoxic Drugs
Citalopram	Present in milk—manufacturer advises avoid
Cladribine	*see* Cytotoxic Drugs

Drug	Comment
Clarithromycin	Manufacturer advises avoid unless potential benefit outweighs risk—present in milk
Clavulanic acid [ingredient]	see Co-amoxiclav, *Timentin*®
Clemastine	*see* Antihistamines
Clindamycin	Amount probably too small to be harmful but bloody diarrhoea reported in 1 infant
Clobazam	*see* Benzodiazepines
Clodronate sodium	*see* Sodium Clodronate
Clomethiazole	Amount too small to be harmful
Clomifene	May inhibit lactation
Clomipramine	*see* Antidepressants, Tricyclic (and related)
Clonazepam	*see* Benzodiazepines
Clonidine	Present in milk—manufacturer advises avoid
Clopidogrel	Manufacturer advises avoid
Clorazepate	*see* Benzodiazepines
Clozapine	Manufacturer advises avoid
Co-amoxiclav	*see* Penicillins
Co-beneldopa	*see* Levodopa
Co-careldopa	*see* Levodopa
Codeine	Amount too small to be harmful
Co-fluampicil	*see* Penicillins
Colchicine	Present in milk but no adverse effects reported; manufacturers advise avoid because of risk of cytotoxicity
Colecalciferol	*see* Vitamin D
Colistin	Present in milk but poorly absorbed from gut; manufacturers advise avoid (or use only if potential benefit outweighs risk)
Contraceptives, oral	Avoid combined oral contraceptives until weaning or for 6 months after birth (adverse effects on lactation); progestogen-only contraceptives do not affect lactation (start 3 weeks after birth or later)
Corticosteroids	Systemic effects in infant unlikely with maternal dose of prednisolone up to 40 mg daily; monitor infant's adrenal function with higher doses—the amount of inhaled drugs in breast milk is probably too small to be harmful
Cortisone acetate	*see* Corticosteroids
Co-trimoxazole	Small risk of kernicterus in jaundiced infants and of haemolysis in G6PD-deficient infants (due to sulfamethoxazole)
Crisantaspase	*see* Cytotoxic Drugs
Cromoglicate	*see* Sodium Cromoglicate
Cyclopenthiazide	*see* Thiazides and Related Diuretics
Cyclophosphamide	Discontinue breast-feeding during and for 36 hours after stopping treatment
Cycloserine	Amount too small to be harmful
Cyclosporin	*see* Ciclosporin
Cyproheptadine	*see* Antihistamines
Cyproterone	Caution; possibility of anti-androgen effects in neonate
Cytarabine	*see* Cytotoxic Drugs
Cytotoxic drugs	Discontinue breast-feeding
Daclizumab	Avoid
Dactinomycin	*see* Cytotoxic Drugs
Dalfopristin [ingredient]	*see Synercid*®
Dalteparin	No information available
Danaparoid	Amount probably too small to be harmful but manufacturer advises avoid
Danazol	No data available but avoid because of possible androgenic effects in infant
Dantrolene	Present in milk—manufacturer advises avoid
Dantron	*see* Anthraquinones
Dapsone	Haemolytic anaemia; although significant amount in milk, risk to infant very small unless infant is G6PD deficient
Darbepoetin	Manufacturer advises avoid—no information available
Daunorubicin	*see* Cytotoxic Drugs
Deferiprone	Manufacturer advises avoid—no information available
Deflazacort	*see* Corticosteroids
Demeclocycline	*see* Tetracyclines
Desferrioxamine	Manufacturer advises use only if potential benefit outweighs risk—no information available
Desloratadine	*see* Antihistamines
Desmopressin	Not known to be harmful
Desogestrel	*see* Contraceptives, Oral
Dexamethasone	*see* Corticosteroids
Dexamfetamine	*see* Amphetamines
Dexketoprofen	Manufacturer advises avoid—no information available
Dextropropoxyphene	Amount too small to be harmful
Diamorphine	Therapeutic doses unlikely to affect infant; withdrawal symptoms in infants of dependent mothers; breast-feeding no longer considered best method of treating dependence in offspring of dependent mothers and should be stopped
Diazepam	*see* Benzodiazepines
Diclofenac	Amount too small to be harmful
Didanosine	Breast-feeding not advised in HIV infection
Diflunisal	Manufacturer advises avoid
Digoxin	Amount too small to be harmful
Dihydrocodeine	Manufacturer advises use only if potential benefit outweighs risk
Dihydrotachysterol	*see* Vitamin D
Diloxanide	Manufacturer advises avoid
Diltiazem	Significant amount present in milk—no evidence of harm but avoid unless no safer alternative
Diphenhydramine	*see* Antihistamines
Dipyridamole	Small amount present in milk—manufacturer advises caution
Disodium etidronate	No information available
Disodium pamidronate	Manufacturer advises avoid
Disopyramide	Present in milk—use only if essential and monitor infant for antimuscarinic effects
Distigmine	No information available
Disulfiram	Manufacturer advises avoid—no information available

Drug	Comment
Docetaxel	*see* Cytotoxic Drugs
Docusate sodium	Present in milk following oral administration—manufacturer advises caution; rectal administration not known to be harmful
Dolasetron	Manufacturer advises avoid—no information available
Domperidone	Amount probably too small to be harmful
Dornase alfa	Amount probably too small to be harmful—manufacturer advises caution
Dosulepin (dothiepin)	*see* Antidepressants, Tricyclic (and related)
Dothiepin	*see* Antidepressants, Tricyclic (and related)
Doxazosin	Accumulates in milk—manufacturer advises avoid
Doxepin	*see* Antidepressants, Tricyclic (and related)
Doxorubicin	*see* Cytotoxic Drugs
Doxycycline	*see* Tetracyclines
Doxylamine	*see* Antihistamines
Drotrecogin alfa (activated)	Manufacturer advises avoid—no information available
Duloxetine	Present in milk in *animal* studies—avoid
Dydrogesterone	Present in milk—no adverse effects reported
Edrophonium	Amount probably too small to be harmful
Efalizumab	May be present in milk—manufacturer advises avoid
Efavirenz	Breast-feeding not advised in HIV infection
Eflornithine	Manufacturer advises avoid—no information available
Eformoterol	*see* Formoterol
Eletriptan	Present in milk—avoid breast-feeding for 24 hours
Emtricitabine	Breast-feeding not advised in HIV infection
Enalapril	Amount probably too small to be harmful
Enfuvirtide	Breast-feeding not advised in HIV infection
Enoxaparin	Manufacturer advises avoid—no information available
Enoximone	Manufacturer advises caution—no information available
Entacapone	Manufacturer advises avoid—present in milk in *animal* studies
Ephedrine	Irritability and disturbed sleep reported
Epinastine	Present in milk in *animal* studies—manufacturer advises caution
Epirubicin	*see* Cytotoxic Drugs
Eplerenone	Manufacturer advises use only if potential benefit outweighs risk
Epoetin	Manufacturers advise avoid—no information available
Eprosartan	Manufacturer advises avoid unless potential benefit outweighs risk
Eptifibatide	No information available—manufacturer advises avoid
Ergocalciferol	*see* Vitamin D
Ergotamine	Avoid; ergotism may occur in infant; repeated doses may inhibit lactation
Ertapenem	Present in milk—manufacturer advises avoid
Erythromycin	Only small amounts in milk—not known to be harmful
Escitalopram	Manufacturer advises avoid—no information available
Esmolol	*see* Beta-blockers
Esomeprazole	Manufacturer advises avoid—no information available
Etamsylate	Significant amount but not known to be harmful
Etanercept	Manufacturer advises avoid—no information available
Ethambutol	Amount too small to be harmful
Ethinylestradiol	*see* Oestrogens
Ethosuximide	Present in milk but unlikely to be harmful; manufacturer advises avoid
Etidronate disodium	*see* Disodium Etidronate
Etodolac	Manufacturer advises avoid
Etomidate	Avoid breast-feeding for 24 hours after administration
Etoposide	*see* Cytotoxic Drugs
Etoricoxib	Manufacturer advises avoid—present in milk in *animal* studies
Etynodiol	*see* Contraceptives, Oral
Ezetimibe	Present in milk in *animal* studies—manufacturer advises avoid
Famciclovir	Manufacturer advises avoid unless potential benefit outweighs risk—present in milk in *animal* studies
Famotidine	Present in milk—not known to be harmful but manufacturer advises avoid
Fansidar®	Small risk of kernicterus in jaundiced infants and of haemolysis in G6PD-deficient infants (due to sulfadoxine)
Felodipine	Present in milk
Fenbufen	Small amount present in milk—manufacturer advises avoid
Fenofibrate	Manufacturer advises avoid—no information available
Fenoprofen	Amount too small to be harmful
Fentanyl	Manufacturer advises avoid
Fenticonazole	Manufacturer advises avoid unless essential—present in milk in *animal* studies
Fexofenadine	*see* Antihistamines
Filgrastim	No information available—manufacturer advises avoid
Flavoxate	Manufacturer advises caution—no information available
Flecainide	Significant amount but not known to be harmful
Flucloxacillin	*see* Penicillins
Fluconazole	Manufacturer advises avoid—present in milk
Flucytosine	Manufacturer advises avoid
Fludarabine	*see* Cytotoxic Drugs
Fluorouracil	*see* Cytotoxic Drugs
Fluoxetine	Present in milk—manufacturer advises avoid
Flupentixol	*see* Antipsychotics

Drug	Comment
Fluphenazine	*see* Antipsychotics
Flurazepam	*see* Benzodiazepines
Flurbiprofen	Amount too small to be harmful
Fluticasone	*see* Corticosteroids
Fluvastatin	*see* Statins
Fluvoxamine	Present in milk—manufacturer advises avoid
Follitropin alfa and beta	Avoid
Fomepizole	Manufacturer advises caution—no information available
Fondaparinux	Present in milk in *animal* studies—manufacturer advises avoid
Formoterol (eformoterol)	Amount in milk probably too small to be harmful but manufacturers advise avoid
Fosamprenavir	Breast-feeding not advised in HIV infection
Fosinopril	Present in milk—manufacturer advises avoid
Fosphenytoin	*see* Phenytoin
Frovatriptan	Present in milk in *animal* studies—withhold breast-feeding for 24 hours
Frusemide	*see* Furosemide
Fulvestrant	Manufacturer advises avoid—present in milk in *animal* studies
Furosemide (frusemide)	Amount too small to be harmful
Fusidic acid	*see* Sodium Fusidate
Gabapentin	Present in milk—manufacturer advises avoid
Galantamine	Manufacturer advises avoid—no information available
Ganciclovir	Avoid
Ganirelix	Manufacturer advises avoid—no information available
Gemcitabine	*see* Cytotoxic Drugs
Gemfibrozil	Manufacturer advises avoid—no information available
Gestodene	*see* Contraceptives, Oral
Gestrinone	Manufacturer advises avoid
Glatiramer	Manufacturer advises caution—no information available
Glibenclamide	*see* Sulphonylureas
Gliclazide	*see* Sulphonylureas
Glimepiride	*see* Sulphonylureas
Glipizide	*see* Sulphonylureas
Gliquidone	*see* Sulphonylureas
Goserelin	Manufacturer advises avoid
Granisetron	Manufacturer advises avoid—no information available
Griseofulvin	Avoid—no information available
Haem arginate	Manufacturer advises avoid unless essential—no information available
Haloperidol	*see* Antipsychotics
Halothane	Present in milk
Hepatitis A vaccine	No information available
Human menopausal gonadotrophins	Avoid
Hydralazine	Present in milk but not known to be harmful; monitor infant
Hydrochlorothiazide	*see* Thiazides and Related Diuretics
Hydrocortisone	*see* Corticosteroids
Hydroflumethiazide	*see* Thiazides and Related Diuretics
Hydromorphone	Manufacturer advises avoid—no information available
Hydroxocobalamin	Present in milk but not known to be harmful
Hydroxycarbamide (hydroxyurea)	*see* Cytotoxic Drugs
Hydroxychloroquine	Avoid—risk of toxicity in infant
Hydroxyurea	*see* Cytotoxic Drugs
Hydroxyzine	*see* Antihistamines
Hyoscine	Amount too small to be harmful
Ibandronic acid	Manufacturer advises caution—present in milk in *animal* studies
Ibuprofen	Amount too small to be harmful but some manufacturers advise avoid (including topical use)
Idarubicin	*see* Cytotoxic Drugs
Idoxuridine	May make milk taste unpleasant
Ifosfamide	*see* Cytotoxic Drugs
Iloprost	Manufacturer advises avoid—no information available
Imatinib	*see* Cytotoxic Drugs
Imidapril	Manufacturer advises avoid—no information available
Imiglucerase	No information available
Imipenem [ingredient]	*see Primaxin*®
Imipramine	*see* Antidepressants, Tricyclic (and related)
Imiquimod	Manufacturer advises no information available
Indapamide	No information available—manufacturer advises avoid
Indinavir	Breast-feeding not advised in HIV infection
Indometacin	Amount probably too small to be harmful but convulsions reported in one infant—manufacturers advise avoid
Infliximab	Avoid; manufacturer advises avoid for at least 6 months after last dose
Influenza vaccine	Not known to be harmful
Insulin	Amount too small to be harmful
Interferons	Manufacturers advise avoid—no information available
Iodine and iodides	Stop breast-feeding; danger of neonatal hypothyroidism or goitre; appears to be concentrated in milk
Iodine, radioactive	Breast-feeding contra-indicated after therapeutic doses. With diagnostic doses withhold breast-feeding for at least 24 hours
Ipratropium	Amount probably too small to be harmful
Irbesartan	Manufacturer advises avoid—no information available
Irinotecan	*see* Cytotoxic Drugs
Isoniazid	Monitor infant for possible toxicity; theoretical risk of convulsions and neuropathy; prophylactic pyridoxine advisable in mother and infant
Isotretinoin	Avoid
Isradipine	Manufacturer advises avoid—present in milk in *animal* studies

Drug	Comment
Itraconazole	Small amounts present in milk—may accumulate; manufacturer advises avoid unless potential benefit outweighs risk
Kaletra®	Breast-feeding not advised in HIV infection
Ketoconazole	Manufacturer advises avoid
Ketoprofen	Amount probably too small to be harmful but manufacturer advises avoid unless essential
Ketorolac	Avoid
Ketotifen	*see* Antihistamines
Labetalol	*see* Beta-blockers
Lacidipine	Manufacturer advises avoid—no information available
Lamivudine	Present in milk—manufacturer advises avoid; breast-feeding not advised in HIV infection
Lamotrigine	Present in milk but limited data suggest no harmful effects on infants
Lanreotide	Manufacturer advises avoid unless potential benefit outweighs risk—no information available
Lansoprazole	Manufacturer advises avoid unless essential—present in milk in *animal* studies
Laronidase	Manufacturer advises avoid—no information available
Latanoprost	May be present in milk—manufacturer advises avoid
Leflunomide	Present in milk—manufacturer advises avoid
Lenograstim	Manufacturer advises avoid—no information available
Lepirudin	Avoid
Lercanidipine	Manufacturer advises avoid
Leuprorelin	Manufacturer advises avoid
Levetiracetam	Manufacturer advises avoid—present in milk in *animal* studies
Levobupivacaine	Likely to be present in milk but risk to infant minimal
Levocabastine	Amount too small to be harmful
Levocetirizine	*see* Antihistamines
Levodopa	May suppress lactation; present in milk—manufacturers advise avoid
Levofloxacin	Manufacturer advises avoid
Levomepromazine (methotrimeprazine)	*see* Antipsychotics
Levonorgestrel	*see* Contraceptives, Oral
Levothyroxine (thyroxine)	Amount too small to affect tests for neonatal hypothyroidism
Lidocaine (lignocaine)	Amount too small to be harmful
Lignocaine	*see* Lidocaine
Linezolid	Manufacturer advises avoid—present in milk in *animal* studies
Liothyronine	Amount too small to affect tests for neonatal hypothyroidism
Lisinopril	No information available—manufacturer advises caution
Lisuride	May suppress lactation
Lithium salts	Present in milk and risk of toxicity in infant—manufacturers advise avoid
Lofepramine	*see* Antidepressants, Tricyclic (and related)
Loperamide	Amount probably too small to be harmful
Lopinavir [ingredient]	*see Kaletra®*
Loprazolam	*see* Benzodiazepines
Loratadine	*see* Antihistamines
Lorazepam	*see* Benzodiazepines
Lormetazepam	*see* Benzodiazepines
Losartan	Manufacturer advises avoid—no information available
Lumefantrine [ingredient]	*see Riamet®*
Lymecycline	*see* Tetracyclines
Macrogols	Manufacturers advise use only if essential—no information available
Malarone®	Manufacturer advises avoid; *see also* Atovaquone and Proguanil
Maprotiline	*see* Antidepressants, Tricyclic (and related)
Mebendazole	Amount too small to be harmful but manufacturer advises avoid
Mebeverine	Amount too small to be harmful
Medroxyprogesterone	Present in milk—no adverse effects reported
Mefenamic acid	Amount too small to be harmful but manufacturer advises avoid
Mefloquine	Present in milk but risk to infant minimal
Meloxicam	No information available—manufacturer advises avoid
Melphalan	*see* Cytotoxic Drugs
Memantine	Avoid
Menotrophin	Avoid
Meprobamate	Avoid; concentration in milk may exceed maternal plasma concentrations fourfold and may cause drowsiness in infant
Meptazinol	Manufacturer advises use only if potential benefit outweighs risk
Mercaptamine	Manufacturer advises avoid
Mercaptopurine	*see* Cytotoxic Drugs
Meropenem	Unlikely to be absorbed (however, manufacturer advises avoid unless potential benefit justifies potential risk)
Mesalazine	Diarrhoea reported but manufacturers advise negligible amounts detected in breast milk
Mesterolone	*see* Androgens
Mestranol	*see* Oestrogens
Metaraminol	Manufacturer advises caution—no information available
Metformin	Manufacturer advises avoid; present in milk
Methadone	Withdrawal symptoms in infant; breast-feeding permissible during maintenance but dose should be as low as possible and infant monitored to avoid sedation
Methenamine	Amount too small to be harmful
Methocarbamol	Present in milk in *animal* studies—manufacturer advises caution
Methotrexate	*see* Cytotoxic Drugs
Methotrimeprazine	*see* Antipsychotics
Methyldopa	Amount too small to be harmful

Drug	Comment
Methylphenidate	No information available—manufacturer advises avoid
Methylprednisolone	*see* Corticosteroids
Methysergide	Manufacturer advises avoid
Metoclopramide	Small amount present in milk; manufacturer advises avoid
Metolazone	*see* Thiazides and Related Diuretics
Metoprolol	*see* Beta-blockers
Metronidazole	Significant amount in milk; manufacturer advises avoid large single doses
Metyrapone	Manufacturer advises avoid—no information available
Mexiletine	Amount too small to be harmful
Mianserin	*see* Antidepressants, Tricyclic (and related)
Miconazole	Manufacturer advises caution—no information available
Midazolam	*see* Benzodiazepines
Mifepristone	No information available—manufacturer advises stop breast-feeding for 14 days after administration
Miglustat	Manufacturer advises avoid—no information available
Milrinone	Manufacturer advises caution—no information available
Minocycline	*see* Tetracyclines
Minoxidil	Present in milk but not known to be harmful
Mirtazapine	Manufacturer advises avoid—present in milk in *animal* studies
Misoprostol	No information available—manufacturer advises avoid
Mitomycin	*see* Cytotoxic Drugs
Mitoxantrone (mitozantrone)	*see* Cytotoxic Drugs
Mitozantrone	*see* Cytotoxic Drugs
Mizolastine	*see* Antihistamines
Moclobemide	Amount too small to be harmful, but patient leaflet advises avoid
Modafinil	Manufacturer advises avoid—no information available
Moexipril	Manufacturer advises avoid—no information available
Montelukast	Manufacturer advises avoid unless essential
Morphine	Therapeutic doses unlikely to affect infant; withdrawal symptoms in infants of dependent mothers; breast-feeding not best method of treating dependence in offspring and should be stopped
Moxifloxacin	Manufacturer advises avoid—present in milk in *animal* studies
Moxonidine	Present in milk—manufacturer advises avoid
Mupirocin	Manufacturer advises avoid unless potential benefit outweighs risk—no information available
Mycophenolate mofetil	Manufacturer advises avoid—present in milk in *animal* studies
Nabilone	Manufacturer advises avoid—no information available
Nabumetone	No information available—manufacturer advises avoid
Nadolol	*see* Beta-blockers
Nafarelin	Manufacturer advises avoid—no information available
Nalidixic acid	Risk to infant very small but one case of haemolytic anaemia reported
Naloxone	No information available
Naproxen	Amount too small to be harmful but manufacturer advises avoid
Naratriptan	Manufacturer advises caution—no information available
Nateglinide	Manufacturer advises avoid—present in milk in *animal* studies
Nebivolol	*see* Beta-blockers
Nedocromil	Unlikely to be present in milk
Nelfinavir	Breast-feeding not advised in HIV infection
Neostigmine	Amount probably too small to be harmful; monitor infant
Nevirapine	Breast-feeding not advised in HIV infection
Nicardipine	Manufacturer advises avoid—no information available
Nicorandil	No information available—manufacturer advises avoid
Nicotine	Present in milk; use only if smoking cessation without nicotine replacement fails; patient information for some products contra-indicates use
Nicotinic acid	Present in milk—avoid
Nicoumalone	*see* Anticoagulants, Oral
Nifedipine	Amount too small to be harmful but manufacturers advise avoid
Nimodipine	No information available
Nisoldipine	Manufacturer advises avoid—no information available
Nitrazepam	*see* Benzodiazepines
Nitrofurantoin	Only small amounts in milk but could be enough to produce haemolysis in G6PD-deficient infants
Nitroprusside	*see* Sodium Nitroprusside
Nizatidine	Amount too small to be harmful
Nonoxynol-9	Present in milk in *animal* studies
Norethisterone	Higher doses may suppress lactation and alter milk composition—use lowest effective dose; *see also* Contraceptives, Oral
Norfloxacin	No information available—manufacturer advises avoid
Norgestimate	*see* Contraceptives, Oral
Norgestrel	*see* Contraceptives, Oral
Nortriptyline	*see* Antidepressants, Tricyclic (and related)
NSAIDs	*see* individual entries
Nystatin	No information available, but absorption from gastro-intestinal tract negligible
Octreotide	Manufacturer advises avoid unless essential—no information available
Oestrogens	Avoid; adverse effects on lactation; *see also* Contraceptives, Oral
Ofloxacin	Manufacturer advises avoid
Olanzapine	Manufacturer advises avoid—present in milk

Drug	Comment
Olmesartan	Manufacturer advises avoid—present in milk in *animal* studies
Olsalazine	Manufacturer advises avoid
Omega-3-acid ethyl esters	Manufacturer advises avoid—no information available
Omeprazole	Present in milk but not known to be harmful
Ondansetron	Manufacturer advises avoid—present in milk in *animal* studies
Opioid analgesics	*see* individual entries
Oral contraceptives	*see* Contraceptives, Oral
Orlistat	Manufacturer advises avoid—no information available
Orphenadrine	Present in milk—manufacturer advises avoid
Oseltamivir	Manufacturer advises use only if potential benefit outweighs risk—present in milk in *animal* studies
Oxaliplatin	*see* Cytotoxic Drugs
Oxazepam	*see* Benzodiazepines
Oxcarbazepine	Present in milk—manufacturer advises avoid
Oxprenolol	*see* Beta-blockers
Oxybutynin	Present in milk—manufacturers advise avoid
Oxycodone	Present in milk—manufacturer advises avoid
Oxytetracycline	*see* Tetracyclines
Paclitaxel	*see* Cytotoxic Drugs
Palonosetron	Manufacturer advises avoid—no information available
Pamidronate disodium	*see* Disodium Pamidronate
Pancuronium	Manufacturer advises avoid unless potential benefit outweighs possble risk—no information available
Pantoprazole	Manufacturer advises avoid unless potential benefit outweighs risk—small amount present in milk in *animal* studies
Papaveretum	*see* Morphine
Paracetamol	Amount too small to be harmful
Paraldehyde	Manufacturer advises avoid unless essential—present in milk
Parecoxib	Manufacturer advises avoid—present in milk in animal studies
Paricalcitol	Manufacturer advises caution—no information available; *see also* Vitamin D
Paroxetine	Present in milk but amount too small to be harmful
Pegfilgrastim	No information available—manufacturer advises avoid
Peginterferon alfa	*see* Interferons
Pemetrexed	*see* Cytotoxic Drugs
Penicillamine	Manufacturer advises avoid unless potential benefit outweighs risk—no information available
Penicillins	Trace amounts in milk
Pentamidine isetionate	Manufacturer advises avoid unless essential
Pentazocine	Small amount present in milk—manufacturer advises caution
Pentostatin	*see* Cytotoxic Drugs
Pergolide	May suppress lactation
Pericyazine	*see* Antipsychotics
Perindopril	Manufacturer advises avoid—no information available
Perphenazine	*see* Antipsychotics
Phenindione	*see* Anticoagulants, Oral
Phenobarbital	Avoid when possible; drowsiness may occur but risk probably small; one report of methaemoglobinaemia with phenobarbital and phenytoin
Phenoxybenzamine	May be present in milk
Phenoxymethylpenicillin	*see* Penicillins
Phentolamine	Manufacturer advises avoid—no information available
Phenytoin	Small amount present in milk; manufacturer advises avoid—but *see* section 4.8.1
Phytomenadione	Present in milk
Pilocarpine	Manufacturer advises avoid—no information available
Pimozide	*see* Antipsychotics
Pindolol	*see* Beta-blockers
Pioglitazone	Manufacturer advises avoid—present in milk in *animal* studies
Piperacillin [ingredient]	*see Tazocin*®
Piperazine	Present in milk—manufacturer advises avoid breast-feeding for 8 hours after dose (express and discard milk during this time)
Piracetam	Manufacturer advises avoid
Piroxicam	Amount too small to be harmful
Pizotifen	Amount probably too small to be harmful, but patient information leaflet advises avoid
Podophyllum	Avoid
Porfimer	No information available—manufacturer advises avoid
Povidone–iodine	Avoid; iodine absorbed from vaginal preparations is concentrated in milk
Pramipexole	May suppress lactation; manufacturer advises avoid—present in milk in *animal* studies
Pravastatin	Small amount present in milk—manufacturer advises avoid
Prazosin	Amount probably too small to be harmful
Prednisolone	*see* Corticosteroids
Pregabalin	Present in milk in *animal* studies—manufacturer advises avoid
Prilocaine	Present in milk but not known to be harmful
Primaxin®	Present in milk but unlikely to be absorbed (however, manufacturer advises avoid)
Primidone	*see* Phenobarbital
Probenecid	No information available
Procainamide	Present in milk—manufacturer advises avoid
Procarbazine	*see* Cytotoxic Drugs
Prochlorperazine	*see* Antipsychotics
Progesterone	Manufacturers advise avoid—present in milk

Drug	Comment
Proguanil	Amount probably too small to be harmful when used for malaria prophylaxis; inadequate for reliable protection against malaria in breast-fed infant, see p. 331
Promazine	*see* Antipsychotics
Promethazine	*see* Antihistamines
Propafenone	Manufacturer advises avoid—no information available
Propantheline	May suppress lactation
Propiverine	Manufacturer advises avoid—present in milk in *animal* studies
Propofol	Present in milk but amount probably too small to be harmful
Propranolol	*see* Beta-blockers
Propylthiouracil	Monitor infant's thyroid status but amounts in milk probably too small to affect infant; high doses might affect neonatal thyroid function
Protirelin	Breast enlargement and leaking of milk reported
Pseudoephedrine	Amount too small to be harmful
Pyrazinamide	Amount too small to be harmful
Pyridostigmine	Amount probably too small to be harmful
Pyrimethamine	Significant amount—avoid administration of other folate antagonists to infant; avoid breast-feeding during toxoplasmosis treatment
Quetiapine	Manufacturer advises avoid—no information available
Quinagolide	Suppresses lactation
Quinapril	No information available—manufacturer advises caution
Quinidine	Significant amount but not known to be harmful
Quinupristin [ingredient]	*see Synercid*®
Rabeprazole	Manufacturer advises avoid—no information available
Raltitrexed	*see* Cytotoxic Drugs
Ramipril	Manufacturer advises avoid—no information available
Ranitidine	Significant amount but not known to be harmful
Ranitidine bismuth citrate	Manufacturer advises avoid—no information available
Rasburicase	Manufacturer advises avoid—no information available
Reboxetine	Manufacturer advises avoid—no information available
Remifentanil	Manufacturer advises caution—present in milk in *animal* studies
Repaglinide	Manufacturer advises avoid—present in milk in *animal* studies
Reteplase	Manufacturer advises avoid breast-feeding for 24 hours after dose (express and discard milk during this time)
Reviparin	No information available
Riamet®	Manufacturer advises avoid breast-feeding for at least 1 week after last dose; present in milk in *animal* studies
Ribavirin	Avoid—no information available
Rifabutin	Manufacturer advises avoid—no information available
Rifampicin	Amount too small to be harmful
Riluzole	Manufacturer advises avoid—no information available
Risedronate sodium	Manufacturer advises avoid
Risperidone	Present in milk—manufacturer advises avoid
Ritonavir	Breast-feeding not advised in HIV infection
Rituximab	Avoid
Rivastigmine	Present in milk in *animal* studies—manufacturer advises avoid
Rizatriptan	Present in milk in *animal* studies—withhold breast-feeding for 24 hours
Rocuronium	Manufacturer advises avoid unless potential benefit outweighs risk—present in milk in *animal* studies
Rosiglitazone	Manufacturer advises avoid—present in milk in *animal* studies
Rosuvastatin	*see* Statins
Salbutamol	Probably present in milk; manufacturer advises avoid unless potential benefit outweighs risk—the amount of inhaled drugs in breast milk is probably too small to be harmful
Salcatonin	*see* Calcitonin (salmon)
Saquinavir	Breast-feeding not advised in HIV infection
Secobarbital	*see* Barbiturates
Selegiline	Manufacturer advises avoid—no information available
Senna	*see* Anthraquinones
Sertindole	Manufacturer advises avoid—no information available
Sertraline	Present in milk but not known to be harmful in short-term use
Sevelamer	Manufacturer advises use only if potential benefit outweighs risk
Sibutramine	Manufacturer advises avoid—no information available
Silver sulfadiazine	*see* Sulphonamides
Simvastatin	*see* Statins
Sirolimus	Discontinue breast-feeding
Sodium aurothiomalate	Caution—present in milk; theoretical possibility of rashes and idiosyncratic reactions
Sodium clodronate	No information available
Sodium cromoglicate	Unlikely to be present in milk
Sodium fusidate	Present in milk—manufacturer advises caution
Sodium nitroprusside	Manufacturer advises caution—no information available
Sodium phenylbutyrate	Manufacturer advises avoid—no information available
Sodium picosulfate	Not known to be present in milk but manufacturer advises avoid
Sodium valproate	*see* Valproate
Solifenacin	Manufacturer advises avoid—present in milk in *animal* studies
Somatropin	No information available
Sotalol	*see* Beta-blockers
Spironolactone	Amount probably too small to be harmful but manufacturer advises avoid

Drug	Comment
Statins	Manufacturers of atorvastatin, fluvastatin, rosuvastatin and simvastatin advise avoid—no information available; *see also* pravastatin
Stavudine	Breast-feeding not advised in HIV infection
Strontium ranelate	Avoid
Sulfadiazine	*see* Sulphonamides
Sulfasalazine	Small amounts in milk (1 report of bloody diarrhoea and rashes); theoretical risk of neonatal haemolysis especially in G6PD-deficient infants
Sulfinpyrazone	No information available
Sulindac	No information available
Sulphonamides	Small risk of kernicterus in jaundiced infants particularly with long-acting sulphonamides, and of haemolysis in G6PD-deficient infants
Sulphonylureas	Theoretical possibility of hypoglycaemia in infant
Sulpiride	Best avoided; present in milk; *see also* Antipsychotics
Sumatriptan	Present in milk—withhold breast-feeding for 24 hours
Suxamethonium	No information available
Synercid®	Manufacturer advises avoid—no information available
Tacalcitol	Manufacturer advises avoid application to breast area—no information available
Tacrolimus	Avoid—present in milk following systemic administration
Tamoxifen	Supresses lactation; manufacturer advises avoid unless potential benefit outweighs risk
Tazarotene	Manufacturer advises avoid—present in milk in *animal* studies
Tazobactam [ingredient]	*see Tazocin*®
Tazocin®	Present in milk—manufacturer advises use only if potential benefit outweighs risk
Tegafur with uracil	*see* Cytotoxic Drugs
Teicoplanin	No information available
Telithromycin	Manufacturer advises avoid—present in milk in *animal* studies
Telmisartan	Manufacturer advises avoid—no information available
Temazepam	*see* Benzodiazepines
Temozolomide	*see* Cytotoxic Drugs
Tenecteplase	Manufacturer advises avoid breast-feeding for 24 hours after dose (express and discard milk during this time)
Tenofovir	Breast-feeding not advised in HIV infection
Tenoxicam	No information available
Terazosin	No information available
Terbinafine	Present in milk—manufacturer advises avoid
Terbutaline	Amount too small to be harmful
Terfenadine	*see* Antihistamines
Terlipressin	Not known to be harmful
Testosterone	*see* Androgens
Tetrabenazine	Manufacturer advises avoid
Tetracaine (amethocaine)	No information available
Tetracyclines	Avoid (although absorption and therefore discoloration of teeth in infant probably usually prevented by chelation with calcium in milk)
Theophylline	Present in milk—irritability in infant reported; modified-release preparations preferable
Thiamine	Severely thiamine-deficient mothers should avoid breast-feeding as toxic methyl-glyoxal present in milk
Thiazides and related diuretics	Amount too small to be harmful; large doses may suppress lactation
Thiopental	Present in milk—manufacturer advises avoid
Thiotepa	*see* Cytotoxic Drugs
Thyroxine	*see* Levothyroxine
Tiagabine	Manufacturer advises avoid unless potential benefit outweighs risk
Tiaprofenic acid	Amount too small to be harmful
Ticarcillin [ingredient]	*see* Penicillins
Tiludronic acid	Manufacturer advises avoid—no information available
Timentin®	*see* Penicillins
Timolol	*see* Beta-blockers
Tinidazole	Present in milk—manufacturer advises avoid breast-feeding during and for 3 days after stopping treatment
Tinzaparin	Manufacturer advises avoid—no information available
Tioguanine	*see* Cytotoxic Drugs
Tiotropium	Amount in milk probably too small to be harmful (present in milk in *animal* studies)—manufacturer advises use only if potential benefit outweighs risk
Tirofiban	Manufacturer advises avoid—no information available
Tizanidine	Manufacturer advises use only if potential benefit outweighs risk—no information available
Tolbutamide	*see* Sulphonylureas
Tolcapone	Manufacturer advises avoid—present in milk in *animal* studies
Tolfenamic acid	Amount too small to be harmful
Tolterodine	Manufacturer advises avoid—no information available
Topiramate	Manufacturer advises avoid
Topotecan	*see* Cytotoxic Drugs
Torasemide	No information available
Tramadol	Amount probably too small to be harmful, but manufacturer advises avoid
Trandolapril	Manufacturers advise avoid
Tranexamic acid	Small amount present in milk—antifibrinolytic effect in infant unlikely
Trastuzumab	Avoid breast-feeding during treatment and for six months after
Travoprost	Present in milk in animal studies; manufacturer advises avoid

Drug	Comment
Trazodone	*see* Antidepressants, Tricyclic (and related)
Treosulfan	*see* Cytotoxic Drugs
Tretinoin	Avoid
Triamcinolone	*see* Corticosteroids
Triamterene	Present in milk—manufacturer advises avoid
Tribavirin	*see* Ribavirin
Triclofos	Avoid
Trifluoperazine	*see* Antipsychotics
Trimeprazine	*see* Antihistamines
Trimethoprim	Present in milk—short-term use not known to be harmful
Trimipramine	*see* Antidepressants, Tricyclic (and related)
Triprolidine	*see* Antihistamines
Triptorelin	Manufacturers advise avoid
Tropisetron	No information available
Trospium	Manufacturer advises caution—no information available
Ursodeoxycholic acid	Not known to be harmful but manufacturer advises avoid
Valaciclovir	No information available; *see also* Aciclovir
Valganciclovir	*see* Ganciclovir
Valproate	Amount too small to be harmful
Valproic acid	*see* Valproate
Valsartan	Manufacturer advises avoid—no information available
Vancomycin	Present in milk—significant absorption following oral administration unlikely
Vasopressin	Not known to be harmful
Vecuronium	No information available
Venlafaxine	Present in milk—manufacturer advises avoid
Verapamil	Amount too small to be harmful
Verteporfin	No information available—manufacturer advises avoid breast-feeding for 48 hours after administration
Vigabatrin	Present in milk—manufacturer advises avoid
Vinblastine	*see* Cytotoxic Drugs
Vincristine	*see* Cytotoxic Drugs
Vindesine	*see* Cytotoxic Drugs
Vinorelbine	*see* Cytotoxic Drugs
Vitamin A	Theoretical risk of toxicity in infants of mothers taking large doses
Vitamin D	Caution with high systemic doses; may cause hypercal-caemia in infant; manufacturer of *topical* calcitriol advises avoid; *see also* Calcipotriol and Tacal-citol
Voriconazole	Manufacturer advises avoid—no information available
Warfarin	*see* Anticoagulants, Oral
Xipamide	No information available
Zafirlukast	Present in milk—manufacturer advises avoid
Zalcitabine	Breast-feeding not advised in HIV infection
Zaleplon	Present in milk—manufacturer advises avoid
Zanamivir	Manufacturer advises avoid—present in milk in *animal* studies
Zidovudine	Breast-feeding not advised in HIV infection
Zoledronic acid	Manufacturer advises avoid—no information available
Zolmitriptan	Manufacturer advises caution—present in milk in *animal* studies
Zolpidem	Small amounts present in milk—manufacturer advises avoid
Zonisamide	Avoid; manufacturer advises avoid breast-feeding for 4 weeks after administration
Zopiclone	Present in milk—manufacturer advises avoid
Zotepine	Manufacturer advises avoid
Zuclopenthixol	*see* Antipsychotics

Appendix 6: Intravenous additives

INTRAVENOUS ADDITIVES POLICIES. A local policy on the addition of drugs to intravenous fluids should be drawn up by a multi-disciplinary team in each Health Authority and issued as a document to the members of staff concerned.

Centralised additive services are provided in a number of hospital pharmacy departments and should be used in preference to making additions on wards.

The information that follows should be read in conjunction with local policy documents.

Guidelines

1. Drugs should only be added to infusion containers when constant plasma concentrations are needed or when the administration of a more concentrated solution would be harmful.
2. In general, only one drug should be added to any infusion container and the components should be compatible. Ready-prepared solutions should be used whenever possible. Drugs should not normally be added to blood products, mannitol, or sodium bicarbonate. Only specially formulated additives should be used with fat emulsions or amino-acid solutions (section 9.3).
3. Solutions should be thoroughly mixed by shaking and checked for absence of particulate matter before use.
4. Strict asepsis should be maintained throughout and in general the giving set should not be used for more than 24 hours (for drug admixtures).
5. The infusion container should be labelled with the patient's name, the name and quantity of additives, and the date and time of addition (and the new expiry date or time). Such additional labelling should not interfere with information on the manufacturer's label that is still valid. When possible, containers should be retained for a period after use in case they are needed for investigation.
6. It is good practice to examine intravenous infusions from time to time while they are running. If cloudiness, crystallisation, change of colour, or any other sign of interaction or contamination is observed the infusion should be discontinued.

Problems

MICROBIAL CONTAMINATION. The accidental entry and subsequent growth of micro-organisms converts the infusion fluid pathway into a potential vehicle for infection with micro-organisms, particularly species of Candida, Enterobacter, and Klebsiella. Ready-prepared infusions containing the additional drugs, or infusions prepared by an additive service (when available) should therefore be used in preference to making extemporaneous additions to infusion containers on wards etc. However, when this is necessary strict aseptic procedure should be followed.

INCOMPATIBILITY. Physical and chemical incompatibilities may occur with loss of potency, increase in toxicity, or other adverse effect. The solutions may become opalescent or precipitation may occur, but in many instances there is no visual indication of incompatibility. Interaction may take place at any point in the infusion fluid pathway, and the potential for incompatibility is increased when more than one substance is added to the infusion fluid.

Common incompatibilities. Precipitation reactions are numerous and varied and may occur as a result of pH, concentration changes, 'salting-out' effects, complexation or other chemical changes. Precipitation or other particle formation must be avoided since, apart from lack of control of dosage on administration, it may initiate or exacerbate adverse effects. This is particularly important in the case of drugs which have been implicated in either thrombophlebitis (e.g. diazepam) or in skin sloughing or necrosis caused by extravasation (e.g. sodium bicarbonate and certain cytotoxic drugs). It is also especially important to effect solution of colloidal drugs and to prevent their subsequent precipitation in order to avoid a pyrogenic reaction (e.g. amphotericin).

It is considered undesirable to mix beta-lactam antibiotics, such as semi-synthetic penicillins and cephalosporins, with proteinaceous materials on the grounds that immunogenic and allergenic conjugates could be formed.

A number of preparations undergo significant loss of potency when added singly or in combination to large volume infusions. Examples include ampicillin in infusions that contain glucose or lactates. The breakdown products of dacarbazine have been implicated in adverse effects.

Blood. Because of the large number of incompatibilities, drugs should not normally be added to blood and blood products for infusion purposes. Examples of incompatibility with blood include hypertonic mannitol solutions (irreversible crenation of red cells), dextrans (rouleaux formation and interference with cross-matching), glucose (clumping of red cells), and oxytocin (inactivated).

If the giving set is not changed after the administration of blood, but used for other infusion fluids, a fibrin clot may form which, apart from blocking the set, increases the likelihood of microbial growth.

Intravenous fat emulsions may break down with coalescence of fat globules and separation of phases when additions such as antibacterials or electrolytes are made, thus increasing the possibility of embolism. Only specially formulated products such as *Vitlipid N®* (section 9.3) may be added to appropriate intravenous fat emulsions.

Other infusions that frequently give rise to incompatibility include amino acids, mannitol, and sodium bicarbonate.

Bactericides such as chlorocresol 0.1% or phenylmercuric nitrate 0.001% are present in some injection solutions. The total volume of such solutions added to a container for infusion on one occasion should not exceed 15 mL.

Method

Ready-prepared infusions should be used whenever available. **Potassium chloride** is usually available in concentrations of 20, 27, and 40 mmol/litre in sodium chloride intravenous infusion (0.9%), glucose intravenous infusion (5%) or sodium chloride and glucose intravenous infusion. **Lidocaine hydrochloride** (lignocaine hydrochloride) is usually available in concentrations of 0.1 or 0.2% in glucose intravenous infusion (5%).

When addition is required to be made extemporaneously, any product reconstitution instructions such as those relating to concentration, vehicle, mixing, and handling precautions should be strictly followed using an aseptic technique throughout. Once the product has been reconstituted, addition to the infusion fluid should be made immediately in order to minimise microbial contamination and, with certain products, to prevent degradation or other formulation change which may occur; e.g. reconstituted ampicillin injection degrades rapidly on standing, and also may form polymers which could cause sensitivity reactions.

It is also important in certain instances that an infusion fluid of specific pH be used (e.g. **furosemide** (frusemide) injection requires dilution in infusions of pH greater than 5.5).

When drug additions are made it is important to mix thoroughly; additions should not be made to an infusion container that has been connected to a giving set, as mixing is hampered. If the solutions are not thoroughly mixed a concentrated layer of the additive may form owing to differences in density. **Potassium chloride** is particularly prone to this 'layering' effect when added without adequate mixing to infusions packed in non-rigid infusion containers; if such a mixture is administered it may have a serious effect on the heart.

A time limit between addition and completion of administration must be imposed for certain admixtures to guarantee satisfactory drug potency and compatibility. For admixtures in which degradation occurs without the formation of toxic substances, an acceptable limit is the time taken for 10% decomposition of the drug. When toxic substances are produced stricter limits may be imposed. Because of the risk of microbial contamination a maximum time limit of 12 hours may be appropriate for additions made elsewhere than in hospital pharmacies offering central additive service.

Certain injections must be protected from light during continuous infusion to minimise oxidation, e.g. amphotericin, dacarbazine, and sodium nitroprusside.

Dilution with a small volume of an appropriate vehicle and administration using a motorised infusion pump is advocated for preparations such as heparin where strict control over administration is required. In this case the appropriate dose may be dissolved in a convenient volume (e.g. 24 to 48 mL) of sodium chloride intravenous infusion (0.9%).

Use of table

The table lists preparations given by three methods:

continuous infusion,
intermittent infusion, and
addition via the drip tubing.

Drugs for **continuous infusion** must be diluted in a large volume infusion. Penicillins and cephalosporins are not usually given by continuous infusion because of stability problems and because adequate plasma and tissue concentrations are best obtained by intermittent infusion. Where it is necessary to administer them by continuous infusion, detailed literature should be consulted.

Drugs that are both compatible and clinically suitable may be given by **intermittent infusion** in a relatively small volume of infusion over a short period of time, e.g. 100 mL in 30 minutes. The method is used if the product is incompatible or unstable over the period necessary for continuous infusion; the limited stability of ampicillin or amoxicillin in large volume glucose or lactate infusions may be overcome in this way.

Intermittent infusion is also used if adequate plasma and tissue concentrations are not produced by continuous infusion as in the case of drugs such as dacarbazine, gentamicin, and ticarcillin.

An in-line burette may be used for intermittent infusion techniques in order to achieve strict control over the time and rate of administration, especially for infants and children and in intensive care units. Intermittent infusion may also make use of the 'piggy-back' technique provided that no additions are made to the primary infusion. In this method the drug is added to a small secondary container connected to a Y-type injection site on the primary infusion giving set; the secondary solution is usually infused within 30 minutes.

Addition *via* the drip tubing is indicated for a number of cytotoxic drugs in order to minimise extravasation. The preparation is added aseptically *via* the rubber septum of the injection site of a fast-running infusion. In general, drug preparations intended for a bolus effect should be given directly into a separate vein where possible. Failing this, administration may be made *via* the drip tubing provided that the preparation is compatible with the infusion fluid when given in this manner.

Table of drugs given by intravenous infusion

Covers addition to *Glucose intravenous infusion* 5 and 10%, *Sodium chloride intravenous infusion* 0.9%, *Compound sodium chloride intravenous infusion* (Ringer's solution), and *Compound sodium lactate intravenous infusion* (Hartmann's solution). Compatibility with glucose 5% and with sodium chloride 0.9% indicates compatibility with *Sodium chloride and glucose intravenous infusion.* Infusion of a large volume of hypotonic solution should be avoided therefore care should be taken if water for injections is used. The information in the Table relates to the proprietary preparations indicated; for other preparations suitability should be checked with the manufacturer

Abciximab (*ReoPro®*)
Continuous *in* Glucose 5% *or* Sodium chloride 0.9%
Withdraw from vial, dilute in infusion fluid and give *via* infusion pump through a non-pyrogenic low protein-binding 0.2, 0.22 or 5 micron filter

Acetylcysteine (*Parvolex®*)
Continuous *in* Glucose 5% or Sodium chloride 0.9%
Glucose 5% is preferable—see Emergency Treatment of Poisoning

Aciclovir (as sodium salt) (*Zovirax IV®*; *Aciclovir IV*, Mayne; *Aciclovir IV*, Genus; *Aciclovir Sodium*, Zurich)
Intermittent *in* Sodium chloride 0.9% *or* Sodium chloride and glucose *or* Compound sodium lactate
For *Zovirax IV®*, *Aciclovir IV* (Genus) initially reconstitute to 25 mg/mL in water for injections or sodium chloride 0.9% then dilute to not more than 5 mg/mL with the infusion fluid; to be given over 1 hour; alternatively, may be administered in a concentration of 25 mg/mL using a suitable infusion pump and given over 1 hour; for *Aciclovir IV* (Mayne) dilute to not more than 5 mg/mL with infusion fluid; give over 1 hour

Agalsidase beta (*Fabrazyme®*)
Intermittent *in* Sodium chloride 0.9%
Reconstitute initially with water for injections (35 mg in 7.2 mL, 5 mg in 1.1 mL) to give 5 mg/mL solution; dilute requisite dose to 500 mL with infusion fluid and give over at least 2 hours

Alemtuzumab (*MabCampath®*)
Intermittent in Glucose 5% *or* Sodium chloride 0.9%
Add requisite dose to 100 mL infusion fluid; infuse over 2 hours

Alfentanil (as hydrochloride) (*Rapifen® preparations*)
Continuous *or* intermittent *in* Glucose 5% *or* Sodium chloride 0.9% *or* Compound sodium lactate

Alprostadil (*Prostin VR®*)
Continuous *in* Glucose 5% *or* Sodium chloride 0.9%
Add directly to the infusion solution avoiding contact with the walls of plastic containers

Alteplase (*Actilyse®*)
Continuous *or* intermittent *in* Sodium chloride 0.9%
Dissolve in water for injections to a concentration of 1 mg/mL and infuse intravenously; alternatively dilute the solution further in the infusion fluid to a concentration of not less than 200 micrograms/mL; not to be infused in glucose solution

Amikacin sulphate (*Amikin®*)
Intermittent *in* Glucose 5% *or* Sodium chloride 0.9% *or* Compound sodium lactate
To be given over 30 minutes

Aminophylline
Continuous *in* Glucose 5% *or* Sodium chloride 0.9% *or* Compound sodium lactate

Amiodarone hydrochloride (*Cordarone X®*)
Continuous *or* intermittent *in* Glucose 5%
Suggested initial infusion volume 250 mL given over 20–120 minutes; for repeat infusions up to 1.2 g in max. 500 mL; infusion in extreme emergency see section 2.7.3; should not be diluted to less than 600 micrograms/mL; incompatible with sodium chloride infusion; avoid equipment containing the plasticizer di-2-ethylhexyphthalate (DEHP)

Amoxicillin (as sodium salt) (*Amoxil®*)
Intermittent *in* Glucose 5% *or* Sodium chloride 0.9%
Reconstituted solutions diluted and given without delay; suggested volume 100 mL given over 30–60 minutes
via drip tubing *in* Glucose 5% *or* Sodium chloride 0.9%
Continuous infusion not usually recommended

Amphotericin (colloidal) (*Amphocil®*)
Intermittent *in* Glucose 5%
Initially reconstitute with water for injections (50 mg in 10 mL, 100 mg in 20 mL), shaking gently to dissolve (fluid may be opalescent) then dilute to a concentration of 625 micrograms/mL (1 volume of reconstituted solution with 7 volumes of infusion fluid); give at a rate of 1–2 mg/kg/hour or slower if not tolerated (initial test dose 2 mg of a 100 microgram/mL solution over 10 minutes); incompatible with sodium chloride or other electrolyte solutions, flush existing intravenous line with glucose 5% or use separate line

Amphotericin (lipid complex) (*Abelcet®*)
Intermittent *in* Glucose 5%
Allow suspension to reach room temperature, shake gently to ensure no yellow settlement, withdraw requisite dose (using 17–19 gauge needle) into one or more 20-mL syringes; replace needle on syringe with a 5-micron filter needle provided (fresh needle for each syringe) and dilute to a concentration of 1 mg/mL (2 mg/mL in fluid restriction); preferably give *via* an infusion pump at a rate of 2.5 mg/kg/hour (initial test dose of 1 mg given over 15 minutes); an in-line filter (pore size no less than 15 micron) may be used; do not use sodium chloride or other electrolyte solutions, flush existing intravenous line with glucose 5% or use separate line

Amphotericin (liposomal) (*AmBisome®*)
Intermittent *in* Glucose 5%
Reconstitute each vial with 12 mL water for injections and shake vigorously to produce a preparation containing 4 mg/mL; withdraw requisite dose from vial and introduce into infusion fluid through the 5 micron filter provided to produce a final concentration of 0.2–2 mg/mL; infuse over 30–60 minutes (initial test dose 1 mg over 10 minutes); incompatible with sodium chloride solutions, flush existing intravenous line with glucose 5% or use separate line

Amphotericin (as sodium deoxycholate complex) (*Fungizone®*)
Intermittent *in* Glucose 5%
Reconstitute each vial with 10 mL water for injections and shake immediately to produce a 5 mg/mL colloidal solution; dilute further in infusion fluid to a concentration of 100 micrograms/mL; pH of the glucose must not be below 4.2 (check each container—consult product literature for details of buffer); infuse over 2–4 hours, or longer if not tolerated (initial test dose 1 mg over 20–30 minutes); begin infusion immediately after dilution and protect from light; incompatible with sodium chloride solutions, flush existing intravenous line with glucose 5% or use separate line; an in-line filter (pore size no less than 1 micron) may be used

Ampicillin sodium (*Penbritin®*)
Intermittent *in* Glucose 5% *or* Sodium chloride 0.9%
Reconstituted solutions diluted and given without delay; suggested volume 100 mL given over 30–60 minutes
via drip tubing *in* Glucose 5% *or* Sodium chloride 0.9% *or* Ringer's solution *or* Compound sodium lactate
Continuous infusion not usually recommended

Amsacrine (*Amsidine*®)
Intermittent in Glucose 5%
Reconstitute with diluent provided and dilute to suggested volume 500 mL; give over 60–90 minutes; use glass syringes; incompatible with sodium chloride infusion

Arsenic trioxide (*Trisenox*®)
Intermittent *in* Glucose 5% *or* Sodium chloride 0.9%
Dilute requisite dose with 100–250 mL infusion fluid; infuse over 1–2 hours (up to 4 hours if vasomotor reactions observed)

Atenolol (*Tenormin*®)
Intermittent *in* Glucose 5% *or* Sodium chloride 0.9%
Suggested infusion time 20 minutes

Atosiban (*Tractocile*®)
Continuous *in* Glucose 5% *or* Sodium chloride 0.9% *or* Compound sodium lactate
Withdraw 10 mL infusion fluid from 100-mL bag and replace with 10 mL atosiban concentrate (7.5 mg/mL) to produce a final concentration of 750 micrograms/mL

Atracurium besilate (*Tracrium*®; *Atracurium besilate injection*, Mayne; *Atracurium injection/infusion*, Genus)
Continuous *in* Glucose 5% *or* Sodium chloride 0.9% *or* Compound sodium lactate
Stability varies with diluent; dilute requisite dose with infusion fluid to a concentration of 0.5–5 mg/mL

Azathioprine (as sodium salt) (*Imuran*®)
Intermittent *in* Sodium chloride 0.9% *or* Sodium chloride and glucose
Reconstitute 50 mg with 5–15 mL water for injections; dilute with 20–200 mL infusion fluid

Aztreonam (*Azactam*®)
Intermittent *in* Glucose 5% *or* Sodium chloride 0.9% *or* Ringer's solution *or* Compound sodium lactate
Dissolve initially in water for injections (1 g per 3 mL) then dilute to a concentration of less than 20 mg/mL; to be given over 20–60 minutes

Basiliximab (*Simulect*®)
Intermittent in Glucose 5% or Sodium chloride 0.9%
Reconstitute 10 mg with 5 mL water for injections then dilute to at least 25 mL with infusion fluid; reconstitute 20 mg with 10 mL water for injections then dilute to at least 50 mL with infusion fluid; give over 20–30 minutes

Benzylpenicillin sodium (*Crystapen*®)
Intermittent *in* Glucose 5% *or* Sodium chloride 0.9%
Suggested volume 100 mL given over 30–60 minutes
Continuous infusion not usually recommended

Betamethasone (as sodium phosphate) (*Betnesol*®)
Continuous *or* intermittent *or via* drip tubing *in* Glucose 5% *or* Sodium chloride 0.9%

Bevacizumab (*Avastin*®)
Intermittent in Sodium chloride 0.9%
Dilute requisite dose in infusion fluid to 100 ml and give over 90 minutes; if initial dose well tolerated give second dose over 60 minutes; if second dose well tolerated give subsequent dose over 30 minutes; incompatible with glucose solutions

Bivalirudin (*Angiox*®)
Continuous *in* Glucose 5% *or* Sodium chloride 0.9%
Reconstitute each 250-mg vial with 5 mL water for injections then withdraw 5 mL and dilute to 50 mL with infusion fluid

Bleomycin sulphate
Intermittent *in* Sodium chloride 0.9%
To be given slowly; suggested volume 200 mL

Bumetanide (*Burinex*®)
Intermittent *in* Glucose 5% *or* Sodium chloride 0.9%
Suggested volume 500 mL given over 30–60 minutes

Busulfan (*Busilvex*®)
Intermittent in Glucose 5% or Sodium chloride 0.9%
Dilute to a concentration of 500 micrograms/mL; give through a central venous catheter over 2 hours

Calcitonin (salmon)/Salcatonin (*Miacalcic*®)
Intermittent *in* Sodium chloride 0.9%
Diluted solution given without delay; dilute in 500 mL and give over at least 6 hours; glass or hard plastic containers should not be used; some loss of potency on dilution and administration

Calcium folinate (*Calcium Leucovorin*®, *Refolinon*®)
Intermittent *in* Sodium chloride 0.9%
Calcium Leucovorin® can also be infused in Glucose 5 and 10% or Compound sodium lactate
Protect from light

Calcium gluconate
Continuous *in* Glucose 5% *or* Sodium chloride 0.9%
Avoid bicarbonates, phosphates, or sulphates

Calcium levofolinate (*Isovorin*®)
Intermittent *in* Glucose 5 and 10% *or* Sodium chloride 0.9% *or* Compound sodium lactate
Protect from light

Carboplatin (*Paraplatin*®)
Intermittent *in* Glucose 5% *or* Sodium chloride 0.9%
Final concentration as low as 500 micrograms/mL; give over 15–60 minutes

Carmustine (*BiCNU*®)
Intermittent *in* Glucose 5% *or* Sodium chloride 0.9%
Reconstitute with solvent provided; give over 1–2 hours

Caspofungin
Intermittent *in* Sodium chloride 0.9% *or* Compound sodium lactate
Allow vial to reach room temperature; initially reconstitute each vial with 10.5 mL water for injections, mixing gently to dissolve then dilute requisite dose in 250 mL infusion fluid (35- or 50-mg doses may be diluted in 100 mL infusion fluid if necessary); give over 60 minutes; incompatible with glucose solutions

Cefotaxime (as sodium salt) (*Claforan*®; *Cefotaxime Injection*, Genus)
Intermittent *in* Glucose 5% *or* Sodium chloride 0.9% *or* Compound sodium lactate *or* Water for injections
Suggested volume 40–100 mL given over 20–60 minutes

Cefradine (*Velosef*®)
Continuous *or* intermittent *in* Glucose 5 and 10% *or* Sodium chloride 0.9% *or* Ringer's solution *or* Compound sodium lactate
Reconstitute 500 mg with 5 mL water for injections or glucose 5% or sodium chloride 0.9% then dilute with infusion fluid

Ceftazidime (as pentahydrate) (*Fortum*®, *Kefadim*®)
Intermittent *or via* drip tubing *in* Glucose 5 and 10% *or* Sodium chloride 0.9% *or* Compound sodium lactate
Dissolve 2 g initially in 10 mL (3 g in 15 mL) infusion fluid; for *Fortum*® dilute further to a concentration of 40 mg/mL; for *Kefadim*® dilute further to a concentration of 20 mg/mL; give over up to 30 minutes

Ceftriaxone (as sodium salt) (*Rocephin*®; *Ceftriaxone Injection*, Genus)
Intermittent *or via* drip tubing *in* Glucose 5 and 10% *or* Sodium chloride 0.9%
Reconstitute 2-g vial with 40 mL infusion fluid; give intermittent infusion over at least 30 minutes (60 minutes in neonates); not to be given with infusion fluids containing calcium

Cefuroxime (as sodium salt) (*Zinacef*®; *Cefuroxime Injection*, Lilly)
Intermittent *or via* drip tubing *in* Glucose 5% *or* Sodium chloride 0.9% *or* Compound sodium lactate
Dissolve initially in water for injections (at least 2 mL for each 250 mg, 15 mL for 1.5 g); suggested volume 50–100 mL given over 30 minutes

Chloramphenicol (as sodium succinate) (*Kemicetine*®)
Intermittent *or via* drip tubing *in* Glucose 5% *or* Sodium chloride 0.9%

Chloroquine sulphate (*Nivaquine*®)
Continuous *in* Sodium chloride 0.9%
See also section 5.4.1

Ciclosporin (*Sandimmun*®)
Continuous *in* Glucose 5% *or* Sodium chloride 0.9%
Dilute to a concentration of 50 mg in 20–100 mL; give over 2–6 hours; not to be used with PVC equipment

Cidofovir (*Vistide*®)
Intermittent *in* Sodium chloride 0.9%
Dilute requisite dose with 100 mL infusion fluid; infuse over 1 hour

Cimetidine (*Tagamet*®)
Continuous *or* intermittent *in* Glucose 5% *or* Sodium chloride 0.9%
For intermittent infusion suggested volume 100 mL given over 30–60 minutes

Cisatracurium (*Nimbex*®, *Nimbex Forte*®)
Continuous *in* Glucose 5% *or* Sodium chloride 0.9%
Solutions of 2 mg/mL and 5 mg/mL may be infused undiluted; alternatively dilute with infusion fluid to a concentration of 0.1–2 mg/mL

Cisplatin (*Cisplatin*, Pharmacia; *Cisplatin injection solution*, Mayne)
Intermittent *in* Sodium chloride 0.9% *or* Sodium chloride and glucose
Reconstitute initially with water for injections to produce 1 mg/mL solution then dilute in 2 litres infusion fluid; give over 6–8 hours

Cladribine (*Leustat*®)
Continuous *in* Sodium chloride 0.9%
Dilute with 100–500 mL; glucose solutions are unsuitable

Clarithromycin (*Klaricid*® *I.V.*)
Intermittent *in* Glucose 5% *or* Sodium chloride 0.9% *or* Ringer's solution *or* Compound sodium lactate
Dissolve initially in water for injections (500 mg in 10 mL) then dilute to a concentration of 2 mg/mL; give over 60 minutes

Clindamycin (as phosphate) (*Dalacin*® *C Phosphate*)
Continuous *or* intermittent *in* Glucose 5% *or* Sodium chloride 0.9%
Give over at least 10–60 minutes (1.2 g over at least 60 minutes; higher doses by continuous infusion)

Clonazepam (*Rivotril*®)
Intermittent *in* Glucose 5 and 10% *or* Sodium chloride 0.9%
Suggested volume 250 mL

Co-amoxiclav *Augmentin*®; *Co-amoxiclav Injection*, CP)
Intermittent *in* Sodium chloride 0.9% *or* Water for injections; see also package leaflet
Suggested volume 50–100 mL given over 30–40 minutes and completed within 4 hours of reconstitution
via drip tubing *in* Glucose 5% *or* Sodium chloride 0.9%

Co-fluampicil (as sodium salts) (*Magnapen*®)
Intermittent *in* Glucose 5% *or* Sodium chloride 0.9%
Reconstituted solutions diluted and given without delay; suggested volume 100 mL given over 30–60 minutes
via drip tubing *in* Glucose 5% *or* Sodium chloride 0.9% *or* Ringer's solution *or* Compound sodium lactate

Colistimethate sodium (*Colomycin*®)
Intermittent *in* Sodium chloride 0.9% *or* Water for injections
Dilute with 50 mL infusion fluid and give over 30 minutes

Co-trimoxazole (*Septrin*® *for infusion*)
Intermittent *in* Glucose 5 and 10% *or* Sodium chloride 0.9% *or* Ringer's solution
Dilute contents of 1 ampoule (5 mL) to 125 mL, 2 ampoules (10 mL) to 250 mL or 3 ampoules (15 mL) to 500 mL; suggested duration of infusion 60–90 minutes (but may be adjusted according to fluid requirements); if fluid restriction necessary, 1 ampoule (5 mL) may be diluted with 75 mL glucose 5% and infused over max. 60 minutes

Cyclophosphamide (*Endoxana*®)
via drip tubing *in* Glucose 5% *or* Sodium chloride 0.9%
Reconstitute with sodium chloride 0.9%

Cyclosporin *see* Ciclosporin

Cytarabine (*Cytosar*®)
Continuous *or* intermittent *or via* drip tubing *in* Glucose 5% *or* Sodium chloride 0.9%
Reconstitute *Cytosar*® with water for injections or with infusion fluid; check container for haze or precipitate during administration

Dacarbazine (*DTIC-Dome*®; *Dacarbazine*, Medac)
Intermittent *in* Glucose 5% *or* Sodium chloride 0.9%
Reconstitute initially with water for injections then for *DTIC-Dome*® dilute in 125–250 mL infusion fluid; for *Dacarbazine* (Medac) dilute in 200–300 mL infusion fluid; give over 15–30 minutes; protect infusion from light

Daclizumab (*Zenapax*®)
Intermittent *in* Sodium chloride 0.9%
Dilute requisite dose in 50 mL infusion fluid; infuse over 15 minutes

Dactinomycin (*Cosmegen Lyovac*®)
Intermittent *or via* drip tubing *in* Glucose 5% *or* Sodium chloride 0.9%
Reconstitute with water for injections

Danaparoid sodium (*Orgaran*®)
Continuous *in* Glucose 5% *or* Sodium chloride 0.9%

Daunorubicin (as hydrochloride) (*Cerubidin*®)
via drip tubing *in* Sodium chloride 0.9%
Reconstitute vial with 4 mL water for injections to give 5 mg/mL solution; dilute requisite dose with infusion fluid to a concentration of 1 mg/mL; give over 20 minutes

Daunorubicin (liposomal) (*DaunoXome*®)
Intermittent *in* Glucose 5%
Dilute to a concentration of 0.2–1 mg/mL; give over 30–60 minutes; incompatible with sodium chloride solutions; in-line filter not recommended (if used, pore size should be no less than 5 micron)

Desferrioxamine mesilate (*Desferal*®)
Continuous *or* intermittent *in* Glucose 5% *or* Sodium chloride 0.9%
Dissolve initially in water for injections (500 mg in 5 mL) then dilute with infusion fluid

Desmopressin (*DDAVP*®)
Intermittent *in* Sodium chloride 0.9%
Dilute with 50 mL and give over 20 minutes

Dexamethasone sodium phosphate
(*Dexamethasone*, Mayne; *Dexamethasone*, Organon)
Continuous *or* intermittent *or via* drip tubing *in* Glucose 5% *or* Sodium chloride 0.9%
Dexamethasone (Organon) can also be infused in Ringer's solution *or* Compound sodium lactate

Diamorphine hydrochloride (*Diamorphine Injection*, CP)
Continuous *in* Glucose 5% *or* Sodium chloride 0.9%
Glucose is preferred as infusion fluid

Diazepam (solution) (*Diazepam*, CP)
Continuous *in* Glucose 5% *or* Sodium chloride 0.9%
Dilute to a concentration of not more than 10 mg in 200 mL; adsorbed to some extent by the plastics of bags and infusion sets

Diazepam (emulsion) (*Diazemuls*®)
Continuous *in* Glucose 5 and 10%
May be diluted to a max. concentration of 200 mg in 500 mL; max. 6 hours between addition and completion of administration; adsorbed to some extent by the plastics of the infusion set
via drip tubing *in* Glucose 5 and 10% *or* Sodium chloride 0.9%
Adsorbed to some extent by the plastics of the infusion set

Diclofenac sodium (*Voltarol*®)
Continuous *or* intermittent *in* Glucose 5% *or* Sodium chloride 0.9%
Dilute 75 mg with 100–500 mL infusion fluid (previously buffered with 0.5 mL sodium bicarbonate 8.4% solution *or* with 1 mL sodium bicarbonate 4.2% solution); for intermittent infusion give 25–50 mg over 15–60 minutes or 75 mg over 30–120 minutes; for continuous infusion give at a rate of 5 mg/hour

Digoxin (*Lanoxin*®)
Intermittent *in* Glucose 5% *or* Sodium chloride 0.9%
To be given over at least 2 hours

Digoxin-specific antibody fragments (*Digibind*®)
Intermittent *in* Sodium chloride 0.9%
Dissolve initially in water for injections (4 mL/vial) then dilute with the sodium chloride 0.9% and give through a 0.22 micron sterile, disposable filter over 30 minutes

Dinoprostone (*Prostin E2*®)
Continuous *or* intermittent *in* Glucose 5% *or* Sodium chloride 0.9%

Disodium folinate (*Sodiofolin*®)
Intermittent *in* Sodium chloride 0.9%
Protect from light
Avoid bicarbonate containing infusions

Disodium pamidronate (*Aredia*®; *Disodium pamidronate*, Britannia, Mayne, Medac)
Intermittent *in* Glucose 5% *or* Sodium chloride 0.9%
For *Aredia*® and *Pamidronate disodium* (Britannia), reconstitute initially with water for injections (15 mg in 5 mL, 30 mg or 90 mg in 10 mL); for *Aredia*®, *Pamidronate disodium* (Britannia), *Disodium pamidronate* (Mayne), dilute with infusion fluid to a concentration of not more than 60 mg in 250 mL; for *Disodium pamidronate* (Medac) dilute with infusion fluid to a concentration of not more than 90 mg in 250 mL; give at a rate not exceeding 1 mg/minute; not to be given with infusion fluids containing calcium

Disopyramide (as phosphate) (*Rythmodan*®)
Continuous *or* intermittent *in* Glucose 5% *or* Sodium chloride 0.9% *or* Ringer's solution *or* Compound sodium lactate
Max. rate by continuous infusion 20–30 mg/hour (or 400 micrograms/kg/hour)

Dobutamine (as hydrochloride) (*Dobutrex*®, *Posiject*®)
Continuous *in* Glucose 5% *or* Sodium chloride 0.9%
Dilute to a concentration of 0.5–1 mg/mL and give *via* a controlled infusion device; give higher concentration (max. 5 mg/mL) with infusion pump; incompatible with bicarbonate

Docetaxel (*Taxotere*®)
Intermittent *in* Glucose 5% *or* Sodium chloride 0.9%
Stand docetaxel vials and diluent at room temperature for 5 minutes; add diluent to produce a concentrate containing 10 mg/mL and allow to stand for a further 5 minutes; dilute the requisite dose with at least 250 mL infusion fluid to a final concentration not exceeding 740 micrograms/mL; infuse over 1 hour

Dolasetron mesilate (*Anzemet*®)
Intermittent *in* Glucose 5% *or* Sodium chloride 0.9% *or* Compound sodium lactate
Suggested volume 50 mL given over 30 seconds–15 minutes

Dopamine hydrochloride
Continuous *in* Glucose 5% *or* Sodium chloride 0.9% *or* Compound sodium lactate
Dilute to max concentration of 3.2 mg/mL; incompatible with bicarbonate

Dopexamine hydrochloride (*Dopacard®*)
Continuous *in* Glucose 5% *or* Sodium chloride 0.9%
Dilute to a concentration of 400 or 800 micrograms/mL; max. concentration *via* large peripheral vein 1 mg/mL, concentrations up to 4 mg/mL may be infused *via* central vein; give *via* infusion pump or other device which provides accurate control of rate; contact with metal should be minimised; incompatible with bicarbonate

Doxorubicin hydrochloride (*Doxorubicin Rapid Dissolution*, *Doxorubicin Solution*) (both Pharmacia)
via drip tubing *in* Glucose 5% *or* Sodium chloride 0.9%
Reconstitute *Doxorubicin Rapid Dissolution* with water for injections or sodium chloride 0.9% (10 mg in 5 mL, 50 mg in 25 mL); give over 2–3 minutes

Doxorubicin hydrochloride (liposomal) (*Caelyx®*)
via drip tubing *in* Glucose 5%
Dilute up to 90 mg in 250 mL infusion fluid and over 90 mg in 500 mL infusion fluid

Enoximone (*Perfan®*)
Continuous *or* intermittent *in* Sodium chloride 0.9% *or* Water for injections
Dilute to a concentration of 2.5 mg/mL; incompatible with glucose solutions; use only plastic containers or syringes

Epirubicin hydrochloride (*Pharmorubicin® Rapid Dissolution*, *Pharmorubicin® Solution*)
via drip tubing *in* Sodium chloride 0.9%
Reconstitute *Pharmorubicin® Rapid Dissolution* with sodium chloride 0.9% or with water for injections (10 mg in 5 mL, 20 mg in 10 mL, 50 mg in 25 mL); give over 3–5 minutes

Epoprostenol (*Flolan®*)
Continuous *in* Sodium chloride 0.9% (but see also below)
Reconstitute using the filter and solvent (glycine buffer diluent) provided to make a concentrate; may be diluted further (consult product literature); for *pulmonary hypertension* dilute further with glycine buffer diluent only, for *renal dialysis* may be diluted further with sodium chloride 0.9%

Ertapenem (*Invanz®*)
Intermittent *in* Sodium chloride 0.9%
Reconstitute 1 g with 10 mL water for injections or sodium chloride 0.9% then dilute in 50 mL infusion fluid; give over 30 minutes; incompatible with glucose solutions

Erythromycin (as lactobionate)
Continuous *or* intermittent *in* Glucose 5% (neutralised with sodium bicarbonate) *or* Sodium chloride 0.9%
Dissolve initially in water for injections (1 g in 20 mL) then dilute to a concentration of 1 mg/mL for continuous infusion and 1–5 mg/mL for intermittent infusion; give intermittent infusion over 20–60 minutes

Esmolol hydrochloride (*Brevibloc®*)
Continuous *or* intermittent *in* Glucose 5% *or* Sodium chloride 0.9%
Dilute to a concentration of 10 mg/mL; for continuous infusion use a suitable infusion control device; incompatible with bicarbonate

Esomeprazole (as sodium salt) (*Nexium®*)
Intermittent *in* Sodium chloride 0.9%
Reconstitute 40 mg with 5 mL sodium chloride 0.9% then dilute with up to 100 mL infusion fluid, give requisite dose over 10–30 minutes

Ethanol
Continuous *in* Glucose 5% *or* Sodium chloride 0.9% *or* Ringer's solution *or* Compound sodium lactate
Dilute to a concentration of 5–10%

Etoposide (*Eposin®*; *Vepesid®*; *Etoposide*, TEVA UK and Mayne)
Intermittent *in* Sodium chloride 0.9%
For *Vepesid®* dilute to a concentration of not more than 250 micrograms/mL and give over not less than 30 minutes; for *Etoposide* (TEVA UK) dilute with either sodium chloride 0.9% or glucose 5% to a concentration of 200 micrograms/mL and give over 30–60 minutes; for *Etoposide* (Mayne) dilute with either sodium chloride 0.9% or glucose 5% to a concentration of not more than 250 micrograms/mL and give over not less than 30 minutes; for *Eposin®* dilute with either sodium chloride 0.9% or glucose 5% to a concentration of 200–400 micrograms/mL and give over at least 30 minutes; check container for haze or precipitate during infusion

Etoposide (as phosphate) (*Etopophos®*)
Intermittent *in* Glucose 5% *or* Sodium chloride 0.9%
Reconstitute with 5–10 mL of either water for injections *or* with infusion fluid then dilute further with infusion fluid to a concentration as low as 100 micrograms/mL and give over 5 minutes to 3.5 hours

Fentanyl (*Sublimaze®*)
Continuous *or* intermittent *in* Glucose 5% *or* Sodium chloride 0.9%

Filgrastim (*Neupogen®*)
Continuous *or* intermittent *in* Glucose 5%
For a filgrastim concentration of less than 1 500 000 units/mL (15 micrograms/mL) albumin solution (human serum albumin) is added to produce a final albumin concentration of 2 mg/mL; should not be diluted to a filgrastim concentration of less than 200 000 units/mL (2 micrograms/mL) and should not be diluted with sodium chloride solution

Flecainide acetate (*Tambocor®*)
Continuous *or* intermittent *in* Glucose 5% *or* Sodium chloride 0.9% *or* Compound sodium lactate
Minimum volume in infusion fluids containing chlorides 500 mL

Flucloxacillin (as sodium salt) (*Floxapen®*)
Intermittent *in* Glucose 5% *or* Sodium chloride 0.9%
Suggested volume 100 mL given over 30–60 minutes
via drip tubing *in* Glucose 5% *or* Sodium chloride 0.9% *or* Ringer's solution *or* Compound sodium lactate
Continuous infusion not usually recommended

Fludarabine phosphate (*Fludara®*)
Intermittent *in* Sodium chloride 0.9%
Reconstitute each 50 mg with 2 mL water for injections and dilute requisite dose in 100 mL; give over 30 minutes

Flumazenil (*Anexate®*)
Continuous *in* Glucose 5% *or* Sodium chloride 0.9%

Fluorouracil (as sodium salt)
Continuous *or* intermittent *or via* drip tubing *in* Glucose 5% *or* Sodium chloride 0.9%
Give intermittent infusion over 30–60 minutes or over 4 hours

Foscarnet sodium (*Foscavir*®)
Intermittent *in* Glucose 5% *or* Sodium chloride 0.9%
Dilute to a concentration of 12 mg/mL for infusion into peripheral vein (undiluted solution *via* central venous line only); infuse over at least 1 hour

Fosphenytoin Sodium (*Pro-Epanutin*®)
Intermittent *in* Glucose 5% *or* Sodium chloride 0.9%
Dilute to a concentration of 1.5–25 mg (phenytoin sodium equivalent)/mL

Furosemide/Frusemide (as sodium salt) (*Lasix*®)
Continuous *in* Sodium chloride 0.9% *or* Ringer's solution
Infusion pH must be above 5.5 and rate should not exceed 4 mg/minute; glucose solutions are unsuitable

Fusidic acid (as sodium salt)
Continuous *in* Glucose 5% (but see below) *or* Sodium chloride 0.9%
Reconstitute with the buffer solution provided and dilute to 500 mL; give through central venous line over 2 hours (or over 6 hours if superficial vein used); incompatible in solution of pH less than 7.4

Ganciclovir (as sodium salt) (*Cymevene*®)
Intermittent *in* Glucose 5% *or* Sodium chloride 0.9% *or* Ringer's solution *or* Compound sodium lactate
Reconstitute initially in water for injections (500 mg/10 mL) then dilute to not more than 10 mg/mL with infusion fluid (usually 100 mL); give over 1 hour

Gemcitabine (*Gemzar*®)
Intermittent *in* Sodium chloride 0.9%
Reconstitute initially with sodium chloride 0.9% (200 mg in at least 5 mL, 1 g in at least 25 mL); may be diluted further with infusion fluid; give over 30 minutes

Gentamicin (as sulphate) (*Cidomycin*®; *Gentamicin Paediatric Injection*, Beacon; *Gentamicin Injection*, Mayne)
Intermittent *or via* drip tubing *in* Glucose 5% *or* Sodium chloride 0.9%
Suggested volume for intermittent infusion 50–100 mL given over 20–30 minutes

Glyceryl trinitrate (*Nitrocine*®, *Nitronal*®, *Tridil*®)
Continuous *in* Glucose 5% *or* Sodium chloride 0.9%
For *Tridil*® dilute to a concentration of not more than 400 micrograms/mL; for *Nitrocine*® suggested infusion concentration 100 micrograms/mL; incompatible with polyvinyl chloride infusion containers such as *Viaflex*® or *Steriflex*®; use glass or polyethylene containers or give *via* a syringe pump

Granisetron (as hydrochloride) (*Kytril*®)
Intermittent *in* Glucose 5% *or* Sodium chloride 0.9% *or* Compound sodium lactate
Dilute 3 mL in 20–50 mL infusion fluid (up to 3 mL in 10–30 mL for children); give over 5 minutes

Haem arginate (*Normosang*®)
Intermittent *in* Sodium chloride 0.9%
Dilute requisite dose in 100 mL infusion fluid in glass bottle and give over at least 30 minutes *via* large antebrachial vein; administer within 1 hour after dilution

Heparin sodium
Continuous *in* Glucose 5% *or* Sodium chloride 0.9%
Administration with a motorised pump advisable

Hydralazine hydrochloride (*Apresoline*®)
Continuous *in* Sodium chloride 0.9% *or* Ringer's solution
Suggested infusion volume 500 mL

Hydrocortisone (as sodium phosphate) (*Efcortesol*®)
Continuous *or* intermittent *or via* drip tubing *in* Glucose 5% *or* Sodium chloride 0.9%

Hydrocortisone (as sodium succinate) (*SoluCortef*®)
Continuous *or* intermittent *or via* drip tubing *in* Glucose 5% *or* Sodium chloride 0.9%

Ibandronic acid (*Bondronat*®)
Intermittent *in* Glucose 5% *or* Sodium chloride 0.9%
Dilute requisite dose in 500 mL infusion fluid and give over 1–2 hours

Idarubicin hydrochloride (*Zavedos*®)
via drip tubing *in* Sodium chloride 0.9%
Reconstitute with water for injections; give over 5–10 minutes

Ifosfamide (*Mitoxana*®)
Continuous *or* intermittent *or via* drip tubing *in* Glucose 5% *or* Sodium chloride 0.9%
For continuous infusion, suggested volume 3 litres given over 24 hours; for intermittent infusion, give over 30–120 minutes

Imiglucerase (*Cerezyme*®)
Intermittent *in* Sodium chloride 0.9%
Initially reconstitute with 5.1 mL water for injections to give 40 units/mL solution; dilute requisite dose in 100–200 mL infusion fluid and give over 1–2 hours *or* at a rate not exceeding 1 unit/kg/minute; administer within 3 hours after reconstitution

Imipenem with cilastatin (as sodium salt) (*Primaxin*®)
Intermittent *in* Sodium chloride 0.9% *or* Sodium chloride and Glucose
Dilute to a concentration of 5 mg (as imipenem)/mL; infuse 250–500 mg (as imipenem) over 20–30 minutes, 1 g over 40–60 minutes
Continuous infusion not usually recommended

Infliximab (*Remicade*®)
Intermittent *in* Sodium chloride 0.9%
Reconstitute each 100-mg vial with 10 mL water for injections; gently swirl vial without shaking to dissolve; allow to stand for 5 minutes; dilute requisite dose with infusion fluid to a final volume of 250 mL and give through a low protein-binding filter (1.2 micron or less) over at least 2 hours; start infusion within 3 hours of reconstitution

Insulin (soluble)
Continuous *in* Sodium chloride 0.9% *or* Compound sodium lactate
Adsorbed to some extent by plastics of infusion set; see also section 6.1.3; ensure insulin is not injected into 'dead space' of injection port of the infusion bag

Insulin aspart
Continuous *in* Sodium chloride 0.9% *or* Glucose 5%
Dilute to 0.05–1 unit/mL with infusion fluid; adsorbed to some extent by plastics of infusion set

Insulin lispro
Continuous *in* Sodium chloride 0.9% *or* Glucose 5%

Interferon alfa-2b (*IntronA®*)
Intermittent *in* Sodium chloride 0.9%
For *IntronA®* solution, dilute requisite dose in 50 mL infusion fluid and administer over 20 minutes; not to be diluted to less than 300 000 units/mL
For *IntronA®* powder, reconstitute with 1 mL water for injections; dilute requisite dose in 100 mL infusion fluid and administer over 20 minutes; not to be diluted to less than 100 000 units/mL

Irinotecan hydrochloride (*Campto®*)
Intermittent *in* Glucose 5% *or* Sodium chloride 0.9%
Dilute requisite dose in 250 mL infusion fluid; give over 30–90 minutes

Iron dextran (*Cosmofer®*)
Intermittent *in* Glucose 5% *or* Sodium chloride 0.9%
Dilute 100–200 mg in 100 mL infusion fluid; give 25 mg over 15 minutes as a test dose initially, then give at a rate not exceeding 3.33 mL/minute; *total dose infusion* diluted in 500 mL infusion fluid and given over 4–6 hours (initial test dose 25 mg over 15 minutes)

Iron sucrose (*Venofer®*)
Intermittent *in* Sodium chloride 0.9%
Dilute 100 mg in up to 100 mL infusion fluid; give 25 mg over 15 minutes as a test dose initially, then give at a rate not exceeding 3.33 mg/minute

Isosorbide dinitrate (*Isoket 0.05%®*, *Isoket 0.1%®*)
Continuous *in* Glucose 5% *or* Sodium chloride 0.9%
Adsorbed to some extent by polyvinyl chloride infusion containers; preferably use glass or polyethylene containers or give *via* a syringe pump; *Isoket 0.05%®* can alternatively be administered undiluted using a syringe pump with a glass or rigid plastic syringe

Itraconazole (*Sporanox®*)
Intermittent *in* Sodium chloride 0.9%
Dilute 250 mg in 50 mL infusion fluid and infuse only **60 mL** through an in-line filter (0.2 micron) over 60 minutes

Ketamine (as hydrochloride) (*Ketalar®*)
Continuous *in* Glucose 5% *or* Sodium chloride 0.9%
Dilute to 1 mg/mL; microdrip infusion for maintenance of anaesthesia

Labetalol hydrochloride (*Trandate®*)
Intermittent *in* Glucose 5% *or* Sodium chloride and glucose
Dilute to a concentration of 1 mg/mL; suggested volume 200 mL; adjust rate with in-line burette

Laronidase (*Aldurazyme®*)
Intermittent *in* Sodium chloride 0.9%
Body-weight under 20 kg, use 100 mL infusion fluid; body-weight over 20 kg use 250 mL infusion fluid; withdraw volume of infusion fluid equivalent to volume of laronidase concentrate being added; give through an in-line filter (0.22 micron) at an initial rate of 2 units/kg/hour then increasing gradually every 15 minutes to max. 43 units/kg/hour

Lenograstim (*Granocyte®*)
Intermittent *in* Sodium chloride 0.9%
Initially reconstitute with 1 mL water for injection provided (do not shake vigorously) then dilute with up to 50 mL infusion fluid for each vial of *Granocyte-13* or up to 100 mL infusion fluid for *Granocyte-34*; give over 30 minutes

Lepirudin (*Refludan®*)
Continuous *in* Glucose 5% *or* Sodium chloride 0.9%
Reconstitute initially with water for injections *or* sodium chloride 0.9% then dilute to a concentration of 2 mg/mL with infusion fluid

Magnesium sulphate
Continuous *in* Glucose 5% *or* Sodium chloride 0.9%
Suggested concentration up to 200 mg/mL

Melphalan (*Alkeran®*)
Intermittent *or via* drip tubing *in* Sodium chloride 0.9%
Reconstitute with the solvent provided then dilute with infusion fluid; max. 90 minutes between addition and completion of administration; incompatible with glucose infusion

Meropenem (*Meronem®*)
Intermittent *in* Glucose 5 and 10% *or* Sodium chloride 0.9%
Dilute in 50–200 mL infusion fluid and give over 15–30 minutes

Mesna (*Uromitexan®*)
Continuous *or via* drip tubing *in* Glucose 5% *or* Sodium chloride 0.9%

Metaraminol (as tartrate) (*Aramine®*)
Continuous *or via* drip tubing *in* Glucose 5% *or* Sodium chloride 0.9%
Suggested volume 500 mL

Methotrexate (as sodium salt) (*Methotrexate*, Lederle)
Continuous *or via* drip tubing *in* Glucose 5% *or* Sodium chloride 0.9% *or* Compound sodium lactate *or* Ringer's solution
Dilute in a large-volume infusion; max. 24 hours between addition and completion of administration

Methylprednisolone (as sodium succinate) (*Solu-Medrone®*)
Continuous *or* intermittent *or via* drip tubing *in* Glucose 5% *or* Sodium chloride 0.9%
Reconstitute initially with water for injections; doses up to 250 mg should be given over at least 5 minutes, high doses over at least 30 minutes

Metoclopramide hydrochloride (*Maxolon High Dose®*)
Continuous *or* intermittent *in* Glucose 5% *or* Sodium chloride 0.9% *or* Compound sodium lactate
Continuous infusion recommended; loading dose, dilute with 50–100 mL and give over 15–20 minutes; maintenance dose, dilute with 500 mL and give over 8–12 hours; for intermittent infusion dilute with at least 50 mL and give over at least 15 minutes

Mexiletine hydrochloride (*Mexitil®*)
Continuous *in* Glucose 5% *or* Sodium chloride 0.9%

Midazolam (*Hypnovel®*)
Continuous *in* Glucose 5% *or* Sodium chloride 0.9%
For neonates and children under 15 kg dilute to a max. concentration of 1 mg/mL

Milrinone (*Primacor®*)
Continuous *in* Glucose 5% *or* Sodium chloride 0.9%
Dilute to a suggested concentration of 200 micrograms/mL

Mitoxantrone/Mitozantrone (as hydrochloride) (*Novantrone*®, *Onkotrone*®)
Intermittent *or via* drip tubing *in* Glucose 5% *or* Sodium chloride 0.9%
For administration *via* drip tubing suggested volume at least 50 mL given over at least 3–5 minutes; for intermittent infusion (*Onkotrone*® only), dilute with 50–100 mL and give over 15–30 minutes

Mivacurium (as chloride) (*Mivacron*®)
Continuous *in* Glucose 5% *or* Sodium chloride 0.9%
Dilute to a concentration of 500 micrograms/mL; may also be given undiluted

Mycophenolate mofetil (as hydrochloride) (*CellCept*®)
Intermittent *in* Glucose 5%
Reconstitute each 500-mg vial with 14 mL glucose 5% and dilute the contents of 2 vials in 140 mL infusion fluid; give over 2 hours

Naloxone (*Min-I-Jet*® *Naloxone Hydrochloride*, *Narcan*®)
Continuous *in* Glucose 5% *or* Sodium chloride 0.9%
Reversal of opioid-induced respiratory depression, dilute to a concentration of 4 micrograms/mL; opioid overdose only, dilute 10 mg in 50 mL glucose 5%, see Emergency Treatment of Poisoning

Netilmicin (as sulphate) (*Netillin*®)
Intermittent *or via* drip tubing *in* Glucose 5 and 10% *or* Sodium chloride 0.9%
For intermittent infusion suggested volume 50–200 mL given over 30–120 minutes

Nimodipine (*Nimotop*®)
via drip tubing *in* Glucose 5% *or* Sodium chloride 0.9% *or* Ringer's solution
Not to be added to infusion container; administer *via* an infusion pump through a Y-piece into a central catheter; incompatible with polyvinyl chloride giving sets or containers; protect infusion from light

Nizatidine (*Axid*®)
Continuous *or* intermittent *in* Glucose 5% *or* Sodium chloride 0.9% *or* Compound sodium lactate
For continuous infusion, dilute 300 mg in 150 mL and give at a rate of 10 mg/hour; for intermittent infusion, dilute 100 mg in 50 mL and give over 15 minutes

Noradrenaline acid tartrate/Norepinephrine bitartrate
Continuous *in* Glucose 5% *or* Sodium chloride and glucose
Give *via* controlled infusion device; for administration *via* syringe pump, dilute 4 mg noradrenaline acid tartrate (2 mL solution) with 48 mL; for administration *via* drip counter dilute 40 mg (20 mL solution) with 480 mL; give through a central venous catheter; incompatible with alkalis

Omeprazole (as sodium salt) (*Losec*®)
Intermittent *in* Glucose 5% *or* Sodium chloride 0.9%
Reconstitute with infusion fluid and dilute to 100 mL; give over 20–30 minutes

Ondansetron (as hydrochloride) (*Zofran*®)
Continuous *or* intermittent *in* Glucose 5% *or* Sodium chloride 0.9% *or* Ringer's solution
For intermittent infusion, dilute 32 mg in 50–100 mL and give over at least 15 minutes

Oxaliplatin (*Eloxatin*®)
Continuous *in* Glucose 5%
Reconstitute with water for injections or glucose 5% to a concentration of 5 mg/mL; dilute with 250–500 mL infusion fluid and give over 2–6 hours

Oxycodone hydrochloride (*OxyNorm*®)
Continuous *or* intermittent *in* Glucose 5% *or* Sodium chloride 0.9%
Dilute to a concentration of 1 mg/mL

Oxytocin (*Syntocinon*®)
Continuous *in* Glucose 5% *or* Sodium chloride 0.9% or Compound sodium lactate *or* Ringer's solution
Preferably given *via* a variable-speed infusion pump in a concentration appropriate to the pump; if given by drip infusion for *induction or enhancement of labour*, dilute 5 units in 500 mL infusion fluid; for *postpartum uterine haemorrhage* dilute 5–30 units in 500 mL; if high doses given for prolonged period (e.g. for inevitable or missed abortion or for postpartum haemorrhage), use low volume of an electrolyte-containing infusion fluid (not Glucose 5%) given at higher concentration than for induction or enhancement of labour; close attention to patient's fluid and electrolyte status essential

Paclitaxel (*Taxol*®)
Continuous *in* Glucose 5% *or* Sodium chloride 0.9%
Dilute to a concentration of 0.3–1.2 mg/mL and give through an in-line filter (0.22 micron or less) over 3 hours; not to be used with PVC equipment (short PVC inlet or outlet on filter may be acceptable)

Pantoprazole (as sodium sesquihydrate) (*Protium*®)
Intermittent *in* Glucose 5 and 10% *or* Sodium chloride 0.9%
Reconstitute 40 mg with 10 mL sodium chloride 0.9% and dilute to 100 mL with infusion fluid

Pemetrexed (*Alimta*®)
Intermittent *in* Sodium chloride 0.9%
Reconstitute 500-mg vial with 20 mL sodium chloride 0.9% to produce a 25 mg/mL solution; dilute requisite dose with infusion fluid to 100 mL; give over 10 minutes

Pentamidine isetionate (*Pentacarinat*®)
Intermittent *in* Glucose 5% *or* Sodium chloride 0.9%
Dissolve initially in water for injections (300 mg in 3–5 mL) then dilute in 50–250 mL; give over at least 60 minutes

Pentostatin (*Nipent*®)
Intermittent *in* Glucose 5% *or* Sodium chloride 0.9%
Reconstitute initially with 5 mL water for injections to produce a 2 mg/mL solution; dilute requisite dose in 25–50 mL infusion fluid (final concentration 180–330 micrograms/mL) and give over 20–30 minutes

Phenoxybenzamine hydrochloride
Intermittent *in* Sodium chloride 0.9%
Dilute in 200–500 mL infusion; give over at least 2 hours; max. 4 hours between dilution and completion of administration

Phentolamine mesilate (*Rogitine*®)
Intermittent *in* Glucose 5% *or* Sodium chloride 0.9%

Phenylephrine hydrochloride
Intermittent *in* Glucose 5% *or* Sodium chloride 0.9%
Dilute 10 mg in 500 mL infusion fluid

Phenytoin sodium (*Epanutin*®)
Intermittent *in* Sodium chloride 0.9%
Flush intravenous line with Sodium chloride 0.9% before and after infusion; dilute in 50–100 mL infusion fluid (final concentration not to exceed 10 mg/mL) and give through an in-line filter (0.22–0.50 micron) at a rate not exceeding 50 mg/minute (neonates, give at a rate of 1–3 mg/kg/minute); complete administration within 1 hour of preparation

Phytomenadione (in mixed micelles vehicle) (*Konakion*® *MM*)
Intermittent *in* Glucose 5%
Dilute with 55 mL; may be injected into lower part of infusion apparatus

Piperacillin with tazobactam (as sodium salts) (*Tazocin*®)
Intermittent *in* Glucose 5% *or* Sodium chloride 0.9% *or* Water for injections
Reconstitute initially with water for injections or sodium chloride infusion 0.9% (2.25 g in 10 mL, 4.5 g in 20 mL) then dilute to at least 50 mL with infusion fluid; give over 20–30 minutes

Potassium chloride
Continuous *in* Glucose 5% *or* Sodium chloride 0.9%
Dilute in a large-volume infusion; mix thoroughly to avoid 'layering', especially in non-rigid infusion containers; use ready-prepared solutions when possible

Procainamide hydrochloride (*Pronestyl*®)
Continuous *or* intermittent *in* Glucose 5%
For maintenance, dilute to a concentration of *either* 2 mg/mL and give at a rate of 1–3 mL/minute *or* 4 mg/mL and give at a rate of 0.5–1.5 mL/minute

Propofol (emulsion) (*Diprivan*®; Abbott; Baxter; *Propofol-Lipuro*®, Braun; Mayne; Fresenius Kabi; Zurich)
1% or 2% emulsion
via drip tubing *in* Glucose 5% *or* Sodium chloride 0.9%
To be administered *via* a Y-piece close to injection site; microbiological filter not recommended
1% emulsion only
Continuous *in* Glucose 5% (*or* Sodium chloride 0.9% for *Propofol-Lipuro*®, Braun, Fresenius Kabi, and Zurich brands only)
Dilute to a concentration not less than 2 mg/mL; microbiological filter not recommended; administer using suitable device to control infusion rate; use glass or PVC containers (if PVC bag used it should be full—withdraw volume of infusion fluid equal to that of propofol to be added); give within 6 hours of preparation; propofol may alternatively be infused undiluted using a suitable infusion pump

Quinine dihydrochloride
Continuous *in* Sodium chloride 0.9%
To be given over 4 hours; see also section 5.4.1

Quinupristin with dalfopristin (*Synercid*®)
Intermittent *in* Glucose 5%
Reconstitute 500 mg with 5 mL water for injections or glucose 5%; gently swirl vial without shaking to dissolve; allow to stand for at least 2 minutes until foam disappears; dilute requisite dose in 100 mL infusion fluid and give over 60 minutes *via* central venous catheter (in an emergency, first dose may be diluted in 250 mL infusion fluid and given over 60 minutes *via* peripheral line); flush line with glucose 5% before and after infusion; incompatible with sodium chloride solutions

Raltitrexed (*Tomudex*®)
Intermittent *in* Glucose 5% *or* Sodium chloride 0.9%
Reconstitute with water for injections; dilute requisite dose in 50–250 mL infusion fluid and give over 15 minutes

Ranitidine (as hydrochloride) (*Zantac*®)
Intermittent *in* Glucose 5% *or* Sodium chloride 0.9% *or* Compound sodium lactate

Rasburicase (*Fasturtec*®)
Intermittent *in* Sodium chloride 0.9%
Reconstitute with solvent provided; gently swirl vial without shaking to dissolve; dilute requisite dose to 50 mL with infusion fluid and give over 30 minutes

Remifentanil (*Ultiva*®)
Intermittent *or via* drip tubing *in* Glucose 5% *or* Sodium chloride 0.9% *or* Water for injections
Reconstitute with infusion fluid to a concentration of 1 mg/mL then dilute further to a concentration of 20–250 micrograms/mL (50 micrograms/mL recommended for general anaesthesia)

Rifampicin (*Rifadin*®, *Rimactane*®)
Intermittent *in* Glucose 5 and 10% *or* Sodium chloride 0.9% *or* Ringer's solution
Reconstitute with solvent provided then dilute with 250 mL (*Rimactane*®) or 500 mL (*Rifadin*®) infusion fluid; give over 2–3 hours

Ritodrine hydrochloride (*Yutopar*®)
Continuous *in* Glucose 5%
Give *via* controlled infusion device, preferably a syringe pump; if syringe pump available dilute to a concentration of 3 mg/mL; if syringe pump not available dilute to a concentration of 300 micrograms/mL; close attention to patient's fluid and electrolyte status essential

Rituximab (*MabThera*®)
Intermittent *in* Glucose 5% *or* Sodium chloride 0.9%
Dilute to 1–4 mg/mL and gently invert bag to avoid foaming

Rocuronium bromide (*Esmeron*®)
Continuous *or via* drip tubing *in* Glucose 5% *or* Sodium chloride 0.9%

Salbutamol (as sulphate) (*Ventolin*® *For Intravenous Infusion*)
Continuous *in* Glucose 5%
For *bronchodilatation* dilute 5 mg with 500 mL glucose 5% or sodium chloride 0.9%; for *premature labour* dilute with glucose 5% to a concentration of 200 micrograms/mL for use in a syringe pump *or* for other infusion methods (preferably *via* controlled infusion device), dilute to a concentration of 20 micrograms/mL; close attention to patient's fluid and electrolyte status essential

Sodium calcium edetate (*Ledclair*®)
Continuous *in* Glucose 5% *or* Sodium chloride 0.9%
Dilute to a concentration of not more than 3%; suggested volume 250–500 mL given over at least 1 hour

Sodium clodronate (*Bonefos*® *Concentrate*, *Loron*®)
Continuous *in* Sodium chloride 0.9%
Dilute 300 mg in 500 mL and give over at least 2 hours or 1.5 g in 500 mL and give over at least 4 hours; *Bonefos*® *Concentrate* can also be diluted in Glucose 5%

Sodium nitroprusside (Mayne)
Continuous *in* Glucose 5%
Reconstitute 50 mg with 2–3 mL glucose 5% then dilute immediately with 250–1000 mL infusion fluid; preferably infuse *via* infusion device to allow precise control; protect infusion from light

Sodium valproate (*Epilim®*)
Continuous *or* intermittent *in* Glucose 5% *or* Sodium chloride 0.9%
Reconstitute with solvent provided then dilute with infusion fluid

Sotalol hydrochloride (*Sotacor®*)
Continuous *or* intermittent *in* Glucose 5% *or* Sodium chloride 0.9%
Dilute to a concentration of between 0.01–2 mg/mL

Streptokinase (*Streptase®*; *Streptokinase*, Braun)
Continuous *or* intermittent *in* Glucose 5% *or* Sodium chloride 0.9%
Reconstitute *Streptase®* with sodium chloride 0.9%, and *Streptokinase* (Braun) with either water for injections or sodium chloride 0.9% then dilute further with infusion fluid

Sulfadiazine sodium
Continuous *in* Sodium chloride 0.9%
Suggested volume 500 mL; ampoule solution has a pH of over 10

Suxamethonium chloride (*Anectine®*)
Continuous *in* Glucose 5% *or* Sodium chloride 0.9%

Tacrolimus (*Prograf®*)
Continuous *in* Glucose 5% *or* Sodium chloride 0.9%
Dilute concentrate in infusion fluid to a final concentration of 4–100 micrograms/mL; give over 24 hours; incompatible with PVC

Teicoplanin (*Targocid®*)
Intermittent *in* Glucose 5% *or* Sodium chloride 0.9% *or* Compound sodium lactate
Reconstitute initially with water for injections provided; infuse over 30 minutes
Continuous infusion not usually recommended

Terbutaline sulphate (*Bricanyl®*)
Continuous *in* Glucose 5%
For *bronchodilatation* dilute 1.5–2.5 mg with 500 mL glucose 5% or sodium chloride 0.9% and give over 8–10 hours; for *premature labour* dilute in glucose 5% and give *via* controlled infusion device preferably a syringe pump; if syringe pump available dilute to a concentration of 100 micrograms/mL; if syringe pump not available dilute to a concentration of 10 micrograms/mL; close attention to patient's fluid and electrolyte status essential

Ticarcillin sodium with clavulanic acid (*Timentin®*)
Intermittent *in* Glucose 5% *or* Water for injections
Suggested volume (depending on dose) glucose 5% 100–150 mL or water for injections 50–100 mL; given over 30–40 minutes

Tirofiban (*Aggrastat®*)
Continuous *in* Glucose 5% *or* Sodium chloride 0.9%
Withdraw 50 mL infusion fluid from 250-mL bag and replace with 50 mL tirofiban concentrate (250 micrograms/mL) to give a final concentration of 50 micrograms/mL

Tobramycin (as sulphate) (*Nebcin®*)
Intermittent *or via* drip tubing *in* Glucose 5% *or* Sodium chloride 0.9%
For adult intermittent infusion suggested volume 50–100 mL (children proportionately smaller volume) given over 20–60 minutes

Topotecan (as hydrochloride) (*Hycamtin®*)
Intermittent *in* Glucose 5% *or* Sodium chloride 0.9%
Reconstitute 4 mg with 4 mL water for injections then dilute to a final concentration of 25–50 micrograms/mL; give over 30 minutes

Tramadol hydrochloride (*Zydol®*)
Continuous *or* intermittent *in* Glucose 5% *or* Sodium chloride 0.9% *or* Ringer's solution *or* Compound sodium lactate

Tranexamic acid (*Cyklokapron®*)
Continuous *in* Glucose 5% *or* Sodium chloride 0.9% *or* Ringer's solution

Trastuzumab (*Herceptin®*)
Intermittent *in* Sodium chloride 0.9%
Reconstitute each 150-mg vial with 7.2 mL water for injections to produce 21 mg/mL solution, swirl vial gently to avoid excessive foaming and allow to stand for approximately 5 minutes; dilute requisite dose in 250 mL infusion fluid

Treosulfan (*Treosulfan*) (Medac)
Intermittent *in* Water for injections
Infusion suggested for doses above 5 g; dilute to a concentration of 5 g in 100 mL

Trisodium edetate (*Limclair®*)
Continuous *in* Glucose 5% *or* Sodium chloride 0.9%
Dilute to a concentration of 10 mg/mL; give over 2–3 hours

Tropisetron (as hydrochloride) (*Navoban®*)
Intermittent *or via* drip tubing *in* Glucose 5% *or* Sodium chloride 0.9% *or* Ringer's solution
Suggested concentration for infusion 50 micrograms/mL

Vancomycin (as hydrochloride) (*Vancocin®*)
Intermittent *in* Glucose 5% *or* Sodium chloride 0.9%
Reconstitute each 500 mg with 10 mL water for injections and dilute with infusion fluid to a concentration of up to 5 mg/mL (10 mg/mL in fluid restriction but increased risk of infusion-related effects); give over at least 60 minutes (rate not to exceed 10 mg/minute for doses over 500 mg); use continuous infusion only if intermittent not feasible

Vasopressin, synthetic (*Pitressin®*)
Intermittent *in* Glucose 5%
Suggested concentration 20 units/100 mL given over 15 minutes

Vecuronium bromide (*Norcuron®*)
Continuous *in* Glucose 5% *or* Sodium chloride 0.9% *or* Ringer's solution
Reconstitute with the solvent provided

Verteporfin (*Visudyne®*)
Intermittent *in* Glucose 5%
Reconstitute each 15 mg with 7 mL water for injections to produce a 2 mg/mL solution then dilute requisite dose with infusion fluid to a final volume of 30 mL and give over 10 minutes; protect from light and administer within 4 hours of reconstitution. Incompatible with sodium chloride infusion

Vinblastine sulphate (*Velbe®*)
via drip tubing *in* Sodium chloride 0.9%
Reconstitute with sodium chloride 0.9%; give over approx. 1 minute

Vincristine sulphate (*Oncovin®*)
via drip tubing *in* Glucose 5% *or* Sodium chloride 0.9%

Vindesine sulphate (*Eldisine®*)
via drip tubing *in* Glucose 5% *or* Sodium chloride 0.9%
Reconstitute with sodium chloride 0.9%; give over 1–3 minutes

Vinorelbine (*Navelbine®*)
Intermittent *in* Glucose 5% *or* Sodium chloride 0.9%
Dilute in 125 mL infusion fluid; give over 20–30 minutes

Vitamins B & C (*Pabrinex® I/V High potency*)
Intermittent *or via* drip tubing *in* Glucose 5% *or* Sodium chloride 0.9%
Ampoule contents should be mixed, diluted, and administered without delay; give over 10 minutes (see CSM advice, section 9.6.2)

Vitamins, multiple
(*Cernevit®*)
Intermittent *in* Glucose 5% *or* Sodium chloride 0.9%
Dissolve initially in 5 mL water for injections (or infusion fluid)
(*Solivito N®*)
Intermittent *in* Glucose 5 and 10%
Suggested volume 500–1000 mL given over 2–3 hours; see also section 9.3

Voriconazole (*Vfend®*)
Intermittent *in* Glucose 5% *or* Sodium chloride 0.9% *or* Compound sodium lactate
Reconstitute each 200 mg with 19 mL water for injections to produce a 10 mg/mL solution; dilute dose in infusion fluid to concentration of 0.5–5 mg/mL; give at a rate not exceeding 3 mg/kg/hour

Zidovudine (*Retrovir®*)
Intermittent *in* Glucose 5%
Dilute to a concentration of 2 mg/mL or 4 mg/mL and give over 1 hour

Zoledronic acid (*Zometa®*)
Intermittent *in* Glucose 5% *or* Sodium chloride 0.9%
Dilute requisite dose with 100 mL infusion fluid; infuse over at least 15 minutes

Appendix 7: Borderline substances

In certain conditions some foods (and toilet preparations) have characteristics of drugs and the Advisory Committee on Borderline Substances advises as to the circumstances in which such substances may be regarded as drugs. Prescriptions issued in accordance with the Committee's advice and endorsed 'ACBS' will normally not be investigated.

> General Practitioners are reminded that the ACBS recommends products on the basis that they may be regarded as drugs for the management of specified conditions. Doctors should satisfy themselves that the products can safely be prescribed, that patients are adequately monitored and that, where necessary, expert hospital supervision is available.

Foods which may be prescribed on FP10, GP10 (Scotland), or when available WP10 (Wales)

NOTE. This is a list of food products which the ACBS has approved. The clinical condition for which the product has approval follows each entry.
Foods included in this Appendix may contain cariogenic sugars and patients should be advised to take appropriate oral hygiene measures.

Alcoholic Beverages
see under Rectified Spirit

Alembicol D® (Alembic Products)
Fractionated coconut oil. Net price 5 kg = £125.55.
For steatorrhoea associated with cystic fibrosis of the pancreas, intestinal lymphangiectasia, surgery of the intestine, chronic liver disease, liver cirrhosis, other proven malabsorption syndromes; in a ketogenic diet in the management of epilepsy; type 1 hyperlipoproteinaemia

Aminex® (Gluten Free Foods Ltd)
Low-protein. Biscuits, net price 200 g = £3.75. Cookies, 150 g = £3.75. Rusks, 200 g = £3.75.
For inherited metabolic disorders, renal or liver failure requiring a low-protein diet

Amino Acid Modules (SHS)
see XLEU Faladon, XMET Homidon, XMTVI Asadon, XPHEN TYR Tyrosidon, or *XPTM Tyrosidon*

Aminogran® (UCB Pharma)
Food Supplement, powder, containing all essential amino acids except phenylalanine, net price 500 g = £39.78. Aminogran PKU tablet (≡ 1 g powder), net price 150-tab pack = £30.00.
For the dietary management of phenylketonuria. Tablets not to be prescribed for any child under 8 years

Analog® (SHS)
see MSUD Analog, XLEU Analog, XLYS Analog, XLYS Low TRY Analog, XMET Analog, XMTVI Analog, XP Analog, XP LCP Analog, XPHEN TYR Analog, XPTM Analog

NOTE. Analog products are generally intended for use in children up to 1 year, see also Flavour Sachets, for use with unflavoured amino acid and peptide products from SHS

Aproten® (Ultrapharm)
Gluten-free. Flour. Net price 500 g = £4.99.
For gluten-sensitive enteropathies including steatorrhoea due to gluten sensitivity, coeliac disease, and dermatitis herpetiformis
Low protein. Low Na^+ and K^+. Net prices: biscuits 180 g (36) = £2.88; bread mix 250 g = £2.17; cake mix 300 g = £2.10; crispbread 260 g = £4.06; pasta (anellini, ditalini, rigatini, spaghetti) 500 g = £4.06; tagliatelle 250 g = £2.16.
For inherited metabolic disorders, renal or liver failure requiring a low-protein diet

L-Arginine (SHS)
Powder, net price 100 g = £8.39.
For use as a supplement in urea cycle disorders other than arginase deficiency, such as hyperammonaemia types I and II, citrullaemia, arginosuccinic aciduria, and deficiency of N-acetyl glutamate synthetase

Arnott® (Ultrapharm)
Rice Cookies, gluten-free. Net price 200 g = £2.06.
For gluten-sensitive enteropathies including steatorrhoea due to gluten sensitivity, coeliac disease, and dermatitis herpetiformis

Baker's Delight®
Gluten-free. Bread, net price 100 g = 80p.
For established gluten enteropathy

Barkat® (Gluten Free Foods Ltd)
Gluten-free. Bread mix, net price 500 g = £4.12. Multi Grain Bread, 450 g = £2.99. Rice bread (sliced), brown or white, 450 g = £2.99. Rice pizza crust, brown or white, 150 g = £2.21.
For gluten-sensitive enteropathies including steatorrhoea due to gluten sensitivity, coeliac disease, and dermatitis herpetiformis

Bi-Aglut® (Novartis Consumer Health)
Gluten-free. Biscuits, net price 180 g = £2.89. Crackers, 150 g = £2.36. Cracker toast, 240 g = £4.18. Pasta (fusilli, macaroni, penne, spaghetti), 500 g = £5.23.
For gluten-sensitive enteropathies including steatorrhoea due to gluten sensitivity, coeliac disease, and dermatitis herpetiformis

Calogen® (SHS)
Emulsion, arachis oil (peanut oil) 50% in water, net price, 250 mL = £4.31 (banana or natural flavour), £4.31 (strawberry flavour); 1 litre = £16.91 (natural flavour), £16.91 (banana or butterscotch flavour).
For disease-related malnutrition, malabsorption states or other conditions requiring fortification with a high-fat supplement with or without fluid and electrolyte restrictions

Caloreen® (Nestlé Clinical)
Powder, water-soluble dextrins, 390 kcal/100 g, with less than 1.8 mmol of Na^+ and 0.3 mmol of K^+/100 g. Gluten-, lactose-, and fructose-free. Net price 500 g = £3.02.
For disease-related malnutrition, malabsorption states or other conditions requiring fortification with a high or readily available carbohydrate supplement

Calshake® (Fresenius Kabi)
Powder, protein 4 g, carbohydrate 58 g, fat 20.4 g, energy 1809 kJ (432 kcal)/87 g. Gluten-free. Strawberry, vanilla, neutral, and banana flavours,

net price 87-g sachet = £1.82; also available chocolate flavour (protein 4 g, carbohydrate 58 g, fat 20.4 g, fibre 1.6 g, energy 1809 kJ (432 kcal)/ 90 g = £1.82.

For disease-related malnutrition, malabsorption states or other conditions requiring fortification with a fat/ carbohydrate supplement

Caprilon® (SHS)

Powder, protein 11.8%, carbohydrate 55.1%, fat 28.3% (medium chain triglycerides 21.3%). Low in lactose, gluten- and sucrose-free. Used as a 12.7% solution. Net price 420 g = £12.46.

For disorders in which a high intake of MCT is beneficial

Carobel, Instant® (Cow & Gate)

Powder, carob seed flour. Net price 135 g = £2.63.

For thickening feeds in the treatment of vomiting

Casilan 90® (Heinz)

Powder, whole protein, containing all essential amino acids, 90% with less than 0.1% Na^+. Net price 250 g = £4.69.

For biochemically proven hypoproteinaemia

Clinutren® **1.5** (Nestlé Clinical)

Liquid, protein 11 g, carbohydrate 42 g, fat 10 g, energy 1260 kJ (300 kcal)/200 mL with vitamins and minerals. Gluten-free; clinically lactose-free. Flavours: apricot, banana, chocolate, coffee, strawberry-raspberry or vanilla, net price 4 × 200-mL pot = £5.60.

For indications see *Clinutren Fruit*

Clinutren® **1.5 Fibre** (Nestlé Clinical)

Liquid, protein 5.7 g, carbohydrate 19 g, fat 5.9 g, fibre 2.6 g, energy 630 kJ (150 kcal)/100 mL with vitamins, minerals and trace elements. Gluten-free; clinically lactose-free. Flavours: vanilla or plum, net price 4 × 200-mL pot = £5.60.

For use as the sole source of nutrition or as a necessary nutritional supplement prescribed on medical grounds for: short-bowel syndrome, intractable malabsorption, pre-operative preparation of undernourished patients, proven inflammatory bowel disease, following total gastrectomy, dysphagia, bowel fistulas, disease-related malnutrition. Not suitable for any child under 3 years; not suitable as a sole source of nutrition for patients under 6 years

Clinutren® **Dessert** (Nestlé Clinical)

Semi-solid, protein 12 g, carbohydrate 19 g, fat 3.3 g, energy 650 kJ (160 kcal)/ 125 g with vitamins and minerals. Gluten-free. Flavours: caramel, chocolate, peach or vanilla, net price 4 × 125-g pot = £4.20.

For use as a nutritional supplement prescribed on medical grounds for: short-bowel syndrome, intractable malabsorption, pre-operative preparation of undernourished patients, proven inflammatory bowel disease, following total gastrectomy, dysphagia, bowel fistulas, disease-related malnutrition, continuous ambulatory peritoneal dialysis (CAPD), haemodialysis. Not suitable for any child under 3 years; maximum of 3 units daily for children aged 3 to 6 years

Clinutren® **Fruit** (Nestlé Clinical)

Liquid, protein 8 g, carbohydrate 54 g, fat less than 0.4 g, energy 1040 kJ (250 kcal)/200 mL with vitamins and minerals. Gluten-free. Low-lactose. Flavours: grapefruit, orange, pear-cherry, or raspberry-blackcurrant, net price 4 × 200-mL cup = £6.00.

For use as a nutritional supplement prescribed on medical grounds for: short-bowel syndrome, intractable malabsorption, pre-operative preparation of undernourished patients, proven inflammatory bowel disease, following total gastrectomy, dysphagia, bowel fistulas, disease-related malnutrition. Not suitable for any child under 3 years; maximum of 3 units daily for children aged 3 to 6 years

Clinutren® **ISO** (Nestlé Clinical)

Liquid, protein 7.6 g, carbohydrate 28 g, fat 6.6 g, energy 840 kJ (200 kcal)/200 mL with vitamins and minerals. Gluten-free. Flavours: chocolate or vanilla, net price 4 × 200-mL pot = £4.72.

For use as a sole source of nutrition or as a necessary nutritional supplement prescribed on medical grounds for: short-bowel syndrome, intractable malabsorption, pre-operative preparation of undernourished patients, proven inflammatory bowel disease, following total gastrectomy, dysphagia, bowel fistulas, disease-related malnutrition. Not suitable for any child under 3 years; not suitable as a sole source of nutrition for patients under 6 years; maximum of 3 units daily for children aged 3 to 6 years

Clinutren® **Thickened Drinks** (Nestlé Clinical)

Liquid, modified maize starch, gluten-free. Flavours: orange, peppermint, and tea, net price 4 × 125 g = £1.96.

Thickening of foods and fluids in dysphagia. Not to be used for children under 3 years

Clinutren® **Thickener** (Nestlé Clinical)

Powder, modified maize starch, gluten-free, net price 300 g = £4.53.

Thickening of foods and fluids in dysphagia. Not to be used for children under 3 years

Colief® (Britannia)

Liquid, lactase 50 000 units/g, net price 7-mL dropper bottle = £7.00

For the relief of symptoms associated with lactose intolerance in infants, provided that lactose intolerance is confirmed by the presence of reducing substances and/or excessive acid in stools, a low concentration of the corresponding disaccharide enzyme on intestinal biopsy or by breath hydrogen test or lactose intolerance test. For dosage and administration details, consult product literature

Comminuted Chicken Meat (SHS)

Suspension (aqueous). Net price 150 g = £2.56.

For carbohydrate intolerance in association with possible or proven intolerance of milk; glucose and galactose intolerance

Corn flour and corn starch

For hypoglycaemia associated with glycogen-storage disease

Dextrose

see Glucose

Dialamine® (SHS)

Powder, essential amino acids 30%, with carbohydrate 62%, energy 1500 kJ (360 kcal)/100 g, with ascorbic acid, minerals, and trace elements. Flavour: orange. Net price 200 g = £25.11.

For oral feeding where essential amino acid supplements are required; e.g. chronic renal failure, hypoproteinaemia, wound fistula leakage with excessive protein loss, conditions requiring a controlled nitrogen intake, and haemodialysis

Dietary Specials (Nutrition Point)

Gluten-free. Bread. Loaf, sliced (brown, white or multigrain) 400 g = £2.50; bread rolls, long (white) 3 = £1.55. Bread mix (brown or white), net price 500 g = £4.75; cracker bread, 150 g = £1.80; cake mix (white), 750 g = £4.75; white or fibre mix, 500 g = £4.75; pastry mix, 600 g = £4.75; digestive biscuits, 150 g = £1.70. Tea biscuits, 220 g = £2.00. Pasta (spaghetti, penne, fusilli), 500 g = £3.20

For gluten-sensitive enteropathies including steatorrhoea due to gluten sensitivity, coeliac disease, and dermatitis herpetiformis

Duobar® (SHS)

Bar, protein-free (phenylalanine nil added), carbohydrate 49.9 g, fat 49.9 g, energy 2692 kJ (648 kcal)/100 g. Low sodium and potassium. Strawberry, toffee, or neutral flavours. Net price 45-g bar = £1.34.

For disease-related malnutrition, malabsorption states or other conditions requiring fortification with fat/carbohydrate supplement

Duocal® (SHS)

Liquid, emulsion providing carbohydrate 23.4 g, fat 7.1 g, energy 661 kJ (158 kcal)/100 mL. Low-electrolyte, gluten-, lactose-, and protein-free. Net price 250 mL = £2.74; 1 litre = £9.77

MCT Powder, carbohydrate 74 g, fat 23.2 g (of which MCT 83%), energy 2042 kJ (486 kcal)/100 g. Low electrolyte, gluten-, protein- and lactose-free. Net price 400 g = £14.69

Super Soluble Powder, carbohydrate 72.7 g, fat 22.3 g, energy 2061 kJ (492 kcal)/100 g. Low electrolyte, gluten-, protein-, and lactose-free. Net price 400 g = £12.36

All for disease-related malnutrition, malabsorption states or other conditions requiring fortification with fat/carbohydrate supplement

Easiphen® (SHS)

Liquid, protein (containing essential and non-essential amino acids, phenylalanine-free) 6.7 g, carbohydrate 5.1 g, fat 2 g, energy 275 kJ (65 kcal)/100 mL with vitamins, minerals, and trace elements. Forest berries or grapefruit flavour, net price 250-mL carton = £6.60.

For the dietary management of proven phenylketonuria. Not to be prescribed for children under 8 years

Elemental 028® (SHS)

028 Powder, amino acids 12%, carbohydrate 70.5–72%, fat 6.64%, energy 1544–1568 kJ (364–370 kcal)/100 g with vitamins and minerals. For preparation with water before use. Net price 100-g box (orange flavoured or plain) = £4.03

For use as the sole source of nutrition or as a nutritional supplement prescribed on medical grounds for: short-bowel syndrome, intractable malabsorption, proven inflammatory bowel disease, bowel fistulas. Not to be prescribed for any child under 1 year; use with caution for children up to 5 years

NOTE. See also Flavour Sachets, for use with unflavoured amino acid and peptide products from SHS

Elemental 028® **Extra** (SHS)

Liquid, amino acids 3 g, carbohydrate 11 g, fat 3.48 g, energy 358 kJ (86 kcal)/100 mL, with vitamins, minerals, and trace elements. Flavours: grapefruit, orange and pineapple, summer fruits. Net price 250-mL carton = £2.51

Powder, amino acids 15%, carbohydrate 59%, fat 17.45%, energy 1860 kJ (443 kcal)/100 g, with vitamins, minerals, and trace elements. For preparation with water before use. Net price 100 g (plain) = £4.88; also available in banana, citrus, or orange flavours (carbohydrate 55%, energy 1793 kJ (427 kcal)/100 g), 100 g = £4.88

All for use as the sole source of nutrition or as a nutritional supplement prescribed on medical grounds for: short-bowel syndrome, intractable malabsorption, proven inflammatory bowel disease, bowel fistulas. Not to be prescribed for any child under 1 year; use with caution for children up to 5 years

NOTE. see also Flavour Sachets, for use with unflavoured amino acid and peptide products from SHS

Emsogen® (SHS)

Powder, amino acids 15%, carbohydrate 60%, fat 16.4%, energy 1839 kJ (438 kcal)/100 g, with vitamins, minerals, and trace elements. For preparation with water before use. Net price 100 g = £5.03; also available orange-flavoured (carbohydrate 55%, energy 1754 kJ (418 kcal)/100 g), 100 g = £5.03.

For use as the sole source of nutrition or as a nutritional supplement prescribed on medical grounds for short-bowel syndrome, intractable malabsorption, proven inflammatory bowel disease, bowel fistulas. Not to be prescribed for any child under 1 year; use with caution for children up to 5 years

Ener-G® (General Dietary)

Gluten-free. Cookies (vanilla flavour), net price 435 g = £4.88. Rice bread (sliced), brown, 474 g = £4.28; white, 456 g = £4.28. Rice loaf (sliced), 612 g = £4.28. Seattle brown loaf, 600 g = £4.93. Tapioca bread (sliced), 480 g = £4.28. Rice pasta (macaroni, shells, small shells, and lasagne), 454 g = £3.98; spaghetti, 447 g = £3.98; tagliatelle, 400 g = £3.98; vermicelli, 300 g = £3.98; cannelloni, 335 g = £3.98. Brown rice pasta: lasagne, 454 g = £3.98; macaroni, 454 g = £3.98; spaghetti, 447 g = £3.98. Xanthan gum, 170 g = £6.76.

For gluten-sensitive enteropathies including steatorrhoea due to gluten sensitivity, coeliac disease, and dermatitis herpetiformis

Gluten-free. Pizza bases, 372 g = £3.75. Six flour bread loaf, 576 g = £3.60. Seattle brown rolls (round or long), 4 x 119 g = £3.00

For established gluten enteropathy with coexisting established wheat sensitivity only

Low protein egg replacer, carbohydrate 94 g, energy 1574 kJ (376 kcal)/100 g. Egg-, gluten- and lactose-free, net price 454 g = £4.05.

For phenylketonuria, similar amino acid abnormalities, renal failure, liver failure and liver cirrhosis.

Low protein pasta (lasagne, macaroni, large shells, small shells, spaghetti), net price 454 g = £5.05.

For phenylketonuria, similar amino acid abnormalities, renal failure, liver failure requiring a low-protein diet

Low protein rice bread, net price 600 g = £4.39.

For inherited metabolic disorders, renal or liver failure requiring a low-protein diet

Energivit® (SHS)

Powder, protein-free, carbohydrate 66.7 g, fat 25 g, energy 2059 kJ, (492 kcal)/100 g with vitamins, minerals and trace elements, net price 400 g = £15.04.

For infants requiring additional enegy, vitamins, minerals and trace elements following a protein restricted diet

Enfamil AR® (Mead Johnson)

AR (Anti-Reflux), powder, protein 13 g, fat 26 g, carbohydrate 56 g, energy 2124 kJ (508 kcal)/100 g with vitamins, minerals and trace elements, net price 400 g = £2.55.

For significant reflux disease. For use not in excess of a 6-month period. Not to be used in conjunction with any other thickener or antacid product.

Enfamil Lactofree® (Mead Johnson)

Powder, protein 11.9 g, fat 28 g, carbohydrate 56 g, energy 2176 kJ (520 kcal)/100 g with vitamins, minerals and trace elements. Lactose- and sucrose-free, net price 400 g = £3.51.

For proven lactose intolerance

Enlive Plus® (Abbott)

Liquid, protein 4.8 g, carbohydrate 32.7 g, energy 638 kJ (150 kcal)/100 mL, with vitamins, minerals and trace elements. Fat- and gluten-free; clinically lactose-free. Flavours: apple, fruit punch, grapefruit, lemon and lime, orange, peach, pineapple, strawberry, net price 220-mL Tetrapak® = £1.66.

For use as a nutritional supplement prescribed on medical grounds for: short-bowel syndrome, intractable malabsorption, pre-operative preparation of undernourished patients, proven inflammatory bowel disease, following total gastrectomy, dysphagia, bowel fistulas, disease-related malnutrition. Not for use in galactosaemia. Not to be prescribed for any child under 1 year; use with caution for children up to 5 years

Enrich® (Abbott)

Liquid with dietary fibre, providing protein 3.8 g, carbohydrate 14 g, fat 3.5 g, fibre 1.4 g, energy 432 kJ (102 kcal)/100 mL with vitamins and minerals. Lactose- and gluten-free. Vanilla flavour. Net price 250-mL can = £2.24.

For use as the sole source of nutrition or as a nutritional supplement prescribed on medical grounds for: short-bowel syndrome, intractable malabsorption, pre-operative preparation of patients who are undernourished, proven inflammatory bowel disease, following total gastrectomy, dysphagia, disease-related malnutrition. Not to be prescribed for any child under 1 year; use with caution for children up to 5 years

Enrich Plus® (Abbott)

Liquid with dietary fibre, providing protein 6.25 g, carbohydrate 20.2 g, fat 4.92 g, fibre 1.25 g, energy 642 kJ (153 kcal)/100 mL with vitamins and minerals. Lactose- and gluten-free. Vanilla, chocolate, fruits of the forest, raspberry, strawberry and banana flavours. Net price 200-mL Tetrapak® = £1.71.

For use as a nutritional supplement for patients with disease-related malnutrition, continuous ambulatory peritoneal dialysis (CAPD), short-bowel syndrome, intractable malabsorption, dysphagia, proven inflammatory bowel disease, bowel fistulas, gastrectomy, and pre-operative preparation of undernourished patients. Not to be prescribed for any child under 1 year; use with caution for children up to 5 years

Ensure® (Abbott)

Liquid, protein 4 g, fat 3.4 g, carbohydrate 13.6 g, energy 423 kJ (100 kcal)/100 mL with minerals and vitamins, lactose- and gluten-free. Vanilla, coffee, eggnog, nut, chicken, mushroom, and asparagus flavours. Net price 250-mL can = £1.92; 500-mL ready-to-hang (vanilla) = £3.74

For use as the sole source of nutrition or as a nutritional supplement prescribed on medical grounds for: short-bowel syndrome, intractable malabsorption, pre-operative preparation of patients who are undernourished, proven inflammatory bowel disease, following total gastrectomy, dysphagia, bowel fistulas, disease-related malnutrition. Not to be prescribed for any child under 1 year; use with caution for children up to 5 years

Ensure Plus® (Abbott)

Liquid, protein 6.3 g, fat 4.9 g, carbohydrate 20.2 g, with vitamins and minerals, lactose- and gluten-free, energy 632 kJ (150 kcal)/100 mL. Vanilla flavour, (formulations may vary slightly). Net price 220-mL Tetrapak® = £1.59; 250-mL can = £2.10; 500-mL ready-to-hang (unflavoured) = £3.91; 1-litre ready-to-hang (unflavoured) = £7.63; 1.5-litre ready-to-hang (unflavoured) = £11.44. Caramel, chocolate, strawberry, banana, fruit of the forest, raspberry, orange, coffee, blackcurrant, peach, vanilla or neutral flavours. Net price 220-mL Tetrapak® = £1.59.

Yoghurt Style, protein 6.3 g, fat 4.9 g, carbohydrate 20.2 g, with vitamins, minerals and trace elements, gluten-free, clinically lactose-free, energy 632 kJ (150 kcal)/100 mL. Peach, pineapple, or strawberry flavour, net price 220-mL Tetrapak® = £1.59.

Both as nutritional supplements prescribed on medical grounds for: short-bowel syndrome, intractable malabsorption, pre-operative preparation of patients who are undernourished, proven inflammatory bowel disease, following total gastrectomy, dysphagia, bowel fistulas, disease-related malnutrition, continuous ambulatory peritoneal dialysis (CAPD), and haemodialysis. Not to be prescribed for any child under 1 year; use with caution for children up to 5 years

Farley's Soya Formula (Heinz)

Powder, providing protein 2%, carbohydrate 7%, fat 3.8% with vitamins and minerals when reconstituted. Gluten-, sucrose-, and lactose-free. Net price 450 g = £3.38.

For proven lactose and associated sucrose intolerance in pre-school children, galactokinase deficiency, galactosaemia, and cow's milk protein intolerance

Fate® (Fate)

Low protein. All-purpose mix, net price 500 g = £5.63; Cake mix, 2 × 250 g = £5.63; Chocolate-flavour cake mix, 2 × 250 g = £5.63.

For inherited metabolic disorders, renal or liver failure requiring a low-protein diet

FlavourPac® (Vitaflo)

Powder, flavours: blackcurrant, lemon, orange, tropical or raspberry, net price 4 × 30 × 4-g sachets = £40.12

For use in conjuntion with Vitaflo's Inborn Error range of protein substitutes

Flavour Sachets (SHS)

Powder, flavours: cherry-vanilla, grapefruit, lemon-lime, net price 20 × 5-g sachets = £8.32.

For use with SHS unflavoured amino acid and peptide products

Foodlink Complete (Foodlink)

Powder, protein 21.9 g, carbohydrate 57.3 g, fat 13.3 g, energy 1838 kJ (436.5 kcal)/100 g with vitamins and minerals, Flavours: banana, chocolate, natural, or strawberry, net price 450-g carton = £3.19; also available, vanilla with fibre, protein 19.5 g, carbohydrate 60.2 g, fat 12.3 g, fibre 8 g, energy 1804 kJ (428 kcal)/100 g = £3.75.

As a nutritional supplement prescribed on medical grounds for: short-bowel syndrome, intractable malabsorption, pre-operative preparation of undernourished patients, proven inflammatory bowel disease, following total gastrectomy, dysphagia, bowel fistulas, disease-related malnutrition. Not to be prescribed for any child under 1 year; use with caution for children up to 5 years

Formance® (Abbott)

Semi-solid, protein 4 g, carbohydrate 27 g, fat 5 g, energy 703 kJ (167 kcal)/113 g with vitamins and minerals. Gluten-free. Vanilla and butterscotch flavours. Net price 113-g pot = £1.40.

As a nutritional supplement prescribed on medical grounds for: short-bowel syndrome, intractable malabsorption, pre-operative preparation of patients who are undernourished, proven inflammatory bowel disease, following total gastrectomy, dysphagia, bowel fistulas, disease-related malnutrition, continuous ambulatory peritoneal dialysis (CAPD), and haemodialysis. Not to be prescribed for any child under 1 year; use with caution for children up to 5 years

Forticreme® (Nutricia Clinical)

Semi-solid, protein 10 g, carbohydrate 19 g, fat 5 g, energy 680 kJ (161 kcal)/100 g with vitamins and minerals. Gluten-free. Vanilla, chocolate, coffee, banana, and forest fruit flavours, net price 4 × 125-g pot = £6.37.

As a nutritional supplement prescribed on medical grounds for: short-bowel syndrome, intractable malabsorption, pre-operative preparation of patients who are undernourished, proven inflammatory bowel disease, following total gastrectomy, dysphagia, bowel fistulas, disease-related malnutrition, continuous ambulatory peritoneal dialysis (CAPD) and haemodialysis. Not to be prescribed for any child under 3 years; use with caution for children aged 3 to 5 years

Fortifresh® (Nutricia Clinical)

Liquid, protein 12 g, carbohydrate 37.4 g, fat 11.6 g, energy 1260 kJ (300 kcal)/200 mL with vitamins, minerals and trace elements. Gluten-free. Flavours: blackcurrant, peach and orange, pineapple, raspberry, and vanilla and lemon, net price 200 mL carton = £1.59.

For use as a nutritional supplement prescribed on medical grounds for: intractable malabsorption, pre-operative preparation of patients who are undernourished, inflammatory bowel disease, dysphagia, disease-related malnutrition. Not to be prescribed for any child under 3 years; use with caution for children aged 3 to 5 years

Fortijuce® (Nutricia Clinical)

Liquid, protein 4 g, carbohydrate 33.5 g, energy 635 kJ (150 kcal)/100 mL, with vitamins, minerals and trace elements. Fat-free. Flavours: apple and pear, apricot, blackcurrant, forest fruits, lemon and lime, peach and orange, pineapple. Net price 200-mL carton = £1.59.

As a nutritional supplement prescribed on medical grounds for: short-bowel syndrome, intractable malabsorption, pre-operative preparation of patients who are undernourished, proven inflammatory bowel disease, following total gastrectomy, dysphagia, bowel fistulas, disease-related malnutrition. Not to be prescribed for any child under 3 years; use with caution for children up to 5 years

Fortimel® (Nutricia Clinical)

Liquid, protein 20 g, carbohydrate 20.8 g, fat 4.2 g, energy 840 kJ (200 kcal)/200 mL with vitamins and minerals. Gluten-free. Vanilla, strawberry, coffee, chocolate, and forest fruits flavours. Net price 200-mL carton = £1.39.

As a nutritional supplement prescribed on medical grounds for: short-bowel syndrome, intractable malabsorption, pre-operative preparation of patients who are undernourished, proven inflammatory bowel disease, following total gastrectomy, dysphagia, bowel fistulas, disease-related malnutrition. Not to be prescribed for any child under 3 years; use with caution for children up to 5 years

Fortini® (Nutricia Clinical)

Liquid, protein 3.4 g, carbohydrate 18.8 g, fat 6.8 g, energy 630 kJ (150 kcal)/100 mL with vitamins, minerals, and trace elements. Gluten- and lactose-free. Flavours: strawberry or vanilla, net price 200 mL = £2.38.

For use as a nutritional supplement prescribed on medical grounds for: disease-related malnutrition, and growth failure. For children between 8–20 kg body-weight

Fortini Multifibre® (Nutricia Clinical)

Liquid, protein 3.4 g, carbohydrate 18.8 g, fat 6.8 g, fibre 1.5 g, energy 630 kJ (150 kcal)/ 100 mL with vitamins, minerals, and trace elements. Gluten- and lactose-free. Flavours: banana, chocolate, strawberry, and vanilla, net price 200-mL = £2.50.

For indications see Fortini liquid

Fortisip® **Bottle** (Nutricia Clinical)

Liquid, protein 12 g, carbohydrate 36.8 g, fat 11.6 g, energy 1260 kJ (300 kcal)/200 mL, with vitamins, minerals and trace elements. Gluten-free; clinically lactose-free. Vanilla, banana, chocolate, orange, strawberry, tropical fruits, toffee, and neutral flavours, net price 200 mL = £1.59.

As a nutritional supplement prescribed on medical grounds for: short-bowel syndrome, intractable malabsorption, pre-operative preparation of patients who are undernourished, proven inflammatory bowel disease, following total gastrectomy, dysphagia, bowel fistulas, disease-related malnutrition. Not to be prescribed for any child under 3 years; use with caution for children aged 3 to 5 years

Fortisip® **Multi Fibre** (Nutricia Clinical)

Liquid, protein 12 g, carbohydrate 36.8 g, fat 11.6 g, fibre 4.5 g, energy 1260 kJ (300 kcal)/200 mL, with vitamins, minerals and trace elements. Gluten-free, clinically lactose-free. Banana, chicken, orange, strawberry, tomato, vanilla flavours; also available chocolate flavour (protein 10 g, carbohydrate 36 g, fat 13 g, fibre 4.5 g, energy 1260 kJ (300 kcal)/ 200 mL, net price 200 mL = £1.64.

As a nutritional supplement prescribed on medical grounds for: short-bowel syndrome, intractable malabsorption, pre-operative preparation of undernourished patients, proven inflammatory bowel disease, following total gastrectomy, dysphagia, disease-related malnutrition. Not to be prescribed for any child under 3 years; use with caution for children aged 3 to 5 years

Fortisip® **Protein** (Nutricia Clinical)

Liquid, protein 10 g, carbohydrate 14.7 g, fat 3.5 g, energy 550 kJ (130 kcal)/100 mL, with vitamins, minerals and trace elements. Gluten-free. Chocolate, forest fruits, strawberry, and vanilla flavour, net price 200 mL = £1.54.

As a nutritional supplement prescribed on medical grounds for: short-bowel syndrome, intractable malabsorption, pre-operative preparation of undernourished patients, proven inflammatory bowel disease, following total gastrectomy, dysphagia, bowel fistulas, disease-related malnutrition. Not to be prescribed for any child under 6 years

Frebini® **Energy** (Fresenius Kabi)

Sip feed, protein 3.75 g, carbohydrate 18.8 g, fat 6.65 g, energy 630 kJ (150 kcal)/100 mL, with vitamins, minerals and trace elements. Gluten-free; clinically lactose-free. Flavours: banana or strawberry. Net price 200-mL carton = £2.16.

Tube feed, protein 3.75 g, carbohydrate 18.75 g, fat 6.7 g, energy 630 kJ (150 kcal)/100 mL, with vitamins, minerals and trace elements. Gluten-free; clinically lactose-free. Flavour: neutral, net price 500-mL EasyBag® = £5.70.

For use as a sole source of nutrition or as a nutritional supplement for children aged 1 to 10 years or 8–30kg with disease-related malnutrition and/or growth failure, proven inflammatory bowel disease, following total gastrectomy, short-bowel syndrome, intractable malabsorption, dysphagia, bowel fistulas, and for pre-operative preparation of malnourished patients. Not to be prescribed for any child under 1 year

Frebini® **Energy Fibre** (Fresenius Kabi)

Sip feed, protein 3.75 g, carbohydrate 18.8 g, fat 6.65 g, fibre 1.1 g, energy 630 kJ (150 kcal)/ 100 mL, with vitamins, minerals and trace elements. Gluten-free; clinically lactose-free. Chocolate flavour, net price 200-mL carton = £2.21.

Tube feed, protein 3.75 g, carbohydrate 18.75 g, fat 6.7 g, fibre 1.13 g, energy 630 kJ (150 kcal)/ 100 mL, with vitamins, minerals and trace elements. Gluten-free, clinically lactose-free. Flavour: neutral, net price 500-mL EasyBag® = £6.10.

For indications see *Frebini Energy*®

Frebini® **Original** (Fresenius Kabi)

Liquid, tube feed, protein 2.5 g, carbohydrate 13.5 g, fat 4 g, energy 420 kJ (100 kcal)/100 mL, with vitamins, minerals and trace elements. Flavour: neutral, net price 500-mL EasyBag® = £4.55

For use as the sole source of nutrition or as a nutritional supplement for children aged 1–10 years or 8–30 kg with short-bowel syndrome, intractable malabsorption, pre-operative preparation of patients who are undernourished, proven inflammatory bowel disease, following total gastrectomy, dysphagia, bowel fistulas, disease-related malnutrition and/or growth failure. Not to be prescribed for any child under 1 year

Frebini® Original Fibre (Fresenius Kabi)

Tube feed, protein 2.5 g, carbohydrate 12.5 g, fat 4.4 g, fibre 750 mg, energy 420 kJ (100 kcal)/100 mL, with vitamins, minerals and trace elements. Gluten-free, clinically lactose-free. Neutral flavour, net price 500-mL EasyBag® = £5.05

For use as a sole source of nutrition or as a nutritional supplement for children aged 1–10 years or 8–30 kg with disease-related malnutrition and/or growth failure, proven inflammatory bowel disease, following total gastrectomy, short-bowel syndrome, intractable malabsorption, dysphagia, bowel fistulas, and pre-operative preparation of malnourished patients. Not to be prescribed for any child under 1 year

Fresubin® Energy (Fresenius Kabi)

Liquid, protein 5.65 g, carbohydrate 18.8 g, fat 5.83 g, energy 630 kJ (150 kcal)/100 mL, with vitamins and minerals. Net price 200-mL carton = £1.55 (flavours: vanilla, strawberry, butterscotch, blackcurrant, banana, orange, pineapple, chocolate-mint, vegetable cream, and neutral): 500-mL bottle = £3.80 (flavour: neutral); 500-mL EasyBag® = £3.88; 1-litre EasyBag® = £7.70.

For use as sole source of nutrition or as a nutritional supplement prescribed on medical grounds for: short-bowel syndrome, intractable malabsorption, pre-operative preparation of undernourished patients, proven inflammatory bowel disease, following total gastrectomy, dysphagia, bowel fistulas, disease-related malnutrition. Not to be prescribed for any child under 1 year; use with caution for children under 5 years

Fresubin® Energy Fibre (Fresenius Kabi)

Sip feed, protein 5.65 g, carbohydrate 18.8 g, fat 5.83 g, fibre 2.5 g, energy 630 kJ (150 kcal)/100 mL, with vitamins, minerals and trace elements. Gluten-free; clinically lactose-free. Flavours: banana, cappucino, chocolate, lemon, strawberry, vanilla. Net price 200-mL carton = £1.70.

For indications see *Fresubin® Energy*

Tube feed, protein 5.6 g, carbohydrate 18.8 g, fat 5.8 g, fibre 2 g, energy 630 kJ (150 kcal)/100 mL, with vitamins, minerals and trace elements. Gluten-free; clinically lactose-free. Unflavoured, net price 500-mL EasyBag® = £4.00; 1-litre EasyBag® = £7.99.

For indications see *Fresubin® Energy*

Fresubin HP Energy® (Fresenius Kabi)

Liquid, protein 7.5 g, carbohydrate 17 g, fat 6 g, energy 630 kJ (150 kcal)/100 mL with vitamins, minerals, and trace elements. Gluten-free and low lactose. Vanilla flavour. Net price 500-mL bottle = £3.67; 500-mL EasyBag® = £3.72; 1-litre EasyBag® = £7.44.

As a nutritional supplement prescribed on medical grounds for: short-bowel syndrome, intractable malabsorption, pre-operative preparation of patients who are undernourished, proven inflammatory bowel disease, following total gastrectomy, dysphagia, bowel fistulas, disease-related malnutrition, continuous ambulatory peritoneal dialysis (CAPD), and haemodialysis. Not to be prescribed for any child under 1 year; use with caution for children up to 5 years

Fresubin® 1000 Complete (Fresenius Kabi)

Liquid, tube feed, protein 5.5 g, carbohydrate 12.5 g, fat 3.1 g, fibre 2 g, energy 420 kJ (100 kcal)/100mL with vitamins, minerals and trace elements. Gluten-free, clinically lactose-free, net price 1-litre EasyBag® = £8.20.

For use as the sole source of nutrition or as a nutritional supplement prescribed on medical grounds for: short-bowel syndrome, intractable malabsorption, pre-operative preparation of undernourished patients, proven inflammatory bowel disease, following total gastrectomy, dysphagia, bowel fistulas, disease-related malnutrition. Not to be prescribed for any child under 1 year; use with caution for children up to 5 years

Fresubin® 1200 Complete (Fresenius Kabi)

Liquid, tube feed, protein 4 g, carbohydrate 10 g, fat 2.7 g, fibre 2 g, energy 336 kJ (80 kcal)/100 mL with vitamins, minerals and trace elements. Gluten-free, clinically lactose-free, net price 1.5-litre EasyBag® = £10.20.

For use as the sole source of nutrition or as a nutritional supplement prescribed on medical grounds for: short-bowel syndrome, intractable malabsorption, pre-operative preparation of undernourished patients, proven inflammatory bowel disease, following total gastrectomy, bowel fistulas, disease-related malnutrition. Not to be prescribed for any child under 5 years

Fresubin® Original (Fresenius Kabi)

Liquid, protein 3.8 g, carbohydrate 13.8 g, fat 3.4 g, energy 420 kJ (100 kcal)/100 mL with vitamins and minerals. Gluten-free, low lactose and cholesterol. Net price 200-mL carton (nut, peach, blackcurrant, chocolate, mocha, and vanilla flavours) = £1.55; 500-mL bottle (neutral flavour) = £3.08; 500-mL EasyBag® = £2.99; 1-litre EasyBag® = £5.97; 1.5-litre EasyBag® = £8.96

For use as the sole source of nutrition or as a nutritional supplement prescribed on medical grounds for: short-bowel syndrome, intractable malabsorption, pre-operative preparation of patients who are undernourished, proven inflammatory bowel disease, following total gastrectomy, dysphagia, bowel fistulas, disease-related malnutrition, and Refsum's disease. Not to be prescribed for any child under 1 year; use with caution for children up to 5 years

Fresubin® Original Fibre (Fresenius Kabi)

Liquid with dietary fibre, protein 3.8 g, carbohydrate 13.8 g, fat 3.4 g, energy 420 kJ (100 kcal)/100 mL, with vitamins and minerals. Flavour: neutral. Net price 500-mL bottle = £3.48; 500-mL EasyBag® = £3.62; 1-litre EasyBag® = £7.24; 1.5-litre EasyBag® = £10.20.

For use as sole source of nutrition or as a nutritional supplement prescribed on medical grounds for: short-bowel syndrome, intractable malabsorption, pre-operative preparation of patients who are undernourished, proven inflammatory bowel disease, following total gastrectomy, dysphagia, disease-related malnutrition. Not to be prescribed for any child under 2 years; use with caution for children up to 5 years

Fresubin Protein Energy Drink (Fresenius Kabi)

Liquid, protein 10 g, carbohydrate 12.4 g, fat 6.7 g, energy 630 kJ (150 kcal)/100 mL, with vitamins, minerals and trace elements. Gluten- and lactose-free. Chocolate, strawberry, and vanilla flavours, net price 200-mL = £1.58.

As a necessary nutritional supplement prescribed on medical grounds for: short-bowel syndrome, intractable malabsorption, pre-operative preparation of undernourished patients, proven inflammatory bowel disease, following total gastrectomy, dysphagia, bowel fistulas, disease-related malnutrition, continuous ambulatory peritoneal dialysis (CAPD), haemodialysis. Not to be prescribed for any child under 1 year; use with caution for children up to 5 years of age

Fructose
(Laevulose)
For proven glucose/galactose intolerance

Gadsby's
Gluten-free. White bread flour, net price 1 kg = £4.99. White sliced bread, 400 g = £2.50. White bread rolls, 4 × 75 g = £2.00
For established gluten enteropathy

Galactomin® 17 (SHS)
Powder, protein 14.5 g, fat 25.9 g, carbohydrate 56.9 g, mineral salts 3.4 g/100 g. Used as a 13.1% solution with additional vitamins in place of milk. Net price 400 g = £11.48.
For proven lactose intolerance in preschool children, galactosaemia and galactokinase deficiency

Galactomin® 19 (SHS)
Powder, protein 14.6 g, fat 30.8 g, carbohydrate 49.7 g (fructose as carbohydrate source), mineral salts 2.1 g/100 g, with vitamins. Used as a 12.9% solution in place of milk. Net price 400 g = £30.24.
For glucose plus galactose intolerance

Generaid® (SHS)
Powder, whey protein and additional branched-chain amino acids (protein equivalent 81%). Net price 200 g (unflavoured) = £20.92. See also Flavour Sachets.
For patients with chronic liver disease and/or porto-hepatic encephalopathy

Generaid Plus® (SHS)
Powder, whey protein and additional branched-chain amino acids (protein equivalent 11%) carbohydrate 62%, fat 19% with vitamins, minerals and trace elements. Net price 400 g = £14.96.
For children over 1 year with hepatic disorders

Glucose
(Dextrose monohydrate)
Net price 100 g = 39p.
For glycogen storage disease and sucrose/isomaltose intolerance

Glutafin® (Nutricia Dietary)
Gluten-free. Biscuits, savoury, 125 g = £1.70; 150 g = £2.32. Biscuits, digestive, sweet or tea, 150 g = £1.70. Biscuits, 200 g = £3.31. Biscuits, shortbread, 100 g = £1.40. Cake mix, 500 g = £5.31. Crackers, 200 g = £2.76. High fibre crackers, 200 g = £2.31. Pasta (penne, shells, spirals, spaghetti), 500 g = £5.36; (lasagne, tagliatelle), 250 g = £2.81. Pizza bases, 2 × 110 g = £3.83.
Select Gluten-free. Fibre loaf (sliced or unsliced), 400 g = £2.73; part-baked, 400 g = £3.06. Fresh Bread, white loaf, (sliced), 400 g = £2.94 Seeded loaf, 400 g = £2.97. White loaf (sliced or unsliced), 400 g = £2.73; part-baked, 400 g = £3.06. Fibre rolls, 4 = £3.06; (part-baked), 4 = £2.97; long, 2 = £3.06. White rolls, 4 = £2.76; (part-baked), 4 = £3.06; long, 2 = £3.06. Mixes (bread, cake, fibre, fibre bread, pastry, and white), 500 g = £5.31
For gluten-sensitive enteropathies including steatorrhoea due to gluten sensitivity, coeliac disease, and dermatitis herpetiformis
Gluten-free, wheat-free, crisp bread, 2 × 125 g = £3.61; crisp roll, 220 g = £3.72. Fibre loaf (sliced or unsliced), 400 g = £2.73. Fibre rolls, 4 = £2.97. White loaf (sliced or unsliced), 400 g = £3.06. White rolls, 4 = £2.97. Mixes (fibre bread, bread, white or fibre), 500 g = £5.31; cake or pastry mix, 500 g = £5.31.
For gluten-sensitive enteropathy with co-existing established wheat sensitivity

Glutano® (Gluten Free Foods Ltd)
Gluten-free, wheat-free. Tea biscuits, net price 125 g = £1.58; wheat-free digestive biscuit, 200 g = £1.58. Shortcake rings, 125 g = £1.12. Crispbread, 125 g = £1.58. Crackers, 150 g = £1.58. Flour mix, 750 g = £4.12. Pasta (animal shapes, spaghetti, spirals, tagliatelle), 250 g = £1.58; macaroni, 500 g = £3.16. White sliced bread (par-baked), 300 g = £1.86. Wholemeal bread (sliced), 500 g = £2.24. Baguette or rolls (par-baked), 200 g = £1.49.
For gluten-sensitive enteropathies including steatorrhoea due to gluten sensitivity, coeliac disease, and dermatitis herpetiformis

HCU Express® (Vitaflo)
Powder, protein (essential and non-essential amino acids except methionine) 15 g, carbohydrate 3.8 g, fat 0.03 g, energy 315 kJ (75.3 kcal)/25 g with vitamins, minerals and trace elements. Unflavoured, net price 30 × 25- g sachets = £225.00
A methionine-free protein substitute for use as a nutritional supplement in patients over 8 years of age with homocystinuria

HCU-gel® (Vitaflo)
Powder, protein (essential and non-essential amino acids except methionine) 10.1 g, carbohydrate 8.6 g, fat 0.03 g, energy 285.5 kJ (68 kcal)/20 g with vitamins, minerals and trace elements. Unflavoured, net price 30 × 20- g sachets = £129.50
For the dietary management of homocystinuria in children between 12 months and 10 years of age

InfaSoy® (Cow & Gate)
Powder, carbohydrate 7.1%, fat 3.6%, and protein 1.8% with vitamins and minerals when used as a 12.7% solution. Net price 450 g = £3.77; 900 g = £7.23.
For proven lactose and associated sucrose intolerance in preschool children, galactokinase deficiency, galactosaemia, and proven whole cow's milk sensitivity

Infatrini® (Nutricia Clinical)
Liquid, protein 2.6 g, carbohydrate 10.3 g, fat 5.4 g, energy 420 kJ (100 kcal)/100 mL with vitamins, minerals and trace elements. Gluten-free. Net price 100 mL = 88p, 200-mL Tetrapak® = £1.75
For use as a sole source of nutrition or as a nutritional supplement prescribed on medical grounds for: failure to thrive, disease-related malnutrition and malabsorption. Manufacturer advises suitable for infants between 1–8 kg body weight

Instant Carobel®
see **Carobel, Instant®**

Isomil® (Abbott)
Powder, protein 1.8%, carbohydrate 6.9%, fat 3.7% with vitamins and minerals when reconstituted. Lactose-free. Net price 400 g = £3.38.
For proven lactose intolerance in preschool children, galactokinase deficiency, galactosaemia, and proven whole cow's milk sensitivity

Isosource® Energy (Novartis Consumer Health)
Liquid, protein 5.7 g, carbohydrate 20 g, fat 6.2 g, energy 660 kJ (160 kcal)/100 mL with vitamins, minerals and trace elements. Gluten-free; clinically lactose-free. Net price 500-mL flexible pouch = £3.72, 1-litre flexible pouch = £7.44.
For indications see *Isosource Standard*

Isosource® Energy Fibre (Novartis Consumer Health)
Liquid, tube feed, protein 4.9 g, carbohydrate 20.2 g, fat 5.5 g, fibre, 1.5 g, energy 630 kJ (150 kcal)/100 mL with vitamins, minerals and trace elements. Gluten-free; clinically lactose-free. Net price 500-mL flexible pouch = £4.04, 1-litre flexible pouch = £8.08.
For use as the sole source of nutrition or as a nutritional supplement prescribed on medical grounds for: short-bowel syndrome, intractable malabsorption, pre-operative preparation of undernourished patients, proven inflammatory bowel disease, following total

gastrectomy, dysphagia, disease-related malnutrition. Not to be prescribed for any child under 1 year; use with caution for children up to 5 years

Isosource® Fibre (Novartis Consumer Health)

Liquid, protein 3.8 g, carbohydrate 13.6 g, fat 3.4 g, fibre 1.4 g, energy 422 kJ (100 kcal)/100 mL with vitamins, minerals and trace elements. Gluten-free; clinically lactose-free. Net price 500-mL flexible pouch = £3.45, 1-litre flexible pouch = £6.90.

For indications see *Isosource Standard*

Isosource® Junior (Novartis Consumer Health)

Liquid, protein 2.7 g, carbohydrate 17 g, fat 4.7 g, energy 512 kJ (122 kcal)/100 mL with vitamins, minerals and trace elements. Gluten-free; clinically lactose-free. Net price 500-mL flexible pouch = £5.17.

Nutritionally complete feed for disease-related malnutrition, short-bowel syndrome, intractable malabsorption, pre-operative preparation of undernourished patients, proven inflammatory bowel disease, following total gastrectomy, dysphagia, bowel fistulas, growth failure, for children aged 1 to 6 years or 8 to 20 kg

Isosource® Standard (Novartis Consumer Health)

Liquid, protein 4.1 g, carbohydrate 14.2 g, fat 3.5 g, energy 441 kJ (105 kcal)/100 mL with vitamins, minerals and trace elements. Gluten-free; clinically lactose-free. Net price 500-mL flexible pouch = £3.03, 1-litre flexible pouch = £6.06.

For use as a sole source of nutrition or as a nutritional supplement prescribed on medical grounds for: short-bowel syndrome, intractable malabsorption, pre-operative preparation of undernourished patients, proven inflammatory bowel disease, following total gastrectomy, dysphagia, bowel fistulas, disease-related malnutrition. Not to be prescribed for any child under 1 year; use with caution for children up to 5 years

Jevity® (Abbott)

Liquid, protein 4 g, fat 3.5 g, carbohydrate 14.8 g, dietary fibre 1.1 g, energy 441 kJ (106 kcal)/ 100 mL, with vitamins and minerals. Gluten-, lactose-, and sucrose-free. Net price 500-mL ready-to-hang = £3.53, 1-litre ready-to-hang = £6.82, 1.5-litre ready-to-hang = £10.23.

For use as the sole source of nutrition or as a nutritional supplement prescribed on medical grounds for: short-bowel syndrome, intractable malabsorption, pre-operative preparation of patients who are undernourished, proven inflammatory bowel disease, bowel fistulas, following total gastrectomy, dysphagia, disease-related malnutrition. Not to be prescribed for any child under 2 years; use with caution for children up to 5 years

Jevity 1.5 kcal® (Abbott)

Liquid, tube feed, protein 6.38 g, carbohydrate 21.1 g, fat 4.9 g, fibre 1.2 g, energy 640 kJ (152 kcal)/100 mL, with vitamins, minerals and trace elements. Gluten- and lactose-free. Net price 500-mL ready-to-hang = £4.42, 1-litre ready-to-hang = £8.20, 1.5-litre ready-to-hang = £12.80.

For use as the sole source of nutrition or as a nutritional supplement prescribed on medical grounds for: short-bowel syndrome, intractable malabsorption, pre-operative preparation of undernourished patients, proven inflammatory bowel disease, bowel fistulas, following total gastrectomy, dysphagia, disease-related malnutrition. Not to be prescribed for any child under 2 years; use with caution for children up to 10 years

Jevity Plus® (Abbott)

Liquid, protein 5.6 g, carbohydrate 16.1 g, fat 3.9 g, dietary fibre 1.2 g, energy 504 kJ (120 kcal)/ 100 mL, with vitamins and minerals. Gluten- and lactose-free. Net price 500-mL ready-to-hang = £4.00, 1-litre ready-to-hang = £8.18, 1.5-litre ready-to-hang = £12.28.

For indications see under *Jevity®*.

Juvela® (SHS)

Gluten-free. Harvest mix, fibre mix, and flour mix, net price 500 g = £5.47. Bread (whole or sliced), 400-g loaf = £2.72; part-baked loaf (with or without fibre), 400g = £2.83. Fibre bread (sliced and unsliced), 400-g loaf = £2.64. Bread rolls, 5 × 85 g = £3.56, fibre bread rolls, 5 × 85 g = £3.56, part-baked rolls (with or without fibre), 5 × 75 g = £3.67. Crispbread, 210 g = £3.45. Pasta (fusilli, macaroni, spaghetti), 500 g = £5.36; lasagne, 250 g = £2.47. Pizza bases, 2 × 180 g = £6.53. Digestive biscuits, 160 g = £2.27. Savoury biscuits, 150 g = £2.84. Tea biscuits, 160 g = £2.27.

For gluten-sensitive enteropathies including steatorrhoea due to gluten sensitivity, coeliac disease, and dermatitis herpetiformis

Low Protein. Mix, net price 500 g = £5.81. Bread (whole or sliced), 400-g loaf = £2.72. Bread rolls, 5 × 70 g = £3.38. Biscuits, orange and cinnamon flavour, 125 g = £5.68; chocolate chip, 130 g = £4.89.

For inherited metabolic disorders, renal or liver failure requiring a low-protein diet

Kindergen® (SHS)

Powder, protein 7.5 g, carbohydrate 60.5 g, fat 26.1 g, energy 2060 kJ (492 kcal)/100 g with vitamins and minerals. Net price 400 g = £19.86.

For complete nutritional support or supplementary feeding for infants and children with chronic renal failure who are receiving peritoneal rapid overnight dialysis

Leucine-Free Amino Acid Mix

see Amino Acid Modules, Xleu Faladon

Lifestyle® (Ultrapharm)

Gluten-free. Brown bread (sliced and unsliced), net price 400 g = £2.63. White bread (sliced and unsliced), 400 g = £2.63. High fibre bread (unsliced), 400 g = £2.63. Bread rolls, 400 g = £2.63.

For gluten-sensitive enteropathies including steatorrhoea due to gluten sensitivity, coeliac disease, and dermatitis herpetiformis

Liquigen® (SHS)

Emulsion, medium chain triglycerides 52%. Net price 250 mL = £6.34; 1 litre = £26.60.

For steatorrhoea associated with cystic fibrosis of the pancreas; intestinal lymphangiectasia, surgery of the intestine; chronic liver disease and liver cirrhosis; other proven malabsorption syndromes; ketogenic diet in the management of epilepsy; type I hyperlipoproteinaemia

Locasol® (SHS)

Powder, protein 14.6 g, carbohydrate 56.5 g, fat 26.1 g, mineral salts 1.9 g, not more than 55 mg of Ca^{2+}/100 g and vitamins. Used as a 13.1% solution in place of milk. Net price 400 g = £15.96.

For calcium intolerance

Lophlex® (SHS)

Powder, protein (containing essential and non-essential amino acids, phenylalanine-free) 20 g, carbohydrate 1.4 g, fat 60 mg, fibre 220 mg, energy 366 kJ (86 kcal)/27.8 g with vitamins, minerals, and trace elements. Flavours: berry, orange or unflavoured, net price 30 x 27.8-g sachets = £198.00.

For use in the dietary management of proven phenylketonuria in older children (over 8 years) and adults (includes use in pregnant women)

Loprofin® (SHS)

Low protein. Sweet biscuits, net price 150 g = £1.82; chocolate cream-filled biscuits, 125 g = £1.82; cookies (chocolate chip or cinnamon), 100 g = £4.82; wafers (orange, vanilla, or chocolate), 100 g = £1.76. Breakfast cereal, 375 g = £5.65. Egg replacer, 500 g = £10.59. Egg-white replacer, 100 g = £6.82. Bread (sliced or whole), 400-g loaf = £2.72. Rolls (part-baked) 4 × 65 g = £2.86. Mix, 500 g = £5.78. Crackers, 150 g = £2.48. Herb crackers, 150 g = £2.48. Pasta (lasagne, macaroni, pasta spirals, spaghetti), 500 g = £6.03. Pasta (vermicelli), 250 g = £3.00. Snack Pot, 47 g = £3.20.

For inherited metabolic disorders, renal or liver failure requiring a low-protein diet

PKU Drink, protein 0.4 g (phenylalanine 10 mg), lactose 9.4 g, fat 2 g, energy 165 kJ (40 kcal)/ 100 mL. Net price 200-mL Tetrapak® = 52p.

For phenylketonuria

Low protein drink (Milupa)

Powder, protein 0.4%, carbohydrate 5.1%, fat 2% when reconstituted. Net price 400 g = £7.23.

For inherited disorders of amino acid metabolism in childhood

NOTE. Termed *Milupa® lpd* by manufacturer

Mapleflex® (SHS)

Powder, essential and non-essential amino acids 35% except isoleucine, leucine, and valine, with carbohydrate 38%, fat 13.5%, vitamins, minerals, and trace elements. Unflavoured. Net price 30 × 29-g sachets = £142.10.

For maple syrup urine disease in children aged 1–10 years

Maxamaid® (SHS)

see *MSUD Maxamaid, XLEU Maxamaid, XLYS Maxamaid, XLYS Low TRY Maxamaid, XMET Maxamaid, XMTVI Maxamaid, XP Maxamaid, XP Maxamaid Concentrate, XPHEN TYR Maxamaid*

NOTE. Maxamaid products are generally intended for use in children aged 1 to 8 years, see also Flavour Sachets, for use with unflavoured amino acid and peptide products from SHS

Maxamum® (SHS)

see *MSUD Maxamum, XMET Maxamum, XMTVI Maxamum, XP Maxamum*

NOTE. Maxamum products are generally intended for use in children over 8 years

Maxijul® (SHS)

Liquid, carbohydrate 50%, with potassium 0.004%, sodium 0.023%. Gluten-, lactose-, and fructose-free. Flavours: blackcurrant, lemon and lime, orange, and natural. Net price 200 mL = £1.12

LE Powder, modification of *Maxijul*® with lower concentrations of sodium and potassium. Net price 200 g = £3.82, 2 kg = £26.62

Super Soluble Powder, glucose polymer, potassium 0.004%, sodium 0.046%. Gluten-, lactose-, and fructose-free. Net price 4 × 132-g sachet pack = £4.41, 200 g = £1.78, 2.5 kg = £15.66, 25 kg = £106.35

All for disease-related malnutrition; malabsorption states or other conditions requiring fortification with high or readily available carbohydrate supplement

Maxipro Super Soluble® (SHS)

Powder, whey protein and additional amino acids (protein equivalent 80%). Net price 200 g = £8.64; 1 kg = £34.66.

For biochemically proven hypoproteinaemia. Not to be prescribed for any child under 1 year; unsuitable as a sole source of nutrition

Maxisorb® (SHS)

Powder, protein 12 g, carbohydrate 9 g, fat 6 g, energy 579 kJ (138 kcal)/30 g with minerals. Vanilla, strawberry and chocolate flavours. Net price 5 × 30-g sachets = £3.63.

For biochemically proven hypoproteinaemia. Not to be prescribed for any child under 1 year; use with caution for children up to 5 years

MCT Oil

Triglycerides from medium chain fatty acids. For steatorrhoea associated with cystic fibrosis of the pancreas; intestinal lymphangiectasia; surgery of the intestine; chronic liver disease and liver cirrhosis; other proven malabsorption syndromes; in a ketogenic diet in the management of epilepsy; in type I hyperlipoproteinaemia

Available from Mead Johnson (net price 950 mL = £12.18); SHS (net price 500 mL = £9.79)

MCT Pepdite® (SHS)

Powder, essential and non-essential amino acids, peptides, medium chain triglycerides, monoglyceride of sunflower oil, with carbohydrate, fat, vitamins, minerals, and trace elements. Flavour Sachets available.

MCT Pepdite. Net price 400 g = £13.96

MCT Pepdite 1+. Net price 400 g = £13.96

Both for disorders in which a high intake of medium chain triglyceride is beneficial

Metabolic Mineral Mixture® (SHS)

Powder, essential mineral salts. Net price 100 g = £8.67.

For mineral supplementation in synthetic diets

Methionine-Free Amino Acid Mix

see Amino Acid Modules, XMET Homidon

Methionine, Threonine, Valine-Free and Isoleucine-Low Amino Acid Mix

see Amino Acid Modules, XMTVI Asadon

Milupa® lpd

see under Low Protein Drink

Milupa® PKU2 and PKU3

see under PKU2 and PKU3

Modulen IBD® (Nestlé)

Powder, protein 18 g, carbohydrate 54 g, fat 23 g, energy 2040 kJ (500 kcal)/100 g with vitamins, minerals and trace elements. Net price 400 g = £9.72.

For use as the sole source of nutrition during the active phase of Crohn's disease and for nutritional support during the remission phase in patients who are malnourished. Not to be prescribed for any child under one year; use with caution for children up to 5 years

May be flavoured with Nestlé Nutrition Flavour Mix (see under *Peptamen*)

Monogen® (SHS)

Powder, protein 11.4 g, carbohydrate 68 g, fat 11.4 g (of which MCT 93%), energy 1772 kJ (420 kcal)/100 g, with vitamins, minerals and trace elements. Net price 400 g = £13.89.

For long-chain acyl-CoA dehydrogenase deficiency (LCAD), carnitine palmitoyl transferase deficiency (CPTD), primary and secondary lipoprotin lipase deficiency

MSUD Aid III® (SHS)

Powder, containing full range of amino acids except isoleucine, leucine, and valine, with vitamins, minerals, and trace elements. Net price 500 g = £127.20.

For maple syrup urine disease and related conditions where it is necessary to limit the intake of branched chain amino acids

MSUD Analog (SHS)
Powder, essential and non-essential amino acids 15.5% except isoleucine, leucine and valine, with carbohydrate, fat, vitamins, minerals, and trace elements. Net price 400 g = £24.62.
For maple syrup urine disease
NOTE. Analog products are generally intended for use in children up to 1 year, see also Flavour Sachets, for use with unflavoured amino acid and peptide products from SHS

MSUD Maxamaid® (SHS)
Powder, essential and non-essential amino acids 30% except isoleucine, leucine, and valine, with carbohydrate, fat less than 0.5%, vitamins, minerals, and trace elements. Net price 500 g = £67.15.
For maple syrup urine disease
NOTE. Maxamaid products are generally intended for use in children aged 1 to 8 years, see also Flavour Sachets, for use with unflavoured amino acid and peptide products from SHS

MSUD Maxamum® (SHS)
Powder, essential and non-essential amino acids 47% except isoleucine, leucine, and valine, with carbohydrate, fat less than 0.5%, vitamins, minerals, and trace elements. Flavours: orange, unflavoured, see also Flavour Sachets. Net price 500 g = £107.65.
For maple syrup urine disease
NOTE. Maxamum products are generally intended for use in children over 8 years

Neocate® (SHS)
Powder, essential and non-essential amino acids, maltodextrin, fat, vitamins, minerals, and trace elements. Net price 400 g = £19.98.
For proven whole protein intolerance, short-bowel syndrome, intractable malabsorption, and other gastro-intestinal disorders where an elemental diet is specifically indicated; for use in children under 1 year

Neocate Advance® (SHS)
Powder, essential and non-essential amino acids, carbohydrate, fat, vitamins, minerals and trace elements. Milk protein-, soy- and lactose-free. Net price 100 g = £4.10; banana-vanilla flavour 15 x 50 g = £33.24.
For proven whole protein intolerance, short-bowel syndrome, intractable malabsorption, and other gastro-intestinal disorders where an elemental diet is specifically indicated; for use in children over 1 year

Nepro® (Abbott)
Liquid, protein 7 g, carbohydrate 20.6 g, fat 9.6 g, energy 840 kJ (200 kcal)/100 mL with vitamins and minerals. Net price 237-mL can = £2.28; 500–mL ready-to-hang = £4.81.
For patients with chronic renal failure who are on haemodialysis or continuous ambulatory peritoneal dialysis (CAPD), or patients with cirrhosis or other conditions requiring a high energy, low fluid, low electrolyte diet

Nestargel® (Nestlé)
Powder, carob seed flour 96.5%, calcium lactate 3.5%. Net price 125 g = £2.99.
For thickening feeds in the treatment of vomiting

Novasource® **Forte** (Novartis Consumer Health)
Liquid, protein 6 g, carbohydrate 18.3 g, fat 5.9 g, fibre 2.2 g, energy 631 kJ (150 kcal)/100 mL with vitamins, minerals and trace elements. Gluten-free; low-lactose, net price 500-mL flexible pouch = £4.36.
For use as a sole source of nutrition or as a nutritional supplement prescribed on medical grounds for: short-bowel syndrome, intractable malabsorption, pre-operative preparation of undernourished patients, proven inflammatory bowel disease, following total gastrectomy, dysphagia, bowel fistulas, disease-related malnutrition, neoplasia-related cachexia. Not to be prescribed for any child under 1 year; use with caution for children up to 5 years

Novasource GI Control® (Novartis Consumer Health)
Liquid, protein 4.1 g, carbohydrate 14.2 g, fat 3.5 g, fibre 2.2 g, energy 440 kJ (100 kcal)/100 mL with vitamins minerals and trace elements. Gluten-free; clinically lactose-free, net price 500-mL bottle = £4.39, 500-mL flexible pouch = £4.70.
For use as a sole source of nutrition or as a nutritional supplement prescribed on medical grounds for: short-bowel syndrome, intractable malabsorption, pre-operative preparation of undernourished patients, proven inflammatory bowel disease, following total gastrectomy, dysphagia, bowel fistulas, disease-related malnutrition. Not to be prescribed for any child under 1 year; use with caution for children up to 5 years

Nutilis® (Nutricia Clinical)
Powder, modified maize starch, gluten- and lactose-free. Net price 225 g = £3.88.
For thickening of foods in dysphagia. Not to be prescribed for children under 3 years

Nutramigen® **1** (Mead Johnson)
Powder, protein 1.9 g, carbohydrate 7.5 g, fat 3.4 g, energy 280 kJ (68 kcal)/100 mL with vitamins and minerals. Gluten-, sucrose-, and lactose-free. Net price 400 g = £7.81.
For disaccharide and/or whole protein intolerance where additional medium chain triglyceride is not indicated

Nutramigen® **2** (Mead Johnson)
Powder, protein 2.3 g, carbohydrate 7.8 g, fat 3.5 g energy 301 kJ (72 kcal) per 100 mL when normal dilution used, with vitamins, minerals and trace elements. Gluten-, sucrose-, and lactose-free, net price 425 g = £7.81.
For disaccharide and/or whole protein intolerance where additional medium chain triglyceride is not indicated. Not suitable for infants under 6 months

Nutrini® (Nutricia Clinical)
Liquid, protein 2.75 g, carbohydrate 12.3 g, fat 4.4 g, energy 420 kJ (100 kcal)/100 mL. Gluten- and sucrose-free; clinically lactose-free. Net price 200-mL bottle = £1.93, 500-mL flexible pack = £4.83.
For use as the sole source of nutrition or as a nutritional supplement prescribed on medical grounds for: short-bowel syndrome, intractable malabsorption, pre-operative preparation of undernourished patients, dysphagia, bowel fistulas, disease-related malnutrition and/or growth failure. For children between 8–20 kg body-weight

Nutrini® **Energy** (Nutricia Clinical)
Liquid, protein 4.1 g, carbohydrate 18.5 g, fat 6.7 g, energy 630 kJ (150 kcal)/100 mL. Gluten- and sucrose-free; clinically lactose-free. Net price 200-mL bottle = £2.38, 500-mL collapsible pack = £5.95.
For use as the sole source of nutrition or as a nutritional supplement prescribed on medical grounds for: disease-related malnutrition and growth failure

Nutrini® **Energy Multi Fibre** (Nutricia Clinical)
Liquid, tube feed, protein 4.1 g, carbohydrate 18.5 g, fat 6.7 g, fibre 0.75 g, energy 630 kJ (150 kcal)/100 mL with vitamins, minerals and trace elements. Gluten- and lactose-free, net price 200-mL bottle = £2.58, 500-mL pack = £6.44.
For short-bowel syndrome, intractable malabsorption, pre-operative preparation of undernourished patients, total gastrectomy, dysphagia, disease-related malnutrition, and growth failure. Not to be prescribed for any child under 1 year

Nutrini® Low Energy Multi Fibre (Nutricia Clinical)

Liquid, tube feed, protein 1.7 g, carbohydrate 10.4 g, fat 3 g, fibre 0.75 g, energy 315 kJ (75 kcal)/ 100 mL with vitamins, minerals and trace elements. Gluten- and lactose-free, net price 200-mL bottle = £1.87, 500-mL pack = £4.71

For indications see *Nutrini Energy Multi Fibre*

Nutrini® Multi Fibre (Nutricia Clinical)

Liquid, protein 2.75 g, carbohydrate 12.3 g, fat 4.4 g, fibre 750 mg, energy 420 kJ (100 kcal)/ 100 mL. Gluten- and sucrose-free; clinically lactose-free. Net price 200-mL bottle = £2.14, 500-mL collapsible pack = £5.35.

For indications see *Nutrini Liquid*

Nutriprem 2® (Cow & Gate)

Powder, protein 2 g, carbohydrate 7.4 g, fat 4.1 g, energy 310 kJ (75 kcal) per 100 mL when reconstituted, with vitamins and minerals. Net price 900 g = £8.80.

For catch-up growth in pre-term infants (less than 35 weeks at birth), and small-for-gestational-age infants, until 6 months corrected age

Nutrison® Energy (Nutricia Clinical)

Liquid, protein 6 g, carbohydrate 18.4 g, fat 5.8 g, energy 640 kJ (150 kcal)/100 mL with vitamins, minerals and trace elements. Gluten- and sucrose-free; clinically lactose-free. Net price 500-mL bottle = £3.77; 500-mL pack = £4.04; 1-litre pack = £7.55; 1.5-litre pack = £11.32.

As a nutritional supplement prescribed on medical grounds for: short-bowel syndrome, intractable malabsorption, pre-operative preparation of undernourished patients, proven inflammatory bowel disease, following total gastrectomy, dysphagia, bowel fistulas, disease-related malnutrition. Not to be prescribed for any child under 1 year; use with caution for children up to 5 years

Nutrison® Energy Multi Fibre (Nutricia Clinical)

Liquid, protein 6 g, carbohydrate 18.5 g, fat 5.8 g, fibre 1.5 g, energy 630 kJ (150 kcal)/100 mL with vitamins, minerals, and trace elements. Gluten-free and clinically lactose-free. Net price 500-mL bottle = £4.20; 500-mL pack = £4.48; 1-litre pack = £8.39; 1.5-litre pack = £13.45.

For use as the sole source of nutrition or as a nutritional supplement prescribed on medical grounds for: short-bowel syndrome, intractable malabsorption, pre-operative preparation of undernourished patients, proven inflammatory bowel disease, following total gastrectomy, dysphagia, disease-related malnutrition. Not to be prescribed for any child under 1 year; use with caution for children up to 6 years

Nutrison MCT® (Nutricia Clinical)

Liquid, protein 5 g, carbohydrate 12.3 g, fat 3.3 g, energy 419 kJ (100 kcal)/100 mL with vitamins, minerals and trace elements. Gluten- and fructose-free, clinically lactose-free. Vanilla flavour. Net price 1-litre pack = £7.05.

For indications see *Nutrison Energy*. Not to be prescribed for any child under 1 year; use with caution for children up to 5 years

Nutrison® Multi Fibre (Nutricia Clinical)

Liquid, protein 4 g, carbohydrate 12.3 g, fat 3.9 g, fibre 1.5 g, energy 420 kJ (100 kcal)/100 mL with vitamins, minerals and trace elements. Gluten- and sucrose-free; clinically lactose-free. Net price 500-mL bottle = £3.40; 500-mL pack = £3.63; 1-litre pack = £6.79; 1.5-litre pack = £10.19.

For indications see *Nutrison Standard* excluding bowel fistulas. Not to be prescribed for any child under 1 year; use with caution for children up to 5 years

Nutrison® Protein Plus (Nutricia Clinical)

Liquid, protein 6.3 g, carbohydrate 14.2 g, fat 4.9 g, energy 525 kJ (125 kcal)/100 mL, with vitamins, minerals and trace elements. Gluten- and lactose-free. Net price l-litre pack = £7.45.

For use in the dietary management of disease-related malnutrition. Not suitable for infants under 1 year; use with caution in children aged 1 to 6 years

Nutrison® Protein Plus Multi Fibre (Nutricia Clinical)

Liquid, protein 6.3 g, carbohydrate 14.2 g, fat 4.9 g, fibre 1.5 g, energy 525 kJ (125 kcal)/100 mL, with vitamins, minerals and trace elements. Gluten- and lactose-free. Net price l-litre pack = £8.29.

For use in the dietary management of disease-related malnutrition. Not suitable for infants under 1 year; use with caution in children aged 1 to 6 years

Nutrison® Soya (Nutricia Clinical)

Liquid, protein 4 g, carbohydrate 12.3 g, fat 3.9 g, energy 420 kJ (100 kcal)/100 mL, with vitamins, minerals and trace elements. Gluten- and sucrose-free; clinically lactose-free. Net price 500-mL bottle = £3.75; 1-litre pack = £7.50.

For indications see *Nutrison Standard*

Nutrison® Standard (Nutricia Clinical)

Liquid, protein 4 g, carbohydrate 12.3 g, fat 3.9 g, energy 425 kJ (100 kcal)/100 mL, with vitamins, minerals and trace elements. Gluten- and sucrose-free; clinically lactose-free. Net price 500-mL bottle = £3.12; 500-mL pack = £3.36; 1-litre pack = £6.09; 1.5-litre pack = £9.14.

For use as the sole source of nutrition or as a nutritional supplement prescribed on medical grounds for: short-bowel syndrome, intractable malabsorption, pre-operative preparation of undernourished patients, proven inflammatory bowel disease, following total gastrectomy, dysphagia, bowel fistulas, disease-related malnutrition. Not to be prescribed for any child under 1 year; use with caution for children up to 5 years

Nutrison® Vitaplus Multi Fibre (Nutricia Clinical)

Liquid, protein 5.5 g, carbohydrate 15 g, fat 4.3 g, energy 505 kJ (120 kcal)/100 mL, with vitamins, minerals and trace elements. Gluten- and lactose-free, net price 500-mL bottle = £4.03; l-litre pack = £8.05; 1.5-litre pack = £12.08.

As a nutritional supplement prescribed on medical grounds for: short-bowel syndrome, intractable malabsorption, pre-operative preparation of undernourished patients, proven inflammatory bowel disease, following total gastrectomy, dysphagia, disease-related malnutrition. Not to be prescribed for any child under 1 year; use with caution for children up to 5 years

Orgran® (Community)

Gluten-free. Pasta: lasagne (corn, rice and maize), 150 g = £2.89; shells (split pea and soya), 200 g = £2.25; spaghetti (corn, rice, rice and maize), 250 g = £2.25; spirals (buckwheat, corn, rice, rice and millet, rice and maize), 250 g = £2.25, spirals (organic brown rice), 250 g = £2.60. Crispbread (corn or rice), 200 g = £2.39. Pizza and pastry mix, 375 g = £3.33.

For gluten-sensitive enteropathies including steatorrhoea due to gluten sensitivity, coeliac disease, and dermatitis herpetiformis

Osmolite® (Abbott)

Liquid, protein 4 g, carbohydrate 13.56 g, fat 3.4 g, energy 424 kJ (100 kcal)/100 mL with vitamins and minerals. Gluten- and lactose-free. Net price 250-mL can = £1.69; 500-mL bottle = £3.10, 1-litre bottle = £5.99, 1.5-litre bottle = £8.99.

For use as the sole source of nutrition or as a nutritional supplement prescribed on medical grounds for: short-bowel syndrome, intractable malabsorption, pre-operative preparation of undernourished patients, proven inflammatory bowel disease, following total gastrectomy, bowel fistulas, disease-related malnutrition, dysphagia. Not to be prescribed for any child under 1 year; use with caution for children up to 5 years

Osmolite Plus® (Abbott)

Liquid, protein 5.6 g, carbohydrate 15.8 g, fat 3.9 g, energy 508 kJ (121 kcal)/100 mL with vitamins, minerals and trace elements. Gluten-free and clinically lactose-free. Net price 500-mL ready-to-hang = £3.73, 1-litre ready-to-hang = £7.20, 1.5-litre ready-to-hang = £10.79.

For indications see *Osmolite*

Paediasure® (Abbott)

Liquid, protein 2.8 g, carbohydrate 11 g, fat 5 g, energy 422 kJ (101 kcal)/100 mL with vitamins and minerals. Gluten-free, clinically lactose-free. Flavours: vanilla (can, ready-to-hang and tetrapaks), strawberry, chocolate and banana (tetrapaks). Net price 250-mL can = £2.34, 500-mL ready-to-hang = £4.69, 200-mL tetrapaks = £1.88.

For use as the sole source of nutrition or as a nutritional supplement prescribed on medical grounds for children aged 1 to 10 years for short-bowel syndrome, intractable malabsorption, pre-operative preparation of undernourished patients, dysphagia, bowel fistulas, and disease-related malnutrition and/or growth failure. Not to be prescribed for any child under 1 year

Paediasure® **with Fibre** (Abbott)

Liquid, protein 2.8 g, carbohydrate 11.16 g, fat 5 g, fibre 520 mg, energy 422 kJ (101 kcal)/100 mL with vitamins and minerals. Gluten-free, clinically lactose-free. Flavours: vanilla (can, ready-to-hang and tetrapak), banana (tetrapak) strawberry (tetrapak). Net price 250-mL can = £2.60, 500-mL ready-to-hang = £5.20, 200-mL tetrapak = £2.08.

For indications see *Paediasure*

Paediasure® **Plus** (Abbott)

Liquid, protein 4.2 g, carbohydrate 16.7 g, fat 7.5 g, energy 632 kJ (151 kcal)/100 mL with vitamins and minerals. Gluten-free, clinically lactose-free. Flavours: vanilla (ready-to-hang and tetrapak), strawberry (tetrapak). Net price 200-mL tetrapak = £2.30, 500-mL ready-to-hang = £5.87.

For indications see *Paediasure liquid*

Paediasure® **Plus with Fibre** (Abbott)

Tube feed, protein 4.2 g, carbohydrate 16.7 g, fat 7.5 g, energy 629 kJ (150 kcal)/100 mL with vitamins and minerals. Gluten-free, clinically lactose-free, net price 500-mL ready-to-hang = £6.25.

As a sole source of nutrition, or as a nutritional supplement for children aged 1 to 10 years with disease-related malnutrition and/or growth failure, short-bowel syndrome, intractable malabsorption, dysphagia, bowel fistulas, pre-operative preparation of undernourished patients. Not to be prescribed for any child under 1 year.

Paediatric Seravit® (SHS)

Powder, vitamins, minerals, low sodium and potassium, and trace elements. Net price 200 g (unflavoured) = £12.24; pineapple flavour, 200 g = £13.04.

For vitamin and mineral supplementation in restrictive therapeutic diets in infants and children

Pepdite® (SHS)

Powder, peptides, essential and non-essential amino acids, with carbohydrate, fat, vitamins, minerals, and trace elements. Flavour Sachets available.
Pepdite. Providing 1925 kJ (472 kcal)/100 g. Net price 400 g = £12.83
Pepdite 1+. Providing 1787 kJ (439 kcal)/100 g. Net price 400 g = £13.48; 15 x 57 g (banana flavour) = £32.70

Both for disaccharide and/or whole protein intolerance, or where amino acids or peptides are indicated in conjunction with medium chain triglycerides

Peptamen® (Nestlé Clinical)

Liquid, protein 4 g, carbohydrate 12.7 g, fat 3.7 g, energy 420 kJ (100 kcal)/100 mL, with vitamins, minerals and trace elements. Lactose- and gluten-free. Flavours: unflavoured (can), vanilla (cup, see also *Flavour Sachets*). Net price 375-mL can = £3.69, 200-mL cup = £2.25; 500-mL (Dripac-Flex) = £4.57, 1-litre = £8.23.

For use as the sole source of nutrition or as a nutritional supplement prescribed on medical grounds for: short-bowel syndrome, intractable malabsorption, proven inflammatory bowel disease, bowel fistulas. Not to be prescribed for any child under 1 year; use with caution for children up to 5 years

Nestlé Nutrition Flavour Mix for use with *Peptamen Liquid* 200-mL cup and *Modulen IBD*. Flavours: banana, chocolate, coffee, lemon and lime, strawberry. Net price 60 g = £5.62

Pepti-Junior® (Cow & Gate)

Powder, protein 15.3 g, fat 28.3 g, carbohydrate 55.1 g, energy 2140 kJ (507 kcal)/100 g with vitamins and minerals. Used as a 13.1% solution in place of milk. Net price 450 g = £8.80.

For disaccharide and/or whole protein intolerance or where amino acids and peptides are indicated in conjunction with medium chain triglycerides

Peptisorb® (Nutricia Clinical)

Liquid, protein 4 g, carbohydrate 17.6 g, fat 1.7 g, energy 420 kJ (100 kcal)/100 mL with vitamins, minerals and trace elements. Gluten-free. Net price 500-mL bottle = £4.86; 500-mL pack = £5.34; 1-litre pack = £9.65.

For use as the sole source of nutrition or as a nutritional supplement prescribed on medical grounds for: short-bowel syndrome, intractable malabsorption, proven inflammatory bowel disease, bowel fistulas. Not to be prescribed for any child under 1 year; use with caution for children up to 5 years

Perative® (Abbott)

Liquid, providing protein 6.67 g, carbohydrate 17.7 g, fat 3.7 g, energy 552 kJ (131 kcal)/100 mL, with vitamins and minerals. Gluten-free, unflavoured. Net price 500-mL ready-to-hang = £5.36, 1-litre ready-to-hang = £10.72.

For use as a nutritional supplement prescribed on medical grounds for: short-bowel syndrome, intractable malabsorption, pre-operative preparation of patients who are undernourished, proven inflammatory bowel disease, following total gastrectomy, bowel fistulas, disease-related malnutrition. Not to be prescribed for any child under 5 years

Phenylalanine, Tyrosine and Methionine-Free Amino Acid Mix

see Amino Acid Modules, XPTM Tyrosidon

Phlexy-10® **Exchange System** (SHS)

Bar, essential and non-essential amino acids except phenylalanine 8.33 g, carbohydrate 20.5 g, fat 4.5 g/42-g bar. Citrus fruit flavour. Net price per bar = £4.16
Capsules, essential and non-essential amino acids except phenylalanine 500 mg/capsule. Net price 200-cap pack = £29.09
Tablets, essential and non-essential amino acids except phenylalanine, 1 g tablet. Net price 75-tab pack = £18.85
Drink Mix, powder, containing essential and non-essential amino acids except phenylalanine 10 g, carbohydrate 8.8 g/20-g sachet. Apple and black-

currant, citrus, or tropical flavour. Net price 20-g sachet = £2.92

All for phenylketonuria

Phlexyvits® (SHS)

Powder, vitamins, minerals and trace elements, net price 30 × 7-g sachets = £48.94.

For use as a vitamin and mineral component of restricted therapeutic diets in older children from the age of around 11 years and over and adults with phenylketonuria and similar amino acid abnormalities

PK Aid 4® (SHS)

Powder, containing essential and non-essential amino acids except phenylalanine. Net price 500 g = £97.78.

For phenylketonuria

PK Foods (Gluten Free Foods Ltd)

Bread, white (sliced), 550 g = £4.00. Crispbread, 75 g = £2.00. Pasta (spirals), 250 g = £2.00.

For phenylketonuria and similar amino acid abnormalities

Cookies (chocolate chip, orange, or cinnamon), 150 g = £3.75. Egg replacer, 350 g = £3.75. Flour mix, 750 g = £6.99. Jelly (orange or cherry flavour), 4 × 80 g = £5.76.

For phenylketonuria

PKU 2® (Milupa)

Granules, containing essential and non-essential amino acids except phenylalanine; with vitamins, minerals, trace elements, 7.1% sucrose. Flavour: vanilla. Net price 500 g = £44.75.

For phenylketonuria

PKU 3® (Milupa)

Granules, containing essential and non-essential amino acids except phenylalanine, vitamins, minerals, and trace elements, with 3.4% sucrose. Flavour: vanilla. Net price 500 g = £44.75.

For phenylketonuria, not recommended for child under 8 years

PKU-Express® (Vitaflo)

Powder, protein (containing essential and non-essential amino acids, phenylalanine-free) 72 g, carbohydrate 15.1 g, energy 1260 kJ (301.5 kcal)/100 g with vitamins, minerals, and trace elements. Lemon, orange, tropical or unflavoured, net price 30 x 25 g sachets = £140.50.

For phenylketonuria, not recommended for children under 8 years

PKU-gel® (Vitaflo)

Powder, protein (containing essential and non-essential amino acids, phenylalanine-free) 10.1 g, carbohydrate 8.6 g, fat 0.03 g, energy 285.5 kJ (68 kcal)/20 g with vitamins, minerals and trace elements. Orange or unflavoured, net price 30 × 20-g sachets = £80.85.

For use as part of the low-protein dietary management of phenylketonuria in children aged 1 to 10 years. Not recommended for children under 1 year

Pleniday® (TOL)

Gluten-free. Bread: loaf (sliced) net price 350 g = £1.80; country loaf (sliced), 500 g = £2.85; rustic loaf (par-baked baguette), 400 g = £2.09; petit pain, 2 × 150 g = £2.02. Pasta (penne), 250 g = £1.27; (rigate), 250 g = £1.50

For gluten-sensitive enteropathies including steatorrhoea due to gluten sensitivity, coeliac disease, and dermatitis herpetiformis

Polial® (Ultrapharm)

Biscuits. Gluten- and lactose-free. Net price 200-g pack = £2.85.

For gluten-sensitive enteropathies including steatorrhea due to gluten sensitivity, coeliac disease, and dermatitis herpetiformis

Polycal® (Nutricia Clinical)

Powder, glucose, maltose, and polysaccharides, providing 1615 kJ (380 kcal)/100 g. Net price 400 g = £3.24

Liquid, glucose polymers providing carbohydrate 61.9 g/100 mL. Low-electrolyte, protein-free. Flavours: orange and neutral. Net price 200 mL = £1.29

Both for disease-related malnutrition; malabsorption states or other conditions requiring fortification with a high or readily available carbohydrate supplement

Polycose® (Abbott)

Powder, glucose polymers, providing carbohydrate 94 g, energy 1598 kJ (376 kcal)/100 g. Net price 350-g can = £3.30.

For disease-related malnutrition; malabsorption states or other conditions requiring fortification with a high or readily available carbohydrate supplement

Prejomin® (Milupa)

Granules, protein 13.5 g, carbohydrate 57 g, fat 24 g, energy 2085 kJ (497 kcal)/100 g, with vitamins and minerals. Gluten-free. For preparation with water before use. Net price 400 g = £9.44.

For disaccharide and/or whole protein intolerance where additional medium chain triglyceride is not indicated

PremCare® (Heinz)

Powder, protein 1.85 g, carbohydrate 7.24 g, fat 3.96 g, energy 301 kJ (72 kcal) per 100 mL when reconstituted, with vitamins and minerals. Gluten-, sucrose-, and lactose-free. Net price 450 g = £3.29.

For catch-up growth in pre-term infants (less than 35 weeks at birth), and small-for-gestational-age infants, until 6 months post-natal age

Pro-Cal® (Vitaflo)

Powder, protein 13.5 g, carbohydrate 26.8 g, fat 56.2 g, energy 2788 kJ (667 kcal)/100 g, net price 25 x 15 g sachets = £11.73, 510 g = £10.86, 1.5 kg = £21.15, 12.5 kg = £140, 25 kg = £250.

For disease-related malnutrition, malabsorption states or other conditions requiring fortification with a fat/carbohydrate supplement. Not to be prescribed for any child under 1 year; use with caution for young children up to 5 years

Promin® (Firstplay Dietary)

Low protein. Cous Cous, 500 g = £5.70. Pasta (alphabets, macaroni, shells, shortcut spaghetti, spirals); Pasta tricolour (alphabets, shells, spirals), net price 500 g = £5.70; Lasagne sheets, 200 g = £2.45. Pasta shells in tomato, pepper and herb sauce, 4 x 72-g sachets = £6.30; Pasta elbows in cheese and broccoli sauce, 4 x 66- g sachets = £6.20. Pasta meal, 500 g = £5.70. Pasta imitation rice, 500 g = £5.70.

For inherited metabolic disorders, renal or liver failure requiring a low-protein diet

ProMod® (Abbott)

Powder, protein 75 g, carbohydrate 7.5 g, fat 6.9 g/100 g. Gluten-free. Net price 275-g can = £8.82.

For biochemically proven hypoproteinaemia

Prosobee® (Mead Johnson)

Powder, protein 15.6%, carbohydrate 51.4%, fat 27.9% with vitamins and minerals. Gluten-, sucrose-, and lactose-free. Net price 400 g = £3.51.

For proven lactose and associated sucrose intolerance in pre-school children, galactokinase deficiency, galactosaemia, and proven whole cow's milk sensitivity

ProSure® (Abbott)

Liquid, protein 6.65 g, carbohydrate 19.4 g, fat 2.56 g, fibre 0.97 g, energy 528 kJ (125 kcal)/100 mL with vitamins, minerals, and trace elements. Gluten-free, clinically lactose-free. Vanilla, orange, or banana flavour, net price, 240-mL Tetrapak® = £2.70; 500-mL ready-to-hang = £5.63 (vanilla only).

As a nutritional supplement for patients with cancer cachexia. Not to be prescribed for children under 1 year; use with caution in children under 4 years

Protifar® (Nutricia Clinical)

Powder, protein 88.5%. Low lactose, gluten- and sucrose-free. Net price 225 g = £6.58.

For biochemically proven hypoproteinaemia

Provide Xtra® (Fresenius Kabi)

Liquid, protein 3.75 g, carbohydrate 27.5 g, energy 525 kJ (125 kcal)/100 mL with vitamins, minerals and trace elements. Gluten-free. Apple, blackcurrant, carrot-apple, cherry, citrus cola, lemon & lime, melon, orange & pineapple, or tomato flavour. Net price 200-mL carton = £1.58.

As a nutritional supplement prescribed on medical grounds for: short-bowel syndrome, intractable malabsorption, pre-operative preparation of patients who are undernourished, proven inflammatory bowel disease, following total gastrectomy, dysphagia, bowel fistulas, disease-related malnutrition. Not to be prescribed for any child under 1 year; use with caution for children up to 5 years

QuickCal® (Vitaflo)

Powder, protein 4.6 g, carbohydrate 17 g, fat 77 g, energy 3260 kJ (780 kcal)/100 g, net price 25 × 13-g sachets = £10.55, 1.5 kg = £16.65.

For disease-related malnutrition, malabsorption states or other conditions requiring fortification with a fat/carbohydrate supplement. Not to be prescribed for any child under 1 year; use with caution for young children up to 5 years

Rectified Spirit

Where the therapeutic qualities of alcohol are required rectified spirit (suitably flavoured and diluted) should be prescribed

Renamil® (KoRa)

Powder, protein 4.7 g, carbohydrate 70.2 g, fat 18.7 g, 1984 kJ (468 kcal)/100 g, with vitamins and minerals. Net price 1 kg = £25.40.

For chronic renal failure. Not suitable for infants and children under 1 year

Renapro® (KoRa)

Powder, whey protein providing protein 92 g, carbohydrate less than 300 mg, fat 500 mg, 1562 kJ (367 kcal)/100 g. Net price 20-g sachet = £2.32.

For dialysis and hypoproteinaemia. Not suitable for infants and children under 1 year

Resource® Benefiber® (Novartis Consumer Health)

Powder, soluble dietary fibre, carbohydrate 19 g, fibre 78 g, energy 323 kJ (76 kcal)/100 g with minerals. Gluten-free; low lactose, net price 250 g pack = £8.76, 16 x 8-g sachets = £5.72.

As a nutritional supplement prescribed on medical grounds for: short-bowel syndrome, intractable malabsorption, pre-operative preparation of undernourished patients, proven inflammatory bowel disease, following total gastrectomy, bowel fistulas, disease-related malnutrition. Not to be prescribed for children under 5 years

Resource® Energy Dessert (Novartis Consumer Health)

Semi-solid, protein 4.8 g, carbohydrate 21.2 g, fat 6.24 g, energy 671 kJ (160 kcal)/100 g with vitamins, minerals, and trace elements. Gluten-free; low lactose. Flavours: caramel, chocolate, or vanilla, net price 125-g cup = £1.35.

For use as a nutritional supplement prescribed on medical grounds for: disease-related malnutrition, short-bowel syndrome, intractable malabsorption, proven inflammatory bowel disease, bowel fistulas, dysphagia, pre-operative preparation of undernourished patients, after total gastrectomy, continuous ambulatory peritoneal dialysis (CAPD), haemodialysis. Not to be prescribed for any child under 1 year; use with caution for children up to 5 years

Resource® Fruit Flavour Drink (Novartis Consumer Health)

Liquid, protein 4 g, carbohydrate 33.5 g, energy 638 kJ (150 kcal)/100 mL with vitamins, minerals, and trace elements. Fat- and gluten-free; low lactose. Flavours: apple, orange, or pineapple, net price 125-g carton = £1.49.

For use as a nutritional supplement prescribed on medical grounds for: disease-related malnutrition, short-bowel syndrome, intractable malabsorption, proven inflammatory bowel disease, bowel fistulas, dysphagia, pre-operative preparation of undernourished patients, after total gastrectomy. Not to be prescribed for any child under 3 years; use with caution for children up to 5 years

Resource® Junior (Novartis Consumer Health)

Liquid, protein 3 g, carbohydrate 20.6 g, fat 6.2 g, energy 631 kJ (150 kcal)/100 mL with vitamins, minerals, and trace elements. Gluten-free; clinically lactose-free. Flavours: chocolate, strawberry, or vanilla, net price 200-mL carton = £1.69.

For use as a sole source of nutrition or as a nutritional supplement prescribed on medical grounds for: disease-related malnutrition, short-bowel syndrome, intractable malabsorption, pre-operative preparation of undernourished patients, proven inflammatory bowel disease, following total gastrectomy, bowel fistulas, and dysphagia. Not to be prescribed for any child under 1 year

Resource® Protein Extra (Novartis Consumer Health)

Liquid, protein 9.4 g, carbohydrate 14 g, fat 3.5 g, energy 530 kJ (125 kcal)/100 mL with vitamins, minerals and trace elements. Gluten-free; low lactose. Flavours: apricot, chocolate, summer fruits, or vanilla. Net price 200-mL carton = £1.29.

For use as a nutritional supplement prescribed on medical grounds for: disease-related malnutrition, short-bowel syndrome, intractable malabsorption, proven inflammatory bowel disease, bowel fistulas, dysphagia, pre-operative preparation of undernourished patients, after total gastrectomy. Not to be prescribed for any child under 1 year; use with caution for children up to 5 years

Resource® Shake (Novartis Consumer Health)

Liquid, protein 5.1 g, carbohydrate 22.6 g, fat 7 g, energy 731 kJ (174 kcal)/100 mL with vitamins, minerals and trace elements. Gluten-free; low lactose. Flavours: banana, chocolate, lemon, strawberry, summer fruits, toffee, or vanilla. Net price 175-mL carton = £1.46.

For use as a nutritional supplement prescribed on medical grounds for: disease-related malnutrition, short-bowel syndrome, intractable malabsorption, proven inflammatory bowel disease, bowel fistulas, dysphagia, pre-operative preparation of undernourished patients, after total gastrectomy. Not to be prescribed for any child under 1 year; use with caution for children up to 5 years

Resource® Thickened Drink (Novartis Consumer Health)

Liquid, carbohydrate 22 g, energy: orange 383 kJ (89 kcal); apple 375 kJ (89 kcal)/100 mL. Syrup and custard consistencies. Gluten-free; clinically lactose free, net price 12 × 114-mL cups = £7.08.

For dysphagia. Not suitable for children under 1 year

Resource® Thickened Squash (Novartis Consumer Health)

Liquid, syrup consistency: carbohydrate 16.9 g, energy 287 kJ (68 kcal)/100 mL; custard consistency: carbohydrate 17.8 g, energy 303 kJ (71 kcal)/100 mL. Gluten-free; clinically lactose-free. Orange and lemon flavour, net price 1.89-litre bottle = £3.99.

For dysphagia. Not suitable for children under 1 year

Resource® ThickenUp® (Novartis Consumer Health)

Powder, modified maize starch. Gluten- and lactose-free, net price 227 g = £3.90; 75 × 6.4-g sachet = £15.75.

For thickening of foods in dysphagia. Not to be prescribed for children under 1 year

Rite-Diet® Gluten-free (Nutricia Dietary)

Gluten-free. White bread (sliced or unsliced), 400 g = £2.75. White loaf (part-baked), 400 g = £3.09. Fibre bread (sliced or unsliced), 400 g = £2.75. Fibre loaf (part-baked), 400 g = £3.09. White rolls, 4 = £2.72; (part-baked) long, 2 = £3.04. Fibre rolls, 4 = £2.72 (part-baked) long, 2 = £2.95. Flour mix (white or fibre), 500 g = £5.22.

For gluten-sensitive enteropathies including steatorrhoea due to gluten sensitivity, coeliac disease, and dermatitis herpetiformis

Rite-Diet® Low-protein (SHS)

Low protein. Baking mix. Net price 500 g = £5.78. Flour mix. 400 g = £4.95.

For inherited metabolic disorders, renal or liver failure requiring a low-protein diet

Scandishake® Mix (Nutricia Clinical)

Powder, protein 11.7 g, carbohydrate 66.8 g, fat 30.4 g, energy 2457 kJ (588 kcal)/serving (serving = 1 sachet reconstituted with 240 mL whole milk). Flavours: banana, caramel, chocolate, strawberry, vanilla, and unflavoured. Net price 85-g sachet = £1.89.

For disease-related malnutrition; malabsorption states or other conditions requiring fortification with a fat/carbohydrate supplement

Schar® (Nutrition Point)

Gluten-free. Bread.(white, sliced), net price 2 x 200 g = £2.65. Baguette (french bread), 400 g = £2.90. Bread rolls, 150 g = £1.60. Lunch rolls, 150 g = £1.85. White bread buns, 200 g = £2.30. Bread mix, 1 kg = £4.75. Ertha brown bread, 2 x 250 g = £3.00. Cake mix, 500 g = £4.50. Flour mix, 1 kg = £4.75. Breadsticks (Grissini), 150 g = £1.95. Cracker toast, 150 g = £2.10. Crackers, 200 g = £2.35. Crispbread, 250 g = £3.50. Pasta (fusilli, penne), 500 g = £3.30; lasagne, 250 g = £3.30; macaroni pipette, 500 g = £3.30; spaghetti, 500 g = £3.30. Pizza bases, 300 g (2 × 150 g) = £4.75. Biscuits, 200 g = £2.00. Savoy biscuits, 200 g = £2.25.

For gluten-sensitive enteropathies including steatorrhoea due to gluten sensitivity, coeliac disease, and dermatitis herpetiformis

SHS Modjul® Flavour System (SHS)

Powder, blackcurrant, orange, and pineapple flavours. Net price 100 g = £8.32.

For use with any unflavoured products based on peptides or amino acids

SMA High Energy® (SMA Nutrition)

Liquid, protein 2 g, carbohydrate 9.8 g, fat 4.9 g, energy 382 kJ (91 kcal)/100mL, with vitamins and minerals. Net price 250 mL = £1.80.

For disease-related malnutrition, malabsorption, and growth failure

SMA LF® (SMA Nutrition)

Powder, protein 1.5 g, carbohydrate 7.2 g, fat 3.6 g, energy 282 kJ (67 kcal)/100 mL, with vitamins and minerals. Net price 430 g = £3.99.

For proven lactose intolerance

SMA Staydown® (SMA Nutrition)

Powder, protein 12.4 g, fat 27.9 g, carbohydrate 54.3 g, energy 2166 kJ (518 kcal)/100g, with vitamins, minerals, and trace elements. Net price 900 g = £5.74.

For significant reflux disease. Not to be used for more than 6 months or in conjunction with any other thickener or antacid product

Sno-Pro® (SHS)

Drink, protein 220 mg (phenylalanine 12.5 mg), carbohydrate 8 g, fat 3.8 g, energy 280 kJ (67 kcal)/100 mL. Net price 200 mL = 85p.

For phenylketonuria, chronic renal failure, and other inborn errors of metabolism

Sondalis Junior® (Nestlé Clinical)

Powder, protein 13.9 g, carbohydrate 62.2 g, fat 18.3 g, energy 1950 kJ (467 kcal)/100 g with vitamins, minerals and trace elements. Gluten-free; clinically lactose-free. Flavour: vanilla, net price 400 g = £9.72.

For use as a sole source of nutrition or as a nutritional supplement prescribed on medical grounds for: short bowel syndrome, intractable malabsorption, pre-operative preparation of undernourished patients, proven inflammatory bowel disease, following total gastrectomy, dysphagia, bowel fistulas, disease-related malnutrition, and growth failure in children aged 1-6 years. Not to be prescribed for any child under 1 year

Sunnyvale® (Everfresh)

Mixed grain bread, gluten-free. Net price 400 g = £1.79.

For gluten-sensitive enteropathies including steatorrhoea due to gluten sensitivity, coeliac disease and dermatitis herpetiformis

Suplena® (Abbott)

Liquid, protein 3 g, carbohydrate 25.5 g, fat 9.6 g, energy 841 kJ (201 kcal)/100 mL. Flavour: vanilla. Net price 237-mL can = £2.28.

For patients with chronic or acute renal failure who are not undergoing dialysis; chronic or acute liver disease with fluid restriction; other conditions requiring a high-energy, low-protein, low-electrolyte, low-volume enteral feed

Survimed OPD® (Fresenius Kabi)

Liquid, protein 4.5 g, carbohydrate 15 g, fat 2.6 g, energy 420 kJ (100 kcal)/100 mL, with vitamins, minerals, and trace elements. Gluten-free, and low lactose. Net price 500-mL EasyBag® = £5.00.

As a nutritional supplement prescribed on medical grounds for: short-bowel syndrome, intractable malabsorption, pre-operative preparation of patients who are undernourished, proven inflammatory bowel disease, following total gastrectomy, dysphagia, bowel fistulas, disease-related malnutrition. Not to be prescribed for any child under 1 year; use with caution for children up to 5 years

Tentrini® (Nutricia Clinical)

Liquid, tube feed, protein 3.3 g, carbohydrate 12.3 g, fat 4.2 g, energy 420 kJ (100 kcal)/100 mL, with vitamins, minerals and trace elements. Gluten- and lactose-free. Unflavoured, net price 500-mL bottle or pack = £4.24

For short-bowel syndrome, intractable malabsorption, pre-operative preparation of undernourished patients, inflammatory bowel disease, total gastrectomy, dysphagia, bowel fistulas, disease-related malnutrition, and growth failure. For children between 21–45 kg body-weight

Tentrini® Energy (Nutricia Clinical)

Liquid, tube feed, protein 4.9 g, carbohydrate 18.5 g, fat 6.3 g, energy 630 kJ (150 kcal)/100 mL, with vitamins, minerals and trace elements.

Gluten- and lactose-free. Unflavoured, net price 500-mL bottle or pack = £5.25

For indications see *Tentrini*

Tentrini® Energy Multi Fibre (Nutricia Clinical)

Liquid, tube feed, protein 4.9 g, carbohydrate 18.5 g, fat 6.3 g, fibre 1.12 g, energy 630 kJ (150 kcal)/100 mL, with vitamins, minerals and trace elements. Gluten- and lactose-free. Unflavoured, net price 500-mL bottle or pack = £5.79

For indications see *Tentrini Multi Fibre*

Tentrini® Multi Fibre (Nutricia Clinical)

Liquid, tube feed, protein 3.3 g, carbohydrate 12.3 g, fat 4.2 g, fibre 1.12 g, energy 420 kJ (100 kcal)/100 mL, with vitamins, minerals and trace elements. Gluten- and lactose-free. Unflavoured, net price 500-mL bottle or pack = £4.66

For short-bowel syndrome, intractable malabsorption, pre-operative preparation of undernourished patients, inflammatory bowel disease, total gastrectomy, dysphagia, disease-related malnutrition, and growth failure. Not to be prescribed for any child under 1 year; use with caution for children under 7 years or 21 kg

Thick and Easy® (Fresenius Kabi)

Powder. Modified maize starch, net price 225-g can = £3.99; 100 × 9-g sachets = £26.35; 4.54 kg = £70.53.

Dairy. Pre-thickened milk, net price 250 mL = £1.38

Thickened Juices, liquid, modified food starch. Flavours: apple, blackcurrant, cranberry, kiwi-strawberry, and orange, net price 118-mL pot = 52p; 1.42-litre bottle = £3.61.

For thickening of foods in dysphagia. Not to be prescribed for children under 1 year except in cases of failure to thrive

Thixo-D® (Sutherland)

Powder, modified maize starch, gluten-free. Net price 375-g tub = £5.79.

For thickening of foods in dysphagia. Not to be prescribed for children under 1 year except in cases of failure to thrive

Tinkyada® (General Dietary)

Gluten-free. Brown rice pasta (elbows, fettucini, fusilli, penne, shells, spaghetti, spirals). Net price 454 g = £3.00.

For gluten-sensitive enteropathies including steatorrhoea due to gluten-sensitivity, coeliac disease and dermatitis herpetiformis

Tritamyl® (Gluten Free Foods Ltd)

Gluten-free. Flour, net price 1 kg = £5.60. Brown bread mix, 1 kg = £5.60. White bread mix, 1 kg = £5.60.

For gluten-sensitive enteropathies including steatorrhoea due to gluten sensitivity, coeliac disease and dermatitis herpetiformis

TYR Gel® (Vitaflo)

Gel, essential and non-essential amino acids (except tyrosine and phenylalanine) 10.1 g, protein equivalent 8.4 g, carbohydrate 8.6 g, fat 0.03 g, energy 285.5 kJ (68 kcal)/20 g, with vitamins, minerals and trace elements. Unflavoured, net price 30 × 20-g sachets = £129.50

A tyrosine- and phenylalanine-free protein substitute for use in the dietary management of tyrosinaemia in children between 12 months and 10 years

L-Tyrosine (SHS)

Powder, net price 100 g = £12.53.

For use as a supplement in maternal phenylketonurics who have low plasma tyrosine concentrations

Ultra® (Ultrapharm)

Gluten-free. Baguette, net price 400 g = £2.46. Bread, net price 400 g = £2.46. High-fibre bread, 500 g = £3.26. Crackerbread, 100 g = £1.77. Pizza base, net price 400 g = £2.65.

For gluten-sensitive enteropathies including steatorrhoea due to gluten sensitivity, coeliac disease and dermatitis herpetiformis

Low protein. PKU bread, 400 g = £2.16. PKU flour, 500 g = £3.07. PKU biscuits, 200 g = £2.21. PKU cookies, 250 g = £2.31. PKU pizza base, 400 g = £2.21. PKU savoy biscuits, 150 g = £2.06.

For inherited metabolic disorders, renal or liver failure requiring a low-protein diet

Valpiform® (Gluten Free Foods Ltd)

Gluten-free. Bread mix, 2 × 500 g = £6.74; country loaf (sliced), 400 g = £3.74. Crac'form toast, 2 × 125 g = £3.52. Crisp rolls, 220 g = £3.60; Maxi baguettes, 2 × 200 g = £4.49. Pastry mix, 2 × 500 g = £6.74. Petites baguettes, 2 × 160 g = £2.99.

For gluten-sensitive enteropathies including steatorrhoea due to gluten sensitivity, coeliac disease and dermatitis herpetiformis

Vita-Bite® (Vitaflo)

Bar, protein 30 mg (less than 2.5 mg phenylalanine), carbohydrate 15.35 g, fat 8.4 g, energy 572 kJ (137 kcal)/25 g. Chocolate flavoured, net price 25 g = 88p.

For inherited metabolic disorders, renal or liver failure requiring a low-protein diet. Not recommended for any child under 1 year

Vitajoule® (Vitaflo)

Powder, glucose polymers, providing carbohydrate 96 g, energy 1610 kJ (380 kcal)/100 g. Net price 125 g = 99p, 200 g = £1.65, 500 g = £3.24, 2.5 kg = £16.15, 25 kg = £99.00.

For disease-related malnutrition; malabsorption states or other conditions requiring fortification with a high or readily available carbohydrate supplement

Vitamins and Minerals

Only for use in the management of actual or potential vitamin or mineral deficiency; not to be prescribed as dietary supplements or 'pick-me-ups'

Vitapro® (Vitaflo)

Powder, whole milk proteins, containing all essential amino acids, 75%. Net price 250 g = £6.49, 2 kg = £50.90.

For biochemically proven hypoproteinaemia

Vitaquick® (Vitaflo)

Powder. Modified maize starch. Net price 100 g = £2.38, 300 g = £5.85; 2 kg = £30.72; 6 kg = £78.60.

For thickening of foods in dysphagia. Not to be prescribed for children under 1 year except in cases of failure to thrive

Vitasavoury® (Vitaflo)

Powder, protein 12 g, carbohydrate 24 g, fat 54 g, energy 2610 kJ (630 kcal)/100 g, net price 10 x 50-g sachets = £14.63, 24 × 33-g ready cups = £24.28. Flavours: chicken, leek and potato, mushroom, vegetable.

As a nutritional supplement for disease-related malnutrition, malabsorption states or other conditions requiring fortification with a fat/carbohydrate supplement. Not to be prescribed for any child under 1 year; use with caution for young children up to 5 years

Wysoy® (Wyeth)

Powder, carbohydrate 6.9%, fat 3.6%, and protein 2.1% with vitamins and minerals when reconstituted. Net price 430 g = £3.98; 860 g = £7.58.

For proven lactose and associated sucrose intolerance in preschool children, galactokinase deficiency, galactosaemia and proven whole cow's milk sensitivity

XLEU Analog (SHS)

Powder, essential and non-essential amino acids 15.5% except leucine, with carbohydrate, fat,

vitamins, minerals, and trace elements. Net price 400 g = £24.62.
For isovaleric acidaemia
Ingredients: include arachis oil (peanut oil)
NOTE. Analog products are generally intended for use in children up to 1 year, see also Flavour Sachets, for use with unflavoured amino acid and peptide products from SHS

XLEU Faladon (SHS)
Powder, essential and non-essential amino acids 93%, except leucine. Net price 200 g = £50.87.
For isovaleric acidaemia

[1]**XLEU Maxamaid** (SHS)
Powder, essential and non-essential amino acids 28.6% except leucine, with carbohydrate, fat less than 0.5%, vitamins, minerals, and trace elements. Net price 500 g = £67.15.
For isovaleric acidaemia

XLYS Analog (SHS)
Powder, essential and non-essential amino acids 15.5% except lysine, with carbohydrate, fat, vitamins, minerals, and trace elements. Net price 400 g = £24.62.
For hyperlysinaemia
NOTE. Analog products are generally intended for use in children up to 1 year, see also Flavour Sachets, for use with unflavoured amino acid and peptide products from SHS

XLYS, Low TRY, Analog (SHS)
Powder, essential and non-essential amino acids 15.5% except lysine, and low tryptophan, with carbohydrate, fat, vitamins, minerals, and trace elements. Net price 400 g = £24.62.
For type 1 glutaric aciduria
NOTE. Analog products are generally intended for use in children up to 1 year, see also Flavour Sachets, for use with unflavoured amino acid and peptide products from SHS

[1]**XLYS, Low TRY, Maxamaid** (SHS)
Powder, essential and non-essential amino acids 30% except lysine, with carbohydrate, fat less than 0.5%, vitamins, minerals, and trace elements. Net price 500 g = £67.15.
For type 1 glutaric aciduria

[1]**XLYS Maxamaid** (SHS)
Powder, essential and non-essential amino acids 30% except lysine, with carbohydrate, fat less than 0.5%, vitamins, minerals, and trace elements. Net price 500 g = £67.15.
For hyperlysinaemia

XMET Analog (SHS)
Powder, essential and non-essential amino acids 15.5% except methionine, with carbohydrate, fat, vitamins, minerals, and trace elements. Net price 400 g = £24.62.
For hypermethioninaemia; homocystinuria
NOTE. Analog products are generally intended for use in children up to 1 year, see also Flavour Sachets, for use with unflavoured amino acid and peptide products from SHS

XMET Homidon (SHS)
Powder, essential and non-essential amino acids 93%, except methionine. Net price 200 g = £49.59.
For homocystinuria or hypermethioninaemia

[1]**XMET Maxamaid** (SHS)
Powder, essential and non-essential amino acids 30% except methionine, with carbohydrate, fat less than 0.5%, vitamins, minerals, and trace elements. Net price 500 g = £67.15
For hypermethioninaemia, homocystinuria

[2]**XMET Maxamum**® (SHS)
Powder, essential and non-essential amino acids 47% except methionine, with carbohydrate, fat less than 0.5%, vitamins, minerals, and trace elements. Unflavoured, see also Flavour Sachets. Net price 500 g = £107.65.
For hypermethioninaemia, homocystinuria

XMTVI Analog (SHS)
Powder, essential and non-essential amino acids 15.5% except methionine, threonine, valine and low isoleucine, with carbohydrate, fat, vitamins, minerals, and trace elements. Net price 400 g = £24.62.
For methylmalonic acidaemia or propionic acidaemia
NOTE. Analog products are generally intended for use in children up to 1 year, see also Flavour Sachets, for use with unflavoured amino acid and peptide products from SHS

XMTVI Asadon (SHS)
Powder, essential and non-essential amino acids 93%, except methionine, threonine, and valine, with trace amounts of isoleucine. Net price 200 g = £50.87.
For methylmalonic acidaemia or propionic acidaemia

[1]**XMTVI Maxamaid** (SHS)
Powder, essential and non-essential amino acids 30% except methionine, threonine, valine and low isoleucine, with carbohydrate, fat less than 0.5%, vitamins, minerals, and trace elements. Net price 500 g = £67.15.
For methylmalonic acidaemia or propionic acidaemia

[2]**XMTVI Maxamum**® (SHS)
Powder, essential and non-essential amino acids 47% except methionine, threonine, valine, and low isoleucine, with carbohydrate, fat less than 0.5%, vitamins, minerals, and trace elements. Unflavoured, see also Flavour Sachets. Net price 500 g = £107.65.
For methylmalonic acidaemia or propionic acidaemia

XP Analog (SHS)
Powder, essential and non-essential amino acids 15.5% except phenylalanine, with carbohydrate, fat, vitamins, minerals, and trace elements. Net price 400 g = £19.67.
For phenylketonuria
NOTE. Analog products are generally intended for use in children up to 1 year, see also Flavour Sachets, for use with unflavoured amino acid and peptide products from SHS

XP LCP Analog (SHS)
Powder, essential and non-essential amino acids except phenylalanine 15.5%, with carbohydrate, fat, vitamins, minerals and trace elements. Gluten- and lactose-free. Net price 400 g = £22.38.
For phenylketonuria in infants and children under 2 years of age
NOTE. See also Flavour Sachets, for use with unflavoured amino acid and peptide products from SHS

[1]**XP Maxamaid** (SHS)
Powder, essential and non-essential amino acids 30% except phenylalanine, with carbohydrate, vitamins, minerals, and trace elements. Net price powder (unflavoured), 500 g = £39.73; (orange-flavoured), 500 g = £39.73.
For phenylketonuria. Not to be prescribed for children under 2 years

1. Maxamaid products are generally intended for use in children aged 1 to 8 years, see also Flavour Sachets, for use with unflavoured amino acid and peptide products from SHS

2. Maxamum products are generally intended for use in children aged over 8 years

XP Maxamaid Concentrate[1] (SHS)
Powder, essential and non-essential amino acids 65% except phenylalanine, with carbohydrate, fat less than 0.5%, vitamins, minerals, and trace elements. Unflavoured. Net price 500 g = £101.72.
For phenylketonuria. Not to be prescribed for children under 2 years
NOTE. See also Flavour Sachets, for use with unflavoured amino acid and peptide products from SHS

XP Maxamum[2]® (SHS)
Powder, essential and non-essential amino acids 47% except phenylalanine, with carbohydrates, vitamins, minerals, and trace elements. Flavours: orange, unflavoured, see also Flavour Sachets. Net price 30 × 50-g sachets = £184.27, 500 g = £61.42.
For phenylketonuria. Not to be prescribed for children under 8 years

XPHEN TYR Analog (SHS)
Powder, essential and non-essential amino acids 15.5% except phenylalanine and tyrosine, with carbohydrate, fat, vitamins, minerals and trace elements. Net price 400 g = £24.62.
For tyrosinaemia
NOTE. Analog products are generally intended for use in children up to 1 year, see also Flavour Sachets, for use with unflavoured amino acid and peptide products from SHS

XPHEN TYR Maxamaid[1] (SHS)
Powder, essential and non-essential amino acids 30% except phenylalanine and tyrosine, with carbohydrate, fat less than 0.5%, vitamins, minerals, and trace elements. Unflavoured. Net price 500 g = £67.15.
For tyrosinaemia

XPHEN TYR Tyrosidon (SHS)
Powder, essential and non-essential amino acids 93%, except phenylalanine and tyrosine. Net price 500 g = £127.20
For tyrosinaemia where plasma methionine concentrations are normal

XPTM Analog (SHS)
Powder, essential and non-essential amino acids 15.5% except phenylalanine, tyrosine and methionine, with carbohydrate, fat, vitamins, minerals and trace elements. Net price 400 g = £24.62.
For tyrosinaemia
NOTE. Analog products are generally intended for use in children up to 1 year, see also Flavour Sachets, for use with unflavoured amino acid and peptide products from SHS

XPTM Tyrosidon (SHS)
Powder, essential and non-essential amino acids 93%, except methionine, phenylalanine, and tyrosine. Net price 500 g = £127.20.
For tyrosinaemia type I where plasma concentrations are above normal

1. Maxamaid products are generally intended for use in children aged 1 to 8 years, see also Flavour Sachets, for use with unflavoured amino acid and peptide products from SHS

2. Maxamum products are generally intended for use in children aged over 8 years

Conditions for which foods may be prescribed on FP10, GP10 (Scotland), or when available, WP10 (Wales)

NOTE. This is a list of clinical conditions for which the ACBS has approved food products. It is essential to check the list of products (above) for availability.

Amino acid metabolic disorders and similar protein disorders

See histidinaemia; homocystinuria; maple syrup urine disease; phenylketonuria; low-protein products; synthetic diets; tyrosinaemia.

Bowel fistulas

Complete foods: Clinutren 1.5 Fibre and Clinutren ISO; Elemental 028 and 028 Extra; Emsogen; Enrich and Enrich Plus; Ensure; Ensure Powder; Foodlink Complete; Frebini, Frebini Energy, Frebini Energy Fibre; Fresubin Energy, Fresubin Original Liquid and Sip feeds, Fresubin 1000, and Fresubin 1200 Complete; Isosource Energy, Standard; Jevity; Modulen IBD; Novasource Forte and GI Control; Nutrini, Nutrini Energy and Fibre; Nutrison Standard and Multifibre; Osmolite Liquid and Plus; Paediasure Liquid and Plus; Peptamen; Peptisorb; Sondalis; Tentrini and Energy.
Nutritional supplements: Clinutren Dessert, Fruit, and 1.5; Enlive Plus; Ensure Plus; Formance; Forticreme; Fortifresh; Fortijuce; Fortimel; Fortisip Bottle; Fortisip Multi Fibre, Protein; Fresubin HP Energy; Nutrison Energy, and MCT; Perative; Provide Xtra; Resource Benefiber, Energy, Dessert, Protein Extra, Shake; Survimed OPD.

Calcium intolerance

Locasol.

Carbohydrate malabsorption

See also synthetic diets; malabsorption states.

(a) *Disaccharide intolerance*: Caloreen; Duocal Super Soluble and Duocal Liquid; Maxijul LE, Liquid, Super Soluble; Nutramigen 1 and 2; Nutrison Soya; Pepdite; Pepti-Junior; Polycal liquid and powder; Polycose powder; Prejomin; Pro-Cal; QuickCal; Vitajoule; Vitasavoury. See also lactose intolerance; lactose with associated sucrose intolerance.
(b) *Isomaltose intolerance*: Glucose (dextrose).
(c) *Glucose and galactose intolerance*: Comminuted Chicken Meat (Cow & Gate); Fructose; Galactomin 19 (fructose formula).
(d) *Lactose intolerance*: Colief; Comminuted Chicken Meat (SHS); Enfamil Lactofree; Farley's Soya Formula; Galactomin 17; InfaSoy; Isomil powder; Nutramigen 1; Nutrison Soya; Pepdite; Prejomin; Prosobee; SMA LF; Wysoy.
(e) *Lactose with associated sucrose intolerance*: Comminuted Chicken Meat (SHS); Farley's Soya Formula; Galactomin 17; InfaSoy; Nutramigen 1; Nutrison Soya; Pepti-Junior; Prejomin; Prosobee; Wysoy.
(f) *Sucrose intolerance*: Glucose (dextrose) and see also synthetic diets; malabsorption states; lactose with associated sucrose intolerance.

NOTE. Lactose or sucrose intolerance is defined as a condition of intolerance to an intake of the relevant disaccharide confirmed by demonstrated clinical benefit of the effectiveness of the disaccharide-free diet, and presence of reducing substances and/or excessive acid in the stools, a low concentration of the corresponding disaccharidase enzyme on intestinal biopsy, or by breath tests or lactose tolerance tests

Carnitine palmitoyl transferase deficiency (CPTD)
Monogen

Coeliac disease
See gluten-sensitive enteropathies.

Continuous Ambulatory Peritoneal Dialysis (CAPD)
See dialysis.

Cystic fibrosis
See malabsorption states.

Dermatitis Herpetiformis
See gluten-sensitive enteropathies.

Dialysis
Nutritional supplements for haemodialysis or continuous ambulatory peritoneal dialysis (CAPD) patients: Clinutren Dessert; Enrich Plus; Ensure Plus; Formance; Forticreme; Fresubin HP Energy, and Fresubin Protein Energy Drink; Kindergen; Nepro; Renapro; Resource Energy Dessert; Suplena.

Disaccharide intolerance
See carbohydrate malabsorption.

Dysphagia
Complete foods: Clinutren 1.5 Fibre and Clinutren ISO; Enfamil AR; Enrich and Enrich Plus; Ensure; Ensure Powder; Foodlink Complete; Frebini Original, Energy Fibre and Energy; Fresubin Energy, Fresubin Energy Fibre (sip and tube feed), Fresubin Original Fibre, Fresubin Original Liquid and Sip Feeds, Fresubin Protein Energy Drink; Fresubin 1000, and Fresubin 1200 Complete; Isosource Energy, Fibre Junior and Standard; Jevity; Novasource GI Control and Forte; Nutrini Fibre and Standard; Nutrison Multi Fibre, Energy Multi Fibre, Soya, Standard and Vitaplus Multifibre; Osmolite Liquid and Plus; Paediasure Liquid, Liquid with fibre and Plus; SMA Staydown; Sondalis; Tentrini, Energy, Energy Multi Fibre, Multi Fibre.
Nutritional supplements: Clinutren Dessert, Fruit, and 1.5; Clinutren Thickened Drinks, Enlive Plus; Ensure Plus and Yoghurt style; Formance; Forticreme; Fortifresh; Fortijuce; Fortimel; Fortisip Bottle, Multi Fibre, Protein; Fresubin HP Energy, and Fresubin Protein Energy Drink; Nutrison Energy and MCT; Provide Xtra; Resource Energy Dessert, Resource Benefiber, Protein Extra, ThickenUp, Thickened Squash, and Shake; Survimed OPD.
Thickeners: Clinutren Thickener, Nutilis; Thick & Easy powder and thickened juices; Thixo-D; Vitaquick.
NOTE. Dysphagia is defined as that associated with intrinsic disease of the oesophagus, e.g. oesophagitis; neuromuscular disorders, e.g. multiple sclerosis and motor neurone disease; major surgery and/or radiotherapy for cancer of the upper digestive tract; protracted severe inflammatory disease of the upper digestive tract, e.g. Stevens-Johnson syndrome and epidermolysis bullosa

Epilepsy (ketogenic diet in)
Alembicol D; Liquigen; Medium-Chain Triglyceride Oil (MCT).

Flavouring
For use with any unflavoured SHS product based on peptides or amino acids: SHS Flavour Modjul; Flavour Sachets

Galactokinase deficiency and galactosaemia
Farley's Soya Formula; Galactomin 17; InfaSoy; Isomil powder; Prosobee; Wysoy

Gastrectomy (total)
Complete foods: Clinutren 1.5 Fibre and Clinutren ISO; Enrich; Enrich Plus; Ensure; Ensure Powder; Foodlink Complete; Frebini Original; Fresubin Energy, Fresubin Energy Fibre (sip and tube feed), Fresubin Original Fibre, Fresubin Original Liquid and Sip Feeds, Fresubin 1000, and Fresubin 1200 Complete; Isosource Energy, Fibre and Standard; Jevity and Plus; Novasource GI Control, and Forte; Nutrison Multi Fibre, Energy Multi Fibre, Soya and Standard; Osmolite Liquid and Plus; Sondalis Junior; Tentrini, Energy, Energy Multi Fibre, Multi Fibre.
Nutritional supplements: Clinutren Dessert, Fruit, and 1.5; Enlive Plus; Ensure Plus; Formance; Fortijuce; Fortimel; Fortipudding; Fortisip Bottle, Multi Fibre, Protein; Fresubin HP Energy, and Fresubin Protein Energy Drink; Nutrison Energy and MCT; Perative; Provide Xtra; Resource Benefiber, Resource Energy Dessert, Protein Extra, and Shake; Survimed OPD.

Glucose/galactose intolerance
See carbohydrate malabsorption.

Glutaric aciduria
XLYS, Low Try Analog; XLYS, Low Try Maxamaid

Gluten-sensitive enteropathies
Aproten flour; Arnott gluten-free rice cookies; Baker's Delight wheat-, gluten- and dairy-free bread; Barkat gluten-free bread mix, brown or white rice bread, Brown or white rice pizza crust; Bi-Aglut biscuits, crackers, cracker toast, lasagne, pasta (fusilli, macaroni, penne, spaghetti); DS Dietary Specials Mixes: brown or white bread, white cake, white or fibre; Ener-G brown and white rice bread, gluten-free tapioca bread, rice loaf, Seattle brown loaf, cookies (vanilla), xanthum gum, gluten-free rice pasta (cannelloni, lasagna, macaroni, shells, small shells, spaghetti, tagliatelli, vermicelli); brown rice pasta (lasagna, macaroni, spaghetti); Gadsby's white bread (sliced or unsliced), white bread flour, white bread rolls; Glutafin bread, multigrain white loaf (sliced or unsliced, white or part-baked), rolls (white or part-baked), fibre bread, mixes (white, multigrain white, fibre, multigrain fibre), biscuits (digestive, savoury, sweet (without chocolate or sultanas), tea), crackers, high fibre crackers and pasta (lasagne, penne, spirals, spaghetti), pizza bases; Glutano gluten-free tea biscuits, crackers, crispbread, flour mix, pastas (animal shapes, macaroni, spaghetti, spirals, tagliatelle), wholemeal bread (sliced or par-baked), baguette or rolls (par-baked), white sliced bread (par-baked); Juvela gluten-free harvest mix, loaf and high-fibre loaf (sliced and unsliced), bread rolls, fibre bread rolls, part-baked rolls with or without fibre, crispbread, mix and fibre mix; digestive biscuits, savoury biscuits and tea biscuits, pizza bases; Lifestyle gluten-free bread rolls, brown and white bread, high-fibre bread or rolls; Pleniday bread and pastas; Polial gluten-free biscuits; Rite-Diet gluten-free fibre rolls, high-fibre bread (sliced and unsliced), white bread (sliced and unsliced), white rolls, part-baked fibre loaf and long rolls; Schar gluten-free bread, bread mix, ertha brown bread, bread rolls and buns, crackers, cake mix, cracker toast, crispbread, flour mix, french

bread (baguette), pasta (fusilli, lasagne, macaroni pipette penne, rigati, rings, shells, spaghetti), pizza base, biscuits, savoy biscuits, white bread buns, wholemeal flour mix; Sunnyvale gluten-free bread; Tinkyada gluten-free brown rice pasta (elbows, fettucini, fusilli, penne, shells, spaghetti, spirals); Tritamyl flour, brown bread mix and white bread mix; Ultra gluten-free baguette, bread, bread rolls, high-fibre bread, crackerbread, pizza base; Valpiform bread mix, country loaf, pastry mix, petites baguettes

Gluten-sensitive enteropathies with coexisting established wheat sensitivity
Ener-G pizza bases, Seattle brown rolls (round or long), Six flour loaf; Glutafin Crisp Bread, Crisp Roll

Glycogen storage disease
Caloreen; Corn Flour or Corn Starch; Glucose (dextrose); Maxijul LE, Liquid (orange flavour), and Super Soluble; Polycal; Polycal Liquid and powder; Polycose; Pro-Cal; QuickCal; Vitajoule; Vitasavoury.

Growth Failure (disease related)
Enrich Plus ready-to-hang; Fortini, Fortini Multifibre; Frebini Original; Infatrini; Nutrini Extra, Multifibre and Standard; Paediasure Liquid and Liquid with fibre and Plus; SMA High Energy; Sondalis Junior; Survimed OPD; Tentrini, Energy, Energy Multi Fibre, Multi Fibre.

Haemodialysis
See dialysis.

Histidinaemia
See low-protein products; synthetic diets.

Homocystinuria
Analog XMet; Methionine-Free Amino Acid Mix; Vitaflo Flavour Pac; HCU Express; HCU gel; XMet Homidon; XMet Maxamaid; XMet Maxamum, and see also low-protein products; synthetic diets.

Hyperlipoproteinaemia type I
Alembicol D; Liquigen; Medium Chain Triglyceride Oil.

Hyperlysinaemia
Analog XLys; XLys Maxamaid

Hypermethioninaemia
XMET Analog; Methionine-Free Amino Acid Mix; XMET Homidon; XMET Maxamaid; XMET Maxamum.

Hypoglycaemia
Corn Flour or Corn Starch; and see also glycogen storage disease.

Hypoproteinaemia
Casilan 90; Dialamine; Maxipro Super Soluble; Maxisorb; ProMod; Protifar; Renapro; Vitapro.

Inflammatory Bowel Disease
Complete foods: Clinutren 1.5 Fibre, and Clinutren ISO; Elemental 028; Elemental 028 Extra; Emsogen; Enrich; Ensure; Ensure Powder; Foodlink Complete; Frebini Original; Fresubin Energy, Fresubin Energy Fibre (sip and tube feed) Fresubin Original Liquid and Sip Feeds, Fresubin 1000, and Fresubin 1200 Complete; Isosource Energy, Fibre and Standard; Jevity and Plus; Novasource GI Control, and Forte; Nutini Extra, and Fibre; Nutrison Multi Fibre, Energy Multi Fibre, Soya and Standard; Osmolite Liquid and Plus; Peptamen, Sondalis Junior; Tentrini, Energy, Energy Multi Fibre, Multi Fibre.
Nutritional supplements: Clinutren Dessert, Fruit and 1.5; Enlive Plus; Ensure Plus; Formance; Forticreme; Fortifresh; Fortijuce; Fortimel; Fortipudding; Fortisip Bottle, Multi Fibre, Protein; Fresubin HP Energy, and Fresubin Protein Energy Drink; Nutrison Energy, MCT and Pepti Powder; Perative; Provide Xtra; Resource Benefiber, Dessert Energy, Protein Extra, and Shake; Survimed OPD.

Intestinal lymphangiectasia
See malabsorption states.

Intestinal surgery
See malabsorption states

Isomaltose intolerance
See carbohydrate malabsorption.

Isovaleric acidaemia
XLEU Analog; XLEU Faladon; XLEU Maxamaid.

Lactose intolerance
See carbohydrate malabsorption.

Lipoprotein lipase deficiency (primary and secondary)
Monogen

Liver failure
Alembicol D; Aminex low-protein biscuits, cookies and rusks; Aproten products (anellini, biscuits, bread mix, cake mix, crispbread, ditalini, rigatini, spaghetti, tagliatelle); Ener-G low protein egg replacer, rice bread; Generaid; Generaid Plus; Juvela low-protein (chocolate chip, orange, and cinnamon flavour) cookies, loaf (sliced and unsliced), bread rolls, mix; Liquigen; Loprofin egg replacer, egg white replacer; Loprofin low-protein bread (sliced and unsliced), bread rolls (part-baked), white rolls, fibre bread (sliced and unsliced), mix, breakfast cereal, pasta (macaroni, penne, spaghetti long, pasta spirals, vermicelli), sweet biscuits, chocolate cream-filled biscuits, crackers, cookies (chocolate chip, cinnamon), wafers (orange, chocolate, vanilla); Medium Chain Triglyceride Oil; Nepro; Promin low-protein pasta (alphabets, macaroni, shells, short-cut spaghetti, spirals), pasta tricolour (alphabets, shells, spirals), pasta meal, Rite-Diet low-protein baking mix, flour mix; Suplena; Ultra low-protein, canned bread (brown and white); Ultra PKU biscuits, bread, cookies, flour, pizza base and savoy biscuits; Valpiform cookies with chocolate nuggets, shortbread biscuits; Vita-Bite.

Long chain acyl-CoA dehydrogenase deficiency (LCAD)
Monogen

Low-protein products
Aminex low-protein biscuits, cookies and rusks; Aproten products (anellini, biscuits, bread mix, cake mix, crispbread, ditalini, rigatini, spaghetti, tagliatelle); Ener-G low protein egg replacer, rice bread; Juvela low-protein (chocolate chip, orange, and cinnamon flavour) cookies, loaf (sliced and unsliced), mix, bread rolls; Loprofin egg replacer, egg white replacer; Loprofin low-protein bread (sliced and unsliced), mix, rolls (part-baked), fibre bread (sliced or unsliced), herb crackers, pasta (macaroni, spaghetti long, pasta spirals, vermicelli); sweet biscuits, chocolate cream-filled biscuits, crackers, cookies (chocolate chip, cinnamon), wafers (orange, chocolate, vanilla), breakfast cereal; PK Foods bread (sliced), crispbread, pasta (spirals); PKU-Gel; Promin low-protein pasta (alphabets, macaroni, shells, shortcut spaghetti, spirals), pasta tricolour (alphabets, shells, spirals), pasta meal, pasta

imitation rice; Rite-Diet low-protein flour mix, baking mix; Ultra low-protein, canned bread (brown and white); Ultra PKU biscuits, bread, cookies, flour, pizza base and savoy biscuits; Valpiform cookies with chocolate nuggets, shortbread biscuits; Vita-Bite.

Malabsorption states

(see also gluten-sensitive enteropathies; liver failure; carbohydrate malabsorption; intestinal lymphangiectasia; milk intolerance and synthetic diets); includes short-bowel syndrome. It should be noted that hyperosmolar feeds should be **avoided** if the short bowel ends in a stoma or the short bowel is anastomosed to the colon.

(a) *Protein sources*: Caprilon; Comminuted Chicken Meat (SHS); Maxipro Super Soluble; Maxisorb; MCT Pepdite; Neocate; Neocate Advance; Pepdite.
(b) *Fat sources*: Alembicol D; Calogen; Caprilon; Liquigen; MCT Pepdite; Medium Chain Triglyceride Oil; Pro-Cal; QuickCal; Vitasavoury.
(c) *Carbohydrate*: Caloreen; Maxijul LE, Liquid, and Super Soluble; Novasource GI Control, and Forte; Nutini Extra and Multifibre, Polycal Liquid and Powder; Polycose; Pro-Cal; QuickCal; Resource Benefiber; Vitajoule; Vitasavoury.
(d) *Fat/carbohydrate sources*: Calshake; Duobar; Duocal Liquid, MCT and Super Soluble; Scandishake; SPS Energy Bar.
(e) *Complete Feeds*: For use as the sole source of nutrition or as a nutritional supplement prescribed on medical grounds: Caprilon; Clinutren 1.5 Fibre and Clinutren ISO; Elemental 028; Elemental 028 Extra; Emsogen; Enrich; Ensure; Ensure Powder; Foodlink Complete; Frebini Original; Fresubin Energy, Fresubin Energy Fibre (sip and tube feed), Fresubin Original Liquid and Sip Feeds, Fresubin 1000, and Fresubin 1200 Complete; Isosource Energy, Fibre and Standard; Jevity, and Plus; MCT Pepdite; Novasource GI Control, and Forte; Nutrini, Extra and Fibre; Nutrison Multi Fibre, Energy Multi Fibre, Soya, Standard, Vitaplus Multi Fibre; Osmolite Liquid and Plus; Paediasure Liquid, Liquid with fibre and Plus; Pepdite; Peptamen; Pepti-Junior; SMA High Energy; Sondalis Junior; Tentrini, Energy, Energy Multi Fibre, Multi Fibre.
(f) *Nutritional supplements*: Nutritional supplements prescribed on medical grounds: Clinutren Dessert, Fruit, Junior, and 1.5; Enlive Plus; Enrich Plus; Ensure Bar and Plus; Formance; Forticreme; Fortifresh; Fortijuce; Fortimel; Fortisip Bottle, Multi Fibre, Protein; Fresubin HP Energy, and Fresubin Protein Energy Drink; Nutrison Energy, MCT, and Pepti Powder; Perative; Provide Xtra; Resource Shake and Benefiber; Survimed OPD.
(g) *Minerals*: Aminogran Mineral Mixture; Metabolic Mineral Mixture.
(h) *Vitamins*: As appropriate, and see synthetic diets.
(i) *Vitamins and Minerals*: Energivit; Paediatric Seravit

Malnutrition (disease-related)

Complete foods: Calogen; Caloreen; Calshake; Duobar; Duocal Liquid, MCT, and Super Soluble; Enrich and Plus; Ensure; Ensure Powder; Foodlink Compete; Frebini Original; Fresubin Energy, Fresubin Energy Fibre (sip and tube feed), Fresubin Original Liquid and Sip Feeds, Fresubin 1000, and Fresubin 1200 Complete; Infatrini; Isosource Energy, Fibre and Standard; Jevity and Plus; Maxijul LE, Liquid and Super Soluble; Novasource GI Control and Forte; Nutrini Extra, Fibre and Standard; Nutrison Multi Fibre, Energy Multi Fibre, Soya, Standard, Vitaplus Multi Fibre; Osmolite Liquid and Plus; Paediasure Liquid, Liquid with fibre and Plus; Polycal Liquid and Powder; Polycose; Scandishake; SMA High Energy; Tentrini, Energy, Energy Multi Fibre, Multi Fibre; Vitajoule.
Nutritional supplements: Clinutren Dessert, Fruit, ISO and 1.5; Enlive Plus; Ensure Plus; Formance; Forticreme; Fortifresh; Fortijuce; Fortimel; Fortini, Fortini Multifibre, Fortipudding; Fortisip Bottle, Multi Fibre, Protein; Fresubin HP Energy; Nutrison Energy and MCT; Perative; ProSure, Provide Xtra; Pro-Cal; Quickcal; Resource Benefiber, Dessert Energy, Protein Xtra, and Shake; Sondalis Junior; Survimed OPD; Vitasavoury.

Maple syrup urine disease

Mapleflex; MSUD Analog; MSUD Maxamaid; MSUD Maxamum; MSUD Aid III, and see also low-protein products; synthetic diets.

Methylmalonic acidaemia

XMTVI Analog; XMTVI Asadon; XMTVI Maxamaid; XMTVI Maxamum.

Milk protein sensitivity

Comminuted Chicken Meat (SHS); Farley's Soya Formula; InfaSoy; Isomil powder; Nutramigen; Prosobee; Wysoy, and see also synthetic diets.

Nutritional support for adults

(a) **Nutritionally complete feeds.** For use as the sole source of nutrition or as a necessary nutritional supplement prescribed on medical grounds:
    (i) Gluten-Free: Foodlink Complete; Fortifresh; Fresubin Liquid and Sip Feeds; Nutrison Multi Fibre, Energy Multi Fibre and Standard; Sondalis Junior.
    (ii) Lactose- and Gluten-Free: Enrich; Ensure, Ensure Powder; Fresubin Original Fibre; Nutrison Soya; Osmolite Liquid and Plus; Sondalis 1.5.
    (iii) Containing fibre: Enrich; Fresubin Energy Fibre (tube and sip feed), Fresubin Original Fibre; Isosource Fibre; Jevity; Novasource GI Control, and Forte; Nutrini Extra, and Fibre; Nutrison Multi Fibre, Energy Multi Fibre; Paediasure with Fibre.
    (iv) Elemental Feeds: Elemental 028; Elemental 028 Extra; Emsogen; Peptamen; Peptisorb.
(b) **Nutritional source supplements**: see synthetic diets; malabsorption states.
    (i) General supplements. Necessary nutritional supplements prescribed on medical grounds: Clinutren range; Enlive Plus; Enrich Plus; Ensure Plus; Foodlink Complete; Formance; Forticreme; Fortijuce; Fortimel; Fortini, Fortini MultiFibre; Fortisip; Fortisip Multi Fibre; Fresubin HP Energy; Fresubin 1000, and 1200 Complete; Maxisorb; Nutrison Energy and MCT; Perative; Provide Xtra; Resource Shake; Survimed OPD.
    (ii) Carbohydrates; lactose-free and gluten-free; [1]Caloreen; [1]Maxijul LE Liquid, and Super

1. Have low electrolyte content

Soluble; [1]Polycal; [1]Polycal Liquid; Polycose; Pro-Cal; QuickCal; Resource Benefiber; Vitajoule; Vitasavoury.
(iii) Fat: Alembicol D; Calogen; Liquigen; MCT Oil.
(iv) Fat/carbohydrate sources: Calshake; Duobar; Duocal Liquid, MCT Powder and Super Soluble (low-electrolyte content); Scandishake, SPS Energy Bar.
(v) Nitrogen sources: Casilan 90 (whole protein based, low-sodium); Maxipro Super Soluble (whey protein based, low-sodium); Maxisorb; Pro-Mod (whey protein based, low-sodium).
(vi) Minerals: Aminogran Mineral Mixture; Metabolic Mineral Mixture.

Phenylketonuria
Aminex low-protein biscuits, cookies and rusks; Aminogran Food Supplement (powder and tablets) and Mineral Mixture; Analog LCP; Analog XP; Aproten products (annellini, biscuits, bread mix, cake mix, crispbread, ditalini, rigatini, spaghetti, tagliatelle); Ener-G low protein egg replacer; Juvela low-protein loaf (sliced and unsliced), bread rolls, cookies (chocolate chip, orange, and cinnamon flavour), mix; Lofenalac; Loprofin egg replacer; Loprofin low-protein bread (sliced and unsliced), breakfast cereal, rolls (part-baked), rolls (white), fibre bread (sliced and unsliced), mix and pasta (macaroni, penne, spaghetti long, pasta spirals, vermicelli), sweet biscuits, chocolate cream-filled biscuits, crackers, cookies (chocolate chip, cinnamon), wafers (orange, chocolate, vanilla); Loprofin PKU drink; Metabolic Mineral Mixture; Milupa PKU2 and PKU3; Phlexy-10 exchange system; Phlexyvits; PK Aid 4; PK Foods bread (sliced), crispbread, pasta (spirals), cookies (chocolate chip, orange, cinnamon), egg replacer, flour mix, jelly (orange, cherry); PKU-Gel; Promin low-protein pasta (alphabets, macaroni, shells, shortcut spaghetti, spirals), pasta tricolour (alphabets, shells, spirals), pasta meal; Rite-Diet low-protein baking mix, flour mix; Sno-Pro; L-Tyrosine supplement; Ultra low-protein, canned white bread; Ultra PKU biscuits, bread, cookies, flour, pizza base, savoy biscuits; Valpiform cookies, shortbread biscuits; XP Maxamaid XP Concentrate Maxamaid; XP Maxamum; and see low-protein products and synthetic diets

Propionic acidaemia
XMTVI Analog; XMTVI Asadon; XMTVI Maxamaid; XMTVI Maxamum.

Protein intolerance
See amino acid metabolic disorders, low-protein products, milk protein sensitivity, synthetic diets, and whole protein sensitivity.

Refsum's Disease
Fresubin Original Liquid and Sip Feeds.

Renal dialysis
See Dialysis.

Renal failure
Aminex low-protein biscuits, cookies and rusks; Aproten products (annellini, biscuits, bread mix, cake mix, crispbread, ditalini, rigatini, spaghetti, tagliatelle); Dialamine; Ener-G low protein egg replacer, rice bread; Juvela low-protein (chocolate chip, orange, and cinnamon flavour) cookies, loaf (sliced and unsliced), bread rolls and flour mix; Kindergen; Loprofin egg replacer, egg white replacer, Loprofin bread (sliced and unsliced), breakfast cereal, rolls (part-baked), rolls (white), fibre bread (sliced and unsliced), mix and pasta (macaroni, penne, spaghetti long, pasta spirals, vermicelli), sweet biscuits, chocolate cream-filled biscuits, crackers, cookies (chocolate chip, cinnamon), wafers (orange, chocolate, vanilla); Nepro; Promin low-protein pasta (alphabets, macaroni, shells, shortcut spaghetti, spirals), pasta tricolour (alphabets, shells, spirals), pasta meal; Renamil; Rite-Diet low-protein flour mix, baking mix, Sno-Pro Drink; Suplena; Ultra low-protein, canned bread (brown and white); Ultra PKU bread, biscuits, cookies, flour, pizza base and savoy biscuits; Valpiform cookies with chocolate nuggets, shortbread biscuits, Vita-Bite

Short-bowel syndrome
See Malabsorption states.

Sicca Syndrome
Bioxtra Moisturising Gel; Glandosane; Luborant; Oralbalance; Saliva Orthana; Salivace; Saliveze; Salivix.

Sucrose intolerance
See Carbohydrate malabsorption.

Synthetic diets
(a) *Fat*: Alembicol D; Calogen; Liquigen; Medium Chain Triglyceride Oil; Pro-Cal; QuickCal; Vitasavoury.
(b) *Carbohydrate*: Caloreen; Maxijul LE, Liquid, Super Soluble; Polycal; Polycal Liquid; Polycose powder; Pro-Cal; QuickCal; Vitasavoury.
(c) *Fat/carbohydrate sources*: Calshake; Duobar; Duocal Liquid, MCT Powder and Super Soluble (low-electrolyte content); Scandishake.
(d) *Minerals*: Aminogran Mineral Mixture; Metabolic Mineral Mixture.
(e) *Protein sources*: see malabsorption states, complete feeds.
(f) *Vitamins*: as appropriate and see malabsorption states, nutritional support for adults.
(g) *Vitamins and Minerals*: Paediatric Seravit; Phlexyvits.

Tyrosinaemia
Analog XPhen, Tyr; Analog XPhen, Tyr, Met; XPhen, Tyr Maxamaid; XPTM Tyrosidon; XPT Tyrosidon.

Urea cycle disorders
L-Arginine supplement

Vomiting in infancy
Instant Carobel, Nestargel.

Whole protein sensitivity
Caprilon; MCT Pepdite; Neocate; Neocate Advance; Nutramigen; Pepdite; Pepti-Junior; Prejomin.
NOTE. Defined as intolerance to whole protein, proven by at least two withdrawal and challenge tests, as suggested by an accurate dietary history

Xerostomia
Bioxtra Moisturising Gel; Glandosane; Luborant; Biotene Oralbalance Dry Mouth Saliva Replacement Gel; Saliva Orthana; Saliveze; Salivix.

1. Have low electrolyte content

Conditions for which toilet preparations may be prescribed on FP10, GP10 (Scotland), WP10 (Wales)

NOTE. This is a list of clinical conditions for which the ACBS has approved toilet preparations. For details of the preparations see Chapter 13.

Birthmarks
See disfiguring skin lesions.

Dermatitis
Aveeno Bath Oil; Aveeno Cream; Aveeno Colloidal; Aveeno Baby Colloidal ; E45 Emollient Bath Oil; E45 Emollient Wash Cream; E45 Lotion; Vaseline Dermacare Cream and Lotion

Dermatitis herpetiformis
See gluten-sensitive enteropathies.

Disfiguring skin lesions (birthmarks, mutilating lesions, scars, vitiligo)
Covermark classic foundation and finishing powder; Dermablend Cover Creme, Leg and Body Cover, and Setting Powder; Dermacolor Camouflage cream and fixing powder; Keromask masking cream and finishing powder; Veil Cover cream and Finishing Powder. (Cleansing Creams, Cleansing Milks, and Cleansing Lotions are excluded)

Disinfectants (antiseptics)
May be prescribed on an FP10 only when ordered in such quantities and with such directions as are appropriate for the treatment of patients, but not for general hygenic purposes.

Eczema
See dermatitis.

Photodermatoses (skin protection in)
Ambre Solaire Total Screen for Sun Intolerant skin SPF 60; Coppertone Ultrashade 23; Delph Sun Lotion SPF 15, SPF 20, SPF 25, and SPF 30; E45 Sun Block SPF 25, and 50; RoC Total Sunblock Cream SPF 25; Spectraban 25, and Ultra; Sunsense Ultra; Uvistat Sun Block Cream Factor 20, and Ultrablock Suncream Factor 30.

Pruritus
See dermatitis.

Appendix 8: Wound management products and elastic hosiery

A8.1 Wound dressings

An overview of the management of *chronic wounds* (including venous ulcers and pressure sores) and the role of different dressings is given below as is the NICE guidance on difficult-to-heal surgical wounds; the notes do not deal with the management of clean surgical wounds which usually heal very rapidly. The correct dressing for wound management depends not only on the type of wound but also on the stage of the healing process. The principal stages of healing are:

- cleansing, removal of debris;
- granulation, vascularisation;
- epithelialisation.

Greater understanding of the requirements of a surgical dressing, including recognition of the benefits of maintaining a moist environment for wound healing, has improved the management of chronic wounds.

The ideal dressing needs to ensure that the wound remains:

- moist with exudate, but not macerated;
- free of clinical infection and excessive slough;
- free of toxic chemicals, particles or fibres;
- at the optimum temperature for healing;
- undisturbed by the need for frequent changes;
- at the optimum pH value.

As wound healing passes through its different stages, variations in dressing type may be required to satisfy better one or other of these requirements. Depending on the type of wound or the stage of the healing process, the functions of dressings may be summarised as follows:

Type of wound	Role of dressing
Dry, necrotic, black	Moisture retention or rehydration
Yellow, sloughy	If dry, moisture retention or rehydration If moist, fluid absorption Possibly odour absorption Possibly antimicrobial activity
Clean, exuding (granulating)	Fluid absorption Thermal insulation Possibly odour absorption Possibly antimicrobial activity
Dry, low exudate (epithelialising)	Moisture retention or rehydration Low adherence Thermal insulation

A decrease in pain and reduction in healing time is achieved to a marked extent with **alginate**, **foam**, **hydrogel** and **hydrocolloid** dressings and also to an important extent with **vapour-permeable films** and **membranes**; dressings such as dry gauze have little place. Practices such as the use of irritant cleansers may be harmful and are largely obsolete; removal of debris and dressing remnants should need minimal irrigation with physiological saline.

Alginate, **foam**, **hydrogel** and **hydrocolloid** dressings are designed to absorb wound exudate and thus to control the state of hydration of a wound. All are claimed to be effective, but as yet there have been few trials able to establish a clear advantage for any particular product. The choice between different dressings may therefore often depend not only on the type and stage of the wound, but also on personal experience, availability of the dressing, patient preference or tolerance and site of the wound.

NICE guidance (debriding agents for difficult-to-heal surgical wounds). The National Institute for Health and Clinical Excellence has stated that alginate, foam, hydrocolloid, hydrogel, and polysaccharide (as beads or paste) dressings as well as maggots may reduce pain from difficult-to-heal surgical wounds. There is insufficient evidence to support one debriding agent over another and choice should be based on patient acceptability (including factors such as comfort and odour control), type and location of the wound, and total cost (including time for changing the dressings).

A8.1.1 Alginate dressings

The gelling characteristics of alginate dressings vary according to the product used. Some products only gel to a limited extent to form a partially gelled sheet that can be lifted off; others form an amorphous gel that can be rinsed off with water or physiological saline. A secondary covering is needed. They are highly absorbent and are therefore suitable for moderately or heavily exuding wounds, but not for eschars or for dry wounds.

ActivHeal® Alginate (MedLogic)

Calcium sodium alginate dressing, sterile, net price 5 cm × 5 cm = 57p, 10 cm × 10 cm = £1.11, 10 cm × 20 cm = £2.73

Uses: moderately to heavily exuding wounds

ActivHeal® Alginate cavity dressing, net price 2 cm × 30 cm = £2.05

Uses: moderately to heavily exuding cavity wounds

Algisite® M (S&N Hlth.)

Calcium alginate fibre, sterile, flat non-woven dressing, net price 5 cm × 5 cm = 80p, 10 cm × 10 cm = £1.66, 15 cm × 20 cm = £4.44

Uses: moderately to heavily exuding wounds

Algisite® M Rope, net price 2 cm × 30 cm = £3.00

Uses: moderately to heavily exuding cavity wounds

Algosteril® (Beiersdorf)

Calcium alginate dressing. Net price 5 cm × 5 cm = 79p, 10 cm × 10 cm = £1.81, 10 cm × 20 cm = £3.07

Uses: moderately to heavily exuding wounds

Algosteril® Rope, net price 2 g, 30 cm = £3.28

Uses: moderately to heavily exuding cavity wounds

Curasorb® (Tyco)

Calcium alginate dressing, net price 5 cm × 5 cm = 69p, 10 cm × 10 cm = £1.46, 10 cm × 14 cm = £2.36, 10 cm × 20 cm = £2.87, 15 cm × 25 cm = £5.05, 30 cm × 61 cm = £26.50 (other sizes NHS)

Curasorb® Plus, calcium alginate dressing, 10 cm × 10 cm = £2.00

Curasorb® Zn, calcium alginate and zinc dressing, 5 cm × 5 cm = 78p, 10 cm × 10 cm = £1.65, 10 cm × 20 cm = £3.24 (other sizes NHS)

Kaltostat® (ConvaTec)

(Alginate Dressing, BP 1993, type C). Calcium alginate fibre, flat non-woven pads, 5 cm × 5 cm, net price = 83p, 7.5 cm × 12 cm = £1.80, 10 cm × 20 cm = £3.50, 15 cm × 25 cm = £6.01, (NHS) 30 cm × 60 cm = £25.13

Uses: moderately to heavily exuding wounds

Kaltostat® Wound Packing, net price 2 g = £3.28

Uses: moderately to heavily exuding cavity wounds

Melgisorb® (Mölnlycke)

Calcium sodium alginate fibre, sterile, highly absorbent, gelling dressing, flat non-woven pads, net price 5 cm × 5 cm = 79p, 10 cm × 10 cm = £1.64, 10 cm × 20 cm = £3.09

Uses: moderately to heavily exuding wounds including leg ulcers, dermal lesions and traumatic wounds

Melgisorb® Cavity, calcium sodium alginate fibre, sterile, highly absorbent, gelling filler ribbon, net price 32 cm × 2.2 cm, 3 pieces (2 g) = £3.11

Uses: moderately to heavily exuding cavity wounds, fistulas, sinuses, pressure sores and deep leg ulcers

SeaSorb® (Coloplast)

SeaSorb® Soft, alginate containing hydrocolloid dressing, sterile, highly absorbent, gelling dressing, 5 cm × 5 cm = 85p, 10 cm × 10 cm = £2.02, 15 cm × 15 cm = £3.83

Uses: heavily exuding wounds including leg ulcers and pressure sores

SeaSorb® Soft Filler, calcium sodium alginate fibre, highly absorbent, gelling filler, 44 cm = £2.38

Uses: moderately to heavily exuding cavity wounds, fistulas, sinus drainage, decubitus and deep leg ulcers

Sorbalgon® (Hartmann)

Calcium alginate dressing, net price 5 cm × 5 cm = 73p, 10 cm × 10 cm = £1.52

Uses: for medium to heavily exuding wounds

Sorbalgon T®, calcium alginate cavity dressing, net price 2 g, 32 cm = £3.11

Uses: for medium to heavily exuding wounds

Sorbsan® (Unomedical)

(Alginate Dressing, BP 1993, type A). Calcium alginate fibre, highly absorbent, flat non-woven pads, 5 cm × 5 cm, net price = 74p, 10 cm × 10 cm = £1.55, 10 cm × 20 cm = £2.90

Uses: moderately to heavily exuding wounds

Sorbsan® Plus, alginate dressing bonded to a secondary absorbent viscose pad, net price 7.5 cm × 10 cm = £1.57, 10 cm × 15 cm = £2.77, 10 cm × 20 cm = £3.53, 15 cm × 20 cm = £4.90

Uses: moderately to heavily exuding shallow wounds and ulcers

Sorbsan® Surgical Packing, 30 cm (2 g) = £3.22

Sorbsan® Ribbon, 40 cm (with 12.5-cm probe) = £1.88

Uses: moderately to heavily exuding cavity wounds

Sorbsan® SA NHS calcium alginate fibre, highly absorbent flat non-woven pads for wound contact bonded to adhesive semi-permeable polyurethane foam. Net price 9 cm × 11 cm = £2.24

Uses: moderately to lightly exuding shallow wounds

Suprasorb A® (Vernon-Carus)

Calcium alginate dressing, sterile, net price 5 cm × 5 cm = 56p, 10 cm × 10 cm = £1.10

Suprasorb A® Rope, net price 2 g × 30 cm = £2.04

Uses: moderate to heavily exuding wounds

Tegagen® (3M)

(Alginate Dressing, BP 1993, type B). Net price 5 cm × 5 cm = 75p, 10 cm × 10 cm = £1.58

Uses: for leg ulcers, pressure sores, second degree burns, post-operative wounds, fungating carcinomas

Tegagen® Rope, net price 2 cm × 30 cm = £2.63

Uses: moderately to heavily exuding cavity wounds

Urgosorb® (Parema)
Alginate containing hydrocolloid dressing without adhesive border, sterile, net price 10 cm × 10 cm = £1.83, 10 cm × 20 cm = £3.35
Urgosorb Rope cavity dressing, net price 30 cm = £2.44

A8.1.2 Foam dressings

Foam dressings vary from products that are suitable for lightly exuding wounds to highly absorbent structures for heavily exuding wounds. They may also be used as secondary dressings. In hypergranulating (or overgranulating) tissue (which may arise from the use of occlusive dressings such as hydrocolloids), changing to a more permeable product such as a foam dressing may be beneficial.

Polyurethane Foam Dressing, BP 1993
Absorbent foam dressing of low adherence, sterile
Lyofoam®, net price 7.5 cm × 7.5 cm = 97p, 10 cm × 10 cm = £1.14, 10 cm × 17.5 cm = £1.78, 15 cm × 20 cm = £2.40, other sizes (NHS) 10 cm × 25 cm = £4.79 (hosp. only), 25 cm × 30 cm = £11.35 (Medlock)
Uses: treatment of burns, decubitus ulcers, donor sites, granulating wounds

Polyurethane Foam Film Dressing, Sterile, with Adhesive Border
(Drug Tariff specification 47)
Allevyn® *Lite Island*, net price 9.75 cm × 16.5 cm = £1.71; 13.5 cm × 13.5 cm = £2.23; 16 cm × 16 cm = £2.65; 13.5 cm × 23.5 cm = £3.41 (S & N Hlth)
Lyofoam® *Extra Adhesive*, net price 9 cm × 9 cm = £1.20; 15 cm × 15 cm = £2.25; 22 cm × 22 cm = £4.44; 30 cm × 30 cm = £6.45; sacral, 15 cm × 13 cm = £1.84; 22 cm × 26 cm = £3.49 (Medlock)
Suprasorb P®, net price 7.5 cm × 7.5 cm = £1.16, 10 cm × 10 cm = £1.25, 15 cm × 15 cm = £2.24 (Vernon-Carus)
Tielle®, net price 11 cm × 11 cm = £2.24; 15 cm × 15 cm = £3.66; 18 cm × 18 cm = £4.67; 7 cm × 9 cm = £1.21; 15 cm × 20 cm = £4.59; *Tielle*® *Sacrum* 18 cm × 18 cm = £3.39 (J&J)
Trufoam®, net price 7 cm × 9 cm = £1.07; 11 cm × 11 cm = £2.04 (Unomedical)
Uses: light to moderately exuding wounds, not recommended for dry superficial wounds

Polyurethane Foam Film Dressing, Sterile, without Adhesive Border
(Drug Tariff specification 47)
Allevyn® *Lite*, net price 5 cm × 5 cm = 98p; 10 cm × 10 cm = £1.77; 10 cm × 20 cm = £3.04; 15 cm × 20 cm = £3.79 (S&N Hlth)
Allevyn® *Thin* (with adhesive border), net price 5 cm × 6 cm = 92p, 10 cm × 10 cm = £1.87, 15 cm × 15 cm = £3.08, 15 cm × 20 cm = £3.73
FlexiPore®, net price 10 cm × 10 cm = £1.73; 10 cm × 30 cm = £3.60 (MedLogic)
Lyofoam® *Extra*, net price 10 cm × 10 cm = £1.91; 17.5 cm × 10 cm = £3.23; 20 cm × 15 cm = £4.19; 25 cm × 10 cm = £3.84; (NHS) 30 cm × 25 cm = £14.35 (Medlock)
Suprasorb P®, net price 5 cm × 5 cm = 90p, 7.5 cm × 7.5 cm = 96p, 10 cm × 10 cm = £1.13, 15 cm × 15 cm = £3.01 (Vernon-Carus)
Transorbent®, net price 5 cm × 7 cm = 94p; 10 cm × 10 cm = £1.78; 15 cm × 15 cm = £3.27; 20 cm × 20 cm = £5.23 (Unomedical)
Uses: light to moderately exuding wounds, not recommended for dry superficial wounds

Polyurethane Foam Film Dressing, Sterile, with Adhesive Border
Tielle® *Lite*, net price 11 cm × 11 cm = £2.15; 7 cm × 9 cm = £1.14; 8 cm × 15 cm = £2.65; 8 cm × 20 cm = £2.80 (J&J)
Uses: light to non-exuding wounds
ActivHeal® *Foam Island*, net price 10 cm × 10 cm = £1.57, 15 cm × 15 cm = £1.92, 20 cm × 20 cm = £4.34 (MedLogic)
Uses: moderate to heavily exuding wounds
Allevyn® *Adhesive*, net price 7.5 cm × 7.5 cm = £1.32, 10 cm × 10 cm = £1.93, 12.5 cm × 12.5 cm = £2.37, 17.5 cm × 17.5 cm = £4.66, 12.5 cm × 22.5 cm = £3.68, 22.5 cm × 22.5 cm = £6.79 (S&N Hlth)
Allevyn® *Plus Adhesive*, net price 12.5 cm × 12.5 cm = £2.90; 17.5 cm × 17.5 cm = £5.60; 12.5 cm × 22.5 cm = £5.14
Allevyn® *Sacrum* shaped, net price 17 cm × 17 cm = £3.49, 22 cm × 22 cm = £5.02
Uses: light to moderately exuding sacral wounds
Biatain® *Adhesive*, net price 12 cm × 12 cm = £2.25, 18 cm × 18 cm = £4.50, 18 cm × 28 cm = £6.79, 23 cm × 23 cm (sacral) = £3.85, 19 cm × 20 cm (heel) = £4.49; 6 cm diameter = £1.50 (Coloplast)
Uses: moderate to heavily exuding wounds
Curafoam® *Island*, net price 10 cm × 10 cm = £1.21, 15 cm × 15 cm = £2.19, 20 cm × 20 cm = £4.34 (Tyco)
Uses: moderate to heavily exuding wounds
Tielle® *Plus*, net price 11 cm × 11 cm = £2.48; 15 cm × 15 cm = £4.05; 15 cm × 20 cm = £5.08; 15 cm × 15 cm (sacrum) = £2.95 (J&J)
Uses: moderate to heavily exuding wounds
Trufoam®, net price 15 cm × 15 cm = £3.41, 15 cm × 20 cm = £4.28 (Unomedical)
Uses: moderate to heavily exuding wounds

Polyurethane Foam Film Dressing, Sterile, without Adhesive Border
ActivHeal® *Foam Non-Adhesive*, net price 5 cm × 5 cm = 72p, 10 cm × 10 cm = £1.09, 20 cm × 20 cm = £3.78 (MedLogic)
Uses: heavily exuding wounds
Advazorb®, net price 5 cm × 7.5 cm = 45p, 10 cm × 10 cm = 80p (Advancis)
Allevyn®, net price 5 cm × 5 cm = £1.11, 9 cm × 9 cm = £3.49 NHS, 10 cm × 10 cm = £2.21, 10 cm × 20 cm = £3.55, 20 cm × 20 cm = £5.92, 10.5 cm × 13.5 cm (heel) = £4.43 (S&N Hlth)
Allevyn® *Compression*, net price 5 cm × 6 cm = £1.08; 10 cm × 10 cm = £2.23; 15 cm × 15 cm = £3.78, 15 cm × 20 cm = £4.24 (S&N Hlth)
Uses: moderately exuding wounds, burns, decubitus ulcers, and leg ulcers
Biatain® *Non-Adhesive*, net price 10 cm × 10 cm = £2.07, 10 cm × 20 cm = £3.49, 15 cm × 15 cm = £3.82, 20 cm × 20 cm = £5.68, circular, 5 cm diameter = £1.07, 8 cm diameter = £1.50 (Coloplast)
Curafoam® *Plus*, net price 6 cm × 6 cm = £1.06, 10 cm × 10 cm = £1.65, 10 cm × 13 cm = £2.05, 10 cm × 20 cm = £3.20, 20 cm × 20 cm = £5.04 (Tyco)
Hydrafoam®, net price 10 cm × 10 cm = £1.73, 10 cm × 20 cm = £3.10, 15 cm × 15 cm = £3.32, 20 cm × 20 cm = £5.15 (Tyco)
3M®, net price 8.9 cm × 8.9 cm (fenestrated) = £2.13, 10 cm × 10 cm = £2.09, 10 cm × 20 cm = £3.54, 20 cm × 20 cm = £5.65, 10 cm × 60 cm = £11.96 (3M)
Tielle® *Plus Borderless*, net price 11 cm × 11 cm = £2.98; 15 cm × 20 cm = £5.40 (J&J)
Trufoam® *NA*, net price 5 cm × 5 cm = £1.02, 10 cm × 10 cm = £1.93, 15 cm × 15 cm = £3.56 (Unomedical)
Uses: moderate to heavily exuding wounds

Allevyn® (S&N Hlth.)

Hydrophilic polyurethane dressing, foam sheets with trilaminate structure, non-adherent wound contact layer, foam based central layer, bacteria- and water-proof outer layer

Allevyn® Plus Cavity Sterile, highly absorbent polyurethane dressing consisting of a vapour-permeable foam matrix, net price 1.5 cm × 20 cm = £1.61, 5 cm × 6 cm = £1.64; 10 cm × 10 cm = £2.73; 15 cm × 20 cm = £5.46

Uses: heavily exuding deep wounds, including deep leg ulcers, decubitus ulcers, abscesses; management of post-operative wounds including pilonidal sinus excision

Allevyn® Cavity, net price circular, 5 cm diameter = £3.64, 10 cm = £8.69, tubular 9 cm × 2.5 cm = £3.53, 12 cm × 4 cm = £6.22

Uses: moderately to heavily exuding cavity wounds including deep pressure sores and leg ulcers, surgical incisions and excisions such as pilonidal sinus excisions

Avance® (Medlock)

Silver impregnated polyurethane foam film dressing

Avance® (without adhesive border), net price 10 cm × 10 cm = £2.59, 10 cm × 17 cm = £4.13, 15 cm × 20 cm = £5.71

Avance®A (with adhesive border), net price 9 cm × 9 cm = £2.18, 12 cm × 12 cm = £3.61, 15 cm × 15 cm = £4.42, 15 cm × 13 cm (sacral) = £3.25

Uses: for exuding wounds

Cavi-Care® (S&N Hlth.)

Soft, conforming cavity wound dressing prepared by mixing thoroughly for 15 seconds immediately before use and allowing to expand its volume within the cavity. Net price 20 g = £17.13

Uses: in the management of open post-operative granulating cavity wounds (with no underlying tracts or sinuses) such as pilonidal sinus excision, dehisced surgical wounds, hydradenitis suppurativa wounds, peri-anal wounds, perineal wounds, pressure sores

A8.1.3 Hydrogel dressings

Hydrogel dressings are most commonly supplied as an amorphous, cohesive material that can take up the shape of a wound. A secondary covering is needed. These dressings are generally used to donate liquid to dry sloughy wounds and facilitate autolytic debridement but they may also have the ability to absorb limited amounts of exudate. Hydrogel sheets are also available which have a fixed structure; such products have limited fluid handling capacity. Hydrogel sheets are best avoided in the presence of infection.

ActiFormCool® (Activa)

Net price 10 cm × 10 cm = £2.29, 10 cm × 15 cm = £3.29

ActivHeal® **Hydrogel** (MedLogic)

Net price 15 g = £1.36

Uses: pressure sores, cavity wounds, leg ulcers, skin donor sites, diabetic foot ulcers

Aquaform® (Unomedical)

(Drug Tariff specification 50) Hydrogel containing modified starch copolymer, net price 8 g = £1.48, 15 g = £1.80

Uses: for dry, sloughy or necrotic wounds, lightly exuding wounds, granulating wounds

Aquaflo® (Tyco)

Net price 3.8 cm diameter = £2.41, 7.5 cm = £2.50, 12 cm = £5.16

Curagel® (Tyco)

Net price 5 cm × 7.5 cm = £1.74, 10 cm × 10 cm = £2.71

Curagel Island (with adhesive border), net price 7.5 cm × 10 cm = £2.47, 12.5 cm × 12.5 cm = £3.58

Debrisan® (Pharmacia)

Beads, dextranomer. Net price 60-g castor = £29.01

Uses: for exudative and infected wounds, decubital ulcers, leg ulcers, hand burns, surgical wounds, post-traumatic wounds, sprinkle onto wound to a thickness of at least 3 mm and cover with appropriate dressing, renew before saturation occurs (usually once or twice daily)

Paste, dextranomer in a soft paste basis. Net price 10-g pouch = £4.99

Uses: for exudative and infected wounds, decubital ulcers, leg ulcers, surgical wounds, post-traumatic wounds, apply to a thickness of at least 3 mm and cover with appropriate dressing, renew before saturation occurs (usually once or twice daily)

Geliperm® (Geistlich)

Gel sheets in wet form, 10 cm × 10 cm = £2.23, 12 cm × 13cm = £4.88 (NHS); 12 cm × 26 cm = £8.73 (NHS)

Uses: wound and ulcer dressing, burns, donor sites

GranuGel® (ConvaTec)

(Drug Tariff Specification 50). Net price 15 g = £2.01

Uses: dry, sloughy or necrotic wounds, lightly exuding wounds, granulating wounds

Hydrosorb® (Hartmann)

Absorbent, transparent, hydrogel sheets containing polyurethane polymers covered with a semi-permeable film

Hydrosorb®, 5 cm × 7.5 cm = £1.80; 10 cm × 10 cm = £2.84; 20 cm × 20 cm = £6.84

Hydrosorb® comfort (with adhesive border, water-proof), 4.5 cm × 6.5 cm = £1.66; 7.5 cm × 10 cm = £2.59; 12.5 cm × 12.5 cm = £3.73

Uses: second degree burns, donor sites; chronic wounds where granulation is unsatisfactory, including leg ulcers, pressure sores

Intrasite Conformable® (S&N Hlth.)

(Drug Tariff specification 50). Soft and easily moulded non-woven dressing impregnated with Intrasite gel, net price 10 cm × 10 cm = £1.56; 10 cm × 20 cm = £2.11; 10 cm × 40 cm = £3.77

Uses: for dry, sloughy or necrotic wounds, lightly exuding wounds; granulating wounds

Intrasite® **Gel** (S&N Hlth.)

(Drug Tariff specification 50). A ready-mixed hydrogel containing modified carmellose polymer applied directly into the wound. Net price 8-g sachet = £1.56, 15-g sachet = £2.09, 25-g sachet = £3.10

Uses: for dry, sloughy or necrotic wounds; lightly exuding wounds; granulating wounds

Iodoflex® (S&N Hlth.)

Paste, iodine 0.9% as cadexomer–iodine in a paste basis with gauze backing, net price 5-g unit = £3.65; 10 g = £7.32; 17 g = £11.58

Uses: for treatment of chronic exuding wounds, such as leg ulcers, apply to wound surface, remove gauze backing and cover; renew when saturated (usually 2–3 times weekly, daily for heavily exuding wounds); max. single application 50 g, max. weekly application 150 g; max. duration up to 3 months in any single course of treatment

Cautions: caution in patients with severe renal impairment or history of thyroid disorders; iodine may be absorbed particularly if large wounds treated

Contra-indications: avoid in thyroid disorders, in those receiving lithium, in pregnancy and breast-feeding and use in children

Iodosorb® (S&N Hlth.)

Ointment, iodine 0.9% as cadexomer–iodine in an ointment basis, net price 10 g = £4.04; 20 g = £8.09

Powder, iodine 0.9% as cadexomer–iodine microbeads, net price 3-g sachet = £1.73
Uses: for treatment of chronic exuding wounds, such as leg ulcers, apply to wound surface to depth of approx. 3 mm and cover; renew when saturated (usually 2–3 times weekly, daily for heavily exuding wounds); max. single application 50 g, max. weekly application 150 g; max. duration up to 3 months in any single course of treatment
Cautions: caution in patients with severe renal impairment or history of thyroid disorders; iodine may be absorbed particularly if large wounds treated
Contra-indications: avoid in thyroid disorders, in those receiving lithium, in pregnancy and breast-feeding, and use in children

Novogel® (Ford)
Sterile, glycerol-based hydrogel sheets, net price 10 cm × 10 cm = £2.95; 30 cm × 30 cm, standard = £12.50, thin = £11.80; 5 cm × 7.5 cm = £1.88; 15 cm × 20 cm = £5.63; 20 cm × 40 cm = £10.73; 7.5 cm diameter = £2.68
Uses: diabetic wounds, burns, leg ulcers, decubitus ulcers, donor sites

Nu-Gel® (J&J)
(Drug Tariff Specification 50). A ready-mixed hydrogel containing alginate, applied directly into wound and covered with secondary dressing. Net price 15 g = £1.97
Uses: dry, sloughy or necrotic, lightly exuding or granulating wounds

Purilon® **Gel** (Coloplast)
(Drug Tariff specification 50). Net price 8 g = £1.52, 15 g = £1.98
Uses: for dry, sloughy or necrotic wounds; lightly exuding wounds; granulating wounds

■ Protease modulating matrix

Promogran® (J&J)
Sterile, collagen and oxidised regenerated cellulose matrix, applied directly to wound and covered with secondary dressing, net price 28 cm² (hexagonal) = £4.80, 123 cm² (hexagonal) = £14.73
Uses: chronic wounds free of necrotic tissue and infection, e.g. leg ulcers, pressure sores, diabetic foot ulcers

A8.1.4 Hydrocolloid dressings

Hydrocolloid dressings are usually presented as an absorbent layer on a vapour-permeable film or foam. Because of their impermeable nature, hydrocolloid dressings facilitate rehydration and autolytic debridement of dry, sloughy, or necrotic wounds; they are also suitable for promoting granulation. Fibrous dressings made from modified carmellose fibres resemble alginate dressings (e.g. *Aquacel*®); these are not occlusive.

ActivHeal® **Hydrocolloid** (MedLogic)
Sterile, semi-permeable polyurethane film backing, hydrocolloid wound contact layer, net price 10 cm × 10 cm = £1.52, 15 cm × 15 cm = £3.31, 15 cm × 18 cm (sacral) = £3.84
Uses: light to moderately exuding wounds

Alione® (Coloplast)
Sterile, semi-permeable hydrocolloid dressing with adhesive border, net price 10 cm × 10 cm = £2.79, 12.5 cm × 12.5 cm = £3.83, 12 cm × 20 cm = £5.04, 15 cm × 15 cm = £4.85, 20 cm × 20 cm = £7.26; without adhesive border 10 cm × 10 cm = £2.79, 12.5 cm × 12.5 cm = £3.83, 12 cm × 20 cm = £5.04, 15 cm × 15 cm = £4.85, 20 cm × 20 cm = £7.26
Uses: chronic and exuding wounds

Aquacel® (ConvaTec)
Soft sterile non-woven pad containing hydrocolloid fibres, net price 5 cm × 5 cm = £1.01; 10 cm × 10 cm = £2.40; 15 cm × 15 cm = £4.51
Uses: moderately to heavily exuding wounds
Aquacel® *Ribbon*, 2 cm × 45 cm = £2.40
Uses: moderately to heavily exuding cavity wounds
Aquacel® *Ag* (silver impregnated), net price 5 cm × 5 cm = £1.68, 10 cm × 10 cm = £4.00, 15 cm × 15 cm = £7.54, 20 cm × 30 cm = £18.70
Uses: moderately to heavily exuding wounds
Aquacel® *Ag Ribbon* (silver impregnated), net price 2 cm × 45 cm = £4.02
Uses: moderately to heavily exuding cavity wounds

Askina® **Biofilm Transparent** (Braun)
Sterile, semi-permeable, polyurethane film dressing with hydrocolloid adhesive, net price, 10 cm × 10 cm = £1.00, 15 cm × 15 cm = £2.27, 20 cm × 20 cm = £2.96

Biofilm S® (Braun) NHS
Hydrocolloid dressing with polyurethane-polyester backing; also in powder form for direct application into wound, net price 10 cm × 10 cm = £1.65, 20 cm × 20 cm = £5.70
Biofilm® powder, 1 sachet = £1.82

CombiDERM® (ConvaTec)
Dressing with hydrocolloid adhesive border and absorbent wound contact pad, net price 10 cm × 10 cm = £1.42; 14 cm × 14 cm = £1.97; 15 cm × 18 cm (triangular) = £3.40; 20 cm × 20 cm = £3.78; 20 cm × 23 cm (triangular) = £4.56
Uses: chronic exuding wounds such as leg ulcers, pressure sores; postoperative wounds
CombiDERM N® Hydrocolloid absorbent dressing, net price 7.5 cm × 7.5 cm = £1.11; 14 cm × 14 cm = £1.98; 15 cm × 25 cm = £4.03
Uses: chronic wounds (e.g. leg ulcers and diabetic ulcers) and exuding wounds (e.g. biopsies), and surgical wounds

Comfeel® (Coloplast)
Soft elastic pad consisting of carmellose sodium particles embedded in adhesive mass; smooth outer layer and polyurethane film backing; available as sheets, powder in plastic blister units and paste for direct application into the wound: ulcer dressing, net price 10 cm × 10 cm = £2.41; 15 cm × 15 cm = £4.83; 20 cm × 20 cm = £7.39; other sizes (NHS): 4 cm × 6 cm = £1.19; powder 6 g = £4.04; paste 12-g sachet = £1.56; 50 g = £5.98

Comfeel® **Plus** (Coloplast)
Hydrocolloid dressings containing carmellose sodium and calcium alginate. Contour dressing, net price 6 cm × 8 cm = £1.92, 9 cm × 11 cm = £3.34; Ulcer Dressing, 4 cm × 6 cm = 83p, 10 cm × 10 cm = £2.13, 15 cm × 15 cm = £4.56, 18 cm × 20 cm (triangular) = £4.96, 20 cm × 20 cm = £6.56; Transparent Dressing, 5 cm × 7 cm = 58p, 5 cm × 15 cm = £1.37, 5 cm × 25 cm = £2.24, 9 cm × 14 cm = £2.11, 9 cm × 25 cm = £3.00, 10 cm × 10 cm = £1.11, 15 cm × 15 cm = £2.89, 15 cm × 20 cm = £2.93, 20 cm × 20 cm = £2.95; Pressure Relieving Dressing, 7 cm diameter = £3.00, 10 cm = £4.02, 15 cm = £6.06

Cutinova® (Beiersdorf)
Cutinova® *Hydro Border* Sterile, highly absorbent semi-transparent two-layered polyurethane dressing with vapour-permeable foam matrix on a semi-permeable film backing, net price 5 cm × 6 cm = £1.09; 10 cm × 10 cm = £2.20; 15 cm × 20 cm = £4.66
Uses: moderately to heavily exuding wounds including burns and decubitus ulcers
Cutinova® *Thin* NHS Sterile, highly absorbent, semi-transparent two-layered polyurethane dressing with two-layered vapour-permeable foam matrix on a semi-permeable film backing, net price

5 cm × 6 cm = £1.16; 10 cm × 10 cm = £1.87; 15 cm × 20 cm = £5.13

Uses: lightly exuding wounds including abrasions, burns, decubitus ulcers, donor sites, skin protection and post-operative wounds

DuoDERM® (ConvaTec)

Extra Thin (formerly *Granuflex® Extra Thin*), net price 5 cm × 10 cm = 66p; 7.5 cm × 7.5 cm = 69p; 10 cm × 10 cm = £1.14; 15 cm × 15 cm = £2.46; NHS 5 cm × 20 cm = £1.38

Uses: minimally exuding wounds, such as abrasions, minor burns or minor surgery

Signal, hydrocolloid dressing with 'Time to change' indicator net price 10 cm × 10 cm = £1.82, 14 cm × 14 cm = £3.20, 20 cm × 20 cm = £6.35, 11 cm × 19 cm (oval) = £2.77, 18.5 cm × 19.5 cm (heel) = £4.47, 22.5 cm × 20 cm (sacral) = £5.22

Uses: leg ulcers, pressure sores, diabetic ulcers, burns, postoperative wounds

Granuflex® (ConvaTec)

Hydrocolloid wound contact layer bonded to plastic foam layer, with outer semi-permeable polyurethane film, net price 10 cm × 10 cm = £2.42, 15 cm × 15 cm = £4.59, 15 cm × 20 cm = £4.97, 20 cm × 20 cm = £6.91, NHS 20 cm × 30 cm = £11.36

Granuflex® Paste (NHS), net price 30 g = £2.73

Granuflex® Bordered Dressing, net price 6 cm × 6 cm = £1.51, 10 cm × 10 cm = £2.88, 15 cm × 15 cm = £5.45, triangular dressing, 10 cm × 13 cm = £3.40, 15 cm × 18 cm = £5.30

Uses: chronic ulcers, pressure sores, open wounds, debridement of wounds; powders, gel, and pastes used with sheet dressings to fill deep or heavily exuding wounds

Hydrocoll® (Hartmann)

Hydrocolloid dressing with adhesive border and absorbent wound contact pad, net price 5 cm × 5 cm = 90p, 7.5 cm × 7.5 cm = £1.48, 10 cm × 10 cm = £2.15, 15 cm × 15 cm = £4.05; Concave dressing, 8 cm × 12 cm = £1.90; Sacral dressing, 12 cm × 18 cm = £3.22; Basic dressing without adhesive border, 10 cm × 10 cm = £2.19; Thin film dressing, 7.5 cm × 7.5 cm = 62p, 10 cm × 10 cm = £1.03, 15 cm × 15 cm = £2.32

Uses: light to medium exuding wounds

NU DERM® (J&J)

Sterile, semi permeable hydrocolloid dressing without adhesive border, net price 5 cm × 5 cm = 80p, 10 cm × 10 cm = £1.50, 15 cm × 15 cm = £3.00, 20 cm × 20 cm = £6.00, 8 cm × 12 cm (heel/elbow) = £3.00, 15 cm × 18 cm (sacral) = £4.20; without adhesive border, thin, 10 cm × 10 cm = £1.00

Replicare Ultra® (S&N Hlth.)

Sterile, adhesive hydrocolloid dressing with outer semi-permeable polyurethane film backing, net price 10 cm × 10 cm = £2.25, 15 cm × 15 cm = £4.48, 20 cm × 20 cm = £6.61; Sacral dressing, 15 cm × 18 cm = £4.24

Uses: lightly to moderately exuding wounds such as leg ulcers, pressure sores; postoperative wounds; superficial burns

Suprasorb H® (Vernon-Carus)

Sterile, semi permeable hydrocolloid dressing, with adhesive border net price 14 cm × 14 cm = £2.23; without adhesive border 10 cm × 10 cm = £1.51, 15 cm × 15 cm = £3.30; without adhesive border, thin 5 cm × 10 cm = 65p, 10 cm × 10 cm = 99p, 15 cm × 15 cm = £2.26

Uses: lightly to moderately exuding wounds

Tegasorb® (3M)

Hydrocolloid dressing with adhesive border, net price 10 cm × 12 cm (oval) = £2.20; 13 cm × 15 cm (oval) = £4.11; without adhesive border 10 cm × 10 cm = £2.24; 15 cm × 15 cm = £4.34

Uses: chronic wounds such as leg ulcers and pressure sores

Tegasorb® Thin Sterile, semi-permeable, clear film dressing with hydrocolloid and adhesive border, net price 10 cm × 12 cm (oval) = £1.46; 13 cm × 15 cm (oval) = £2.74; without adhesive border 10 cm × 10 cm = £1.47

Uses: low to moderately exuding wounds including leg ulcers, abrasions, burns, and donor sites

Ultec Pro® (Tyco)

Sterile, semi-permeable hydrocolloid dressing with adhesive border, net price 10.5 cm × 10.5 cm = £1.39, 14 cm × 14 cm = £2.24, 21 cm × 21 cm = £4.49, 15 cm × 18 cm (sacral) = £3.17, 19.5 cm × 23 cm (sacral) = £4.88; without adhesive border 10 cm × 10 cm = £2.19, 15 cm × 15 cm = £4.27, 20 cm × 20 cm = £6.43

Uses: lightly to moderately exuding wounds

Versiva® (ConvaTec)

Sterile, semi-permeable hydrocolloid dressing with adhesive border, net price 9 cm × 9 cm = £2.26, 11 cm × 19 cm (oval) = £4.00, 14 cm × 14 cm = £4.22, 19 cm × 19 cm = £6.57, 19 cm × 24 cm = £7.93, 19 cm × 17.7 cm (sacral) = £5.59, 21 cm × 22.5 cm (sacral) = £7.93, 19.5 cm × 18.5 cm (heel) = £6.74

Uses: chronic and acute exudating wounds

■ Keloid dressings

Silicone gel and gel sheets are used to reduce and prevent hypertrophic and keloid scarring. They should not be used on open wounds. Application times should be increased gradually. Silicone sheets can be washed and reused.

Cica-Care® (S&N Hlth.)

Soft, self-adhesive, semi-occlusive silicone gel sheet with backing. Net price, 6 cm × 12 cm = £12.66; 15 cm × 12 cm = £24.68

Dermatix® (Valeant)

Silicone gel, net price 15 g = £19.00, 60 g = £57.00

Mepiform® (Mölnlycke)

Self-adhesive silicone gel sheet with polyurethane film backing, net price 5 cm × 7.5 cm = £3.24, 10 cm × 18 cm = £13.15, 4 cm × 30 cm = £9.26

Silgel® (Nagor)

Silicone gel sheet, net price 10 cm × 10 cm = £13.50; 20 cm × 20 cm = £40.00; 40 cm × 40 cm = £144.00; 10 cm × 5 cm = £7.50; 15 cm x 10 cm = £19.50; 30 cm × 5 cm = £19.50; 10 cm × 30 cm = £31.50; 25 cm × 15 cm (submammary) = £21.12; 46 cm × 8.5 cm (abdominal) = £39.46; 5 cm diameter (circular) = £4.00

Silgel® STC-SE silicone gel, net price, 20-mL tube = £19.00

■ Hyaluronic acid

Hyalofill® (ConvaTec)

Hyalofill-F, NHS flat, non-woven, absorbent fibrous fleece of *Hyaff* (an ester of hyaluronic acid), net price 5 cm × 5 cm = £9.98, 10 cm × 10 cm = £27.68

Uses: for treatment of chronic or acute wounds, place on surface of lesion and cover with sterile dressing, renew daily or when saturated (at least every 2–3 days)

Hyalofill-R, NHS absorbent fibrous rope of *Hyaff* (an ester of hyaluronic acid), net price 500 mg = £27.68

Uses: for treatment of chronic or acute wounds, position gently inside cavity and cover with sterile dressing, renew daily or when saturated (at least every 2–3 days)

A8.1.5 Vapour-permeable films and membranes

Vapour-permeable films and membranes allow the passage of water vapour and oxygen but not of water or micro-organisms, and are suitable for mildly exuding wounds. They are highly conformable, convenient to use, provide a moist healing environment, and some may permit constant observation of the wound. However, water vapour loss may occur at a slower rate than exudate is generated, so that fluid accumulates under the dressing, which can lead to tissue maceration and to wrinkling at the adhesive contact site (with risk of bacterial entry). Newer versions have increased moisture vapour permeability; some also contain water-soluble antimicrobials. Despite these advances vapour-permeable films and membranes remain less suitable for large heavily exuding wounds and are probably not suitable for chronic leg ulcers. They are most commonly used as secondary dressings over alginates or gels; they are also sometimes used to protect fragile skin of patients at risk of developing minor skin damage.

Vapour-permeable Adhesive Film Dressing, BP 1993
(Semi-permeable Adhesive Dressing)

Sterile, extensible, waterproof, water vapour-permeable polyurethane film coated with synthetic adhesive mass; transparent. Supplied in single-use pieces.

ActivHeal® Film, net price 6 cm × 7 cm = 31p, 10 cm × 12.7 cm = 73p, 15 cm × 17.8 cm = £1.78 (MedLogic)

Alldress®, net price 10 cm × 10 cm = 83p, 15 cm × 15 cm = £1.82, 15 cm × 20 cm = £2.25 (Mölnlycke)

Bioclusive®, net price 10.2 cm × 12.7 cm = £1.45 (J&J)

Blisterfilm®, net price 5 cm × 8 cm = 40p, 9 cm × 10 cm = 70p, 10 cm × 13 cm = 90p, 14 cm × 15 cm = £1.23 (Tyco)

C-View®, net price 6 cm × 7 cm = 37p, 10 cm × 12 cm = £1.02, 12 cm × 12 cm = £1.18, 15 cm × 20 cm = £2.33, 20 cm × 30 cm = £3.53 (NHS) (Unomedical)

Hydrofilm®, net price 6 cm × 9 cm = 50p, 10 cm × 15 cm = £1.32, 12 cm × 25 cm = £2.37 (Hartmann)

Mefilm®, net price 6 cm × 7 cm = 40p, 10 cm × 12.7 cm = £1.08, 10 cm × 25 cm = £2.11, 15 cm × 21.5 cm = £2.67 (Mölnlycke)

Mepore® Ultra, net price 6 cm × 7 cm = 27p, 9 cm × 10 cm = 58p, 9 cm × 15 cm = 87p, 9 cm × 20 cm = £1.31, 9 cm × 25 cm = £1.45, 9 cm × 30 cm = £2.39 (Mölnlycke)

OpSite® Flexigrid, net price 6 cm × 7 cm = 34p, 12 cm × 12 cm = 98p, 15 cm × 20 cm = £2.47, 12 cm × 25 cm = £3.20 (NHS), 10 cm × 12 cm = £2.06 (NHS), *OpSite® Plus*, 5 cm × 5 cm = 27p, 9.5 cm × 8.5 cm = 76p, 10 cm × 12 cm = £1.04, 10 cm × 20 cm = £1.75, 35 cm × 10 cm = £2.89 (S&N Hlth)

Polyskin® II, net price 4 cm × 4 cm = 35p, 5 cm × 7 cm = 38p, 10 cm × 12 cm = 99p, 10 cm × 20 cm = £1.96, 15 cm × 20 cm = £2.26, 20 cm × 25 cm = £3.95 (Tyco)

Polyskin® MR, net price 5 cm × 7 cm = 40p, 10 cm × 12 cm = £1.08, 15 cm × 20 cm = £2.53 (Tyco)

Suprasorb F®, net price 5 cm × 7 cm = 30p, 10 cm × 12 cm = 72p, 15 cm × 20 cm = £2.25, 10 cm × 25 cm = £3.44 NHS (Vernon-Carus)

Tegaderm®, net price 6 cm × 7 cm = 38p, 12 cm × 12 cm = £1.23, 15 cm × 20 cm = £2.34 (3M)
Uses: postoperative dressing, donor sites, superficial decubitus ulcers, amputation stumps, stoma care; protective cover to prevent skin breakdown

Omiderm® (Chemical Search) NHS

Sterile, water-vapour permeable polyurethane film (plain and meshed versions). Net price 5 cm × 7 cm = £2.00; 8 cm × 10 cm = £3.50, meshed = £4.75; 18 cm × 10 cm = £6.40, meshed = £9.50; 60 cm × 10 cm = £23.50; 21 cm × 31 cm = £24.00, meshed = £32.00; meshed 23 cm × 39 cm = £48.75
Uses: ulcers; donor sites; superficial and partial thickness burns; meshed: donor sites, skin grafts

A8.1.6 Low adherence dressing and wound contact materials

Low adherence dressings and wound contact materials are used as interface layers under secondary absorbent dressings.

Tulle dressings are manufactured from cotton or viscose fibres which are impregnated with white or yellow soft paraffin to prevent the fibres from sticking, but this is only partly successful and it may be necessary to change the dressings frequently. The paraffin reduces absorbency of the dressing. Dressings with a reduced content of soft paraffin (i.e. *Paratulle®* and *Unitulle®*) are less liable to interfere with absorption; those containing the traditional amount (such as *Jelonet®*) have been considered more suitable for skin graft transfer.

Medicated tulle dressings are not generally recommended for wound care. Although hypersensitivity is unlikely with **chlorhexidine gauze dressing**, its antibacterial efficacy has not been established.

Povidone–iodine fabric dressing is a knitted viscose dressing with povidone–iodine incorporated in a hydrophilic polyethylene glycol basis; this facilitates diffusion of the iodine into the wound and permits removal of the dressing by irrigation. The iodine has a wide spectrum of antimicrobial activity but it is rapidly deactivated by wound exudate; systemic absorption of iodine may occur.

Perforated film absorbent dressings partially overcome the problems of adherence but they are suitable only for wounds with mild to moderate amounts of exudate; they are **not** appropriate for leg ulcers or for other lesions that produce large quantities of viscous exudate.

Knitted viscose primary dressing is an alternative to tulle dressings for exuding wounds; it is sometimes used as the initial layer of multi-layer compression bandaging.

Absorbent Cellulose Dressing with Fluid Repellent Backing

Exu-Dry®, net price 10 cm × 15 cm = 97p, 15 cm × 23 cm = £1.99, 23 cm × 38 cm = £4.62 (S&N Hlth)
Uses: primary or secondary dressing for medium to heavily exuding wounds

Mesorb® cellulose wadding pad with gauze wound contact layer and non-woven repellent backing, net price 10 cm × 10 cm = 55p, 10 cm × 15 cm = 71p, 10 cm × 20 cm = 87p, 15 cm × 20 cm = £1.24, 20 cm × 25 cm = £1.97, 20 cm × 30 cm = £2.23 (Mölnlycke)
Uses: post-operative use for heavily exuding wounds

Absorbent Perforated Dressing with Adhesive Border

Low adherence dressing consisting of viscose and rayon absorbent pad with adhesive border.

Cosmopor E®, net price 5 cm × 7.2 cm = 7p, 6 cm × 10 cm = 13p, 8 cm × 10 cm = 15p, 6 cm × 15 cm = 17p, 8 cm × 15 cm = 24p, 8 cm × 20 cm = 33p, 10 cm × 20 cm = 40p, 10 cm × 25 cm = 49p, 10 cm × 35 cm = 69p (Hartmann)

Medipore® + *Pad*, net price 5 cm × 7.2 cm = 7p, 10 cm × 10 cm = 15p, 10 cm × 15 cm = 23p, 10 cm × 20 cm = 36p, 10 cm × 25 cm = 44p, 10 cm × 35 cm = 61p (3M)

Mepore®, net price 7 cm × 8 cm = 9p, 10 cm × 11 cm = 19p, 11 cm × 15 cm = 32p, 9 cm × 20 cm = 39p, 9 cm × 25 cm = 53p, 9 cm × 30 cm = 61p, 9 cm × 35 cm = 67p (Mölnlycke)

Neosafe® , net price 9 cm × 10 cm = 16p, 9 cm × 20 cm = 34p (Neomedic)

Primapore®, net price 6 cm × 8.3 cm = 16p, 8 cm × 10 cm = 17p, 8 cm × 15 cm = 29p, 10 cm × 20 cm = 37p, 10 cm × 25 cm = 42p, 10 cm × 30 cm = 54p, 12 cm × 35 cm = 89p (S&N Hlth)

Sterifix®, net price 5 cm × 7 cm = 18p, 7 cm × 10 cm = 29p, 10 cm × 14 cm = 52p (Hartmann)

Telfa® *Island*, net price 5 cm × 10 cm = 8p, 10 cm × 12.5 cm = 26p, 10 cm × 20 cm = 34p, 10 cm × 25.5 cm = 43p, 10 cm × 35 cm = 60p (Tyco)

Uses: lightly exuding and post-operative wounds

Absorbent Perforated Plastic Film Faced Dressing

(Drug Tariff specification 9). Low-adherence dressing consisting of 3 layers.

Cutilin®, net price 5 cm × 5 cm = 13p, 10 cm × 10 cm = 21p, 10 cm × 20 cm = 40p (Beiersdorf)

Interpose®, net price 5 cm × 5 cm = 9p, 10 cm × 10 cm = 15p, 10 cm × 20 cm = 32p (Frontier)

Melolin®, net price 5 cm × 5 cm = 15p, 10 cm × 10 cm = 24p, 20 cm × 10 cm = 46p (S&N Hlth)

Release®, net price 5 cm × 5 cm = 14p, 10 cm × 10 cm = 22p, 20 cm × 10 cm = 42p (J&J)

Skintact®, net price 5 cm × 5 cm = 10p, 10 cm × 10 cm = 17p, 20 cm × 10 cm = 34p (Robinson)

Solvaline N®, net price 5 cm × 5 cm = 9p, 10 cm × 10 cm = 16p, 10 cm × 20 cm = 32p (Vernon-Carus)

Telfa®, net price 5 cm × 7.5 cm = 12p, 10 cm × 7.5 cm = 15p, 15 cm × 7.5 cm = 17p, 20 cm × 7.5 cm = 28p (Tyco)

Where no size specified by the prescriber, the 5 cm × 5 cm size to be supplied

Uses: dressing for post-operative and low exudate wounds; low adherence property and low absorption capacity

Knitted Viscose Primary Dressing, BP 1993

Warp knitted fabric manufactured from a bright viscose monofilament.

N-A Dressing®, net price 9.5 cm × 9.5 cm = 33p, 9.5 cm × 19 cm = 63p (J&J)

N-A Ultra® (silicone-coated), net price 9.5 cm × 9.5 cm = 32p, 9.5 cm × 19 cm = 60p (J&J)

Paratex®, net price 9.5 cm × 9.5 cm = 25p (Parema)

Robinson Primary®, net price 12.5 cm × 14.5 cm = 39p (Robinsons)

Tricotex®, net price 9.5 cm × 9.5 cm = 29p (S&N Hlth)

Uses: low adherence wound contact layer for use on ulcerative and other granulating wounds with superimposed absorbent pad

Paraffin Gauze Dressing, BP 1993

(Tulle Gras). Fabric of leno weave, weft and warp threads of cotton and/or viscose yarn, impregnated with white or yellow soft paraffin, sterile, 10 cm × 10 cm, net price (light loading) = 27p; (normal loading) = 35p (most suppliers including Vernon-Carus—*Paranet*® (light loading); Aventis Pharma—*Unitulle*® (light loading); S&N Hlth—*Jelonet*® (normal loading))

Uses: treatment of abrasions, burns, and other injuries of skin, and ulcerative conditions; postoperatively as penile and vaginal dressing and for sinus packing; heavier loading for skin graft transfer

Chlorhexidine Gauze Dressing, BP 1993

Fabric of leno weave, weft and warp threads of cotton and/or viscose yarn, impregnated with ointment containing chlorhexidine acetate, sterile, 5 cm × 5 cm, net price = 25p; 10 cm × 10 cm = 53p (S&N Hlth—*Bactigras*®)

Povidone–iodine Fabric Dressing

(Drug Tariff specification 43). Knitted viscose primary dressing impregnated with povidone–iodine ointment 10%, net price 5 cm × 5 cm = 30p; 9.5 cm × 9.5 cm = 45p (J&J—*Inadine*®)

Uses: wound contact layer for abrasions and superficial burns

Atrauman® (Hartmann)

Non-adherent knitted polyester primary dressing impregnated with neutral triglycerides, 5 cm × 5 cm = 24p, 7.5 cm × 10 cm = 25p, 10 cm × 20 cm = 56p

Uses: abrasions, burns, and other injuries of skin, and ulcerative conditions; postoperatively for granulating wounds

Mepilex® (Mölnlycke)

Absorbent soft silicone dressing with polyurethane foam film backing, net price 10 cm × 10 cm = £2.33, 10 cm × 20 cm = £3.84, 15 cm × 15 cm = £4.33, 20 cm × 20 cm = £6.41

Mepilex® *Border*, with soft silicone adhesive border, net price 7.5 cm × 7.5 cm = £1.35, 10 cm × 10 cm = £2.45, 15 cm × 15 cm = £4.00, 15 cm × 20 cm = £5.01

Mepilex® *Lite*, thin absorbent soft silicone dressing, net price 6 cm × 8.5 cm = £1.60, 10 cm × 10 cm = £1.91, 15 cm × 15 cm = £3.71

Mepilex® *Transfer*, soft silicone exudate transfer dressing, net price, 15 cm × 20 cm = £9.33, 20 cm × 50 cm = £23.84

Mepitel® (Mölnlycke)

Soft silicone wound contact dressing. Net price 5 cm × 7 cm = £1.44, 8 cm × 10 cm = £2.88, 12 cm × 15 cm = £5.83, 20 cm × 30 cm = £14.99

Uses: leg ulcers, decubitus ulcers, burns, fixation of skin grafts; should be covered with simple absorbent secondary dressing

Physiotulle® (Coloplast)

Non-adherent soft polymer wound contact dressing, net price 10 cm × 10 cm = £1.98, 15 cm × 20 cm = £6.02

Uses: leg ulcers, pressure sores, burns, postoperative wounds, donor sites, skin abrasions

[1]**Surgipad**® (J&J) NHS

Absorbent pad of absorbent cotton and viscose in sleeve of non-woven viscose fabric, sterile, net price pouch 12 cm × 10 cm = 18p, 20 cm × 10 cm = 25p, 20 cm × 20 cm = 30p, 40 cm × 20 cm = 41p; non-sterile, net price pack 12 cm × 10 cm = 5p, 20 cm × 10 cm = 10p, 20 cm × 20 cm = 17p, 40 cm × 20 cm = 28p

Uses: for heavily exuding wounds requiring frequent dressing changes

1. NHS Except in Sterile Dressing Pack with Non-woven Pads

Tegapore® (3M)

Non-adherent soft polymer wound contact dressing, net price 7.5 cm × 10 cm = £2.13, 7.5 cm × 20 cm = £4.17, 20 cm × 25 cm = £10.16

Urgotul® (Parema)
Non-adherent soft polymer wound contact dressing, net price 10 cm × 10 cm = £2.38, 10 cm × 40 cm = £9.34, 15 cm × 20 cm = £7.23
Urgotul® SSD (silver impregnated), net price 10 cm × 12 cm = £2.84, 15 cm × 20 cm = £7.17

A8.1.7 Odour absorbent dressings

These dressings have an important role in absorbing the odour of infected wounds. Some dressings may also benefit wound healing by binding bacteria, but this effect awaits confirmation.

Actisorb® Silver 200 (J&J)
(formerly Actisorb® Plus) Knitted fabric of activated charcoal, with one-way stretch, with silver residues, within spun-bonded nylon sleeve. Net price 6.5 cm × 9.5 cm = £1.55, 10.5 cm × 10.5 cm = £2.44, 10.5 cm × 19 cm = £4.43

CarboFLEX® (ConvaTec)
Dressing in 5 layers: wound-facing absorbent layer containing alginate and hydrocolloid; water-resistant second layer; third layer containing activated charcoal; non-woven absorbent fourth layer; water-resistant backing layer. Net price 10 cm × 10 cm = £2.74, 8 cm × 15 cm = £3.29, 15 cm × 20 cm = £6.23

Carbonet® (S&N Hlth.) NHS
Activated charcoal dressing, net price 10 cm × 10 cm = £3.13, 10 cm × 20 cm = £6.10

Carbopad® VC (Vernon-Carus)
Activated charcoal non-absorbent dressing, net price 10 cm × 10 cm = £1.59, 10 cm × 20 cm = £2.15

CliniSorb® Odour Control Dressings (CliniMed)
Layer of activated charcoal cloth between viscose rayon with outer polyamide coating. Net price 10 cm × 10 cm = £1.65, 10 cm × 20 cm = £2.20, 15 cm × 25 cm = £3.54

Lyofoam C® (Medlock)
Lyofoam sheet with layer of activated charcoal cloth and additional outer envelope of polyurethane foam. Net price 10 cm × 10 cm = £2.69, 15 cm × 20 cm = £6.11, 25 cm × 10 cm = £5.39

A8.1.8 Dressing packs

The role of dressing packs is very limited. They are used to provide a clean or sterile working surface; packs shown below include cotton wool balls, but they are not recommended for use on wounds.

Non-Drug Tariff Specification Sterile Dressing Pack
Contains paper towel, disposable bag, softswabs, dressing pad, softdrape, net price = 60p (Richardson — *Dress-it®*)

Sterile Dressing Pack
(Drug Tariff specification 10). Contains gauze and cotton tissue pad, gauze swabs, absorbent cotton wool balls, absorbent paper towel, water repellent inner wrapper. Net price per pack = 79p (Vernon-Carus—*Vernaid®*)

Sterile Dressing Pack with Non-woven Pads
(Drug Tariff specification 35). Contains non-woven fabric covered dressing pad, non-woven fabric swabs, absorbent cotton wool balls, absorbent paper towel, water repellent inner wrapper. Net price per pack = 78p (Vernon-Carus—*Vernaid®*)

A8.1.9 Surgical absorbents

Surgical absorbent dressings, applied directly to the wound, have many disadvantages, since they adhere to the wound, shed fibres into it, and dehydrate it; they also permit leakage of exudate ('strike through') with an associated risk of infection. Surgical absorbents may be used as secondary absorbent layers in the management of heavily exuding wounds.

Absorbent Cotton, BP
Carded cotton fibres of not less than 10 mm average staple length, available in rolls and balls, 25 g, net price = 65p; 100 g = £1.49; 500 g = £5.01 (most suppliers). 25-g pack to be supplied when weight not stated
Uses: general purpose cleansing and swabbing, pre-operative skin preparation, application of medicaments; supplementary absorbent pad to absorb excess wound exudate

Absorbent Cotton, Hospital Quality
As for absorbent cotton but lower quality materials, shorter staple length etc. 100 g, net price = £1.03; 500 g = £3.26 (most suppliers)
Drug Tariff specifies to be supplied only where specifically ordered
Uses: suitable only as general purpose absorbent, for swabbing, and routine cleansing of incontinent patients; not for wound cleansing

Gauze and Cotton Tissue, BP 1988
Consists of absorbent cotton enclosed in absorbent cotton gauze type 12 or absorbent cotton and viscose gauze type 2. 500 g, net price = £6.35 (most suppliers, including Robinsons—*Gamgee Tissue®* (blue label))
Uses: absorbent and protective pad, as burns dressing on non-adherent layer

Gauze and Cotton Tissue
(Drug Tariff specification 14). Similar to above. 500 g, net price = £4.64 (most suppliers, including Robinsons—*Gamgee Tissue®* (pink label))
Drug Tariff specifies to be supplied only where specifically ordered
Uses: absorbent and protective pad, as burns dressing on non-adherent layer

Absorbent Lint, BPC
Cotton cloth of plain weave with nap raised on one side from warp yarns. 25 g, net price = 81p; 100 g = £2.48; 500 g = £10.44 (most suppliers). 25-g pack supplied where no quantity stated
NOTE. Not recommended for wound management

Absorbent Cotton Gauze, BP 1988
Cotton fabric of plain weave, in rolls and as swabs (see below), usually Type 13 light, sterile. 90 cm (all) × 1 m, net price = 98p; 3 m = £2.04; 5 m = £3.19; 10 m = £6.10 (most suppliers). 1-m packet supplied when no size stated
Uses: pre-operative preparation, for cleansing and swabbing
NOTE. Drug Tariff also includes unsterilised absorbent cotton gauze, 25 m roll, net price = £13.98

Absorbent Muslin, BP 1988 NHS
Fabric of plain weave, warp threads of cotton, weft threads of cotton and/or viscose
Uses: wet dressing, soaked in 0.9% sterile sodium chloride solution

Absorbent Cotton Ribbon Gauze, BP 1993 NHS
Cotton fabric of plain weave in ribbon form with fast selvedge edges
Uses: post-surgery cavity packing for sinus, dental, throat cavities etc.

Absorbent Cotton and Viscose Ribbon Gauze, BP 1993

Woven fabric in ribbon form with fast selvedge edges, warp threads of cotton, weft threads of viscose or combined cotton and viscose yarn, sterile. 5 m (both) × 1.25 cm, net price = 74p; 2.5 cm = 82p

Uses: post-surgery cavity packing for sinus, dental, throat cavities etc.

Gauze Swab, BP 1988

Consists of absorbent cotton gauze type 13 light or absorbent cotton and viscose gauze type 1 folded into squares or rectangles of 8-ply with no cut edges exposed, net price sterile, 7.5 cm × 7.5 cm 5-pad packet = 36p; non-sterile, 10 cm × 10 cm 100-pad packet = £5.73 (most suppliers)

Filmated Gauze Swab, BP 1988

As for Gauze Swab, but with thin layer of Absorbent Cotton enclosed within, net price non-sterile, 10 cm × 10 cm, 100-pad packet = £7.87 (Vernon-Carus—*Cotfil*®)

Uses: general swabbing and cleansing

Non-woven Fabric Swab

(Drug Tariff specification 28). Consists of non-woven fabric folded 4-ply; alternative to gauze swabs, type 13 light, net price sterile, 7.5 cm × 7.5 cm, 5-pad packet = 23p; non-sterile, 10 cm × 10 cm, 100-pad packet = £2.69 (J & J—*Topper 8*®); 100-pad pack = £2.74 (CliniMed)

Uses: general purpose swabbing and cleansing; absorbs more quickly than gauze

Filmated Non-woven Fabric Swab

(Drug Tariff specification 29). Film of viscose fibres enclosed within non-woven viscose fabric folded 8-ply, net price non-sterile, 10 cm × 10 cm, 100-pad packet = £5.82 (J & J—*Regal*®)

Uses: general purpose swabbing and cleansing

A8.1.10 Capillary dressings

Capillary dressings consist of an absorbent core of hydrophilic fibres sandwiched between two low-adherent wound-contact layers. Wound exudate is taken up by the dressing and retained within the highly absorbent central layer.

The dressing may be applied intact to relatively superficial areas, but for deeper wounds or cavities it may be cut to shape to ensure good contact with the wound base. Multiple layers may be applied to heavily exuding wounds to further increase the fluid-absorbing capacity of the dressing.

Capillary dressings can be applied to a variety of wounds but they are contra-indicated for heavily bleeding wounds or arterial bleeding.

Advadraw® (Advancis)

Non-adherent, sterile dressing consisting of a soft viscose and polyester absorbent pad with central wicking layer between two perforated permeable wound contact layers. Net price 5 cm × 7.5 cm = 55p, 10 cm × 10 cm = 85p, 10 cm × 15 cm = £1.15

Advadraw Spiral®, net price 0.5 cm × 40 cm = 79p

Vacutex® (Hybrand)

Low-adherent dressing consisting of two external polyester wound contact layers with central wicking polyester/cotton mix absorbent layer. Net price 5 cm × 5 cm = 94p, 10 cm × 10 cm = £1.66, 10 cm × 15 cm = £2.23, 10 cm × 20 cm = £2.68, 15 cm × 20 cm = £3.14, 20 cm × 20 cm = £4.28

A8.2 Bandages and adhesives

According to their structure and performance bandages are used for dressing retention, for support, and for compression.

A8.2.1 Non-extensible bandages

Bandages made from non-extensible woven fabrics have generally been replaced by more conformable products, therefore their role is now extremely limited. Triangular calico bandage has a role as a sling.

Open-wove Bandage, BP 1988

Cotton cloth, plain weave, warp of cotton, weft of cotton, viscose, or combination, one continuous length. Type 1, 5 m (all): 2.5 cm, net price = 32p; 5 cm = 53p; 7.5 cm = 75p; 10 cm = 98p (most suppliers) 5 m × 5 cm supplied when size not stated

Uses: protection and retention of absorbent dressings; support for minor strains, sprains; securing splints

Triangular Calico Bandage, BP 1980

Unbleached calico right-angled triangle. 90 cm × 90 cm × 1.27 m, net price = £1.17 (most suppliers)

Uses: sling

Domette Bandage, BP 1988 NHS

Fabric, plain weave, cotton warp and wool weft (hospital quality also available, all cotton). Net price 5 m (all): 5 cm = 54p; 7.5 cm = 81p; 10 cm = £1.08; 15 cm = £1.61 (Bailey, Robert)

Uses: protection and support where warmth required

Multiple Pack Dressing No. 1

(Drug Tariff). Contains absorbent cotton, absorbent cotton gauze type 13 light (sterile), open-wove bandages (banded). Net price per pack = £3.71

A8.2.2 Light-weight conforming bandages

Lightweight conforming bandages are used for dressing retention, with the aim of keeping the dressing close to the wound without inhibiting movement or restricting blood flow. The elasticity of **conforming-stretch bandages** (also termed contour bandages) is greater than that of **cotton conforming bandages**.

Cotton Conforming Bandage, BP 1988

Cotton fabric, plain weave, treated to impart some elasticity to warp and weft. Net price 3.5 m (all): type A, 5 cm = 67p, 7.5 cm = 83p, 10 cm = £1.02, 15 cm = £1.39 (S&N Hlth— *Crinx*®)

Knitted Polyamide and Cellulose Contour Bandage, BP 1988

Fabric, knitted warp of polyamide filament, weft of cotton or viscose, fast edges, one continuous length. 4 m stretched (all):

K-Band®, net price 5 cm = 19p, 7 cm = 25p, 10 cm = 27p, 15 cm = 47p (Parema)

Knit-Band®, net price 5 cm = 11p, 7 cm = 16p, 10 cm = 18p, 15 cm = 33p (CliniMed)

Knit Fix®, net price 5 cm = 13p, 7 cm = 18p, 10 cm = 19p, 15 cm = 36p (Bailey, Robert)

Polyamide and Cellulose Contour Bandage, BP 1988

(formerly Nylon and Viscose Stretch Bandage) Fabric, plain weave, warp of polyamide filament, weft of cotton or viscose, fast edges, one continuous length. 4 m stretched (all):

Acti-Wrap®, net price cohesive, 6 cm = 39p, 8 cm = 57p, 10 cm = 68p; latex-free 6 cm = 45p, 8 cm = 65p, 10 cm = 77p (Activa)

Stayform®, net price 5 cm = 31p, 7.5 cm = 39p, 10 cm = 44p, 15 cm = 74p (Robinsons)

Slinky®, net price 5 cm = 41p, 7.5 cm = 59p, 10 cm = 71p, 15 cm = £1.01 (Medlock)

Easifix®, net price 5 cm = 36p, 7.5 cm = 44p, 10 cm = 51p, 15 cm = 87p (S&N Hlth)

Conforming Bandage (Synthetic)

Fabric, plain weave, warp of polyamide, weft of viscose. 4 m stretched (all):

Hospiform® (formerly *Peha Crepp*® E), net price 6 cm = 13p, 8 cm = 16p, 10 cm = 19p, 12 cm = 23p (Hartmann)

A8.2.3 Tubular bandages

Tubular bandages are available in different forms, according to the function required of them. Some are used under orthopaedic casts and some are suitable for protecting areas to which creams or ointments (other than those containing potent corticosteroids) have been applied. The conformability of the elasticated versions makes them particularly suitable for retaining dressings on difficult parts of the body or for soft tissue injury, but their use as the only means of applying pressure to an oedematous limb or to a varicose ulcer is not appropriate, since the pressure they exert is inadequate. Compression hosiery (section A8.3.1) reduces the recurrence of venous leg ulcers and should be considered after wound healing.

Cotton Stockinette, Bleached, BP 1988

Knitted fabric, cotton yarn, tubular, net price 1 m × 2.5 cm = 32p; 5 cm = 48p; 7.5 cm = 59p; 6 m × 10 cm = £3.99 (J&J, Medlock)

Uses: 1 m lengths, basis (with wadding) for Plaster of Paris bandages etc.; 6 m length, compression bandage

Elasticated Tubular Bandage, BP 1993

(formerly Elasticated Surgical Tubular Stockinette). Knitted fabric, elasticated threads of rubber-cored polyamide or polyester with cotton or cotton and viscose yarn, tubular. Lengths 50 cm and 1 m, widths 6.25 cm, 6.75 cm, 7.5 cm, 8.75 cm, 10 cm, 12 cm (other sizes NHS); Shiloh—*Comfigrip*®; Easigrip—*EasiGRIP*®; Sallis—*Eesiban*®; Sigma—*Sigma ETB*®; S&N Hlth—*Tensogrip*® NHS; JLB—*Textube*®; Medlock—*Tubigrip*®. Where no size stated by prescriber the 50 cm length should be supplied and width endorsed

Uses: retention of dressings on limbs, abdomen, trunk

Elasticated Surgical Tubular Stockinette, Foam padded

(Drug Tariff specification 25). Fabric as for Elasticated Tubular Bandage with polyurethane foam lining. Net price heel, elbow, knee, small = £2.63, medium = £2.83, large = £3.03; sacral, small, medium, and large (all) = £13.55 (Medlock—*Tubipad*®)

Uses: relief of pressure and elimination of friction in relevant area; porosity of foam lining allows normal water loss from skin surface

Elasticated Viscose Stockinette

(Drug Tariff specification 46). Lightweight plain-knitted elasticated tubular bandage.

Acti-Fast®, net price 3.5 cm red line (small limb), length 1 m = 74p; 5 cm green line (medium limb), length 1 m = 80p, 3 m = £2.27, 5 m = £3.89; 7.5 cm blue line (large limb), length 1 m = £1.06, 3 m = £2.99, 5 m = £5.22; 10.75 cm yellow line (child trunk), length 1 m = £1.70, 3 m = £4.86, 5 m = £8.36; 17.5 cm beige line (adult trunk), length 1 m = £2.15 (Activa)

Comfifast®, net price 3.5 cm red line (small limb), length 1 m = 64p; 5 cm green line (medium limb), length 1 m = 68p, 3 m = £1.94, 5 m = £3.33; 7.5 cm blue line (large limb), length 1 m = 92p, 3 m = £2.56, 5 m = £ 4.47; 10.75 cm yellow line (child trunk), length 1 m = £1.46, 3 m = £4.17, 5 m = £7.16; 17.5 cm beige line (adult trunk), length 1 m = £1.84 (Shiloh)

Coverflex®, net price 3.5 cm red line (small limb), length 1 m = 73p; 5 cm green line (medium limb), length 1 m = 76p, 3 m = £2.24, 5 m = £3.87; 7.5 cm blue line (large limb), length 1 m = £1.07, 3 m = £2.54, 5 m = £ 5.04; 10.75 cm yellow line (child trunk), length 1 m = £1.68, 3 m = £4.83, 5 m = £8.50; 17.5 cm beige line (adult trunk), length 1 m = £2.24 (Hartmann)

Tubifast®, net price 3.5 cm red line (small limb), length 1 m = 80p; 5 cm green line (medium limb), length 1 m = 87p, 3 m = £2.48, 5 m = £4.23; 7.5 cm blue line (large limb), length 1 m = £1.16, 3 m = £3.26, 5 m = £5.68; 10.75 cm yellow line (child trunk), length 1 m = £1.85, 3 m = £5.30, 5 m = £9.11; 17.5 cm beige line (adult trunk), length 1 m = £2.34; vest, 6–24 months = £10.07, 2–5 years = £13.43, 5–8 years = £15.10, 8–11 years = £16.78, 11–14 years = £16.78; tights (pair) 6–24 months = £10.07; leggings (pair) 2–5 years = £13.43, 5–8 years = £15.10, 8–11 years = £16.78, 11–14 years = £16.78; socks (pair) = £4.20 (Medlock)

Uses: retention of dressings

Ribbed Cotton and Viscose Surgical Tubular Stockinette, BP 1988

Knitted fabric of 1:1 ribbed structure, singles yarn spun from blend of two-thirds cotton and one-third viscose fibres, tubular. Length 5 m (all):

type A (lightweight): net price arm/leg (child), arm (adult) 5 cm = £2.26; arm (OS adult), leg (adult) 7.5 cm = £2.97; leg (OS adult) 10 cm = £3.94; trunk (child) 15 cm = £5.68; trunk (adult) 20 cm = £6.55; trunk (OS adult) 25 cm = £7.84 (SSL)

type B (heavyweight): sizes as for type A, net price £2.26–£7.84 (Sallis—*Eesiban*®)

Drug Tariff specifies various combinations of sizes to provide sufficient material for part or full body coverage

Uses: protective dressings with tar-based and other non-steroid ointments

Tubular Gauze Bandage, Seamless NHS

Unbleached cotton yarn, positioned with applicators. Net price 20 m roll (all): 00 = £2.95; 01 = £3.55; 12 = £4.60; 34 = £6.75; 56 = £9.35; 78 = £10.75; T1 = £14.75; T2 = £19.00 (Medlock—*Tubegauz*®)

Uses: retention of dressings on limbs, abdomen, trunk

A8.2.4 Support bandages

Light support bandages, which include the various forms of crepe bandage, are used in the prevention of oedema; they are also used to provide support for mild sprains and joints but their effectiveness has not been proven for this purpose. Since they have limited extensibility, they are able to provide light support without exerting undue pressure. For a warning against injudicious compression see section A8.2.5.

Crepe Bandage, BP 1988
Fabric, plain weave, warp of wool threads and crepe-twisted cotton threads, weft of cotton threads; stretch bandage. Net price 4.5 m stretched (all): 5 cm = 93p; 7.5 cm = £1.31; 10 cm = £1.72; 15 cm = £2.49 (most suppliers)
Uses: light support system for strains, sprains, compression over paste bandages for varicose veins

Cotton Crepe Bandage
light support bandage, net price 4.5 m stretched (all): 5 cm = 48p; 7.5 cm = 67p; 10 cm = 87p; 15 cm = £1.27 (Bailey, Robert– *Hospicrepe 239*)

Cotton Crepe Bandage, BP 1988
Fabric, plain weave, warp of crepe-twisted cotton threads, weft of cotton and/or viscose threads; stretch bandage. Net price 4.5 m stretched (both): 7.5 cm = £2.93; 10 cm = £3.77; other sizes NHS (most suppliers)
Uses: light support system for strains, sprains, compression over paste bandages for varicose ulcers

Cotton, Polyamide and Elastane Bandage
Fabric, cotton, polyamide, and elastane; light support bandage (Type 2). 4.5 m stretched (all): 5 cm, net price = 59p, 7.5 cm = 79p, 10 cm = 99p (Neomedic—*Neosport*®); 5 cm, net price = 68p, 7.5 cm = 97p, 10 cm = £1.24, 15 cm = £1.78 (S&N Hlth —*Soffcrepe*®); 10 cm, net price = £1.18 (Medlock—*Setocrepe*®)
Uses: light support for sprains and strains; retention of dressings

Cotton Stretch Bandage, BP 1988
Fabric, plain weave, warp of crepe-twisted cotton threads, weft of cotton threads; stretch bandage, lighter than cotton crepe. Net price 4.5 m stretched (all): 5 cm = 56p; 7.5 cm = 78p; 10 cm = £1.04; 15 cm = £1.48 (Bailey, Robert—*Hospicrepe 233*)
Uses: light support system for strains, sprains, compression over paste bandages for varicose veins

Cotton Suspensory Bandage
(Drug Tariff). Type 1: cotton net bag with draw tapes and webbing waistband; net price small, medium, and large (all) = £1.62, extra large = £1.72. Type 2: cotton net bag with elastic edge and webbing waistband; small = £1.79, medium = £1.85, large = £1.91, extra large = £1.99. Type 3: cotton net bag with elastic edge and webbing waistband with elastic insertion; small, medium, and large (all) = £1.94; extra large = £2.00. Type supplied to be endorsed
Uses: support of scrotum

Knitted Elastomer and Viscose Bandage
Knitted fabric, viscose and elastomer yarn. Type 2 (light support bandage) 4.5 m stretched (all):
Knit-Firm®, net price 5 cm = 39p, 7 cm = 55p, 10 cm = 72p, 15 cm = £1.04 (Bailey, Robert)
Ultra Lite®, net price 5 cm = 52p, 7 cm = 73p, 10 cm = 95p, 15 cm = £1.37 (Parema)
Uses: light support for sprains and strains
Type 3a (light compression bandage):
Elset®, 6 m stretched, net price 10 cm = £2.55, 15 cm = £2.76; 8 m stretched, 10 cm = £3.26 (Medlock)
Elset® *S*, 12 m stretched, net price 15 cm = £5.48 (Medlock)
Mill Plus®, 6 m stretched, net price 10 cm = £1.34; 8.7 m stretched, 10 cm = £1.81 (Bailey, Robert)
Ultra Plus®, net price 8.7 m stretched, 10 cm = £2.05 (Parema)

A8.2.5 High compression bandages

High compression products are used to provide the high compression needed for the management of gross varices, post-thrombotic venous insufficiency, venous leg ulcers, and gross oedema in average-sized limbs. Their use calls for an expert knowledge of the elastic properties of the products and experience in the technique of providing careful graduated compression. Inappropriate application can lead to uneven and inadequate pressures or to hazardous levels of pressure. In particular, injudicious use of compression in limbs with arterial disease has been reported to cause severe skin and tissue necrosis (in some instances calling for amputation). Doppler testing is required before treatment with compression. Pentoxifylline (section 2.6.4.1) may be of benefit if a chronic venous leg ulcer does not respond to compression bandaging [unlicensed indication].

■ High compression bandages

PEC High Compression Bandage
(Drug Tariff specification 52). Polyamide, elastane, and cotton compression (high) extensible bandage, 3.5 m unstretched (both): net price 7.5 cm = £2.68; 10 cm = £3.46 (Medlock—*Setopress*®)

VEC High Compression Bandage
(Drug Tariff specification 52). Viscose, elastane, and cotton compression (high) extensible bandage, 3 m unstretched (both); net price 7.5 cm = £2.70; 10 cm = £3.47 (S&N—*Tensopress*®)

High Compression Bandage
(Drug Tariff specification 52). Cotton, viscose, nylon, and Lycra® extensible bandage, 3 m (unstretched), 10 cm = £3.41 (ConvaTec—*Sure-Press*®); 3.5 m (unstretched), 10 cm = £1.95 (Advancis—*Adva-Co*®)

ProGuide® (S&N Hlth.)
Two layer system, for ankle circumference 18–22 cm (red), net price = £9.23, 22–28 cm (yellow) = £9.74, 28–32 cm (green) = £10.24
NOTE. Second layer is orthopaedic padding; to be used with any High Compression bandage

■ Short Stretch Compression Bandage

Short stretch bandages help to reduce oedema and promote healing of venous leg ulcers. They are also used to reduce swelling associated with lymphoedema. They are applied at full stretch over padding (*see* Sub-compression Wadding Bandage below) which protects areas of high pressure and sites at high risk of pressure damage.

Actiban® (Activa)
Net price (all 5 m), 8 cm = £3.22; 10 cm = £3.46; 12 cm = £4.21

Actico® (Activa)
Cohesive, net price 6 m × 10 cm = £3.21

Comprilan® (Beiersdorf)
Net price (all 5 m) 6 cm = £2.68; 8 cm = £3.15; 10 cm = £3.39; 12 cm = £4.13

Rosidal K® (Vernon-Carus)
Net price (all 5 m) 8 cm = £3.08; 10 cm = £3.36; 12 cm = £4.08; NHS 6 cm = £2.58

Silkolan® (Parema)
Net price (all 5 m) 8 cm = £3.20; 10 cm = £3.62

■ Sub-compression Wadding Bandage

Advasoft® (Advancis)
Net price 3.5 m unstretched, 10 cm = 39p

Cellona® **Undercast Padding** (Vernon-Carus)
Net price 2.75 m unstretched (all): 7.5 cm = 37p; 10 cm = 46p; 15 cm = 59p

Flexi-Ban® (Activa)
Padding, net price 3.5 m unstretched, 10cm = 48p

K-Soft® (Parema)
Net price 3.5 m unstretched, 10 cm = 43p

Ortho-Band Plus® (Bailey, Robert)
Net price 10 cm × 3.5 cm unstretched = 40p

Profore® **#1** (S&N Hlth.)
Natural fleece, net price 3.5 m unstretched, 10 cm = 66p
(Formerly *Soffban*® *Natural*)

Softexe® (Medlock)
Net price 3.5 m unstretched, 10 cm = 62p

SurePress® (ConvaTec)
Absorbent padding, net price 3 m unstretched, 10 cm = 52p

Ultra Soft® (Robinsons)
Soft absorbent bandage, net price 3.5 m unstretched, 10 cm = 42p

Velband® (J&J)
Absorbent padding, net price 4.5 m unstretched, 10 cm = 72p

A8.2.6 Extra-high performance compression bandages

These bandages are capable of applying pressures even higher than those of high compression bandages, therefore the same stringent warnings apply. Their use is reserved for the largest and most oedematous limbs. Extra-high performance compression bandages are poorly tolerated by patients.

Elastic Web Bandage, BP 1993
(Also termed Blue Line Webbing). Characteristic fabric woven ribbon fashion, warp threads of cotton and rubber with mid-line threads coloured blue, weft threads of cotton or combined cotton and viscose; may be dyed skin colour; with or without foot loop. Per m (both) 7.5 cm, net price = 80p; 10 cm = £1.15; with foot loop (Drug Tariff specification 2a) 7.5 cm = £4.62
Uses: provision of support and high compression over large surface

Elastic Web Bandage without Foot Loop
(Also termed Red Line Webbing) (Drug Tariff specification 2b) (Scott-Curwen). Characteristic fabric woven ribbon fashion, warp threads of cotton and rubber with mid-line threads coloured red, weft threads of cotton or combined cotton and viscose. 7.5 cm × 2.75 m (2.5 m unstretched), net price = £3.65; 7.5 cm × 3.75 m (3.5 m unstretched) = £4.41
Uses: provision of support and high compression over large surfaces

Heavy Cotton and Rubber Elastic Bandage, BP 1993
Heavy version of above with one end folded as foot loop; fastener also supplied. 1.8 m unstretched × 7.5 cm, net price = £12.40 (SSL, S&N Hlth—*Elastoweb*®).
Uses: provision of high even compression over large surface

A8.2.7 Adhesive bandages

Elastic adhesive bandages are used to provide compression in the treatment of varicose veins and for the support of injured joints; they should no longer be used for the support of fractured ribs and clavicles. They have also been used with **zinc paste bandage** in the treatment of venous ulcers, but they can cause skin reactions in susceptible patients and may not produce sufficient pressures for healing (significantly lower than those provided by other compression bandages).

Elastic Adhesive Bandage, BP 1993
Woven fabric, elastic in warp (crepe-twisted cotton threads), weft of cotton and/or viscose threads spread with adhesive mass containing zinc oxide. 4.5 m stretched (all): 5 cm, net price = £3.46; 7.5 cm = £5.00; 10 cm = £6.65 (Robinsons—*Flexoplast*®; S&N Hlth—*Elastoplast*® Bandage). 7.5 cm width supplied when size not stated
Uses: compression for chronic leg ulcers; compression and support for swollen or sprained joints

A8.2.8 Cohesive bandages

Cohesive bandages adhere to themselves, but not to the skin, and are useful for providing support for sports use where ordinary stretch bandages might become displaced and adhesive bandages are inappropriate. Care is needed in their application, however, since the loss of ability for movement between turns of the bandage to equalise local areas of high tension carries the potential for creating a tourniquet effect. They should not be used if arterial disease is suspected.

■ Cohesive extensible bandages

These elastic bandages adhere to themselves and not to skin; this prevents slipping during use.
Uses: support of sprained joints; outer layer of multi-layer compression bandaging

Coban® (3M)
Net price 6 m stretched, 10 cm = £2.95; other sizes NHS 4.5 m stretched (all): 2.5 cm = £1.29; 5 cm = £1.81; 7.5 cm = £2.74; 10 cm = £3.61; 15 cm = £5.33

Ultra Fast® (Robinsons)
Latex-free, net price 6.3 m stretched, 10 cm = £2.82

A8.2.9 Medicated bandages

Zinc Paste Bandage remains one of the standard treatments for leg ulcers and can be left on undisturbed for up to a week; it is often used in association with compression for treatment of venous ulcers.

Zinc paste bandages are also used with **coal tar** or **ichthammol** in chronic lichenified skin conditions such as chronic eczema (ichthammol often being preferred since its action is considered to be milder). They are also used with **calamine** in milder eczematous skin conditions (but the inclusion of **clioquinol** may lead to irritation in susceptible subjects).

Zinc Paste Bandage, BP 1993
Cotton fabric, plain weave, impregnated with suitable paste containing zinc oxide; requires additional bandaging. Net price 6 m × 7.5 cm = £3.28 (Medlock—*Steripaste*® (15%), *excipients: include* polysorbate 80); £3.23 (Medlock—*Zincaband*® (15%), *excipients: include* hydroxybenzoates); £3.37 (S&N Hlth—*Viscopaste PB7*® (10%), *excipients: include* hydroxybenzoates)

Zinc Paste and Calamine Bandage
(Drug Tariff specification 5). Cotton fabric, plain weave, impregnated with suitable paste containing calamine and zinc oxide; requires additional

bandaging. Net price 6 m × 7.5 cm = £3.33 (Medlock—*Calaband*®)

Zinc Paste and Ichthammol Bandage, BP 1993
Cotton fabric, plain weave, impregnated with suitable paste containing zinc oxide and ichthammol; requires additional bandaging. Net price 6 m × 7.5 cm = £3.24 (Medlock—*Icthaband*® (15/2%), *excipients: include* hydroxybenzoates; S&N Hlth—*Ichthopaste*® (6/2%)
Excipients: none as listed in section 13.1.3 *Uses:* see section 13.5

■ Medicated stocking

Zipzoc® (S&N Hlth.)
Sterile rayon stocking impregnated with ointment containing zinc oxide 20%. Net price 4-pouch carton = £12.50; 10-pouch carton = £31.26
Uses: chronic leg ulcers; can be used under appropriate compression bandages or hosiery in chronic venous insufficiency

A8.2.10 Multi-layer compression bandaging

Multi-layer compression bandaging systems are an alternative to High Compression Bandages (section A8.2.5) for the treatment of venous leg ulcers. Compression is achieved by the combined effects of two or three extensible bandages applied over a layer of orthopaedic wadding.

Hospifour® (Bailey, Robert)
Hospifour® # 1 (Ortho-Band Plus®—see Sub-compression Wadding Bandage); *Hospifour*® # 2 (*Hospicrepe 239*®—see Cotton Crepe Bandage); *Hospifour*® # 3 (*Mill Plus*® —see Knitted Elastomer and Viscose Bandage); *Hospifour*® # 4 (*AAA-Flex*®), net price 10 cm × 6.3 m (stretched) = £1.93

K-Four® (Parema)
K-Four® # 1 (*K-Soft*®—see Sub-compression Wadding Bandage); *K-Four*® # 2 (*Ultra Lite*®—see Knitted Elastomer and Viscose Bandage); *K-Four*® # 3 (*Ultra Plus*®—see Knitted Elastomer and Viscose Bandage); *K-Four*® # 4 (*Ko-Flex*®), net price 10 cm × 6 m (unstretched) = £2.90
Multi-layer compression bandaging kit, four layer system, for ankle circumference 18–25 cm, net price = £6.67

Profore® (S&N Hlth.)
Profore® wound contact layer (*Tricotex*®—see Knitted Viscose Primary Dressing); *Profore*® *#1* (see Sub-compression Wadding bandage); *Profore*® *#2* (*Soffcrepe*®—see Cotton, Polyamide and Elastane Bandage); *Profore*® *#3* (*Litepress*®—see Knitted Elastomer and Viscose Bandage); *Profore*® *#4* (*Co-Plus*®—see Cohesive bandages); *Profore*® *Plus* = £3.46
Multi-layer compression bandaging kit, four layer system, for ankle circumference up to 18 cm, net price = £9.58, 18–25 cm = £8.92, 25–30 cm = £7.40, above 30 cm = £11.09

System 4® (Medlock)
System 4® wound contact layer (*Setoprime*® 9.5 cm × 9.5 cm; *System 4*® *#1* (*Softexe*®—see Sub-compression Wadding Bandage), *System 4*® *#2* (*Setocrepe*®—see Cotton, Polyamide and Elastane Bandage); *System 4*® *#3* (*Elset*®—see Knitted Elastomer and Viscose Bandage); *System 4*® *#4* (*Coban*®—see Cohesive bandages)
Multi-layer compression bandaging kit, four layer system, for ankle circumference 18–25 cm, net price = £8.29

Ultra Four® (Robinsons)
Ultra Four® wound dressing 14.5 cm × 12.5 cm; *Ultra Four*® *#1* (Robinsons—*Ultra Soft*®—see Sub-compression Wadding Bandage); *Ultra Four*® *#2* (Parema—*Ultra Lite*®—see Knitted Elastomer and Viscose Bandage); *Ultra Four*® *#3* (Parema—*Ultra Plus*®—see Knitted Elastomer and Viscose Bandage); *Ultra Four*® *#4* (Robinsons—*Ultra Fast*®—see Cohesive bandages)
Multi-layer compression bandaging kit, four layer system, for ankle circumference 18–25 cm, net price = £6.16

A8.2.11 Surgical adhesive tapes

Adhesive tapes are useful for retaining dressings on joints or awkward body parts. These tapes, particularly those containing rubber, can cause irritant and allergic reactions in susceptible patients; synthetic adhesives have been developed to overcome this problem, but they, too, may sometimes be associated with reactions. Adhesive tapes that are occlusive may cause skin maceration. Care is needed not to apply these tapes under tension, to avoid creating a tourniquet effect. If applied over joints they need to be orientated so that the area of maximum extensibility of the fabric is in the direction of movement of the limb.

Permeable adhesive tapes

Zinc Oxide Adhesive Tape, BP 1988
(Zinc Oxide Plaster). Fabric, plain weave, warp and weft of cotton and /or viscose, spread with an adhesive containing zinc oxide. 5 m (all): 1.25 cm, net price = 88p; 2.5 cm = £1.27; 5 cm = £2.15; 7.5 cm = £3.23 (most suppliers)
Uses: securing dressings and immobilising small areas

Strappal (BSN Medical)
Zinc oxide adhesive tape. Net price 5 m (all): 1.25 cm = 86p, 2.5 cm = £1.24, 5 cm = £2.10, 7.5 cm = £3.15; other sizes NHS

Permeable Woven Synthetic Adhesive Tape, BP 1988
Non-extensible closely woven fabric, spread with a polymeric adhesive. Net price 5 m (all): 1.25 cm = 72p; 2.5 cm = £1.06; 5 cm = £1.84 (Beiersdorf—*Leukosilk*®)
Uses: securing dressings for patients with skin reactions to other plasters and strapping, which require use for long periods

Elastic Adhesive Tape, BP 1988
(Elastic Adhesive Plaster). Woven fabric, elastic in warp (crepe-twisted cotton threads), weft of cotton and/or viscose threads, spread with adhesive mass containing zinc oxide. Net price 4.5 m stretched × 2.5 cm = £1.55 (Robinsons—*Flexoplast*®; S&N—*Elastoplast*®)
Uses: securing dressings
For 5 cm width, see Elastic Adhesive Bandage

Permeable Non-woven Synthetic Adhesive Tape, BP 1988
Backing of paper-based or non-woven textile material spread with a polymeric adhesive mass. 5 m (all):
Clinipore®, net price 1.25 cm = 35p, 2.5 cm = 59p, 5 cm = 99p (Clinisupplies)
Leukofix®, net price 1.25 cm = 51p, 2.5 cm = 81p, 5 cm = £1.42 (BSN Medical)
Leukopor®, net price 1.25 cm = 45p, 2.5 cm = 70p, 5 cm = £1.23 (Beiersdorf)

Mediplast®, net price 1.25 cm = 30p, 2.5 cm = 50p (Neomedic)
Micropore®, net price 1.25 cm = 60p, 2.5 cm = 89p, 5 cm = £1.57 (3M)
Scanpor®, net price 1.25 cm = 40p, 2.5 cm = 64p, 5 cm = £1.11 (BioDiagnostics)
Where no brand stated by prescriber, net price of tape supplied not to exceed 35p (1.25 cm), 59p (2.5 cm), 99p (5 cm)
Uses: securing dressings; skin closures for small incisions for patients with skin reactions to other plasters and strapping, which require use for long periods

Permeable, Apertured Non-Woven Synthetic Adhesive Tape, BP 1988
Non-woven fabric with a polyacrylate adhesive.
Hypafix®, net price 10 m (all): 2.5 cm = £1.51, 5 cm = £2.39, 10 cm = £4.18, 15 cm = £6.19, 20 cm = £8.21, 30 cm = £11.87 (BSN Medical)
Mefix®, net price 5 m (all): 2.5 cm = 90p, 5 cm = £1.58; 10 cm = £2.53, 15 cm = £3.45, 20 cm = £4.42, 30 cm = £6.34 (Mölnlycke)
Omnifix®, net price 10 m (all): 5 cm = £2.15, 10 cm = £3.62, 15 cm = £5.34 (Hartmann)
Uses: securing dressings

Occlusive adhesive tapes

Impermeable Plastic Adhesive Tape, BP 1988
Extensible water-impermeable plastic film spread with an adhesive mass. Net price 2.5 cm × 3 m = £1.23; 2.5 cm × 5 m = £1.84; 5 cm × 5 m = £2.33; 7.5 cm × 5 m = £3.39 (Robinsons; Medlock—*Setoplast*®; S&N Hlth)
Uses: securing dressings; covering site of infection where exclusion of air, water, and water vapour is required

Impermeable Plastic Synthetic Adhesive Tape, BP 1988
Extensible water-impermeable plastic film spread with a polymeric adhesive mass. Net price 5 m (both): 2.5 cm = £1.72; 5 cm = £3.27 (3M—*Blenderm*®)
Uses: isolating wounds from external environment; covering sites where total exclusion of water and water vapour required; securing dressings and appliances

A8.2.12 Adhesive dressings

Adhesive dressings (also termed 'island dressings') have a limited role for minor wounds only. The inclusion of an antiseptic is not particularly useful and may cause skin irritation in susceptible subjects.

Permeable adhesive dressings

Elastic Adhesive Dressing, BP 1993 NHS
Wound dressing or dressing strip, pad attached to piece of extension plaster, leaving suitable adhesive margin; both pad and margin covered with suitable protector; pad may be dyed yellow and may be impregnated with suitable antiseptic (see below); extension plaster may be perforated or ventilated
Uses: general purpose wound dressing
NOTE. Permitted antiseptics are aminoacridine hydrochloride (aminacrine hydrochloride), chlorhexidine hydrochloride (both 0.07–0.13%), chlorhexidine gluconate (0.11–0.20%); domiphen bromide (0.05–0.25%)

Permeable Plastic Wound Dressing, BP 1993 NHS
Consisting of an absorbent pad, which may be dyed and impregnated with a suitable antiseptic (see under Elastic Adhesive Dressing), attached to a piece of permeable plastic surgical adhesive tape, to leave a suitable adhesive margin; both pad and margin covered with suitable protector (most suppliers)
Uses: general purpose wound dressing, permeable to air and water

Vapour permeable adhesive dressings

Vapour-permeable Waterproof Plastic Wound Dressing, BP 1993
(former Drug Tariff title: Semipermeable Waterproof Plastic Wound Dressing). Consists of absorbent pad, may be dyed and impregnated with suitable antiseptic (see under Elastic Adhesive Dressing), attached to piece of semi-permeable waterproof surgical adhesive tape, to leave suitable adhesive margin; both pad and margin covered with suitable protector. 8.5 cm × 6 cm, net price = 34p (S&N Hlth—*Elastoplast Airstrip*®)
Uses: general purpose waterproof wound dressing, permeable to air and water vapour

Occlusive adhesive dressings

Impermeable Plastic Wound Dressing, BP 1993 NHS
Consists of absorbent pad, may be dyed and impregnated with suitable antiseptic (see under Elastic Adhesive Dressing), attached to piece of impermeable plastic surgical adhesive tape, to leave suitable adhesive margin; both pad and margin covered with suitable protector (most suppliers)
Uses: protective covering for wounds requiring an occlusive dressing

A8.2.13 Skin closure dressings

Skin closure strips are used as an alternative to sutures for minor cuts and lacerations.

Skin closure strips, sterile
Leukostrip®, 6.4 mm × 76 mm, 3 strips per envelope. Net price 10 envelopes = £5.46 (Beiersdorf)
Steri-strip®, 6 mm × 75 mm, 3 strips per envelope. Net price 12 envelopes = £8.52; NHS 3 mm × 75 mm, 12 envelopes = £8.32; 12 mm × 100 mm, 12 envelopes = £8.52 (3M)
Drug Tariff specifies that these are specifically for personal administration by the prescriber

A8.3 Elastic hosiery

Before elastic hosiery can be dispensed, the quantity (single or pair), article (including accessories), and compression class (I, II or III) must be specified by the prescriber; all dispensed articles must state on the packaging that they conform with Drug Tariff technical specification No. 40, for further details see Drug Tariff.
NOTE. Graduated compression tights are NHS.

A8.3.1 Graduated compression hosiery

Class 1 Light Support

Hosiery, compression at ankle 14–17 mm Hg, thigh length or below knee with knitted in heel. Net price per pair, circular knit (standard), thigh length = £7.02, below knee = £6.41; light weight elastic net (made-to-measure), thigh length = £18.79, below knee = £14.67

Uses: superficial or early varices, varicosis during pregnancy

Class 2 Medium Support

Hosiery, compression at ankle 18–24 mm Hg, thigh length or below knee with knitted in heel. Net price per pair, circular knit (standard), thigh length = £10.43, below knee = £9.37, (made-to-measure), thigh length = £34.85, below knee = £21.80; net (made-to-measure), thigh length = £18.79, below knee = £14.67; flat bed (made-to-measure, only with closed heel and open toe), thigh length = £34.85, below knee = £21.80

Uses: varices of medium severity, ulcer treatment and prophylaxis, mild oedema, varicosis during pregnancy

Class 3 Strong Support

Hosiery, compression at ankle 25–35 mm Hg, thigh length or below knee with open or knitted in heel. Net price per pair, circular knit (standard), thigh length = £12.36, below knee = £10.63, (made-to-measure) thigh length = £34.85, below knee = £21.80; flat bed (made-to-measure, only with open heel and open toe), thigh length = £34.85, below knee = £21.80

Uses: gross varices, post thrombotic venous insufficiency, gross oedema, ulcer treatment and prophylaxis

A8.3.2 Accessories

Suspender

Suspender, for thigh stockings, net price = 61p, belt (specification 13), = £4.68, fitted (additional price) = 61p

A8.3.3 Anklets

Class 2 Medium Support

Anklets, compression 18–24 mm Hg, circular knit (standard and made-to-measure), net price per pair = £6.14; flat bed (standard and made-to-measure) = £12.76; made-to-measure = £12.76

Uses: soft tissue support

Class 3 Strong Support

Anklets, compression 25–35 mm Hg, circular knit (standard and made-to-measure), net price per pair = £8.57; flat bed (standard) = £8.57; made-to-measure = £12.76

Uses: soft tissue support

A8.3.4 Knee caps

Class 2 Medium Support

Kneecaps, compression 18–24 mm Hg, circular knit (standard and made-to-measure), net price per pair = £6.14; flat bed (standard and made-to-measure) = £12.76; net made-to-measure = £10.03

Uses: soft tissue support

Class 3 Strong Support

Kneecaps, compression 25–35 mm Hg, circular knit (standard and made-to-measure), net price per pair = £8.19; flat bed (standard) = £8.19; made-to-measure = £12.76

Uses: soft tissue support

Appendix 9: Cautionary and advisory labels for dispensed medicines

Numbers following the preparation entries in the BNF correspond to the code numbers of the cautionary labels that pharmacists are recommended to add when dispensing. It is also expected that pharmacists will counsel patients when necessary.

Counselling needs to be related to the age, experience, background, and understanding of the individual patient. The pharmacist should ensure that the patient understands how to take or use the medicine and how to follow the correct dosage schedule. Any effects of the medicine on driving or work, any foods or medicines to be avoided, and what to do if a dose is missed should also be explained. Other matters, such as the possibility of staining of the clothes or skin by a medicine should also be mentioned.

For some preparations there is a special need for counselling, such as an unusual method or time of administration or a potential interaction with a common food or domestic remedy, and this is indicated where necessary.

ORIGINAL PACKS. Most preparations are now dispensed in unbroken original packs (see Patient Packs, p. xi) that include further advice for the patient in the form of patient information leaflets. Label 10 may be of value where appropriate. More general leaflets advising on the administration of preparations such as eye drops, eye ointments, inhalers, and suppositories are also available.

SCOPE OF LABELS. In general no label recommendations have been made for injections on the assumption that they will be administered by a healthcare professional or a well-instructed patient. The labelling is not exhaustive and pharmacists are recommended to use their professional discretion in labelling new preparations and those for which no labels are shown.

Individual labelling advice is not given on the administration of the large variety of antacids. In the absence of instructions from the prescriber, and if on enquiry the patient has had no verbal instructions, the directions given under 'Dose' should be used on the label.

It is recognised that there may be occasions when pharmacists will use their knowledge and professional discretion and decide to omit one or more of the recommended labels for a particular patient. In this case counselling is of the utmost importance. There may also be an occasion when a prescriber does not wish additional cautionary labels to be used, in which case the prescription should be endorsed 'NCL' (no cautionary labels). The exact wording that is required instead should then be specified on the prescription.

Pharmacists label medicines with various wordings in addition to those directions specified on the prescription. Such labels include 'Shake the bottle', 'For external use only', and 'Store in a cool place', as well as 'Discard . . . . days after opening' and 'Do not use after . . . .', which apply particularly to antibiotic mixtures, diluted liquid and topical preparations, and to eye-drops. Although not listed in the BNF these labels should continue to be used when appropriate; indeed, 'For external use only' is a legal requirement on external liquid preparations, while 'Keep out of the reach of children' is a legal requirement on all dispensed medicines. Care should be taken not to obscure other relevant information with adhesive labelling.

It is the usual practice for patients to take standard tablets with water or other liquid and for this reason no separate label has been recommended.

The label wordings recommended by the BNF apply to medicines dispensed against a prescription. Patients should be aware that a dispensed medicine should never be taken by, or shared with, anyone other than for whom the prescriber intended it. Therefore, the BNF does not include warnings against the use of a dispensed medicine by persons other than for whom it was specifically prescribed.

The label or labels for each preparation are recommended after careful consideration of the information available. However, it is recognised that in some cases this information may be either incomplete or open to a different interpretation. The Executive Editor will therefore be grateful to receive any constructive comments on the labelling suggested for any preparation.

Recommended label wordings

Wordings which can be given as separate warnings are labels 1-19 and labels 29-33. Wordings which can be incorporated in an appropriate position in the directions for dosage or administration are labels 21-28. A label has been omitted for number 20.

If separate labels are used it is recommended that the wordings be used without modification. If changes are made to suit computer requirements, care should be taken to retain the sense of the original.

1 **Warning. May cause drowsiness**
To be used on *preparations for children* containing antihistamines, or other preparations given to children where the warnings of label 2 on driving or alcohol would not be appropriate.

2 **Warning. May cause drowsiness. If affected do not drive or operate machinery. Avoid alcoholic drink**
To be used on *preparations for adults that can cause drowsiness*, thereby affecting the ability to drive and operate hazardous machinery; label 1 is more appropriate for children. *It is an offence to drive while under the influence of drink or drugs.*
Some of these preparations only cause drowsiness in the first few days of treatment and some only cause drowsiness in higher doses.

In such cases the patient should be told that the advice applies until the effects have worn off. However many of these preparations can produce a slowing of reaction time and a loss of mental concentration that can have the same effects as drowsiness.
Avoidance of alcoholic drink is recommended because the effects of CNS depressants are enhanced by alcohol. Strict prohibition however could lead to some patients not taking the medicine. Pharmacists should therefore explain the risk and encourage compliance, particularly in patients who may think they already tolerate the effects of alcohol (see also label 3). Queries from patients with epilepsy regarding fitness to drive should be referred back to the patient's doctor.
Side-effects unrelated to drowsiness that may affect a patient's ability to drive or operate machinery safely include *blurred vision, dizziness, or nausea*. In general, no label has been recommended to cover these cases, but the patient should be suitably counselled.

3 **Warning. May cause drowsiness. If affected do not drive or operate machinery**
To be used on *preparations containing monoamine-oxidase inhibitors*; the warning to avoid alcohol and dealcoholised (low alcohol) drink is covered by the patient information leaflet.
Also to be used as for label 2 but where alcohol is not an issue.

4 **Warning. Avoid alcoholic drink**
To be used on *preparations where a reaction such as flushing may occur if alcohol is taken* (e.g. metronidazole and chlorpropamide). Alcohol may also enhance the hypoglycaemia produced by some oral antidiabetic drugs but routine application of a warning label is not considered necessary.

5 **Do not take indigestion remedies at the same time of day as this medicine**
To be used with label 25 on *preparations coated to resist gastric acid* (e.g. enteric-coated tablets). This is to avoid the possibility of premature dissolution of the coating in the presence of an alkaline pH.
Label 5 also applies to drugs such as ketoconazole *where the absorption is significantly affected by antacids*; the usual period of avoidance recommended is 2 to 4 hours.

6 **Do not take indigestion remedies or medicines containing iron or zinc at the same time of day as this medicine**
To be used on *preparations containing ofloxacin and some other quinolones, doxycycline, lymecycline, minocycline, and penicillamine*. These drugs chelate calcium, iron and zinc and are less well absorbed when taken with calcium-containing antacids or preparations containing iron or zinc. These incompatible preparations should be taken 2-3 hours apart.

7 **Do not take milk, indigestion remedies, or medicines containing iron or zinc at the same time of day as this medicine**
To be used on *preparations containing ciprofloxacin, norfloxacin or tetracyclines that chelate, calcium, iron, magnesium, and zinc* and are thus less available for absorption; these incompatible preparations should be taken 2-3 hours apart. Doxycycline, lymecycline and minocycline are less liable to form chelates and therefore only require label 6 (see above).

8 **Do not stop taking this medicine except on your doctor's advice**
To be used on *preparations that contain a drug which is required to be taken over long periods without the patient necessarily perceiving any benefit* (e.g. antituberculous drugs).
Also to be used on *preparations that contain a drug whose withdrawal is likely to be a particular hazard* (e.g. clonidine for hypertension). Label 10 (see below) is more appropriate for corticosteroids.

9 **Take at regular intervals. Complete the prescribed course unless otherwise directed**
To be used on *preparations where a course of treatment should be completed* to reduce the incidence of relapse or failure of treatment.
The preparations are antimicrobial drugs given by mouth. Very occasionally, some may have severe side-effects (e.g. diarrhoea in patients receiving clindamycin) and in such cases the patient may need to be advised of reasons for stopping treatment quickly and returning to the doctor.

10 **Warning. Follow the printed instructions you have been given with this medicine**
To be used particularly on *preparations containing anticoagulants, lithium and oral corticosteroids*. The appropriate treatment card should be given to the patient and any necessary explanations given.
This label may also be used on other preparations to remind the patient of the instructions that have been given.

11 **Avoid exposure of skin to direct sunlight or sun lamps**
To be used on *preparations that may cause phototoxic or photoallergic reactions* if the patient is exposed to ultraviolet radiation. Many drugs other than those listed (e.g. phenothiazines and sulphonamides) may on rare occasions cause reactions in susceptible patients. Exposure to high intensity ultraviolet radiation from sunray lamps and sunbeds is particularly likely to cause reactions.

12 **Do not take anything containing aspirin while taking this medicine**
To be used on *preparations containing probenecid and sulfinpyrazone* whose activity is reduced by aspirin. Label 12 should not be used for anticoagulants since label 10 is more appropriate.

13 **Dissolve or *mix with water* before taking**
To be used on *preparations that are intended to be dissolved in water* (e.g. soluble tablets) or *mixed with water* (e.g. powders, granules) before use. In a few cases other liquids such as fruit juice or milk may be used.

14 **This medicine may colour the urine**
To be used on *preparations that may cause the patient's urine to turn an unusual colour*. These include phenolphthalein (alkaline urine pink), triamterene (blue under some lights), levodopa (dark reddish), and rifampicin (red).

15 **Caution flammable: keep away from fire or flames**
To be used on *preparations containing sufficient flammable solvent to render them flammable if exposed to a naked flame*.

16 **Allow to dissolve under the tongue. Do not transfer from this container. Keep tightly closed. Discard eight weeks after opening**
To be used on *glyceryl trinitrate tablets* to remind the patient not to transfer the tablets to plastic or less suitable containers.

17 **Do not take more than . . . in 24 hours**
To be used on *preparations for the treatment of acute migraine* except those containing ergotamine, for which label 18 is used. The dose form should be specified, e.g. tablets or capsules.
It may also be used on preparations for which no dose has been specified by the prescriber.

18 **Do not take more than . . . in 24 hours or . . . in any one week**
To be used on preparations containing ergotamine. The dose form should be specified, e.g. tablets or suppositories.

19 **Warning. Causes drowsiness which may continue the next day. If affected do not drive or operate machinery. Avoid alcoholic drink**
To be used on *preparations containing hypnotics (or some other drugs with sedative effects) prescribed to be taken at night*. On the rare occasions (e.g. nitrazepam in epilepsy) when hypnotics are prescribed for daytime administration this label would clearly not be appropriate. Also to be used as an *alternative to the label 2 wording* (the choice being at the discretion of the pharmacist) *for anxiolytics prescribed to be taken at night*.
It is hoped that this wording will convey adequately the problem of residual morning sedation after taking 'sleeping tablets'.

21 **. . . with or after food**
To be used on *preparations that are liable to cause gastric irritation, or those that are better absorbed with food*.
Patients should be advised that a *small amount of food is sufficient*.

22 **. . . half to one hour before food**
To be used on some preparations *whose absorption is thereby improved*.
Most oral antibacterials require label 23 instead (see below).

23 **. . . an hour before food or on an empty stomach**
To be used on *oral antibacterials whose absorption may be reduced by the presence of food and acid in the stomach.*

24 **. . . sucked or chewed**
To be used on *preparations that should be sucked or chewed.*
The pharmacist should use discretion as to which of these words is appropriate.

25 **. . . swallowed whole, not chewed**
To be used on *preparations that are enteric-coated or designed for modified-release.*
Also to be used on *preparations that taste very unpleasant or may damage the mouth* if not swallowed whole.

26 **. . . dissolved under the tongue**
To be used on *preparations designed for sublingual use.* Patients should be advised to hold under the tongue and avoid swallowing until dissolved. The buccal mucosa between the gum and cheek is occasionally specified by the prescriber.

27 **. . . with plenty of water**
To be used on *preparations that should be well diluted* (e.g. chloral hydrate), *where a high fluid intake is required* (e.g. sulphonamides), or *where water is required to aid the action* (e.g. methylcellulose). The patient should be advised that 'plenty' means at least 150 mL (about a tumblerful). In most cases fruit juice, tea, or coffee may be used.

28 **To be spread thinly . . .**
To be used on *external preparations* that should be applied sparingly (e.g. corticosteroids, dithranol).

29 **Do not take more than 2 at any one time. Do not take more than 8 in 24 hours**
To be used on containers of dispensed *solid dose preparations containing paracetamol for adults when the instruction on the label indicates that the dose can be taken on an 'as required' basis.* The dose form should be specified, e.g. tablets or capsules.
This label has been introduced because of the serious consequences of overdosage with paracetamol.

30 **Do not take with any other paracetamol products**
To be used on all containers of dispensed *preparations containing paracetamol.*

31 **Contains aspirin and paracetamol. Do not take with any other paracetamol products**
To be used on all containers of dispensed *preparations containing aspirin and paracetamol.*

32 **Contains aspirin**
To be used on containers of dispensed *preparations containing aspirin when the name on the label does not include the word 'aspirin'.*

33 **Contains an aspirin-like medicine**
To be used on containers of dispensed *preparations containing aspirin derivatives.*

Products and their labels

Products introduced or amended since publication of BNF No. 49 (March 2005) are underlined.
Proprietary names are in *italic.*
C = counselling advised; see BNF = consult product entry in BNF

Abacavir, C, hypersensitivity reactions, see BNF
Abilify, C, driving
Acamprosate, 21, 25
Acarbose, C, administration, see BNF
Accolate, 23
Acebutolol, 8
Aceclofenac, 21
Acemetacin, 21, C, driving
Acenocoumarol, 10, anticoagulant card
Acetazolamide, 3
Acetazolamide m/r, 3, 25
Aciclovir susp and tabs, 9
Acipimox, 21
Acitretin, 10, patient information leaflet, 21
Acorvio Plus, 28
Acrivastine, C, driving, alcohol, see BNF
Actinac, 28
Actiq, 2
Actonel, C, administration, food and calcium, see BNF
Acupan, 2, 14, (urine pink)
Adalat LA, 25
Adalat Retard, 25
Adalimumab, C, tuberculosis
Adcal, 24
Adcal-D_3, 24
Adcortyl with Graneodin, 28
Adipine MR, 21, 25
Adipine XL, 25
Adizem preps, 25
AeroBec, 8, C, dose
AeroBec Forte, 8, 10, steroid card, C, dose
Agenerase caps, 5
Agenerase oral solution, 4, 5
Airomir, C, dose, change to CFC-free inhaler, see BNF
Albendazole, 9
Alclometasone external preps, 28
Aldara, 10, patient information leaflet
Aldomet, 3, 8
Alendronic acid, C, administration, see BNF
Alfuzosin, 3, C, dose, see BNF
Alfuzosin m/r, 3, 21, 25, C, dose, see BNF
Alimemazine, 2
Allegron, 2
Allopurinol, 8, 21, 27
Almogran, 3
Almotriptan, 3
Alphosyl HC, 28
Alphaderm, 28
Alprazolam, 2
Alvedon, 30
Alvesco, 8, C, dose
Alvercol, 25, 27, C, administration, see BNF
Amantadine, C, driving
Aminophylline m/r, see preps
Amiodarone, 11
Amisulpride, 2
Amitriptyline, 2
Amitriptyline m/r, 2, 25
Amobarbital, 19
Amorolfine, 10, patient information leaflet
Amoxapine, 2
Amoxicillin, 9
Amoxicillin chewable tabs, 9, 10, patient information leaflet
Amoxicillin dispersible sachets, 9, 13
Amoxil, 9
Amoxil dispersible sachets, 9, 13
Amoxil paed susp, 9, C, use of pipette
Amphotericin loz, 9, 24, C, after food
Amphotericin mixt (g.i.), 9, C, use of pipette
Amphotericin mixt (mouth), 9, C, use of pipette, hold in mouth, after food
Amphotericin tabs, 9
Ampicillin, 9, 23
Amprenavir caps, 5
Amprenavir oral solution, 4, 5
Amytal, 19
Anafranil, 2
Anafranil m/r, 2, 25
Anagrelide, C, driving
Anakinra, C, blood disorder symptoms
Androcur, 21
Andropatch, C, administration, see BNF
Angettes-75, 32
Angiopine 40 LA, 21, 25

Angitil SR, 25
Angitil XL, 25
Anhydrol Forte, 15
Antabuse, 2, C, alcohol reaction, see BNF
Antacids, see BNF dose statements
Antepsin, 5
Anthranol preps, 28
Anticoagulants, oral, 10, anticoagulant card
Antihistamines, (see individual preparations)
Anturan, 12, 21
Apomorphine sublingual tabs, C, driving
Arava, 4
Aripiprazole, C, driving
Aromasin, 21
Arpicolin, C, driving
Artane, C, before or after food, driving, see BNF
Artemether with lumefantrine, 21, C, driving
Arythmol, 21, 25
Arthrotec, 21, 25
Asacol MR tabs, 5, 25, C, blood disorder symptoms, see BNF
Asacol enema and supps, C, blood disorder symptoms, see BNF
Asasantin Retard, 21, 25
Ascorbic acid, effervescent, 13
Ascorbic acid tabs (500mg), 24
Asendis, 2
Asmabec preps, 8, 10, steroid card (high-dose preparations only), C, dose
Asmanex, 8, 10, steroid card, C, dose
Asmasal, C, dose, see BNF
Aspav, 2, 13, 21, 32
Aspirin and papaveretum dispersible tabs, 2, 13, 21, also 32 (if 'aspirin' not on label)
Aspirin dispersible tabs, 13, 21, also 32 (if 'aspirin' not on label)
Aspirin effervescent, 13, also 32 (if 'aspirin' not on label)
Aspirin e/c, 5, 25, also 32 (if 'aspirin' not on label)
Aspirin m/r, 25, also 32 (if 'aspirin' not on label)
Aspirin tabs, 21, also 32 (if 'aspirin' not on label)
Aspirin, paracetamol and codeine tabs, 21, 29, also 31 (if 'aspirin' and 'paracetamol' not on label)
Atarax, 2
Atazanavir, 5, 21
Atenolol, 8
Atorvastatin, C, muscle effects, see BNF
Atovaquone, 21
Atrovent inhalations, C, dose, see BNF
Augmentin susp and tabs, 9
Augmentin Duo, 9
Augmentin dispersible tabs, 9, 13
Auranofin, 21, C, blood disorder symptoms, see BNF
Aureocort, 28
Avandamet, 21
Avelox, 6, 9, C, driving
Avloclor, 5, C, malaria prophylaxis, see BNF
Avodart, 25
Avomine, 2
Azathioprine, 21
Azithromycin caps, 5, 9, 23
Azithromycin susp, 5, 9

Baclofen, 2, 8
Balsalazide, 21, 25
Baratol, 2
Baxan, 9
Beclazone, 8, 10, steroid card (250-microgram only), C, dose
Becloforte preps, 8, 10, steroid card, C, dose
Beclometasone external preps, 28
Beclometasone inhalations, 8, 10, steroid card (high-dose preparations only), C, dose
Becodisks, 8, 10, steroid card (high-dose preparation only), C, dose
Becotide preps, 8, C, dose
Benemid, 12, 21, 27
Benperidol, 2
Benquil, 2
Benzatropine, 2
Benzoin tincture, cpd, 15
Beta-Adalat, 8, 25
Betacap, 15, 28
Beta-Cardone, 8
Betahistine, 21
Betaloc, 8
Betaloc-SA, 8, 25
Betamethasone inj, 10, steroid card
Betamethasone tab, 10, steroid card, 21
Betamethasone external preps, 28
Betamethasone scalp application, 15, 28
Bethanechol, 22
Betim, 8
Betnelan, 10, steroid card, 21
Betnesol injection, 10, steroid card
Betnesol tabs, 10, steroid card, 13, 21
Betnovate external preps, 28
Betnovate scalp application, 15, 28
Betnovate-RD, 28
Bettamousse, 28
Bezafibrate, 21
Bezalip, 21
Bezalip-Mono, 21, 25
Biorphen, C, driving
Bisacodyl tabs, 5, 25
Bisoprolol, 8
Bondronat tabs, C, administration, see BNF
Bonefos caps and tabs, C, food and calcium, see BNF
Brexidol, 21
Bricanyl inhalations, C, dose, see BNF
Bricanyl SA, 25
Britlofex, 2
Broflex, C, before or after food, driving, see BNF
Bromocriptine, 21, C, hypotensive reactions, see BNF
Brufen, 21
Brufen gran, 13, 21
Brufen Retard, 25, 27
Buccastem, 2, C, administration, see BNF
Budenofalk, 5, 10, steroid card, 22, 25
Budesonide inhalations, 8, 10, steroid card (high-dose preparations only), C, dose
Budesonide caps, 5, 10, steroid card, 22, 25
Buprenorphine, 2, 26
Bupropion, 25
Burinex K, 25, 27, C, posture, see BNF
Buserelin nasal spray, C, nasal decongestants, see BNF
Buspar, C, driving
Buspirone, C, driving
Butobarbital, 19

Cabaser, 21, C, driving, hypotensive reactions, see BNF
Cabergoline, 21, C, driving, hypotensive reactions, see BNF
Cacit, 13
Cacit D3, 13
Cafergot, 18, C, dosage
Calceos, 24
Calcicard CR, 25
Calcichew preps, 24
Calcisorb, 13, 21, C, may be sprinkled on food
Calcium-500, 25
Calcium acetate tabs, 21, 25
Calcium carbonate tabs, chewable, 24
Calcium carbonate tabs and gran effervescent, 13
Calcium gluconate tabs, 24
Calcium phosphate sachets, 13
Calcium Resonium, 13
Calcium and ergocalciferol tabs, C, administration, see BNF
Calcort, 5, 10, steroid card
Calfovit D3, 13, 21
Calmurid HC, 28
Calpol susp, 30
Camcolit 250 tabs, 10, lithium card, C, fluid and salt intake, see BNF
Camcolit 400 tabs, 10, lithium card, 25, C, fluid and salt intake, see BNF
Campral EC, 21, 25
Canesten HC, 28
Canesten spray, 15
Capecitabine, 21
Caprin, 5, 25, 32
Carbaglu, 13
Carbamazepine chewable, 3, 8, 21, 24, C, blood, hepatic or skin disorder symptoms (see BNF), driving (see BNF)

Carbamazepine liq, supps and tabs, 3, 8, C, blood, hepatic or skin disorder symptoms (see BNF), driving (see BNF)
Carbamazepine m/r, 3, 8, 25, C, blood, hepatic or skin disorder symptoms (see BNF), driving (see BNF)
Carbimazole, C, blood disorder symptoms, see BNF
Cardene SR, 25
Cardilate MR, 25
Cardinol, 8
Cardura XL, 25
Carglumic acid, 13
Carisoma, 2
Carisoprodol, 2
Carvedilol, 8
Carylderm lotion, 15
Catapres, 3, 8
Cedocard Retard, 25
Cefaclor, 9
Cefaclor m/r, 9, 21, 25
Cefadroxil, 9
Cefalexin, 9
Cefixime, 9
Cefpodoxime, 5, 9, 21
Cefprozil, 9
Cefradine, 9
Cefuroxime susp, 9, 21
Cefuroxime sachets, 9, 13, 21
Cefuroxime tab, 9, 21, 25
Cefzil, 9
Celance, C, driving, hypotensive reactions, see BNF
Celectol, 8, 22
Celevac (constipation or diarrhoea), C, administration, see BNF
Celevac tabs (anorectic), C, administration, see BNF
Celiprolol, 8, 22
Centyl K, 25, 27, C, posture, see BNF
Ceporex caps, mixts, and tabs, 9
Cerivastatin, C, muscle effects, see BNF
Cetirizine, C, driving, alcohol, see BNF
Chemydur 60XL, 25
Chloral hydrate, 19, 27
Chloral paed elixir, 1, 27
Chloral mixt, 19, 27
Chlordiazepoxide, 2
Chloroquine, 5, C, malaria prophylaxis, see BNF
Chlorphenamine, 2
Chlorpromazine mixts and supps, 2, 11
Chlorpromazine tabs, 2, 11
Chlorpropamide, 4
Cholera vaccine (oral), C, administration
Ciclesonide, 8, C, dose
Ciclosporin, C, administration, see BNF
Cimetidine chewable tabs, C, administration, see BNF
Cinacalcet, 21
Cinnarizine, 2
Cipralex, C, driving
Cipramil drops, C, driving, administration
Cipramil tabs, C, driving
Ciprofloxacin, 7, 9, 25, C, driving
Ciproxin susp and tabs, 7, 9, 25, C, driving
Citalopram drops, C, driving, administration
Citalopram tabs, C, driving
Citramag, 10, patient information leaflet, 13, C, administration
Clarithromycin, 9
Clarithromycin m/r, 9, 21, 25
Clemastine, 2
Clindamycin, 9, 27, C, diarrhoea, see BNF
Clinoril, 21
Clobazam, 2 or 19, 8, C, driving (see BNF)
Clobetasol external preps, 28
Clobetasol scalp application, 15, 28
Clofazimine, 8, 14, (urine red), 21
Clomethiazole, 19
Clomipramine, 2
Clomipramine m/r, 2, 25
Clonazepam, 2, 8, C, driving (see BNF)
Clonidine, *see Catapres*
Clonidine m/r, 3, 8, 25
Clopixol, 2
Clorazepate, 2 or 19
Clotrimazole spray, 15
Clozapine, 2, 10, patient information leaflet
Clozaril, 2, 10, patient information leaflet
Coal tar paint, 15
Co-amoxiclav, 9
Co-amoxiclav dispersible tabs, 9, 13
Cobadex, 28
Co-beneldopa, 14, (urine reddish), C, driving
Co-beneldopa dispersible tabs, 14, (urine reddish), C, administration, driving, see BNF
Co-beneldopa m/r, 14, (urine reddish), 25, C, driving
Co-Betaloc, 8
Co-careldopa, 14, (urine reddish), C, driving
Co-careldopa m/r, 14, (urine reddish), 25, C, driving
Co-codamol, see preps
Co-codaprin dispersible tabs, 13, 21, 32
Codafen Continus, 2, 21, 25
Codalax, 14, (urine red)
Co-danthramer, 14, (urine red)
Co-danthrusate, 14, (urine red)
Codeine phosphate syr and tabs, 2
Codipar, 2, 29, 30
Co-dydramol, 21, 29, 30
Co-fluampicil, 9, 22
Cogentin, 2
Colazide, 21, 25
Colestid, 13, C, avoid other drugs at same time, see BNF
Colestipol preps, 13, C, avoid other drugs at same time, see BNF
Colestyramine, 13, C, avoid other drugs at same time, see BNF
Collodion, flexible, 15
Colofac, C, administration, see BNF
Colofac MR, 25, C, administration, see BNF
Colpermin, 5, 25
Combivent, C, dose
Co-methiamol, 29, 30
Comtess, 14, (urine reddish-brown), C, driving
Concerta XL, 25
Condyline, 15
Convulex, 8, 25, C, blood or hepatic disorder symptoms (see BNF), driving (see BNF)
Copegus, 21
Co-prenozide, 8, 25
Co-proxamol, 2, 10, patient information leaflet, 29, 30
Coracten preps, 25
Cordarone X, 11
Corgard, 8
Corticosteroid external preps, 28
Corticosteroid tabs, 10, steroid card, 21
Corticosteroid injections (systemic), 10, steroid card
Cortisone tab, 10, steroid card, 21
Cosalgesic, 2, 10, patient information leaflet, 29, 30
Co-tenidone, 8
Co-triamterzide, 14, (urine blue in some lights), 21
Co-trimoxazole mixts and tabs, 9
Co-trimoxazole dispersible tabs, 9, 13
Creon preps, C, administration, see BNF
Crixivan, 27, C, administration, see BNF
Cromogen Easi-Breathe, 8
Cuplex, 15
Cyclizine, 2
Cyclophosphamide, 27
Cycloserine caps, 2, 8
Cymbalta, 2
Cymevene, 21
Cyproheptadine, 2
Cyprostat, 21
Cyproterone, 21
Cystrin, 3

Daktacort, 28
Daktarin oral gel, 9, C, hold in mouth, after food
Dalacin C, 9, 27, C, diarrhoea, see BNF
Dalmane, 19
Dantrium, 2
Dantrolene, 2
Dapsone, 8
DDAVP tabs and intranasal, C, fluid intake, see BNF

Deferiprone, 14, C, blood disorders
Deflazacort, 5, 10, steroid card
Deltacortril e/c, 5, 10, steroid card, 25
Deltastab inj, 10, steroid card
Demeclocycline, 7, 9, 11, 23
De-Noltab, C, administration, see BNF
Denzapine, 2, 10, patient information leaflet
Depakote, 25
Depixol, 2
Depo-Medrone (systemic), 10, steroid card
Dermestril, C, administration, see BNF
Dermovate cream and oint, 28
Dermovate scalp application, 15, 28
Dermovate-NN, 28
Deseril, 2, 21
Desmopressin tabs and intranasal, C, fluid intake, see BNF
Desmospray, C, fluid intake, see BNF
Desmotabs, C, fluid intake, see BNF
Destolit, 21
Deteclo, 7, 9, 11, 23, C, posture
Detrunorm, 3
Detrusitol m/r, 25
Dexamethasone inj, 10, steroid card
Dexamethasone tabs and solution, 10, steroid card, 21
Dexamfetamine, C, driving
Dexedrine, C, driving
Dexketoprofen, 22
Dextropropoxyphene, 2
DF118 Forte, 2, 21
DHC Continus, 2, 25
Diamicron MR, 25
Diamorphine preps, 2
Diamox tabs, 3
Diamox SR, 3, 25
Diazepam, 2 or 19
Diclofenac dispersible tabs, 13, 21
Diclofenac e/c, 5, 25
Diclofenac m/r, 21, 25
Dicloflex Retard, 21, 25
Diclomax 75 mg SR and Retard, 21, 25
Diconal, 2
Didanosine e/c caps, 25, C, administration
Didanosine tabs, 23, C, administration
Didronel, C, food and calcium, see BNF
Didronel PMO, 10, patient leaflet, C, food and calcium, see BNF
Diflucan 50 and 200mg, 9
Diflucan susp, 9
Diflucortolone external preps, 28
Diflunisal, 21, 25, C, avoid aluminium hydroxide
Digoxin elixir, C, use of pipette
Dihydrocodeine, 2, 21
Dihydrocodeine m/r, 2, 25
Dilcardia SR, 25
Diloxanide, 9
Diltiazem, 25
Dilzem preps, 25
Dindevan, 10, anticoagulant card, 14, (urine pink or orange)
Dioderm, 28
Dipentum, 21, C, blood disorder symptoms, see BNF
Diphenhydramine, 2
Diprosalic, 28
Diprosone, 28
Dipyridamole, 22
Dipyridamole m/r, 21, 25
Disipal, C, driving
Disodium etidronate, C, food and calcium, see BNF
Disopyramide m/r, 25
Disprin CV, 25, 32
Disprol, 30
Distaclor, 9
Distaclor MR, 9, 21, 25
Distalgesic, 2, 10, patient information leaflet, 29, 30
Distamine, 6, 22, C, blood disorder symptoms, see BNF
Distigmine, 22
Disulfiram, 2, C, alcohol reaction, see BNF
Dithranol preps, 28
Dithrocream preps, 28
Dithrolan, 28
Ditropan, 3
Dolmatil, 2
Dolobid, 21, 25, C, avoid aluminium hydroxide
Doloxene, 2
Doloxene Compound, 2, 21, 32
Domperamol, 17, 30
Doralese, 2
Dostinex, 21, C, hypotensive reactions, see BNF
Dosulepin, 2
Dovobet, 28
Doxazosin m/r, 25
Doxepin, 2
Doxepin topical, 2, 10, patient information leaflet
Doxycycline caps, 6, 9, 11, 27, C, posture, see BNF
Doxycycline dispersible tabs, 6, 9, 11, 13
Doxycycline tabs, 6, 11, 27, C, posture, see BNF
Dozic, 2
Driclor, 15
Droleptan, 2
Dromadol XL, 2, 25
Dukoral, C, administration
Dulcolax tabs, 5, 25
Duloxetine, 2
Dumicoat, 10, patient information leaflet
Duofilm, 15
Duovent inhalations, C, dose
Duraphat toothpaste, C, administration
Durogesic, 2
Dutasteride, 25
Dutonin, 3
Dyazide, 14, (urine blue in some lights), 21
Dyspamet tabs, C, administration, see BNF
Dytac, 14, (urine blue in some lights), 21
Dytide, 14, (urine blue in some lights), 21

Econacort, 28
Edronax, C, driving
Efcortelan external preps, 28
Efcortesol, 10, steroid card
Efexor, 3, 21, C, driving
Efexor XL, 3, 21, 25, C, driving
Elantan preps, 25
Elleste Solo MX patches, C, administration, see BNF
Elocon, 28
Emcor preps, 8
Emeside, 8, C, blood disorder symptoms (see BNF), driving (see BNF)
Emflex, 21, C, driving
En-De-Kay mouthwash, C, food and drink, see BNF
Endoxana, 27
Enfuvirtide, C, hypersensitivity reactions, see BNF
Entacapone, 14, (urine reddish-brown), C, driving, avoid iron-containing preparations at the same time of day
Entocort CR, 5, 10, steroid card, 22, 25
Epanutin caps, 8, 27, C, administration, blood or skin disorder symptoms (see BNF), driving (see BNF)
Epanutin Infatabs, 8, 24, C, blood or skin disorder symptoms (see BNF), driving (see BNF)
Epanutin susp, 8, C, administration, blood or skin disorder symptoms (see BNF), driving (see BNF)
Epilim Chrono, 8, 25, C, blood or hepatic disorder symptoms (see BNF), driving (see BNF)
Epilim e/c tabs, 5, 8, 25, C, blood or hepatic disorder symptoms (see BNF), driving (see BNF)
Epilim crushable tabs, liquid and syrup, 8, C, blood or hepatic disorder symptoms (see BNF), driving (see BNF)
Eprosartan, 21
Equanil, 2
Equasym XL, 25
Ergotamine, 18, C, dosage
Erymax, 5, 9, 25
Erythrocin, 9
Erythromycin caps, 5, 9, 25
Erythromycin ethyl succinate, 9
Erythromycin ethyl succinate gran, 9, 13
Erythromycin stearate tabs, 9
Erythromycin tabs, 5, 9, 25
Erythroped, 9

Erythroped A tabs, 9
Escitalopram, C, driving
Esomeprazole, C, administration, see BNF
Estracombi, C, administration, see BNF
Estracyt, 23, C, dairy products, see BNF
Estraderm MX, C, administration, see BNF
Estraderm TTS, C, administration, see BNF
Estradiol vaginal ring, 10, patient information leaflet
Estradot, C, administration, see BNF
Estrapak-50, C, administration, see BNF
Estramustine, 23, C, dairy products, see BNF
Estring, 10, patient information leaflet
Estriol, 25
Ethambutol, 8
Ethosuximide, 8, C, blood disorder symptoms (see BNF), driving (see BNF)
Etidronate, C, food and calcium, see BNF
Etodolac m/r, 25
Etonogestrel implant, C, see patient information leaflet
Etoposide caps, 23
Eucardic, 8
Eumovate external preps, 28
Eurax-Hydrocortisone, 28
Evorel preps, C, administration, see BNF
Exelon caps, 21, 25
Exelon solution, 21
Exemestane, 21

Famciclovir, 9
Famvir, 9
Farlutal 500-mg tabs, 27
Fasigyn, 4, 9, 21, 25
Faverin, C, driving, see BNF
Fefol, 25
Fefol-Vit, 25
Felbinac foam, 15
Feldene caps, 21
Feldene dispersible tabs, 13, 21
Feldene Melt, 10, patient information leaflet, 21
Felodipine m/r, 25
Fematrix, C, administration, see BNF
Femapak, C, administration, see BNF
FemSeven, C, administration, see BNF
Fenbid, 25
Fenbufen, 21
Fenofibrate, 21
Fenofibrate m/r, 21, 25
Fenogal, 21
Fenoprofen, 21
Fenopron, 21
Fentanyl patches and lozenges, 2
Fentazin, 2
Feospan, 25
Ferriprox, 14, C, blood disorders
Ferrograd, 25
Ferrograd C, 25
Ferrograd Folic, 25
Ferrous salts m/r, see preps
Ferrous sulphate paed mixt, 27
Fexofenadine, C, driving, see BNF
Fibrelief, 13, C, administration, see BNF
Flagyl S, 4, 9, 23
Flagyl supps, 4, 9
Flagyl tabs, 4, 9, 21, 25, 27
Fleet Phospho-soda, 10, patient information leaflet, C, administration
Flixotide, 8, 10, steroid card (high-dose preparations only), C, dose
Flixotide Evohaler, 8, C, dose, change to CFC-free inhaler (see BNF), 10, steroid card (250-*Evohaler* only)
Flomax MR, 25
Florinef, 10, steroid card
Floxapen, 9, 23
Fluanxol, 2, C, administration, driving, see BNF
Flucloxacillin, 9, 23
Fluconazole 50 and 200mg, 9
Fluconazole susp, 9
Fludrocortisone, 10, steroid card
Fludroxycortide external preps, 28
Fluocinolone external preps, 28
Fluocinonide external preps, 28
Fluocinonide scalp lotion, 15, 28
Fluocortolone external preps, 28
Fluorigard mouthwash, C, food and drink, see BNF
Fluoxetine, C, driving, see BNF
Flupentixol, see preps
Fluphenazine, 2
Fluprednidene, 28
Flurazepam, 19
Flurbiprofen, 21
Flurbiprofen m/r, 21, 25
Fluticasone inhalations, 8, 10, steroid card (high-dose preparations only), C, dose
Fluticasone inhalations (CFC-free), 8, C, dose, change to CFC-free inhaler (see BNF), 10, steroid card (high-dose preparations only)
Fluvastatin, C, muscle effects, see BNF
Fluvastatin m/r, 25, C, muscle effects, see BNF
Fluvoxamine, C, driving, see BNF
Foradil, C, dose, see BNF
Formoterol fumarate, C, dose, see BNF
Fortipine LA 40, 21, 25
Fortovase, 21
Fortral caps and tabs, 2, 21
Fortral supps, 2
Fosamax, C, administration, see BNF
Franol, 21
Franol Plus, 21
Frisium, 2 or 19, 8, C, driving (see BNF)
Froben, 21
Froben SR, 21, 25
Frovatriptan, 3
Frusene, 14, (urine blue in some lights), 21
Fucibet, 28
Fucidin susp, 9, 21
Fucidin tabs, 9
Fucidin H, 28
Full Marks lotion, mousse, 15
Fungilin loz, 9, 24, C, after food
Fungilin susp (g.i.), 9, C, use of pipette
Fungilin susp (mouth), 9, C, use of pipette, hold in mouth, after food
Fungilin tabs, 9
Furadantin, 9, 14, (urine yellow or brown), 21
Furamide, 9
Fuzeon, C, hypersensitivity reactions, see BNF
Fybogel, 13, C, administration, see BNF
Fybogel Mebeverine, 13, 22, C, administration, see BNF

Gabapentin, 3, 5, 8, C, driving (see BNF)
Gabitril, 21
Galake, 21, 29, 30
Galantamine, 3, 21
Galantamine m/r, 3, 21, 25
Gamanil, 2
Ganciclovir, 21
Gastrobid Continus, 25
Gemfibrozil, 22
Gliclazide m/r, 25
Glucobay, C, administration, see BNF
Glucophage, 21
Glucophage SR, 21, 25
Glyceryl trinitrate patch, see preps
Glyceryl trinitrate m/r, 25
Glyceryl trinitrate tabs, 16
Griseofulvin spray, 15
Griseofulvin tabs, 9, 21, C, driving
Grisol, 15
Grisovin, 9, 21, C, driving
GTN 300 mcg, 16

Haelan, 28
Halciderm Topical, 28
Halcinonide external preps, 28
Haldol, 2
Half-Inderal LA, 8, 25
Half-Securon SR, 25
Half-Sinemet CR, 14, (urine reddish), 25
Haloperidol, 2
HeliClear, 5, 9, 25
Heminevrin, 19
Hiprex, 9
Humira, C, tuberculosis

Hydrocortisone inj, 10, steroid card
Hydrocortisone external preps, 28
Hydrocortisone tabs, 10, steroid card, 21
Hydrocortisone butyrate external preps, 28
Hydrocortisone butyrate scalp lotion, 15, 28
Hydrocortistab inj, 10, steroid card
Hydrocortone, 10, steroid card, 21
Hydromorphone caps, 2, C, administration, see BNF
Hydromorphone m/r, 2, C, administration, see BNF
Hydroxychloroquine, 5, 21
Hydroxyzine, 2
Hyoscine hydrobromide, 2, (patches 19)
Hypolar Retard, 25
Hypovase, 3, C, initial dose, see BNF
Hytrin, 3, C, dose, see BNF

Ibandronic acid tabs, C, administration, see BNF
Ibumousse, 15
Ibuprofen, 21
Ibuprofen gran, 13, 21
Ibuprofen m/r, 25, 27
Ibuspray, 15
Idarubicin caps, 25
Idrolax, 13
Imazin XL, 25, 32
Imdur, 25
Imigran, 3, 10, patient information leaflet
Imigran RADIS, 3, 10, patient information leaflet
Imipramine, 2
Imiquimod, 10, patient information leaflet
Imodium Plus, 24
Implanon, C, see patient information leaflet
Imunovir, 9
Imuran, 21
Indapamide m/r, 25
Inderal-LA, 8, 25
Indinavir, 27, C, administration, see BNF
Indolar SR, 21, 25, C, driving
Indometacin caps and mixt, 21, C, driving
Indometacin m/r, see preps
Indometacin supps, C, driving
Indomod, 25, C, driving
Indoramin, 2
Industrial methylated spirit, 15
Inegy, C, muscle effects, see BNF
Infacol, C, use of dropper
Infliximab, 10, Alert card, C, tuberculosis and hypersensitivity reactions
Inosine pranobex, 9
Insulin, C, see BNF
Intal Spincaps and inhalers, 8
Invirase, 21
Iodine Solution, Aqueous, 27
Ionamin, 25, C, driving
Ipocol, 5, 25, C, blood disorder symptoms, see BNF
Ipratropium inhalations, C, dose, see BNF
Isib 60XL, 25
Ismo Retard, 25
Ismo tabs, 25
Isocarboxazid, 3, 10, patient information leaflet
Isodur XL, 25
Isogel, 13, C, administration, see BNF
Isoket Retard, 25
Isomide CR, 25
Isoniazid elixir and tabs, 8, 22
Isosorbide dinitrate m/r, 25
Isosorbide mononitrate, 25
Isosorbide mononitrate m/r, 25
Isotard XL, 25
Isotretinoin, 10, patient information leaflet, 11, 21
Isotretinoin gel, 10, patient information leaflet
Isotrex, 10, patient information leaflet
Isotrexin, 10, patient information leaflet
Ispagel, 13, C, administration, see BNF
Ispaghula, 13, C, administration, see BNF
Itraconazole caps, 5, 9, 21, 25
Itraconazole liq, 9, 23

Junifen, 21

Kaletra, 21
Kalspare, 14, (urine blue in some lights), 21
Kalten, 8
Kapake caps and tabs, 2, 29, 30
Kapake effervescent, 2, 13, 29, 30
Kay-Cee-L, 21
Keflex, 9
Kemadrin, C, driving
Kenalog (systemic), 10, steroid card
Kentera, C, administration, see BNF
Keppra, 8
Keral, 22
Ketek, 9
Ketoconazole tabs and susp, 5, 9, 21
Ketoprofen caps, 21
Ketoprofen CR, 21, 25
Ketoprofen m/r caps, 21, 25
Ketotifen, 2, 8, 21
Ketorolac tabs, 17, 21
Ketovail, 21, 25
Kineret, C, blood disorder symptoms
Kinidin Durules, 25
Kivexa, C, hypersensitivity reactions, see BNF
Klaricid, 9
Klaricid sachets, 9, 13
Klaricid XL, 9, 21, 25
Klean-Prep, C, administration, see BNF
Kloref, 13, 21
Konakion tabs, 24

Labetalol, 8, 21
Lamictal dispersible tabs, 8, 13, C, driving (see BNF)
Lamictal tabs, 8, C, driving (see BNF)
Lamisil, 9
Lamotrigine dispersible tabs, 8, 13, C, driving (see BNF)
Lamotrigine tabs, 8, C, driving (see BNF)
Lanoxin-PG elixir, C, use of pipette
Lansoprazole caps, 5, 25
Lansoprazole oro-dispersible tabs, 5, C, administration, see BNF
Lansoprazole susp, 5, 13
Larapam SR, 2, 25
Largactil, 2, 11
Lariam, 21, 25, 27, C, driving, malaria prophylaxis, see BNF
Lasikal, 25, 27, C, posture, see BNF
Lasix + K, 25, 27, C, posture, see BNF
Lederfen, 21
Ledermycin, 7, 9, 11, 23
Leflunomide, 4
Lercanidipine, 22
Lescol, C, muscle effects, see BNF
Lescol XL, 25, C, muscle effects, see BNF
Levetiracetam, 8
Levocetirizine, C, driving
Levodopa, 14, (urine reddish), 21, C, driving
Levofloxacin, 6, 9, 25, C, driving
Levomepromazine, 2
Librium, 2
Li-Liquid, 10, lithium card, C, fluid and salt intake, see BNF
Linezolid susp and tabs, 9, 10, patient information leaflet
Lioresal, 2, 8
Lipantil, 21
Lipitor, C, muscle effects, see BNF
Lipostat, C, muscle effects, see BNF
Liquid paraffin, C, administration, see BNF
Liskonum, 10, lithium card, 25, C, fluid and salt intake, see BNF
Lisuride, 21, C, hypotensive reactions, see BNF
Litarex, 10, lithium card, 25, C, fluid and salt intake, see BNF
Lithium carbonate, 10, lithium card, C, fluid and salt intake, see BNF
Lithium carbonate m/r, 10, lithium card, 25, C, fluid and salt intake, see BNF
Lithium citrate liq, 10, lithium card, C, fluid and salt intake, see BNF
Lithium citrate m/r, 10, lithium card, 25, C, fluid and salt intake, see BNF

Lithonate, 10, lithium card, 25, C, fluid and salt intake, see BNF
Loceryl, 10, patient information leaflet
Locoid cream, oint, and topical emulsion, 28
Locoid scalp lotion, 15, 28
Locoid C, 28
Lofepramine, 2
Lofexidine, 2
Lopid, 22
Loprazolam, 19
Lopresor, 8
Lopresor SR, 8, 25
Loratadine, C, driving, alcohol, see BNF
Lorazepam, 2 or 19
Lormetazepam, 19
Loron tabs, 10, patient information leaflet, C, food and calcium, see BNF
Losec, C, administration, see BNF
Lotriderm, 28
Ludiomil, 2
Lugol's solution, 27
Lustral, C, driving, see BNF
Lyclear Dermal cream, 10, patient information leaflet
Lymecycline, 6, 9
Lyrica, 3, 8, C, driving
Lysovir, C, driving

Macrobid, 9, 14, (urine yellow or brown), 21, 25
Macrodantin, 9, 14, (urine yellow or brown), 21
Madopar, 14, (urine reddish), C, driving
Madopar dispersible tabs, 14, (urine reddish), C, administration, driving, see BNF
Madopar CR, 5, 14, (urine reddish), 25, C, driving
Magnapen, 9, 22
Magnesium citrate effervescent pdr, 10, patient information leaflet, 13, C, administration
Magnesium sulphate, 13, 23
Malarivon, 5, C, malaria prophylaxis
Malarone, 21
Manerix, 10, patient information leaflet, 21
Manevac, 25, 27
Maprotiline, 2
Marevan, 10, anticoagulant card
Maxalt, 3
Maxalt Melt, 3, C, administration
Maxepa, 21
Maxolon paed liquid, C, use of pipette
Maxolon SR, 25
Maxtrex (methotrexate), C, NSAIDs (see BNF)
Mebeverine, C, administration, see BNF
Mecysteine, 5, 22, 25
Medrone tabs, 10, steroid card, 21
Mefenamic acid caps, paed susp, and tabs, 21
Mefloquine, 21, 25, 27, C, driving, malaria prophylaxis, see BNF
Meloxicam tabs, 21
Menoring 50, 10, patient information leaflet
Mepacrine, 4, 9, 14, 21
Meprobamate, 2
Meptazinol, 2
Meptid, 2
Mesalazine e/c, see preps
Mesalazine m/r, see preps
Mesalazine enema and supps, C, blood disorder symptoms, see BNF
Mesalazine gran, see preps
Mesren MR, 5, 25, C, blood disorder symptoms, see BNF
Metformin, 21
Metformin m/r, 21, 25
Methadone, 2
Methadose, 2
Methenamine, 9
Methocarbamol, 2
Methotrexate tabs, C, NSAIDs (see BNF)
Methylcellulose (constipation or diarrhoea), C, administration, see BNF
Methylcellulose tabs (anorectic), C, administration, see BNF
Methyldopa, 3, 8
Methylphenidate m/r, 25
Methylprednisolone external preps, 28
Methylprednisolone inj, 10, steroid card
Methylprednisolone tabs, 10, steroid card, 21
Methysergide, 2, 21
Metirosine, 2
Metoclopramide paed liquid, C, use of pipette
Metoclopramide m/r, see preps
Metopirone, 21, C, driving
Metoprolol, 8
Metoprolol m/r, see preps
Metosyn cream and oint, 28
Metosyn scalp lotion, 15, 28
Metrogel, 10, patient information leaflet
Metrolyl supps, 4, 9
Metronidazole gel, see preps
Metronidazole mixt, 4, 9, 23
Metronidazole supps, 4, 9
Metronidazole tabs, 4, 9, 21, 25, 27
Metyrapone, 21, C, driving
Mianserin, 2, 25
Micanol, 28
Miconazole denture lacquer, 10, patient information leaflet
Miconazole oral gel, 9, C, hold in mouth, after food
Miconazole tabs, 9, 21
Midrid, 30, C, dosage
Mifegyne, 10, patient information leaflet
Mifepristone, 10, patient information leaflet
Migard, 3
Migraleve, 2, (pink tablets), 17, 30
Migravess, 13, 17, 32
Migravess Forte, 13, 17, 32
Migril, 2, 18, C, dosage
Mildison, 28
Mimpara, 21
Minocin, 6, 9, C, posture, see BNF
Minocin MR, 6, 25
Minocycline, 6, 9, C, posture, see BNF
Minocycline m/r, 6, 25
Mintec, 5, 22, 25
Mintezol, 3, 21, 24
Mirapexin, C, hypotensive reactions, driving, see BNF
Mirtazapine oral solution, 2
Mirtazapine orodispersible tablets, 2, C, administration, see BNF
Mirtazapine tabs, 2, 25
Mizolastine, 25, C, driving
Mizollen, 25, C, driving
Mobic tabs, 21
Mobiflex, 21
Moclobemide, 10, patient information leaflet, 21
Modisal XL, 25
Moditen, 2
Modrasone, 28
Modrenal, 21
Moducren, 8
Mogadon, 19
Molipaxin, 2, 21
Mometasone cream, 28
Mometasone inhaler, 8, 10, steroid card, C, dose
Mometasone ointment, 28
Mometasone scalp lotion, 28
Mono-Cedocard, 25
Monocor, 8
Monomax SR, 25
Monomax XL, 25
Monosorb XL, 25
Monotrim, 9
Montelukast chewable tabs, 24
Morcap SR, 2, C, administration, see BNF
Morphine preps, 2
Morphine m/r susp, 2, 13
Morphine m/r caps and tabs, see preps
Motifene, 25
Motival, 2
Movicol, 13
Movicol-Half, 13
Moxifloxacin, 6, 9, C, driving
Moxisylyte, 21
Moxonidine, 3
MST Continus susp, 2, 13
MST Continus tabs, 2, 25
MXL, 2, C, administration, see BNF
Myambutol, 8
Mycobutin, 8, 14, (urine orange-red), C, soft lenses
Mynah, 8, 23
Myocrisin inj, C, blood disorder symptoms, see BNF

Myotonine Chloride, 22
Mysoline, 2, 8, C, driving (see BNF)

Nabilone, 2, C, behavioural effects, see BNF
Nabumetone, 21
Nabumetone dispersible tabs, 13, 21
Nabumetone susp, 21
Nadolol, 8
Nafarelin spray, 10, patient information leaflet, C, nasal decongestants, see BNF
Naftidrofuryl, 25, 27
Nalcrom, 22, C, administration, see BNF
Nalidixic acid, 9, 11
Napratec, 21
Naprosyn EC, 5, 25
Naprosyn tabs and susp, 21
Naproxen e/c, 5, 25
Naproxen tabs and susp, 21
Naramig, 3
Naratriptan, 3
Nardil, 3, 10, patient information leaflet
Natrilix SR, 25
Navoban, 23
Nebilet, 8
Nebivolol, 8
Nedocromil sodium inhalation, 8
Nefopam, 2, 14, (urine pink)
Negram, 9, 11, 23
Nelfinavir tabs, 21
Nelfinavir powder, 21, C, administration, see BNF
Neo-Medrone, 28
Neo-Mercazole, C, blood disorder symptoms, see BNF
Neo-NaClex-K, 25, 27, C, posture, see BNF
Neoral, C, administration, see BNF
Neotigason, 10, patient information leaflet, 21
Nerisone, 28
Nerisone Forte, 28
Neulactil, 2
Neurontin, 3, 5, 8, C, driving (see BNF)
Nevirapine, C, hypersensitivity reactions, see BNF
Nexium, C, administration, see BNF
Niaspan, 21, 25
Nicardipine m/r, 25
Nicorette Microtab, 26
Nicotine (sublingual), 26
Nicotinell lozenges, 24
Nicotinic acid tabs, 21
Nicotinic acid m/r, see preps
Nidazol, 4, 9, 21, 25, 27
Nifedipine m/r, see preps
Nifedipress MR, 25
Nifedotard, 25
Nifelease, 25
Niferex elixir, C, infants, use of dropper
NiQuitin CQ lozenges, 24
Nisoldipine, 22, 25
Nitrazepam, 19
Nitrofurantoin, 9, 14, (urine yellow or brown), 21
Nitrofurantoin m/r, 9, 14, (urine yellow or brown), 21, 25
Nivaquine, 5, C, malaria prophylaxis, see BNF
Nizoral, 5, 9, 21
Nootropil, 3
Norfloxacin, 7, 9, 23, C, driving
Noritate, 10, patient information leaflet
Normacol preps, 25, 27, C, administration, see BNF
Normax, 14, (urine red)
Norprolac, 21, C, hypotensive reactions, see BNF
Nortriptyline, 2
Norvir, 21, C, administration, see BNF
Nozinan, 2
Nuelin SA preps, 25
Nurofen for children, 21
Nu-Seals Aspirin, 5, 25, 32
Nycopren, 5, 25
Nystadermal, 28
Nystaform-HC, 28
Nystan pastilles, 9, 24, C, after food
Nystan susp (g.i.), 9, C, use of pipette
Nystan susp (mouth), 9, C, use of pipette, hold in mouth, after food
Nystan tabs, 9
Nystatin mixt (g.i.), 9, C, use of pipette
Nystatin mixt (mouth), 9, C, use of pipette, hold in mouth, after food
Nystatin pastilles, 9, 24, C, after food
Nystatin tabs, 9

Occlusal, 15
Ocusert Pilo, C, method of use
Oestrogel, C, administration, see BNF
Ofloxacin, 6, 9, 11, C, driving
Olanzapine tabs, 2
Olanzapine orodispersible tabs, 2, C, administration, see BNF
Olbetam, 21
Olsalazine, 21, C, blood disorder symptoms, see BNF
Omacor, 21
Omega-3-acid ethyl esters, 21
Omeprazole caps, 5, C, administration, see BNF
Omeprazole tabs, 25
Ondansetron (freeze-dried tablets), C, administration, see BNF
Opilon, 21
Optimax, 3
Oramorph preps, 2
Oramorph SR, 2, 25
Orap, 2
Orbenin, 9, 23
Orelox, 5, 9, 21
Orovite Comploment B6, 25
Orphenadrine, C, driving
Orudis caps, 21
Oruvail, 21, 25
Oseltamivir, 9
Ovestin, 25
Oxazepam, 2
Oxcarbazepine, 3, 8, C, see BNF
Oxerutins, 21
Oxis, C, dose, see BNF
Oxprenolol, 8
Oxprenolol m/r, 8, 25
Oxybutynin tabs and elixir, 3
Oxybutynin patch, C, administration, see BNF
Oxycodone caps and liq, 2
Oxycodone m/r, 2, 25
OxyContin, 2, 25
OxyNorm, 2
Oxytetracycline, 7, 9, 23

Palladone, 2, C, administration, see BNF
Palladone SR, 2, C, administration, see BNF
Paludrine, 21, C, malaria prophylaxis, see BNF
Panadeine, 29, 30
Panadeine effervescent, 13, 29, 30
Panadol tabs, 29, 30
Panadol Soluble, 13, 29, 30
Panadol susp, 30
Pancrease preps, C, administration, see BNF
Pancreatin, C, administration, see BNF
Pancrex gran, 25, C, dose, see BNF
Pancrex V Forte tabs, 5, 25, C, dose, see BNF
Pancrex V caps, 125 caps and pdr, C, administration, see BNF
Pancrex V tabs, 5, 25, C, dose, see BNF
Pantoprazole, 25
Paracetamol liq and supps, 30
Paracetamol tabs, 29, 30
Paracetamol tabs, soluble, 13, 29, 30
Paracodol, 13, 29, 30
Paradote, 29, 30
Paramax sachets, 13, 17, 30
Paramax tabs, 17, 30
Pariet, 25
Parlodel, 21, C, hypotensive reactions, see BNF
Paroven, 21
Paroxetine, 21, C, driving, see BNF
Penbritin caps, 9, 23
Penicillamine, 6, 22, C, blood disorder symptoms, see BNF
Pentasa tabs and gran, C, administration, blood disorder symptoms, see BNF
Pentasa enema and supps, C, blood disorder symptoms, see BNF
Pentazocine caps and tabs, 2, 21
Pentazocine supps, 2
Pentoxifylline m/r, 21, 25

Peppermint oil caps, 5, 22, 25
Percutol, C, administration, see BNF
Pergolide, C, driving, hypotensive reactions, see BNF
Periactin, 2
Pericyazine, 2
Periostat, 6, 11, 27, C, posture, see BNF
Permethrin dermal cream, 10, patient information leaflet
Perphenazine, 2
Persantin, 22
Persantin Retard, 21, 25
Pethidine, 2
Phenelzine, 3, 10, patient information leaflet
Phenergan, 2
Phenindione, 10, anticoagulant card, 14, (urine pink or orange)
Phenobarbital elixir and tabs, 2, 8, C, driving (see BNF)
Phenothrin lotion, mousse, 15
Phenoxymethylpenicillin, 9, 23
Phentermine m/r, 25, C, driving
Phenytoin caps and tabs, 8, 27, C, administration, blood or skin disorder symptoms (see BNF), driving (see BNF)
Phenytoin chewable tabs, 8, 24, C, blood or skin disorder symptoms (see BNF), driving (see BNF)
Phenytoin susp, 8, C, administration, blood or skin disorder symptoms (see BNF), driving (see BNF)
Phosex, 21, 25
Phosphate-Sandoz, 13
Phyllocontin Continus, 25
Physeptone, 2
Physiotens, 3
Phytomenadione, 24
Picolax, 10, patient information leaflet, 13, C, solution, see BNF
Pilocarpine tabs, 21, 27, C, driving
Pimozide, 2
Pindolol, 8
Piperazine powder, 13
Piracetam, 3
Piriton, 2
Piroxicam caps and tabs, 21
Piroxicam dispersible tabs, 13, 21
Pivmecillinam, 9, 21, 27, C, posture, see BNF
Pizotifen, 2
Plaquenil, 5, 21
Plendil, 25
Podophyllin paint cpd, 15, C, application, see BNF
Ponstan, 21
Potaba caps and tabs, 21
Potaba Envules, 13, 21
Potassium chloride m/r, see preps
Potassium citrate mixt, 27
Potassium effervescent tabs, 13, 21
Pramipexole, C, hypotensive reactions, driving, see BNF
Pranoxen Continus, 25
Pravastatin, C, muscle effects, see BNF
Praxilene, 25, 27
Prazosin, 3, C, initial dose, see BNF
Prednesol, 10, steroid card, 13, 21
Prednisolone inj, 10, steroid card
Prednisolone tabs, 10, steroid card, 21
Prednisolone e/c, 5, 10, steroid card, 25
Pregabalin, 3, 8, C, driving
Preservex, 21
Prestim, 8
Priadel liq, 10, lithium card, C, fluid and salt intake, see BNF
Priadel tabs, 10, lithium card, 25, C, fluid and salt intake, see BNF
Primidone, 2, 8, C, driving (see BNF)
Prioderm lotion, 15
Pripsen, 13
Pro-Banthine, 23
Probenecid, 12, 21, 27
Procarbazine, 4
Prochlorperazine, 2
Prochlorperazine buccal tabs, 2, C, administration, see BNF
Prochlorperazine sachets, 2, 13
Procyclidine, C, driving
Prograf, 23, C, driving, see BNF
Proguanil, 21, C, malaria prophylaxis, see BNF
Progynova TS preps, C, administration, see BNF
Promazine, 2
Promethazine, 2
Propaderm, 28
Propafenone, 21, 25
Propantheline, 23
Propiverine hydrochloride, 3
Propranolol, 8
Propranolol m/r, 8, 25
Protelos, 5, 13, C, administration, see BNF
Prothiaden, 2
Protionamide, 8, 21
Protium, 25
Protopic, 4, 11, 28
Prozac, C, driving, see BNF
Psorin, 28
Pulmicort, 8, 10, steroid card, C, dose
Pulmicort LS, 8, C, dose
Pulmicort Respules, 8, 10, steroid card, C, dose
Pylorid, C, discoloration (tongue and faeces), see BNF
Pyrazinamide, 8

Questran preps, 13, C, avoid other drugs at same time, see BNF
Quetiapine, 2
Quinagolide, 21, C, hypotensive reactions, see BNF
Quinidine m/r, 25
Quinocort, 28
Quinoderm with Hydrocortisone, 28
Qvar preps, 8, 10, steroid card (high-dose preparations only), C, dose

Rabeprazole, 25
Ranitidine bismuth citrate, C, discoloration (tongue and faeces), see BNF
Ranitidine effervescent tabs, 13
Rapamune, C, administration
Rebetol, 21
Reboxetine, C, driving
Regulan, 13, C, administration, see BNF
Regurin, 23
Relifex, 21
Relifex dispersible tablets, 13, 21
Relifex susp, 21
Remedeine, 2, 21, 29, 30
Remedeine effervescent tabs, 2, 13, 21, 29, 30
Remicade, 10, Alert card, C, tuberculosis and hypersensitivity reactions
Reminyl, 3, 21
Reminyl XL, 3, 21, 25
Renagel, 25, C, with meals
Requip, 21, C, driving, see BNF
Resonium A, 13
Restandol, 21, 25
Retrovir syrup, C, use of oral syringe
Revanil, 21, C, hypotensive reactions, see BNF
Reyataz, 5, 21
Rheumacin SR, 21, 25, C, driving
Rhumalgan, 5, 25
Riamet, 21, C, driving
Ribavirin caps and tabs, 21
Ridaura, 21, C, blood disorder symptoms, see BNF
Rifabutin, 8, 14, (urine orange-red), C, soft lenses
Rifadin, 8, 14, (urine orange-red), 22, C, soft lenses
Rifampicin caps and mixt, 8, 14, (urine orange-red), 22, C, soft lenses
Rifater, 8, 14, (urine orange-red), 22, C, soft lenses
Rifinah, 8, 14, (urine orange-red), 22, C, soft lenses
Rilutek, C, blood disorders, driving
Rimactane, 8, 14, (urine orange-red), 22, C, soft lenses
Rimactazid, 8, 14, (urine orange-red), 22, C, soft lenses
Risedronate sodium, C, administration, food and calcium, see BNF
Risperdal, 2
Risperidone, 2
Ritonavir, 21, C, administration, see BNF
Rivastigmine, 21, 25
Rivotril, 2, 8, C, driving (see BNF)
Rizatriptan tabs, 3

Rizatriptan wafers, 3, C, administration
Roaccutane, 10, patient information leaflet, 11, 21
Robaxin, 2
Ropinirole, 21, C, driving, see BNF
Rowachol, 22
Rowatinex caps, 25
Rozex, 10, patient information leaflet
Rythmodan Retard, 25

Sabril sachets, 3, 8, 13, C, driving (see BNF)
Sabril tabs, 3, 8, C, driving (see BNF)
Safapryn, 5, 25
Safapryn-Co, 5, 25
Salactol, 15
Salagen, 21, 27, C, driving
Salatac, 15
Salazopyrin, 14, (urine orange-yellow), C, blood disorder symptoms and soft lenses, see BNF
Salazopyrin EN-tabs, 5, 14, (urine orange-yellow), 25, C, blood disorder symptoms and soft lenses, see BNF
Salbulin, C, dose, change to CFC-free inhaler, see BNF
Salbutamol inhalations, C, dose, see BNF
Salbutamol inhalations (CFC-free), C, dose, change to CFC-free inhaler, see BNF
Salbutamol m/r, 25
Salicylic acid collodion, 15
Salicylic acid lotion, 15
Salmeterol, C, dose, see BNF
Salofalk enema and supps, C, blood disorder symptoms, see BNF
Salofalk gran, C, administration, blood disorder symptoms, see BNF
Salofalk tabs, 5, 25, C, blood disorder symptoms, see BNF
Sandimmun, C, administration, see BNF
Sandrena, C, administration, see BNF
Sando-K, 13, 21
Sandocal, 13
Sanomigran, 2
Saquinavir, 21
Scopoderm TTS, 19, C, administration, see BNF
Sebomin MR, 6, 25
Secadrex, 8
Secobarbital, 19
Seconal, 19
Sectral, 8
Securon SR, 25
Selegiline (freeze-dried tablets), C, administration, see BNF
Selexid, 9, 21, 27, C, posture, see BNF
Semprex, C, driving, alcohol, see BNF
Septrin susp and tabs, 9
Septrin dispersible tabs, 9, 13
Serc, 21
Serenace, 2
Seretide, 8, 10, steroid card (250- and 500-*Accuhaler* only), C, dose
Seretide Evohaler, 8, C, dose, change to CFC-free inhaler (see BNF), 10, steroid card (125- and 250-*Evohaler* only)
Serevent, C, dose, see BNF
Seroquel, 2
Seroxat liq and tabs, 21, C, driving, see BNF
Sertraline, C, driving, see BNF
Sevelamer, 21
Sevredol, 2
Simeticone, see paediatric prep
Simvastatin, C, muscle effects, see BNF
Sinemet CR, 14, (urine reddish), 25, C, driving
Sinemet preps, 14, (urine reddish), C, driving
Sinequan, 2
Singulair chewable tabs, 24
Sinthrome, 10, anticoagulant card
Sirolimus, C, administration
Skelid, C, food and calcium
Slofedipine XL, 25
Slo-Indo, 21, 25, C, driving
Slo-Phyllin, 25 or C, administration, see BNF
Sloprolol, 8, 25
Slow Sodium, 25
Slow-Fe, 25
Slow-Fe Folic, 25
Slow-K, 25, 27, C, posture, see BNF
Slow-Trasicor, 8, 25
Slozem, 25
Sodium Amytal, 19
Sodium aurothiomalate, C, blood disorder symptoms, see BNF
Sodium cellulose phosphate, 13, 21, C, may be sprinkled on food
Sodium chloride m/r, 25
Sodium chloride tabs, 13
Sodium chloride and glucose oral pdr, cpd, 13
Sodium chloride solution-tabs, 13
Sodium clodronate, C, food and calcium, see BNF
Sodium cromoglicate (oral), 22, C, administration, see BNF
Sodium cromoglicate inhalations, 8
Sodium fusidate susp, 9, 21
Sodium fusidate tabs, 9
Sodium picosulfate pdr, 10, patient information leaflet, 13, C, see BNF
Sodium valproate e/c, 5, 8, 25, C, blood or hepatic disorder symptoms (see BNF), driving (see BNF)
Sodium valproate m/r, 8, 25, C, blood or hepatic disorder symptoms (see BNF), driving (see BNF)
Sodium valproate crushable tabs, liquid and syrup, 8, C, blood or hepatic disorder symptoms (see BNF), driving (see BNF)
Solian, 2
Solifenacin, 3
Solpadol caps and caplets, 2, 29, 30
Solpadol Effervescent, 2, 13, 29, 30
Solu-Cortef, 10, steroid card
Solu-Medrone, 10, steroid card
Solvazinc, 13, 21
Somnite, 19
Sonata, 2
Soneryl, 19
Sotacor, 8
Sotalol, 8
Sporanox caps, 5, 9, 21, 25
Sporanox liq, 9, 23
Stalevo, 14, (urine reddish-brown), C, driving, avoid iron-containing preparations at the same time of day
Stelazine syrup and tabs, 2
Stelazine Spansule, 2, 25
Stemetil, 2
Stemetil Eff, 2, 13
Sterculia, C, administration, see BNF
Stilnoct, 19
Striant SR, C, administration, see BNF
Strontium, 5, 13, C, administration, see BNF
Stugeron, 2
Stugeron Forte, 2
Subutex, 2, 26
Sucralfate, 5
Sudafed Plus, 2
Suleo-M, 15
Sulfadiazine, 9, 27
Sulfasalazine, 14, (urine orange-yellow), C, blood disorder symptoms and soft lenses, see BNF
Sulfasalazine e/c, 5, 14, (urine orange-yellow), 25, C, blood disorder symptoms and soft lenses, see BNF
Sulfinpyrazone, 12, 21
Sulindac, 21
Sulpiride, 2
Sulpitil, 2
Sulpor, 2
Sumatriptan, 3, 10, patient information leaflet
Suprax, 9
Supralip, 21, 25
Suprecur, C, nasal decongestants, see BNF
Suprefact nasal spray, C, nasal decongestants, see BNF
Surgam tabs, 21
Surgam SA, 25
Surgical spirit, 15
Surmontil, 2
Suscard Buccal, C, administration, see BNF
Sustac, 25
Symbicort, C, dose, 10, steroid card

Symmetrel, C, driving
Synalar external preps, 28
Synarel, 10, patient information leaflet, C, nasal decongestants, see BNF
Synflex, 21
Syscor MR, 22, 25

Tacrolimus caps, 23, C, driving, see BNF
Tacrolimus topical, 4, 11, 28
Tamiflu, 9
Tamsulosin m/r, 25
Tarka, 25
Tarivid, 6, 9, 11, C, driving
Tasmar, 14, 25
Tavanic, 6, 9, 25, C, driving
Tavegil, 2
Tegretol Chewtabs, 3, 8, 21, 24, C, blood, hepatic or skin disorder symptoms (see BNF), driving (see BNF)
Tegretol liq, supps and tabs, 3, 8, C, blood, hepatic or skin disorder symptoms (see BNF), driving (see BNF)
Tegretol Retard, 3, 8, 25, C, blood, hepatic or skin disorder symptoms (see BNF), driving (see BNF)
Telfast, C, driving, see BNF
Telithromycin, 9
Temazepam, 19
Temgesic, 2, 26
Temodal, 23, 25
Temozolomide, 23, 25
Tenben, 8
Tenif, 8, 25
Tenofovir, 21, C, administration, see BNF
Tenoret 50, 8
Tenoretic, 8
Tenormin, 8
Tenoxicam tabs, 21
Tensipine MR, 21, 25
Terazosin, 3, C, dose, see BNF
Terbinafine, 9
Terbutaline inhalations, C, dose, see BNF
Terbutaline m/r, 25
Terfenadine, C, driving, alcohol
Testim, C, administration, see BNF
Testogel, C, administration, see BNF
Testosterone buccal tablets, C, administration, see BNF
Testosterone gel, C, administration, see BNF
Testosterone patch, C, administration, see BNF
Testosterone undecanoate caps, 21, 25
Tetrabenazine, 2
Tetracycline, 7, 9, 23, C, posture
Tetracycline mouthwash, see BNF
Tetralysal preps, 6, 9
Teveten, 21
Theophylline, 21
Theophylline m/r, see preps
Tiabendazole, 3, 21, 24
Tiagabine, 21
Tiaprofenic acid m/r, 25
Tiaprofenic acid tabs, 21
Tilade, 8
Tildiem preps, 25
Tilolec, 14, 25, C, driving (see BNF)
Tiludronic acid, C, food and calcium
Timodine, 28
Timolol, 8
Tinidazole tabs, 4, 9, 21, 25
Tizanidine, 2
Tofranil, 2
Tolcapone, 14, 25
Tolterodine m/r, 25
Topamax Sprinkle, 3, 8, C, administration, driving (see BNF)
Topamax tabs, 3, 8, C, driving (see BNF)
Topiramate Sprinkle caps, 3, 8, C, administration, driving (see BNF)
Topiramate tabs, 3, 8, C, driving (see BNF)
Toradol tabs, 17, 21
Tramacet, 2, 25, 29, 30
Tramadol, 2
Tramadol m/r, 2, 25
Tramadol sachets, 2, 13
Tramadol soluble, 2, 13
Tramake, 2
Tramake Insts, 2, 13
Trandate, 8, 21
Tranxene, 2 or 19
Trasicor, 8
Trasidrex, 8, 25
Traxam foam, 15
Trazodone, 2, 21
Trazodone m/r, 2, 21, 25
Trental m/r, 21, 25
Treosulfan, 25
Tretinoin caps, 21
Tri-Adcortyl external preps, 28
Triamcinolone inj, 10, steroid card
Triamcinolone tabs, 10, steroid card, 21
Triamterene, 14, (urine blue in some lights), 21
Triapin preps, 25
Triclofos sodium, 19
Trientine, 6, 22
Trifluoperazine, 2
Trihexyphenidyl, C, before or after food, driving, see BNF
Trileptal, 3, 8, C, see BNF
Trilostane, 21
Trimethoprim mixt and tabs, 9
Trimipramine, 2
Trimopan, 9
Trimovate, 28
Tripotassium dicitratobismuthate, C, administration, see BNF
Triprolidine m/r, 2, 25
Triptafen preps, 2
Trizivir, C, hypersensitivity reactions, see BNF
Tropisetron, 23
Tropium, 2
Trospium chloride, 23
Truvada, 21, C, administration, see BNF
Tryptophan, 3
Tuinal, 19
Tylex caps, 2, 29, 30
Tylex effervescent tabs, 2, 13, 29, 30
Typhoid vaccine, oral, 23, 25, C, administration, see BNF

Ubretid, 22
Ucerax, 2
Ultralanum Plain, 28
Uniphyllin Continus, 25
Univer, 25
Uprima, C, driving
Urdox, 21
Uriben, 9, 11
Ursodeoxycholic acid, 21
Ursogal, 21
Ursofalk, 21
Utinor, 7, 9, 23, C, driving

Valaciclovir, 9
Valcyte, 21
Valganciclovir, 21
Valium, 2 or 19
Vallergan, 2
Valoid, 2
Valproic acid, see individual preparations
Valtrex, 9
Vancocin caps, 9
Vancomycin caps, 9
Velosef, 9
Venlafaxine, 3, 21, C, driving
Venlafaxine m/r, 3, 21, 25, C, driving
Ventmax SR, 25
Ventodisks, C, dose, see BNF
Ventolin Evohaler, C, dose, change to CFC-free inhaler, see BNF
Ventolin inhalations, C, dose, see BNF
Vepesid caps, 23
Verapamil m/r, 25
Verapress, 25
Vertab SR, 25
Vesanoid, 21
Vesicare, 3
Vfend, 11, 23
Viazem XL, 25
Vibramycin caps, 6, 9, 11, 27, C, posture, see BNF
Vibramycin-D, 6, 9, 11, 13
Videx, 23, C, administration, see BNF
Videx e/c caps, 25, C, administration
Videx tabs, 23, C, administration
Vigabatrin sachets, 3, 8, 13, C, driving (see BNF)
Vigabatrin tabs, 3, 8, C, driving (see BNF)
Vioform-Hydrocortisone, 28
Viracept powder, 21, C, administration, see BNF
Viracept tabs, 21

Viramune, C, hypersensitivity reactions, see BNF
Viread, 21, C, administration, see BNF
Visclair, 5, 22, 25
Viskaldix, 8
Visken, 8
Volmax, 25
Voltarol dispersible tabs, 13, 21
Voltarol 75mg SR and Retard, 21, 25
Voltarol tabs, 5, 25
Voriconazole, 11, 23

Warfarin, 10, anticoagulant card
Warfarin WBP, 10, anticoagulant card
Warticon, 15
Welldorm, 19, 27
Wellvone, 21

Xagrid, C, driving
Xanax, 2
Xatral, 3, C, dose, see BNF
Xatral XL, 3, 21, 25, C, dose, see BNF
Xeloda, 21
Xepin, 2, 10, patient information leaflet
Xismox XL, 25
Xyzal, C, driving

Yentreve, 2

Zaditen, 2, 8, 21
Zadstat supps, 4, 9
Zafirlukast, 23
Zaleplon, 2
Zamadol, 2
Zamadol SR, 2, 25
Zanaflex, 2
Zanidip, 22
Zantac effervescent tabs, 13
Zaponex, 2, 10, patient information leaflet
Zarontin, 8, C, blood disorder symptoms (see BNF), driving (see BNF)
Zavedos caps, 25
Zelapar, C, administration, see BNF
Zemon XL, 25
Zemtard XL, 25
Ziagen, C, hypersensitivity reactions, see BNF
Zidovudine syrup, C, use of oral syringe
Zimovane, 19
Zinamide, 8
Zinc sulphate, see preps
Zinnat susp, 9, 21
Zinnat tabs, 9, 21, 25
Zispin SolTab, 2
Zithromax caps, 5, 9, 23
Zithromax susp, 5, 9
Zocor, C, muscle effects, see BNF
Zofran Melt, C, administration, see BNF
Zoleptil, 2
Zolmitriptan orodispersible tabs, C, administration, see BNF
Zolpidem, 19
Zomig Rapimelt, C, administration, see BNF
Zomorph, 2, 25
Zonegran, 3
Zonisamide, 3
Zopiclone, 19
Zotepine, 2
Zoton caps, 5, 25
Zoton FasTab, 5, C, administration, see BNF
Zoton susp, 5, 13
Zovirax susp and tabs, 9
Zuclopenthixol, 2
Zyban, 25
Zydol, 2
Zydol soluble, 2, 13
Zydol SR, 2, 25
Zydol XL, 2, 25
Zyloric, 8, 21, 27
Zyomet, 10, patient information leaflet
Zyprexa tabs, 2
Zyprexa Velotab, 2, C, administration, see BNF
Zyvox susp and tabs, 9, 10, patient information leaflet

Dental Practitioners' Formulary

List of Dental Preparations

The following list has been approved by the appropriate Secretaries of State, and the preparations therein may be prescribed by dental practitioners on form FP10D (GP14 in Scotland, WP10D in Wales).

Sugar-free versions, where available, are preferred.

- Aciclovir Cream, BP
- Aciclovir Oral Suspension, BP, 200 mg/5 mL
- Aciclovir Tablets, BP, 200 mg
- Amoxicillin Capsules, BP
- Amoxicillin Oral Powder, DPF[1]
- Amoxicillin Oral Suspension, BP
- Amphotericin Lozenges, BP
- Amphotericin Oral Suspension, BP
- Ampicillin Capsules, BP
- Ampicillin Oral Suspension, BP
- Artificial Saliva, DPF[2]
- Artificial Saliva Substitutes as listed below (to be prescribed only for indications approved by ACBS[3]):
  - AS Saliva Orthana®
  - Glandosane®
  - Biotene Oralbalance®
  - BioXtra®
  - Saliveze®
  - Salivix®
- Ascorbic Acid Tablets, BP
- Aspirin Tablets, Dispersible, BP[4]
- Azithromycin Oral Suspension, 200 mg/5 mL, DPF
- Benzydamine Mouthwash, BP 0.15%
- Benzydamine Oromucosal Spray, BP 0.15%
- Carbamazepine Tablets, BP
- Carmellose Gelatin Paste, DPF
- Cefalexin Capsules, BP
- Cefalexin Oral Suspension, BP
- Cefalexin Tablets, BP
- Cefradine Capsules, BP
- Cefradine Oral Solution, DPF
- Chlorhexidine Gluconate 1% Gel, DPF
- Chlorhexidine Mouthwash, BP
- Chlorhexidine Oral Spray, DPF
- Chlorphenamine Tablets/Chlorpheniramine Tablets, BP
- Choline Salicylate Dental Gel, BP
- Clindamycin Capsules, BP
- Diazepam Oral Solution, BP, 2 mg/5 mL
- Diazepam Tablets, BP
- Diflunisal Tablets, BP
- Dihydrocodeine Tablets, BP, 30 mg
- Doxycycline Capsules, BP, 100 mg
- Doxycycline Tablets, 20 mg, DPF
- Ephedrine Nasal Drops, BP
- Erythromycin Ethyl Succinate Oral Suspension, BP
- Erythromycin Ethyl Succinate Tablets, BP
- Erythromycin Stearate Tablets, BP
- Erythromycin Tablets, BP
- Fluconazole Capsules, 50 mg, DPF
- Fluconazole Oral Suspension, 50 mg/5 mL, DPF
- Hydrocortisone Cream, BP, 1%
- Hydrocortisone Oromucosal Tablets, BP
- Hydrocortisone and Miconazole Cream, DPF
- Hydrocortisone and Miconazole Ointment, DPF
- Hydrogen Peroxide Mouthwash, BP
- Ibuprofen Oral Suspension, BP, sugar-free
- Ibuprofen Tablets, BP
- Lidocaine 5% Ointment/Lignocaine 5% Ointment, DPF
- Menthol and Eucalyptus Inhalation, BP 1980[5]
- Metronidazole Oral Suspension, DPF
- Metronidazole Tablets, BP
- Miconazole Oromucosal Gel, BP
- Mouthwash Solution-tablets, DPF
- Nitrazepam Tablets, BP
- Nystatin Ointment, BP
- Nystatin Oral Suspension, BP
- Nystatin Pastilles, BP
- Oxytetracycline Tablets, BP
- Paracetamol Oral Suspension, BP[6]
- Paracetamol Tablets, BP
- Paracetamol Tablets, Soluble, BP
- Penciclovir Cream, DPF
- Pethidine Tablets, BP
- Phenoxymethylpenicillin Oral Solution, BP
- Phenoxymethylpenicillin Tablets, BP
- Promethazine Hydrochloride Tablets, BP
- Promethazine Oral Solution, BP
- Sodium Chloride Mouthwash, Compound, BP
- Sodium Fluoride Oral Drops, BP
- Sodium Fluoride Tablets, BP
- Sodium Fusidate Ointment, BP
- Temazepam Oral Solution, BP
- Temazepam Tablets, BP
- Tetracycline Tablets, BP
- Triamcinolone Dental Paste, BP
- Vitamin B Tablets, Compound, Strong, BPC

Preparations in this list which are not included in the BP or BPC are described on p. 842

1. Amoxicillin Dispersible Tablets are no longer available
2. Supplies may be difficult to obtain
3. Indications approved by the ACBS are: patients suffering from dry mouth as a result of having (or having undergone) radiotherapy or sicca syndrome
4. The BP directs that when soluble aspirin tablets are prescribed, dispersible aspirin tablets should be dispensed
5. This preparation does not appear in subsequent editions of the BP
6. The BP directs that when Paediatric Paracetamol Oral Suspension or Paediatric Paracetamol Mixture is prescribed and no strength stated Paracetamol Oral Suspension 120 mg/5 mL should be dispensed

Details of DPF preparations

Preparations on the List of Dental Preparations which are specified as DPF are described as follows in the DPF.

Although brand names have sometimes been included for identification purposes preparations on the list should be prescribed by non-proprietary name.

Amoxicillin Oral Powder PoM (proprietary product: *Amoxil Sachets SF*), amoxicillin (as trihydrate) 750 mg[1] and 3 g sachet

1. 750-mg sachets are no longer available

Artificial Saliva, (proprietary product: *Luborant*) consists of sorbitol 1.8 g, carmellose sodium (sodium carboxymethylcellulose) 390 mg, dibasic potassium phosphate 48.23 mg, potassium chloride 37.5 mg, monobasic potassium phosphate 21.97 mg, calcium chloride 9.972 mg, magnesium chloride 3.528 mg, sodium fluoride 258 micrograms/60 mL, with preservatives and colouring agents

Azithromycin Oral Suspension 200 mg/5 mL PoM (proprietary product: *Zithromax*); azithromycin (as dihydrate) 200 mg/5 mL when reconstituted with water

Carmellose Gelatin Paste (proprietary product: *Orabase Oral Paste*), gelatin, pectin, carmellose sodium, 16.58% of each in a suitable basis

Cefradine Oral Solution PoM (proprietary product: *Velosef Syrup*), cefradine 250 mg/5mL when reconstituted with water

Chlorhexidine Gluconate 1% Gel (proprietary product: *Corsodyl Dental Gel*), chlorhexidine gluconate 1%

Chlorhexidine Oral Spray (proprietary product: *Corsodyl Oral Spray*), chlorhexidine gluconate 0.2%

Doxycycline Tablets 20 mg PoM (proprietary product: *Periostat*), doxycycline (as hyclate) 20 mg

Fluconazole Capsules 50 mg PoM (proprietary product: *Diflucan*), fluconazole 50 mg

Fluconazole Oral Suspension 50 mg/5 mL PoM (proprietary product: *Diflucan*), fluconazole 50 mg/5 mL when reconstituted with water

Hydrocortisone and Miconazole Cream PoM (proprietary product: *Daktacort Cream*), hydrocortisone 1%, miconazole nitrate 2%

Hydrocortisone and Miconazole Ointment PoM (proprietary product: *Daktacort Ointment*), hydrocortisone 1%, miconazole nitrate 2%

Lidocaine 5% Ointment/Lignocaine 5% Ointment lidocaine 5% in a suitable basis

Metronidazole Oral Suspension PoM (proprietary product: *Flagyl S*), metronidazole (as benzoate) 200 mg/5mL

Mouthwash Solution-tablets consist of tablets which may contain antimicrobial, colouring and flavouring agents in a suitable soluble effervescent basis to make a mouthwash suitable for dental purposes

Penciclovir Cream PoM (proprietary product: *Vectavir Cream*), penciclovir 1%

Changes to Dental Practitioners' Formulary since September 2004

Deletion

Povidone-Iodine Mouthwash, BP, 1%
Rofecoxib Tablets, DPF
Zinc Sulphate Mouthwash, DPF

Nurse Prescribers' Formulary

Nurse Prescribers' Formulary for Community Practitioners

Nurse Prescribers' Formulary Appendix (Appendix NPF). List of preparations approved by the Secretary of State which may be prescribed on form FP10P (form HS21(N) in Northern Ireland, form GP10(N) in Scotland, forms FP10(CN) and FP10(PN) in Wales or when available WP10CN and WP10PN in Wales (ordered as WP10CN and WP10PN)) by Nurses for National Health Service patients

Medicinal Preparations

Preparations on this list which are not included in the BP or BPC are described on p. 846

Almond Oil Ear Drops, BP
Arachis Oil Enema, NPF
[1]Aspirin Tablets, Dispersible, 300 mg, BP
Bisacodyl Suppositories, BP (includes 5-mg and 10-mg strengths)
Bisacodyl Tablets, BP
Cadexomer-Iodine Ointment, NPF
Cadexomer-Iodine Paste, NPF
Cadexomer-Iodine Powder, NPF
Catheter Maintenance Solution, Chlorhexidine, NPF
Catheter Maintenance Solution, Sodium Chloride, NPF
Catheter Maintenance Solution, 'Solution G', NPF
Catheter Maintenance Solution, 'Solution R', NPF
Choline Salicylate Dental Gel, BP
Clotrimazole Cream 1%, BP
Co-danthramer Capsules, NPF
Co-danthramer Capsules, Strong, NPF
Co-danthramer Oral Suspension, NPF
Co-danthramer Oral Suspension, Strong, NPF
Co-danthrusate Capsules, BP
Co-danthrusate Oral Suspension, NPF
Crotamiton Cream, BP
Crotamiton Lotion, BP
Dimeticone barrier creams containing at least 10%
Docusate Capsules, BP
Docusate Enema, NPF
Docusate Enema, Compound, BP
Docusate Oral Solution, BP
Docusate Oral Solution, Paediatric, BP
Econazole Cream 1%, BP
Emollients as listed below:
- Aqueous Cream, BP
- Arachis Oil, BP
- Cetraben® Emollient Cream
- Decubal® Clinic
- Dermamist®
- Diprobase® Cream
- Diprobase® Ointment
- Doublebase®
- E45® Cream
- Emulsifying Ointment, BP
- [2]Epaderm®
- Gammaderm® Cream
- Hydromol® Cream
- Hydromol® Ointment
- Hydrous Ointment, BP
- Keri® Therapeutic Lotion
- LactiCare® Lotion
- Lipobase®
- Liquid and White Soft Paraffin Ointment, NPF
- Neutrogena® Dermatological Cream
- Oilatum® Cream
- Paraffin, White Soft, BP
- Paraffin, Yellow Soft, BP
- Ultrabase®
- Unguentum M®
- Zerobase® Cream

Emollient Bath Additives as listed below:
- Alpha Keri® Bath Oil
- Ashbourne Emollient Medicinal Bath Oil
- [3]Balneum®
- Cetraben® Emollient Bath Additive
- Dermalo® Bath Emollient
- Diprobath®
- Hydromol® Emollient
- Imuderm® Bath Oil
- Oilatum® Emollient
- Oilatum® Fragrance Free
- Oilatum® Gel

Folic Acid 400 micrograms/5 mL Oral Solution, NPF
Folic Acid Tablets 400 micrograms, BP
Glycerol Suppositories, BP
[4]Ibuprofen Oral Suspension, BP
[4]Ibuprofen Tablets, BP
Ispaghula Husk Granules, BP
Ispaghula Husk Granules, Effervescent, BP
Ispaghula Husk Oral Powder, BP
Lactulose Solution, BP
Lidocaine Gel/Lignocaine Gel, BP
Lidocaine Ointment/Lignocaine Ointment, BP
Lidocaine and Chlorhexidine Gel/Lignocaine and Chlorhexidine Gel, BP
Macrogol Oral Powder, NPF
Macrogol Oral Powder, Compound, NPF
Macrogol Oral Powder, Compound, Half-strength, NPF
Magnesium Hydroxide Mixture, BP
Magnesium Sulphate Paste, BP
Malathion alcoholic lotions containing at least 0.5%

1. Max. 96 tablets; max. pack size 32 tablets

2. Included in the Drug Tariff, Scottish Drug Tariff, and Northern Ireland Drug Tariff

3. Except pack sizes that are not to be prescribed under the NHS (see Part XVIIIA of the Drug Tariff, Part XI of the Northern Ireland Drug Tariff)

4. Except for indications and doses that are PoM

Malathion aqueous lotions containing at least 0.5%
Mebendazole Oral Suspension, NPF
Mebendazole Tablets, NPF
Methylcellulose Tablets, BP
Miconazole Cream 2%, BP
Miconazole Oromucosal Gel, BP
Mouthwash Solution-tablets, NPF
Nicotine Inhalation Cartridge for Oromucosal Use, NPF
Nicotine Lozenge, NPF
Nicotine Medicated Chewing Gum, NPF
Nicotine Nasal Spray, NPF
Nicotine Sublingual Tablets, NPF
Nicotine Transdermal Patches, NPF
Nystatin Oral Suspension, BP
Nystatin Pastilles, BP
Olive Oil Ear Drops, BP
Paracetamol Oral Suspension, BP (includes 120 mg/5 mL and 250 mg/5 mL strengths—both of which are available as sugar-free formulations)
[1]Paracetamol Tablets, BP
[1]Paracetamol Tablets, Soluble, BP (includes 120-mg and 500-mg tablets)
Permethrin Cream, NPF
Phenothrin Alcoholic Lotion, NPF
Phenothrin Aqueous Lotion, NPF
Phosphate Suppositories, NPF
Phosphates Enema, BP
Piperazine and Senna Powder, NPF
Povidone–Iodine Solution, BP
Senna Granules, Standardised, BP
Senna Oral Solution, NPF
Senna Tablets, BP
Senna and Ispaghula Granules, NPF
Sodium Chloride Solution, Sterile, BP
Sodium Citrate Compound Enema, NPF
Sodium Picosulfate Capsules, NPF
Sodium Picosulfate Elixir, NPF
Spermicidal contraceptives as listed below:
- Gynol II® Jelly
- Ortho-Creme® Cream
- Orthoforms® Pessaries

Sterculia Granules, NPF
Sterculia and Frangula Granules, NPF
Streptokinase and Streptodornase Topical Powder, NPF
Thymol Glycerin, Compound, BP 1988
Titanium Ointment, BP
Water for Injections, BP
Zinc and Castor Oil Ointment, BP
Zinc Cream, BP
Zinc Ointment, BP
Zinc Oxide and Dimeticone Spray, NPF
Zinc Oxide Impregnated Medicated Stocking, NPF
Zinc Paste Bandage, BP 1993
Zinc Paste and Calamine Bandage
Zinc Paste, Calamine and Clioquinol Bandage BP 1993
Zinc Paste and Ichthammol Bandage, BP 1993

1. Max. 96 tablets; max. pack size 32 tablets

Appliances and Reagents (including Wound Management Products)

> In the Drug Tariff Appliances and Reagents which may **not** be prescribed by Nurses are annotated (**Nx** in the Scottish Drug Tariff and in the Northern Ireland Drug Tariff)

Applicators, Vaginal as listed in Part IXA of the Drug Tariff (Part 3 of the Scottish Drug Tariff, not prescribable by nurses in Northern Ireland)

Atomizers, Hand Operated as listed in Part IXA of the Drug Tariff (Part 3 of the Scottish Drug Tariff, not prescribable by nurses in Northern Ireland)

Auto Inflation Device (for treatment of glue ear) as listed in Part IXA of the Drug Tariff (Part 3 of the Scottish Drug Tariff, Part III of the Northern Ireland Drug Tariff)

Breast Reliever as listed in Part IXA of the Drug Tariff (Part 3 of the Scottish Drug Tariff, not prescribable by nurses in Northern Ireland)

Breast Shields as listed in Part IXA of the Drug Tariff (not prescribable by nurses in Scotland or Northern Ireland)

Chemical Reagents
The following as listed in Part IXR of the Drug Tariff (Part 9 of the Scottish Drug Tariff, Part II of the Northern Ireland Drug Tariff):
- Detection Strips for Glycosuria
- Detection Strips for Ketonuria
- Detection Strips for Proteinuria
- Detection Strips for Blood Glucose
- Detection Strips for Blood Ketones (not prescribable by nurses in Northern Ireland)
- Detection Strips for Determination of International Normalised Ratio (INR) (not prescribable by nurses in Northern Ireland)

Catheter Accessories as listed in Part IXA of the Drug Tariff (Part 3 of the Scottish Drug Tariff, Part III of the Northern Ireland Drug Tariff)

Catheter Maintenance Solutions as listed in Part IXA of the Drug Tariff (Part 3 of the Scottish Drug Tariff, Part III of the Northern Ireland Drug Tariff)

Catheters, Urethral Sterile as listed under Catheters in Part IXA of the Drug Tariff (Part 3 of the Scottish Drug Tariff, Part III of the Northern Ireland Drug Tariff)

Cervical Collar, Soft Foam as listed in Part IXA of the Drug Tariff (Part 3 of the Scottish Drug Tariff, not prescribable by nurses in Northern Ireland)

Chiropody Appliances as listed in Part IXA of the Drug Tariff (Part 2 of the Scottish Drug Tariff (except for Corn Plasters), not prescribable by nurses in Northern Ireland)

Contraceptive Devices as listed in Part IXA of the Drug Tariff (Part 3 of the Scottish Drug Tariff, Part III of the Northern Ireland Drug Tariff (fertility (ovulation) thermometers only))

Douches (with vaginal and rectal fittings) as listed in Part IXA of the Drug Tariff (Part 3 of the Scottish Drug Tariff, not prescribable by nurses in Northern Ireland)

Droppers as listed in Part IXA of the Drug Tariff (Part 3 of the Scottish Drug Tariff, not prescribable by nurses in Northern Ireland)

Dry Mouth Products as listed in part IXA of the Drug Tariff (Part 3 of the Scottish Drug Tariff, not prescribable by nurses in Northern Ireland)

Ear Wax Softening Medical Devices as listed in Part IXA of the Drug Tariff (Part 3 of the Scottish Drug Tariff, Part III of the Northern Ireland Drug Tariff)
Elastic Hosiery including accessories as listed in Part IXA of the Drug Tariff (Part 4 of the Scottish Drug Tariff, Part III of the Northern Ireland Drug Tariff)
Emollients as listed in Part IXA of the Drug Tariff (Part 3 of the Scottish Drug Tariff, Part III of the Northern Ireland Drug Tariff)
Eye Baths as listed in Part IXA of the Drug Tariff (Part 3 of the Scottish Drug Tariff, not prescribable by nurses in Northern Ireland)
Eye-drop Dispensers as listed in Part IXA of the Drug Tariff (Part 3 of the Scottish Drug Tariff, Part III of the Northern Ireland Drug Tariff)
Eye Shades as listed in Part IXA of the Drug Tariff (Part 3 of the Scottish Drug Tariff, not prescribable by nurses in Northern Ireland)
Finger Cots as listed in Part IXA of the Drug Tariff (Part 3 of the Scottish Drug Tariff, not prescribable by nurses in Northern Ireland)
Finger Stalls as listed in Part IXA of the Drug Tariff (Part 3 of the Scottish Drug Tariff, not prescribable by nurses in Northern Ireland)
Head Lice Device as listed in Part IXA of the Drug Tariff (Part 3 of the Scottish Drug Tariff, Part III of the Northern Ireland Drug Tariff)
Hypodermic Equipment as listed in Part IXA of the Drug Tariff (Part 3 of the Scottish Drug Tariff, Part III of the Northern Ireland Drug Tariff (with some exceptions))
Incontinence Appliances as listed in Part IXB of the Drug Tariff (Part 5 of the Scottish Drug Tariff, Part III of the Northern Ireland Drug Tariff)
Inhaler, Spare Tops as listed in Part IXA of the Drug Tariff (Part 3 of the Scottish Drug Tariff, not prescribable by nurses in Northern Ireland)
Insufflators as listed in Part IXA of the Drug Tariff (Part 3 of the Scottish Drug Tariff, not prescribable by nurses in Northern Ireland)
Irrigation Fluids as listed in Part IXA of the Drug Tariff (Part 2 of the Scottish Drug Tariff, Part III of the Northern Ireland Drug Tariff)
Latex Foam, Adhesive as listed in Part IXA of the Drug Tariff (not prescribable by nurses in Scotland or Northern Ireland)
Lubricating Jelly as listed in Part IXA of the Drug Tariff (Part 2 of the Scottish Drug Tariff, not prescribable by nurses in Northern Ireland)
Nasal Device (nasal dilator) as listed in Part IXA of the Drug Tariff (Part 3 of the Scottish Drug Tariff, Part III of the Northern Ireland Drug Tariff)
Nipple Shields, Plastic as listed in Part IXA of the Drug Tariff (Part 3 of the Scottish Drug Tariff, not prescribable by nurses in Northern Ireland)
Oral Film Forming Agents as listed in Part IXA of the Drug Tariff (Part 3 of the Scottish Drug Tariff, not prescribable by nurses in Northern Ireland)
Peak Flow Meters as listed in Part IXA of the Drug Tariff (Part 3 of the Scottish Drug Tariff, not prescribable by nurses in Northern Ireland)
Pessaries as listed in Part IXA of the Drug Tariff (Part 3 of the Scottish Drug Tariff, Part III of the Northern Ireland Drug Tariff (with some exceptions))
Protectives as listed in Part IXA of the Drug Tariff (Part 2 of the Scottish Drug Tariff, Part III of the Northern Ireland Drug Tariff (EMA Disposable Film Gloves only))
Stoma Appliances and Associated Products as listed in Part IXC of the Drug Tariff (Part 6 of the Scottish Drug Tariff, Part III of the Northern Ireland Drug Tariff)
Suprapubic Belts (replacements only) as listed in Part IXA of the Drug Tariff (Part 3 of the Scottish Drug Tariff, not prescribable by nurses in Northern Ireland)
Suprapubic Catheters as listed in Part IXA of the Drug Tariff (Part 3 of the Scottish Drug Tariff, not prescribable by nurses in Northern Ireland)
Synovial Fluid as listed in Part IXA of the Drug Tariff (Part 3 of the Scottish Drug Tariff, not prescribable by nurses in Northern Ireland)
Syringes (Bladder/Irrigating, Ear, Enema, Spare Vaginal Pipes) as listed in Part IXA of the Drug Tariff (Part 3 of the Scottish Drug Tariff, not prescribable by nurses in Northern Ireland)
Test Tubes as listed in Part IXA of the Drug Tariff (Part 3 of the Scottish Drug Tariff, not prescribable by nurses in Northern Ireland)
Tracheostomy and Laryngectomy Appliances as listed in Part IXA of the Drug Tariff (Part 2 of the Scottish Drug Tariff, not prescribable by nurses in Northern Ireland)
Trusses as listed in Part IXA of the Drug Tariff (Part 3 of the Scottish Drug Tariff, not prescribable by nurses in Northern Ireland)
Vacuum Pumps and Constrictor Rings for Erectile Dysfunction as listed in Part IXA of the Drug Tariff (Part 3 of the Scottish Drug Tariff, Part III of the Northern Ireland Drug Tariff)—prescribing restrictions may apply (see Drug Tariff)
Vaginal Moisturisers as listed in Part IXA of the Drug Tariff (Part 3 of the Scottish Drug Tariff)
Wound Management and Related Products (including bandages, dressings, gauzes, lint, stockinette, etc)
The following as listed in Part IXA of the Drug Tariff (Part 2 of the Scottish Drug Tariff, Part III of the Northern Ireland Drug Tariff):
- Absorbent Cellulose Dressing with Fluid Repellent Backing
- Absorbent Cottons
- Absorbent Cotton Gauzes
- Absorbent Cotton and Viscose Ribbon Gauze, BP 1988
- Absorbent Dressing Pads, Sterile
- Absorbent Lint, BPC
- Absorbent Perforated Dressing with Adhesive Border
- Absorbent Perforated Plastic Film Faced Dressing
- Arm Slings
- Belladonna Adhesive Plaster BP 1980
- Boil Dressing Pack
- Cellulose Wadding, BP 1988
- Chlorhexidine Gauze Dressing, BP
- Conforming Bandage (Synthetic)
- Cotton Conforming Bandage, BP 1988
- Cotton Crêpe Bandage, BP 1988
- Cotton Crêpe Bandage, Hospicrepe 239
- Cotton, Polyamide and Elastane Bandage
- Cotton Stretch Bandage, BP 1988
- Crêpe Bandage, BP 1988
- Elastic Adhesive Bandage, BP

Elastic Web Bandages
Elastomer and Viscose Bandage, Knitted
Gauze and Cotton Tissues
Gauze Dressings (Impregnated)
Heavy Cotton and Rubber Elastic Bandage, BP
High Compression Bandages (Extensible)
Knitted Polyamide and Cellulose Contour Bandage, BP 1988
Knitted Viscose Primary Dressing, BP, Type 1
Multi-layer Compression Bandaging
Multiple Pack Dressing No. 1
Open-wove Bandage, BP 1988, Type 1
Paraffin Gauze Dressing, BP
Plaster of Paris Bandage BP 1988
Polyamide and Cellulose Contour Bandage, BP 1988
Polyester Primary Dressing with Neutral Triglycerides, Knitted
Povidone–Iodine Fabric Dressing, Sterile
Short Stretch Compression Bandage
Skin Adhesive, Sterile
Skin Closure Strips, Sterile
Standard Dressings
Sterile Dressing Packs
Stockinettes
Sub-compression Wadding Bandage
Surgical Adhesive Tapes
Surgical Sutures (absorbable and non-absorbable)
Suspensory Bandages, Cotton
Swabs
Triangular Calico Bandage, BP 1980
Vapour-permeable Adhesive Film Dressing, BP (including with absorbent pad)
Vapour-permeable Waterproof Plastic Wound Dressing, BP, Sterile
Venous Ulcer Compression System
Wound Drainage Pouch
Wound Management Dressings (including activated charcoal, alginate, capillary-action, cavity, collagen, hydrocolloid, hydrogel, foam, polyurethane matrix, protease modulating matrix, silicone, silver-coated and silver-impregnated, and soft polymer dressings)
Zinc Paste Bandages (including both plain and with additional ingredients)—see also under Medicinal Preparations

In the Drug Tariff Appliances and Reagents which may **not** be prescribed by Nurses are annotated (**Nx** in the Scottish Drug Tariff and in the Northern Ireland Drug Tariff)

Details of NPF preparations

Preparations on the Nurse Prescribers' Formulary which are not included in the BP or BPC are described as follows in the Nurse Prescribers' Formulary.

Although brand names have sometimes been included for identification purposes, it is recommended that non-proprietary names should be used for prescribing medicinal preparations in the NPF except where a non-proprietary name is not available.

Arachis Oil Enema
(proprietary product: *Fletchers' Arachis Oil Retention Enema*), arachis oil

Cadexomer–Iodine Ointment
(proprietary product: *Iodosorb Ointment*), cadexomer–iodine containing iodine 0.9% in an ointment basis

Cadexomer–Iodine Paste PoM
(proprietary product: *Iodoflex*), cadexomer–iodine containing iodine 0.9% in a paste basis

Cadexomer–Iodine Powder PoM
(proprietary product: *Iodosorb Powder*), cadexomer–iodine containing iodine 0.9%

Catheter Maintenance Solution, Chlorhexidine
(proprietary products: *Uro-Tainer Chlorhexidine*; *Uriflex C*), chlorhexidine 0.02%

Catheter Maintenance Solution, Sodium Chloride
(proprietary products: *Uro-Tainer Sodium Chloride*; *Uriflex-S*), sodium chloride 0.9%

Catheter Maintenance Solution, 'Solution G'
(proprietary products: *Uro-Tainer Suby G*, *Uriflex G*), citric acid 3.23%, magnesium oxide 0.38%, sodium bicarbonate 0.7%, disodium edetate 0.01%

Catheter Maintenance Solution, 'Solution R'
(proprietary products: *Uro-Tainer Solution R*, *Uriflex R*), citric acid 6%, gluconolactone 0.6%, magnesium carbonate 2.8%, disodium edetate 0.01%

Co-danthramer Capsules PoM
co-danthramer 25/200 (dantron 25 mg, poloxamer '188' 200 mg)

Co-danthramer Capsules, Strong PoM
co-danthramer 37.5/500 (dantron 37.5 mg, poloxamer '188' 500 mg)

Co-danthramer Oral Suspension PoM
(proprietary product: *Codalax*), co-danthramer 25/200 in 5 mL (dantron 25 mg, poloxamer '188' 200 mg/5 mL)

Co-danthramer Oral Suspension, Strong PoM
(proprietary product: *Codalax Forte*), co-danthramer 75/1000 in 5 mL (dantron 75 mg, poloxamer '188' 1 g/5 mL)

Co-danthrusate Oral Suspension PoM
(proprietary product: *Normax*), co-danthrusate 50/60 (dantron 50 mg, docusate sodium 60 mg/5 mL)

Dimeticone barrier creams
(proprietary products: *Conotrane Cream*, dimeticone '350' 22%; *Siopel Barrier Cream*, dimeticone '1000' 10%; *Vasogen Barrier Cream*, dimeticone 20%), dimeticone 10–22%

Docusate Enema
(proprietary product: *Norgalax Micro-enema*) docusate sodium 120 mg in 10 g

Folic Acid Oral Solution 400 micrograms/5 mL
(proprietary product: *Folicare*), folic acid 400 micrograms/5 mL

Liquid and White Soft Paraffin Ointment
liquid paraffin 50%, white soft paraffin 50%

Macrogol Oral Powder
(proprietary product: *Idrolax*), macrogol '4000' (polyethylene glycol '4000') 10 g/sachet

Macrogol Oral Powder, Compound
(proprietary product: *Movicol*), macrogol '3350' (polyethylene glycol '3350') 13.125 g, sodium bicarbonate 178.5 mg, sodium chloride 350.7 mg, potassium chloride 46.6 mg/sachet

Macrogol Oral Powder, Compound, Half-strength
(proprietary product: *Movicol-Half*), macrogol '3350' (polyethylene glycol '3350') 6.563 g, sodium bicarbonate 89.3 g, sodium chloride 175.4 mg, potassium chloride 23.3 mg/sachet

Malathion alcoholic lotions
(proprietary products: *Prioderm Lotion*; *Suleo-M Lotion*), malathion 0.5% in an alcoholic basis

Malathion aqueous lotions
(proprietary products: *Derbac-M Liquid*; *Quellada M Liquid*), malathion 0.5% in an aqueous basis

Mebendazole Oral Suspension PoM
(proprietary product: *Vermox*), mebendazole 100 mg/5 mL

[1]**Mebendazole Tablets** PoM
(proprietary products: *Ovex*, *Vermox*), mebendazole 100 mg

Mouthwash Solution-tablets
consist of tablets which may contain antimicrobial, colouring and flavouring agents in a suitable soluble effervescent basis to make a mouthwash

[2]**Nicotine Inhalation Cartridge for Oromucosal Use**
(proprietary products: *Nicorette Inhalator*, *Boots Nicotine Inhalator*), nicotine 10 mg

Nicotine Lozenge
nicotine (as bitartrate) 1 mg (proprietary product: *Nicotinell Mint Lozenge*) or nicotine (as polacrilex) 2 mg or 4 mg (proprietary product: *NiQuitin CQ Lozenges*)

Nicotine Medicated Chewing Gum
(proprietary products: *Nicorette Gum*, *Nicorette Plus Gum*, *Nicotinell Gum*, *Nicotinell Plus Gum*, *NiQuitin CQ Gum*, *Boots Nicotine Gum*), nicotine 2 mg or 4 mg

Nicotine Nasal Spray
(proprietary product: *Nicorette Nasal Spray*), nicotine 500 micrograms/metered spray

[3]**Nicotine Sublingual Tablets**
(proprietary product: *Nicorette Microtab*), nicotine (as a cyclodextrin complex) 2 mg

[4]**Nicotine Transdermal Patches**
releasing in each 16 hours, nicotine approx. 5 mg, 10 mg, or 15 mg (proprietary product: *Nicorette Patch*) or releasing in each 24 hours nicotine approx. 7 mg, 14 mg, or 21 mg (proprietary products: *Nicotinell TTS*, *NiQuitin CQ*, *Boots NRT Patch*)

Permethrin Cream
(proprietary product: *Lyclear Dermal Cream*), permethrin 5%

Phenothrin Alcoholic Lotion
(proprietary product: *Full Marks Lotion*), phenothrin 0.2% in a basis containing isopropyl alcohol

Phenothrin Aqueous Lotion
(proprietary product: *Full Marks Liquid*), phenothrin 0.5% in an aqueous basis

Phosphate Suppositories
(proprietary product: *Carbalax*), sodium acid phosphate (anhydrous) 1.3 g, sodium bicarbonate 1.08 g

1. For PoM exemption, see p. 340

2. For use with inhalation mouthpiece; to be prescribed as either a starter pack (6 cartridges with inhalator device and holder) or refill pack (42 cartridges with inhalator device)

3. To be prescribed as either a starter pack (2 x 15-tablet discs with dispenser) or refill pack (7 x 15-tablet discs)

4. Prescriber should specify the brand to be dispensed

Piperazine and Senna Powder
(proprietary product: *Pripsen Oral Powder*), piperazine phosphate 4 g, sennosides 15.3 mg/sachet

Senna Oral Solution
(proprietary product: *Senokot Syrup*), sennosides 7.5 mg/5 mL

Senna and Ispaghula Granules
(proprietary product: *Manevac Granules*), senna fruit 12.4%, ispaghula 54.2%

Sodium Citrate Compound Enema
(proprietary products: *Micolette Micro-enema*; *Micralax Micro-enema*; *Relaxit Micro-enema*), sodium citrate 450 mg with glycerol, sorbitol and an anionic surfactant

Sodium Picosulfate Capsules
(proprietary products: *Dulco-lax Perles*), sodium picosulfate 2.5 mg

Sodium Picosulfate Elixir
(proprietary products: *Dulco-lax Liquid*, *Laxoberal* NHS), sodium picosulfate 5 mg/5 mL

Sterculia Granules
(proprietary product: *Normacol Granules*), sterculia 62%

Sterculia and Frangula Granules
(proprietary product: *Normacol Plus Granules*), sterculia 62%, frangula (standardised) 8%

Streptokinase and Streptodornase Topical Powder PoM
(proprietary product: *Varidase Topical*), streptokinase 100 000 units, streptodornase 25 000 units

Zinc Oxide and Dimeticone Spray
(proprietary product: *Sprilon*), dimeticone 1.04%, zinc oxide 12.5% in a pressurised aerosol unit

Zinc Oxide Impregnated Medicated Stocking
(proprietary product: *Zipzoc*), sterile rayon stocking impregnated with ointment containing zinc oxide 20%

Nurse Prescribers' Extended Formulary

List of preparations which may be prescribed by Extended Formulary Nurse Prescribers on Form FP10P, for NHS patients in England (Form HS21(N) in Northern Ireland, Form GP10(N2) in Scotland).

Independent nurse prescribers who have completed the necessary training and are authorised to prescribe from the Nurse Prescribers' Extended Formulary list may prescribe all General Sales List and Pharmacy medicines currently prescribable by GPs, together with specified Prescription Only Medicines. In addition they may prescribe all items in the nurse prescribing list for Community Practitioners on p. 843. The Committee on Safety of Medicines and the Medicines Commission advise that Extended Formulary Nurse Prescribers should prescribe medicines (including pharmacy-only and general sales list medicines) **only** for the medical conditions specified below. This advice is reinforced in Extending Independent Nurse Prescribing within the NHS in England: a guide for implementation (available on the Department of Health website, www.dh.gov.uk). Nurses should **not** prescribe independently for conditions other than those on the list.

Medical Conditions

	BNF section[1]
Central Nervous System	
Acute dystonias	4.9.2
Acute severe pain after trauma	4.7.2
Changing painful dressings	15.2
Nausea and vomiting	4.6
Prophylaxis and treatment of nausea and vomiting in the postoperative period	4.6
Recurrent generalised tonic-clonic seizures	4.8.2
Circulatory	
Acute myocardial infarction	2.10
Acute pulmonary oedema associated with cardiac failure	2.2.2
Angina pectoris	2.6
Fluid replacement and potassium replacement (hypovolaemia and dehydration)	9.2.2.1
Haemorrhoids	1.7.1, 1.7.2
Phlebitis, superficial	-
Plasma substitutes for patients with a low blood volume	9.2.2.2
Thromboprophylaxis—defined as prophylaxis against venous thrombosis (including congestive heart failure, in bed-bound patients, and perioperatively) and for acute coronary syndrome	2.8.1
Ventricular fibrillation or pulseless ventricular tachycardia	2.7.3
Ear	
Furuncle	-
Otitis externa	12.1.1
Otitis media	12.1.2
Wax in ear	12.1.3
Endocrine	
Hyperglycaemia	6.1.1
Hypoglycaemia	6.1.4
Eye	
Blepharitis	11.3.1
Conjunctivitis, allergic	11.4.2
Conjunctivitis, infective	11.3.1
Corneal trauma	11.7
Diagnostic use in ophthalmology	11.5
Local anaesthetic for ophthalmic conditions	11.7
Tear deficiency	11.8.1
Gastro-intestinal conditions	
Constipation	1.6
Gastro-enteritis	1.4
Heartburn	1.1
Infantile colic	1.1.1
Pre-surgery prophylaxis against acid aspiration	1.3.1, 1.3.5
Worms—threadworms	5.5.1
Immunisations	
Routine childhood and specific vaccinations	14.1, 14.4
Infections	
Emergency treatment of suspected meningococcal septicemia or meningococcal meningitis	5.1 (table 1)
Spreading cellulitis usually of a limb with a risk of, or an established, lymphangitis	5.1 (table 1)
Tetanus prophylaxis and treatment	14.4, 14.5
Musculoskeletal	
Back pain, acute uncomplicated	4.7.1, 10.1.1
Neck pain, acute uncomplicated	4.7.1, 10.1.1
Pain and inflammation	10.1.1
Soft tissue injuries	4.7.1, 10.1.1, 10.3.2
Sprains	4.7.1, 10.1.1, 10.3.2
Oral conditions	
Aphthous ulcer	12.3.1
Candidiasis, oral	12.3.2
Dental abscess	4.7.1, 10.1.1
Dental infections	5.1 (table 1)
Gingivitis	12.3.4
Stomatitis	-
Poisoning	
Poisoning	Emergency treatment of poisoning
Respiratory	
Acute attacks of asthma	3.1
Acute exacerbation of chronic bronchitis	5.1 (table 1)
Acute nasopharyngitis (coryza)	12.2.2
Acute reversible airways obstruction (acute severe asthma or acute exacerbation of chronic obstructive pulmonary disease)	3.1
Anaphylaxis	3.4.3
Conditions requiring oxygen supplementation (e.g. hypoxaemia)	3.6
Croup	3.1
Laryngitis	12.3.1
Pharyngitis	12.3.1
Rhinitis, allergic	3.4.1, 12.2.1, 12.2.2
Sinusitis, acute	3.4.1
Tonsillitis	12.2.2, 12.3.1
Skin	
Abrasions	13.10.5
Acne	13.6
Animal and human bites	5.1 (table 1)
Boil/carbuncle	13.10.5
Burn/scald	13.11, App. 8
Candidiasis, skin	13.10.2
Chronic skin ulcer	13.11.7, 13.10.1
Dermatitis, atopic	13.5.1
Dermatitis, contact	13.5.1
Dermatitis, seborrhoeic	13.5.1
Dermatophytosis of the skin (ringworm)	13.10.2
Herpes labialis	13.10.3
Impetigo	5.1 (table 1), 13.10.1
Insect bite/sting	13.3
Lacerations	13.11, App. 8
Local anaesthetic for occasions when procedure requires it	15.2

1. BNF sections appropriate to the listed conditions are shown. However, not all drugs in these sections are prescribable by nurses. Also, in some cases preparations (including General Sales List and Pharmacy medicines) in other BNF sections may be suitable. Before choosing a Prescription Only Medicine, nurses need to check the Nurse Prescribers' Extended Formulary list and to satisfy themselves that the product is licensed for the condition they wish to prescribe for and that the condition falls within the remit of the Nurse Prescribers' Extended Formulary.

Local anaesthetic for suturing of lacerations	15.2
Molluscum contagiosum	-
Nappy rash	13.2.2
Pediculosis (head lice)	13.10.4
Pruritus in chicken pox	13.3
Psoriasis	13.5.2
Scabies	13.10.4
Urticaria	3.4.1
Warts (including verrucas)	13.7
Substance Dependence	
Acute alcohol withdrawal	4.10
Smoking cessation	4.10
Urinary system	
Urinary tract infection (women) —lower, uncomplicated	5.1 (table 1), 7.4.3
Female genital system	
Bacterial vaginosis	5.1.11, 7.2.2
Candidiasis, vulvovaginal	7.2.2
Contraception	7.3
Dysmenorrhoea	4.7.1, 10.1.1
Emergency contraception	7.3
Laboratory-confirmed uncomplicated genital chlamydia infection (and the sexual partners of these patients)	5.1 (table 1)
Menopausal vaginal atrophy	7.2.1
Preconceptual counselling	9.1.2
Trichomonas vaginalis infection (and the sexual partners of these patients)	5.4.3
Male genital system	
Balanitis	13.10.2
Palliative Care of patients with advanced progressive illness	
Anxiety	4.1.2
Bowel colic	Prescribing in palliative care
Candidiasis, oral	12.3.2
Confusion	Prescribing in palliative care
Constipation	Prescribing in palliative care
Convulsions and restlessness	Prescribing in palliative care
Cough	Prescribing in palliative care
Dry mouth	Prescribing in palliative care
Excessive respiratory secretions	Prescribing in palliative care
Fungating malodorous tumours	13.10.1.2
Muscle spasm	Prescribing in palliative care
Nausea and vomiting	Prescribing in palliative care
Neuropathic pain in palliative care	Prescribing in palliative care
Pain control	Prescribing in palliative care

Nurse Prescribers' Extended Formulary

- All licensed P and GSL Medicines prescribable on the NHS
- Prescription Only Medicines from the list below by the route or form specified
- See above for the list of those medical conditions for which nurses may prescribe independently

List of prescription only medicines for prescribing by extended formulary nurse prescribers

Oral antibacterials marked *—see separate list below for indications

Drug	Route of administration, use or pharmaceutical form
Acetylcysteine	Parenteral
Aciclovir	External
Acrivastine	Oral
Adapalene	External
Adrenaline	Parenteral
Alclometasone dipropionate	External
Alimemazine tartrate (trimeprazine tartrate)	Oral
Alteplase	Parenteral
Amiodarone	Parenteral
Amitriptyline hydrochloride	Palliative care—oral
Amorolfine hydrochloride	External
Amoxicillin trihydrate*	Oral
Aspirin	Oral
Azelaic acid	External
Azelastine hydrochloride	Ophthalmic, nasal
Azithromycin dihydrate*	Oral
Baclofen	Palliative care—oral
Beclometasone dipropionate	External, nasal, inhalation
Bemiparin sodium	Parenteral
Benzatropine mesilate	Parenteral
Benzylpenicillin sodium	Parenteral
Betamethasone sodium phosphate	Aural, nasal
Betamethasone valerate	External, rectal
Budesonide	Nasal, inhalation
Calcipotriol	External
Calcitriol	External
Carbamazepine	Palliative care—oral, rectal
Carbaryl	External
Carbenoxolone sodium	Mouthwash
Cefotaxime sodium	Parenteral
Ceftriaxone sodium	Parenteral
Certoparin sodium	Parenteral
Cetirizine hydrochloride	Oral
Chloramphenicol	Ophthalmic
Chlorphenamine maleate	Parenteral
Cimetidine	Oral, parenteral
Cinchocaine hydrochloride	Rectal
[1]Clavulanic acid	Oral
Clindamycin phosphate	External, vaginal
Clobetasone butyrate	External
Clotrimazole	External
Codeine phosphate	Oral
Conjugated oestrogens (equine)	External
Co-phenotrope	Oral
Cyclizine hydrochloride	Oral
Cyclizine lactate	Parenteral
Dalteparin sodium	Parenteral
Dantrolene sodium	Palliative care—oral
Dantron	Oral
[2]Desogestrel	Oral
Desoximetasone	External
Dexamethasone	Aural
Dexamethasone isonicotinate	Nasal

Footnotes—see p. 851

Dexamethasone sodium phosphate	Oral
Dextran 70	Parenteral
Diazepam	Oral, parenteral and rectal
Diclofenac diethylammonium	External
Diclofenac potassium	Oral
Diclofenac sodium	Oral, rectal, ophthalmic
Dihydrocodeine tartrate	Oral
Dolasetron mesilate	Oral and parenteral
Domperidone	Oral and rectal
Domperidone maleate	Oral
Doxycycline*	Oral
Doxycycline hyclate*	Oral
Econazole nitrate	External, vaginal
Emedastine	Ophthalmic
Enoxaparin	Parenteral
Erythromycin*	External, oral
Erythromycin ethyl succinate*	Oral
Erythromycin stearate*	Oral
Estradiol	External
Estriol	External
[2]Ethinylestradiol	Oral
Etonogestrel	Implant
[2]Etynodiol diacetate	Oral
Famotidine	Oral
Felbinac	External
Fenticonazole nitrate	Vaginal
Fexofenadine hydrochloride	Oral
Flucloxacillin magnesium*	Oral
Flucloxacillin sodium*	Oral, parenteral
Fluconazole	Oral
Fludroxycortide (flurandrenolone)	External
Flumazenil	Parenteral
Flumetasone pivalate	Aural
Flunisolide	Nasal
Fluocinolone acetonide	External
Fluocinonide	External
Fluocortolone hexanoate	External, rectal
Fluocortolone pivalate	External, rectal
Flurbiprofen	Lozenges
Fluticasone propionate	External, nasal
Furosemide	Oral, parenteral
Fusidic acid	External
Gabapentin	Palliative care—oral
Gelatin 3.5–4%	Parenteral
Gentamicin sulphate	Aural
[2]Gestodene	Oral
Glucagon hydrochloride	Parenteral
Glucose	Parenteral
Glucose 5%	Parenteral
Glucose 5% with Potassium (K^+ 40 mmol/L) ready-made infusion bag	Parenteral
Granisetron hydrochloride	Parenteral
Heparin	Parenteral
Heparin sodium	Parenteral for the purpose of cannulae flushing
Hexastarch	Parenteral
Human soluble insulin	Parenteral
Hydrocortisone	External including rectal
Hydrocortisone acetate	External, aural
Hydrocortisone butyrate	External
Hydrocortisone sodium succinate	Lozenges, parenteral
Hydroxyethl starch	Parenteral
Hyoscine	Palliative care—transdermal
Hyoscine butylbromide	Palliative care—parenteral
Hyoscine hydrobromide	Palliative care—oral, parenteral
Ibuprofen	External, oral
Ibuprofen lysine	Oral
Imipramine hydrochloride	Palliative care—oral

Ipratropium bromide	Nasal, inhalation
Isotretinoin	External
Ketoconazole	External
Ketoprofen	External
Levocabastine hydrochloride	Nasal and ophthalmic
Levomepromazine (including levomepromazine (methotrimeprazine) maleate and levomepromazine (methotrimeprazine) hydrochloride	Oral, parenteral
[2]Levonorgestrel	Oral
Lidocaine hydrochloride	External, parenteral
Lithium succinate	External
Lodoxamide trometamol	Ophthalmic
Loperamide hydrochloride	Oral
Loratadine	Oral
Lorazepam	Oral, parenteral
Lymecycline*	Oral
Mebendazole	Oral
[2]Medroxyprogesterone acetate	Injection
[2]Mestranol	Oral
Metoclopramide hydrochloride	Oral and parenteral
Metronidazole*	Oral, external, vaginal, rectal
Metronidazole benzoate*	Oral
Miconazole	Dental lacquer
Miconazole nitrate	External, vaginal
Midazolam	Parenteral
Minocycline hydrochloride*	Oral
Mizolastine	Oral
Mometasone furoate	External, nasal
Naloxone	Parenteral
Nedocromil sodium	Ophthalmic
Nefopam hydrochloride	Oral
Neomycin sulphate	Aural
Neomycin undecanoate	Aural
Nitrofurantoin*	Oral
Nizatidine	Oral
[2]Norethisterone	Oral
[2]Norethisterone acetate	Oral
[2]Norethisterone enanthate	Parenteral
[2]Norgestimate	Oral
[2]Norgestrel	Oral
Nortriptyline hydrochloride	Palliative care—oral
Nystatin	External, local mouth treatment, vaginal
Omeprazole	Oral
Omeprazole sodium	Parenteral
Ondansetron hydrochloride	Oral, parenteral
Oxybuprocaine hydrochloride	Ophthalmic
Oxytetracycline dihydrate*	Oral
Paracetamol	Oral
Penciclovir	External
Pentastarch	Parenteral
Piroxicam	External
Prednisolone	Oral
Prednisolone hexanoate	Rectal
Prednisolone sodium phosphate	Aural, oral
Prilocaine	External, parenteral
Prochlorperazine mesilate	Oral, rectal
Prochlorperazine maleate	Oral, rectal, buccal
Proxymetacaine hydrochloride	Ophthalmic
Ranitidine hydrochloride	Oral, parenteral
Reteplase	Parenteral
Salbutamol sulphate	Inhalation
Silver sulfadiazine	External
Sodium chloride 0.9%	Parenteral, for reconstitution of injections and for the purpose of cannulae flushing
Sodium chloride 0.9% & Glucose 5% ready-made infusion bag	Parenteral

Footnotes—see p. 851

Sodium chloride 0.45% & Glucose 5% ready-made infusion bag	Parenteral
Sodium chloride 0.9% with Potassium (K^+ 40 mmol/litre) ready-made infusion bag	Parenteral
Sodium chloride 0.45% and Glucose 5% with Potassium 20 mmol per 500 mL ready-made infusion bag	Parenteral
Sodium cromoglicate	Ophthalmic
Sodium fusidate	External
Streptodornase	External
Streptokinase	External, parenteral
Sulconazole nitrate	External
Tacalcitol	External
Tenecteplase	Parenteral
Terbinafine hydrochloride	External
Terbutaline sulphate	Inhalation
Tetanus immunoglobulin	Parenteral
Tetracaine	External
Tetracycline hydrochloride*	External, oral
Tinzaparin sodium	Parenteral
Tretinoin	External
Triamcinolone acetonide	Aural, external, nasal, oral paste
Trimethoprim*	Oral
Tropicamide	Ophthalmic
Tropisetron hydrochloride	Parenteral
[3]Tuberculin PPD	Injection
[3]Vaccine, Adsorbed Diphtheria	Injection
[3]Vaccine, Adsorbed Diphtheria and Tetanus	Injection
[3]Vaccine, Adsorbed Diphtheria and Tetanus for Adults and Adolescents	Injection
[3]Vaccine, Adsorbed Diphtheria for Adults and Adolescents	Injection
[3]Vaccine, Adsorbed Diphtheria, Tetanus and Pertussis	Injection
[3]Vaccine, Adsorbed Diphtheria, Tetanus Toxoid and Pertussis (Acellular Component)	Injection
[3]Vaccine, BCG	Injection
[3]Vaccine, BCG Percutaneous	Injection
Vaccine, Combined Tetanus, Diphtheria, Acellular Pertussis, Inactivated Poliomyelitis and Haemophilus Influenza Type B	Parenteral
[3]Vaccine, Haemophilus Influenzae Type B (Hib)	Injection
[3]Vaccine, Haemophilus Influenzae Type B (Hib) with Diphtheria, Tetanus and Pertussis	Injection
[3]Vaccine, Haemophilus Influenzae Type B, (Hib) with Diphtheria, Tetanus and Acellular Pertussis	Injection
[4]Vaccine, Hepatitis A	Injection
[4]Vaccine, Hepatitis A with Typhoid	Injection
[4]Vaccine, Hepatitis A, Inactivated, with recombinant (DNA) Hepatitis B	Injection
[4]Vaccine, Hepatitis B	Injection
Vaccine, Inactivated Poliomyelitis	Parenteral
[4]Vaccine, Influenza	Injection
[3]Vaccine, Live Measles, Mumps and Rubella (MMR)	Injection
[3]Vaccine, Meningococcal Group C Conjugate	Injection
[3 or 4]Vaccine, Meningococcal Polysaccharide A and C	Injection
Vaccine, Meningococcal Polysaccharide A, C, W135 and Y	Parenteral
[4]Vaccine, Pneumococcal	Injection
[3]Vaccine, Poliomyelitis, Live (Oral)	Oral
[3]Vaccine, Rubella, Live	Injection
[4]Vaccine, Tetanus, Adsorbed	Injection
Vaccine, Typhoid, Live Attenuated (Oral)	Oral
[4]Vaccine, Typhoid, Polysaccharide	Injection
Water for Injections	Parenteral

*** Oral antibacterials and indications considered suitable for nurse prescribing**

Drug	Indication
[5]Amoxicillin trihydrate	Lower urinary-tract infection (women), animal and human bites, acute exacerbation of chronic bronchitis, dental infections
Azithromycin dihydrate	Laboratory-confirmed uncomplicated genital chlamydial infection, plus sexual partners of these patients
Doxycycline hyclate	Acne, animal and human bites, laboratory-confirmed uncomplicated genital chlamydial infection, plus sexual partners of these patients
Doxycycline monohydrate	Acne, animal and human bites, laboratory-confirmed uncomplicated genital chlamydial infection, plus sexual partners of these patients
Erythromycin	Impetigo, animal and human bites, laboratory-confirmed uncomplicated genital chlamydial infection, plus sexual partners of these patients, spreading cellulitis usually of a limb with a risk of, or an established lymphangitis, dental infections
Erythromycin ethyl succinate	Impetigo, animal and human bites, laboratory-confirmed uncomplicated genital chlamydial infection, plus sexual partners of these patients, spreading cellulitus usually of a limb with a risk of, or an established lymphangitis, dental infections
Erythromycin stearate	Impetigo, animal and human bites, laboratory-confirmed uncomplicated genital chlamydial infection, plus sexual partners of these patients, spreading cellulitus usually of a limb with a risk of, or an established lymphangitis, dental infections
Flucloxacillin magnesium	Impetigo, spreading cellulitus usually of a limb with a risk of, or an established lymphangitis
Flucloxacillin sodium	Impetigo, spreading cellulitus usually of a limb with a risk of, or an established lymphangitis
Lymecycline	Acne
Metronidazole	Animal and human bites; fungating malodorous tumours; bacterial vaginosis; *trichomonas vaginalis* infection plus sexual partners of these patients, dental infections
Metronidazole benzoate	Animal and human bites, dental infections
Minocycline hydrochloride	Acne
Nitrofurantoin	Lower urinary-tract infection (women)
Oxytetracycline dihydrate	Acne, animal and human bites, acute exacerbation of chronic bronchitis
Tetracycline hydrochloride	Acne
Trimethoprim	Lower urinary-tract infection (women)

1. Present as potassium clavulanate in co-amoxiclav
2. Nurse Prescribers in Family Planning Clinics—where it is not appropriate for nurse prescribers in family planning clinics to prescribe contraceptive drugs using form FP10(P) (forms FP10(CN) and FP10(PN), or when available WP10CN and WP10PN, in Wales), they may prescribe using the same system as doctors in the clinic.
3. Centrally supplied vaccine excluded from reimbursement via prescription route
4. High Volume Personally Administered Vaccine. Claims for these vaccines should be ordered on form FP34D
5. With Clavulanic acid (as co-amoxiclav) for animal and human bites

Index of manufacturers

3M
3M Health Care Ltd
3M House
Morley St, Loughborough
Leics, LE11 1EP.
Tel: (01509) 611611
Fax: (01509) 237288

A&H
Allen & Hanburys Ltd
See GSK.

Abbott
Abbott Laboratories Ltd
Abbott House
Norden Rd, Maidenhead, Berks
SL6 4XE.
Tel: (01628) 773 355
Fax: (01628) 644 185

Acorus
Acorus Therapeutics Ltd
High Crane Lodge
Hamsterley, Bishop Auckland,
Durham DL13 3QS.
Tel: (01388) 710 505
Fax: (01388) 710 770
enquiries@acorus-therapeutics.com

Actelion
Actelion Pharmaceuticals UK Ltd
BSi Building, 13th Floor
389 Chiswick High Rd, London
W4 4AL.
Tel: (020) 8987 3333
Fax: (020) 8987 3322

Activa
Activa Healthcare
1 Lancaster Park
Newborough Rd, Needwood,
Burton-upon-Trent, Staffs
DE13 9PD.
Tel: (0845) 060 6707
Fax: (01283) 576 808
advice@activahealthcare.co.uk

Adams Hlth.
Adams Healthcare Ltd
Lotherton Way
Garforth, Leeds LS25 2JY.
Tel: (0113) 232 0066
Fax: (0113) 287 1317
enquiries@adams-healthcare.co.uk

Advancis
Advancis Medical Ltd
Lowmoor Business Park
Kirkby-in-Ashfield, Nottingham
NG17 7JZ.
Tel: (01623) 751 500
Fax: (01623) 757 636
enquiries@advancis.co.uk

Aguettant
Aguettant Ltd
Bishops House
Bishops Rd, Claverham, Somerset
BS49 4NF.
Tel: (01934) 835 694
Fax: (01934) 876 790
info@aguettant.co.uk

Air Products
Air Products plc
Medical Group
2 Millennium Gate, Westmere
Drive, Crewe
Cheshire, CW1 6AP.
Tel: (0800) 373 580
Fax: (0800) 214 709

Alcon
Alcon Laboratories (UK) Ltd
Pentagon Park
Boundary Way, Hemel Hempstead,
Herts HP2 7UD.
Tel: (01442) 341 234
Fax: (01442) 341 200

Alembic Products
Alembic Products Ltd
River Lane
Saltney, Chester, Cheshire
CH4 8RQ.
Tel: (01244) 680 147
Fax: (01244) 680 155

ALK-Abelló
ALK-Abelló (UK) Ltd
1 Tealgate
Hungerford, Berks RG17 0YT.
Tel: (01488) 686 016
Fax: (01488) 685 423
info@uk.alk-abello.com

Allergan
Allergan Ltd
Coronation Rd
High Wycombe, Bucks HP12 3SH.
Tel: (01494) 444 722
Fax: (01494) 473 593

Allergy
Allergy Therapeutics Ltd
Dominion Way
Worthing, West Sussex BN14 8SA.
Tel: (01903) 844 702
Fax: (01903) 844 744
infoservices@allergytherapeutics.
com

Alliance
Alliance Pharmaceuticals Ltd
Avonbridge House
2 Bath Rd, Chippenham, Wilts
SN15 2BB.
Tel: (01249) 466 966
Fax: (01249) 466 977
info@alliancepharma.co.uk

Alpharma
Alpharma Ltd
Whiddon Valley
Barnstaple, Devon EX32 8NS.
Tel: (01271) 311 257
Fax: (01271) 346 106
med.info@alpharma.co.uk

Alphashow
Alphashow Ltd
35A High Street
Marlborough, Wiltshire SN8 1LW.
Tel: (0870) 240 2775
Fax: (0870) 240 2775
info@alphashow.co.uk

Altana
Altana Pharma Ltd
Three Globeside Business Park
Fieldhouse Lane, Marlow, Bucks
SL7 1HZ.
Tel: (01628) 646 400
Fax: (01628) 646 401
medinfo@altanapharma.co.uk

Amdipharm
Amdipharm plc
Regency House
Miles Gray Rd, Basildon, Essex
SS14 3AF.
Tel: (0870) 777 7675
Fax: (0870) 777 7875
info@amdipharm.com

Amgen
Amgen Ltd
240 Cambridge Science Park
Milton Rd, Cambridge CB4 0WD.
Tel: (01223) 420 305
Fax: (01223) 426 314
infoline@uk.amgen.com

Anglian
Anglian Pharma Sales & Marketing
Titmore Court
Titmore Green, Little Wymondley,
Hitchin
Herts, SG4 7XJ.
Tel: (01438) 743 070
Fax: (01438) 743 080
mail@anglianpharma.com

Anpharm
See Antigen.

Antigen
See Goldshield

APS
See TEVA UK

Ardana
Ardana Bioscience Ltd
58 Queen St
Edinburgh EH2 3NS.
Tel: (0131) 226 8550
Fax: (0131) 226 8551
info@ardana.co.uk

Ardern
Ardern Healthcare Ltd
Pipers Brook Farm
Eastham, Tenbury Wells, Worcs
WR15 8NP.
Tel: (01584) 781 777
Fax: (01584) 781 788
info@ardernhealthcare.com

AS Pharma
AS Pharma Ltd
PO Box 181
Polegate, East Sussex BN26 6WD.
Tel: (08700) 664 117
Fax: (08700) 664 118
info@aspharma.co.uk

Ashbourne
Ashbourne Pharmaceuticals Ltd
Victors Barns
Northampton Rd, Brixworth,
Northampton NN6 9DQ.
Tel: (01604) 883 100
Fax: (01604) 881 640

AstraZeneca
AstraZeneca UK Ltd
Horizon Place
600 Capability Green, Luton, Beds
LU1 3LU.
Tel: 0800 7830 033
Fax: (01582) 838 003
medical.informationuk@
astrazeneca.com

Auden Mckenzie
Auden Mckenzie (Pharma Division)
Ltd
30 Stadium Business Centre
North End Rd, Wembley, Middx
HA9 0AT.
Tel: (020) 8900 2122
Fax: (020) 8903 9620

Aurum
Aurum Pharmaceuticals Ltd
Hubert Rd
Brentwood, Essex CM14 4LZ.
Tel: (01277) 266600
Fax: (01277) 848 976
info@martindalepharma.co.uk

Aventis Pasteur
Aventis Pasteur MSD Ltd
See Sanofi Pasteur.
Tel: (01628) 685 291
Fax: (01628) 671 722

Aventis Pharma
See Sanofi-Aventis

Bailey, Robert
Robert Bailey Healthcare Ltd
Unit 6
Heapham Rd Industrial Estate,
Gainsborough, Lincs DN21 1RZ.
Tel: (01427) 677 559
Fax: (01427) 677 654
rbsales@cottonwool.uk.com

Bard
Bard Ltd
Forest House
Brighton Rd, Crawley, West Sussex
RH11 9BP.
Tel: (01293) 527 888
Fax: (01293) 552 428

Bausch & Lomb
Bausch & Lomb UK Ltd
106 London Rd
Kingston-upon-Thames, Surrey
KT2 6TN.
Tel: (020) 8781 2900
Fax: (01344) 8781 2901

Baxter
Baxter Healthcare Ltd
Wallingford Rd
Compton, Newbury
Berks, RG20 7QW.
Tel: (01635) 206 345
Fax: (01635) 206 071
surecall@baxter.com

Baxter BioScience
See Baxter.

Bayer
Bayer plc
Pharmaceutical Division
Bayer House, Strawberry Hill,
Newbury, Berks RG14 1JA.
Tel: (01635) 563 000
Fax: (01635) 563 393
medical.science@bayer.co.uk

Bayer Consumer Care
See Bayer.

Bayer Diagnostics
Bayer plc
Diagnostics Division
Bayer House, Strawberry Hill,
Newbury, Berks RG14 1JA.
Tel: (01635) 563 000
Fax: (01635) 563 393

BCM Specials
BCM Specials Manufacturing
D10 First 114
Nottingham NG90 2PR.
Tel: 0800 952 1010
Fax: 0800 085 0673
bcm-specials@bcm-ltd.co.uk

Beacon
Beacon Pharmaceuticals Ltd
85 High St
Tunbridge Wells TN1 1YG.
Tel: (01892) 506 958
Fax: (01892) 610 397
info@beaconpharma.co.uk

Becton Dickinson
Becton Dickinson UK Ltd
Between Towns Rd
Cowley, Oxford, Oxon OX4 3LY.
Tel: (01865) 748 844
Fax: (01865) 717 313

Beiersdorf
Beiersdorf UK Ltd
3500 Parkside
Birmingham Business Park,
Birmingham B37 7YS.
Tel: (0121) 329 8800
Fax: (0121) 329 8801

Bell and Croyden
John Bell and Croyden
50-54 Wigmore St
London W1U 2AU.
Tel: (020) 7935 5555
Fax: (020) 7935 9605
jbc@johnbellcroyden.co.uk

Berk
See TEVA UK.

BHR
BHR Pharmaceuticals Ltd
41 Centenary Business Centre
Hammond Close, Attleborough
Fields, Nuneaton
Warwickshire, CV11 6RY.
Tel: (024) 7635 3742
Fax: (024) 7632 7812
info@bhr.co.uk

Bioenvision
Bioenvision Ltd
11-12 Charles II St
Savanah House, London
SW1Y 4QU.
Tel: (020) 7451 2488
Fax: (020) 7451 2469
info@bioenvision.com

Biogen
Biogen Ltd
5d Roxborough Way
Foundation Park, Maidenhead
Berks, SL6 3UD.
Tel: (01628) 501 000
Fax: (01628) 501 010

Biolitec
Biolitec Pharma Ltd
Unit 2, Broomhill Business Park
Broomhill Rd, Tallaght
Dublin 24, Ireland.
Tel: (00353) 14637415
Fax: (00353) 14637411
medical.info@biolitec.com

Biosurgical Research
Biosurgical Research Unit
Surgical Materials Testing
Laboratory
Princess of Wales Hospital, Coity
Rd, Bridgend, Mid Glamorgan
South Wales, CF31 1RQ.
Tel: (01656) 752 820
Fax: (01656) 752 830
maggots@smtl.co.uk

Blackwell
Blackwell Supplies Ltd
Medcare House
Centurion Close, Gillingham
Business Park, Gillingham
Kent, ME8 0SB.
Tel: (01634) 877 620
Fax: (01634) 877 621

Blake
Thomas Blake & Co
The Byre House
Fearby, Nr. Masham
North Yorks, HG4 4NF.
Tel: (01765) 689 042
Fax: (01765) 689 042
sales@veilcover.com

BOC
BOC Medical
The Priestley Centre,
10 Priestley Rd, Surrey Research Park
Guildford, Surrey, GU2 7XY.
Tel: 0800 111 333
Fax: 0800 111 555

Boehringer Ingelheim
Boehringer Ingelheim Ltd
Ellesfield Ave
Bracknell
Berks, RG12 8YS.
Tel: (01344) 424 600
Fax: (01344) 741 444
medinfo@bra.boehringer-ingelheim.com

Boots
Boots The Chemists
Medical Services
Thane Rd, D90 East S10
Nottingham, NG90 1BS.
Tel: (0115) 959 5168
Fax: (0115) 959 2565

Borg
Borg Medicare
PO Box 99
Hitchin
Herts, SG5 2GF.
Tel: (01462) 442 993
Fax: (01462) 441 293

BPC 100
The Bolton Pharmaceutical 100 Ltd
2 Chapel Drive
Ambrosden, Oxfordshire
OX25 2RS.
Tel: (0845) 602 3907
Fax: (0845) 602 3908
info@bpc100.com

BPL
Bio Products Laboratory
Dagger Lane
Elstree, Herts WD6 3BX.
Tel: (020) 8258 2200
Fax: (020) 8258 2601

Braun
B Braun (Medical) Ltd
Brookdale Rd
Thorncliffe Park Estate,
Chapeltown, Sheffield S35 2PW.
Tel: (0114) 225 9000
Fax: (0114) 225 9111
enquiry@bbmuk.demon.co.uk

Braun Biotrol
See Braun.

Bray
Bray Health & Leisure
1 Regal Way
Faringdon
Oxon, SN7 7BX.
Tel: (01367) 240 736
Fax: (01367) 242 625
info@bray.co.uk

Bristol
Bristol Laboratories Ltd
Unit 3, Canalside
Northbridge Rd, Berkhamsted
Herts, HP4 1EG.
Tel: (01442) 200 922
Fax: (01442) 873 717
info@bristol-labs.co.uk

Bristol-Myers Squibb
Bristol-Myers Squibb Pharmaceuticals Ltd
Uxbridge Business Park
Sanderson Rd, Uxbridge
Middx, UB8 1DH.
Tel: (01895) 523 000
Fax: (01895) 523 010
medical.information@bms.com

Britannia
Britannia Pharmaceuticals Ltd
41-51 Brighton Rd, Redhill
Surrey, RH1 6YS.
Tel: (01737) 773 741
Fax: (01737) 762 672
medicalservices@forumgroup.co.uk

British Biocell
British Biocell International
Golden Gate, Ty Glas Avenue
Llanishen, Cardiff CF14 5DX.
Tel: (02920) 747 232
Fax: (02920) 747 242
info@bbigold.co.uk

Brodie & Stone
Brodie and Stone International plc
51 Calthorpe St
London, WC1X 0HH.
Tel: (020) 7278 9597
Fax: (020) 7278 2458
mailbox@brodieandstone.com

BSIA
See Torbet.

BSN Medical
BSN Medical Ltd
PO Box 258
Willerby, Hull HU10 6WT.
Tel: (0845) 1223 600
Fax: (0845) 1223 666

C D Medical
C D Medical Ltd
Aston Grange
Oker, Matlock DE4 2JJ.
Tel: (01629) 733 860
Fax: (01629) 733 414

Cambridge
Cambridge Laboratories
Deltic House, Kingfisher Way
Silverlink Business Park, Wallsend,
Tyne & Wear NE28 9NX.
Tel: (0191) 296 9369
Fax: (0191) 296 9368
enquries@camb-labs.com

Castlemead
Castlemead Healthcare Ltd
2nd Floor
The Maltings, Bridge St
Hitchin, Herts, SG5 2DE.
Tel: (01462) 454 452
Fax: (01462) 435 684

Cell Therapeutics
Cell Therapeutics (UK) Ltd
100 Pall Mall
London SW1Y 5HP.
Tel: (0031) 6 5164 1765
Fax: (0031) 24360 8075
celltherapeuticseurope@vwbintermedical.com

Celltech
See UCB Pharma.

Centrapharm
Centrapharm Ltd
Dale House
Suckley Rd, Knightwick
Worcs, WR6 5QE.
Tel: (01886) 822 116
Fax: (01886) 822 125
info@centrapharm.co.uk

Cephalon
Cephalon UK Ltd
11-13 Frederick Sanger Rd
Surrey Research Park, Guildford
Surrey, GU2 7YD.
Tel: 0800 783 4869
Fax: (01483) 453 324
ukmedinfo@cephalon.com

Ceuta
Ceuta Healthcare Ltd
Hill House
41 Richmond Hill, Bournemouth
Dorset, BH2 6HS.
Tel: (01202) 780 558
Fax: (01202) 780 559

Chauvin
Chauvin Pharmaceuticals Ltd
106 London Rd
Kingston-Upon-Thames, Surrey
KT2 6TN.
Tel: (020) 8781 2900
Fax: (020) 8781 2901

Chefaro UK
Chefaro UK Ltd
Unit 1, Tower Close
St. Peter's Industrial Park,
Huntingdon
Cambs, PE29 7DH.
Tel: (01480) 421 800
Fax: (01480) 434 861

Chemical Search
Chemical Search International Ltd
29th floor
1 Canada Square, Canary Wharf
London, E14 5DY.
Tel: (020) 7712 1758
Fax: (020) 7712 1759
info@chemicalsearch.co.uk

Chemidex
Chemidex Pharma Ltd
Chemidex House
Egham Business Village, Crabtree Rd, Egham
Surrey, TW20 8RB.
Tel: (01784) 477 167
Fax: (01784) 471 776
info@chemidex.co.uk

Chiron
Chiron Corporation Ltd
Symphony House
7 Cowley Business Park, High St, Cowley
Uxbridge, UB8 2AD.
Tel: (020) 8580 4000
Fax: (020) 8580 4001
medicalinfo-europe@chiron.com

Chiron Vaccines
Chiron Vaccines Ltd
Gaskill Rd
Speke, Liverpool L24 9GR.
Tel: (08457) 451 500
Fax: (0151) 7055 669
serviceuk@chiron.com

CHS
Cambridge Healthcare Supplies Ltd
14D Wendover Rd
Rackheath Industrial Estate, Rackheath
Norwich, NR13 6LH.
Tel: (01603) 735 200
Fax: (01603) 735 217
customerservices@typharm.com

Chugai
Chugai Pharma UK Ltd
Mulliner House, Flanders Rd
Turnham Green, London W4 1NN.
Tel: (020) 8987 5680
Fax: (020) 8987 5661

Clement Clarke
Clement Clarke International Ltd
Edinburgh Way
Harlow
Essex, CM20 2TT.
Tel: (01279) 414 969
Fax: (01279) 456 304
resp@clement-clarke.com

CliniMed
CliniMed Ltd
Cavell House, Knaves Beech Way
Loudwater, High Wycombe
Bucks, HP10 9QY.
Tel: (01628) 850 100
Fax: (01628) 850 331
enquires@clinimed.co.uk

Clinisupplies
Clinisupplies Ltd
9 Crystal Way
Elmgrove Rd, Harrow
Middx, HA1 2HP.
Tel: (020) 8863 4168
Fax: (020) 8426 0768
info@clinisupplies.co.uk

Clonmel
Clonmel Healthcare Ltd
Waterford Rd
Clonmel, Co. Tipperary
Ireland
Tel: (00353) 52 77777
Fax: (00353) 52 77799
info@clonmelhealthcare.com

Colgate-Palmolive
Colgate-Palmolive Ltd
Guildford Business Park
Middleton Rd, Guildford
Surrey, GU2 5LZ.
Tel: (01483) 302 222
Fax: (01483) 303 003

Coloplast
Coloplast Ltd
Peterborough Business Park
Peterborough PE2 6FX.
Tel: (01733) 392 000
Fax: (01733) 233 348
gbcareteam@coloplast.com

Community
Community Foods Ltd
Micross, Brent Terrace
London, NW2 1LT.
Tel: (020) 8450 9411
Fax: (020) 8208 1803
email@communityfoods.co.uk

Concord
Concord Pharmaceuticals Ltd
Bishops Weald House
Albion Way, Horsham RH12 1AH.
Tel: (0870) 241 2330
Fax: 0870 241 2335
enquiries@concordpharma.com

ConvaTec
ConvaTec Ltd
Harrington House, Milton Rd
Ickenham, Uxbridge
Middx, UB10 8PU.
Tel: (01895) 628 400
Fax: (01895) 628 456

Cow & Gate
See Nutricia Clinical.
Tel: (01225) 768 381
Fax: (01225) 768 847

CP
See Wockhardt.

Crawford
Crawford Pharmaceuticals
Furtho House
20 Towcester Rd, Milton Keynes
MK19 6AQ.
Tel: (01908) 262 346
Fax: (01908) 567 730

Crookes
Crookes Healthcare Ltd
D80 Building
Nottingham NG90 1LP.
Tel: (0115) 953 9922
Fax: (0115) 968 8722
medicalinfo@crookes.co.uk

DDD
DDD Ltd
94 Rickmansworth Rd
Watford
Herts, WD18 7JJ.
Tel: (01923) 229 251
Fax: (01923) 220 728

De Vilbiss
De Vilbiss Health Care UK Ltd
High Street
Wollaston, West Midlands
DY8 4PS.
Tel: (01384) 446 688
Fax: (01384) 446 699

De Witt
E C De Witt & Co Ltd
Tudor Rd
Manor Park, Runcorn
Cheshire, WA7 1SZ.
Tel: (01928) 579 029
Fax: (01928) 579 712
ecdewitt@ecdewitt.com

Denfleet
Denfleet Pharmaceuticals Ltd
260 Centennial Park
Elstree Hill South, Elstree
Herts, WD6 3SR.
Tel: (020) 8236 0000
Fax: (020) 8236 3501
medical.information@denfleet.com

Dental Health
Dental Health Products Ltd
60 Boughton Lane
Maidstone
Kent, ME15 9QS.
Tel: (01622) 749 222
Fax: (01622) 744 672

Dentsply
Dentsply Ltd
Hamm Moor Lane
Addlestone, Weybridge
Surrey, KT15 2SE.
Tel: (01932) 837 279
Fax: (01932) 858 970

Dermal
Dermal Laboratories Ltd
Tatmore Place
Gosmore, Hitchin
Herts, SG4 7QR.
Tel: (01462) 458 866
Fax: (01462) 420 565

Dexcel
Dexcel-Pharma Ltd
1 Cottesbrooke Park
Heartlands Business Park, Daventry
Northamptonshire, NN11 5YL.
Tel: (01327) 312 266
Fax: (01327) 312 262
office@dexcelpharma.co.uk

DiagnoSys
DiagnoSys Medical
Cams Hall
Fareham, Hants PO16 8AB.
Tel: 0800 085 8808
Fax: (01329) 227 599

Dimethaid
Dimethaid International
c/o Benoliel Partners
Linden House, Ewelme,
Oxfordshire OX10 6HQ.
Tel: (01491) 825 016
Fax: (01491) 834 592
medinfo@dimethaid.com

Dista
Dista Products Ltd
See Lilly.

Dr Falk
Dr Falk Pharma UK Ltd
Bourne End Business, Cores End Rd
Bourne End, Bucks SL8 5AS.
Tel: (01628) 536 600

DuPont
See Bristol-Myers Squibb.

Durbin
Durbin plc
180 Northolt Rd
South Harrow
Middx, HA2 0LT.
Tel: (020) 8869 6500
Fax: (020) 8869 6565
info@durbin.co.uk

Easigrip
Easigrip Ltd
Unit 13, Scar Bank
Millers Rd, Warwick
Warwickshire, CV34 5DB.
Tel: (01926) 497 108
Fax: (01926) 497 109
enquiry@easigrip.co.uk

Egis
Egis Pharmaceuticals UK Ltd
127 Shirland Rd
London W9 2EP.
Tel: (020) 7266 2669
Fax: (020) 7266 2702
enquiries@medimpexuk.com

Eisai
Eisai Ltd
3 Shortlands
Hammersmith, London W6 8EE.
Tel: (020) 8600 1400
Fax: (020) 8600 1401
Lmedinfo@eisai.net

Elida Fabergé
Elida Fabergé Ltd
Coal Rd
Seacroft
Leeds, LS14 2AR.
Tel: (0113) 222 5000
Fax: (0113) 222 5362

ENTACO
ENTACO Ltd
Royal Victoria Works,
Birmingham Rd, Studley,
Warwickshire B80 7AP.
Tel: (01527) 852 306
Fax: (01527) 857 447
sales@entaco.com

Epiderm
Epiderm Ltd
Wass Lane
Sotby, Market Rasen LN8 5LR.
Tel: (01507) 343 091
Fax: (01507) 343 092
djjcovermarkcryo@aol.com

Espire
Espire Healthcare Ltd
The Search Offices
Main Gate Road, The Historic
Dockyard
Chatham, ME4 4TE.
Tel: (01634) 812 144
Fax: (01634) 813 601
info@espirehealth.com

Ethicon
Ethicon Ltd
P.O. Box 1988
Simpson Parkway, Kirkton Campus
Livingston, EH54 0AB.
Tel: (01506) 594 500
Fax: (01506) 460 714

Everfresh
Everfresh Natural Foods
Gatehouse Close
Aylesbury
Bucks, HP19 3DE.
Tel: (01296) 425 333
Fax: (01296) 422 545

Exelgyn
Exelgyn Laboratories
PO Box 4511
Henley-on-Thames, Oxon
RG9 5ZQ.
Tel: (01491) 642 137
Fax: (0800) 731 6120

Fabre
Pierre Fabre Ltd
Hyde Abbey House
23 Hyde St, Winchester
Hampshire, SO23 7DR.
Tel: (01962) 856 956
Fax: (01962) 874 413
PFabreUK@aol.com

Farillon
Farillon Ltd
Ashton Rd
Harold Hill, Romford
Essex, RM3 8UE.
Tel: (01708) 379 000
Fax: (01708) 376 554

Fate
Fate Special Foods
Unit E2
Brook Street Business Centre, Brook
St, Tipton
West Midlands, DY4 9DD.
Tel: (01215) 224 433
Fax: (01215) 224 433

Fenton
Fenton Pharmaceuticals Ltd
4J Portman Mansions
Chiltern St, London W1U 6NS.
Tel: (020) 7224 1388
Fax: (020) 7486 7258
mail@Fent-Pharm.co.uk

Ferndale
Ferndale Pharmaceuticals Ltd
Unit 605, Thorp Arch Estate
Wetherby, West Yorks LS23 7BJ.
Tel: (01937) 541 122
Fax: (01937) 849 682
info@ferndalepharma.co.uk

Ferraris
Ferraris Medical Ltd
4 Harforde Court
John Tate Rd, Hertford
Herts, SG13 7NW.
Tel: (01992) 526 300
Fax: (01992) 526 320
info@fre.ferrarisgroup.com

Ferring
Ferring Pharmaceuticals (UK)
The Courtyard
Waterside Drive, Langley
Berks, SL3 6EZ.
Tel: (01753) 214 800
Fax: (01753) 214 801

Firstplay Dietary
Firstplay Dietary Foods Ltd
338 Turncroft Lane
Offerton, Stockport
Cheshire, SK1 4BP.
Tel: (0161) 474 7576
Fax: (0161) 474 7576

Florizel
Florizel Ltd
PO Box 138
Stevenage SG2 8YN.
Tel: (01462) 436 156
Fax: (01462) 457 402

Flynn
Flynn Pharma Ltd
2nd Floor, The Maltings
Bridge St, Hitchin
Herts, SG5 2DE.
Tel: (01462) 458 974
Fax: (01462) 450 755

Foodlink
Foodlink (UK) Ltd
2B Plymouth Rd
Plympton, Plymouth PL7 4JR.
Tel: (01752) 344 544
Fax: (01752) 342 412
info@foodlinkltd.co.uk

Ford
Ford Medical Associates Ltd
8 Wyndham Way
Orchard Heights, Ashford
Kent, TN25 4PZ.
Tel: (01233) 633 224
Fax: (01223) 646 595
enquiries@fordmedical.co.uk

Forest
Forest Laboratories UK Ltd
Bourne Rd
Bexley, Kent DA5 1NX.
Tel: (01322) 550 550
Fax: (01322) 555 469
medinfo@forest-labs.co.uk

Fournier
Fournier Pharmaceuticals Ltd
19-20 Progress Business Centre
Whittle Parkway
Slough, SL1 6DQ.
Tel: (01753) 740 400
Fax: (01753) 740 444

Fox
C. H. Fox Ltd
22 Tavistock St
London WC2E 7PY.
Tel: (020) 7240 3111
Fax: (020) 7379 3410

FP
Family Planning Sales Ltd
28 Kelburne Rd
Cowley, Oxford OX4 3SZ.
Tel: (01865) 772 486
Fax: (01865) 748 746

Fresenius Kabi
Fresenius Kabi Ltd
Hampton Court
Tudor Rd, Manor Park, Runcorn
Cheshire, WA7 1UF.
Tel: (01928) 594 200
Fax: (01928) 594 314
med.info-uk@fresenius-kabi.com

Frontier
Frontier Multigate
Newbridge Rd Industrial Estate
Blackwood
South Wales, NP12 2YL.
Tel: (01495) 233 050
Fax: (01495) 233 055
multigate@frontier-group.co.uk

Fujisawa
Fujisawa Ltd
Lovett House
Lovett Rd, Staines TW18 3AZ.
Tel: (01784) 419 615
Fax: (01784) 419 401
medinfo@fujisawa.co.uk

Galderma
Galderma (UK) Ltd
Galderma House
Church lane, Kings Langley
Herts, WD4 8JP.
Tel: (01923) 291 033
Fax: (01923) 291 060

Galen
Galen Ltd
Seagoe Industrial Estate
Craigavon, Northern Ireland
BT63 5UA.
Tel: (028) 3833 4974
Fax: (028) 3835 0206

Garnier
Laboratoires Garnier
255 Hammersmith Rd,
LondonW6 8AZ.
Tel: (020) 8762 4000
Fax: (020) 8762 4001

GBM
GBM Healthcare Ltd
Beechlawn House
Hurtmore Rd, Godalming
Surrey, GU7 2RA.
Tel: (01483) 860 881
Fax: (01483) 425 715
mba_gbm@compuserve.com

GE Healthcare
GE Healthcare
The Grove Centre, White Lion Rd
Amersham, Bucks HP7 9LL.
Tel: (01494) 544 000

Geistlich
Geistlich Pharma
Newton Bank
Long Lane, Chester CH2 2PF.
Tel: (01244) 347 534
Fax: (01244) 319 327

General Dietary
General Dietary Ltd
PO Box 38
Kingston upon Thames
Surrey, KT2 7YP.
Tel: (020) 8336 2323
Fax: (020) 8942 8274

Generics
Generics (UK) Ltd
Albany Gate
Darkes Lane, Potters Bar
Herts, EN6 1AG.
Tel: (01707) 853 000
Fax: (01707) 643 148

Genus
Genus Pharmaceuticals
Benham ValenceNewbury
Berks, RG20 8LU.
Tel: (01635) 568 400
Fax: (01635) 568 401
enquiries@genuspharma.com

Genzyme
Genzyme Biosurgery
4620 Kingsgate
Cascade Way, Oxford Business Park
South
Oxford, OX4 2SU.
Tel: (01865) 405 200
Fax: (01865) 774 172

Gilead
Gilead Sciences
The Flowers Building
Granta Park, Great Abington
Cambs, CB1 6GT.
Tel: (01223) 897 300
Fax: (01223) 897 282
ukmedinfo@gilead.com

GlaxoSmithKline
See GSK.

Glenwood
Glenwood Laboratories Ltd
Jenkins Dale
Chatham
Kent, ME4 5RD.
Tel: (01634) 830 535
Fax: (01634) 831 345
g.wooduk@virgin.net

Gluten Free Foods Ltd
Gluten Free Foods Ltd
Unit 270 Centennial Park
Centennial Ave, Elstree,
Borehamwood
Herts, WD6 3SS.
Tel: (020) 8953 4444
Fax: (020) 8953 8285
info@glutenfree-foods.co.uk

Goldshield
Goldshield Pharmaceuticals Ltd
NLA Tower
12-16 Addiscombe Rd, Croydon
CR0 0XT.
Tel: (020) 8649 8500
Fax: (020) 8686 0807

GP Pharma
GP Pharma
ARC Progress
Beckerings Park Rd, Lidlington
Beds, MK43 0RD.
Tel: (01525) 288 588
Fax: (01525) 289 339
info@gppharma.co.uk

Grünenthal
Grünenthal Ltd
Aston Court
Kingsmead Business Park,
Frederick Place
High Wycombe, Bucks, HP11 1LA.
Tel: (0870) 351 8960

Grifols
Grifols UK Ltd
72 St Andrew's Rd
Cambs CB4 1GS.
Tel: (01223) 446 900
Fax: (01223) 446 911
reception.uk@grifols.com

GSK
GlaxoSmithKline
Stockley Park West
Uxbridge
Middx, UB11 1BT.
Tel: 0800 221 441
Fax: (020) 8990 4328
customercontactuk@gsk.com

GSK Consumer Healthcare
GlaxoSmithKline Consumer Healthcare
GSK House
980 Great West Rd, Brentford
Middx, TW8 9GS.
Tel: (0500) 888 878
Fax: (020) 8047 6860
customer.relations@gsk.com

Hameln
Hameln Pharmaceuticals
Glevum Works
Upton St, Gloucester GL1 4LA.
Tel: (01452) 522 255
Fax: (01452) 306 051
enquiries@hameln.co.uk

Hartmann
Paul Hartmann Ltd
Unit P2, Parklands
Heywood Distribution Park,
Pilsworth Rd, Heywood
Lancs, OL10 2TT.
Tel: (01706) 363 200
Fax: (01706) 363 201
info@uk.hartmann.info

Hawgreen
Hawgreen Ltd
The Maltings, 2nd Floor
Bridge St, Hitchin
Herts, SG5 2DE.
Tel: (01462) 441 831
Fax: (01462) 435 868

Heinz
H. J. Heinz Company Ltd
South Building
Hayes Park, Hayes UB4 8AL.
Tel: (020) 8573 7757
Fax: (020) 8848 2325
Farleys_Heinz@Heinz.co.uk

Henleys
Henleys Medical Supplies Ltd
Brownfields
Welwyn Garden City
Herts, AL7 1AN.
Tel: (01707) 333 164
Fax: (01707) 334 795

Hillcross
AAH Pharmaceuticals Ltd
Sapphire Court
Walsgrave Triangle, Coventry
CV2 2TX.
Tel: (024) 7643 2000
Fax: (024) 7643 2001

HK Pharma
HK Pharma Ltd
PO Box 105
Hitchin
Herts, SG5 2GG.
Tel: (01462) 433 993
Fax: (01462) 450 755

Hoechst Marion Roussel
See Aventis Pharma.

Huntley
Huntley Pharmaceuticals Ltd
PO Box 2752
Marlborough, Wilts SN8 1ZH.
Tel: (0870) 240 2723
Fax: (01672) 514 187
info@huntley-pharma.co.uk

Hybrand
Hybrand Ltd
Eagle House, The Ring
Bracknell, Berks RG12 1HB.
Tel: (08700) 114 545
Fax: (08700) 114 646
customer.services@hybrand.com

Hypoguard
Hypoguard Ltd
Dock Lane
Melton, Woodbridge
Suffolk, IP12 1PE.
Tel: (01394) 387 333
Fax: (01394) 380 152
enquiries@hypoguard.com

IDIS
IDIS World Medicines
171-185 Ewell Rd
Millbank House, Surbiton
Surrey, KT6 6AX.
Tel: (020) 8410 0700
Fax: (020) 8410 0800
idis@idispharma.com

Infai
Infai UK Ltd
Innovation Centre
University of York Science Park,
University Rd
Heslington, York, YO10 5DG.
Tel: (01904) 435 228
Fax: (01904) 435 229
paul@infai.co.uk

Intrapharm
Intrapharm Laboratories Ltd
60 Boughton Lane
Maidstone
Kent, ME15 9QS.
Tel: (01622) 749 222
Fax: (01622) 744 672
sales@intraphamlabs.com

Invicta
See Pfizer.

Ipsen
Ipsen Ltd
190 Bath Rd
Slough, Berks SL1 3XE.
Tel: (01753) 627 777
Fax: (01753) 627 778
medical.information@ipsen.com

IVAX
IVAX Pharmaceuticals UK Ltd
IVAX Quay, Albert Basin
Royal Docks, London E16 2QJ.
Tel: (08705) 020 304
Fax: (08705) 323 334

J&J
Johnson & Johnson Ltd
Foundation Park
Roxborough Way, Maidenhead
Berks, SL6 3UG.
Tel: (01628) 822 222
Fax: (01628) 821 222

J&J Medical
Johnson & Johnson Medical
Coronation Rd
Ascot
Berks, SL5 9EY.
Tel: (01344) 871 000
Fax: (01344) 872 599

J&J MSD
Johnson & Johnson MSD
See McNeil.
Tel: (01494) 450 778
Fax: (01494) 450 487

Janssen-Cilag
Janssen-Cilag Ltd
PO Box 79
Saunderton, High Wycombe
Bucks, HP14 4HJ.
Tel: (01494) 567 567
Fax: (01494) 567 568

JHC
JHC Healthcare Ltd
The Maltings, 2nd Floor
Bridge St, Hitchin
Herts, SG5 2DE.
Tel: (01462) 432 533
Fax: (01462) 432 535

JLB
B. Braun JLB Ltd
Unit 2A
St Columb Industrial Estate, St Columb Major
Cornwall, TR9 6SF.
Tel: (01637) 880 065
Fax: (01637) 881 549

K/L
K/L Pharmaceuticals Ltd
21 Macadam Place
South Newmoor, Irvine
Ayrshire, KA11 4HP.
Tel: (01294) 215 951
Fax: (01294) 221 600

Kestrel
Kestrel Ltd
Ashfield House
Resolution Rd, Ashby de la Zouch
Leics, LE65 1HW.
Tel: (01530) 562 301
Fax: (01530) 562 430
kestrel@ventiv.co.uk

King
King Pharmaceuticals Ltd
3 Ash Street
Leicester LE5 0DA.
Tel: (01462) 434 366
Fax: (01462) 450 755

KoRa
KoRa Healthcare Ltd
Frans Maas House
Swords Business Park, Swords, Co. Dublin
Ireland, .Tel: (00353) 1890 0406
Fax: (00353) 1890 3016
Kora@ireland.com

Kyowa Hakko
Kyowa Hakko UK Ltd
258 Bath Rd
Slough
Berks, SL1 4DX.
Tel: (01753) 566 020
Fax: (01753) 566 030

LAB
Laboratories for Applied Biology
91 Amhurst Park
London N16 5DR.
Tel: (020) 8800 2252
Fax: (020) 8809 6884
enquiries@cerumol.com

Lederle
See Wyeth.

Leo
Leo Pharma
See LEO.
Tel: (01844) 347 333
Fax: (01844) 342 278
medical-info.uk@leo-pharma.com

LEO
LEO Pharma
Longwick Rd
Princes Risborough, Bucks
HP27 9RR.
Tel: (01844) 347 333
Fax: (01844) 342 278
medical-info.uk@leo-pharma.com

LifeScan
LifeScan
50-100 Holmers Farm Way
High Wycombe, Bucks HP12 4DP.
Tel: (01494) 658 750
Fax: (01494) 658 751

Lilly
Eli Lilly & Co Ltd
Lilly House
Priestley Rd, Basingstoke
Hampshire, RG24 9NL.
Tel: (01256) 315 999
Fax: (C 256) 775 858

Linderma
Linderma Ltd
Canon Bridge House
Canon Bridge, Madley
Hereford, HR2 9JF.
Tel: (01981) 250 124
Fax: (01981) 251 412
linderma@virgin.net

Link
Link Pharmaceuticals Ltd
Bishops Weald House
Albion Way, Horsham
West Sussex, RH12 1AH.
Tel: (01403) 272 451
Fax: (01403) 272 455
medical.information@linkpharm.co.uk

LPC
LPC Medical (UK) Ltd
30 Chaul End Lane
Luton, Beds LU4 8E2.
Tel: (01582) 560 393
Fax: (01582) 560 395
info@lpcpharma.com

Lundbeck
Lundbeck Ltd
Lundbeck House
Caldecotte Lake Business Park,
Caldecotte, Milton Keynes
Bucks, MK7 8LF.
Tel: (01908) 649 966
Fax: (01908) 647 888
ukmedicalinformation@lundbeck.com

Mölnlycke
Mölnlycke Health Care Ltd
The Arenson Centre
Arenson Way, Dunstable
Beds, LU5 5UL.
Tel: (0870) 606 0766
Fax: (0870) 608 1888
info.uk@molnlycke.net

Manx
Manx Healthcare
1 Hawkes Drive
Heathcote Industrial Estate,
Warwick
Warickshire, CV34 6LX.
Tel: (01926) 461 628
Fax: (01926) 461 621
info@manxhealthcare.com

Martindale
Martindale Pharmaceuticals Ltd
Hubert Rd
Brentwood, Essex CM14 4LZ.
Tel: (01277) 266 600
Fax: (01277) 848 976
info@martindalepharma.co.uk

MASTA
MASTA
Moorfield Rd
Yeadon
Leeds, LS19 7BN.
Tel: (0113) 238 7500
Fax: (0113) 238 7501
medical@masta.org

Mayne
Mayne Pharma plc
Queensway
Royal Leamington Spa,
Warwickshire CV31 3RW.
Tel: (01926) 820 820
Fax: (01926) 821 041
medinfouk@uk.maynepharma.com

McNeil
McNeil Ltd
Enterprise House, Station Rd
Loadwater, High Wycombe, Bucks
HP10 9UF.
Tel: (01494) 450 778
Fax: (01494) 450 487

MDE
MDE Diagnostics Europe Ltd
The Surrey Technology Centre
40 Occam Rd, Surrey Research Park, Guildford
Surrey, GU2 7YG.
Tel: (01483) 688 400info@mdediagnostic.co.uk

Mead Johnson
Mead Johnson Nutritionals
Uxbridge Business Park
Sanderson Rd, Uxbridge
Middx, UB8 1DH.
Tel: (00800) 8834 2568
Fax: (01895) 523 103

Meadow
Meadow Laboratories Ltd
18 Avenue Rd
Chadwell Heath, Romford
Essex, RM6 4JF.
Tel: (020) 8597 1203enquiries@meadowlabs.fsnet.co.uk

Meda
Meda Pharmaceuticals Ltd
Regus House, Herald Way
Pegasus Business Park, Castle Donnington
Derbyshire, DE74 2TZ.
Tel: (01332) 638 033
Fax: (01332) 638 192
information@uk.meda.se

Medac
Medac (UK)
Scion House, Stirling University
Stirling FK9 4NF.
Tel: (01786) 458 086
Fax: (01786) 458 032
info@medac-uk.co.uk

Medical House
The Medical House plc
199 Newhall Rd
Sheffield S9 2QJ.
Tel: (0114) 261 9011
Fax: (0114) 243 1597
info@themedicalhouse.com

Medigas
Medigas Ltd
Enterprise Drive
Four Ashes, Wolverhampton
WV10 7DF.
Tel: (01902) 791 944
Fax: (01902) 791 125

MediSense
MediSense
Abbott Laboratories Ltd
Mallory House, Vanwall Business Park
Maidenhead, Berks, SL6 4UD.
Tel: (01628) 678 900
Fax: (01628) 678 805

Medix
See Clement Clarke.

Medlock
Medlock Medical Ltd
Tubiton House
Medlock St., Oldham OL1 3HS.
Tel: (0161) 621 2100
Fax: (0161) 627 0932
medical.information@
medlockmedical.com

MedLogic
MedLogic Global Ltd
Western Wood Way
Langage Science Park, Plympton
Plymouth, Devon, PL7 5BG.
Tel: (01752) 209 955
Fax: (01752) 209 956
enquiries@mlgl.co.uk

Menarini
A. Menarini Pharma UK SRL
Menarini House
Mercury Park, Wycombe Lane,
Wooburn Green
Bucks, HP10 0HH.
Tel: (01628) 856 400
Fax: (01628) 856 402

Menarini Diagnostics
A. Menarini Diagnostics
Wharfedale Rd
Winnersh, Wokingham
Berks, RG41 5RA.
Tel: (0118) 944 4100
Fax: (0118) 944 4111

Merck
Merck Pharmaceuticals
Harrier House
High St, West Drayton
Middx, UB7 7QG.
Tel: (01895) 452 307
Fax: (01895) 452 296
medinfo@merckpharma.co.uk

Merck Consumer Health
See Seven Seas.

Merck Sharp & Dohme
See MSD.

Micro Medical
Micro Medical Ltd
Quayside
Chatham Maritime, Chatham
Kent, ME4 4QY.
Tel: (01634) 893 500
Fax: (01634) 893 600
sales@micromedical.co.uk

Milupa
Milupa Ltd
White Horse Business Park
Trowbridge, Wilts BA14 0XQ.
Tel: (01225) 711 511
Fax: (01225) 711 970

Molar
Molar Ltd
The Borough Yard
The Borough, Wedmore
Somerset, BS28 4EB.
Tel: (01934) 710 022
Fax: (01934) 710 033
info@molar.ltd.uk

MSD
Merck Sharp & Dohme Ltd
Hertford Rd
Hoddesdon
Herts, EN11 9BU.
Tel: (01992) 467 272
Fax: (01992) 451 066

Myogen
Myogen GmbH
PO Box 122
Richmond, North Yorks DL10 5YA.
Tel: (01748) 828 812
Fax: (01748) 828 801
info@myogen.de

Nagor
Nagor Ltd
PO Box 21, Global House
Isle of Man Business Park, Douglas
Isle of Man, IM99 1AX.
Tel: (01624) 625 556
Fax: (01624) 661 656
enquiries@nagor.com

Napp
Napp Pharmaceuticals Ltd
Cambridge Science Park
Milton Rd, Cambs CB4 0GW.
Tel: (01223) 424 444
Fax: (01223) 424 441

Neolab
Neolab Ltd
57 High St
Odiham, Hampshire RG29 1LF.
Tel: (01256) 704 110
Fax: (01256) 701 144
info@neolab.co.uk

Neomedic
Neomedic Ltd
2a Crofters Rd
Northwood, Middx HA6 3ED.
Tel: (01923) 836 379
Fax: (01923) 840 160
marketing@neomedic.co.uk

Nestlé
Nestlé UK Ltd
St. George's House
Park Lane, Croydon
Surrey, CR9 1NR.
Tel: (020) 8686 3333
Fax: (020) 8686 6072

Nestlé Clinical
Nestlé Clinical Nutrition
St George's House
Park Lane, Croydon
Surrey, CR9 1NR.
Tel: (020) 8667 5130
Fax: (020) 8667 6061
nutrition@uk.nestle.com

Network
Network Health & Beauty
Network House
41 Invincible Rd, Farnborough
Hants, GU14 7QU.
Tel: (01252) 533 333
Fax: (01252) 533 344
networkm@globalnet.co.uk

Neutrogena
See J&J.

Nordic
Nordic Pharma UK Ltd
Abbey House
1650 Arlington Business Park,
Theale
Reading, RG7 4SA.
Tel: (0118) 929 8233
Fax: (0118) 929 8234
info@nordicpharma.co.uk

Norgine
Norgine Ltd
Chaplin House
Moorhall Rd, Harefield
Middx, UB9 6NS.
Tel: (01895) 826 600
Fax: (01895) 825 865

Nova
Nova Laboratories Ltd
Martin House
Gloucester Crescent, Wigston
Leicester, LE18 4YL.
Tel: (0116) 223 0099
Fax: (0116) 223 0120
sales@novalabs.co.uk

Novartis
Novartis Pharmaceuticals UK Ltd
Frimley Business Park
Frimley, Camberley
Surrey, GU16 7SR.
Tel: (01276) 692 255
Fax: (01276) 692 508

Novartis Consumer Health
Novartis Consumer Health
Wimblehurst Rd
Horsham
West Sussex, RH12 5AB.
Tel: (01403) 210 211
Fax: (01403) 323 939
medicalaffairs.uk@ch.novartis.com

Novo Nordisk
Novo Nordisk Ltd
Broadfield Park
Brighton Rd, Crawley
West Sussex, RH11 9RT.
Tel: (01293) 613 555
Fax: (01293) 613 535
customercareuk@novonordisk.com

Nutricia Clinical
Nutricia Clinical Care
Nutricia Ltd
White Horse Business Park,
Trowbridge
Wilts, BA14 0XQ.
Tel: (01225) 711 688
Fax: (01225) 711 798
cndirect@nutricia.co.uk

Nutricia Dietary
Nutricia Dietary Care
see Nutricia Clinical.
Tel: (01225) 711 801
Fax: (01225) 711 567

Nutrition Point
Nutrition Point Ltd
13 Taurus Park
Westbrook, Warrington
Cheshire, WA5 7ZT.
Tel: (07041) 544 044
Fax: (07041) 544 055
info@nutritionpoint.co.uk

Nycomed
Nycomed UK Ltd
The Magdalen Centre
Oxford Science Park, Oxford
UX4 4GA.
Tel: (01865) 784 500
Fax: (01865) 784 501
nycomed.uk@nycomed.com

Octapharma
Octapharma Ltd
6 Elm Court
Copse Drive, Meriden Green,
Coventry CV5 9RG.
Tel: (01676) 521 000
Fax: (01676) 521 200
octapharma@octapharma.co.uk

Omron
Omron Healthcare (UK) Ltd
Opal Drive
Fox Milne, Milton Keynes
MK15 0DG.
Tel: (0870) 750 2771
Fax: (0870) 750 2772
info.omronhealthcare.uk@eu.omron.com

Opus
See Trinity.

Oral B Labs
Oral B Laboratories Ltd
Gillette Corner
Great West Rd, Isleworth
Middx, TW7 5NP.
Tel: (020) 8847 7800
Fax: (020) 8847 7828

Organon
Organon Laboratories Ltd
Cambridge Science Park
Milton Rd, Cambs CB4 0FL.
Tel: (01223) 432 700
Fax: (01223) 424 368
medrequest@organon.co.uk

Orion
Orion Pharma (UK) Ltd
Leat House, Overbridge Square
Hambridge Lane, Newbury
Berks, RG14 5UX.
Tel: (01635) 520 300
Fax: (01635) 520 319
medicalinformation@orionpharma.com

Orphan Europe
Orphan Europe (UK) Ltd
Isis House
43 Station Rd, Henley-on-Thames
Oxon, RG9 1AT.
Tel: (01491) 414 333
Fax: (01491) 414 443
info.uk@orphan-europe.com

Ortho Biotech
Ortho Biotech
PO Box 79
Saunderton, High Wycombe
Bucks, HP14 4HJ.
Tel: (0800) 389 2926
Fax: (01494) 567 568

Otsuka
Otsuka Pharmaceutical (UK) Ltd
BSi Tower
389 Chiswick High Rd, London
W4 4AJ.
Tel: (020) 8742 4300
Fax: (020) 8994 8548
medinfo@otsuka.co.uk

Owen Mumford
Owen Mumford Ltd
Brook Hill
Woodstock, Oxford OX20 1TU.
Tel: (01993) 812 021
Fax: (01993) 813 466
customerservices@owenmumford.co.uk

Paines & Byrne
Paines & Byrne Ltd
Lovett House
Lovett Rd, Staines
Middx, TW18 3AZ.
Tel: (01784) 419 620
Fax: (01784) 419 401

Parema
Parema Ltd
Sullington Rd
Shepshed, Loughborough
Leics, LE12 9JJ.
Tel: (01509) 502 051
Fax: (01509) 650 898

Pari
PARI Medical Ltd
Enterprise House
Station Approach, West Byfleet
Surrey, KT14 6NE.
Tel: (01932) 341 122
Fax: (01932) 341 134
parimedical@compuserve.com

Parke-Davis
See Pfizer.

Parkside
Parkside Healthcare
12 Parkside Ave
Salford M7 4HB.
Tel: (0161) 795 2792
Fax: (0161) 795 4076

Peckforton
Peckforton Pharmaceuticals Ltd
Crewe Hall
Crewe
Cheshire, CW1 6UL.
Tel: (01270) 582 255
Fax: (01270) 582 299
info@peckforton.com

Penn
Penn Pharmaceuticals Services Ltd
Unit 23 & 24, Tafarnaubach
Industrial Estate
Tredegar
Gwent, NP22 3AA.
Tel: (01495) 711 222
Fax: (01495) 711 225
penn@pennpharm.co.uk

Pfizer
Pfizer Ltd
Walton Oaks
Dorking Rd, Walton-on-the-Hill
Surrey, KT20 7NS.
Tel: (01304) 616 161
Fax: (01304) 656 221

Pfizer Consumer
Pfizer Consumer Healthcare
Walton Oaks
Dorking Rd, Walton-on-the-Hill
Surrey, KT20 7NS.
Tel: (01304) 616 161
Fax: (01304) 656 221

Pharma-Global
Pharma-Global Ltd
SEQ Ltd, Nerin House
26 Ridgeway St, Douglas, Isle of
Man IM1 1EL.
Tel: (01624) 692 999
Fax: (01624) 613 998

Pharmacia
see Pfizer
Tel: (01304) 616 161
Fax: (01304) 656 221

Pharmasol
Pharmasol Ltd
North Way, Walworth Industrial
Estate
Andover, Hampshire SP10 5AZ.
Tel: (01264) 363 117
Fax: (01264) 332 223
info@pharmasol.co.uk

Pharmion
Pharmion Ltd
Riverside House
Riverside Walk, Windsor
Berks, SL4 1NA.
Tel: (01753) 240 600
Fax: (01753) 240 656
info-UK@pharmion.com

Pickles
J. Pickles Healthcare
Beech House
62 High St, Knaresborough
N. Yorks, HG5 0EA.
Tel: (01423) 867 314
Fax: (01423) 869 177

Pinewood
Pinewood Healthcare
Ballymacabry
Clonmel, Co Tipperary, Eire.Tel:
(00353) 523 6253
Fax: (00353) 523 6311
info@pinewood.ie

PLIVA
PLIVA Pharma Ltd
Vision House
Bedford Rd, Petersfield
Hampshire, GU32 3QB.
Tel: (01730) 710900
Fax: (01730) 710901
medinfo@pliva-pharma.co.uk

Procter & Gamble
Procter & Gamble UK
The Heights
Brooklands, Weybridge
Surrey, KT13 0XP.
Tel: (01932) 896 000
Fax: (01932) 896 200

Procter & Gamble Pharm.
Procter & Gamble Technical
Centres
Medical Dept
Rusham Park, Whitehall Lane
Egham, Surrey, TW20 9NW.
Tel: (01784) 474 900
Fax: (01784) 474 705

Profile
Profile Pharma Ltd
Heath Place
Bognor Regis, West Sussex
PO22 9SL.
Tel: (0870) 770 2025
Fax: (0870) 770 2224
info@profilepharma.com

Profile Respiratory
Profile Respiratory Systems Ltd
Heath Place
Bognor Regis, West Sussex
PO22 9SL.
Tel: (0870) 770 3434
Fax: (0870) 770 3433
info@profilehs.com

Provalis
Provalis Healthcare Ltd
Newtech Square
Deeside Industrial Park, Deeside
Flintshire, CH5 2NT.
Tel: (01244) 288 888
Fax: (01244) 280 342
enquiries@provalis.plc.uk

R&C
See Reckitt Benckiser.

Ransom
Ransom Consumer Healthcare
104 Bancroft
Hitchin, Herts SG5 1LY.
Tel: (01462) 437 615
Fax: (01462) 443 512
info@williamransom.com

Reckitt Benckiser
Reckitt Benckiser Healthcare
Dansom Lane
Hull HU8 7DS.
Tel: (01482) 326 151
Fax: (01482) 582 526
miu@reckittbenckiser.com

Recordati
Recordati Pharmaceuticals Ltd
Ash House
Fairfield Avenue, Staines
Middx, TW18 4AB.
Tel: (01784) 224 237
Fax: (01784) 224 312

Rhône-Poulenc Rorer
See Aventis Pharma.

Richardson
Richardson Healthcare
Richardson House
Crondal Rd, Coventry
Warwickshire, CV7 9NH.
Tel: (08700) 111 126
Fax: (08700) 111 127

Robinsons
Robinson Healthcare Ltd
Lawn Rd
Carlton-in-Lindrick Industrial
Estate, Worksop
Notts, S81 9LB.
Tel: (01909) 735 001
Fax: (01909) 731 103
enquiries@robinsoncare.com

Roche
Roche Products Ltd
Hexagon Place
6 Falcon Way, Shire Park, Welwyn
Garden City
Herts, AL7 1TW.
Tel: (0800) 328 1629
Fax: (01707) 384 555
medinfo.uk@roche.com

Roche Consumer Health
See Bayer.

Roche Diagnostics
Roche Diagnostics Ltd
Bell Lane
Lewes
East Sussex, BN7 1LG.
Tel: (01273) 480 444
Fax: (01273) 480 266

Rosemont
Rosemont Pharmaceuticals Ltd
Rosemont House
Yorkdale Industrial Park, Braithwaite
St
Leeds, LS11 9XE.
Tel: (0113) 244 1999
Fax: (0113) 246 0738
info@rosemontpharma.com

Rowa
Rowa Pharmaceuticals Ltd
Bantry
Co Cork, Ireland.
Tel: (00 353 27) 50077
Fax: (00 353 27) 50417
rowa@rowa-pharma.ie

Rybar
See Shire.

S&N Hlth.
Smith & Nephew Healthcare Ltd
Healthcare House
Goulton St, Hull HU3 4DJ.
Tel: (01482) 222 200
Fax: (01482) 222 211
advice@smith-nephew.com

Sallis
E. Sallis Ltd
Vernon Works
Waterford St, Basford
Nottingham, NG6 0DH.
Tel: (0115) 978 7841
Fax: (0115) 942 2272

Sandoz
Sandoz Ltd
37 Woolmer Way
Bordon, Hants GU35 9QE.
Tel: (01420) 478 301
Fax: (01420) 474 427

Sankyo
Sankyo Pharma UK Ltd
Sankyo House
Repton Place, White Lion Rd,
Amersham
Bucks, HP7 9LP.
Tel: (01494) 766 866
Fax: (01494) 766 557
medinfo@sankyo.co.uk

Sanochemia
Sanochemia Diagnostics UK Ltd
Argentum
510 Bristol Business Park,
Coldharbour Lane
Bristol, BS16 1EJ.
Tel: (0117) 906 3562
Fax: (0117) 906 3709

Sanofi-Aventis
Sanofi-Aventis Ltd
1 Onslow St
Guildford
Surrey, GU1 4YS.
Tel: (01483) 505 515
Fax: (01483) 535 432
uk-medicalinformation@sanofi-aventis.com

Sanofi Pasteur
Sanofi Pasteur MSD Ltd
Mallards Reach
Bridge Avenue, Maidenhead
Berks, SL6 1QP.
Tel: (01628) 785 291
Fax: (01628) 671 722

Sanofi-Synthelabo
See Sanofi-Aventis

Schering Health
Schering Health Care Ltd
The Brow
Burgess Hill
West Sussex, RH15 9NE.
Tel: (0845) 609 6767
Fax: (01444) 465 878
customer.care@schering.co.uk

Schering-Plough
Schering-Plough Ltd
Shire Park
Welwyn Garden City
Herts, AL7 1TW.
Tel: (01707) 363 636
Fax: (01707) 363 763
medical.info@spcorp.com

Schwarz
Schwarz Pharma Ltd
Schwarz House
East St, Chesham
Bucks, HP5 1DG.
Tel: (01494) 797 500
Fax: (01494) 774 960
medinfo@schwarzpharma.co.uk

Searle
See Pfizer.

Serono
Serono Pharmaceuticals Ltd
Bedfont Cross
Stanwell Rd, Feltham
Middx, TW14 8NX.
Tel: (020) 8818 7200
Fax: (020) 8818 7222
serono_uk@serono.com

Servier
Servier Laboratories Ltd
Gallions
Wexham Springs, Framewood Rd
Wexham, SL3 6RL.
Tel: (01753) 662 744
Fax: (01753) 663 456

Seven Seas
Seven Seas Ltd
Hedon Rd
Marfleet, Hull HU9 5NJ.
Tel: (01482) 375 234
Fax: (01482) 374 345

Shiloh
Shiloh Healthcare Ltd
Lion Mill
Fitton St, Royton
Oldham, OL2 5JX.
Tel: (0161) 624 5641
Fax: (0161) 627 0902
enquiry@shiloh.co.uk

Shire
Shire Pharmaceuticals Ltd
Hampshire International Business Park
Chineham, Basingstoke
Hants, RG24 8EP.
Tel: (01256) 894 000
Fax: (01256) 894 708

SHS
SHS International Ltd
100 Wavertree Boulevard
Wavertree Technology Park,
Liverpool L7 9PT.
Tel: (0151) 228 8161
Fax: (0151) 230 5365
seve@shsint.co.uk

Sigma
Sigma Pharmaceuticals plc
PO Box 233
Unit 1-7 Colonial Way, Watford
Herts, WD24 4YR.
Tel: (01923) 444 999
Fax: (01923) 444 998
info@sigpharm.co.uk

Sinclair
Sinclair Pharmaceuticals Ltd
Borough Rd
Godalming
Surrey, GU7 2AB.
Tel: (01483) 426 644
Fax: (01483) 860 927
info@sinclairpharma.com

SMA Nutrition
See Wyeth.

SNBTS
Scottish National Blood Transfusion Service
Protein Fractionation Centre
Ellen's Glen Rd, Edinburgh
EH17 7QT.
Tel: (0131) 536 5700
Fax: (0131) 536 5781

Solvay
Solvay Healthcare Ltd
Mansbridge RdWest End
Southampton, SO18 3JD.
Tel: (023) 8046 7000
Fax: (023) 8046 5350
medinfo.shl@solvay.com

Sovereign
Sovereign Medical
Sovereign House
Miles Gray Rd, Basildon
Essex, SS14 3FR.
Tel: (01268) 535 200
Fax: (01268) 535 299

Special Products
Special Products Ltd
Orion House
49 High Street, Addlestone
Surrey, KT15 1TU.
Tel: (01932) 820 666
Fax: (01932) 850 444
graham.march@specprod.co.uk

Specials Laboratory
The Specials Laboratory Ltd
Unit 1, Regents Drive
Lower Prudhoe Industrial Estate,
Northumberland NE42 6PX.
Tel: (0800) 028 4925
Fax: (0800) 083 4222

Squibb
See Bristol-Myers Squibb.

SSL
See Medlock.

STD Pharmaceutical
STD Pharmaceutical Products Ltd
Plough Lane
Hereford HR4 0EL.
Tel: (01432) 373 555
Fax: (01432) 373 556
enquiries@stdpharm.co.uk

Sterling Health
See GSK Consumer Healthcare.

Sterwin
See Winthrop.

Stiefel
Stiefel Laboratories (UK) Ltd
Holtspur Lane
Wooburn Green, High Wycombe
Bucks, HP10 0AU.
Tel: (01628) 524 966
Fax: (01628) 810 021
general@stiefel.co.uk

Strakan
Strakan Ltd
Buckholm Mill
Galashiels TD1 2HB.
Tel: (01896) 668 060
Fax: (01896) 668 061
medinfo@strakan.com

Sutherland
Sutherland Health Ltd
Unit 1, Rivermead
Pipers Way, Thatcham
Berks, RG19 4EP.
Tel: (01635) 874 488
Fax: (01635) 877 622

Swedish Orphan
Swedish Orphan International (UK) Ltd
The White House
Wilderspool Park, Greenalls Ave,
Stockton Heath, Warrington
Cheshire, WA4 6HL.
Tel: (01925) 438 028
Fax: (01925) 438 001

Syner-Med
Syner-Med (Pharmaceutical Products) Ltd
Beech House
840 Brighton Rd, Purley CR8 2BH.
Tel: (0845) 634 2100
Fax: (0845) 634 2101
mail@syner-med.com

Takeda
Takeda UK Ltd
Takeda House, Mercury Park
Wycombe Lane, Wooburn Green
High Wycombe, Bucks, HP10 0HH.
Tel: (01628) 537 900
Fax: (01628) 526 615

Taro
Taro Pharmaceuticals (UK) Ltd
1st Floor, Prince of Wales House
3 Bluecoats Ave, Hertford
SG14 1PB.
Tel: (01992) 557 445
Fax: (01992) 557 447
customerservice@taropharma.co.uk

Tarus
See Chemidex.

Teva
Teva Pharmaceuticals Ltd
Barclays House
1 Gatehouse Way, Aylesbury
Bucks, HP19 8DB.
Tel: (01296) 719 768
Fax: (01296) 719 769
info@tevapharma.co.uk

TEVA UK
TEVA UK Ltd
Brampton Rd
Hampden Park, Eastbourne, East
Sussex BN22 9AG.
Tel: (01323) 501 111
Fax: (01323) 520 306

TheraSense
TheraSense UK
Centaur House
Ancells Business Park, Ancells Rd,
Fleet
Hants, GU51 2UJ.
Tel: (01252) 761 392
Fax: (01252) 761 393

Thornton & Ross
Thornton & Ross Ltd
Linthwaite Laboratories
Huddersfield, HD7 5QH.
Tel: (01484) 842 217
Fax: (01484) 847 301
mail@thorntonross.com

Tillomed
Tillomed Laboratories Ltd
3 Howard Rd
Eaton Socon, St Neots, Cambs
PE19 3ET.
Tel: (01480) 402 400
Fax: (01480) 402 402
info@tillomed.co.uk

TOL
Tree of Life
Coaldale Rd
Lymedale Business Park, Newcastle
Under Lyme
Staff, ST5 9QX.
Tel: (01782) 567 100
Fax: (01782) 567 199
health@tol-europe.com

Torbet
Torbet Laboratories Ltd
14D Wendover Rd
Rackheath Industrial Estate, Rackheath
Norwich, NR13 6LH.
Tel: (01603) 735 200
Fax: (01603) 735 217
torbet@typharm.com

Trinity
Trinity Pharmaceuticals Ltd
See Trinity-Chiesi.

Trinity-Chiesi
Trinity-Chiesi Pharmaceuticals Ltd
The Old Exchange
12 Compton Rd, Wimbledon
London, SW19 6QD.
Tel: (020) 8944 9443
Fax: (020) 8947 9325

TSL
Tissue Science Laboratories plc
Victoria House
Victoria Rd, Aldershot
Hants, GU11 1EJ.
Tel: (01252) 333 002
Fax: (01252) 333 010
enquiries@tissuescience.com

Tyco
Tyco Healthcare
154 Fareham Rd
Gosport
Hants, PO13 0AS.
Tel: (01329) 224 000

Typharm
Typharm Ltd
14D Wendover Rd
Rackheath Industrial Estate,
Rackheath
Norwich, NR13 6LH.
Tel: (01603) 735 200
Fax: (01603) 735 217
customerservices@typharm.com

UCB Pharma
UCB Pharma Ltd
208 Bath Rd
Slough SL1 3WE.
Tel: (01753) 534 655
Fax: (01753) 536 632
medicaluk@ucb-group.com

Ultrapharm
Ultrapharm Ltd
Centenary Business Park
Henley-on-Thames
Oxon, RG9 1DS.
Tel: (01491) 578 016
Fax: (01491) 570 001
orders@glutenfree.co.uk

Univar
Univar Ltd
International House
Zenith, Paycocke Rd, Basildon
Essex, SS14 3DW.
Tel: (01268) 594 400
Fax: (01268) 594 481
trientine@univareurope.com

Unomedical
Unomedical Ltd
Thornhill Rd
Redditch B98 7NL.
Tel: (01527) 587 700
Fax: (01527) 592 111

Valeant
Valeant Pharmaceuticals Ltd
Cedarwood
Chineham Business Park, Crockford
Lane, Basingstoke
Hants, RG24 8WD.
Tel: (01256) 707 744
Fax: (01256) 707 334
valeantuk@valeant.com

Vernon-Carus
Vernon-Carus Ltd
Penwortham Mills
Preston
Lancs, PR1 9SN.
Tel: (01772) 744 493
Fax: (01772) 748 754
mail@vernon-carus.co.uk

Viatris
Viatris Pharmaceuticals Ltd
Building 2000, Beach Drive
Cambridge Research Park,
Waterbeach, Cambs CB5 9PD.
Tel: (01223) 205 999
Fax: (01223) 205 998
info@viatrisuk.co.uk

Vitaflo
Vitaflo Ltd
11 Century Building
Brunswick Business Park, Liverpool
L3 4BL.
Tel: (0151) 709 9020
Fax: (0151) 709 9727
vitaflo@vitaflo.co.uk

Vitaline
Vitaline Pharmaceuticals UK Ltd
8 Ridge Way
Drakes Drive, Crendon Business
Park
Long Crendon, Bucks, HP18 9BF.
Tel: (01844) 202 044
Fax: (01844) 202 077
vitalineinfo@aol.com

Vitalograph
Vitalograph Ltd
Maids Moreton
Buckingham, MK18 1SW.
Tel: (01280) 827 110
Fax: (01280) 823 302
sales@vitalograph.co.uk

W-L
Warner Lambert UK Ltd
See Pfizer.

Wallace Mfg
Wallace Manufacturing Chemists Ltd
Wallace House
New Abbey Court, 51-53 Stert St,
Abingdon
Oxon, OX14 3JF.
Tel: (01235) 538 700
Fax: (01235) 538 800
info@alinter.co.uk

Wanskerne
Wanskerne Ltd
44 Broomfield Drive
Billingshurst RH4 9TN.
Tel: (01403) 783 214
Fax: (01403) 783 214

Warner Lambert
See Pfizer.

Winthrop
Winthrop Pharmaceuticals UK Ltd
PO Box 611
Guildford, Surrey GU1 4YS.
Tel: (01483) 554 101
Fax: (01483) 554 810
sterwin.sales@sterwin.com

Wockhardt
Wockhardt UK Ltd
Ash Rd North
Wrexham Industrial Estate,
Wrexham LL13 9UF.
Tel: (01978) 661 261
Fax: (01978) 660 130

Wyeth
Wyeth Pharmaceuticals
Huntercombe Lane South
Taplow, Maidenhead
Berks, SL6 0PH.
Tel: (01628) 604 377
Fax: (01628) 666 368
ukmedinfo@wyeth.com

Wynlit
Wynlit Laboratories
153 Furzehill Rd
Borehamwood, Herts WD6 2DR.
Tel: (07903) 370 130
Fax: (020) 8292 6117

Wyvern
Wyvern Medical Ltd
PO Box 17
Ledbury
Herefordshire, HR8 2ES.
Tel: (01531) 631 105
Fax: (01531) 634 844

Yamanouchi
Yamanouchi Pharma Ltd
Lovett House
Lovett Rd, Staines
Middx, TW18 3AZ.
Tel: (01784) 419 615
Fax: (01784) 419 401

Zeal
G. H. Zeal Ltd
Deer Park Rd
London SW19 3UU.
Tel: (020) 8542 2283
Fax: (020) 8543 7840
scientific@zeal.co.uk

Zeneus
Zeneus Pharma Ltd
Abel Smith House
Gunnels Wood Rd, Stevenage, Herts
SG1 2BT.
Tel: (01438) 731 731
Fax: (01438) 765 080
medinfo@zeneuspharma.com

Zeroderma
Zeroderma Ltd
The Manor House
Victor Barns, Northampton Rd,
Brixworth
Northampton, NN6 9DQ.
Tel: (01604) 889 855
Fax: (01604) 883 199
info@ixlpharma.com

ZLB
ZLB Bioplasma UK Ltd
Breckland House
St. Nicholas St, Thetford
Norfolk, IP24 1BT.
Tel: (01842) 755 025
Fax: (01842) 755 174
info-uk@zlb.com

ZLB Behring
ZLB Behring UK Ltd
Hayworth House
Market Place, Haywards Heath
West Sussex, RH16 1DB.
Tel: (01444) 447 400
Fax: (01444) 447 401
medinfo@zlbbehring.com

Zurich
See Trinity.

Special-order manufacturers

The following **companies** manufacture 'special-order' products: BCM Specials, Fresenius, Martindale, Nova Laboratories, Phoenix, Rosemont, Special Products, The Specials Laboratory (see Index of Manufacturers for contact details).

Hospital manufacturing units also manufacture 'special-order' products, details may be obtained from any of the centres listed below.

> It should be noted that when a product has a licence the *Department of Health recommends that the licensed product should be ordered* unless a specific formulation is required

England

East Anglian and Oxford

Mr G. Hanson,
Production Manager
Pharmacy Manufacturing Unit
Ipswich Hospital NHS Trust
Heath Rd
Ipswich, IP4 5PD.
Tel: (01473) 703 603
Fax: (01473) 703 609
con.hanson@ipswichhospital.nhs.uk

London

Mr M. Lillywhite,
Director of Technical Services
Barts and the London NHS Trust, St. Bartholomew's Hospital
West Smithfield
London, EC1A 7BE.
Tel: (020) 7601 7491
Fax: (020) 7601 7486
mike.lillywhite@bartsandthelondon.nhs.uk

Mr P. Forsey,
Production Manager
Guy's and St. Thomas' Hospital Trust
St. Thomas' Hospital,
Lambeth Palace Rd
London, SE1 7EH.
Tel: (020) 7118 4992
Fax: (020) 7118 5013
paul.forsey@gstt.sthames.nhs.uk

Mr C. Evans,
Production Manager
Pharmacy Department
St. George's Hospital
Blackshaw Rd
Tooting, London SW17 0QT.
Tel: (020) 8725 1770
Fax: (020) 8725 3690
chris.evans@stgeorges.nhs.uk

Mr A. Krol,
Director of Commercial Services
Pharmaceutical Manufacturing Unit
Moorfields Eye Hospital NHS Trust
34 Nile St
London, N1 7LX.
Tel: (020) 7684 8561 / 8562
Fax: 0800 328 8191
alan.krol@moorfields.nhs.uk

North West

Mr M.D. Booth,
Production & Aseptic Services Manager
Stockport Pharmaceuticals
Stepping Hill Hospital
Poplar Grove
Stockport, Cheshire SK2 7JE.
Tel: (0161) 419 5657
Fax: (0161) 419 5664
mike.booth@stockport-tr.nwest.nhs.uk

Northern

Mr Ian Smeaton
Production and Quality Control Unit
Royal Victoria Infirmary
Queen Victoria Rd
Newcastle-upon-Tyne, NE1 4LP.
Tel: (0191) 282 0377
Fax: (0191) 282 0376
pharmacy.tpn@nuth.northy.nhs.uk

South East

Mr F. Brown,
Production Manager
Pharmacy Production Unit
St Peter's Hospital
Guildford Rd
Chertsey, Surrey KT16 OPZ.
Tel: (01932) 722 520
Fax: (01932) 873 632
fraser.brown@asph.nhs.uk

Ms G. Middlehurst,
Production Manager
Pharmacy Manufacturing Unit
Queen Alexandra Hospital
Cosham
Portsmouth, Hants PO6 3LY.
Tel: (02392) 286 335
Fax: (02392) 378 288
gillian.middlehurst@porthosp.nhs.uk

South Western

Mr P. S. Bendell,
Principal Pharmacist
Unit Manager, Torbay PMU
South Devon Healthcare
Long Rd
Paignton, Devon TQ4 7TW.
Tel: (01803) 664 707
Fax: (01803) 664 354
phil.bendell@sdevonhc-tr.swest.nhs.uk

Trent

Mr R.W. Brookes,
Production Pharmacist
Royal Hallamshire Hospital
Glossop Rd, Sheffield, S10 2JF.
Tel: (0114) 271 3104
Fax: (0114) 271 2783
roger.brookes@sth.nhs.uk

West Midlands

Mr A. Broad,
Principal Pharmacist
Sterile Fluids Manufacturing Unit
Queen Elizabeth Medical Centre
Edgbaston, Birmingham, B15 2TH.
Tel: (0121) 627 2326
Fax: (0121) 627 2168
alan.broad@uhb.nhs.uk

Mr P.G. Williams,
Principal Pharmacist
Pharmacy Manufacturing Unit
Queens Hospital
Burton Hospitals NHS Trust,
Belvedere Rd, Burton-on-Trent,
DE13 0RB.
Tel: (01283) 566 333/511 511
Extn 5138
Fax: (01283) 593 036
paul.williams@burtonh-tr.wmids.nhs.uk

Yorkshire

Dr J. Harwood,
Production Manager
Pharmacy Manufacturing Unit
Huddersfield Royal Infirmary
Lindley, Huddersfield, West Yorks
HD3 3EA.
Tel: (01484) 342 421
Fax: (01484) 342 074
john.harwood@cht.nhs.uk

Northern Ireland

Principal Pharmacist
Victoria Pharmaceuticals
The Royal Hospitals
77 Boucher Cres, Belfast,
BT12 6HU.
Tel: (028) 9055 3407
Fax: (028) 9055 3498

Scotland

Mr J.A. Cook,
Principal Pharmacist—Production
Tayside Pharmaceuticals
Ninewells Hospital
Dundee, DD1 9SY.
Tel: (01382) 632 273
Fax: (01382) 632 060
jon.a.cook@tuht.scot.nhs.uk

Wales

Mr P. Spark,
Principal Pharmacist
Pharmacy Department
Cardiff and Vale NHS Trust
Heath Park, Cardiff, CF14 4XW.
Tel: (029) 2074 4828
Fax: (029) 2074 3114
paul.spark@cardiffandvale.wales.nhs.uk

Index

Principal page references are printed in **bold** type. Proprietary (trade) names and names of organisms are printed in *italic* type; where the BNF does not include a full entry for a branded product, the non-proprietary name is shown in brackets.

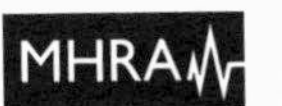

In Confidence

SUSPECTED ADVERSE DRUG REACTIONS

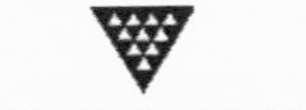

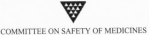

COMMITTEE ON SAFETY OF MEDICINES

If you suspect that an adverse reaction may be related to a drug, or a combination of drugs, you should complete this Yellow Card or complete a report on the website at www.yellowcard.gov.uk. For *intensively monitored medicines* (identified by ▼) report **all** suspected reactions (including any considered not to be serious). For *established drugs* and *herbal remedies* report **all serious** adverse reactions in adults; report **all serious and minor** adverse reactions in **children** (under 18 years). You do not have to be certain about causality: if in doubt, please report. Do not be put off reporting just because some details are not known. See BNF (page 10) or the MHRA website (http://medicines.mhra.gov.uk) for additional advice.

PATIENT DETAILS Patient Initials: ______ Sex: M / F Weight if known (kg): ______

Age (at time of reaction): ______ Identification (Your Practice / Hospital Ref.)*: ______

SUSPECTED DRUG(S)

Give brand name of drug and batch number if known	Route	Dosage	Date started	Date stopped	Prescribed for

SUSPECTED REACTION(S)

Please describe the reaction(s) and any treatment given:

Outcome

Recovered ☐
Recovering ☐
Continuing ☐
Other ☐

Date reaction(s) started: ______ Date reaction(s) stopped: ______

Do you consider the reaction to be serious? Yes / No

If *yes*, please indicate why the reaction is considered to be serious (please tick all that apply):

Patient died due to reaction ☐ Involved or prolonged inpatient hospitalisation ☐
Life threatening ☐ Involved persistent or significant disability or incapacity ☐
Congenital abnormality ☐ Medically significant; please give details:

* This is to enable you to identify the patient in any future correspondence concerning this report

Please attach additional pages if necessary

Please list other drugs taken in the last 3 months prior to the reaction (including self-medication & herbal remedies)

Was the patient on any other medication? Yes / No

If *yes*, please give the following information if known:

Drug (Brand, if known)	Route	Dosage	Date started	Date stopped	Prescribed for

Additional relevant information e.g. medical history, test results, known allergies, rechallenge (if performed), suspected drug interactions. For congenital abnormalities please state all other drugs taken during pregnancy and the date of the last menstrual period.

REPORTER DETAILS

Name and Professional Address: __________

Post code: __________ Tel No: __________

Speciality: __________

Signature: Date:

CLINICIAN (if not the reporter)

Name and Professional Address: __________

Post code: __________

Tel No: __________ Speciality: __________

If you would like information about other adverse reactions associated with the suspected drug, please tick this box ☐

Send to **Medicines and Healthcare Products Regulatory Agency, CSM FREEPOST, LONDON SW8 5BR** or if you are in one of the following NHS regions:

to **CSM Mersey, FREEPOST, Liverpool L3 3AB**
or **CSM Northern, FREEPOST 1085, Newcastle upon Tyne NE1 1BR**
or **CSM West Midlands, FREEPOST SW2991, Birmingham B18 7BR**
or **CSM Scotland, CARDS, FREEPOST NAT3271, Edinburgh EH16 4BR**
or **CSM Wales, FREEPOST, Cardiff CF4 1ZZ**

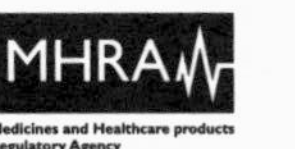

In Confidence

SUSPECTED ADVERSE DRUG REACTIONS

COMMITTEE ON SAFETY OF MEDICINES

If you suspect that an adverse reaction may be related to a drug, or a combination of drugs, you should complete this Yellow Card or complete a report on the website at www.yellowcard.gov.uk. For *intensively monitored medicines* (identified by ▼) report **all** suspected reactions (including any considered not to be serious). For *established drugs* and *herbal remedies* report **all serious** adverse reactions in adults; report **all serious and minor** adverse reactions in **children** (under 18 years). You do not have to be certain about causality: if in doubt, please report. Do not be put off reporting just because some details are not known. See BNF (page 10) or the MHRA website (http://medicines.mhra.gov.uk) for additional advice.

PATIENT DETAILS Patient Initials: ____________ Sex: M / F Weight if known (kg): ____________

Age (at time of reaction): ____________ Identification (Your Practice / Hospital Ref.)*: ____________

SUSPECTED DRUG(S)

Give brand name of drug and batch number if known	Route	Dosage	Date started	Date stopped	Prescribed for

SUSPECTED REACTION(S)

Please describe the reaction(s) and any treatment given:

Outcome

- Recovered ☐
- Recovering ☐
- Continuing ☐
- Other ☐

Date reaction(s) started: ____________ Date reaction(s) stopped: ____________

Do you consider the reaction to be serious? Yes / No

If *yes*, please indicate why the reaction is considered to be serious (please tick all that apply):

- Patient died due to reaction ☐
- Life threatening ☐
- Congenital abnormality ☐
- Involved or prolonged inpatient hospitalisation ☐
- Involved persistent or significant disability or incapacity ☐
- Medically significant; please give details:

* This is to enable you to identify the patient in any future correspondence concerning this report

Please attach additional pages if necessary

Please list other drugs taken in the last 3 months prior to the reaction (including self-medication & herbal remedies)

Was the patient on any other medication? Yes / No

If *yes*, please give the following information if known:

Drug (Brand, if known)	Route	Dosage	Date started	Date stopped	Prescribed for

Additional relevant information e.g. medical history, test results, known allergies, rechallenge (if performed), suspected drug interactions. For congenital abnormalities please state all other drugs taken during pregnancy and the date of the last menstrual period.

REPORTER DETAILS

Name and Professional Address: ______________________

Post code: ____________ Tel No: ____________

Speciality: ______________________

Signature: Date:

CLINICIAN (if not the reporter)

Name and Professional Address: ______________________

Post code: ____________

Tel No: ____________ Speciality: ____________

If you would like information about other adverse reactions associated with the suspected drug, please tick this box ☐

Send to **Medicines and Healthcare Products Regulatory Agency, CSM FREEPOST, LONDON SW8 5BR** or if you are in one of the following NHS regions:

to **CSM Mersey, FREEPOST, Liverpool L3 3AB**
or **CSM Northern, FREEPOST 1085, Newcastle upon Tyne NE1 1BR**
or **CSM West Midlands, FREEPOST SW2991, Birmingham B18 7BR**
or **CSM Scotland, CARDS, FREEPOST NAT3271, Edinburgh EH16 4BR**
or **CSM Wales, FREEPOST, Cardiff CF4 1ZZ**

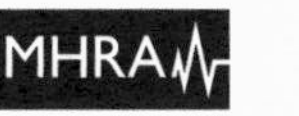

In Confidence

SUSPECTED ADVERSE DRUG REACTIONS

COMMITTEE ON SAFETY OF MEDICINES

If you suspect that an adverse reaction may be related to a drug, or a combination of drugs, you should complete this Yellow Card or complete a report on the website at www.yellowcard.gov.uk. For *intensively monitored medicines* (identified by ▼) report **all** suspected reactions (including any considered not to be serious). For *established drugs* and *herbal remedies* report **all serious** adverse reactions in adults; report **all serious and minor** adverse reactions in **children** (under 18 years). You do not have to be certain about causality: if in doubt, please report. Do not be put off reporting just because some details are not known. See BNF (page 10) or the MHRA website (http://medicines.mhra.gov.uk) for additional advice.

PATIENT DETAILS Patient Initials: ____________ Sex: M / F Weight if known (kg): ____________

Age (at time of reaction): ____________ Identification (Your Practice / Hospital Ref.)*: ____________

SUSPECTED DRUG(S)

Give brand name of drug and batch number if known	Route	Dosage	Date started	Date stopped	Prescribed for

SUSPECTED REACTION(S)

Please describe the reaction(s) and any treatment given:

Outcome

Recovered ☐
Recovering ☐
Continuing ☐
Other ☐

Date reaction(s) started: ____________ Date reaction(s) stopped: ____________

Do you consider the reaction to be serious? Yes / No

If *yes*, please indicate why the reaction is considered to be serious (please tick all that apply):

Patient died due to reaction ☐
Life threatening ☐
Congenital abnormality ☐
Involved or prolonged inpatient hospitalisation ☐
Involved persistent or significant disability or incapacity ☐
Medically significant; please give details:

* This is to enable you to identify the patient in any future correspondence concerning this report

Please attach additional pages if necessary

Please list other drugs taken in the last 3 months prior to the reaction (including self-medication & herbal remedies)

Was the patient on any other medication? Yes / No

If *yes*, please give the following information if known:

Drug (Brand, if known)	Route	Dosage	Date started	Date stopped	Prescribed for

Additional relevant information e.g. medical history, test results, known allergies, rechallenge (if performed), suspected drug interactions. For congenital abnormalities please state all other drugs taken during pregnancy and the date of the last menstrual period.

REPORTER DETAILS

Name and Professional Address: ____________

Post code: ________ Tel No: ________

Speciality: ____________

Signature: Date:

CLINICIAN (if not the reporter)

Name and Professional Address: ____________

Post code: ________

Tel No: ________ Speciality: ________

If you would like information about other adverse reactions associated with the suspected drug, please tick this box ☐

Send to **Medicines and Healthcare Products Regulatory Agency, CSM FREEPOST, LONDON SW8 5BR** or if you are in one of the following NHS regions:

to **CSM Mersey, FREEPOST, Liverpool L3 3AB**
or **CSM Northern, FREEPOST 1085, Newcastle upon Tyne NE1 1BR**
or **CSM West Midlands, FREEPOST SW2991, Birmingham B18 7BR**
or **CSM Scotland, CARDS, FREEPOST NAT3271, Edinburgh EH16 4BR**
or **CSM Wales, FREEPOST, Cardiff CF4 1ZZ**

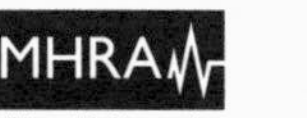

In Confidence

SUSPECTED ADVERSE DRUG REACTIONS

COMMITTEE ON SAFETY OF MEDICINES

If you suspect that an adverse reaction may be related to a drug, or a combination of drugs, you should complete this Yellow Card or complete a report on the website at www.yellowcard.gov.uk. For *intensively monitored medicines* (identified by ▼) report **all** suspected reactions (including any considered not to be serious). For *established drugs* and *herbal remedies* report **all serious** adverse reactions in adults; report **all serious and minor** adverse reactions in **children** (under 18 years). You do not have to be certain about causality: if in doubt, please report. Do not be put off reporting just because some details are not known. See BNF (page 10) or the MHRA website (http://medicines.mhra.gov.uk) for additional advice.

PATIENT DETAILS Patient Initials: ______ Sex: M / F Weight if known (kg): ______

Age (at time of reaction): ______ Identification (Your Practice / Hospital Ref.)*: ______

SUSPECTED DRUG(S)

Give brand name of drug and batch number if known	Route	Dosage	Date started	Date stopped	Prescribed for

SUSPECTED REACTION(S)

Please describe the reaction(s) and any treatment given:

Outcome

- Recovered ☐
- Recovering ☐
- Continuing ☐
- Other ☐

Date reaction(s) started: ______ Date reaction(s) stopped: ______

Do you consider the reaction to be serious? Yes / No

If *yes*, please indicate why the reaction is considered to be serious (please tick all that apply):

- Patient died due to reaction ☐
- Life threatening ☐
- Congenital abnormality ☐
- Involved or prolonged inpatient hospitalisation ☐
- Involved persistent or significant disability or incapacity ☐
- Medically significant; please give details:

* This is to enable you to identify the patient in any future correspondence concerning this report

Please attach additional pages if necessary

Please list other drugs taken in the last 3 months prior to the reaction (including self-medication & herbal remedies)

Was the patient on any other medication? Yes / No

If *yes*, please give the following information if known:

Drug (Brand, if known)	Route	Dosage	Date started	Date stopped	Prescribed for

Additional relevant information e.g. medical history, test results, known allergies, rechallenge (if performed), suspected drug interactions. For congenital abnormalities please state all other drugs taken during pregnancy and the date of the last menstrual period.

REPORTER DETAILS

Name and Professional Address: ______

Post code: ______ Tel No: ______

Speciality: ______

Signature: Date:

CLINICIAN (if not the reporter)

Name and Professional Address: ______

Post code: ______

Tel No: ______ Speciality: ______

If you would like information about other adverse reactions associated with the suspected drug, please tick this box ☐

Send to **Medicines and Healthcare Products Regulatory Agency, CSM FREEPOST, LONDON SW8 5BR** or if you are in one of the following NHS regions:

to **CSM Mersey, FREEPOST, Liverpool L3 3AB**
or **CSM Northern, FREEPOST 1085, Newcastle upon Tyne NE1 1BR**
or **CSM West Midlands, FREEPOST SW2991, Birmingham B18 7BR**
or **CSM Scotland, CARDS, FREEPOST NAT3271, Edinburgh EH16 4BR**
or **CSM Wales, FREEPOST, Cardiff CF4 1ZZ**

Cardiovascular Risk Prediction Charts

J Hum Hypertens 2004; **18**: 139–85

low to use the Cardiovascular Risk Prediction Charts or Primary Prevention

nese charts are for estimating cardiovascular disease (CVD) risk (non-fatal myocardial farction and stroke, coronary and stroke death and new angina pectoris) for individuals no have **not** already developed coronary heart disease (CHD) or other major herosclerotic disease. They are an aid to making clinical decisions about how tensively to intervene on lifestyle and whether to use antihypertensive, lipid lowering nd anti-platelet medication, but should **not replace clinical judgment**.

The use of these charts is **not appropriate** for patients who have existing diseases which already put them at high risk such as:

- coronary heart disease or other major atherosclerotic disease;
- familial hypercholesterolaemia or other inherited dyslipidaemias;
- renal dysfunction including diabetic nephropathy;
- type 1 and 2 diabetes mellitus.

The charts should **not** be used to decide whether to introduce antihypertensive medication when blood pressure is persistently at or above 160/100 mmHg or when target organ damage due to hypertension is present. In both cases antihypertensive medication is recommended regardless of CVD risk. Similarly the charts should **not** be used to decide whether to introduce lipid-lowering medication when the ratio of serum total to HDL cholesterol exceeds 7. Such medication is generally then indicated regardless of estimated CVD risk.

To estimate an individual's absolute 10-year risk of developing CVD choose the chart for his or her gender, lifetime smoking status and age. Within this square identify the level of risk according to the point where the coordinates for systolic blood pressure and the ratio of total cholesterol to high density lipoprotein (HDL) cholesterol meet. If no HDL cholesterol result is available, then assume this is 1.0 mmol/litre and the lipid scale can be used for total cholesterol alone.

Higher risk individuals (red areas) are defined as those whose 10-year CVD risk exceeds 20%, which is approximately equivalent to the coronary heart disease risk of > 15% over the same period.

The chart also assists in identifying individuals whose 10-year CVD risk is moderately increased in the range 10–20% (orange areas) and those in whom risk is lower than 10% over 10 years (green areas).

Smoking status should reflect lifetime exposure to tobacco and not simply tobacco use at the time of assessment. For example, those who have given up smoking within 5 years should be regarded as current smokers for the purposes of the charts.

The initial blood pressure and the first random (non-fasting) total cholesterol and HDL cholesterol can be used to estimate an individual's risk. However, the decision on using drug therapy should generally be based on repeat risk factor measurements over a period of time.

(Continued over)

- Men and women do not reach the level of risk predicted by the charts for the thre age bands until they reach the ages 49, 59, and 69 years respectively. The charts w overestimate current risk most in the under 40s. Clinical judgement must be exercise in deciding on treatment in younger patients. However, it should be recognised th blood pressure and cholesterol tend to rise most and HDL cholesterol to decline mo in younger people already with adverse levels. Left untreated, their risk at the age 4 years is likely to be higher than the projected risk shown on the age-under-50-yea chart. From age 70 years the CVD risk, especially for men, is usually ≥ 20% over 1 years and the charts will underestimate true total CVD risk.

- These charts (and all other currently available methods of CVD risk prediction) ar based on groups of people with **untreated** levels of blood pressure, total choleste and HDL cholesterol. In patients already receiving antihypertensive therapy in who the decision is to be made about whether to introduce lipid-lowering medication, c vice versa, the charts can only act as a guide. Unless recent pre-treatment risk fact values are available it is generally safest to assume that CVD risk is higher than th predicted by current levels of blood pressure or lipids on treatment.

- CVD risk is also higher than indicated in the charts for:
    - those with a family history of premature CVD or stroke (male first-degree relative aged < 55 years and female first-degree relatives aged < 65 years) which increase the risk by a factor of approximately 1.5;
    - those with raised triglyceride levels (> 1.7 mmol/litre);
    - women with premature menopause;
    - those who are not yet diabetic, but have impaired fasting glycaemi (6.1–6.9 mmol/litre) or impaired glucose tolerance (2 hour glucose ≥ 7.8 mmol/litr but < 11.1 mmol/litre in an oral glucose tolerance test).

- The charts have not been validated in ethnic minorities and in some may underestimat CVD risk. For example, in people originating from the Indian subcontinent it is safest t assume that the CVD risk is higher than predicted from the charts (1.5 times).

- An individual can be shown on the chart the direction in which his or her risk of CV can be reduced by changing smoking status, blood pressure, or cholesterol, but should be borne in mind that the estimate of risk is for a group of people with simila risk factors and that within that group there will be considerable variation in risk. should also be pointed out in younger people that the estimated risk will generally n be reached before the age of 50, if their current blood pressure and lipid levels remai unchanged. The charts are primarily to assist in directing intervention to those wh typically stand to benefit most.

(Continued over

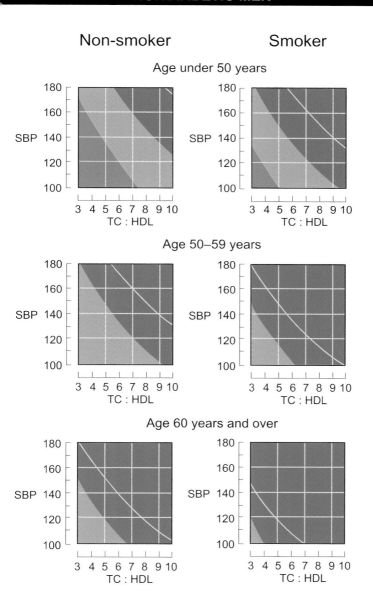

NONDIABETIC MEN

Non-smoker | Smoker

Age under 50 years

SBP 180 160 140 120 100

3 4 5 6 7 8 9 10
TC : HDL

SBP 180 160 140 120 100

3 4 5 6 7 8 9 10
TC : HDL

Age 50–59 years

SBP 180 160 140 120 100

3 4 5 6 7 8 9 10
TC : HDL

SBP 180 160 140 120 100

3 4 5 6 7 8 9 10
TC : HDL

Age 60 years and over

SBP 180 160 140 120 100

3 4 5 6 7 8 9 10
TC : HDL

SBP 180 160 140 120 100

3 4 5 6 7 8 9 10
TC : HDL

CVD risk <10% over next 10 years
CVD risk 10-20% over next 10 years
CVD risk >20% over next 10 years

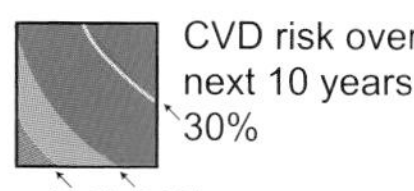

SBP = systolic blood pressure mmHg
TC : HDL = serum total cholesterol to HDL cholesterol ratio

(Continued over)

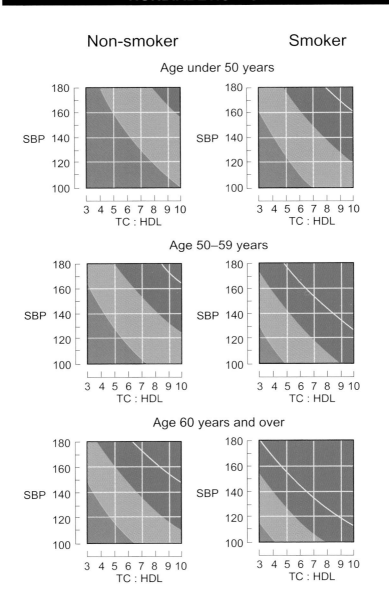

NONDIABETIC WOMEN

Non-smoker | Smoker

Age under 50 years

SBP 180 160 140 120 100

TC : HDL 3 4 5 6 7 8 9 10

Age 50–59 years

SBP 180 160 140 120 100

TC : HDL 3 4 5 6 7 8 9 10

Age 60 years and over

SBP 180 160 140 120 100

TC : HDL 3 4 5 6 7 8 9 10

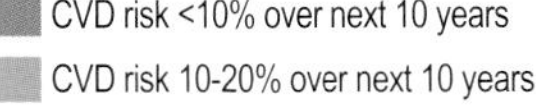

CVD risk <10% over next 10 years

CVD risk 10-20% over next 10 years

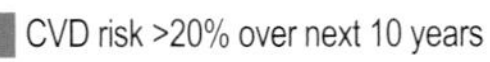

CVD risk >20% over next 10 years

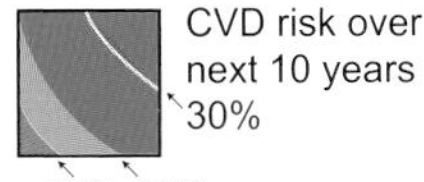

CVD risk over next 10 years

30%

10% 20%

SBP = systolic blood pressure mmH

TC : HDL = serum total cholesterol : HDL cholesterol ratio

ADULT ADVANCED LIFE SUPPORT

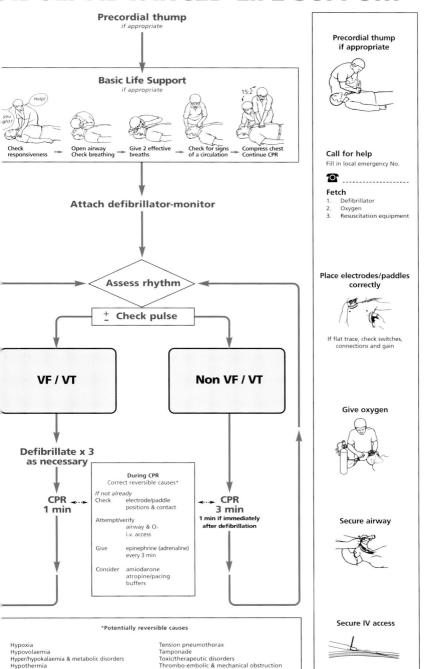

Precordial thump
if appropriate

↓

Basic Life Support
if appropriate

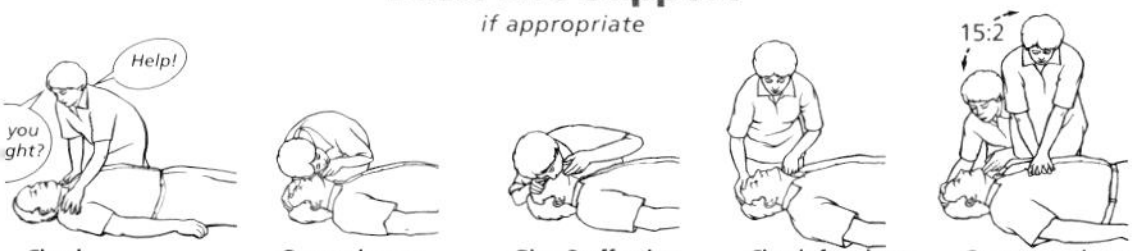

Check responsiveness → Open airway Check breathing → Give 2 effective breaths → Check for signs of a circulation → Compress chest Continue CPR

↓

Attach defibrillator-monitor

↓

Assess rhythm

± **Check pulse**

VF / VT | **Non VF / VT**

VF / VT:

↓

Defibrillate x 3 as necessary

↓

CPR 1 min

Non VF / VT:

↓

CPR 3 min
1 min if immediately after defibrillation

During CPR
Correct reversible causes*

If not already

Check	electrode/paddle positions & contact
Attempt/verify	airway & O_2 i.v. access
Give	epinephrine (adrenaline) every 3 min
Consider	amiodarone atropine/pacing buffers

***Potentially reversible causes**

Hypoxia	Tension pneumothorax
Hypovolaemia	Tamponade
Hyper/hypokalaemia & metabolic disorders	Toxic/therapeutic disorders
Hypothermia	Thrombo-embolic & mechanical obstruction

Precordial thump if appropriate

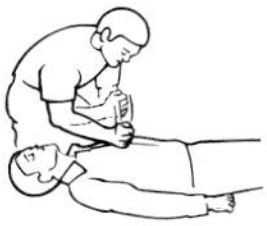

Call for help
Fill in local emergency No.

☎ --------------------

Fetch
1. Defibrillator
2. Oxygen
3. Resuscitation equipment

Place electrodes/paddles correctly

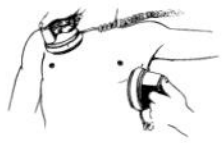

If flat trace, check switches, connections and gain

Give oxygen

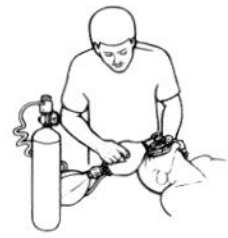

Secure airway

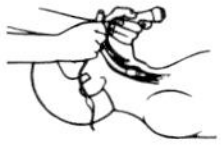

Secure IV access

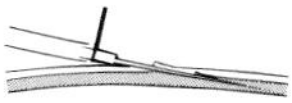

2001
ions courtesy of Laerdal
5 ERC rev D

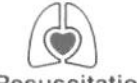

European Resuscitation Council In co-operation with

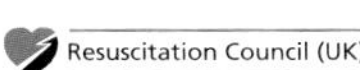

Available from:
LAERDAL MEDICAL LTD.
Laerdal House, Orpington,
Kent BR6 OHX,
Tel. 01689 876634, Fax. 01689 873800

proximate conversions and units

kg	stones	kg	mL	fl oz
0.45	1	6.35	50	1.8
0.91	2	12.70	100	3.5
1.36	3	19.05	150	5.3
1.81	4	25.40	200	7.0
2.27	5	31.75	500	17.6
2.72	6	38.10	1000	35.2
3.18	7	44.45		
3.63	8	50.80		
4.08	9	57.15		
4.54	10	63.50		
4.99	11	69.85		
5.44	12	76.20		
5.90	13	82.55		
6.35	14	88.90		
	15	95.25		

ngth

etre (m)		= 1000 millimetres (mm)
ntimetre (cm)		= 10 mm
ch (in)		= 25.4 mm
ot (ft)	=12 inches	= 304.8 mm

ss

ogram (kg)	= 1000 grams (g)
am (g)	= 1000 milligrams (mg)
lligram (mg)	= 1000 micrograms
crogram	= 1000 nanograms
nogram	= 1000 picograms

lume

re	= 1000 millilitres (mL)
llilitre (1 mL)	= 1000 microlitres
nt	≈ 568 mL

her units

ocalorie (kcal)	= 4186.8 joules (J)
kilocalories (kcal)	= 4.1868 megajoules (MJ)
gajoule (MJ)	= 238.8 kilocalories (kcal)
llimetre of mercury mmHg)	= 133.3 pascals (Pa)
opascal (kPa)	= 7.5 mmHg (pressure)

asma-drug concentrations in the BNF are pressed in mass units per litre (e.g. mg/litre). The proximate equivalent in terms of amount of subnce units (e.g. micromol/litre) is given in brackets.

Prescribing in children

Age	Ideal body-weight kg	Ideal body-weight lb	Height cm	Height inch	Body-surface m^2
Newborn*	3.5	7.7	50	20	0.23
1 month*	4.2	9	55	22	0.26
3 months*	5.6	12	59	23	0.32
6 months	7.7	17	67	26	0.40
1 year	10	22	76	30	0.47
3 years	15	33	94	37	0.62
5 years	18	40	108	42	0.73
7 years	23	51	120	47	0.88
12 years	39	86	148	58	1.25
Adult					
Male	68	150	173	68	1.80
Female	56	123	163	64	1.60

* The figures relate to full term and not preterm infants who may need reduced dosage according to their clinical condition.

Recommended wording of cautionary and advisory labels

For details see Appendix 9

1 Warning. May cause drowsiness
2 Warning. May cause drowsiness. If affected do not drive or operate machinery. Avoid alcoholic drink
3 Warning. May cause drowsiness. If affected do not drive or operate machinery
4 Warning. Avoid alcoholic drink
5 Do not take indigestion remedies at the same time of day as this medicine
6 Do not take indigestion remedies or medicines containing iron or zinc at the same time of day as this medicine
7 Do not take milk, indigestion remedies, or medicines containing iron or zinc at the same time of day as this medicine
8 Do not stop taking this medicine except on your doctor's advice
9 Take at regular intervals. Complete the prescribed course unless otherwise directed
10 Warning. Follow the printed instructions you have been given with this medicine
11 Avoid exposure of skin to direct sunlight or sun lamps
12 Do not take anything containing aspirin while taking this medicine
13 Dissolve or mix with water before taking
14 This medicine may colour the urine
15 Caution flammable: keep away from fire or flames
16 Allow to dissolve under the tongue. Do not transfer from this container. Keep tightly closed. Discard 8 weeks after opening
17 Do not take more than ... in 24 hours
18 Do not take more than ... in 24 hours or ... in any one week
19 Warning. Causes drowsiness which may continue the next day. If affected do not drive or operate machinery. Avoid alcoholic drink
21 ... with or after food
22 ... half to one hour before food
23 ... an hour before food or on an empty stomach
24 ... sucked or chewed
25 ... swallowed whole, not chewed
26 ... dissolved under the tongue
27 ... with plenty of water
28 To be spread thinly ...
29 Do not take more than 2 at any one time. Do not take more than 8 in 24 hours
30 Do not take with any other paracetamol products
31 Contains aspirin and paracetamol. Do not take with any other paracetamol products
32 Contains aspirin
33 Contains an aspirin-like medicine

THE HILLBILLIES

BY

PETER HARRISON

First published by Barny Books

ISBN No: 978.1.903172.89.6

Publishers: Barny Books
Hough on the Hill
Grantham
Lincolnshire
NG32 2BB

Tel: 01400 250246
www.barnybooks.biz

Other books written by this author:

Hovis Brown

Dedicated to

My daughters

Lynne & Eve

Acknowledgments:

To the power-brokers behind
Barny Books:

Molly Burkett and Jayne Thompson
whose help, guidance and energy proved
they're the real Spice Girls.

Agnes Bailey looked at the clock. She couldn't wait any longer. "Roy," she said, "get upstairs. Wash your face and clean your teeth. I'll be five minutes."

The boy scampered out of sight, laughing and shouting with pleasure, "South Shields! We're going to South Shields!"

Minutes later and Agnes reached the back door of her neighbour's house. She looked resignedly at the property, knocked at the door and entered. "Rebecca! You there?" she called out. There was no answer. Agnes walked through the kitchen, her features pinched and grim at the acrid, overpowering smell that wafted over her.

"Charlie", she said, her voice lower, softer, as she peered into the living-room. The curtains had been closed but it couldn't hide the mess and mayhem of the place. She saw the boy in the gloom huddled in the big old arm-chair.

"Oh Charlie!" she whispered. Charlie Hill started to sob. Agnes approached the lad, eased her large frame onto the arm of the chair, her fingers gently touching the nape of his neck. "Where's your mother, Charlie?"

"Gone, Missus."

"Where, Charlie?" she asked resignedly.

The boy kept his head down, "Don't know, Missus Bailey."

Agnes shook her head, her emotions held in check, her tone soft, "How long this time, Charlie?"

"Two days," he stammered and began sobbing, his face hidden in his grubby hands, "two full days!"

Agnes asked carefully, "You know what today is Charlie?"

"School outing, Missus Bailey," he replied, wiping his shirt-sleeve across his running nose, "me and Roy are supposed to be going to South Shields."

The woman stood, sucking in air, a determined look on her stout face. "Right," she said, resolutely, "we're still going!"

The boy looked up for the first time, attempted to dry his eyes as he gasped, "Nothing's ready, Missus, no money, nothing!"

Agnes grasped the lad's hand and eased him out of the chair, cuddled him like he was her very own. "Where's your Dad, Charlie?" she said, pulling a huge handkerchief from the sleeve of her blouse. Licking one corner of the material, she proceeded brusquely to clean his face.

"Bed, Missus," said Charlie, grimacing, "he's in night-shift." His fingers tightened on hers, "Can't wake him, Missus, he's in a bad mood with Ma. She took all the money again." Charlie didn't mention the beatings he'd suffered at the hands of his demented father. "Took all the wages again and left nothing for us!"

"You eaten Charlie?"

His face puckered with grief, his head lowered and slowly eased into the pendulous midriff of the woman, whispered, "Haven't even stayed off school, Missus. Teacher said anyone staying off school couldn't go on the school trip. Didn't stay for school dinners, Missus, Ma didn't leave any money for me so I just came home at dinner time and sat until it was time to go back. Didn't tell anyone, not even Roy."

"Bugger this!" said a determined Agnes Bailey.

"Missus?"

"Get your coat, Charlie, or we'll miss the bus!"

"I've got no spending-money, Missus Bailey," and he started sobbing softly, "not a penny!"

"I've got plenty to spare, my love," she answered and swept the child into her arms, "now come on, or Roy will get upset!"

"What about my dad?" cried Charlie, "shouldn't I leave him a note and explain? He might go mad if he doesn't know where I'm at?"

"Leave your father to me, pet," soothed the woman, bustling towards the door, "I'll sort it out later."

It was the best day of Charlie's life. The sun burned all day long, the resort bursting with folk determined to enjoy the day, better than the Costa Del Sol. South Shields, sand, sea and uninterrupted sunshine! Glorious. The Easington crowd were game for anything and everything, Mid-morning and the fourth year pupils, parents and tutors were all in the park watching the local brass band bursting with confidence, very loud and occasionally out-of-tune, like an inebriated Temperance Seven as they blew and battered their instruments with gay abandon, intoxicated with a head mix of alcohol and atmosphere and nobody cared a damn. Then the finale; the climax of the show: the singing contest announced over a squeaky, echoing microphone and Agnes, always eager for a laugh and a good time, volunteered their little group as first in line for the gala, dragging two fearful boys with her onto the rickety stage. Agnes, Charlie and Roy, aka, Shakin'Stevens and his backing group, Agnes lead vocalist and after a hesitant, nervous start, the boys dutifully followed her lead and the winning song - This Ole House - would have made Rosemary Clooney proud. Charlie cried with laughter.

Afternoon saw the school party descend on to the beach. After an hour on the hot sands, someone suggested a swim. Almost as one the group started stripping off their clothes, only Charlie wavered and dithered. It was as if a cloud had settled over him.

Agnes, still in over-sized knickers and bra, knew something was wrong. "You okay, Charlie!" she said, trying to nudge him into action, "something wrong, pet?"

"No trunks, Missus!" He looked crest-fallen and embarrassed, his features turning crimson, "no swimming-trunks!"

Agnes Bailey chortled and said, "It's nothing to worry about, Charlie," playfully raking her fingers through his hair. "Leave your underpants on, no one will care."

Charlie looked mortified, "Got none, Missus Bailey," he stammered, eyes glared morosely at the sands. "Ma said they're a waste of money." He started to sob with humiliation.

There was just the touch of the parent in her tone. "That's enough of that," she said firmly. Striding to the oversized bag, Agnes fished about before pulling out Roy's underpants. Bright red! "Right my boy! We're sorted!"

Roy ran into view. "Ma!" he cried with outrage, "they're mine!"

"Shut your gob!" said Agnes Bailey, feigning irritation, grabbed at the youngsters and cuddled them fondly, "it's time for a swim."

Charlie had a wonderful day.

The evening, however, was a different matter. Eight o-clock and the two figures sat opposite each other, not a sound in the room, save for the spluttering of the coal-fire, total silence between father and son, each alone with their own thoughts. Charlie, worn out with the excitement of the day ached for sleep but couldn't move, he'd been ordered to sit still and not to speak a word and he knew he had to obey. It was eight-o-clock, another hour and Adam Hill would have to leave. He was in a sour mood anyway. Night-shift! He hated night-shift. He glowered at the boy; hating him, hating his mother, full of anger and frustration, his huge hands unconsciously gripped the arms of the chair. She'd been gone two days. Two bloody days! Up to her usual tricks, no doubt, raided his pockets too, even took the change. He thought of the long night ahead without any bait. Adam was starving, hadn't eaten a bite of food all day, not a bloody scrap anywhere in the house! That bloody woman! Two days missing, how the hell was he going to get through the shift?

"Bed," he ordered, the tone venomous and threatening, "this minute!"

The boy walked quickly out of the room, his head down. When he reached the staircase, Charlie belted up the steps, ran into his bedroom and bolted the door, slumped on to the unmade bed, put his hands together and started to say a prayer for his mother. Same prayer he'd said the previous night. He wanted his mother home. Drunk, sober, it didn't matter, couldn't bear the thought of another night without her, worrying about her, wondering where she was, wondering what she was doing.

"Our father, who art in heaven," could never remember the next word - was it 'Hello' be thy name or 'Hi'- neither sounded right as he bit his lip and concentrated. Charlie improvised, "Dear Jesus, please bring my mother home safely. Please ask her to come home tonight because my dad is really worried about her." He started sobbing so he pulled blankets over his face to muffle the sound, didn't want his dad running up the stairs again, leather belt in hand, didn't want any more punishment, "Ma," he gasped, tears streaming over his face, "I want my Ma, God, I'm frightened on my own!"

****

CHAPTER ONE

A cold morning mist clung to the deserted streets. Old Ben Russell drove the milk-float through the rows of council houses; he parked the vehicle, grasped the few bottles and made his way into the small cul-de-sac. Striding back to the van minutes later, his arms full of empties Ben inadvertently glanced at the middle house, at the upstairs window damaged months earlier in a domestic dispute, still in need of repair, curtains fluttering wildly at the inrush of air. He shook his head, used to deliver to the house, not any more, even though he was still owed money. Not worth the bother, not worth the harassment from the nightmare Hill family.

It started to rain. The milk float moved away towards the western perimeter of the village, towards the big church and the single row of terraced houses called *Clappersgate.* Ben was already soaked to the skin as he hurried into the small back-yard, not seeing the figure standing motionless. With a shriek loud enough to wake the dead, the old man dropped the bottles. The din was horrendous. “Hell’s Teeth!” he shouted.

The youth stood before him. Harry Shannon, five feet two, twenty stone plus, a huge dressing-gown draped untidily over his obese frame and adorning his huge skull was a large, battered fedora, a cascade of golden locks fell to his shoulders almost hiding the whiskered jowls. Harry Shannon was concentrating on the overcast, leaden heavens, head arched up towards the grey morning. With an almost inaudible grunt and the faintest hint of a frown he turned his attention to the newcomer.

“Good morning, Mister Russell,” he said in an almost childlike voice.

“Jesus, Harry,” was all Ben could muster as he looked at the mess of glass and liquid strewn over the yard, “look at the mess!”

Harry Shannon sighed, whispered, “Mother said the sunrise can be lovely” and gazed again at the dull skies seemingly oblivious to the broken bottles that tattooed the place. Bemused and confused he continued, “But there’s no sun, Mr. Russell?”

The old man calmed, being annoyed with Harry was like being angry with an infant. Harry was brain-damaged; born that way.

“I’ll get some more,” Ben said and left the yard.

The back-door of the house squeaked open. It was Ruby, Harry’s long-suffering mother. She’d been pretty once but that was a long time ago. The burden of her son had left its mark. She was old for her years and heavy now, almost as wide as her son.

Ruby Shannon scolded, “Harry?”

“Ma?” said the innocent, bewildered youth.

“What have you done now?”

“Ma,” said Harry naively, “it was Mister Russell’s fault.”

Ben hurried back to the scene, tried to apologise as he handed over new bottles to the mother. Ruby smiled resignedly, handed the milk to her gaping son, ordered him gently back into the house, found a broom and started to clean the mess.

“I’m sorry Ben,” she muttered, “he can’t help it.”

****

Hours later and the rain stopped. Tantalizing fingers of sun tapped over rooftops and streets. Charlie opened his eyes. He’d been dreaming of his grandparents again. He gazed about the bedroom, at the broken window and the curtains slapping noisily like abandoned flags. In those long distant days, his grandparent's house had been a warm and comfortable home. Charlie had been carried daily to the place, had a vague picture of his mother laughing as she helped with the household chores, still remembered the smell of polish always wafting about the place as his mother cleaned and cared for her parents' home. Everybody happy then, apart from his dad; always moaning, always something wrong, couldn't understand the bond between daughter and parents. It was a pig-sty now. There were times when he missed the old home, two streets away and like a thousand miles. His first house was okay, not too bad in fact, once; clean enough to invite his friends in to play. Charlie closed his eyes, reminiscing. His grandparents had died within eight weeks of each other and his mother demanded they all move from their old home into her parent's house, couldn't bear the thought of someone else living there. Ma had been born there and wanted to spend the rest of her life there. *Comforting,* she said to dad, *Please Adam,* she pleaded, *do it for me!* Dad was livid, he'd spent a fortune on the old house and was adamant that under no circumstances were they moving.

He lost the battle and they moved lock, stock and barrel into his grandparent's house. Then slowly, inextricably, things seemed to go downhill after that. Dad was unhappy about starting over and Ma, well, that was the turning-point in Mother's life. She changed as a person. Little things at first, things you'd hardly notice. After meals, for example, where once she would be taking away plates and dishes and start cleaning and washing, full of bounce and energy, *Spick and span,* she would say, *a place for everything and everything in its place,* she started leaving the washing-up. *I'll do it soon enough,* she'd comment. *The washing-up will be there when I'm not,* her head in the clouds, miles away some days, hardly making conversation at all, from chatterbox, always fussing and loving to silent brooding clown. She'd forget to vacuum, ask Charlie - who wasn't as big as the *Hoover* - to finish the task and after a while she wouldn't even ask but look at him with those big blank eyes, only she wasn't looking at him, she was miles away and he couldn't help. He didn't think anyone could help. Ma changed, not immediately, but slowly, surely, over weeks and months. She became a different person, as if she were drowning in her own despair, in a quicksand of sorrow and mourning of her own making, pulling down those closest to her.

Charlie stirred; it was Saturday, best day of the week. He smiled to himself, knowing that both parents were present for once. His Dad was snoring loudly from the other bedroom and the occasional clatter downstairs meant that Ma was around. Week five and Rebecca Hill hadn't vanished, hadn't disappeared into the night only to resurface days, sometimes weeks later, filled with regret and misery, disorientated and despondent, always promising never to wander again, never again to drink. *On my word, son,* she'd always say, *that's the last time! May God strike me down dead if I touch another drink!* Some days she'd swear it on the rosary. Charlie missed his mother when she was gone, nobody knew the pain he suffered. Week five and she was still around, couldn't believe his good fortune. He ran down the stairs, filled with optimism and good cheer.

"Ma," he greeted her, then attempted to grasp the cigarette packet from his mother's hand.

Rebecca winked, a rare smile filled her face. She threw the pack at her son. "Don't take liberties," she said, "one only, you hear?"

Charlie pulled out two fags and stuck them in his mouth, grabbing a box of matches from the fireplace he lit them both together, seen it done at the movies, the ancient black and white films. Jimmy Cagney, tough guy with cool moves. "Ma," he said and handed one to his mother, said cautiously, "You okay?"

Rebecca nodded her reply, gazed at her son, a myriad thoughts clouding her head. With a loud sigh she rose on unsteady feet, alcohol still washing around her system, felt nauseous and queasy and moody enough to sour vinegar.

"I'll make some breakfast," she muttered and wandered towards the kitchen, wondered if she'd make it through the day.

The upstairs door banged out an ugly tune and the landing groaned like an out-of-tune piano as the big man thumped his way down the staircase. Adam Hill walked into view, squatted heavily in the big arm-chair that had just been vacated by his wife, stretched out a thick arm towards Charlie and demanded the smoke. "Pass it over!" he grunted arrogantly.

Charlie fired back immediately, "Get lost!"

"Give it here," demanded the older man, "if you know what's good for you."

Rebecca shouted from the other room. "For Christ's sake!"

Charlie relented, still fearful of his old man, handed over the cigarette and growled, "Hope it chokes you!" and joined his mother in the kitchen, didn't want to push his luck.

Rebecca handed her cigarette to her pouting son. She grasped the cup and drank greedily at the dark contents.

Charlie naively said, "No milk again, Ma?" remembered the old days when the milkman would call daily. Long gone.

"There's a bit of milk left for you and him" and gestured towards the living-room where Adam sat and waited for his breakfast.

Rebecca Hill looked at the remainder in the cup; the *Guinness* looked like coffee, tasted like nectar. With one long swig she drained the liquid. "That's better!" she said with a satisfied, smug look.

"Breakfast!" shouted Adam Hill from the other room. "You'll feed me before that brat!"

"Ma!" whined Charlie. "It's me first!"

"When you get a bloody job," bawled Adam, "you might be first in line, until then, it's me first! You hear?"

"Ma!"

Rebecca Hill shook her head and stared sullenly out of the window, wanted to run away, run a million miles away from everything and everyone.

****

Edward Aaron Priestley had, for the past thirty years, swept his thick black hair back off his pasty face. For the last ten years he had relied on a fortnightly rinse to keep the grayness in check. He had a reputation to keep and appearances counted. He could not perfect the smirk of the King but he persevered, same initials as the King of Rock and Roll: *Elvis Aron Presley* and if Elvis had once ruled the charts then he ruled Easington.

He was 55 years of age and he was wealthy; richer than most folk in the area. Elvis had tried his hand at every mortal thing since leaving school all those years ago and his most enduring characteristic, his one saving-grace was his obstinacy, skin as thick and tough as a rhinoceros. Elvis had tried pit-work. Left school at fourteen on the Friday and was grafting at Easington Colliery on the Monday. Five years he lasted and he hated every damn shift. Elvis knew nothing else, there was precious little else for a naïve and young lad to aspire to, especially without qualifications, it was either the pit or one of the few factories in Peterlee.

The explosion at the mine was his wake-up call: *Lucky bastard*, said his father. Wrong shift that day or he definitely would have met his maker. Elvis didn't go back to the pit, not even to collect his work clothes and boots. Eighty odd men killed, *Stick that*, mused Elvis Priestley, *stick that for a lark!*

The next year saw him working as a car mechanic at nearby Horden, quite liked it too, but a spot of bad luck meant he had to leave sharpish. Still, he'd made a penny or two flogging spare parts to the daft lads in the area and that was a real eye-opener, a genuine piece of good fortune which led Elvis on to his next enterprise. A few of these dodgy characters owned Army surplus wagons with engines big enough to haul loads up the steep inclines that snaked from the nearby colliery beaches. Easington, Horden and Blackhall collieries all tipped their waste into the sea, not only stone and shale but coal too, tons of coal. The shoreline was literally covered with a beautiful mix of muck and money - fine coal nuggets, black gold. Elvis's ears flapped like a bat as he heard all about the magic of the ocean currents allowing the heavier stone to sink and the lighter black stuff being pushed by the tide towards the shore. Some nights the entire coastline was piled high with beautiful coal, free for the taking. If you had the gumption, the grit and the vehicles to haul it up the treacherous cliffs- easy pickings and a tax-free booty for the audacious pit pirates.

Elvis persevered with the newness. Although he worked with the local skip-rats, Elvis always wanted to branch out on his own, knew enough about life to know self-employment was the only way to guarantee riches. Ignoring the threats from the other, more established crews, he bought his very own wagon, found his own piece of shore-line and set up shop. Within two years, the newcomer had bought a second wagon and even hired a few local idiots as casual labour. His biggest competitor, mouth-almighty, Reggie Brown, who always boasted, '*This beach belongs to me, Priestley!* had left the scene permanently after a suspicious accident and was wheel-chair bound. Someone had doctored the brakes on his truck. Elvis was a rising star and he was gaining respect.

He was the first in the area to purchase an automated coal delivery wagon for home deliveries. Early sixties and almost every home was driven by coal or coke. Coal was King then and it was going to last forever. *Forever*! What a salesman he was, had the gift of the gab and who couldn't be convinced that, unlike all the other merchants who personally bagged their own sacks of coal, his was the real deal. Automated coal wagon with exact weight in every sack! *Look at the instruments*, he would brag, *look at counters*, he would say and because he owned the only automated delivery wagons in the Easington district he quickly became the dominant force in the whole area. *I'm the only damn one who gives proper weight in every bag of coal*. Of course, the opposite was true, Elvis was an enterprising entrepreneur and a scoundrel to boot and grew richer by the year.

By 1960 Elvis owned three beach wagons, two motors for home deliveries and a small grocery shop just north of the colliery - run by his late wife Janet and their daughter Irene. Two years previously, Elvis had bought a garage on the outskirts of the village. He'd bought the business for a song, the despondent owner finally giving-up on the loss-making venture. Poor sales and the constant break-ins and wanton vandalism (all paid for by Elvis Priestley) meant the final price was well-below market price. Elvis was well pleased with the acquisition, not only could he repair all of his motors behind closed doors but he could also buy and sell anything too hot to be viewed openly by the public. Word soon spread about the garage. It was always busy, one way or another.

Another decade saw the fellow sell the garage at the village for double its purchase price. The Government was re-routing the A19 and the small lock-up was compulsory purchased. A gut-feeling and a perfect set of timing also saw the fellow dispose of his coal business for a sizeable sum in the same year. He'd read the ominous signs of change, guessed within his lifetime that the black gold would be replaced with a cleaner and cheaper alternative. *Gas*, he thought wisely, *gas would be the new energy king.* Elvis purchased one of the two garages situated in the town-centre of Peterlee in the same year. The new town had tremendous potential thought the entrepreneur; he also bought his first fast-food outlet in one of the large housing estates of the town, bought it cheaply too. The previous owner could no longer afford the insurance premiums; the nightly vandalism was costing him a fortune in repair bills. He was pleased to sell it to the chunky entrepreneur. *Fortuitous*, said the new owner. Elvis had the knack of being in the right place at the right time and the hidden shekels to pay miscreants to cause mayhem. The following year he acquired a lock-up, leasehold property in Horden selling pizza, fish and chips, whatever. *'Gimme the recipe,'* said the porky proprietor, *'and I'll sell it!'* Elvis purchased a delivery-car for use between both of his fast-food stores, first in the whole county of Durham to advertise a delivery-service. He was a devious, dangerous, man, who would stop at nothing to get his own way………..

Noon and Elvis was about to leave the grocery store. He stood in the doorway, filled the doorway, matter of fact, unconsciously patting his enormous stomach and looked at the two sullen figures standing inside the gloomy store, sighed loud and long, thinking unkindly, *Every picture tells a story!*

The man's daughter, Irene, had managed the small grocery store for the past five years since the sudden death of Elvis's wife. Irene, 45 years old, plump and permanently sour (she still rankled over her absent husband, Ronnie Oliver, running off with Ivy Lochrane; the Colliery Clubs's chief barmaid) stood, arms folded with a definite look of defiance over her round flat face. Seventeen years since Ronnie had bolted; sixteen years since Irene had followed him to Blackpool hoping for reconciliation. *Not a hope in Hell*, said Ronnie Oliver, so Irene had a night on the town and the result, standing next to her, was Sheryl, a fifteen year old incarnation of Halle Berry, slim, gorgeous and as black as the coal he once loved.

Elvis barked with obvious irritation, "What's the matter now?" as if he didn't know. How he missed his wife, Janet: God rest her soul, she would work all the hours under the sun, for free and yet his only daughter was the opposite, constantly whining and bemoaning her lot. Only happy when she was twisting, even demanding minimum wages, as if she wasn't family, didn't matter that she and her black mistake were living rent-free in the bungalow next to the grocery-store. *Part and parcel of the job*, she would moan, *I work night and day, blah, blah, blah!*

"It's Saturday!" pleaded Sheryl, all pouting and pleading.

The grandfather said gruffly, “Is that a fact!”

“Elvis” pleaded the granddaughter, “please!”

The man did not want reminding of his age; hence the fitted shirts and the hair-dye, always insisted that his granddaughter call him by his preferred name. She was fifteen. Pretty too and she knew it. All her friends would be out, parading up and down Peterlee town-centre, posing and posturing and hearing the latest gossip. Sheryl glanced at the big clock on the wall. She could be sitting in *Weatherspoon's* checking out the talent and scowled at her miserable tight-fisted grandpa as if she suffered toothache.

The older woman, Irene, intervened. “Eddie, it's quiet. I can manage on my own for a few hours.”

Elvis was adamant, his voice was raised, his tone severe, tore strips off both of them. *So ungrateful*, he thought petulantly, his features stone as he bellowed, “Don't know how lucky you are!” then he stormed away.

Sheryl begged, “Ma?”

“Two hours, baby,” replied the mother. “Make sure you're back before him.”

The year-old Jaguar sped through the village. Elvis was on his way to the garage. He passed the crowd of youngsters sauntering across the road. *The hunting trip,* thought the man and grinned mischievously. All the teenagers carried air-rifles. He recognised the natural leader of the group, Charlie Hill. Stood out a mile, reminded Elvis of himself: *charismatic,* the others hovered around him like flies around shit.

The man had known Charlie a while, caught the little thief weeks ago nicking sweets from his shop and was dumbstruck by the arrogance of the youth, showed no fear, even when he was physically carried out of the grocery shop and clouted to boot. *Tough guy,* thought Elvis at the time, *a regular Al Pacino, a little hard-case. He* won Elvis over with his resilience, didn't shout for his parents or the cops like most kids, took his punishment like a grown-up.

Elvis watched the group of would-be hunters clamber over a fence and hurry across the field. *Up to no damn good,* he thought, watched again as Charlie Hill sauntered after his gang. The memories flooded back...............

"A Mars-bar," the youth adamant, "it was just a bloody Mars bar."

"Three actually," shouted Elvis as he dragged the youth out of the shop, "not learn to count at school, kid?"

"You'll not do that when I'm bigger!" yelled Charlie Hill venomously, not a tear in sight. Defiant and bold as he shrugged his slim shoulders with a youthful rebelliousness.

Elvis was incredulous. "I should call the bloody police!" he yelled and he pushed at the lad who stumbled and fell.

On his feet in a second, the youth lifted his fists in the mock stance of a boxer.

"Give it a break, lad," Elvis chuckled, "or I'll huff and I'll puff..."

"Any time you're ready!"

Elvis paused by the shop-door. He asked, "You like this all the time," and started to smile. "What's your name, son?"

"Sugar Ray Leonard!"

"Wrong colour, lad."

"So?"

Elvis relented, pulling the stolen confectionary from his pocket; he threw a chocolate bar to the boy. He had an idea, might be able to use the lad.

"Truce?" asked Elvis.

"Okay Mister."

"Now," asked the older man. "What's your name?"

That was the first meeting of Charlie Hill and the King. The first of many.

The boy told him all about himself, left some things out, naturally. Turned out that Elvis knew his parents, especially the boy's mother. Rebecca was a looker once, quiet sort of a girl. Elvis could remember her coming into his shop. Rebecca and little Jimmy Shannon. Years ago, made for each other, that was the chat, then he buggered off with someone else. Had a bairn too, kid had something wrong with it, he recalled, lived in the village. *Little Jimmy Shannon,* Elvis had almost forgotten the man. Dead now, neither use nor ornament. When he was alive he was permanently drunk. Walked home one night, pissed out of his brains, ignored the path and followed the white dotted lines in the centre of the road, first car knocked him clean onto the other side of the road, a second car, driving in the opposite direction, finished off the job. *Waste of space,* thought Elvis, *a piss-artist!*

Then Rebecca married Adam Hill. A strange pairing if ever there was one. Adam Hill, one of life's losers, known throughout the area as a psycho; big as an ox and some would say as dumb - but never to his face - short-tempered, fast hands and a heavy drinker to boot. Worked at the mine still, couldn't see the industry was obsolete and dying the death, no one in the land who could match Thatcher, not even Scargill, *Mr. Throw-Over* himself.

Elvis listened and nodded as the kid droned on about his family. *Not a hope in hell,* thought the man, *not coming from that background, the lad had been dealt a cruel hand. Prison fodder, put money on it, boy'll end up dealing or injecting.*

Hillbillies, born and bred, guaranteed at least one family of crackerjacks in every village.

"Still at school then?"

"Not for long," said Charlie, "leave next month."

"And then?"

"Easington pit," said it like he was proud.

Elvis tried to explain the economics of the situation, told him that he'd be unemployed by the time he was eighteen. It was like talking to a stone, the lad was adamant; he was going to work at the colliery. Elvis tried a different tactic, asked the youth if he wanted to make some *pocket-money,* smiled when he suggested it.

"Suppose so."

"Fancy part-time work then?" *Anything like his parents and I'm laughing*, thought Elvis.

"Nah, couldn't work in a shop," retorted the lad.

Elvis smiled, threw over another chocolate bar to the lad, started talking about himself, about his businesses, never bored talking about Elvis Aaron Priestley, talk till the cows came home could Elvis. He mentioned casually how he needed the occasional favour doing and how he paid good money, especially to people who could keep their traps shut.

"Money," asked Charlie, "what kind of money we talking?"

"Big money, son."

"Kind of business we talking about?"

"Well," sniggered Elvis, nudging the kid, "sort of naughty business, stuff you keep to yourself, kind of business that would put you out of circulation for a while … if you were dumb enough to get caught, or stupid enough to boast about it. You gotta understand son, no one can be trusted. Tell one person and the secret is no longer a secret. Prisons, young-offenders institutions are full of mugs who made the ultimate mistake … they told someone, who told someone, who told someone else! You get my drift?"

"I'm all ears, Mister," laughed Charlie Hill.

Elvis Priestley smiled like Fagin and wondered if Charlie Hill could be another Artful Dodger, *Do you have the bottle, my dear, do you have the bottle?*

CHAPTER TWO

When they were all present and correct, the gang numbered eight, all had the gang's name *Angels* tattooed across the palm of their hands. Charlie's idea, remembered the movie *The Wanderers,* left a huge impression on him, *The Young Savages* was another whopper and Jimmy Dean - who could touch *Rebel?* American films were so cool! It was Saturday, a few of the boys had gone to Sunderland to watch the match, a few still in bed and couldn't be roused so half the group were missing. It mattered less. It was the weekend, the sun was out and it didn't matter that a chill easterly wind blew. The youths were sweating buckets as they hurried across the farmer's field, reached the safety of the trees and slowed their pace, still heading for the distant beach at Hawthorn, a mile north of Easington. The earlier panic was starting to ease. Charlie's fault of course, *If it moves shoot it*, was his motto, pity he had shot the farm cat. *'It's no big deal!'* he bawled at the group, full to the brim with false bravado. The others were in a right stew waiting for the expected appearance of the incensed farmer with his shotgun at the ready, could feel the icy blast of buckshot on their backsides. *'Black for luck,'* Charlie Hill chortled, expert at hiding his feelings, scoffing at their weakness.

"Just a bloody moggy," he chided, fighting the urge to glance again at the disappearing farm-yard. Charlie was in luck. Being Saturday the local Mart was being held at the nearby village of Haswell. It was always well-attended by local farmers, the general public and the usual assortment of riff-raff trying to flog anything and everything that some luckless punter would foolishly purchase. The farm would be unattended until tea-time and the gang would be miles away by then.

"You said it was a rabbit," grunted Billy Nord. The lad towered over the entire group, been the hard-case of the school once, until the third year when he and Charlie Binns had been in one hell of a scrap. The fight was long and ferocious and the bigger youth was gradually winning the bloody contest, well on the way to keeping his title until Charlie desperately sunk his teeth into Billy's flesh. Like a pit-bull, wouldn't let go. Finished Billy Nord, good and proper, on the grass weeping like a girl, everyone thought it was over, not Charlie, wanted no come-back so he lashed out viciously with his boot, kicked out Billy's front teeth. Game over, Charlie won by a unanimous knock-out.

"Thought it was!" answered an adamant Charlie, "either a rabbit or a hare!"

"Black rabbit, eh," chortled Nelly, the baby of the bunch could get away with blue murder, wide as he was tall, lovable by nature, he offered no threat to anyone. John Nellis slapped Charlie on the shoulder, smile as wide as his face, "Just killed us a bunny-cat?"

A pair of fat slow-moving wood-pigeons suddenly appeared on the horizon. They were heading towards the group. The gang froze and waited for the order. "Now!" cried Charlie and five assorted weapons were lifted to the heavens; explosions cracking, booming and shattering the peace of the place. The birds flew on, unharmed. They blamed each other and all felt foolish.

Alan Mounter, wall-eyed and carrot-topped quickly re-loaded his air-rifle, took careful aim and shot at the nearest tree-trunk. "Gotcha!" he yelled, trying to ease the tension.

Ten minutes later and Charlie was on top of the world. The gang was skirting the woods in single file, guns at the ready when a huge cock pheasant shrieked its frantic call and scrambled from the sanctuary of the trees and through the centre of the group. The suddenness and the speed of the fowl scattered most of the youths. Charlie stood his ground and aimed the rifle as the bird struggled to gain height. *Bang!* A cloud of feathers burst from its body, one of its wings was bent and damaged and the fowl spiralled from the sky and landed awkwardly. Instinct made the wounded bird struggle to its feet and scurry away from the howling and excited predators.

Charlie watched as the group chased the demented bird. He re-loaded and waited, laughing loudly at the spectacle, half a dozen youths screaming and shrieking as they gave chase, like a scene from a *Keystone Cops* movie and about as funny, running and firing their slug-guns at the shrieking, scampering chicken. Nelly, frustrated at his lack of prowess, his gun empty and useless, gave an almighty yell and flung the rifle high in the sky. The weapon, spinning like a boomerang, lifted high in the sky and then crashed on to the poor bird, killing it instantly.

More shocked than buoyant, the chunky teenager stopped dead in his tracks and raised his arm triumphantly, started singing at the top of his voice, '*My boomerang won't come back, my boomerang won't come back...*' cackling at his good fortune, prodding both arms at the group of smirking lads, '*What about that, eh?*'

"Pick it up, Nelly," demanded Charlie, "we'll have it for dinner!"

Gingerly approaching the feathered corpse, John Nellis leaned over the silent bird, carefully prodding it with his shoe, "Reckon it's dead, then?" before squeamishly grasping the fowl's stiff claws, glanced at the waiting crew, "anybody fancy carrying it then?"

Half an hour later and the juvenile mafia had reached the deserted shore-line. A huge fire was started and the unlucky pheasant was dutifully cremated, alongside two sea-gulls and a hedgehog.

****

Jenny Bruce, pretty as a picture, lived with her parents in the heart of the colliery. She was an only child. Her father, Albert, worked at Easington pit, rotund, mild-mannered and prematurely old, he doted on his daughter. The Bruce family was close and caring; Jenny had always been a good girl, mature for her years and always considerate towards her parents. She had brought no scandal to their door, not a smidgen, not even a whiff of mischief.

Both parents, however, were worried about her seeing Charlie Hill. He was a year younger than Jennie, always on his best behaviour. *Please* and *Thank you*, all the time, couldn't fault the lad and yet there was something about him, looked so aggressive and tetchy, covered in tattoos and him only sixteen, a chip on his shoulder so big it stood out a mile. What kind of family allowed such behavior? Albert had seen Charlie's dad, knew his reputation, working the same seam at the pit he was bound to hear the gossip. Albert didn't work at the coal-face, he was in no condition, too fond of his grub was Albert Bruce, always out of breath, so he worked the transfer-points, occasionally picking up his shovel and cleaning around the conveyor-belts: mopping up spillages. Long shifts working on his own and sometimes, sick of his own company, Albert would wander along to the coal-face and share a few minutes with the power-loaders and coal-hewers. He'd asked about Adam Hill. Curious about the fellow, like any concerned parent would be, idle chit-chat and gossip about the man and what he'd heard hadn't pleased him. *Crackerjack* he was told and by more than one, had a short fuse; too quick to use his fists. Most of the tittle-tattle blamed his missus, well on the way to being an alcoholic she was and the lad, according to the gossip-mongers, was as wild as his father.

He'd met him once and once was enough. The pit-showers were a warm, loud and comfortable place. End of the shift brought blessed relief for the colliers, always a load of daft banter and camaraderie and despite the uncertain future, there was always good cheer. Albert was in the shower-cubicle, bent double, trying to scrub the dirt from his feet, gasping and heaving as he struggled with the almost impossible task. He glanced up at the gawking stare from the big stranger.

"How do?" said Albert, knew who it was. He stood upright and smiled anxiously at the towering figure.

"You got a problem?" said the man.

"Pardon?" mild-mannered Albert started to quake.

"Asking a lot of questions about me?" Adam Hill stared coldly at the naked man.

"Hold on a minute," blustered Albert as he attempted to switch off the shower, desperately tried to think of an excuse, couldn't find one, "no harm meant."

The big man wouldn't let go, "Waiting for an answer," lifted both arms and rested them on either side of the cubicle.

"Just concerned is all," said Albert Bruce, his chest clanking like an old drum.

The big stranger smirked and muttered, "Concerned?"

"The bairn, my daughter Jenny," replied Albert, "she's walking out with your Charlie."

"Walking out?" shook his head, could think of a better way of putting it.

"Charlie and Jenny," said Albert humbly, "they're courting. I was just asking about, that's all."

"Should keep your old nose out of it," he growled, his tone intimidating, the warning ominous, "expect Charlie sees many a young filly." He gazed contemptuously at the naked, obese figure. "You'll not catch me checking on Charlie's conquests or their parents for that matter, I've better things to do with my time!"

Albert could never allow anyone to call his daughter, no matter the size or the age of the aggressor. The earlier fear left him as he answered curtly, "Cut that out, you hear, my daughter is no filly and she's certainly no conquest!"

Adam Hill smirked, his eyes cold. "Let the bairns have their bit of fun. Keep your nose out of their doings and keep your nose out of mine!" With that the collier turned and strode away from the shower-room.

Albert stepped out of the cubicle, his body still red with the sting of hot water, shouted after the man with growing resentment and anger, "And if he thinks my Jenny is a bloody conquest then he has another think coming!" past caring now, "you hear me, Adam Hill, you bloody hear me!"

The commotion acted like a magnet, a dozen heads abruptly appeared in unison from various parts of the shower-room, some covered in a heavy white lather of soap-suds; others still tar-babies.

Someone shouted in mock annoyance, *'Steady-on, Albert,'* cheers and cat-calls erupted through the place, *'tha's a bit old for that kind of behaviour!'*

****

Jenny skipped down the stairs and hurried past her parents. She was in her underwear, floppy dressing-gown flapping like pigeon's wings, her arms full of soiled work-clothes. The clothing-basket was in a large roomy cupboard in the kitchen. She smiled at her parents and asked if they wanted tea. Both nodded and Jenny disappeared into the other room.

"What do you think, father?" whispered Nancy Bruce.

Albert grimaced. "Suppose so, I'll have a word," his brow furrowed and he started rubbing his fingers together.

Nancy persisted, "Now's a good time, love."

Albert stalled, couldn't hurt his daughter, not for all the tea in China. "Listen, Nancy, should we not wait awhile, let it run its course, it might fizzle out?"

"That Charlie is no good......" the words died in her mouth.

Jenny stood at the door; she was holding a large plastic kettle, the look on her face said it all, "Go on, mother!"

"Pet," said Albert defensively, "your mother means no harm."

The girl's eyes never left her quarry, "Mother?"

Nancy took a deep breath, "It's about Charlie, love. We've heard some bad reports about him, that's all."

Jenny pouted, her features like thunder as she asked, "Such as?"

The older woman turned to her husband for help but Albert's nerve faltered and he could only stare uncomfortably at the floor.

Jenny persisted, "Mother?"

Nancy Bruce found the courage, looked her daughter straight in the eye and said defensively, "Alice Nord said he's trouble, love, said Charlie almost killed her Billy at school, had to take him to hospital. She was even going to report Charlie to the police."

Jenny shook her head in disbelief, "Mother, that was almost a year ago and it wasn't even Charlie's fault!"

Nancy was on her feet now, arms on hips she continued. "Right, my girl, then what about last Saturday?"

"What about it?" retorted the girl, her young face scrunched with annoyance.

"Thought you had a date with Charlie Hill," she spluttered contemptuously. "He didn't even turn up for you!"

Jenny's face calmed, tightened the dressing gown about her body and walked to the arm-chair, flopped down and watched her mother join her father on the sofa opposite.

"You're right, mother," said the girl, her voice was softer but still determined. "Charlie didn't show and yes I was hurt. And I cried because I thought he didn't want to see me." She glanced at the troubled face of her father. "There's something else I didn't tell you. I didn't go to Anne Hunter's house when Charlie didn't show." She paused, "I'm sorry that I had to lie to you."

Albert spoke for the first time. "You went to see Charlie?"

"Walked all the way to the Village, thought he was out because the house was dark and no one answered the door. I knew I couldn't go home, had to see for myself." Jenny bit her lip, "The door wasn't locked. I went in." She stopped speaking, didn't know how to continue.

Nancy looked at Albert. The room was silent. Albert Bruce shifted uneasily on the sofa, his features turning waxen with worry.

"He was sitting next to the fire," continued the girl. "Charlie had the fire-guard covered with his washing, shirt and socks, almost on top of the fire … stupid really because the fire was out. Didn't have any sticks to light it. He was trying to dry his clothes because he didn't have anything else to wear because his horrible parents were out and he wanted clean clothes." Tears were falling and her voice started to falter, "He wanted to look good for me, you understand?"

Albert was won over, shook his head slowly, feeling her pain. "Never mind, flower, we all know where the fault lies."

Nancy was resolute, the parental instinct too strong. "There's nothing good can come from this, Jenny," she struggled to her feet and straightened her skirt, glancing at her husband she said, "Your father had words with Charlie's dad." There was an edge to her voice. "Tell her, Albert, tell her what he said to you".

"Leave it mother," said Albert Bruce. He left the sofa. "Can we not leave it for now?"

****

It was four-o-clock when he reached the village. Charlie had left the others at the beach, still feasting and frolicking and causing mayhem. Saturday night was always a special night for the couple, Jenny and him, had been for months, the two of them, doing nothing special, being together, that was happiness enough. Charlie felt good; maybe things were changing long term at home, perhaps this time his mother really meant the things she said and wasn't going to leave him again. *Please God*, he thought, *let things stay normal.*

Charlie hurried along Laburnum Crescent, a few more streets and he'd be home, saw the familiar figure working in the garden of number 26, head and shoulders bigger than Charlie now. A gentle giant was Roy Bailey. The two childhood friends had drifted apart when they moved to the

Secondary Modern. The school was different again from their Junior School in the Village, rough and tough was the Comprehensive, full of hooligans from the colliery, a different breed from anything they had ever seen, wild as wolves and Charlie Hill was in his element, gave as good as he got, in his nature; too many beatings from his dad had made him as hard as metal. He joined the new crowd and flourished. Poor Roy, as big as he was, could not cope with the changes, took a back-seat, found the few friends who were more docile than the majority and survived. Teacher's pet really, did what he was told, always completed his homework and never back-answered the staff. Roy became a model pupil and the natural target for bullies. The bond of childhood however still held the pair close and Charlie watched over him, protected him.

Roy glanced up and saw his friend, waved a greeting. "Charlie, how are you?" saw the shoulder-bag, "shot anything?"

Charlie paused by the fence, telling tall tales, making Roy laugh, then he moved off saying, "You should come some time, Roy," but he knew it would be out-of-bounds for his old pal. Charlie had a reputation; he was bad news for most.

Turning the corner of the street, Charlie was shocked to see his parents leaving the cul-de-sac. *What the hell*, he thought and started running up the street. Charlie bellowed and the pair stopped, his mother waved a greeting.

Reaching them he spluttered, "What's up, Ma?"

"Father is taking me to the Leek Show at the Club," said Rebecca, looking pleased, Adam by her side proud as punch and preening like a peacock.

One hell of a drinking session, thought the youth. Said sullenly, "Okay then." At least they were going out together for a change, perhaps things were really on the mend long term.

"We'll not be too long, son," said the woman, turned and locked arms with a grinning Adam and the pair sauntered off. "Make your own tea, pet," shouted Rebecca as an afterthought, "there's a good boy."

The couple reached the main road, Rebecca paused and searched her hand-bag, irritation began to spread across her face. "*Lambert and Butler*, Adam, I've forgotten them," shoved coins into the man's hands, "be a love, will you?" Rebecca walked the few paces to the council-bench and eased her thin frame onto the wooden surface.

The man grunted with annoyance then turned and back-tracked to Greaney's corner-shop. Rebecca found the hand-mirror and carefully inspected her face, satisfied, she replaced the glass. A figure approached the bench, a strange sight indeed, short and squat and as wide as a barrel. The young man closed on Rebecca. He was dressed bizarrely; long overcoat almost touched the ground, on his head the wide battered fedora perched perilously over long, shoulder-length locks. The woman realized who it was and felt the pain of yesteryear like a punch in the chest, closed her eyes for a moment, her head full of memories. Jimmy Shannon, all those years ago, Little Jimmy and her mind danced with the tender images. *All for nothing*, she sighed. *All gone now and Jimmy in Heaven. Such a mess, such a terrible mess.*

"Hello," greeted the youth. He sat close to her, so close that the heavy frame touched her.

Rebecca took a deep breath. Sitting next to her, Jimmy Shannon's son. She croaked an almost inaudible reply.

"It's a lovely day?" said the boy, staring intently at the woman, eyes big and innocent.

“Hello, Harry,” answered Rebecca, regaining her composure; she looked at him and smiled.

“Are you tired, lady,” he asked, “is that why you’re sitting down?”

“Waiting for someone, Harry,” said Rebecca and she gazed at the warm, open face.

The chunky youth asked, “Where are you going?”

“Going for a drink, Harry.”

“Are you thirsty, then?” replied the boy.

Adam Hill strode up to the seat, his face masked in anger. He knew the youth, flung the cigarettes into the lap of the woman. Rebecca, caught off-guard, jumped with alarm.

Harry Shannon smiled at the big man. “Hello, Mister,” he said and he brushed aside the long golden locks that touched his face. “It’s a lovely day?”

“You ready, Rebecca?” grunted Adam, ignoring the boy, his face crunched with annoyance. He knew the imbecile, had known his father once, hated the man, detested the late Jimmy Shannon.

“Are you thirsty, Mister,” asked the youth naively, “are you going for a drink too?”

Rebecca left the bench and joined her retreating husband, as they walked away she turned and waved at the gaping, childlike figure.

“Bye, Missus!” he grinned and returned the wave.

“Straighten your face, Adam,” said Rebecca, “the bairn’s harmless.”

“Bloody idiot!” muttered Adam under his breath, “should have been drowned at birth!”

The woman shook her head slowly. Adam would never forget Jimmy Shannon. She sighed, *Need a drink*, she thought, *a bloody long drink!*

They walked towards the Workingmen's' Club, two troubled, tortured souls.

****

Charlie hid the rifle behind the settee, threw his jacket across the arm-chair and walked into the kitchen. He winced at the accumulated mess that littered the table, moved to the larder and cursed loudly. *Empty!* not a bite to eat in the house so he decided to visit Greaney's grocery. He started searching for money. All the usual places were empty, moved to the stairwell and began looking through the coat-pockets of his parents, found only scrap copper.

Then he remembered and bounded up the stairs and into the big bedroom. His dad always kept a stash under the mattress. He lifted the bedding and groaned. *Not a penny-piece,* he mused, *what to do?* He knew where the big money was hidden, had known about the place for a year, smiled at the memory. His mother, recently returned from one of her jaunts and desperate to re-stock and disappear before Adam returned from work told Charlie to wait downstairs, threatened him and then staggered up the stairs on unsteady inebriated legs, forgetting to look back as the self-appointed voyeur duly followed his mother step by step all the way to the treasure-trove.

Charlie hesitated for a moment, recalled the severity of the beating metered out by his dad, his mother laid-up for days afterwards because of the theft of his savings, black and blue from the assault. He sucked in air, stooped and pulled back the carpet, the loose floor-board was lifted and the solitary note was pulled from the roll. It would never be missed. At that very moment the back-door slammed shut, only the wind playing tricks with his imagination, but Charlie imagined his father was returning to the house, with a single bound he ran from the room and closed the door behind him, hurried down the stairs away from possible confrontation. The bedroom carpet had been forgotten, left crumpled and adrift from the wall, several floor-boards were on show for all to see.

Minutes later and Charlie bustled into the shop. Old Jack Greaney was alone and that suited the youth, better chance to steal the odd item when Jack wasn't looking. He liked Jack Greaney, he was always nice to Charlie, always gave him respect. The proprietor used to work at Horden pit until his accident, made him ever so slow and gullible.

"Now Charlie?" said the man.

The boy felt a stab of conscience. He decided to be good and not steal a single thing. "Hi, Mr. Greaney," he smiled, "how's Missus Greaney?"

Alice Greaney was a teacher at the Secondary. She taught English, had a soft spot for Charlie, always kind to him perhaps that was why Charlie never disrupted her lessons.

"What can I buy for £5, Mister Greaney?" asked the lad.

"£5 did you say, son?" a faint hint of a smile began to cover his wrinkled features. The kid normally brought in a handful of change, pilfered, no doubt, from his parent's pockets. "Not all in bronze is it?"

Charlie waved the crisp note like a magic wand across the counter, mischievous grin on his freckled face, "Pocket-money, Mr. Greaney!"

Brought a smile to the old man's face, "Buy whatever you want Charlie."

****

Eight-o-clock and the young couple sat in front of the large television screen. Charlie was gazing down the contents page of the *Northern Echo*. B.B.C. was showing *Some like it Hot*: Tyne Tees was advertising *Witness*. Jenny had no interest in either Monroe or Ford, Charlie wasn't too keen on game-shows or the power base of Robert Mugabe, blamed it all on Jenny's tight-fisted father, Albert Bruce for refusing to buy a *Sky* package. '*Waste of money*,' he would whine, *'too much choice already!'* Jenny appeared ill at ease, so unlike her, especially on a Saturday night. Her folks always visited the Colliery Club at the weekend: few pints and a game of bingo, their one night out, Saturday night.

The girl snuggled up close to the youth, touched and fondled his fingers. "Been some trouble, Charlie," she said carefully.

"Let me guess," he answered sarcastically, "grown-ups?"

"Mam and dad."

"Talking about me?'

"Billy Nord's mam was chatting about you, you know, when you and Billy had a fight?"

"Old news, Jenny," said Charlie, "and you know Billy started it."

"That what I told Ma."

"So what's the problem?"

"Ma's worried about me. The usual stuff, no one is good enough for their little girl." She glanced at the youth, knew him inside and out, could see past the outer shell, the swagger, the posturing, all an act. Behind the bombastic, aggressive stance was a gentle, affectionate and caring person, her Charlie, her special love, someone she would die for.

"Does it really matter what people think about me ...about us?" His tone was quiet and soft. He gripped her hand and squeezed it lovingly. "It should be about me and you and no one else……"

He was stopped in his tracks as the kitchen door crashed open and the two adults hurried inside. Albert and Nancy Bruce, full of bile and bite.

"Jenny," called out the mother, "are you in the other room?"

The daughter hurried to the adults leaving Charlie confused and a little anxious sitting on the sofa. He listened with baited breath as the discussion started.

"I've never been so insulted in all of my life!" whined the woman.

"Ma," asked Jenny, glancing at both of her parents, "what on earth is the matter?"

Albert threw his jacket over the back of a chair, found a cigarette, struck a match and sucked at the smoke like his life depended on it. "Called in to see the Leek Show, didn't we, Nancy, pet?"

"Bloody Leek Show!" spat the wife, livid with anger and embarrassment.

"Charlie's parents were havin' a blazing row," said Albert, pulled at the chair and squatted, cigarette-ash fell over the table-surface, another long suck on the smoke before he continued. "Hell for leather, the pair of them!"

Jenny asked, "What about?"

Albert told Jenny. There had been a loud and verbal battle between Adam and Rebecca Hill, pushing and prodding one another, not caring that dozens of incredulous members were watching. '*About someone dead and buried*,' said Albert.

"You're kidding," queried Jenny, "someone dead and buried?"

“Jimmy Shannon,” interrupted Nancy Bruce, “used to live at the village, knocked over about ten years ago. Always drunk, married Ruby Wright. They had a backward bairn?”

“Harry Shannon,” said Charlie standing at the doorway, “year older than me.” He watched as all eyes devoured him, silence as they waited for more. He focused on the seated figure, “They were talking about Harry’s dad?”

“Aye, lad,” said Albert, “they were havin’ a right ding-dong”.

Charlie could only shake his head, *No wonder people don’t like me,* he thought.

“Your mother stormed out,” continued Albert. Little drops of perspiration covered leaden jowls. He was ill at ease, “Your dad was in a right stew, needed ta vent his temper. That’s when he saw me…..”

“He’s a bully,” said Nancy, her eyes burrowed into her daughter. “Your dad is not well, Jenny, he’s had angina for years, certainly doesn’t need some …..brute to shout and threaten him.” She stole a glance at Charlie.

“Why would he do that, Missus?” asked a crestfallen Charlie.

“He was rude to Jenny’s dad,” barked Nancy Bruce, “made snide remarks about …… you and Jenny.”

“I think, under the circumstances,” said Albert, lighting a second cigarette, glancing at the youth, “that maybe you should leave, let things cool for a while, eh?”

“Don’t you talk to Charlie like that, Dad!” Jenny’s voice was raised with emotion, “it’s not Charlie’s fault he’s got crazy…….” realized too late the error, the severity of her words, knew immediately the hurt that would be felt by Charlie.

The youth could only stare at them, his head bursting with a thousand excuses for his parent's behaviour. He loved his parents, hated them, so confused, how could he possibly explain why they acted the way they did. With his head bowed with embarrassment, the lad walked to the door.

"Don't go!" cried Jenny, "Charlie, I'm sorry," she grabbed at his arm.

"Let him go Jenny," said Nancy Bruce.

"You'll be pleased then, Missus?" grunted Charlie, stealing a glance at the rotund, smirking figure.

"Cheeky young pup!" barked a pouting Nancy Bruce.

"Don't, Charlie!" begged Jenny. She was crying now.

"Jenny," shouted Albert, "do as your mother says!"

He pushed away her hand and left the house. Once outside he bolted away into the night, wanting to be alone, needing only his own company. Charlie slowed to a walking pace when he reached the main road, Seaside Lane, which snaked through the colliery. He walked along the gentle decline towards the coast and the colliery buildings. A cruel biting breeze swept off the shore and made him shiver. The streets were deserted. Charlie stood and stared at the distant outlines of the mine, the faint wafting sounds as the big wheel intermittently turned and pulled the black bounty to the surface, the *thump thump* as the colliery locomotive dragged the big mining-cars across the huge expanse of yard.

He recalled Elvis's warnings about the demise of the industry. *Two years*, he had warned, *three years maximum.* The youth wasn't stupid, knew things would change, only hoped that the change would take longer, much longer. He had spoken to his dad, told him what Elvis Priestley had said about the pits. Adam had spat venom at the dire warnings, did not take kindly to anyone who didn't work in the mines, had an innate, immediate, unwarranted distrust of so called *strangers,* told his son that the government was attempting to close the mines because of the debacle with Ted Heath years earlier. '*Debacle means bloody shambles, Charlie, they learn you bugger all at the school?'* the explanation filled with sarcasm. The miners had beaten the Prime Minister fair and square despite his underhand tactics at introducing the three-day working week. The Conservatives had neither forgiven nor forgotten the colliers and wouldn't be happy until Scargill - the union leader - was crucified and the industry destroyed. *Three hundred years of coal under the North Sea*, Adam boasted and *there's thirty years of gas.* He told Charlie to stop fretting.

The school examinations had been taken over a month ago by the majority of the fifth-year pupils. Charlie, always a disruptive influence in most lessons, had missed much of his basic education, detention was the norm; the *sin-bin* was visited almost daily because of his rowdy, anti-social behaviour. Charlie wasn't evil, more immature. He always tried to avert being barred from the school, hated being at home for long periods. He played the fool and tended to fire the bullets given by other, more devious, trouble-makers. He had taken no G.C.S.E.s. Where could Charlie find employment, the Coal Board was still hiring and his dad had connections with the union. Charlie had decided to work at the colliery despite the warnings.

Charlie found himself wandering slowly back to the Bruce's home. He had calmed and wanted to see Jenny. He reached the rear-yard of the terraced property, last house in the steep incline, stood and listened as the racket of the argument wafted over him. All about Charlie. Charlie's family too. He cringed with embarrassment.

He walked away and reached Avon Street, several rows up from Jenny's home and turned left onto the steep decline, noticed the open gate and the street light gleaming over the *Honda* motor-bike propped against the wall, stopped him like a magnet. Charlie glanced around, no one about, the place deserted; the only noise came from the house itself; the television blasting out a garbled tune. He stepped into the rear-yard, his heart pounding, couldn't believe his eyes, there was no locking-chain on the bike. Moments later and the youth and the machine were hurtling silently down the heavy incline, turning left at the bottom of the street, Charlie glided the motor-bike towards the coast, manipulated the machine under the loco-bridge only stopping when he was safely out of sight. Wet with perspiration and fear, he fumbled at the large bunch of keys that he kept on his belt, a recent present from Elvis Priestley, Elvis with the lovely and available granddaughter, Sheryl Priestley; *She could be in the movies*, he thought, *Sheryl the wildcat.*

Key number 10 opened the box, the ignition turned and with one press of a button the bike roared to life then he was gone from the place. Charlie headed south, towards Horden Colliery, avoiding the main streets of Easington, decided to make a detour and drive in a huge circle through the outskirts of Horden, touching the edges of the town, head for the farming hamlet of Little Thorpe and the rough quarry road that was a back-door route to the Waterworks. Charlie Hill was ecstatic; the motor-bike had been stolen and delivered in less than ten minutes. He left the bike in Elvis's back-yard, walked away like he'd scooped the pools, wondered how much Priestley would pay for such a pristine machine.

Hurrying from the place, Charlie followed the unmade back-lane that was wedged between the primary school and the council houses. It wasn't too late. He guessed 10.30, smiled at himself when he saw the lights shining brightly from his home, imagined his parents home early. *'Definitely on the mend,'* mused the boy, *'at least on the home-front.'*

Adam Hill was waiting behind the door, the fellow demented with anger knowing his son had stolen some of his money. Charlie was caught off-guard and beaten to an inch of his life, his body covered with bruises and swellings from the vicious assault. Like a rat caught in a trap, the youngster had little chance of defending himself, the speed and ferocity caught Charlie by surprise and he was knocked unconscious in seconds. Adam Hill had never lost a battle in his entire life, in fact, few stood up to him. Charlie was one of the few. Over the past year he had had fought back twice, always took a hiding, mattered little to him; once the fists started the boy seemed to go trance-like, the pain masked by the rush of adrenalin as he fought his father, the battle surreal and dreamlike as Charlie appeared to observe himself battling his father in slow motion. The earlier fights used to last only seconds but as he grew older the seconds turned to minutes and he knew one day he would be victorious. But not that night.

Charlie was stunned, staggering blindly, the bombshell of the first blow sending a kaleidoscope of stars through his head, the second whack as the heavy frying-pan smashed again into his skull felled him and he collapsed like a clown as the blackness enveloped him. Hours later he managed to crawl to his bedroom and stayed there all of the next day, visited once by a subdued and repentant father, listening grimly as his son tried to explain why the money was taken. He could barely talk so severe was the facial damage. There was more bleak news. His mother had gone again. Charlie reckoned that the argument witnessed by Jenny's parents must have escalated into something more serious, perhaps that was why his father had been in such a foul mood and the reason for the brutal beating. '*Gone again,*' moaned Adam. *'We've had an almighty row!'* leaving young Charlie to fret and worry, forgot about the assault, his mother's image never leaving his thoughts, cared too much, that was probably the worst part for him, fretted and ached for her. His Ma was dreadful when she was intoxicated, intoxicated and in a foul mood she was liable to do anything. Anything!

Charlie clung to his home for most of the first week. Some nights he ventured out and wandered the Village. The nights were drawing shorter and he felt more comfortable hidden by the blackness. Two long weeks, busted and bruised, riddled with aches and pains, didn't seek company, didn't want anyone to see the state of his battered features. Jenny finally showed at the end of the week. Her initial reaction was of anger then shock, the girl thinking Charlie had been up to mischief. When he explained about the beating, she mellowed, started to fuss over him but she couldn't get close to him, no one could. Jenny didn't stay long; the talk one-sided; she took the hint and left him to wallow in the mire of self-pity.

At the end of the second week, Charlie started to feel better. He visited Elvis who slipped him a wad of money, payment for the stolen bike. *'Bull's Eye, Elvis!'* he said, his spirits lifting as he counted his ill-gotten gains, *'keep me in mind for the next job!'* The youth thought that thieving wasn't so bad after all and the rewards were excellent.

He decided to return to school, needed something to distract his head, better busy and in company than sitting wallowing with his finger on the self-destruct button. His Ma would return soon, she'd been missing a fortnight and her record away from the family home was three weeks. She always tended to resurface when all of the money disappeared, one thing guaranteed.

****

CHAPTER THREE

Charlie hurried from the house. He had fifteen minutes to reach school and his friend, Roy Bailey, would be waiting for him at the bottom of the Village. The boys, friends since childhood still walked to school together but Roy, nervous by nature, was always fidgeting and pacing the pavement outside of his home anxiously waiting Charlie's arrival, couldn't bear the thought of being late or the thought of incurring the wrath of any teacher. Charlie scurried from the cul-de-sac when he saw the lone figure slowly approaching, felt his heart skip a beat as he recognized the unsteady, meandering gait of his mother. He stopped dead in his tracks and called out to her, '*Mother, you're back,*' and hurried to her side, smelled the stale stench of alcohol oozing from her. '*Ma, where have you been?*', not that he cared, she was home and that was all that mattered, putting his arm around her for support, the youth half-carried his mother towards their home. From a nearby house, curtains flickered and lifted: prying neighbours loving the spectacle.

Rebecca Hill spotted the voyeur and despite the nausea and discomfort of the hangover she pointed an angry fist towards the council house. Down but not out, she yelled defiantly, *'Have a bloody good look, you old bastard!'* clinging perilously on to her son, wanting to reach the sanctuary of her home, aching for rest and sleep. Charlie tried to ease his struggling mother into their backyard, with Rebecca still valiantly tussling, gesticulating and verbally abusing the snooping neighbour. Soon the couple was inside their home and the boy carefully eased his mother on to the settee. Arranging pillows, Charlie lowered his protesting mother on to the stained and ancient couch, took off her shoes and made her comfortable. Finding one of his mother's overcoats, Charlie gently covered her. Rebecca's eyes closed immediately. The boy hurried to the kitchen to make the tea, the kettle filled in an instant, a solitary cup hastily washed, then he heard the sound of slumber, loud guttural snoring filled the room and Charlie waited. The noise continued unabated. His mother was fast asleep; he left the tea-making, glanced quickly at the crumpled, moaning figure of his wayward parent then slipped out of the home, he would return at lunch-time and look after her properly, a bit of love and attention before his dad returned from work. Last thing he wanted was fireworks, had to somehow pacify his old man, ease him down a peg or two, try and arrange a temporary truce.

Charlie ran as fast as his legs would carry him, almost at the school entrance when he saw his friend. Roy Bailey clearly irritated at the long fruitless wait, shouted, *'Charlie, where were you?'* as they hurried through the entrance of Easington Comprehensive, the smaller youth, buoyant about the return of his mother, calmly explained his delay. The pair reached the big hall with only minutes to spare, the interior already filled to capacity with over two hundred bored and weary youngsters: Year Five pupils and the Headmaster, Lancelot Mearman, already strutting aggressively on the small stage with eight tutors standing in an untidy line behind him. Open aggression roared from the moustachioed, twitching mouth of the Headmaster, his little arms gesticulated wildly, angry that his prolonged and fevered attempts at establishing a school uniform with the more senior of his pupils had proved an unmitigated disaster, doomed to failure. Before him, for the most part, a rag-bag army of delinquents and tearaways, who cared little for his authority or for his school.

The small dapper figure pounded a fist against open palm. *'The reputation of this school will not falter,'* he shrieked. *'I will not have louts, yes louts, coming into my school dressed in any manner of stupid clothing! We have a policy concerning school uniforms!'* His gaze searched frantically at the older pupils. He could see perhaps a dozen or so youths sporting something resembling a uniform. He had long ago given up on a school-blazer or even regulation-grey trousers and as a last resort he had opted for a simple pullover - grey or blue - but even this simple request had fallen, for the most part, on deaf ears. His eyes found one immaculately dressed boy, a god-send for the tutor, *'You lad!'* he bellowed and a wicked finger beckoned, *'Come!'*

A whimpering twig of a lad, lost in some pleasant pubescent daydream, was prodded by his crony. Suddenly wide awake, he quaked at his friend, *'What have I done?'* then he began the stumbling walk towards the demon headmaster, turning for the fleetest of moments towards his disappearing friend, he mimed again, *What have I done*? climbed the few wooden steps on to the stage, his face a bright shade of red. Faint with fear he stood transfixed and waiting for the expected reprimand.

Archibald Harvey, a short, squat man of middle years, closed on him, grasping the boy's collar he started to drag the terrified youth to the centre of the stage.

"A've done nowt!" he protested.

"Shut up, stupid boy!" grunted the tutor. "Stand to attention, fool!" then backtracked and joined his motley crew of colleagues at the rear of the stage.

The Headmaster took over. "See this!" he thundered. "This is what I mean!" His strong, wiry fingers grasped the coat-lapels.

The fifth-year pupil closed his eyes and waited for the beating.

Lancelot Mearman continued. “This is what I mean, this boy is a fine example, an asset to the entire school!”

Jackie Thompson opened his eyes, truly amazed at his good fortune, focused on his friend, big goofy smile over his perplexed features, scratching anxiously at his wild feral hair, looking like a youthful version of Stan Laurel, minus the bowler-hat.

Near to the back of the hall Charlie rubbed his face with his hands, trying to stay focused, trying to forget the baboon parading as a teacher on the stage, thinking of his mother and praying she would sleep until he returned from school, dreading the afternoon and worrying about his dad’s reaction to the homecoming.

The headmaster spotted the youth. “Front and centre, Hill!” he shrieked.

Charlie sauntered to the front of the hall, tried not to show fear, climbed on to the stage and walked purposefully towards the Headmaster, reaching him; he swivelled away from the irate tutor and faced the audience, cool as a cucumber, faking confidence like a stage magician, a seemingly confident smile blossomed over his young face.

Lancelot Mearman lost his temper. He began stamping up and down and shouting like a madman, could not abide arrogant, insolent youths who thought they could show disrespect to anyone in authority. ‘*Dumb insolence*,’ he shrieked to the heavens as he tried to manhandle Charlie from the stage, other teachers joined in the fiasco and the youth was pulled and prodded and dragged to the main office. Later, when the assembly was at an end and Mearman had chance to collect himself, Charlie was verbally admonished and threatened with further punishment if he did not improve his behaviour. '*I smiled,*' said Charlie, '*nothing more.*' Perhaps the Headmaster realised the mistake of losing his temper in front of the entire school, always a dangerous ploy in front of so many witnesses, it took only one phone call from some agitated parent and County Hall bigwigs descended and created mayhem for him. The Hill clan was a different kettle of fish; worst that could happen was some verbal onslaught from the wild parents. Grateful for small mercies the tutor admonished Charlie but kept his tone and his threats to a minimum, then he sent him on his way. The boy could not believe his luck.

He headed for the hall and his Music Lesson. Only weeks before leaving school and they were still subjected to such irrelevant and superficial tutorials, small wonder the class was disruptive and argumentative. Peering through the windows Charlie observed the two crescent-shaped lines of chairs surrounding the ancient piano. Mister Ireland - Paddy behind his back - was shouting abuse at the lethargic class. Monday morning and *Music* and not another instrument in sight, never had been. Music lessons sounded superior to singing lessons, because that's all it was; half an hour of mayhem. *Like Jools Holland with a hangover,* commented Charlie Hill as Paddy pounded out his golden tunes, pushed open the door and moved towards the group. Ireland glared at the newcomer. The little book was grasped by the youth, the page found and the lad waited to begin miming the words.

Paddy Ireland started pounding frantically at the piano and then he raised his arm for the introduction, started to sing loudly and lovingly. *'Singing is a joy! Singing is a joy!'* so enthusiastic about his lessons, playing the old instrument single-handed whilst gesticulating with his free hand, the middle-aged tutor singing like there was no tomorrow. '*Singing is a joy!*' stared at the sullen class with incredulity, '*Sing! Sing!*' he bellowed frantically, left the piano and moved between the rows of pupils. About half were singing, the others were miming, it resembled a pantomime. Charlie wouldn't sing, couldn't sing to save his life, might have attempted the odd note if it were sing-a-long with *Madonna* or *Sinead* or even *The Bangles* but never this rubbish. Ireland closed on him. Charlie continued with the sham until only inches separated the two.

"Still can't hear!" bawled the tutor.

Charlie closed his eyes with growing frustration as tiny droplets of spittle danced across Charlie face and the youth grimaced and turned away from the onslaught of germs and bad breath, lifted the hymn book and held it like a barrier in front of the teacher. The book, despite being waved like a miniature umbrella, proved to be an inadequate barrier against the flying globules. Ireland was incensed at the youth's behaviour and dragged a protesting Charlie to the Headmaster's office, but the punishment - much to the annoyance of Ireland - was a paltry 200 lines. He was ordered back to the hall but made to stand outside for the remainder of the time.

The next lesson was Charlie's favourite: P.E. He excelled in all types of sport - football; cross-country; gymnastics. The spanner in the works was the fool in charge. Allan Cunningham thought he was *Arnold Schwarzenegger,* acted the part, always throwing his weight around and in Charlie's opinion, the man was an arrogant swollen-headed fool. The queue of pupils waited impatiently in an untidy line outside the gymnasium, it had started to rain, a light drizzle but it was putting a dampener on the lesson. The young gym teacher was having a quick fag and a cup of tea, a common occurrence. Suddenly the doors opened with a clash and the lads hurried inside and without a word said, the entire class started undressing. Only Charlie waited, forgotten his kit again, an excuse, in truth, the shorts and shirt were still in his bedroom, a permanent fixture and still in need of a good wash.

"I might have guessed," snapped the brute of a teacher, "away from school again and still you return empty-handed!"

No washing-powder sir, thought Charlie, his face grim and uncompromising. *No soap even. And the bloody washing-machine hasn't worked since I was thirteen! Tell you what Cunningham: I'll go down to the river with my washing-board and there's a history lesson tackled too.*

Charlie said stoically, "Sorry Sir, forgot them again," lowered his head and stared at the floor.

A powerful push caught Charlie off-guard and he was catapulted back into the crowd of boys. Poor Roy Bailey, half-undressed fell headfirst into the backside of Alan Mounter who clashed awkwardly into the steel locker. Up in a flash, Alan, with his good eye honed in on a quaking Roy and his other eye gaping into the retreating lads, lashed out at Charlie's mate. Down like a collapsed deck-chair, poor weak Roy shrieking with fear, covering his face to stop any more blows then began wheezing and blowing, his asthma erupting and the more he fought for breath, the more he laboured.

Like a rocket, a maddened Charlie threw himself at the aggressor. The first punch caught Alan flush on the jaw; the second slammed into the unprotected stomach, out like a light, Mounter fell on top of the struggling Roy. A moment's bedlam and then total silence as the rest of the class watched and waited for the expected reprisals.

The tutor was in his element. A trained body-builder and an avid follower of the martial arts, he lifted and threw a hapless Charlie Hill across the room. His temper broken the youth rose and ran at the teacher, an impossible task. *David against Goliath,* only the Bible wasn't on Charlie's side, with a quick side-step, the tutor had the boy in a secure head-lock, with the lad's arm painfully cranked up his back. Charlie was frog-marched from the room screaming with anger, howled all the way to the Headmaster's office.

After sitting for twenty minutes in the secretary's office Charlie was called into the Headmaster's study. Lancelot Mearman felt like throwing in the towel. *It wasn't worth it*, he thought, *it really wasn't worth it,* glanced at the boy's neck and noticed the bruising was starting to disappear, he would have strong words with Cunningham, but later, perhaps after lunch, the situation needed a period of calm. He looked again at the boy's face, still at school and the lad had the look of a street fighter, all pocked with battle scars. *What a bloody nightmare family,* mused Mearman then decided on diplomacy as the best course of action, the last thing he wanted on this earth was another head to head with either one of the warring parents.

"Now Charlie," he began cautiously, "this is your third visit to my office and it's not even lunch-time?"

"Not my fault, sir," answered the surly, subdued youth.

Probably not, thought Mearman. *But what on earth do I do?*

"Sir," repeated Charlie, the headmaster seemed preoccupied, "it really wasn't my fault".

"Last warning, Hill," replied a blustering headmaster, "now off you go!"

Lancelot Mearman decided to have strong words with the gymnastics tutor, the fellow was getting a little to cocky for his boots, needed putting in his place. *After lunch*, thought the Headmaster*, I'll leave it until after lunch.*

The third and last lesson of the morning was Art. Charlie sauntered from the main block and crossed the small back-road towards the solitary brick building housing the Art; metal-work and wood-work departments. Charlie was aching for a smoke and was about to scamper behind the buildings for a quick fag when he saw the car turn sharply into the school drive. He watched as the lone vehicle neared, recognized the car, the ancient silver Volvo belonged to Agnes Bailey. The car slowed then stopped next to the youth.

"What happened, Charlie?" said the troubled woman.

Charlie told her about the incident, couldn't understand why she was visiting the school, perhaps to make a complaint? It was all sorted, he told her, Roy would have no more bother with Alan Mounter, he would see to that.

"Going to the hospital, Charlie," she replied. "Roy is still poorly. He's still in the Medical Room, not very well at all, they said."

And to prove she was a liar, her son stomped into view, his face masked with a deep brooding frown. Charlie waved greeting to his approaching friend, said his farewells to the woman and hurried into the school building, forgot all about his smoke.

Roy Bailey nodded a greeting to his mother and climbed into the car, his features still pale from the beating.

"Off we go, son," purred Agnes and the motor eased away from the place, "straight to Hartlepool General."

After some moments Roy felt able to speak. "I give him what-for mother," gulped noisily, "he didn't think I'd retaliate." He didn't look at his mother but continued to stare out of the window, lost in thought.

Pull the other one my love, she thought, replied softly, "Don't you worry about it, son. It's over now, just let it go."

"What did Charlie say, Ma?" asked Roy and glanced nervously at his mother, hoping that his friend hadn't said too much about the incident, last thing he wanted was being called a liar, or worse still, a coward.

"Not a lot, son," said Agnes loyally, "said you'd been in a fight with someone," couldn't hurt his feelings, her only son, only wished he had the gumption of young Charlie Hill, still, push come to shove, Roy was a good boy, brought no sorrow or trouble to her door, he'd never see the inside of a prison cell, run a mile from felony or fault would Roy.

"Alan Mounter will think twice about me in future, Ma," pouted the relieved youth, "showed him up good and proper! Charlie had to pull me off him! Honest Ma, he had to pull me off him or I would have killed him for sure!"

"That's my boy," answered Agnes, her head still focusing on Rebecca's son. Poor Charlie didn't have a hope in hell of salvation, not with those two as parents.

Midday and Charlie sprinted towards the colliery. The lunch break was an hour long, time enough to visit Jenny who worked at the co-operative store on Seaside Lane, spend a few precious minutes with her, maybe sort out their differences, see if her parents had calmed about him and then, if he really hurried he'd have time to see to his mother and sort out her problems. He took a breathless five minutes to reach the store, only stopped for air when the huge and festooned Co-op window was reached. Jenny was standing next to the cash register talking to a woman. Charlie tapped loudly against the pane; both women turned simultaneously and looked at him. Jenny was with her mother. *Hell's Teeth*, thought the youth and feigned an apologetic smile. It didn't work, not even a glimmer of a smile came back to him. Desperately Charlie beckoned the girl, didn't have a lot of time and wanted a few moments with her, put things right again. Torn emotionally Jenny hesitated too long and watched, miserably, as the youth turned and hurried away.

Reaching home, Charlie had a brief panic attack, his mother was no longer on the settee; he bundled through all of the down-stairs rooms. Empty. The boy was about to bolt out of the door in search of her - first step would have been a quick reconnoitre around the nearest pubs - when he realized that he hadn't checked the bedrooms, up the stairs like rocket-man and Charlie found her wrapped in an untidy bundle of blankets, in his bed. Didn't matter one jot, she was still home and safe, the woman snoring like a piglet but to the lad it was the sweetest sound in the world, he touched and toyed the sweaty mop of matted hair, fondled it, pleased that his mother was home again, tried to rearrange the bedding to make it more comfortable but the unconscious figure clung to the blankets; deep in dreams, safe with the cushion of cloth about her, words fell from her dry lips, soft and distant gibberish; foreign to all but her, leaned closer vainly trying to understand her messages but they proved impossible to decipher.

Charlie retraced his steps, searched the living-room for pen and paper, found the remains of a pencil but no writing paper so he used the old stand-by - a discarded cigarette packet, tearing it open, Charlie used the inside cover, scrawled a message to his Dad, wanting to pacify him so that he might leave his mother in peace. *Mother not well, dad,* he wrote. *I've put her to bed. Don't wake her. I'll make your tea.'* There was no logic behind the desperate note, nothing edible in the house and no money to buy any food, but that was another problem, he would sort it out, somehow. A final cuddle, a gentle stroke of her hair and he hurried back to school.

Charlie was late for registration, got a right mouthful from his form-teacher but Jack Daniels (Arthur Daniels actually) was all wind and water, all bark and not a bad old fart really. Charlie felt better, so pleased his mother was still at home and a little bonus to follow registration; a double lesson with Alice Greaney. English was one of his best lessons, brought out the best in Charlie.

In most other lessons the class attempted bedlam and riot, it mattered little that they were usually punished, the boys could almost smell the end of their school days and most were game for anything, all wanted to be the class clowns, all wanted to boast of the mayhem and disruption they'd instigated that day. *St. Trinians* was definitely on even par with Easington Comprehensive's non-academic fifth year. For example, that morning's Art lesson. The topic: *Great People of the Past*: choose someone who was known and admired. Alan Whiley; budding artiste, painted a full body drawing of Joan of Arc, nude, even down to the copious pubic hair! Brilliant, until the tutor saw it. He was given his marching-orders by Smedley, the Welsh teacher who tore the picture into a thousand shreds and threw the remains over the protesting youth before sending him to the sin-bin. Happy days!

There was something calming about Alice Greaney. Unlike most teachers, she rarely raised her voice and she always listened to her pupils as if she really cared. Alice gave every last one her undivided attention, plus buckets of respect and what she got back was love and attention - although none of the toughs in the class would ever admit to such tender emotion. Almost all teachers were classed as the enemy, some were tolerated, one or two respected. Alice Greaney was top of the heap, always commenced the lesson with a little idle chatter, buzzing around the sea of faces she would listen to the banter and sometimes offer advice but always with a smile. She was a one-off.

Alice ventured to the black-board and chalked the heading for the lesson. *Games people play and* the class pondered for several moments. The tutor waited patiently, not in any hurry, wanting a class discussion first, followed by some attempt at written work. She was a miracle-worker.

"Fun or serious, Miss?" asked John Nellis.

The tutor's arms went up in mock surrender. "Whatever, the choice is up to you."

"Miss," chortled Nelly, "when I was little".

The tutor scratched the words, *Childhood* and *Infant* on to the black-board.

"My dad used to work in the hospital," continued the boy, "doing odd-jobs."

Porter appeared on the board.

"Ryhope Hospital, Miss, near Sunderland," said Nelly, "before some of it was knocked down."

Another word, *Demolished.*

"Dad forgot his lunch, so my mother drove me to the hospital." John Nellis smiled as the memory came back. "Dad took me on a guided tour, Miss; even saw where they kept the dead bodies."

And again, *Mortuary.*

"Miss," said Nelly. "Honest Miss and this no word of a lie, when we were walking around the coffin place, one of the dead ones farted!" His eyes gazed about the classroom, "Honest to God!"

Alice Greaney wrote the word, *Flatulence,* then she turned to a beaming youth and asked him to write all of the words from the black-board into his writing-book. She rubbed out the words, ready for the next volunteer.

Martin Bradley was first with his hand up. Every finger had a letter tattooed on it. On a bad day Big Marty would battle anyone, but not this day, he too talked about his childhood and the tutor scribbled more words on to the black-board. "Miss," said Marty, "I used to have a pet tortoise."

"What was his name!" shouted someone at the back of the room.

"Speedy!" said the youth, chortling, "it was a boy."

Everybody laughed, including the teacher.

Marty Bradley didn't tell the class about the large penis he'd drawn on to the belly of his pet tortoise with a felt-tip pen. He never found out if the creature was male or female, didn't have it long enough, his idea of a joke and anyway, how could you tell the teacher that? He continued, "Mother shouted us in for dinner, me and my big brother. He was always nasty to me."

"Big brothers tend to be," sympathized the woman.

"I was eating my dinner when our Reg came in. He started being nice to me for a change, said my tortoise had a terrible headache so I ran back into the garden!" Marty took a deep breath. "Cut its head off, Miss, teased its head out of its shell with a lettuce leaf and used my scissors to chop off its head!" The big lad shook his head from side to side.

The last word Alice wrote was *Decapitated.*

It was Charlie's turn. He kept it light. They were nine years old at the time; Charlie and Roy and it was the summer holidays. They'd spent the morning playing on a swing in the nearby Little Thorpe **dene** then in the afternoon, bored out of their heads and wandering the streets of the village, they had decided to join with a bunch of girls playing with a skipping-rope. The rope itself was long and had probably been stolen from the stores of the local mine. It stretched the full width of the cul-de-sac and the two oldest girls worked the twine round and round and faster and faster. The group had been divided into two teams, with the two boys each on different sides. All had to run into the huge spinning circle of rope and attempt as many skips as was possible, then scamper away from the swirling rope. Time after time the unfortunate Roy let his side down, never quick enough to escape the twine, always getting whacked and losing points, he even managed to trip and fall.

Emotions grew, tempers raged as the game became more and more fractious, especially with Roy Bailey's team as they cat-called and belittled his clumsy attempts, then all hell broke loose as the embarrassed, incensed boy finally lost his temper. Perhaps Roy thought he had a chance against the females. Had the game involved boys, Roy Bailey would have controlled his growing anger, the youth hated confrontation, was mortified at the thought of physical force but with girls? Charlie remembered his friend jumping up and down in a fit of pique he'd never seen before, shrieking at some girl and perhaps it would have ended there if Roy hadn't pushed the female.

The tutor was busily scribbling notes on the black-board. But Charlie was finished with the reminiscences, he would conclude by spinning some yarn to end the story. There was no way he was going to tell her what occurred next...............

Anne Marie Hickson, slightly taller than Roy, suddenly attacked with determined venom that took everyone by surprise. Her fists battered and scratched the retreating boy who immediately crashed to the road, but the shrieking Anne Marie was not finished as she launched herself on to the squirming, screaming Roy who tried vainly to struggle to his feet and escape. The fight was totally one-sided. Charlie could wait no longer, blood was oozing from his friend's face so he rushed into the fracas and started to drag the hysterical female from a weeping Roy. A hard back-hand knocked him sideways but Charlie was not to be thwarted and he locked on to Anne Marie's hair and with all of his might he managed to separate the two. Roy was on his feet immediately and ran from the scene. Charlie was left alone to face the crazed female. The fight started and Charlie was surprised at the strength and ferocity of the girl, he hadn't intended to retaliate but as soon as he was bloodied, he defended himself. All the other girls ran from the place, shouting and crying and adding to the drama. Minutes later and a victorious Charlie clambered to his feet.

Grown-ups sprung from nowhere, bawling and prodding at a protesting boy, fussing over a distraught Anne Marie. What an actress as she blamed an increasingly scared Charlie, then the girl's mother was on the scene, shouting and bawling like a lunatic as she whacked at the retreating boy until his temper snapped, pulled out his favourite *Rambo* hunting knife - a recent birthday present - and jabbed at the woman, stopped her in her tracks. Then it was Charlie's turn to make a hasty retreat. For the rest of the day the lad could still remember the long and lonely nightmare of police and parents inside Peterlee Police Station. It was sorted out eventually but the girl's family never looked at Charlie again and Anne Marie verbally tortured him at every opportunity, knowing he could never retaliate without paying the consequences.

Poor Roy, it took him weeks to show his face, so embarrassed at the beating he took from the girl and for months afterwards he was ridiculed and barracked by both girls and boys. Only Charlie stuck by his side and Charlie was the only one to make him face the world again. Eventually things got better for both of them.....................

Alice Greaney was talking to him, smiling at him. Charlie started to copy all of the words that she'd written on the black-board. The tutor moved along the line of boys, waiting patiently for the next reminiscence to blossom forth. It had been a good lesson, talking about the incident: thinking again about the past, brought it all back, good times and bad, then the clanking bell signalled the end of English. The boys filed out of the room in an orderly fashion. Alice Greaney beamed as they left, the woman loved her job, loved her pupils, turning to the blackboard, she started to clean away the assorted notes, still smiling at all the beautiful memories.

The last lesson of the day was Mathematics with Percy Poulson. He was a sadist. Inflicted verbal and physical punishment daily, no matter how trivial the misdemeanor, the tutor ruled the classroom with zealous tyrannical streak, middle-aged and uncomfortable with it, tall and skinny and with a stupid wrap-over hairstyle to hide his bald pate. He was nick-named Charlton and he was as skilled with his biting sarcastic wit, as was Bobby with a football.

The boys filed into the classroom. Nelly reached his seat and broke wind, loud and long. Immediately Poulson was on him, slapping and pushing the protesting youth until he was outside.

"It was all those corpses, Sir!" screamed John Nellis. "Honest, Sir, brought it all back again….in the English lesson, didn't mean to have flatulence!"

The whole class erupted with laughter.

CHAPTER FOUR

Seven-o-clock and the chocolate-coloured Ford Fiesta chugged along the cobbled lane that served Low Row. Arnold Anders had already checked the *Shoulder of Mutton* pub, not a soul inside, stopped outside the *Kings Head* and hurried inside. There were a few brave regulars in the gloomy bar. Wiping rain from his head, Arnie moved to the counter and ordered a beer. The juke-box stood next to a blazing coal-fire. He warmed himself then fed several tokens into the machine, took a long swig, licked his lips, found the nearest seat to the fire. Don Mclean belted out one of his favourite tunes and Arnie mimed along: *Drove my chevy to the levee but the levee was dry,* took a deep breath, felt better already, knew he could face Elvis now, took another drink, thinking, *What the hell is a levee?*

Arnold Anders worked on a casual basis for Elvis Priestley. He was a time-served motor mechanic and had a bit more savvy about engines than his boss. He had worked for Paddy Burns at Peterlee Town Centre, served his apprenticeship under the old tyrant. Arnie was a good tradesman thanks to his employer's tenacity and determination. Trouble with Arnold, his *Achilles' Heel*, was his fondness for the booze, enjoyed a tipple or two, missed the occasional Monday morning, got the odd warning now and then but ignored them, thought he was indispensable, thought wrong, got the boot. Life was a bitch.

When Elvis Priestley bought Paddy's garage, Arnold had managed to secure casual work, worked when he was wanted, did the odd bit of dodgy work for Priestley - strip the occasional hot motor; find an engine, swap a gear-box, the usual tricks of the trade and all cash-in-hand, Arnie need the money, four kids and a fat wife to support, needed the money and some!

When he was really desperate, Arnie could be bribed to do mucky stuff, naughty stuff. The money was excellent but the consequences were dire if the shit ever hit the fan. The previous evening was a prime example, *'Only a bit of arson,'* soothed Elvis, man had a tongue that could make Jesus sin, *'piece of cake, Arnie, nothing to it!'* He had to leave his motor at Lowhills Road in Peterlee and walk a mile or so, risk life and limb running over the busy A19, then across scrub land and fields, which wasn't too difficult. A simple stroll towards the nearby landscaped bulge that once was the pit-heap of Shotton Colliery, follow the broad sweep around the base of the artificial mound and hit Broxon's garage.

Piece of cake, my arse! thought Arnie when the episode was over. *Yeah, try it in the dark with a bloody heavy canister of fuel and no lights to guide you.* The number of times he'd fallen, slipped and tripped in cow-shit; shallow pools and a multitude of holes, cracks and crannies was beyond belief. Covered in sweat and assorted crap Arnie had finally reached his destination and then he was confronted with bloody dogs, a whole pack of ferocious wolves roaming the blackened yard waiting to eat him alive. *No thank you, Elvis, not for any price!*

He finished his drink and made for the bar-counter, grabbed another pint and sauntered back to his seat, paused at the mirror above the open fire; it was the horn-rimmed spectacles and the thin features. *Yes, Buddy Holly wasn't dead. He was alive and well and working as a mechanic,* Arnie had a final look, if only he had some bloody hair! He collapsed on to chair, finished the drink in one long guzzle and smiled at himself. It was a hoot really; Buddy waiting for Elvis, he chortled and the two near the bar looked at him curiously. Arnie lifted an empty glass towards them.

"Cheers!" he said, "here's to Ritchie Valens and the Big Bopper!" Morons didn't have a clue what he was talking about.

After his third pint, Arnie decided to move. As he left the room he shouted at the bar-man, "If Eddie Priestley asks for me. I've been and gone!"

When the door clanked shut, Henry Bower, up to his neck with alcohol, turned and said to Peter Cassidy, the bar-man, "He's the bloody double of that fella used ta be on the television years ago? What's his name, pretended he was in the army, liked a flutter?"

"A was thinkin' the same!" Peter broke wind loudly.

"Bilko!"

"Sergeant Bilko," chortled Peter Bower, "bloody double."

Leaving his faithful jalopy parked outside of the pub, the man hurried across the busy road and made for the *Liberality Tavern,* he would sample the nectar before heading for home, pushed open the swing-doors and saw the solitary figure propping up the bar. Elvis glowered at him, had been waiting for well over an hour for Arnie Anders, he looked sour enough to explode.

Arnie faked a smile, "Elvis, I've been waiting in the *King's Head.*"

"My arse!" grunted an incensed Elvis, turned towards the pretty bar-maid and ordered drinks.

Arnold Anders tried to keep it light, knew all about Eddie's temper. "Could be Las Vegas, eh?" He gave a little laugh.

"What do you mean?"

"Elvis meets Buddy?"

It didn't go down well. "Arnie", grunted the shorter man, 'the only thing that you've got in common with bloody Buddy Holly is bad breath!"

"Buddy had bad breath?"

"Halitosis," insisted the chunky entrepreneur, "big time!"

The drinks were paid for, a tip was left for the pretty barmaid and the two men headed for the far end of the room, didn't want anyone listening. The banter began, all one-sided, as Arnie explained about the failed mission. Elvis was not amused.

"But there was no one in the bloody house!" snorted the boss-man.

"Dogs, dozens of them were running about loose in the yard. I thought…."

Elvis interrupted him, "You're not paid to think, Arnold!"

"Steady on, Elvis," whined the taller man, "there's no need to get personal!"

Elvis Priestley took a sip of ale. *Plan A* had gone belly-up; he would have to think of *Plan B.* Something needed doing to Norman Broxon, he was making headway into Elvis's customers and needed stopping, permanently. Broxon was buggering the profit margins as customers turned away from Elvis and used the competitor's garage. Cheaper servicing, cheaper second-hand motors, it couldn't be allowed to continue.

"Get the drinks in, Arnie," said Elvis, "let me think of something."

****

Hours earlier, a few streets south, Charlie was stomping away from his home, infuriated and irate. *Abandoned again,* he thought, both parents out of sight, waited for an age hoping at least one of them would show, he'd not eaten all day, wanted money for food and the longer he paced his home, the angrier he became, six-o-clock and his patience had broken, his mood foul as he ran away from the Village towards the nearby Colliery.

The Jepson twins, Monty and Patton, were waiting outside the café. Like Charlie they had been barred from the shop. Both brothers were feeding their faces with assorted junk. Charlie Hill, never the shy one - followed the dictum, squeaking doors get oiled, which worked every time - grunted, *'Pass them over, Monty, don't be a greedy cow.'*

The packet was handed over. The contents wolfed down by a ravenous Charlie.

"Here," offered Pat, wanting to keep on the good side of Charlie, the bottle of coke was pressed into the open palm, "might as well wash it down?"

The twins were good mates, knew, but didn't speak about Charlie's life, heard all the tittle-tattle, all the shitty gossip about the boy's riotous and brutish lifestyle, warned many times to stay clear of him by their worried parents. They cared less, he was okay was Charlie, a good friend, dependable and the natural leader of their pack. The trio moved off and searched or called for their friends. Within half-an-hour they had been joined by Billy Nord, Nelly and a sheepish Alan Mounter. Alan's face still bore the swelling from the earlier fracas with Charlie. Nothing was mentioned about the disagreement, over and done with, past and forgotten. Charlie and Alan buddies again, part of the gang as they roamed the Colliery looking for fun and excitement. *The Angels,* tough guys.

Reaching the library the gang spotted the noisy group of older youths lounging on the council bench. It was always a problem of status as to the course of action to take. If the lads had been the same age as Charlie's gang then it would have been no contest. The *Angels* were top dogs at the Comprehensive School, would have scattered the group and occupied the bench. Not this time, these youths were right tearaways, all worked at the colliery, older by a few years, bigger and tougher. Cautiously they closed in on the newcomers, the loud banter started, especially from the leader of the band. Charlie's group immediately bounced back with the jibes, tit for tat for as long as they dared. Alfie Hogg, self-appointed leader, centred on Charlie. He was the biggest, meanest thug of the group.

"Charlie Hill," he spat, "still leader of the kiddies?"

"Now Alfie," smiled the younger lad, hiding the growing feeling of unease that gripped him, stomach churning with fear, "how's pit work?"

The strapping figure, a dead ringer for *Meatloaf*, smirked, thick jowls puckered and Alfie Hogg snorted loudly; spat a huge wedge of phlegm towards Charlie. It landed short. Charlie grinned bravely, stood his ground and waited for more abuse. The taunting would soon be over and then he'd be on his way.

"Fancy a laugh?" asked the older youth, an evil smile on his face.

"Meeting people, Alfie," answered the youth, "at the Waterworks, calling on Jimmy Archer," a truism but irrelevant. Charlie glanced at his group and gestured, a signal for them to move away from the growing tension between the two gangs.

"Come on, Charlie," laughed the man-mountain, "just a laugh!"

Charlie faced his aggressor, nothing else to do. "Okay, Alfie."

"It's like this, Charlie," said Alfie Hogg. "My lot likes to keep in shape, even when we have a daft carry-on … keep in shape."

Charlie thinking, *The one who needs to keep in shape is you,* said resignedly, "Okay, Alfie, I'm easy."

"We've got this game, see," a glint of malice flickered across his thick features, his thick brow furrowed menacingly, the smile wicked. "Bit of a laugh, really."

"Game?" Charlie wanted so much to run for his life, knew he could not, everyone watching, waiting, his reputation on the line.

"Aye," said Alfie and elbowed his way from the mix of bodies, he stood and looked down at the diminutive figure.

Charlie asked boldly, "What kind of game?"

A thick finger tapped at the air and seemed to be pointing towards the heavens. "You got *Sky*, kid?" asked the bully.

Charlie frowned, shook his head, *Not even a television, Alfie*, he thought sadly, *not since Ma kicked in the screen*.

"*Run of the Arrow,* Charlie," said Alfie Hogg. "On the Movie Channel last night*?"*

Unable to speak the youth could only shake his head. *He wants to play Cowboys and Indians on the open range of Easington*? He waited and wondered, *Run of the arrow?*

"Rod Steiger," teased the older youth, "captured by the Apaches, given a chance to escape?" Alfie Hogg teased, "surely you've seen the movie, Charlie, been out donkey's years. The Indians fire an arrow and Rod is given that distance to run before they give chase"

"Who's the Indians, Alf?"

"Guess, Charlie?"

"And who is *Rod Steiger*, Alf?"

The bigger youth sniggered gleefully, "You are, Charlie!"

Charlie looked quickly at his friends who appeared to be melting into the night.

"Ten seconds, Charlie," bellowed the giant, "then we give chase. Got no bows and arrows you understand, so we gotta improvise?" and he lowered his bulk and grasped the piece of wood that lay on the council bench.

Like a rabbit chased by a pack of wild dogs Charlie Hill scorched a path towards the heart of the colliery, the gap between them only yards; there had been no ten-second count. Nothing. Time enough for the gang to grab assorted weaponry and bolt after their terrified prey. Slowly and painfully the youngster eased away, he was running for his life, his heart banging like a huge pump as the screaming horde attempted to catch him. Reaching *The Diamond* Pub, Charlie took a sharp right and ran towards the recreational grounds, out of sight for only a moment the youth made a split-second decision. Ahead, the park. To the left, allotments. To the right, farmers' fields, he made a split-second choice, the path of most resistance and ran towards the quagmire of the farmer's fields.

Up the grassy incline and over the barbed-wire fence, Charlie landed heavily on the wet, clinging soil, slowly and carefully he followed the line of fencing eastwards, making a parallel journey up the long incline of the colliery street. Soon the baying screams and threats lessened in velocity and volume as the quarry made his getaway. Despite the nearness of the perimeter fence there was little firm ground and Charlie was very soon up to his ankles in the squelching bog. He wanted to scream with rage, his only shoes were ruined.

After what seemed an age, the youth left the safety of the fields. The main road loomed ahead. Charlie was opposite the old *Rialto* cinema now metamorphosised into *Dallas Carpets,* cursing Rod bloody Steiger and Alfie Hogg, he walked slowly and hesitantly to the council seat and squatted on its wet surface. His feet ached, soaked with a mix of mud, grit and water, pulled off his shoes and battered them against the pavement, misery covering his features as the oozing contents littered the roadway. *'My best shoes,'* he moaned. *'My only shoes!'* sighed with rage as he struggled into his foot-wear, at least the madness of the game was over.

Then the anguish in his head resurfaced as he heard the slapping and stamping of approaching runners. Charlie stood ready to bolt then stared at the wet mire that clung to his lower body. He had taken enough. He sat and waited, the running was over. The band of loons faltered. To a man they looked at Alfie Hogg, not knowing quite what to do next. The cat-calls commenced, but nothing else. *Wasn't Charlie supposed to run*? *Shouldn't he be frightened?* The seated youth glowered at the mob.

The weapon held by man-mountain was raised then hurled at Charlie Hill. It flew wide of the target. Still Charlie held his ground.

"Little Big Man?" shouted the gorilla.

Charlie answered aggressively, "Leave off, Alfie!"

"Leave off!" shouted the incensed and venomous youth. "Leave off!" No one ever disrespected Alfie Hogg, not unless they wanted a spell in hospital.

Charlie raised his arms in mock surrender, said determinedly, grimly, "You win, Alfie, okay!"

Man-mountain had his reputation to think about. “Run!” he bellowed, “or be damaged,” strode towards the council-seat, all huffing and puffing, arms gesticulating wildly.

His cronies followed: all noise, all swagger.

Charlie stood his ground, too late to do anything else, he blustered loudly, “I’m not after any bother, Alfie”

The human gorilla cackled. “You’re not big enough to cause bother!” *Meatloaf* was spoiling for a fight.

“Alfie,” offered the seated figure, “you’re too big for me.”

“Very true!” snarled Alfie contemptuously. “I could eat you for breakfast!” He looked at his trusting crew, they all had dubious reputations. “You!” and he beckoned a tall scrawny specimen to step forward. He looked smugly at Charlie. “Fancy your chances with Joe?”

Charlie slowly rose. He had little choice, if he ran, he’d be battered by them all, if he stayed, he might only cop a bruising. He slowly took off his jacket; despite the coolness of the evening he only wore a tee-shirt which highlighted his thick, muscled torso, brawny tattooed arms added to the effect, made him look fierce.

Joe Barton was taken aback. Always the bully, he was used to his victims cowering, allowing him to look good, couldn’t remember anyone ever fighting back. Quick as a flash he grunted, “Too easy for me, he’s just a school-kid!”

The school-kid did not say a word, gave an icy stare. *He was Dorothy looking at the Cowardly Lion*

“Weapons,” snorted Joe Barton, head and shoulders bigger than Charlie, he couldn’t lose, “give the bairn a fighting chance!”

Man-mountain chuckled; it was going to be fun. He fumbled with his coat-collar and pulled out a bicycle-chain.

The weapon was handed to his pal. One of the cronies threw another bike-chain at Charlie. It landed at his feet.

"Off the main-street!" ordered Alfie like some demented sergeant-major.

The group all trooped away from the lighted street and into the back-lane, seemed like a procession of juvenile undertakers, not a word spoken between them, single file as they followed the leader, reached the small walled enclosure; gateway to half-a-dozen aged miners' cottages and walked silently into the big expanse of lawn.

"Make a circle!" ordered Alfie Hogg, leaving Charlie and Joe Barton marooned between the wide loop of fascinated bodies.

"I'll count to three," said Alfie, his voice lifting with emotion, "then it starts!"

Unwilling to be caught out twice in one night by the same ploy Charlie Hill launched himself at the mesmerized opponent, *'Three!'* he screamed. The chain tore through the air and whipped across the unprotected head of the bigger youth. A fountain of crimson erupted over Joe Barton's face, blood spurting like a geyser, the youth tried to speak but choked and retched then collapsed in a dead faint. Silence enveloped the gory scene. All looked in awe at the spectacle, no one knew what to do then a door squeaked open and an old man appeared.

The aged-miner, shouted angrily, "Will you piss off and let me watch the bloody television!" Then he saw the crumpled body on the grass and the group of boys close by. "Jesus," he gasped, "what the hell has happened?"

The gang scattered in all directions, leaving only Charlie Hill and the unconscious Joe Barton. Then the youth walked slowly from the place and threw the weapon away. *Not so tough after all*, he thought, *especially with a chain to help,* reached Seaside Lane and started to run homewards, didn't stop until he had reached the Village, gave him time to take stock, realize the implications of his actions. Dreaded the future, Joe Barton was one crazy individual, bound to be repercussions. *Come tomorrow,* thought Charlie and *Joe will kill me for what I've done!* Another thought struck home. *What if Joe's mother calls the police, I'll be locked up for sure!*

****

CHAPTER FIVE

Charlie stayed away from school, couldn't face the gossip, worried sick about the previous evening's *entertainment* and the possible conclusion. The sun was up and warm and both parents were back, spoke to them the preceding night, waiting for him, filled with drink and full of false cheer, frivolous trivial talk, wanting him to share the beer, even his Dad was in a good mood, giddy with alcohol, offered Charlie money time and time again. *Take it, Charlie*, he'd said, *I've got plenty and* the youth finally obliged.

The following morning he was in Greaney's Grocery, first customer of the day. Old Jack was alone. Alice, his wife, would have left for school ages ago; she was always an early bird. Charlie filled the carrier-bag and hurried home. He ate alone: jam and bread, tea and a full packet of ginger-snaps, sumptuous and succulent for a sixteen year old, couldn't wake his mother for love nor money and his dad was in first-shift. By eleven-o-clock Charlie was sick of his own company, moving to the bottom of the cul-de-sac, the lad jumped over the ancient fence, strolled to the nearby quarry, past assorted litter and debris as the buzz of insects tapped out a distant continuous tune. At the top of the quarry stood the old abandoned motor, no doors, no wheels, just a shell, been a permanent fixture since he'd been a kid. Charlie squatted on the sun-warmed bonnet, sat relaxed with arms folded and head facing the beautiful heavens.

There were visitors close by. Three small urchins scurried about in the midst of the deep, rancid crater, occasionally a small body launched itself into view followed by two noisy chasers, in a fantasy land of make-believe and mayhem then, as suddenly as they burst on the scene, they were gone, back into the abyss, bursting through the land of wonderment, oblivious to the world around them. Close by stood the few lines of private houses that bordered the wilderness of the quarry. Charlie watched as a girl busied herself filling the washing-line, recognized her, Linda Macdonald, trim and pretty and with a smidgeon of a reputation as a good-time girl.

Minutes passed and Charlie was still chameleon-like, rigid and rapturous with the growing heat of the day, soaking in the sunlight. Sometimes he thought about the bother that would surely result from the fight, wondered when he would have a visit from the police, worst still, a call from an angry and battered Joe Barton, spoiling for revenge. Nothing had occurred and it was mid-morning, not even a knock on the door from irate parents, not a whiff of trouble. Nothing! Zilch! Perhaps Joe Barton had kept his mouth shut and was biding his time. He opened his eyes when footsteps alerted him. It was the girl, Linda Macdonald, a big smile creased her face and an even bigger chest beckoned. She was struggling with a large heavy plastic sack.

"Charlie Hill," she said, "off school then?"

He said, "Something like that."

The girl swung the bag in a wide arc then released it, watched it spiral then disappear into the bowels of the quarry then joined Charlie on the bonnet. "It's a right dump, this place."

Charlie nodded; his head was starting to fill with lurid thoughts.

"Mother is always complaining to the Council," said the female, "about people chucking their rubbish. The wind blows it all over the place, it's a disgrace!"

Charlie pondered, chuckled softly and said, 'But you've just thrown a sack in the quarry."

"I know that," retorted the adamant female, "but we live here, we're allowed."

The youth nodded and said dryly,"Logical, eh?"

The sarcasm was lost on the girl. "Last week," said Linda, "our Tommy brought in a dead cat, asked my dad if he could keep it! Dad was drunk, said he would stuff it and put it in the bedroom, upset Ma when he said it would make a nice change, said he hadn't seen a pussy for a long time!" Linda Macdonald giggled and glanced at Charlie, teasing, tantalising.

Suddenly the place erupted with the arrival of the three tots. One of them, with nose streaming like a yellow liquid candle, hurried to the girl's side.

"Our Linda!" he squawked, "what you doing here?"

"Come for you, haven't I," she answered sternly, "bath-time!"

The ploy worked and the ragged urchin scampered back into the quarry, shouting, "Not yet, our Linda, we're playing *Star Wars!"* The youngsters vanished out of sight.

"Fancy a cuppa, Charlie?"

"Don't know about that," and he glanced towards the girls' home.

"Don't worry, Charlie, there's no one in," her big eyes feasted on him, inviting him, "come on, nothing spoiling is there?"

Like a puppy, the boy followed her the short distance to the home. They entered the living-room, the place littered with a vast array of tasteless bric-a-brac, a blossoming infestation of plastic and china and cloth, loud and garish.

"Do you like it?" asked the girl, "mum is always dusting."

Do I care? Not one jot. "Is she?"

"Yes." laughed the female, leading him with a short sweet rope of temptation, "but I've got to clean my own room. I'll show you, if you want?"

Together they started to climb the stairs. He wanted to burst into song. *I should be so lucky,* but he held his tongue and his breath as they entered the small box-room. Almost all of the wall-space was filled with posters, large and small. *Rick Astley*. *Jason Donovan,* big toothy grins feasted on the would-be lovers. A brooding *Michael Jackson* scowled from a huge poster. Next to *Jacko* was a picture of the *Pet Shop Boys.* Charlie smiled, *Hell of a photo*, he thought, then suddenly his conscience pricked him, made him realize the predicament he was in, his head in a spin, bouncing with hormones, should he, shouldn't he? If Jenny found out there'd be hell to pay. Charlie Hill had never looked at another girl since he'd met Jenny Bruce.

"Charlie, are you alright?" her young eyes feasted over him.

He couldn't resist, his resilience and reluctance lasted seconds as he leaned close and pecked at her open mouth, watched breathlessly as she grinned, returned the kiss and slowly eased on to the small bed. Charlie was smitten he closed on her, as she melted on to the mattress, soft arms covered him, fingers caressed and played with him, beads of sweat trickled and ran over his trembling body, her gaze never leaving his; coaxing and willing him. With clumsy and awkward movements Charlie began to caress the girl, now her eyes closed as pleasure seeped through her young body, soft, gasping moans spilt from her lips. With expert ease, she arched her firm torso and began to pull her skirt up over her thighs. The youth watched with a look of incredulity and wonder, mouth open, unable to speak as he gaped at the taut, beautiful legs of the temptress.

Linda Macdonald whispered softly, "Like what you see, Charlie?"

He nodded, his whole body trembling with emotion.

Smiling coyly, the girl closed her eyes and said, "Do it then, Charlie."

In the nearby quarry the children had been joined by their new friend. He was older, a grown-up, but different. He was nice to them all, gave them sweets and chocolates. He was the oldest spaceman they'd ever met. He owned his own ray-gun and he wanted to be called *Darth Vader*. Harry Shannon didn't own a proper helmet but said his felt hat would suffice, smiled and giggled when Billy Macdonald said it looked like a cowboy hat. They began to play their new game.

Little Billy shrieked, "I'm *Han Solo!"* and he burned up a mighty dusk cloud as he was chased across the quarry.

"I'm *Luke Skywalker*!" cried his friend and he too gave chase.

The smallest of the trio screamed, "I'm *R2D2*!" He followed slowly because he was a robot, tried to make a noise like a robot but he sounded like the *road-runner*: *Beep! Beep,* he cried loudly, *Beep! Beep!*

****

Between the coastal mine and the village stood the Waterworks, so named because of the size and proximity of the *Sunderland and South Shields Water Company*. The miscellaneous buildings, warehouses and offices stood in several unkempt acres off the main road. Feeding from the sprawl was the huge bulge of council houses and the odd smattering of private accommodation. One solitary grocery store, owned by Elvis Priestley and one fish-shop served the area.

Rebecca Hill left her home shortly before noon; half a cup of Guinness had eased her into the new day, the woman plodded her way to Priestley's store. She had been using the place for a while. The owners gave short-term credit but no more, after seven days, payment in full was expected; there was no bending of the rules. Rebecca knew were she stood. The woman had recently stopped visiting the Village shop. It was Jack Greaney's fault. He wasn't a good businessman. *Too bloody soft*, she thought. It was his error that her bills had steadily grown. He was not strict enough, too lenient, tell Jack a sob story and the credit was stuck on to another week. Now she owed the man a bloody fortune and it was embarrassing the way he was now barracking her for payment. Rebecca had offered a little bit of cash every week, her way of pacifying him. It hadn't worked so she stayed away. His loss.

A policeman had called that morning. Banging the door like it was a big drum. '*Wake the dead with your clatter*,' she'd scolded, soon put him in his place, young pup that he was, barely out of school and all that nonsense about her boy. Her Charlie putting someone in hospital, '*Load of rubbish*,' she'd bawled. '*A lad three years older than Charlie in hospital! Pull the other one!*' Her boy was innocent, totally innocent, told the bobby in no uncertain terms that her boy had been home with her all night.

The young copper had been persistent, wanted a word with Charlie, demanded a word with Charlie. '*Then go to the bloody pathetic school and interview him*,' she'd barked defiantly. '*You'll get the same answers*.' Cheeky begger, had the nerve to say he'd visited the school that very morning and Charlie was not present. Her temper had snapped, Rebecca pushed him out of her home, barracking and prodding, '*Bugger off and go catch some proper criminals instead of harassing kids!*'

Rebecca entered the store. Eddie Priestley stood behind the counter lost in the pages of the Northern Echo. They chattered for a while, swapping gossip, told him about her boy, about the bother and the visit by the policeman. The owner gave a big beefy grin, nonchalant and casual, his only comment, '*Kids, eh, worse by the year!*' She passed over her brief note and waited as the groceries were filled into the carrier bag.

She had a fond spot for the man. He was good to her, sold her naughty stuff, under-the-counter stuff. Always a subtle hint, '*Anything else, Rebecca,*' he'd say, a little wink and a smile. Like today, a little bottle of *Gordon's Gin,* just the stuff to keep her spirits up. The purchase was wrapped well and well-hidden in the bag. Rebecca promised to pay soon.

"Saturday, Becky!" smiled the man. "Don't you forget!"

"You're a good man, Eddie," answered Rebecca. "Don't you worry."

"Saturday, Becky," smiled when he said it, but the smile was cold.

"Saturday on the dot, Eddie," assured the woman. *Not bad-looking,* thought Rebecca, eyeing the proprietor up and down as she left the store, *Man must be worth a fortune!*

****

The short walk from the allotment to his home was getting to be a bit of a struggle for Albert Bruce. He needed to lose weight and fast. He'd confided in no-one about the occasional chest pains. Always a stubborn man, Albert thought that it could be indigestion, or heart-burn, that's what he told himself. An hour digging at his allotment had tired him. He was looking forward to a cup of tea and a few hours rest before work. Albert hated night-shift.

He heard the women gossiping moments before he stepped into the back-yard. Then silence from the pair of hens as he approached, nodded a greeting to the neighbour, planted the small sack of fresh vegetables next to the back door and entered the house. Moments later and his wife appeared. Married for a lifetime and Albert could sense what was coming. *Idle gossip.* He spread the Sunderland Echo across the full width of the small table, found the fags and waited. Tea was served and the miner took a deep draught of smoke, arched his head and blew a thick column of muck towards the ceiling.

"Come on, woman," he said quietly, "get it off your chest."

"Joan Barton," returned Nancy, "on the boil about Charlie Hill. Apparently her Joe is in hospital through that scallywag! Hit Joe with a stick or something. He's been stitched from his brow to his neck. Top of his head was split in two!"

Albert nodded, took a smoke and glanced at the newspaper. It was worse than he thought. He answered, "That's it, then?"

"Albert Bruce, you'll not sit there and say nothing! That animal was seeing our Jenny!"

Still reading, Albert said. "So what's the problem, love?" took a heavy drag on the ciggy, "our Jenny hasn't seen him for weeks." He thought about his only child, worried sick about her, knew the pain she was in, fretting after Charlie Hill.

The woman's tea-cup was clashed on to the table and liquid spilt over the newspaper. There was silence for some moments then the man quietly folded the paper, smoothed it and looked at his wife.

"Love," he said in soft voice, "gettin' upset will not fix the situation. You've seen the state of Jenny, spat her dummy out and can't find it."

"He's no good!" whined the woman. "I think you should tell her about the things he's gettin' up to, make her see sense about the lad."

"Jenny has only got eyes for young Charlie. She's besotted, look at the tantrums we've had since that argument. Jenny was never like this. Never." Albert took stock. "Best to say nowt, let sleeping dogs lie?"

"A'll tell you for nothin'," replied an incensed Nancy, "that Charlie Hill will never cross this door again, bloody animal, putting that lad in hospital!"

"He's just a bairn, half the bloody time he'll not know right from wrong." The cigarette was stubbed out on the saucer. "Most lads go through a funny spell at his age, always was the case … get a bit mixed up, think they're men one minute, boys the next, run with the crowd. Get a taste for the beer and the like. Tend to come out of it okay." He inspected the packet of *Benson and Hedges*. "Doesn't help with the family he's lumbered with?"

"So that's it!" her voice lifted in anger, "after all he's done to poor Joan Barton's son!"

Albert lit another cigarette. There was more than a hint of sarcasm in his tone as he said, "That's not the same family that you've cursed these last ten years? Don Barton, who's pissed his wages down the Colliery Club's toilet every bloody night? Who every other week gives his precious Joan a good slappin' when the drink sends him loopy? And as for their bloody worthless son! Is this the same precious Joe who wrecked

Jonty Blackburn's car with a cricket bat because his daughter ditched him? Talk sense, love."

"Wasn't even a fair fight, Albert!" retorted Nancy indignantly.

"Really?" He gazed at his wife with candour, "you were there?"

"I'm just…"

"Gossiping, Nancy, nothing more, nothing less. Let me tell you I've heard a very different story and from the horse's mouth." He fumbled with the cigarette-packet and continued with his story. "Mojo Hogg?"

"Can't stand the man," paused then said, "go on, Albert!"

"Mojo Hogg's son, Alfie? He's as daft as a brush, nineteen and still hangs around the bloody street with his cronies. Apparently one of his pack - Joe Barton - decided he wanted to sort out young Charlie. Wouldn't fight him proper, used a weapon. Charlie beat the hell out of him." He smiled at Nancy, "So much for gossip?"

"In other words," whined the woman. "You think it's right?"

"Temporary madness, love," he sucked at the cigarette. "Few years time and they'll all be married and settled down."

****

Elvis shook his pelvis and got to work. It wasn't just the chat from Charlie's mother that prompted action, there had been a queue that morning in the shop and all buzzing about the same incident and every time the story was told it grew in horror, folks adding their little bit of gory detail. Young Charlie needed a little help but, more importantly, Elvis had need of the young tearaway, saw potential in the brash, arrogant youth, already made good money out of Charlie's thieving ways. The lad had courage and mettle by the bucketful. The last thing the guru needed was internment for his pupil.

Despite the wailing protest from his granddaughter, Elvis left the store, stood for a moment and surveyed his latest purchase: a gleaming *BMW*. Top of the range. He smiled at the motor. *Not bad for an ex-miner*, he thought. Soon he was buzzing down the road to the colliery houses.

Mojo Hogg acquired his name because of his daft hairstyle. The diminutive figure - he stood a shade over five foot without shoes - sported a basin-cut very similar to that worn by Moe. *The Three Stooges Moe*! His real name was Joe Hogg and he was a shot-firer at Easington pit. He had three sons: Henry, Joe and the youngest, Alfie. Three giants. *Good stuff comes from little bundles*, he would say.

Eddie Priestley had known Mojo for years. They had worked together at the mine. Good pals, been through some scrapes together, always helped each other.

"Mojo." greeted Elvis and he smiled his warmest smile, "need a favour," entered the small terraced home. Despite the warmth of the day, a huge crackling coal-fire had turned the kitchen into a furnace. Mojo, sporting jeans and a grubby vest did not seem to notice.

The little miner smiled a toothless grin at his old pal, "Anything, Eddie."

"It's about your Alfie".

"What's the bugger done now?"

"Bit of bother."

Mojo chortled mischievously, "What's new!"

Within two hours, Mojo's son had paid a visit to all of his pals. The Hogg Gang had been given new instructions if and when, the slow-coach police questioned them. *'Tell them this, tell them that,'* ordered the gang-leader. Young Alfie made his final call to Joe Barton's home, put the weasel into the picture, told him what to say, told him to change his statement when the bobbies next called. '*Say you were in shock*,' he demanded. '*Didn't know what you were saying!'* Alfie could be very persuasive, *'And stay well away from Charlie Hill. It's over, you hear me, Joe?'*

****

CHAPTER SIX

It was a pleasant shock to see his mother; it was an even greater surprise to see her cooking. Charlie sat in the hovel that professed to be a kitchen, pushed aside soiled cups, some grimy plates and assorted junk, checked the two packets of cigarettes that stood side by side, next to the half-empty bottle of milk. Empty.

"Ma?" and he shook the empty packets at her smiling face.

Rebecca handed over a cigarette, cleared the table and set out the meal: a fry-up and only a little burned, *Things can only get better*, thought the boy, the conversation one-sided as Charlie's mother slowly and determinately worked her way through the meal, appeared to be in a world of her own, day-dreaming and only answering when prompted by her son.

"What's up, Ma?" asked the concerned youth.

"Things are going to change, Charlie," said Rebecca, looking about the small room and shaking her head with an obvious look of shame and sorrow, glanced in her son's direction, puppy-dog eyes, "I'm sorry, Charles," she muttered, "you don't deserve this."

Charlie couldn't bear to see her so distressed, tore at his heart-strings when she acted so pitifully, never knew quite what to say to ease her, lift her spirits. He rose and cleared the table, even picked up the sauce bottles that tended to have a permanent squat at the corner of the table.

"You're a good boy, Charlie," she offered quietly, "my treasure."

The putrid sink was full to the brim and the lad couldn't find the vigour to help with the washing-up. Hesitantly Charlie said, "Ma, you think I should go to school?" The afternoon session lasted only a few hours and the strange mood of his mother bothered him, thought it better to leave her on her own for a few hours, give her time to unwind, maybe sort out her troubled head. "What do you think, Ma?"

Rebecca nodded, moved close to him and pecked him lightly on the cheek, squeezed him lovingly, "Might be a good idea, Charles, shall I write you a note for the teacher?"

"Tomorrow, Ma," said the boy, "I'll take a letter tomorrow."

She watched him stroll away from the street, smiled as he glanced momentarily back at the house, knowing she was watching, tears welled in her eyes as the reminiscences swamped her again, emotions that she had fought all her adult life, shook her very soul and when these times came she was utterly ashamed and engulfed with remorse. Rebecca stared as Charlie disappeared from view, her beautiful boy, so loving and true, a boy to be proud of, neglected, abandoned, pushed aside while she rode the nightmare of doubt and self-pity. And Adam too, a husband betrayed, belittled, tortured by her. Adam Hill who, in his own way, loved her deeply, knew that, knew it more than anything. He'd stayed when he should have run from her, broken him time and time again and still he remained by her side, shouted at her, shrieked and bellowed like a madman at her and rightly so. Words! Words meant nothing, his love was boundless, taking all the bile she could throw and more, knocked him down with the pain, time and time again, tortured him, hurt him so much with lies and betrayal and still he persevered. Adam Hill had stayed because he loved her. Rebecca knew that and was truly ashamed.

She was such a fool, a sick, sad twisted fool of a woman and still worshipped by them, despite everything: the mayhem and chaos, the confrontations and hostilities she conjured out of spite, fear and self-loathing. Her eyes filled with tears and Rebecca Hill wept bitterly, moaning loudly as the pain torched her.

"I need help," she wailed, "I need help!" but no one was listening. No one had ever listened.

She returned to the chair and closed her eyes, remembered another time, younger then and beautiful, the whole world at her feet and being pursued by the most handsome young man in the whole of Easington. Jimmy Shannon who could have had his pick of any girl wanted her, Rebecca Hancock. A perfect gentleman who had the nerve to knock on her parent's door and ask permission - *permission* - to walk out with their daughter. Remembered as if it were yesterday, frightened at the time and yet bursting with pride as she watched her father open the door. *'Mr. Hancock, I wonder if I could have a word,'* he'd said, cocksure and with that twinkle in his eyes. *'Mrs. Hancock too, if you don't mind.'* Charm the birds off the trees could Jimmy Shannon. Little Jimmy he was called but what he lacked in height he more than made up with a giant personality. *'It's about your daughter, Rebecca,'* he said ever so sincerely, *'I would like your permission to see her, don't want to go behind your back and cause upset in the family, I've too much respect for your daughter. With your permission I'd like to walk out with Rebecca?'*

Loved him and lost him, a lifetime ago and still haunted by the consequences.

****

The Village was a quiet and peaceful backwater of streets and lanes, then, suddenly: chaos and calamity, like an atom bomb had fallen near the Comprehensive and hundreds of milling, shouting, running, frantic pupils were bolting from the scene as if there very lives depended on it. Charlie stood impatiently next to the Art Block and watched as the multitude fought their way home. He was waiting for his pal, Roy, the pair always walked home together. A motor chugged into the school driveway, its horn working overtime as it pushed its way through the impatient teenagers. It chugged to a standstill next to the youth, the door was opened, the loud voice gruff and familiar.

Elvis Priestley, clever-clogs himself, said dryly, "John Conteh?"

Charlie leaned in close and smiled at the squat, grinning figure.

"Or is it Sugar Ray today?" Elvis beckoned the lad to get into the car, enormous smile on his face.

"Waiting for Roy."

"To hell with Roy!" said the driver, chuckling but with a hint of impatience in his voice.

Charlie clambered into the vehicle and it moved towards the exit-gate, horn blasting a passage through the mob. Elvis gave him the good news, told him he's squared everything with Alfie Hogg's father, told it straight, *'There'll be no come-back, nothing to worry your pretty face about,'* his cheery face beaming proudly.

"Owe you one, Elvis."

"It wasn't much of a problem," said Elvis pausing deliberately, "but if you want, you can help me sort out a little difficulty."

Charlie Hill, quick as a flash, said, "How much?"

"Cheeky young bugger," the man laughed, "let's go for a little drive," as cigarettes were handed over. "Ever been to Shotton Colliery?" asked the hoodlum

"No," said Charlie, opened up the *Lambert and Butler* packet and was soon sucking on the cigarette, "but I've seen where the pit-heap used to be."

"Like Krakatoa, once," smiled Elvis.

Charlie wasn't the brightest of sparks when it came to history or geography. "What's Krakatoa, Elvis?" he asked.

Elvis started the history lesson, "1883, Indonesia!"

"Where's that, then?"

Irritated, Elvis continued, "Between Java and Sumatra."

"You've lost me there, Elvis. What's the connection between Shotton and Krakatoa?"

"Loudest bang in history .... heard 3000 miles away!"

"I don't follow, Elvis?"

"Shotton Colliery is next in line for the big bang!"

****

Charlie was dropped off behind the Official's Club in Shotton at ten-o-clock that evening. Elvis gave him directions. '*Left through the allotments, skirt the airfield and follow the gentle mound that was once the pit-heap. Down towards the road, pass the coal-yard and straight across the highway to the garage and bungalow. Any movement or traffic ... squat and wait until it's quiet.*' Elvis didn't want any witnesses driving past when the boy was lugging gear across the road. Better safe than sorry.

The weather was on the lad's side, black dark and the occasional hint of rain. A sharp wind tormented him as he inched his way over the undulating fields, took an age to reach the dim lifting outline of the man-made hill. It had once been an enormous eyesore of coal slag, filling the skyline with a malignant splendour, a mighty tribute to the God of Coal, now a shadow of it's former self, a grassy hillock the only reminder of the once perpetual smoking man-made mountain of muck and debris. Slowly Charlie inched his way down the blackness towards the base of the hill to the roadway, stumbled several times and fell as he walked on to stones and boulders. In the murky distance, he could make out vague shapes of horses with their heads to the ground, munching on the grasses, impervious and unafraid of the darkness and gloom of the night. He reached the coal-merchant's premises, frantically scanning the area, then saw the bungalow situated on the opposite side of the road. It was in shadow; the garage and the cars would be situated behind the building. Charlie Hill scurried across the lonely road and headed for the pathway that followed the eastern boundary of the property. He could see the definite shapes of half a dozen motors next to the large garage.

New sounds touched him, the movement and occasional yapping of dogs. Charlie squatted and took deep breaths, knew he had to stay calm, kept focusing on the reward money offered by Elvis Priestley, knew that if he were successful he'd have spending-money for months. Slowly he unpacked the meal, four pieces in total, succulent pieces of steak, *'Don't think about having a nibble of the beef, son',* Elvis giving good advice, *'it's been laced with strychnine!'* Leaving the haversack propped against a large boulder, Charlie carefully approached the compound, the breeze was in his favour: the dogs would not catch his scent. One after another, the silent missiles flew into the depths of the yard and both Rottweilers, large and black and hungry, fought one another for the precious meal. Charlie retreated.

The compound itself was an untidy mixture of old and new. The bungalow was large and modern with a semi-circle of block-paving separated the living-quarters from the business, a grey light, attached to one side of the garage shone a dim and murky probe across the perimeter of the yard. The floor-area of the compound appeared to have a liberal coating of engine oil; the entire surface was awash with a sea of dust and grime. The line of vehicles stood side by side against the southern wall of the garage, a wide gap between them that led to the double-doors of the garage. *Wooden doors*, mused Charlie. Elvis had done his homework.

Charlie opened the haversack and pulled out the four heavy bottles, all corked with petrol-soaked cloth, remembered the instructions: *Light one*; *aim and throw it. Watch where it falls. The second attempt will be more accurate as your aim will have been adjusted. Remember, son,* Elvis had pushed home the point, *don't just fling the missiles anywhere! Do you understand, or the whole night will be wasted*! *Look! Adjust*! *The first attempt might be too long; too wide. Not important, not the first one. That's the dummy-run! The others will do the damage. Understand?*

Charlie was close to the compound. His hands were shaking so much that the bottle had to be wedged into a mound of soil and sod as he struggled with the lighter. It burst into flames. *In for a penny*, he thought, *in for a pound and* the bottle was hurled at the wagons. Beginners' luck for the youth as the missile shattered the side-window of a vehicle. With an almighty roar, the interior of the car exploded in flames. Charlie's nerve snapped, he knew he would not be able to light any more of the weapons so he grabbed the remaining bottles and flung them at the burning motor. Two hit their target and shattered. Petrol ignited and the yard became an inferno.

Charlie Hill grabbed the empty haversack and ran for his life across the open fields.

The following day, Eddie Priestley, together with two other local reprobates was interviewed by the police and released. The most vocal and indignant, amongst them was, of course, Eddie Priestley. He was furious at the questioning; he was, after all, a friend of Norman Broxon. '*Yes I own a garage. Was that a problem, officer? We've known each other for years. Bad blood,*' cried Elvis full of indignation and bile. '*Not in the least. Well if he said that about me I'm more than surprised. I'm also very hurt at the insinuations. Alibi, officer? You've been watching too much American garbage. Don't you mean witnesses, officers? I was home all evening! I'll repeat, constable. Broxon and myself are not rivals. We're miles apart. My business is choc-a-bloc. I can't handle any more trade. Second-hand motors? Of course I deal in second-hand motors. Like Norman Broxon.*' Elvis concluded his interview with guile and cunning befitting his natural instincts, took a detective to one side and, having been promised complete confidentiality and anonymity, gave the police a long list of would-be suspects. Killed two birds with one stone, settled a few old scores with old rivals.

Charlie Hill blissfully asleep in his bed until well after lunch, awoke ravenous and grabbed what little food there was, ate in silence, his head full of the previous night's escapade, elated, one moment, terrified, the next, like being in a movie. For some time he paced the house, waiting for something to happen. No mother, no father anywhere in sight, no one to confide in, no knock at the door from the police, walked from room to room in a trance-like state, even thought about visiting

Elvis but decided it was too dangerous. Charlie grabbed his coat and fled.

The Village was quiet and peaceful. There weren't too many people about, thought of school, another day missed, bound to be bother. Where was his mother, why had she not woken him? His Dad would be at work. Then Jenny blossomed in his head, hadn't seen her in ages, maybe she knew about him, perhaps had heard the gossip, his head was bursting, probably spend years in prison, deserved it too. What a fool he'd been.

The boy slowed when he had reached the top of the Village Green. In the shadow of the huge church was the large, deserted council seat, its canopy protection against the elements. When he was young he used to ride to the place on his bike. He remembered the bicycle, a gift from his parents for being a good boy …one of the best pupils at the junior school. And he was a good son, good enough to receive the brand new bike. Charlie smiled as he pictured the distant scene: on his dad's shoulders; touching the skies as they hurried to the Co-op for his special present. All of his friends were so envious of him; he was the only six year old with a brand-new bike.

The memories wouldn't go, like it was yesterday, he remembered the routine on school-days. Seven-thirty on the dot and his mother would fuss with his hair and gently ease him into the day and they'd sit together at the kitchen-table- the same kitchen-table that had witnessed so much upheaval and change - and eat the lovely breakfasts. Never burnt then. They'd talk and plan the day and when he was dressed she would always check him thoroughly: his clothes; his appearance, even down to the little dab of *Brylcreem* that made his hair special. A little star he was.

And if the days were sunny, he would be allowed to take out his bike, with strict instructions to watch the traffic. Charlie smiled. '*Traffic! Watch out for the cars, Charlie,'* his mother would say, then off he'd go, across the deserted streets, feeling the sun on his face and legs, cycling to the top of the village, perhaps pausing for some moments at the bench before starting the slow zig-zag down through the streets again and always the big church clock to tell him when his time was up, informing him that school beckoned. Wondrous days for Charlie.

He left the seat and strolled through *Clappersgate*, saw the youth watching him. Charlie gave a nod at the figure, *Daft Harry* was his name, that's what everyone called him, or *Harry the Hat.* When Charlie was younger he would sometimes chase the lad, occasionally grab his hat, just for the devilment, then you saw another side to Harry. Like Jekyll and Hyde, instantly hysterical and as mad as a hatter. Frightening. Charlie glanced back and saw the beady eyes of the youth following him, surely, he couldn't remember him, not after so many years, another backward glance and Harry Shannon was gone, the yard empty.

He paused at the bottom of the lane, spoilt for choice: left and it was the *Half Moon* pub, the Village Green and then home, couldn't face anyone yet so he turned right onto *Durham Road* and started following the signs for *Haswell,* moments later saw Charlie passing the small graveyard. He stopped by the railings, thought about the funeral of his grandparents and his demented and frantic mother, a truly awful day when everyone was weepy and miserable. Charlie gazed across the well-tended lawns at the myriad of marble gravestones, searched for the special spot. Too far away. On an impulse Charlie entered the place.

Memories of his grandfather and grandmother were hazy. He still thought of them and always his mother was in the image, part of the picture. Charlie walked through the expanse of grass, looking at the words on the headstones. He still remembered some names. *Albert Barker*: blacksmith by trade and Charlie recalled sneaking into the big yard and watching the man shoe the horses. *Thomas Tully*: five years old, *sleeping,* proclaimed the headstone, but Charlie had different memories …. *squashed* Tommy Tully, more like. Charlie remembered clearly holding hands with his mother, the two of them hurrying from the Co-op and the bedlam and noise of the howling brakes as the truck hit the little bike and Tommy disappearing under the huge wheels of the juggernaught. *What was left of Tommy Tully*. Charlie could still feel his mother's hands pawing at his disbelieving face trying to shield him from the horror.

He found his grandparent's graves, side by side and Charlie gasped with astonishment. All neat and tidy, both draped with the beautiful garland of flowers, both bouquets fresh and new. Charlie gazed at the vivid colours, couldn't believe it, who could have put flowers on their graves. *Ma,* he thought, *it had to be Ma* and a wave of sadness swamped Charlie, his mother still visited, after all this time and she told no one. Charlie would have understood, would have walked with her, Charlie loved his grandparents. He eased on to the warm earth, stroked at the grass, looked again at the flowers and saw the card, half-hidden between colours, the little note. Charlie prized out the message, read it again and again and started to weep. His mother leaving notes on his grandparent's graves!

He stayed for an age, couldn't leave, recalled the old folks sitting around the crackling fire: little Charlie snug on his grandma's lap and granddad spinning tales of wonder. Charlie listening, captivated with wonder, eyes wide with the tales from yesteryear, believing it all: loving it. Grandad the War hero: The *Audie Murphy* of his day, capturing entire battalions of German troops single-handed, the most decorated man in Durham and Charlie's mother laughing and shaking her head at her naive small son, captivated by another exploit, another tale of valour. Years earlier and his Grandpa saving hundreds of passengers from the sinking *Titanic,* what a giant of a man, time and time again as he launched himself into the freezing waters of the Atlantic, with Herculean strength saving countless lives, *'Honest, grandpa,'* he gasped, *'you really saved all those people? And the iceberg was as big as a skyscraper?'* And earlier still, his grandfather fighting alongside real cowboys. '*Not in America, Charlie, no, the real west was in Australia. Ned Kelly was the most dastardly outlaw of his day.'* Grandpa was one of the Ned Kelly Gang, cradled little Charlie Hill and whispered, '*It's our secret! Charlie, I designed Ned's tin helmet, honest. Cross my heart and hope to die.'*

"Son," said the nearby stranger, his tone wary and puzzled and Charlie immediately lifted from his stupor. "Son," repeated the man benevolently, "are you all right?"

The grey-haired man was leaning against his shovel, next to him; the large barrow filled with old and decaying flowers and wreaths. The council gardener looked quizzically at the seated youth, his earlier frown turning into a compassionate smile as the fellow comprehended.

"You related to the Hancock's then?" asked the kindly man, gesturing towards his grandparent's headstones. "I knew them, you know, nice old couple." His eyes suddenly sparkled with recognition, "They had a daughter … you must be Rebecca's kid?"

Too embarrassed and flustered to reply, Charlie hurried from the place.

****

Five-o-clock, the lad pushed open the kitchen-door. His mother smiled and busied herself with the food. *Too much*, thought Charlie, *present, correct and cooking.* Throwing off his jacket, he sat at the kitchen-table, now was the time to talk to his mother, questions to be asked, but how to start the conversation. *Ma, I've been to the graveyard.* No, that would never do. *Ma, I was thinking about Granddad?* Maybe that would be a good opener, then the door opened for a second time and his father waltzed into view. *Another time,* thought Charlie Hill.

The permanent frown that was etched on the man's face melted away when he saw his wife. His wife at home! All it took was some semblance of kindness or show of caring from his wife and Adam was back to his old self, all the doubts, aches and pain pushed aside in moments as he witnessed normality, couldn't stop himself from grinning manically. All he ever wanted, something like family life, even the simple meal meant everything, her presence at home was enough. His emotions were like a yoyo, up and down, heaven and hell and nothing in between.

Playfully slapping the newspaper over his son's head, he said, "How do," and handed over the journal. Like his son, Adam Hill removed his coat, placed it on the back of a chair and sat at the table, pointed a grubby finger at the headlines, "Front page, Charlie, been a hell of a fire!"

Ashen-faced, the youth read the article; the news burned him with conscience and fear, believed beyond doubt he was destined for prison.

"It'll be low-life scum," said his father, took a cigarette from behind his ear, found matches and scorched a line of sulpher across the table-top, the matchstick flared into life and the man sucked at the cigarette, "says as much in the paper!"

Charlie wasn't listening, too busy reading, trying to assimilate all of the news, his eyes flitting through line after line. The attack had wiped out the proprietor, his wagons, his livelihood up in smoke, the whole yard a smouldering ruin, his home was gutted. He was ruined. They'd even killed his guard-dogs. *They! They!* Charlie read on trying to reach the outcome: the conclusion, praying with all his heart that he would not be discovered, his breath laboured, his chest pounding, couldn't breathe properly. The final few lines: *police were appealing for witnesses!* His eyes closed with relief.

His meal was bolted and then he was away, hurrying from his home, needing to see Elvis, his emotions like a yoyo, riding the Big Dipper, as mixed as a cuckoo chick. He needed to talk with Priestley and listen to his advice. Perhaps he'd be alright, out of the woods, scot-free. Charlie started to feel better.

"Charlie!" called Jenny Bruce. The girl was walking into the cul-de-sac, her features pulled tight, grimacing.

The youth paused and tried to make conversation but his head was elsewhere. He needed to sort out things, mentioned Priestley's shop and how he had to see the owner.

"There's been talk, Charlie," said Jenny, as if she wanted to kick-start a conversation and when Charlie nodded, she added sarcastically, "about you and Linda Macdonald?"

Any other time and the boy would have flustered and his lies would have been etched clearly on his face. Perhaps the events of the past few days had hardened his emotions and no tell-tale flush touched his features. Charlie was pleasantly surprised the way he had hidden his deceit. He asked her to explain, matter-of-fact, as if he had nothing to hide.

"There's talk, Charlie," said a distraught Jenny Bruce. "Linda is making her mouth go, she's telling people you're seeing her!"

The lies came out as if he'd rehearsed them. He'd been in the quarry, on his own. Three toddlers playing when one of them had an accident. Charlie carried him home and guess who came to the door. Of course, Linda Macdonald, '*And before you ask, no, I wouldn't touch her with a barge-pole,'* feigned annoyance and impatience with her. It worked.

Jenny eased, her fingers brushed lightly against his. She apologized then she added, "Ma doesn't want me to see you again, Charlie, she heard all about Joe Barton. Dad stuck up for you, Charlie," said in a rush of emotion, "I'm grounded, Charlie, not allowed out because I said I'd never give you up."

"How come you're here?" he queried, a smirk on his face, "if you're grounded?"

"I came straight from work, Charlie," she gasped. "I had to see you."

He was lost for words, too much going on in his head. "I'll walk with you to the Waterworks, Mr. Priestley wants to see me. You can walk the rest of the way home on your own, okay?"

They walked away from the cul-de-sac and headed south.

"Joe Barton's mother called in to see Ma again."

"She's full of wind!"

The girl nodded in agreement, "Knocked on the door again, yesterday. She was saying that her son had been threatened and told to forget all that he'd said to the police. Blamed you and your cronies, Charlie!"

Good old Elvis, thought Charlie*, he's like the Godfather.*

"Joe changed his story, Charlie. He said he was all confused with the beating, told the police a bunch of strangers - thinks they came from Horden - whacked him with sticks, said you were there Charlie, mentioned that you tried to help him."

"I'm the hero, now?" he chuckled and shook his head.

"Stop it Charlie," said the girl, "Dad told me what really happened."

They continued on their way without either of them speaking. When the couple neared the grocery shop they stopped. It felt awkward for both of them, both hesitant, searching for the right words, glancing at one another, each one waiting for the other to start some conversation.

"It's going to be hard for me to see you, Charlie," said Jenny softly, "but no matter how long they keep me grounded, I'll not change my mind about you. I love you." Her eyes were wet with emotion. She turned and hurried away.

Charlie walked towards the rear of the shop, his head cabbaged with the news, his mood crabby, mixed-up emotionally, reached the back-yard and viewed the large brick garage that filled most of the ground space. The doors squeaked loudly in protest as he pushed his way into the garage. It was deserted apart from a pair on thin legs that protruded from beneath the white gleaming *Primera.* He waited for some moments until the clashing stopped.

"Seen Elvis?" he shouted at the legs.

A quick shuffle, a little manipulation and the man dragged himself from beneath the motor and struggled to his feet. He looked middle-aged, wasted and weary, sported enormous thick-rimmed spectacles. He was bald and covered in dirt and grease. A slight nod was given.

"Elvis," repeated Charlie, "need to see him."

"Important?'

Charlie showed his irritation, barked his reply, "Yeah!"

Arnold Anders smiled, the work could wait, any excuse to venture into the property and see Elvis's beautiful granddaughter. *Dionne Warwick's baby sister*, thought Arnie Anders. *Jail-bait, but worth it*. The fellow had a penchant for ripe young girls and Sheryl was a star to behold.

"And you are," Arnold acting the cool dude, wiping away the grime on to an oily rag, "you gotta name?"

"Charlie Hill".

"Aye," laughed Arnie, "Elvis has told me all about you."

He walked to the back-door and rapped loudly, looked back at the smiling youth then stepped inside the home, collided headlong into Sheryl who was struggling with an empty crate of pop bottles.

"Arnold," bawled the female contemptuously and she pushed the fellow aside, "watch where you're walking!"

The bald, leering man backed away and allowed the youngster to squeeze past him; lecherous eyes bulged with pleasure as he watched Sheryl plant the plastic crate in one corner of the yard.

Mister Flirt chortled, "What a sight!"

Sheryl snorted indignantly, "Give it a rest, Arnie!"

"You know, Sheryl," said Arnold and he gazed lovingly at the huge bee-hive hairstyle that clung like a living volcano to her head, "you know who you look like … absolute double, matter of fact!"

"Surprise me."

"*Diana Ross,*" smiled the happy chap. "Come on then, Sheryl, a little *Chain Reaction* for Arnie?"

"Cheeky bugger," grunted the girl, "she's an old woman!" She was about to leave when she caught sight of the youth, a brief wave, a coming smile and she tap-tapped her stiletto heels towards Charlie Hill.

"*Dionne Warwick*!" Arnie Anders was always persistent, skin as thick as an elephant, "*Anyone who had a heart*," loved his music, could have been a D.J.

"On your bike, Arnie," Sheryl had other things on her mind, always had a fancy for Charlie.

"Only if you'll ride pillion," chortled Arnold, wouldn't give up, "what you say, eh?"

Then the back door opened and the smile froze on Arnold's face.

"Back to work," growled Elvis as he glowered at his hired-help. His gaze zoomed in on his wayward granddaughter. Sheryl and Charlie were standing so close they were sharing the same airspace. "And you!" Sheryl stopped her obvious flirtation as if caught by a magnet. "Get inside!"

Father and granddaughter faced one another, same stance: same pout, wrong colour, but only one in charge. With an audible groan, the female stomped into the shop, leaving the *Three Amigos* alone.

Arnie backed off, said, "The lad wants a word with you."

Elvis growled belligerently, "Right!"

"Better get back to work then?"

"Right!"

"I was changing the exhaust, Elvis?"

“What are you waiting for?” barked the chubby proprietor.

Arnie Anders disappeared under the motor muttering to himself.

Elvis Priestley gestured at youth, “Better come in to the kitchen. We’ll have a bit of a chat?”

A big grin covered Charlie’s face as he trooped to the home. *Money, money, money*, he thought.

****

Easington and District Working Mens’ Club, Mecca of the North-East. Mid-week special: bingo in the Snug, seven-o-clock until seven thirty, followed by Handicap dominoes and in the lounge, sing-a-long with the Reg Prentice Band. The warmness of the evening had boosted the attendance figures. There must have been at least thirty couples sweating to win the meagre prizes, Rebecca was on a high, sweetly dazed with booze as she played the game of chance, sweated on the first two games and then won the large tin of biscuits, nearly missed the paltry prize because she was at the counter ordering a refill. The win made the chat flow between the inebriated woman and those close to her.

Full of good cheer, Rebecca decided to mooch and she waltzed from the room and headed for the lounge, fancied a bit of light relief, a little entertainment, maybe listen to the music. The room was dimly lit; smoke clung to the air like a low threatening cloud. There was a cheerful crowd clinging to the tables as the group tried their hardest to destroy song after song. The woman found places at a table nearest the stage, convenient for the bar but a mite painful on the ears, too close for comfort, reach up and stretch and you could touch the drums and Barty Smith was heavy-handed, still thought he was swinging a pickaxe for the Council. Robby Glasgow, wearing his best jam-jar spectacles, thought he was Easingtons' answer to Bert Weedon. Self-praise, they say. Reg Prentice - Toneless Reg behind his back - thought he was the reincarnation of Guy Mitchell. He sported heavy stubble to hide his lifelong affliction to acne and an enormous beer-gut.

The band struggled though their version of *Stranger in Paradise*. Tony Bennett would have sued and won. A final drum roll and the song stuttered to an end. The trio relaxed, guzzled at their drinks and decided on the next crucifixion. Becky nodded at the folks around her, only recognized Dizzy and Joan Armstrong, knew Joan from her schooldays; nervous, until she was full of drink then she was a bugger for trouble. Dizzy, her third husband was really called Derek until one day underground, using a mechanical pneumatic wind-drill, wrongly positioned it and cut a perfect passage through his pit-boot. Lost a toe then it went all downhill fast. Still screaming, Dizzy manages to pull free the drill only to drop it exactly dead-centre onto his other boot. The *Enola Gay* couldn't have picked a better target, spot-on, stigmata of the foot! Dizzy by name, Dizzy by nature.

Joan was well away, talking like a parrot, the life and soul of the party as she sipped her sixth Bacardi and coke of the evening, spotted Becky and immediately moved places and sat next to her. Their voices rose as the hottest band in town struck up with a Reg Prentice favourite.

"All together now," bellowed an inebriated Reg, "Guy Mitchell's best ever number," glanced at the other band members, nodded expertly, shouted, "one and two and three …. *She wears Red Feathers….*"

The two girls grinned mischievously and burst into song and *a Hula Hula skirt*..... thought they were *Connie Francis* and *Rosemary Clooney,* sounded like a couple with dementia.

****

CHAPTER SEVEN

They made the Colliery Co-op with five minutes to spare, wouldn't have mattered either way, Elvis had made a quick telephone call to Ronny Spellman, the devious manager of the store, who bought rejected stock and any returned clothing for a song. Both men made the odd penny from the scam. The kid was all ears when Elvis had suggested the new deal. '*Any way, Charlie,*' he'd said. *'either take the cash,'* and the money was pulled out of his pocket for effect, *'or go another route. One: Cash; but nothing else. Two: settle your mother's bill at the shop; which amounted to a pretty penny. Three: A drive to the Co-op and get a full rig-out: the works; shoes; jeans; shirt.* Elvis Priestley, conman extraordinaire. *'Up to you Charlie-boy.'*

Charlie Hill, innocent in business dealings but quick-witted and intelligent, learning fast the dubious underhand ways of the chunky proprietor, wavered momentarily, didn't want to rock the apple-cart, said, tongue-in-cheek, "Only way is one, two, or three," his face cracking into a mischievous grin, "why not mix and match, Elvis?"

The little bastard, thought Priestley but said with faked sadness and a morose shake of his head, "Go on, son, ruin my day."

"Numbers two and three," retorted the youth brashly, told himself he'd settled Elvis's dirty work for peanuts, worked like a professional and was headlines in newspapers, knew what he was really worth. Young kid maybe, but with an old head on his shoulders, a hard glance at Priestley, adding audaciously, "Plus twenty pounds cash," knew the Co-op sold good gear and he was desperate for shoes and his mother would be ever so pleased when she discovered her debt with Elvis had been settled. "Do that and I'll work for you again?"

They reached the store, deserted, apart from the obese and middle-aged chap who struggled with the bolt on the big doors, the man reeking of sweat and after-shave, ushered them unceremoniously into the clothing section. Big, tired eyes gazed over Charlie's torso, a brief spit of questions about the youth's waist, inside-leg, chest and shoe-size then he was gone. Six-thirty and well after closing-time, the three emerged from the store. Charlie was right chuffed with all of the gear and when he was driven home Elvis Priestley pushed the few notes into his hand. *What a guy*, thought the boy, *the best,* then to cap it all the older man shook Charlie's hand, like they were equals, made the lad's day.

The youth hurried into his home, the bundle close to his chest; the money still clenched in his fist, couldn't wait to tell his Ma that he'd cleared her debt. Adam Hill squatted close to the fire, a cup of tea in one hand and a fag in the other, looked ill at ease, took a long drag of his cigarette before greeting the youth.

"Now, Charlie," he whispered and his gaze returned to the crackling fire, "everything okay then?" his mind elsewhere.

Adam Hill subdued and introverted, always an ominous sign of trouble: a threatening storm or a passing squall - depression or violence - depended on the wind's direction and the muck it carried. Charlie knew instinctively what it was about; only one person drove his father into such depths of despair.

"Where's Ma?"

"God knows," said the adult glumly, glanced at the clock on the mantelpiece; it was a little after seven-o-clock. "I've sat here since six."

"Not eaten?"

"No food", replied the man sullenly, "just tea-bags, milk and sugar, found a *Kit Kat* but I ate it."

"I'll go to Greaney's shop, they're open till nine," Charlie stuck his hand in his pocket, the notes would be put to use, "I've got some money, dad," and he turned to leave.

"Charlie," said his father and handed over a £10 note, "here you are, you don't have to spend your cash," pondered a moment, took a long breath and added sullenly, "while you're out, have a quick look in the *Mutton* and the *Kings Head,* see if you can see your Mother?"

An hour later and Charlie was hurrying towards the colliery, he'd pushed aside his father's brooding, made worse when he'd reported neither sight nor sound of his absent mother. The boy's heartstrings were tugging as he thought of Jenny Bruce, missed her and wanted to see her. Shaking with trepidation, Charlie knew he would have to speak to Jenny's parents if the situation was to be resolved, decided to tell them the truth about the trouble with Joe Barton, cards on the table, knowing, hoping, that they would realize he had not instigated the fracas and had initially been the intended victim of the Hogg Gang. It was going to be embarrassing and, knowing the extent of distrust from Jenny's mother, he was going to eat lots of humble pie, but Charlie wanted to see Jenny, no matter what.

He was decked out in the shoes and shirt provided by Elvis Priestley, the jeans were too long in the leg and he'd have to find cotton and thread the following day and alter them, not for the first time he'd had to make do and mend. He felt good, like a million dollars, reached the start of the colliery and spied the crowd on the seat next to the library, took a long breath and carried on his way expecting cat-calls, maybe worse, *Here we go,* thought Charlie, *get ready for fireworks.* He was surprised by the reception.

"Mad Charlie," called Alfie Hogg. There was no bitterness or malice in his tone, "join us!"

No one refused an invitation from Big Alfie. Reluctantly he strolled towards the older lads, walked with an enforced swagger trying to hide his gut-wrenching fear of reprisal. A deft movement of a heavy back-hand and two of Alfie's cronies made a space for the newcomer.

"Take a pew, Charlie," said the *Meatloaf* double.

There was a definite hint of a smile across the broad features of the older youth. Charlie Hill took a seat next to the older youth and waited for the worst. A bottle of spirit appeared from the milling crowd of miscreants. One after another, the bottle was tasted and passed. Alfie took a long swig, coughed violently as the whiskey burned his throat and then handed it to Charlie. Tongue against the bottle-neck, Charlie faked the ritual without a trickle of liquid touching his throat. He crunched his face like a professional and returned it to the gang leader.

"You're alright, Charlie Hill," said Man-Mountain, "you're one of the boys."

Charlie nodded, wondered if a punch-line was to follow the praise, or maybe a punch, sucked in air and waited with growing unease for what was about to follow.

"Sorted the job for you," said Alfie, "had a word with Joe Barton," didn't mention the threats from his father, it wouldn't have looked good for one so feared to be coerced by a diminutive, puny-looking parent, "put our heads together… me and the boys, got our story right. Horden gang paid a flying visit, tooled-up they were, chased us, caught Joe, give him a right going-over. Knock on the head sent him doolally daft, made him say all kinds of rubbish." A beefy grin from the bear and an elbow into Charlie's side, "You okay with that?"

"Thanks, Alf," replied a thankful Charlie, knew for certain he'd not be coerced, threatened or thrashed that night and he was truly relieved. He rose to make an exit, "Got to go, Alfie, girl trouble, you know how it is."

Desperate Dan didn't know anything about girl trouble, never been that fortunate with the opposite sex, Alfie Hogg was nineteen and still a virgin, hadn't told a living soul, not the kind of story that could ever see the light of day, didn't stop him acting like the colliery lothario. "Understand exactly."

The bottle of spirit was lifted at the youngster as a kind of tribute. "Cheers, Charlie Hill, I was wrong about you," took a long swig. "Got a few more bottles if you change your mind."

Charlie couldn't believe it, he was accepted, felt like Christmas Eve and Alfie was a surreal Santa Claus. With a little wave, Charlie was off again on his journey, felt a surge of affection for the big guy. Alfie Hogg was okay and he was much better looking than *Meatloaf's Marvin Lee Aday,* better by far.

Deep, deep breath as he stepped into the yard, silently he edged to the back-door of the Bruce's home. Needn't have worried about making a noise because *World War Three* was taking place inside. It was *Blitzkrieg* all over again so he stood, transfixed not knowing what to do especially when all he could hear was his name mocked, ridiculed and derided. He should have had the courage to knock on the door and face the accusers but his strength failed him. Charlie Hill turned and hurried away into the night.

Charlie retraced his steps across the colliery street and joined up with the wild bunch themselves, the notorious *Hogg Gang* and had a good time, in fact, fuelled by the copious draughts of alcohol, a smashing time was had by all. Two cars damaged and a futile attempt to steal a Toyota *Starlett* meant that the pit-posse was chased through the back-street of Tombstone by one irate miner with a pick-axe handle for back-up. Later, after they'd skirted the entire boundary of the colliery, they landed back at their favourite haunt where, for pure devilment, a large litter-bin was removed and found a new home in the library via the large plate-glass window.

Wanton vandalism, fuelled by an endless supply of booze and a sick sense of bravado, the infamous *Hogg Gang* and one solitary member of the *Angels*, ran riot that night. By ten-o'clock they had wearied and one by one, they drifted to their homes, leaving only Charlie and Alfie alone to reminisce and boast.

"Hell of a night," gushed the inebriated Charlie Hill.

"Best night's work for ages," chuckled Alfie, "almost got us a Toyota … could have taken a ride around the other collieries, caused more bother, eh?" He pondered for some moments then grabbed and hugged the young kid, "You're okay, Charlie Hill," said Alfie, "be seein' you!" Then he was gone.

Charlie started to walk home then, on a whim, changed direction, the alcohol giving him false courage. He could still hear the words of wrath from Jenny's parents ricocheting around his head. Time to confront them, tell them the truth, put them in their place; they had no right to talk about his family like that, time to knock them down a peg or two.

****

The Workingmen's Club was full to capacity, the cabaret continued apace. Nostalgia Night and the band was on top form or seemed to be, judging by the riotous applause and the good humour of the crowd, or maybe it was more to do with the huge amount of alcohol consumed, no matter. The Reg Prentice Band, fuelled with a continuous drip-feed of *Federation Best* became more and more adventurous, thought they were *Bill Haley and the Comets* as they pranced about the small stage.

The centre of the large room was cleared so that the folks could dance. The band abandoned the fifties and rocked off with *Chubby Checker*, only the half-dozen participants couldn't twist if their lives depended on it. A quick drum-roll, a tap-tap on the microphone and the amazing band metamorphosised into *Cliff Richard and the Shadows.* With beer-glasses knocking in harmony on the wet, wooden table, the girls, Rebecca and Joan, sang out loud, '*Got myself a crying, talking, sleeping, walking ... Living Doll!'* staggered on to the dance-floor and started to jive, beer glasses still in their greedy hands, '*Got to do my best to please, just 'cos she's a Living Doll ...'*

Charlie neared the Workingmen's Club, wondered if his mother would be in the place. *Take a chance*, thought the youth, pushing open the heavy double-doors the lad entered and spotted the old man sitting in the foyer. Jack Greaney was absorbed in the sporting section of the newspaper. Jack was Doorman at the Club, part-time, took him away from the humdrum boredom of the shop; a bit of company for the old man.

Charlie said, "Mister Greaney."

A look of puzzlement touched the old mans' face, "Hello, son."

"Seen Ma?"

Jack folded the newspaper, said, “Playing bingo a while back.” Non-members were not allowed unless signed in by a current member and younguns, no chance, not worth his job, he moved off sharply saying, “Stay there, Charlie.”

The lad could hear the music escaping from the room, music and the buzz of people, took a chance and made his move. The large room was awash with happy, boisterous folk, smoke and music swirled over the heads of gyrating couples, the bar area was crowded with men folk: talking; listening; shouting; gesticulating as if their lives depended on prolonging the irrelevant banter.

The music ended and the aged crooner started introducing the next act. ‘*Ladies and gentlemen,*’ he said, then spotted Charlie Hill gaping at the door, past caring he continued, ‘*and children, let’s have a big round of applause for Dizzy Armstrong!*’

Derek Armstrong stumbled drunkenly towards the microphone, full of mirth and good cheer, started howling into the mike, ‘*I married Joan! What a girl! What a whirl! What a wife!*’ pointed wickedly at the two women dancing nearest to the bandstand. One of the women waved a hand in recognition, still grasping the empty glass in the other and then with a quick twirl, proceeded to unfasten her blouse with her other hand, two mounds of firm breast, flimsily wrapped in a bright pink bra burst into view and a loud cheer exploded as several conservative souls hurried to her side and helped hide the offending chest.

Charlie recognized the strippers’ companion. His mother was laughing hysterically as she waltzed back to the table, grabbing her arm he shouted out her name. Rebecca turned and smiled vacantly at her son, smothered him with loving arms and pulled him towards her drinking companions.

Turning to his mother, Charlie tried to tell her about his argument with Jenny's parents: the accusations, the threats, the nastiness and name-calling, explained again as Joan Armstrong tottered towards the boy, stifling him with kisses and cuddles. '*Will you listen to me*, *Ma?*' he demanded hysterically, told the females how the row escalated, with Albert Bruce trying to push Charlie out of the yard and with only the slightest retaliation from him, *'I only shoved him, honest Ma!'* the older man collapsing to the ground. Rebecca and Joan were intoxicated, unable to comprehend, two pairs of dazed, bloodshot eyes trying to follow the story, slopping down the ale as they nodded with little apparent interest.

Their drinking companion joining them, Dizzy Armstrong, out of this world with a heady mixture of spirits and ale trying to drape his arms about the boy: smacking wet lips over his protesting face, on a high since his brief stint on stage, fondled and scratched at his head, kind words from the inebriated trio as they tried to placate and mollify the boy. A last desperate attempt by Charlie to motivate his mother failed.

"Ma!" he yelled above the racket. "Come home, will you, Dad is in a hell of a mood!"

"Tell him to come and join us," laughed Joan Armstrong.

No one budged, too soaked in an alcoholic haze to listen or even care and when the Reg Prentice Band started their rendition of *Singing the Blues* he could only watch as his mother joined Joan in the rousing sing-a-long. He turned and stormed from the place.

****

Lately, the boy had started to leave his home during the night, his mother did not seem to mind any more, always appeared to be drowsy and exhausted in the evenings. Ruby Shannon never used to be so distant or tired, always a live-wire, all the time in the world for Harry, her only son. Once, they would sit together and read his special books or watch the television and talk, always talking, discussing all manner of things and for hours at a time. Harry Shannon and his Ma, no one else mattered, no one else in the world but Harry and Ruby.

She started drinking the special drink. It was her medicine from the tall thin bottle. Harry was told never to touch it. '*Don't you dare drink it, Harry. It will make you so ill. You'll probably die if you touch it!*' And always she would go to sleep and leave Harry on his own. He hated having to undress himself and pull on his pajamas so, occasionally when the big moon in the sky was bright, he would leave the house and wander all over the Village. Harry never got lost, not any more. He was a big boy now.

Harry Shannon stood transfixed in the heart of the quarry. A gentle breeze covered him; he wore his favourite hat and his long overcoat, like a little chunky statue, hardly breathing, waiting for all of natures' creatures to show themselves, just like television or his picture-books, only better because it was real.

He detected movement and the slightest of sounds to the right of his rigid body. Only his eyes registered and focused on the place. '*Fluffy bunnies,*' his Ma called them. A small line of rabbits scampered towards him then paused, twitching their small heads this way and that, so close to Harry that he could have reached out and touched their soft bodies. Big rabbits and baby rabbits and all in a line. The youth heard a noise above his head, there was movement above him, the faintest fanning in the luminous skies. His eyes lifted and Harry saw the white bird: like a living, flapping, silent cloud, slowly following the scampering creatures. It was an owl. *A barn owl,* mused the youth, he'd seen pictures of them in his nature book. He was hypnotized; amazed, watching the scenes unravel before his eyes, could hardly believe the show. *The big owl is watching the rabbits just like me!*

The rodent's journey continued and soon the column of rabbits had disappeared from sight but not the flying creature. It flew noiselessly in wider circles and seemed to be watching the ground around where Harry stood, then, suddenly, unexpectedly, the big bird swooped towards the earth, the youth gulped with apprehension as he heard the distant thump, the almost inaudible scuffle and the brief cry of pain before silence returned over the barren, murky landscape.

Harry Shannon waited and watched until his body protested; still he endured the discomfort, wanting nature's show to start again. Nothing else stirred. An age passed. Finally, apparently satisfied that the spectacles were over for the night, he sauntered and shuffled his way from the quarry. It was time to return home.

"Time to go to bed," he said to himself, "time for Harry to go to sleep."

****

CHAPTER EIGHT

At school the following day, Billy Nord told Charlie about the blather and hearsay that had spread like wildfire around the colliery of the brawl between old Albert Bruce and the young trouble-maker, not an inkling of truth but a spreading fabrication of innuendo and intimation as tittle-tattle and gossip hit the streets, not the disagreement but the assault, not a word about the pushing match or the bad words only the violent attack by the young drunken hooligan against the older, weaker man. The news spiralled out of control. According to Billy, who had heard his mother nattering to a next-door neighbour, Albert Bruce had been rushed to hospital with a suspected heart-attack and that his working-days were over.

Lunch-time and the youth was hurrying towards the Colliery, he needed to see Jenny and tell her the truth about the quarrel between himself and her parents, face to face, tell it like it happened, a verbal spat, a heated wrangle, nothing more. Charlie Hill had only glimpsed her momentarily the previous evening when he had called at their home demanding to talk to her parents. Her startled face as she answered the door to him, the disbelief at the lateness of the hour and the state he was in, *'Charlie, what on earth do you want. Do you know what time it is? Have you been drinking? Stop shouting Charlie, you'll waken everyone!'* Then she was gone, dragged inside by an incensed mother, followed by an appearance of a bedraggled, confused Albert Bruce intervening in the growing fracas, confusion and chaos as the two men commenced a verbal, bitter argument in the rear yard of the colliery house, rowing, recriminations and then finally the older man remonstrating with Charlie. *'Enough! No more! Get away from my home!*

Stay away from my daughter, you hear me!' and pushing Charlie. The youth refusing to leave, standing his ground, a retaliatory shove, nothing more and the old man buckling and falling to the floor.

Jenny needed to know the truth, his fault for calling so late, guilty of arguing, the alcohol making him loud and aggressive in his manner and attitude but, as for physical violence, nothing could be further from the truth. She had to be told the facts. He needed to apologise, both to her and her parents. He was waiting, still breathless from the journey, as Jenny Bruce left the shop. The shock of seeing him was too much for her, she bolted, left him standing rooted to the spot and not a word had passed between them, no time for explanations, assurances, admissions of immature behaviour. The meeting over in seconds, *'I'm sorry, Jenny',* whispered to the wind as he watched her scurrying away. Crestfallen, embarrassed, Charlie mooched his way back to the Comprehensive, head down, wallowing in the depths of depression, mumbling incoherently, didn't notice nor care as passing strangers occasionally glanced nervously at the youngster's antics as he meandered sullenly through the streets. The following day was a repeat performance from the young girl, with one exception, she screamed at Charlie to leave, unconcerned as shoppers turned and stared as the one-sided fracas erupted. *'Go away! Leave me alone!'* she howled, stamped her feet with uncontrollable rage, *'My father is in hospital because of you! Go away, Charlie!* then Jenny was off running again, leaving the youth humiliated and inconsolable.

Success came on day three, a partial success. The young couple did engage in conversation for several minutes but Jenny was adamant. Her mother would never lie to her, she said. If her mother said that Charlie had attacked her dad, well, enough said. She believed her mother's version of the events of that night, reminded him, in no uncertain terms that he was drunk when he called, not only very drunk, but loud and extremely aggressive. The youth would not let her escape without some attempt at putting his side of the story. Charlie held her and would not release her until she listened. She had little choice, with big eyes blazing and mouth tightly closed, Jenny was forced to pay attention and listen to the events of that night.

"I told them Jenny," he pleaded, "I wasn't to blame for my parents. Told them it wasn't fair to keep us apart because of that!"

"So now it's your mother and father who are at fault, Charlie," said a sardonic Jenny Bruce.

"Something like that," murmured the boy, trying desperately to find the right words.

"I understand, Charlie, foolish of me," chided the girl.

"You understand?" Charlie stuck fast in a quagmire, nodding desperately.

"Of course! It's the booze to blame. You've told me so many times, haven't you!" started mimicking Charlie's countless apologies for his parent's outrageous and infamous reputation as rabble-rousers, *'They're not bad, you know, Jenny! When they're sober they're lovely, just like anyone else.'* The girl wide-eyed with anger and frustration. *'It's when they've had too much too drink! Jekyll and Hyde,'* you said. *'Jekyll and Hyde!'*

"Stop it, Jenny!"

"Stop what? The truth, Charlie?" shouted the girl venomously. "Who are you today, Charlie … Jekyll or Hyde?" her face distorted with indignation and rage, "and tomorrow, Charlie, who will you blame tomorrow?" She slapped him suddenly; the blow unrehearsed and wanton, the noise embarrassingly loud. She turned and hurried away. "It's over, Charlie!" she cried. "It's over between you and me!"

****

Montgomery Jepson had a date that night. Sixteen years old and his first real outing with a female, biggest day of his life, date number-one and the girl in question was a scorcher. Lynne James, same age and with a tawdry and tarnished reputation to match her best friend, Linda Macdonald. Monty was in deep trouble because of his naive brother, Patton. The twins - named after Second World War Generals by a proud and patriotic father - was determined to go the match. Patton didn't want to see Linda Macdonald. '*I've got free tickets for Hartlepool United*,' Pat had said adamantly. '*Free tickets!*' screamed his infuriated and enraged brother. '*Who the hell wants free tickets when he had the chance of a free fuck!*'

It took all afternoon to persuade Charlie to double-date. Two hours of gentle pleading from Monty and Charlie Hill succumbed. He kept thinking about Jenny Bruce, his mind in turmoil, kept remembering Jenny's final words, the reality sinking in. Maybe their relationship was at an end. Irreparable. At 3.00pm he weakened. *Why not,* he reasoned, he was a free agent; Jenny wasn't coming back on to the scene, knew that for a fact and Montgomery Jepson was persistent, persuasive and vocal. *'Come on, Charlie,'* he begged, '*Let's have a ball, it'll be a laugh!*'

He was at the Jepson home just after six-o-clock. Minutes later and they were safe in Montgomery's bedroom. Charlie pulled out the bottle of gin - his mother's gin - and his friend grabbed a handful of records.

“There’s some orange downstairs,” said Monty. “We’ll mix the booze. I’ll get some glasses”

“Party time!” laughed Charlie.

He flipped through the records, took only one and placed in the machine, set it for repeat play with the volume as high as it would go: *New Kids on the Block,* smiled as the disc blasted through the terraced house. *You got it.* Charlie took a long swig from the bottle, the noise of the record, the vocals started to ease his tension, *‘What the hell,’* he muttered and took another drink from the bottle, started laughing softly, maybe Jenny’s words were prophetic, perhaps it was all in the genes, *‘Like father like son, eh?’*

The James house was situated to the rear of the *Diamond Pub,* behind Seaside Lane. At seven-thirty the boys arrived, well and truly under the influence, the alcohol easy on the throat, like guzzling soft drinks, didn’t feel the effects until they left Monty’s home then suddenly the pair were unsteady on their feet, incessantly loud and full of merriment and good spirits, deliriously happy, all haze and uncertainty and infantile wit. What a night in store for the drunken adolescents and heavenly bliss waiting in the form of two gorgeous and willing females. Nine-thirty and it was time to call it a day, reluctantly for all but Lynne James’s mother would be returning soon, despite the protests and the arguments to prolong the evening, the two boys had to cease their cavorting and leave. *‘Mother finds out I’ve had boys in the house and it’ll be goodbye babysitting for ever,’* Lynne reading the riot act to the inebriated lads. *‘Come on you two, better safe than sorry. There’ll be other times!’* Montgomery, smiling like the cat that had found the cream was left on the doorstep talking to the love of his life. Charlie and Linda Macdonald, arm in arm, headed for the Village, both of them were talkative and loud, both sodden with booze and good cheer. *'Good night, Charlie,'* said Linda coyly, *'maybe do it again?'* knew what she wanted and was determined to succeed, whatever it took. Charlie Hill was some catch.

They turned at the *Diamond* corner and staggered along the gentle incline towards the distant Waterworks, still laughing and horsing around. Full of high spirits they stumbled headlong into a couple hurrying in the opposite direction. Mother and daughter, arms linked in a loving bond, chattering incessantly as they made their way home. At first, there were quick apologies all round and then the sudden realization, the smack of reality, as voices and faces were recognized. A numbing silence engulfed the quartet as Nancy Bruce stared from Charlie to Linda then back to her daughter. Charlie and Jenny locked eyes on one another for what seemed an eternity. All the emotions captured in moments: deceit, despair and so much damage; all the hurt and embarrassment squeezed into those few brief seconds. Apologies, excuses, explanations sucked into a terrible and silent void as the couples backed away from one another and stumbled on their separate ways.

He couldn't remember the walk home, felt the rain falling on him and the coolness of the evening, couldn't recall Linda Macdonald's words as she tried to pull aside the stupor that had engulfed him. Charlie Hill was bombarded with a myriad of mixed emotions; guilt, shame, embarrassment and a deep sense of humiliation, clear-headed and sober with the unexpected confrontation with Jennie Bruce. *It's over now, Charlie,* he thought bitterly, *well and truly over,* there was no way on earth the damage could be repaired.

****

"Please mother", begged Charlie, "let me come with you."

Rebecca Hill sat at the kitchen table, the small bathroom mirror propped against the squat tea-pot. About the surface of the table lay the miscellaneous collection of toiletries: bric-a-brac, ancient and new, jumbled and strewn haphazardly over the bureau. The female was middle-aged and the daily abuse was starting to leave its mark; skin prematurely aged, permanently lined and with the dull lacklustre markings common to alcoholics, Rebecca knew this, the mirror couldn't lie and so she applied the liberal coating of powder and paint to mask the damage. Occasionally the woman would pause at her task and reach out for the small tumbler of refreshment, lifted and swallowed in one expert movement and then immediately refilled.

"Can I, mother," whined the boy pathetically, "please?"

The grizzled features stared long and hard into the mirror, the thin garish lips puckered. "Charles," muttered the female, "be a love, fetch the rest of my make-up," her tone dead-pan and distant as if her thoughts were elsewhere.

"I'll do that mother," answered the lad, "if you'll let me come with you?"

Becky Hill looked her son up and down. "Charles, you're a big boy now, you'll be safe on your own. Mother will be out for only a little while." She toyed with her untidy thatch of hair, "I can't stay out too long, your father will need his tea," a little glance at her boy's troubled features. "I'm only going to the colliery for your father's wages, it's pay-day, Charlie," patted his head as if he were the family pet. "I promise, Charles, I'll be straight home." The woman took another swig from the glass.

"Please mother." The boy was desperate; he couldn't have stayed at home, not alone, not with his father. Adam Hill, like his wife, was a heavy drinker, but different, prone to violent mood swings and Charlie tended to end up a punch-bag. Charlie had scars to prove it. Big scars!

"But I'm coming straight home, Charles."

The lad knew better, could have written a book about his mother's lies and half-truths. Twice that year, Rebecca had collected her husband's wages then promptly disappeared and for weeks at a time, returning only when the funds had dried up, leaving Charlie alone to face the nightmare and wrath of his demented father.

"Ma," he took a deep breath, "the last time you took the pay, you stayed away for a full week!"

"I had a spot of bother, Charles."

"Ma, there was no food left," he whimpered, "had to eat Chappie, Ma!" There were three tins of dog-meat in the cupboard, he remembered, couldn't forget, wept buckets when he ate it.

"Don't lie, Charles!"

"Honest Ma," he began to weep, "Dad wouldn't give me any money, said he wanted me to suffer like he was suffering!"

"That dog had to go," insisted the female indignantly. "I couldn't afford him!" Booze came before damn mutts!

"Had half a tin of Chappie every day, Ma," said the boy, thought about the dog, hated his mother when she took it to Tommy Jamieson. Killed it for a miserly quid! Butch was a lovely animal, used to keep him company when he was left on his own.

"You must stop lying, Charles." Rebecca cackled at the mirror, "dog meat indeed!" glanced at her sniffling son. "You didn't tell anyone, did you Charles?"

"Don't tell anyone about us, Ma"

The woman relented, smiled at the mirror, her new dentures were perfect. "Promise to be good, Charles?"

The boy attempted to grasp at his mother, tried to kiss her face. "Promise, Mother," he whispered happily.

She pushed him aside, growling, "You little idiot! Stop it, you'll ruin my make-up!"

Charlie's lip began to quiver and his eyes filled with tears, all he wanted was her arms around him, missed the comfort and reassurance of a mother's love.

"Start if you dare" and she wagged a finger at his puckered face, "and you'll stay at home!"

Young Charlie waited patiently. Although he held the comic-book, he did not read the print, instead he watched the long line of people waiting to be served. His mother was in the queue, next to the counter. The boy stared as the pay-slip was handed over and the money counted out into the outstretched palm, saw his mother hurry towards the door without any acknowledgement to her son. Charlie scampered after the retreating figure. They waited for public transport, mother and son standing apart from the rest of the folks. There was chatter and gossip bandied about from the others but no one bothered talking to Rebecca Hill, the woman seemingly impervious about the exclusion, not bothered by the chitchat, in a world of her own.

The double-decker arrived and the boy and his mother climbed to the upper-deck. Charlie's wish. He loved to sit and view the passing sights, like a real picture-show, he said. The ticket-collector buzzed onto the deck, whistling and singing softly to himself, the fare collected and the ticket handed over. The boy sat mortified, something was wrong, knew enough about the price of tickets for the short journey from the colliery to the Village. They were going on a journey and it was not to their home. Charlie sat sullen. He could never get used to deceit.

Finally, as the vehicle roared away from the district and along the coast road away from Easington, he asked, "Ma, where are we going?"

The bus picked up the solitary fare next to the dog-track stadium, north of the Village, then rumbled down the steep decline that would take them past Hawthorn and on to Seaham. Rebecca was miles away. Eventually, after a gentle elbow from the boy, the question was repeated.

The mother, clearly irritated, barked her reply, "What Charles?" paused momentarily then added whimsically, "oh, didn't I say? We're going to Sunderland, I have bills to pay!"

Charlie grimaced, knew he would have to watch his mother like a hawk, be vigilant at all times. His young body ached with foreboding and fear, couldn't understand why his mother acted the way she did, hurt him so much so often, told so many lies, time and time again. The boy grimaced and held his tongue, his head shouting out a warning, 'She's going to dump you again, Charlie. Mother's going to deceive you and leave you! Watch her, Charlie! On your guard, Charlie!' He reached out and held her hand.

After a weary hour, the pair reached their destination. The town was heaving with people and traffic. Charlie followed his parent like a lap-dog, never leaving her side. In shops, paying bills, store after store, the boy starting to believe her story. After some time, the tension between the two was lifting and the chatter became light and frivolous. It seemed like the old days again, the closeness between the mother and son, Rebecca even treated him to an ice-cream and tea and a Mars

Bar. Charlie was beginning to enjoy himself, enjoyed Sunderland, loved the hustle and bustle of town life, it was so exciting.

Then, as always, the woman weakened, suddenly, out of the blue she said poignantly, "Charles, mother needs a little drink."

The boy visibly slumped, "Ma", he wailed, "you promised!"

"Don't start, Charles," Rebecca was adamant, "you've had your refreshment, now it's my turn!" her gaze fell on the nearby public-house, like a magnet to the female as the smell and the laughter spilled into the street. Gesturing to the nearby public seat, Rebecca Hill ordered him to wait outside. "I'll only be a few minutes, Charles. Just one little drink."

"Ma," he pleaded. "Please don't leave me!"

She held his hand and looked at him with a sweet smile. "Charles. I won't let you down again, I promise!" Coins were taken from her purse, pointing to the corner shop, she said softly, "Go and buy another ice-cream, Charles, go on, son." Gestured again, fondling his hair she eased him on his way, "By the time you've eaten it, I'll be finished." The woman gave a final caress and said, "I promise, Charles."

"Why can't I come in with you, Ma?" He was scowling at her, his head in turmoil, heard the deceit so many times.

"Not allowed, son," and moved away towards the open door, gave him a little wave as she disappeared into the pub.

And always, at the start of her drinking-sessions, Rebecca would keep her word. Half an hour, maybe more and she would totter out into the bright sunlight, happy with the world, content with her lot and every time she made the brief appearance, she would feed her boy with coins, then, away again and they would waltz along the streets until she found another place. The exercise and the excuses would be regurgitated and it wouldn't be half an hour the second or the third time ... maybe an hour and sometimes longer, as the day became haze and the pubs became havens as more and more alcohol was consumed. As the day progressed, the woman became reluctant to leave the heady atmosphere of the inns, enticed by the camaraderie and the cheer, the child ignored and all but abandoned and when Charlie complained he was chided and threatened.

Charlie Hill, like a lost puppy: an infant soldier patrolling his solitary patch outside of some noisy, filthy crowded den, marching up and down the pathway, ever watchful, eyes focused on the open doorway, vigilant and conscientious as he waited for his mother to reappear. Always ended the same way for the boy, on his own, frightened, worried; for himself; and for his wayward parent, desperate for an end to it, weary for the bus-ride home next to his intoxicated parent.

But this day was to be different. Early evening and his wait outside some tavern was becoming an endurance test. Hours had passed and Charlie was beginning to fret. He had twice been approached by strangers who appeared too interested in him. Fear, like some spark on a barren fire was about to explode. Charlie was becoming desperate. Then the man staggered from the public-house.

He was his father's age, tall and thin, with a thick crop of graying hair. He approached Charlie directly, as if he knew him, held money in his hand. It was for the boy, from his mother. Charlie stood rigid and solemn, not believing.

"You have to take it home," the man said, "give it to your father."

"Tell Ma," begged the delirious child, tears welling in his eyes, "tell Ma to come out now!"

The stranger persisted; he was becoming impatient with the lad, missing good drinking-time, knowing that to stay away too long from the boy's mother might cost the good time she'd promised. She was like a bitch in heat and she owed him. He had spent a pretty packet on her, glanced back at the pub, worried in case some stranger had taken his place.

"Here!" he insisted and stuffed the remains of the hard-earned wages into the boy's breast-pocket. "Bloody take it, will you!" rummaged around in deep pockets and flushed out a handful of coins, "Here," he said, feeling discomfort as he stared at the quaking moppet, "bus fare, now bloody leave!"

The boy started to cry. It was all too much for Charlie Hill.

"Son," the stranger's voice mellowed, he wasn't the Tin-Man, still felt the tug of heart-strings, knew what the kid was going through, "your mother left the pub a long time ago. She told me to wait a while before seeing you. Honest, lad, she's long gone." His eyes etched a deep sorrow, pointed along the highway, "Follow that road, son, can't miss the bus station. Someone will help you there. Go on, lad," turned and without looking back, disappeared into the murky interior, entered the lounge. Sure enough, the bitch was surrounded and, judging by the laughter, loving it.

****

Charlie looked at the clock that stood above the fire-place. It was past midnight, he sat and sniffed and stared into the dying ambers of the fire, head aching still from the beating: his body a mass of weal's from the leather strap, his father's favourite weapon. The boy cried quietly for his mother. The monster called Dad slept soundly in bed upstairs and woe betide anyone waking him!

Charlie had been punished twice that evening. As soon as his father had entered the home after finishing his shift at the pit he was beaten. Awful but expected. Most of Adam Hill's wages had vanished, so had his wife so Charlie had become the kicking-block. Then, hours later, after the fellow's head was well and truly festered, he had dragged the boy out of his bedroom and thrashed him again, taking all of his venom and frustration out on his son, the assault prolonged with only brief respites while Adam tried in vain to illicit information as to the whereabouts of his wife. Adam acting manically, "Where's your bloody mother? Tell me or I'll thrash you again!" The man demented with grief, "Who was she with this time, tell me or I'll whip you!" And the boy, as always, remained mute, always loyal to his mother, dragged, pushed, prodded and beaten but never a word from Charlie. Then it would start all over again. The pleading and the weeping disregarded as the man filled with pain and uncontrollable anger.

Hours had past since the last assault and now he waited, alone, praying for the return of his mother, his father, unconscious and drugged with alcohol, slept. Suddenly the pull of slumber was pushed aside as Charlie heard the faint tap-tap of footsteps, recognized the distinctive rhythm of stiletto heels and he bolted to the rear-door.

Rebecca Hill shuffled into the warmth of the house, then she paused, swaying like some virgin deck-hand, her coat, hanging dejectedly from her body, her clothing dishevelled, her features blank and big, morose, eyes rolling at her son.

"Charles," she gasped, "it's your mother. Charles, help me!"

The young boy struggled heroically as he slowly and carefully manoeuvred the wavering adult towards the settee. Rebecca stumbled and fell headlong on to the sofa, took the boy with her and they crashed into the comfort of the ancient settee.

"My son," gushed the drunken woman and she attempted to kiss Charlie.

The boy saw the open, drooling mouth, noticed that her new dentures were missing but didn't have the courage to tell her. Her eyes flickered and dimmed, deeply exhausted after the daylong intoxicating binge, Rebecca immediately fell into a deep and uncomfortable sleep. Charlie took off her shoes. Searching her pockets, he found the dentures wrapped in a soiled handkerchief, took them to the kitchen sink, washed them and left them to dry. Quietly, he eased to the bottom of the stairs and took an overcoat from the rack and covered his sleeping mother with the garment.

He snuggled next to her, felt her warmth. The woman struggled into consciousness, "I'm so sorry, my baby."

"Ma, you promised," held on to her like some precious doll.

Rebecca started to weep, "I'm sorry, Charles," she mumbled.

"It's alright, Ma," he cuddled into her. "Ma, I was so scared!"

"Mother will make it up to you, baby," sniffled the woman.

"You promised, Ma," he cried.

"No more, Charles," she whispered almost incoherently, "I'll never hurt you again," eyes rolled and her head started spinning like a wheel.

"Promise, Ma," begged the boy, "promise on the Holy Bible!" Now he was crying.

"On the Holy Bible, Charles," she gasped, "never again."

"Kiss and promise, Ma?"

The drunkard kissed and caressed the child. "Sorry, baby, I never mean to hurt you, Charles."

Rebecca Hill fell into a deep sleep, the boy snuggled into her, his arms around her vice-like, held her all night, never sleeping more than a few minutes at a time, didn't want her leaving him again, said his prayers, thanked Jesus for bringing his Mother back safely.

****

CHAPTER NINE

Months later

The five young miners stood beside the exit door of the lamp cabin, all loud and boisterous, talking the talk, no big deal taking the vertical tram-ride into the bowels of the earth. To a man, scared to death, worried sick about entering the pit-cage for the very first time and plunging hundreds of feet into the hellish black hole. Five trainee colliers standing resolutely and stoically on the bank-top of Easington pit, one of the biggest and deepest of the coastal mines in the North-east. Suddenly, unexpectedly, from a nearby open door came a bustling stream of soiled and unkempt figures, tar babies of all shapes and sizes: black and white minstrels; excitable and full of good cheer, their shift at an end and the relief evident, their pit-boots echoing through the place like some giant metal centipede. Some of the older miners grinned at the boys, their teeth pearl-white against their ebony features. The rag-bag platoon marched their way towards the waiting shower block.

The youngsters waited and watched as a crippled figure hobbled towards them, the stranger wearing the regulation hard-hat and overalls. One of his arms was bent and stiff, one of his legs shorter than the other. The lads could only wait and watch with growing incredulity, all thinking the same thought: who was this fellow and was he approaching their group? He could not possibly be employed at the colliery!

"It's the Hunchback of Notre Dame," whispered Pat Jepson.

"Wearing a pit-hat and overalls?" queried Charlie Hill.

Everyone in the group went silent, staring and gaping at the loping, shuffling frightening figure. He neared them and stopped, a lop-sided smile greeted them.

"Now lads," uttered the man, his voice soft, kind. His name was Arthur Ridley, his body crippled; his mind good and whole. Born with cerebral palsy, Arthur had worked all his adult life at the colliery, in the lamp-cabin, a cushy-number for some, a struggle for the courageous cripple. Brave as they come was Arthur Ridley, ignored his infirmity with a permanent smile and benign resignation "You'll be wanting these," he said and doled out the regulation tokens to the trainees: two per person.

The group took the offerings in total silence. A brief nod from the older, scary figure, kindly words of advice, 'Take care, boys, first shift downstairs is always the worst,' then he turned, gave a little wave and limped away into the workshops.

Two miners approached. One was as tall as a tree, well over six feet in height and solemn, his companion, much shorter and stout, beamed a friendly smile at all the group.

"How do?" said the chubby figure, stuck a thick finger at himself and announced, "I'm Theo Williams," then he gestured at his lanky mate, "and this is Dennis Paine. Paine by name: pain by nature!" A little joke to ease the group. The youths laughed with Theo, the tall man shook his weary head.

Theo Williams asked for Charlie and Montgomery Jepson. They stepped forward. A gentle smile, a little nod of the head and the two boys followed the fellow into the lamp-cabin, moments later and the two were donned in hard-hat and safety light. Their supervisor then took their tokens, given to them moments earlier by the crippled employee and pocketed them.

"The disks," asked Charlie, "don't understand?"

“Two tokens, colour-coded,” explained the grinning official, “before you get in the cage to go underground, you give one to the man who operates the cage. End of the shift, come back up, give him the other one” Another smile from Theo, “Easy way of checking people in and out of the pit, simple method of keeping tabs on people. No one can go missing.”

Monty asked, “Then why’ve you taken them?”

“I’ll not lose them,” he said sardonically, turned and hurried off, “come on you two or we’ll miss the cage.

Up the steel steps and along the enclosed corridor, steel doors opened and the little man gesticulated towards them. They quickened their pace and entered the enclosed tunnel. Theo Williams clamped shut the door and their ear-drums cracked at the change in air pressure, walked a few paces and the second door was opened with a loud clanking sound and they were facing the huge and ugly contraption that was the double-decked, man-riding cage. The door closed behind them and the heavy, cool draught whacked them. Theo saw their eyes on him.

“Ventilation,” he said gruffly, “I’ll explain later,” and he shuffled towards the double-decked structure.

The cage was full of miners waiting to descend into the depths of the earth; the upper-deck was chocker-bloc full so Theo moved them to the bottom compartment.

“Make way for the lads!” yelled the supervisor. A yell went up from the cage, all directed at Theo. Harmless banter and the diminutive figure grinned broadly as he approached the check-man, who stood like some deranged doorman, fitted out in ancient clothes, cloth-hat askew on his tousled head and his grubby hand outstretched. The tokens were handed over. Theo squashed into the crowded steel structure and gestured for the boys to follow, stood close to the boys, knew how they'd feel, still remembered his first ride underground, only one word to describe the feeling as they hurled downwards into the blackness…terrified!

Charlie looked at Montgomery and was about to speak when the huge ventilation doors banged open. Figures hurried towards the cage. It was Dennis Paine, the second official, striding towards them: their friends meekly followed in single file behind him. Minutes later and the lower deck was jam-packed. An ugly, jarring rattle and the perforated steel doors were clamped shut, a definite jolt as the man-riding cage was freed for descent: a sudden, fearful stutter then down it hurtled like a vertical train-ride to hell.

"Hang on boys," shouted Dennis Paine to his little group of trainees, "nothing to worry about."

Some comedian amongst the colliers yelled frantically, "Not unless the rope snaps!"

"Fuck me!" moaned Monty Jepson and he closed his eyes and said a silent prayer.

"Jesus," gasped Billy Nord as he lost control and wet himself, couldn't hold his tongue, "I've pissed my pants!"

The howl went up from all of the miners.

****

Elvis reached the Peterlee garage within minutes, switched off the motor and let it free-wheel silently to the rear of the building. Ages since he'd had a laugh at Arnold's expense, man was a shirker and a lay-about, needed an occasional jolt to keep him on his toes, wanted to see what the idiot was up to when he was left to his own devices. Leaving the motor, the man silently stepped to the side-window and glanced inside his workshop, grunted a silent oath. *You can lead a horse to water……*

"How the hell can I make any money," he bellowed as he entered the premises, "when I can't get workers to work!"

Arnold Anders almost fell off the chair, the *girlie* magazine flung out of his grimy hands as if jolted by a surge of electricity, on his feet in an instant as he jumped and faced his boss, flustered and gawking awkwardly, lost for words.

"You playing with yourself again!" bawled Elvis.

Protesting bitterly, Arnie whined, "It's the first time I've stopped today," and hurried to the open bonnet of the *Escort.*

"It's only nine-o-clock, you idle bastard!"

"Steady on, Elvis," protested the bald employee and he grasped the adjustable spanner for the first time that day.

Elvis Priestly smiled, threw the package towards the man. "Couple of pies for our breakfast," he said, chortling, adding, "make a cup of tea." He moved to the bench and retrieved the juicy magazine. Still gazing at the pictures, he said casually, "We're going for a little ride."

Arnold asked curiously, "Anywhere nice?"

"Back to the Waterworks," said Elvis.

Arnold Anders groaned, "Not another job you've got lined up?"

"You got a problem with that, Arnie?"

"Elvis," protested the mechanic, "I'm getting a bit long in the tooth for the naughty stuff!"

"This," assured the chunky proprietor, "is a piece of cake."

"Same kind of cake like the Shotton fiasco," retorted Arnie, pouting like a child, "crawling on all fours through bloody fields to be confronted by a pack of pit-bulls!"

"Yeah, tell me about it, hubble-bubble toil and trouble, eh?"

"I don't follow?"

"Job was done and dusted by someone else, wasn't it," said a solemn Elvis, almost mentioned the kid, then decided against it, some things better left unsaid, lied when he said matter-of-fact, "Same man said it was a doddle."

"Good for him," said a petulant Arnold Anders, thought about the money he'd forgone not completing the business at Coxon's, "If he's that good how come you're asking me to do some naughty?"

"Loyalty, Arnie," said a devious, indignant Elvis Priestley, thinking, *Two's better than one. Lose one and there's always a spare!*

****

It had started to rain, gentle at first, then harder and more persistent. The two women sauntered out of *Woolworths* carrying parcels, stood in the doorway and watched the rain. Joan Armstrong pulled out cigarettes and offered one to her companion.

"First day down the pit, eh?" said Joan.

"Bit nervous," answered Rebecca. "It's his father's fault, put the fear of God in him! Deeper than Hell, he said and five miles out in the North Sea!"

"He said that?"

Rebecca nodded. "That's Adam, all or nothing. Hardly speaks for days on end then he's all mouth, non-stop about everything!"

"Men," cackled Joan, "read them like a book."

Rebecca continued, shaking her head despondently, "Then he caps it all by telling Charlie about Willy Pearson!"

"Wheelchair Willy?"

"The one and only," said Rebecca, sucked at the cigarette and looked at the grey skies. "Bloody weather! Anyway, Adam and Willy were mates at the pit when he had the accident. It was Adam who pulled him free."

"It was a tree trunk!" uttered Joan, remembering the incident. "John, my first husband, he told me about the solidified trunk. *Like a torpedo* he said. *Straight from the roof.* Didn't have a chance, poor sod!"

"Broke his back," mouthed Rebecca, "snapped in two. Pity, you know. Willy was a good-looking man. Once!"

"Wears a bag," lectured Joan, "you know the kind I mean?"

"A colostomy-bag?"

"That's the one," said Joan, her face contorting at the image. "You imagine that … talking a shit out of your stomach?"

"Let's change the subject, eh?

"Rumour is the Queen Mother wears one, has done for years."

"Lucky for her she's get servants to change it!"

Joan muttered poignantly, "Poor Willy Pearson, poor bugger."

"I know what you mean, bad enough wearing a colostomy. Then his wife threw in the towel and left him. Bad business."

"Blamed the smell, said she couldn't bear to be near him."

"Mary Pearson was a trained nurse," said Rebecca sardonically, "between you and me I think that was an excuse."

"Poor Willy!"

"Thing was," continued Rebecca Hill, reverting back to the gossip about her son, "my Charlie thought his Dad was taking the water. You know, about the tree, so clever-clogs Adam gives him a geography lesson on bloody coal!"

"Teacher now, eh?" laughed Joan.

"Bloody idiot, scared Charlie to death!"

Joan Armstrong stepped out on to the street. The rain had eased, "Fancy a look around *Safeway?*" she asked.

"Why not," said her companion, "all the time in the world."

"Then maybe a quick drink," asked Joan, "a glass of stout?"

"I'm in enough trouble with Adam already," chortled Becky, "keeps threatening to leave, not be satisfied till I'm teetotal. Teetotal" mouthed Rebecca ironically, "his very words!"

"Men!" muttered Joan. "There's a law for them and a law for us!"

"Tell me about it, Joan."

"Okay for them to drink when the mood takes them!"

"Which is most weekends!"

"I say," said Joan mockingly, "what's good for the goose!"

"You're damned right!"

"Anyway," Joan retorted, a mischievous smile touching her face, "speaking as such …you've got to see the bar-man in the *Gamecock,* he's gorgeous, a bit young, but lovely all the same."

Rebecca replied, "Nothing wrong in having a look."

Like two teenagers talking about their first date, the pair *tap-tapped* along the shopping parade.

****

It didn't seem as it should, not to Charlie. He stood with dozens of miners and gazed about the huge gallery at the shaft-bottom. It was more like an enormous iron and timber work-place: ceiling stretching way up high; held in place with steel arched girders, like some surreal, half-completed warehouse. Between the girders, hiding most of the rock and stone was a multitude of wooden struts, like bizarre building blocks, one clamped on top of the other in perfect symmetry: dark and soiled with a lifetime of grime and soot. Powerful electric lights were fastened on to these wooden frames like giant torches blazing artificial light on the ground below. A constant breeze fanned their waiting bodies, irritating and chilly as it raced past and was sucked into the nearby shaft.

It was so different to all that Charlie Hill had ever imagined, more akin to a huge and weird factory, all around him was noise and bustle and organized chaos. The man-riding cage that had secreted the colliers underground now opened its doors and, with the aid of noisy hydraulics, was being fed whopping tubs of coal, both decks chock-full and straining with the weight, alarm-bells howling, followed by an almighty *whoosh* and the cage with its bounty disappeared, whisked away, hoisted up the spine of the shaft towards the distant surface. Minutes later and the empty cage reappeared and the process was repeated endlessly. Close by, big locomotives shunted back and forth, with seemingly endless lines of tubs banging and smacking one another as they were pulled and pushed by these mechanical monsters to and from the zone. The shaft-area was all commotion and never-ending activity as the colliery buzzed with activity.

Theo Williams nudged him, "Not what you thought, kid?"

"Unbelievable," replied Charlie Hill.

The youth stood and watched, mesmerized by it all until the entire group began slowly to move towards huge ventilation doors. The enormous steel doors were pushed open and the collier, followed by the trainees, clonked into a long dusty passageway; a moment's wait as the doors were eased shut, the irritation as ear-drums protested as air pressure slapped at them, then other doors situated at the opposite end of the corridor were flung ajar and the band of men stomped onwards. The place became darker now, smaller and claustrophobic, more like a mine with smaller, dimly-lit passageways snaking off in every direction. The older pitmen oblivious to it all, chatting to one another, now that the bedlam of the shaft-bottom had been left behind as they made their way up the dusty, debris-ridden incline. Warmer now, the temperature rising with every step they strode up the gentle sloping roadway until they reached a wide landing. Snaking out before them was the man-riding set. As the miners hopped into the small tubs (two facing one way; one straddled between them) the head-lamps were extinguished. The place slowly dimmed and darkened, until only three torches flickered their lonely beams at the cascading dust particles.

Theo Williams struggled into the steel tub: the two trainees followed.

"Lights out, lads," he said, "don't want to blind anyone, eh?" Total pitch enveloped the landing. A little chug and a gentle forward movement and the train started its journey. It buzzed and buckled away into the inky blackness. "Close your eyes, boys," chuckled the older man, "have a nap."

"How far, Theo?" asked Montgomery Jepson, his eyes were tightly closed.

Theo said lethargically, "Few miles is all."

Charlie, staring at the darkness feeling the warm breeze on his face asked, "How long, Theo?"

Theo Williams pulled the pit-helmet over his eyes. "Shh, Charlie," he answered, "we'll get there soon enough."

Montgomery shouted above the din, "It's hard to believe but we're under the sea!"

Charlie persisted, "Theo!"

"What now?"

"How far does the train go?"

"Five, maybe six miles," he replied and started to yawn, always enjoyed the ride, slept like a log.

The train tapped out its gentle rhythmic tune as it snaked its way to a distant destination.

Charlie Hill closed his eyes and pictured the mighty North Sea above his terrified head, thought about the myriad solidified tree-trunks waiting to crash at any moment onto the snaking, rumbling train, said a little prayer and cursed his father.

****

The vehicle slowed as it approached the line of council houses. *Hazel Terrace* situated in the centre of the Waterworks sprawl. Both men silently started mouthing the numbers from the properties. The pair saw the council house and stared at the boarded-up bedroom window.

Elvis Priestly said softly, "Easy enough, Arnie?" and continued driving, added sarcastically, "not the kind of thing you'd miss?"

"It's too close to your shop," whined Arnold Anders, "it's a stone's throw away."

"Problem with that?" queried Elvis then he started to chuckle. "Stone's throw, you're wasted, Arnie, bloody comedian."

Arnold wasn't amused by the humour, said anxiously, "I'll be seen for definite!"

The car made a right turn, then another right, up another long grey line of homes, now they were a street behind but running parallel to *Hazel Terrace*. Elvis stopped the car, pulled down the window, nodded at the nearest house. "Easy as pie, walk down that path, across the garden, jump the fence and bingo, straight ahead."

"The one with the broken window!"

"When can you do it?"

Arnold answered, "You're the boss, Elvis," and grimaced. "You tell me," thinking, *I'm the bloody slave, like I have a choice*.

"He owes four weeks money! They both work! They've been threatened!" pulled out the cigarettes and handed one to his passenger. "They need a lesson!"

"This week?"

"This week," agreed Elvis. The motor moved off. "I'm going to Peterlee, spot of business, fancy a ride?"

"Not more bother?" whined Arnold, "gimme a break, Elvis!"

"Show you something", replied the boss-man, "nice surprise."

I'll sit here all day, *Elvis,* thought Arnie. *Anything beats work.*

Arnold Anders said, "Surprise?" and smiled, "you gonna tell me about it?"

If the pair of low-life gangsters had waited just one minute and back-tracked along the street in question, then they would have been surprised at the sight of Ernie Beint struggling into view with the big ladders. Moments later and the young miner was clambering up the ladder one-handed: held the hammer and chisel with his free hand. *'Work to be done,'* he muttered morosely, *'all my own bloody fault!'* Ernie had taken a shift off work the previous week and spent an eventful day at Doncaster Races, a bit of fun and relaxation with the boys, a day of gambling and losing money like there was no tomorrow, tossing money after the donkeys … definitely weren't damn horses he'd backed, pack-mules more like. Got back late, didn't he, lost his bloody key, threw a little stone at the window to wake the missus, didn't know his own strength. What a clatter when he smashed the bedroom window. Damn neighbours up in arms.

****

"Charlie!" called a distant voice, he'd fallen asleep and felt so embarrassed as he struggled out of his slumber.

"Charlie," said Theo Williams, "we're here," and he heaved his overweight, wheezing body out of the tub.

Montgomery Jepson was too busy gazing about the landing-station to notice the awaking figure next to him.

Out like a gazelle, the youth landed with a clatter next to the overseer. "Just waiting of you, Theo," he said then moved towards his pal.

The trio stood and watched as the colliers drifted away from the man-riding set and walked into a wide arched tunnel. Several dozen light-beams splattered from the crowd as they disappeared from sight. A distant bellow from the driver of the loco and the train began its journey back to the shaft-bottom, leaving the small group alone.

Monty said, "Aren't we going with them, Theo?"

Theo Williams clamped his light on to his hard-hat; fastened the light-cable to the string on the back of the hat and muttered lethargically, "We could, if you want," pulled out the small tin, unfastened the screw top, nipped finger and thumb into the contents and sniffed the muck up his nostrils. A second later and the man sneezed violently. “Snuff!” he explained, “clears the dust from your nose.”

“What now?” asked Charlie Hill.

“We’ll walk in-bye, give us a chance to talk.”

“How far?” Monty was knackered already; it was so warm and dry.

“About a mile,” replied Theo, like it was no distance.

They followed the tracks of the miners and reached a second landing-point. Another long dark passageway stretched away into the distance, the faint rumbling of the departing train touched them as tiny dust particles danced before their beams. The slow walk commenced, with Theo Williams leading the way, chattering happily, explaining the general set-up …what to do, what not to do, no pressure from Theo, not like a boss, more like a mate, telling the trainees all about pit-work in general.

Theo Williams was a colliery lad, born and bred, knew the Jepson family well, drank with Montgomery’s dad, lived two streets away. *‘Small world,’* he said, *‘your dad enjoys the greyhounds, made some money on those dogs of his.’* He’d heard of Adam Hill, Charlie’s dad, knew he worked in the five-quarter seam, but made no personal comment about him, only his work-place. *‘It’s above this one*,’ said Theo, then he explained to the youths that they were in the deepest seam in the whole pit, *‘This is called The Low-Main,’* said the overseer which was all confusing to the lads. They plodded away in silence for some time before Theo casually, mentioned Charlie’s reputation, took the lad by surprise. Theo kept it light: didn’t dig too deep but seemed to know all about Charlie’s disagreement with Joe Barton and even the tussle with old Albert Bruce, said, in a roundabout but firm way, that

Charlie had to behave, hold his temper, put emphasis on the colliery management's style of containing trouble. '*Any physical stuff, son,*' said Theo, '*and it's instant dismissal.*'

Charlie, shocked and smarting at Theo's insinuations, nodded obediently but said stubbornly, "You've not heard the truth, Theo, wrong on both counts ….."

Montgomery interrupted Charlie, boisterous with his praises for his pal, told Theo the truth about the incident with Albert Bruce, made light of it, *'Think about it, Theo, a sixteen year old swinging punches at an old man! Load of bollocks! Charlie wanted to see Albert's daughter and Albert would have none of it, pushed him out of the yard. First bit of exercise he'd done in years, give him a bloody heart attack,"* the explanation brought a benign smile from Theo.

Charlie Hill intervened, still rankled him the way he behaved that night. "My fault, Monty," he said with regret in his voice, "should have stayed away. Been in Albert's shoes, reckon I'd have done the same. I was full of booze, out of my head." He turned and glanced at the older figure, "Truth, Theo, I never hit him. He started pushing and prodding and I shouda walked away; instead I locked arms with him. Fella was out of condition, couldn't get his breath and he fell to his knees. Honest to God, I never done what they said. He was always good to me was Albert."

"I believe you, son," replied Theo, started to like the kid, big enough to own up to his own failings, shrugged his wide shoulders, "these things happen, eh?"

Monty continued, mentioned in detail about the antics of Joe Barton and the fracas with Charlie. Theo nodded agreeably, said he knew the Barton family well, shared the occasional drink with Don Barton. Theo had heard different versions of the disagreement between the two youths, didn't overtly voice any opinion but was minded to side with his young protégé. Not many people liked young Joe Barton, heard more than once he was a braggart and a bully.

"I've heard he's a bit of an arse," said Theo, opening up his bait-can, "bit like his dad. Don Barton is a piss artist and a gob-shite. Son's probably a chip off the old block."

"He knocks about with Alfie Hogg," said Montgomery, the un-official colliery chatterbox, "now he's some piece of dangerous work!"

"Big bugger, mind you," said Theo, nodding his head in agreement, "like his brothers."

"Alfie's okay," said a subdued Charlie Hill, still taken aback that Theo knew all about him, wondered how much gossip he'd heard about his parents.

"Know his dad well," said Theo, "bloody midget is Mojo Hogg, barely five feet in his cotton socks and all his sons are giants. Mind you," added Theo, "there's few in the colliery who could stand up to Mojo," glanced at Charlie and smiled warmly, thinking of the boy's father, added impishly, "perhaps one or two!"

Some time later and the little band had reached their place of work. They were exhausted with the long trek, wet with sweat, thirsty as hell and needed to sit awhile, squatted happily in the soft mattress of stone-dust. Theo Williams pulled out the pocket-watch; nodded agreeably, the shift was already half-over.

"We'll eat now, boys," he said matter-of-fact, "maybe half an hour to recover then we'll start work. Okay with that?"

He'd start the afternoon showing the pups how to clean the conveyor-belt, it was all about pacing oneself and Theo Williams held an honours degree in lethargy. If time allowed he might have a slow wander to the coal-face, introduce the boys to the stars of the show, the coal-hewers, the stone-men, the real miners on whom everything and everyone else depended. Work-horses they were, worth their weight in gold, deserved every penny they earned.

"But we haven't started work yet, Theo?" quizzed Monty.

"Plenty of time, son," said the boss, "now eat!"

Moments past as both trainees pulled out their lunches, jam and bread for Charlie and a tin bottle of water; corned-beef, lettuce and salad cream for Montgomery and a large bottle of ice-cream soda.

"Swap, if you want, Charlie?" asked his pal, feeling guilty at the discrepancy in the menus, "sick to death of corned-dog!"

"Naw, I'm fine, Monty," replied the youth, a gentle flush of discomfort touching his features.

Montgomery Jepson was a true friend, one in a million, pals for years, always trying to look after him.

"Tell the truth," said the youth, "I'm not that hungry."

In reality, Charlie Hill was sick to death of bloody jam and bread, day in, day out, tired of making his own bait, knew for a fact he'd end up like his father and forgo lunch altogether. There were times when he hated his mother the way she treated him and his dad.

"Theo," asked Charlie quizzically, anxious to change the subject, "do you get many fallin' trees comin' through the roof?"

"Pardon me, son," replied the overseer, "trees, did you say?"

"Trees?" asked a puzzled Montgomery, "you feelin' okay?"

"Tree-trunks," prompted Charlie Hill, "solidified tree-trunks!"

***

Noon and the two women were intoxicated. They'd been in the *Gamecock* for an hour and the alcohol was starting to take effect. Rebecca felt calm, good, at ease with the world, looked at the clock perched above the bar, knowing she had plenty time to get back home for Adam's tea, glanced at her image in the long mirror opposite. *'Still a beauty,'* she thought and smiled.

"Two Guinness, please!" she said to the bar-man, "and one for yourself, son." Joan was right, the youngster was gorgeous.

The pub doors momentarily swung open, spraying the room with a heady dollop of sunshine. Two men stepped into the bar and headed for the counter. Rebecca Hill recognized one of the men and smiled roguishly.

"Eddie," shouted Rebecca, "over here!" and she turned again to the young man across the counter, "can you add two bottles of *Newcastle Brown* to that order, son?"

Joan Armstrong viewed the strangers, fancying her chances she stuck out her ample chest. "I'll have the little one with the hair and the sideburns," started grinning like someone who'd lost a penny and found a shilling.

Rebecca said, "That's Elvis Priestley."

"Heard about him", said Joan, pulling in her waist, "worth some money I've heard."

"Tighter than *Scrooge!*" commented Rebecca dryly.

"Bit of a gangster, if you believe all the rumours," said Joan. She smiled a winning smile. "Not so keen on yours, Rebecca?"

Rebecca glanced at the tall, bespectacled, bald companion and winced visibly, "Thanks, Joan," she muttered, "you're all heart."

“Honey,” said Joan, expelling air, allowing her girth to blossom, hoping all interested eyes would be focused on her breasts, “looks are skin deep.”

“You want to exchange?”

“You’ve got no chance,” said a buoyant Joan Armstrong, eyeing the chunky, arrogant smaller chap, liked what she saw, especially the obvious bulge in his trousers.

Rebecca quizzed, “The fella with the specs?”

“What about him?” asked Joan, glancing at the gangling, grinning figure of Arnold Anders.

“Remind you of someone?”

“If he were younger and a mite thicker, yeah!”

“Tip of my tongue,” said Rebecca Hill.

“Sergeant Bilko,” uttered Joan, “the absolute double!”

“Pass the playing-cards,” said Rebecca, voice as sour as vinegar.

****

CHAPTER TEN

What started out as a good day jerked to a halt as soon as Charlie walked through the door. Excited and as happy as a kid first in line at the ice-cream van, the youth buzzing with enthusiasm after his very first trip underground at Easington mine, couldn't wait to share his joy with his parents, '*Ma, I'm back,*' he called out, '*what a day!*' words dried in his mouth as he surveyed the morose, miserable couple, shook his head despondently. *Here we go again,* he thought, the atmosphere in the house was as cold as ice, could have carved the word *frost* with a knife and the one holding the carving knife was his mother, the master-butcher. His father, looking so sour he could curdle, sat stiffly at the kitchen table waiting for his food, not a word of greeting for his son as he waited and watched the antics of his errant spouse busying herself preparing the meal.

Father and son in the same shift but Adam, with legs up to his neck, easily won the race home, maybe that was why he was agitated and angry. He'd followed his wife into his home, his wilful, rebelious and inebriated wife. Out all day, doing who knows what, with who knows who! His head hurt with a silent, contained rage, his chest thumped and churned with physical pain, Adam Hill down in the dumps of despair, all he wanted was a normal life; all he ever wanted was his family, all he got was mental torture and continuous grief from his wife. The fellow bit his lip, shook his tired head and forced his eyes towards his son, managed a glum nod, '*How do, son,*' he whispered, was looking forward to the banter, kid's first day in the mucky backwater of *Second-South*, his old work place years ago, so many tales to tell, waited all day for the chat and then to come home and find Rebecca tottering in the house, dressed to kill and reeking of booze! *Where to go,* he thought, *what to do?*

And with two sets of eyes focused on her, Rebecca struggled with the meal. *Damn Joan*, thought the woman. *Bloody Joan,* wanted to leave the pub in good time, knew what Adam would be like. *Damn and blast that woman!* Her head ached with the alcohol and all she wanted to do was sleep for a few hours, gritting her teeth, she persevered with the cooking, occasionally glancing in Adam's direction. Man was like a bear with a sore head, in an awful mood. Rebecca knew she'd have to be careful, play it by ear, as wily as a coyote because he wouldn't believe her story, wouldn't let her even finish. It was worse than walking on hot stones, having to act as if nothing was a problem, no big thing, after all, she'd only been to Joan Armstrong's house. '*You know what Joan is like, Adam. No! I haven't been out at all! Bugger you, Adam Hill! Believe what you want to believe!* Time and time again she bawled her response, no use back-tracking now. *I was in Joan's house, you stupid bugger! So what! You want me to refuse a drink from her? Trouble with you, Adam Hill,* she attacked, *you've got such a bloody wicked mind! You want me to cook or not? Last time I'll ask!*

The burnt offerings were place on the table. Two pots of scalding tea followed. Rebecca beat a hasty retreat into the living-room and waited for the fire-works to start, the battle to commence, stood anxiously with bated breath, mentally cursing her best friend for keeping her so long at the pub. *Bloody Joan Armstrong! Never again!* then she heard the chatter from the kitchen, strained at first, then gradually building as the two men discussed Charlie's day underground.

The woman breathed a sigh of relief, perhaps Adam half-believed her story after all.

****

At six-thirty youths entered the *Trust* in Horden. Word had spread that the pub was easy on under-aged boozers so it enjoyed brisk business and, so far, the local police hadn't cottoned-on as there had been little bother from the drinkers. The big and brassy juke-box stood waiting to be fed; two lads hovered with their coins, eyes scanning the long record list. Charlie stood with Abby Baxter. Abby, big and friendly; face full of freckles and spots, was a dead ringer for *Tony Curtis,* a tubby, teenage Tony Curtis. The two had met when they joined groups during basic training at Horden Colliery. Abby was a quiet, soft-spoken individual, happy with his life, full of fun and good to be around. The youth, easy-going and passive lived in *Grants Houses*, a hamlet of about one hundred plus homes, located between Easington Colliery and Horden, a stone's throw from Easington but classed according to the post-code, as part of Horden. Abby had attended the small primary school in Horden and then Dene House Comprehensive in Peterlee, never met one another until they found employment at their respective collieries. All the pit trainees in the area were temporarily drafted to Horden to learn the basics of mining. The two had ended up good friends.

"There'll be no trouble, then?" asked the rotund Abby Baxter.

"Not a chance," replied a confident Charlie Hill, knew everyone who was important in the colliery. "It's gonna be a good night, trust me!"

Charlie understood his concern, after all, Abby was venturing into foreign territory. He might be working at Easington pit, having transferred after training, but he was still classed as an outsider - a Horden lad - and therefore an intruder and with all the alcohol consumed and the youthful exuberance and immaturity of the participants, evenings tended to end with the usual fist-a-cuffs and squabbles. But Charlie had persisted, insisted, Abby had to come to the opening night of the Easington Colliery Welfare dance. It had never been held on a Monday night before. In the past, the place had opened Fridays, occasionally Saturdays, but never at the start of the week. *'Keep the kids off the streets,'* Jake Foster, Chairman of the Committee, argued at the welfare-meeting. *'Give it a bloody try, there's no harm done, might stop the vandalism and the graffiti artists. Open the place for a month, kids are okay, so long as they've got something to occupy themselves with. Come on, let's have a show of hands.'*

"If you're sure, Charlie," Abby succumbing at last, "and you'll stick with me?"

"Like glue!"

"No leaving me if you get fixed up?"

"We'll search for pairs, eh, hit the jackpot, we'll leave together!"

Coins were fed into the machine. Charlie's choice : *You win again*: *It's a sin*. Abby Baxter's choice: *Don't leave me this way: Relax*. What a selection! The atmosphere jumped into life. The beer started flowing. Charlie was going to enjoy himself, wanted to forget all the trouble from home. He started singing, *Relax, don't do it.......*

Abby blurted out valiantly, bravely, *When you wanna come .....*

****

"You out again tonight?" Terri Anders scowled, moved away from the window of the house in Basingstoke Road, plodded across the living-room and placed a laden tea-tray on the coffee-table.

Dulcie and Bethany sat either side of their father, eyes riveted to the television screen. Without looking at his wife, Arnold nodded impatiently, nod but did not speak.

Anna, the oldest and full of brass, barked, "Ma, can't see the television! Move!"

Terri persevered, sick and tired of struggling night after night on her own with the brood of kids, "How long this time, Arnie?" she asked grudgingly, thought she heard a grunt from her husband, prodded again, voice raised in anger, "well?"

"Elvis wants me to do some work for him, Terri," said Arny reluctantly, "maybe a bit of cash in hand, you know?" Arnold thinking glumly, *Breaking a few windows, that's all. Clearing a bad debt, kind of work that's advertised in the job-centre!*

"You spend more time with that man than me!"

"Just trying to earn an honest crust, love," said Arnold Anders.

"Then get a proper job instead of working for that man," she spat venomously, "Jesus, you're a qualified mechanic."

Terri hated Peterlee, hated Basingstoke Road. The woman was deeply unhappy with her lot, with her life. She comfort-ate to compensate. Terri had been a shapely seven-stone beauty when she met Arnold, fell in love with the man, believed his lies and his promises and married him, wouldn't listen to her parents' advice, head over heels then. Another lifetime then, she sylph-like and Arnold with a thick head of hair, another life, another planet! Her weight had blossomed annually and now she was the shape of a whale, didn't need reminding, mirrors couldn't hide the fact, past caring, Terri was in serious need of counselling, required help badly but she had few friends. Her parents lived five miles away in Haswell. Five miles without transport, could have been fifty, occasionally visited but was dependent on Arnold for a lift, everything depended on Arnold. Four children too and that was some chore, took up most of her days. Anna, Bethany, Camilla and Dulcie, four toddlers in five years and that was it, over. Didn't want the hockey-team to stop at Zelda so Terri had the cut and tuck.

Golden-haired Camilla bounced into sight, carried the comic-book tight to her chest, no one was reading it until she'd finished with the paperback, took one look at the offerings and guffawed with alarm and distaste, whined, "Ma, sandwiches," squatted on the carpet in front of Anna, "I'm not eating bread again!"

Anna shrieked, "Shift! Our Camilla! " Now she definitely couldn't see the little screen. "Shift!"

"Get lost, Anna," retorted an indignant Camilla, "it's not your television!"

The round puckered features of the mother winced with frustration, she turned and retreated to the kitchen. There were tears in her eyes.

"Ma," howled Anna Anders, "I want you now!"

Hate my life, Terri thought. *I really do hate my life.*

****

At nine the dance-floor was heaving with the gyrating bodies. Between the dancers, standing like two opposing factions, were the gaping males and the equally anxious, but not too obvious, females. Occasionally, a brave soul, sometimes accompanied with a rather nervous mate, ventured across *no-mans land,* through the bouncing, bopping melee, hoping to score, praying that they would not be rejected. Nothing hurt worse than the embarrassment of failure when making the return journey with all of your pals watching and gloating. Charlie stood with a large crew of youths. Standing next to him; over-shadowing him, was his old pal, Roy Bailey. Charlie was chuffed that his friend had ventured out; it was getting to be a rare sight seeing Roy other than near his home. Immaculately dressed; standing out like a tailor's dummy, next to the wild bunch. '*Take off the bloody tie, Roy,'* insisted Charlie. Roy Bailey naturally obeyed and then clung, literally, to Charlie's shirt-tails.

They had bumped into one another in the lavatories. Charlie, dazed with a skin-full of alcohol was stumbling away from the long line of fellow drunks: all with heads bowed as they relieved themselves and there was Roy Bailey, stepping out of the toilet cubicle. Good old Roy, never could pee if someone was next to him, too shy by half. They cuddled like they were Stanley and Livingstone ...it was a bit like a jungle in the Welfare Hall! Charlie, dazed and happy with the alcohol, Roy as sober as a judge, what a mix and match, didn't matter at all and felt like old times. Then, later that night, Charlie striding towards the line of beauties and shy Roy *tut-tutting* after him, following close behind was the nervous Abby Baxter. Charlie acting like he ruled the world: full of confidence; Abby living in high expectation of catching from the bevy of delightful females and Roy: ecstatic with joy to be with his old friend.

"Charlie Hill?" said the tall striking blonde, standing confidently between two pouting, diminutive and rather dowdy companions.

The female had a beautiful smile and showed a perfect set of sparkling teeth. Charlie grinned mischievously, greeted her warmly at the same time trying in vain to place a name to the beauty, shook his head as Roy Bailey nudged him. Heads almost touching as the tall companion told Charlie the news.

"Anne Marie Hickson!" laughed the youth, his fuddled brain trying to connect the name with someone from his distant past, "name rings a bell."

He remembered, not seen her in years, changed beyond all recognition, thirteen year old to seventeen was some time span. '*Anne Marie Hickson*,' he muttered, '*you've changed some!*' Charlie jumbled with drink, annoyed that he hadn't immediately recognised her. *Anne Marie*, he recalled clearly now, *the psycho with the skipping rope. Thrashed Roy and almost killed me*. The long day held like a criminal inside Peterlee Police Station because he *assaulted* her? *Assaulted* her? Anne Marie almost killed him. He carried scars weeks after the confrontation and poor Roy, he became a recluse for months because of the humiliation.

Charlie looked around the immediate vicinity, the girl could have a giant companion and still might hold a grudge, recalled the countless times after the conflict when Anne Marie chided and ridiculed him for hitting her and it didn't last weeks … months of abuse from her, so much hatred had been dredged up because of the melee, enough for both families to stop communicating and then suddenly it ceased. Anne Marie and her family left the village and moved half a mile away to the Waterworks, stayed only months before leaving Easington altogether.

"I'm sorry Charlie," she said loudly above the din of the records.

Charlie Hill said, "It's not a problem."

Roy Bailey, quaking in his shoes backed away slowly, tripped over an ever cautious Abby Baxter. Both youths watched and waited with bated breath.

Anne Marie stepped forward a pace, away from her friends and closed on the youth, Charlie glanced back at the nervous pair behind him, smiled genuinely, concentrated on Roy, 'It's okay, honest,' he mimed above the din of music.

"Can we talk?" asked Anne Marie.

"Not the place really?" replied Charlie Hill, shouting above the racket.

"I understand, Charlie," Anne Marie said, "you must hate me." Disappointment touched her features as she repeated, "I do understand."

A gaggle of noisy exuberant females suddenly shouldered their way past the small group. One of the girls stopped so suddenly that others around her stumbled and cursed. Charlie stared with disbelief. Jenny gasped as their eyes locked on one another. Almost a year since they'd seen one another, Charlie Hill and Jenny Bruce, suddenly reunited and the sparks of emotion and passion burst into a torrid flame.

"Jenny?" he spluttered and watched as she grinned joyfully at him.

"Hello Charlie," said Jenny Bruce, glanced at the tall companion standing close, recognized him immediately, "Roy Bailey!"

Roy nodded gleefully, it was like old times.

An inebriated Abby Baxter muttered despondently, "Someone introduce me!"

"Shh," chided Roy and nudged his new friend, "tell you later."

Charlie Hill remembered Anne Marie and turned to face her, saw the disappointment etched on her face, wanting to apologise, dazed and confused with alcohol as his head flustered and flapped. *Old friends! Girl-friends! Old enemies! What next tonight?* struggling from the swamp of intoxication he looked at his old adversary, trying to make allowances for the past and the present predicament, blurted out innocuously, *'Anne Marie, I'm out with friends Saturday night, probably around the Village. Could we talk then, it's awkward at the moment,"* glanced at Jenny Bruce and tried to introduce both females, *'Jenny, this is an old friend from my primary school,'* then to Anne Marie, *'Meet Jenny, we ... we were friends once,'* the embarrassment growing by the moment.

They left the place shortly afterwards. Charlie and Jenny, arm in arm as they stepped from the dance floor and not a word of protest from either Abby Baxter or Roy Bailey, both youths relaxed in one another's company. As the couple wandered aimlessly through the back streets of the colliery they talked about everything and anything, her family, his family, Jenny's work at the co-op, Charlie's new employment at the colliery, irrelevant yet delicious pieces of gossip; old news mixing and merging with the more recent succulent revelations, a beautiful mishmash of hearsay and rumour as the couple tried to complete the jigsaw of the missing months apart.

She asked about Linda MacDonald, without bitterness or malice, more curious than cutting and Charlie masked the truth as best he could, told mistruths and made light of the events, not wishing to hurt Jenny with his prolonged unfaithfulness. *'The night we bumped into you and your Ma? I was with Linda, remember? That was the very first time. Honest to God. Monty and Patton had a date with Lynne James and Linda Mac. Patton backed off, so Monty asked me as a favour, you understand? Monty and Lynne. Linda and me.'* Jenny understood, told him so. '*Charlie, we were no longer an item. I knew and I told you, that the tussle you had with dad and the way Ma disliked you, I knew it was all over. I still wanted to see you, but I wasn't allowed out of the house. It's just.... when I saw you* with *Linda MacDonald, laughing and enjoying her company, well I was hurt. Shocked.*' Then she added poignantly. '*It gave Ma a field day! Your ears must have been burning!*'

Jenny said she had been seeing someone for months. Wayne Tully was his name, worked at the newsprint factory *Metro Mail,* he was nice, she confided, fussed over her a lot. Nancy, Jenny's mother liked him. '*Do I love him, Charlie*? *Not like I loved you*.' She was so honest. '*Nobody in the whole world like you, Charlie*. *You still take my breath away*.' Then she mentioned her parents again. '*They're not keen on you, Charlie, Ma won't even mention your name. It's taboo.*' She added poignantly, '*Charlie*, *I was grounded for two months. I was only allowed out if I promised not to see you again. You do understand, Charlie*?' The youth tried to smile and hide his obvious disappointment, he'd foolishly imagined that the evening would have cumulated with their reunion. He still missed her, she was the only one he'd ever loved, but when Jenny started talking about Wayne Tully, he immediately clamped up his true feelings. '*Nobody quite like you, Charlie.*' she'd insisted, as if she had waited forever for his return. *True love,* thought a confused Charlie Hill and *it only lasts months?*

Charlie was utterly bewildered, suddenly he started talking, confessing his inner feelings, couldn't stop himself. '*Don't you know how I feel, Jenny*? *Don't you know I'm still waiting for you*? *I love you Jenny. I really do*.' And she looked at him for an age, caressed and held him like he was something precious. *'Would have been nice, Charlie. You and me. It's was too much for me. Ma was so determined there'd be no contact between us that she was always waiting outside the Co-op when I'd finished work. Mother walked me home!'* Jenny stared through moist, sad eyes. *'Walked me home every night! You ever been chaperoned, Charlie and threatened with eviction from my own home if I saw you again? I was out of my head, Charlie. Especially when I knew you were seeing someone else.'*

Like an emotional tennis match. Charlie would talk and give his views and opinions then Jenny would retort with her feelings and frustrations, this way and that until they exhausted themselves. Charlie bemused, asked, *'At the dance, Jenny, why did you stop and talk to me? Couldn't you have walked away and pretended not to see me?'* She replied candidly, *'Can't explain, saw you again and my heart skipped a beat. Honestly, Charlie. Saw you and I lost my breath. I had to speak to you again. Charlie. I'll never meet anyone like you again. You were my first love.'*

They made love for the first time that night. *'I really want to, Charlie,* she'd whispered. *'I've always wanted to make love to you.'*

He was helpless, hopeless and weak, "Let me see you again, Jenny. Now and again, let's keep in touch?"

Jenny was adamant, wouldn't change her mind. The young couple shared paradise for a brief moment then parted, both hurt, guilty and confused. The bond between them finally over.

****

It was midnight when Arnold Anders parked his motor near the *Diamond* pub, set off walking at a brisk pace, full of confidence and self-assurance, wasn't so stupid as not to have a contingency plan. If there was bother, if he was discovered, rumbled, whatever, he knew where to bolt for safety. Across the road from the pub was the Welfare Hall and beyond the Hall was the safety of the recreation grounds with its acres of fields, walkways and bowling-greens, a perfect hidey-hole. The sky was brightly lit with a full and sparkling moon that dominated the heavens, a star-spangled sky which made the inept criminal somewhat anxious but Arnold had thought of everything, his shining dome hidden with the black woolen balaclava, a perfect disguise for the hoodlum. Only one problem with the hat, it was hot and uncomfortable and made him sweat buckets.

By the time he'd reached the Waterworks, he was drenched, had to remove the damp helmet to wipe away the wetness, even his spectacles were fogged. He slowed his pace and started searching for anything that could be used as a weapon. The closer he got to the street, the more he panicked, his head in overdrive, *Must have been a 'Keep Britain Tidy' campaign going on with the Council,* he imagined. Arnold had an idea, hurried to the nearby back-yard of the grocery shop owned by Priestley, always open, because everyone was scared of Elvis. Plenty of missiles about and Arnie pulled two empty milk-bottles out of the nearest crate, *'Cool under crisis',* he whispered, *'that's the name of the game!'* His journey continued.

The entire street was deserted, not one light could be seen. Arnie took a deep breath and proceeded along the garden-path. The moon was like a beacon guiding him, crept gingerly past the darkened home and into the rear garden, the wire fence was for midgets and the tall man eased his frame over and heard the agonizing sound of his trousers tearing, *Rip!* his best pants were caught on something. Swearing silently, Arnold manoeuvered his frame into the neighbouring garden, *Rip!* his trousers shredded for the second time, couldn't stop himself from cursing out loud, *'Bastard! Bastard!'*

A few doors away a hound started to bark. Too late to retreat, the bespectacled phantom hurried across the lawns, unaware of the childs' bicycle abandoned many hours earlier, walked headlong into the steel frame and was immediately propelled airborne, instantly transformed into a human cannonball. With a stifled shriek and the faintest of cries, the fellow catapulted into a large bed of roses. A myriad cuts and scratches blossomed across his face and chest as he staggered to his feet determined to finish the task, only his pride forced him onwards.

Johnny Ridley, working the late shift at *Walker's Crisps*, had been dropped off at the Village by the works-bus. Johnny was always the first home from that particular shift, the other passengers would be dropped off in a long circular route that took the bus to Hawthorn, South Hetton, Haswell, then finally to Shotton Colliery, one of the perks of night-shift was the free ride home. The man hurried into his back-yard, looked up at the bedroom-window, the home in darkness, his wife and kids asleep, smiled at the thought of the dinner waiting for him, piping-hot in the oven, a relaxing hour eating and watching the television with no distractions. Then he saw the shadow close to his door. With a shout, the man charged up the yard.

Arnold was transformed into a human greyhound as he bolted blindly across the rear garden, jumped free of the bike; threw himself over the fence and away. Almost made it. Sheer vexation made Johnny Ridley hurl his empty vacuum-flask after the burglar, didn't have time to aim the missile, instinct was the guiding force and it caught Arnold square on his bald head, opened it like a can-opener and down he stumbled: headlong into the garden, spread-eagled like a corpse, dazed and hurt.

Lady-luck was on Arnie's side because Johnny Ridley was no hero. He'd done enough, imagined the would-be burglar carrying some weapon … knife, hammer, maybe a gun, heard enough news stories to make turn tail and run back towards his house, almost destroyed the door-lock as he tried to gain access. Dithering wildly he took many seconds to find the right key, wailing softly with a growing panic before he stumbled headlong into his home. *'He's got a gun! A bloody knife!'* he screamed, howled for his wife, then calmed enough to reach for the phone and dial for *Emergency Services*. He would let them deal with the maniac.

With a long, low moan Arnie struggled to his feet and half-ran, half-stumbled up the long street, reached *Paradise Crescent* and turned into the dirt-track that led to the recreation grounds. Safe now, he took deep agonizing breaths and walked into the darkness of the park. He cursed long and loud, knowing the jibes that would surely come from Elvis. Bad enough. But the thought of his wife, his beloved Terri, especially when she saw the state of his clothes and the bruising and damage to his head! Jesus Christ, being out after midnight was one thing, but dishevelled and torn clothes! What on earth would Terri think. She'd have his life!

"This is the bloody end!" he grunted as he limped through the deserted grounds. "This is definitely the finish!"

****

CHAPTER ELEVEN

Theo Williams gave out the simple instructions, like he was a proper boss. "Come on, Monty," pleaded the overseer, "we've got to do something or I'll be in bother," his voice unusually loud due to the proximity of the noisy transfer-point.

That'll be the day, Theo, thought Montgomery Jepson unkindly, lowered his head so that the torch attached to his helmet scanned the newspaper's sports section, fidgeted as he tried to find level ground and ease the discomfort to his rump from the undulating, gravelled floor. *It's only dinner-time, gimme a break!*

Charlie Hill wandered slowly into view, been missing a while, told Theo he was desperate for the lavatory which had some truth to it, peeing however, took seconds and sometimes the youth seemed to disappear from the district for an age as he wandered along old abandoned roadways, fascinated at the character and the atmosphere of the mine, discovered ancient corridors, long since discarded, the black bounty long gone; old, ruined driveways with buckled girders twisted into grotesque mosaics as pressure from above pushed and forced the rusted steel down towards the floor. Some days Charlie would be halted on his travels as the aged roadway before him slipped gently and turned into a flooded, eerie river of smudge, an underground lake, silent, muck encrusted water that appeared to stretch forever before him.

"How's tricks, Charlie?" asked a desperate Theo, increasingly concerned in case a Deputy wandered into the area. Some of the officials could be right buggers and cause no end of bother.

"Better thanks, Theo," replied the youth.

"Then you'll not mind doin' a spot of graft?" said Theo Williams, looking more and more harassed, his tone unusually high-pitched and scolding.

The boys relented, accepted the haranguing, understood the limits, didn't want to push their luck too far, the look on the overseer's trouble features enough to cause their consciences to prick and scratch. They started to feel sorry for old Theo, the shift half-over and they'd done very little work, picking up their shovels they walked towards the rumbling conveyor-belt, Theo directing and explaining exactly what was expected of them.

"Back in an hour," said Theo, grabbed his jacket and plodded out of sight.

The old man decided to take a slow wander to the neighbouring district, *Second-North,* knew Timmy Coxon would be there, spend a bit of time with his old mate, pass an hour before returning and checking on the lads, let his temper cool, last thing he wanted was a heart attack. He had made his mark and felt better, knew the two lads would spend an hour cleaning the spillages from the conveyor-belt.

Charlie followed the motion of the conveyor, decided to clean the opposite side, threw his shovel over the moving stretch of rubber, placed both hands firmly on the coal and dust of the slow-moving belt and with an expert forward movement he bounced on then off the device, landing flat-footed on the other side. He immediately retrieved his shovel and attacked the debris and dust that grew in buckets from the floor with gusto, kept his back bent all the time, only his arms moving in a steady motion. '*Better that way,*' instructed Theo, ages ago. '*Shovel and throw on to the belt, shovel and throw! Keep your back bent for as long as you can!* Within minutes he was drenched with running perspiration.

As Charlie toiled, a lethargic Montgomery watched for some time before finally moving further into the belt-line, slowly and methodically scraping the shovel under the conveyor-belt and across the surface of the steel supporting table on which it was positioned. Easy work, no hurry, in and out as his shovel collected the dust and the coal spillages and threw it on to the moving belt. Minutes later and his shovel retrieved an ancient newspaper, probably someone's ancient lunch-wrapping, disposed of years ago. Montgomery immediately forgot about work, threw down his shovel and re-positioned his helmet allowing the bright beam to highlight the yellowed pages.

The youth moved along the highway and close to his companion, stopping when he was on the opposite side of the conveyor-belt, shouted over the racket, "*New Musical Express*, Charlie!" He scanned the filthy pages and a puzzled look touched his features as he found the front cover of the newspaper. "Bloody hell, Charlie, it's really old.....1955!"

Charlie lifted his body and gasped for breath, his face lined with sweat, called out, "Any of the old ones in there," he quizzed, "Elvis, Little Richard, Jerry Lee?"

Monty flipped page after page. "Weird, it's all bloody foreign stuff!" started shouting out names he'd never heard of before. "*David Whitfield, Jimmy Young, Alma Cogan, Chris Barber*. The youth suddenly recalled the familiar name, "He's on Radio Two ... *Jimmy Young,* didn't know he used to be a singer?" He scanned the lists of records, said bemused, "Jimmy Young, number one in the charts! *The Man from Laramie* ... thought that was a cowboy film?"

Charlie shouted, "Pass it over!"

"Look here", Montgomery fascinated, calling out as he flipped the page, "Here's another cowboy! *Tennessee Ernie Ford!"*

"Pass it then!"

Montgomery on a roll, chuckled, "*Winifred Atwell,* who the hell was she?"

A miner hurried towards them, black as the night, wearing only shorts, boots and hard-hat, covered in coal-dust, zebra-striped with heavy sweat-lines running down his grimy torso. The collier was short in stature but muscular and tight without an ounce of body fat.

"Played the Honky-tonk," shouted the stranger. "Brilliant she is, black as me but she could never wash it off!"

"How do?" said Montgomery Jepson.

The man stopped and smiled a greeting, "Busy?"

"Naw," said Charlie, "belt-cleanin' for Theo Williams. He's our boss."

"Theo, eh," uttered the diminutive miner, "where's he at then?"

"Sleeping somewhere," said a bemused Charlie.

"Listen", said the man, "you two fancy helpin' us out?"

The youths nodded eagerly, anything was better than belt-cleaning. The man explained that the two men whose job it was to load and haul girders and timber up the coal-face were absent and the gear was badly needed. He clomped back into the darkness of the passageway and grasped at the suspended mono-rail table, pulled it slowly into view.

"Know what this is?" didn't wait for an answer but grasped a long, heavy piece of timber and eased it on to the swaying steel-frame. "Has to be filled! Load the timber first, okay? I'll go out-bye and get us a pony to help you haul it to the coal-face." He pointed at the huge mound of materials,

“Okay, can you do that, boys?” He didn’t wait for an answer but hurried away along the roadway.

Charlie finished his work and was over the man-riding belt in seconds. The pair walked to the stacks of timber, each grabbing one end of a heavy chock of timber and started to hoist it on to the swaying steel contraption. It was like lifting lead, the long batons were so heavy they soon paused for breath.

“That little fella lifted one on his own!”

“Mighty Atom!”

Half an hour later and the task was completed. They squatted amongst the rubble and dust, exhausted and drained of energy.

The clip-clip noise of the approaching pit-pony pushed them to their feet, a brief greeting and the collier guided the animal to the front of the laden mono-rail table, the harness adjusted; steel chains clamped to the front bar. He told them what to do, slowly and methodically, Charlie with the pony by his side, guiding and goading the animal; Montgomery behind the contraption, pushing when the inclines proved too stressful for the animal.

“Easy as fuck!” he concluded, was about to take his leave when, as an afterthought, he asked, “what’s your name, kid?”

“Charlie Hill”

“Know your father,” he chuckled, “he’s a big bugger!” neared Charlie, clouted him playfully, “know you, got a temper like your Dad!”

“Who are you, then?”

“Mojo Hogg,” said the collier, “Alfie’s Dad. He’s told me all about you.”

“Alfie Hogg but he’s ….” couldn’t find the courage to finish the sentence, didn’t want to upset the stranger. Alfie was so big, nothing like the under-sized collier next to him.

“Bloody giant and he’s got brothers bigger!” proud as punch he was. “Dynamite for spunk,” he chortled.

“Opposite’s happened to me,” groaned Charlie, “bloody runt compared to my dad!”

“Good stuff in little bundles,” said the man, aimed a huge wad of phlegm at the floor-bottom, a cheeky grin over his blackened face, “look at me! I’ve never lost a fight in my life! It’s not the size of the man that matters, it’s the size of the heart in the man!”

Montgomery, feeling like a leper the way he’d been ignored, joined in the banter, “Monty Jepson is my name. Patton is my brother, my dad is….”

“A bloody drunk,” the little man interrupted, laughed out loud, “and tell him Mojo said!” turned away from the boys and started striding away into the dim passageway, returning to the coal-face. “Can’t get lost,” he called out, “follow me,” then he stopped suddenly, turned and shouted at Charlie, “tell Elvis he’s an ugly bugger!” He disappeared from view.

“Right,” shouted Charlie and nodded at Montgomery standing at the rear, “you ready?”

“Been ready ten minutes,” answered the agitated youth, “just kick the horse, Charlie, that’ll make it move!”

“You can’t mistreat the pony!” said an adamant Charlie Hill. “Gee-up!” he yelled frantically. “Git-up!” and he tugged again at the reins. The animal refused to budge, was as stubborn as a mule

“Kick the bloody horse, Charlie,” cried Monty, “or we’ll be here ‘till Friday!”

“Gee-up!” yelled the youth and got the same result. Ziltch, not a hint of movement, his temper broke and he aimed a kick at the animal’s stomach. “Gee-up!” Another boot and the startled pony suddenly came to life, jerked forward, straining with all its might and the slow journey commenced.

Montgomery was ecstatic, yelled out, “Remember that song, Charlie!”

“Which one?”

“About workin’ down the pit?”

They both started singing in unison, ‘*Working in the coal-mine, going down down……*’ laughing and singing as they struggled towards the coal-face.

Lee Dorsey would have been proud.

****

At eleven twenty Charlie Hill slipped noiselessly out of the house. It was too easy; his father was working night shift and had left a few hours earlier, his mother, intoxicated and fast asleep on the settee. Charlie had sat alone in his bedroom most of the evening as the battle raged between his parents, his mother deserving all the barracking from his incensed father as Rebecca sat mute, without a trace of shame or sorrow as the man tore strips off her, immune to it all, long past caring. She’d re-surfaced early that evening sullen and sour, having been gone two long days and nights and without a word of apology or explanation.

Frustrated and boiling with a jealous fury, Adam Hill had finally exhausted himself and grudgingly left for work at 9.30. Almost immediately the woman had continued her binge, Charlie, upstairs and alert, listened at the clink of the bottles: the *glug, glug* as the liquid was transferred to the tumbler. He was all mixed up inside: pleased she had returned because deep inside he always held on to the memory of the person he loved, still naively believed his mother would somehow, miraculously, change back to that person. He hated the creature that she had spent years perfecting. She was a drunk, a whore, knew it in his heart. When his mother was desperate enough, she would do anything, loved alcohol more than him, more than his dad, more than life and Charlie believed she would do anything to satisfy the craving.

He stepped out of the bedroom and walked slowly down the stairs, detesting his mother more than he loved her, into the living-room, past the snorting corpse that held the empty bottle close to her chest and in to the kitchen, the stinking, filthy kitchen that hadn't been cleaned in years, found the knife and retraced his steps until he stood over her, touched her with the blade: played the weapon across her wheezing throat, listened and wondered about her dreams and tried to understand, always tried to understand, knew he could not take her life. The knife was flung across the room and he stormed from the house.

He took the long route, walked to the neck of the cul-de-sac, jumped the fence and turned left and marched along the fringe of the field towards the Waterworks, didn't want anyone seeing him wandering the streets so late. He had memorized the address: 20 *Hazel Terrace,* Elvis wanted someone taught a lesson: wanted the property of a bad debtor damaged. '*A window will do, Charlie. There's twenty quid for you, take you five minutes.*' Elvis in a stinking mood, had a major fall-out with Arnie Anders. '*Doesn't concern you, Charlie. Now, will you do the job*?' Charlie had agreed, better to break a window or two, easier than an arson job, never again would he be tempted to undertake such dreadful jobs. Elvis or no Elvis, no matter the size of the bounty.

At the eastern boundary of the field, the youth jumped the barbed wire and started walking up the incline that led to the bulge of council houses, kept repeating the address, took the two missiles out of his pocket, made him smile, grin like a Cheshire cat. '*I knew they'd come in handy,*' he said. They'd been stolen from his old school years earlier, two cork tennis balls, rock-hard, perfect for the job in hand. He was close now and he started to run.

Elvis had hinted as to how he should fulfil the task. Too complicated for the boy: '*Next street, Charlie, through the back-garden, over a fence: another garden, down a path and throw.*' Charlie thinking, *From about twenty yards, pull the other one, Elvis, this is not American Football and my aim is far from perfect.* The gangster adamant and pushy, Mr. Know-It-All himself, '*Pretend you're Ian Botham, Charlie.*' The reference to the cricketer had jolted Charlie's memory, recalled his school days and the P.E. lessons, school cricket and the stolen balls. '*Thanks, Elvis. I'll pretend I'm throwing petrol-bombs again.*'

He saw the house and without a second thought the youth flung the first missile at the big window, the sound as the ball whacked at the frame was alarming. Cursing his ill-fortune, Charlie released the final ball. *Bang! Crash!* like a grenade exploding as the whole window shattered, adrenalin smacked at him and he bolted along the quiet street, laughing hysterically, on a high at the apparent ease of the task.

The small police-car turned down routinely into *Hazel Terrace* as fate lent a hand. Pure instinct made Charlie jump the garden fence and run between the houses. Seconds later and the vehicle squealed to a halt, one of the officers clambered out and gave chase, the patrol-car then shot away along the road, hoping to catch the criminal as he made his way towards the rear street.

The lad was thinking and running, cold and calculating as he burned through the darkened gardens, knew instinctively that the police would try and block his escape with a pincer movement. Out for a moment on the opposite side, Charlie ran across the lawns, down a path and doubled-back on himself then slowed and listened. He could hear the stamping labouring noises from the chasing officer in the next yard. Like a cat, the boy hurried back to Hazel Terrace, crossed the road and ran through the terraced properties. A man was standing by the street-light, dressed in pyjamas and barefoot, it was Charlie's victim and he howled like a demented soul as he tried to give chase, lasted seconds before his exposed feet caught some sharp object and he pulled up sharp, squealing in pain.

The youth bolted down the street, across the main road, didn't stop until he was safely in the farmer's fields and only then did he began to walk, his pace slow and cumbersome as he struggled with the lack of vision in the pitch-black fields. Charlie decided to loiter about the nearby quarry in case the police-vehicle was already patrolling the streets near his home, didn't wish to be seen or recognized and decided to wait a while until the danger had passed. Minutes later and he was gazing into the inky quarry, sat on the moist earth and tried to gather his thoughts. He decided that this would be the last time he would work for Elvis Priestley. It was too dangerous and his conscience was bothering him. He was hurting people that had done him no wrong.

Charlie Hill did not see the lone figure that stood statuesque next to the clump of gnarled bushes, so close to the seated figure he could hear his heavy breathing, not making the slightest sound, he watched intently as the stranger finally rose to his feet and made the short journey towards the distant houses. Harry Shannon was watching the fellow with mixed emotions, knowing him from a lifetime ago, still frightened of the man who used to ridicule and chase him, who shouted abuse and who stole from him. '*Took my hat! Stole my hat!*' he would cry to his anxious mother. Soon the intruder was gone but Harry still gazed into the blackness. Harry Shannon remembered well, forgot nothing, pictured his mother sympathizing as he wept miserable tears, fearful to walk alone lest the boy taunted him again, his beautiful mother comforting, crying with him, telling Harry not to worry and that his father was watching over him, his father, a distant memory, would, nevertheless, always protect and care for him. '*Because your daddy has changed into an Angel, Harry. He lives in Heaven and he's always watching over you.*' Harry's dad: Jimmy Shannon, his very own Guardian Angel. His mother even showed him how to pray, how to talk to him and to this day the boy talked to his father.

Harry Shannon had stood in the heart of the quarry for hours. It had been worth it. Minutes earlier, Harry had witnessed an extraordinary sight. He had observed the fox, his first real encounter with such a creature, smaller than he had imagined: more delicate than in the picture-books, a wild little terrier but with a glorious bushy tail, hurrying back to its lair; carrying the struggling prey in its clamped jaws, oblivious to the figure that silently observed then, suddenly recognizing danger, the fox dropped the injured weasel and scurried away into the night, pausing momentarily, unsure, with beady eyes locked on the nearby shape. Hesitation as the fox wavered and dithered then the creature turned away and bolted into the night, its prize lost way, scampering across the quarry leaving Harry alone with his thoughts, smiling broadly. Better than television, better than his tapes or his picture books, real life happening before his very eyes! A magical musical from Mother Nature.

He gazed up to the heavens and pictured his father. *'I've seen a fox, dad, with something in its mouth. I think it was its dinner,'* he paused and pondered before adding softly, *'seen Charlie Hill too. He was the one who always stole my hat. Ma says he was a naughty boy, daddy, for pinching my hat. He's still a bad boy, daddy. I've been watching him. He's been hiding from someone. I think he's stolen someone's hat!'*

Harry Shannon slowly eased his way towards the discarded prey, inches away from the small animal he stopped and gingerly lowered his enormous bulk to the ground, nervous and a little frightened because the weasel was definitely alive and extremely agitated. In the past, the youth had found many a dead creature in the quarry and he had always taken them home to show his mother. Hedgehogs, birds, rabbits, rats, all manner of creature were proudly exhibited and Ruby, his mother, would wrap them in beautiful material and leave them close to their home while she escorted her son inside and explain all about the creatures. They were always gone the next day. His mother explained that they had gone to heaven to join his daddy.

He'd never found a live animal before and he was unsure about handling it. He prodded the furry creature to check on its progress. It was alive still because it squirmed. He decided to take it home, thinking optimistically that his mother would be able to make it better, wrap it in bandages, give it some medicine and then he'd have his very own pet. Harry smiled. He would be able to play with the animal. He reached out and grasped the weasel only to have his fingers bitten by the demented creature. With a startled wail, Harry whacked at the writhing animal and it immediately became docile and limp. He placed it carefully in his pocket, struggled to his feet and left the quarry, climbed the rickety fence and hurried along Thorpe Road. It started to rain but Harry Shannon wasn't bothered, in fact he was ecstatic with his find.

Almost at the house and the creature, badly crippled and in pain tried to escape from the coat and Harry had to slap at his pocket to silence the mutt. Not knowing his own strength he knocked it unconscious. *'Shh!'* he whispered, didn't want his mother to know about his little friend until the morning, didn't want it departing to heaven overnight. He sneaked into the house and hurried up the stairs away from his mother's watchful eyes.

"Harry?" shouted Ruby Shannon, placed her drink out of sight and heaved her enormous bulk off the sofa and waddled towards the door.

Harry was already upstairs in his very own sanctuary. Stripping off his overcoat and his beloved hat, the imbecile glanced about his cluttered room. Satisfied that his mother had not disturbed anything, he bounced down the protesting staircase and squatted next to the large television, ravenous with hunger he asked for something to eat.

An hour later and Ruby Shannon was asleep on the sofa, drunk. Harry climbed the staircase and entered his bedroom, cleared the bed of all the assorted paraphernalia, straightened the bedspread and propped up the large garish pillowcase. From the cupboard, Harry pulled out the beautiful doll. Carefully he arranged it on the bedspread so that it appeared to be sitting, lounging against the pillow and facing him, next, he fished out the dazed creature and placed it on the bed. He started a conversation with the doll. *She must still be fast asleep*, thought Harry. Locked tightly in his own world of fun and fantasy, he leaned across and stroked at the doll's golden locks, gently manipulating the tiny head in an upward motion. The puppet opened her eyes. *'Hello, Norah Jane,'* he whispered, *'I've brought you a friend,'* and lifted the creature, placing it on the doll's lap. The weasel awoke, its small damp body was screaming with pain and in a last desperate effort lunged forward and sunk its fangs into the body of the doll and started savaging the puppet.

"No! No!" Harry screamed.

He grasped hold of the animal and when the beast refused to release its grip on the beautiful mannequin, the man attacked with a terrible force. Yelping and squealing in agony the weasel was dragged away from his favourite doll and ripped apart like a Christmas-cracker, the two bloodied halves of the corpse were flung across the bedroom. Both sections of the animal landed either side of the door.

"Ma!" he wailed. Harry wanted his mother to take away the horrible creature and wrap it in cloth and send it immediately to heaven. God could glue it together again and give it to his daddy. He definitely didn't want it.

****

CHAPTER TWELVE

It had been a quiet day at the shop, old Jack Greaney had got through the *Northern Echo* before ten-o-clock, even read every memorial, death notice and advertisement in the damn paper, never been as quiet, could have been Cup-Final Day. He'd brushed out the shop, which was a stupid thing to do because no-one had been inside the bloody place; dusted all the shelves, polished the counters, knew there were people about because he watched them walk past the shop-window, thought about putting a notice on the door. *All stock, free!*

He walked to *Brison's* Newspaper Shop, took all of five minutes, purchased the Hartlepool Mail and the Sunderland Echo, still had hours to go before closing and needed the reading material. Back safely at his store, started flicking through the paper, reached page three and saw the first piece of local gossip ... house in Hazel Terrace, Easington Colliery, subjected to damage; living-room window broken by several missiles and police still investigating: '*Have you seen this man?*' said the headlines, the police had compiled an identikit picture of the culprit, even gave his possible height and weight - wrong on both accounts - and Charlie Hill was not a suspect, thanks to Ernie Beint's poor vision, the victim adamant about the culprit: *Average height: average size; black hair!*

Gladys Harriman struggled into the shop. Big spender Gladys. Jack Greaney pushed the newspapers to one side, forced a smile and waited. Minutes later and Jack was again on his own. Now he could retire on his takings: dependable Gladys Harriman, last of the big spenders, '*Two rashers of side-bacon, Jack, one egg and one small loaf of bread,*' Jack now serious about giving up work, retiring to Barbados or the

Canary Islands. '*Thank Christ for Gladys,*' he groused, '*she's made my day!*'

There was worse to come. Tea-time and his wife Alice would give him a few hours break which he normally enjoyed. Not today, the couple had spent the previous evening discussing Rebecca Hill and her outstanding bill and Alice had decided that the problem had to be resolved. It was agreed that the husband would be approached. Jack would call that evening and have a talk with Adam Hill. '*It's not a problem, pet,*' he said to his wife, '*nothing to worry about!*' Truth be told, he'd rather face a firing-squad than call at the madhouse.

It was five-o-clock and Jack Greaney approached the cul-de-sac with a terrible dread, his stomach churned and his heart pounded as he neared the house, called weeks earlier and had talked to the woman, the aggressive, inebriated witch of a woman. It had been a complete waste of time trying to reason with Rebecca and he had left with his tail between his legs, embarrassed, humiliated and hurt because of her stinging rebuke, transpired that it was all Jack's fault for allowing the debt to mount so high! '*You're an old fool, Jack,*' she'd scolded, '*shouldn't even be in business!*'

The aged proprietor stepped into back-yard shaking with trepidation, notice something different about the place, glanced upwards, saw the improvement, the broken window had been repaired after years of damage and it looked as if the room now possessed curtains. Jack wondered if his luck was about to change,

'*Deep breath, Jack,*' he whispered bravely and he knocked quietly at the door, didn't want to upset anyone, didn't want to see the woman, especially the woman. The door squeaked ajar.

"It's you again!" barked Rebecca Hill.

Jack was resigned to defeat, thinking, *Not a chance in hell!*

"Hello, Becky, love," giving it his best shot, there was a lot of money at stake, "it's about the unpaid bill."

Sober for once, Rebecca stood her ground, adamant that the bill was not of immediate concern, it would be paid eventually.

There was movement behind the woman and old Jack prayed for an appearance from Adam Hill. It was the wayward son, Charlie. *Bugger and blast*, mused the old man but managed to smile at the youngster.

"Jack!" said Charlie and he flicked the remains of a cigarette on to the garden.

The lad looked good, still needing a bit of horse-muck in his shoes; he was turning into a handsome lad, looked clean and tidy too. Work and the touch of maturity had worked wonders on the youth; he had a twinkle in his eyes, something nice about him, nothing like his obnoxious mother. Surprisingly, Charlie took control of the situation, talking to his mother like an equal, smiling and calming her, said he would sort out the problem. With a stubborn pout blossoming across Rebecca's features and muttering obscenities under her breath, she turned and disappeared into the house.

Jack Greaney turned as if to leave. *At least he had tried*, he thought and then the strangest thing, he was told to wait. *'Hang on, Jack!'* said the youth and the door closed for a short time, perhaps minutes, then a smiling Charlie reappeared, stepped outside, closed the door behind him and pulled out a wad of money, could have knocked Jack down with a feather. The youth counted out the money, big silly grin etched across his face as if he was enjoying the exercise. Debt settled. No big deal.

"I'm working now, Jack," said the lad, cock-sure and brimming with confidence.

Minutes earlier the lad had read avidly the account of the vandalism and breakage at the nearby Waterworks and had seen the identikit picture of the wanted felon. He was home and dry and in excellent spirits.

The man was dumbfounded, couldn't believe his good fortune, said weakly, 'Charlie, I don't know what to say," he had tears in his eyes.

Charlie, suddenly stung with conscience at the stock he'd pinched from the shop said, "Sorry about Ma, she doesn't mean it, Jack."

The proprietor, still numb with the gentle shock of kindness, grasped hold of Charlie's hand, shook it limply, turned and started to walk away, dumbfounded with delight. Then he stopped, faced the youth, managed a smile and a nod of gratitude and, without a word, walked quickly away.

"Ma!" shouted a beaming Charlie as he closed the door on Jack Greaney, "guess what I've done?"

The lavatory flushed noisily. Rebecca appeared, her features showing her mood, glowered at her naïve son. "I don't believe it, Charlie!"

The youth was crestfallen. "Paid Greaney's bill Ma, thought you'd be pleased?"

"The old bugger could have waited for his money," whined Rebecca, thinking about all the potential beer-money gone to waste. "He's loaded, Charlie, there was no need to settle it all, could have slipped him a few quid to keep his face straight."

"Thanks, Ma," muttered Charlie, disgusted at her attitude.

****

Low Main: Second South and the pair had finished their break and were preparing to begin the last half of their shift. Montgomery had the usual stomach-ache; not surprising really, like a pig in a trough when it came to his food, not only the volume but the speed at which it was consumed. *Stomach-ache,* thought Charlie Hill, *a bloody glutton!* His mate devoured grub like every meal was his last.

"Hurry up, then!" said an impatient Charlie.

"Stomach cramps!" moaned Montgomery.

"Just say you want a good shite," said Charlie, "for Christ's sake!" couldn't walk ten yards in any direction without passing Monty's droppings and the lingering smell was obnoxious!

The youth hurried away into the sanctuary of the darkness carrying a magazine. Theo Williams was squatting nearby on a seat made from timber struts, he'd completed an hours belt-cleaning already and was well and truly exhausted. The whole place was warm, oppressive even and there was little ventilation, didn't take long before Theo's strength was sapped. Charlie approached and smiled when he heard the rhythmatic wheezing lifting from the old man. He was sound asleep again.

Charlie eased past the still figure and made his way into the heading. The mono-rail table had already been filled to capacity with arch-girders, the pony was strapped and ready for the off. The youth began stroking the animal, it was a little work-horse and so strong. It was called *Midnight* and it was white! *Bloody daft miners*, thought Charlie, fed the remains of his lunch to the animal, jam and bread and best butter, lovely grub for the animal. *Midnight* almost took off his fingers. "Steady on, boy!" It was female but no one gave a damn.

Montgomery, now relieved of his stomach-ache, joined him and with Charlie guiding the still-chomping beast and Monty at the rear holding on to the swaying portable table, the intrepid pair moved forward towards the distant coal-face leaving Theo Williams still fast asleep, snorting like an infant.

Thirty minutes later and the boys paused for breath, covered in heavy running perspiration, all exhausted, including the wheezing pony. They gulped greedily from their water-bottles then Charlie poured water across the open mouth of the animal. The youths eased onto the ground, too tired to make conversation, they sat in silence and relaxed.

Boom! The whole place seemed to shake. *Boom! Boom!* A distant muffled echo touched them, louder and longer than normal, gave them opportunity to speak.

"Shot-firing," grunted Montgomery, "seemed a bit loud?"

Charlie stood and gazed into the passageway. "Never known the bloody place to shake before" started to chuckle, *Not unless I'm too close to Monty when he's having a crap!*

A dust cloud came at them like a thick blanket of soot which totally covered them for some minutes; a continuous veil of dancing particles sparkled through their torch-beams and enveloped the trainees. Overwhelmed by the debris and muck the pair covered their mouths but so thick and continuous was the smog that they both started coughing and retching. It seemed never-ending, unsettling and a little scary.

"Hell's teeth!" gasped a frightened Charlie as he struggled for breath.

Then, as suddenly as it came, the muck and dust lifted then cleared, it was normal again. Both boys looked at one another, unsure as to what to do.

Monty asked, "What now?"

"Seems okay," answered Charlie Hill, "probably the shot-firer having a bad day."

"Too much bloody dynamite!"

Their journey was about to continue when they noticed approaching lights, dozens of dancing flashing beams. Men were approaching. Running men! Then they heard the shouting and a fear swamped them, knew instantly something was wrong, something had happened at the coal-face. The noise grew in intensity as miners swarmed over the place, scrambling past them, hysterical with panic.

"Run! Run!" someone screamed at them as he bundled and fought to pass the stationary youths.

"The whole face has gone up!" cried another as he shot past.

Charlie clung on to the pony that was growing more and more agitated. He had to grip the harness with all of his might to stop the animal from bolting.

"What shall we do?" Charlie bellowed over the growing din. "What shall…." looked frantically for Montgomery. His friend had vanished. *Jesus Christ! Jesus Christ!* he thought.

Charlie was alone, he tore at the chains that held the pony to the mono-rail, dragged the nervous animal about-face so that he was facing away from the distant coal-face and aiming a hefty kick at the pony's rump, sent it scurrying out-bye then he ran for his life.

Theo was waiting for him, pacing up and down like a man in a maternity ward. He was alone. In the distance came the faint echoes of shouting and commotion as miners ran from the threat.

"We'd better go, son." gasped a nervous Theo.

They set off at an agonisingly slow pace, there was no alternative, Theo Williams was not in the best of health and

Charlie was not about to leave him. The main landing point was a mile away. Five minutes into the journey and the pony was spotted. *Midnight* stood still, nervously watching them: mouth open and tongue hanging out. The lad spoke soft words as he cautiously approached the edgy pit-pony, touching and stroking its wet coat and gently led it towards Theo. He told Theo what he wanted him to do, Charlie strong and resolute with the older collier. After a moments hesitation and, with the boy's help, Theo managed to scramble on to the back of the animal. Charlie set off jogging; the pony pulled behind him, Theo clinging on for dear life, no one speaking as they ran from the place. After what seemed an eternity they reached the main arterial trunk-way, full to bursting with panicky, anxious colliers. Few were talking: almost all were bellowing and shouting at one another, scurrying this way and that: going nowhere, waiting impatiently for the man-riding set to appear, desperate for the life-line to pull them to the safety of the mine-shaft.

In 1951, eighty-odd men had perished in a horrific nightmare of fire-damp and gas. Same mine, different seam. There were many present who had lost friends and family in the disaster and all saw the same horrible scenario occurring again. One of the officials was grabbed and threatened. '*Where's the loco!''* shrieked the miner. '*Why is it taking so long!'*

Charlie helped Theo Williams climb off the animal. The overseer was as white as the pony as he slid to the dusty ground, sick with fear, there was an awful smell coming from his body. The boy knelt next to him, knew that Theo Williams had lost a brother in the fifties catastrophe. There were tears in Theo's eyes.

"Jesus Christ," he quaked, "I've shit myself, Charlie!"

Charlie had an inner strength that surprised him and said with a laugh, “Who gives a fuck!” grabbed at the straps that hung from the animal’s headgear, “Theo, I’m taking the donkey to the stables”

“Leave it, Charlie!”

The big stables were about half a mile out-bye, on the same route as the man-riding set. Charlie’s idea was simple, return the animal to the stable-block and wait for the loco to pass him on its return journey then jump into one of the vacant tubs. He was resolute, knew if he left the pony at the landing it would either die from the escaping gas, wander away into the labyrinth of passageways or the loco would knock it down as it followed the scent from the distant stables. There was no other way.

“Tell the driver to slow down when he passes the stables, Theo,” the youth turned and hurried along the wide tunnel and was soon out of sight.

Hysteria was breaking out amongst the colliers. Amos Brenkley was to blame. The Deputy had been radioed instructions from the surface, it was all systems go! The man-riding set was still racing to them. If the men wanted to leave that was okay, soothed Amos, but management was seeking volunteers. Sand-bags were going to be used to block both main and tail gates of the coal face, the entry and exit passageways, the bags were being loaded on the surface that very moment and would arrive within a short time.

Amos stood fidgeting next to the phone, nodding at the instructions coming from the surface, glancing nervously at the crowds close by, attempting unsuccessfully to restore order, calling to the milling anxious colliers.

“Volunteers, that’s all I said,” croaked the Deputy, “What the hell have I said wrong?”

"When the set comes in," shrieked Johnny Knowles, still in shorts and vest and missing a boot, "nobody is waiting, you hear me Amos!"

Amos Brenkley was no hero, knew enough not to mess with the pack, tried again, this time his tone was less confrontational, asking for help, pleading almost. "Volunteers, he pleaded, "a few volunteers is all?"

The deafening noise of the big loco as it clanked into view shuttling the dozens of man-riding tubs into the wide landing, stopped all conversation. The din was horrific but at least it brought some order. All the colliers clambered on board. There was silence as the lone official tried one last time.

Theo Williams put his head in his hands, said a silent prayer, fifty years of age and he'd shit himself with fear, he thought of Charlie Hill and he felt ashamed of himself, knew what he had to do. Taking a deep breath he rose on unsteady feet and hauled himself back out of the train, slowly tramped past the line of stationary tubs to the side of Amos Brenkley.

"Thanks, Theo," said the official.

Two more colliers left the safety of the train.

One last effort from Amos, "Just a few more, fellas, one or two to help with the sand-bags?"

Danny Longstaff stood up, grappled with his tin water-bottle and pulled it free of his coat-pocket, threw it with all his might at the deputy. "Pull the friggin' wire Amos before I choke you!"

Amos Brenkley managed to dodge the missile, which splattered inches from his face. Clearly intimidated he waved at the loco-driver, "Take it away," he cried heroically, "get these men out of here!"

With a bump and a clatter the train left the station.

Charlie stood ready. He had waited only minutes, his timing perfect; the animal was safely in its stall, fed and watered; now he waited as the noisy man-riding train trundled past the stables on its way to the shaft. It didn't slow! Theo Williams must have forgotten to pass on the information. The youth knew what he had to do, running alongside the line of screaming tubs Charlie judged his speed, said a silent prayer and jumped between two empty tubs. His feet gripped at the buffers, a deft movement and the lad stumbled into the tiny rumbling tub. He'd done it, succeeded! Switching off his light, Charlie Hill made himself comfortable, closed his eyes and tried not to dwell on the calamitous events, miles before they would reach the safety of the shaft-bottom, Charlie Hill said another prayer.

****

At six-thirty Charlie left his house, still on a high with the events of the day, pleased as punch that both parents were home, sober too which allowed him to repeat the story to the interested pair, made him feel good for once as his exploits were re-told and only slightly exaggerated. He walked arm in arm with Linda Macdonald. The pair were visiting the colliery, calling at Lynne James's home. Her parents were out for the evening. Monty Jepson already had his feet under the table which made a pleasant change, it was usually the girl's bedroom after a few hours. The evening was warm, despite the shortening hours and the darkening skies and there were few people about. One stood out, Harry Shannon, larger than life, standing on his own, filling the pavement on the opposite side of the street wearing the regulation trench coat and the silly fedora perched on his head, he appeared to be scrutinising them.

Full of mischief, Charlie Hill called out, "Harry, lend me your hat, I think it's going to rain."

The poor lad looked puzzled and started to shake his head with alarm, whispered, "Shut up, you!"

Charlie countered, "I'm coming to get that hat, Harry!"

Charlie Hill spouting and acting the clown, adrenalin still awash in his system because of the momentous day, trying to impress the girl with his immature, intimidating antics, started to beckon and prod his hands at the cowering figure. Charlie Hill, comedian, *'Coming to get you, Harry!'* he cried.

"Stop it, Charlie!" said Linda, clearly agitated at the sick humour.

Harry Shannon grabbed at his hat, bundled it into his coat and hurried away, plainly upset by the youth.

"Neither use nor ornament!" uttered the youth, gaping at the retreating figure.

"Charlie," said Linda, "what's your problem, Harry's not well in the head, he's harmless, couldn't hurt a fly."

"Has the bloody brain of a fly. If I had a giant fly-catcher I'd squash him!" Charlie started chuckling to himself.

Linda sighed, something was wrong, Charlie never acted so selfishly, had to be the scare at the colliery, scrambled his head. *That was it,* she decided, *hell, that's all he's talked about!* Linda Mac had known little Harry all her life and found him a gentle, lost soul living in a world of his own, the last thing he needed was bullying. She decided to steer the conversation away from the unfortunate youth and from the colliery incident, smiled as she recalled Charlie's explanation about the Monday night dance at the Welfare Hall. Rumours were bouncing off every wall about him for days; *Linda, have you heard about Charlie chatting to Anne Marie Hickson. Linda, guess who was like an octopus around your Charlie ... none other than Jenny Bruce!* Charlie Hill talking to this girl, that girl, Mister Flirtation himself.

"Jenny Bruce was there," grilled the girl, smiling broadly, wondered if Charlie's head was still centred on Harry or the colliery, or on other more personal things, saw the change in his expression. "Is she okay then?" colliery gossip coming to the fore, slipped in like an expert quiz hostess by Linda Macdonald.

"Fine. Okay," Charlie stammering, wondering what she'd heard.

"That's nice."

"Jenny's seeing someone," gasped the youth, better half a truth than blatant lies, "serious too … can't remember his name."

Linda didn't draw breath, moved the interrogation along nicely. "And Anne Marie, how was she?"

"Anne Marie Hickson," said a bemused Charlie, "you know her?"

"All my life," said the girl, "we were friends once, close friends."

"Bloody wildcat she was," Charlie reminisced, "wicked temper, almost killed poor Roy Bailey," explained the bruising confrontation between himself and Anne Marie Hickson. "Last year of the juniors when it happened, ended up defending him, Anne Marie was demented; the police were called ….."

Linda interrupted, her voice grim, *'Anne Marie was abused by her father,'* saw the look of disbelief on Charlie's face, *'you honestly didn't know?'* spent the rest of the journey talking all about the girl, reached their destination and Lynne James at the doorstep appeared like some blistered incarnation of a living *Barbie,* which, despite the liberal layers of makeup, couldn't camouflage the blossoming army of acne. The couple were ushered inside but Charlie's head was elsewhere, the evening's entertainment ruined, all he could think about was the dreadful images of Anne Marie, now he understood the manic outbursts, the aggression, the mood-swings, should have recognized the tell-tale symptoms.

Anne Marie and Charlie had something in common, both had been abused, physically and mentally ....

****

"Please open the door, Charlie," said the stranger. "No one is going to hurt you."

"I want to go home!" demanded the boy.

"Charlie," pleaded the fellow. "Open the door. If you open the door we can at least talk about our little problem. Please, son."

"Go away Mister," muttered the lad. He held his breath and waited. Seconds passed before the sounds of footsteps echoed. The man was leaving.

Charlie Hill squatted next to the door, his thin frame acting like a wedge. The strangers might return and attempt to force open the door, sat for an age, only moving when the numbness had enveloped his body. Still he waited and listened, they were not coming back, not for a while.

He wandered about the large spartan room. It was huge and cold, the floor was without carpet and the thin decrepit linoleum showed the long protruding lines of the floorboards underneath. A solitary table, old and dark and scuffed with age stood beside the long window. A metal grid covered the entire surface of the window-pane, security against attempted escape. There were no curtains to hide the grimness and the reality of the place. Charlie Hill climbed on to the table and stared out into the night. Shadows of trees and shrubs oozed before his young and frightened eyes. He could see the occasional lights beyond the large gardens as traffic hurried past the grounds, felt completely alone in the world. It started to rain, the noise sudden and loud against the window.

He did not know why he was in the large house. It had happened so quickly that very day. Two strangers at the door, inquisitive, wanting information that he could not give, demanding to see his parents, barracking him, as he fumbled and stumbled his guarded replies, made him cry. Then the people forced their way into his home, searched about the rooms until Charlie became hysterical, calling at the top of his voice for his mother. Still more questions, personal questions, one after another until his head ached and he could take no more, goading him until his temper snapped, ran at them, screaming abuse and threatening the strangers. He was grabbed and hoisted aloft, like a captive puppet, carried from his home, thrashing and kicking for all he was worth and bundled into the waiting vehicle, their words scaring and confusing him, telling Charlie that it was for his own good, that he needed protection, over and over the pair repeated the words. He needed protection, had to be looked after, the adults trying to calm him, but achieving the opposite as he howled dementedly for his mother, shrieked and begged to be released.

An age passed and still Charlie stood and stared out of the big window. Then footsteps echoed louder and louder as someone approached. With a single bound he was off the table and running to the door, his body planted firmly behind it.

"Charles," said the female, her tone soft and kind. "Charles, please open the door, no one is going to hurt you. I promise, Charles."

"Missus," wavered the boy, "I want Ma."

She persevered, asked, "Charles, are you hungry?"

Charlie Hill had not eaten since the previous evening when he'd tucked into a full tin of spaghetti, eaten cold and straight from the tin, stolen that very day from the Co-op. The realization hit him like a brick. He was locked up because someone had reported the theft. He groaned at the realization.

The woman repeated, "Charles, would you like something to eat?"

"Missus," whimpered the boy, stricken with grief, "it wasn't me who stole the spaghetti, honest, Missus."

Moments passed and then the perplexed lady said, "Charles, I don't understand ... what are you're talking about?"

Charlie swore under his breath, she obviously didn't have a clue about the incident at the Co-op. Now he was even more confused about his predicament, could not understand why he was being held in such a place. His head was aching.

"I'm hungry, Missus."

He heard the gentle laughter. "If you take the bolt out of the door, Charles, perhaps we can eat?"

Charlie unlocked the door, opened it slowly, it squeaked in protest. The small tousled head peered nervously across the wide stairway. A woman was leaning against the far wall and grinning at the frightened lad.

"That door," she chuckled, "definitely needs some oil." She stayed propped against the wall, not wishing to alarm the newcomer, knew that any sudden movements and the lad would bolt back into the room. "Well, Charles, shall we eat?"

They walked through passageways, down long flights of stairs, then through several dormitories and down more stairs. The home had an empty, eerie feel about it. They stopped before an enormous kitchen. A massive wooden table filled the centre of the room, there were chairs cluttered untidily around the table; three large cookers, on which stood a jumble of pots and pans, stood along one entire wall and at the opposite end of the room was a giant-sized coal fire. It blazed and cackled a noisy welcome.

"Jack and the Beanstalk!" gasped Charlie. "Like the Giant's kitchen."

The lady laughed. She laughed a lot, thought Charlie. He started to relax.

"Abbot and Costello," she answered. "Good film."

She gestured for Charlie to find a seat, but the numerous chairs proved too great a choice so he stood hesitantly and gazed at the woman. She pulled noisily at the nearest chair and gesticulated for him to sit.

"How many live here, Miss?"

"At the moment, only a few lads. We had a dozen staying with us until last week, but several have moved since then." She moved to the cooker and started turning dials and knobs.

"Moved, Miss?"

"Yes, Charles, they moved back with their parents."

Charlie visibly brightened at the news, knew he had the strength to persevere for a few days, closed his eyes momentarily. He had to remain strong, he would show them what a good boy he could be. Charlie ate until he could eat no more. The female sat close to him, the talk light-hearted and didn't worry him at all. She didn't force the conversation. Finally, fully gorged, the boy pushed aside the dinner-plate.

She introduced herself, "My name is Rose, I'll be here as long as you are under my supervision." The woman was a house-parent one year out from her basic training. Her fingers lightly touched the grubby paws of the newest inmate, "Please don't think that your stay with us will be a long one, it's not a permanent arrangement. We all want you back with your parents as soon as possible."

"How long, Miss?"

"Charles, the courts have only your interests at heart," the female hesitated, "the courts want your parents to behave. They want your mum and dad to look after you properly." She glanced sympathetically at the waif.

Charlie sighed with relief. It was no big deal after all, only people checking on his Ma. That was easily explained.

"Missus," he said optimistically, "Ma wasn't at home when those people called today. She was shopping is all. My dad, he was at work, see? That's why she wasn't at home. Ma was shopping, for grub for our tea." He gave Rose his best smile, "That's the truth, Missus. Ma is okay."

"Okay, Charles."

"So if you take me home now, Ma will definitely be back." Probably dead drunk, thought Charlie whimsically. "And she'll be making my tea. Honest, Missus."

Rose Newman tried to smile, it was a strain trying to keep the lad buoyant. She pushed on, attempting to hold the boy's confidence, mentioned the once-a-week visits that were allowed and saw the dark despair settle over his face. The realization stung him like a bee and Charlie Hill started to weep. When Rose put her arm around him he sobbed uncontrollably.

"Please let me see my Ma," he pleaded, "please, Missus."

Minutes passed and slowly the crying subsided. The boy composed himself, dried his face on his coat-sleeves.

The woman continued, her voice warm, "You'll be treated as one of the family, Charles. This will be your home for a little while until things are sorted, you'll soon get used to the new routine. There's a school nearby which you'll attend."

"Miss," interrupted Charlie, shaking his head with alarm, "don't hardly ever go to school."

She had read the case-files. The boy was regularly barred from the infant school because of his disruptive and aggressive behavior, most of his teachers thought Charles Hill was beyond help. Before Rose could reply, the house erupted with the arrival of the residents. Charlie shook with fear and gazed helplessly at the house-parent. She smiled, stood next to him and tightly grasped his hand.

"Come on, Charles, I'll introduce you," and she led him through the council-home.

A door swung open and a huge man was strolling towards them. Charlie recognized the fat man. His feelings towards the stranger were still hostile. He did not trust him.

"So, my dear," laughed the man, "you've finally come out of your hiding-place?"

Charlie could only glower at the man.

"Say hello to David," said the woman.

Charlie pulled away from the female and folded his arms over his chest, defiant to the end.

The big man turned and retreated, beckoning the pair to follow. "These things come to try us," he muttered under his breath.

Rose followed with a hesitant Charlie lagging behind. They entered a large and dingy living-room, several thread-bare arm-chairs and settees were dotted about the room, a solitary television stood in the farthest corner. The fat man was engaged in conversation with three youths, one was about the same age as Charlie, perhaps younger, the other two were much older, perhaps fourteen or fifteen years old.

Charlie stood close to the female. He felt uneasy and threatened by the strange youths. Rose stooped and began telling Charlie about his room-mates. Fred was the oldest, the woman pointed at the biggest youth, who stole a long, cold look at Charlie. He was as tall as a tree, bony and covered with a liberal display of acne, sported a thick dot tattoo on his cheekbone; his hair was carrot-red and cropped short. Next to him was Ted, not quite as tall as his companion but much chunkier. He flashed a bitter smile at Charlie. Ted looked odd, brilliant-white hair was swept back from his face and showed the almost invisible blond eyelashes; his eyes reminded Charlie of a rat, a dull crimson colour. The newcomer visibly shuddered. The smallest of the trio, Albert, waved a hesitant hand at Rose. He was about the same size as Charlie, fair-haired and painfully thin.

The big man gestured at Rose Newman who began walking towards him, together they strode from the room, the woman turned and gave Charlie a little wave, then the adults were gone. The oldest youths left the room, leaving Charlie alone with Albert.

"Where you from, then?" Albert's tone was soft and hesitant.

"Easington Village."

"Where's that?" asked Albert.

A moment's careful thought before Charlie ventured, "Next to Easington Colliery."

Half an hour later and Charlie Hill was starting to feel a lot better. Albert talked about his life. He originated from a small village near Durham called Pity Me. Charlie thought he was talking foolish, coming from such a place, but Albert insisted, Pity Me was his very own village.

Albert could talk under water, thought Charlie. He never took breath, talked about everything and nothing, so pleased to have someone his own age to talk to, loved science-fiction, books, cinema and television. He switched on the television-set and sat through an entire episode of Star-Trek, talked to Charlie and watched the television at the same time, head like a yoyo.

"Doctor Who is my favourite on the T.V.", he admitted. "At the pictures I like the Alien pictures the best, Sigourney Weaver is brilliant!" Albert pronounced Sigourney as Ziggy. "Have you seen Dune, what about Tremors?" talked like an express-train.

"I liked Star Wars," replied Charlie, "remember that big monkey-man?"

"Chewbacca," corrected Albert, "brilliant. You seen Dark Crystal?"

"No," said Charlie, he stood and wandered around the room, turned his body away from Albert and thought about home and his mother. He momentarily closed his eyes, Ma, the words echoed through his mind. 'Ma, come and get me, please.'

"Are you okay?" Albert was standing close to him.

Charlie almost jumped out of his skin, stared wide-eyed at the boy for some moments before he could compose himself, "Headache is all," he blustered.

"Hard to get tablets, Charlie," said Albert.

"Tablets?"

"For your headache, they think you'll store them for an overdose or sell them for cash"

Charlie Hill asked, "How long have you been here, Albert?"

"Years!"

"How long, really?"

"Six weeks."

"Why you here?"

"Think it was the neighbours," answered Albert sullenly, "they didn't like Ma having boy-friends." He pondered for several moments before adding, "Said they couldn't get any sleep for the noise."

"Honest?"

Albert nodded, then he asked, "What about you?"

"Haven't a clue."

Albert squatted in the old arm-chair, almost disappeared from view. He attempted to place his feet on to a small table opposite the chair but couldn't quite reach, instead he stuck his hands deep inside his trouser-pockets, said anxiously, "Horrible in here. That man - David - is a right bully, tells you what to do and you have to jump to it, doesn't take any lip, even the big lads are scared of him."

"Why they here?"

"Ted is a right thief, kept getting caught though. Woolworths took him to court. Sick of him." He thought a while then said, "He's says he's from Hetton, but I heard David talking about him once, called him an Albino....reckon he's a foreigner."

"What about Fred?"

"Hit his mother with a brick," he snorted with alarm, "she wouldn't give him any pocket-money."

"Honest?"

Albert stood, took a deep breath and continued. "I'll tell you something else about those two...." the words died in his throat as the door opened and the two older youths strolled into the room. They approached Charlie Hill, towered over him. Silence descended over the room. The youngster watched and waited nervously like rabbits caught between two sets of car-beams.

"What's the matter, squirt?" said the rat-faced Ted.

Charlie stared, too frightened to reply.

"Scared, or what?" asked Fred and he gave Charlie a shove.

"Get off, will you!" tough-guy Charlie, stuck his chin out defiantly.

The sound of approaching feet stopped the confrontation. Rose Newman popped her head through the door, misread the situation. "That's what I like to see, boys." she said and walked towards the small group, "getting to know one another?"

"Yes Miss," said Fred.

"Good. Good. Right then, shall we eat?" grinned at Charlie, "Not you, eh, think you eaten enough for everyone?" turned and tapped her way out of the room. Three of the boys followed. Charlie kept his head down until they'd gone.

At nine-o-clock, the house-master appeared. David Lane glanced about the room, looked at his wrist-watch and then snapped his fingers together. Like Pavlov's dogs, three of the boys rose as one and hurried to the door, Charlie followed. Without a word the man turned and hurried away, the small troupe followed, reaching a stairwell the man paused, stood aside and allowed the boys to pass.

"Oldest first," pronounced the fellow solemnly, "oldest two bathroom ... other two, bedroom!" and stood, sentry-like, with arms folded and watched as the boys scattered.

Albert led Charlie to the bedroom. It looked comfortable, the best room he had viewed all day. Six beds filled the room: three either side, all with small cabinets next to them, all identical, a single line of carpet ran down the entire length of the room.

"That's your bed, Charlie," and the boy pointed to the end bed. He nodded at the tall steel locker and added, "Pyjamas are in there."

Charlie couldn't remember the last time he had possessed pyjamas, hurried to the locker and found a single pair, grabbed them and went to his bedside.

Albert said. "When you wake up tomorrow, you put your pyjamas in your cabinet, okay?"

Charlie asked. "And we wash every night?"

"Every night."

"Hot water?" asked Charlie, fearing the worst.

"Red-hot!"

"Brilliant," said Charlie.

"Not a chance!" muttered Albert Decker, pouting, "we all share the same bath and those two bastards piss in the bath when they've done!"

Ten-o-clock and a distant bell clanked out a faint tune. The two youngsters sat together on Charlie's bed, both were reading comic-books.

"Lights out," whispered Albert and he hurried away to his bed.

The lights flickered then died. The room was pitch-black.

The door squeaked ajar and David Lane appeared. The lights from the hallway filtered over his huge frame.

"Goodnight, boys," he growled.

The reply was returned and in perfect harmony. The man observed the place for some moments, then turned and snapped the door shut.

Charlie closed his eyes and thought about his mother, she would be worried about him. Charlie said a little prayer to God, told him to watch over his Ma, promised himself that he would behave. He had to get out of the strange place as soon as possible, had to get home to Ma. Footsteps closed on the bed and fear gripped Charlie, couldn't speak or move, bed sheets were pulled aside, the eerie charcoal face of Ted loomed over him.

"Push over!" demanded the older youth and he began to climb into the bed.

"Get lost!" Charlie Hill spluttered and he tried to push the larger boy away.

A fist caught him flush on the face, the force of the blow knocked Charlie on to his back. As he raised a hand to repel the attack, his fingers were grabbed and twisted, Charlie squirmed and moaned in panic.

"Had enough," grunted the aggressor, "do you want more?"

Charlie croaked, "I'll tell! I'll tell!" He lashed out at Ted and was beaten soundly.

An arm wedged across his neck and the pressure made him gasp and retch, still he attempted to fight the older youth but was too small and too weak. Charlie Hill was grasped and forced on to his belly. The bully heaved his bulk on to his back, Charlie was hysterical with grief, now he was begging and pleading with his tormentor, crying softly as his small legs were prized apart, rough hands squeezed at his flesh, kneading and nipping and hurting him, pulling and prodding at his thin buttocks, a frenzy of lust overpowering the older lad.

"Please don't," whined a demented Charlie, "please leave me alone!"

A powerful hand gripped and covered his open mouth. Charlie could smell the odour and sweat as the fingers tore at his face, now he was gasping for air, unable to cry out as the horrible, excruciating pain burrowed deep into him……..

Time passed. Charlie lay still, his eyes wide and wet as he stared into the blackness. A figure approached and the breath left him, mortified and mute with fear, he watched and waited.

"It's me," whispered Albert as he eased his scrawny frame on to the bed. "It'll be okay, honest, Charlie."

"Want to go home," gasped Charlie Hill, felt Albert's arm cover him, comfort him. He fell asleep wrapped around his new friend.

Charlie's first taste of a Council Home, his home for the next twelve months.

****

CHAPTER THIRTEEN

Kenny Tupling was laying down the law to the two tearaways, the trio was out-bye in the district of *Seventh - North*. The two youths were brassed-off, didn't like the new set-up one bit, hated the big gruff Deputy who was always on their backs, twice during the shift he'd left the coal-face to check on the trainees.

"Stop takin' bloody liberties," he said loudly, "this is friggin' twice I've caught you!"

Charlie wondered if the moron could string a sentence together without swearing. *'What's up?'* he replied angrily, still rested on to the big shovel, trying to give the Deputy the impression he'd actually been working, both mouse-traps had been quickly hidden when they'd seen the approaching figure. The official kicked at the shovel, clearly exasperated at the pair if shirkers. *'Don't mess with me, youngun',* he bawled, *'you've both been sittin' on yer arses,'* pointed at the underside of the conveyor-belt where coal-dust lay inches deep either side of the spinning rollers, *'clean the damn belt or find another job!'* Kenny Tupling stormed off, muttering profanities at the top of his voice, at his wit's end with the trainees.

"Better do some work, eh?" asked Montgomery.

Charlie reluctantly agreed. He missed Theo, missed the easy-going atmosphere of *Second-South.* The old district was now closed, sand-bagged, sealed-off, big noisy machinery installed to suck out the poisonous gases. The pair had regularly visited the place over the past weeks, checking out the progress, maybe that was why *Tut-Tut* had kicked off and barracked them constantly. The boys assumed they'd be left to their own devices like before, but the Deputy was a different kettle of fish to Theo Williams.

'*Gotta* do *this, do that. Gotta keep busy, gotta make money,*' always moaning was Kenny Tupling. '*Mrs Thatcher tryin ta shut us down, don't you understand?*'

They started to work, forgot about the mouse-traps that they had purchased from *Lennie Barber's* hardware shop, the continuous clacking and whine of the conveyor-belt muffled the squeaking of the trapped vermin. They had caught four mice and tied them by their tails to the belt trip-wire, good fun for the trainees.

One-o-clock and two colliers approached carrying a piece of equipment. They paused next to the trainees who, thinking they were officials, were working hell for leather. One of the strangers spoke.

"Gotta job for you boys," said Rex Harrison, power-loader. His real name was George.

"This gear," said Micky Stamp, Rex's mate, "needs to be taken to bank… to the surface."

"Take it to the Mechanics' Stores," intervened Rex, "next to the lamp-cabin."

"When?" Charlie asked, "because Kenny Tupling doesn't give us time to piss!"

Both Charlie and Montgomery were well and truly knackered after grafting for two hours.

"Take no notice of Kenny Tut-tut, he's not too bad for a deputy," laughed Rex, "all wind, worries too much," he took out the small tin of snuff and offered it to the boys. There were no takers. "Thinks if we make money, we'll keep the pit open."

"We'll all be out of a job in a few years," laughed Micky Stamp, "but some buggers just won't face reality. Kenny is one of them."

Monty asked, "If we take the machinery to bank how much wages do we lose?" He needed every penny as he was saving for his first motor.

"Daft bugger," said Rex, sneezed loudly then blew his nose through his fingers and wiped the grime on to his shorts. "Kenny Tupling will clock your cards at the end of the shift."

"You're jokin," said Monty incredulously, "we take some broken machinery to the surface and then we can go home?"

"It's only one-o-clock?" said Charlie, he was starting to feel good.

"Go down to the landing, the man-riding set is waiting." said Micky, "don't forget, when you get to bank take this equipment directly to the Mechanics Shops."

"Where's that again?" asked Monty.

"Next to the clocking-in cabin," answered Rex Harrison, smiling, "you want me to draw a fuckin' map?"

Two-o-clock and the boys were in the showers, two-thirty and Charlie Hill, full of the joys of life, was strolling towards his home. He saw the Jaguar reversing out of his cul-de-sac, knowing it was Priestley he waved but the car eased away. The youth entered his home.

"Ma," he shouted, saw his mother and Joan Armstrong busy opening bottles of ale. He grimaced with anger.

"Hello son," said Becky. She was inebriated and happy.

"My favourite boy," laughed Joan, as she emptied the contents into tumblers.

"Early, aren't we?" said Rebecca.

There was a carrier-bag propped on the table-top. There must have been half a dozen bottles of beer showing their necks through the bag. Charlie shook his head at his mother and walked into the living-room, intending to make his own tea then he changed his mind and confronted the pair.

"Elvis wanted me, did he?" he spat out the words.

His mother looked puzzled, didn't answer, started sipping at the nectar.

"Wanted me, more like!" giggled Joan Armstrong and she nudged at her breasts with her free arm, "not bad for my age, Charlie?"

Rebecca almost spilled her beer as she started laughing with her friend.

It was all too much for the boy, he lunged at the carrier-bag and strode to the door, with one deft sweep of his arm, Charlie threw the package high in to the sky and watched it as it opened like a miniature parachute, bottles mushroomed every way and then came crashing down to earth like a handful of grenades, broken glass and liquid littered the yard. Several of the missiles almost caught Charlie, landing so close to his feet as to soak him.

"Done and dusted!" grunted the youth, a look of self-satisfaction on his young face.

A riot started. Hysterical at the loss of their recently-purchased ale, the women attacked the boy with a savage fury that shocked and bewildered him, punching and pushing at him until he was almost forced out of his home, manic as they howled their protestations at the startled youth, scratching, clawing and bloodying the retreating figure. Charlie retaliated, his temper broken. With powerful hands the lad grasped Joan Armstrong by the hair and hurled her out through the open door, away she scattered, down the steps and into the yard, on her back-side and into the puddles of beer and broken glass, screaming like a demented clown as she struggled to regain her feet, her clothing soiled and wet with the alcohol. Next, he grabbed at his mother, ducking and flinching from her wild swinging arms, dragged her away from the door and on to the steps, a powerful kick at her rump and Rebecca was propelled into the garden. She landed awkwardly in a clump of nettles with her dress up to her thighs, screamed loud and long as the stinging plants ripped pain into her legs. The door was slammed shut, the key turned, the women locked out of the house.

Slowly Charlie climbed the stairs, didn't stop when he heard the door battered and the windows being smashed, entered his bedroom and lay on the bed, filled with frustration and dismay. Only minutes earlier he was full of bounce and optimism having finished his shift hours early, so happy at the unexpected early conclusion of his shift and then all of this, pandemonium within minutes of his arrival, bloody bedlam. He cursed his mother, cursed his miserable life and stayed in his room for hours, in a state of flux, not knowing quite what to do. Finally, a little before five-o-clock, Charlie eased off the bed and hurried down the stairs, unlocked the door then stood waiting for his father to appear.

"What happened, Charlie?" Adam said stoically, almost casually.

Damaged windows, yard full of broken bottles and bloody imprints everywhere, Adam Hill accepting the carnage as if it were an everyday occurrence, listened intently as his son tried to explain the tale of woe. Charlie talking and pacifying his father and at the same time making a simple meal for both of them. Charlie telling tall-tales, omitting most of the physical stuff, knowing Jesus on the Cross wouldn't save him mentioned the assault on his mother.

“Shouldn’t be drinking, Dad, not during the day, not with that Armstrong woman. It’s not fair,” kept glancing at his father, waiting for a reaction.

None came, it was if Adam Hill was past caring. All he said, more as an afterthought really. “Did you see which way they went, Charlie, did they leave together. What do yer reckon, Charlie, think Ma will be out long?” his voice resigned and tinged with sadness.

Charlie calmed his Dad, then ever so gently changed the topic, moved to safer grounds and started talking again about his working day, told his father about his short shift at the pit, about the new deputy, gave Adam Hill something to beef about, maybe moan about the new Deputy rather than his missing mum.

Adam Hill knew of Kenny Tupling, known him for years, a wry smile came over his features as he pushed aside bleak thoughts.

“Kenny Tupling, you say?” said Adam, “fancy that!”

“Big mouth,” replied Charlie sharply,” all he did was shout!”

“You know why he’s like that, don’t you,” said the father sardonically, “he’s a homosexual!”

Charlie couldn’t follow the reasoning, shot a puzzled look at his Dad, “So if you shout you’re queer?”

“Aggression, over the top with it,” said Adam, “tries too hard to act like a man, shoutin’ and cursin’. Just an act, went to school with Kenny, soft as butter and just as shy, always playing with the girls he was.” He pondered and studied for some moments before adding, “He still lives with his mother,” sniggered and said, “come the week-end he’ll be in Newcastle in the bloody queer bars! Daft beggar even wears a bloody cravat!”

"Cravat?" Charlie didn't even possess a tie, never mind the fancy scarves.

Adam laughed, "Bloody wide tie worn by homosexuals!" The ignorant man thought he was hilarious, said, "Next time he shouts at you, tell him to watch his back," Adam Hill as comical as an under-taker.

Charlie walked to the table and put down the two plates, smiling proudly at his attempts. "There we are, dinner is served!"

"Beans on toast again," whined Adam Binns, "Jesus Christ!"

"Dad," muttered the lad, "there's nowt else to eat!"

"That bloody woman!" grunted Adam Hill, his mind back on his wayward missus, shook his head despondently, looked around for utensils. "Charlie, wash a few forks, eh?"

****

Joan Armstrong had relations in Sunderland. When married life started to depress her the woman would often spend days, sometimes weeks, away from her Derek. He didn't appear to mind and if the truth were spoken, Dizzy Armstrong had little control over his beloved wife, thought the sun shone through her tight shapely backside. Joan did pretty much as she pleased. Days earlier, after the fracas with Charlie, both females called at Joan's home and collected clothing. The girls were about the same height; although Joan had a much bigger bust. They still managed to equip themselves with several days attire. The tin-box - the Armstrong Fund - hidden under the bed, was raided and a good sum of money borrowed. '*We need some drinking-money*,' Joan had insisted. '*Won't Derek mind if you take the money*?' asked a bemused Becky Hill. '*Dizzy does as he's told,*' Joan had replied seriously, '*or he'd be shown the door.*' Derek Armstrong, like most colliers, took only pocket-money and relied on his spouse to look after all the bills and out-goings and holidays. Joan ruled the roost.

Six-o-clock and the girls were well and truly established in the lounge of the Palatine Hotel in the heart of the town. They had hardly touched the money, so generous were the many clients who frequented the place, the two flirted and toyed with the locals until Elvis Priestley and Arnold Anders entered the bar. Rebecca, remembering that her son had seen the Jaguar leaving their home earlier in the week, spoke of her concern. *'Charlie isn't stupid, Elvis, he might put two and two together!'*

Elvis brushed aside her apprehension, "He'll think I've got work for him," he said casually, thought young Charlie Hill had spunk and grit, "stop worrying and have another drink."

****

Saturday morning and still his mother had not returned. Adam had questioned him again about the incident and prudently Charlie again omitted the physical outburst. Once again, there was an uneasy calm about the home. The longer the absence, the more his father retreated into a shell, conversation dried up as the older figure lost himself in a world of his own. He would never admit it to anyone but the man was pining for his wife, desperate for her return: his head centred only on her.

The previous evening Charlie had left the house at six-o-clock, had a date with Linda Mac. They were visiting the cinema in Hartlepool, spoilt for choice: *Goodfellas or Ghost,* the couple spun a coin and Charlie won. The gangster movie was chosen and Linda sulked all evening. 10.30pm and Charlie breezed through the door only to find his father seated in the same chair and the house in total silence, still in abject misery. Adam was suffering dreadfully. Charlie Hill made his excuses and took to his bed.

The week-end arrived bright and breezy and full of promise. Charlie, mainly to pacify an agitated Linda Mac, had agreed to take her to Sunderland. '*You always see me on a Saturday night, Charlie. Why can't you see your friends another night? I always feel second-best, Charlie.'* They were visiting the town and still she was pouting and acting like a spoilt child. '*What more do you want, Linda? I hate shopping, but I'm here with you and spending my money on you. Keep on with the twisty face and I'll go home.'* He continued with the pretence, '*I'm going out with the boys tonight,'* he lied, '*like it or lump it!* Truth was, he wanted to see Anne Marie Hickson.

****

Kenny Tupling: *Mister Cravat* himself, together with a young male friend, was seated in the Bar area of the *Seaburn Hotel*. Kenny had spent the previous evening prowling the bars and night-clubs in Newcastle and had almost given up hope of finding Morris Hepplewhite. The very last watering-hole and there he was. The two had met in the summer. Kenny, with his beloved mother, had spent a lonely week in Benidorm. On the very last evening and purely on a whim, Morris had ventured out alone, walked the sea-shore: called in to a bar and met another equally lonely soul, beautiful Morris: perfume and pan-stick and so effeminate. It was heaven for both of them: big, rough good-looking Kenny Tupling and the small, petite and gorgeous Morris*: like Rock Hudson and Jimmy Dean,* commented Kenny, swapped addresses and agreed to meet when the season was over.

A Jaguar saloon pulled up outside the entrance to the hotel. The driver climbed out and Kenny almost choked on his drink. It was Eddie Priestley, Eddie Priestley from Easington! *Jesus!* he thought. *Mary, Mother of God!* jumped off the bar-stool and told Morris to wait, hurried to the foyer and exit- area, couldn't think straight, had to disappear until it was safe to show his face. He'd lose everything if his secret came out - job, house, everything - have to scarper to another part of the country and he'd only known pit-work! *Jesus! Jesus!*

He need not have worried. Elvis Priestley and another man, tall and bald, were helping out two female companions. Kenny recognized the women, made him smile with wicked glee. *Well! Fancy that! Fancy bloody that!* his mind working overtime and always wanting to be on top of the game, made his move, knowledge was power and it didn't hurt his cause one little bit to have one or two or three people in his pocket!

Kenny Tupling stepped out in to the sunlight, waved a greeting at the group, said loudly, "Coming in for a drink? Mother still talks about you, Eddie," focused on the females, saw the terror smudge their features. "Rebecca! Joan! Nice to see you!" and he grinned like a fox. *Wait 'till I see Adam and Dizzy*!

Elvis grimaced then casually returned to the driver's door. All of his companions scrambled back into the darkness of the limousine and watched as Elvis stared at the stranger, lifted a lone finger to his lips, wanting their secret kept, *'Another time, Kenny,'* he mimed, gave a knowing wink. The car sped towards Sunderland and home.

The collier smiled broadly. '*Thank you, Jesus,*' he thought and he returned to the hotel, felt as horny as a hamster in heat. '*Morris! Morris! I want you so badly!*'

"Hell!" said Joan, staring out of the car window, watching the gloating figure of Kenny Tupling.

Rebecca said guardedly, "He drinks with Adam!"

Elvis put on a brave face. "Don't have to worry, Kenny won't say a word. Do you think for one moment that his mother is in the hotel, give me a break, he'll have one of his boy-friends in the bloody lounge!" He looked at the ashen-faces and kept on pushing, "The only time his mother leaves the house is for the bingo and he has to escort her … she's as deaf as a post!" glanced back and glowered at the females, "one word from me about his little secret and his life is over."

Arny offered his pennyworth. "He's right, girls, Elvis is right!"

"Shut your mouth!" growled Rebecca.

"Yeah," agreed Joan, "why don't you button it?"

"Well," snapped Arnold Anders. "If that's your attitude!"

****

Charlie was through with the shopping lark, time to take a slow walk towards the bus depot. The streets were crowded with shoppers; the roads choc-a-bloc with traffic. It was nice to put aside all the worries and meander through the place. Linda had calmed, perhaps the obligatory gifts had gone some way to stop her whining, better still, Charlie had promised to call on her after he'd left the pub. She felt better now, laughed at her earlier jealousy, Charlie wouldn't deceive her otherwise why had he promised to see her later that evening? '*Screw your head on girl,*' she thought to herself, '*or you might lose him.*'

Linda slipped her arm through his, gave a playful tug and smiled lovingly at him.

The traffic slowed bumper to bumper and Charlie thought he recognized the big Jaguar, couldn't see the registration but the colour was the same as the Priestley car. Pulling at the girl he hurried forward and was about to rap against the car when it pulled away quickly. He hollered out for Elvis as the two rear passengers in the plush vehicle slid out of sight, but the car did not stop or even slow, on the contrary, Charlie watched it tear along the busy road, zig-zagging through traffic, putting distance between them.

"There were two women in the back," said Linda sniggering.

The youth did not answer, his eyes following the disappearing vehicle. He thought he recognized one of the figures in the rear of the vehicle then he laughed out loud, his head was playing games with him. *Wasn't Elvis,* thought the youth, *he would have stopped.*

****

Eight-o-clock that same evening saw Charlie Hill standing between the taller Jepson brothers propping up the bar at the *Shoulder of Mutton*. Montgomery was filling the juke-box with coins and Patton was ordering drinks. The brothers wanted to visit the colliery club. Saturday evening and it always guaranteed a full house, bingo in the lounge: group in the singing-end, something for everyone.

"The *Flying Pickets* are on, Charlie," moaned Pat Jepson, "*Only You!*"

"Prefer *Yazoo*," said Charlie. What he really preferred was a meeting with Anne Marie Hickson. They had tramped around the pubs in the Village for the past hour without success.

"Right," said Monty returning to their side, "we'll finish these drinks and it's off to the colliery then?"

Three girls walked into the pub and made a bee-line for the bar, one, the tallest, was beaming at Charlie Hill. The Jepson boys glanced at their pal. *Still waters*, thought Monty. *Still Waters*.

They greeted one another: Charlie and Anne Marie. Like clockwork dolls, both brothers shook their heads in feigned annoyance, already they were grinning, same thoughts buzzing through their heads: three girls; three fellas. Charlie introduced the Jepson twins. Anne Marie introduced Lucy and Irene Bower, sisters but more like identical twins with their look-alike and unconventional mode of dress; short and frumpy and with a style reminiscent of the singer *Bjork*, the females acted flirtatiously and engaged immediately with the Jepson boys in light-hearted banter. The atmosphere lifted to the stratosphere.

Hours later and the young couple talked quietly at the end of Thorpe Road, at the southern perimeter of the Village. They stood close together at the apex of the small decline. Myriad twinkling lights of Peterlee shone in the distance. On one side of the road the darkness and murkiness of empty fields, on the other, the abandoned quarry, no one else around but the boy and the girl. It was very late and house lights were being extinguished one by one along the private terraced street.

The bubbly, vivacious foursome: the Jepson twins and the Bower girls had left them at nine-thirty, anxious to see the final session at the Colliery Club. '*The Flying Pickets are a class act*,' said Pat Jepson as he playfully caressed the rather inflated bottom of Lucy Bowers. '*For the last time, Charlie, are you staying or going?'* The couple was left alone in the almost deserted bar at the *Shoulder of Mutton*.

Anne Marie was not what he had expected. She was mature and comfortable in his company, charming, pleasing, funny at times, dry and witty, in other words, captivating, fascinating company, choosing neither to dwell in the past nor to dredge up old memories which had initially perplexed Charlie. Her charm and vivacity was apt compensation and he had enjoyed her presence. '*Like a breath of fresh air*,' he had confided prior to leaving the pub and it was so true, women normally bored him with their pettiness and inbuilt small-mindedness. Anne Marie reminded Charlie of Jenny Bruce. She made him laugh, talked to him as an equal, wanted to listen as well as being listened to, spoke as an equal, eleven-o-clock, still alive with conversation and genuine dialogue, the pair strolled arm in arm away from the place. It was Anne Marie's idea to show Charlie her old home, unburdening and confiding now, no bitterness in her tone as she spoke of the awful time when her world was disintegrating, never once condemning nor denouncing. She spoke with compassion and fortitude, her maturity was evident as she re-lived the awful times.

"It's life, Charlie," she said with a resilience beyond her years. "If you can survive then you become stronger. I was suffering because my mother was destroying all of us, not only my dad but me too. My mother was a party-animal, lived for the week-ends, enjoyed the night-life; the drinking and the flirting. Dad was a home-bird, slippers and television. *Match of the Day* was Dad's idea of enjoyment. My father loved my mother, despite all her faults and indiscretions; he never stopped loving her, even when it became obvious what she was doing. Mother tortured and tormented him with her socialising and entertaining. She'd return home if and when the mood took her, flaunting and flirting, ridiculed my father for being weak."

"You must hate your mother then?"

"Once," replied the girl, "when I was small." Anne Marie paused and shook her head morosely, "I can see both sides now," she whispered, "can you believe that? It's so sad."

Charlie Hill said, "But your father shouldn't have done….."

"I really don't want to talk about it, Charlie," retorted the girl firmly. "Dad was out of his mind, literally, he was on medication, depressed, all he had was me and we would sit and cuddle. Then he started drinking, drinking until his mind was gone." Her voice became a whisper as she said, "Do you know what it's like to see your father cry, Charlie, to watch a grown man cry for his wife, can you imagine what it was like. There were no winners, Charlie. We all suffered in our own ways." Anne Marie looked at the youth and smiled bravely, "My father was imprisoned; Ma had to move away because of all the hateful gossip. She's not happy, she's drunk more than she's sober, deep down I know she feels some responsibility for Dad, I suppose Dad will carry the guilt to his grave."

Charlie asked, "Your father … is he still in prison?"

"He's out, Charlie, released a few years ago," replied Anne Marie, "lives in Stockton, written a few letters to me. He can't really visit us again can he? I do write to him." She shrugged her shoulders, "He's still my father after all, but his life is over." The girl stopped talking for some minutes then added apologetically, "Maybe that's why I was so nasty to you and Roy when we were kids. I think all of my pain and frustration was focused on others and made me so aggressive," she glanced at him, "I'm sorry."

Charlie made light of it, chuckled nervously, said, “I’ve still got the scars to prove it.”

The girl continued, her features resolute and tenacious, “After a time, you start to think *Why Me,* why is it happening to me, but there’s no rhyme nor reason to it. It’s life … good, bad, whatever. People have different ways of coping. Some seem to take all the knocks in their stride, no matter what is thrown at them, you understand what I’m saying, Charlie. When my parents married they must have thought it was forever … the good times, everything new and exciting, two people ready to face all the challenges.” She sighed and glanced into the night sky. When she resumed, her voice was softer, her tone lower, “I don’t condemn anyone anymore. My mother loved my father in her own way, but she wanted more, though not at first. I’m talking years of good times when I was a toddler, normal family life, the ups and downs, the struggles and then things changed, slowly at first, nothing much at all. Ma arguing, wanting more than changing nappies and the occasional night out with my Dad. Slowly drifting apart. Maybe my mother saw life passing her by, looked in the mirror one day and didn’t like what she saw, thought there was a better life to be had somewhere other than in the home and maybe Dad didn’t agree. Perhaps Ma didn’t want to get old, wanted to squeeze every last bit of goodness out of each day. *‘It’s not a rehearsal,’* she’d say when they argued. *‘You only get the one chance, so let’s enjoy it!’* but sitting in the Workingman’s Club or partying at the nightclubs was not my Dad’s way.” Anne Marie sighed loudly, “Everyone copes differently, Charlie. For some, it’s sticking your head in the sand and hoping things will get better, others seem to have the mettle to cope with whatever comes their way. For Ma it was the make-believe world of revelry and drink. Drink to make her happy, to make her sad …. coping. For my father it was muddling through each day, dealing with it in his way, calling at the doctors, taking the odd prescription. Then turning to the bottle, drinking at home, on his own. He was never like that, Charlie, he was never a drinker." The girl looked directly at the youth and said unemotionally, "I always remember my father talking to me, not as a daughter, more as an adult, blunt and matter of fact. *'Annie,'* he said, *'you understand that life is hell, every day pain and purgatory and how much we can endure, but when we die we find peace. Heaven, Annie, heaven for everyone.'* I didn't understand what he meant at the time, Charlie, but I do now."

"I'm sorry," whispered the youth.

"Let's find a telephone, Charlie," she said, as if suddenly exhausted by the confessional, "I'll phone for a taxi." She slipped her arm around his and started walking towards the bustle of the village.

"Are you okay?" asked the youth, lovingly squeezing her arm.

"I'm fine, Charlie?"

"You've gone quiet?"

"I was thinking of you actually," said Anne Marie. "You've had an awful life, Charlie."

He smiled and nodded, "Bit of a roller-coaster."

"You've done okay, Charlie Hill," she whispered, "I'm proud of you," she stopped and pulled him close, looked deeply into his eyes, wanting to say so much, then kissed him tenderly on the lips.

They walked on until they reached a public telephone. Anne Marie phoned for a taxi and waited an age before the cab arrived, neither was concerned, as they had more time to talk and discover more about each other. Anne Marie was living in

Peterlee, renting a corporation flat in the *Little Eden* estate in the town, worked at Sca Packaging on the North West Industrial Estate. She was a clerk in the accounts department of the firm, attending Peterlee College once a week and hoping to obtain her G.C.S.E. in book-keeping and accounts.

"I'll try anything, Charlie," she said. "I want to do so much, I didn't take qualifications at school, no interest, but now, why not?"

Always the pessimist, Charlie said, "What if you fail, Anne Marie, people might laugh at you."

She laughed out loud, "It's a long time since I've been bothered about what people say about me, I've had a lifetime of gossip thrown at me. I couldn't care less. One life, Charlie and it's there for the taking.

He smiled, "Maybe you're right, Anne Marie. I never thought like that before."

"We'll talk some more?" she said as the taxi screeched alongside.

"Can't wait," he replied and pecked her on the cheek, "take care."

"Goodnight, Charlie," she said and climbed in the cab.

CHAPTER FOURTEEN

Rebecca lay in bed, Adam next to her, fast asleep, his breathing deep and melodic, the only sounds echoing around the home. Charlie had risen earlier. She'd listened as her son busied himself preparing the coal-fire without a mutter or a moan, the dust and ash disposed outside, kitchen noises followed as he quietly made breakfast. Minutes past and then the door reverberated as the youth left and silence returned. Rebecca grimaced as she pictured her boy. Charlie was a good son, deserved a better life than the one he endured, merited a decent mother. All her fault, knew more than anything she was in the wrong, closed her eyes and thought about the previous day's momentous events and wondered if her secret liaisons with Elvis Priestley had been detected.

Seeing Charlie wandering along the high street in Sunderland with his girlfriend and his frantic efforts to gain Elvis's attention, had unnerved Rebecca so much that at eight-o-clock that evening she had left the others still bothered with the near-catastrophic meeting with her son, wondering if he had recognized his mother in the back of the Jaguar, the feeling of bitter humiliation and shame as she crumpled out of sight was too much to bear. The others in the group were clearly unhappy. Joan especially, her tone sardonic and mocking, *'I don't understand, Becky, you're going home. It's early!'* looked at her with incredulity, *'and what the hell am I supposed to do now?'* gesturing at her two leering companions, *'share them?'*

Rebecca was reluctantly dropped off a safe distance from her home. The house was dark and empty but Adam had left the door unlocked, hoping his wife would return. The reality made her cringe with shame, for no matter how badly Rebecca dishonoured her husband, he always forgave her. In the distant past Adam had been physically abusive towards her, slapped and bruised her and Rebecca had always retaliated by howling her protests but deep inside she knew the chastisement was deserved. Other men would have battered her, thrashed her within an inch of her life, would have given up on her and left, she fully merited the punishment, knew it for a fact even though it had been years since she had been manhandled and hurt by Adam, perhaps he was resigned to the misery inflicted on him, perhaps she had destroyed the soul of her poor husband.

She had waited an hour, hoping that someone would return to the house. Adam, Charlie, it didn't matter, she needed their company. One long hour before she weakened, then walked through the streets and reached the sanctuary of the *Southside Social Club,* sat alone with a glass of Guinness, the only customer in the place. *'There's a hell of a band playing at the Colliery Club,"* said Jonty Brightwell, the barman, damned if he could recall their name. *'They used to be famous!'* Rebecca wasn't listening, wasn't too keen on the barman and certainly didn't want his company, so she sat in the far corner of the room, morose and deep in thought. Rebecca was reminiscing, images from the past haunting and troubling her ....

Becky had been a sweet and innocent girl. Like thousands of others, wanting the normal things in life, dollops of happiness and security and love, most of all love. She found it when she met Jimmy Shannon, everyone called him Little Jimmy, but what he lacked in height he more than made up for it in stunning looks and vibrant personality. Jimmy Shannon had the world at his feet and he chose Rebecca. They became engaged and were going to be married. Rebecca was in heaven, ignored the gossip, disregarded her parents, blissfully in love, totally smitten with Jimmy Shannon. Until the knock at the door that changed her world. It had to change. The young girl at the door was noticeably pregnant and hysterical with grief. All the commotion, all the pain and the certain knowledge that Becky was never going to be with the man she loved.

And a full year later, working nights at the Kings Head pub, grieving and still in mourning and then meeting Adam Hill for the first time. Big powerful Adam, a loner and so different from Jimmy; mysterious and deep and with a reputation for violence, a man with a short fuse, the pair like chalk and cheese. Adam at the bar, pint glass in one hand, awkward, silent for most of the time and only the occasional nervous gestures and fawning and always watching and listening, as if he were guarding and protecting her. Rebecca was quite flattered by the attention. After some time she finally succumbed to the quiet charms of the big man and started walking out with Adam Hill. Of course it wasn't the same, it couldn't be, not after the charm and charisma of Jimmy Shannon. She was never on Cloud Nine, never dreamed of Adam like she used to dream of Jimmy. But she started to feel safe again, started to feel wanted.

Rebecca saw Jimmy Shannon again. Not instigated by her, she wasn't that kind of girl. Jimmy had married and moved near to the big church on the Village green, Clappersgate, the same village green that bordered Low Row with its smattering of shops and pubs. One of the pubs was the Kings Head.

The first time Jimmy Shannon walked into the bar, Becky almost fainted, only a smile of recognition from the man and she felt the acute pain of lost love, cut her like a knife, almost a year since they had last met and when Jimmy spoke to her Becky could hardly reply. With her eyes full of tears she listened to his excuses and his lies, as conniving and cunning as he bantered and pouted like a little cockerel. She listened knowing she shouldn't, listened because she wanted to believe. He walked her home. It was wrong, she was betraying Adam but she was flesh and blood and the love she held for Jimmy Shannon was too much to bear. They walked the short journey to her home, the girl overjoyed as he charmed and enticed her and by the time they had reached her destination Rebecca was laughing out loud. He had the personality to charm the birds off the trees and he knew it. They made love that night, violently, passionately, two souls enjoined. Blissfully happy, confused, uncertain, the girl arranged a second meeting.

It did not happen. Days later and Rebecca waited at the rendezvous, inconsolable when he did not show. The walk home was slow and agonizing, the pain of another rejection burned into her soul. She had been a fool, a complete and utter fool. Her mind was made up. Rebecca was angry and felt humiliated, felt used and abused, became resolute, the past had to stay in the past and her future was with Adam Hill. Adam loved her, she was certain of that and in time she would love him and she was determined to start rebuilding her life. Within months and pregnant herself, she married the man who adored her……………………………..

"Rebecca, love," said Jonty Brightwell carefully, "it's closing-time, okay if I take your glass, love?"

Rebecca Hill stirred from the stupor of the past, nodded approval and without a word spoken, walked unsteadily from the room, her head pounding like a drum, filled with regret and sorrow about the past and the present, all she wanted to do was forget, return to her home and sleep.

"Goodnight, love," said Jonty and he started to clean the table.

The barman heard the outer door clash. He was alone at last, few minutes and he'd be out of the place. It had been a long and boring evening. "Too quiet for a Saturday night," he said gruffly, then remembered the band playing at the Colliery Club, "bloody *Flying Pickets!* No wonder!"

The kitchen light had been left on, the leaden spray of light was sufficient for Rebecca to see the outline of the steps. The remains of smashed particles of glass still radiated from the path days after the heated argument with her son. Her footsteps crunched and cracked against the crumbs and grains of debris as she stepped into her home, told herself that the paths would be cleaned the next day. Tomorrow, she promised herself, she would sweep the place tomorrow. *It's always tomorrow*, she mused.

The house was quiet. She walked from the kitchen to the living-room. A warm cheerful fire blazed in the grate, switched on the ceiling light, then immediately clicked it off. The place felt more comfortable with the fire glowing and the kitchen light filtering through, looked like it used to be, warm and cozy, a million years ago, nice and snug. Rebecca walked to the bottom of the stairs and called for her husband. The mattress groaned as the man altered his position and began to cough and moaned incoherently, made her smile, Adam was waiting for her, knew he would bark and growl and threaten when she slipped into the bed, knew that when she attempted to hold him he would bluster and push her away, only words, all a sham as he moved as far away from her as possible, cursing and belittling her. No contact or comfort from him, didn't love her, the marriage was over, he was leaving her, for definite this time. He'd said it over and over, lovely Adam, who would patiently wait until she slept and then would wrap his big powerful arms around her and gently caress her, loved her so much it hurt.

****

Linda MacDonald worked for *Spick-n-Span* home cleaners. There were six cleaners in total: four worked the Peterlee district and two females, Linda Macdonald and her mother, covered the Easington area. Linda was working in the Holme-Hill estate, a large private working-class estate situated on high ground overlooking the colliery and the sea. Like the young in general, Linda could not bear the sounds of silence and so the radio or television blasted incessantly, the girl unable to concentrate when it was quiet. *Jive Bunny* blasted relentlessly through the terraced property loud and clear despite the vacuum howling its presence. Linda was working and checking her wrist-watch, determined to see Charlie Hill. *Mister Recluse*, as she called him these days. He was definitely seeing someone and she had a shrewd idea it was his old flame, Jenny Bruce, she still recalled one of the last conversations she had with him, Charlie mentioning that he had *bumped* into Jenny at the dance, found out later, from Norma Jane Bradshaw, *Miss Poison-Tongue* of the colliery, that Charlie and Jenny had left the dance together.

At five-o-clock Linda left the house and hurried down the decline towards Seaside Lane, made a sharp left and headed along the steep colliery A streets … Avon, Argent … the pit buildings closing on her as the girl veered towards the shower-block. She wanted a face-to-face, needed to know the truth, if their relationship was over, fine. It would be nice to be told instead of waiting around like a pathetic wallflower, walked the floors for two whole weeks waiting from an appearance from Charlie Hill, declined offers from Henry Clarkson and his mate Eddie Cummins and she was waiting no longer. Henry Clarkson, taller and more handsome than his pal, was two years older than her, worked as a mechanic in one of the Peterlee factories and owned a brand new Fiesta, besotted he was, probably liked her more than Charlie Hill. Linda hadn't wept for a week, maybe her mother was right when she ridiculed her antics. *'There's a Jack for every Jill, our Linda, so stop bloody moping!'*

"Charlie?" she shouted as the group of colliers strolled from the pit-head baths.

A painful smile covered Charlie's features as he sauntered away from his friends. Linda was prepared, spent a lifetime watching and learning her mother's spoiling tactics whenever her parents battled, had seen her Ma on numerous occasions win arguments over her so-called wily, scheming husband. *'Pretend you know more than you know,'* said Sharon Macdonald to her bemused daughter. Always worked too, her dad, Micky MacDonald rarely won an argument with his wife.

"Linda!" Charlie's face chalked in stone, the grin now a definite grimace, lost for words, in a terrible quandary.

"I know all about it," she snapped, "been told by too many people!" stood in front of him, her arms placed aggressively on her hips, tousled head stuck high in the air. "Why didn't you tell me, Charlie, why should someone else have to tell me?"

He shrugged in defeat and the girl suddenly felt weak, eyes locked on one another. Charlie was the first to look away, shamefaced as he rubbed at imaginary stubble.

"Well," she barked, her body trembling, couldn't believe it was actually happening, dug a hole so deep for herself that she seemed unable to climb out. Standing so close to Charlie Hill, beautiful, sweet Charlie Hill and Henry Clarkson no longer seemed a proper substitute. Linda said, "I know who it is."

"I'm sorry, Linda."

"I heard about the farce at the dance!"

The youth was perplexed, "The dance?" he asked.

Linda said sarcastically, "The Welfare Dance, Charlie, don't treat me like a fool! I do know!"

He sighed and blew like a straining mule, his head downcast with embarrassment.

"Can't you say her name?" barked Linda Macdonald, thinking, *What do you see in Jenny Bruce?*

"I'm sorry, Linda," his reply soft and filled with remorse.

"You know how many times I've called at your house?" snapped Linda. "All the time I've known you, it's never been bolted!"

Charlie Hill shrugged his shoulders and looked away.

"Your door is never locked," she seethed, her tone venomous, her temper breaking, "nothing much to steal!"

The youth looked at her with a cold icy stare, his eyes wide, nodding slowly he said quietly, "Suppose you're right."

Linda Mac on a roll, past caring, "Always an open house in case mummy returns after one of her trips!"

Charlie Hill stiffened, glowering he hissed, "I should have told you about Anne Marie," then he turned and walked away.

Linda MacDonald stood frozen with shock and watched him go.

****

The argument between Adam and Becky Hill started with the smallest spark of whisper and innuendo. They'd had far worse over the long difficult years of their marriage. Sunday afternoon and the couple had just returned from an afternoon binge around the village, consumed their usual mid-day quota and were only slightly intoxicated. Rebecca was attempting to prepare a late lunch. She had not taken any drink midweek telling Adam she was a changed woman and would only socialize in future with her husband by her side. *'Joan was a mistake, Adam,'* said an indignant Rebecca, *'she nothing but trouble!'* The reality of the situation was more related to the fact that Joan Armstrong, her drinking companion, had disappeared off the radar screen. Rebecca's fault really. Weeks ago when she had imagined her son had seen her in Elvis's car she had bade a hasty retreat from her companions and lay low hoping the clouds of suspicion would eventually blow away. The nagging doubts, however, were all in her head because no one, least of all her son, had ever mentioned her absence or asked after her whereabouts.

"Spaghetti on toast," cried Adam, "so much for a Sunday lunch!"

Say another word! thought Becky Hill but said with a strained smile, "Eat up, Adam and I'll make something later."

For some unknown reason Adam started talking about Charlie. Their son was rarely at home these days, which, from Rebecca's point of view, was something of a blessing. When Charlie wasn't present there were few arguments between the two men. When her son was at home, the men constantly squabbled whenever the television was in operation. Charlie loved sport - any sport - and Adam enjoyed the *Soaps*. Rebecca wondered how long the television truce would last this time. *Last as long as he's courting,* thought the woman.

“I think he’s seeing someone” said Rebecca, prized open a bottle of stout and filled two glasses,” in fact, I know he is.”

“What’s new about that,” replied the husband as he accepted the drink, “he’s been sniffin’ around Micky MacDonald’s daughter for months.” Adam had a subtle way with words.

“Actually,” said Rebecca, “he’s seeing Betty Hickson’s daughter.”

“Charlie is seein’ Teddy’s bairn?”

“Anne Marie,” answered Becky, “poor bairn, all she went through with that pervert of a father.

Adam said, “Not her who was abused?”

“Yes,” retorted Becky, “Anne Marie.”

“Bloody hell,” said Adam Hill ruefully, shook his head, lifted the glass to his mouth and drank thirstily, studied a while then repeated the process, wiping his lips, the man said sarcastically, “takes after his mother then?”

“Who does?”

“Charlie,” mouthed Adam, a smirk filled his features.

“Charlie?” Rebecca couldn’t follow her husband’s logic, thought she might take a nap for a few hours, the break would do her good, Adam was becoming a pain.

“Seeing two at once,” snapped Adam Hill, supping noisily at the dregs in the glass, “two girls at the same time, does he not realize?”

“Spit it out, Adam,” said Rebecca, “say what you mean and don’t talk in riddles.”

“You know,” said Adam, an ugly glint in his eyes, “like his mother all those years ago. Surely you haven’t forgotten Becky, when *we* were courtin?” He emphasized *we.* “Becky and Adam and when Adam’s back was turned, it was Becky and Jimmy Shannon.”

She could only scowl, too many years had passed for her to become embroiled in any of the old arguments, a bloody lifetime ago - eighteen/nineteen years - and he still suffered. *'He walked me home, Adam. Nothing happened. He said he was sorry for hurting me and walked me home.'* The first few years of their marriage and her indiscretion was regularly vomited up with a vengeance by Adam and her defence always the same, '*How do you know that?'* she would ask. '*Who the hell told you that he walked me home, you followed didn't you, Adam, you were stalking me!* Then it would always stop, the recriminations repressed.

But not this day, for some unknown reason the man continued, perhaps a lifetime of festering and doubting came to the surface like a cauldron of spite and suppressed anger.

"If he was only walking you home, Rebecca," said Adam, uncharacteristically subdued, "how come you had arranged to meet him again, why would you want to meet Jimmy Shannon for a second time?"

Her features clouded with guilt. 'You knew, all these years and you knew*?'* Rebecca gulped unconsciously, her mouth suddenly dry. *God, the man knows……….*

She managed to gasp, "Why on earth would you want to talk about Jimmy Shannon, he's dead and buried!"

"The thought of Charlie playing with two lives," said the man grudgingly, "Linda and Anne Marie. The scallywag doesn't realise the sufferin' he's inflictin' on those girls," grasped the packet of cigarettes and took two out, one was handed to Rebecca. She took the cigarette thinking that it was a signal for the cessation of the feuding. The woman was wrong, Adam continued. "Brought it all back, you and me, thought we were an item and that you'd forgotten the little swine then he breezes back into your life and snaps his fingers and you run to him!" The man shook his head. "And you agreed to meet him again, never a thought about me."

She was beaten, too tired of denials. Rebecca lit her cigarette and sucked heavily, stared at her husband, mute, waiting.

"How long did you wait for your lover, Becky," he didn't pause for an answer, "shall I tell you, you want to know … two hours. I was there, watching."

She continued to stare morosely. *God,* she thought, *he knows it all.*

"You want to know why he didn't show, Becky?" said Adam, his smile manic, "I put him in hospital…….."

The door banged open and Charlie appeared. He was in a hurry; Elvis Priestley wanted to see him but Charlie had decided he no longer wanted to work for the man, the jobs were too dangerous and Charlie was determined to stop his criminal ways, wanting the relationship with Anne Marie to be permanent; he didn't wish to spoil it with any illegal activities and wanted to start afresh. She was a wonderful girl, never met anyone like her and he felt so in love. They had been sleeping together at Anne Marie's flat for weeks and the ecstasy between the pair was spiralling to the heavens. The feeling was electric, surreal and he had decided to tell his parents.

"Okay?" he grinned at the grim couple. There was no response from his parents. *Nothing changes*, he thought. *Easington's own Vietnam!*

Adam Hill eased off the seat and stood head and shoulders above the diminutive youth, glowered at Charlie, wanting to say so much, then turned without speaking and left the room. The staircase groaned as the man thumped his way to the bedroom.

"Happy Families, Ma?" he said whimsically.

“Happy bloody families, Charlie!” seethed the woman, walked into the kitchen and grabbed another beer, returned to the living-room and sat heavily in the arm-chair next to the fireplace. She fumbled at the packet of cigarettes, visibly annoyed. *Twenty bloody years,* she thought and *the bastard still can’t let it die!* Rebecca Hill sucked hard on the smoke and glared at the spitting coals, could not find the strength to speak.

“Ma,” said the youth, “what’s wrong with the old man?”

“You don’t want to know son,” she whispered, “you don’t want to know.”

“What’s up, Ma?”

Why the hell can’t you grow a few more inches, Charlie, thought Rebecca, *Just a few more inches.*

****

CHAPTER FIFTEEN

Sheryl brought in the refreshments and placed the steel tray, laden with two large mugs of steaming tea and an assortment of snacks, on the small table next to the seated figure of Charlie. The couple sat in the small living-room adjoining the shop. Elvis, Sheryl's grandfather, was in the lavatory, complained earlier of an upset stomach. Ten long minutes the youth had waited before Sheryl finally poured refreshments, purposely stooped so close to Charlie to display her ample cleavage, teasing the lad, wearing her favourite pink bra which contrasted against the dark skin. The beautiful girl tantalizing as she flaunted and paraded in front of a besotted Charlie, the garish undergarment glowing seductively against the young tanned skin, eyes meeting, the young couple smiling at one another. Sheryl the seductress, winning every time.

"The real Elvis died on the lavatory," said the youth, immediately regretting his choice of conversation, the girl causing all manner of problems to his head, couldn't think straight, his body pumping with a heady mix of adrenalin and hormones as he tried to fight off his natural bodily urges. *You're supposed to love Anne Marie,* words shouted inside his head, *why are you thinking about Sheryl's breasts? Concentrate, Charlie! Concentrate!* He leaned forwards and rested his elbows on his thighs, mortified by a growing and very obvious erection.

"Granddad lives in the toilet," Sheryl answered softly, her eyes focused provocatively on the youth, "can't blame him," she smiled warmly and showed dazzling white teeth, "the amount of food he puts away in one day could feed an African for a month. Have you seen the size of his waist?"

"Can't say I've noticed," spluttered Charlie Hill, a faint hue of colour filtered across his features.

Sheryl stood erect, patting her minuscule waistline, "You think I've got a nice waist Charlie?" she purred, flattered by his attention.

The conversation ceased as the bulky figure of Elvis Priestley strolled in to the room; the man glanced knowingly at his precious black pearl, forced a smile and then told her to help her mother in the shop. Sheryl momentarily ignored the order, she was as feisty as her granddad when the mood took her.

Sheryl said haughtily, "I was telling Charlie that you'd written to that agency in Newcastle," and she grinned mischievously, glancing from her grandfather to the boy. "Tell him grandpa!"

It was only a little white lie and her way of broadcasting the news, old enough to know she could turn heads at the drop of a hat, old and young, knew she had the looks and the voluptuous body to fill any sleazy magazine, had her eyes set on a modelling career and would do anything to achieve her goal. Anything. A child with a head mature enough to recognise the power she wielded over the opposite sex and despite her lack of stature she oozed confidence, personality and sexual chemistry. Sheryl was going places and her rich granddad had the necessary financial clout to place her on the first rung of the commercial ladder.

"Another time, Sheryl," smiled Elvis as he struggled to place his bulk in to the chair, "Charlie and I are talking business."

"He knows Gordon Sumner," she pouted proudly, glanced at the older figure, "don't you, Granddad?"

Elvis hated being reminded of his looming old age. "What have I said about my name, Sheryl, for Christ's Sake!"

"Sorry. Elvis," replied the girl taking her leave, "but tell Charlie about Gordon Sumner, you said he was a personal friend?"

"Gordon Sumner?" asked the youth. *Who the hell is Gordon Sumner?*

"Sting," said Elvis, told more lies than Pinocchio when he had to prove a point. "*The Police?*" anything to pacify Sheryl, "now go and help your mother!"

"Tell him about Robson Green out of *Casualty*?" continued the girl, propping open the shop-door, work was the last thing on her young mind. "You know, the actor."

Elvis had read somewhere that the artist lived near Newcastle. Damn and blast if he could remember where. Months ago, after a particularly heavy drinking session at Newcastle's Quayside, he blurted out that he'd been drinking with the fellow, never thinking he'd be queried about his fictitious drinking companion, never short of an answer he had blurted out, *'Jesmond. Robson has a place just north of the city!'* could have said black was white and people believed him. *'Robson Green, a genuine man, salt of the earth!'* No one questioned him after telling tall tales so easily. Name-dropping was becoming a regular pass-time for Elvis, especially when the conversation dried-up, lied out of his teeth and no one queried him, that's what driving a top-of-the-range Jaguar, owning properties and a pocketful of money in the bank did for you; suckers believed anything; money talks.

"Little Robson," sighed the chubby proprietor, then he barked with frustration, "Sheryl, will you please bugger off and leave me to do some business!"

The female stormed out of the room, almost taking the door off its hinges, so infuriated with her grandfather. Sheryl had a short fuse.

Elvis started the patter. It would be, he assured Charlie, the last time he would ask a favour. The job was a doddle, easy-peasy. All the lad had to do was sit in Elvis's car while he drove to Crook.

'*Crook*,' said Charlie. '*Where the hell is that?*' Charlie's C.V. was limited to arson, criminal damage and G.B.H. Elvis explained that it was only a short drive away - west of Durham and all the lad had to do was collect the car and drive it back to Elvis's shop.

'*It's money for old rope, Charlie,*' said a conniving Elvis Priestley. '*All you have to do is drive the car back to Easington.*'

The vehicle was a beautiful *B.M.W.* and as black as his granddaughter and just as stunning. He had sold the car eighteen months ago, long enough for the link between him and the vehicle to be forgotten. As a matter of business acumen Elvis always had extra keys cut and labelled for possible future reference. '*Good business practice*,' spouted the hoodlum, wanted Charlie to take the vehicle from the driveway of the property and deliver it to the rear of Elvis's shop. He had a garage large enough to house a *Sherman* tank, so the *B.M.W.* would not be a problem. '*Come on, Charlie. One more for old Elvis*.' He was so persuasive, especially when he handed over the wad of cash.

'*I'll get caught, Elvis*,' protested the youth, '*and then I'll be in shit-creek*.'

But Elvis had the gift of the gab, could sell sand to the Arabs, explained that the unfortunate couple who were about to lose their vehicle were on holiday in America so there was virtually no risk. '*The house-lights will be on, but they're on a bloody timer, Charlie. Trust me?*'

"I'll do it, Elvis," said Charlie hesitantly, like a qualified bank-teller, as he expertly counted the cash. "What time do you want me?"

"Call back in a few hours," said Elvis.

****

Eight-o-clock and Adam was still sulking upstairs. Her son, Charlie had disappeared, probably whisked away by his new love, the blonde and feisty, Anne Marie. *Knows what she wants and gets it*, thought the woman as she sat quietly in the living-room. *Strange,* thought Rebecca, *the way some folks, despite all the damage and muck thrown at them, come out unscathed. Nothing stuck, like water off a duck's back, no mess, no memories ... what did the Americans call it, Teflon, that was it. Anne Marie was covered in it,* made her feel jealous. She pictured Anne Marie lying awake in bed at night, wondered if the demons still visited her like they visited Rebecca. She sighed, her mind made up; she was going out for a few drinks, there was no point in attempting to ambush Adam into an armistice, knew well enough how the ploy would end, no doubt about the outcome … both in the double bed for a ten-minute play, fine for Adam but all that sweat and groaning and feigning falseness followed by the washing and changing. Thanks, but no thanks, Adam wanted to spit out his dummy, fine! Rebecca washed her face, applied make-up and left the house, walked slowly through the streets of the village thinking about her husband. All of those years together and not once had he admitted knowledge about her indiscretion with Jimmy Shannon. '*I put him in hospital,*' that's what he'd admitted, '*Put Jimmy in hospital*.' No wonder he didn't show, but how on earth did Adam find out, must have followed them from the *Kings Head* every step of the way. She reminisced, remembered how Jimmy Shannon had walked her to the back-door of her parent's home, out of sight of the road, the pair of them pressed tight against the wall as Jimmy seduced her, said he loved only her, only ever wanted to marry Rebecca. *'She's pregnant, Becky. Ruby is three months pregnant. I've got to do the right thing*.' Jimmy married his little Ruby: Becky married Adam. *Bloody life*, thought Becky and she pushed open the pub door, *'two boys born so close together, one as daft as a brush, the other, so perfect. The bloody irony of it all!'*

****

The Jaguar pulled to a stop in the centre of Crook. It was a little after ten and the street lights shone murky strobes of light about the deserted junction. Charlie Hill could see the lines of shops following the main highway, no large supermarkets only small shops boxed tight next to each other. Elvis pointed to the side road snaking north from the crossroads, told him to walk along the road until he reached the restaurant. Mohammed Khan, the owner of the desired *B.M.W.* lived above the small rooms. The Khans, however, were on holiday and the lights were operated by a timer. Elvis handed Charlie the single key, still giving instructions to the lad, *'Take your time, Charlie and keep to the speed limits and remember, lights and indicators, use them!'*

The lights shone a hazy shadow against the heavy drapes. The big car was parked with its off-side wheels over the small path. Charlie's head was screaming with fear and panic, imagining at any moment someone intervening and grabbing him. *Do it now! Put the key in the door and get in the car.* He eased into the vehicle, his body trembling and running with perspiration, fingers shaking uncontrollably as he struggled to fit the key. The engine purred into life. He engaged the gears and drove slowly away, no shouting or screaming followed; no whining sirens echoed over the lonely streets. He headed for Durham and home.

Half-an-hour later and he turned off Seaside Lane and into the Waterworks council houses, drove past the grocery shop and slowed the *B.M.W.* The vehicle purred like some magnificent sleek beast, Charlie Hill ecstatic and jubilant that the evening had ended so well. As he turned in to the back street his entry into Elvis's rear yard and garage was blocked by the revving taxi-cab, cursing his ill-fortune, Charlie was forced to temporarily park further along the lane. He saw Irene, Elvis's ancient daughter struggle out of the vehicle. *Booze or bingo*, thought the youth as he passed her, walked into the yard and knocked at the door. Irene was still paying the fare when Elvis Priestley opened the door. He was in his dressing-gown and looked so old without the armour and disguise of clothing. Irene bustled past nodding and scowling at the two men, grunted something inaudible to her father and disappeared into the interior of the place.

"Everything okay, Charlie?" asked the proprietor gingerly, looking over the youth's shoulder.

"Fine," said the youth, "but the motor is further down the street. Irene's taxi was blocking the way into your garage."

"Not a problem, son," said the wheezing figure then his breath stopped and his mouth dropped with alarm.

A big police cruiser eased past the rear entrance of the shop. It started slowing as it past the rear entrance, brake lights glowing and indicators signalling.

"Damn," muttered Elvis as he dragged the boy into the kitchen, closed the door and extinguished the light, "you must have been followed!"

Charlie was incredulous at the insinuation, "Not a chance, Elvis," he grunted, heart racing against his chest, "I checked all the way back. No one followed me at all; I swear, nothing was behind me!"

Elvis scratched at his head, pushing aside the terror, trying to think logically. "The black bastard," he said angrily, "that bloody Mohammed must have installed a tracker device!"

"What we gonna do," Charlie in turmoil as he started to panic, "I ain't ready for jail!"

"Right," said a resolute Elvis. "I've got a plan." He eyeballed the youth, said tenaciously, "and it'll work if you've got the balls to do it!"

Charlie listened wide-eyed as he was bundled through the home and into the shop, the door was carefully opened and Charlie was free. '*It all depends on you Charlie,'* Elvis's last words as the shop-door closed on the youth. Charlie Hill walked slowly and casually from the premises, his head down, hands pushed deep inside coat-pockets away from the premises and headed in a wide circle for the back lane and the stolen vehicle, his young head bursting with fear. *It all depends on you, Charlie. It all depends on you.*

The two uniformed officers radioed for information. They had followed the vehicle from Durham, stayed well back and out of sight so as not to create panic amongst the thieves, followed the tracking device right into the heart of the small coastal colliery. It was parked up near to the top of a back lane. The *B.M.W.* was empty and the thief or thieves were somewhere close. They waited only minutes before they stepped from the police-vehicle, both had been directed to the small grocery store at the end of the street. Edward Priestley owned the business. He was a known criminal, thief, arsonist and a very violent man, the luckiest man on the planet, never even collected a parking ticket. One of the officers smiled, thinking the low-life had finally used up his nine lives. One policeman entered the rear yard of the premises, the other walked purposefully past the house, turned a hard left and started hurrying up the small incline, left again and he'd be at the front shop, blocking any attempt at escape, neither of the constables paid any attention to the approaching youth, too interested in snaring the big fish that was Edward Aaron Priestley.

Elvis was in his granddaughter's bedroom. Sheryl was wide awake and still watching television. Elvis had already warned his daughter Irene to stay in her room, now he was priming his lovely and receptive black pearl. Elvis offered Sheryl everything and anything, whatever her heart desired he would deliver. The girl believed her grandpa, followed his instructions to the letter. Elvis waited outside her bedroom door as she stripped out of her dowdy pajamas and pulled on her risqué see-through negligee, told not to wear any undergarments.

With Elvis standing stiff as a wheezing statue, trying unsuccessfully to hold his breath, Sheryl waltzed past him, smiling broadly; this was one show she would relish. The girl breezed to the rear door. The officer had been knocking for some moments and was becoming more agitated by the slow response from the residents. *Can't hide the evidence this time, Eddie. It's parked up outside*, thought the uniformed man, smiling broadly as the door opened and the light flickered on.

"D.C. O'Brian, love…" and the words died in his mouth. Before him stood an angel, a beautiful black and near naked angel from heaven. The girl was young; fourteen, fifteen, who could tell these days and wore the flimsiest of nightshirts, so sheer that the gaping officer could plainly see the full firm shape of her breasts, the dark luxuriant foliage between her thighs at the top of her very long and slender legs. He tried to look away but was mesmerized by the beautiful sight before him.

Sheryl rubbed at her eyes, looking so weary and confused and such an actress as she pushed fingers through her thick crinkled locks, lifting her nightdress in the process, exposing, for the briefest of moments, her thick pubic hair. The policeman almost swooned with pleasure as he feasted on the prize, couldn't stop himself from moaning under his breath.

"What's the matter, mister," muttered a well-rehearsed Sheryl, "what do you want?"

"Could I have a word with your Dad, love?" asked the officer, at last regaining some of his composure.

"My Dad," mumbled Sheryl, looking perplexed, "I've never ever seen my Dad in my whole life!" She folded her arms defensively.

The door at the front of the shop was hammered noisily, as if on cue, the girl turned her back on the policeman and slid away from the rear door towards the shop-front. "You'd better come in," she said sleepily and then added, "will you please close the door after you?"

D.C. O'Brian stepped into the kitchen but forgot to close the door, followed the siren like a lost puppy through the winding maze of interior rooms, his eyes locked on the small tight rump. Sheryl unlocked the shop-door and allowed the second officer - a novice P.C. - into the premises. P.C. Stoker looked hungrily at the young girl and then at his senior partner. He was speechless.

"I'll wake up my Granddad," sighed Sheryl, sleepily, "he's not very well."

Outside, in the dark of the back road, Charlie was on his hands and knees searching for the key. His jittery nerves had got the better of him and as he had opened the door of the vehicle he had fumbled and then dropped the car-key. Like panning for hidden gold, the youth scraped at the road surface vainly searching for the missing object, tears in his eyes, moaning incoherently, convinced he was about to be arrested. Then his fingers touched the prize and he was back in business. He jumped into the limo and in his haste to drive away, revved the motor. Cursing loudly, the youth skidded and roared down the street. The noise of the disappearing car echoed through the silent house as a bedraggled Elvis made an appearance before the officers. Without a word of explanation the two uniforms bolted for the back-door and ran wildly through the rear yard. Elvis grasped at the girl, cuddled her like he had never done before. "I owe you one, love," he whispered, "I'll never forget what you've done for me."

The big police vehicle screamed after the disappearing tail-lights of the stolen car, along the street they shot, shouting into the radio for back-up. Charlie, out of sight for a few seconds, turned the vehicle left and double-backed on the police-car, driving parallel but in the opposite direction. He knew the car had a *tracker* so he had to ditch the car within minutes otherwise he would be caught.

His lights were left out purposefully. As he tore up the quiet street he could see the police vehicle roaring in the converse direction: lights cascading: siren blaring. He had to get out of the housing estate. Reaching the apex of the road Charlie turned and drove as fast as he could towards the main coastal road, skidded wildly into Seaside Lane and headed for *Pearce's Garage* which bordered the road to the west of the colliery. Into the deserted blackened forecourt the *B.M.W.* was swiftly manoeuvered. Charlie pulled off one of his shoes, dragged off a sock and proceeded to wipe away all the evidence from the interior of the motor, out of the vehicle, the youth scrubbed wildly at the door-handle, the windows, everything touchable was scoured manically. In the near distance he could hear the approaching police-cruiser, grabbing and fumbling with his shoe, the youth ran for his life, the sock still in his hand, across the deserted forecourt, scrambling into the terraced back-lane, up the steep incline, across a minor road and away towards the nearby village.

The police-car overshot the garage, P.C. Stoker screaming at the top of his voice, 'There it is, there's the *B.M.W.!*' the cruiser skidding and bouncing across the road. D.C. O'Brian bawled out to his apprentice to examine the stolen car, check the garage and listen for any unusual noises. *'Do it now! Go!'* the senior officer driving swiftly towards the coastal colliery, determined to catch the criminal gang no matter how long it took. Two miles away, on the coastal road, a second police vehicle, travelling in the opposite direction, summoned from Peterlee, raced towards Easington, the officers determined they would apprehend the crooks.

Charlie Hill, walking now, soaked with perspiration, entered his back yard, breathless but euphoric after evading capture, the youth vowed never again to commit further criminal acts, it was finally over, Elvis could do his own dirty work in future, walked through the door to be confronted by the distressing sight of his father.

"Ma's gone again," he moaned, "it's my fault this time, son."

Adam didn't seem to notice the state of the youngster whose face was blotchy and reddened, features running with sweat; even the flimsy jacket was stained and discoloured under the armpits. Adam Hill preoccupied and in a deep state of depression could only think about his missing wife. Charlie squatted on the kitchen-chair, kicked off a shoe and pulled on the sock. The shoe was replaced, the older man oblivious to the distress of the youth.

"Your mother…." he lifted the pint glass to his lips and drained it in noisy gulps.

"Right, dad, I understand," muttered Charlie, removed his jacket and wiped his face with the garment, "Ma's gone again!"

****

CHAPTER SIXTEEN

The door burst open and whacked noisily against the kitchen wall, Rebecca, so intoxicated and exhausted almost stumbled to the floor, she staggered into the living-room, eyes glazed and dull, spittle covered her lips, drunk, demonised and spoiling for a fight.

"Have you missed me, boys," she gasped spitefully and glared at her son and her husband, "although it's only been a day, hasn't it?"

Charlie was weary and the last thing he wanted was an argument. He needed to go to bed. "Ma," he said wearily, "I'll make you some tea."

Rebecca bawled, "I don't want any tea!"

Charlie Hill said resignedly, "I'm goin' to bed, Ma," glanced at his scowling father and added hopefully, "see you tomorrow," and strode towards the stairs.

"You'll stay and hear what I have to say," whined Rebecca, "and you," her tone lifted with anger and frustration as she looked daggers at Adam, "it's about time you had the courage of your convictions for once in your bloody life!"

Charlie glanced at his mother then his father, curious enough to stay and listen.

"Nowt to say!" muttered Adam, stood and back-pedalled towards the kitchen.

Rebecca looked at her perplexed son, said coldly, "The row the other night concerned you Charlie!"

The youth shrugged his shoulders and replied sarcastically, "Does there have to be a reason for the pair of you to argue?"

The woman smirked and glowered at her son, “You’ll want to know, Charlie,” she grunted, “you’ll really want to know!”

Charlie shrugged his shoulders, almost seventeen years of age he’d known little else but trouble and strife between his warring parents. He had imagined the earlier argument was simply a spat between his parents, the usual tit-for tat squabble with his mother usually losing the battle; naturally, it was almost always her fault. Rebecca strode after her husband beckoning Charlie to follow. The boy obeyed.

“Adam, haven’t you got something you want to get off your chest?” she shouted.

Adam Hill eased past his fuming spouse, returned to the living-room, flopped into an arm-chair and stared into the embers of the fire. He started to shake his head from side to side and refused to be drawn into the fracas. Rebecca stood swaying, glowering at her husband. Charlie glanced from one to the other, perplexed. He was so tired, *Jesus,* he thought, *another night!* His mother motioned for him to sit and he reluctantly squatted on the edge of the sofa.

Rebecca said bitterly, “Not angry enough to start barking, Adam, not had enough beer down your gullet to start with the poison?”

“Let it go, woman.”

“Ma?”

“You won’t talk, Adam Hill,” spluttered Rebecca, ignoring her son, “even though you’ve tortured me for almost twenty years? Tell him, Adam; tell Charlie what you really think of him! Go on, Adam. You’ve punished him since he was a bairn, any excuse and you were there like a bloody devil with a stick or a strap!”

Charlie was starting to feel uneasy; he'd never known an argument manipulated in such a way. Past quarrels concerning him tended to be about his bad behaviour - brawling, stealing, infuriated neighbours and ultimately his involvement with the police - the usual antics of an immature and out-of-control youth. This time it was different. Charlie could sense it, stole a glance at his dad whose head appeared permanently bowed with the weight of grief.

"Ma," he asked, "what's happened?"

"You'd better start talking, Adam Hill," said the woman, strode from the room and entered the kitchen.

Both men could hear the bottle-opener being used, the distinct sound as beer was poured into a glass.

Adam spoke at last, his words laconic and almost inaudible. "Charlie, take no notice of your mother, she's had too much to drink."

Push come to shove and the man was lukewarm about rekindling old wounds, regretting the earlier confrontation with his wife; Adam Hill wanted to take the heat out of the ancient squabble, glanced momentarily at the boy and remembered why he had erupted again, why the past had been resurrected, with all the associated bile and hatred spilling from his lips. It had been about Charlie, Charlie messing with people, intentionally or otherwise, hurting two decent girls; Linda Macdonald and Anne Marie Hickson. Did Charlie not realize the pain he was inflicting on innocent lives?

The woman returned with added fire in her belly, twenty years of simmering and holding-back, the eruption imminent as she stood smouldering between them. She drained her glass in one go.

"When I married your father, Charlie", her words came out soft yet resolute. "I thought I loved someone else." Rebecca waited for any response, glancing from one adult to the other. Her son was staring strangely at her; Adam, seemingly lost in the dying flames of the fire, his hands clenched tightly into fists. "No, that's a lie. I did love someone else. He was my very first love; we were going to be married…."

"Ma," stuttered Charlie, "Where is this goin'?"

"His name was Jimmy Shannon," said Rebecca, growing in confidence. She faced her son, "You'll know his family, Charlie. He had a son … brain-damaged at birth. Harry Shannon? Ruby Wright is his mother, well, Ruby Shannon now." She was gawking at her son, the alcohol controlling and guiding and she no longer cared about the consequences. "Charlie, I was engaged to Jimmy Shannon; we were going to be married and do you know what happened, shall I tell you what happened, Charlie?"

"Let it go, woman!" grunted Adam and he tried to stand.

Like someone possessed, Rebecca was next to him, forcing him back on the chair, threatening him. Adam squirmed uncomfortably and stared wilfully at his wife but he remained seated, his hands gripping both corners of the chair.

"Jimmy Shannon married someone else!" rasped the man defiantly.

"Shut up!" shrieked Rebecca so loud that Charlie jumped with shock. "Shut up! It wasn't like that!"

"Get on with it, then," muttered a chastened Adam. "Get on with the bloody story."

"Ruby was pregnant with Jimmy's bairn, so he called off our wedding and married her," shrieked the woman, her voice breaking with emotion. "That was the kind of man he was! Loyal!"

Adam could not contain himself any longer, jumping to his feet he screamed, “Tell the truth woman, he was a ladies-man; chase anythin’ in a skirt, the little bastard!”

Charlie felt his skin crawl at the mention of the fellow’s size. The dawning realization cut him; he grimaced and squirmed with discomfort, wanted to run away but couldn’t move.

“He loved me!” said Rebecca proudly.

“He used you,” retorted Adam Hill, “a bloody married man still interested in you!” He guffawed and added, “And what did *you* do, woman?” Adam took a deep breath, “Jimmy Shannon shows up out of the blue, talks his usual bullshit and waltzes you home!” His voice rose in anger, “You were with *me!* It was supposed to be you and me! And then … and then arrange *another* bloody meeting with him!” Adam started stomping about the room. “Supposed to be with me and you arrange to see the little bastard again!”

It was as if Charlie was no longer present as both adults attacked one another.

“You made damn sure he couldn’t see me again, Adam Hill!”

“I should have broken his damn neck not his legs!” replied Adam willfully.

“Didn’t stop you crucifying me for the next twenty bloody years!”

“Maybe I had cause enough?”

“Say what you really mean, Adam,” her tone softened suddenly, tainted with sarcasm, “lost your nerve, Adam Hill, haven’t you got something to say to Charlie?”

The adult flushed the colour of crimson, looked as if he would burst; his eyes were wide and bright with anger, glared at the woman and then the youth, mute with frustration and vexation, his eyes moved again to the boy, his hand involuntary clawed at his mouth, his courage failed him and he could not say the words he wanted to say. *I don't know if you are my son, Charlie!* His head screamed with the nightmare, *I want you to be my son, but I don't know!* tortured with uncertainty, Adam Hill said nothing.

Charlie Hill, tough as old boots, started to weep; he stood and left the room, grabbed his coat and stumbled disoriented and confused from the house, his mind dancing out of control in a terrified state of flux. It was no longer his home. He didn't want them as parents, they had abused and deprived him and made him what he was today, a violent, arrogant, ignorant rogue, disliked and despised by most people. He walked slowly and purposefully through the lonely streets of the village, reached the telephone-kiosk, his hands shaking as he lifted the receiver. For some moments Charlie could not remember the girl's name. He began to shake with panic and then it came to him: Anne Marie Hickson. He started to dial her telephone number then paused, couldn't recall her number. The same girl he telephoned each night, her personal number imprinted in his head, but his mind was a blank, *'Anne Marie!'* he called out aloud, *'Anne Marie!'* trying to jog his memory, but couldn't recall a single digit.

Charlie needed her company badly, wanted to share his dilemma with her, missed Anne Marie so much. Over the past weeks she had hinted that their relationship could develop if they started living together. He'd laughed initially but the more he thought about it the more he welcomed the idea. He really needed her tonight. *'What the hell is your number!'* he cried, held the phone tightly in his hands so confused, so many things happening so fast, it scared him. Charlie slowly replaced the receiver.

He walked to the apex of the Village green; saw the looming outline of the huge Minster with Clappersgate to the left of the church and the *Seven-Sisters* public house to the right and, in front of the youth, the large council-bench with its canopied roof. Charlie strode towards the beloved seat, slumped heavily on the bench and gazed down across the empty Village; his head in turmoil, *My dad is not really my dad? My mother has been a drunk for most of her life because she married someone she didn't love, had a child to another man? Ma out of her mind because she lost someone but still had his child? Was that child me, Charlie Hill is really Charlie Shannon, who had a brother, an older brother! The same Harry Shannon who I've ridiculed and tormented since I was a kid? Harry and me, we're the same blood?*

He could not rest. The big clock on the church tower said it was midnight and he realized his weariness had disappeared and his exhaustion replaced with so much energy he was unable to stay still. Charlie began manically pacing back and forth, couldn't stop himself, unable to rest, burning with adrenalin. *'What can I do*, he mused, *where do I go?* Knew he couldn't stay in the Village and had to get as far away from his parents as possible, annoyed that he had forgotten Anne Marie's telephone number. *'I'll walk to her house,'* he shouted triumphantly. Peterlee was a little over a mile away, the journey straightforward, past Clappersgate, the *Half-Moon* pub and then he would skirt the A19, it would take ten, fifteen minutes at the most. He needed to walk and think.

As he turned the corner that led past the church he froze in his tracks. Harry Shannon was outside his home, leaning lethargically against the gate, gazing into the heavens. Harry Shannon of all people, striped pajamas and the regulation battered hat stuck on top of his tousled head staring at the stars.

Charlie did not know what to do, his mind dancing with all kinds of weird images. Fate playing cruel tricks on him as he stood welded to the ground staring at the lonely figure, confused and concerned and hesitant.

Harry Shannon came out of his self-imposed stupor and glanced alarmingly at the stranger. Fearing the worst, he grasped his fedora from his head and held it to his chest, stalemate and stillness between the two youths as their eyes locked on one another, then some inner resolve returned to Charlie and he started walking slowly along the street towards the older lad, spoke to Harry Shannon, calling him by his name, the rudeness and immaturity of yesteryear replaced with kind words and reassurances. Harry, sceptical and frightened, stood stiff watching his old adversary close on him.

Too much for the chubby imbecile, Harry Shannon abruptly shrieked in panic, howled for his mother and bolted for the back door of his home. A door cracked open and a huge figure, with nightshirt and dressing-gown flapping wildly, waddled bravely to the boy's aid. Ruby Shannon was irritated and alarmed at the stranger's presence and immediately began barking and threatening the unwelcome visitor. Charlie Hill lifted both arms in a calming gesture and started walking away then stopped, suddenly steadfast and tenacious he faced the irate woman. He started talking, unable to stop himself; it was as if someone was inside his head and speaking for him. Harry disappeared into the safety of his home leaving Ruby Shannon open-mouthed with incredulity, listening to the young stranger, who, after some frantic minutes of initial panic, started nodding acknowledgement. She recognized the lad, *'It's Rebecca Hill's son',* she said. *'Young Charlie.'*

She took him into her home; the woman had heard enough of the rambling almost incoherent sermon from Charlie and pulled him gently into the warmth of her house, all the while calming him, shaking her head in sympathy, *'Shh! It's not true, honey,'* Ruby Shannon comforted the distraught lad with soothing words, *'all these thing you've heard are wrong. Come inside, I'll make some tea and I'll tell you the truth.'*

They sat in the cluttered kitchen, opposite one another, drinking tea; Harry was safely upstairs in his bedroom, watching television. Ruby said, "Harry can't sleep much. Whenever he gets the chance he wanders, sometimes for hours. I used to worry sick about him, but not anymore. He's a good boy really," decided not to steer the conversation away from her boy, wasn't important to mention his occasional lapses, some things were best left unsaid. She looked at Charlie Hill, such a fine-looking boy, saw the pain and despair in his eyes and decided to open her heart to the youth. Ruby had told few people the truth about her late husband, or their sham of a marriage. He needed to know everything, for his own well-being. Charlie Hill should hear the true story about the infamous Jimmy Shannon. ....

'All the things your father said about my late husband were true. Jimmy was not a nice man. He was cruel and selfish, full of his own self-importance. He had the looks and the charm of a film star. Knew it too, maybe that was his downfall, thought he was something special. I was seeing someone else when Jimmy came on the scene. He was a good man and I left him for Jimmy Shannon. I couldn't resist all the attention and adoration that he heaped on me, Charlie. It was the biggest mistake of my life.' She stood and walked to a large bureau, pulled open a drawer and fished out a photograph and handed it to the youth. It was old and the edges had yellowed with age. A young attractive couple smiled at the camera: two happy people. Charlie reckoned the man was Jimmy Shannon.

'*That's us*,' she said and the boy looked again at the dark-haired girl beauty with the svelte-like figure, then he glanced up at the bloated figure; at the moon-shaped and blotched face. It was hard to believe Ruby had ever been so stunning.

'I was pregnant and I honestly thought Jimmy was the father.' Ruby looked at the youth. '*I called to see your mother. I knew she was engaged to Jimmy Shannon but I was pregnant! I called at your home Charlie, told her the situation, thought there'd be hell to pay. Not a word from your Ma. Only tears.*' The woman took the photo from the boy and inspected it closely as if drawing from the memory. '*And that was an end of it all or so I thought. I can't remember when, but your father came to see me, told me Jimmy had been trying to resurrect the relationship between your mother and him. I knew nothing about it, didn't have a clue. Your father was angry, left word for Jimmy to stay away from your mother, or else! When I told Jimmy that Adam Hill had called he laughed, made light of it, denied everything. A few days later Jimmy was involved in an accident, well, that's what he told me at the time. In hospital for weeks, two broken legs and cracked ribs! Thought he'd been hit by a bus!* Ruby sighed loudly. *'He was always an arrogant little man.* The woman shook her head resignedly and bit her lip. *I heard later that Rebecca had married Adam Hill and then you were born Charlie. I thought everything was okay.'*

Charlie stammered and spluttered his way through his mother's anguished confessional. *'Ma thinks I'm a Shannon not a Hill,'* said the youth, his head downcast with shame. *'Ma said your husband is my father!'* He was burning with discomfort and embarrassment.

The woman smiled warmly and touched his hand trying to comfort and ease him. *'Nothing could be further from the truth, Charlie. You see, my husband wanted more children, especially after the disappointment of Harry. Three years we tried and he kept blaming me, even hit me once. I went to see the specialist at Dryburn Hospital. Not a thing wrong with me! It was him! He found out that he was sterile, not one little tadpole to his name! Apparently the hospital checked all of his old medical records and he'd contacted mumps when he was twelve, wiped him clean. He was impotent.'* Charlie looked amazed. Ruby continued. *'Jimmy was livid and told the doctors they were a bunch of idiots, told them that he had a son - Harry - and that's when we found out the truth. Harry wasn't his son. I thought he was. I honestly thought Harry was Jimmy's son. I'd just ended an affair with Tommy Russell ... you'll know his father, Ben Russell, the milk-man? I thought my world was over, thought Jimmy would leave and start afresh but he stayed. That's when the drinking got out of hand.'* Ruby grimaced, *'Do you understand what I'm saying, Charlie. My boy Harry is Tommy Russell's son! I could never understand why Jimmy Shannon stayed with me, bad enough knowing someone isn't your flesh and blood, but Harry was born brain-damaged. It was a heavy burden for Jimmy to carry ... too much for him. His drinking went from bad to worse, every night he was out on the town, enjoying himself, paralytic most nights.'* She concluded. *'You'll know the rest. Walked in front of a car one night and was killed instantly.'*

"Ma seemed to think he was a decent man," said Charlie

'Tell your mother,' said Ruby, *'when Jimmy Shannon was married to me he never once stopped chasing women. Even before he found out about Harry he had countless affairs. He used people, Charlie, cared about no one but himself. Your mother would have been another casualty.'* Ruby stood, asked Charlie if he would like more refreshment. The youth refused,

too interested in the history lesson, she returned to her seat and continued with the reminiscences. *'I remember one night coming back from the hospital after visiting Jimmy and Maurice Johnstone was waiting at the gate. Maurice and Milly,'* explained Ruby, *'were good friends years ago, we used to do the usual socialising. The four of us would call at the Workingman's Club every Saturday night. Milly and I would often shop together ... good friends they were. Well, this particular night Maurice was in a right state, not at all his usual self. Told me all about Jimmy and Milly gallivanting! I couldn't believe it,'* her voice trailed off, *'that was Jimmy Shannon, couldn't resist the temptation. Needless to say that was the end of that friendship.'* Ruby took a deep breath, *'Tell your mother, son, Jimmy Shannon was scum; he would have tortured any woman he married ... in his nature, he couldn't help himself, he had wandering eyes, Charlie.'*

They walked to the door and, for a moment stood uncomfortable with their own thoughts and misgivings, the youngster and the adult, two lives intertwined because of innuendo and mistruths, suddenly, spontaneously, they came together and held each other close, drawing comfort and strength from one another.

"Take care, Charlie," the woman said and gave him a loud smacking kiss on the cheek, "and tell your mother…." hesitating, unsure, prised the boy out of her arms, looked lovingly into his eyes and repeated, "take care, son."

The youth nodded and walked away into the night. He heard the unmistakable sound of a door being closed then bolted, glanced back and saw the upstairs lights spew brightness into the yard. Ruby Shannon safe inside her sanctuary, weary, exhausted, heading for the comfort of her bed. Soon he had reached his home. The lights were out, his parents asleep. Charlie stood for an age, hesitant and undecided then he turned and walked away from his home. He felt resolute and strong, strode purposefully through the sleeping village. He would walk to the distant town and call on Anne Marie Hickson, maybe tomorrow see his parents, maybe tomorrow put the record straight.

Other books written by Peter Harrison:

Hovis Brown

Set in the North East in the early Eighties. Jackie 'Hovis' Brown, a virtual giant of a man, is clinging to the gutter of life. A bully and an enforcer, he was imprisoned for blindly obeying the woman he loved, Anna Belling, then set free to slide into a life of crime, longing to find a true love.

Anna was abused from the age of four and grew up a cold and calculating woman. Manipulating and damaging all who come under her spell. A conniving and cunning vixen who will stop at nothing in her pursuit of personal gain.

Ryan Dimonti – criminal and drug lord. Uses people like Jackie Brown to inflict terror and loyalty in his domain. Cruel and calculating, just like Anna Belling who wins a way into his heart.

The three are thrown together in their daily lives where each one's desires delivers a cruel twist of fate.

£4.99 ISBN: 978.1.903172.91.9

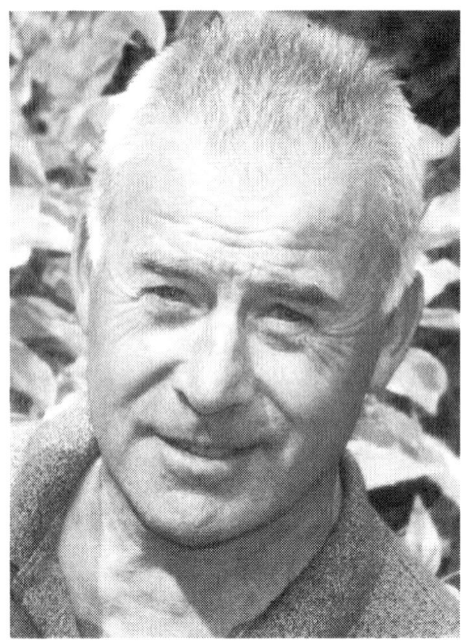

This is Peter Harrison's second novel.
Peter lives in the North East and now spends his time researching and writing novels.